Dear Students and Faculty

We are pleased to bring you the 8th edition of a book that has been the foundational nursing textbook for generations of nurses. What is now considered fundamental to the practice of nursing was unimaginable to those nurses who practiced during the years of the first edition. Although the language and devices you will see in this edition differ immensely from those used by nurses before us and before you, the systematic nature of gathering data to determine health challenges and designing, implementing, and evaluating care, has not changed.

As authors, we have met the challenge of scanning the environment to determine the core knowledge and skills you need to deliver timely, sensitive, quality, and personal care to the individuals and communities with whom you work. To bring the reality of practice to you, in this edition we have introduced several new features. The *Real World Reflection* and *Real World Practice* features allow you to hear experiences of other real students and nurses relevant to the topics being covered in the chapters in their own words. Two other new features are *Anatomy & Physiology Review* and *Drug Capsules*. We know that your learning is enhanced when you revisit concepts and apply them in new situations. So, we build on your anatomy and physiology course backgrounds, plus some chemistry and pharmacology, in teaching concepts such as pain, elimination, and circulation. We hope you find these new teaching tools useful.

We have been nurse educators for many years and have taught students in their first classroom nursing courses, in clinical and in the skills lab. We have taught associate degree, baccalaureate, and graduate nursing students. We know from first hand and current experience what students find the most challenging in beginning their nursing profession. Many other faculty who teach beginning nursing students review your textbook and provide confirmation that it reflects the standards they see in their settings.

We are grateful to the original authors of this textbook, Barbara Kozier and the late Glenora Erb, for setting the standard for all the editions that have followed. This book is known for being comprehensive and yet honed down to key content presented in a way novice students understand and find useful. We encourage both students and faculty who use this book to give us feedback on it. Feel free to email us directly at NursingExcellence@prenhall.com. You are the next generation of nursing excellence!

Audrey Berman
Shirlee Snyder

Nursing Excellence
for the Next Generation. . .

Nursing Excellence Starts Here!

Kozier & Erb's Fundamentals of Nursing continues to set the foundation for nursing excellence. Now in it's eighth edition, *Kozier & Erb* is designed for success in today's classroom and to prepare tomorrow's nurses.

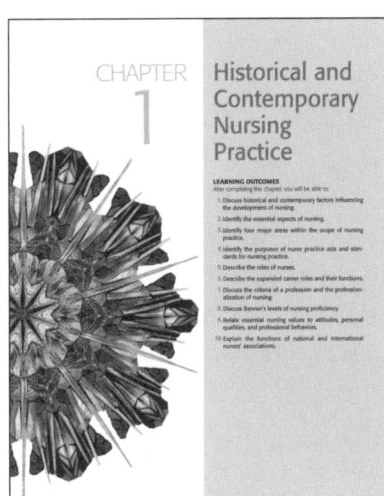

Excellence from the Start...

Start by reviewing learning outcomes and key terms.

◀ **Learning Outcomes** help identify critical concepts.

Key Terms provide a ▶ study tool for learning new vocabulary. Page numbers are included for easy reference.

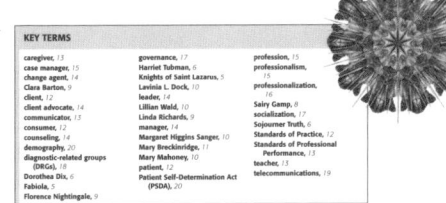

...To the Finish

The end of each chapter summarizes and applies chapter information.

Chapter highlights focus your attention and review critical concepts.

Test Your Knowledge helps you prepare for the NCLEX-RN® exam. Alternative-style questions are also included.

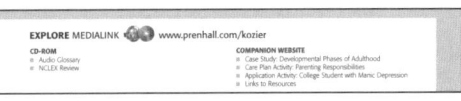

▲

Explore MediaLink lets you know what you will find on the *Prentice Hall Nursing MediaLink DVD-ROM* and the Companion Website that accompany this book.

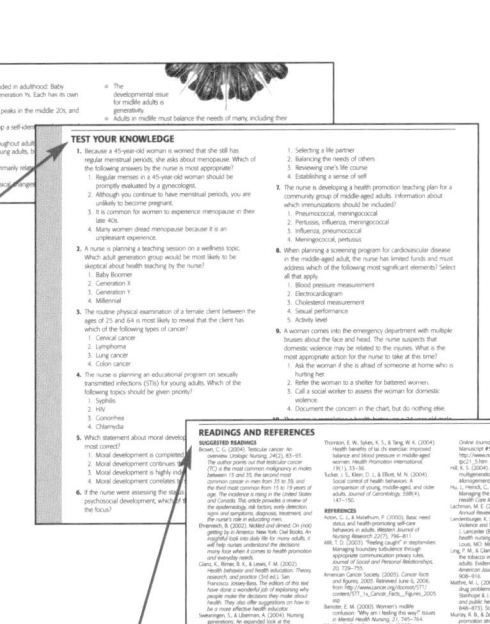

Readings and References give you a source for supporting and evidence-based material and additional information.

And Everything

Anatomy & Physiology Reviews offer a quick reminder and direct application of anatomy and physiology to chapter topics. *New to this edition!*

ANATOMY AND PHYSIOLOGY REVIEW Glaucoma

Glaucoma is a group of diseases of the eye caused by increased intraocular pressure that can lead to optic nerve damage and eventual vision loss (see Part D). Review Part A for the normal anatomy of the eye.

A clear liquid, the aqueous humor, circulates inside the front portion of the eye nourishing the lens and cornea. To maintain a normal level of pressure in the eye, the body constantly produces a small amount of aqueous humor and an equal amount flows out of the eye through a drainage system at the junction of the iris and the cornea (Halvorson, 2005, p. 42). It is at this angle that the fluid passes through a trabecular meshwork and drains into the Canal of Schlemm and enters into the bloodstream in the back of the eye.

In acute open-angle glaucoma, the anterior chamber angle remains open but drainage of the aqueous humor through the Canal of Schlemm is impaired. This causes a slow rise of the intraocular pressure. The eye's drainage angle becomes less efficient as a person ages and the risk of developing chronic open-angle glaucoma increases. The cause is unknown.

In acute closed-angle glaucoma, the drainage angle narrows and closes or becomes blocked by the iris. The intraocular pressure can rise quickly and cause an acute attack.

A

A, The normal anatomy of the eye.

ASSESSMENT INTERVIEW Determining the Risk for Medication Nonadherence

- Are you having side effects from any of your medications?
- Do you think your medications are helping?
- Do you have "tools" to remind you to take your medication? Examples could be an alarm or environmental cues (e.g., 6:00 news).
- Is there someone at home who helps you with your medications?
- How many times per day are your medications prescribed?

- How many pills do you take every day?
- Are there any special storage requirements for your medications?
- How much do your medication requirements interfere with your lifestyle?
- How well are you able to follow special dosing requirements?
- How many doses of your medications have you missed over the last 3 days?

◄ **Assessment Interview** boxes help you learn the type and range of what to ask in particular situations.

Culturally Competent Care boxes focus on how situations may have different approaches when considering the client's cultural background.

CULTURALLY COMPETENT CARE Hmong Elders

In the 1970s the Hmong arrived in the United States as refugees taking advantage of resettlement opportunities. The largest numbers of Hmong live in California, Minnesota, and Wisconsin.

Spiritual beliefs join their beliefs related to health and illness. The Hmong of Laos believe that a person has multiple souls and that health results from the souls living in harmony. Spiritual illness results when one or more of the souls leave the physical body. Healing ceremonies are performed to call and retrieve the lost soul(s).

In Laos, Hmong elders are treated with great respect. Others consult the elders because they have acquired wisdom and insight from their experiences. Many older Hmong in the United States do not speak English, and an interpreter will be needed. Avoiding di-

rect eye contact and speaking in a calm, caring manner will facilitate communication.

Among the Hmong who practice traditional beliefs, confusion and memory impairment of an older adult may be treated with herbal teas and a spiritual ceremony conducted by a shaman. Hmong families living in the United States may seek out both their traditional healers and Western medicine health professionals to help the older adult(s) in their family. Nurses need to honor traditional beliefs while providing Western medical care.

Note: From "Chronic Confusion and Memory Impairment in Hmong Elders," by L. A. Gerdner, S. V. Xiong, and D. Cha, 2006, *Journal of Gerontological Nursing, 32*(3), pp. 23–31.

in Between!

HOME CARE ASSESSMENT
Infection

CLIENT AND ENVIRONMENT

- *Self-care abilities for wound care:* Understanding of rationale for wound care as well as wound care technique; ability to gather and use supplies for clean or aseptic technique to change dressings or care for wounds
- *Self-care abilities for hygiene and toileting:* Understanding of rationale for hygiene in the home setting; ability to contain potentially infectious material, such as that from coughing or sneezing, and body fluids (urine, stool, drainage); ability to cleanse hands and implement any required isolation practices
- *Self-care abilities for medication administration:* Understanding of medication therapy, expected outcomes, and potential side effects; physical dexterity to take pills, administer intravenous antibiotics, and store medications safely
- *Facilities:* Presence of running water, trash containers and disposal, bathroom to facilitate wound care and contain potentially infectious materials

FAMILY

- *Caregiver availability, skills, and responses:* Understanding of rationale for wound care as well as wound care technique; persons able to assist with wound care, medication administration, and shopping if client has restricted activity; people able to comprehend infection control activities without excessive personal anxiety
- *Other susceptible cohabitants:* Presence and immunization status of children, elders, or others who may be at risk of infection from the client

COMMUNITY

- *Resources:* Availability of and familiarity with possible sources of assistance for finances, supplies, and home health aid (such as public health department and visiting nurses)

◀ **Home Care Assessment** and **Home Care Considerations** boxes help you think beyond the hospital room and consider client issues for successful home recovery and living.

▼

HOME CARE CONSIDERATIONS
Specimen Collection

- If specimen collection is done on an outpatient basis or in the home, the nurse teaches the client how to obtain the specimens. Provide written instructions and specimen containers to ensure correct and safe performance of the procedure.
- Ensure that the laboratory knows where to send the test results.

Lifespan Considerations highlight how nursing care is adapted for infants, children, adolescents, and elders. ▼

LIFESPAN CONSIDERATIONS
International Adoption

CHILDREN

International adoption of children by families in the United States is increasing, with over 150,000 children adopted in the past 14 years. These children present many challenges, and the care given by pediatric health providers can strongly influence the success with which they are assimilated into their new families. Understanding and assessing adopted children's potential issues early and intervening appropriately can lead to stronger family bonds. Children who arrive in the United States should be evaluated within 10 to 14 days for the following:

- Immunization history (blood titers may be appropriate)
- Infectious disease, parasites, general health (CBC, thyroid, liver function, and other blood work)
- Tuberculosis exposure (PPD)
- Developmental history and status, including speech, language, motor, and social development
- Vision and hearing
- Dental health

Note: Adapted from "International adoption: A health and developmental prospective," by P. Mason & C. Narad, 2005, *Seminars in Speech and Language, 26*(1), 1–9.

CLIENT TEACHING Developing
Written Teaching Aids

- Keep language level at or below the fifth-grade level.
- Use active, not passive, voice.
- Use easy, common words of one or two syllables (e.g., *use* instead of *utilize,* or *give* instead of *administer*).
- Use the second person (*you*) rather than the third person (*the client*).
- Use a large type size (14 to 16 point).
- Write short sentences.
- Avoid using all capital letters.
- Place priority information first and repeat more than once.
- Use bold for emphasis.
- Use simple pictures, drawings, or cartoons, if appropriate.
- Leave plenty of white space.
- Obtain feedback from nurses and clients.

◀ **Client Teaching** boxes give tips and tools to help clients facilitate self-care, monitor potential problems, perform prescribed therapies, and assist in other client teaching experiences.

Client-Focused Nursing Evidence-

▶ **Nursing Care Plans** help you approach care from the nursing process perspective.

Sensory-Perception Disturbance

ASSESSMENT DATA	NURSING DIAGNOSIS	DESIRED OUTCOMES*
Nursing Assessment Julia Hagstrom is an 80-year-old widow who has recently become a resident of an extended care facility. Just prior to her admission she underwent surgery for the removal of cataracts and also experienced more difficulty with hearing. Her children were concerned about her physical safety and lack of socialization and urged her to enter a nursing home. Mrs. Hagstrom had cared for herself independently for 15 years in her own home. Three days after admission the nurse finds the client somewhat confused and disoriented to place, and time. She appears restless and withdrawn. She states, "I'm afraid of all of these strange creatures in this orphanage."	*Disturbed Sensory Perception (Sensory Overload)* related to change in environment, and hearing loss (as evidenced by disorientation to time and place; restlessness; and altered behavior)	**Cognitive Orientation** [0901] as evidenced by not compromised: ■ Identifies significant other(s) ■ Identifies current place ■ Identifies correct season **Hearing Compensation Behavior** [1610] as evidenced by often demonstrated: ■ Positions self to advantage hearing ■ Reminds others to use techniques that advantage hearing ■ Eliminates background noise ■ Uses hearing supportive devices
Physical Examination **Diagnostic Data** Height: 160 cm (5'3") Chest x-ray, CBC, and urinalysis Weight: 55.3 kg (122 lb) all negative Temperature: 37°C (98.6°F) Pulse: 72 BPM Respirations: 18/minute Blood Pressure: 128/74 mm Hg Rinne test: negative		

▶ **Applying Critical Thinking** questions come at the end of each sample Nursing Care Plan to encourage further reflection and analysis.

APPLYING CRITICAL THINKING

1. What assumptions does the nurse make when deciding that using a standardized care plan for *Deficient Fluid Volume* is appropriate for this client?
2. Identify an outcome in the care plan and its nursing intervention that contribute to discharge care planning. What evidence supports your choice?
3. Consider how the nurse shares the development of the care plan and outcomes with the client.

4. Not every intervention has a time frame or interval specified. It may be implied. Under what circumstances is this acceptable practice?
5. In Table 13–1, *Ineffective Airway Clearance* is Amanda's highest priority nursing diagnosis. Under what conditions might this diagnosis be of only moderate priority in Amanda's case?

See Critical Thinking Possibilities in Appendix A. ∞

▶ **Identifying Nursing Diagnoses, Outcomes, and Interventions** boxes provide guidelines for establishing diagnoses, outcomes, and interventions for situations and conditions.

IDENTIFYING NURSING DIAGNOSES, OUTCOMES, AND INTERVENTIONS
The Preoperative Client

DATA CLUSTER Mr. Taylor, 62 years old, has disabling osteoarthritis and is scheduled for a total knee replacement tomorrow. This is his first surgical experience and he is asking many questions about what to expect before and after surgery. He says, "The more I know, the less anxious I feel."

NURSING DIAGNOSIS/ DEFINITION	SAMPLE DESIRED OUTCOME*/ DEFINITION	INDICATORS	SELECTED INTERVENTIONS*/ DEFINITION	SAMPLE NIC ACTIVITIES
Deficient Knowledge (Surgery)/*Absence or deficiency of cognitive information related to a specific topic*	Knowledge: Treatment Procedure(s) [1814]/ *Extent of understanding conveyed about procedure(s) required as part of a treatment regimen*	Substantial: ■ Description of steps of procedure (e.g., preoperative process) ■ Description of treatment procedures (e.g., deep breathing and coughing, leg exercises)	Teaching: Preoperative [5610]/ *Assisting a patient to understand and mentally prepare for surgery and the postoperative recovery period*	■ Provide time for the client to ask questions and discuss concerns ■ Describe the preoperative routines (e.g., anesthesia, diet, tests/lab, voiding, IV therapy, family waiting area) as appropriate ■ Instruct the client on the technique of splinting his/her incision, coughing, and deep breathing ■ Evaluate the client's ability to return demonstrate leg exercise

*The NOC # for desired outcomes and the NIC # for nursing interventions are listed in brackets following the appropriate outcome or intervention. Outcomes, indicators, interventions, and activities selected are only a sample of those suggested by NOC and NIC and should be further individualized for each client.

Care, Critical Thinking and Based Practice!

Critical Thinking Checkpoints provide a brief case study followed by questions that encourage students to analyze, compare, contemplate, interpret and evaluate information.

CRITICAL THINKING CHECKPOINT

You have just interviewed for two nursing positions and are trying to decide which job to pursue. During your first interview for a team member position, the nurse manager, Mr. Caruso, was cheerful, spoke highly of his current staff and complimented them for their ability to set goals and participate in decision making, listened to your ideas, and explored ways in which you could contribute to this team's effectiveness. The second nurse manager, Mrs. Turner, was also cheerful and talkative. She provided you with a job description as a primary nurse caregiver, explained her expectations of you as a new employee, and spoke of new programs she was attempting to implement. Both nurse managers talked about changes taking place in their facilities and the need for employees to remain flexible.

1. Based on the brief data provided, speculate about the leadership style of each of these nurse managers.
2. Think about managers (or leaders) you have known and admired. What characteristics did they have that you would like to integrate into your own management style should you become a nurse manager?
3. Both nurse managers spoke of changes that were taking place in their facility. As a nurse, how can you assist your peers who are unhappy and seem to resist change even when it is positive?
4. How might the delegation of tasks to other nurses or UAPs be different in the two settings?

See Critical Thinking Possibilities in Appendix A.

RESEARCH NOTE   How Can Nurses Help Prevent Childhood Obesity?

The prevalence rate of obesity among children in the United States has been rising in recent years. Crawford and colleagues' (2004) pilot study aimed to improve the self-efficacy of staff counseling clients enrolled in the Women, Infants, and Children (WIC) program about childhood obesity. The study compared a sample of 51 WIC employees split into an intervention group that received educational sessions to help them identify ways to make changes in eating habits, activity information, and pedometers to promote the 10,000-steps-per-day program, and a control group. The intervention group was more likely to make healthy food choices when supported by the environment, to make positive changes in counseling parents about their children's weight issues, and to feel more confident in encouraging the WIC clients to be physically active with their own children.

IMPLICATIONS

Evidence suggests that overweight children have at least one associated biochemical or cardiovascular risk factor. The need for effective programs to help control America's growing waistline among our youngest citizens is becoming imperative. Chronic health issues such as obesity require the establishment of long-term supportive relationships between the nurse and the client. Nurses can contribute and encourage lifestyle alterations to improve client health by modeling behaviors, providing educational materials, and counseling.

Note: From "Walking the Talk: Fit WIC Wellness Programs Improve Self-Efficacy in Pediatric Obesity Prevention Counseling," by P. B. Crawford, W. Gosliner, P. Strode, S. E. Samuels, L. Craypo, C. Burnett, et al., 2004, *American Journal of Public Health, 94*, pp. 1480–1485.

Research Notes focus on evidence-based practice. These boxes highlight relevant nursing journal articles and implications for nursing care.

Concept Maps! *Completely revised* sample concept maps throughout the textbook provide a visual representation of the nursing process, nursing care plans, and the relationships in different concepts.

Use the **NEW Concept Mapping** tool provided on the *Prentice Hall Nursing MediaLink DVD-ROM* that accompanies the textbook and the end-of-unit exercises for concept mapping practice!

Excellence in the

Step-by-step skills. A NEW easy-to-follow, two-column format helps students understand techniques and practice sequence.

▼

Clearly labeled **Delegation** boxes assist you in assigning tasks appropriately.

Includes a complete **Equipment** list for easy preparation.

---

806 UNIT VIII / Integral Components of Client Care

SKILL 34-1

OBTAINING A CAPILLARY BLOOD SPECIMEN TO MEASURE BLOOD GLUCOSE

PURPOSES
- To determine or monitor blood glucose levels of clients at risk for hyperglycemia or hypoglycemia
- To promote blood glucose regulation by the client
- To evaluate the effectiveness of insulin administration

ASSESSMENT
- Before obtaining a capillary blood specimen, determine
- The frequency and type of testing.
- The client's understanding of the procedure.
- The client's response to previous testing.
- Assess the client's skin at the puncture site to determine if it is intact and the circulation is not compromised. Check color, warmth, and capillary refill.
- Review the client's record for medications that may prolong bleeding such as anticoagulants.
- Assess the client's self-care abilities that may affect accuracy of test results, such as visual impairment and finger dexterity.

PLANNING

Delegation
Check the applicable nurse practice act and the facility policy and procedure manual to determine who can perform this skill. It is usually considered an invasive technique and one that requires problem solving and application of knowledge. It is the responsibility of the nurse to know the results of the test.

Equipment
- Blood glucose meter (glucometer)
- Blood glucose reagent strip compatible with the meter
- 2 × 2 gauze
- Warm cloth or other warming device (optional)
- Antiseptic swab
- Disposable gloves
- Sterile lancet
- Lancet injector

IMPLEMENTATION
Preparation
Review the type of meter and the manufacturer's instructions. Assemble the equipment at the bedside.

Performance
1. Prior to performing the procedure, introduce self and verify the client's identity using agency protocol. Explain to the client what you are going to do, why it is necessary, and how he or she can cooperate. Discuss how the results will be used in planning further care or treatments.
2. Perform hand hygiene and observe other appropriate infection control procedures (e.g., gloves).
3. Provide for client privacy.
4. Prepare the equipment.
   - Calibrate the meter and run a control sample according to the manufacturer's instructions.
5. Select and prepare the vascular puncture site.
   - Choose a vascular puncture site (e.g., the side of an adult's finger). Avoid sites beside bone. Wrap the finger first in a warm cloth, or hold a finger in a dependent position. If the earlobe is used, rub it gently with a small piece of gauze. **Rationale:** These actions increase the blood flow to the area, ensure an adequate specimen, and reduce the need for a repeat puncture.
   - Clean the site with the antiseptic swab or soap and water and allow it to dry completely. **Rationale:** Alcohol can affect accuracy and the site burns when punctured when wet with alcohol.
6. Obtain the blood specimen.
   - Put on gloves.
   - Place the injector, if used, against the site, and release the needle, thus permitting it to pierce the skin. Make sure the lancet is perpendicular to the site. **Rationale:** The lancet is designed to pierce the skin at a specific depth when it is in a perpendicular position relative to the skin. ❶

❶ Place the injector against the site.

or
- Prick the site with a lancet or needle.
- Gently squeeze (but do not touch) the large drop of blood forms. The size vary depending on the meter. Som as 0.3 mL (Passanza, 2001) or not n riod at the end of this sentence (Me
- Hold the reagent strip under the pun blood covers the indicator square. The and a chemical reaction will occur. D **Rationale:** This will cause an inaccura ters wick the blood by just touching th strip.
- Ask the client to apply pressure to the a 2 × 2 or 4 × 4. **Rationale:** Pressure
7. Expose the blood to the test strip for th ner specified by the manufacturer. As placed on the test strip:

CHAPTER 34 / Diagnostic Testing **807**

SKILL 34-1

OBTAINING A CAPILLARY BLOOD SPECIMEN TO MEASURE BLOOD GLUCOSE *continued*

❷ Gently squeeze a drop of blood onto the reagent strip.

❸ The glucose meter will display the glucose reading.

- Follow the manufacturer's recommendations on the glucose meter and monitor for the amount of time indicated by the manufacturer. **Rationale:** The blood must remain in contact with the test pad for a prescribed time to obtain accurate results. Some glucometers have the test strip placed in the machine before the specimen is obtained.
8. Measure the blood glucose.
   - Place the strip into the meter according to the manufacturer's instructions. Some devices require that the strip be wiped or blotted after a designated period of time before being inserted in the meter. Other strips do not require blotting or wiping. Refer to the specific manufacturer's recommendations for the specific procedure.
- After the designated time, most glucose meters will display the glucose reading automatically. Correct timing ensures accurate results ❸
- Turn off the meter and discard the test strip and 2 × 2 gauze in a biohazard container. Discard the lancet into a sharps container.
9. Document the method of testing and results on the client's record. If appropriate, record the client's understanding and ability to demonstrate the technique. The client's record may also include a flow sheet on which capillary blood glucose results and the amount, type, route, and time of insulin administration are recorded.
10. Check for orders for sliding scale insulin based on capillary blood glucose results. Administer insulin as prescribed.

EVALUATION
- Compare glucose meter reading with normal blood glucose level, status of puncture site, and motivation of the client to perform the test independently.
- Relate blood glucose reading to previous readings and the client's current health status.
- Report abnormal results to the primary care provider.
- Conduct appropriate follow-up such as asking the client to explain the meaning of the results and/or demonstrating the procedure at the next scheduled test.

Critical steps are visually represented with full-color **photos** and **illustrations**!

Easy-to-find **rationales** give you a better understanding of why things are done.

Clinical Alerts ▶ highlight special information such as safety issues.

CLINICAL ALERT

When a client falls, the nurse's first duty is to the client. First, assess for injuries. Then, notify the primary care provider. ■

Clinical Manifestations. ▶
New to this edition! These boxes are a quick resource to learn key signs and symptoms of illness.

CLINICAL MANIFESTATIONS
SENSORY DEPRIVATION

- Excessive yawning, drowsiness, sleeping
- Decreased attention span, difficulty concentrating, decreased problem solving
- Impaired memory
- Periodic disorientation, general confusion, or nocturnal confusion
- Preoccupation with somatic complaints, such as palpitations
- Hallucinations or delusions
- Crying, annoyance over small matters, depression
- Apathy, emotional lability

Clinical Setting!

Practice Guidelines ▶ provide instant-access summaries of clinical do's and don'ts.

PRACTICE GUIDELINES **Preventing Falls in Health Care Agencies**

- On admission, orient clients to their surroundings and explain the call system.
- Carefully assess the client's ability to ambulate and transfer. Provide walking aids and assistance as required.
- Closely supervise the clients at risk for falls, especially at night.
- Encourage the client to use the call bell to request assistance. Ensure that the bell is within easy reach.
- Place beside tables and overbed tables near the bed or chair so that clients do not overreach and consequently lose their balance.

- Always keep hospital beds in the low position and wheels locked when not providing care so that clients can move in or out of bed easily.
- Encourage clients to use grab bars mounted in toilet and bathing areas and railings along corridors.
- Make sure nonskid bath mats are available in tubs and showers.
- Encourage the client to wear nonskid footwear.
- Keep the environment tidy; especially keep light cords from underfoot and furniture out of the way.
- Use individualized interventions (e.g., alarm sensitive to client position) rather than side rails for confused clients.

DRUG CAPSULE **Client Taking Medication for Glaucoma** *travoprost (Travatan)*

Travoprost is an anti-glaucoma drug that decreases intraocular pressure in open-angle glaucoma

NURSING RESPONSIBILITIES
- Assess eye for inflammation, exudate, and pain.
- Note iris color.

CLIENT AND FAMILY TEACHING
- Use once daily as directed.
- Do not let the tip of the dropper touch any part of the eye.
- It may be used with other eye products to lower intraocular pressure. If more than one medication, administer 5 minutes apart.

- Inform of risk of darkening of the iris, eyelashes, or skin around the eye.
- Do not administer while wearing contact lenses. Remove contact lens and wait 15 minutes after instilling eyedrop before reinserting contact lens.
- Discard the container within 6 weeks of removing it from the sealed pouch.

◀ **Drug Capsules.** *New to this edition!* These boxes provide a brief overview of drug information, nursing responsibilities, and client teaching to help you understand implications in different situations.

Real World Practice offers insight from today's ▶ excellent nurses. Chosen from magnet hospitals across the U.S., these nurses offer their perspectives on learning and what to expect in the clinical environment. *New to this edition!*

REAL WORLD PRACTICE

One of the biggest changes you'll see as you progress from being a novice nurse to becoming an expert nurse is your willingness to "trust your gut"—You know, that little voice in your head saying, "something isn't right here." There may be no change in your client's vital signs, no change in his or her mental status, nothing concrete you can put your finger on, no *numbers* you can report to the physician (oh, how we all love *numbers*). But in your heart, in your gut, you *know* there's something wrong.

What do you do? As a novice nurse, you are likely to talk yourself out of this feeling. You will think you are just overreacting, hearing hoofbeats and thinking zebras instead of horses. You may mention this feeling in passing to a trusted co-worker, but that's about as far as you'll take it.

As you progress through your career, you will find yourself acting on the advice of that little voice more and more often. You'll find yourself calling physicians at 2:00 in the morning because your little voice is telling you that something is wrong. ~~You~~ know you have arrived, however, when you call a ~~physician~~ at 2 A.M. who tells you, "I'll be right there because I ~~trust your~~ little voice."

— *Tina Saiani, RN*
The Children's Hospital at the
Medical Center of Central Georgia

Real World Reflections give student accounts of real student clinical experiences. *New to this edition!*

▼

 REAL WORLD REFLECTION

THE STORY: "ALL THIS AND CALVIN KLEINS TOO"

This was my first shift in the Neonatal Intensive Care Unit (NICU). The infant I was caring for was born around 34 weeks gestation. She was being evaluated because she was small for her gestational age. The infant had a nasogastric tube and was being gavaged to meet the minimum daily intake, but also was doing well at bottle feeding. The nurse showed me how to check for residuals from the last feeding.

The infant had been hospitalized for about one month, and now she was ready for discharge the following day. While I was interested in the infant's medical condition, I was most interested in the mother's psychosocial status. She was very passive about holding her baby, and indicated that the infant's grandmother would be taking care of the baby when she came home because of her need to return to work. The mother didn't seem interested in participating in any teaching/learning before discharge. She did request a prescription for a specialized formula so she could obtain it from a public assistance program. I am sure that the special formula is expensive, but I also noticed that this young (probably late teens) mom was in full make-up, hair, and Calvin Klein jeans.

STUDENT REFLECTION

As the evening progressed the parents went home and the lights dimmed in the NICU. I continued assessing, feeding, changing, and comforting my clients. As I look back on this experience, I think

most about my inclination to judge the parents and think that they are responsible for the infant's medical problems. As I talked with other nurses they stressed that even moms who do everything right can find their baby in the NICU for a short or extensive stay. I know that there are many risks in pregnancy and delivery, but looking at these tiny babies fighting to live made me want to blame someone.

I also assumed that all parents would want to be with their baby day in and out if they were in the NICU. While some parents do spend as much time as possible with their child, many of the infants are in the NICU for weeks or months making a parental vigil nearly impossible.

FACULTY REFLECTION

Jennifer did a great job on reflecting on how she felt while caring for this infant and mother. She recognized the feeling in herself of assigning blame for what she considered an injustice, and yet, she did not know where to direct that blame. As nurses we may verbally say to ourselves and others that we don't judge our clients. But often our nonverbal language is "screaming" something to the contrary. Until we recognize, name, and understand those feelings in ourselves, we cannot effectively deliver caring and compassionate care.

— *Student: Jennifer Trucke*
Faculty member: Deb Filer, RN, PhD
College of St. Catherine, St. Paul, MN

Additional Student Resources for Nursing Excellence

Clinical Handbook for Fundamentals of Nursing, 8e
ISBN 0-13-188933-8
This clinical companion serves as a portable, quick reference to the fundamentals of nursing that students can bring into any clinical setting. Topics include lab values, diagnostic tests, standard precautions, documentation, NANDA diagnoses, and MORE!

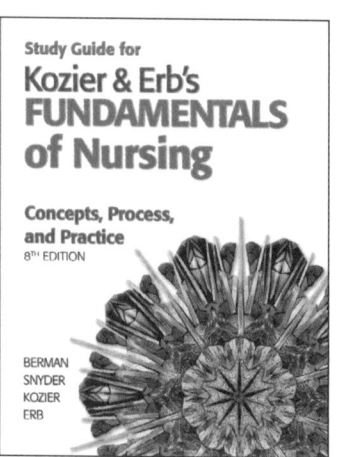

Study Guide for Fundamentals of Nursing, 8e
ISBN 0-13-188938-9
The study guide that accompanies the textbook includes case studies, NCLEX® review, and other exercises. MediaLinks refer students to activities on the *Prentice Hall Nursing MediaLink DVD-ROM* and the Companion Website.

ADDITIONAL ILLUSTRATED SKILL RESOURCES!

Kozier & Erb's Techniques in Clinical Nursing, 5e
Kozier, Erb, Berman & Snyder
ISBN 0-13-114229-1

Clinical Nursing Skills, 7e
Smith, Duell, & Martin
ISBN 0-13-224355-5

Prentice Hall Nursing MediaLink DVD-ROM
This DVD-ROM comes packaged with every textbook. It provides an interactive study program with NCLEX®-style review questions complete with comprehensive rationales. Also included are animations and videos, concept mapping end-of-unit exercises and NEW concept mapping software, a review of dosage calculations, and skill checklists. *CD-ROM versions are available for those who cannot use the DVD-ROM version. ISBN 0-13-159800-3*

Companion Website www.prenhall.com/berman
This online study guide contains additional NCLEX®-style review questions, case studies, application activities, and care plan activities organized by chapter. This site also contains additional tools, weblinks and more that help explore and apply concepts presented in the textbook.

◄ **MediaLink and EXPLORE MediaLink**
The **EXPLORE MediaLink** section lists chapter specific case studies, animations, websites, and additional information that can be found on the *Prentice Hall Nursing MediaLink DVD-ROM* or the Companion Website. Special **MediaLink** tabs appear throughout the chapters in the margins, prompting students to use specific media resources for specific activities and applications for that chapter. **MediaLink** helps foster critical thinking and builds upon knowledge gained from the textbook.

Anatomical Landmarks Animation

MediaLink

Instructor Resources
for Nursing Excellence

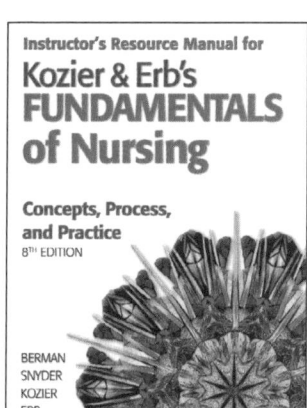

Instructor Resource Manual
ISBN 0-13-188936-2

This manual contains a wealth of material to help faculty plan and manage the Fundamentals of Nursing course. It includes chapter overviews, detailed lecture outlines, teaching activities, PowerPoint outlines, and a complete NCLEX®-style test bank.

Instructor's Resource Manual for
Kozier & Erb's
FUNDAMENTALS
of Nursing
Concepts, Process, and Practice
8TH EDITION

BERMAN
SNYDER
KOZIER
ERB

Instructor's Resource DVD-ROM
ISBN 0-13-188940-0

This DVD-ROM includes all the textbook resources instructors need to teach fundamental nursing courses—

- Comprehensive PowerPoint presentation that integrates lecture slides, images, animations, videos, and other resources
- Classroom Response System questions set in PowerPoint slides (ask your Prentice Hall representative for more information about hardware to enhance your presentation)
- First Day of Class presentation to show your students how to use this textbook
- Complete Image Gallery in PowerPoint
- TestGen Test Item File with over 3,000 questions in all NCLEX-RN® formats, including questions mapped to chapter learning objectives and clinical competencies
- Link to the Prentice Hall Instructors Resource Center for additional resources

CD-ROM versions are available to faculty who cannot use the DVD-ROM version.

OneKey Online Course Management Systems

Prentice Hall OneKey is an integrated online resource that brings a variety of resources together in one convenient place for faculty and students using Blackboard, WebCT, and CourseCompass platforms, including:

- NCLEX-RN® Review questions
- Case studies
- MediaLinks
- Application Activities
- Test Item Files
- PowerPoint Presentations
- Media Gallery resources

For a demonstration, please contact your Prentice Hall sales representative or go online to
www.prenhall.com/nursing

Brief Table of Contents

Kozier & Erb's

FUNDAMENTALS OF NURSING

Concepts, Process, and Practice

8th Edition

Audrey Berman, PhD, RN, AOCN

Shirlee J. Snyder, EdD, RN

Barbara Kozier, MN, RN

Glenora Erb, BSN, RN

PEARSON

Prentice Hall

Upper Saddle River, New Jersey 07458

Library of Congress Cataloging-in-Publication Data
Fundamentals of nursing : concepts, process, and practice / Audrey
   Berman . . . [et al.]. – 8th ed.
      p. ; cm.
   Barbara Kozier's name appears first on earlier ed.
   Includes bibliographical references and index.
   ISBN 0-13-171468-6
   1. Nursing.   I. Berman, Audrey.
   [DNLM: 1. Nursing Process. 2. Nursing Care. 3. Nursing Theory. WY 100 F97984 2008]
RT41.F8813 2008
610.73—dc22   2006029312

Publisher: Julie Levin Alexander
Publisher's Assistant: Regina Bruno
Editor-in-Chief: Maura Connor
Senior Acquisitions Editor: Kelly Trakalo
Editorial Assistant: JulieAnn Oliveros
Development Editor: Teri Zak
Managing Editor, Development: Marilyn Meserve
Managing Production Editor: Patrick Walsh
Production Liaison: Cathy O'Connell
Production Editor: Emily Bush, Carlisle Publishers Services
Manufacturing Manager: Ilene Sanford
Design Director and Cover Designer: Cheryl Asherman
Photographer: Patrick Watson
Director of Marketing: Karen Allman
Senior Marketing Manager: Francisco Del Castillo
Marketing Coordinator: Michael Sirinides
Marketing Assistant: Patricia Linard
Associate Editor: Michael Giacobbe
Media Development Editor: John J. Jordan
Media Production Manager: Amy Peltier
New Media Project Manager: Tina Rudowski
Composition: Carlisle Publishers Services, Inc.
Printer/Binder: Courier Kendalville
Cover Printer: Phoenix Color
Cover photo: Kaleidoscopic XXII: September 11, 2002 © Paula Nadelstern

Pearson Education LTD.
Pearson Education Australia PTY, Limited
Pearson Education Singapore, Pte. Ltd
Pearson Education North Asia Ltd
Pearson Education Canada, Ltd.

Pearson Educación de Mexico, S.A. de C.V.
Pearson Education—Japan
Pearson Education Malaysia, Pte. Ltd
Pearson Education, Upper Saddle River, NJ

10 9 8 7 6 5 4 3 2

ISBN 978-0-13-206674-7

Audrey Berman dedicates this edition to the real heroes in nursing education: the faculty. These men and women elect to spend their professional energies transmitting their knowledge, skills, and caring not just to clients, but to the extensions of their arms and minds—the generations of nurses to come. They are my colleagues, my friends, and my family.

Shirlee Snyder dedicates this edition to her husband, Terry J. Schnitter, for his unconditional love and support, and to her stepdaughter Kelly, an awesome young woman, and caring mother, wife, and daughter who is diligently working on achieving her goal of becoming a nurse.

About the Authors

Audrey Berman received her BSN from the University of California–San Francisco and later returned to that campus to obtain her MS in physiologic nursing and her PhD in nursing. Her dissertation was entitled *Sailing a Course through Chemotherapy: The Experience of Women with Breast Cancer*. She worked in oncology at Samuel Merritt Hospital prior to beginning her teaching career in the diploma program at Samuel Merritt Hospital School of Nursing in 1976. As a faculty member, she participated in the transition of that program into a baccalaureate degree and in the development of the master of science in nursing program. Over the years, she has taught a variety of medical-surgical nursing courses in the prelicensure programs. She currently serves as the dean of nursing at Samuel Merritt College (an affiliate of Sutter Health).

Dr. Berman has traveled extensively, visiting nursing and health care institutions in Germany, Israel, Spain, Korea, Botswana, Australia, Japan, and Brazil. She serves on the board of directors for the Bay Area Tumor Institute. She is a member of the American Nurses Association and Sigma Theta Tau and is a site visitor for the Commission on Collegiate Nursing Education. She has twice participated as an NCLEX-RN item writer for the National Council of State Boards of Nursing. She is certified as an advanced oncology nurse and as an AIDS educator and has presented locally, nationally, and internationally on topics related to nursing education, breast cancer, and technology in health care.

Dr. Berman authored the scripts for more than 35 nursing skills videotapes in the 1990s. She was a coauthor of the sixth and seventh editions of *Fundamentals of Nursing* and, with Shirlee Snyder, coauthor of the fifth edition of *Kozier & Erb's Techniques in Clinical Nursing*.

Shirlee J. Snyder graduated from Columbia Hospital School of Nursing in Milwaukee, Wisconsin, and subsequently received a bachelor of science in nursing from University of Wisconsin–Milwaukee. Because of an interest in cardiac nursing and teaching, she earned a master of science in nursing with a minor in cardiovascular clinical specialist and teaching from the University of Alabama in Birmingham. A move to California resulted in becoming a faculty member at Samuel Merritt Hospital School of Nursing in Oakland, California. Shirlee was fortunate to be involved in the phasing out of the diploma and ADN programs and development of a baccalaureate intercollegiate nursing program. She held numerous positions during her 15-year tenure at Samuel Merritt College, including curriculum coordinator, assistant director–instruction, dean of instruction, and associate dean of the Intercollegiate Nursing Program. She is an associate professor alumnus at Samuel Merritt College. Her interest and experiences in nursing education resulted in Shirlee obtaining a doctorate of education focused in curriculum and instruction from the University of San Francisco.

Dr. Snyder moved to Portland, Oregon, in 1990 and taught in the ADN program at Portland Community College for 8 years. During this teaching experience she became interested in computer-assisted instruction (CAI) and initiated Web-based assessment testing for student learning. She presented locally and nationally on topics related to using multimedia in the classroom and promoting ethnic and minority student success.

Another career opportunity in 1998 led her to the Community College of Southern Nevada in Las Vegas, Nevada, where Dr. Snyder was the nursing program director with responsibilities for the associate degree and practical nursing programs for 5 years. During this time she became involved in coauthoring the fifth edition of *Kozier & Erb's Techniques in Clinical Nursing* with Audrey Berman.

In 2003, Dr. Snyder returned to baccalaureate nursing education. She embraced the opportunity to be one of the nursing faculty teaching the first nursing class in the baccalaureate nursing program at the first state college in Nevada, which opened in 2002. She is currently the associate dean of the School of Nursing at Nevada State College in Henderson, Nevada.

Dr. Snyder is an advisory board member for the Nevada Geriatric Education Center and a member of the American Nurses Association, Sigma Theta Tau, and a variety of task groups addressing the Southern Nevada nursing shortage. She has been a site visitor for the National League for Nursing Accrediting Commission and the Northwest Association of Schools and Colleges.

Dr. Snyder's experiences in nursing education and teaching keep her current in nursing and nursing education. She appreciates all she learns from the students she has taught and her past and present faculty colleagues.

Barbara Kozier was educated in Vancouver, British Columbia, Canada. After obtaining a bachelor of arts degree from the University of British Columbia, she entered the nursing program at that institution. After 4 years of study she graduated with a bachelor's degree in nursing. She obtained a position at Bella Bella, an aboriginal settlement on the northern coast of British Columbia. She then nursed with the Victorian Order of Nurses providing home care. Following a position with a large general hospital as an acute care nurse in a medical surgical unit, she taught medical and surgical nursing, pediatric nursing, psychiatric nursing, and community nursing courses at the Vancouver General Hospital School of Nursing. Ms. Kozier then enrolled at the University of Washington where she studied for 2 years, taught part time, and obtained her master of nursing title.

Barbara is a member of three honor societies: Sigma Theta Tau (nursing), Pi Lambda Theta (education), and Delta Sigma Pi (Canadian Honor Society for University Women). Barbara was a member and a chair of many nursing and government committees. She wrote a number of texts and collaborated with Glenora Erb on four books: *Techniques of Clinical Nursing, Fundamentals of Nursing, Concepts and Issues in Nursing Practice*, and *Essentials of Nursing Practice*.

Glenora Lea Erb was born in Calgary, Alberta, Canada. All of her schooling took place in Calgary and, with her identical twin sister, she attended the Nursing School of Calgary General Hospital. She was awarded a gold medal when she graduated and was recognized as an outstanding bedside nurse.

Following 2 years traveling in Asia, Europe, India, Australia, and New Zealand, Ms. Erb returned to Vancouver and taught nursing at St. Paul's Hospital School of Nursing, and later at a 2-year program at the British Columbia Institute of Technology. At this time she also coauthored textbooks on *Fundamentals of Nursing, Techniques of Clinical Nursing, Concepts and Issues in Nursing Practice*, and *Essentials of Nursing Practice*.

Glen died at home December 24, 2001 of breast cancer. Her death has meant that nursing has lost a highly skilled clinical nurse and her friends and family have lost a sensitive and giving person.

Preface

The practice of nursing continues to evolve ... the practice of caring is timeless.

Nurses today must be able to grow and evolve to meet the demands of a dramatically changing health care system. They need skills in technology, communication, and interpersonal relations to be effective members of the collaborative health care team. They need to think critically and be creative in implementing nursing strategies with clients of diverse cultural backgrounds in increasingly varied settings. They need skills in teaching, leading, managing, and the process of change. They need to be prepared to provide home- and community-based nursing care to clients across the life span—especially to the increasing numbers of elders. They need to understand holistic healing modalities and complementary therapies. And, they need to continue their unique role that demands a blend of nurturance, sensitivity, caring, empathy, commitment, and skill founded on a broad base of knowledge.

Kozier & Erb's Fundamentals of Nursing: Concepts, Process, and Practice, eighth edition, addresses the concepts of contemporary professional nursing. These concepts include but are not limited to caring, wellness, health promotion, disease prevention, holistic care, multiculturalism, nursing theories, nursing informatics, nursing research, ethics, and advocacy. With this edition, every chapter has been extensively revised. The content has been updated to reflect the latest nursing research and the increasing emphasis on aging, wellness, and home- and community-based care. Many of the changes are in response to suggestions and comments from reviewers and nursing students using the text. We developed this text so that it can be used with a variety of nursing theories and conceptual frameworks.

ORGANIZATION

The detailed table of contents at the beginning of the book makes its clear organization easy to follow. Continuing with a strong focus on nursing care, the eighth edition of this book is divided into 10 units.

Unit 1, The Nature of Nursing, clusters five chapters that provide comprehensive coverage of introductory concepts of nursing.

In Unit 2, Contemporary Health Care, four chapters cover contemporary health care topics such as health care delivery systems, community-based care, home care, and informatics.

Unit 3 is now The Nursing Process. Six chapters introduce students to this important framework with each chapter dedicated to a specific step of the nursing process. Chapter 10 applies critical thinking and the nursing process. A Nursing in Action case study is used as the frame of reference for applying content in all phases of the nursing process in Chapter 11, Assessing; Chapter 12, Diagnosing; Chapter 13, Planning; and Chapter 14, Implementing and Evaluating. Chapter 15 covers documenting and reporting. Starting in this unit and incorpo-

rated throughout the book, we refer to the new NANDA 2007–2008 diagnoses.

In Unit 4, Health Beliefs and Practices, four chapters cover health-related beliefs and practices for individuals and families from a variety of different cultural backgrounds.

Unit 5, Life Span Development, consists of five chapters that discuss life span and development from conception to elders. Chapter 23 is a new chapter devoted specifically to promoting health in elders.

Unit 6, Integral Aspects of Nursing, discusses topics such as caring; communicating; teaching; and leading, managing, and delegating. These topics are all crucial elements for providing competent nursing care. In the eighth edition a new chapter (Chapter 26) has been dedicated to communicating.

Unit 7, Assessing Health, covers vital signs and health assessment in two separate chapters, so beginning students can understand normal assessment techniques and findings. Chapter 29, Vital Signs, begins to introduce students to the clinical procedures that they need to learn to perform.

In Unit 8, Integral Components of Client Care, the focus shifts to those components of client care that are universal to all clients, including asepsis, safety, hygiene, diagnostic testing, medications, wound care, and preoperative care.

Unit 9, Promoting Psychosocial Health, includes six chapters that cover a wide range of areas that affect one's health. Sensory perception, self-concept, sexuality, spirituality, stress, and loss are all things that a nurse needs to consider to properly care for a client.

Unit 10, Promoting Physiologic Health, discusses a variety of physiologic concepts that provide the foundations for nursing care. These include activity and exercise; sleep; pain; nutrition; elimination; oxygenation; circulation; and fluid, electrolyte, and acid–base balance.

Features

For years, *Kozier & Erb's Fundamentals of Nursing* has been a gold standard that helps students embark on their careers in nursing. This new edition retains many of the features that have made this textbook the number-one choice of nursing students and faculty. The walk-through at the beginning of the textbook illustrates these features.

To further enhance this popular fundamentals textbook, we invited nursing faculty and students to provide suggestions. Based on their recommendations, we added several new features to make this edition of *Kozier & Erb's Fundamentals of Nursing* a current and engaging textbook that helps all students succeed in their first nursing courses. These new features are illustrated in the walk-through at the beginning of the book and include Real World Reflections, Real World Practice, Drug Capsule boxes, Anatomy & Physiology Reviews, and Clinical Manifestation boxes.

Supplements that Inspire Success for the Student and the Instructor

To supplement the textbook and facilitate active student learning, we include a variety of student learning aids in our comprehensive supplements package.

PRENTICE HALL NURSING MEDIALINK DVD-ROM. A DVD-ROM comes packaged with every textbook. It provides an interactive study program that allows students to practice answering NCLEX®-style questions with rationales for right and wrong answers. It also contains an audio glossary, animations, videos, skill checklists, and a link to the Companion Website. New to this edition is a dosage calculation module and a software tool for building your own concept maps along with end-of-unit activities for creating concept maps that relate to unit topics.

STUDY GUIDE. This workbook includes case studies, NCLEX® review, and other review exercises. MediaLinks refer students to activities on the **Prentice Hall Nursing MediaLink DVD-ROM** and Companion Website.

CLINICAL HANDBOOK. This handy reference serves as a portable, quick-reference to fundamentals of nursing. Topics include lab values, diagnostic tests, infection control documentation, NANDA diagnoses, and much more. This handbook allows students to bring the information they learn from class into any clinical setting.

COMPANION WEBSITE. Access to an online study guide, at http://www.prenhall.com/berman, is provided with every textbook. The Companion Website is designed to help students apply the concepts presented in the book. Each chapter-specific module features learning outcomes, an audio glossary of terms, NCLEX® review questions, case studies, care plan activities, application activities, web links, and more.

INSTRUCTOR'S RESOURCE MANUAL. This manual contains a wealth of material to help faculty plan and manage the Fundamentals of Nursing course. It includes chapter overviews, detailed lecture suggestions and outlines, learning outcomes, a complete test bank, teaching tips, and more for each chapter.

INSTRUCTOR'S RESOURCE DVD-ROM. This cross-platform DVD-ROM provides an all-new set of PowerPoint presentations for use in classroom lectures. It also contains an electronic test bank and animations and videos from the **Prentice Hall Nursing MediaLink DVD-ROM.** This supplement is available to faculty on adoption of the textbook.

ONLINE COURSE MANAGEMENT SYSTEMS. Also available are online companions for schools using WebCT, Blackboard, or CourseCompass course management systems. The online course management solutions feature interactive modules, electronic test banks, PowerPoint images and text slides, animations, assessment activities, and more. For more information about adopting an online course management system to accompany *Kozier & Erb's Fundamentals of Nursing, eighth edition,* please contact your Prentice Hall Health sales representative. Or go online to the appropriate website below and select Courses and Nursing to access a free preview of our online course companions:

WebCT: **http://cms.prenhall.com/webct/index.html**

Blackboard: **http://cms.prenhall.com/blackboard/index.html**

CourseCompass: **http://cms.prenhall.com/coursecompass/**

ACKNOWLEDGMENTS

We wish to extend a sincere thank you to the talented team involved in the eighth edition of this book: the contributors and reviewers who provide content and very helpful feedback; the nursing students, for their questioning minds and motivation; and the nursing instructors, who provided many valuable suggestions for this edition.

We would like to thank the editorial team at Prentice Hall including Kelly Trakalo, senior acquisitions editor, for keeping our noses to the grindstone; Marilyn Meserve, managing editor, who can multitask with the best of them; and Teri Zak, development editor, for her dedication and attention to detail that promoted an excellent outcome. Many thanks to the production team of Patrick Walsh, production manager; Cathy O'Connell, production liaison; and Emily Bush, production editor, for producing this book with precision, and to the design team led by Cheryl Asherman, creative director, for providing a truly beautiful design for this textbook. Many of the new photos in the eighth edition were photographed by Patrick Watson, setting courtesy of the School of Nursing at Nevada State College.

Finally, the kaleidoscope image used on the cover and throughout this textbook was designed by Paula Nadelstern. A kaleidoscope is an ever changing piece of art with its colors, light, and form. As a kaleidoscope turns, it represents new opportunities for beautiful new designs. Seeking light and reflections to form new shapes allows you to open your mind to all of the possibilities a kaleidoscope has to offer. It is more expansive than you first imagined. As a nursing student begins on the path of a career in nursing, he or she also finds new opportunities unfolding as a light from within that brightens the path ahead. As students learn more about the field of nursing, they will explore and pursue areas of the field that they may have never imagined at the beginning of their journey. Now is your beginning—open your eyes and your mind to all of the wonderful opportunities in the field of nursing that are waiting to be pursued. You are the next generation of nursing.

Audrey Berman
Shirlee Snyder

Contributors

CHAPTER CONTRIBUTORS

Paul Arnstein, RN, PhD, APRN-BC
Associate Professor
Boston College
Boston, Massachussetts
Chapter 46 Pain Management

Jean Benzel-Lindley, PhD, RN
Course Coordinator
Nevada State College School of Nursing
Henderson, Nevada
Chapter 6 Health Care Delivery Systems
Chapter 7 Community Nursing and Care
*   Continuity*
Chapter 8 Home Care
Chapter 9 Nursing Informatics
Chapter 12 Diagnosing
Chapter 17 Health, Wellness, and Illness
Home Care Considerations
Teaching: Home Care
Home Care Assessment

Sherrilyn Coffman, DNS, RN, CPN
Associate Professor
Nevada State College School of Nursing
Henderson, Nevada
Chapter 25 Caring

Barbara D'Anna, DSL, RN, MSN, CNOR
Assistant Professor
Anne Arundel Community College
Arnold, Maryland
Chapter 37 Perioperative Nursing

Karen DeAngelis, RN, BSN, MSN, EdD
Acting Director of Nursing 2004
Lanier Village Estates
Gainesville, Georgia
Chapter 38 Sensory Perception

Ardys Dunn, PhD, PNP
Professor
Samuel Merritt College
Oakland, California

Chapter 20 Concepts of Growth and
*   Development*
Chapter 21 Promoting Health from
*   Conception to Adolescence*
LifeSpan Considerations

Karen Fontaine, RN, MSN
Professor
Purdue University Calumet
Hammond, Indiana
Chapter 19 Complementary and Alternative
*   Healing Modalitites*
Chapter 40 Sexuality

Cory Hartley, MSN, BSN
3M Company
San Ramon, California
Chapter 36 Skin Integrity and Wound Care
Chapter 49 Fecal Elimination

Judith Herrman, PhD, MS, BSN
Assistant Director and Assistant Professor of
Nursing
University of Delaware
Newark, Delaware
Chapter 35 Medications

Chris Jackson, PhD, MSN, BSN
Associate Professor
Eastern University
St. David's, Pennsylvania
Chapter 44 Activity and Exercise

Jackie Jones, RN, MSN, EdD
Assistant Professor
North Georgia College and State University
Dahlonega, Georgia
Chapter 52 Fluid, Electrolyte, and
*   Acid–Base Balance*

Lindsay McCrea, MS, CS, CWOCN, FNP
Assistant Professor
Samuel Merritt College
Oakland, California
Chapter 48 Urinary Elimination

Helda Pinzon-Perez, PhD, CHES, RMT
Associate Professor
California State University
Fresno, California
Chapter 18 Culture and Heritage

Ann Rogers, PhD, RN, FAAN
Associate Professor
University of Pennsylvania School of
Nursing
Philadelphia, Pennsylvania
Chapter 45 Sleep

Barbara Steuble, PhD, MSN, BSN
Assistant Professor
Samuel Merritt College
Sacramento, California
Chapter 50 Oxygenation

Elizabeth Taylor, PhD
Associate Professor
Loma Linda College
Loma Linda, California
Chapter 41 Spirituality

Tamara Zurakoski, PhD, CRNP
Lecturer/Clinical Specialist
University of Pennsylvania School of
Nursing
Henderson, Nevada
Philadelphia, Pennsylvania
Chapter 22 Promoting Health in Young and
*   Middle-Aged Adults*
Chapter 23 Promoting Health in Elders

REAL WORLD PRACTICE CONTRIBUTORS

Ann Fekete, RN, CCRN, CRNI
UCD General Clinical Research Center
Sacramento VA Medical Center
Mather, California

Kelly Flavin, RN, PCCN
OSF Saint Francis Medical Center
Peoria, Illinois

Sherrie Hatch, RN, BSN, CCRN
UC Davis Medical Center
Sacramento, California

Teresa Hsieh, BSN, RN
Children's Memorial Hospital
Chicago, Illinois

Jan Knudsen, RN, MSN, CCRN
Saint Elizabeth Regional Medical Center
Lincoln, Nebraska

Patricia Larson, RN
La Porte Hospital
La Porte, Indiana

Marie Lasater, RN, MSN, CCRN
Barnes Jewish Hospital
St. Louis, Missouri

Constance Lemley, MSN
La Porte Hospital
La Porte, Indiana

Ann Ohmann, RNC, ONC
St Cloud Hospital
St. Cloud, Minnesota

Carol Olff, RN, MSN, CCRN
John Muir Health
Walnut Creek, California

Joy Plamann, RN, BSN, BC
St. Cloud Hospital
St. Cloud, Minnesota

Mary Catherine Rawls, RN, MS, BC
Dartmouth-Hitchcock Medical Center
Lebanon, New Hampshire

Jane Reintges, RN, MS, CRRN, APRN-bc
Washington Hospital Healthcare Systems
Fremont, California

Tina Saiani, RN
The Children's Hospital at the Medical
Center of Central Georgia
Macon, Georgia

Danene Shannon, MS Ed, BSN, BA, RN
Advocate Lutheran General Hospital
Park Ridge, Illinois

Toni Stamps, RN, BSN
University Medical Center
Tucson, Arizona

Susan Sullivan, RN, BSN, CCRN
The Rehabilitation Institute of Chicago
Chicago, Illinois

Catherine Tieva, RN, OCN
St Cloud Hospital
St. Cloud, Minnesota

REAL WORLD REFLECTION CONTRIBUTOR LIST

Scott Eddy, Student
College of St. Catherine
St. Paul, Minnesota

Lisa Lindley, Student
College of St. Catherine
St. Paul, Minnesota

Jennifer Trucke, Student
College of St. Catherine
St. Paul, Minnesota

SUPPLEMENT AND MEDIA CONTRIBUTORS

Jane Benedict, RN, BSN, MSN
Assistant Professor
Pennsylvania College of Technology
Williamsport, Pennsylvania
*Classroom Response System Questions for
    Instructor Resource Manual*

Melissa Black, MSN, RN, FNP
Greenville Technical College
Greenville, South Carolina
*NCLEX-RN® Questions for Prentice Hall
    Nursing MediaLink DVD-ROM*

Mary Boylston BSN, MSN, EdD
Chair, Associate Professor & Nursing
Informatics Coordinator
Eastern University
St. David's, Pennsylvania
Companion Website

Michelle Buchman, RN, BSN, BC
Manager
Educational Support Services
Springfield, Missouri
Student Study Guide

Joanna E. Cain, BSN, RN
Auctorial Pursuits
Wilmington, North Carolina
*NCLEX-RN® Questions for Prentice Hall
    Nursing MediaLink DVD-ROM*

Marian Doyle, RN, BS, MS
Northampton Community College
Bethlehem, Pennsylvania
*NCLEX-RN® Questions for Prentice Hall
    Nursing MediaLink DVD-ROM*

Pamela Fowler, MS, RN, C
Assistant Professor
Rogers State University
Claremore, Oklahoma
Test Bank for Instructor Resource Manual

Patricia B. Lisk, BSN
Instructor
Augusta Technical College
Augusta, Georgia
Test Bank for Instructor Resource Manual

Kathryn G. Magorian, MSN, RN
Mount Mary College
Yankton, South Dakota
Test Bank for Instructor Resource Manual

Tammy Owens, MSN, RN
Assistant Professor
West Kentucky community and Technical
School
Paducah, Kentucky
Test Bank for Instructor Resource Manual

Lillian Rafeldt, RN, BSN, MA
Assistant Professor
Three Rivers Community College
Norwich, Connecticut
*NCLEX-RN® Questions for Prentice Hall
    Nursing MediaLink DVD-ROM*

Linda Robertson PhD, CRNP
Associate Professor
La Roche College Pittsburgh
Pittsburgh, Pennsylvania
Instructor Resource Manual

Deborah Rushing RN, MSN
Assistant Professor
Troy University School of Nursing
Troy, Alabama
Student Study Guide

Thank You

We would like to extend our heartfelt thanks to more than 90 of our colleagues from schools of nursing across the country who have given their time generously over the last few years to help us create this learning package. These individuals helped us develop this textbook and supplements by reviewing chapters, art, and media, and by answering a myriad of questions right up until the time of publication. *Kozier & Erb's Fundamentals of Nursing, 8e* has benefited immeasurably from their efforts, insights, suggestions, objections, encouragement and inspiration, as well as from their vast experience as teachers and nurses. Thank you again for helping us set the foundation for nursing excellence.

REVIEWERS

Nell Ard, PhD, CNS, RNC
Director of Nursing
Collin County Community College District

Elaine Beaupre, RN, Med, MSN
Quincy College

Eva Beliveau, RN, MSN
Northern Essex Community College

Julie Bliss, RN, EdD
Associate Professor and Chair
William Paterson University

Teri Boese, RN, MSN
Assistant Professor Clinical Learning
University of Iowa College of Nursing

Paula Bostwick, RN, MSN
Program Chair
Ivy Tech Community College

Wendy Burr, MSN, RN
Stephen F. Austin State University

Jeanie Burt, MSN, MS, RN
Assistant Professor
Harding University College of Nursing

Steve Campbell, RN, BSN, MSN, CCRN
Polk Community College

Mary M. Cimador, RN, MSN
Professor
Community College of Allegheny County

Pattie Clark, RN, MSN
Associate Professor, Nursing Outreach
Coordinator
Abraham Baldwin College

Diane Cline, RN, MSN
Professor
Victor Valley College

Traudel B. Cline, RN, MSN
Milwaukee Area Technical College

Carol L. Collins, RN, MS
Assistant Professor
Wilson School of Nursing Midwestern State
University

Patsy Cornelius, RN, MHSA, MSN
Assistant Professor
Texarkana College

Kathleen R. Crane, MSN, RN BC
Assistant Professor
Texas A&M University

Susan Cristoferi, MSN, RN
Professor
St Clair County Community College

**Barbara Daniel, CRNP, MeD, MS,
RPRN, BC**
Professor
Cecil Community College

Sandra Deveny, MSN, RNC, WHCNP
Truckee Meadows Community College

Colette Dieujuste, MSN, RN
Assistant Professor
Simmons College

Kathleen Dolin, RN, MSN
Assistant Professor
Northampton Community College

Barbara Douglas, RN, MSN, CNOR
Assistant Professor
West Virginia University Institute of
Technology

Nancy Duphily, MS, RNC, CCE, IBCLC
Professor
Mount Wauchusett Community College

Judy Eng, GNP, RN, CS
Assistant Professor
Borough of Manhattan Community College

Carol L. Esche, RN, ND, MA, CNA
Assistant Professor
University Of Maryland School of Nursing

Karen Faison, PhD, APRN, CNE
Director of Nursing
Virginia State University

Debbie Freyman, RN, MA, MSN
National Park Community College

Stefanie Gatica, RN, BSN, BA
Des Moines Area Community College

Shirley Girouard, RN, PhD, FAAN
Associate Professor
Southern Connecticut State University

Cornelia Gordon, RN, BSN, MA
McLennan Community College

Teresa Graham, RN
Holmes County College

Annette Gunderman, DEd, MSN, RN
Bloomsburg University

Kathleen Guyett, RN, MS
Professor
Genesee Community College

Debbie Hackler, RN, MSN
Department Chair, Allied Health Director of
Nursing
Hutchinson Community College

**Dr. K. Toby Haghenbeck, PhD, APRN,
BC, FNP, RN, CCRN**
Assistant Professor
Lienhard School of Nursing Pace University

Mark Hand, RN, MSN
Durham Technical Community College

Phyllis Hayes, RN, BSN
Halifax Community College

Linda Haynes, PhD, RN
Associate Professor
University of Northern Colorado School of
Nursing

Teresa Heemsbergen, RN, BS, MS
McLennan Community College

Karen Heys, MN, RN
Chair-Nursing Department
Everette Community College

Beth Hickey, RN, MSN, CRRN, CNA
Assistant Professor
Northern Kentucky University School of
Nursing and Health Professions

Ruby Houldson, RN, MSN, MS
Professor
Lincoln Trail College

Dr. Susan E. Jackson, RN, EdD, CEN, CCRN
Assistant Professor
William Paterson University

Ann-Marie John, RN, MS
Monroe Community College

Juanita Johnson, PhD, RN
Adjunct Professor
Oklahoma Baptist University

Karen Kearcher, MS, ARNP
Lower Columbia College

Heidi Loucks, MS, RN, CNE
Casper College

Susan Madson, RN, MSN
Professor
Horry-Georgetown Technical College

Pamela Mahon, PhD, RN
Associate Professor
Kingsborough Community College

Sharon Marquard, RNC, MS, CRRN
Assistant Professor
St. Ambrose University

Claire Martino Maze, PhD, RN
Director Nursing Resource Center, Assistant
Professor
Barry University

Louise McGee, RN, MS
Professor
Tompkins Cortland Community College

Glenna McMinn, MS, RN
Professor
Tompkins Cortland Community College

MaryEllen Miller, MSN, RN
Texas A & M University

Christina Olson, RN, MSN
Assistant Professor
San Antonio College

Cynthia O'Neal, MSN, RN
Assistant Professor
Texas Tech University Health Sciences Center

Robin Pattillo, RN, PhD
Associate Professor
Auburn University School of Nursing

Michael Perlow, DNS, RN
Professor
Murray State University

Linda Picklesimer, RN, MSN
Greenville Technical College

Susan Piva, MS, RN
Associate Professor
Brevard Community College

Barbara Poremba, EdD, MPH, MSN, RNCS, ANP
Professor
Salem State College

Karla Randall, RN, PhD
Assistant Professor
University of Southern Maine

Susan Randol, RN, MSN
University of Louisiana at Lafayette

Rhonda Roxanna Rash, BSN, MS, EdD
Professor
Cecil Community College

Marysue Rayno, RN, MSN, EdD(c)
Luzerne County Community College

Pamela Read, RN, MSN
Assistant Professor
Georgia Perimeter College

Donna Richards, RN, PhD
Professor and Chair Department of Nursing
Horry-Georgetown Technical College

Diane Roberson, RN, MSN
Aiken Technical College

Nancy Rymut, RN, MS, CEN
Professor
Three Rivers Community College

Kay Sackett, EdD, RN
Clinical Associate Professor
University at Buffalo State University of
New York

Cheryl Sadler, PhD, RN
Associate Professor
University of Akron

Karen Schaefer, DNSc, RN
Director Undergraduate Program, Assistant
Professor
Temple University

Lee Schmidt, RN, PhD
Assistant Professor
Loyola University Chicago

Michelle Schutt, MSN, RN
Auburn University Montgomery School

Maria Seidel, MS, ARNP
Associate Professor
Indian River Community College

Sally Shultz, MSN, RN
Fox Valley Technical College

Lorie Sigmon, RN, MSN, FNP
Nash Community College

Roxanne Sparks, RN, BSN, LNC
Assistant Director Vocational Nursing Program
Merced College

Doris Stone, MAHSM, MAHRD, MSN
Associate Professor
Jefferson Community College

Jeanie Stroud, RN, MS
Professor
Imperial Valley College

Karen Tarnow, RN, PhD
Clinical Assistant Professor
University of Kansas

Barbara Taylor, RN, MSN
Professor
Chipola College Health Science Department

Patricia Durham Taylor, RN PhD
Truckee Meadows Community College

Laura Thelen, RN, MSN
Assistant Professor
Oakton Community College

Nancy Torre, RN, MS
Jones County Junior College

Constance Twyman, RN, MSN, CS
Assistant Professor
Alvernia College

Barbara E. Vickers, RN, MS, CCRN
Professor
Erie Community College

Amanda White, RN, BSN
Nash Community College

Sue Wojciechowski, RN, MSN
Westmoreland County Community College

Joanne Woods, MSN, RN, NP-C
McLennan Community College

Dolores Zygmont, PhD, RN
Associate Professor
Temple University

STUDENT REVIEWERS

Lorna Benoit
Essex Community College

Lori Bunalski
The College of New Jersey

Jessica Kramer
The College of New Jersey

Kristina Smith
University of Maryland

Emily Watson
The College of New Jersey

Melissa Whitty
The College of New Jersey

Special Features

CLINICAL MANIFESTATIONS

CONCEPT MAP

CRITICAL PATHWAY

CRITICAL THINKING CHECKPOINT

CULTURALLY COMPETENT CARE

DRUG CAPSULE

HOME CARE ASSESSMENT

HOME CARE CONSIDERATIONS

IDENTIFYING NURSING DIAGNOSES, OUTCOMES, AND INTERVENTIONS

LIFESPAN CONSIDERATIONS

NURSING CARE PLAN

PRACTICE GUIDELINES

RESEARCH NOTES

SKILLS

Table of Contents

UNIT 1

The Nature of Nursing

Throughout its distinguished history, nursing has had a significant effect on people's lives. As rapid change continues to transform the profession of nursing and the health care system with which it is intricately linked, nurses embrace broader opportunities to influence human well-being. Today, nurses bring knowledge, leadership, spirit, and vital expertise to expanding roles that afford increased participation, responsibility, and rewards. However nursing continues to evolve, underlying all is a time-honored, fervent, and profound commitment to caring.

CHAPTER 1

Historical and Contemporary Nursing Practice

LEARNING OUTCOMES

After completing this chapter, you will be able to:

1. Discuss historical and contemporary factors influencing the development of nursing.

2. Identify the essential aspects of nursing.

3. Identify four major areas within the scope of nursing practice.

4. Identify the purposes of nurse practice acts and standards for nursing practice.

5. Describe the roles of nurses.

6. Describe the expanded career roles and their functions.

7. Discuss the criteria of a profession and the professionalization of nursing.

8. Discuss Benner's levels of nursing proficiency.

9. Relate essential nursing values to attitudes, personal qualities, and professional behaviors.

10. Explain the functions of national and international nurses' associations.

MediaLink **MWW** Evolution of Nursing Case Study

KEY TERMS

caregiver, *13*

case manager, *15*

change agent, *14*

Clara Barton, *9*

client, *12*

client advocate, *14*

communicator, *13*

consumer, *12*

counseling, *14*

demography, *20*

diagnostic-related groups (DRGs), *18*

Dorothea Dix, *6*

Fabiola, *5*

Florence Nightingale, *9*

governance, *17*

Harriet Tubman, *6*

Knights of Saint Lazarus, *5*

Lavinia L. Dock, *10*

leader, *14*

Lillian Wald, *10*

Linda Richards, *9*

manager, *14*

Margaret Higgins Sanger, *10*

Mary Breckinridge, *11*

Mary Mahoney, *10*

patient, *12*

Patient Self-Determination Act (PSDA), *20*

profession, *15*

professionalism, *15*

professionalization, *16*

Sairy Gamp, *8*

socialization, *17*

Sojourner Truth, *6*

Standards of Practice, *12*

Standards of Professional Performance, *13*

teacher, *13*

telecommunications, *19*

Nursing today is far different from nursing as it was practiced years ago, and it is expected to continue changing during the 21st century. To comprehend present-day nursing and at the same time prepare for the future, one must understand not only past events but also contemporary nursing practice and the sociological and historical factors that affect it.

HISTORICAL PERSPECTIVES

Nursing has undergone dramatic change in response to societal needs and influences. A look at nursing's beginnings reveals its continuing struggle for autonomy and professionalization. In recent decades, a renewed interest in nursing history has produced a growing amount of related literature. This section highlights only selected aspects of events that have influenced nursing practice. Recurring themes of women's roles and status, religious (Christian) values, war, societal attitudes, and visionary nursing leadership have influenced nursing practice in the past. Many of these factors still exert their influence today.

Women's Roles

Traditional female roles of wife, mother, daughter, and sister have always included the care and nurturing of other family members. From the beginning of time, women have cared for infants and children; thus, nursing could be said to have its roots in "the home." Additionally, women, who in general occupied a subservient and dependent role, were called on to care for others in the community who were ill. Generally, the care provided was related to physical maintenance and comfort. Thus, the traditional nursing role has always entailed humanistic caring, nurturing, comforting, and supporting.

Religion

Religion has also played a significant role in the development of nursing. Although many of the world's religions encourage benevolence, it was the Christian value of "love thy neighbor as thyself" and Christ's parable of the Good Samaritan that had a significant impact on the development of Western nursing. Dur-

ing the third and fourth centuries, several wealthy matrons of the Roman Empire, such as **Fabiola,** converted to Christianity and used their wealth to provide houses of care and healing (the forerunner of hospitals) for the poor, the sick, and the homeless. Women were not, however, the sole providers of nursing services.

The Crusades saw the formation of several orders of knights, including the Knights of Saint John of Jerusalem (also known as the Knights Hospitalers), the Teutonic Knights, and the Knights of Saint Lazarus (Figure 1-1 ■). These brothers in arms provided nursing care to their sick and injured comrades. These orders also built hospitals, the organization and management of which set a standard for the administration of hospitals throughout Europe at that time. The **Knights of Saint Lazarus** dedicated themselves to the care of people with leprosy, syphilis, and chronic skin conditions.

Figure 1-1 ■ The Knights of Saint Lazarus (established circa 1200) dedicated themselves to the care of people with leprosy, syphilis, and chronic skin conditions. From the time of Christ to the mid-13th century, leprosy was viewed as an incurable and terminal disease.

(CORBIS Images.)

The deaconess groups, which had their origins in the Roman Empire of the third and fourth centuries, were suppressed during the Middle Ages by the Western churches. However, these groups of nursing providers resurfaced occasionally throughout the centuries, most notably in 1836 when Theodore Fliedner reinstituted the Order of Deaconesses and opened a small hospital and training school in Kaiserswerth, Germany. Florence Nightingale received her "training" in nursing at the Kaiserswerth School.

Early religious values, such as self-denial, spiritual calling, and devotion to duty and hard work, have dominated nursing throughout its history. Nurses' commitment to these values often resulted in exploitation and few monetary rewards. For some time, nurses themselves believed it was inappropriate to expect economic gain from their "calling."

War

Throughout history, wars have accentuated the need for nurses. During the Crimean War (1854–1856), the inadequacy of care given to soldiers led to a public outcry in Great Britain. The role Florence Nightingale played in addressing this problem is well known. She was asked by Sir Sidney Herbert of the British War Department to recruit a contingent of female nurses to provide care to the sick and injured in the Crimea. Nightingale and her nurses transformed the military hospitals by setting up sanitation practices, such as hand washing and washing clothing regularly. Nightingale is credited with performing miracles; the mortality rate in the Barrack Hospital in Turkey, for example, was reduced from 42% to 2% (Donahue, 1996, p. 197).

During the American Civil War (1861–1865), several nurses emerged who were notable for their contributions to a country torn by internal strife. **Harriet Tubman** and **Sojourner Truth** (Figures 1-2 ■ and 1-3 ■) provided care and safety to slaves fleeing to the North on the Underground Railroad. Mother Biekerdyke and Clara Barton searched the battlefields and gave care to injured and dying soldiers. Noted authors Walt Whitman and

Figure 1-3 ■ Sojourner Truth (1797–1883), abolitionist, Underground Railroad agent, preacher, and women's rights advocate, was a nurse for over 4 years during the Civil War and worked as a nurse and counselor for the Freedmen's Relief Association after the war.

(Randall Studio (1805–1875) Sojourner Truth (c. 1797–18--), abolitionist. © 1870. Photograph, Albumen Silver Print. Copyright National Portrait Gallery, Smithsonian Institution/Art Resources, NY.)

Louisa May Alcott volunteered as nurses to give care to injured soldiers in military hospitals. Another woman leader who provided nursing care during the Civil War was **Dorothea Dix** (Figure 1-4 ■). She became the Union's Superintendent of Female Nurses responsible for recruiting nurses and supervising the nursing care of all women nurses working in the army hospitals.

The arrival of World War I resulted in American, British, and French women rushing to volunteer their nursing services. These nurses endured harsh environments and treated injuries not seen before. A monument, entitled "The Spirit of Nursing," stands in Arlington National Cemetery (Figure 1-5 ■). It honors the nurses

Figure 1-2 ■ Harriet Tubman (1820–1913) was known as "The Moses of Her People" for her work with the Underground Railroad. During the Civil War (1861–1865), she nursed the sick and suffering of her own race.

(© CORBIS.)

Figure 1-4 ■ Dorothea Dix (1802–1887) was the Union's Superintendent of Female Nurses during the Civil War.

(CORBIS Images.)

A

B

C

Figure 1-5 ■ *A*, Section 21 in Arlington National Cemetery honors the nurses who served in the Armed Services in World War I. *B*, The "Spirit of Nursing" monument that stands in Section 21. *C*, Monument plaque.

(Photo by Sherrilyn Coffman, PhD, RN.)

who served in the U.S. Armed Services in World War I, many of whom are buried in Section 21 which is also called the "Nurses Section" (Military District of Washington, n.d.). Progress in health care occurred during World War I, particularly in the field of surgery. For example, there were advancements in the use of anesthetic agents, infection control, blood typing, and prosthetics (Holder, 2004, p. 915).

World War II casualties created an acute shortage of caregivers, and the Cadet Nurse Corps was established in response to a marked shortage of nurses (Figure 1-6 ■). Also at that time, auxiliary health care workers became prominent. "Practical" nurses, aides, and technicians provided much of the actual nursing care under the instruction and supervision of better prepared nurses. Medical specialties also arose at that time to meet the needs of hospitalized clients.

During the Vietnam War, approximately 90% of the 11,000 American military women stationed in Vietnam were nurses. Most of them volunteered to go to Vietnam right after they graduated from nursing school. This made them the youngest group of medical personnel ever to serve in wartime (Vietnam Women's Memorial Foundation, n.d.). Near the Vietnam Veterans Memorial ("The Wall") stands the Vietnam Women's

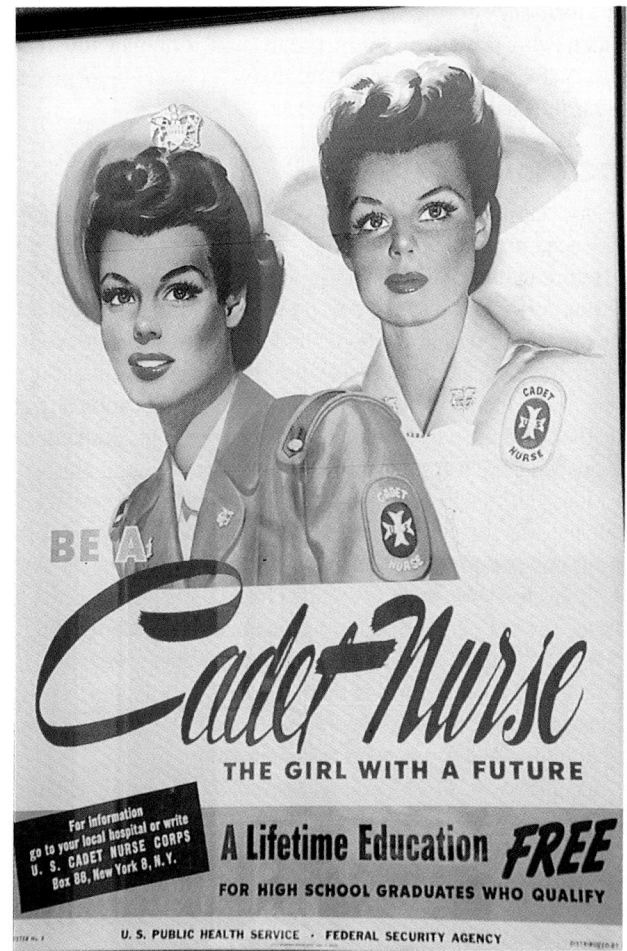

Figure 1-6 ■ Recruiting poster for the Cadet Nurse Corps during World War II.

(Courtesy of Illinois State University.)

Figure 1-7 ■ Vietnam Women's Memorial. Four figures include a nurse tending to the chest wound of a soldier, another woman looking for a helicopter for assistance, and a third woman (behind the other figures) kneeling while staring at an empty helmet in grief.
(Photo by Sherrilyn Coffman, PhD, RN.)

Figure 1-8 ■ Sairy Gamp, a character in Dickens' book *Martin Chuzzlewit,* represented the negative image of nurses in the early 1800s.
(CORBIS Images.)

Memorial (Figure 1-7 ■). This monument was established to "honor the women who served and also for the families who lost loved ones during the war . . . to let them know about the women who provided comfort, care and a human touch for those who were suffering and dying" (Vietnam Women's Memorial Foundation, n.d.).

Societal Attitudes

Society's attitudes about nurses and nursing have significantly influenced professional nursing.

Before the mid-1800s, nursing was without organization, education, or social status; the prevailing attitude was that a woman's place was in the home and that no respectable woman should have a career. The role for the Victorian middle-class woman was that of wife and mother, and any education she obtained was for the purpose of making her a pleasant companion to her husband and a responsible mother to her children. Nurses in hospitals during this period were poorly educated; some were even incarcerated criminals. Society's attitudes about nursing during this period are reflected in the writings of Charles Dickens. In his book *Martin Chuzzlewit* (1896), Dickens reflected his attitude toward nurses through his character **Sairy Gamp** (Figure 1-8 ■). She "cared" for the sick by neglecting them, stealing from them, and physically abusing them (Donahue, 1996, p. 192). This literary portrayal of nurses greatly influenced the negative image and attitude toward nurses up to contemporary times.

In contrast, the *guardian angel* or *angel of mercy* image arose in the latter part of the 19th century, largely because of the work of Florence Nightingale during the Crimean War. After Nightingale brought respectability to the nursing profession, nurses were viewed as noble, compassionate, moral, religious, dedicated, and self-sacrificing.

Another image arising in the early 19th century that has affected subsequent generations of nurses and the public and other professionals working with nurses is the image of *doctor's handmaiden.* This image evolved when women had yet to obtain the right to vote, when family structures were largely paternalistic, and when the medical profession portrayed increasing use of scientific knowledge that, at that time, was viewed as a male domain. Since that time, several images of nursing have been portrayed. The *heroine* portrayal evolved from nurses' acts of bravery in World War II and their contributions in fighting poliomyelitis—in particular, the work of the Australian nurse Elizabeth Kenney. Other images in the late 1900s include the nurse as sex object, surrogate mother, tyrannical mother, and body expert.

During the past few decades, the nursing profession has taken steps to improve the image of the nurse. In the early 1990s, the Tri-Council for Nursing (the American Association of Colleges of Nursing, the American Nurses Association, the American Organization of Nurse Executives, and the National League for Nursing) initiated a national effort (titled "Nurses of America") to improve the image of nursing. More recently, the Johnson & Johnson corporation contributed $20 million in 2002 to launch a "Campaign for Nursing's Future" to promote nursing as a positive career choice (Anonymous, 2003; Fitzpatrick, 2002). In addition, nursing schools and hospitals are targeting men in their recruitment efforts (Meyers, 2003).

Nursing Leaders

Florence Nightingale, Clara Barton, Lillian Wald, Lavinia Dock, Margaret Sanger, and Mary Breckinridge are among the leaders who have made notable contributions both to nursing's history and to women's history. These women were all politically astute pioneers. Their skills at influencing others and bringing about change remain models for political nurse activists today. Contemporary nursing leaders, such as Virginia Henderson, who created a modern worldwide definition of nurs-

Figure 1-9 ■ Considered the founder of modern nursing, Florence Nightingale (1820–1910) was influential in developing nursing education, practice, and administration. Her publication, *Notes on Nursing: What It Is, and What It Is Not*, first published in England in 1859 and in the United States in 1860, was intended for all women.
(© Bettman/CORBIS.)

Figure 1-10 ■ Clara Barton (1812–1912) organized the American Red Cross, which linked with the International Red Cross when the U.S. Congress ratified the Geneva Convention in 1882.
(© Bettman/CORBIS.)

ing, and Martha Rogers, a catalyst for theory development, are discussed in Chapter 3. ∞

Nightingale (1820–1910)

Florence Nightingale's contributions to nursing are well documented. Her achievements in improving the standards for the care of war casualties in the Crimea earned her the title "Lady with the Lamp." Her efforts in reforming hospitals and in producing and implementing public health policies also made her an accomplished political nurse: She was the first nurse to exert political pressure on government. Through her contributions to nursing education—perhaps her greatest achievement—she is also recognized as nursing's first scientist-theorist for her work *Notes on Nursing: What It Is, and What It Is Not* (1860/1969).

Nightingale (Figure 1-9 ■) was born to a wealthy and intellectual family. She believed she was "called by God to help others . . . [and] to improve the well-being of mankind" (Schuyler, 1992, p. 4). She was determined to become a nurse in spite of opposition from her family and the restrictive societal code for affluent young English women. As a well-traveled young woman of the day, she visited Kaiserswerth in 1847, where she received 3 months' training in nursing. In 1853 she studied in Paris with the Sisters of Charity, after which she returned to England to assume the position of superintendent of a charity hospital for ill governesses.

When she returned to England from the Crimea, a grateful English public gave Nightingale an honorarium of £4500. She later used this money to develop the Nightingale Training School for Nurses, which opened in 1860. The school served as a model for other training schools. Its graduates traveled to other countries to manage hospitals and institute nurse-training programs.

Nightingale's vision of nursing, which included public health and health promotion roles for nurses, was only partially addressed in the early days of nursing. The focus tended to be on developing the profession within hospitals.

Barton (1821–1912)

Clara Barton (Figure 1-10 ■) was a schoolteacher who volunteered as a nurse during the American Civil War. Her responsibility was to organize the nursing services. Barton is noted for her role in establishing the American Red Cross, which linked with the International Red Cross when the U.S. Congress ratified the Treaty of Geneva (Geneva Convention). It was Barton who persuaded Congress in 1882 to ratify this treaty so that the Red Cross could perform humanitarian efforts in time of peace.

Richards (1841–1930)

Linda Richards (Figure 1-11 ■) was America's first trained nurse. She graduated from the New England Hospital for Women and Children in 1873. Richards is known for introducing nurse's notes and doctor's orders. She also initiated the practice of nurses wearing uniforms (American Nurses Association, 2006a). She is credited for her pioneer work in psychiatric and industrial nursing.

Figure 1-11 ■ Linda Richards (1841–1930) was America's first trained nurse.
(National Library of Medicine)

Figure 1-12 ■ Mary Mahoney (1845–1926) was the first African American trained nurse.

(Schomburg Center for Research in Black Culture, New York Public Library.)

Mahoney (1845–1926)

Mary Mahoney (Figure 1-12 ■) was the first African American professional nurse. She graduated from the New England Hospital for Women and Children in 1879. She constantly worked for the acceptance of African Americans in nursing and for the promotion of equal opportunities (Donahue, 1996, p. 271). The American Nurses Association (2006b) gives a Mary Mahoney Award biennially in recognition of significant contributions in interracial relationships.

Wald (1867–1940)

Lillian Wald (Figure 1-13 ■) is considered the founder of public health nursing. Wald and Mary Brewster were the first to offer trained nursing services to the poor in the New York slums. Their home among the poor on the upper floor of a tenement, called the Henry Street Settlement and Visiting Nurse Service, provided nursing services, social services, and organized educational and cultural activities. Soon after the founding of the

Figure 1-13 ■ Lillian Wald (1867–1940) founded the Henry Street Settlement and Visiting Nurse Service (circa 1893), which provided nursing and social services and organized educational and cultural activities. She is considered the founder of public health nursing. .

(Schevill, William Valentine (1864–1951) Lillian D. Wald (1867–1940). Public health nurse, social worker. 1919. Oil on Cardboard. Copyright National Portrait Gallery, Smithsonian Institution/Art Resources, NY.)

Figure 1-14 ■ Nursing leader and suffragist Lavinia L. Dock (1858–1956) was active in the protest movement for women's rights that resulted in the U.S. Constitution amendment allowing women to vote in 1920.

(Courtesy of Teachers College, Columbia University.)

Henry Street Settlement, school nursing was established as an adjunct to visiting nursing.

Dock (1858–1956)

Lavinia L. Dock (Figure 1-14 ■) was a feminist, prolific writer, political activist, suffragette, and friend of Wald. She participated in protest movements for women's rights that resulted in the 1920 passage of the 19th Amendment to the U.S. Constitution, which granted women the right to vote. In addition, Dock campaigned for legislation to allow nurses rather than physicians to control their profession. In 1893, Dock, with the assistance of Mary Adelaide Nutting and Isabel Hampton Robb, founded the American Society of Superintendents of Training Schools for Nurses of the United States and Canada, a precursor to the current National League for Nursing.

Sanger (1879–1966)

Margaret Higgins Sanger (Figure 1-15 ■), a public health nurse in New York, has had a lasting impact on women's health care.

Figure 1-15 ■ Nurse activist Margaret Sanger, considered the founder of Planned Parenthood, was imprisoned for opening the first birth control information clinic in Baltimore in 1916.

(© Bettman/CORBIS.)

Figure 1-16 ■ Mary Breckinridge, a nurse who practiced midwifery in England, Australia, and New Zealand, founded the Frontier Nursing Service in Kentucky in 1925 to provide family-centered primary health care to rural populations.
(Courtesy of Frontier Nursing Service, Inc., Wandover, KY.)

Imprisoned for opening the first birth control information clinic in America, she is considered the founder of Planned Parenthood. Her experience with the large number of unwanted pregnancies among the working poor was instrumental in addressing this problem.

Breckinridge (1881–1965)

After World War I, **Mary Breckinridge** (Figure 1-16 ■), a notable pioneer nurse, established the Frontier Nursing Service (FNS). In 1918, she worked with the American Committee for Devastated France, distributing food, clothing, and supplies to rural villages and taking care of sick children. In 1921, Breckinridge returned to the United States with plans to provide health care to the people of rural America. In 1925, Breckinridge and two other nurses began the FNS in Leslie County, Kentucky. Within this organization, Breckinridge started one of the first midwifery training schools in the United States.

CONTEMPORARY NURSING PRACTICE

An understanding of contemporary nursing practice includes a look at definitions of nursing, recipients of nursing, scope of nursing, settings for nursing practice, nurse practice acts, and current standards of clinical nursing practice.

Definitions of Nursing

Florence Nightingale defined nursing nearly 150 years ago as "the act of utilizing the environment of the patient to assist him in his recovery" (Nightingale, 1860-1969). Nightingale considered a clean, well-ventilated, and quiet environment essential for recovery. Often considered the first nurse theorist, Nightingale raised the status of nursing through education. Nurses were no longer untrained housekeepers but people educated in the care of the sick.

Virginia Henderson was one of the first modern nurses to define nursing. She wrote, "The unique function of the nurse is to assist the individual, sick or well, in the performance of those activities contributing to health or its recovery (or to peaceful death) that he would perform unaided if he had the necessary strength, will, or knowledge, and to do this in such a way as to help him gain independence as rapidly as possible" (Henderson, 1966, p. 3). Like Nightingale, Henderson described nursing in relation to the client and the client's environment. Unlike Nightingale, Henderson saw the nurse as concerned with both healthy and ill individuals, acknowledged that nurses interact with clients even when recovery may not be feasible, and mentioned the teaching and advocacy roles of the nurse.

In the latter half of the 20th century, a number of nurse theorists developed their own theoretical definitions of nursing. Theoretical definitions are important because they go beyond simplistic common definitions. They describe what nursing is and the interrelationship among nurses, nursing, the client, the environment, and the intended client outcome: health (see Chapter 3). ∞

Certain themes are common to many of these definitions:

- Nursing is caring.
- Nursing is an art.
- Nursing is a science.
- Nursing is client centered.
- Nursing is holistic.
- Nursing is adaptive.
- Nursing is concerned with health promotion, health maintenance, and health restoration.
- Nursing is a helping profession.

Professional nursing associations have also examined nursing and developed their definitions of it. In 1973, the American Nurses Association (ANA) described nursing practice as "direct, goal oriented, and adaptable to the needs of the individual, the family, and community during health and illness" (ANA, 1973, p. 2). In 1980, the ANA changed this definition of nursing to this: "Nursing is the diagnosis and treatment of human responses to actual or potential health problems" (ANA, 1980, p. 9). In 1995, the ANA recognized the influence and contribution of the science of caring to nursing philosophy and practice. Their most recent definition of professional nursing is much broader and states: "Nursing is the protection, promotion, and optimization of health and abilities, preventions of illness and injury, alleviation of suffering through the diagnosis and treatment of human response, and advocacy in the care of individuals, families, communities, and populations" (ANA, 2003, p. 6).

Research to explore the meaning of caring in nursing has been increasing. For example, Coffman (2004) conducted a metasynthesis of qualitative studies describing cultural caring in nursing practice. Likewise, Graber and Mitcham (2004) sought to identify actions, interventions, and interpersonal relationships that demonstrated caring and compassion. Details about caring are discussed in Chapter 25. ∞ See also Watson's "Assumptions of Caring" (Box 3–1) in Chapter 3. ∞

Recipients of Nursing

The recipients of nursing are sometimes called consumers, sometimes patients, and sometimes clients. A **consumer** is an individual, a group of people, or a community that uses a service or commodity. People who use health care products or services are consumers of health care.

A **patient** is a person who is waiting for or undergoing medical treatment and care. The word *patient* comes from a Latin word meaning "to suffer" or "to bear." Traditionally, the person receiving health care has been called a patient. Usually, people become patients when they seek assistance because of illness or for surgery. Some nurses believe that the word *patient* implies passive acceptance of the decisions and care of health professionals. Additionally, with the emphasis on health promotion and prevention of illness, many recipients of nursing care are not ill. Moreover, nurses interact with family members and significant others to provide support, information, and comfort in addition to caring for the patient.

For these reasons, nurses increasingly refer to recipients of health care as *clients*. A **client** is a person who engages the advice or services of another who is qualified to provide this service. The term *client* presents the receivers of health care as collaborators in the care, that is, as people who are also responsible for their own health. Thus, the health status of a client is the responsibility of the individual in collaboration with health professionals. In this book, *client* is the preferred term, although *consumer* and *patient* are used in some instances.

Scope of Nursing

Nurses provide care for three types of clients: individuals, families, and communities. Theoretical frameworks applicable to these client types, as well as assessments of individual, family, and community health, are discussed in Chapters 7 and 24. ∞

Nursing practice involves four areas: promoting health and wellness, preventing illness, restoring health, and caring for the dying.

Promoting Health and Wellness

Wellness is a process that engages in activities and behaviors that enhance quality of life and maximize personal potential (Anspaugh, Hamrick, & Rosata, 2003, p. 490). Nurses promote wellness in clients who are both healthy and ill. This may involve individual and community activities to enhance healthy lifestyles, such as improving nutrition and physical fitness, preventing drug and alcohol misuse, restricting smoking, and preventing accidents and injury in the home and workplace. See Chapter 16 for details. ∞

Preventing Illness

The goal of illness prevention programs is to maintain optimal health by preventing disease. Nursing activities that prevent illness include immunizations, prenatal and infant care, and prevention of sexually transmitted disease.

Restoring Health

Restoring health focuses on the ill client, and it extends from early detection of disease through helping the client during the recovery period. Nursing activities include the following:

- Providing direct care to the ill person, such as administering medications, baths, and specific procedures and treatments
- Performing diagnostic and assessment procedures, such as measuring blood pressure and examining feces for occult blood
- Consulting with other health care professionals about client problems
- Teaching clients about recovery activities, such as exercises that will accelerate recovery after a stroke
- Rehabilitating clients to their optimal functional level following physical or mental illness, injury, or chemical addiction

Caring for the Dying

This area of nursing practice involves comforting and caring for people of all ages who are dying. It includes helping clients live as comfortably as possible until death and helping support persons cope with death. Nurses carrying out these activities work in homes, hospitals, and extended care facilities. Some agencies, called *hospices,* are specifically designed for this purpose.

Settings for Nursing

In the past, the acute care hospital was the main practice setting open to most nurses. Today many nurses work in hospitals, but increasingly they work in clients' homes, community agencies, ambulatory clinics, long-term care facilities, health maintenance organizations (HMOs), and nursing practice centers (see Figure 1-17 ■).

Nurses have different degrees of nursing autonomy and nursing responsibility in the various settings. They may provide direct care, teach clients and support persons, serve as nursing advocates and agents of change, and help determine health policies affecting consumers in the community and in hospitals. For information about the models for delivery of nursing, see Chapter 6. ∞

Nurse Practice Acts

Nurse practice acts, or legal acts for professional nursing practice, regulate the practice of nursing in the United States and Canada. Each state in the United States and each province in Canada has its own act. Although nurse practice acts differ in various jurisdictions, they all have a common purpose: to protect the public. Nurses are responsible for knowing their state's nurse practice act as it governs their practice. For additional information, see Chapter 4. ∞

Standards of Nursing Practice

Establishing and implementing standards of practice are major functions of a professional organization. The purpose of the ANA **Standards of Practice** is to describe the responsibilities for

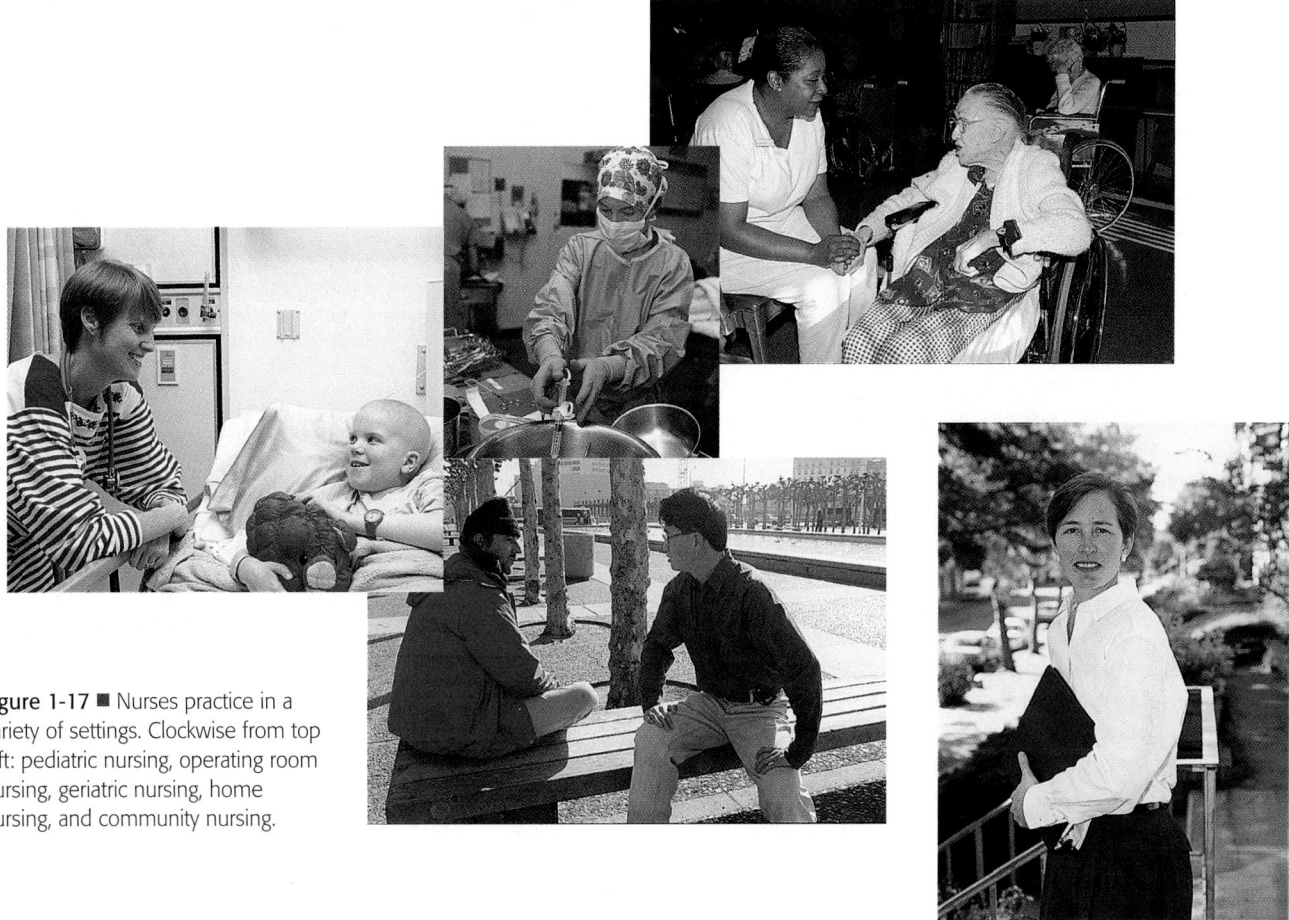

Figure 1-17 ■ Nurses practice in a variety of settings. Clockwise from top left: pediatric nursing, operating room nursing, geriatric nursing, home nursing, and community nursing.

which nurses are accountable (Box 1–1). The American Nurses Association developed standards of nursing practice that are generic in nature, by using the nursing process as a foundation, and provide for the practice of nursing regardless of area of specialization. Various specialty nursing organizations have further developed specific standards of nursing practice for their area. For nurses in Canada, each province or territory establishes its own standards of practice. The ANA **Standards of Professional Performance** (see Box 1–1) describe behaviors expected in the professional nursing role.

ROLES AND FUNCTIONS OF THE NURSE

Nurses assume a number of roles when they provide care to clients. Nurses often carry out these roles concurrently, not exclusively of one another. For example, the nurse may act as a counselor while providing physical care and teaching aspects of that care. The roles required at a specific time depend on the needs of the client and aspects of the particular environment.

Caregiver

The **caregiver** role has traditionally included those activities that assist the client physically and psychologically while preserving the client's dignity. The required nursing actions may in-

volve full care for the completely dependent client, partial care for the partially dependent client, and supportive-educative care to assist clients in attaining their highest possible level of health and wellness. Caregiving encompasses the physical, psychosocial, developmental, cultural, and spiritual levels. The nursing process provides nurses with a framework for providing care (see Chapters 10–14 ∞). A nurse may provide care directly or delegate it to other caregivers.

Communicator

Communication is integral to all nursing roles. Nurses communicate with the client, support persons, other health professionals, and people in the community.

In the role of **communicator,** nurses identify client problems and then communicate these verbally or in writing to other members of the health team. The quality of a nurse's communication is an important factor in nursing care. The nurse must be able to communicate clearly and accurately in order for a client's health care needs to be met (see Chapters 15 and 26 ∞).

Teacher

As a **teacher,** the nurse helps clients learn about their health and the health care procedures they need to perform to restore or maintain their health. The nurse assesses the client's learning needs and readiness to learn, sets specific learning goals in conjunction with

---

BOX 1–1   ANA Standards

Standards of Practice for the Registered Nurse—describe a competent level of nursing care as demonstrated by the nursing process.

1. Assessment
   Collects comprehensive data pertinent to the patient's health or the situation.
2. Diagnosis
   Analyzes the assessment data to determine the diagnoses or issues.
3. Outcomes Identification
   Identifies expected outcomes for a plan individualized to the patient or the situation.
4. Planning
   Develops a plan that prescribes strategies and alternatives to attain expected outcomes.
5. Implementation
   Implements the identified plan.
   5A. Coordination of care
   5B. Health teaching and health promotion
   5C. Consultation
        The advanced practice registered nurse and the nursing role specialist provide consultation to influence the identified plan, enhance the abilities of others, and effect change.
   5D. Prescriptive authority and treatment
        The advanced practice registered nurse uses prescriptive authority, procedures, referrals, treatments, and therapies in accordance with state and federal laws and regulations.
   5E. Treatment and evaluation
6. Evaluation
   Evaluates progress towards attainment of outcomes.
   Standards of Professional Performance—describe a competent level of behavior in the professional role.

7. Quality of practice
   Systematically enhances the quality and effectiveness of nursing practice.
8. Education
   Attains knowledge and competency that reflects current nursing practice.
9. Professional practice evaluation
   Evaluates one's own nursing practice in relation to professional practice standards and guidelines, relevant statutes, rules, and regulations.
10. Collegiality
    Interacts with and contributes to the professional development of peers and colleagues.
11. Collaboration
    Collaborates with patient, family, and others in the conduct of nursing practice.
12. Ethics
    Integrates ethical provisions in all areas of practice.
13. Research
    Integrates research findings into practice.
14. Resource utilization
    Considers factors related to safety, effectiveness, cost, and impact on practice in the planning and delivery of nursing services.
15. Leadership
    Provides leadership in the professional practice setting and the profession.

Note: Reprinted with permission from American Nurses Association, *Nursing: Scope and Standards of Practice,* © 2004 Nursebooks.org, Silver Spring, MD..

---

the client, enacts teaching strategies, and measures learning. Nurses also teach unlicensed assistive personnel (UAP) to whom they delegate care, and they share their expertise with other nurses and health professionals. See Chapter 27 for additional details about the teaching/learning process. ∞

Client Advocate

A **client advocate** acts to protect the client. In this role the nurse may represent the client's needs and wishes to other health professionals, such as relaying the client's wishes for information to the physician. They also assist clients in exercising their rights and help them speak up for themselves (see Chapter 5 ∞).

Counselor

Counseling is the process of helping a client to recognize and cope with stressful psychologic or social problems, to develop improved interpersonal relationships, and to promote personal growth. It involves providing emotional, intellectual, and psychologic support. The nurse counsels primarily healthy individuals with normal adjustment difficulties and focuses on helping the person develop new attitudes, feelings, and behaviors by encouraging the client to look at alternative behaviors, recognize the choices, and develop a sense of control.

Change Agent

The nurse acts as a **change agent** when assisting clients to make modifications in their behavior. Nurses also often act to make changes in a system, such as clinical care, if it is not helping a client return to health. Nurses are continually dealing with change in the health care system. Technological change, change in the age of the client population, and changes in medications are just a few of the changes nurses deal with daily. See Chapter 28 for additional information about change. ∞

Leader

A **leader** influences others to work together to accomplish a specific goal. The leader role can be employed at different levels: individual client, family, groups of clients, colleagues, or the community. Effective leadership is a learned process requiring an understanding of the needs and goals that motivate people, the knowledge to apply the leadership skills, and the interpersonal skills to influence others. The leadership role of the nurse is discussed in Chapter 28. ∞

Manager

The nurse manages the nursing care of individuals, families, and communities. The nurse **manager** also delegates nursing activities to ancillary workers and other nurses, and supervises and evaluates their performance. Managing requires knowledge about organizational structure and dynamics, authority and accountability, leadership, change theory, advocacy, delegation, and supervision and evaluation. See Chapter 28 for additional details. ∞

Case Manager

Nurse case managers work with the multidisciplinary health care team to measure the effectiveness of the case management plan and to monitor outcomes. Each agency or unit specifies the role of the nurse **case manager.** In some institutions, the case manager works with primary or staff nurses to oversee the care of a specific caseload. In other agencies, the case manager is the primary nurse or provides some level of direct care to the client and family. Insurance companies have also developed a number of roles for nurse case managers, and responsibilities may vary from managing acute hospitalizations to managing high-cost clients or case types. Regardless of the setting, case managers help ensure that care is oriented to the client, while controlling costs.

Research Consumer

Nurses often use research to improve client care. In a clinical area, nurses need to (a) have some awareness of the process and language of research, (b) be sensitive to issues related to protecting the rights of human subjects, (c) participate in the identification of significant researchable problems, and (d) be a discriminating consumer of research findings.

Expanded Career Roles

Nurses are fulfilling expanded career roles, such as those of nurse practitioner, clinical nurse specialist, nurse midwife, nurse educator, nurse researcher, and nurse anesthetist, all of which allow greater independence and autonomy (see Box 1–2).

CRITERIA OF A PROFESSION

Nursing is gaining recognition as a profession. **Profession** has been defined as an occupation that requires extensive education or a calling that requires special knowledge, skill, and preparation. A profession is generally distinguished from other kinds of occupations by (a) its requirement of prolonged, specialized training to acquire a body of knowledge pertinent to the role to be performed; (b) an orientation of the individual toward service, either to a community or to an organization; (c) ongoing research; (d) a code of ethics; (e) autonomy; and (f) a professional organization.

Two terms related to profession need to be differentiated: professionalism and professionalization. **Professionalism** refers to professional character, spirit, or methods. It is a set of attributes, a way of life that implies responsibility and commitment.

BOX 1–2 **Selected Expanded Career Roles for Nurses**

NURSE PRACTITIONER
A nurse who has an advanced education and is a graduate of a nurse practitioner program. These nurses are certified by the American Nurses Credentialing Center in areas such as adult nurse practitioner, family nurse practitioner, school nurse practitioner, pediatric nurse practitioner, or gerontology nurse practitioner. They are employed in health care agencies or community-based settings. They usually deal with nonemergency acute or chronic illness and provide primary ambulatory care.

CLINICAL NURSE SPECIALIST
A nurse who has an advanced degree or expertise and is considered to be an expert in a specialized area of practice (e.g., gerontology, oncology). The nurse provides direct client care, educates others, consults, conducts research, and manages care. The American Nurses Credentialing Center provides national certification of clinical specialists.

NURSE ANESTHETIST
A nurse who has completed advanced education in an accredited program in anesthesiology. The nurse anesthetist carries out preoperative visits and assessments, and administers general anesthetics for surgery under the supervision of a physician prepared in anesthesiology. The nurse anesthetist also assesses the postoperative status of clients.

NURSE MIDWIFE
An RN who has completed a program in midwifery and is certified by the American College of Nurse Midwives. The nurse gives prenatal and postnatal care and manages deliveries in normal pregnancies. The midwife practices in association with a health care agency and can obtain medical services if complications occur. The nurse midwife may also conduct routine Papanicolaou smears, family planning, and routine breast examinations.

NURSE RESEARCHER
Nurse researchers investigate nursing problems to improve nursing care and to refine and expand nursing knowledge. They are employed in academic institutions, teaching hospitals, and research centers such as the National Institute for Nursing Research in Bethesda, Maryland. Nurse researchers usually have advanced education at the doctoral level.

NURSE ADMINISTRATOR
The nurse administrator manages client care, including the delivery of nursing services. The administrator may have a middle management position, such as head nurse or supervisor, or a more senior management position, such as director of nursing services. The functions of nurse administrators include budgeting, staffing, and planning programs. The educational preparation for nurse administrator positions is at least a baccalaureate degree in nursing and frequently a master's or doctoral degree.

NURSE EDUCATOR
Nurse educators are employed in nursing programs, at educational institutions, and in hospital staff education. The nurse educator usually has a baccalaureate degree or more advanced preparation and frequently has expertise in a particular area of practice. The nurse educator is responsible for classroom and often clinical teaching.

NURSE ENTREPRENEUR
A nurse who usually has an advanced degree and manages a health-related business. The nurse may be involved in education, consultation, or research, for example.

RESEARCH NOTE **What Are New Nurses' Perceptions of Nursing Practice?**

The purpose of this study was to assess new nurses' perceptions of nursing practice and their expectations for meeting professional goals. The authors' rationale was that nurses who are satisfied with their working environment will stay longer, and retention of satisfied nurses will increase quality patient care.

The sample consisted of 67 new nurses hired within a 12-month period. The nurses were from baccalaureate, associate degree, and practical nursing programs. They completed a questionnaire that consisted of items relating to their work environment and interpersonal relationships. Two open-ended questions asked the nurses to comment on their personal experiences in nursing practice.

The results indicated that approximately half of the new nurses felt that the transition from novice to professional nurse was somewhat difficult. A longer orientation period was desired by new nurses in the more specialized units. Continuing education programs, both in and outside the organization, were ranked as very important by the majority. The preceptor was considered most supportive by 31% of the new nurses; however, the majority reported positive experiences with other staff nurses. The main area of anxiety for the new nurses related to communication with physicians. They did not believe they had the knowledge or experience to discuss patients with the doctors. They feared that the physician would ask questions that they could not answer.

IMPLICATIONS

Because of the nursing shortage, it is important for hospitals to recruit and retain competent nursing staff. The findings of this study assisted the hospital to improve orientation policies and the preceptorship program and to adopt strategies to improve nurse–physician communication. Using the results of studies such as this one allows hospitals to implement new strategies to ease the transition from novice to professional nurse with the outcome of increased quality of patient care and nursing retention—a win-win for all.

Note: From S. Boswell, L. Lowry, & K. Wilboit, "New Nurses' Perceptions of Nursing Practice and Quality Patient Care," *Journal of Nursing Care Quality, 19*(1), pages 76–81. Copyright © 2004 Lippincott, Williams & Wilkins. Reprinted with permission.

Nursing professionalism owes much to the influence of Florence Nightingale. **Professionalization** is the process of becoming professional, that is, of acquiring characteristics considered to be professional.

Specialized Education

Specialized education is an important aspect of professional status. In modern times, the trend in education for the professions has shifted toward programs in colleges and universities. Many nursing educators believe that the undergraduate nursing curriculum should include liberal arts education in addition to the biologic and social sciences and the nursing discipline.

In the United States today, there are five means of entry into registered nursing: hospital diploma, associate degree, baccalaureate degree, master's degree, and doctoral degree. These programs are discussed in Chapter 2. ∞ The ANA recommends the baccalaureate degree as the entry level for professional practice. Conversely, the National Organization for Associate Degree Nursing (N-OADN) supports ADN preparation as the entry level into registered nursing (N-OADN, 2005).

Body of Knowledge

As a profession, nursing is establishing a well-defined body of knowledge and expertise. A number of nursing conceptual frameworks (discussed in Chapter 3) contribute to the knowledge base of nursing and give direction to nursing practice, education, and ongoing research. ∞

Service Orientation

A service orientation differentiates nursing from an occupation pursued primarily for profit. Many consider altruism (selfless concern for others) the hallmark of a profession. Nursing has a tradition of service to others. This service, however, must be guided by certain rules, policies, or codes of ethics. Today, nursing is also an important component of the health care delivery system.

Ongoing Research

Increasing research in nursing is contributing to nursing practice. In the 1940s, nursing research was at a very early stage of development. In the 1950s, increased federal funding and professional support helped establish centers for nursing research. Most early research was directed to the study of nursing education. In the 1960s, studies were often related to the nature of the knowledge base underlying nursing practice. Since the 1970s, nursing research has focused on practice-related issues. Nursing research as a dimension of the nurse's role is discussed further in Chapter 2. ∞

Code of Ethics

Nurses have traditionally placed a high value on the worth and dignity of others. The nursing profession requires integrity of its members; that is, a member is expected to do what is considered right regardless of the personal cost.

Ethical codes change as the needs and values of society change. Nursing has developed its own codes of ethics and in most instances has set up means to monitor the professional behavior of its members. See Chapter 5 for additional information on ethics. ∞

Autonomy

A profession is autonomous if it regulates itself and sets standards for its members. Providing autonomy is one of the purposes of a professional association. If nursing is to have professional status, it must function autonomously in the formation of policy and in the control of its activity. To be autonomous, a professional group must be granted legal authority to define the scope of its practice, describe its particular functions and roles, and determine its goals and responsibilities in delivery of its services.

To practitioners of nursing, autonomy means independence at work, responsibility, and accountability for one's actions. Autonomy is more easily achieved and maintained from a position of authority. Therefore, some nurses seek administrative positions rather than expanded clinical competence as a means to ensure their autonomy in the workplace.

Professional Organization

Operation under the umbrella of a professional organization differentiates a profession from an occupation. **Governance** is the establishment and maintenance of social, political, and economic arrangements by which practitioners control their practice, their self-discipline, their working conditions, and their professional affairs. Nurses, therefore, need to work within their professional organizations.

The American Nurses Association is a professional organization that "advances the nursing profession by fostering high standards of nursing practice, promoting the economic and general welfare of nurses in the workplace, projecting a positive and realistic view of nursing, and by lobbying the Congress and regulatory agencies on health care issues affecting nurses and the public" (ANA, 2005).

SOCIALIZATION TO NURSING

The standards of education and practice for the profession are determined by the members of the profession, rather than by outsiders. The education of the professional involves a complete socialization process, more far reaching in its social and attitudinal aspects and its technical features than is usually required in other kinds of occupations.

BOX 1–3   Benner's Stages of Nursing Expertise

STAGE I, NOVICE
No experience (e.g., nursing student). Performance is limited, inflexible, and governed by context-free rules and regulations rather than experience.

STAGE II, ADVANCED BEGINNER
Demonstrates marginally acceptable performance.
Recognizes the meaningful "aspects" of a real situation. Has experienced enough real situations to make judgments about them.

STAGE III, COMPETENT
Has 2 or 3 years of experience. Demonstrates organizational and planning abilities. Differentiates important factors from less important aspects of care. Coordinates multiple complex care demands.

STAGE IV, PROFICIENT
Has 3 to 5 years of experience. Perceives situations as wholes rather than in terms of parts, as in Stage II. Uses maxims as guides for what to consider in a situation. Has holistic understanding of the client, which improves decision making. Focuses on long-term goals.

STAGE V, EXPERT
Performance is fluid, flexible, and highly proficient; no longer requires rules, guidelines, or maxims to connect an understanding of the situation to appropriate action. Demonstrates highly skilled intuitive and analytic ability in new situations. Is inclined to take a certain action because "it felt right."

Note: Benner, Patricia, from *Novice to Expert: Excellence and Power in Clinical Nursing Practice, Commemorative Edition,* 1st ed. © 2001. Electronically reproduced by permission of Pearson Education, Inc., Upper Saddle River, New Jersey.

REAL WORLD PRACTICE

One of the biggest changes you'll see as you progress from being a novice nurse to becoming an expert nurse is your willingness to "trust your gut"—You know, that little voice in your head saying, "something isn't right here." There may be no change in your client's vital signs, no change in his or her mental status, nothing concrete you can put your finger on, no *numbers* you can report to the physician (oh, how we all love *numbers*). But in your heart, in your gut, you *know* there's something wrong.

What do you do? As a novice nurse, you are likely to talk yourself out of this feeling. You will think you are just overreacting, hearing hoofbeats and thinking zebras instead of horses. You may mention this feeling in passing to a trusted co-worker, but that's about as far as you'll take it.

As you progress through your career, you will find yourself acting on the advice of that little voice more and more often. You'll find yourself calling physicians at 2:00 in the morning because your little voice is telling you that something is wrong.

You'll know you have arrived, however, when you call a physician at 2 A.M. who tells you, "I'll be right there because I trust your little voice."

— *Tina Saiani, RN*
The Children's Hospital at the
Medical Center of Central Georgia

Socialization can be defined simply as the process by which people (a) learn to become members of groups and society and (b) learn the social rules defining relationships into which they will enter. Socialization involves learning to behave, feel, and see the world in a manner similar to other persons occupying the same role as oneself (Hardy & Conway, 1988, p. 261). The goal of professional socialization is to instill in individuals the norms, values, attitudes, and behaviors deemed essential for survival of the profession.

Various models of the socialization process have been developed. Benner's model (2001) describes five levels of proficiency in nursing based on the Dreyfus general model of skill acquisition. The five stages, which have implications for teaching and learning, are novice, advanced beginner, competent, proficient, and expert. Benner writes that experience is essential for the development of professional expertise (see Box 1–3).

One of the most powerful mechanisms of professional socialization is interaction with fellow students. Within this student culture, students collectively set the level and direction of their scholastic efforts. They develop perspectives about the situation in which they are involved, the goals they are trying to achieve, and the kinds of activities that are expedient and proper, and they establish a set of practices congruent with all of these. Students become bound together by feelings of mutual cooperation, support, and solidarity.

BOX 1—4 **National Student Nurses' Association, Inc., Code of Academic and Clinical Conduct**

PREAMBLE

Students of nursing have a responsibility to society in learning the academic theory and clinical skills needed to provide nursing care. The clinical setting presents unique challenges and responsibilities while caring for human beings in a variety of health care environments.

The Code of Academic and Clinical Conduct is based on an understanding that to practice nursing as a student is an agreement to uphold the trust with which society has placed in us. The statements of the Code provide guidance for the nursing student in the personal development of an ethical foundation and need not be limited strictly to the academic or clinical environment but can assist in the holistic development of the person.

A CODE FOR NURSING STUDENTS

As students are involved in the clinical and academic environments we believe that ethical principles are a necessary guide to professional development. Therefore within these environments we:

1. Advocate for the rights of all clients.
2. Maintain client confidentiality.
3. Take appropriate action to ensure the safety of clients, self, and others.
4. Provide care for the client in a timely, compassionate and professional manner.
5. Communicate client care in a truthful, timely and accurate manner.
6. Actively promote the highest level of moral and ethical principles and accept responsibility for our actions.
7. Promote excellence in nursing by encouraging lifelong learning and professional development.
8. Treat others with respect and promote an environment that respects human rights, values and choice of cultural and spiritual beliefs.

9. Collaborate in every reasonable manner with the academic faculty and clinical staff to ensure the highest quality of client care.
10. Use every opportunity to improve faculty and clinical staff understanding of the learning needs of nursing students.
11. Encourage faculty, clinical staff, and peers to mentor nursing students.
12. Refrain from performing any technique or procedure for which the student has not been adequately trained.
13. Refrain from any deliberate action or omission of care in the academic or clinical setting that creates unnecessary risk of injury to the client, self, or others.
14. Assist the staff nurse or preceptor in ensuring that there is full disclosure and that proper authorizations are obtained from clients regarding any form of treatment or research.
15. Abstain from the use of alcoholic beverages or any substances in the academic and clinical setting that impair judgment.
16. Strive to achieve and maintain an optimal level of personal health.
17. Support access to treatment and rehabilitation for students who are experiencing impairments related to substance abuse and mental or physical health issues.
18. Uphold school policies and regulations related to academic and clinical performance, reserving the right to challenge and critique rules and regulations as per school grievance policy.

Note: Adopted by the NSNA House of Delegates, Nashville, TN, on April 6, 2001. Reprinted with permission.

Critical Values of Nursing

It is within the nursing educational program that the nurse develops, clarifies, and internalizes professional values. Specific professional nursing values are stated in nursing codes of ethics (see Chapter 5), in standards of nursing practice (discussed earlier in this chapter), and in the legal system itself (see Chapter 4 ∞). Additionally, in 2001, the National Student Nurses' Association (NSNA) adopted a code of academic and clinical conduct (see Box 1–4).

FACTORS INFLUENCING CONTEMPORARY NURSING PRACTICE

To understand nursing as it is practiced today and as it will be practiced tomorrow requires an understanding of some of the social forces currently influencing this profession. These forces usually affect the entire health care system, and nursing, as a major component of that system, cannot avoid the effects.

Economics

Greater financial support provided through public and private health insurance programs has increased the demand for nurs-

ing care. As a result, people who could not afford health care in the past are increasingly using such health services as emergency department care, mental health counseling, and preventive physical examinations.

Costs of health care have also increased during the past two decades. In 1982, the Medicare payment system to hospitals and physicians was revised to establish reimbursement fees according to the client's medical diagnosis. This classification system is known as **diagnostic-related groups (DRGs).** The system has categories that establish pretreatment diagnosis billing categories. With the implementation of this legislation, clients in hospitals are more acutely ill than before and clients once considered sufficiently ill to be hospitalized are now treated at home; however, health care costs continue to rise.

These changes present challenges to nurses. Currently, the health care industry is shifting its emphasis from inpatient to outpatient care with preadmission testing, increased outpatient same-day surgery, post-hospitalization rehabilitation, home health care, health maintenance, physical fitness programs, and community health education programs. As a result, more nurses are being employed in community-based health settings, such as home health agencies, hospices, and community clinics. These changes in employment for nurses have implications for nursing education, nursing research, and nursing practice.

Consumer Demands

Consumers of nursing services (the public) have become an increasingly effective force in changing nursing practice. On the whole, people are better educated and have more knowledge about health and illness than in the past. Consumers also have become more aware of others' needs for care. The ethical and moral issues raised by poverty and neglect have made people more vocal about the needs of minority groups and the poor.

The public's concepts of health and nursing have also changed. Most now believe that health is a right of all people, not just a privilege of the rich. The media emphasize the message that individuals must assume responsibility for their own health by obtaining a physical examination regularly, checking for the seven danger signals of cancer, and maintaining their mental well-being by balancing work and recreation. Interest in health and nursing services is therefore greater than ever. Furthermore, many people now want more than freedom from disease—they want energy, vitality, and a feeling of wellness.

Increasingly, the consumer has become an active participant in making decisions about health and nursing care. Planning committees concerned with providing nursing services to a community usually have active consumer membership. Recognizing the legitimacy of public input, many state nursing associations and regulatory agencies have consumer representatives on their governing boards.

Family Structure

New family structures are influencing the need for and provision of nursing services. More people are living away from the extended family and the nuclear family, and the family breadwinner is no longer necessarily the husband. Today, many single men and women rear children, and in many two-parent families both parents work. It is also common for young parents to live at great distances from their own parents. These young families need support services, such as day-care centers. For additional information about the family, see Chapter 24. ∞

Adolescent mothers also need specialized nursing services, both while they are pregnant and after their babies are born. These young mothers usually have the normal needs of teenagers as well as those of new mothers. Many teenage mothers are raising their children alone with little, if any, assistance from the child's father. This type of single-parent family is especially vulnerable because motherhood compounds the difficulties of adolescence. And because many of these families live in poverty, the children often do not receive preventive immunizations and are at increased risk for nutritional and other health problems.

Science and Technology

Advances in science and technology affect nursing practice. For example, people with acquired immune deficiency syndrome (AIDS) are receiving new drug therapies to prolong life and delay the onset of AIDS-associated diseases. Nurses must be knowledgeable about the action of such drugs and the needs of clients receiving them. Biotechnology is affecting health care.

For example, nurses are exposed to emerging genetic technology such as the field of cancer gene therapy (Cashion, Driscoll, & Sabek, 2004; Liu, 2003). Nurses will need to expand their knowledge base and technical skills as they adapt to meet the new needs of clients.

In some settings, technological advances have required that nurses be highly specialized. Nurses frequently have to use sophisticated computerized equipment to monitor or treat clients. As technologies change, nursing education changes, and nurses require increasing education to provide effective, safe nursing practice.

The space program has developed advanced technologies for space travel based on the need for long-distance monitoring of astronauts and spacecraft, lighter materials, and miniaturization of equipment. Health care has benefited as this new technology has been adapted in such health care aids as Viewstar (an aid for the visually impaired), the insulin infusion pump, the voice-controlled wheelchair, magnetic resonance imaging, laser surgery, filtering devices for intravenous fluid control devices, and monitoring systems for intensive care.

Information and Telecommunications

The information superhighway or Internet has already affected health care, with more and more clients becoming well informed about their health concerns. People with chronic health conditions or battling life-threatening disease are the hungriest information seekers (DeLenardo, 2004). As a result, nurses may need to interpret Internet sources of information for clients and their families. Because not all of the Internet-based information is accurate, nurses need to become information brokers so they can help people to access high-quality, valid websites; interpret the information; and then help clients evaluate the information and determine if it is useful to them.

Telecommunications is the transmission of information from one site to another, using equipment to transmit information in the form of signs, signals, words, or pictures by cable, radio, or other systems (Chaffee, 1999, p. 27). Greenberg (2000) explains that terms with the prefix *tele*, meaning distance, are used to describe the many health care services provided via telecommunications. The common denominators of teleservices are distance and technology (p. 220).

Telehealth uses telecommunication technology to provide long-distance health care. It can include using videoconferencing, computers, or telephones. Telenursing occurs when the nurse delivers care through a telecommunication system. Examples of telenursing include the nurse who telephones clients at home to assess their progress or to answer questions, the nurse who participates in a video teleconference where consultants or experts at various sites discuss a client's health care plan, and the nurse who uses videophone technology to assess a client living in a rural area.

Telehealth recognizes no state boundaries and, subsequently, licensure issues have been raised. For example, if a nurse licensed in one state provides health information to a client in another state, does the nurse need to maintain licensure in both states? The National Council of State Boards of Nursing endorses a change from single-state licensure to a mutual recognition model. Many state legislatures have adopted mutual recognition language into statute and are currently implementing it (see Chapter 4). ∞

Legislation

Legislation about nursing practice and health matters affects both the public and nursing. Legislation related to nursing is discussed in Chapter 4. ∞ Changes in legislation relating to health also affect nursing. For example, the **Patient Self-Determination Act (PSDA)** requires that every competent adult be informed in writing on admission to a health care institution about his or her rights to accept or refuse medical care and to use advance directives. See Chapter 4 ∞ for more information about the PSDA and advance directives. This law, which in many institutions is implemented by nurses, affects the nurse's role in supporting clients and their families.

Demography

Demography is the study of population, including statistics about distribution by age and place of residence, mortality (death), and morbidity (incidence of disease). From demographic data, needs of the population for nursing services can be assessed. For example:

- The total population in North America is increasing. The proportion of elderly people has also increased, creating an increased need for nursing services for this group.
- The population is shifting from rural to urban settings. This shift signals an increased need for nursing related to problems caused by pollution and by the effects on the environment of concentrations of people. Thus, most nursing services are now provided in urban settings.
- Mortality and morbidity studies reveal the presence of risk factors. Many of these risk factors (e.g., smoking) are major causes of death and disease that can be prevented through changes in lifestyle. The nurse's role in assessing risk factors and helping clients make healthy lifestyle changes is discussed in Chapter 16. ∞

The Current Nursing Shortage

The multiple factors influencing the current nursing shortage (see Box 1–5) are different from previous nursing shortages. Registered nurses make up the largest group of health care providers. Fewer nurses, however, are entering the workforce, and certain geographic areas are experiencing acute nursing shortages. The supply is inadequate to meet the demand, especially for specialized nurses (e.g., critical care), and it is anticipated to worsen during the next 20 years (National League for Nursing, 2005).

Addressing the nursing shortage requires collaborative activities among health care systems, policy makers, nursing educators, and professional organizations. Recommendations include but are not limited to these:

- Develop mechanisms for nursing students to progress to and through educational programs more efficiently and quickly.

BOX 1–5 Factors Affecting the Nursing Shortage

AGING NURSE WORKFORCE
- Number of nurses under 30 decreasing
- Number of nurses age 40–49 increasing with 40% older than 50 by 2010
- New graduates entering workforce at an older age and will have fewer years to work

AGING OF NURSING FACULTY
- As nursing faculty retire, nursing programs may have fewer faculty to educate future nurses

REDUCED ENTRY OF YOUNGER PEOPLE INTO NURSING
- Reduction in nursing program enrollments

AGING POPULATION
- Individuals 65 and older to double between 2000 and 2030
- Increasing health care needs of aging population

INCREASED DEMAND FOR NURSES
- Increased acuity of hospital clients requiring skilled and specialized nurses
- Shorter hospital stays resulting in transfer of clients to long-term care and community settings, creating increased demand for nurses in the community

WORKPLACE ISSUES
- Inadequate staffing
- Heavy workloads
- Increased use of overtime
- Lack of sufficient support staff
- Inadequate wages
- Difficulty recruiting and retaining nurses

- Recruit young people to nursing early (e.g., grade school).
- Improve the nurse's work environment: Provide greater flexibility in work hours, reward experienced nurses who serve as mentors, ensure adequate staffing, and increase salaries.
- Increase nursing education funding.

Collective Bargaining

More nurses are using collective bargaining to deal with their concerns. The ANA participates in collective bargaining on behalf of nurses through its economic and general welfare programs. Today, some nurses are joining other labor organizations that represent them at the bargaining table. Nurses have gone on strike over economic concerns and over issues about safe care for clients and safety for themselves.

Nursing Associations

Professional nursing associations have provided leadership that affects many areas of nursing. Voluntary accreditation of nursing education programs by the National League for Nursing Accrediting Commission (NLNAC) and Commission on Collegiate Nursing Education (CCNE) has also influenced nursing. Many nursing programs have steadily improved to meet the standards for accreditation over the years. As a result, nurse graduates are better prepared to meet the demands of society.

To influence policy making for health care, a group of professional nurses organized formally to promote political action in the nursing and health care arenas. Nurses for Political Action (NPA) formed in 1971 and became an arm of the ANA in 1974, when its name changed to Nurses Coalition for Action in Politics (N-CAP). In 1986, the name was changed to American Nurses Association—Political Action Committee (ANA-PAC). Through this group, nurses have lobbied actively for legislation affecting health care. A number of nursing leaders hold positions of authority in government. Attaining such positions is essential if nurses hope to exert ongoing political influence.

NURSING ORGANIZATIONS

As nursing has developed, an increasing number of nursing organizations have formed. These organizations are at the local, state, national, and international levels. The organizations that involve most North American nurses are the American Nurses Association, the Canadian Nurses Association, the National League for Nursing, the International Council of Nurses, and the National Student Nurses' Association. The number of nursing specialty organizations is also increasing, for example, the Academy of Medical Surgical Nursing, the American Association of Nurse Anesthetists, the National Black Nurses Association, and the National Association of Pediatric Nurse Practitioners. Participation in the activities of nursing associations enhances the growth of involved individuals and helps nurses collectively influence policies affecting nursing practice.

American Nurses Association

The American Nurses Association (ANA) is the national professional organization for nursing in the United States. It was founded in 1896 as the Nurses Associated Alumnae of the United States and Canada. In 1911 the name was changed to the American Nurses Association. It was a charter member of the International Council of Nurses, along with organizations in Great Britain and Germany, in 1899. The purposes of the ANA are to foster high standards of nursing practice and to promote the educational and professional advancement of nurses so that all people may have better nursing care.

In 1982, the organization became a federation of state nurses' associations. Individuals participate in the ANA by joining their state nurses' associations. The official journal of the ANA is the *American Journal of Nursing,* and *American Nurse* is the official newspaper.

Canadian Nurses Association

The Canadian Nurses Association (CNA) is the national nursing association in Canada. Nurses do not join the CNA independently but obtain membership by paying a fee to the provincial chapters. The CNA has developed standards and a code of ethics,

and it offers support to all provincial associations. The CNA prepares licensure examinations and offers research grants, fellowships, and scholarships to Canadian nurses. The official journal of the CNA, *The Canadian Nurse,* is published monthly.

National League for Nursing

The National League for Nursing (NLN), formed in 1952, is an organization of both individuals and agencies. Its objective is to foster the development and improvement of all nursing services and nursing education. People who are not nurses but have an interest in nursing services, for example, hospital administrators, can be members of the league. This feature of the NLN— involving non-nurse members, consumers, and nurses from all levels of practice—is unique.

The NLN presents continuing education workshops and seminars for its members. For schools of nursing, the NLN offers testing services including preadmission testing for potential students, and achievement testing throughout the program. The NLN also conducts yearly surveys of nursing schools, newly registered nurses, and post-basic graduates. These surveys serve as a primary source of research data about nursing education in the United States. The National League for Nursing Accrediting Commission, an independent body within the NLN, provides voluntary accreditation for educational programs in nursing. The official journal of the NLN is *Nursing and Health Care Perspectives.*

International Council of Nurses

The International Council of Nurses (ICN) was established in 1899. Nurses from Great Britain, the United States, and Canada were among the founding members. The council is a federation of national nurses' associations, such as the ANA and CNA.

The ICN provides an organization through which member national associations can work together for the mission of representing nursing worldwide, advancing the profession, and influencing health policy. The five core values of the ICN are visionary leadership, inclusiveness, flexibility, partnership, and achievement (ICN, 2005). The official journal of the ICN is *International Nursing Review.*

National Student Nurses' Association

The National Student Nurses' Association (NSNA) is the official preprofessional organization for nursing students. Formed in 1953 and incorporated in 1959, the NSNA originally functioned under the aegis of the ANA and NLN; however, in 1968 the NSNA became an autonomous body, although it communicates with the NLN and the ANA. To qualify for membership in the NSNA, a student must be enrolled in a state-approved nursing education program. The official organ of the NSNA is *Imprint* magazine.

In Canada, nursing students have a similar organization, the Canadian University Student Nurses Association. The provincial student nurses' associations also have programs related to the needs of nursing students and to concerns within the health field in general.

MediaLink Sigma Theta Tau Application

International Honor Society: Sigma Theta Tau

Sigma Theta Tau, the international honor society in nursing, was founded in 1922 and is headquartered in Indianapolis, Indiana. The Greek letters stand for the Greek words *storga, tharos,* and *tima,* meaning "love," "courage," and "honor." The society is a member of the Association of College Honor Societies. The society's purpose is professional rather than social. Membership is attained through academic achievement. Students in baccalau-reate programs in nursing and nurses in master's, doctoral, and postdoctoral programs are eligible to be selected for membership. Potential members, who hold a minimum of a bachelor's degree and have demonstrated achievement in nursing, can apply for membership as a nurse leader in the community.

The official journal of Sigma Theta Tau, *Journal of Nursing Scholarship,* is published quarterly. The journal publishes scholarly articles of interest to nurses. The society also publishes *Reflections,* a quarterly newsletter that provides information about the organization and its various chapters.

CHAPTER 1 **REVIEW**

CHAPTER HIGHLIGHTS

- Historical perspectives of nursing practice reveal recurring themes or influencing factors. For example, women have traditionally cared for others, but often in subservient roles. Religious orders left an imprint on nursing by instilling such values as compassion, devotion to duty, and hard work. Wars created an increased need for nurses and medical specialties. Societal attitudes have influenced nursing's image. Visionary leaders have made notable contributions to improve the status of nursing.
- The scope of nursing practice includes promoting wellness, preventing illness, restoring health, and caring for the dying.
- Although traditionally the majority of nurses were employed in hospital settings, today the numbers of nurses working in home health care, ambulatory care, and community health settings are increasing.
- Nurse practice acts vary among states, and nurses are responsible for knowing the act that governs their practice.
- Standards of nursing practice provide criteria against which the effectiveness of nursing care and professional performance behaviors can be evaluated.
- Every nurse may function in a variety of roles that are not exclusive of one another; in reality, they often occur together and serve to clarify the nurse's activities. These roles include caregiver, communicator, teacher, client advocate, counselor, change agent, leader, manager, case manager, and research consumer.
- With advanced education and experience, nurses can fulfill advanced practice roles such as clinical nurse specialist, nurse practitioner, nurse midwife, nurse anesthetist, educator, administrator, and researcher.

- A desired goal of nursing is professionalism, which necessitates specialized education; a unique body of knowledge, including specific skills and abilities; ongoing research; a code of ethics; autonomy; a service orientation; and a professional organization.
- Socialization is a lifelong process by which people become functioning participants of a society or a group. It is a reciprocal learning process that is brought about by interaction with other people and established boundaries of behavior. Socialization to professional nursing practice is the process whereby the values and norms of the nursing profession are internalized into the nurse's own behavior and self-concept. The nurse acquires the knowledge, skill, and attitudes characteristic of the profession.
- Although several models of the socialization process have been developed, Benner's five stages of novice, advanced beginner, competent, proficient, and expert may serve as guidelines to establish the phase and extent of an individual's socialization.
- Contemporary nursing practice is influenced by economics, changing demands for nurses, consumer demand, family structure, science and technology, information and telecommunications, legislation, demographic and social changes, the nursing shortage, collective bargaining, and the work of nursing associations.
- Participation in the activities of nursing associations enhances the growth of involved individuals and helps nurses collectively influence policies that affect nursing practice.

TEST YOUR KNOWLEDGE

1. Which of the following women made significant contributions to the nursing care of soldiers during the Civil War? Select all that apply.
 1. Harriet Tubman
 2. Florence Nightingale
 3. Fabiola
 4. Dorothea Dix
 5. Sojourner Truth

2. Health promotion is best represented by which of the following activities?
 1. Administering immunizations
 2. Giving a bath
 3. Preventing accidents in the home
 4. Performing diagnostic procedures

3. Who are America's first two trained nurses?
 1. Barton and Wald
 2. Dock and Sanger
 3. Richards and Mahoney
 4. Henderson and Breckinridge

4. A nurse with 2 to 3 years of experience who has the ability to coordinate multiple complex nursing care demands is at which stage of Benner's states of nursing expertise?
 1. Advanced beginner
 2. Competent
 3. Proficient
 4. Expert

5. Which professional organization developed a code for nursing students?
1. ANA
2. NLN
3. AACN
4. NSNA

6. Which of the following social forces is most likely to significantly impact the future supply and demand for nurses?
1. Aging
2. Economics
3. Science/technology
4. Telecommunications

See Answers to Test Your Knowledge in Appendix A. ∞

EXPLORE MEDIALINK **www.prenhall.com/berman**

DVD-ROM
▦ Audio Glossary
▦ NCLEX Review
▦ Video: History of Nursing

COMPANION WEBSITE
▦ Additional NCLEX Review
▦ Case Study: Evolution of Nursing
▦ Application Activities:
  Florence Nightingale
  American Association of Colleges of Nursing
  Sigma Theta Tau
▦ Links to Resources

READINGS AND REFERENCES

SUGGESTED READINGS

Dossey, B. M., Selanders, L. C., Beck, D., & Attewell, A. (2005). *Florence Nightingale today. Healing, leadership, global action.* Silver Spring, Maryland: American Nurses Association.
The authors are three nursing scholars and the director of the Florence Nightingale Museum who present an insightful portrait of Florence Nightingale. The book is divided into four parts. The first three parts are Nightingale's Tenets—Healing, Leadership, and Global Action. The fourth part contains unedited letters and an essay written by Nightingale.

Houweling, L. (2004). Image, function, and style. A history of the nursing uniform. *American Journal of Nursing, 104*(4), 40–48.
The author describes how the nurse's uniform is linked to the history of the nursing profession. The photographs of the various nurse's uniforms, including caps and shoes, add to the historical narrative. The written and art depiction of the uniform for the future is thought provoking.

REFERENCES

American Nurses Association. (1973). *Standards of nursing practice.* Kansas City, MO: Author.

American Nurses Association. (1980). *Nursing: A social policy statement.* Kansas City, MO: Author.

American Nurses Association. (2003). *Nursing's social policy statement.* Washington, DC: American Nurses Publishing.

American Nurses Association. (2004). *Nursing: Scope and standards of practice.* Washington, DC: Author.

American Nurses Association. (2005). About ANA. Retrieved June 19, 2006, from http://nursingworld.org/about/index.htm

American Nurses Association. (2006a). *ANA hall of fame.* Retrieved April 23, 2006, from http://www.ana.org/hof/richla.htm

American Nurses Association. (2006b). *ANA hall of fame.* Retrieved April 23, 2006, from http://www.ana.org/hof/mahome.htm

Anonymous. (2003). Image change boosts US nurse recruitment. *Australian Nursing Journal, 11*(3), 16.

Anspaugh, D. J., Hamrick, M. H., & Rosata, F. D. (2003). *Wellness: Concepts and applications.* New York: McGraw-Hill.

Benner, P. (2001). *From novice to expert: Excellence and power in clinical nursing practice* (commemorative ed.). Upper Saddle River, NJ: Prentice Hall Health.

Cashion, A.K., Driscoll, C.J., & Sabek, O. (2004). Emerging genetic technologies in clinical and research settings. *Biological Research for Nursing, 5*(3), 159–167.

Chaffee, M. (1999). A telehealth odyssey. *American Journal of Nursing, 99*(7), 27–32.

Coffman, M. J. (2004). Cultural caring in nursing practice: A meta-synthesis of qualitative research. *Journal of Cultural Diversity, 11*(3), 100–109.

DeLenardo, C. (2004). Web-based tools steer patient-focused care. *Nursing Management, 35*(12), 60–64.

Donahue, M. P. (1996). *Nursing: The finest art. An illustrated history* (2nd ed.). St. Louis, MO: Mosby.

Fitzpatrick, M. A. (2002). "I" is for image. *Nursing Management, 33*(6), 6.

Graber, D. R., & Mitcham, M. D. (2004). Compassionate clinicians: Take patient care beyond the ordinary. *Holistic Nursing Practice, 18*(2), 87–94.

Greenberg, M. E. (2000). The domain of telenursing: Issues and prospects. *Nursing Economics, 18*(4), 220–223.

Hardy, M. E., & Conway, M. E. (1988). *Role theory: Perspectives for healthy professionals* (2nd ed.). Norwalk, CT: Appleton & Lange.

Henderson, V. (1966). *The nature of nursing: A definition and its implications for practice, research, and education.* New York: Macmillan.

Holder, V. L. (2004). From handmaiden to right hand—World War I and advancements in medicine. *AORN Journal, 80*(5), 911–923.

International Council of Nurses. (2005). *About the International Council of Nurses.* Retrieved June 19, 2006, from http://www.icn.ch/abouticn.htm

Liu, K. (2003). Breakthroughs in cancer gene therapy. *Seminars in Oncology Nursing, 19*(3), 217–226.

Meyers, S. (2003). Real men choose nursing. *Hospitals & Health Networks, 77*(6), 72–77.

Military District of Washington. (n.d.). *The Nurses Memorial at Arlington Cemetery section 21.* Retrieved January 23, 2005, from http://www.mdw.army.mil/content/anmviewer.aspa-39

National League for Nursing. (2005). Tri-Council for Nursing policy statement: Strategies to reverse the new nursing shortage. Retrieved June 19, 2006, from http://www.nln.org/aboutnln/news_tricouncil2.htm

National Organization for Associate Degree Nursing. (2005). *Position statement in support of associate degree as preparation for the entry-level registered nurse. Retrieved June 19, 2006, from* http://www.noadn.org/pdfs/ Entry%20Level%20Position%20 Statement%20rev.pdF

National Student Nurses' Association House of Delegates. (2001). *The code of academic and clinical conduct.* Nashville, TN: Author.

Nightingale, F. (1969). *Notes on nursing: What it is, and what it is not.* New York: Dover. (Original work published 1860)

Schuyler, C. B. (1992). Florence Nightingale. In F. Nightingale, *Notes on nursing: What it is, and what it is not* (commemorative ed., pp. 3–17). Philadelphia: Lippincott.

Vietnam Women's Memorial Foundation. (n.d.). *During the Vietnam era. . . .* Retrieved June 19, 2006, from http://www.vietnamwomensmemorial.org/pages/frames/vwmp.html

SELECTED BIBLIOGRAPHY

Aiken, L. H., Buchan, J., Sochalski, J., Nichols, B., & Powell, M. (2004). Trends in international nurse migration. *Health Affairs, 23*(3), 69–77.

American Association of Colleges of Nursing. (2005). *Nursing shortage fact sheet.* Retrieved June 19, 2006, from http://www.aacn.nche.edu/Media/FactSheets/NursingShortage.htm

Battey, L. (2004). The struggle for lives in Iraq. *RN, 67*(12), 32.

Burge, P., Price, C., Cronin, S. N., Dolan, L., Kramer, J., & Ober, J. (2004). "Grow your own": A responsible approach to addressing the nursing shortage. *Nursing Economics, 22*(3), 155–156.

Doyle, R. (2005). Nurses in short supply. *Scientific American, 292*(1), 32.

Dowling, M. (2004). Exploring the relationship between caring, love and intimacy in nursing. *British Journal of Nursing, 13*(21), 1289–1292.

Evans, G. D. (2003). Clara Barton: Teacher, nurse, Civil War heroine, founder of the American Red Cross. *International History of Nursing Journal, 7,* 75–82.

Fest, G. (2003, October 13). Shining light. *Mountain West Nurse Week,* pp. 14–16.

Fest, G. (2003, October 27). A beacon of change. *Mountain West Nurse Week,* pp. 10–13.

Girard, N. J. (2003). Men and nursing. *AORN Journal, 77*(4), 728–730.

Godkin, J., & Godkin, L. (2004). Caring behaviors among nurses: Fostering a conversation of gestures. *Health Care Management Review, 29*(3), 258–267.

Gordon, S., & Nelson, S. (2005). An end to angels. Moving away from the virtue script toward a knowledge-based identity for nurses. *American Journal of Nursing, 105*(5), 62–69.

Holder, V. L. (2003). From hand maiden to right hand: The Civil War. *AORN Journal, 78*(3), 448–464.

Honor Society of Nursing, Sigma Theta Tau International. (2001). *Nurses for a healthier tomorrow. Facts about the nursing shortage.* Retrieved June 19, 2006, from http://www.nursesource.org/facts_shortage.html

Howard, V. B., & Tasota, R. J. (2004). How to spell relief for the nursing shortage: S-t-u-d-e-n-t-s. *Nursing, 34*(9), 32hn14 – 32hn16.

Mee, C. L. (2004). Postcards from the past: A salute to nursing specialties. *Nursing, 34*(1), 43–44.

Nelson, R. (2004). The nurse poachers. *Lancet, 364,* 1743.

Stein, M., & Deese, D. (2004). Addressing the next decade of nursing challenges. *Nursing Economics, 22*(5), 272–279.

Whitten, P., Doolittle, G., Mackert, M., & Rush, T. (2003). Telehospice: End-of-life care over the lines. *Nursing Management, 34*(11), 36–39.

Nursing Education, Research, and Evidence-Based Practice

LEARNING OUTCOMES

After completing this chapter, you will be able to:

1. Describe the different types of educational nursing programs.

2. Discuss aspects of entry to professional nursing practice.

3. Explain the importance of continuing nursing education.

4. Identify ways the nurse can participate in research activities in practice.

5. Differentiate the quantitative approach from the qualitative approach in nursing research.

6. Describe the nurse's role in protecting the rights of human subjects in research.

7. Identify the steps of the research process.

KEY TERMS

confidentiality, *33*	independent variable, *33*	reliability, *34*
continuing education (CE), *30*	in-service education, *30*	researchability, *33*
dependent variable, *33*	mean, *35*	right of self-determination, *33*
descriptive statistics, *35*	measures of central tendency, *35*	risk of harm, *33*
empirical data, *34*	measures of variability, *35*	sample, *34*
ethnography, *36*	median, *35*	significance, *33*
evidence-based practice (EBP), *30*	mode, *35*	standard deviation, *35*
feasibility, *33*	operational definitions, *34*	statistically significant, *35*
full disclosure, *33*	phenomenology, *36*	validity, *34*
grounded theory, *36*	population, *34*	variance, *35*
hypothesis, *34*	range, *35*	

Nursing education is controlled from within the profession through state boards of nursing and national accrediting bodies. The traditional focus of nursing education was to teach the knowledge and skills that would enable a nurse to practice in the hospital setting. However, as nursing responds to new scientific knowledge and technological, cultural, political, and socioeconomic changes in society, nursing education curricula are revised to meet the needs of nurses working in a changing environment. Programs of nursing study are increasingly based on a broad knowledge of biologic, social, and physical sciences as well as the liberal arts and humanities. Nursing curricula now have a greater focus on critical thinking and the application of nursing and supporting knowledge to health promotion, health maintenance, and health restoration as provided in both community and hospital settings (see Figure 2-1 ■).

Nursing research entails developing and expanding knowledge about human responses to actual or potential health problems and investigating the effects of nursing actions on those responses. The major goal of nursing research is to improve client care.

NURSING EDUCATION

At the present time, there are two types of entry-level generalist nurses: the registered nurse (RN), and the licensed practical or vocational nurse (LPN, LVN). Responsibilities and licensure differ for these two levels. The majority of new RNs graduate from diploma, associate degree, or baccalaureate nursing programs. There are also generic master's and doctoral programs that lead to eligibility for RN licensure. For example, students entering a generic master's program already have a baccalaureate degree from a discipline other than nursing. On completion of the program, generally 2–3 years in length, the graduates obtain their initial professional degree in nursing. Graduates of these master's programs are eligible to take the licensure examinations to become an RN and may continue into specialty roles such as nurse practitioner or educator.

Although these programs vary considerably, all RNs in the United States take the same licensing examination. The National Council Licensure Examination (NCLEX-RN) is administered in each state. The successful candidate becomes licensed in that particular state even though the examinations are of national origin. To practice nursing in another state, the nurse must receive reciprocal licensure by applying to that state's board of nursing. Some state legislatures are creating a regulatory model called *mutual recognition* that allows for multistate licensure under one license (see Chapter 4 ∞). Nurses from other countries may be granted registration by endorsement after successfully completing the NCLEX. Both licensure and registration must be renewed regularly to remain valid. For additional information about licensure and registration, see Chapter 4. ∞

The legal right to practice nursing requires not only passing the licensing examination but also verification that the graduate has completed a prescribed course of study in nursing. Individual states may have additional requirements. All U.S. nursing programs require approval by their state board of nursing.

In addition to state approval, the National League for Nursing Accrediting Commission (NLNAC) provides accreditation for all levels of nursing programs, and the Commission on Collegiate Nursing Education (CCNE) accredits baccalaureate and graduate degree nursing programs. Accredited programs meet standard requirements evaluated periodically through written self-studies and on-site visitation by examiners.

Figure 2-1 ■ Nursing students learn to care for clients in community settings.

TYPES OF EDUCATIONAL PROGRAMS

Educational programs available for nurses include practical or vocational, registered nursing, graduate nursing, continuing education, and in-service.

Licensed Practical (Vocational) Nursing Programs

Practical or vocational nursing programs are provided by community colleges, vocational schools, hospitals, or other independent health agencies. These programs usually last 9 or 12 months and provide both classroom and clinical experiences. At the end of the program, the graduate takes the NCLEX-PN to obtain a license as a practical or vocational nurse.

Licensed practical nurses practice under the supervision of a registered nurse in a hospital, nursing home, rehabilitation center, or home health agency. LPNs (LVNs) usually provide basic direct technical care to clients. The registered nurse, who has the knowledge and skill to make more sophisticated nursing judgments, is responsible for assessing the client's condition, planning care, and evaluating the effect of the care provided.

Registered Nursing Programs

Currently, three major educational routes lead to RN licensure: diploma, associate degree, and baccalaureate programs.

Diploma Programs

After Florence Nightingale established the Nightingale Training School for Nurses at St. Thomas's Hospital in England in 1860, the concept traveled quickly to North America. Hospital administrators welcomed the idea of training schools as a source of free or inexpensive staffing for the hospital. Nursing education in the early years largely took the form of apprenticeships. With little formal classroom instruction, students learned by doing, that is, by providing care to clients in hospitals. There was no standardization of curriculum and no accreditation. Programs were designed to meet the service needs of the hospital, not the educational needs of the students.

The 3-year diploma programs were the dominant nursing programs from the late 1800s and were the major source of graduates until the mid-1960s. Today's diploma nursing programs have changed markedly from the original Nightingale model. In the United States, diploma programs are hospital-based educational programs that provide a rich clinical experience for nursing students. These programs are often associated with colleges or universities.

Almost 70 NLNAC accredited diploma programs in 18 states provide this avenue for students desiring an education in nursing (NLNAC, 2005). The number of diploma nursing programs has declined since the ANA resolution in 1965 which recommended that "education for those who work in nursing should be placed in institutions of learning within the general system of education," that "minimal preparation for beginning professional nursing practice at the present time should be the baccalaureate degree education in nursing," and that "associate

degree education in nursing should be the minimum preparation for beginning technical nursing practice" (ANA, 1965, p. 107).

Community College/ Associate Degree Programs

Community college/associate degree nursing programs, which arose in the early 1950s, were the first and only educational programs for nursing that were systematically developed from planned research and controlled experimentation. Several trends and events influenced the development of these programs: (a) the Cadet Nurse Corps, (b) the community college movement, (c) earlier nursing studies, and (d) Dr. Mildred Montag's proposal for an associate degree.

The Cadet Nurse Corps of the United States was legislated and financed during World War II to provide additional nurses to meet both military and civilian nursing needs. The corps proved that qualified nurses could be educated in less time than the traditional 3 years.

After World War II, the number of community colleges in the United States grew rapidly. The low tuition and open-door policy of these colleges made higher education more accessible to all by offering the first 2 years of a 4-year college program.

Studies of nursing education, such as the Goldmark report in 1923, the Committee on the Grading of Schools of Nursing in 1934, and the Brown report in 1948, also had a significant influence on the development of 2-year programs. The recommendations in all of these reports supported independent schools of nursing in institutions of higher learning separate from hospitals.

In the United States, associate degree programs were started after Mildred Montag published her doctoral dissertation in 1951, "The Education of Nursing Technicians," which proposed a 2-year education program for RNs in the community colleges. Dr. Montag made the suggestion as a solution to the acute shortage of nurses that came about because of World War II. She conceptualized a "nursing technician" or "bedside nurse" able to perform nursing functions broader than those of the practical nurse and smaller in scope than those of the professional nurse. At the end of 2 years, the student was to be awarded an associate degree in nursing and be eligible to take the state board examination for registered nurse licensure. The first associate degree in nursing (ADN) program started at Columbia University Teachers' College in 1952 under the direction of Mildred Montag. The number of ADN programs has grown from seven in 1958 to more than 880 in 2004 (National Organization for Associate Degree Nursing, 2005).

Dr. Montag's original idea that these graduates be nursing technicians and that the degree become a terminal one did not last, however. In 1978, the ANA proposed a resolution that associate degree programs were no longer to be considered terminal but part of a career upward-mobility plan. Today many students enter an associate degree program with the intention of continuing their education in nursing to the baccalaureate or higher level.

Associate degree programs are offered in the United States primarily in community colleges although some 4-year colleges also have ADN programs. The graduating student receives an ADN or an associate of arts (AA), associate of science (AS), or associate in applied science (AAS) degree with a major in nursing.

Because ADN-prepared and bachelor of science in nursing (BSN)-prepared nurses currently function under the same practice acts, the need for differentiated competencies has been debated for years. Brady et al. (2001) pointed out that clear and specific information about the type of knowledge, skills, and abilities of each type of nursing education program would "assure that the right nurse with the right competencies is in the right job at the right cost" (p. 34).

The Pew Health Professions Commission (O'Neil, 1998) developed a set of competencies needed by all health professional groups for successful practice in the 21st century (see Box 2–1). In addition, the Pew commission challenges nursing to address a number of issues, among them, to define the various competencies for each educational level. On another front, the Robert Wood Foundation funded 20 nationwide Colleagues in Caring (CIC) projects to "facilitate a statewide collaborative approach to nursing workforce development" (Brady et al., 2001, p. 30). The various CIC projects focus on providing seamless articulation, in which graduates of one nursing program type can easily transition to the next educational level, or on differentiating competencies between the nursing educational levels.

Baccalaureate Degree Programs

The first school of nursing in a university setting was established at the University of Minnesota in 1909. This program's curriculum, however, differed little from a 3-year hospital program. It was not until 1919 that the University of Minnesota established its undergraduate baccalaureate degree in nursing. Most of the early baccalaureate programs were 5 years in length. They consisted of the basic 3-year diploma program in addition to 2 years of liberal arts.

In the 1960s, the number of students enrolled in these baccalaureate programs increased markedly. Almost 700 baccalaureate programs of nursing are in existence in the United States.

Today baccalaureate nursing programs are located in senior colleges and universities and are generally 4 years in length. The curricula offer courses in the liberal arts, sciences, humanities, and nursing. Graduates must fulfill both the degree requirements of the college or university and the nursing program before being awarded a baccalaureate degree. The usual degree awarded is a bachelor of science in nursing (BSN). Partially in response to the significant shortage of RNs, U. S. schools have also established accelerated BSN programs. The programs may include summer semesters in order to shorten the length of time required to complete the curriculum or may be a modified curriculum especially designed for students who already have a baccalaureate degree in another field. These "second-degree" or "fast-track" BSN programs (of which there are over 200 in the United States) can be completed in 12 to 18 months of continuous study.

Many baccalaureate programs also admit registered nurses who have diplomas or associate degrees. Some programs have a special curriculum to meet the needs of these students. Some universities also offer nursing students the opportunity to pursue a self-paced, independent study, or an online program. Many accept transfer credits from other accredited colleges and universities and offer students the opportunity to take challenge examinations when the students believe they have the knowledge or skills taught in a course. These programs are referred to as BSN completion, BSN transition, 2 + 2, or RN-BSN programs.

Because of changes in the practice environment, the nurse who holds a baccalaureate degree is beginning to experience greater autonomy, responsibility, participation in institutional decision making, and career advancement. In addition, the American Nurses Credentialing Center requires a baccalaureate degree for initial basic certification in most nursing specialties. These changes provide an incentive for nurses with diplomas and associate degrees to continue their formal preparation in baccalaureate completion (transition) programs.

Graduate Nursing Education

Most graduate programs are conducted by departments within the graduate school of a university, and the applicant must first meet requirements established by the graduate school. Although graduate schools differ, common requirements for admission to graduate programs in nursing include the following:

- The applicant must be a registered nurse licensed or eligible for licensure within the program's state.
- The applicant generally must hold a baccalaureate degree in nursing from an approved college or university and have had an acceptable upper division major in nursing at the baccalaureate level. Some master's degree programs accept applicants with only an ADN.

BOX 2–1 Twenty-One Competencies for the 21st Century

- Embrace a personal ethic of social responsibility and service.
- Exhibit ethical behavior in all professional activities.
- Provide evidence-based, clinically competent care.
- Incorporate the multiple determinants of health in clinical care.
- Apply knowledge of the new sciences.
- Demonstrate critical thinking, reflection, and problem-solving skills.
- Understand the role of primary care.
- Rigorously practice preventive health care.
- Integrate population-based care and services into practice.
- Improve access to health care for those with unmet health needs.
- Practice relationship-centered care with individuals and families.
- Provide culturally sensitive care to a diverse society.
- Partner with communities in health care decisions.
- Use communication and information technology effectively and appropriately.
- Work in interdisciplinary teams.
- Ensure care that balances individual, professional, system, and societal needs.
- Practice leadership.
- Take responsibility for quality of care and health outcomes at all levels.
- Contribute to continuous improvement of the health care system.
- Advocate for public policy that promotes and protects the health of the public.
- Continue to learn and help others learn.

Note: From Recreating Health Professional Practice for a New Century, by E. H. O'Neil and the Pew Health Professions Commission, 1998, San Francisco: Pew Health Professionals. Reprinted with permission.

- The applicant must give evidence of scholastic ability (usually a minimum grade point average of 2.7 to 3.0 on a 4.0 scale).
- The applicant must demonstrate satisfactory achievement on a qualifying examination, such as the Graduate Record Examination (GRE) or the Miller Analogy Test (MAT).
- The applicant must have letters of recommendation from supervisors, nursing faculty, or nursing colleagues indicating the applicant's ability to do graduate study.

Master's Programs

The growth of university nursing programs encouraged the development of graduate study in nursing. In 1953, the newly established National League for Nursing encouraged educators to develop programs for master's degrees in nursing. The major emphasis of the programs was to be research and specialization for teaching and administration. The first "clinical" master's degree (in psychiatric nursing) was offered at Rutgers University in New Jersey in 1954.

Today master's programs generally take from 1.5 to 2 years to complete. Degrees granted are the master of arts (MA), master in nursing (MN), master of science in nursing (MSN), and master of science (MS).

Master's degree programs provide specialized knowledge and skills that enable nurses to assume advanced roles in practice, education, administration, and research (see Figure 2-2 ■).

Doctoral Programs

Doctoral programs in nursing, which award the degrees of doctor of philosophy (PhD), doctor of nursing science (DNS or DNSc), or nursing doctorate (ND), began in the 1960s in the United States. These programs further prepare the nurse for advanced clinical practice, administration, education, and research. Before 1960, nurses acquired doctoral degrees in such related fields as psychology, sociology, physiology, and education. In 2004, the American Association of Colleges of Nursing (AACN) approved a move to prepare advanced practice nurses (nurse practitioners, nurse anesthetists, nurse midwives, and clinical nurse specialists) at the doctoral level—awarding a doctor of nursing practice (DNP) and phasing out the DNS and ND designations (AACN, 2005).

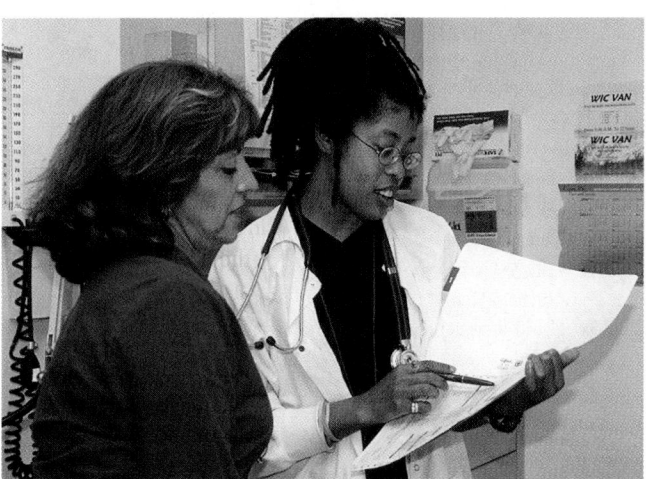

Figure 2-2 ■ A nurse practitioner holds a master's degree and assumes an advanced practice role.

Content and approach vary among doctoral programs. Some focus on the usual clinical areas, such as medical-surgical nursing, and others emphasize such nontraditional areas as transcultural nursing. Some programs emphasize theory development, but all emphasize research.

Entry to Practice

In 1985, the ANA endorsed the BSN as the entry level for professional practice. According to the ANA's proposal, only the baccalaureate graduate would be licensed under the legal title registered nurse. The graduate with an associate degree in nursing would be considered a technical nurse and be licensed under the legal title associate nurse (AN).

The ANA proposal sparked sharp debates among graduates, students, and educators, some of whom perceive that it undervalues associate degree (AD) graduates. As a result, the National League for Nursing (NLN) has suggested that the title of associate nurse be replaced by registered associate nurse. However, this suggestion has not eliminated the controversy; many argue that AD graduates have held the title registered nurse since the inception of these ADN programs and should retain that title.

As a professional organization, the ANA cannot legislate these changes. It is the responsibility of each state to define the legal boundaries of nursing practice and to designate the title to be used by those practitioners who meet the individual state's criteria for licensure. If the ANA's proposal is to be accepted nationally, each state will need to adopt the proposal and implement its own changes in its licensure law.

If the ANA proposal is implemented, a grandfather clause would need to be considered for registered nurses who were educated in associate degree or diploma programs before the date of change. Under a grandfather clause, these nurses would continue to be licensed and practice as registered nurses provided that their performance meets established standards. Note, however, that a grandfather clause would protect only the nurse's license. If, for example, an institution required a minimum of a baccalaureate degree for the position of head nurse, an RN who is currently employed as a head nurse but who does not hold the baccalaureate degree would have no guarantee of retaining that position.

Licensure law changes also have major implications for diploma nurses and LPNs because their status is not discussed in the proposal. In addition, this proposal entails that new standardized examinations must be developed to test the two levels of competence.

Perspectives about entry into practice are changing. For example, the AACN (2005) provides a fact sheet that informs of AACN's support for articulation. The organization supports articulation from associate degree programs to baccalaureate and higher degree programs and desires to strengthen collaboration between ADN and BSN programs. In addition, the AACN is testing models of a new category of nurse, the clinical nurse leader (CNL).

In practice, the CNL oversees the care coordination of a distinct group of patients and actively provides direct patient care in complex situations. This master's degree-prepared clinician puts evidence-based practice into action to ensure that patients benefit from the latest innovations in care delivery. The CNL evaluates patient outcomes,

RESEARCH NOTE **Does Education of the Nurse Affect Client Survival?**

This landmark study aimed to determine how the proportion of nurses with BSN degrees was associated with the deaths of surgical clients. Charts for 232,342 surgical clients in 168 Pennsylvania hospitals over 20 months were examined for many characteristics—including mortality and complication rates. Hospital data included size (number of beds), whether it was a teaching facility, existence of technology, presence of certified surgeons, nurses' years of experience, and nurse–client ratios. Findings showed a significant relationship between the proportion of BSN and MSN nurses and client mortality. For every 10% increase in proportion of higher-degree nurses there was a 5% reduction in mortality. Nurse staffing and certified surgeons also were statistically significant in reducing mortality. Years of nursing experience did not correlate with client survival. The authors noted limitations of their study, including that hospitals in only one state were included.

IMPLICATIONS

In addition to an overall shortage of nurses nationwide, fewer nurses are currently prepared initially at the BSN or higher level than at the diploma or ADN level. Policy decisions related to funding of nursing programs, incentives for nurses to continue their education beyond the associate degree level, and hospital preference for nurses with specific educational levels should consider reliable data that indicate cost-effectiveness of choices made.

Note: From "Educational Levels of Hospital Nurses and Surgical Patient Mortality," by L. H. Aiken, S. P. Clarke, R. B. Cheung, D. M. Sloane, & S. H. Silber, 2003, *Journal of the American Medical Association, 290,* pp. 1617–1623.

assesses cohort risk, and has the decision-making authority to change care plans when necessary. The CNL is a leader in the health care delivery system, and the implementation of this role will vary across settings (AACN, 2005).

Continuing Education

The term **continuing education (CE)** refers to formalized experiences designed to enlarge the knowledge or skills of practitioners. Compared to advanced education programs, which result in an academic degree, CE courses tend to be more specific and shorter. Participants may receive certificates of completion or specialization.

Continuing education is the responsibility of each practicing nurse. Constant updating and growth are essential to keep abreast of scientific and technological change and changes within the nursing profession. A variety of educational and health care institutions conduct continuing education programs. They are usually designed to meet one or more of the following needs: (a) to keep nurses abreast of new techniques and knowledge; (b) to help nurses attain expertise in a specialized area of practice, such as intensive care nursing; and (c) to provide nurses with information essential to nursing practice, for example, knowledge about the legal aspects of nursing.

Some state laws require nurses to obtain a certain number of CE credits to renew their licenses. In these states, required CE contact hours vary from 15 to 30 hours for every 2-year relicensure period. All, some, or none of these hours may be acquired through home study. Some home study courses are offered through professional journals. The ANA offers online CE programs to nurses. A few states also require a certain number of hours of practice, either independently or in lieu of study hours, before license renewal.

In-Service Education

An **in-service education** program is administered by an employer; it is designed to upgrade the knowledge or skills of employees. For example, an employer might offer an in-service program to inform nurses about a new piece of equipment, specific isolation practices, or methods of implementing a nurse theorist's conceptual framework for nursing. Some in-service programs are mandatory, such as cardiopulmonary resuscitation and fire safety programs.

NURSING RESEARCH AND EVIDENCE-BASED PRACTICE

Today, nurses are actively generating, publishing, and applying research in practice to improve client care and enhance nursing's scientific knowledge base. The *Scope and Standards of Practice* published by the ANA (2004) include research as one of the standards of professional performance (see Box 2–2). Recently, there has been increased emphasis on the importance of **evidence-based practice (EBP),** that is, the use of some form of substantiation in making clinical decisions. This substantiation, or evidence, can arise from tradition, authority, experience, trial

BOX 2–2 American Nurses Association's Standards of Professional Performance Pertaining to Research

STANDARD 13: RESEARCH
The registered nurse integrates research findings into practice.

Measurement Criteria
The registered nurse:

Utilizes best available evidence, including research findings, to guide practice decisions.
Actively participates in research activities at various levels appropriate to the nurse's level of education and position. Such activities may include:

- Identifying clinical problems specific to nursing research (patient care and nursing practice).
- Participating in data collection (surveys, pilot projects, and formal studies).
- Participating in a formal committee or program.
- Sharing research activities and/or findings with peers and others.
- Conducting research.
- Critically analyzing and interpreting research for application to practice.
- Using research findings in the development of policies, procedures, and standards of practice in patient care.
- Incorporating research as a basis for learning.

and error, logic or reason, or research. For example, nurses can learn from the Agency for Healthcare Research and Quality's Effective Health Care Program, which has three approaches to publishing research on the comparative effectiveness of different treatments and clinical practices:

■ Review and synthesize knowledge. The Evidence-Based Practice Centers systematically review published and unpublished scientific evidence.

■ Promote and generate knowledge. The DEcIDE (Developing Evidence to Inform Decisions about Effectiveness) Research Network studies new scientific evidence and analytic tools in an accelerated and practical format.

■ Compile the findings and translate knowledge. The Clinical Decisions and Communications Science Center compiles the research results into a variety of useful formats for stakeholders.

Although the focus for all nurses is use of research findings in practice, the degree of participation in research depends on the nurse's educational level, position, experience, and practical environment. In March 2006, the AACN approved a revised position statement on nursing research that delineates the expectations and competencies of graduates of each level of nursing education from baccalaureate through postdoctoral programs (AACN, 2006). As early as 1854, Florence Nightingale demonstrated the importance of research in the delivery of nursing care. When Nightingale arrived in the Crimea in November 1854, she found the military hospital barracks overcrowded, filthy, rat and flea infested, and lacking in food, drugs, and essential medical supplies.

As a result of these conditions, men died from starvation and such diseases as dysentery, cholera, and typhus. By systematically collecting, organizing, and reporting data, Nightingale was able to institute sanitary reforms and significantly reduce mortality rates from contagious disease.

Although the Nightingale tradition influenced the establishment of American nursing schools, the research approach did not take hold until the beginning of the 20th century.

The journal *Nursing Research* was established in 1952 to serve as a vehicle to communicate nurses' research and scholarly productivity. The publication of many other nursing research journals followed, some dedicated to research and others combining clinical and research manuscripts (see Box 2–3). The breadth and diversity of nursing research is reflected in the examples of recent nursing studies shown in Box 2–4.

In 1985, the U.S. Congress passed a bill creating a National Center for Nursing Research in the National Institutes of Health (NIH) to house the research activities conducted by the Division of Nursing at the Department of Health and Human Services (DHHS). In 1993, the Center for Nursing Research was pro-

---

BOX 2–3 Nursing Research Journals

EXAMPLES OF RESEARCH JOURNALS IN NURSING

Advances in Nursing Science
Applied Nursing Research
Evidence-Based Nursing
International Journal of Nursing Studies
Journal of Nursing Scholarship
Nursing Research
Research in Nursing and Health
Scholarly Inquiry for Nursing Practice
Western Journal of Nursing Research

EXAMPLES OF CLINICAL AND SPECIALTY NURSING JOURNALS THAT PUBLISH RESEARCH

American Journal of Critical Care
American Journal of Nursing
Heart and Lung
Journal of Gerontologic Nursing
Journal of Neuroscience Nursing
Journal of Nursing Administration
Journal of Nursing Education
Journal of Pediatric Nursing
Journal of Professional Nursing
MedSurg Nursing
Nursing Administration Quarterly
Nursing Outlook
Oncology Nursing Forum

BOX 2–4 Examples of Nursing Studies

■ Baumann (2004) compared six research studies on the experience of hope in Japan, Taiwan, Sweden, Finland, and the United States. While the structure of the experience of hope was similar, some differences were found that enhance nursing practice and guide further study.

■ Hicks, Rantz, Petroski, and Mukamel (2004) examined the relationship between cost and quality of care in nursing homes using quality indicator measures of resident outcomes. Although each individual quality measure makes only small contributions to costs, when considered across the facility, quality could have a substantial financial impact on the operations of the home.

■ Survey data from pairs of nursing students in their and second semesters indicated that they felt their understanding and perceptions of nursing had changed following their first clinical experience (Sand-Jecklin & Schaffer, 2006). The statistically significant difference between semester scores seemed logical on some items e.g., that they had a more accurate view of what nurses do, while others were counterintuitive and invite further study e.g., they agreed less in semester two that nursing offers many career opportunities and that nurses are intelligent and creative than they did in semester one.

■ As part of a randomized clinical trial, Sutters et al. (2005) found no differences in the frequency of moderate-to-severe side effects with around-the-clock (ATC) dosing of acetaminophen with codeine, compared with as-needed (prn) dosing in the first 3 days after tonsil surgery. Children in the ATC groups reported a statistically significant decrease over time in vomiting ($p = .001$) and feeling lightheaded or dizzy ($p = .003$), and a significant increase in constipation ($p = .018$). Except for daytime sedation, changes, over time, in the frequency of moderate-to-severe side effects were not observed in the prn group.

■ Researchers at Johns Hopkins University (Vetter, Bristow, & Ahrens, 2004) conducted a randomized clinical trial to test the effect of nurse case management and community health worker interventions on diabetes control among inner-city African Americans. The results demonstrated that the greatest improvement occurred when nurse case managers and community health workers worked together.

moted to the National Institute for Nursing Research (NINR), gaining equal status with other institutes within the NIH. Research opportunities identified by NINR for the years 2000 to 2004 are listed in Box 2–5.

Approaches to Nursing Research

There are two major approaches in nursing research to investigating diverse phenomena. These approaches originate from different philosophical perspectives and use different methods for collection and analysis of data.

Quantitative Research

Quantitative research progresses through systematic, logical steps according to a specific plan to collect information, often under conditions of considerable control, that is analyzed using statistical procedures. The quantitative approach is most frequently associated with positivism or logical positivism, a philosophical doctrine that emphasizes the rational and the scientific (Polit & Beck, 2005). Quantitative research is often viewed as "hard" science and uses deductive reasoning and the measurable attributes of human experience.

BOX 2–5 Research Opportunities of the National Institute of Nursing Research for 2000–2004

Support research opportunities and provide leadership in:

- *End of life/palliative care research.* NINR is currently the lead institute at NIH for this area of research and is focusing on clinical management of physical and psychological symptom management, communication, ethics and clinical decision making, caregiver support, and care delivery issues.
- *Chronic illness experiences,* such as managing symptoms, avoiding complications of disease and disability, supporting family caregivers, promoting adherence and self-management activities, and promoting healthy behaviors within the context of the chronic condition.
- *Cultural and ethnic considerations* in health and illness, including culturally sensitive interventions to decrease *health disparities* among groups by focusing upon health promotion activities and chronic illness management strategies.
- *Health promotion and disease prevention research,* particularly as it relates to lifestyle changes and healthy behavior maintenance across the life span.
- *Implications of genetic advances,* including reducing factors that increase risk of disease, issues related to genetic screening, and subsequent gene therapy techniques.
- *Quality of life and quality of care,* to include cost savings for the patient, health care system, and society.
- *Symptom management* of illness and treatment, such as pain, cognitive impairment, fatigue, nausea and vomiting, and sleep problems.
- *Telehealth interventions and monitoring* or other emerging technologies to promote patient education and treatment.

Note: From *"Mission of the National Institute of Nursing Research. Scientific Goals and Objectives (Objective 1.1),"* by National Institute of Nursing Research, 2000. Retrieved March 13, 2006, from http://ninr.nih.gov/ninr/research/diversity/mission.html. Reprinted with permission.

The following are examples of research questions that lend themselves to a quantitative approach:

- What are the differential effects of continuous versus intermittent application of negative pressure on tracheal tissue during endotracheal suctioning?
- Is the auscultatory method effective in validating the location of a feeding tube?

Qualitative Research

The qualitative approach is often associated with naturalistic inquiry, which explores the subjective and complex experiences of human beings. "Naturalistic investigation emphasizes understanding the human experience as it is lived, usually through careful collection and analysis of qualitative materials that are narrative and subjective" (Polit & Beck, 2005, p. 16). Data collection and its analysis occur concurrently. Using the inductive method, data are analyzed by identifying themes and patterns to develop a theory or framework that helps explain the processes under observation. The qualitative approach would be appropriate for the following types of research questions:

- What is the bereavement process in spouses of clients with terminal cancer?
- What is the nature of coping and adjustment after a radical prostatectomy?
- As experienced by the caregiver, what is the process of family caregiving for elderly relatives with Alzheimer's dementia?

Protecting the Rights of Human Subjects

Because nursing research usually focuses on humans, a major nursing responsibility is to be aware of and to advocate on behalf of clients' rights. All clients must be informed and understand the consequences of consenting to serve as research participants (Figure 2-3 ■). The client needs to be able to assess

Figure 2-3 ■ It is important for clients to be fully informed before they participate in a research study.

whether an appropriate balance exists between the risks of participating in a study and the potential benefits, either to the client or to the development of knowledge.

For many years, adults have been the focus of much health care research conducted on human subjects. The American Academy of Pediatrics has identified the need to conduct pediatric research so that children can benefit from advances in medical science. At the same time, because children are so vulnerable, extra precautions must be taken to ensure their rights are upheld and they are not harmed. It is critical to have pediatric expertise on panels that review prospective research studies and in research development. All nurses who practice in settings where research is being conducted with human subjects or who participate in such research play an important role in safeguarding the following rights.

Right Not to Be Harmed

The **risk of harm** to a research subject is exposure to the possibility of injury going beyond everyday situations. The risk can be physical, emotional, legal, financial, or social. For instance, withholding standard care from a client in labor for the purpose of studying the course of natural childbirth clearly poses a potential physical danger. Risks can also involve psychologic factors, such as exposure to stress or anxiety, or social factors, such as loss of confidentiality or loss of privacy.

Right to Full Disclosure

Even though it may be possible to collect data about a client as part of everyday care without the client's particular knowledge or consent, to do so is considered unethical. **Full disclosure,** the act of making clear the client's role in a research situation, is a basic right. It means that deception, either by withholding information about a client's participation in a study or by giving the client false or misleading information about what participating in the study will involve, must not occur.

Right of Self-Determination

Many dependent clients, such as people in long-term care facilities, feel pressured to participate in studies. They believe that they must please the doctors and nurses who are responsible for their treatment and care. The **right of self-determination** means that participants should feel free from constraints, coercion, or any undue influence to participate in a study. Hidden inducements—for instance, suggesting to potential participants that by taking part in the study they might become famous, make an important contribution to science, or receive special attention—must be strictly avoided.

Right of Privacy and Confidentiality

Privacy enables a client to participate without worrying about later embarrassment. The anonymity of a study participant is ensured if even the investigator cannot link a specific person to the information reported. **Confidentiality** means that any information a participant relates will not be made public or available to others without the participant's consent. Investigators must inform research participants about the measures that provide for these rights. Such measures may include the use of pseudonyms or code numbers or reporting only aggregate or group data in published research.

The Quantitative Research Process

Polit and Beck (2005) define research as "systematic inquiry that uses disciplined methods to answer questions or solve problems" (p. 3). Research is the application of the scientific approach to generate empirical knowledge. The steps in the quantitative research process are discussed next.

State a Research Question or Problem

The investigator's initial task is to narrow a broad area of interest to a circumscribed problem that specifies exactly the intent of the study. The ideas for research may arise from recurrent problems encountered in practice, questions that are difficult to resolve because of contradictions in the literature, or areas in which minimal or no research has been done.

In formulating a research problem, Polit and Beck (2005) suggest that four criteria be used: significance, researchability, feasibility, and interest to the researcher. A research problem has **significance** if it has the potential to contribute to nursing science by enhancing client care, testing or generating a theory, or resolving a day-to-day clinical problem. The question "So what?" must be answered adequately to determine if a research problem is significant.

Researchability means that the problem can be subjected to scientific investigation. Many significant problems that produce ambiguity and uncertainty in clinical situations may not be amenable to research. For instance, "Should nurses be allowed to go on strike?" is a relevant, timely, and difficult question, but it cannot be answered through research.

Feasibility pertains to the availability of time as well as the material and human resources needed to investigate a research problem or question. Conducting a study involves the use of space, money, equipment, supplies, computers, subjects, research assistants, and consultants.

A researcher spends much time and energy while conducting a research project. It is important, therefore, that the researcher be genuinely interested in the research problem because the researcher's enthusiasm can be a factor for successful completion of the research.

Quantitative research problems address the relationships between dependent and independent variables, except for descriptive research, which has no dependent variables. The **dependent variable** is the behavior, characteristic, or outcome that the researcher wishes to explain or predict. The **independent variable** is the presumed cause of or influence on the dependent variable. As an example, a research problem might be "Do people who lose weight on a low-carbohydrate diet maintain their weight loss longer than those people who lose weight on a low-calorie diet?"

Define the Study's Purpose or Rationale

The statement of the study's purpose indicates what the researcher intends to do with the research problem identified. The study purpose includes what the researcher will do, who the participants will be, and where the data will be collected. Continuing the previous example, the purpose might be to "Collect data from adult obese persons in the state of Iowa who have lost weight on either a low-carbohydrate or low-calorie diet and compare how long they maintain their weight loss."

Review the Related Literature

Before progressing with the development of the research design, the investigator determines what is known and what is not known about the problem. A thorough review of the literature provides the foundation on which to build new knowledge. Through a literature review, a researcher may also acquire information about available techniques, instruments, and methods of data analysis that have been used in prior research, as well as potential flaws or problems and how to avoid them.

Formulate Hypotheses and Define Variables

A **hypothesis** is a prediction of the relationship among two or more variables. Some studies are intended to develop hypotheses, whereas others are intended to test hypotheses using statistical procedures. Hypothesis formulation requires not only sufficient knowledge about a topic to predict the outcome of the study but also **operational definitions**, definitions that specify the instruments or procedures by which concepts will be measured. In our example, one hypothesis might be "Obese persons are equally likely to maintain their weight loss whether they have lost weight using a low-carbohydrate or low-calorie diet."

Select a Research Design to Test the Hypothesis

A research design is the overall plan for conducting the study to answer the research questions or test the research hypotheses. The research design includes the study setting, the sample, and the type of data to be collected, as well as strategies to control extraneous variables and reduce bias. There are three major types of research design:

■ *Experimental design.* The investigator manipulates the independent variable by administering an experi-

mental treatment to some participants while withholding it from others.
■ *Quasi-experimental design.* The investigator manipulates the independent variable but without either the randomization or control that characterizes true experiments.
■ *Nonexperimental design.* The investigator does no manipulation of the independent variable.

Select the Population, Sample, and Setting

At this stage, the researcher chooses the study population, selects a sample, and decides on the setting where the sample can be found. The **population** includes all possible members of the group who meet the criteria for the study. The **sample** is the segment of the population from whom the data will actually be collected.

Conduct a Pilot Study

A pilot study is a "dress rehearsal" before the actual study begins. A trial run of the research procedure is conducted on a few participants to assess the adequacy and feasibility of the data collection plan. By identifying any problems or flaws during the pilot study, the investigators can refine the proposed plan and strengthen the research methodology.

Collect the Data

The research process relies on **empirical data,** or information collected from the observable world. Conclusions and generalizations are derived from collected data. The most commonly used methods of collecting data in nursing are questionnaires, rating scales, interviews, observation, and biophysical measures.

The validity and reliability of measurement tools need to be established prior to the start of data collection. **Validity** is the degree to which an instrument measures what it is supposed to measure. If a nurse measures anxiety, how would the nurse be sure that what is being measured is not fear or stress, which are related concepts? **Reliability** is the degree of consistency with which an instrument measures a concept or variable. If an in-

REAL WORLD PRACTICE

Approximately seven years ago when I was working in the cardiac intensive care unit, I was asked by my nurse manager if I would like to start a research project. She had someone who could provide the research background if I could provide the clinical expertise. Well I didn't know anything about research or the IRB (International Review Board) at that time, let alone the time requirements. I mulled over the request for several weeks before I crazily consented to try it.

The woman who was to provide the research background was an art therapist. She was wonderfully supportive even though I was clueless. We came up with a study on "Relaxation and Guided Imagery with Cardiac Patients." Our decision to study subjective data was not the smartest move. To prove clinical significance you have to have very large numbers and you have to decrease variables as much as possible. Five years and at least three major trips

to the IRB later, we completed our study. My art therapist retired after about four years into the study, but I was able to find another nurse with research experience to help.

The relationship with the art therapist and the nurse research associate turned into wonderful lifelong friendships. The study results were presented as a poster at NTI (National Training Institute), a very prestigious nursing seminar. Last but not least, I was given a job at the General Clinical Research Center. It is a job I really love!

My point is . . . don't be afraid to venture into the unknown. You might be surprised at what wonderful open doors await you.

—Anne Fekete, RN, CCRN, CRNI,
General Clinical Research Center,
University of California, Davis Medical Center

strument is reliable, repeated measurement of the same variable should yield similar or nearly similar results.

Analyze the Data

In this step, the collected data are organized, coded, and analyzed for the purpose of answering the research question or testing the hypotheses. Even before data collection is initiated, a systematic plan must be in place for analyzing the results. Data analysis may involve descriptive or inferential statistics. **Descriptive statistics,** procedures that summarize large volumes of data, are used to describe and synthesize data, showing patterns and trends. Descriptive statistics include measures of central tendency and measures of variability.

Measures of central tendency describe the center of a distribution of data, denoting where most of the subjects lie. These include the **mean, median,** and **mode. Measures of variability** indicate the degree of dispersion or spread of the data. These include the **range, variance,** and **standard deviation.** See Box 2–6 for definitions of these measures. Typically in a research report, the mean (a measure of central tendency) and standard deviation (a measure of variability) are reported together to give the reader an idea of the nature of the data distribution. The following is an example:

Systolic blood pressure
130 ± 30 mm Hg

The two statistics reported are the mean and the standard deviation. The number 130 indicates the mean systolic blood pressure, whereas 30 represents 1 standard deviation (SD) from the mean. Hence, 1 SD from the mean would include blood pressure from 100 mm Hg to 160 mm Hg (1 SD below to 1 SD above the mean).

After data have been analyzed, nurse researchers attempt to determine whether the results were **statistically significant**—unlikely to have occurred by chance. Underlying this statement

is the notion of probability. By convention, p (probability) less than .05 is considered the acceptable level of significance. A p value greater than .05 is considered statistically nonsignificant. In research, the desire is to generalize beyond the sample, so there is a need to determine the probability that the results were due to chance rather than a true occurrence in the population. Hence, a p value of .05 means that the probability of the findings being caused by chance alone is 5 in 100.

Communicate Conclusions and Implications

Implicit in conducting research is the requirement to share the knowledge generated with others, either through publication in professional journals or by reporting the results at professional conferences. Interpreting the results, communicating the findings, and suggesting directions for further study conclude the research process. The summary reports of research also include a discussion of any limitations in applying the particular findings to the broader population.

Evidence-Based Practice

In EBP, the nurse integrates research findings with clinical experience, the client's preferences, and available resources in planning and implementing care. Such practice can help control cost by focusing on substantiated yet individualized approaches to care. A significant source of EBP data is the Cochrane Database of Systematic Reviews. The data found in this resource often combine research to increase the power of the findings of numerous studies, each too small to produce reliable results individually. The Cochrane Collaboration is an international not-for-profit organization dedicated to making up-to-date, accurate information about the effects of health care readily available worldwide. Other major resources for information on EBP are the Healthlinks search engine at the University of Washington, the Academic Center for Evidence-Based Nursing at the University of Texas Health Science Center at San Antonio, and the National Guideline Clearinghouse (www.guideline.gov), a public resource for evidence-based clinical practice guidelines.

Not all health care providers believe that EBP is the ideal approach to client care. Some are concerned that it creates a hierarchy of evidence in which the strictest controlled research studies are viewed as better indicators of proper care than are descriptive studies or expert opinions. Others believe that EBP focuses on problems rather than people and de-emphasizes creative, personalized care created through nurses' critical thinking (Parse, 2004). It is the nurse's responsibility to be aware of findings published in the literature, to question practice so it can be continuously improved, and to participate in investigating better ways to improve health.

The Qualitative Research Process

Qualitative research is not linear like quantitative research. Qualitative researchers do not use independent and dependent variables or manipulate some aspect of the study to test a hypothesis. The intent of qualitative research is to thoroughly describe and explain a phenomenon. The researchers collect narrative data through interviews or observation. These data are transcribed and often result in hundreds of pages that need to be organized

---

BOX 2–6 Definitions of Measures of Central Tendency and Variability

CENTRAL TENDENCY

mean A measure of central tendency, computed by summing all scores and dividing by the number of subjects; commonly symbolized as $\bar{x}$ or M.

median A measure of central tendency, representing the exact middle score or value in a distribution of scores; the median is the value above and below which 50% of the scores lie.

mode The score or value that occurs most frequently in a distribution of scores.

VARIABILITY

range A measure of variability, consisting of the difference between the highest and lowest values in a distribution of scores.

variance A measure of variance or dispersion, equal to the square of the standard deviation.

standard deviation The most frequently used measure of variability, indicating the average to which scores deviate from the mean; commonly symbolized as SD or S.

and interpreted. These narrative data may be organized around some type of categorization scheme such as concepts, actions, or themes. Finally, the themes of the data are integrated to present a description or theory.

There are three common qualitative research traditions:

- **Ethnography:** Research that provides a framework to focus on the culture of a group of people.
- **Phenomenology:** Research that investigates people's life experiences and how they interpret those experiences.
- **Grounded theory:** Research to understand social structures and social processes. This method focuses on generation of categories or hypotheses that explain patterns of behavior of the people in the study.

CRITIQUING RESEARCH REPORTS

If nurses are to use research, they must conduct a critical appraisal of research reports published in the literature. A research critique enables the nurse, as a research consumer, to evaluate the scientific merit of the study and decide how the results may be useful in practice. A critique involves intensive scrutiny of a study, including its strengths and weaknesses, statistical and clinical significance, and the generalizability of the results.

Polit and Beck (2005) propose that the following elements be considered in a critique of quantitative research: substantive and theoretical dimensions, methodologic dimensions, ethical dimensions, interpretive dimensions, and presentation and stylistic dimensions.

- *Substantive and theoretical dimensions.* For these dimensions, the nurse needs to evaluate the significance of the research problem, the appropriateness of the concep-

tualizations and the theoretical framework of the study, and the congruence between the research question and the methods used to address it.

- *Methodologic dimensions.* The methodologic dimensions pertain to the appropriateness of the research design, the size and representativeness of the study sample as well as the sampling design, validity and reliability of the instruments, adequacy of the research procedures, and the appropriateness of data analytic techniques used in the study.
- *Ethical dimensions.* The nurse must determine whether the rights of human subjects were protected during the course of the study and whether any ethical problems compromised the scientific merit of the study or the well-being of the subjects.
- *Interpretive dimensions.* For these dimensions, the nurse needs to ascertain the accuracy of the discussion, conclusions, and implications of the study results. The findings must be related back to the original hypotheses and the conceptual framework of the study. The implications and limitations of the study should be reviewed, together with the potential for replication or generalizability of the findings to similar populations.
- *Presentation and stylistic dimensions.* The manner in which the research plan and results are communicated refers to the presentation and stylistic dimensions. The research report must be detailed, logically organized, concise, and well written.

Reports of qualitative research are critiqued for their relevance to other persons or situations with the same characteristics as those studied and for usefulness in extending theory and nursing knowledge. A well-done qualitative study will have results that "ring true" to the reader.

CRITICAL THINKING CHECKPOINT

A friend, knowing that you are a nursing student, tells you that he or she is considering nursing school and wants your advice.

1. What questions would you ask before responding?
2. What went into your decision making to choose your nursing educational program?

3. How would the research process described in this chapter be potentially useful for someone considering entering nursing?

See Critical Thinking Possibilities in Appendix A. ∞

CHAPTER 2 **REVIEW**

CHAPTER HIGHLIGHTS

- Nursing education curricula are continually undergoing revisions in response to new scientific knowledge and technological, cultural, political, and socioeconomic changes in society.
- Nursing education has changed dramatically since the mid-1800s. Early apprenticeship programs established in the 1800s were designed to meet the service needs of the hospital, not the educational needs of the students. Today, nursing education is provided primarily in college and university settings independent of

hospitals' needs—a concept proposed by Florence Nightingale.
- Growth of ADN programs in community colleges began in the 1950s after Mildred Montag's proposal supported a 2-year education program for RNs.

- Some professional organizations have recommended that minimum entry into practice be at the baccalaureate or master's degree level.
- Continuing education is the responsibility of each practicing nurse to keep abreast of scientific and technological change and changes within the nursing profession.
- Nursing research began in North America in the early 1900s. Since that time, the concept of research has been introduced into nursing education programs, research journals in nursing have

been developed, and the National Institute for Nursing Research has been established.
- All nurses practicing in settings where research is conducted have a role in safeguarding their clients' rights.
- Both quantitative and qualitative research involve identifying a research problem/question, collecting data, and analyzing the data. Quantitative studies are reported using descriptive and analytic statistics, and qualitative studies are reported in narrative format.

TEST YOUR KNOWLEDGE

1. Which of the following is an example of continuing education for nurses?
    1. Attending the hospital's orientation program
    2. Talking with a company representative about a new piece of equipment
    3. Completing a workshop on ethical aspects of nursing
    4. Obtaining information about the facility's new computer charting system

2. Which of the following is a nursing responsibility when critiquing published nursing research?
    1. Assume that the research was properly conducted since it has been published.
    2. Evaluate whether the findings are applicable to the nurse's specific clients.
    3. Implement the research findings if at least two studies have shown the same results.
    4. Request the raw data from the researchers so that the nurse can analyze the statistics again.

3. Quantitative research is most appropriate for which of the following studies?
    1. A study measuring the effects of sleep deprivation on wound healing
    2. A study examining the bereavement process in spouses of clients with terminal cancer

3. A study exploring factors influencing weight control behavior
4. A study examining a client's feelings before and after a bone marrow aspiration

4. The use of a qualitative research process is most appropriate for which of the following studies?
    1. A study measuring nutrition and weight loss or gain in clients with cancer
    2. A study examining oxygen levels after endotracheal suctioning
    3. A study examining client reactions to stress after open heart surgery
    4. A study measuring differences in blood pressure before, during, and after a procedure

5. An 85-year-old client in a nursing home tells a nurse, "Because the doctor was so insistent, I signed the papers for that research study. Also, I was afraid he would not continue taking care of me." Which client right is being violated?
    1. Right not to be harmed
    2. Right to full disclosure
    3. Right of privacy and confidentiality
    4. Right of self-determination

See Answers to Test Your Knowledge in Appendix A.

EXPLORE MEDIALINK www.prenhall.com/berman

DVD-ROM
- Audio Glossary
- NCLEX Review
- Video: LPN/LUN

- Application Activity: Entry into Practice
- Links to Resources

COMPANION WEBSITE
- Additional NCLEX Review
- Case Study: Nursing Profession

READINGS AND REFERENCES

SUGGESTED READINGS
Goodwin, J. A. (2004). Patient advocacy: Witnessing informed consent for research in acute care. *MedSurg Nursing, 31,* 227–231. *This article describes the two different perspectives on the nurse's role in the signing of consents to participate in research: (a) confirming that the proper person is signing the consent and (b) confirming that the nurse observed the process of informed consent.*
Sigma Theta Tau International Evidence-Based Practice Task Force. (2004). Evidence-based

nursing: Rationale and resources. *Worldviews on Evidence-Based Nursing, 1,* 69–75. *This task force of the international nursing honor society offers definitions of EBP, evidence-based nursing, and the various sources of information used in EBP. The society favors EBP, and this article presents detailed responses to what it considers the three greatest misconceptions about EBP: that it ignores client preferences, overemphasizes clinical trials research, and is not theory based. A variety of international sources of EBP data are described.*

BMJ Publishing Group, *Clinical Evidence* and *Clinical Evidence Concise.*
This publication summarizes the current state of knowledge and uncertainty about the prevention and treatment of clinical conditions, based on thorough searches and appraisal of the literature. It describes the best available evidence, and if there is no good evidence it says so. The full version and a smaller summary handbook are published in print twice each year and include both CD-ROM and online access. Free copies are available to developing countries and through the United Health Foundation in the United States.

REFERENCES

Aiken, L. H., Clarke, S. P., Cheung, R. B., Sloane, D. M., & Silber, S. H. (2003). Educational levels of hospital nurses and surgical patient mortality. *Journal of the American Medical Association, 290*, 1617–1623.

American Association of Colleges of Nursing. (2002). *Fact sheet: Articulation agreements among nursing education programs.* Retrieved March 13, 2006, from http://www.aacn.nche.edu/Media/FactSheets/AA.htm

American Association of Colleges of Nursing. (2004). *AACN position statement on the practice doctorate in nursing.* Retrieved March 13, 2006, from http://www.aacn.nche.edu/DNP/pdf/DNP.pdf

American Association of Colleges of Nursing. (2005). *Fact sheet: The Clinical Nurse Leader.* Retrieved March 13, 2006, from http://www.aacn.nche.edu/Media/FactSheets/CNLFactSheet.htm

American Association of Colleges of Nursing. (2006). *AACN position statement on nursing research.* Retrieved March 13, 2006, from http://www.aacn.nche.edu/Publications/positions/rscposst.htm

American Nurses Association. (1965). ANA's first position on education for nursing. *American Journal of Nursing, 65*(12), 106–111.

American Nurses Association. (2004). *Nursing: Scope and standards of practice.* Washington, DC: Author.

Baumann, S. L. (2004). Similarities and differences in experiences of hope. *Nursing Science Quarterly, 17*, 339–344.

Brady, M., Leuner, J. D., Bellack, J. P., Loquist, R. S., Cipriano, P. F., & O'Neil, E. H. (2001). A proposed framework for differentiating the 21 Pew competencies by level of nursing education. *Nursing and Health Care Perspectives, 22*(1), 30–35.

Brown, E. L. (1948). *Nursing for the future: A report prepared for the National Nursing Council.* New York: Russell Sage Foundation.

Committee on the Grading of Nursing Schools. (1934). *Nursing schools today and tomorrow.* New York: National League of Nursing Education.

Goldmark, J. (1923). *Nursing and nursing education in the United States.* New York: Macmillan.

Hicks, L. L., Rantz, M. J., Petroski, G. F., & Mukamel, D. B. (2004). Nursing home costs and quality of care outcomes. *Nursing Economics, 22*, 178–192.

Montag, M. L. (1951). *The education of nursing technicians.* New York: Putnam.

National Institute of Nursing Research. (2000). *About NINR. Mission of the National Institute of Nursing Research. Scientific goals and objectives* (Objective 1.1). Retrieved March 13, 2006, from http://ninr.nih.gov/ninr/research/diversity/mission.html

National League for Nursing Accrediting Commission. (2005). *Directory of accredited nursing programs.* New York: Author.

National Organization for Associate Degree Nursing. (2005). *Associate degree nursing (ADN) facts.* Retrieved March 13, 2006, from http://www.noadn.org/pdfs/Associate Degree Nursing.pdf

O'Neil, E. H., & the Pew Health Professions Commission. (1998). *Recreating health professional practice for a new century.* San Francisco: Pew Health Professions Commission.

Parse, R. R. (2004). Person-centered care. *Nursing Science Quarterly, 17*, 193.

Polit, D. F., & Beck, C. T. (2005). *Essentials of nursing research: Methods, appraisal, and utilization* (6th ed.). Philadelphia: Lippincott, Williams & Wilkins.

Sand-Jecklin, K. E., & Schaffer, A. J. (2006). Nursing students' perceptions of their chosen profession. *Nursing Education Perspectives, 27*, 130–136.

Sutters, K. A., Miaskowski, C., Holdridge-Zeuner, D., Waite, S., Paul, S. M., Savedra, M. C., et al. (2005). Time-contingent dosing of an opioid analgesic after tonsillectomy does not increase moderate-to-severe side effects in children. *Pain Management Nursing, 6*, 49–57.

Vetter, M. J., Bristow, L., & Ahrens, J. (2004). A model for home care clinician and home health aide collaboration: Diabetes care by nurse case managers and community health workers. *Home Healthcare Nurse, 22*, 645–648.

Woodham-Smith, C. (1950). *Florence Nightingale.* London: Constable & Co.

SELECTED BIBLIOGRAPHY

American Association of Colleges of Nursing. (1998). *The essentials of baccalaureate education for professional nursing practice.* Washington, DC: Author.

American Nurses Association, Cabinet on Nursing Research. (1985). *Directions for nursing research: Toward the twenty-first century.* Kansas City, MO: Author.

ANA delegates vote to limit RN title to BSN grads: "Associate nurse" wins vote for technical level. (1985). *American Journal of Nursing, 85*(9), 1016, 1017, 1020, 1022, 1024, 1025.

Donahue, M. P. (1996). *Nursing: The finest art.* St. Louis, MO: Mosby.

Fondiller, S. H. (2001). From the archives: Nursing's pioneers in the associate degree movement. *Nursing and Health Care Perspectives, 22*(4), 172–174.

Granger, B. B. (2003). How to make nursing research work for you. *Nursing, 33*(11), 47–49.

Malloch, K., & Porter-O'Grady, T. (2005). *Introduction to evidence-based practice in nursing and health care.* Sudbury, MA: Jones & Bartlett.

Melnyk, B. M., & Fineout-Overholt, E. (2004). *Evidence-based practice in nursing and healthcare.* Philadelphia: Lippincott Williams & Wilkins.

Mills, N. M., Haun, L. L., & Daldrup, D. (2000). Kansas City colleagues in caring: Giving new meaning to networking. *Journal of Nursing Education, 39*(2), 54–56.

National Commission on Nursing Implementation Project (NCNIP). (1987). *Timeline for transition into the future: Nursing education system for two categories of nurse.* Milwaukee, WI: Author.

National League for Nursing. (2000). *Educational competencies for graduates of associate degree nursing programs.* Sudbury, MA: Jones & Bartlett.

Overbay, J. D., & Aaltonen, P. M. (2001). A comparison of NLNAC and CCNE accreditation. *Nurse Educator, 26*(1), 17–22.

Wooten, J. M., & Ross, V. M. (2005). How to make sense of clinical research. *RN, 68*(1), 22–27.

Nursing Theories and Conceptual Frameworks

LEARNING OUTCOMES

After completing this chapter, you will be able to:

1. Differentiate the terms *concept, conceptual framework, theory, paradigm*, and *metaparadigm for nursing.*

2. Identify the purposes of nursing theory in nursing education, research, and clinical practice.

3. Identify the components of the metaparadigm for nursing.

4. Describe the major purpose of theory in the sciences and practice disciplines.

5. Identify one positive and one negative effect of using theory to understand clinical practice.

As a profession, nursing is involved in identifying its own unique body of knowledge essential to nursing practice—nursing science. To identify this knowledge base, nurses must develop and recognize concepts and theories that are specific to nursing. Because theories in some other disciplines were developed and used much before most nursing theories, it is helpful to briefly explore how theory has been used by those disciplines before considering theory in nursing.

INTRODUCTION TO THEORIES

Theory has been defined as a supposition or system of ideas that is proposed to explain a given phenomenon. For now, think of theory as a major, very well-articulated idea about something important. Theories are also used to describe, predict, and control phenomena.

Four influential theories from the 20th century were Marx's theory of alienation, Freud's theory of the unconscious, Darwin's theory of evolution, and Einstein's theory of relativity. Most undergraduate students are introduced to the major theories in their disciplines. Psychology majors study Freud and Jung's theories of the unconscious, Sullivan and Piaget's theories of development, and Skinner's theory of behaviorism. Psychology majors are also introduced to critiques of those theories. Sociology majors study Marx's theory of alienation and Weber's theories of modern work, as well as the critiques of their theories. Biology majors are introduced to Darwin's theory of evolution, but also to Stephen Jay Gould's critique and modification of evolutionary theory. Physics majors are introduced to a historical progression of theorists including Copernicus, Newton, Einstein, and newer theorists in quantum mechanics.

The extent to which theories build on or modify previous theories varies with the discipline, as does the importance of theory in the discipline. Undergraduate music and art majors often take some courses in theory, but these students generally focus on creating art or performing music. This is also true of students in nursing, teaching, and management. Management students study management theories, but the relationship between the theory of management and the practice of management is not nearly as strong as the relationship between the theory of physics and the practice of physics. This is because the practice of physics *is* theory and research, whereas the practice of management, teaching, nursing, art, music, law, clinical psychology, and pastoral care is something else entirely. The term **practice discipline** is used for fields of study in which the central focus is performance of a professional role (nursing, teaching, management, music). Practice disciplines are differentiated from the disciplines that have research and theory development as their central focus, for example, the natural sciences. In the practice disciplines, the main function of theory (and research) is to provide new possibilities for understanding the discipline's practice (music, art, management, nursing).

Context for Theory Development in American Universities

In the 19th century, Florence Nightingale thought that the people of Great Britain needed to know more about how to maintain healthy homes and to care for sick family members. Nightingale's *Notes on Nursing: What It Is, and What It Is Not* (1860/1969) was our first textbook on home care and community health. However, the audience for that text was the public at large, not a separate discipline or profession. To Nightingale, the knowledge to provide good nursing was neither unique nor specialized. Rather, Nightingale viewed nursing as a central human activity grounded in observation, reason, and commonsense health practices. Nightingale's theory is further described on page 43.

In the 20th century, nursing education in the United States took a different path from nursing education in Great Britain and Europe. The drive to establish nursing departments in colleges and universities exposed American nursing to the dominant ideas and pressures in American higher education at the time. During the latter half of the 20th century, disciplines seeking to establish themselves in universities had to demonstrate something that Nightingale had not envisioned for nursing—a unique body of theoretical knowledge.

The natural and technological sciences were often seen as role models in this regard. Theories in the natural sciences provided a foundation and direction for research. Research in these disciplines often produced tangible results: knowledge that could be used in our efforts to control nature, disease, and foreign threats. Scientifically produced knowledge resulted in a stronger national security and economy.

The term *practice discipline* was not in common use until the very end of the 20th century. Disciplines without a strong theory and research base were referred to as "soft," a negative comparison with the "hard" natural sciences. Many of the soft disciplines attempted to emulate the sciences, so theory and scientific research became a more important part of academic life, both in the practice disciplines and in the humanities.

In practice disciplines, theories work like lenses through which we are invited to interpret things like market forces, industrial efficiency, the human mind, pain, and suffering. Their usefulness comes from helping us interpret phenomena from unique perspectives, building new understandings, relationships, and possibilities.

Defining Terms

Concepts are often called the building blocks of theories. Concepts are hard to define because the definition has to include everything from the speed of light to the unconscious. Concepts are easier to understand by example. Einstein's theory of relativity consists of a beautiful mathematical relationship between three concepts in physics: mass, energy, and the speed of light. However, theories are not always built like houses out of block-like concepts. Freud's theory of the unconscious not only required some new concepts, it required a completely new model. Freud needed a model for the mind that could bring a host of human experiences together under one mental roof: dreams, wishes, decisions, behaviors, feelings, anxieties, and sexuality. Freud's theory of the mind included three new concepts: the ego, the id, and the superego. It would not be right to say that Freud's theory of the unconscious evolved out of these concepts. Rather, these new concepts helped him create a model in which his larger idea, the unconscious, might be understood.

A **conceptual framework** is a group of related ideas, statements, or concepts. Freud's structure of the mind (id, ego, superego) could be considered a conceptual framework or model. The term *conceptual model* is often used interchangeably with conceptual framework, and sometimes with **grand theories,** those that articulate a broad range of the significant relationships among the concepts of a discipline (Fitzpatrick & Whall, 2005).

No scientific theory is purely objective, because each is developed in cultures and expressed in language. Theories offer ways of looking at or conceptualizing the central interests of a discipline. In the natural sciences, theories are often expressed in mathematical terms, but Darwin's *Origin of Species* theory is a short book. In the social and behavioral sciences, theories attempt to explain relationships between concepts. The conceptualization is often complex. Other authors build on, explain, and critique the original work.

Broadly speaking, a **paradigm** refers to a pattern of shared understandings and assumptions about reality and the world. Paradigms include our notions of reality that are largely unconscious or taken for granted. However, the term *paradigm* is used in a variety of ways by different authors, and its everyday usage varies considerably.

We become aware of paradigms when realities clash. The paradigm of 16th-century Europe, informed largely by established religious doctrines and practices, clashed with the emerging discoveries in astronomy. The Industrial Revolution clashed with the long-standing feudal order, disrupting social and class relationships. In the 20th century, the ideals of socialism clashed with ideals of capitalism, and religious fundamentalism clashed with evolution. The next paradigm clash is likely to be between commonsense notions of space and time and the emerging field of quantum mechanics.

THE METAPARADIGM FOR NURSING

In the late 20th century, much of the theoretical work in nursing focused on articulating relationships among four major concepts: person, environment, health, and nursing. Because these four concepts can be superimposed on almost any work in nursing, they are sometimes collectively referred to as a **metaparadigm** for nursing. The term originates from two Greek words: *meta,* meaning "with," and *paradigm,* meaning "pattern."

Many consider the following four concepts to be central to nursing.

1. Person or **client,** the recipient of nursing care (includes individuals, families, groups, and communities).
2. **Environment,** the internal and external surroundings that affect the client. This includes people in the physical environment, such as families, friends, and significant others.
3. **Health,** the degree of wellness or well-being that the client experiences.
4. **Nursing,** the attributes, characteristics, and actions of the nurse providing care on behalf of, or in conjunction with, the client.

The work of American nurse theorists reflects a wide range of ideas about people, health, values, and the world. Each nurse theorist's definitions of these four major concepts vary in accordance with scientific and philosophical orientation, experience in nursing, and the effects of that experience on the theorist's view of nursing.

Nursing theories fall into one of two paradigms. One view reflects prevailing understandings in medicine and the health care system. The other view reflects emerging understandings in transpersonal psychology. Hood and Leddy (2003) refer to the dominant view as the "stability model" containing theories that use systems or stress/adaptation as frameworks, and the emerging view as the "growth model" with theories using caring or complexity as frameworks. Hood and Leddy place the theories of Imogene King, Betty Neuman, and Callista Roy in the stability model and the theories of Dorothea Orem, Jean Watson, Hildegard Peplau, Martha Rogers, and Rosemarie Parse in the emerging growth model.

Nursing theorists have built on the metaparadigm and on the work of Nightingale, whether or not they were conscious of doing so. In addition, other theories foundational to many nursing theories include interactive, systems, and developmental theory (see Figure 3-1 ■).

PURPOSES OF NURSING THEORY

Direct links exist among theory, education, research, and clinical practice. In many cases, nursing theory guides knowledge development and directs education, research, and practice although each influences the others (Fitzpatrick & Whall, 2005). The interface between nursing experts in each area helps to ensure that work in the other areas remains relevant, current, useful, and ultimately influences health.

In Education

Because nursing theory was used primarily to establish the profession's place in the university, it is not surprising that nursing theory became more firmly established in academia than in clinical practice. In the 1970s and 1980s, many nursing programs identified the major concepts in one or two nursing models, organized

MediaLink

The Growth of Nursing Theory Application

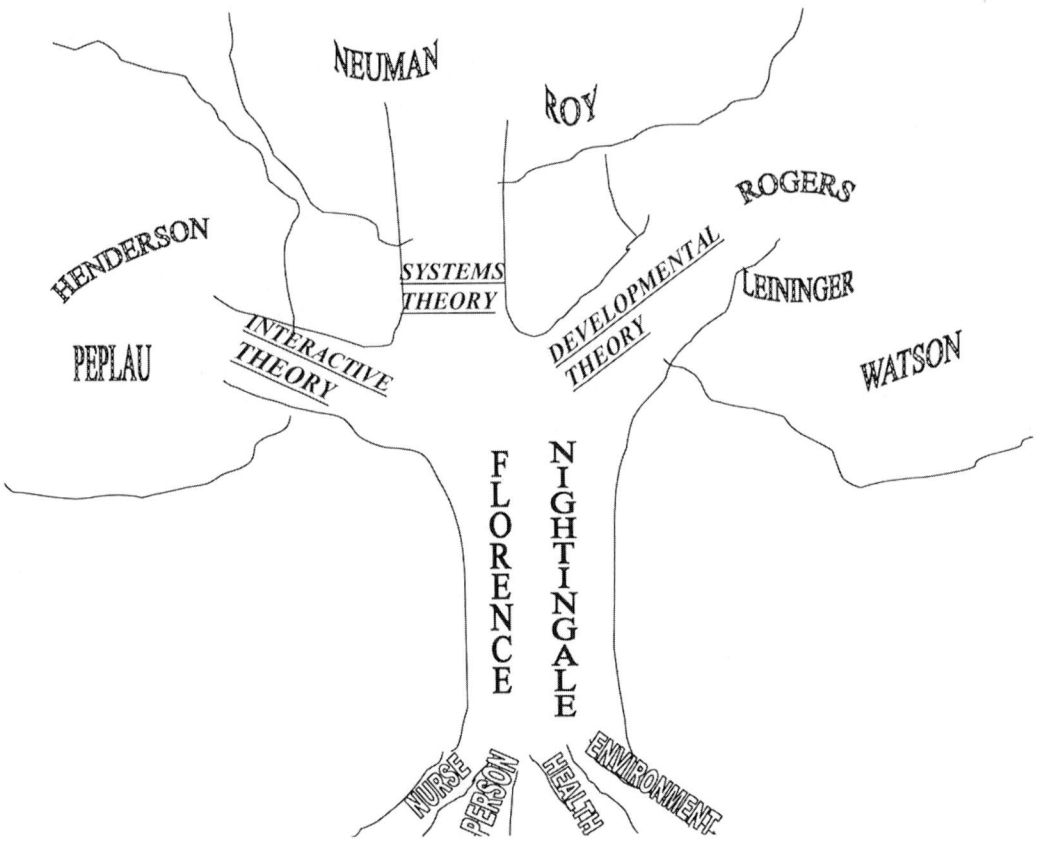

Figure 3-1 ■ The living tree of nursing theories.

(*Note:* From "The Living Tree of Nursing Theories" by C. Tourville & K. Ingalls, 2003, *Nursing Forum, 38,*(3) p. 23. Copyright © 2003 Blackwell Publishers. Reprinted with permission.)

these concepts into a conceptual framework, and built the entire curriculum around that framework. The unique language in these models was typically introduced into program objectives, course objectives, course descriptions, and clinical performance criteria. The purpose was to elucidate the central meanings of the profession and to improve the status of the profession. Although all nursing programs are organized around concepts, many nursing programs have abandoned theory-driven conceptual frameworks.

In Research

Nurse scholars have repeatedly insisted that nursing research identifies the philosophical assumptions or conceptual frameworks from which it proceeds. That is because all thinking, writing, and speaking is based on previous assumptions about people and the world. New theoretical perspectives provide an essential service by identifying gaps in the way we approach specific fields of study such as symptom management or quality of life. Different conceptual perspectives can also help generate new ideas, research questions, and interpretations.

Because of their breadth, grand theories only occasionally direct nursing research. Nursing research is more often informed by **midlevel theories** that focus on the exploration of concepts such as pain, self-esteem, learning, and hardiness. Qualitative research in nursing and the social sciences can also be grounded in theories from philosophy or the social sciences. For example, the term **critical theory** is used in academia to de-

scribe theories that help elucidate how social structures affect a wide variety of human experiences from art to social practices. In nursing, critical theory research helps explain how these structures such as race, gender, sexual orientation, and economic class affect patient experiences and health outcomes.

In Clinical Practice

Where nursing theory has been employed in a clinical setting, its primary contribution has been the facilitation of reflecting, questioning, and thinking about what nurses do. For example, a recent publication described application of Leininger's transcultural nursing theory for developing culturally congruent strategies useful to professionals working with suspected child maltreatment cases (Campbell, 2005). Because nurses and nursing practice are often subordinate to powerful institutional forces and traditions, the introduction of any framework that encourages nurses to reflect on, question, and think about what they do provides an invaluable service.

As described in Chapter 2, evidence-based practice involves the recognition of which knowledge is appropriate for application to client care. Practice theories, those that describe the relationships among variables as applied to specific clinical situations (e.g., theory of postpartum depression), are important contributors to effective evidence-based practice.

An increasing body of theoretical scholarship in nursing practice has been outside the framework of the formal theories presented in the next section. Philosophy is used to explore both clinical and theoretical issues in the journal *Nursing Philosophy*. Family theorists and critical theorists have encouraged the profession to move the focus from individuals to families and social structures. Debates about the role of theory in nursing practice provide evidence that nursing is maturing, both as an academic discipline and as a clinical profession.

OVERVIEW OF SELECTED NURSING THEORIES

The nursing theories discussed in this chapter vary considerably (a) in their level of abstraction; (b) in their conceptualization of the client, health/illness, environment, and nursing; and (c) in their ability to describe, explain, or predict phenomena. Some theories are broad in scope; others are limited. The works presented in this chapter are primarily classified as philosophies, nursing models, or nursing theories using the categorizations of Tomey and Alligood (2006). A **philosophy** is a belief system, often an early effort to define nursing phenomena, and serves as the basis for later theoretical formulations. Examples of philosophies are those of Nightingale, Henderson, and Watson. Nursing models include those of Neuman, Orem, Rogers, Roy, and King, whereas nursing theories are those of Peplau, Leininger, and Parse. Only brief summaries of the author's central theme and basic assumptions are included here (and presented in chronological order).

Nightingale's Environmental Theory

Florence Nightingale, often considered the first nurse theorist, defined nursing almost 150 years ago as "the act of utilizing the environment of the patient to assist him in his recovery" (Nightingale, 1860/1969). She linked health with five environmental factors: (1) pure or fresh air, (2) pure water, (3) efficient drainage, (4) cleanliness, and (5) light, especially direct sunlight. Deficiencies in these five factors produced lack of health or illness.

These environmental factors attain significance when one considers that sanitation conditions in the hospitals of the mid-1800s were extremely poor and that women working in the hospitals were often unreliable, uneducated, and incompetent to care for the ill. In addition to those factors, Nightingale also stressed the importance of keeping the client warm, maintaining a noise-free environment, and attending to the client's diet in terms of assessing intake, timeliness of the food, and its effect on the person.

Nightingale set the stage for further work in the development of nursing theories. Her general concepts about ventilation, cleanliness, quiet, warmth, and diet remain integral parts of nursing and health care today.

Peplau's Interpersonal Relations Model

Hildegard Peplau, a psychiatric nurse, introduced her interpersonal concepts in 1952. Central to Peplau's theory is the use of a therapeutic relationship between the nurse and the client.

Nurses enter into a personal relationship with an individual when a need is present. The nurse–client relationship evolves in four phases:

1. *Orientation.* During this phase, the client seeks help, and the nurse assists the client to understand the problem and the extent of the need for help.
2. *Identification.* During this phase, the client assumes a posture of dependence, interdependence, or independence in relation to the nurse (relatedness). The nurse's focus is to assure the person that the nurse understands the interpersonal meaning of the client's situation.
3. *Exploitation.* In this phase, the client derives full value from what the nurse offers through the relationship. The client uses available services based on self-interest and needs. Power shifts from the nurse to the client.
4. *Resolution.* In this final phase, old needs and goals are put aside and new ones adopted. Once older needs are resolved, newer and more mature ones emerge.

To help clients fulfill their needs, nurses assume many roles: stranger, teacher, resource person, surrogate, leader, and counselor. Peplau's model continues to be used by clinicians when working with individuals who have psychologic problems.

Henderson's Definition of Nursing

In 1966, Virginia Henderson's definition of the unique function of nursing was a major stepping stone in the emergence of nursing as a discipline separate from medicine. Like Nightingale, Henderson describes nursing in relation to the client and the client's environment. Unlike Nightingale, Henderson sees the nurse as concerned with both healthy and ill individuals, acknowledges that nurses interact with clients even when recovery may not be feasible, and mentions the teaching and advocacy roles of the nurse.

Henderson (1966) conceptualizes the nurse's role as assisting sick or healthy individuals to gain independence in meeting 14 fundamental needs:

1. Breathing normally
2. Eating and drinking adequately
3. Eliminating body wastes
4. Moving and maintaining a desirable position
5. Sleeping and resting
6. Selecting suitable clothes
7. Maintaining body temperature within normal range by adjusting clothing and modifying the environment
8. Keeping the body clean and well groomed to protect the integument
9. Avoiding dangers in the environment and avoiding injuring others
10. Communicating with others in expressing emotions, needs, fears, or opinions
11. Worshipping according to one's faith
12. Working in such a way that one feels a sense of accomplishment

13. Playing or participating in various forms of recreation
14. Learning, discovering, or satisfying the curiosity that leads to normal development and health, and using available health facilities

Henderson has published many works and continues to be cited in current nursing literature. Her emphasis on the importance of nursing's independence from, and interdependence with, other health care disciplines is well recognized.

Rogers's Science of Unitary Human Beings

Martha Rogers first presented her theory of unitary human beings in 1970. It contains complex conceptualizations related to multiple scientific disciplines (e.g., Einstein's theory of relativity, Burr and Northrop's electrodynamic theory of life, von Bertalanffy's general systems theory, and many other disciplines, such as anthropology, psychology, sociology, astronomy, religion, philosophy, history, biology, and literature).

Rogers views the person as an irreducible whole, the whole being greater than the sum of its parts. *Whole* is differentiated from *holistic,* the latter often used to mean only the sum of all parts. She states that humans are dynamic energy fields in continuous exchange with environmental fields, both of which are infinite. The "human field image" perspective surpasses that of the physical body. Both human and environmental fields are characterized by pattern, a universe of open systems, and four dimensionality. According to Rogers, unitary man

- Is an irreducible, four-dimensional energy field identified by pattern.
- Manifests characteristics different from the sum of the parts.
- Interacts continuously and creatively with the environment.

- Behaves as a totality.
- As a sentient being, participates creatively in change.

Nurses applying Rogers's theory in practice (a) focus on the person's wholeness, (b) seek to promote symphonic interaction between the two energy fields (human and environment) to strengthen the coherence and integrity of the person, (c) coordinate the human field with the rhythmicities of the environmental field, and (d) direct and redirect patterns of interaction between the two energy fields to promote maximum health potential.

Nurses' use of noncontact therapeutic touch is based on the concept of human energy fields. The qualities of the field vary from person to person and are affected by pain and illness. Although the field is infinite, realistically it is most clearly "felt" within several feet of the body. Nurses trained in noncontact therapeutic touch claim they can assess and feel the energy field and manipulate it to enhance the healing process of people who are ill or injured.

Orem's General Theory of Nursing

Dorothea Orem's theory, first published in 1971, includes three related concepts: self-care, self-care deficit, and nursing systems. Self-care theory is based on four concepts: self-care, self-care agency, self-care requisites, and therapeutic self-care demand. Self-care refers to those activities an individual performs independently throughout life to promote and maintain personal well-being. Self-care agency is the individual's ability to perform self-care activities. It consists of two agents: a self-care agent (an individual who performs self-care independently) and a dependent care agent (a person other than the individual who provides the care). Most adults care for themselves, whereas infants and people weakened by illness or disability require assistance with self-care activities.

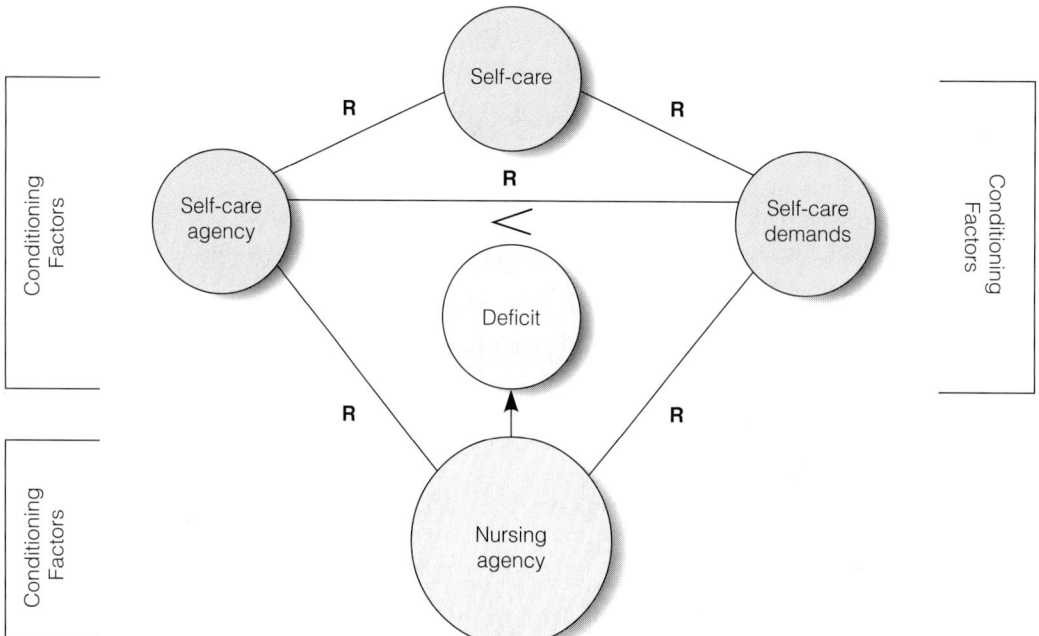

Figure 3-2 ■ The major components of Orem's self-care deficit theory. R indicates a relationship between components; < indicates a current or potential deficit where nursing would be required.

Self-care requisites, also called self-care needs, are measures or actions taken to provide self-care. There are three categories of self-care requisites:

1. Universal requisites are common to all people. They include maintaining intake and elimination of air, water, and food; balancing rest, solitude, and social interaction; preventing hazards to life and well-being; and promoting normal human functioning.
2. Developmental requisites result from maturation or are associated with conditions or events, such as adjusting to a change in body image or to the loss of a spouse.
3. Health deviation requisites result from illness, injury, or disease or its treatment. They include actions such as seeking health care assistance, carrying out prescribed therapies, and learning to live with the effects of illness or treatment.

Therapeutic self-care demand refers to all self-care activities required to meet existing self-care requisites, or in other words, actions to maintain health and well-being (see Figure 3-2 ■).

Self-care deficit results when self-care agency is not adequate to meet the known self-care demand. Orem's self-care deficit theory explains not only when nursing is needed but also how people can be assisted through five methods of helping: acting or doing for, guiding, teaching, supporting, and providing an environment that promotes the individual's abilities to meet current and future demands.

Orem identifies three types of nursing systems:

1. Wholly compensatory systems are required for individuals who are unable to control and monitor their environment and process information.
2. Partly compensatory systems are designed for individuals who are unable to perform some, but not all, self-care activities.
3. Supportive-educative (developmental) systems are designed for persons who need to learn to perform self-care measures and need assistance to do so.

The five methods of helping discussed for self-care deficit can be used in each nursing system.

Figure 3-3 ■ King's conceptual framework for nursing: dynamic interacting systems.

(*Note:* From *A Theory for Nursing: Systems, Concepts, Process* (p. 11), by I. M. King, 1981, Albany, NY: Delmar. Copyright Imogene M. King. Used with permission.)

King's Goal Attainment Theory

Imogene King's theory of goal attainment (1981) was derived from her conceptual framework (Figure 3-3 ■). King's framework shows the relationship of operational systems (individuals), interpersonal systems (groups such as nurse–patient), and social systems (such as educational system, health care system). She selected 15 concepts from the nursing literature (self, role, perception, communication, interaction, transaction, growth and development, stress, time, personal space, organization, status, power, authority, and decision making) as essential knowledge for use by nurses.

Ten of the concepts in the framework were selected (self, role, perception, communication, interaction, transaction, growth and development, stress, time, and personal space) as essential knowledge for use by nurses in concrete nursing situations. Within this theory, a transaction process model was designed (Figure 3-4 ■). This process describes the nature of and standard for nurse–patient interactions that lead to goal attainment—that nurses purposefully interact and mutually set, explore, and agree to means to achieve

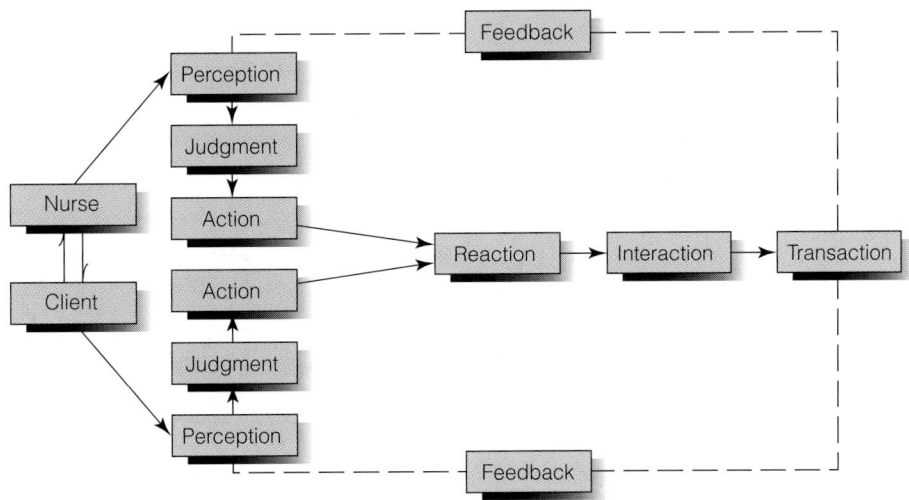

Figure 3-4 ■ King's model of transactions.

(*Note:* From *A Theory for Nursing: Systems, Concepts, Process* (p. 11), by I. M. King, 1981, Albany, NY: Delmar. Copyright Imogene M. King. Reprinted with permission.)

goals. Goal attainment represents outcomes. When this information is recorded in the patient record, nurses have data that represent evidence-based nursing practice.

King's theory offers insight into nurses' interactions with individuals and groups within the environment. It highlights the importance of a client's participation in decisions that influence care and focuses on both the process of nurse–client interaction and the outcomes of care. King believes that her theory, used in evidence theory-based practice, blends the art and the science of nursing (2006).

Neuman's Systems Model

Betty Neuman (Neuman & Fawcett, 2002), a community health nurse and clinical psychologist, developed a model based on the individual's relationship to stress, the reaction to it, and reconstitution factors that are dynamic in nature. Reconstitution is the state of adaptation to stressors.

Neuman views the client as an open system consisting of a basic structure or central core of energy resources (physiologic, psychologic, sociocultural, developmental, and spiritual) surrounded by two concentric boundaries or rings referred to as lines of resistance (see Figure 3-5 ■). The lines of resistance represent internal factors that help the client defend against a stressor; one example is an increase in the body's leukocyte count to combat an infection. Outside the lines of resistance are two lines of defense. The inner or normal line of defense, depicted as a solid line, represents the person's state of equilibrium or the state of adaptation developed and maintained over time and considered normal for that person.

The flexible line of defense, depicted as a broken line, is dynamic and can be rapidly altered over a short period of time. It is a protective buffer that prevents stressors from penetrating the normal line of defense. Certain variables (e.g., sleep deprivation) can create rapid changes in the flexible line of defense.

Neuman categorizes stressors as intrapersonal stressors, those that occur within the individual (e.g., an infection); interpersonal stressors, those that occur between individuals (e.g., unrealistic role expectations); and extrapersonal stressors, those that occur outside the person (e.g., financial concerns). The individual's reaction to stressors depends on the strength of the lines of defense. When the lines of defense fail, the resulting reaction depends on the strength of the lines of resistance. As part of the reaction, a person's system can adapt to a stressor, an effect known as reconstitution. Nursing interventions focus on retaining or maintaining system stability. These interventions are carried out on three preventive levels: primary, secondary, and tertiary.

1. Primary prevention focuses on protecting the normal line of defense and strengthening the flexible line of defense.
2. Secondary prevention focuses on strengthening internal lines of resistance, reducing the reaction, and increasing resistance factors.
3. Tertiary prevention focuses on readaptation and stability and protects reconstitution or return to wellness following treatment.

Betty Neuman's model of nursing is applicable to a variety of nursing practice settings involving individuals, families,

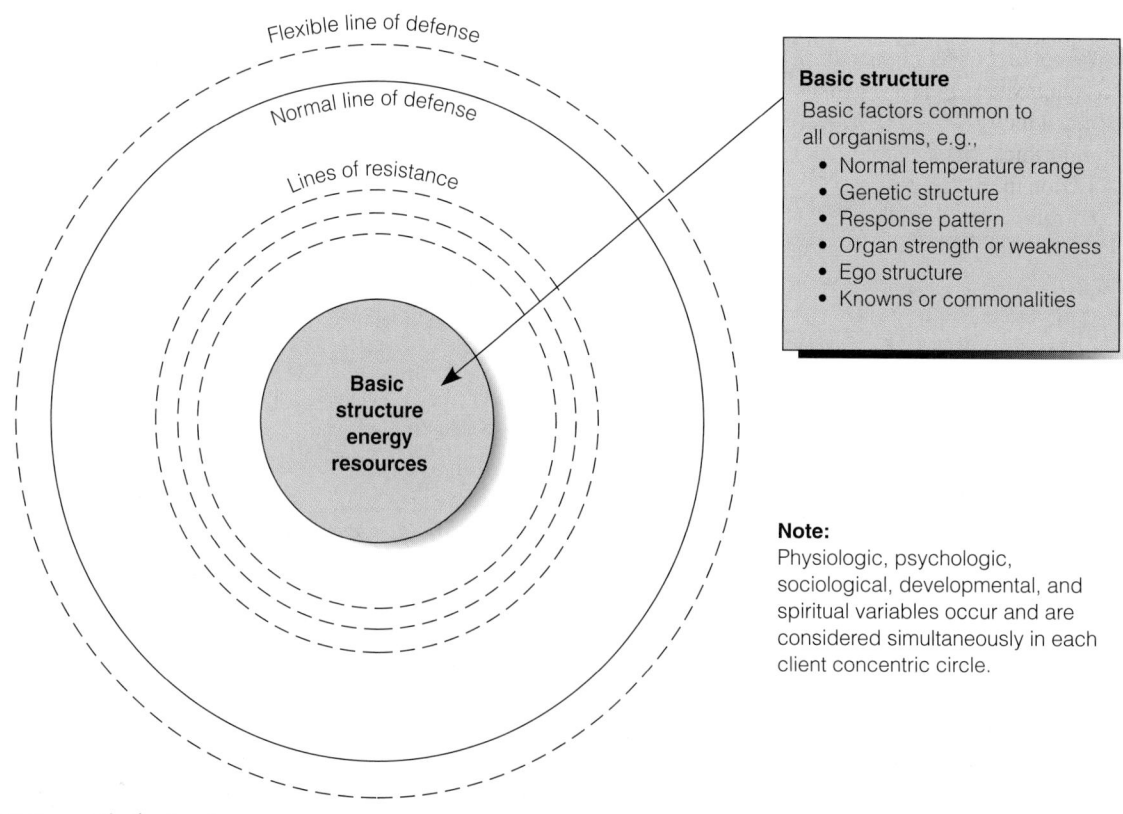

Figure 3-5 ■ Neuman's client system.

(*Note:* From *The Neuman Systems Model*, 4th ed. (p. 15), by B. Neuman and J. Fawcett, 2002, Upper Saddle River, NJ: Prentice Hall. Reprinted with permission.)

groups, and communities. The model is used in many countries and to direct nursing administration and research programs.

Roy's Adaptation Model

Sister Callista Roy (1997) defines adaptation as "the process and outcome whereby the thinking and feeling person uses conscious awareness and choice to create human and environmental integration" (p. 44). Roy's work focuses on the increasing complexity of person and environment self-organization, and on the relationship between and among persons, universe, and what can be considered a supreme being or God. Her philosophical assumptions have been refined using major characteristics of "creation spirituality"—a view that "persons and the earth are one, and that they are in God and of God" (p. 46).

Roy focuses on the individual as a biopsychosocial adaptive system that employs a feedback cycle of input (stimuli), throughput (control processes), and output (behaviors or adaptive responses). Both the individual and the environment are sources of stimuli that require modification to promote adaptation, an ongoing purposive response. Adaptive responses contribute to health, which she defines as the process of being and becoming integrated; ineffective or maladaptive responses do not contribute to health. Each person's adaptation level is unique and constantly changing.

The goal of Callista Roy's model is to enhance life processes through adaptation in four adaptive modes. Individuals respond to needs (stimuli) in one of the four modes:

1. The physiologic mode involves the body's basic physiologic needs and ways of adapting with regard to fluid and electrolytes, activity and rest, circulation and oxygen, nutrition and elimination, protection, the senses, and neurologic and endocrine function.
2. The self-concept mode includes two components: the physical self, which involves sensation and body image, and the personal self, which involves self-ideal, self-consistency, and the moral-ethical self.
3. The role function mode is determined by the need for social integrity and refers to the performance of duties based on given positions within society.
4. The interdependence mode involves one's relations with significant others and support systems that provide help, affection, and attention.

In evolving her work since the early 1980s, Roy has expanded the model for application with families and clients in relationships. She developed the assumption she named *veritivity*, which refers to purposefulness of humans in interactions with others and transcending materialism to support caring (see, for example, Dobratz, 2004).

Leininger's Cultural Care Diversity and Universality Theory

Madeleine Leininger, a nurse anthropologist, put her views on transcultural nursing in print in the 1970s and then in 1991 published her book *Culture Care Diversity and Universality: A Theory of Nursing.*

Leininger states that care is the essence of nursing and the dominant, distinctive, and unifying feature of nursing. She em-

phasizes that human caring, although a universal phenomenon, varies among cultures in its expressions, processes, and patterns; it is largely culturally derived. Leininger produced the Sunrise model to depict her theory of cultural care diversity and universality. This model emphasizes that health and care are influenced by elements of the social structure, such as technology, religious and philosophical factors, kinship and social systems, cultural values, political and legal factors, economic factors, and educational factors. These social factors are addressed within environmental contexts, language expressions, and ethnohistory. Each of these systems is part of the social structure of any society; health care expressions, patterns, and practices are also integral parts of these aspects of social structure (Leininger & McFarland, 2002). In order for nurses to assist people of diverse cultures, Leininger presents three intervention modes:

- Culture care preservation and maintenance
- Culture care accommodation, negotiation, or both
- Culture care restructuring and repatterning

Leininger states that her theory is the only one that "searches for comprehensive and holistic care data relying on social structure, worldview, and multiple factors in a culture in order to get a holistic knowledge base about care" (Leininger, 2006, p. 319).

Watson's Human Caring Theory

Jean Watson (2005) believes the practice of caring is central to nursing; it is the unifying focus for practice. Her major assumptions about caring are shown in Box 3–1. Nursing interventions related to human care originally referred to as *carative factors*

BOX 3–1 Watson's Assumptions of Caring

- Human caring in nursing is not just an emotion, concern, attitude, or benevolent desire. Caring connotes a personal response.
- Caring is an intersubjective human process and is the moral ideal of nursing.
- Caring can be effectively demonstrated only interpersonally.
- Effective caring promotes health and individual or family growth.
- Caring promotes health more than does curing.
- Caring responses accept a person not only as they are now, but also for what the person may become.
- A caring environment offers the development of potential while allowing the person to choose the best action for the self at a given point in time.
- Caring occasions involve action and choice by nurse and client. If the caring occasion is transpersonal, the limits of openness expand, as do human capacities.
- The most abstract characteristic of a caring person is that the person is somehow responsive to another person as a unique individual, perceives the other's feelings, and sets one person apart from another.
- Human caring involves values, a will and a commitment to care, knowledge, caring actions, and consequences.
- The ideal and value of caring is a starting point, a stance, and an attitude that has to become a will, an intention, a commitment, and a conscious judgment that manifests itself in concrete acts.

Note: From J. Watson, personal communication, September 22, 2002. Also see her website: http://www2.uchsc.edu/son/caring/content/default.asp

MediaLink Theories Case Study

have now been translated into clinical caritas processes (Watson, 2006):

1. Formation of humanistic-altruistic system of values, becomes: "practice of loving-kindness and equanimity within context of caring consciousness."
2. Instillation of faith-hope, becomes: "being authentically present, and enabling and sustaining the deep belief system and subjective life world of self and one-being-cared-for."
3. Cultivation of sensitivity to one's self and to others, becomes: "cultivation of one's own spiritual practices and transpersonal self, going beyond ego self."
4. Development of a helping-trusting, human caring relationship, becomes: "developing and sustaining a helping-trusting, authentic caring relationship."
5. Promotion and acceptance of the expression of positive and negative feelings, becomes: "being present to, and supportive of the expression of positive and negative feelings as a connection with deeper spirit of self and the one-being-cared-for."
6. Systematic use of a creative problem-solving caring process, becomes: "creative use of self and all ways of knowing as part of the caring process; to engage in artistry of caring-healing practices."
7. Promotion of transpersonal teaching-learning, becomes: "engaging in genuine teaching-learning experience that attends to unity of being and meaning attempting to stay within other's frame of reference."
8. Provision for a supportive, protective, and/or corrective mental, physical, societal, and spiritual environment, becomes: "creating healing environment at all levels (physical as well as non-physical), subtle environment of energy and consciousness, whereby wholeness, beauty, comfort, dignity, and peace are potentiated."
9. Assistance with gratification of human needs, becomes: "assisting with basic needs, with an intentional caring consciousness, administering 'human care essentials,' which potentiate alignment of mindbodyspirit, wholeness, and

unity of being in all aspects of care," tending to both embodied spirit and evolving spiritual emergence.
10. Allowance for existential-phenomenological-spiritual forces, becomes: "opening and attending to spiritual-mysterious, and existential dimensions of one's own life-death; soul care for self and the one-being-cared-for."

Watson's theory of human caring has received worldwide recognition and is a major force in redefining nursing as a caring-healing health model. Watson has also explored how her theory and that of Rogers can be integrated and synthesized to form a Unitary Caring Science (Watson & Smith, 2002).

Parse's Human Becoming Theory

Parse (1999) proposes three assumptions about *human becoming*:

1. Human becoming is freely choosing personal meaning in situations in the intersubjective process of relating value priorities.
2. Human becoming is cocreating rhythmic patterns or relating in mutual process with the universe.
3. Human becoming is cotranscending multidimensionally with the emerging possibles (p. 6).

These three assumptions focus on meaning, rhythmicity, and cotranscendence.

- Meaning arises from a person's interrelationship with the world and refers to happenings to which the person attaches varying degrees of significance.
- Rhythmicity is the movement toward greater diversity.
- Cotranscendence is the process of reaching out beyond the self.

Parse's model of human becoming emphasizes how individuals choose and bear responsibility for patterns of personal health. Parse contends that the client, not the nurse, is the authority figure and decision maker. The nurse's role involves helping individuals and families in choosing the possibilities for changing the health process. Specifically, the nurse's role consists of

---

RESEARCH NOTE **How Can the Use of a Nursing Model Affect Clients' Condition?**

In this study, nursing faculty in Turkey studied 52 clients with moderate hypertension to determine if care provided by researchers trained in the use of Watson's caring model and 10 carative factors had an influence on the clients' blood pressure. This was a simple pretest/posttest design and no control group was used. The researchers visited the clients weekly and provided support, client teaching, and blood pressure measurement. The clients did not take their condition seriously; they thought that it would just go away. The rationale for the emphasis on using the Watson model was the researchers' belief that if the care providers truly demonstrated their emotional caring and concerns for the clients, they might implement the recommended treatments. After 6 months, there were statistically significant decreases in blood pressure and increases in quality of life measured by mean scores of the total quality-of-life scale, medical interaction, physical symptom and activity, and general well-being.

IMPLICATIONS

This study used a small sample and is of limited generalizability to other clients. It is difficult to state whether similar findings might have resulted if the researchers had been trained in any other supportive model or even if merely visiting the clients so often would have the same outcome. These limitations were noted by the researchers. However, in order to advance nursing knowledge, theories and models must be applied and tested in clinical practice. It is not unexpected, also, that Watson's model has applicability to clients from non-American cultures although it cannot be assumed to apply to all cultures.

Note: From "The Effectiveness of Watson's Caring Model on the Quality of Life and Blood Pressure of Patients with Hypertension," by B. Erci, A. Sayan, G. Tortumluoglu, D. Kiliç, O. Sahin, & Z. Güngörmüs, 2003, *Journal of Advanced Nursing, 41,* pp. 130–139.

illuminating meaning (uncovering what was and what will be), synchronizing rhythms (leading through discussion to recognize harmony), and mobilizing transcendence (dreaming of possibilities and planning to reach them). The goal of nursing from the human becoming perspective is quality of life (Parse, 2006).

The Parse nurse uses "true presence" in the nurse–client process. "In true presence the nurse's whole being is immersed with the client as the other illuminates the meanings of his or her situation and moves beyond the moment" (Parse, 1994, p. 18).

CRITIQUE OF NURSING THEORY

Several nurse scholars have developed strong critiques of 20th-century nursing theories, choosing to ground their work in philosophy or the social sciences (Munhall, 2006). The best theories in philosophy and the social sciences are often used in the humanities for the insights and perspectives that can be brought to literature and art. So far, other disciplines have not discovered a sufficiently unique or interesting perspective on the human condition in nursing theories.

Nursing scholars continue to debate whether grounding our research in the best theories from other disciplines is good or bad. Some think this detracts from the development of nursing as a separate discipline; others argue that nursing research becomes more relevant when informed by scholarship that addresses larger social concerns.

Most things in the world have both positive and negative implications. Technology can be used for good or for evil. Theory can be used to broaden our perspectives in nursing and facilitate the altruistic and humanistic values of the profession. At the same time, rational and predictive theory can produce language and social practices that are superimposed onto the lives of vulnerable patients and do violence to the fragility of human dignity. As a lens, theory can either illuminate or obscure. As a tool, theory can either liberate or enslave.

CRITICAL THINKING CHECKPOINT

Tony is a 32-year-old man with HIV. His first AIDS-defining illness caused his weight to drop from 175 to 116 pounds due to intractable diarrhea. The physician thought caloric intake was of primary importance and urged Tony to eat whatever he wanted. The physician also prescribed tincture of opium for the diarrhea, but Tony hated the tincture of opium because it made him feel out of control. Because Tony was getting worse, his nurse argued that he needed intravenous nutrition and should eat only bananas, rice, applesauce, and weak tea until the diarrhea stopped. The nurse suggested adding other foods one at a time and only as tolerated. Tony's family and friends offered to take control of Tony's food preparation.

The physician compared AIDS to advanced cancer and argued he would not prescribe intravenous nutrition for advanced cancer. The nurse argued that this was Tony's first AIDS infection and that his prognosis was better than someone with advanced cancer. The nurse's primary focus was on stopping the diarrhea, and supplementing nutrition with IVs. Tony's friends preferred the nurse's approach, but Tony was not as easily convinced.

1. What concepts are present in this case?
2. What appear to be the perspectives or views represented by the physician and the nurse (how might you say they are defining the metaparadigm)?
3. How might Florence Nightingale analyze this situation?
4. Which of the nursing models in this chapter best supports the nurse's plan of care?

See Critical Thinking Possibilities in Appendix A.

CHAPTER 3 REVIEW

CHAPTER HIGHLIGHTS

- In the natural sciences, the main function of theory is to guide research. In the practice disciplines, the main function of theory (and research) is to provide new possibilities for understanding the discipline's focus (music, art, management, nursing).
- To Nightingale, the knowledge required to provide good nursing was neither unique nor specialized. Rather, Nightingale viewed nursing as a central human activity grounded in observation, reason, and commonsense health practices.
- During the latter half of the 20th century, disciplines seeking to establish themselves in universities had to demonstrate something that Nightingale had not envisioned for nursing—a unique body of theoretical knowledge.
- Theories articulate significant relationships between concepts in order to point to something larger, such as gravity, the unconscious, or the experience of pain.

- Paradigms include our notions of reality that are largely unconscious or taken for granted. Most theories reflect the dominant paradigm of a culture, although some may grow out of a developing rival paradigm.
- In the late 20th century, much of the theoretical work in nursing focused on articulating relationships between four major concepts: person, environment, health, and nursing. Because these four concepts can be superimposed on almost any work in nursing, they are sometimes collectively referred to as a "metaparadigm" for nursing.
- Debates about the role of theory in nursing practice provide evidence that nursing is maturing, as both an academic discipline and a clinical profession.

TEST YOUR KNOWLEDGE

1. "A supposition or system of ideas that is proposed to explain a given phenomenon" best defines which of the following?
   1. A concept
   2. A conceptual framework
   3. A theory
   4. A paradigm

2. "A group of related ideas or statements" best defines which of the following?
   1. A philosophy
   2. A conceptual framework
   3. A theory
   4. A paradigm

3. "A set of shared understandings and assumptions about reality and the world" is a definition for which of the following?
   1. A concept
   2. A conceptual framework
   3. A practice discipline
   4. A paradigm

4. Which of the following provides the best explanation for describing nursing as a practice discipline?
   1. Nursing focuses on performing the professional role.
   2. It takes time and experience to become a competent nurse.
   3. Research and theory development is a central focus.
   4. Nurses function as members of a team who form a practice group.

5. Person, environment, health and nursing constitute the metaparadigm for nursing because of which of the following?
   1. Provide a framework for implementing the nursing process
   2. Can be utilized in any setting when caring for a client
   3. Can be utilized to determine applicability of a research study
   4. They focus on the needs of a group of clients

See Answers to Test Your Knowledge in Appendix A.

EXPLORE MEDIALINK www.prenhall.com/berman

DVD-ROM
- Audio Glossary
- NCLEX Review

COMPANION WEBSITE
- Additional NCLEX Review
- Case Study: Theories
- Application Activities:
  The Growth of Nursing Theory
  Shaping Watson's Theory
- Links to Resources

READINGS AND REFERENCES

SUGGESTED READINGS

Fawcett, J., Watson, J., Neuman, B., Walker, P. H., & Fitzpatrick, J. (2001). On nursing theories and evidence. *Journal of Nursing Scholarship, 33,* 115–119.
This classic article, written by five of the most prominent nurses in the field of nursing theory, challenges the reader to engage in considering what is required to state that practice is guided by theory and based on research. They propose that there are four patterns of nursing knowledge and each can be considered a type of theory: empirics, ethics, personal, and aesthetics. Further, each requires unique approaches to gathering, interpreting, and naming evidence. Their perspective is significantly broader than that which generally limits evidence to the results of empirical study.

Marrs, J., & Lowry, L. W. (2006). Nursing theory and practice: Connecting the dots. *Nursing Science Quarterly, 19,* 44–50.
Based on the perception that nursing has evolved with a disconnect between theory and practice, the authors recommend adoption of an expanded conceptual-theoretical-empirical (CTE) structure for nursing knowledge. They propose this structure based on the work of Fawcett, who described a hierarchy of nursing knowledge with the metaparadigm as the most abstract, followed by philosophies, conceptual models, grand theories, middle-range theories, practice theories, and finally, empirical indicators.

RELATED RESEARCH

Mahon, N. E., Yarcheski, A., & Yarcheski, T. J. (2004). Social support and positive health practices in early adolescents: A test of mediating variables. *Clinical Nursing Research, 13,* 216–236. *This study used Peplau's interpersonal relations model to examine the relationship between social support and positive health practices in early adolescents, and to test two variables, loneliness and hopefulness, that theoretically mediate this relationship.*

REFERENCES

Campbell, E. T. (2005). Child abuse recognition, reporting and prevention: A culturally congruent approach. *Journal of Multicultural Nursing & Health, 11*(2), 35–40.

Dobratz, M. C. (2004). Life-closing spirituality and the philosophic assumptions of the Roy adaptation model. *Nursing Science Quarterly, 17,* 335–338.

Erci, B., Sayan, A., Tortumluoglu, G., Kiliç, D., Sahin, O., & Güngörmüs, Z. (2003). The effectiveness of Watson's caring model on the quality of life and blood pressure of patients with hypertension. *Journal of Advanced Nursing, 41,* 130–139.

Fitzpatrick, J. J., & Whall, A. L. (2005). *Conceptual models of nursing: Analysis and application* (4th ed.). Upper Saddle River, NJ: Pearson Prentice Hall.

Henderson, V. A. (1966). *The nature of nursing: A definition and its implications for practice, research, and education.* Riverside, NJ: Macmillan.

King, I. M. (1981). *A theory for nursing: Systems, concepts, process.* Albany, NY: Delmar.

King, I. M. (2006). Imogene M. King's theory of goal attainment. In M. E. Parker, *Nursing*

theories and nursing practice (2nd ed., pp. 235–244). Philadelphia: F. A. Davis.

Hood, L. J., & Leddy, S. (2003). *Leddy & Pepper's conceptual bases of professional nursing* (5th ed.). Philadelphia: Lippincott.

Leininger, M. M. (Ed.). (1991). *Culture care diversity and universality: A theory of nursing.* New York: National League for Nursing Press.

Leininger, M., & McFarland, M. R. (2002). *Culture care diversity and universality: A theory of nursing* (3rd ed.). New York: McGraw-Hill.

Leininger, M. M. (2006). Madeline M. Leininger's theory of culture care diversity and universality. In M. E. Parker, *Nursing theories and nursing practice* (2nd ed., pp. 309–320). Philadelphia: F. A. Davis.

Munhall, P. L. (Ed.). (2006). *Nursing research: A qualitative perspective* (4th ed.). Boston: Jones & Bartlett.

Neuman, B., & Fawcett, J. (2002). *The Neuman systems model* (4th ed.). Upper Saddle River, NJ: Prentice Hall.

Nightingale, F. (1969). *Notes on nursing: What it is, and what it is not.* New York: Dover. (Original work published 1860)

Orem, D. E. (1971). *Nursing: Concepts of practice.* Hightstown, NJ: McGraw-Hill.

Parse, R. R. (1994). Quality of life: Sciencing and living the art of human becoming. *Nursing Science Quarterly, 7*(1), 16–21.

Parse, R. R. (Ed.). (1999). *Illumination: The human becoming theory in practice and research.* Boston: Jones & Bartlett.

Parse, R. R. (2006). Rosemarie Rizzo Parse's human becoming school of thought. In M. E. Parker, *Nursing theories and nursing practice* (2nd ed., pp.187–194). Philadelphia: F. A. Davis.

Peplau, H. E. (1952). *Interpersonal relations in nursing.* New York: Putnam.

Rogers, M. E. (1970). *An introduction to the theoretical basis of nursing.* Philadelphia: F. A. Davis.

Roy, C. (1997). Future of the Roy model: Challenge to redefine adaptation. *Nursing Science Quarterly, 10*(1), 42–48.

Tomey, A. M., & Alligood, M. R. (2006). *Nursing theorists and their work* (6th ed.). St. Louis, MO: Mosby.

Tourville, C., Ingalls, K. (2003). The living tree of nursing theories. *Nursing Forum, 38,* 21–30, 36.

Watson, J. (2005). *Caring science as sacred science.* Philadelphia: F. A. Davis.

Watson, J. (2006). From carative factors to clinical caritas processes. Retrieved March 18, 2006, from http://www2.uchsc.edu/son/caring/content/evolution.asp

Watson, J., & Smith, M. C. (2002). Caring science and the science of unitary human beings: A trans-theoretical discourse for nursing knowledge development. *Journal of Advanced Nursing, 37,* 452–461.

SELECTED BIBLIOGRAPHY

Fawcett, J. (2005). *Contemporary nursing knowledge: Analysis and evaluation of nursing models and theories* (2nd ed.). Philadelphia: F. A. Davis.

Freud, S. (1949). *An outline of psycho-analysis* (J. Strachey, Trans.). New York: W.W. Norton. (Original work published 1940)

Henderson, V. A. (1991). *The nature of nursing: Reflections after 25 years.* New York: National League for Nursing Press.

Lasiuk, G. C., & Ferguson, L. (2005). From practice to midrange theory and back again: Beck's theory of postpartum depression. *Advances in Nursing Science, 28,* 127–136.

Orem, D. E., Taylor, S. G., & Renpenning, K. M. (2001). *Nursing: Concepts of practice* (6th ed.). St. Louis, MO: Mosby.

Powers, B. A., & Knapp, T. R. (2005). *Dictionary of nursing theory and research* (3rd ed.). New York: Springer.

Rogers, M. E. (1994). The science of unitary human beings: Current perspectives. *Nursing Science Quarterly, 7*(1), 33–35.

Rosenberg, S. (2006). Utilizing the language of Jean Watson's caring theory within a computerized clinical documentation system. *Computers, Informatics, Nursing, 24,* 53–56.

Roy, C. (1999). *The Roy adaptation model* (2nd ed.). Upper Saddle River, NJ: Prentice Hall.

Watson, J. (2006-7 in process). *Nursing: The philosophy and science of caring. Revised & updated edition.* Boulder: University Press of Colorado.

CHAPTER 4

Legal Aspects of Nursing

LEARNING OUTCOMES

After completing this chapter, you will be able to:

1. List sources of law and types of laws.

2. Describe ways nurse practice acts, standards of care, and agency policies and procedures affect the scope of nursing practice.

3. Compare and contrast the state-based licensure model and the mutual recognition model for multistate licensure.

4. Describe the purpose and essential elements of informed consent.

5. Describe the purpose of the following legislated acts: Good Samaritan acts and Americans with Disabilities Act.

6. Discuss the impaired nurse and available diversion or peer assistance programs.

7. Recognize the nurse's legal responsibilities with selected aspects of nursing practice.

8. Differentiate crimes from torts and give examples in nursing.

9. Discriminate between negligence and malpractice.

10. Delineate the elements of malpractice.

11. Compare and contrast intentional torts (assault/battery, false imprisonment, invasion of privacy, defamation) and unintentional torts (negligence, malpractice).

12. Describe the four specific areas of the Health Insurance Portability and Accountability Act (HIPAA) and their impact on nursing practice.

13. Describe the purpose of professional liability insurance.

14. List information that needs to be included in an incident report.

15. Identify ways nurses and nursing students can minimize their chances of liability.

Nursing practice is governed by many legal concepts. It is important for nurses to know the basics of legal concepts, because nurses are accountable for their professional judgments and actions. Accountability is an essential concept of professional nursing practice and the law. Knowledge of laws that regulate and affect nursing practice is needed for two reasons:

1. To ensure that the nurse's decisions and actions are consistent with current legal principles.
2. To protect the nurse from liability.

GENERAL LEGAL CONCEPTS

Law can be defined as "the sum total of rules and regulations by which a society is governed. As such, law is created by people and exists to regulate all persons" (Guido, 2006, p. 16).

Functions of the Law in Nursing

The law serves a number of functions in nursing:

- It provides a framework for establishing which nursing actions in the care of clients are legal.
- It differentiates the nurse's responsibilities from those of other health professionals.
- It helps establish the boundaries of independent nursing action.

- It assists in maintaining a standard of nursing practice by making nurses accountable under the law.

Sources of Law

The legal system in the United States has its origin in the English common law system. Figure 4-1 ■ provides an overview of the primary sources of law (i.e., how laws are created): constitutions, statutes, administrative agencies, and decisions of courts (common law).

Constitutional Law

The Constitution of the United States is the supreme law of the country. It establishes the general organization of the federal government, grants certain powers to the government, and places limits on what federal and state governments may do. The constitution creates legal rights and responsibilities and is the foundation for a system of justice. For example, the constitution ensures each U.S. citizen the right to due process of law.

Legislation (Statutory Law)

Laws enacted by any legislative body are called **statutory laws.** When federal and state laws conflict, federal law supersedes. Likewise, state laws supersede local laws.

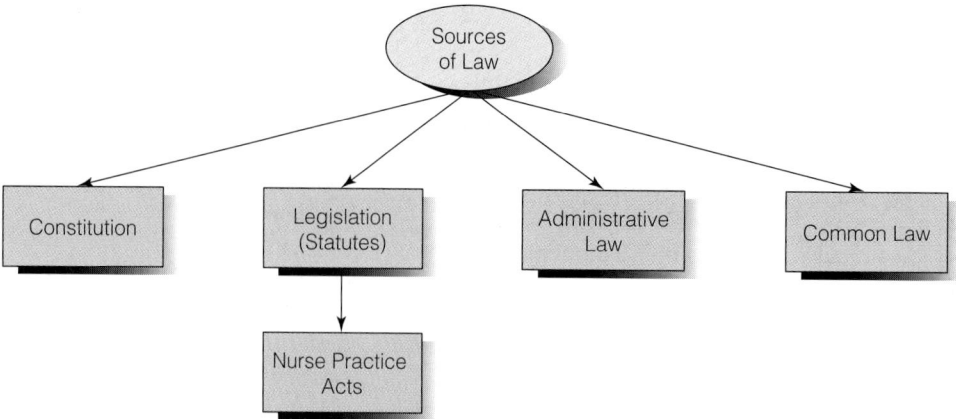

Figure 4-1 ■ Overview of sources of law.

The regulation of nursing is a function of state law. State legislatures pass statutes that define and regulate nursing, that is, nurse practice acts. These acts, however, must be consistent with constitutional and federal provisions.

CLINICAL ALERT

It is important for nurses to keep their legislators informed about nursing because it is the legislature that passes laws that affect nursing practice. ■

Administrative Law

When a state legislature passes a statute, an administrative agency is given the authority to create rules and regulations to enforce the statutory laws. For example, state boards of nursing write rules and regulations to implement and enforce a nurse practice act, which was created through statutory law (Guido, 2006).

Common Law

Laws evolving from court decisions are referred to as **common law.** In addition to interpreting and applying constitutional or statutory law, courts also are asked to resolve disputes between two parties. Common law is continually being adapted and expanded. In deciding specific controversies, courts generally adhere to the doctrine of *stare decisis*— "to stand by things decided"—usually referred to as "following precedent." In other words, to arrive at a ruling in a particular case, the court applies the same rules and principles applied in previous, similar cases.

Types of Laws

Laws can be further classified into different types. The two main types are public law and private or civil law.

Public law refers to the body of law that deals with relationships between individuals and the government and governmental agencies. An important segment of public law is **criminal law,** which deals with actions against the safety and welfare of the public. Examples are homicide, manslaughter, and theft. Crimes

can be classified as either felonies or misdemeanors, which are described in more detail later in this chapter.

Private law, or **civil law,** is the body of law that deals with relationships among private individuals. It can be categorized into a variety of legal specialties such as contract law and tort law. **Contract law** involves the enforcement of agreements among private individuals or the payment of compensation for failure to fulfill the agreements. **Tort law** defines and enforces duties and rights among private individuals that are not based on contractual agreements. Some examples of tort laws applicable to nurses are negligence and malpractice, invasion of privacy, and assault and battery, which are discussed in more detail later in this chapter. See Table 4–1 for selected categories of law affecting nurses.

TABLE 4–1 Selected Categories of Laws Affecting Nurses

CATEGORY	EXAMPLES
Constitutional	Due process
	Equal protection
Statutory (legislative)	Nurse practice acts
	Good Samaritan acts
	Child and adult abuse laws
	Living wills
	Sexual harassment laws
	Americans with Disabilities Act
Criminal (public)	Homicide, manslaughter
	Theft
	Arson
	Active euthanasia
	Sexual assault
	Illegal possession of controlled drugs
Contracts (private/civil)	Nurse and client
	Nurse and employer
	Nurse and insurance
	Client and agency
Torts (private/civil)	Negligence/malpractice
	Libel and slander
	Invasion of privacy
	Assault and battery
	False imprisonment
	Abandonment

Kinds of Legal Actions

There are two kinds of legal actions: civil or private actions and criminal actions. **Civil actions** deal with the relationships among individuals in society; for example, a man may file a suit against a person who he believes cheated him. Civil actions that are of concern to nurses include the torts and contracts listed in Table 4–1. **Criminal actions** deal with disputes between an individual and the society as a whole; for example, if a man shoots a person, society brings him to trial. The major difference between civil and criminal law is the potential outcome for the defendant. If found guilty in a civil action, such as malpractice, the defendant will have to pay a sum of money. If found guilty in a criminal action, the defendant may lose money, be jailed, or be executed and, if a nurse, could lose his or her license. The action of a lawsuit is called **litigation,** and lawyers who participate in lawsuits may be referred to as litigators.

The Civil Judicial Process

The judicial process primarily functions to settle disputes peacefully and in accordance with the law. A lawsuit has strict procedural rules. There are generally five steps:

1. A document, called a **complaint,** is filed by a person referred to as the **plaintiff,** who claims that his or her legal rights have been infringed on by one or more other persons or entities, referred to as **defendants.**
2. A written response, called an **answer,** is made by the defendants.
3. Both parties engage in pretrial activities, referred to as **discovery,** in an effort to obtain all the facts of the situation.
4. In the **trial** of the case, all the relevant facts are presented to a jury or only to a judge.
5. The judge renders a **decision,** or the jury renders a **verdict.** If the outcome is not acceptable to one of the parties, an appeal can be made for another trial.

During a trial, a plaintiff must offer evidence of the defendant's wrongdoing. This duty of proving an assertion of wrongdoing is called the **burden of proof.** See Figure 4-2 ■ for a diagram of the judicial process.

Nurses as Witnesses

A nurse may be called to testify in a legal action. It is advisable that any nurse who is asked to testify in such a situation seek the advice of an attorney before providing testimony. In most cases, the attorney for the employer will provide support and counsel during the legal case. If the nurse is the defendant, however, it is advisable for the nurse to retain an attorney to protect the nurse's own interests.

A nurse may also be asked to provide testimony as an expert witness. An **expert witness** has special training, experience, or skill in a relevant area and is allowed by the court to offer an opinion on some issue within his or her area of expertise. The nurse's credentials and expertise help a judge or jury understand the appropriate standard of care. The nurse expert, thus, has the ability to analyze the facts or evidence and draw inferences (e.g., was the standard of care met).

REGULATION OF NURSING PRACTICE

Protection of the public is the legal purpose for defining the scope of nursing practice, licensing requirements, and standards of care. Nurses who know and follow their nurse practice act and standards of care provide safe, competent nursing care.

Nurse Practice Acts

Each state has a nurse practice act, which protects the public by legally defining and describing the *scope of nursing practice.* State nurse practice acts also legally control nursing practice through licensing requirements. For advanced nursing practice, many states require a different license or have an additional clause that pertains to actions that may be performed only by nurses with advanced education. For example, an additional license may be required to practice as a nurse midwife, nurse anesthetist, or nurse practitioner. The advanced practice nurse also requires a license to prescribe medication or order treatments from physical therapists or other health professionals.

Nurse practice acts, while similar, do differ from state to state. For example, they may differ in their scope of practice definition and in licensing and license renewal requirements. It is the nurse's responsibility to know the nurse practice act of the state in which he or she practices nursing. A state's nurse practice act is easily accessed at the specific state board of nursing's website.

Credentialing

Credentialing is the process of determining and maintaining competence in nursing practice. The credentialing process is one way in which the nursing profession maintains standards of practice and accountability for the educational preparation of its members. Credentialing includes licensure, certification, and accreditation.

Licensure

A **license** is a legal permit that a government agency grants to individuals to engage in the practice of a profession and to use a particular title. Nursing licensure is mandatory in all states. For a profession or occupation to obtain the right to license its members, it generally must meet three criteria:

1. There is a need to protect the public's safety or welfare.
2. The occupation is clearly delineated as a separate, distinct area of work.
3. There is a proper authority to assume the obligations of the licensing process, for example, in nursing, state boards of nursing.

Each state has a mechanism by which licenses can be revoked for just cause (e.g., incompetent nursing practice, professional misconduct, or conviction of a crime such as using illegal drugs or selling drugs illegally). In each situation, a committee at a hearing reviews all the facts. Nurses are entitled to be represented

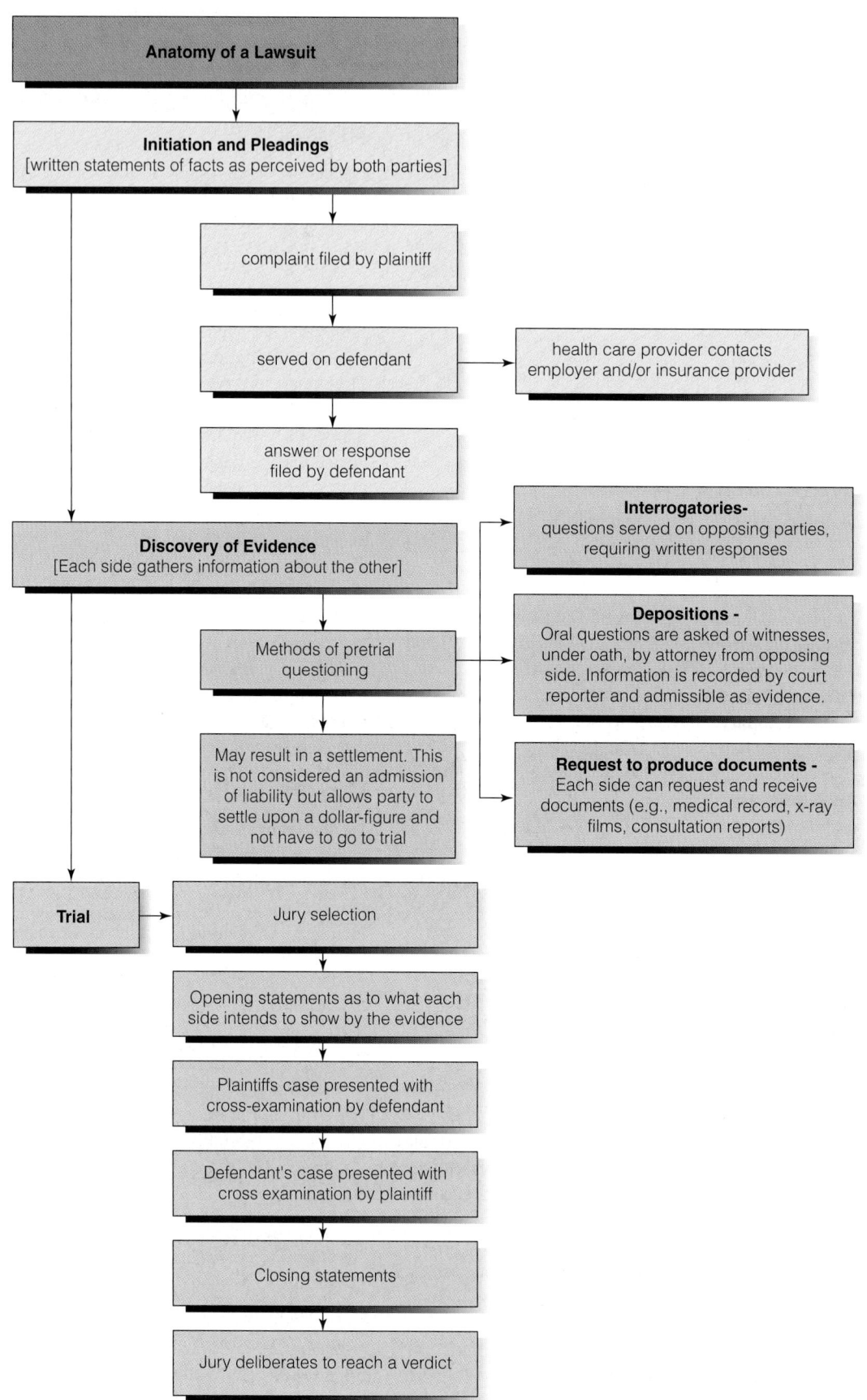

Figure 4-2 ■ Anatomy of a lawsuit.

Note: Adapted from *Legal and Ethical Issues in Nursing* by G. W. Guido, (2006), (4th ed.). Upper Saddle River, N.J.: Prentice-Hall, Inc. pp 38–46.

by legal counsel at such a hearing. If the nurse's license is revoked as a result of the hearing, either the nurse can appeal the decision to a court of law or, in some states, an agency is designated to review the decision before any court action is initiated.

Mutual Recognition Model

Historically, licensure for nurses has been state based; that is, the state's board of nursing has licensed all nurses practicing in the state. Changes, however, in health care delivery and telecommunication technology advances (e.g., telehealth) have raised questions about the state-based model. Telehealth is the delivery of health services over distances and is used to describe the wide range of services delivered by all health-related disciplines (Greenberg, 2000, p. 220). Thus, according to the state-based model, a nurse who electronically interacts with a client in another state to provide health information or intervention is practicing across state lines without a license in the other state.

In response, the National Council of State Boards of Nursing (NCSBN) developed a new regulatory model named the **mutual recognition model,** which allows for multistate licensure. With mutual recognition, a nurse who is not under discipline can practice in person or electronically across state lines under one license. For example, a nurse who lives on the border of a state can practice in both states under one license *if* the adjoining states have an interstate compact. A nurse who practices nursing in a state other than his or her primary state of residence must still contact the other state's board of nursing and provide proof of licensure.

An **interstate compact** called the Nurse Licensure Compact (NLC) (an agreement between two or more states) is the mechanism used to create mutual recognition among states. The state legislature initiates and decides on the establishment of an interstate compact or NLC. As of 2006, 20 states have implemented the Nurse Licensure Compact for RNs and LVN/LPNs, and two states are pending implementation. Only those states who have adopted the RN and LPN/LVN Nurse Licensure Compact may implement a compact for advanced practice registered nurses (APRNs). Utah and Iowa have adopted the APRN compact as of 2006. The NCSBN website provides current information about the number of states that have passed NLC legislation. See Box 4–1 for additional information about the mutual recognition model.

Certification

Certification is the voluntary practice of validating that an individual nurse has met minimum standards of nursing competence in specialty areas such as maternal–child health, pediatrics, mental health, gerontology, and school nursing. National certification may be required to become licensed as an advanced practice nurse. Certification programs are conducted by the American Nurses Association (ANA) and by specialty nursing organizations.

Accreditation/Approval of Basic Nursing Education Programs

One of the functions of a state board of nursing is to ensure that schools preparing nurses maintain minimum standards of educa-

---

BOX 4–1 Mutual Recognition Model

- Each state has to enter into an interstate compact, called the Nurse Licensure Compact (NLC), that allows nurses to practice in more than one state.
- Multistate licensure privilege means the authority to practice nursing in another state that has signed an interstate compact. It is not an additional license.
- A nurse must have a license in his or her primary state of legal residency, if it is an NLC state.
- The states continue to have authority in determining licensure requirements and disciplinary actions.
- The nurse is held accountable for knowing and practicing the nursing practice laws and regulations in the state where the client is located at the time of care.
- Enactment does not change a state's nurse practice act.
- Complaints and/or violations would be addressed by the home state (place of residence) and the remote (practice) state.
- RNs and LPNs/LVNs are included in the interstate compact or NLC. Since 2002, there is now a separate APRN Compact. A state must be a member of the NLC for RNs and LPNs before entering into the APRN Compact. A state must adopt both compacts to cover LPNs/RNs and APRNs for mutual recognition.

Note: From "Frequently Asked Questions Regarding the National Council of State Boards of Nursing (NCSBN) Nurse Licensure Compact (NLC)," by Nurse Licensure Compact Administrators, 2004. Retrieved April 29, 2006, from www.ncsbn.org/pdfs/FrequentlyAskedQuestions.pdf.

---

tion. Depending on the state, a state board of nursing must either approve or accredit a nursing program. This is a legal requirement.

Nursing programs can also choose to seek voluntary accreditation from a private organization such as the National League for Nursing Accrediting Commission (NLNAC) and the Commission on Collegiate Nursing Education (CCNE). Maintaining voluntary accreditation is a means of informing the public and prospective students that the nursing program has met certain criteria.

All states require approval/accreditation by the state board of nursing. Some states require that nursing programs be both state approved/accredited and accredited by a national accrediting agency such as NLNAC or CCNE.

Standards of Care

The purpose of standards of care is to protect the consumer. **Standards of care** are the skills and learning commonly possessed by members of a profession (Guido, 2006, p. 55). These standards are used to evaluate the quality of care nurses provide and, therefore, become legal guidelines for nursing practice.

Nursing standards of care can be classified into two categories: internal and external standards. Internal standards of care include "the nurse's job description, education, and expertise as well as individual institutional policies and procedures" (Guido, 2005, p. 64).

External standards consist of the following:

- Nurse practice acts
- Professional organizations (e.g., ANA)

- Nursing speciality-practice organizations (e.g., Emergency Nurses Association, Oncology Nursing Society)
- Federal organizations and federal guidelines (e.g., Joint Commission on Accreditation of Healthcare Organizations [JCAHO] and Medicare)

It is important, therefore, for nurses to know their institution's policies and procedures and nurse practice act. They also need to remain competent through reading professional journals and attending continuing education and in-service programs. Again, the purpose of knowing and practicing nursing's standards of care is to protect the client/consumer.

CONTRACTUAL ARRANGEMENTS IN NURSING

A contract is the basis of the relationship between a nurse and an employer—for example, a nurse and a hospital or a nurse and a physician. A **contract** is an agreement between two or more competent persons, on sufficient consideration (remuneration), to do or not to do some lawful act. A contract may be written or oral. An oral contract is as equally binding as a written contract. The terms of the oral contract, however, may be more difficult to prove in a court of law. A written contract cannot be changed legally by an oral agreement. If two people wish to change some aspect of a written contract, the change must be written into the contract, because one party cannot hold the other to an oral agreement that differs from the written one.

A contract is considered to be *expressed* when the two parties discuss and agree, orally or in writing, to terms and conditions during the creation of the contract. For example, a nurse will work at a hospital for a stated length of time and under stated conditions. An **implied contract** is one that has not been explicitly agreed to by the parties but that the law nevertheless considers to exist. For example, the nurse is expected to be competent and to follow hospital policies and procedures even though these expectations were not written or discussed. Likewise, the hospital is expected to provide the necessary supplies and equipment needed to provide competent nursing care.

A lawful contract requires the following four features (Guido, 2006):

1. Promise or agreement between two or more persons for the performance of an action or restraint from certain actions
2. Mutual understanding of the terms and meaning of the contract by all
3. A lawful purpose (the activity must be legal)
4. Compensation in the form of something of value—in most cases, compensation is monetary

Legal Roles of Nurses

Nurses have three separate, interdependent legal roles, each with rights and associated responsibilities: provider of service, employee or contractor for service, and citizen.

Provider of Service

The nurse is expected to provide safe and competent care. Implicit in this role are several legal concepts: liability, standards of care, and contractual obligations.

Liability is the quality or state of being legally responsible for one's obligations and actions and to make financial restitution for wrongful acts. A nurse, for example, has an obligation to practice and direct the practice of others under the nurse's supervision so that harm or injury to the client is prevented and standards of care are maintained. Even when a nurse carries out treatments ordered by the physician, the responsibility for the nursing activity belongs to the nurse. When a nurse is asked to carry out an activity that the nurse believes will be injurious to the client, the nurse's responsibility is to refuse to carry out the order and report this to the nurse's supervisor.

The standards of care by which a nurse acts or fails to act are legally defined by nurse practice acts and by the rule of reasonable and prudent action—what a reasonable and prudent professional with similar preparation and experience would do in similar circumstances. **Contractual obligations** refer to the nurse's duty of care, that is, duty to render care, established by the presence of an expressed or implied contract.

Employee or Contractor for Service

A nurse who is employed by an agency works as a representative of the agency, and the nurse's contract with clients is an implied one. However, a nurse who is employed directly by a client, for example, a private nurse, may have a written contract with that client in which the nurse agrees to provide professional services for a certain fee. A nurse might be prevented from carrying out the terms of the contract because of illness or death. However, personal inconvenience and personal problems, such as the nurse's car failure, are not legitimate reasons for failing to fulfill a contract.

Contractual relationships vary among practice settings. An independent nurse practitioner is a contractor for service whose contractual relationship with the client is an independent one. The nurse employed by a hospital functions within an employer–employee relationship in which the nurse represents and acts for the hospital and therefore must function within the policies of the employing agency. This type of legal relationship creates the ancient legal doctrine known as ***respondeat superior*** ("let the master answer"). In other words, the master (employer) assumes responsibility for the conduct of the servant (employee) and can also be held responsible for malpractice by the employee. By virtue of the employee role, therefore, the nurse's conduct is the hospital's responsibility.

This doctrine does not imply that the nurse cannot be held liable as an individual. Nor does it imply that the doctrine will prevail if the employee's actions are extraordinarily inappropriate, that is, beyond those expected or foreseen by the employer. For example, if the nurse hits a client in the face, the employer could disclaim responsibility because this behavior is beyond the bounds of expected behavior. Criminal acts, such as assisting with criminal abortions or taking tranquilizers from a client's supply for personal use, would also be considered extraordinarily inappropriate behavior. Nurses can be held liable for failure to act as well. For example, a nurse who sees another nurse hitting a client and fails to do anything to protect the client may be considered negligent.

The nurse in the role of employee or contractor for service has obligations to the employer, the client, and other personnel.

The nursing care provided must be within the limitations and terms specified. The nurse has an obligation to contract only for those responsibilities that the nurse is competent to discharge. For example, the nurse must practice according to the state's nurse practice act and the policies and procedures of the facility or organization.

The nurse is expected to respect the rights and responsibilities of other health care participants. For example, although the nurse has a responsibility to explain nursing activities to a client, the nurse does not have the right to comment on medical practice in a way that disturbs the client or denounces the physician. At the same time, the nurse has the right to expect reasonable and prudent conduct from other health professionals.

Citizen

The rights and responsibilities of the nurse in the role of citizen are the same as those of any individual under the legal system. Rights of citizenship protect clients from harm and ensure consideration for their personal property rights, rights to privacy, confidentiality, and other rights discussed later in this chapter. These same rights apply to nurses.

Nurses move in and out of these roles when carrying out professional and personal responsibilities. An understanding of these roles and the rights and responsibilities associated with them promotes legally responsible conduct and practice by nurses. A **right** is a privilege or fundamental power to which an individual is entitled unless it is revoked by law or given up voluntarily; a **responsibility** is the obligation associated with a right. See Table 4–2 for examples of the responsibilities and rights associated with each role.

Collective Bargaining

Collective bargaining is the formalized decision-making process between representatives of management (employer) and representatives of labor (employee) to negotiate wages and conditions of employment, including work hours, working environment, and fringe benefits of employment (e.g., vacation time, sick leave, and personal leave). Through a written agreement, both management and employees legally commit themselves to observe the terms and conditions of employment.

The collective bargaining process involves the recognition of a certified bargaining agent for the employees. This agent can be a union, a trade association, or a professional organization. The agent represents the employees in negotiating a contract with management. The ANA, through its state constituent associations (e.g., MSNA—Michigan State Nurses Association), has represented the interests of nurses within individual states.

When collective bargaining breaks down because an agreement cannot be reached, the employees usually call a strike. A **strike** is an organized work stoppage by a group of employees to express a grievance, enforce a demand for changes in conditions of employment, or solve a dispute with management.

Because nursing practice is a service to people who are often ill or vulnerable, striking presents a moral dilemma to many nurses. Actions taken by nurses can affect the safety of people. When faced with a strike, each nurse must make an individual decision to cross or not to cross a picket line. Nursing students may also be faced with decisions about crossing picket lines in

the event of a strike at a clinical agency used for learning experiences. The ANA supports striking as a means of achieving economic and general welfare.

SELECTED LEGAL ASPECTS OF NURSING PRACTICE

Nurses need to know and apply legal aspects in their many different roles. For example, as client advocates, nurses ensure the client's right to informed consent or refusal, and they identify and report violent behavior and neglect of vulnerable clients. Legal aspects also include the duty to report the nurse suspected of chemical impairment.

Informed Consent

Informed consent is an agreement by a client to accept a course of treatment or a procedure after being provided complete information, including the benefits and risks of treatment, alternatives to the treatment, and prognosis if not treated by a health care provider. Usually the client signs a form provided by the agency. The form is a *record* of the informed consent, *not* the informed consent itself.

There are two types of consent: express and implied. **Express consent** may be either an oral or written agreement. Usually, the

TABLE 4–2 Legal Roles, Rights, and Responsibilities

ROLE	RESPONSIBILITIES	RIGHTS
Provider of service	To provide safe and competent care commensurate with the nurse's preparation, experience, and circumstances To inform clients of the consequences of various alternatives and outcomes of care To provide adequate supervision and evaluation of others for whom the nurse is responsible To remain competent	Right to adequate and qualified assistance as necessary Right to reasonable and prudent conduct from clients (e.g., provision of accurate information as required)
Employee or contractor for service	To fulfill the obligations of contracted service with the employer To respect the employer To respect the rights and responsibilities of other health care providers	Right to adequate working conditions (e.g., safe equipment and facilities) Right to compensation for services rendered Right to reasonable and prudent conduct by other health care providers
Citizen	To protect the rights of the recipients of care	Right to respect by others of the nurse's own rights and responsibilities Right to physical safety

more invasive a procedure and/or the greater the potential for risk to the client, the greater the need for written permission. **Implied consent** exists when the individual's nonverbal behavior indicates agreement. For example, clients who position their bodies for an injection or cooperate with the taking of vital signs infer implied consent. Consent is also implied in a medical emergency when an individual cannot provide express consent because of physical condition.

Obtaining informed consent for specific medical and surgical treatments is the responsibility of the person who is going to perform the procedure. Generally it is the physician; however, it could also be a nurse practitioner, nurse anesthetist, nurse midwife, clinical nurse specialist, or physician's assistant who is performing procedures in their advanced practices.

Informed consent also applies to nurses who are not independent practitioners and are performing direct nursing care for such procedures as nasogastric tube insertion or medication administration. The nurse relies on orally expressed consent or implied consent for most nursing interventions. It is imperative to remember the importance of communicating with the client by explaining nursing procedures, ensuring the client understands, and obtaining permission.

The law says that a "reasonable amount" of information required for the client to make an informed decision is what any other reasonable physician or practitioner would disclose under similar circumstances (Quallich, 2005). General guidelines include the following:

- The diagnosis or condition that requires treatment
- The purposes of the treatment
- What the client can expect to feel or experience
- The intended benefits of the treatment
- Possible risks or negative outcomes of the treatment
- Advantages and disadvantages of possible alternatives to the treatment (including no treatment)

There are three major elements of informed consent:

1. The consent must be given voluntarily.
2. The consent must be given by a client or individual with the capacity and competence to understand.
3. The client or individual must be given enough information to be the ultimate decision maker.

To give informed consent voluntarily, the client must not feel coerced. Sometimes fear of disapproval by a health professional can be the motivation for giving consent; such consent is not voluntarily given. Coercion invalidates the consent. It is important, therefore, for the person obtaining the consent to invite and answer client questions.

Cultural perspective also needs to be considered when clients are asked to make decisions about a procedure or treatment. For example, informed consent in the United States is based on the principle of autonomy. That is, each person has the right to decide what can or cannot be done to his or her person. It is expected that the competent adult client will have the autonomy to make his or her own health care decisions. In contrast to this individual perspective, people from other cultures (e.g., Southeast Asia, American Indian) may have a group perspective for decision making. They may believe that another member of

their family or group or tribe should make the decision. The nurse can provide culturally competent care by asking clients if there is someone they would like to be present when information or discussion of their health care treatment occurs.

It is also important that the client understand. Illiteracy in the United States continues to present a challenge as it pertains to recognizing and understanding words commonly used in consent forms. According to Crane, Cody, and McSweeney (2004), the Department of Education's National Adult Literacy Survey reported that 40 million to 44 million individuals in the United States are in the lowest level of literacy and cannot understand basic written material (pp. 41–42). As a result, technical words and language barriers can inhibit understanding and may encourage a signature without discussion of its actual meaning when the client has a lower literacy level (Quallich, 2005, p. 50). If a client cannot read, the consent form must be read to the client and the client must state understanding before the form is signed. If the client does not speak the same language as the health professional who is providing the information, an interpreter must be present. However, even with an interpreter, it is important to remember that potential interpretation errors can occur (see Culturally Competent Care).

If given sufficient information, a competent adult can make decisions regarding health. A competent adult is a person over 18 years of age who is conscious and oriented. A client who is confused, disoriented, or sedated is not considered functionally competent. A legal guardian or representative can provide or refuse consent for the incompetent adult.

Informed consent regulations were originally written with acute care settings in mind. Nonetheless, ensuring informed consent is equally important in providing nursing care in the home. Because the provision of home care often occurs over an extended period of time, the nurse has multiple opportunities to ensure that the client agrees to the plan of treatment. A challenge to informed consent in the home, however, is that the plan may affect other members of the family and, if so, they need to be consulted.

Exceptions

Three groups of people cannot provide consent. The first is minors. In most areas, a parent or guardian must give consent before minors can obtain treatment. The same is true of an adult who has the mental capacity of a child and who has an appointed guardian. In some states, however, minors are allowed to give consent for such procedures as blood donations, treatment for substance abuse, treatment for mental health problems, and treatment for reproductive health concerns such as sexually transmitted diseases or pregnancy (Brent, 2001). In addition, certain groups of minors are often legally permitted to provide their own consent. These include those who are married, pregnant, parents, members of the military, or emancipated (living on their own). These statutes may vary by state.

The second group is persons who are unconscious or injured in such a way that they are unable to give consent. In these situations, consent is usually obtained from the closest adult relative if existing statutes permit. In a life-threatening emergency, if consent cannot be obtained from the client or a relative, then the law generally agrees that consent is implied to provide necessary care for the client's emergency condition.

CULTURALLY COMPETENT CARE
Overcoming a Language Barrier

Health institutions have a legal responsibility—and an ethical obligation—to ensure a means of communication for the increasing number of U.S. residents who report not being able to speak English well or at all. Using an interpreter is one means to do this. However, using an interpreter is not foolproof. For example, Higginbotham (2003) described one study that found that more than half of medical interpretation errors involved the omission of a word or phrase used by the clinician or client. In addition, the incorrect use of a word or a phrase for which there was no direct translation accounted for other errors. The study found that both professional and nonprofessional (e.g., friend or family) interpreters made errors, and the nonprofessionals were more likely to make errors that could significantly affect the outcome for the client. For example, friends or family members are more likely to add their own thoughts when translating because they believe they are doing so in the best interest of the client. Using a family member can also compromise the client's right to confidentiality.

Higginbotham recommends the following steps to minimize translation errors:

- The ideal choice is to use a professional translator who has been trained in medical terminology. If one is not available, a telephone translation service should be considered. The larger services provide 24-hour access. A nonprofessional interpreter should only be used as a last resort.
- Brief the interpreter on the purpose of the translation, the subject(s) to be covered, and the scope of the services needed.
- Inform the interpreter that it is important to translate the words of all parties as literally as possible.
- Ask the interpreter if she or he knows of any cultural beliefs that could affect the encounter.
- Verify that the translater has signed a form requiring confidentiality of the client's health information. If you have to use a family member, you need to tell them that the information disclosed by the client is considered confidential.
- Introduce the interpreter to the client. Check your agency's policy as it may require that the client provide consent to use an interpreter.
- Speak directly to the client. . . . not to the interpreter.
- Take your time. Speak slowly and pause frequently to give the interpreter time to express what you have said.
- Observe the body language of the client and ask questions based on your observations as appropriate.
- Ask the client if he or she has any questions. Ask the client to repeat any instructions to confirm understanding.
- Document in the client's chart that the client gave consent to use an interpreter, the full name and title of the translator, and the translation service. Document if the interpreter is a family member or a nonprofessional.

Note: Reprinted with permission from, *RN* vol. 60, no. 10, pp. 67–69. *RN* is a copyrighted publication of Advanstar Communications Inc. All rights reserved.

The third group is mentally ill persons who have been judged by professionals to be incompetent. State and provincial mental health acts or similar statutes generally provide definitions of mental illness and specify the rights of the mentally ill under the law as well as the rights of the staff caring for such clients.

Nurse's Role

Often the nurse is asked to obtain a signed consent form. The nurse is not responsible for explaining the procedure but for witnessing the client's signature on the form (see Figure 4-3 ■). The nurse's signature confirms three things:

- The client gave consent voluntarily.
- The signature is authentic.
- The client appears competent to give consent.

The nurse advocates for the client by verifying that the client received enough information to give consent. If the client has questions or if the nurse has doubts about the client's understanding, the nurse must notify the health provider. Again, the nurse is not responsible for explaining the medical or surgical procedure. In fact, the nurse could be liable for giving incorrect or incomplete information or interfering with the client–provider relationship.

CLINICAL ALERT

Ask clients to state in their own words what they have been told about the procedure or treatment. ■

According to Guido (2006), the right of consent also involves the right of refusal. Remind clients that they can change their minds and cancel the procedure at any time because the right to refuse continues even after signing the consent. Similar to informed consent, it is important to verify that the client is aware of the pros and cons of refusal and is making an informed decision. The nurse needs to notify the health provider of the client's refusal and document the refusal in the chart.

Documentation is an important aspect to informed consent. A client's concerns or questions must be documented along with the notification of the health care provider. Equally important is documenting when the client states understanding. Record any teaching as a result of nursing-related questions by the client. Any special circumstances, such as use of an interpreter, should be documented. When documenting the use of an interpreter, include the interpreter's full name and title.

Figure 4-3 ■ Obtaining informed consent is the responsibility of the person performing the procedure. The nurse may be asked to witness the client's signature on the consent form.

Delegation

The American Nurses Association (1997) defines **delegation** as "the transfer of responsibility for the performance of an activity from one person to another while retaining accountability for the outcome." Competent unlicensed assistive personnel (UAP) can be of assistance to the nurse, which allows the nurse to perform those functions appropriate to the nurse's scope of practice. From a legal perspective, however, the nurse's authority to delegate is based on laws and regulations. Therefore, nurses must be familiar with their nurse practice act (NPA). Sheehan (2001) states that the nurse needs to determine the answers to these questions:

- Does the NPA permit delegation?
- Does the NPA include a list of what the nurse can delegate?
- Has the state board of nursing issued any guidelines explaining the nurse's responsibilities when delegating?

Nurses must know not only their own scope of practice but also the scope of practice of the UAP, which may vary depending on the facilities' policies and procedures. Thus, the nurse must know the employer's policies and procedures for delegation, the UAP's job description, and the UAP's skill level. Is the UAP competent to perform the delegated task? The NCSBN has provided "five rights of delegation" to help nurses make delegation decisions (see Chapter 28 ∞). It is important to remember that the nurse may delegate a task to a UAP; however, the responsibility for action or inaction of the nurse and UAP remains with the nurse (Zimmermann & Jackson, 2004).

Violence, Abuse, and Neglect

Violent behavior can include domestic violence, child abuse, elder abuse, and sexual abuse. Neglect is the absence of care necessary to maintain the health and safety of a vulnerable individual such as a child or elder. Nurses, in their many roles (e.g., home health nurse, pediatric nurse, emergency department nurse), can often identify and assess cases of violence against others. As a result, they are often included as **mandated reporters.** Brent (2001) states that "when an identified instance of injury appears to be present and the result of abuse, neglect or exploitation, the mandated reporter must report the situation to the proper authorities" (p. 281). See Chapter 21 for additional information about child abuse and Chapter 23 for elder abuse. ∞

The Americans with Disabilities Act

The Americans with Disabilities Act (ADA), passed by the U.S. Congress in 1990 and fully implemented in 1994, prohibits discrimination on the basis of disability in employment, public services, and public accommodations. The purposes of the act are as follows:

- To provide a clear and comprehensive national mandate for eliminating discrimination against individuals with disabilities

---

BOX 4–2 Meeting ADA Eligibility

The employee or applicant for employment must show:

- A disability
- A physical or mental impairment that substantially limits one or more major life activities
- A record of the impairment *or* be regarded as having the impairment
- Ability to perform the essential functions of the position

Note: From *Legal and Ethical Issues in Nursing,* 4th ed. (pp. 356–357), by G. W. Guido, 2006, Upper Saddle River, NJ: Prentice Hall. Reprinted with permission.

- To provide clear, strong, consistent, enforceable standards addressing discrimination against individuals with disabilities
- To ensure that the federal government plays a central role in enforcing standards established under the act

The ADA is about productivity, economic independence, and the ability to move about freely in society. The nurse plays a key part in helping individuals with disabilities comprehend the opportunities provided by the law (Watson, 2000, p. 199). For example, nurses working in a variety of settings may be involved in educating clients with disabilities about accessing and using public transportation, communicating through telecommunications devices for individuals with speech and hearing impairments, and patronizing public accommodations such as grocery stores, restaurants, and theaters. Furthermore, an employer may not refuse to hire a nurse with disabilities if the nurse is qualified and able to fulfill the essential functions of the work role. Box 4–2 lists the criteria for ADA eligibility. The ADA also enables individuals of normal intelligence who have a physical or learning disability to pursue a nursing curriculum through alternative learning methods.

Court cases have challenged the definition of a qualified individual with a disability. For example, early challenges to the ADA concerned HIV-infected individuals. A landmark 1998 Supreme Court decision, *Bragdon v. Abbott,* ruled that an asymptomatic HIV-positive individual is considered to have a disability and is protected by the ADA (Guido, 2006). In contrast, courts have also held that a variety of conditions do not constitute a disability under ADA. Examples include a lifting disability, depression and anxiety, inability to handle the stress of a specific job, migraine headaches, nonlatex allergies, and pregnancy (Guido, 2006).

It is the employer's responsibility to provide reasonable accommodations that would allow the person with a disability to perform the job satisfactorily. The employer, however, can claim undue hardship if the accommodation is extremely expensive or difficult to implement.

Controlled Substances

U.S. laws regulate the distribution and use of controlled substances such as narcotics, depressants, stimulants, and hallucinogens. Misuse of controlled substances leads to criminal penalties (see Chapter 35). ∞

The Impaired Nurse

The term **impaired nurse** refers to a nurse whose ability to perform the functions of a nurse is diminished by chemical dependency on drugs, alcohol, or mental illness (Blair, 2002). Chemical dependence in health care workers has become a problem with many causes including, but not limited to, the high levels of stress involved in many health care settings, increased workloads, decreased staffing, fatigue, isolation, and the easy access to addictive drugs. Approximately 3% to 6% of nurses may practice while impaired because of chemical dependency or psychiatric illness, and alcohol is the number-one substance abused (Trossman, 2003, p. 27). In addition, more than half of impaired nurses began abusing drugs, including alcohol, before they finished their nursing education (Danis, 2004). As a result, professional organizations such as the American Nurses Association (ANA), the American Association of Nurse Anesthetists (AANA), the International Nurses Society on Addictions (IntNSA), and the National Student Nurses Association (NSNA) have passed resolutions to ensure that nurses and student nurses with chemical dependencies receive treatment and support, not discipline and derision (Trossman, 2003).

Employers must have sound policies and procedures for identifying and intervening in situations involving a possibly impaired nurse. The primary concern is for the protection of clients, but it is also critically important that the nurse's problem be identified quickly so that appropriate treatment may be instituted. Box 4–3 lists behaviors that may be seen in the impaired nurse. The Practice Guidelines box on page 75 can be used to report the nurse suspected of chemical impairment.

CLINICAL ALERT

It is important that student nurses and nurses become knowledgeable about the risk factors of chemical abuse and its early identification and interventions. ∎

A variety of programs have been developed to assist impaired nurses to recover. The Intervention Project for Nurses (IPN), an affiliate of the Florida Nurses Association, is the oldest and most comprehensive program. It provides swift interventions and close monitoring and advocacy for impaired nurses (IPN, 2005). In many states, impaired nurses who voluntarily enter a diversion program (sometimes called a peer assistance program) do not have their nursing license revoked if they follow treatment requirements. Their practice, however, is closely supervised within specific guidelines (e.g., working on a general nursing unit versus critical care area, no overtime, work only day shift, not allowed to administer or have access to narcotics). The programs require counseling and ongoing participation in support groups with periodic progress reports that may include random drug screening. The nurse may petition the state board of nursing for reinstatement of full licensure after a specified amount of time and evidence of recovery as determined by the state board. Diversion programs allow for rehabilitation of the nurse while still being able to work in the

profession. They also allow the state board to protect the public while complying with the ADA. According to Brent (2001), "the nurse who is in a treatment program or has successfully completed one is protected under the ADA as an individual with a disability" (p. 352).

Sexual Harassment

Sexual harassment is a violation of the individual's rights and a form of discrimination. In 1987, the law prohibiting sexual discrimination was clarified to apply to all educational and employing institutions receiving federal funding. The Equal Employment Opportunity Commission (EEOC) defines sexual harassment as "unwelcome sexual advances, requests for sexual favors, and other verbal or physical conduct of a sexual nature" occurring in the following circumstances (EEOC, 2000, section 1604.11):

BOX 4–3 **Warning Signs of Impairment**

CLUES TO NURSES WITH PROBLEMS

Alcoholic Nurse
- Irritability, mood swings
- Elaborate excuses for behavior; unkempt appearance
- Blackouts (periods of temporary amnesia)
- Impaired motor coordination, slurred speech, flushed face, bloodshot eyes
- Numerous injuries, burns, bruises, etc., with vague explanations
- Smell of alcohol on breath, or excessive use of mouthwash, mints, etc.
- Increased isolation from others

Drug-Addicted Nurse
- Rapid mood and/or performance changes
- Frequent absence from unit; frequent use of restroom
- May work a lot of overtime, usually arriving early and staying late
- Increased somatic complaints necessitating prescriptions of pain medications
- Consistently signs out more or larger amounts of controlled drugs than anyone else; excessive wasting of drugs
- Often medicates others' clients; may wear long sleeves all of the time
- Increased isolation from others
- Clients complain that pain medication is not effective or they deny receiving medication
- Excessive discrepancies in signing and documentation procedures of controlled substances

Mentally-Ill Nurse
- Depressed, lethargic, unable to focus or concentrate, apathetic
- Makes many mistakes at work
- Erratic behavior or mood swings
- Inappropriate or bizarre behavior or speech
- May also exhibit some of the same or similar characteristics as chemically dependent nurses

---

** It is most important to look for **patterns** or **changes** in behavior. Not all characteristics need to be present to indicate that a problem exists.

Note: From "Texas Peer Assistance Program for Nurses," by Texas Nurses Association. Retrieved April 29, 2006, from www.texasnurses.org/tpapn/ warningsigns.htm. Reprinted with permission.

- When submission to such conduct is considered, either explicitly or implicitly, a condition of an individual's employment
- When submission to or rejection of such conduct is used as the basis for employment decisions affecting the individual
- When such conduct interferes with an individual's work performance or creates an "intimidating, hostile, or offensive working environment."

The victim or the harasser may be male or female. The victim does not have to be of the opposite sex. Nurses must develop skills of assertiveness to deter sexual harassment in the workplace. In addition, nurses must be familiar with the sexual harassment policy and procedures that must be in place in every institution. These will include information regarding the reporting procedure, to whom incidents should be reported, the investigative process, and how confidentiality will be protected to the extent possible.

Abortions

Abortion laws provide specific guidelines for nurses about what is legally permissible. In 1973, when the *Roe v. Wade* and *Doe v. Bolton* cases were decided, the Supreme Court of the United States held that the constitutional rights of privacy give a woman the right to control her own body to the extent that she can abort her fetus in the early stages of pregnancy.

In 1989, the Supreme Court's decision in *Webster v. Reproductive Health Services* upheld a Missouri law banning the use of public funds or facilities for performing or assisting with abortions. In 1992, President Clinton rescinded the *Rust v. Sullivan* 1991 decision, dubbed the "gag rule," that prevented health care providers from discussing abortion services with clients in nonprofit agencies. The Supreme Court and state legislatures continue to struggle with the issue of abortion.

Many statutes also include conscience clauses, upheld by the Supreme Court, designed to protect nurses and hospitals. These clauses give hospitals the right to deny admission to abortion clients and give health care personnel, including nurses, the right to refuse to participate in abortions. When these rights are exercised, the statutes also protect the agency and employee from discrimination or retaliation.

Death and Related Issues

The nurse's role in legal issues related to death is prescribed by the laws of the region and the policies of the health care institution. For example, in some states, a feeding tube cannot be removed from a person in a persistent vegetative state without a prior directive from the client, but in other states the removal is allowed at the family's request or a physician's order. Some facilities permit do-not-resuscitate orders or protocols that specify the extent of invasive life-sustaining measures. Caring for dying clients who have agreed to organ donation can also be complex in terms of determining which medications, treatments, or equipment must be continued until the time for harvesting the organs has arrived. Many of these legal issues stimulate strong ethical concerns. It is important that the nurse have support from other team members in understanding and providing appropriate care to clients facing death.

Advance Health Care Directives

Advance health care directives include a variety of legal and lay documents that allow persons to specify aspects of care they wish to receive should they become unable to make or communicate their preferences. The Patient Self-Determination Act implemented in 1991 requires all health care facilities receiving Medicare and Medicaid reimbursement to (a) recognize advance directives, (b) ask clients whether they have advance directives, and (c) provide educational materials advising clients of their rights to declare their personal wishes regarding treatment decisions, including the right to refuse medical treatment. Clients and families often have difficulty making advance treatment decisions for end-of-life matters. They need to be reassured that even if they make a decision and have an advance directive, they will always have the option to change their decision. For example, clients may have decided not to have ventilator support if they were terminally ill, but if and when the actual situation occurred, they have the right to change their mind or take more time to make the decision.

Nurses need to assess if clients and families have an accurate understanding of life-sustaining measures. They may misunderstand what actually sustains life and base their decisions on that. Nurses need to incorporate teaching in this area and continue to be supportive of clients' decisions.

There are two types of advance health care directives: the living will and the health care proxy or surrogate. The **living will** provides specific instructions about what medical treatment the client chooses to omit or refuse (e.g., ventilatory support) in the event that the client is unable to make those decisions.

The **health care proxy,** also referred to as a *durable power of attorney for health care,* is a notarized or witnessed statement appointing someone else (e.g., a relative or trusted friend) to manage health care treatment decisions when the client is unable to do so. Figure 4-4 ■ shows an example of an advance health care directive that combines a living will declaration and the durable power of attorney for health care. A form specific to the state in which you live can be obtained from the National Hospice and Palliative Care Organization.

Nurses should learn the law regarding patient self-determination for the state in which they practice, as well as the policy and procedures for implementation in the institution where they work. The legally binding nature and specific requirements of advance medical directives are determined by individual state legislation. In most states, advance directives must be witnessed by two people but do not require review by an attorney. Some states do not permit relatives, heirs, or physicians to witness advance directives. As a client advocate, it is important for the nurse to facilitate family discussion about end-of-life concerns and decisions.

Autopsy

An **autopsy** or **postmortem examination** is an examination of the body after death. It is performed only in certain cases. The law describes under what circumstances an autopsy must be performed, for example, when death is sudden or occurs within 48 hours of admission to a hospital. The organs and tissues of the body are examined to establish the exact cause of death, to

POWER OF ATTORNEY FOR HEALTH CARE

(1) **DESIGNATION OF AGENT:** I designate the following individual as my agent to make health care decisions for me: _____

_____
(Name of individual you choose as agent)

_____
(address) (city) (state) (zip code)

_____
(home phone) (work phone)

OPTIONAL: If I revoke my agent's authority or if my agent is not willing, able, or reasonably available to make a health-care decision for me, I designate as my first alternate agent:

_____
(Name of individual you choose as first alternate agent)

_____
(address) (city) (state) (zip code)

_____
(home phone) (work phone)

OPTIONAL: If I revoke the authority of my agent and first alternate agent or if neither is willing, able, or reasonably available to make a health care decision for me, I designate as my second alternate agent:

_____
(Name of individual you choose as second alternate agent)

_____
(address) (city) (state) (zip code)

_____
(home phone) (work phone)

(2) **AGENT'S AUTHORITY:** My agent is authorized to make all health care decisions for me, including decisions to provide, withhold, or withdraw artificial nutrition and hydration, and all other forms of health care to keep me alive, **except** as I state here:

(3) **WHEN AGENT'S AUTHORITY BECOMES EFFECTIVE:** My agent's authority becomes effective when my primary physician determines that I am unable to make my own health care decisions unless I mark the following box. If I mark this box [ ], my agent's authority to make health care decisions for me takes effect immediately.

(4) **AGENT'S OBLIGATION:** My agent shall make health care decisions for me in accordance with this power of attorney for health care, any instructions I give below, and my other wishes to the extent known to my agent. To the extent my wishes are unknown, my agent shall make health care decisions for me in accordance with what my agent determines to be in my best interest. In determining my best interest, my agent shall consider my personal values to the extent known to my agent.

(5) **AGENT'S POSTDEATH AUTHORITY:** My agent is authorized to make anatomical gifts, authorize an autopsy, and direct disposition of my remains, except as I state here or elsewhere in this form:

INSTRUCTIONS FOR HEALTH CARE
Strike any wording you do not want.

(6) **END-OF-LIFE DECISIONS:** I direct that my health care providers and others involved in my care provide, withhold, or withdraw treatment in accordance with the choice I have marked below: **(Initial only one box)**
[ ] (a) **Choice NOT To Prolong Life**
I do not want my life to be prolonged if (1) I have an incurable and irreversible condition that will result in my death within a relatively short time, (2) I become unconscious and, to a reasonable degree of medical certainty, I will not regain consciousness, or (3) the likely risks and burdens of treatment would outweigh the expected benefits, **OR**
[ ] (b) **Choice To Prolong Life**
I want my life to be prolonged as long as possible within the limits of generally accepted health care standards.

(7) **RELIEF FROM PAIN:** Except as I state in the following space, I direct that treatment for alleviation of pain or discomfort should be provided at all times even if it hastens my death:

DONATION OF ORGANS AT DEATH
(8) Upon my death: (mark applicable box)
[ ] (a) I give any needed organs, tissues, or parts,
OR
[ ] (b) I give the following organs, tissues, or parts only: _____
[ ] (c) My gift is for the following purposes:
(strike any of the following you do not want)
(1) Transplant
(2) Therapy
(3) Research
(4) Education

(9) **EFFECT OF COPY:** A copy of this form has the same effect as the original.

(10) **SIGNATURE:** Sign and date the form here:

_____   _____
(date)   (sign your name)

_____   _____
(address)   (print your name)

_____   _____
(city)   (state)

(11) **WITNESSES:** This advance health care directive will not be valid for making health care decisions unless it is either: (1) signed by two (2) qualified adult witnesses who are personally known to you and who are present when you sign or acknowledge your signature; or (2) acknowledged before a notary public.

Figure 4-4 ■ Sample advance health care directive.

learn more about a disease, and to assist in the accumulation of statistical data.

It is the responsibility of the physician or, in some instances, of a designated person in the hospital to obtain consent for an autopsy. Consent must be given by the decedent (before death) or by the next of kin. Laws in many states and provinces prioritize the family members who can provide consent as follows: surviving spouse, adult children, parents, and siblings. After an autopsy, hospitals cannot retain any tissues or organs without the permission of the person who consented to the autopsy.

Certification of Death

The formal determination of death, or pronouncement, must be performed by a physician, a coroner, or a nurse. The granting of the authority to nurses to pronounce death is regulated by the state or province. It may be limited to nurses in long-term care, home health, and hospice agencies or to advanced practice nurses. By law, a death certificate must be made out when a person dies. It is usually signed by the attending physician and filed with a local health or other government office. The family is usually given a copy to use for legal matters, such as insurance claims.

Do-Not-Resuscitate Orders

Physicians may order "no code" or **"do not resuscitate" (DNR)** for clients who are in a stage of terminal, irreversible illness or expected death. A DNR order is generally written when the client or proxy has expressed the wish for no resuscitation in the event of a respiratory or cardiac arrest. Many physicians are reluctant to write such an order if there is any conflict between the client and family members or among family members. A DNR order is written to indicate that the goal of treatment is a comfortable, dignified death and that further life-sustaining measures are not indicated. If it is contrary to the nurse's personal beliefs to carry out a DNR order, the nurse should consult the nurse manager for a change in assignment.

The ANA (2003) makes the following recommendations related to DNR orders:

- The competent client's values and choices should always be given highest priority, even when these wishes conflict with those of the family or health care providers.
- When the client is incompetent, an advance directive or the proxy decision makers acting for the client should make health care treatment decisions.
- A DNR decision should always be the subject of explicit discussion between the client, the client's family, any designated decision maker acting on the client's behalf, and the health care team.
- DNR orders must be clearly documented, reviewed, and updated periodically to reflect changes in the client's condition. Such documentation is required to meet standards of the Joint Commission on Accreditation of Healthcare Organizations.
- A DNR order is separate from other aspects of a client's care and does not imply that other types of care should be withdrawn, for example, nursing care to ensure comfort or medical treatment for chronic but non-life-threatening illnesses.

The ANA also recommends that each health care organization put into place mechanisms to resolve conflicts between clients, their families, and health care professionals, or between different health care professionals. Institutional ethics committees usually deal with such conflicts. It is important that nurses be represented on these institutional ethics committees so that nursing perspectives can be heard and nurses can be involved in developing DNR policies.

Many states (but not all) permit clients living at home to arrange special orders so that emergency technicians called to the home in the event of a cardiopulmonary arrest will respect the client's wish not to be resuscitated. Some emergency medical services have written policies specifying that staff may withhold CPR if the client has a signed order or approved form or wears a MedicAlert DNR medallion. Nurses should be familiar with the federal and state or provincial laws and the policies of their agency concerning withholding life-sustaining measures.

Euthanasia

Euthanasia is the act of painlessly putting to death persons suffering from incurable or distressing disease. It is sometimes referred to as "mercy killing." Regardless of compassion and good intentions or moral convictions, euthanasia is legally wrong in the United States and can lead to criminal charges of homicide or to a civil lawsuit for withholding treatment or providing an unacceptable standard of care. Because advanced technology has enabled the medical profession to sustain life almost indefinitely, people are increasingly considering the meaning of quality of life. For some people, the withholding of artificial life-support measures or even the withdrawal of life support is a desired and acceptable practice for clients who are terminally ill or who are incurably disabled and believed unable to live their lives with some happiness and meaning.

Voluntary euthanasia refers to situations in which the dying individual desires some control over the time and manner of death. All forms of euthanasia are illegal except in states where right-to-die statutes and living wills exist. In 1994, the state of Oregon approved the first U.S. physician-assisted suicide law, the Death with Dignity Act, which permits physicians to prescribe lethal doses of medications. The law took effect in November 1997. Through 2004, a total of 302 prescriptions were written and 208 persons died from the prescriptions they obtained under the act (Department of Human Services, 2005). Since Oregon's action, a number of states have proposed right-to-die laws. Right-to-die statutes legally recognize the client's right to refuse treatment.

Inquest

An **inquest** is a legal inquiry into the cause or manner of a death. When a death is the result of an accident, for example, an inquest is held into the circumstances of the accident to determine any blame. The inquest is conducted under the jurisdiction of a coroner or medical examiner. A **coroner** is a public official, not necessarily a physician, appointed or elected to inquire into the causes of death, when appropriate. A **medical examiner** is a physician and usually has advanced education in pathology or forensic medicine. Agency policy dictates who is responsible for reporting deaths to the coroner or medical examiner.

Organ Donation

Under the Uniform Anatomical Gift Act and the National Organ Transplant Act in the United States, people 18 years or older and of sound mind may make a gift of all or any part of their own bodies for the following purposes: for medical or dental education, research, advancement of medical or dental science, therapy, or transplantation. The donation can be made by a provision in a will or by signing a card-like form. This card is usually carried at all times by the person who signed it. In most states and provinces, the person can revoke the gift, either by destroying the card or by revoking the gift orally in the presence of two witnesses. Nurses may serve as witnesses for people consenting to donate organs.

In early 2004, the American Organ Donation and Recovery Improvement Act was signed, authorizing funds through 2009 for projects and activities to increase public awareness of and willingness to participate in organ donation. In almost every case, there is a greater need for transplantation than there are available organs. Thus, in many states, if there is no valid donor document, health care workers are required to discuss with survivors of a potential organ donor the option to make an anatomical gift. Survivors are obliged to grant or withhold donation in accordance with their knowledge of the donor's views on anatomical gifts. The details regarding this process of requesting donation from family members and other legal aspects of organ donation vary by state. The nurse needs to be familiar with the appropriate legislation.

AREAS OF POTENTIAL LIABILITY IN NURSING

Nursing liability is usually involved with tort law. It is important for the nurse to know the differences between malpractice (an unintentional tort) and intentional torts. Nurses must also recognize those nursing situations in which negligent actions are most likely to occur, and take measures to prevent them.

Crimes and Torts

A **crime** is an act committed in violation of public (criminal) law and punishable by a fine or imprisonment. A crime does *not* have to be intended in order to be a crime. For example, a nurse may accidentally give a client an additional and lethal dose of a narcotic to relieve discomfort.

Crimes are classified as either felonies or misdemeanors. A **felony** is a crime of a serious nature, such as murder, punishable by a term in prison. In some areas, second-degree murder is called **manslaughter.** A nurse who accidentally gives an additional and lethal dose of a narcotic can be accused of manslaughter.

Crimes are punished through criminal action by the state against an individual. A **misdemeanor** is an offense of a less serious nature and is usually punishable by a fine or short-term jail sentence, or both. A nurse who slaps a client's face could be charged with a misdemeanor.

A **tort** is a civil wrong committed against a person or a person's property. Torts are usually litigated in court by civil action between individuals. In other words, the person or persons claimed to be responsible for the tort are sued for damages. Tort liability almost always is based on fault, which is something that was done incorrectly (an unreasonable act of commission) or something that should have been done but was not (an act of omission).

Torts may be classified as unintentional or intentional.

Unintentional Torts

Negligence and malpractice are examples of unintentional torts that may occur in the health care setting. **Negligence** is misconduct or practice that is below the standard expected of an ordinary, reasonable, and prudent person. Such conduct places another person at risk for harm. Both nonmedical and professional persons can be liable for negligent acts. **Gross negligence** involves extreme lack of knowledge, skill, or decision making that the person clearly should have known would put others at risk for harm. **Malpractice** is "professional negligence," that is, negligence that occurred while the person was performing as a professional. Malpractice applies to physicians, dentists, lawyers, and generally includes nurses. Six elements must be present for a case of nursing malpractice to be proven.

- **Duty.** The nurse must have (or should have had) a relationship with the client that involves providing care and following an acceptable standard of care. Such duty, for example, is evident when the nurse has been assigned to care for a client in the home or hospital. A nurse also has a general duty of care, even if not specifically assigned to a client, if the client needs help.

CLINICAL ALERT

It is a nurse's duty to respond to all clients' call lights, not just those of assigned clients. ■

- **Breach of duty.** There must be a standard of care that is expected in the specific situation but that the nurse did not observe. For example, something was done that should not have been done or nothing was done when it should have been done. This is the failure to act as a reasonable, prudent nurse under the circumstances. The standard can come from documents published by national or professional organizations, boards of nursing, institutional policies and procedures, or textbooks or journals, or it may be stated by expert witnesses.
- **Foreseeability.** A link must exist between the nurse's act and the injury suffered.
- **Causation.** It must be proved that the harm occurred as a direct result of the nurse's failure to follow the standard of care and the nurse could have (or should have) known that failure to follow the standard of care could result in such harm.
- **Harm or injury.** The client or plaintiff must demonstrate some type of harm or injury (physical, financial, or emotional) as a result of the breach of duty owed the client. The plaintiff will be asked to document physical injury, medical costs, loss of wages, "pain and suffering," and any other damages.

■ **Damages.** If malpractice caused the injury, the nurse is held liable for damages that may be compensated. The goal of awarding damages is to assist the injured party to his or her original position so far as financially possible (Guido, 2006).

CLINICAL ALERT

The best defense against a malpractice claim is to know your nursing responsibilities and the scope of practice of members of your health team (e.g., LPN/LVN, UAP). ■

Several legal doctrines or principles are related to negligence. One such doctrine is *respondeat superior*. A lawsuit for a negligent act performed by a nurse will also name the nurse's employer. In addition, employers may be held liable for negligence if they fail to provide adequate human and material resources for nursing care, fail to properly educate nurses on the use of new equipment or procedures, or fail to orient nurses to the facility. Another doctrine or principle is *res ipsa loquitur* ("the thing speaks for itself"). In some cases, the harm cannot be traced to a specific health care provider or standard but does not normally occur unless there has been a negligent act. An example is harm that results when surgical instruments or bandages are accidentally left in a client during surgery.

To defend against a malpractice lawsuit, the nurse must prove that one or more of the six required elements is not met. There is also a limit to the amount of time that can pass between recognition of harm and the bringing of a suit. This is referred to as the statute of limitations. The exact time limitation varies by type of suit and state, but typically plaintiffs have 1 to 2 years from the time that they knew of the injury or had reason to believe that an injury was sustained to file a malpractice lawsuit. In some cases, an additional defense is "contributory or comparative negligence" on the part of the injured client. In these situations, the client was at least partly responsible for his or her own injury. When clients choose not to follow health care advice, such as remaining in bed while recovering from a treatment, the court may reduce any verdict against the nurse by an amount considered to be the plaintiff's own contribution.

To avoid charges of malpractice, nurses must recognize those nursing situations in which negligent actions are most likely to occur, and take measures to prevent them (see Box 4–4). The most common situation is the *medication error*. Because of the large number of medications on the market today and the variety of methods of administration, these errors may be on the increase. Nursing errors include failing to read the medication label, misreading or incorrectly calculating the dosage, failing to correctly identify the client, preparing the wrong concentration, or administering a medication by the wrong route (e.g., intravenously instead of intramuscularly). Some medication errors are very serious and can result in death. For example, administering dicumarol, an anticoagulant, to a client recently returned from surgery could cause the client to have a hemorrhage. Nurses always must check medications very carefully. Even after checking, the nurse is wise to recheck the med-

---

BOX 4–4 Categories of Negligence that Result in Malpractice

Failure to follow standards of care, including failure to
■ Perform a complete admission assessment or design a plan of care.
■ Adhere to standardized protocols or institutional policies and procedures (e.g., using an improper injection site).
■ Follow a physician's verbal or written orders.

Failure to use equipment in a responsible manner, including failure to
■ Follow the manufacturer's recommendations for operating the equipment.
■ Check equipment for safety prior to use.
■ Place equipment properly during treatment.
■ Learn how equipment functions.

Failure to communicate, including failure to
■ Notify a physician in a timely manner when conditions warrant it.
■ Listen to a client's complaints and act on them.
■ Communicate effectively with a client (e.g., inadequate or ineffective communication of discharge instructions).
■ Seek higher medical authorization for a treatment.

Failure to document, including failure to note in the patient's medical record
■ A client's progress and response to treatment.
■ A client's injuries.
■ Pertinent nursing assessment information (e.g., drug allergies).
■ A physician's medical orders.
■ Information on telephone conversations with physicians, including time, content of communication between nurse and physician, and actions taken.

Failure to assess and monitor, including failure to
■ Complete a shift assessment.
■ Implement a plan of care.
■ Observe a client's ongoing progress.
■ Interpret a client's signs and symptoms.

Failure to act as a patient advocate, including failure to
■ Question discharge orders when a client's condition warrants it.
■ Question incomplete or illegible medical orders.
■ Provide a safe environment.

Note: From "Nurses, Negligence, and Malpractice," by E. M. Croke, 2003, *American Journal of Nursing, 103*(9), pp. 54–63.

---

ication order and the medication before administering it if the client states, for example, "I did not have a green pill before."

CLINICAL ALERT

To be a client advocate, you must know about the medications being administered. Know why the client is receiving the medication, the dosage range, possible adverse effects, toxicity levels, and contraindications. ■

Clients often fall accidentally, sometimes with resultant injury. Some falls can be prevented by elevating the side rails on the cribs, beds, and stretchers of babies and small children and, when necessary, of adults. If a nurse leaves the rails down or leaves a baby unattended on a bath table, that nurse is guilty of malpractice if the client falls and is injured as a direct result. Most hospitals and nursing homes have policies regarding the use of safety devices. The nurse needs to be familiar with these policies and to take indicated precautions to prevent injuries (see Chapter 32). ∞

CLINICAL ALERT

Assess clients for fall potential. Document all nursing measures taken to protect the client (e.g., instructed client how to use the call light). ∎

In some instances, ignoring a client's complaints can constitute malpractice. This type of malpractice is termed *failure to observe and take appropriate action*. The nurse who does not report a client's complaint of acute abdominal pain is negligent and may be found guilty of malpractice if ensuing appendix rupture and death occur. By failing to take the blood pressure and pulse and to check the dressing of a client who has just had abdominal surgery, a nurse omits important assessments. If the client hemorrhages and dies, the nurse may be held responsible for the death as a result of this malpractice.

CLINICAL ALERT

Monitor both physical and psychosocial status of the client. Document observations and interventions. ∎

Incorrectly identifying clients is a problem, particularly in busy hospital units. Unfortunate occurrences, such as removal of a healthy gallbladder from the wrong person, have resulted from nurses preparing the wrong client for surgery. Cases of *mistaken identity* are costly to the client and render the nurse liable for malpractice.

According to the National Practitioner Data Bank (NPDB), the number of nurses being named in malpractice suits is increasing (Croke, 2003; NPDB, 2004). This increase is related to several factors, including delegation of tasks to unlicensed assistive personnel (UAP), early discharge of clients, the nursing shortage, advances in technology, increased autonomy and responsibility of hospital nurses, better informed consumers, and expanded legal definitions of liability (Croke, 2003, p. 55). See Practice Guidelines later in this chapter for steps to help nurses reduce potential liability.

Intentional Torts

Several differences distinguish unintentional torts from intentional torts. Unintentional torts (e.g., negligence, malpractice) do not require intent but do require the element of harm. In contrast, with intentional torts, the defendant executed the act on purpose or with intent. No harm need be caused by intentional torts for liability to exist. Also, since no standard is involved, no expert witnesses are needed. Four intentional torts related to nursing will be discussed: assault/battery, false imprisonment, invasion of privacy, and defamation (libel/

slander). Figure 4-5 ∎ provides an overview of the types of law in nursing.

The terms *assault* and *battery* are often heard together, but each has its own meaning. **Assault** can be described as an attempt or threat to touch another person unjustifiably. Assault precedes battery; it is the act that causes the person to believe a battery is about to occur. For example, the person who threatens someone by making a menacing gesture with a club or a closed fist is guilty of assault. A nurse who threatens a client with an injection after the client refuses to take the medication orally would be committing assault.

Battery is the willful touching of a person (or the person's clothes or even something the person is carrying) that may or may not cause harm. To be actionable at law, however, the touching must be wrong in some way; for example, touching done without permission, that is embarrassing, or that causes injury. In the previous example, if the nurse followed through on the threat and gave the injection without the client's consent, the nurse would be committing battery. Liability applies even though the physician ordered the medication or the activity and even if the client benefits from the nurse's action.

Consent is required before procedures are performed. Battery exists when there is no consent, even if the plaintiff was not asked for consent. Unless there is implied consent, such as in life-threatening emergencies, a procedure performed on an unconscious client without informed consent is battery. Another requirement for consent is that the client be competent to give consent. It can be very difficult to determine if clients who are elderly, who have specific mental disorders, or who take particular medications are competent to agree to treatments. If the nurse is uncertain whether a client refusing a treatment is competent, the supervisor and physician should be consulted so that ethical treatment that does not constitute battery can be provided. Determination of competency is not a medical decision; it is one made through court hearings.

False imprisonment is the "unjustifiable detention of a person without legal warrant to confine the person" (Guido, 2006, p. 98). False imprisonment accompanied by forceful restraint or threat of restraint is battery.

Although nurses may suggest under certain circumstances that a client remain in the hospital room or in bed, the client must not be detained against the client's will. The client has a right to insist on leaving even though it may be detrimental to health. In this instance, the client can leave by signing an AWA (absence without authority) or AMA (against medical advice) form. As with assault or battery, client competency is a factor in determining whether there is a case of false imprisonment or a situation of protecting a client from injury. To guide nurses in such dilemmas, agencies usually have clear policies regarding the application of restraints (see Chapter 32). ∞

Invasion of privacy is a direct wrong of a personal nature. It injures the feelings of the person and does not take into account the effect of revealed information on the reputation of the person in the community. The right to privacy is the right of individuals to withhold themselves and their lives from public scrutiny. It can also be described as the right to be left alone. Liability can result if the nurse breaches confidentiality by

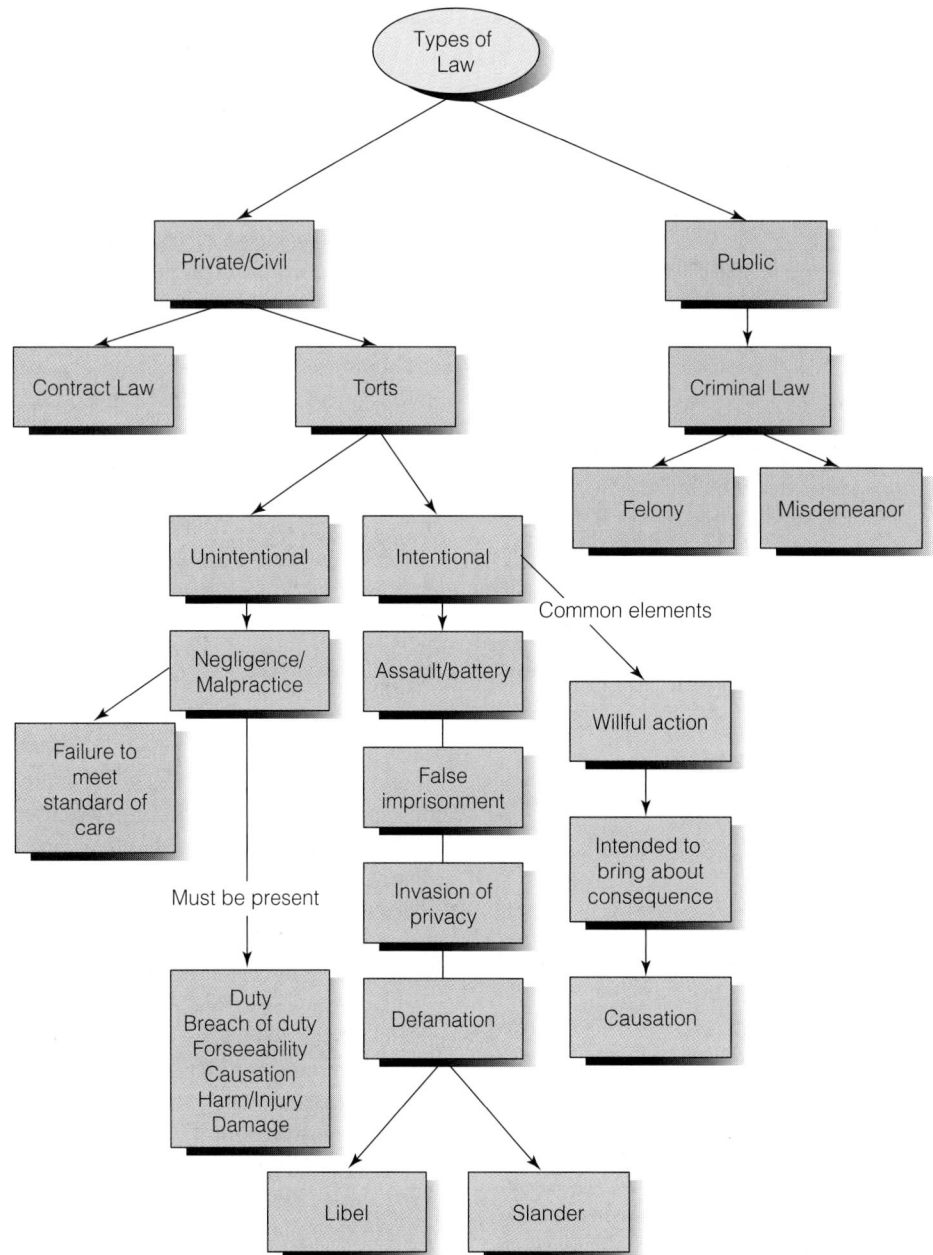

Figure 4-5 ■ An overview of the types of law in nursing practice.

passing along confidential client information to others or intrudes into the client's private domain.

In this context, there is a delicate balance between the need of a number of people to contribute to the diagnosis and treatment of a client and the client's right to confidentiality. In most situations, necessary discussion about a client's medical condition is considered appropriate, but unnecessary discussions and gossip are considered a breach of confidentiality. Necessary discussion involves only those engaged in the client's care.

Most jurisdictions of the country have a variety of statutes that impose a duty to report certain confidential client information. Four major categories are (a) vital statistics, such as births and deaths; (b) infections and communicable diseases, such as diphtheria, syphilis, and typhoid fever; (c) child or elder abuse; and (d) violent incidents, such as gunshot wounds and knife wounds.

The client must be protected from four types of invasion:

■ *Use of the client's name or likeness for profit, without consent.* This refers to use of identifiable photographs or names such as advertising for the health care agency or provider without the client's permission.

■ *Unreasonable intrusion.* This involves observation of client care (such as by nursing students) or taking of photographs for any purpose without the client's consent.

■ *Public disclosure of private facts.* Private information is given to others who have no legitimate need for that information.
■ *Putting a person in a false light.* This type of invasion involves publishing information that is normally considered offensive but which is not true.

Defamation is communication that is false, or made with a careless disregard for the truth, and results in injury to the reputation of a person. Both libel and slander are wrongful actions that come under the heading of defamation. **Libel** is defamation by means of print, writing, or pictures. Writing in the nurse's notes that a physician is incompetent because he didn't respond immediately to a call is an example of libel. **Slander** is defamation by the spoken word, stating unprivileged (not legally protected) or false words by which a reputation is damaged. An example of slander would be for the nurse to tell a client that another nurse is incompetent.

Only the person defamed may bring the lawsuit. The defamatory material must be communicated to a third party such that the person's reputation may be harmed. For example, a comment made in private criticizing that person's competence is not defamation since a third party did not hear it.

Nurses have a qualified privilege to make statements that could be considered defamatory, but only as a part of nursing practice and only to a physician or another health team member caring directly for the client. The communication must be made in good faith with the intent to protect the quality of client care—for example, when a nurse manager provides a prospective employer with information about a nurse's professional practice.

Privacy of Clients' Health Information

Protecting clients' confidentiality has always been an important responsibility of nursing. Recent changes in the laws regarding privacy have implications for health care providers and organizations. The Health Insurance Portability and Accountability Act of 1996 (HIPAA) is the first nationwide legislation to protect privacy for health information. It is important to be aware of identifying information that is protected under HIPAA but may not be initially perceived as health information. Examples include social security number, name, address, phone number, website address, and fingerprints. Wimberley et al. (2005) point out that consideration is given to age also because age becomes an identifier in the population older than age 89.

HIPAA includes four specific areas (Phoenix Health Systems, 2005):

1. *Electronic transfer of information* among organizations. Instead of each health provider using its own electronic format to transact claims, etc., HIPAA implements a national uniform standard to simplify such transactions.
2. *Standardized numbers* for identifying providers, employers, and health plans. Instead of each health care organization using different formats for identification, HIPAA published standard identifiers. For example, an employer's tax ID number or employer identification number is the standard for electronic transactions.

3. *Security rule* which provides for a uniform level of protection of all health information. This rule requires health care organizations and providers to ensure the confidentiality, integrity, and availability of all electronic protected health information (ePHI).
4. *Privacy rule* which sets standards defining appropriate disclosure of protected health information. This rule also gives clients new rights to understand and control how their health information is used (i.e., how to access their medical records, restrict access by others, request changes, and learn how they have been accessed).

See Box 4–5 for examples of how HIPAA compliance affects nursing practice.

Loss of Client Property

Loss of client property, such as jewelry, money, eyeglasses, and dentures, is a constant concern to hospital personnel. Today, agencies are taking less responsibility for property and are generally requesting clients to sign a waiver on admission relieving the hospital and its employees of any responsibility for property. Situations arise, however, in which the client cannot sign a waiver and the nursing staff must follow prescribed policies for safeguarding the client's property. Nurses are expected to take reasonable precautions to safeguard a client's property, and they can be held liable for its loss or damage if they do not exercise reasonable care.

Unprofessional Conduct

According to most nurse practice acts, unprofessional conduct is considered one of the grounds for action against the nurse's license. **Unprofessional conduct** includes incompetence or gross negligence, conviction for practicing without a license, falsification of client records, and illegally obtaining, using, or possessing controlled substances. Having a personal relationship with a client, especially a vulnerable client, may be considered unprofessional conduct because the *Code of Ethics for*

BOX 4–5 Examples of HIPAA Compliance and Nursing Practice

■ A client's name cannot be posted near or on the room door.
■ Charts should be in a secure, nonpublic location to prevent the public from viewing or accessing confidential health information.
■ Printed copies of protected health information should not be left unattended at a printer or fax machine.
■ Access to protected health information is limited to those authorized to obtain the information.
■ Health care providers will need a password to access a client's electronic chart.
■ A notice informing clients of their rights about privacy and their health information should be posted or provided.
■ Voice levels should be lowered to minimize disclosure of information (e.g., when discussing a client's condition over the telephone, giving a report, reading information aloud from a computer screen or chart).
■ Health care providers must stay current with HIPAA regulations.

Nurses states that nurses are responsible for retaining their professional boundaries (ANA, 2001, p.11). Certain acts may constitute a tort or crime in addition to being unprofessional conduct.

Unethical conduct may also be addressed in nurse practice acts. Unethical conduct includes violation of professional ethical codes, breach of confidentiality, fraud, or refusing to care for clients of specific socioeconomic or cultural origins (see Chapter 5). ∞

Nurses at all levels of nursing practice, can be reported to national data banks. The Healthcare Integrity and Protection Data Bank (HIPDB) was created for the reporting of civil judgments or criminal convictions related to health care and licensure or certification actions. Another data bank, the National Practitioner Data Bank (NPDB), was established to identify incompetent and unprofessional health care practitioners. The information in these two data banks is not accessible by the public. It can be accessed, however, by state licensing boards, HMOs, hospitals, and professional organizations. The data banks are examples of a nationwide effort to protect the public and to identify and track professionals found liable of malpractice or actions taken against their license. NPDB annual reports of group data are available at their website.

LEGAL PROTECTIONS IN NURSING PRACTICE

Laws and strategies are in place to protect the nurse against litigation. Good Samaritan acts are an example of laws designed to help protect nurses when assisting at the scene of an emergency. Providing safe, competent practice by following the nurse practice act and standards of practice is a major legal safeguard for nurses. Accurate and complete documentation is also a critical component of legal protection for the nurse.

Good Samaritan Acts

Good Samaritan acts are laws designed to protect health care providers who provide assistance at the scene of an emergency against claims of malpractice unless it can be shown that there was a gross departure from the normal standard of care or willful wrongdoing on their part. Gross negligence usually involves further injury or harm to the person. For example, an automobile may strike an injured child left on the side of the road when the nurse leaves to obtain help.

Most state statutes do not require citizens to render aid to people in distress. Such assistance is considered more of an ethical than a legal duty. To encourage citizens to be Good Samaritans, most states have now enacted legislation releasing a Good Samaritan from legal liability for injuries caused under such circumstances, even if the injuries resulted from negligence of the person offering emergency aid. It is important, however, to check your state's statute since some states (e.g., Vermont) require people to stop and aid persons in danger.

It is generally believed that a person who renders help in an emergency, at a level that would be provided by any reasonably prudent person under similar circumstances, cannot be held liable. The same reasoning applies to nurses, who are among the people best prepared to help at the scene of an accident. If the level of care a nurse provides is of the caliber that would have been provided by any other nurse, then the nurse will not be held liable.

Guidelines for nurses who choose to render emergency care are as follows:

- Limit actions to those normally considered first aid, if possible.
- Do not perform actions that you do not know how to do.
- Offer assistance, but do not insist.
- Have someone call or go for additional help.
- Do not leave the scene until the injured person leaves or another qualified person takes over.
- Do not accept any compensation.

Professional Liability Insurance

Because of the increase in the number of malpractice lawsuits against health professionals, nurses are advised to carry their own liability insurance. Most hospitals have liability insurance that covers all employees, including all nurses. However, some smaller facilities, such as walk-in clinics, may not. Thus, the nurse should always check with the employer at the time of hiring to see what coverage the facility provides. A physician or a hospital can be sued because of the negligent conduct of a nurse, and the nurse can also be sued and held liable for negligence or malpractice. Because hospitals have been known to countersue nurses when they have been found negligent and the hospital was required to pay, nurses are advised to provide their own insurance coverage and not rely on hospital-provided insurance.

Additionally, nurses often provide nursing services outside of employment-related activities, such as being available for first aid at children's sport or social activities or providing health screening and education at health fairs. Neighbors or friends may seek advice about illnesses or treatment for themselves or family members. In the latter situation, the nurse may be tempted to give advice; however, it is always advisable for the nurse to refer the friend or neighbor to their family physician. The nurse may be protected from liability under Good Samaritan acts when nursing service is volunteered; however, if the nurse receives any compensation or if there is a written or verbal agreement outlining the nurse's responsibility to the group, the nurse needs liability coverage for legal expenses in the event that the nurse is sued.

Liability insurance coverage usually defrays all costs of defending a nurse, including the costs of retaining an attorney. The insurance also covers all costs incurred by the nurse up to the face value of the policy, including a settlement made out of court. In return, the insurance company may have the right to make the decisions about the claim and the settlement.

Nursing faculty and nursing students are also vulnerable to lawsuits. Students and teachers of nursing employed by community colleges and universities are not likely to be covered by the insurance carried by hospitals and health agencies. It is advisable for nursing students to check with their school about the coverage that applies to them. Increasingly, faculty carry their own malpractice insurance. Liability insurance can be obtained through the ANA or private insurance companies. Nursing students can also obtain insurance through the National Student Nurses' Association. In some states, hospitals do not allow nursing students to provide nursing care without liability insurance or a signed disclaimer placing the responsibility of the student's actions while in the clinical setting on the student.

Carrying Out a Physician's Orders

Nurses are expected to analyze procedures and medications ordered by the physician. It is the nurse's responsibility to seek clarification of ambiguous or seemingly erroneous orders from the prescribing physician. Clarification from any other source is unacceptable and regarded as a departure from competent nursing practice.

If the order is neither ambiguous nor apparently erroneous, the nurse is responsible for carrying it out. For example, if the physician orders oxygen to be administered at 4 liters per minute, the nurse must administer oxygen at that rate, and not at 2 or 6 liters per minute. If the orders state that the client is not to have solid food after a bowel resection, the nurse must ensure that no solid food is given to the client.

There are several categories of orders that nurses must question to protect themselves legally:

■ *Question any order a client questions.* For example, if a client who has been receiving an intramuscular injection tells the nurse that the doctor changed the order from an injectable to an oral medication, the nurse must recheck the order before giving the medication.

■ *Question any order if the client's condition has changed.* The nurse is considered responsible for notifying the physician of any significant changes in the client's condition, whether the physician requests notification or not. For example, if a client who is receiving an intravenous infusion suddenly develops a rapid pulse, chest pain, and a cough, the nurse must notify the physician immediately and question continuance of the ordered rate of infusion. If a client who is receiving morphine for pain develops severely depressed respirations, the nurse must withhold the medication and notify the physician.

■ *Question and record verbal orders to avoid miscommunications.* In addition to recording the time, the date, the physician's name, and the orders, the nurse documents the circumstances that occasioned the call to the physician, reads the orders back to the physician, and documents that the physician confirmed the orders as the nurse read them back.

■ *Question any order that is illegible, unclear, or incomplete.* Misinterpretations in the name of a drug or in dose, for example, can easily occur with handwritten orders. The nurse is responsible for ensuring that the order is interpreted the way it was intended and that it is a safe and appropriate order.

Providing Competent Nursing Care

Competent practice is a major legal safeguard for nurses. Nurses need to provide care that is within the legal boundaries of their practice and within the boundaries of agency policies and procedures. Nurses therefore must be familiar with their various job descriptions, which may be different from agency to agency. Every nurse is responsible for ensuring that his or her education and experience are adequate to meet the responsibilities delineated in the job description.

Competency also involves care that protects clients from harm. Nurses need to anticipate sources of client injury, educate clients about hazards, and implement measures to prevent injury.

Application of the nursing process is another essential aspect of providing safe and effective client care. Clients need to be assessed and monitored appropriately and involved in care decisions. All assessments and care must be documented accurately. Effective communication can also protect the nurse from negligence claims. Nurses need to approach every client with sincere concern and include the client in conversations. In addition, nurses should always acknowledge when they do not know the answer to a client's questions, telling the client they will find out the answer and then follow through.

Methods of legal protection are summarized in the accompanying Practice Guidelines.

PRACTICE GUIDELINES   **Legal Protection for Nurses**

■ Function within the scope of your education, job description, and nurse practice act.
■ Follow the procedures and policies of the employing agency.
■ Build and maintain good rapport with clients.
■ Always check the identity of a client to make sure it is the right client.
■ Observe and monitor the client accurately. Communicate and record significant changes in the client's condition to the physician.
■ Promptly and accurately document all assessments and care given.
■ Be alert when implementing nursing interventions, and give each task your full attention and skill.
■ Perform procedures correctly and appropriately.

■ Make sure the correct medications are given in the correct dose, by the right route, at the scheduled time, and to the right client.
■ When delegating nursing responsibilities, make sure that the person who is delegated a task understands what to do and that the person has the required knowledge and skill.
■ Protect clients from injury.
■ Report all incidents involving clients.
■ Always check any order that a client questions.
■ Know your own strengths and weaknesses. Ask for assistance and supervision in situations for which you feel inadequately prepared.
■ Maintain your clinical competence. For students, this demands study and practice before caring for clients. For graduate nurses, it means continued study to maintain and update clinical knowledge and skills.

Documentation

The client's medical chart is a legal document and can be produced in court as evidence. Often, the chart is used to remind a witness of events surrounding a lawsuit, because several months or years usually elapse before the suit goes to trial. The effectiveness of a witness's testimony can depend on the accuracy of the nurse's documentation of nursing care. Nurses, therefore, need to provide accurate and complete documentation of the nursing care provided to clients. Failure to properly document can constitute negligence and be the basis for tort liability. Insufficient or inaccurate assessments and documentation can hinder proper diagnosis and treatment and result in injury to the client (see Figure 4-6 ■). See Chapter 15 for types of records and facts about recording. ∞

The Incident Report

An incident report (also called an unusual occurrence report) is an agency record of an accident or unusual occurrence. Incident reports are used to make all the facts available to agency personnel, to contribute to statistical data about accidents or incidents, and to help health personnel prevent future incidents or accidents. All accidents are usually reported on incident forms. Some agencies also report other incidents, such as the occurrence of client infection or the loss of personal effects.

The nurse includes the following information in an incident report:

- Identify the client by name, initials, and hospital or identification number.
- Give the date, time, and place of the incident.
- Describe the facts of the incident. Avoid any conclusions or blame. Describe the incident as you saw it even if your impressions differ from those of others.
- Incorporate the client's account of the incident. State the client's comments by using direct quotes.
- Identify all witnesses to the incident.
- Identify any equipment by number and any medication by name and dosage.

Figure 4-6 ■ Clear and accurate documentation is the nurse's best defense against potential liability.

The report should be completed as soon as possible and filed according to agency policy. Because incident reports are not part of the client's medical record, the facts of the incident should also be noted in the medical record. Do not record in the client record that an incident report has been completed because the facts are already documented in the chart. The purpose of the report form is to alert the risk manager to the event.

The person who identifies that the incident occurred should complete the incident report. This may not be the same person actually involved with the incident. For example, the nurse who discovers that an incorrect medication has been administered completes the form even if it was another nurse who administered the medication. In addition, all witnesses to an incident, such as a client fall, are listed on the incident form even if they were not directly involved.

Incident reports are often reviewed by an agency risk management committee, which decides whether to investigate the incident further. Nurses may be required to answer such questions as what they believe precipitated the accident, how it could have been prevented, and whether any equipment should be adjusted.

When an accident occurs, the nurse should first assess the client and intervene to prevent injury. If a client is injured, nurses must take steps to protect the client, themselves, and their employer. Most agencies have policies regarding accidents. It is important to follow these policies and not to assume one is negligent. Although negligence may be involved, accidents can and do happen even when every precaution has been taken to prevent them.

REPORTING CRIMES, TORTS, AND UNSAFE PRACTICES

Nurses may need to report nursing colleagues or other health professionals for practices that endanger the health and safety of clients. For instance, alcohol and drug use, theft from a client or agency, and unsafe nursing practice should be reported. Reporting a colleague is not easy. The person reporting may feel disloyal, incur the disapproval of others, or perceive chances for promotion are endangered. When reporting an incident or series of incidents, the nurse must be careful to describe observed behavior only and not make inferences as to what might be happening. The accompanying Practice Guidelines box can be used for reporting a crime, tort, or unsafe practice.

Reporting these events is referred to as "whistle-blowing." Many states have laws that prevent wrongful termination of whistle-blowers by employers. In some states, it is mandatory for a nurse with knowledge of unprofessional conduct to report that behavior to the state board of nursing. In addition, reporting illegal, unethical, or incompetent performance is an expectation found in the ANA code of ethics.

LEGAL RESPONSIBILITIES OF STUDENTS

Nursing students are responsible for their own actions and liable for their own acts of negligence committed during the course of

PRACTICE GUIDELINES
Reporting a Crime, Tort, or Unsafe Practice

- Write a clear description of the situation you believe you should report.
- Make sure that your statements are factual and complete.
- Make sure you are credible.
- Obtain support from at least one trustworthy person before filing the report.
- Report the matter starting at the lowest possible level in the agency hierarchy.
- Assume responsibility for reporting the individual by being open about it. Sign your name to the letter.
- See the problem through once you have reported it.

clinical experiences. When they perform duties that are within the scope of professional nursing, such as administering an injection, they are legally held to the same standard of skill and competence as a registered professional nurse. Lower standards are not applied to the actions of nursing students.

CLINICAL ALERT

Students do not practice on their instructor's or another nurse's license. Each nurse and nursing student is responsible and accountable for providing safe client care. ■

Nursing students are not considered employees of the agencies in which they receive clinical experience because these nursing programs contract with agencies to provide clinical experiences for students. In cases of negligence involving such students, the hospital or agency (e.g., public health agency) and the educational institution will be held potentially liable for neg-

ligent actions by students. Some nursing schools require students to carry individual professional liability insurance.

Nursing students need to be aware that most state boards of nursing require a reporting of prior criminal history when applying for licensure. A person with past felony and some misdemeanor offenses may be denied licensure even though that individual graduated from an approved nursing program. Nursing students who are unsure of their personal situation are advised to contact their state board of nursing for more information.

Students in clinical situations must be assigned learning experiences within their capabilities and be given reasonable guidance and supervision. Nursing instructors are responsible for assigning students to the care of clients and for providing reasonable supervision. Failure to provide reasonable supervision or the assignment of a client to a student who is not prepared and competent can be a basis for liability.

To fulfill responsibilities to clients and to minimize chances for liability, nursing students need to:

- Make sure they are prepared to carry out the necessary care for assigned clients.
- Ask for additional help or supervision in situations for which they feel inadequately prepared.
- Comply with the policies of the agency in which they obtain their clinical experience.
- Comply with the policies and definitions of responsibility supplied by the school of nursing.

Students who work as part-time or temporary nursing assistants or aides must also remember that legally they can perform only those tasks that appear in the job description of a nurse's aide or assistant. Even though a student may have received instruction and acquired competence in administering injections or suctioning a tracheostomy tube, the student cannot legally perform these tasks while employed as an aide or assistant. While acting as a paid employee, the student is covered for negligent acts by the employer, not the school of nursing.

LIFESPAN CONSIDERATIONS The Omnibus Budget Reconciliation Act

CHILDREN

The Omnibus Budget Reconciliation Act of 1993 (OBRA 93) created the Pediatric Vaccine Distribution Program (known as Vaccines for Children [VFC] Program). States are required to establish a program for purchase and distribution of pediatric vaccines to program-registered providers. These providers, in turn, immunize certain specified groups of children without charge for the vaccine. Children specified under the law must be 18 years or younger, eligible for Medicaid, uninsured by any form of health insurance, uninsured for the vaccines, recipients of vaccines from a federally qualified or rural health clinic, or Native American Indians.

ELDERS

The Omnibus Budget Reconciliation Act (OBRA) was passed in 1990 and lists requirements for ensuring quality of care in skilled nursing facilities. These requirements mainly affect elders, but also pertain to any resident in a long-term or skilled nursing facility. These standards were developed to enhance the quality of life of each resident and to focus on achieving the highest practical physical, mental, and psy-

chosocial well-being for residents of these facilities. Some of the important requirements from OBRA include the following:

- A quality assessment and assurance committee must meet at least quarterly to discuss the resident's condition and make appropriate revisions.
- A physician is to visit every 30 days for 3 months, and then every 90 days.
- The facility must employ a registered nurse who works there 40 hours a week.
- Rehabilitation services and activities must be available for each resident.
- Nurse aides must have special training and also be given information concerning abuse and neglect.
- Social work requirements were increased.
- The use of psychotropic drugs is strictly monitored and reevaluated at regular intervals. Documentation of behaviors is required to support the need for prescribing these drugs.
- Residents' rights must be recognized and honored.

CRITICAL THINKING CHECKPOINT

A female adult client, who has been blind since birth, is admitted to the surgical unit. She is to have surgery the next morning. The physician has written an order for the client to sign the surgical consent form. The husband is in the client's room when the nurse approaches the client to sign the consent form. The husband says that he will sign for his wife.

1. What question(s) should the nurse ask before addressing the signing of the form?

2. Can someone who is blind give consent?
3. How can the nurse ensure that the client is aware of what she is signing?
4. What else should the nurse consider when obtaining a signature?
5. What would the nurse include in the documentation?

See Critical Thinking Possibilities in Appendix A.

CHAPTER 4 **REVIEW**

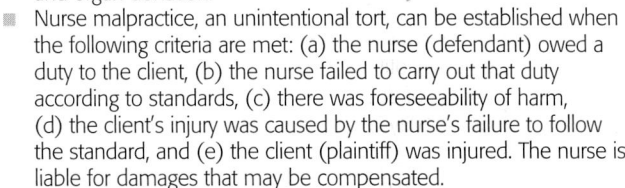

CHAPTER HIGHLIGHTS

- Accountability is an essential concept of professional nursing practice under the law.
- Nurses need to understand laws that regulate and affect nursing practice to ensure that the nurses' actions are consistent with current legal principles and to protect themselves from liability.
- Nurse practice acts legally define and describe the scope of nursing practice that the law seeks to regulate.
- Competence in nursing practice is determined and maintained by various credentialing methods, such as licensure, certification, and accreditation, that protect the public's welfare and safety.
- Standards of practice published by national and state nursing associations, agency policies and procedures, and job descriptions further delineate the scope of a nurse's practice.
- The nurse has specific legal obligations and responsibilities to clients and employers. As a citizen, the nurse has the rights and responsibilities shared by all individuals in the society.
- Collective bargaining is one way nurses can improve their working conditions and economic welfare.
- Informed consent implies that (a) the consent was given voluntarily, (b) the client was of age and had the capacity and competency to understand, and (c) the client was given enough information on which to make an informed decision.
- The Americans with Disabilities Act of 1990 prohibits discrimination on the basis of disability in employment, public services, and public accommodations. Nurses need to know how the ADA affects nursing practice.
- Chemical dependence in health care workers is a problem, in part, because of the high levels of stress involved in many health care settings and the easy access to addictive drugs. Chemical impairment includes abuse of alcohol and addictive drugs. The nurse needs to know the proper reporting of nursing colleagues whose practice is chemically impaired.
- Nurses must be knowledgeable of their responsibilities about legal issues surrounding death: advance directives, autopsies, certification of death, DNR orders, euthanasia, inquests, and organ donation.
- Nurse malpractice, an unintentional tort, can be established when the following criteria are met: (a) the nurse (defendant) owed a duty to the client, (b) the nurse failed to carry out that duty according to standards, (c) there was foreseeability of harm, (d) the client's injury was caused by the nurse's failure to follow the standard, and (e) the client (plaintiff) was injured. The nurse is liable for damages that may be compensated.
- Nurses can be held liable for intentional torts, such as assault and battery, false imprisonment, invasion of privacy, and defamation.
- The Health Insurance Portability and Accountability Act of 1996 (HIPAA) is the first nationwide legislation to protect privacy for health information. HIPAA includes four specific areas: a uniform standard for electronic transfer of information among organizations; standardized numbers for identifying providers, employers, and health plans; a security rule; and a privacy rule.
- Good Samaritan acts protect health professionals from claims of malpractice when they offer assistance at the scene of an emergency, provided that there is no willful wrongdoing or gross departure from normal standards of care.
- Nursing students and practicing nurses can obtain professional liability insurance through professional nursing associations.
- When a client is accidentally injured or involved in an unusual situation, the nurse's first responsibility is to take steps to protect the client and then to notify appropriate agency personnel.
- Nursing students are held to the same standard as licensed nurses and, therefore, need to make certain that they are prepared to provide the necessary care to assigned clients. It is important that students ask for help or supervision in situations for which they feel inadequately prepared.

TEST YOUR KNOWLEDGE

1. A primary care provider's orders indicate that a surgical consent form needs to be signed. Since the nurse was not present when the primary care provider discussed the surgical procedure, which statement best illustrates the nurse fulfilling the client advocate role?

1. "The doctor has asked that you sign this consent form."
2. "Do you have any questions about the procedure?"
3. "What were you told about the procedure you are going to have?"
4. "Remember that you can change your mind and cancel the procedure."

2. Although the client refused the procedure, the nurse insisted and inserted a nasogastric tube in the right nostril. The administrator of the hospital decides to settle the lawsuit because the nurse is most likely to be found guilty of which of the following?
   1. An unintentional tort
   2. Assault
   3. Invasion of privacy
   4. Battery

3. A nurse discovers that a primary care provider has prescribed an unusually large dosage of a medication. Which of the following is the most appropriate action?
   1. Administer the medication.
   2. Notify the prescriber.
   3. Call the pharmacist.
   4. Refuse to administer the medication.

4. A primary care provider prescribes one tablet, but the nurse accidently administers two. After notifying the primary care provider, the nurse monitors the client carefully for untoward effects of which there are none. Is the client likely to be successful in suing the nurse for malpractice?
   1. No, the client was not harmed.
   2. No, the nurse notified the physician.
   3. Yes, a breach of duty exists.
   4. Yes, foreseeability is present.

5. A nursing student is employed and working as an unlicensed assistive personnel (UAP) on a busy surgical unit. The nurses know that the UAP is enrolled in a nursing program and will be graduating soon. A nurse asks the UAP if he has performed a urinary catheterization on clients while in the nursing program. When the UAP says "Yes," the nurse asks him to help her out by doing a urinary catheterization on a postsurgical client. What is the best response by the UAP?
   1. "Let me get permission from the client first."
   2. "Sure. Which client is it?"
   3. "I can't do it unless you supervise me."
   4. "I can't do it. Is there something else I can help you with?"

6. The primary care provider wrote a do not resuscitate (DNR) order. The nurse recognizes that which of the following applies in the planning of nursing care for this client?
   1. The client may no longer make decisions regarding his or her own health care.
   2. The client and family know that the client will most likely die within the next 48 hours.

3. The nurses will continue to implement all treatments focused on comfort and symptom management.
4. A DNR order from a previous admission is valid for the current admission.

7. The nurse's partner/spouse undergoes exploratory surgery at the hospital where the nurse is employed. Which of the following practices is most appropriate?
   1. Because the nurse is an employee, access to the chart is allowed.
   2. The relationship with the client provides the nurse special access to the chart.
   3. Access to the chart requires a signed release form.
   4. The nurse can ask the surgeon to discuss the outcome of the surgery.

8. Following a motor vehicle accident, a nurse stops and offers assistance. Which of the following actions is/are most appropriate? Select all that apply.
   1. The nurse needs to know the Good Samaritan Act for the state.
   2. The nurse is not held liable unless there is gross negligence.
   3. After assessing the situation, the nurse can leave to obtain help.
   4. The nurse can expect compensation for helping.
   5. The nurse offers to help but cannot insist on helping.

9. The nurse notices that a colleague's behaviors have changed during the past month. Which of the following behaviors could indicate signs of impairment? Select all that apply.
   1. Increased absences from the nursing unit during the shift
   2. Interacts well with others
   3. "Forgets" to sign out for administration of controlled substances
   4. Offers to administer prn opioids for other nurse's clients
   5. Is able to say "no" to requests to work more shifts

10. Which of the following nursing actions could result in malpractice? Select all that apply.
    1. Learns about a new piece of equipment
    2. Forgets to complete the assessment of a client
    3. Does not follow up on client's complaints
    4. Charts client's drug allergies
    5. Questions physician about an illegible order

See Answers to Test Your Knowledge in Appendix A.

EXPLORE MEDIALINK www.prenhall.com/berman

DVD-ROM
- Audio Glossary
- NCLEX Review
- Video:
  Understanding Legal and Ethical Issues
  Collective Bargaining

COMPANION WEBSITE
- Additional NCLEX Review
- Case Study: Legal Aspects of Obstetrics
- Application Activities:
  Nurse Practice Act
  Collective Bargaining
  Good Samaritan Act

READINGS AND REFERENCES

SUGGESTED READINGS

Croke, E. M. (2003). Nurses, negligence, and malpractice. *American Journal of Nursing, 103*(9), 54–63. *The author analyzed over 250 malpractice cases against nurses, including the actions and issues that caused the charge of negligence and the practice areas of nursing cited most frequently. The article describes several factors that contribute to the increasing number of malpractice suits, the major categories that result in malpractice suits, and steps to reduce the nurse's potential liability.*

Priest, C. (2005). Held liable. *Reflections on Nursing Leadership, 31*(1), 20–22, 36. *The concept of client advocacy, including assertive communication, is expected nursing practice in the Western Hemisphere. The author reviews studies documenting cultural differences among countries in the way nurses perceive their duties. The article points out that the majority of non-U.S. graduates working in the United States were trained in countries where assertive advocacy and clients' rights are not usual expectations of the nurse's role. As a result, the foreign graduate nurses may find themselves in a legal and cultural dilemma. The article concludes with ideas to resolve this dilemma and maintain a safe environment for client care.*

Reynolds, P. (2004). The keys to identity. *Health Management Technology, 25*(12), 12–16. *The article addresses how the need for HIPAA-compliancy and client privacy concerns is causing health care organizations to adopt greater security standards. The pros and cons of the following six biometric technologies are described: hand geometry verification, fingerprint verification, iris recognition, facial recognition, voice verification, and signature verification.*

RELATED RESEARCH

Johnson, C. E., Dobalian, A., Burkhard, J., Hedgecock, D. K., & Harman, J. (2004). Factors predicting lawsuits against nursing homes in Florida 1997–2001. *Gerontologist, 44*(3), 339–347.

Lipson, A. R., Hausman, A. J., Higgins, P. A., & Burant, C. J. (2004). Knowledge, attitudes, and predictors of advance directive discussions of registered nurses. *Western Journal of Nursing Research, 26*(7), 784.

REFERENCES

American Nurses Association. (1997). *The American Nurses Association position statement on registered nurse utilization of unlicensed personnel.* Kansas City, MO: Author. Retrieved June 20, 2006, from http://www.nursingworld.org/readroom/position/uap/uapuse.htm

American Nurses Association. (2001). *Code of ethics for nurses with interpretive statements.* Washington, DC: Author.

American Nurses Association. (2003). *Position statement on nursing care and do-not-resuscitate (DNR) decisions.* Retrieved April 30, 2006, from http://nursingworld.org/readroom/position/ethics/etdnr.htm

Blair, P. D. (2002). Report impaired practice—stat. *Nursing Management, 33*(1), 24–25.

Brent, N. J. (2001). *Nurses and the law* (2nd ed.). Philadelphia: W. B. Saunders.

Crane, P. B., Cody, M., & McSweeney, J. C. (2004). Informed consent. A process to facilitate older adults' participation in research. *Journal of Gerontological Nursing, 30*(4), 40–44.

Danis, S. J. (2004). The impaired nurse. *Nursing Spectrum.* Retrieved April 29, 2006, from http://www2.nursingspectrum.com/CE/Self-Study_modules/syllabus.html?ID=251

Department of Human Services, Health Services, State of Oregon. (2005). *Seventh annual report on Oregon's Death with Dignity Act.* Retrieved April 30, 2006, from http://www.oregon.gov/DHS/ph/pas/docs/year7.pdf

Equal Employment Opportunity Commission. (2000). *Guidelines on discrimination because of sex* (Section 1604.11, Sexual harassment. Code of Federal Regulations, Title 29, Vol. 4). Retrieved April 29, 2006, from http://www.access.gpo.gov/nara/cfr/waisidx_99/29cfr1604_99.html

Greenberg, M. E. (2000). The domain of telenursing: Issues and prospects. *Nursing Economics, 18*(4), 220–222.

Guido, G. W. (2006). *Legal and ethical issues in nursing* (4th ed.). Upper Saddle River, NJ: Prentice Hall.

Higginbotham, E. (2003). How to overcome a language barrier. *RN, 66*(10), 67–69.

Intervention Project for Nurses (IPN). (2005). *Intervention project for nurses.* Retrieved April 29, 2006, from http://www.ipnfl.org

National Council of State Boards of Nursing. (1995). *Delegation concepts and decision-making process.* Retrieved June 5, 2006, from http://www.ncsbn.org/resources/complimentary_ncsbn_Delegation_asp

National Council of State Boards of Nursing. (2004). *Nurse licensure compact.* Retrieved April 29, 2006, from http://www.ncsbn.org/nlc/index.asp

National Practitioner Data Bank. (2004). *NPDB 2003 annual report.* Retrieved April 29, 2006, from http://www.npdb-hipdb.com/pubs/stats/2004_NPDB_Annual_Report.pdf

Phoenix Health Systems. (2005). *HIPAA primer.* Retrieved April 29, 2006, from http://www.hipaadvisory.com/regs/HIPAAprimer.htm

Quallich, S. A. (2005). The practice of informed consent. *Dermatology Nursing, 17*(1), 49–51.

Sheehan, J. P. (2001). Legally speaking: Delegating to UAPs—a practical guide. *RN, 64*(11), 65–66.

Sloan, A. (2001). Legally speaking: The national data bank nurses need to know about. *RN, 64*(7), 65–69.

Texas Nurses Foundation/Texas Nurses Association. (2004). *Warning signs.* Retrieved April 29, 2006, from http://www.texasnurses.org/tpapn/warningsigns.htm

Trossman, S. (2003). Nurses' addictions. *American Journal of Nursing, 103*(9), 27–28.

Watson, P. G. (2000). The Americans with Disabilities Act: More rights for people with disabilities. *Rehabilitation Nursing, 25*(4), 145–147.

Wimberley, P., Isaacson, J., Walden, D., Wiggins, N., Miller, R., & Stacy, A. (2005). HIPAA and nursing education: How to teach in a paranoid health care environment. *Journal of Nursing Education, 44*(11), 489–492.

Zimmermann, P. G., & Jackson, M. (2004). Delegating to unlicensed assistive personnel. *Nursing Spectrum.* Retrieved April 29, 2006, from http://www2.nursingspectrum.com/CE/Self-Study_modules/syllabus.html?ID=42

SELECTED BIBLIOGRAPHY

Austin, S. (2004). Respect the scope of your license and practice. *Nursing Management, 35*(12), 18, 20, 89.

Berry, M. (2004). Saying the right thing when things go wrong. *RN, 67*(4), 59, 61, 63.

Brous, E. A. (2004). 7 tips on avoiding malpractice claims. *Nursing, 34*(6), 16–18.

Brown, B. (2003). The history of advance directives. A literature review. *Journal of Gerontological Nursing, 29*(9), 4–14.

Clark, A. P. (2004). What's all the HIPAA hype? Source book for Advanced Practice Nurses, 6–7, 10–11.

DiBenedetto, D. V. (2003). Ensuring safe nursing practice across state lines. *Continuing Care, 22*(5), 18–19.

Dowd, S., & Davidhizar, R. (2003). Sexuality, sexual harassment, and sexual humor: Guidelines for the workplace in health care. *Health Care Manager, 22*(2), 144–151.

Fletcher, C. E. (2004). Experience with peer assistance for impaired nurses in Michigan. *Journal of Nursing Scholarship, 36*(1), 92–93.

Frank-Stromberg, M. (2002). How HIPAA will change your practice. *Nursing, 32*(9), 54–57.

Gallagher, P. M. (2004). Maintain privacy with electronic charting. *Nursing Management, 35*(2), 16–17.

Garvis, M. S. (2003). Staying safe when understaffed. *RN, 66*(12), 67–69.

Grace, P. J., & McLaughlin, M. (2005). When consent isn't informed enough. *American Journal of Nursing, 105*(4), 79–84.

Hodge, J. G., & Gostin, K. G. (2004). Challenging themes in American health information privacy and the public's health: Historical and modern assessments. *Journal of Law, Medicine & Ethics, 32*(4), 670–679.

Klein, C. A. (2004). When patients refuse treatment. *Nurse Practitioner, 29*(3), 43.

Leech, E. E. (2005). When your patient threatens to walk. *RN, 68*(9), 56–59.

National Council of State Boards of Nursing. (2004). *Frequently asked questions regarding the National Council of State Boards of Nursing (NCSBN) nurse licensure compact (NLC).* Retrieved April 29, 2006, from http://www.ncsbn.org/pdfs/FrequentlyAskedQuestions.pdf

National Council of State Boards of Nursing. (2004). *Nurse licensure compact.* Retrieved April 29, 2006, from http://www.ncsbn.org/nlc/rnlpvncompact_mutual_recognition_nurse.asp

Nelson, R. (2005). Nurses with disabilities. *American Journal of Nursing, 105*(6), 25–26.

Quallich, S. A. (2004). The practice of informed consent. *Urologic Nursing, 24*(6), 513–515.

Ryan, B. (2004). Advance directives: Your role. *RN, 67*(5), 59–62.

Showers, J. L. (2000). What you need to know about negligence lawsuits. *Nursing, 30*(2), 45–48.

Sullivan, G. H. (2003). Incident reports are a must. *RN, 66*(11), 71–73.

U.S. Department of Health & Human Services. (2003). *Protecting the privacy of patients' health information.* Retrieved April 29, 2006, from http://www.hhs.gov/news/facts/privacy.html

Valente, S. M., & Bullough, V. (2004). Sexual harassment of nurses in the workplace. *Journal of Nursing Care Quality, 19*(3), 234–241.

Weiss, B. (2005). Winning the battle with addiction. *RN, 68*(7), 63–66.

Wirshing, D. A., Sergi, M.J., & Mintz, J. (2005). A videotape intervention to enhance the informed consent process for medical and psychiatric treatment research. *American Journal of Psychiatry, 162*(1), 186–188.

Values, Ethics, and Advocacy

LEARNING OUTCOMES

After completing this chapter, you will be able to:

1. Explain how cognitive development, values, moral frameworks, and codes of ethics affect moral decisions.

2. Explain how nurses use knowledge of values to make ethical decisions and facilitate ethical decision making by clients.

3. When presented with an ethical situation, identify the moral issues and principles involved.

4. Explain the uses and limitations of professional codes of ethics.

5. Discuss common ethical issues currently facing health care professionals.

6. Describe ways in which nurses can enhance their ethical decision making and practice.

7. Discuss the advocacy role of the nurse.

In their daily work, nurses deal with intimate and fundamental human events such as birth, death, and suffering. They must decide the morality of their own actions when they face the many ethical issues that surround such sensitive areas. Because of the special nurse–client relationship, nurses are the ones who are there to support and advocate for clients and families who are facing difficult choices, and for those who are living the results of choices that others make for and about them.

The present environment of cost containment and the nursing shortage tends to emphasize business values. This creates new moral problems and intensifies old ones, making it more critical than ever for nurses to make sound moral decisions. Therefore, nurses need to (a) develop sensitivity to the ethical dimensions of nursing practice, (b) examine their own and clients' values, (c) understand how values influence their decisions, and (d) think ahead about the kinds of moral problems they are likely to face. This chapter explores the influences of values and moral frameworks on the ethical dimensions of nursing practice and on the nurse's role as a client advocate.

VALUES

Values are enduring beliefs or attitudes about the worth of a person, object, idea, or action. Values are important because they influence decisions and actions, including nurses' ethical decision making. Even though they may be unspoken and perhaps even unconsciously held, questions of value underlie all moral dilemmas. Of course, not all values are moral values. For example, people hold values about work, family, religion, politics, money, and relationships, to name just a few. Values are often taken for granted. In the same way that people are not aware of their breathing, they usually do not think about their values; they simply accept them and act on them.

A **value set** is the small group of values held by an individual. People organize their set of values internally along a continuum from most important to least important, forming a **value system.** Value systems are basic to a way of life, give direction to life, and form the basis of behavior—especially behavior that is based on decisions or choices.

Values consist of beliefs and attitudes, which are related, but not identical, to values. People have many different beliefs and attitudes, but only a small number of values. **Beliefs** (or opinions) are interpretations or conclusions that people accept as true. They are based more on faith than fact and may or may not be true. Beliefs do not necessarily involve values. For example, the statement "If I study hard I will get a good grade" expresses a belief that does not involve a value. By contrast, the statement "Good grades are really important to me. I must study hard to obtain good grades" involves both a value and a belief.

Attitudes are mental positions or feelings toward a person, object, or idea (e.g., acceptance, compassion, openness). Typically, an attitude lasts over time, whereas a belief may last only briefly. Attitudes are often judged as bad or good, positive or negative, whereas beliefs are judged as correct or incorrect. Attitudes have thinking and behavioral aspects. Attitudes vary greatly among individuals. For example, some clients may feel strongly about their need for privacy, whereas others may dismiss it as unimportant.

Values Transmission

Values are learned through observation and experience. As a result, they are heavily influenced by a person's sociocultural environment—that is, by societal traditions; by cultural, ethnic, and religious groups; and by family and peer groups. For example, if a parent consistently demonstrates honesty in dealing with others, the child will probably begin to value honesty. Nurses should keep in mind the influence of values on health (see Chapter 17 ∞). For example, some cultures value treatment by a folk healer over that by a physician. For additional information about cultural values related to health and illness, see Chapter 18. ∞

Personal Values

Although people derive values from society and their individual subgroups, they internalize some or all of these values and perceive them as **personal values.** People need societal values to feel accepted, and they need personal values to have a sense of individuality.

TABLE 5–1 Essential Nursing Values and Behaviors

VALUES	PROFESSIONAL BEHAVIORS
Altruism is a concern for the welfare and well-being of others. In professional practice, altruism is reflected by the nurse's concern for the welfare of patients, other nurses, and other health care providers. *Autonomy* is the right to self-determination. Professional practice reflects autonomy when the nurse respects patients' rights to make decisions about their health care. *Human dignity* is respect for the inherent worth and uniqueness of individuals and populations. In professional practice, human dignity is reflected when the nurse values and respects all patients and colleagues. *Integrity* is acting in accordance with an appropriate code of ethics and accepted standards of practice. Integrity is reflected in professional practice when the nurse is honest and provides care based on an ethical framework that is accepted within the profession. *Social justice* is upholding moral, legal, and humanistic principles. This value is reflected in professional practice when the nurse works to ensure equal treatment under the law and equal access to quality health care.	■ Demonstrates understanding of cultures, beliefs, and perspectives of others. ■ Advocates for patients, particularly the most vulnerable. ■ Takes risks on behalf of patients and colleagues. ■ Mentors other professionals. ■ Plans care in partnership with patients. ■ Honors the right of patients and families to make decisions about health care. ■ Provides information so patients can make informed choices. ■ Provides culturally competent and sensitive care. ■ Protects the patient's privacy. ■ Preserves the confidentiality of patients and health care providers. ■ Designs care with sensitivity to individual patient needs. ■ Provides honest information to patients and the public. ■ Documents care accurately and honestly. ■ Seeks to remedy errors made by self or others. ■ Demonstrates accountability for own actions. ■ Supports fairness and nondiscrimination in the delivery of care. ■ Promotes universal access to health care. ■ Encourages legislation and policy consistent with the advancement of nursing care and health care.

Note: From *The Essentials of Baccalaureate Education for Professional Nursing Practice* (pp. 8–9), American Association of Colleges of Nursing, 1998, Washington, DC. Reprinted with permission.

Professional Values

Nurses' **professional values** are acquired during socialization into nursing from codes of ethics, nursing experiences, teachers, and peers. The American Association of Colleges of Nursing (AACN, 1998) identified five values essential for the professional nurse: altruism, autonomy, human dignity, integrity, and social justice. Table 5–1 lists the values and professional behaviors associated with these values.

Values Clarification

Values clarification is a process by which people identify, examine, and develop their own individual values. A principle of values clarification is that no one set of values is right for everyone. When people can identify their values, they can retain or change them and thus act based on freely chosen, rather than unconscious, values. Values clarification promotes personal growth by fostering awareness, empathy, and insight. Therefore, it is an important step for nurses to take in dealing with ethical problems.

One widely used theory of values clarification was developed by Raths, Harmin, and Simon (1978). They described a "valuing process" of thinking, feeling, and behavior that they termed "choosing," "prizing," and "acting" (see Box 5–1). Often, values clarification is an internal process not apparent to the person. In some cases, a values clarification exercise can be useful in helping individuals or groups to become more aware of their values and how they may influence their actions. For example, asking a client to agree or disagree with a list of statements or to rank in order of importance a list of beliefs can assist the nurse and client

to make the client's values more open so they can be considered in planning the client's care. See Table 5–2 for an example of a general values clarification exercise.

BOX 5–1 Values Clarification

Choosing (cognitive)   Beliefs are chosen
- Freely, without outside pressure
- From among alternatives
- After reflecting and considering consequences

Example: A person learns about energy resources, production, and consumption; the greenhouse effect; and other environmental issues, including ways to minimize use of and to recycle limited resources.

Prizing (affective)   Chosen beliefs are prized and cherished

Example: The person is proud of the belief that he or she has an obligation to participate in some way in reducing environmental waste.

Acting (behavioral)   Chosen beliefs are
- Affirmed to others
- Incorporated into one's behavior
- Repeated consistently in one's life

Example: The person participates in the city recycling program for household waste, uses public transportation rather than driving a personal car when possible, helps organize recycling in the workplace, and is active in legislative and political activities related to environmental issues.

Note: From *Values and Teaching*, 2nd ed. (p. 47), by L. Raths, M. Harmin, and S. Simon, copyright 1978. Adapted and reprinted with permission of the authors.

Clarifying the Nurse's Values

Nurses and nursing students need to examine the values they hold about life, death, health, and illness. One strategy for gaining awareness of personal values is to consider one's attitudes about specific issues such as abortion or euthanasia, asking: "Can I accept this, or live with this?" "Why does this bother me?" "What would I do or want done in this situation?" Nurses use critical thinking (see Chapter 10 ∞) to reflect on various viewpoints and previous experiences that may have influenced their own current values.

TABLE 5–2   Questionnaire for Values Clarification

1 = Things I value very much   2 = Things I value   3 = Things I don't value very much

	Help Society	Do something which contributes to improving the world we live in
	Help Others	Be directly included in helping other people, either individually or in small groups
	Work Ethics	Feeling satisfied from a job well done
	Enjoyment of Life	Enjoying life, having fun in life
	Honesty	Being able to tell people what I really think and believe; having them be honest with me.
	Approval	Having other people like me
	Competition	Engage in activities which pit my abilities against others
	Make Decisions	Have the power to decide courses of action
	Respect	Having other people think highly of me and hold me in good esteem
	Leadership	Be in a position to influence the attitudes or opinions of other people
	Knowledge	Understanding gained through study and/or experience
	Work Mastery	Become an expert in whatever work I do
	Peace	Living in a peaceful, harmonious society and environment
	Creativity	Have the opportunity to create new things, ideas, products, works of art
	Freedom	Being able to do or say what I want.
	Good Character	Knowing inside that I do the right, moral, just thing
	Loyalty	Sticking with people who are close to me and/or believe what I do
	Justice	Being fair and just and having others treat me fairly and justly
	Stability	Have a routine and duties that are largely predictable
	Safety	Be assured of being safe and free from harm
	Recognition	Be publicly recognized
	Children	Having happy, healthy children
	Excitement	Experience a high degree of (or frequent) excitement
	Adventure	Have duties which require frequent risk-taking
	Power	Having authority over others
	Economic Security	Having enough money to buy whatever I want.
	Leisure	Having time for hobbies, sports, other activities
	Inner harmony	Being at peace with one's self
	Wealth	Profit, gain, making a lot of money
	Trustworthiness	Having people trust me and being able to trust them
	Challenge	Do activities that use my physical and/or mental capabilities
	Independence	Be able to determine the nature of my day without significant direction from others
	Change and Variety	Varied, frequently changing responsibilities and settings
	Moral Fulfillment	Feel that whatever I do contributes to a set of moral standards that I feel are very important
	Community	Being a part of a close and supportive community
	Caring	Experiencing love and affection daily
	Health	Being free from disease or sickness, feeling good physically
	Religion/Spirituality	Doing what's right according to my religious and/or spiritual beliefs
	Family	Making sure my family members are healthy and safe
	Friendship	Having good, reliable friends I can count on

Now, list your top five essential values (from those rated 1 above).

MY 5 MOST ESSENTIAL VALUES
1.   4.
2.   5.
3.

Note: (From Johns Hopkins University Center for Communication Programs.)

Clarifying Client Values

To plan effective care, nurses need to identify clients' values as they influence and relate to a particular health problem. For example, a client with failing eyesight will probably place a high value on the ability to see, and a client with chronic pain will value comfort. Normally, people take such things for granted. For information about health beliefs and values, see Chapter 17. ∞ When clients hold unclear or conflicting values that are detrimental to their health, the nurse should use values clarification as an intervention. Examples of behaviors that may indicate the need for clarification of health values are listed in Table 5–3.

The following process may help clients clarify their values.

1. *List alternatives.* Make sure that the client is aware of all alternative actions. Ask "Are you considering other courses of action?" "Tell me about them."
2. *Examine possible consequences of choices.* Make sure the client has thought about possible results of each action. Ask "What do you think you will gain from doing that?" "What benefits do you foresee from doing that?"
3. *Choose freely.* To determine whether the client chose freely, ask "Did you have any say in that decision?" "Do you have a choice?"
4. *Feel good about the choice.* To determine how the client feels, ask "How do you feel about that decision (or action)?" Because some clients may not feel satisfied with their decision, a more sensitive question may be "Some people feel good after a decision is made; others feel bad. How do you feel?"
5. *Affirm the choice.* Ask "How will you discuss this with others (family, friends)?"
6. *Act on the choice.* To determine whether the client is prepared to act on the decision, ask, for example, "Will it be difficult to tell your wife about this?"
7. *Act with a pattern.* To determine whether the client consistently behaves in a certain way, ask "How many times have you done that before?" or "Would you act that way again?"

When implementing these seven steps to clarify values, the nurse assists the client to think each question through, but does not impose personal values. The nurse rarely, if ever, offers an opinion when the client asks for it—and then only with great care or when the nurse is an expert in the content area. Since each situation is different, what the nurse would choose in his or her own life may not be relevant to the client's circumstances.

Thus, if the client asks the nurse "What would you have done in my situation?" it is best to redirect the question back to the client rather than answering from the nurse's personal view.

MORALITY AND ETHICS

The term **ethics** has several meanings in common use. It refers to (a) a method of inquiry that helps people to understand the morality of human behavior (i.e., it is the study of morality), (b) the practices or beliefs of a certain group (e.g., medical ethics, nursing ethics), and (c) the expected standards of moral behavior of a particular group as described in the group's formal code of professional ethics. Nurses have been viewed as the most ethical professionals in most of the recent Gallup polls (Gallup, 2005). **Bioethics** is ethics as applied to human life or health (e.g., to decisions about abortion or euthanasia). **Nursing ethics** refers to ethical issues that occur in nursing practice. The American Nurses Association (ANA) revised *Scope and Standards of Practice* (2003) hold nurses accountable for their ethical conduct. Professional Performance Standard 12 relates to ethics (see Box 5–2).

BOX 5–2 ANA Standards of Professional Performance

STANDARD 12: ETHICS

Measurement Criteria

- Uses the Code for Nurses with Interpretive Statements (ANA, 2001) to guide practice.
- Delivers care in a manner that preserves patient autonomy, dignity, and rights.
- Maintains patient confidentiality within legal and regulatory parameters.
- Serves as a patient advocate assisting patients in developing skills for self-advocacy.
- Maintains a therapeutic and professional patient–nurse relationship with appropriate professional role boundaries.
- Demonstrates a commitment to practicing self-care, managing stress, and connecting with self and others.
- Contributes to resolving ethical issues of patients, colleagues, or systems as evidenced in such activities as participating on ethics committees.
- Reports illegal, incompetent, or impaired practices.

Note: Reprinted with permission from American Nurses Association, *Nursing: Scope and Standards of Practice* © 2004 Nursebooks.org, Silver Spring, MD 20910.

TABLE 5–3 Behaviors that May Indicate Unclear Values

BEHAVIOR	EXAMPLE
Ignoring a health professional's advice	A client with heart disease who values hard work ignores advice to exercise regularly.
Inconsistent communication or behavior	A pregnant woman says she wants a healthy baby, but continues to drink alcohol and smoke tobacco.
Numerous admissions to a health agency for the same problem	A middle-aged, obese woman repeatedly seeks help for back pain but does not lose weight.
Confusion or uncertainty about which course of action to take	A woman wants to obtain a job to meet financial obligations, but also wants to stay at home to care for an ailing husband.

Morality (or morals) is similar to ethics, and many use the terms interchangeably. **Morality** usually refers to private, personal standards of what is right and wrong in conduct, character, and attitude. Sometimes the first clue to the moral nature of a situation is an aroused conscience or an awareness of feelings such as guilt, hope, or shame. Another indicator is the tendency to respond to the situation with words such as *ought, should, right, wrong, good,* and *bad.* Moral issues are concerned with important social values and norms; they are not about trivial things.

Nurses should distinguish between morality and law. Laws reflect the moral values of a society, and they offer guidance in determining what is moral. However, an action can be legal but not moral. For example, an order for full resuscitation of a dying client is legal, but one could still question whether the act is moral. On the other hand, an action can be moral but illegal. For example, if a child at home stops breathing, it is moral but not legal to exceed the speed limit when driving to the hospital. Legal aspects of nursing practice are covered in Chapter 4. ∞

Nurses should also distinguish between morality and religion as they relate to health practices, although the two concepts are related. For example, according to some religious beliefs, women should undergo procedures such as female circumcision that may cause physical mutilation. Other religions or groups may consider this practice to be an ethical violation of human right to self-determination (Hellsten, 2004). Additional common instances of differences in moral perspectives on health involving religious beliefs include blood transfusions, abortion, sterilization, and contraceptive and safer sex counseling.

CLINICAL ALERT

Many Chinese people are members of either the Confucian or the Buddhist religion. Confucian religious beliefs do not consider a fetus a human being. However, Buddhists believe the fetus is a form of human life. As a result, Chinese people may vary from each other in their views on abortion, depending on their religious affiliation. ■

Moral Development

Ethical decisions require persons to think and reason. Reasoning is a cognitive function and is, therefore, developmental. **Moral development** is the process of learning to tell the difference between right and wrong and of learning what ought and ought not to be done. It is a complex process that begins in childhood and continues throughout life.

Theories of moral development attempt to answer questions such as these: How does a person become moral? What factors influence the way a person behaves in a moral situation? Two well-known theorists of moral development are Lawrence Kohlberg (1969) and Carol Gilligan (1982). Kohlberg's theory emphasizes rights and formal reasoning; Gilligan's theory emphasizes care and responsibility, although it points out that people use the concepts of both theorists in their moral reasoning. For a full discussion of these two theories, see Chapter 21. ∞

Moral Frameworks

Moral theories provide different frameworks through which nurses can view and clarify disturbing client care situations. Nurses can use moral theories in developing explanations for their ethical decisions and actions and in discussing problem situations with others. Three types of moral theories are widely used, and they can be differentiated by their emphasis on (a) consequences, (b) principles and duties, or (c) relationships.

Consequence-based (teleological) theories look to the outcomes (consequences) of an action in judging whether that action is right or wrong. **Utilitarianism,** one form of consequentialist theory, views a good act as one that brings the most good and the least harm for the greatest number of people. This is called the principle of **utility.** This approach is often used in making decisions about the funding and delivery of health care. Teleological theories focus on issues of fairness.

Principles-based (deontological) theories involve logical and formal processes and emphasize individual rights, duties, and obligations. The morality of an action is determined not by its consequences but by whether it is done according to an impartial, objective principle. For example, following the rule "Do not lie," a nurse might believe he or she should tell the truth to a dying client, even though the physician has given instruction not to do so. There are many deontological theories; each justifies the rules of acceptable behavior differently.

Relationships-based (caring) theories stress courage, generosity, commitment, and the need to nurture and maintain relationships. Unlike the two preceding theories, which frame problems in terms of justice (fairness) and formal reasoning, caring theories (see Chapter 25 ∞) judge actions according to a perspective of caring and responsibility. Principles-based theories stress individual rights, but caring theories promote the common good or the welfare of the group.

A moral framework guides moral decisions, but it does not determine the outcome. Imagine a situation in which a frail, elderly client has made it clear that he does not want further surgery, but the family and surgeon insist. Three nurses have each decided that they will not help with preparations for surgery and that they will work through proper channels to try to prevent it. Using consequence-based reasoning, Nurse A thinks, "Surgery will cause him more suffering; he probably will not survive it anyway, and the family may even feel guilty later." Using principles-based reasoning, Nurse B thinks, "This violates the principle of autonomy. This man has a right to decide what happens to his body." Using caring-based reasoning, Nurse C thinks, "My relationship to this client commits me to protecting him and meeting his needs, and I feel such compassion for him. I must try to help the family understand that he needs their support." Each of these perspectives is based on the nurse's moral framework.

Moral Principles

Moral principles are statements about broad, general, philosophical concepts such as autonomy and justice. They provide the foundation for **moral rules,** which are specific prescriptions for actions. For example, the rule "People should not lie" is based on the moral principle of respect for persons (autonomy). Principles are useful in ethical discussions because even if people disagree about which action is right in a situation, they may be able to agree on the principles that apply. Such an agreement can serve as the basis for a solution that is acceptable to all parties. For example, most people would agree to the principle that nurses are obligated to respect their clients, even if they disagree as to whether the nurse should deceive a particular client about his or her prognosis.

Autonomy refers to the right to make one's own decisions. Nurses who follow this principle recognize that each client is unique, has the right to be what that person is, and has the right to choose personal goals. People have "inward autonomy" if they have the ability to make choices; they have "outward autonomy" if their choices are not limited or imposed by others.

Honoring the principle of autonomy means that the nurse respects a client's right to make decisions even when those choices seem to the nurse not to be in the client's best interest. It also means treating others with consideration. In a health care setting, this principle is violated, for example, when a nurse disregards clients' subjective accounts of their symptoms (e.g., pain). Finally, respect for autonomy means that people should not be treated as an impersonal source of knowledge or training. This principle comes into play, for example, in the requirement that clients provide informed consent before tests, procedures, or participating as a research subject can be carried out. See "Informed Consent" in Chapter 4. ∞

Nonmaleficence is duty to "do no harm." Although this would seem to be a simple principle to follow, in reality it is complex. Harm can mean intentionally causing harm, placing someone at risk of harm, and unintentionally causing harm. In nursing, intentional harm is never acceptable. However, placing a person at risk of harm has many facets. A client may be at risk of harm as a known consequence of a nursing intervention that is intended to be helpful. For example, a client may react adversely to a medication. Unintentional harm occurs when the risk could not have been anticipated. For example, while catching a client who is falling, the nurse grips the client tightly enough to cause bruises to the client's arm. Caregivers do not always agree on the degree of risk that is morally permissible in order to attempt the beneficial result.

Beneficence means "doing good." Nurses are obligated to do good, that is, to implement actions that benefit clients and their support persons. However, doing good can also pose a risk of doing harm. For example, a nurse may advise a client about a strenuous exercise program to improve general health, but should not do so if the client is at risk of a heart attack.

Justice is often referred to as fairness. Nurses often face decisions in which a sense of justice should prevail. For example, a nurse making home visits finds one client tearful and depressed, and knows she could help by staying for 30 more minutes to talk. However, that would take time from her next client, who is a diabetic who needs a great deal of teaching and observation. The nurse will need to weigh the facts carefully in order to divide her time justly among her clients.

Fidelity means to be faithful to agreements and promises. By virtue of their standing as professional caregivers, nurses have responsibilities to clients, employers, government, and society, as well as to themselves. Nurses often make promises such as "I'll be right back with your pain medication" or "I'll find out for you." Clients take such promises seriously, and so should nurses.

Veracity refers to telling the truth. Although this seems straightforward, in practice choices are not always clear. Should a nurse tell the truth when it is known that it will cause harm? Does a nurse tell a lie when it is known that the lie will relieve anxiety and fear? Lying to sick or dying people is rarely justified. The loss of trust in the nurse and the anxiety caused by not knowing the truth, for example, usually outweigh any benefits derived from lying.

Nurses must also have professional accountability and responsibility. According to the *Code of Ethics for Nurses* (ANA, 2001), **accountability** means "answerable to oneself and others for one's own actions," while **responsibility** refers to "the specific accountability or liability associated with the performance of duties of a particular role." Thus, the ethical nurse is able to explain the rationale behind every action and recognizes the standards to which he or she will be held.

NURSING ETHICS

In the past, nurses looked on ethical decision making as the physician's responsibility. However, no one profession is responsible for ethical decisions, nor does expertise in one discipline such as medicine or nursing necessarily make a person an expert in ethics. As situations become more complex, input from all caregivers becomes increasingly important.

Ethical standards of the Joint Commission on Accreditation of Healthcare Organizations (JCAHO) mandate that health care institutions provide ethics committees or a similar structure to write guidelines and policies and to provide education, counseling, and support on ethical issues (JCAHO, 2006). These multidisciplinary committees include nurses and can be asked to review a case and provide guidance to a competent client, an incompetent client's family, or health care providers. They ensure that relevant facts of a case are brought out, provide a forum in which diverse views can be expressed, provide support for caregivers, and can reduce the institution's legal risks. In some settings, ethics rounds are held. In these meetings, ethical dilemmas from real or simulated cases are presented from a more theoretical perspective, introducing those present to the issues and processes used in analyzing such dilemmas (see Figure 5-1 ■).

Nursing Codes of Ethics

A **code of ethics** is a formal statement of a group's ideals and values. It is a set of ethical principles that (a) is shared by members of the group, (b) reflects their moral judgments over time, and (c) serves as a standard for their professional actions. Codes of ethics usually have higher requirements than legal standards, and they are never lower than the legal standards of the profession. Nurses are responsible for being familiar with the code that governs their practice.

Figure 5-1 ■ An ethics committee contemplates all aspects of the case being considered.

(Mark Richards/PhotoEdit)

International, national, and state nursing associations have established codes of ethics. The International Council of Nurses (ICN) first adopted a code of ethics in 1953, and the most recent revisions (2005) are shown in Box 5–3. The ANA first adopted a *Code for Nurses* in 1950. The current version (Box 5–4) reflects several major changes in the code (now called the *Code of Ethics for Nurses*). A statement on compassion has been added, and the duty to protect patients has been broadened to include all patient rights. Several previous provisions have been collapsed, and the provision on delegation has been significantly enhanced to reflect the increased use of unlicensed assistive personnel.

Nursing codes of ethics have the following purposes:

1. Inform the public about the minimum standards of the profession and help them understand professional nursing conduct.
2. Provide a sign of the profession's commitment to the public it serves.
3. Outline the major ethical considerations of the profession.
4. Provide ethical standards for professional behavior.
5. Guide the profession in self-regulation.
6. Remind nurses of the special responsibility they assume when caring for the sick.

BOX 5–3 International Council of Nurses Code of Ethics

PREAMBLE

Nurses have four fundamental responsibilities: to promote health, to prevent illness, to restore health and to alleviate suffering. The need for nursing is universal.

Inherent in nursing is respect for human rights, including cultural rights, the right to life and choice, to dignity and to be treated with respect. Nursing care is respectful of and unrestricted by considerations of age, colour, creed, culture, disability or illness, gender, sexual orientation, nationality, politics, race or social status.

Nurses render health services to the individual, the family and the community and coordinate their services with those of related groups.

THE ICN CODE

The *ICN Code of Ethics for Nurses* has four principal elements that outline the standards of ethical conduct.

Elements of the Code

1. Nurses and People

The nurse's primary professional responsibility is to people requiring nursing care.

In providing care, the nurse promotes an environment in which the human rights, values, customs and spiritual beliefs of the individual, family and community are respected.

The nurse ensures that the individual receives sufficient information on which to base consent for care and related treatment.

The nurse holds in confidence personal information and uses judgement in sharing this information.

The nurse shares with society the responsibility for initiating and supporting action to meet the health and social needs of the public, in particular those of vulnerable populations.

The nurse also shares responsibility to sustain and protect the natural environment from depletion, pollution, degradation and destruction.

2. Nurses and Practice

The nurse carries personal responsibility and accountability for nursing practice, and for maintaining competence by continual learning.

The nurse maintains a standard of personal health such that the ability to provide care is not compromised.

The nurse uses judgement regarding individual competence when accepting and delegating responsibility.

The nurse at all times maintains standards of personal conduct which reflect well on the profession and enhance public confidence.

The nurse, in providing care, ensures that use of technology and scientific advances are compatible with the safety, dignity and rights of people.

3. Nurses and the Profession

The nurse assumes the major role in determining and implementing acceptable standards of clinical nursing practice, management, research and education.

The nurse is active in developing a core of research-based professional knowledge.

The nurse, acting through the professional organization, participates in creating and maintaining safe, equitable social and economic working conditions in nursing.

4. Nurses and Co-workers

The nurse sustains a co-operative relationship with co-workers in nursing and other fields.

The nurse takes appropriate action to safeguard individuals, families and communities when their health is endangered by a co-worker or any other person.

Note: From *The ICN Code of Ethics for Nurses,* International Council of Nurses, 2006, Geneva: Imprimeries Populaires. Reprinted with permission.

BOX 5–4 **American Nurses Association Code of Ethics for Nurses (Approved July 2001)**

1. The nurse, in all professional relationships, practices with compassion and respect for the inherent dignity, worth, and uniqueness of every individual, unrestricted by considerations of social or economic status, personal attributes, or the nature of health problems.
   1.1 Respect for human dignity
   1.2 Relationships to patients
   1.3 The nature of health problems
   1.4 The right to self-determination
   1.5 Relationships with colleagues and others
2. The nurse's primary commitment is to the patient, whether an individual, family, group, or community.
   2.1 Primacy of patient's interests
   2.2 Conflict of interest for nurses
   2.3 Collaboration
   2.4 Professional boundaries
3. The nurse promotes, advocates for, and strives to protect the health, safety, and rights of the patient.
   3.1 Privacy
   3.2 Confidentiality
   3.3 Protection of participants in research
   3.4 Standards and review mechanisms
   3.5 Acting on questionable practice
   3.6 Addressing impaired practice
4. The nurse is responsible and accountable for individual nursing practice and determines the appropriate delegation of tasks consistent with the nurse's obligation to provide optimum patient care.
   4.1 Acceptance of accountability and responsibility
   4.2 Accountability for nursing judgment and action
   4.3 Responsibility for nursing judgment and action
   4.4 Delegation of nursing activities
5. The nurse owes the same duties to self as to others, including the responsibility to preserve integrity and safety, to maintain competence, and to continue personal and professional growth.
   5.1 Moral self-respect
   5.2 Professional growth and maintenance of competence
   5.3 Wholeness of character
   5.4 Preservation of integrity

6. The nurse participates in establishing, maintaining, and improving healthcare environments and conditions of employment conducive to the provision of quality healthcare and consistent with the values of the profession through individual and collective action.
   6.1 Influence of the environment on moral virtues and values
   6.2 Influence of the environment on ethical obligations
   6.3 Responsibility for the healthcare environment
7. The nurse participates in the advancement of the profession through contributions to practice, education, administration, and knowledge development.
   7.1 Advancing the profession through active involvement in nursing and healthcare policy
   7.2 Advancing the profession by developing, maintaining, and implementing professional standards in clinical, administrative, and educational practice
   7.3 Advancing the profession through knowledge development, dissemination, and application to practice
8. The nurse collaborates with other health professionals and the public in promoting community, national, and international efforts to meet health needs.
   8.1 Health needs and concerns
   8.2 Responsibilities to the public
9. The profession of nursing, as represented by associations and their members, is responsible for articulating nursing values, for maintaining the integrity of the profession and its practice, and for shaping social policy.
   9.1 Assertion of values
   9.2 The profession carries out its collective responsibility through professional associations
   9.3 Intraprofessional integrity
   9.4 Social reform

Note: Reprinted with permission from American Nurses Association, *Code of Ethics for Nurses with Interpretive Statements,* © 2001 Nursesbooks.org, Silver Spring, MD 20910.

Origins of Ethical Problems in Nursing

Nurses' growing awareness of ethical problems has occurred largely because of (a) social and technological changes and (b) nurses' conflicting loyalties and obligations.

Social and Technological Changes

Social changes, such as the women's movement and a growing consumerism, also expose problems. The large number of people without health insurance, the high cost of health care, and workplace redesign under managed care all raise issues of fairness and allocation of resources.

Technology creates new issues that did not exist in earlier times. Before monitors, respirators, and parenteral feedings, there was no question about whether to "allow" an 800-gram premature infant to die. Before organ transplantation, death did not require a legal definition that might still permit viable tissues to be removed and given to other living persons. Advances in the ability to decode and control the growth of tissues through gene manipulation pre-

sent new potential ethical dilemmas related to cloning organisms and altering the course of hereditary diseases and biological characteristics. Today, with treatments that can prolong and enhance biologic life, these questions arise: Should we do what we know we can? Who should be treated—everyone, only those who can pay, only those who have a chance to improve?

Conflicting Loyalties and Obligations

Because of their unique position in the health care system, nurses experience conflicts among their loyalties and obligations to clients, families, primary care providers, employing institutions, and licensing bodies. Client needs may conflict with institutional policies, primary care provider preferences, needs of the client's family, or even laws of the state. According to the nursing code of ethics, the nurse's first loyalty is to the client. However, it is not always easy to determine which action best serves the client's needs. For instance, the nurse may be aware that marijuana has been shown to be effective for a condition a client has that has not responded to mainstream therapies. Although legal issues are involved, the nurse must determine if, ethically, the client should be made aware of a potentially effective alternative. Another example is individual nurses' decisions regarding honoring picket lines during employee strikes. The nurse may experience conflict among feeling the need to support co-workers in their efforts to improve working conditions, feeling the need to ensure clients receive care and are not abandoned, and feeling loyalty to the hospital employer.

Making Ethical Decisions

Responsible ethical reasoning is rational and systematic. It should be based on ethical principles and codes rather than on emotions, intuition, fixed policies, or precedent (that is, an earlier similar occurrence). Two decision-making models are shown in Box 5–5.

A good decision is one that is in the client's best interest and at the same time preserves the integrity of all involved. Nurses have ethical obligations to their clients, to the agency that employs them, and to primary care providers. Therefore, nurses must weigh competing factors when making ethical decisions. See Box 5–6 for examples. Although ethical reasoning is principle based and has the client's well-being at center, being involved in ethical problems and dilemmas is stressful for the

---

BOX 5–5 Ethical Decision-Making Models

THOMPSON AND THOMPSON (1985)
- Review the situation to determine health problems, decision needs, ethical components, and key individuals.
- Gather additional information to clarify the situation.
- Identify the ethical issues in the situation.
- Define personal and professional moral positions.
- Identify moral positions of key individuals involved.
- Identify value conflicts, if any.
- Determine who should make the decision.
- Identify range of actions with anticipated outcomes.
- Decide on a course of action and carry it out.
- Evaluate/review results of decision/action.

CASSELLS AND REDMAN (1989)
- Identify the moral aspects of nursing care.
- Gather relevant facts related to a moral issue.
- Clarify and apply personal values.
- Understand ethical theories and principles.
- Utilize competent interdisciplinary resources.
- Propose alternative actions.
- Apply nursing codes of ethics to help guide actions.
- Choose and implement resolutive action.
- Participate actively in resolving the issue.
- Apply state and federal laws governing nursing practice.
- Evaluate the resolutive action taken.

Note: From *Bioethical Decision-Making for Nurses* (p. 99), by J. B. Thompson and H. O. Thompson, 1985, Norwalk, CT: Appleton-Century-Croft; and "Preparing Students to be Moral Agents in Clinical Nursing Practice," by J. Cassells and B. Redman, 1989, *Nursing Clinics of North America, 24*(2), pp. 463–473. Reprinted with permission.

BOX 5–6 Examples of Nurses' Obligations in Ethical Decisions

- Maximize the client's well-being.
- Balance the client's need for autonomy with family members' responsibilities for the client's well-being.
- Support each family member and enhance the family support system.
- Carry out hospital policies.
- Protect other clients' well-being.
- Protect the nurse's own standards of care.

---

nurse. The nurse may feel torn between obligations to the client, the family, and the employer. What is in the client's best interest may be contrary to the nurse's personal belief system. In settings in which ethical issues arise frequently, nurses should establish support systems such as team conferences and use of counseling professionals to allow expression of their feelings.

Many nursing problems are not moral problems at all, but simply questions of good nursing practice. An important first step in ethical decision making is to determine whether a moral situation exists. The following criteria may be used:

- A difficult choice exists between actions that conflict with the needs of one or more persons.
- Moral principles or frameworks exist that can be used to provide some justification for the action.
- The choice is guided by a process of weighing reasons.
- The decision must be freely and consciously chosen.
- The choice is affected by personal feelings and by the particular context of the situation.

Box 5–7 presents an example of ethical decision making.

Although the nurse's input is important, in reality several people are usually involved in making an ethical decision. The client, family, spiritual support persons, and other members of the health care team work together in reaching ethical decisions (see Figure 5-2 on page 90 ■). Therefore, collaboration, communication, and compromise are important skills for health professionals. When nurses do not have the autonomy to act on their moral or ethical choices, compromise becomes essential.

CLINICAL ALERT

Ethical behavior is contextual—what is an ethical action or decision in one situation may not be ethical in a different situation. ■

Strategies to Enhance Ethical Decisions and Practice

Several strategies help nurses overcome possible organizational and social constraints that may hinder the ethical practice of nursing and create moral distress for nurses. You as a nurse should do the following:

- Become aware of your own values and the ethical aspects of nursing.

BOX 5–7 Application of a Bioethical Decision-Making Model

SITUATION

Mrs. L, a 67-year-old woman, is hospitalized with multiple fractures and lacerations caused by an automobile accident. Her husband, who was killed in the accident, was taken to the same hospital. Mrs. L, who had been driving the automobile, constantly questions her primary nurse about her husband. The surgeon has told the nurse not to tell Mrs. L about the death of her husband; however, the surgeon does not give the nurse any reason for these instructions. The nurse expresses concern to the charge nurse, who says the surgeon's orders must be followed—that the surgeon will decide when Mrs. L should be told. However, the nurse is not comfortable with this and wonders what should be done.

Nursing Actions	*Considerations*
1. Identify the moral aspects. See the criteria provided on page 88 to determine whether a moral situation exists.	The alternative actions are to tell the truth or withhold it. The moral principles involved are honesty and loyalty. These principles conflict because the primary nurse wants to be honest with Mrs. L without being disloyal to the surgeon and the charge nurse. The nurse will weigh reasons in making a freely and consciously chosen choice. The choice will probably be affected by feelings of concern for Mrs. L and a context that includes the surgeon's incomplete communication with the client and the nurse.
2. Gather relevant facts that relate to the issue.	Data should include information about the client's health problems. Determine who is involved, the nature of their involvement, and their motives for acting. In this case, the people involved are the client (who is concerned about her husband), the husband (who is deceased), the surgeon, the charge nurse, and the primary nurse. Motives are not known. Perhaps the nurse wishes to protect his or her therapeutic relationship with Mrs. L; possibly the physician believes this action protects Mrs. L from psychologic trauma and consequent physical deterioration.
3. Determine ownership of the decision. For example, for whom is the decision being made? Who should decide and why?	In this case, the decision is being made for Mrs. L. The surgeon obviously believes that a physician should be the one to decide, and the charge nurse agrees. It would be helpful if caregivers agreed on criteria for deciding who the decision maker should be.
4. Clarify and apply personal values.	We can infer from this situation that Mrs. L values her husband's welfare, that the charge nurse values policy and procedure, and that the nurse seems to value a client's right to have information. The nurse needs to clarify his or her own and the surgeon's values, as well as confirm the values of Mrs. L and the charge nurse.
5. Identify ethical theories and principles.	For example, failing to tell Mrs. L the truth can negate her autonomy. The nurse would uphold the principle of honesty by telling Mrs. L. The principles of beneficence and nonmaleficence are also involved because of the possible effects of the alternative actions on Mrs. L's physical and psychologic well-being.
6. Identify applicable laws or agency policies.	Because the surgeon simply "gave instructions" rather than an actual order, agency policies might not require the nurse to follow the instructions. The nurse should clarify this with the charge nurse and be familiar with the nurse practice act in that state.
7. Use competent interdisciplinary resources.	In this case, the nurse might consult literature to find out whether clients are harmed by receiving bad news when they are injured and might also consult with the chaplain.
8. Develop alternative actions and project their outcomes on the client and family. Possibly because of the limited time available for ethical deliberations in the clinical setting, nurses tend to identify two opposing, either-or alternatives (e.g., to tell or not to tell) instead of generating multiple options. This creates a dilemma even when none exists.	Two alternative actions, with possible outcomes, follow (others may also be appropriate): 1. Follow the charge nurse's advice and do as the surgeon says. Possible outcomes: (a) Mrs. L might become anxious and angry when she finds out that information has been withheld from her; or (b) by waiting until Mrs. L is stronger to give her the bad news, the health care team may avoid harming Mrs. L's health. 2. Discuss the situation further with the charge nurse and surgeon, pointing out Mrs. L's right to autonomy and information. Possible outcomes: (a) The surgeon acknowledges Mrs. L's right to be informed, or (b) the surgeon states that Mrs. L's health is at risk and insists that she not be informed until a later time. Regardless of whether the action is congruent with the nurse's personal value system, Mrs. L's best interests take precedence.
9. Apply nursing codes of ethics to help guide actions. (Codes of nursing usually support autonomy and nursing advocacy.)	If the nurse believes strongly that Mrs. L should hear the truth, then as a client advocate, the nurse should choose to confer again with the charge nurse and surgeon.
10. For each alternative action, identify the risk and seriousness of consequences for the nurse. (Some employers may not support nursing autonomy and advocacy in ethical situations.)	If the nurse tells Mrs. L the truth without the agreement of the charge nurse and surgeon, the nurse risks the surgeon's anger and a reprimand from the charge nurse. If the nurse follows the charge nurse's advice, the nurse will receive approval from the charge nurse and surgeon; however, the nurse risks being seen as unassertive, and the nurse violates a personal value of truthfulness. If the nurse requests a conference, the nurse may gain respect for assertiveness and professionalism, but the nurse risks the surgeon's annoyance at having the instructions questioned.

(continued)

BOX 5–7 **Application of a Bioethical Decision-Making Model** *continued*	
Nursing Actions	***Considerations***
11. Participate actively in resolving the issue. Recommend actions that can be ethically supported, recognizing that all actions have positive and negative aspects.	The appropriate degree of nursing input varies with the situation. Sometimes nurses participate in choosing what will be done; sometimes they merely support a client who is making the decision. In this situation, if an action cannot be agreed on, the nurse must decide whether this issue is important enough to merit the personal risks involved.
12. Implement the action.	The nurse will carry out one of the actions developed in step 8.
13. Evaluate the action taken. Involve the client, family, and other health members in the evaluation, if possible.	The nurse can begin by asking, "Did I do the right thing?" Would the nurse make the same decisions again if the situation were repeated? If the nurse is not satisfied, the nurse can review other alternatives and work through the process again.

Figure 5-2 ■ When there is a need for ethical decisions or client advocacy, many different persons contribute to the final outcome.
(A. Ramsey/PhotoEdit)

- Be familiar with nursing codes of ethics.
- Seek continuing education opportunities to stay knowledgeable about ethical issues in nursing.
- Respect the values, opinions, and responsibilities of other health care professionals that may be different from your own.
- Participate in or establish ethics rounds. Ethics rounds use hypothetical or real cases that focus on the ethical dimensions of client care rather than the client's clinical diagnosis and treatment.
- Serve on institutional ethics committees.
- Strive for collaborative practice in which nurses function effectively in cooperation with other health care professionals.

SPECIFIC ETHICAL ISSUES

Some of the ethical problems nurses encounter most frequently are issues in the care of HIV/AIDS clients, abortion, organ transplantation, end-of-life decisions, cost-containment issues that jeopardize client welfare and access to health care (resource allocation), and breaches of client confidentiality (e.g., computerized information management).

Acquired Immune Deficiency Syndrome (AIDS)

Because of its association with sexual behavior, illicit drug use, and physical decline and death, AIDS bears a social stigma. According to an ANA position statement, the moral obligation to care for an HIV-infected client cannot be set aside unless the risk exceeds the responsibility (ANA, 1994).

Other ethical issues center on testing for HIV status and for the presence of AIDS in health professionals and clients. Questions arise as to whether testing of all providers and clients should be mandatory or voluntary and whether test results should be released to insurance companies, sexual partners, or caregivers. As with all ethical dilemmas, there are both positive and negative implications of each possibility for specific individuals.

Abortion

Abortion is a highly publicized issue about which many people feel very strongly. Debate continues, pitting the principle of sanctity of life against the principle of autonomy and the woman's right to control her own body. This is an especially volatile issue because no public consensus has yet been reached.

Most state and provincial laws have provisions known as conscience clauses that permit individual physicians and nurses, as well as institutions, to refuse to assist with an abortion if doing so violates their religious or moral principles. However, nurses have no right to impose their values on a client. Nursing codes of ethics support clients' rights to information and counseling in making decisions.

Organ Transplantation

Organs for transplantation may come from living donors or from donors who have just died. Many living people choose to become donors by giving consent under the Uniform Anatomical Gift Act (see Chapter 43 ∞). Ethical issues related to organ transplantation include allocation of organs, selling of body parts, involvement of children as potential donors, consent, clear definition of death, and conflicts of interest between potential donors and recipients. In some situations, a person's religious belief may also present conflict. For example, certain

How Do Nurses Feel about Abortion Based on the Reasons for Aborting?

There are many reasons why women decide to terminate a pregnancy. Some of these reasons include physiological impairment in the fetus, conditions life-threatening to the mother, the mother's desire not to have the child, and preference for a specific gender of the child. The researchers found few existing studies of nurses' attitudes about abortion. The ANA *Code of Ethics* supports the nurse's choice to avoid participation in an abortion under ethical opposition reasons. The purpose of this study was to determine how often nurses refused to care for patients choosing an abortion and for what reasons. Of the 153 labor and delivery nurses in California surveyed, 75 returned the instrument. The majority of respondents said they would care for a woman having an abortion for fetal death (95%) and when fetal defects were incompatible with life (77%). Between 20% and 37% would care for a client with fetal birth defects compatible with life, and between 8% and 29% for clients choosing to reduce the number of fetuses in multifetal pregnancies, depending on how far along was the pregnancy. Although 32% of nurses would care for a client terminating the pregnancy in the first trimester for personal reasons, only 4% would do so during the third trimester. Less than 5% of the nurses would partici-pate in an abortion being done for gender selection at any time in the pregnancy. Nurses listed a variety of influences on their decisions to care or not care for these clients, including ethical beliefs (57%), spiritual beliefs (48%), and previous work experiences with termination and grief/loss (28%).

IMPLICATIONS

Although ethical guidelines permit nurses to refuse care in nonemergency situations for ethical reasons, little is known about when, why, and how this occurs. Nurses face ethical challenges when there is no other provider available who can provide competent care for the client. Nurses must consider their ethical beliefs when accepting assignments to work in areas known to commonly experience particular ethical issues and, very importantly, must communicate their willingness or refusal to provide care to the team so that safe client care can be assured.

Note: From "Nurses' Attitudes Toward Pregnancy Termination in the Labor and Delivery Setting," by M. J. Marek, 2004, *Journal of Obstetric, Gynecologic, and Neonatal Nursing, 33,* pp. 472–479.

religions forbid the mutilation of the body, even for the benefit of another person.

End-of-Life Issues

The increase in technological advances and the growing number of elderly people have expanded the ethical dilemmas faced by elders and the health care professions. Providing them with information and professional assistance, as well as the highest quality of care and caring, is of the utmost importance during these times. Some of the most frequent disturbing ethical problems for nurses involve issues that arise around death and dying. These include euthanasia, assisted suicide, termination of life-sustaining treatment, and withdrawing or withholding of food and fluids.

Advance Directives

Many moral problems surrounding the end of life can be resolved if clients complete advance directives. Presently, all 50 of the United States have enacted advance directive legislation. Advance directives direct caregivers as to the client's wishes about treatments, providing an ongoing voice for clients when they have lost the capacity to make or communicate their decisions. See Chapter 43 ∞ for a full discussion of advance directives.

Euthanasia and Assisted Suicide

Euthanasia, a Greek word meaning "good death," is popularly known as "mercy killing." **Active euthanasia** involves actions to bring about the client's death directly, with or without client consent. An example of this would be the administration of a lethal medication to end the client's suffering. Regardless of the caregiver's intent, active euthanasia is forbidden by law and can result in criminal charges of murder.

A variation of active euthanasia is **assisted suicide**, or giving clients the means to kill themselves if they request it (e.g., pro-viding pills or a weapon). Some countries or states have laws permitting assisted suicide for clients who are severely ill, who are near death, and who wish to commit suicide. Although some persons may disagree with the concept, in January 2006, the

 REAL WORLD PRACTICE

A brief example of what ethical nurse advocacy might look like follows: At our rehabilitation facility, we were working with a middle aged (50) gentleman who had suffered a stroke. He was medically stable and able to participate fully in his therapies. However, he requested that he be made a DNR (do not resuscitate). His reasoning was that if he had another stroke or cardiac arrest he could lose much more cognitive and motor function and that if he was resuscitated, it would place too heavy a burden of care on his family. Day after day he and his family asked about the DNR order. Day after day we asked the attending physician for an order and day after day the physician said that the client did not need a DNR order—he was stable and he, the physician, had never lost a client. Finally the primary nurse went to the ethics council with the problem and that physician reviewed the chart, spoke with the client and family and entered the DNR order. The client and his family were so thankful and grateful that someone had listened to them and respected their wishes. The client had no further medical crises and was ultimately discharged home.

No one likes to go around or above the attending physician, but in this case the client's wishes demanded a difficult ethical intervention on the part of the nurse. The nurse had a clear, unbiased understanding of her client's wishes and values, as well as a solid rapport, and acted according to the code of nursing ethics by ensuring that the client's wishes for a DNR order were obtained.

—Susan Sullivan, RN, BSN, CRRN
The Rehabilitation Institute of Chicago

U.S. Supreme Court ruled to uphold the assisted suicide regulations in the state of Oregon (see Chapter 4 ∞). In any case, the nurse should recall that legality and morality are not the same thing. Determining whether an action is legal is only one aspect of deciding whether it is ethical. The questions of suicide and assisted suicide are still controversial in our society. The American Nurses Association's position statement on assisted suicide (ANA, 1995) states that active euthanasia and assisted suicide are in violation of the *Code for Nurses.*

Passive euthanasia, more commonly referred to now as withdrawing or withholding life-sustaining therapy (WWLST), involves the withdrawal of extraordinary means of life support, such as removing a ventilator or withholding special attempts to revive a client (e.g., giving the client "no code" status) and allowing the client to die of the underlying medical condition. WWLST is both legally and ethically more acceptable to most persons than assisted suicide (Ersek, 2005).

Termination of Life-Sustaining Treatment

Antibiotics, organ transplants, and technological advances (e.g., ventilators) help to prolong life, but not necessarily to restore health. Clients may specify that they wish to have life-sustaining measures withdrawn, they may have advance directives on this matter, or they may appoint a surrogate decision maker. However, it is usually more troubling for health care professionals to withdraw a treatment than to decide initially not to begin it. Nurses must understand that a decision to withdraw treatment is not a decision to withdraw care. As the primary caregivers, nurses must ensure that sensitive care and comfort measures are given as the client's illness progresses. When the client is at home, nurses often provide this type of education and support through hospice services (see Chapter 43 ∞ for more information regarding hospice and end-of-life care).

It is difficult for families to withdraw treatment, which makes it very important that they fully understand the treatment. They often have misunderstandings about which treatments are life sustaining. Keeping clients and families well informed is an ongoing process, allowing them time to ask questions and discuss the situation. It is also essential that they understand that they can reevaluate and change their decision if they wish.

Withdrawing or Withholding Food and Fluids

It is generally accepted that providing food and fluids is part of ordinary nursing practice and, therefore, a moral duty. However, when food and fluids are administered by tube to a dying client, or are given over a long period to an unconscious client who is not expected to improve, then some consider it to be an extraordinary, or heroic, measure. A nurse is morally obligated to withhold food and fluids (or any treatment) if it is determined to be more harmful to administer them than to withhold them. The nurse must also honor competent and informed clients' refusal of food and fluids. The ANA *Code of Ethics for Nurses* (2001) supports this position through the nurse's role as a client advocate and through the moral principle of autonomy.

CULTURALLY COMPETENT CARE
Variations in Applying Moral Principles

Although a moral principle may exist and be valued in different cultures, the degree to which it is valued and the manner by which it is used in health care may be quite variable. Nurses must become familiar with how moral principles are viewed within the cultural groups with which they practice.

Principle	Examples of Ethnic/Cultural Variations
Autonomy	Family members, rather than the client, receive information on the client's condition and take primary responsibility for decision making. The family and community are viewed as affected by the client's condition and decisions as much as the individual is affected: Chinese, Koreans, Mexican Americans, Bosnian Americans.
Veracity	Prefer client not to be told directly of a life-threatening condition: Hispanics, Asians, Pakistanis, Bosnian Americans, Italian Americans, Canadian Aboriginals.
Nonmaleficence	Discussion of advance directives and issues such as Cardiopulmonary resuscitation are viewed as physically and emotionally harmful to the client: Filipino, Native American, Chinese.
Beneficence	Health care providers should promote client well-being and hope: Asian cultures, Native Americans, Russians.

Note: From "Bioethics for Clinicians: 18 Aboriginal Cultures," by J. H. Ellerby, J. McKenzie, S. McKay, G. J. Gariepy, & J. M. Kaufert, 2000, *Canadian Medical Association Journal, 163,* pp. 845-850; "Cultural Diversity at the End of Life: Issues and Guidelines for Family Physicians," by H. R. Searight & J. Gafford, 2005, *American Family Physician, 71,* 515-522; "It's Like Playing with Your Destiny: Bosnian Immigrants' Views of Advance Directives and End-of-Life Decision-Making," by H. R. Searight & J. Gafford, 2005, *Journal of Immigrant Health, 7,* pp. 195 – 203.

Allocation of Scarce Health Resources

Allocation of limited supplies of health care goods and services, including organ transplants, artificial joints, and the services of specialists, has become an especially urgent issue as medical costs continue to rise and more stringent cost-containment measures are implemented. The moral principle of autonomy cannot be applied if it is not possible to give each client what he or she chooses. In this situation, health care providers may use the principle of justice—attempting to choose what is most fair to all.

Nursing care is also a health resource. Most institutions have been implementing "workplace redesign" in order to cut costs. As a result, nursing units may be staffed with fewer RNs and more unlicensed caregivers. Some nurses are concerned that staffing in their institutions is not adequate to give the level of care they value. California is the first state to enact legislation mandating specific nurse-to-client ratios in hospitals and other health care settings. With a nationwide shortage of nurses, an ethical dilemma arises when, in order to provide adequate staffing, facilities must turn away needy clients. Nurses must continue to look for ways to balance economics and caring in the allocation of health resources.

Management of Personal Health Information

In keeping with the principle of autonomy, nurses are obligated to respect clients' privacy and confidentiality. Privacy is both a legal and ethical mandate. The Health Insurance Portability and Accountability Act of 1996 (HIPAA) includes standards protecting the confidentiality, integrity, and availability of data, and standards defining appropriate disclosures of identifiable health information and client rights protection. Clients must be able to trust that nurses will reveal details of their situations only as appropriate and will communicate only the information necessary to provide for their health care. Computerized client records make sensitive data accessible to more people and accent issues of confidentiality. Nurses should help develop and follow security measures and policies to ensure appropriate use of client data.

ADVOCACY

When people are ill, they are frequently unable to assert their rights as they would if they were healthy. An **advocate** is one who expresses and defends the cause of another. The health care system is complex, and many clients are too ill to deal with it. If they are to keep from "falling through the cracks," clients need an advocate to cut through the layers of bureaucracy and help them get what they require. Values basic to client advocacy are shown in Box 5–8. Clients may also advocate for themselves. Today, clients are seeking more self-determination and control over their own bodies when they are ill.

If a client lacks decision-making capacity, is legally incompetent, or is a minor, these rights can be exercised on the client's behalf by a designated surrogate or proxy decision maker. It is important, however, for the nurse to remember that client control over health decisions is a Western view. In other societies, such decisions may normally be made by the head of the family or another member of the community. The nurse must ascertain the client's and family's views and honor their traditions regarding the locus of decision making.

To help make clients' rights more explicit to both the client and the health care provider, several versions of a patient's bill of

rights have been published by consumer organizations. The most commonly used was originally adopted by the American Hospital Association in 1973 and last revised into The Patient Care Partnership: Understanding Expectations, Rights, and Responsibilities in 2003 (see Box 5–9).

A national bill, H.R. 4628 "Patients' Bill of Rights Act of 2004," is based on the 2001 bipartisan Senate-passed bill that was introduced in the House but never passed. Under the bill, clients would be guaranteed certain rights under their health insurance plans, including the following:

- Basic standards for access to care, including clinical trials
- The ability to gain access to their own doctor, and doctors able to communicate with the client without fear of insurance company retaliation
- The assurance that medical decisions about client care will be made by doctors according to sound medical principles
- A fair, independent external review process if needed care is denied by their insurance company
- The right to hold their health plan accountable if a negligent medical decision resulted in injury or harm

The Advocate's Role

The overall goal of the client advocate is to protect clients' rights. An advocate informs clients about their rights and provides them with the information they need to make informed decisions.

An advocate supports clients in their decisions, giving them full or at least mutual responsibility in decision making when they are capable of it. The advocate must be careful to remain objective and not convey approval or disapproval of the client's choices. Advocacy requires accepting and respecting the client's right to decide, even if the nurse believes the decision to be wrong.

In mediating, the advocate directly intervenes on the client's behalf, often by influencing others. An example of acting on behalf of a client is asking a primary care provider to review with the client the reasons for and the expected duration of therapy because the client says he always forgets to ask the primary care provider.

Advocacy in Home Care

Although the goals of advocacy remain the same, home care poses unique concerns for the nurse advocate. For example, while in the hospital, people may operate from the values of the nurses and primary care providers. When they are at home, they tend to operate from their own personal values and may revert to old habits and ways of doing things that may not be beneficial to their health. The nurse may see this as noncompliance; nevertheless, client autonomy must be respected.

In home care, limited resources and a lack of client care services may shift the focus from client welfare to concerns about resource allocation. Financial considerations can limit the availability of services and materials, making it difficult to ensure that client needs are met.

Professional and Public Advocacy

Advocacy is needed for the nursing profession as well as for the public. Gains that nursing makes in developing and improving health policy at the institutional and government levels help to achieve better health care for the public.

MediaLink Ethics Committee Case Study

BOX 5–8   Values Basic to Client Advocacy

- The client is a holistic, autonomous being who has the right to make choices and decisions.
- Clients have the right to expect a nurse–client relationship that is based on shared respect, trust, collaboration in solving problems related to health and health care needs, and consideration of their thoughts and feelings.
- It is the nurse's responsibility to ensure the client has access to health care services that meet health needs.

BOX 5–9 The Patient Care Partnership: Understanding Expectations, Rights and Responsibilities

When you need hospital care, your doctor and the nurses and other professionals at our hospital are committed to working with you and your family to meet your health care needs. Our dedicated doctors and staff serve the community in all its ethnic, religious and economic diversity. Our goal is for you and your family to have the same care and attention we would want for our families and ourselves.

The sections explain some of the basics about how you can expect to be treated during your hospital stay. They also cover what we will need from you to care for you better. If you have questions at any time, please ask them. Unasked or unanswered questions can add to the stress of being in the hospital. Your comfort and confidence in your care are very important to us.

WHAT TO EXPECT DURING YOUR HOSPITAL STAY

■ *High quality hospital care.* Our first priority is to provide you the care you need, when you need it, with skill, compassion, and respect. Tell your caregivers if you have concerns about your care or if you have pain. You have the right to know the identity of doctors, nurses and others involved in your care, and you have the right to know when they are students, residents or other trainees.

■ *A clean and safe environment.* Our hospital works hard to keep you safe. We use special policies and procedures to avoid mistakes in your care and keep you free from abuse or neglect. If anything unexpected and significant happens during your hospital stay, you will be told what happened, and any resulting changes in your care will be discussed with you.

■ *Involvement in your care.* You and your doctor often make decisions about your care before you go to the hospital. Other times, especially in emergencies, those decisions are made during your hospital stay. When decision-making takes place, it should include:

● *Discussing your medical condition and information about medically appropriate treatment choices.* To make informed decisions with your doctor, you need to understand:
  ● The benefits and risks of each treatment.
  ● Whether your treatment is experimental or part of a research study.
  ● What you can reasonably expect from your treatment and any long-term effects it might have on your quality of life.
  ● What you and your family will need to do after you leave the hospital.
  ● The financial consequences of using uncovered services or out-of-network providers.
  Please tell your caregivers if you need more information about treatment choices.

● *Discussing your treatment plan.* When you enter the hospital, you sign a general consent to treatment. In some cases, such as surgery or experimental treatment, you may be asked to confirm in writing that you understand what is planned and agree to it. This process protects your right to consent to or refuse a treatment. Your doctor will explain the medical consequences of refusing recommended treatment. It also protects your right to decide if you want to participate in a research study.

● *Getting information from you.* Your caregivers need complete and correct information about your health and coverage so that they can make good decisions about your care. That includes:
  ● Past illnesses, surgeries or hospital stays.
  ● Past allergic reactions.
  ● Any medicines or dietary supplements (such as vitamins and herbs) that you are taking.

● Any network or admission requirements under your health plan.

● *Understanding your health care goals and values.* You may have health care goals and values or spiritual beliefs that are important to your well-being. They will be taken into account as much as possible throughout your hospital stay. Make sure your doctor, your family and your care team know your wishes.

● *Understanding who should make decisions when you cannot.* If you have signed a health care power of attorney stating who should speak for you if you become unable to make health care decisions for yourself, or a "living will" or "advance directive" that states your wishes about end-of-life care; give copies to your doctor, your family and your care team. If you or your family need help making difficult decisions, counselors, chaplains and others are available to help.

■ *Protection of your privacy.* We respect the confidentiality of your relationship with your doctor and other caregivers, and the sensitive information about your health and health care that are part of that relationship. State and federal laws and hospital operating policies protect the privacy of your medical information. You will receive a Notice of Privacy Practices that describes the ways that we use, disclose and safeguard patient information and that explains how you can obtain a copy of information from our records about your care.

■ *Preparing you and your family for when you leave the hospital.* Your doctor works with hospital staff and professionals in your community. You and your family also play an important role in your care. The success of your treatment often depends on your efforts to follow medication, diet and therapy plans. Your family may need to help care for you at home.

You can expect us to help you identify sources of follow-up care and to let you know if our hospital has a financial interest in any referrals. As long as you agree that we can share information about your care with them, we will coordinate our activities with your caregivers outside the hospital. You can also expect to receive information and, where possible, training about the self-care you will need when you go home.

■ *Help with your bill and filing insurance claims.* Our staff will file claims for you with health care insurers or other programs such as Medicare and Medicaid. They also will help your doctor with needed documentation. Hospital bills and insurance coverage are often confusing. If you have questions about your bill, contact our business office. If you need help understanding your insurance coverage or health plan, start with your insurance company or health benefits manager. If you do not have health coverage, we will try to help you and your family find financial help or make other arrangements. We need your help with collecting needed information and other requirements to obtain coverage or assistance.

While you are here, you will receive more detailed notices about some of the rights you have as a hospital patient and how to exercise them. We are always interested in improving. If you have questions, comments, or concerns, please contact _____.

Nurses who function responsibly as professional and public advocates are in a position to effect change. To act as an advocate in this arena, the nurse needs an understanding of the ethical issues in nursing and health care, as well as knowledge of the laws and regulations that affect nursing practice and the health of society (see Chapter 4).

Being an effective client advocate involves the following:

- Being assertive
- Recognizing that the rights and values of clients and families must take precedence when they conflict with those of health care providers

- Being aware that conflicts may arise over issues that require consultation, confrontation, or negotiation between the nurse and administrative personnel or between the nurse and primary care provider
- Working with community agencies and lay practitioners
- Knowing that advocacy may require political action—communicating a client's health care needs to government and other officials who have the authority to do something about these needs.

CRITICAL THINKING CHECKPOINT

A 79-year-old man with severe peripheral vascular disease has been told that a nonhealing lesion on his foot must be treated with either vascular bypass surgery or amputation of the foot. Although the surgeon believes the foot can be saved with bypass, the man elects to have the amputation. His main reason is that the site will heal more quickly and allow him to resume normal activities sooner. He asks for the nurse's opinion.

1. What values and beliefs does the client seem to embrace?
2. What additional information might the nurse need to gather from the client or the surgeon?
3. What is the nurse's ethical/moral responsibility in this instance?
4. What conflicting loyalties and obligations does the nurse face?
5. Of what value is the *Code of Ethics for Nurses* to the nurse in solving this dilemma?

See Critical Thinking Possibilities in Appendix A.

CHAPTER 5 **REVIEW**

CHAPTER HIGHLIGHTS

- Values are enduring beliefs that give direction and meaning to life and guide a person's behavior.
- Values clarification is a process in which people identify, examine, and develop their own values.
- Nursing ethics refers to the moral problems that arise in nursing practice and to ethical decisions that nurses make.
- Morality refers to what is right and wrong in conduct, character, or attitude.
- Moral issues are those that arouse conscience, are concerned with important values and norms, and evoke words such as *good, bad, right, wrong, should,* and *ought.*
- Three common moral frameworks (approaches) are consequence-based (teleological), principles-based (deontological), and relationships-based (caring-based) theories.
- Moral principles (e.g., autonomy, beneficence, nonmaleficence, justice, fidelity, and veracity) are broad, general philosophical concepts that can be used to make and explain moral choices.
- A professional code of ethics is a formal statement of a group's ideals and values that serves as a standard and guideline for the group's professional actions and informs the public of its commitment.
- Ethical problems are created as a result of changes in society, advances in technology, conflicts within nursing itself, and nurses'

conflicting loyalties and obligations (e.g., to clients, families, employers, primary care providers, and other nurses).
- Nurses' ethical decisions are influenced by their moral theories and principles, levels of cognitive development, personal and professional values, and nursing codes of ethics.
- The goal of ethical reasoning, in the context of nursing, is to reach a mutual, peaceful agreement that is in the best interests of the client; reaching the agreement may require compromise.
- Nurses are responsible for determining their own actions and for supporting clients who are making moral decisions or for whom decisions are being made by others.
- Nurses can enhance their ethical practice and client advocacy by clarifying their own values, understanding the values of other health care professionals, becoming familiar with nursing codes of ethics, and participating in ethics committees and rounds.
- Client advocacy involves concern for and actions on behalf of another person or organization in order to bring about change.
- The functions of the advocacy role are to inform, support, and mediate.

TEST YOUR KNOWLEDGE

1. When an ethical issue arises, one of the most important nursing responsibilities in managing client care situations is which of the following:
1. Be able to defend the morality of one's own actions
2. Remain neutral and detached when making ethical decisions
3. Ensure that a team is responsible for deciding ethical questions
4. Follow the client and family wishes exactly

2. Which of the following situations is most clearly a violation of the underlying principles associated with professional nursing ethics?
1. The hospital policy permits use of internal fetal monitoring during labor. However, there is literature to both support and refute the value of this practice.
2. When asked about the purpose of a medication, a nurse colleague responds, "Oh, I never look them up. I just give what is prescribed."
3. The nurses on the unit agree to sponsor a fund-raising event to support a labor strike proposed by fellow nurses at another facility.
4. A client reports that he didn't quite tell the doctor the truth when asked if he was following his therapeutic diet at home.

3. Following a motor vehicle accident, the parents refuse to permit withdrawal of life support from the child with no apparent brain function. Although the nurse believes the child should be allowed to die and organ donation considered, the nurse supports their decision. Which moral principle provides the basis for the nurse's actions?

1. Respect for autonomy
2. Nonmaleficence
3. Beneficence
4. Justice

4. Which of the following statements would be *most* helpful when a nurse is assisting clients in clarifying their values?
1. "That was not a good decision. Why did you think it would work?"
2. "The most important thing is to follow the plan of care. Did you follow all your doctor's orders?"
3. "Some people might have made a different decision. What led you to make your decision?"
4. "If you had asked me, I would have given you my opinion about what to do. Now, how do you feel about your choice?"

5. After recovering from her hip replacement, an elderly client wants to go home. The family wants the client to go to a nursing home. If the nurse were acting as a client advocate, the nurse would perform the following:
1. Inform the family that the client has a right to decide on her own.
2. Ask the primary care provider to discharge the client to home.
3. Suggest the client hire a lawyer to protect her rights.
4. Help the client and family communicate their views to each other.

See Answers to Test Your Knowledge in Appendix A. ∞

EXPLORE MEDIALINK www.prenhall.com/berman

DVD-ROM
- Audio Glossary
- NCLEX Review
- End of Unit Concept Map Activity

COMPANION WEBSITE
- Additional NCLEX Review
- Case Study: Ethics Committee
- Applications Activities:
    AIDS Resources
    Privacy
- Links to Resources

READINGS AND REFERENCES

SUGGESTED READINGS
Liaschenko, J., & Peter, E. (2004). Nursing ethics and conceptualizations of nursing: Profession, practice, and work. *Journal of Advanced Nursing, 46*, 488-495.
The authors take a novel approach in suggesting that viewing nursing as work rather than as a profession focuses the discipline better on current social and ethical issues.

RELATED RESEARCH
Volker, D. L. (2003). Is there a unique nursing ethic? *Nursing Science Quarterly, 16*, 207–211.

REFERENCES
American Association of Colleges of Nursing. (1998). *The essentials of baccalaureate education for professional nursing practice.* Washington, DC: Author.

American Hospital Association. (2003). *The patient care partnership: Understanding expectations, rights and responsibilities.* Washington, DC: Author.
American Nurses Association. (1994). *Position statement: Risk versus responsibility in providing nursing care.* Retrieved February 12, 2006, from http://nursingworld.org/readroom/position/ethics/etrisk.htm
American Nurses Association. (1995). Position statement on assisted suicide. *Health Care Law Ethics, 10*(1–2), 125–127.
American Nurses Association. (2001). *Code of ethics for nurses.* Kansas City, MO: Author. Retrieved February 11, 2006, from http://www.nursingworld.org/ethics/code/protected_nwcoe303.htm
American Nurses Association. (2003). *Nursing: Scope and standards of practice.* Washington, DC: Author.

Cassells, J., & Redman, B. (1989). Preparing students to be moral agents in clinical nursing practice. *Nursing Clinics of North America, 24*, 463–473.
Ellerby, J. H., McKenzie, J., McKay, S., Gariepy, G. J., & Kaufert, J. M. (2000). Bioethics for clinicians: 18. Aboriginal cultures. *Canadian Medical Association Journal, 163*, 845–850.
Ersek, M. (2005). Assisted suicide: Unraveling a complex issue. *Nursing, 35*(4), 48–52.
Gallup Organization. (2005). *Nurses remain atop honesty and ethics list.* Princeton, NJ: Author. Retrieved February 11, 2006, from http://poll.gallup.com/content/?ci=20254
Gilligan, C. (1982). *In a different voice.* Cambridge, MA: Harvard University Press.
Hellsten, S. K. (2004). Rationalising circumcision: From tradition to fashion, from public health to individual freedom—critical notes on cultural

persistence of the practice of genital mutilation. *Journal of Medical Ethics, 30,* 248–253.

International Council of Nurses. (2006). *The ICN code for nurses.* Geneva, Switzerland: Author.

Joint Commission on Accreditation of Healthcare Organizations. (2006). 2006 *Comprehensive accreditation manual for hospitals.* Oakbrook Terrace, IL: Author.

Kohlberg, L. (1969). Stage and sequence: The cognitive-developmental approach to socialization. In D. A. Goslin, (Ed.), *Handbook of socialization theory and research* (pp. 347–480). Chicago: Rand McNally.

Marek, M. J. (2004). Nurses' attitudes toward pregnancy termination in the labor and delivery setting. *Journal of Obstetric, Gynecologic, and Neonatal Nursing, 33,* 472–479.

Mathes, M. M. (2004). Assisted suicide and nursing ethics. *MedSurg Nursing, 13,* 261–264.

Raths, L., Harmin, M., & Simon, S. (1978). *Values and teaching: Working with values in the classroom* (2nd ed.). Columbus, OH: Merrill.

Searight, H. R., & Gafford, J. (2005). Cultural diversity at the end of life: Issues and guidelines for family physicians. *American Family Physician, 71,* 515–522.

Searight, H. R., & Gafford, J. (2005). It's like playing with your destiny: Bosnian immigrants' views of advance directives and end-of-life decision-making. *Journal of Immigrant Health, 7,* 195–203.

Thompson, J. B., & Thompson, H. O. (1985). *Bioethical decision-making for nurses.* Norwalk, CT: Appleton-Century-Crofts.

SELECTED BIBLIOGRAPHY

Aiken, T. D. (2003). *Legal, ethical and political issues in nursing* (2nd ed.). Philadelphia: F. A. Davis.

Bandman, E., & Bandman, B. (2002). *Nursing ethics through the life span* (4th ed.). Upper Saddle River, NJ: Prentice Hall.

Canadian Nurses Association. (2002). *Code of ethics for registered nurses.* Ottawa, ON: Author.

Fry, A. T., & Veatch, R. M. (2000). *Case studies in nursing ethics* (2nd ed.). Boston: Jones & Bartlett.

Guido, G. W. (2006). *Legal and ethical issues in nursing* (4th ed.). Upper Saddle River, NJ: Prentice Hall.

Johnstone, M-J. (2004). *Bioethics: A nursing perspective* (4th ed.). Marrickville, NSW, Australia: Churchill-Livingstone.

Haddad, A. (2003). Ethics in action: Fess up to patients. *RN, 66*(9), 27–30.

Haddad, A. (2004). Ethics in action: End-of-life decisions: The family's role. *RN, 67*(1), 25–26, 28.

Haddad, A. (2004). Ethics in action: Warning a patient. *RN, 67*(3), 21–22, 24.

Milton, C. M. (2004). Stories: Implications for nursing ethics and respect for another. *Nursing Science Quarterly, 1,* 208–211.

Tschudin, V. (2003). *Ethics in nursing: The caring relationship.* St. Louis, MO: Elsevier.

Veatch, R. M. (2003). *The basics of bioethics* (2nd ed.). Upper Saddle River, NJ: Prentice Hall.

UNIT 2

Contemporary Health Care

To be effective within a dynamic, complex health care system and to help clients achieve outcomes, nurses need to be knowledgeable, resourceful, and able to work well with other health care practitioners. The nurse is a key participant within interdisciplinary teams whose members share expertise, establish collaborative strategies, and use information technology to support quality care. Nursing care requires even greater flexibility and creativity as it continues to move beyond the hospital into outpatient centers, client homes, and community settings.

Health Care Delivery Systems

LEARNING OUTCOMES

After completing this chapter, you will be able to:

1. Differentiate health care services based on primary, secondary, and tertiary disease prevention categories.

2. Describe the functions and purposes of the health care agencies outlined in this chapter.

3. Identify the roles of various health care professionals.

4. Describe the factors that affect health care delivery.

5. Compare various systems of payment for health care services.

A **health care system** is the totality of services offered by all health disciplines. It is one of the largest industries in the United States. Previously, the major purpose of a health care system was to provide care to the ill and injured. However, with increasing awareness of health promotion, illness prevention, and levels of wellness, health care systems are changing, as are the roles of nurses in these areas. The services provided by a health care system are commonly categorized according to type and level.

TYPES OF HEALTH CARE SERVICES

Health care services are often described in a way correlated with levels of disease prevention: (a) primary prevention, which consists of health promotion and illness prevention, (b) secondary prevention, which consists of diagnosis and treatment, and (c) tertiary prevention, which consists of rehabilitation, health restoration, and palliative care.

Primary Prevention: Health Promotion and Illness Prevention

Based on the notion of maintaining an optimum level of wellness, the World Health Organization (WHO) developed a project called Healthy People. The U.S. Department of Health and Human Services (2000) project that evolved from the original work is called *Healthy People 2010* and has two primary goals: (a) increase quality and years of healthy life and (b) eliminate health disparities.

Health promotion was slow to develop until the 1980s. Since that time more and more people are recognizing the advantages of staying healthy and avoiding illness. Primary prevention programs address areas such as adequate and proper nutrition, weight control and exercise, and stress reduction. Health promotion activities emphasize the important role clients play in maintaining their own health and encourage them to maintain the highest level of wellness they can achieve.

CLINICAL ALERT

As insurance companies have realized that keeping people healthy is less expensive than treating illnesses, their insurance plans have begun to pay for preventive health care activities. ∎

Illness prevention programs may be directed at the client or the community and involve such practices as providing immunizations, identifying risk factors for illnesses, and helping people take measures to prevent these illnesses from occurring. Illness prevention also includes environmental programs that can reduce the incidence of illness or disability. For example, steps to decrease air pollution include requiring inspection of automobile exhaust systems to ensure acceptable levels of fumes. Environmental protective measures are frequently legislated by governments and lobbied for by citizens groups.

Secondary Prevention: Diagnosis and Treatment

In the past, the largest segment of the health care services has been dedicated to the diagnosis and treatment of illness. Hospitals and physicians' offices have been the major agencies offering these complex secondary prevention services. Hospitals continue to focus significant resources on patients requiring emergency, intensive, and around-the-clock acute care.

Freestanding diagnostic and treatment facilities have also evolved and serve ever-growing numbers of clients. For example, magnetic resonance imaging (MRI) and related radiological diagnostic procedures are commonly performed at physician- or corporate-owned centers. Similar structures exist in outpatient surgical units (surgi-centers).

Also included as a health promotion service is early detection of disease. This is accomplished through routine screening of the population and focused screening of those at increased risk of developing certain conditions. Examples of early detection services include regular dental exams from childhood throughout life and bone density studies for women at menopause to evaluate for early osteoporosis. Community-based agencies have become instrumental in providing these services. For example, clinics in some communities provide mammograms and education regarding the early detection of cancer of the breast. Voluntary HIV testing and counseling is another example of the shift in services to community-based agencies. Some malls and shopping centers have walk-in clinics that provide diagnostic tests, such as screening for cholesterol and high blood pressure.

Tertiary Prevention: Rehabilitation, Health Restoration, and Palliative Care

The goal of tertiary prevention is to help people move to their previous level of health (i.e., to their previous capabilities) or to the highest level they are capable of given their current health status. Rehabilitative care emphasizes the importance of assisting clients to function adequately in the physical, mental, social, economic, and vocational areas of their lives. For example, someone with an injured neck or back from an automobile crash may have restrictions in the ability to perform work or daily activities. If the injury is temporary, rehabilitation can assist in return to former function. If the injury is permanent, rehabilitation assists the client in adjusting how to perform activities in order to achieve maximum abilities. Rehabilitation may begin in the hospital, but will eventually lead clients back into the community for further treatment and follow-up once health has been restored.

Sometimes, people cannot be returned to health. A growing field of nursing and tertiary prevention services is that of palliative care—providing comfort and treatment for symptoms. End-of-life care may be conducted in many settings, including the home.

TYPES OF HEALTH CARE AGENCIES AND SERVICES

Health care agencies and services in the United States and Canada are both varied and numerous. Some health care agencies or systems provide services in different settings; for example, a hospi-

tal may provide acute inpatient services, outpatient clinic or ambulatory care services, and emergency room services. Hospice services may be provided in the hospital, in the home, or in another agency within the community (see Figure 6-1 ■). Because the array of health care agencies and services is so great, nurses often need to help clients choose that which best suits their needs. Clients may be seen by any number and type of nurses and other providers, depending on their care and ability to pay for the services.

Public Health

Government (official) agencies are established at the local, state, and federal levels to provide public health services. Health agencies at the state, county, or city level vary according to the need of the area. Their funds, generally from taxes, are administered by elected or appointed officials. Local health departments have responsibility for developing programs to meet the health needs of the people, providing the necessary nursing and other staff and facilities to carry out these programs, continually evaluating the effectiveness of the programs, and monitoring changing needs. State health organizations are responsible for assisting the local health departments. In some remote areas, state departments also provide direct services to people.

The Public Health Service (PHS) of the U.S. Department of Health and Human Services is an official agency at the federal level. Its functions include conducting research and providing training in the health field, providing assistance to communities in planning and developing health facilities, and assisting states and local communities through financing and provision of

Figure 6-1 ■ Various health care settings.

trained personnel. Also at the national level in the United States are research institutions such as the National Institutes of Health (NIH). The National Institute on Drug Abuse, the National Institute on Alcohol Abuse and Alcoholism, and the National Institute of Mental Health work with federal, regional, and state agencies. The Centers for Disease Control and Prevention (CDC) in Atlanta, Georgia, administer a broad program related to surveillance of diseases and behaviors that lead to disease and disability. By means of laboratory and epidemiological investigations, data are made available to the appropriate authorities. The CDC also publishes recommendations about the prevention and control of infections and administers a national health program. The federal government also administers a number of Veterans Affairs (VA) services in the United States.

Physicians' Offices

In North America, the physician's office is a primary care setting. The majority of physicians either have their own offices or work with several other physicians in a group practice. Clients usually go to a physician's office for routine health screening, illness diagnosis, and treatment. People seek consultation from physicians when they are experiencing symptoms of illness or when a significant other considers the person to be ill.

In some medical office practices, such as those of family practice physicians or specialists such as dermatologists or surgeons, nurse practitioners practice alongside physicians. Often, physicians' offices do not require the expertise of registered nurses. Where there are RNs, they have a variety of roles and responsibilities, including client registration, preparing the client for an examination, obtaining health information, and providing information. Other functions may include obtaining specimens, assisting with procedures, and providing some treatments. In offices without RNs, these tasks may be performed by medical assistants.

Ambulatory Care Centers

Ambulatory care centers are used frequently in many communities. Most ambulatory care centers have diagnostic and treatment facilities providing medical, nursing, laboratory, and radiological services, and they may or may not be associated with an acute care hospital. Some ambulatory care centers provide services to people who require minor surgical procedures that can be performed outside the hospital. After surgery, the client returns home, often the same day. These centers offer two advantages: They permit the client to live at home while obtaining necessary health care, and they free costly hospital beds for seriously ill clients. The term *ambulatory care center* has replaced the term *clinic* in many places.

Occupational Health Clinics

The industrial (occupational) clinic is gaining importance as a setting for employee health care. Employee health has long been recognized as important to productivity. Today, more companies recognize the value of healthy employees and encourage healthy lifestyles by providing exercise facilities and coordinating health promotion activities.

Community health nurses in the occupational setting have a variety of roles. Worker safety has always been a concern of occupational nurses. Today, nursing functions in industrial health care include work safety and health education, annual employee health screening for tuberculosis, and maintaining immunization information. Other functions may include screening for such health problems as hypertension and obesity, caring for employees following injury, and counseling.

Hospitals

Hospitals vary in size from the 12-bed rural hospital to the 1,500-bed metropolitan hospital. Hospitals can be classified according to their ownership or control as governmental (public) or nongovernmental (private). In the United States, governmental hospitals are either federal, state, city, or county hospitals. The federal government provides hospital facilities for veterans and merchant mariners (VA hospitals). Military hospitals provide care to military personnel and their families. Private hospitals are often operated by churches, companies, communities, and charitable organizations. Private hospitals may be for-profit or not-for-profit. Although hospitals are chiefly viewed as institutions that provide care, they have other functions, such as providing sources for health-related research and teaching.

Hospitals are also classified by the services they provide. General hospitals admit clients requiring a variety of services, such as medical, surgical, obstetric, pediatric, and psychiatric services. Other hospitals offer only specialty services, such as psychiatric or pediatric care. An acute care hospital provides assistance to clients whose illness and need for hospitalization are relatively short term, for example, several days.

The variety of health care services hospitals provide usually depends on their size and location. The large urban hospitals usually have inpatient beds, emergency services, diagnostic facilities, ambulatory surgery centers, pharmacy services, intensive and coronary care services, and multiple outpatient services provided by clinics. Some large hospitals have other specialized services such as spinal cord injury and burn units, oncology services, and infusion and dialysis units. In addition, some hospitals have substance abuse treatment units and health promotion units. Small rural hospitals often are limited to inpatient beds, radiology and laboratory services, and basic emergency services. The number of services a rural hospital provides is usually directly related to its size and its distance from an urban center.

Hospitals in the United States have undergone organizational changes in order to contain costs or to attract clients. Some hospitals have merged with other hospitals or have been purchased by large multihospital for-profit corporations (e.g., Columbia/HCA Healthcare Corporation, Humana, and Tenet, Inc.). Other hospitals are providing innovative outpatient services, such as fitness classes, day care for elderly people, nutrition classes, and alternative birth centers.

Subacute Care Facilities

Subacute care is a variation of inpatient care designed for someone who has an acute illness, injury, or exacerbation of a disease process. Clients may be admitted after, or instead of, may allow them to provide primary care, prescribe medications, and receive third-party (insurance) reimbursement directly for their services.

Alternative (Complementary) Care Provider

Alternative or complementary health care refers to those practices not commonly considered part of Western medicine. See Chapter 19 ∞ for detailed description of these. Chiropractors, herbalists, acupuncturists, massage therapists, reflexologists, holistic health healers, and other health care providers are playing increasing roles in the contemporary health care system. These providers may practice alongside Western health care providers, or clients may use their services in conjunction with, or in lieu of, Western therapies.

Case Manager

The case manager's role is to ensure that clients receive fiscally sound, appropriate care in the best setting. This role is often filled by the member of the health care team who is most involved in the client's care. Depending on the nature of the client's concerns, the case manager may be a nurse, a social worker, an occupational therapist, a physical therapist, or any other member of the health care team.

Dentist

Dentists diagnose and treat dental problems. Dentists are also actively involved in preventive measures to maintain healthy oral structures (e.g., teeth and gums). Many hospitals, especially long-term care facilities, have dentists on staff.

Dietitian or Nutritionist

A dietitian, often a registered dietitian, has special knowledge about the diets required to maintain health and to treat disease. Dietitians in hospitals generally are concerned with therapeutic diets, may design special diets to meet the nutritional needs of individual clients, and supervise the preparation of meals to ensure that clients receive the proper diet.

A nutritionist is a person who has special knowledge about nutrition and food. The nutritionist in a community setting recommends healthy diets and gives broad advisory services about the purchase and preparation of foods. Community nutritionists often function at the preventive level. They promote health and prevent disease, for example, by advising families about balanced diets for growing children and pregnant women.

Occupational Therapist

An occupational therapist (OT) assists clients with impaired function to gain the skills to perform activities of daily living. For example, an occupational therapist might teach a man with severe arthritis in his arms and hands how to adjust his kitchen utensils so that he can continue to cook. The occupational therapist teaches skills that are therapeutic and at the same time provide some fulfillment. For example, weaving is a recreational activity but also exercises the arthritic man's arms and hands.

Paramedical Technologist

Laboratory technologists, radiological technologists, and nuclear medicine technologists are just three kinds of paramedical technologists in the expanding field of medical technology. *Paramedical* means having some connection with medicine. Laboratory technologists examine specimens such as urine, feces, blood, and discharges from wounds to provide exact information that facilitates the medical diagnosis and the prescription of a therapeutic regimen. The radiological technologist assists with a wide variety of x-ray film procedures, from simple chest radiography to more complex fluoroscopy. The nuclear medicine technologist uses radioactive substances to provide diagnostic information and can administer therapeutic doses of radioactive materials as part of a therapeutic regimen.

Pharmacist

A pharmacist prepares and dispenses pharmaceuticals in hospital and community settings. The role of the pharmacist in monitoring and evaluating the actions and effects of medications on clients is becoming increasingly prominent. A clinical pharmacist is a specialist who guides physicians in prescribing medications. A pharmacy assistant is also recognized in some states. This person administers medications to clients or works in the pharmacy under the direction of the pharmacist.

CLINICAL ALERT

Significant overlap may occur among those providers who can perform certain health care activities. For example, an anesthesiologist (MD), a neonatal care nurse, or a respiratory therapist may be responsible for assisting a newborn baby with breathing problems. All providers perform client teaching. ■

Physical Therapist

The licensed physical therapist (PT) assists clients with musculoskeletal problems. Physical therapists treat movement dysfunctions by means of heat, water, exercise, massage, and electric current. The physical therapist's functions include assessing client mobility and strength, providing therapeutic measures (e.g., exercises and heat applications to improve mobility and strength), and teaching new skills (e.g., how to walk with an artificial leg). Some physical therapists provide their services in hospitals; however, independent practitioners establish offices in communities and serve clients either at the office or in the home. Physical therapy aides also work with PTs and clients.

Physician

The physician is responsible for medical diagnosis and for determining the therapy required by a person who has a disease or injury. The physician's role has traditionally been the treatment of disease and trauma (injury); however, many physicians are now including health promotion and disease prevention in their practice. Some physicians are general practitioners (also known as primary care or family practitioners), while others are dermatologists, neurologists, oncologists, orthopedists, pediatricians, psychiatrists, radiologists, or surgeons—to name a few.

Physician Assistant

Physician assistants (PAs) perform certain tasks under the direction of a physician. They diagnose and treat certain diseases, conditions, and injuries. In many states, nurses are not legally permitted to follow a PA's orders unless they are cosigned by a physician. In some settings, PAs and nurse practitioners have similar job descriptions.

Podiatrist

Doctors of podiatric medicine (DPM) diagnose and treat foot conditions. They are licensed to perform surgery and prescribe medications.

Respiratory Therapist

A respiratory therapist is skilled in therapeutic measures used in the care of clients with respiratory problems. These therapists are knowledgeable about oxygen therapy devices, intermittent positive pressure breathing respirators, artificial mechanical ventilators, and accessory devices used in inhalation therapy. Respiratory therapists administer many of the pulmonary function tests.

Social Worker

A social worker counsels clients and their support persons regarding problems, such as finances, marital difficulties, and adoption of children. It is not unusual for health problems to produce problems in day-to-day living and vice versa. For example, an elderly woman who lives alone and has a stroke resulting in impaired walking may find it impossible to continue to live in her third-floor apartment. Finding a more suitable living arrangement can be the responsibility of the social worker if the client has no support network in place.

Spiritual Support Personnel

Chaplains, pastors, rabbis, priests, and other religious or spiritual advisors serve as part of the health care team by attending to the spiritual needs of clients. In most facilities, local clergy volunteer their services on a regular or on-call basis. Hospitals affiliated with specific religions, as well as many large medical centers, have full-time chaplains on staff. They usually offer regularly scheduled religious services. The nurse is often instrumental in identifying the client's desire for spiritual support and notifying the appropriate person.

Unlicensed Assistive Personnel

Unlicensed assistive personnel (UAPs) are health care staff who assume delegated aspects of basic client care. These tasks include bathing, assisting with feeding, and collecting specimens. UAP titles include certified nurse assistants, hospital attendants, nurse technicians, patient care technicians, and orderlies. Some of these categories of provider may have standardized education and job duties (e.g., certified nurse assistants), while others do not. The parameters regarding nurse delegation to UAPs are delineated by the state boards of nursing.

FACTORS AFFECTING HEALTH CARE DELIVERY

Today's health care consumers have greater knowledge about their health than in previous years, and they are increasingly influencing health care delivery. Formerly, people expected a physician to make decisions about their care; today, however, consumers expect to be involved in making any decisions. Consumers have also become aware of how lifestyle affects health. As a result, they desire more information and services related to health promotion and illness prevention. A number of other factors affect the health care delivery system.

Increasing Number of Elderly

By the year 2020 it is estimated that the number of U.S. adults over the age of 65 years will be more than 53 million (U.S. Census Bureau, 2004). Long-term illnesses are prevalent among this group, and they frequently require special housing, treatment services, financial support, and social networks. The frail elderly, considered to be people over age 85, are projected to be the fastest growing population in the United States and will number over 76.5 million by 2020 and almost 90 million by 2030 (U.S. Census Bureau). Because only 5% of older people are institutionalized with health problems, substantial home management and nursing support services are required to assist those living in their homes and communities.

Older people also need to feel they are part of a community even though they are approaching the end of their lives. The feeling of being a useful, wanted, and productive citizen is essential to every person's health. Special programs are being designed in communities so that the talents and skills of this group will be used and not lost to society.

Advances in Technology

Scientific knowledge and technology related to health care are rapidly increasing. Improved diagnostic procedures and sophisticated equipment permit early recognition of diseases that might otherwise have remained undetected. New antibiotics and medications are continually being manufactured to treat infections and multiple drug-resistant organisms. Surgical procedures involving the heart, lungs, and liver that were nonexistent 20 years ago are common today. Laser and microscopic procedures streamline the treatment of diseases that required surgery in the past.

Computers, bedside charting, and the ability to store and retrieve large volumes of information in databases are commonplace in health care organizations. In addition, as a result of the Internet and World Wide Web access from numerous public and private locations, clients now have access to medical information similar to that of health care providers (although not all websites provide accurate information). One example of a reliable source of health care information for clients is the Agency for Healthcare Research and Quality (AHRQ) website: *Guide to Health Care Quality* (2005).

These discoveries have changed the profile of the client. Clients are now more likely to be treated in the community, utilizing resources, technology, and treatments outside the hospital. For example, years ago a person having cataract surgery had to remain in bed in the hospital for 10 days; today, most cataract removals are performed on an outpatient basis in outpatient surgery centers.

Technological advances and specialized treatments and procedures may come, unfortunately, with a high price tag. Some diagnostic equipment may cost millions of dollars. Due to this expenditure plus the expense of training specialized personnel to perform the tests, each procedure can cost consumers hundreds or thousands of dollars.

Economics

Paying for health care services is becoming a greater problem. The health care delivery system is very much affected by a country's total economic status. According to the Centers for Medicaid and Medicare Services (CMS, 2006), health spending in 2004 was $1.8 trillion in the United States and projected to reach $3.6 trillion by 2014, increasing an average of 7.1% per year. This is currently equal to over $5,000 per year for every man, woman, and child and will more than double to $11,000 by 2014. About 33% are inpatient hospital expenses, 21% physician office and clinic expenses, 15% prescription drug expenses, and the remainder emergency department, home care, dental, and related services. Approximately 42% of these costs are paid through private insurance, 45% through public programs, and 14% out-of-pocket (paid directly by the person) (Kashihara & Carper, 2005).

The major reasons for cost increases are as follows:

- Existing equipment and facilities are continually becoming obsolete as research uncovers new and better methods in health care. Health care providers and patients want the newest and the best, and these cost more each year.
- Inflation increases all costs.
- The total population is growing, especially the segment of older adults who tend to have greater health care needs than younger persons.
- As more people recognize that health is everyone's right, large numbers of people are seeking assistance in health matters. The average American sees a doctor three times per year, but infants less than 12 months of age and elders over 65 average almost seven visits per year (Hing, Cherry, & Woodwell, 2005).
- The relative number of people who provide health care services has increased.
- The numbers of uninsured persons are increasing: approximately 25% of persons under age 65 are uninsured at some time during a year and 13% are uninsured for the entire year (Rhoades, 2006a). Although these percentages have not changed dramatically in the past decade, since the population has increased, the total number of persons affected is rising.
- The cost of prescription drugs is increasing. As of January 2006, Medicare recipients are eligible for prescription drug coverage to help cover some basic and catastrophic medication costs.

Women's Health

The women's movement has been instrumental in changing health care practices. Examples are the provision of childbirth services in more relaxed settings such as birthing centers, and the provision of overnight facilities for parents in children's hospitals. Until recently, women's health issues focused on the reproductive aspects of health, disregarding many health care concerns that are unique to women. Investigators are beginning to recognize the need for research that examines women equally to men in health issues such as osteoporosis, heart disease, and responses to various treatment modalities. Current provision of health care shows an increased emphasis on the psychosocial aspects of women's health, including the impact of career, delayed childbearing, role of caregiver to older family members, and extended life span.

Uneven Distribution of Services

Serious problems in the distribution of health services exist in the United States. Two facets of this problem are (a) uneven distribution and (b) increased specialization. In some areas, particularly remote and rural locations, there are insufficient health care professionals and services available to meet the health care needs of individuals. Rural clients may need to drive large distances to obtain the services they require. Uneven distribution is evidenced by the relatively higher number of nurses per capita in the New England states and the lowest number in California and Nevada (see Figure 6-3 ■). Physicians are also unevenly distributed: In 2003, Mississippi, Idaho, Iowa, and Oklahoma had the fewest physicians per 100,000 people, whereas the District of Columbia, Massachusetts, Maryland, and Vermont had the most (National Center for Health Statistics, 2005).

An increasing number of health care personnel provide specialized services. Specialization can lead to fragmentation of care and, often, increased cost of care. To clients, it may mean receiving care from 5 to 30 people during their hospital experience. This seemingly endless stream of personnel and paperwork required is often confusing and frightening.

Access to Health Insurance

Another problem plaguing individuals is access to health insurance. Data from 2004 show that one in seven Whites, one in five Blacks, and more than one in three Hispanics are uninsured (Rhoades, 2006b). Lack of health insurance is related to income. Persons with incomes below or near the poverty level are at least three times as likely to have no health insurance coverage as those with incomes twice the poverty level or higher (National Center for Health Statistics, 2005). Low income has been associated with relatively higher rates of infectious diseases (e.g., tuberculosis, AIDS), problems with substance abuse, rape, violence, and chronic diseases. Thus, those with the greatest need for health care are often those least able to pay for it. Even though some government assistance is available, eligibility for government insurance programs and benefits varies considerably from state to state and is continually being reevaluated. Other aspects of variations in health beliefs and practices among people of different cultures are found in Chapter 18. ∞

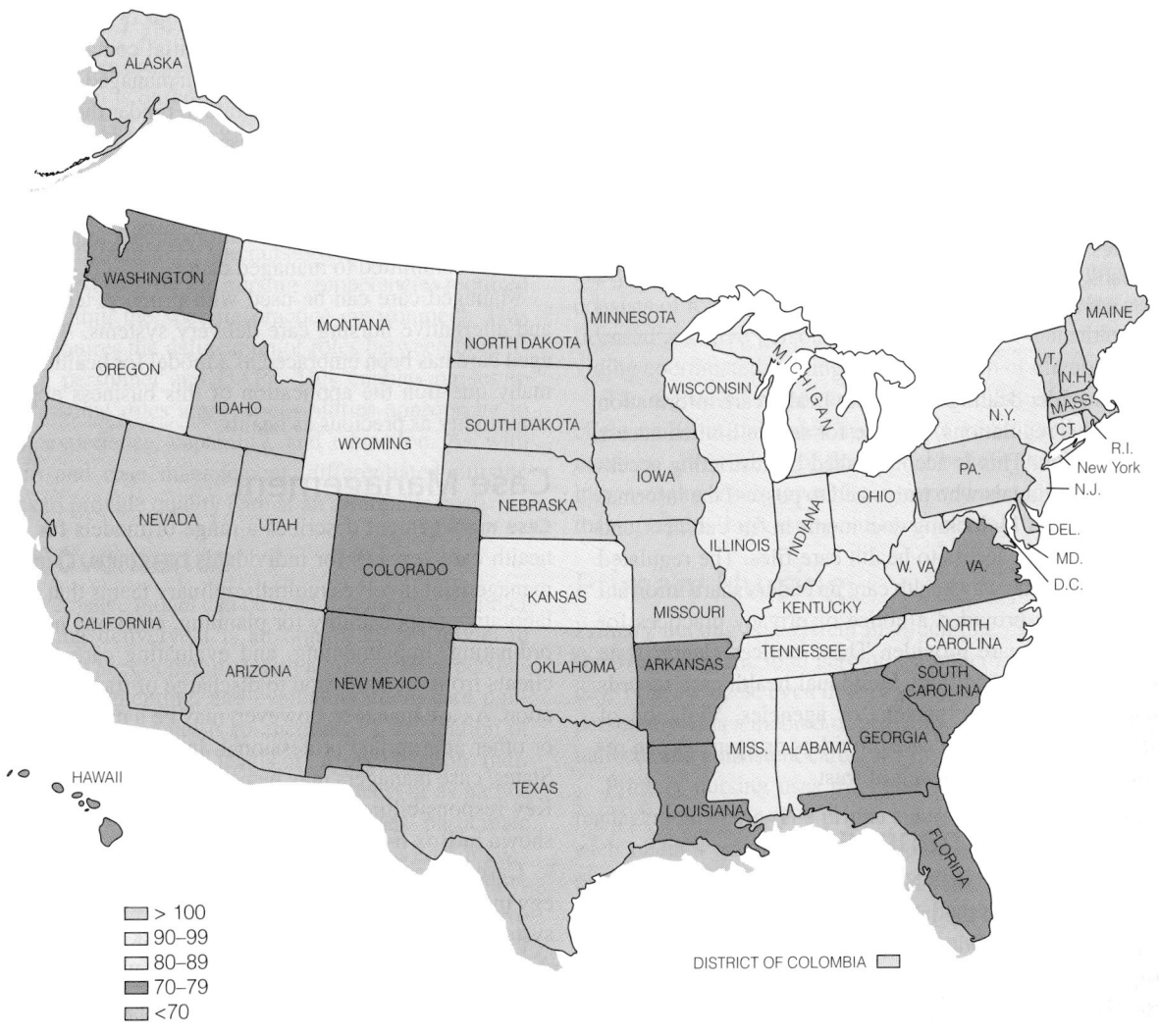

Figure 6-3 ■ Number of nurses per 100,000 population map.

Source: Data from Department of Health & Human Services, Bureau of Health Professions, Division of Nursing. (2004). *The registered nurse population: National sample survey of registered nurses March 2004. Preliminary findings.* Retrieved January 11, 2006, from http://bhpr.hrsa.gov/healthworkforce/reports/rnpopulation/preliminaryfindings.htm

The Homeless and the Poor

Because of the conditions in which homeless people live (in shelters, on the streets, in parks, in tents, under temporary covers and dwellings, in transportation terminals, or in cars), their health problems are often exacerbated and sometimes become chronic. Physical, mental, social, and emotional factors create health care challenges for the homeless and the poor (see Box 6–1). These persons may lack convenient or timely transportation to health care facilities—especially if repeated visits are necessary. Limited access to health care services significantly contributes to the general poor health of the homeless and poor in the United States.

Health Insurance Portability and Accountability Act (HIPAA)

One of the major alterations in how health care is practiced in this country may be attributed to the Health Insurance Portability and Accountability Act of 1996 (HIPAA). These new regulations were instituted to protect the privacy of individuals by safeguarding individually identifiable health care records, in-

cluding those housed in electronic media (see Box 6–2). Protection of individual medical records extends not only to clinical health care sites but also to all ancillary health care providers such as pharmacies, laboratories, and third-party payers. Each

---

BOX 6–1 Factors Contributing to Health Problems of the Homeless and the Poor

- Poor physical environment resulting in increased susceptibility to infections
- Inadequate rest and privacy
- Improper nutrition
- Poor access to facilities for personal hygiene
- Exposure to the elements
- Lack of social support
- Few personal resources
- Questionable personal safety (physical assault is a constant threat for the homeless)
- Inconsistent health care
- Difficulty with adherence to treatment plans

READINGS AND REFERENCES

SUGGESTED READINGS

DeLenardo, C. (2004). Web-based tools steer patient-focused care. *Nursing Management, 35*(12), 60–64.
This article depicts methods to utilize Web-based information to improve understanding of potential treatment venues to cancer patients.

Frist, W. H. (2005). Overcoming disparities in U.S. health care. *Health Affairs, 24*, 445–451.
The many dimensions of health disparities include race, ethnicity, socioeconomic status, and geography. This article suggests strategies for policy makers to address health security for all regardless of socioeconomic characteristics.

RELATED RESEARCH

Agency for Healthcare Research and Quality. (2004). Hospital nurse staffing and quality of care. *Research in Action, Issue 14.* AHRQ Publication No. 04-0029. Retrieved June 9, 2006, from http://www.ahrq.gov/research/nursestaffing/nursestaff.htm

Furaker, C., Hellstrom-Muhli, U., & Walldal, E. (2004). Quality of care in relation to a critical pathway from the staff's perspective. *Journal of Nursing Management, 12*, 309–316.

Short, P. F., & Graefe, D. R. (2003). Battery-powered health insurance? Stability in coverage of the uninsured. *Health Affairs, 22*, 244–255.

REFERENCES

Agency for Healthcare Research and Quality. (2005). *Guide to health care quality.* Retrieved June 24, 2006, from http://www.ahrq.gov/consumer/guidetoq

Department of Health & Human Services, Bureau of Health Professions, Division of Nursing. (2004). *Preliminary findings: 2004 national sample survey of registered nurses.* Retrieved June 25, 2006, from http://bhpr.hrsa.gov/healthworkforce/reports/rnpopulation/preliminaryfindings.htm

Cawley, J., & Simon, K. I. (2005). Health insurance coverage and the macroeconomy. *Journal of Health Economics, 24*, 299–315.

Centers for Medicaid and Medicare Services (CMS). (2006). *National health expenditure data.* Retrieved June 11, 2006, from http://www.cms.hhs.gov/NationalHealth ExpendData/03_NationalHealthAccounts Projected.asp#TopOfPage

Gordon, J. A., Emond, J. A., & Camargo, C. A. (2005). The State Children's Health Insurance Program: A multicenter trial of outreach through the emergency department. *American Journal of Public Health, 95,* 250–253.

Hall, L. M., Doran, D., & Pink, G. H. (2004). Nurse staffing models, nursing hours, and patient safety outcomes. *Journal of Nursing Administration, 34,* 41–45.

Hing, E., Cherry, D. K., & Woodwell, D. A. (2005). National ambulatory medical care survey: 2003 summary. *Advance data from vital and health statistics;* No. 3645. Retrieved June 25, 2006, from http://www.cdc.gov/nchs/data/ad/ad365.pdf

Jennings, C. P. (2004). Insuring America's health: Principles and recommendations: IOM report. *Policy, Politics, and Nursing Practice, 5,* 100–101.

Kashihara, D., & Carper, K. (2005). *National health care expenses in the U.S. civilian noninstitutionalized population, 2003.* Statistical Brief No. 103. Rockville, MD: Agency for Healthcare Research and Quality. Retrieved June 25, 2006, from http://www.meps.ahrq.gov/papers/st103/stat103.pdf

National Center for Health Statistics. (2005). *Health: United States, 2005.* Hyattsville, MD: Author.

Rhoades, J. A. (2006a). *The uninsured in America, 1996–2005: Estimates for the U.S. civilian noninstitutionalized population under age 65.* Statistical Brief #130. Rockville, MD: Agency for Healthcare Research and Quality. Retrieved June 25, 2006, from http://www.meps.ahrq.gov/papers/st130/stat130.pdf

Rhoades, J. A. (2006b). *The uninsured in America, First half of 2005: Estimates for the U.S. civilian noninstitutionalized population under age 65.* Statistical Brief No. 129. Rockville, MD: Agency for Healthcare Research and Quality. Retrieved June 25, 2006, from http://www.meps.ahrq.gov/papers/st129/stat129.pdf

U.S. Census Bureau. (2004). *U.S. interim projections by age, sex, race, and Hispanic origin.* Retrieved June 24, 2006, from http://www.census.gov/ipc/www/usinterimproj/natprojtab02a.pdf

U.S. Department of Health and Human Services. (2000). *Healthy people 2010: Understanding and improving health* (2nd ed.). Washington, DC: U.S. Government Printing Office.

SELECTED BIBLIOGRAPHY

American Association of Colleges of Nursing. (1995). *A model for differentiated nursing practice.* Washington, DC: Author.

Brown, G. (2004). Nursing and its future status. *Minority Nurse Newsletter, 11*(1), 1.

Cutler, D. M. (2004). *Your money or your life: Strong medicine for America's health care system.* New York: Oxford University Press.

Erickson, J. I., & Miller, S. (2005). Caring for patients while respecting their privacy: Renewing our commitment. *Online Journal of Issues in Nursing, 10*(2), Manuscript 2. Retrieved June 11, 2006, from http://www.nursingworld.org/ojin/topic27/tpc27_1.htm

Feuer, L. (2004). The growing population of uninsured: Are you prepared for the challenge? *Case Manager, 15,* 19–21.

Hall, L., & Doran, D. (2004). Nurse staffing, care delivery model, and patient care quality. *Journal of Nursing Care Quality, 19*(1), 27–33.

Harrington, C., & Estes, C. L. (Eds.). (2004). *Health policy and nursing: Crisis and reform in the U.S. health care delivery system* (4th ed.). Boston: Jones & Bartlett.

Institute of Medicine. (2004). *Uninsured in America.* Retrieved June 6, 2006, from http://www.iom.edu/Object.File/Master/21/040/0.pdf

Kovner, A. R., & Knickman, J. R. (2005). *Jonas & Kovner's health care delivery in the United States* (8th ed.). New York: Springer.

Simpson, S. H., Majumdar, S. R., & Marrie, T. J. (2003). Physician-related barriers to the adoption of a critical pathway for community-acquired pneumonia: A qualitative analysis. *Journal of General Internal Medicine, 18* (Suppl. 1), 275–280.

Community Nursing and Care Continuity

LEARNING OUTCOMES

After completing this chapter, you will be able to:

1. Discuss factors influencing health care reform.

2. Describe community-based health care, including the Pew Health Professions Commission recommendations for health competencies for future health practitioners.

3. Describe various community-based frameworks, including integrated health care systems, community initiatives and conditions, and case management.

4. Differentiate community health care settings from traditional settings.

5. Differentiate community-based nursing from traditional institutional-based nursing.

6. Discuss competencies community-based nurses need for practice.

7. Explain essential aspects of collaborative health care: definitions, objectives, benefits, and the nurse's role.

8. Identify various types of communities.

9. Describe the role of the nurse in providing continuity of care.

The health care system is undergoing change. Escalating health care costs, expanding technology, changing patterns of demographics, shorter hospital stays, increased client acuity, and limited access to health care are some of the factors motivating change. The location of client care is expanding out of traditional settings into the community and neighborhoods. For example, health care activities such as intravenous fluid administration or mechanical ventilation, once considered safe only in hospital settings, are now available for clients in their homes (see Chapter 8 ∞) and in ambulatory surgical, rehabilitation, and dialysis centers.

Many things influence whether clients select to have their care in hospitals or in community settings. Some variables include clients' knowledge and awareness of community resources, cost, availability of home care, and perceived safety of home care. Research is needed to show whether there are differences in health outcomes based on location of care.

It is difficult to document care shifting from hospitals to the community. One resource to track changes is the annual survey of health care dollar expenditures conducted by the U.S. government. The most recent data show a decrease in the percent of total health care dollars that were spent in hospitals and an increase in dollars spent for home care (National Center for Health Statistics, 2005). Although hospitals and other health care institutions remain key components of the health care system, the trend is toward an integrated health care system—one that is community based. The shift from institutional to community care also brings changes in the roles and responsibilities of health care professionals.

THE MOVEMENT OF HEALTH CARE TO THE COMMUNITY

Both consumers and health care professionals have had major dissatisfaction about the current health care system which focuses on acute, hospital-based care. Although plans to reform the health care system have been proposed nationally and internationally, no single plan has been adopted. Drafts of legislative reform in the United States include initiatives directed at cost control through managed care competition, providing health insurance for the poor, and transforming the insurance industry.

Nurses, professional organizations, and consumers influence health care reform. Nurses provide a unique perspective on the health care system because of their constant presence in a variety of settings and their contact both with consumers who receive the benefits of the system's most complex services and

with those who have problems with the system's inefficiencies. Greater numbers of advanced practice nurses in recent years have resulted in the provision of primary care to many consumers who had previously been neglected—those living in rural areas, the poor, older adults, and women and infants.

Through nurses' major organizations, nursing has presented a strong voice in describing what a new system should include and what nursing's contributions should be. In 1991, the American Nurses Association (ANA) published *Nursing's Agenda for Health Care Reform,* which set forth the ANA's recommendations for health care reform. These recommendations are summarized in Box 7–1. Although the agenda called for "immediate" changes, the majority of the recommendations have still not been implemented over 15 years later.

Consumers are also effecting major changes in health care delivery systems. Consumers are adopting health-related values that include the following:

- Health means more than the absence of disease; it encompasses well-being and quality of life.
- Quality of life is related to a healthy community that includes healthy families and a healthy environment.

BOX 7–1 Nursing's Agenda for Health Care Reform

- A restructured health care system that (a) enhances consumer access to services by delivering primary health care in community-based settings, (b) fosters consumer responsibility for personal health, self-care, and informed decision making in selecting health care services, and (c) facilitates using the most cost-effective providers and therapeutic options in the most appropriate settings
- A federally defined standard package of essential health care services available to all citizens and residents of the United States, provided and financed through an integration of public and private plans and sources
- A phase-in of essential services
- Planned change to anticipate health service needs that correlate with changing national demographics
- Steps to reduce health care costs
- Case management for those with continuing health care needs
- Provisions for long-term care
- Insurance reforms to improve access to coverage

Note: Reprinted with permission from American Nurses Association, *Nursing's Agenda for Health Care Reform,* © 2001 Nursesbooks.org, Silver Spring, MD 20910.

- Individuals can actively participate in promoting and maintaining their health through behavior and lifestyle changes.
- Disease prevention is important.

These values indicate that consumers support an increased emphasis on health care services and programs that promote wellness and restoration and prevent disease.

Primary Health Care and Primary Care

Another major influence promoting health care reform has been the work on *Healthy People 2000* and *Healthy People 2010* (U.S. Department of Health and Human Services [USDHHS], 2000). These projects present health-related objectives that provide a framework for national health promotion, health protection, and disease prevention. Details of *Healthy People 2010* are discussed in Chapter 16. ∞

The forerunner of *Healthy People 2000* and *Nursing's Agenda for Health Care Reform* was the 1978 World Health Organization (WHO) report *Primary Health Care.* The term *primary health care* (PHC) was coined in the World Health Assembly by WHO and the United Nations International Children's Emergency Fund (UNICEF).

Primary health care (PHC) is defined as

essential health care based on practical, scientifically sound and socially acceptable methods and technology made universally accessible to individuals and families in the community through their full participation and at a cost that the community and country can afford to maintain at every stage of their development in the spirit of self-reliance and self-determination. (WHO, 1978, p. 35)

Primary health care incorporates five principles:

- Equitable distribution
- Appropriate technology
- A focus on health promotion and disease prevention
- Community participation
- A multisectoral approach

Deep concern about health care for the majority of the world's population, specifically low life expectancies and high mortality rates among children, led to the global health strategy of primary health care. The WHO declaration emphasized health or well-being as a fundamental right and a worldwide social goal. It attempted to address inequality in health status of persons in all countries and to target government responsibility for policies that would promote economic, social, and health development. Both economic and social development were considered basic to the achievement of health for all. Thus, PHC extends beyond the boundaries of traditional health care services. It involves issues of the environment, agriculture, housing, and other social, economic, and political issues such as poverty, transportation, unemployment, economic development to sustain the population, and so on. A major feature of PHC is that consumers, governments, and public institutions such as public health departments and city councils should be involved in the planning and delivery of health care.

PHC differs from primary care (PC). Primary care addresses personal health services and not population-based public health services. **Primary care (PC),** according to the Institute of Medicine (IOM), is "the provision of integrated, accessible health care services by clinicians who are accountable for addressing a large majority of personal health services, developing a sustained partnership with patients, and practicing in the context of family and community" (IOM, 1994, p. 15).

PHC is community based and driven and requires active community involvement in making decisions to improve health. PC, on the other hand, is expert driven and involves health professionals who advise individuals and communities about what is best for their health. Other differences are shown in Table 7–1.

There are also similarities between PHC and PC. Both acknowledge the prevention and promotion components of health and well-being. Both strive for universal access to and affordability of health care, support empowerment of the client, and target those at risk for preventable health problems.

COMMUNITY-BASED HEALTH CARE

Community-based health care (CBHC) is a PHC system that provides health-related services within the context of people's daily lives—that is, in places where people spend their time, for example, in the home, in shelters, in long-term care residences, at work, in schools, in senior citizens' centers, in ambulatory settings, and in hospitals. The care is directed toward a specific group within the geographic neighborhood (see Figure 7-1 ■). The group may be established by a physical boundary, an employer, a school district, a managed care insurance provider, or a specific medical need or category. In contrast to the traditional health care system that focuses primarily on the ill and the injured, community-based care is holistic. It involves a broad

TABLE 7–1 **Differences between Primary Care and Primary Health Care**	
PRIMARY CARE	**PRIMARY HEALTH CARE**
■ Community participation is provider directed.	■ Community participation is client directed.
■ The professional's role is expert, provider, authority, and team leader.	■ The professional's role is facilitator, consultant, and resource.
■ Collaboration occurs among members of the health care team.	■ Collaboration goes beyond the health care sector.
■ The individual or family is the focus.	■ The community or some aggregate is the focus.
■ Access is limited.	■ Access is universal.
■ Health care is available within given health care institutions.	■ Health care is available where people live and work.
■ Empowerment is a provider-assisted process.	■ Empowerment is a collaborative, enabling process.

Note: Reprinted from *Nursing Outlook, 43*(1), D. Barnes, et al., "Primary Health Care and Primary Care: A Confusion of Philosophies," pp. 7–16. Copyright 1995, with permission of Elsevier.

Figure 7-1 ■ Communities may consist of several types of neighborhoods. (*Frank Siteman, PhotoEdit Inc.*)

1. *Production, distribution, and consumption of goods and services.* These are the means by which the community provides for the economic needs of its members. This function includes not only the supplying of food and clothing but also the provision of water, electricity, and police and fire protection and the disposal of refuse.
2. *Socialization.* Socialization refers to the process of transmitting values, knowledge, culture, and skills to others. Communities usually contain a number of established institutions for socialization: families, churches, schools, media, voluntary and social organizations, and so on.
3. *Social control.* Social control refers to the way in which order is maintained in a community. Laws are enforced by the police; public health regulations are implemented to protect people from certain diseases. Social control is also exerted through the family, church, and schools.
4. *Social interparticipation.* Social interparticipation refers to community activities that are designed to meet people's needs for companionship. Families and churches have traditionally met this need; however, many public and private organizations also serve this function.
5. *Mutual support.* Mutual support refers to the community's ability to provide resources at a time of illness or disaster. Although the family is usually relied on to fulfill this function, health and social services may be necessary to augment the family's assistance if help is required over an extended period.

range of services designed not only to restore health but also to promote health, prevent illness, and protect the public.

To be truly effective, a CBHC system needs to (a) provide easy access to care, (b) be flexible in responding to the care needs that individuals and families identify, (c) promote care between and among health care agencies through improved communication mechanisms, (d) provide appropriate support for family caregivers, and (e) be affordable.

As far back as 1992 (de Tornyay), an ideal health care system was described that would need to:

■ Be more oriented to health and emphasize health promotion and disease prevention.
■ Focus on individual responsibility for health practices and behavior.
■ Be population based and focus more attention on risk factors in the physical and social environment.
■ Use electronic information systems for client histories and research findings to support diagnostic decisions and treatment recommendations.
■ Have a stronger focus on consumers who would have increased information and be informed participants in decisions about their health care.
■ Base decisions on outcomes.
■ Provide care more efficiently by means of integrated or coordinated teams of providers.
■ Balance technology with nontechnical interventions and weigh the benefits against its effects on human values and interpersonal processes.
■ Have health care providers who will be increasingly accountable to consumers and society for a wider range of outcomes of care.

COMMUNITY HEALTH

A **community** is a collection of people who share some attribute of their lives and interact with each other in some way. They may live in the same locale, attend a particular church, or even share a particular interest such as art. Groups that constitute a community because of common member interests are often referred to as *communities of interest* (e.g., religious and cultural groups). A community can also be defined as a social system in

which the members interact formally or informally and form networks that operate for the benefit of all people in the community. Five of the main functions of a community are described in Box 7–2. In community health, the community may be viewed as having a common health problem, such as a high incidence of infant mortality or of tuberculosis, HIV infection, or another communicable disease. Box 7–3 lists the characteristics of a healthy community. A **population** is composed of people who

A HEALTHY COMMUNITY
■ Is one in which members have a high degree of awareness of being a community
■ Uses its natural resources while taking steps to conserve them for future generations
■ Openly recognizes the existence of subgroups and welcomes their participation in community affairs
■ Is prepared to meet crises
■ Is a problem-solving community; it identifies, analyzes, and organizes to meet its own needs
■ Possesses open channels of communication that allow information to flow among all subgroups of citizens in all directions
■ Seeks to make each of its systems' resources available to all members
■ Has legitimate and effective ways to settle disputes that arise within the community
■ Encourages maximum citizen participation in decision making
■ Promotes a high level of wellness among all its members

RESEARCH NOTE · Are Public Health Nurses Really Doing Public Health Nursing?

In this research study, 289 of the 383 eligible public health nurses (PHNs) in five California counties returned a survey questionnaire regarding their demographics, employment, education, and scope of practice. Due to California regulations, most of the nurses had at least a BSN. Nurses were asked how frequently they performed specific interventions aimed at the individual-family, the community, and the health care system.

Overall, the PHNs regularly performed interventions aimed at the individual-family. The most often performed intervention (91% of the nurses said they did this frequently or extensively) was case management of individuals/families. Few nurses reported frequently performing interventions at the community or the health care system level.

The researchers concluded that the PHNs were not really fulfilling their role since "The focus of PHN is not on providing direct care to individuals in community settings" (American Public Health Association, 1996) but rather on promoting the health of populations. They state that a major obstacle preventing the PHNs from following their community focus included that reimbursement for services is tied to individual client measurable outcomes. They also believe that the current method of educating RNs focuses on preparing generalists with inadequate emphasis on community and public health practice.

IMPLICATIONS

It is important to realize that definitions and roles change over time. The most current description of the PHN role is from the Quad Council of Public Health Nursing Organizations (Quad Council, 2003). Current member organizations are the Association of State and Territorial Directors of Nursing, the American Nurses Association Council on Nursing Practice and Economics, the Association of Community Health Nursing Educators, and the Section of Public Health Nursing of the American Public Health Association. Although their PHN competencies "were developed with the understanding that public health practice is population-focused and public health nursing is also population-focused, one of the unique contributions of public health nurses is the ability to apply these principles at the individual and family level *within the context of population-focused practice*" (original emphasis) (Quad Council, 2003). Thus, emphasis on PHN practice at the individual-family, the community, and the health care system levels remains important.

Note: From "How Much Public Health in Public Health Nursing Practice," by K. Grumbach, J. Miller, E. Mertz, and L. Finocchio, 2004, *Public Health Nursing, 21,* pp. 266–276.

---

share some common characteristic but who do not necessarily interact with each other. **Community health nursing** focuses on promoting and preserving the health of population groups.

Communities, like individuals and families, are living entities. As such, the nurse will need to carry out an assessment of this community as the client. Several community assessment frameworks have been devised. Students who enroll in a community health nursing course will study these in some detail. As one example, Anderson and McFarlane (2004) identified eight subsystems of the community for analysis. The subsystems are illustrated around a core, which consists of the people and their characteristics, values, history, and beliefs. The first stage in assessment is to learn about the people in the community. These community-level subsystems may be thought of as analogous to the physiological subsystems of an individual. Figure 7-2 ■ shows some of the major components of the community core. Surrounding the core are the eight subsystems. Box 7–4 shows major aspects of a community assessment. Box 7–5 shows sources of community data that the nurse may draw on to help identify health care concerns and to aid in intervention planning for any acknowledged community health issues.

Planning community health may be oriented toward improved crisis management, disease prevention, health maintenance, or health promotion. The responsibility for planning at the community level is usually broadly based and needs to include as many of the community partners as possible. The exact resources and skills of members of the community often depend on the size of the community. A broadly based planning group is most likely to create a plan that is acceptable to members of the community. Also, people who are involved in planning become educated about the problems, the resources, and the interrelationships within the system.

When setting priorities, health planners must work with consumers, interest groups, or other involved persons to prioritize health problems. It is important to take into consideration the values and interests of community members, the severity of the problems, and the resources available to identify and act on

Figure 7-2 ■ The community assessment wheel, the assessment segment of the community-as-partner model.

Note: From *Community as Partner: Theory and Practice in Nursing,* 4th ed. (p. 170), by E. T. Anderson and J. McFarlane, 2004, Philadelphia: Lippincott Williams & Wilkins. Reprinted with permission.

BOX 7–4 Major Aspects of a Community Assessment

PHYSICAL ENVIRONMENT

Consider the natural boundaries, size, and population density; types of dwellings; and incidence of crime, vandalism, and substance abuse.

EDUCATION

Consider educational facilities; existing school health facilities; type and amount of health services handled by the school; school lunch programs; extracurricular sports, libraries, and counseling services; continuing education or extended education programs; and extent of parental involvement in the schools.

SAFETY AND TRANSPORTATION

Consider fire, police, and sanitation services; sources of water and its treatment; quality of the air; garbage disposal service; availability and safety of public transportation; and availability of ambulance services.

POLITICS AND GOVERNMENT

Consider kind of government; organizations active in the community; influential people in the community; issues that have recently appeared on local ballots; and the average election turnout.

HEALTH AND SOCIAL SERVICES

Consider existing hospitals, health care facilities, and health care services; number, type, and routine caseloads of community health professionals; geographic, economic, and cultural accessibility to health care services; sources of health information; level of immunization

among children and adults; life expectancy in the community; availability of home health care and long-term care services; and availability of transportation service to all major health facilities.

COMMUNICATION

Consider local newspapers; radio and TV stations, postal services, Internet access, and telephone services; frequency of public forums; and presence of informal bulletin boards.

ECONOMICS

Consider the main industries and occupations; percentage of the population employed or attending school; income levels and quality and type of housing; occupational health programs; and major employers in the community.

RECREATION

Consider recreational facilities in the community and outside the community; theaters and movie houses; number and types of church and religious services; number and utilization of playgrounds, pools, parks, and sports facilities; level of participation in various church programs; and number and types of social committees, organizations, and clubs available.

Note: From *Community as Partner: Theory and Practice in Nursing,* 4th ed. (pp. 172–173), by E. T. Anderson and J. McFarlane, 2004, Philadelphia: Lippincott Williams & Wilkins. Adapted with permission.

BOX 7–5 Sources of Community Assessment Data

- City maps to locate community boundaries, roads, churches, schools, parks, hospitals, and so on
- State census data for population composition and characteristics
- Chamber of commerce for employment statistics, major industries, and primary occupations
- County or state health departments for location of health facilities, occupational health programs, numbers of health professionals, numbers of welfare recipients, and so on
- City or regional health planning boards for health needs and practices
- Telephone book for location of social, recreational, and health organizations, committees, and facilities
- Public and university libraries for district social and cultural research reports
- Health facility administrators for information about employee caseloads, prevalent types of problems, and dominant needs
- Recreational directors for programs provided and participation levels
- Police department for incidence of crime, vandalism, and drug addiction
- Teachers and school nurses for incidence of children's health problems and information on facilities and services to maintain and promote health
- Local newspapers for community activities related to health and wellness, such as health lectures or health fairs
- Online computer services that may provide access to public documents related to community health

the problems. Because any plan is likely to result in change, members of the planning group should understand and use planned change theory.

In community health, evaluation determines whether the planned interventions have led to the achievement of the established goals and objectives; for example, was the immunization rate of preschool children improved? Because community health is usually a collaborative process between health providers, community leaders, politicians, and consumers, all may be involved in the evaluation process. Often the community health nurse is the agent of evaluation, collecting and assessing the data that determine the effectiveness of implemented programs.

Community-Based Frameworks

Various approaches are emerging to address community health. Some of these are an integrated health care system, community initiatives, community coalitions, managed care, case management, and outreach programs using lay health workers.

An **integrated health care system** makes all levels of care available in an integrated form—primary care, secondary care, and tertiary care (see Figure 7-3■). Its goals are to facilitate care across settings, recovery, positive health outcomes, and the long-term benefits of modifying harmful lifestyles through health promotion and disease prevention. In many parts of the country, hospitals are reflecting this concept by changing their names to *health care organization* or *integrated health care*

Figure 7-3 ■ Model of an integrated health care delivery system.

system. This type of system is sometimes referred to as *seamless care.*

Community initiatives are being sponsored by some hospitals or local community agencies. These initiatives, called *healthy cities* and *healthier communities,* involve members of the community to establish health priorities, set measurable goals, and determine actions to reach these goals. If a community agency is initiating this project, the associated hospital generally contributes human resources to assist in this endeavor.

Community coalitions bring together individuals and groups for the shared purpose of improving the community's health. Nurses are major participants and contributors in these coalitions and often assume leadership positions. Community coalitions may focus on a single or multifaceted problem. Examples include establishment of an abuse program, a gang prevention program, an older adults assessment program, or an immunization program for a high-risk group.

In managed care, which is a common model in health care restructuring, health care providers (hospitals, physicians, nurse practitioners, insurance carriers, and so on) join to meet health needs across the care continuum. The managed care organization serves as a "go-between" or "gatekeeper" with the client, provider, and payer. Providers are organized into groups, and the client must select one from the group to which he or she belongs. Managed care aims in this way to enhance the quality and cost-effectiveness of health care.

Case management is an integrative health care model that tracks clients' needs and services through a variety of care settings to ensure continuity. The case manager is familiar with the clients' health needs and resources available through their insurance coverage so they can receive cost-effective care. Another important aspect of case management is assisting the client and family to understand and navigate their way through the health care system.

Outreach programs using lay health workers are a method of linking underserved or high-risk populations with the formal health care system. They can minimize or reduce barriers to health care, increase access to services, and thus improve the health status of the community. They involve partnerships between nurses and members of the community. Interested and committed lay health workers are identified who will assist their neighbors through outreach networks. Nurses provide training, consultation, and support to these individuals.

Community-Based Settings

Traditionally, community nursing services have been provided in county and state health departments (public health nursing), in schools (school nursing), in workplaces (occupational nursing), and in homes (home health care and hospice nursing). Over the years, numerous other settings have been established, including day-care centers, senior centers, storefront clinics, homeless shelters, mental health centers, crisis centers, drug rehabilitation programs, and ambulatory care centers. More recent settings for community nursing practice include nurse-managed community nursing centers, parish nursing, and telehealth projects.

Community Nursing Centers

Community nursing centers provide primary care to specific populations and are staffed by nurse practitioners and community health nurses. Although the nurses are the primary providers of care to clients visiting the center, a physician's consultation is available as needed. Nursing centers may be located in schools, workplaces, or other community agencies, or be free standing. Nursing centers must interface with nurse-managed services in other settings across the health care continuum, that is, services being provided to clients in their home, hospital, or long-term care facility. There are various categories of community nursing centers:

- *Community outreach centers.* Relatively small free-standing clinics providing services similar to those traditionally provided by large public health clinics but focused on a narrower population.
- *Institution-based centers.* Associated with a large parent organization such as a hospital, corporation, or university or college.
- *School-based centers.* Placed within school facilities from kindergarten through college level to provide services such as emergency first aid, diagnosis of acute illnesses, health promotion and maintenance programs, as well as health education to school-age populations.
- *Wellness centers.* Provide services such as health promotion, health maintenance, education, counseling, and screening. In some settings, wellness centers are staffed by members of the health care team other than nurses (e.g., physical therapists or occupational therapists).

Parish Nursing

Parish nursing was founded in the United States in Illinois in the mid-1980s by Reverend Granger Westberg (Smith, 2003) and became a specialty recognized by the ANA in 1998. The International Parish Nurse Resource Center describes the roles of the parish nurse as follows:

- Personal health counselor who discusses health issues and problems with individuals and makes home, hospital, and nursing home visits as needed
- Health educator who educates and supports individuals through health education activities that promote an understanding of the relationship between values, attitudes, lifestyle, faith, and well-being
- Referral source who acts as a liaison to other congregational and community resources
- Facilitator who recruits and coordinates volunteers within the congregation and develops support groups
- Integrator of faith and health

An estimated 3,000 parish nurses serve churches, synagogues, and temples in the United States (see Figure 7-4 ■). Most parish nurses are volunteers, but some are employees paid by the congregation or an affiliated institution such as a health system or community agency. Parish nursing is nondenominational and includes nurses of all religious faiths. Parish nursing is one of the few community-based nursing roles found with a similar structure and focus in nations around the world.

Telehealth

Telehealth projects use communication and information technology to provide health information and health care services to people in rural, remote, or underserved areas. Video confer-

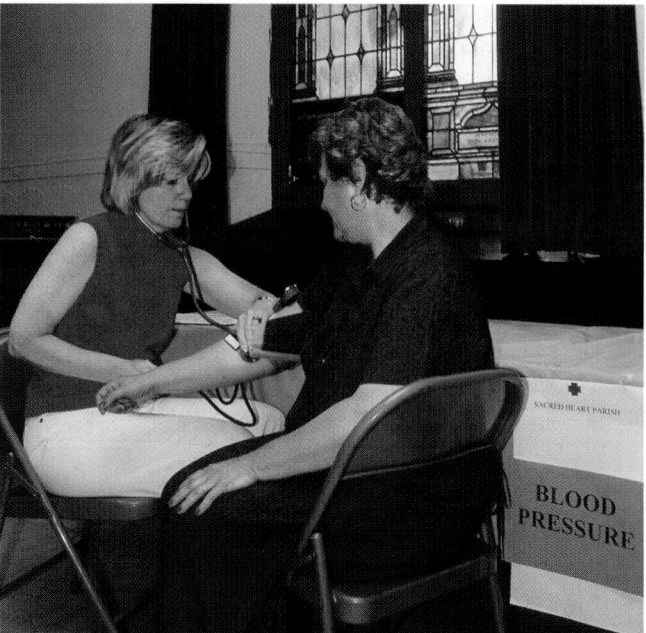

Figure 7-4 ■ Some parish-based health services provide care to community residents in addition to members of the congregation.

ences or "video clinics" enable health care workers to provide distant consultation to assess and treat ambulatory clients who have a variety of health care needs. These video conferences are similar to any outpatient clinic visit except that the client and health care specialist are miles apart. A related development to telehealth is telenursing, in which nurses provide client teaching and health promotion to distant clients.

COMMUNITY-BASED NURSING

Community-based nursing (CBN) is nursing care directed toward specific individuals. However, community-based nursing involves nursing care that is not confined to one practice setting. It extends beyond institutional boundaries and involves a network of nursing services: nursing wellness centers, ambulatory care, acute care, long-term care nursing services, telephone advice, home health, school health, and hospice services. For example, a nurse case manager may be involved in (a) visiting a newly admitted client in the hospital to take a detailed nursing history, confer with the primary nurse, and begin discharge planning; (b) making several home visits to monitor a client recently transferred from a hospital to a long-term care agency to discuss the client's progress with the nursing staff; or (c) making consultative telephone calls to other health professionals (physicians, social workers, respiratory therapists, and so on) and to clients who are managing self-care independently but who may need support.

CLINICAL ALERT

Community-based nursing and community health nursing are not the same concept. Community-based nursing focuses on care of individuals in geographically local settings, whereas community health nursing emphasizes the promotion and preservation of the health of groups (populations or aggregates). ■

Other nurses who work in community-based settings, such as case managers, occupational health nurses, school nurses, and public health department nurses, need to be prepared to make home visits. Home visits can provide information that is not obtainable in other ways.

Competencies Required for Community-Based Care

Nurses practicing in community-based integrated health care systems need to have specific knowledge and skills. In 1991, the Pew Health Professions Commission, in a report entitled *Healthy America: Practitioners for 2005* (as cited in de Tornyay, 1992), identified 17 competencies (skills) that future health professionals would require (see Box 7–6). These competencies have given direction to schools preparing future health professionals for practice. To achieve these competencies, nurses need the following knowledge: (a) determinants of a healthy community; (b) primary and secondary preventive strategies for people of all ages; (c) health promotion strategies for individuals, families, and communities; (d) how to participate in collaborative and interdisciplinary teamwork; (e) determinants of an accessible, cost-effective, integrated health care system; (f) decision-making processes that involve active participation by consumers and balance cost and quality care; and (g) concepts of information management. Community-based nurses also require up-to-date clinical skills and knowledge of complex technology, public health policy, and strategies to influence and effect change.

Collaborative Health Care

Collaboration among health care professionals becomes increasingly important as more practitioners specialize in pro-gressively more narrow areas of expertise while others take on the generalist role. Over time, the boundaries and legal scope of practice of each health care profession may change. To deliver optimal health care for the client, nurses must work as a member of the team providing comprehensive health care.

In 1992, the ANA Congress on Nursing Practice adopted the following operational definition of the concept of collaboration:

> **Collaboration** means a collegial working relationship with another health care provider in the provision of (to supply) patient care. Collaborative practice requires (may include) the discussion of patient diagnosis and cooperation in the management and delivery of care. Each collaborator is available to the other for consultation either in person or by communication device, but need not be physically present on the premises at the time the actions are performed. The patient-designated health care provider is responsible for the overall direction and management of patient care. (ANA, 1992)

The Nurse as a Collaborator

Nurses collaborate with nurse colleagues and other health care professionals. They frequently collaborate about client care but may also be involved, for example, in collaborating on bioethical issues, on legislation, on health-related research, and with professional organizations. Box 7–7 outlines selected aspects of the nurse's role as a collaborator.

To fulfill a collaborative role, nurses need to assume accountability and increased authority in practice areas. Education

---

BOX 7–6 **Pew Commission Competencies for Future Practitioners**

1. Care for the community's health.
2. Expand access to effective care.
3. Provide contemporary clinical care.
4. Emphasize primary care.
5. Participate in coordinated care.
6. Ensure cost-effective and appropriate care.
7. Practice prevention.
8. Involve patients and families in decision-making processes.
9. Promote healthy lifestyles.
10. Access and use technology appropriately.
11. Improve the health care system.
12. Manage information.
13. Understand the role of the physical environment.
14. Practice counseling on ethical issues.
15. Accommodate expanded accountability.
16. Participate in a racially and culturally diverse society.
17. Continue to learn.

Note: From "Reconsidering Nursing Education: The Report of the Pew Health Professional Commission," by R. De Tornyay, 1992, *Journal of Nursing Education, 31,* pp. 296–301. Adapted with permission.

BOX 7–7 **The Nurse as a Collaborator**

WITH NURSE COLLEAGUES
- Shares personal expertise with other nurses and elicits the expertise of others to ensure quality client care.
- Develops a sense of trust and mutual respect with peers that recognizes their unique contributions.

WITH OTHER HEALTH CARE PROFESSIONALS
- Recognizes the contribution that each member of the interdisciplinary team can make by virtue of his or her expertise and view of the situation.
- Listens to each individual's views.
- Shares health care responsibilities in exploring options, setting goals, and making decisions with clients and families.
- Participates in collaborative interdisciplinary research to increase knowledge of a clinical problem or situation.

WITH PROFESSIONAL NURSING ORGANIZATIONS
- Seeks opportunities to collaborate with and within professional organizations.
- Serves on committees in state (or provincial) and national nursing organizations or specialty groups.
- Supports professional organizations in political action to create solutions for professional and health care concerns.

WITH LEGISLATORS
- Offers expert opinions on legislative initiatives related to health care.
- Collaborates with other health care providers and consumers on health care legislation to best serve the needs of the public.

is integral to ensuring that the members of each professional group understand the collaborative nature of their roles, specific contributions, and the importance of working together. Each professional needs to understand how an integrated delivery system centers on the client's health care needs rather than on the particular care given by one group.

Competencies Basic to Collaboration

Key elements necessary for collaboration include effective communication skills, mutual respect, trust, and a decision-making process.

COMMUNICATION Collaborating to solve complex problems requires effective communication skills. Effective communication can occur only if the involved parties are committed to understanding each other's professional roles and appreciating each other as individuals. Additionally, they must be sensitive to differences among communication styles. Instead of focusing on distinctions, a group of professionals needs to center on their common ground: the client's needs.

MUTUAL RESPECT AND TRUST Mutual respect occurs when two or more people show or feel honor or esteem toward one another. Trust occurs when a person is confident in the actions of another person. Both mutual respect and trust imply a mutual process and outcome. They must be expressed both verbally and nonverbally.

DECISION MAKING The decision-making process at the team level involves shared responsibility for the outcome. To create a solution the team must follow each step of the decision-making process, beginning with a clear definition of the problem. Team decision making must be directed at the objectives of the specific effort. It requires full consideration and respect of diverse viewpoints. Members must be able to verbalize their perspectives in a nonthreatening environment.

An important aspect of decision making is satisfied when the interdisciplinary team focuses on the client's priority needs and organizing interventions accordingly. The discipline best able to address the client's needs is given priority in planning and is responsible for providing its interventions in a timely manner. For example, a social worker may first direct attention to a client's social needs when these needs interfere with the client's ability to respond to therapy. Nurses, by the nature of their holistic practice, are often able to help the team identify priorities and areas requiring further attention.

CONTINUITY OF CARE

A major responsibility of the nurse is to ensure continuity of care. **Continuity of care** is the coordination of health care services by health care providers for clients moving from one health care setting to another and between and among health care professionals. Continuity ensures uninterrupted and consistent services for the client from one level of care to another. When coordinated appropriately, it maintains client-focused individualized care and helps optimize the client's health status. To provide continuity of care, nurses need to accomplish the following:

- Initiate discharge planning for all clients when they are admitted to any health care setting.

- Involve the client and the client's family or support persons in the planning process.
- Collaborate with other health care professionals as needed to ensure that biopsychosocial, cultural, and spiritual needs are met.

However, achieving continuity assumes that needed client data are shared with other providers while implementing strategies to protect client privacy. The Health Insurance Portability and Accountability Act (HIPAA) requires that health information about clients be secured in such a way that only those with the right and need to acquire the information are able to do so. In the computer age, this has become a complex requirement since standards for coding and transmitting data are not universal and authentication of authority to access may be breached. The privacy aspect of HIPAA will result in a balance between protecting disclosure of confidential client information and the need for certain data to be released to specific agencies. Ultimately, clients will have increased control over their own information, and those who violate the rule face significant penalties. Community nursing practice has altered in the face of the HIPAA regulations. Case managers and public health nurses need to maintain vigilance to protect the privacy of client health care information when sending and receiving telephone messages, faxes, and electronic documentation when in field settings as well as within health care facilities.

Care Across the Life Span

The majority of children and elders receive their health care in their communities rather than in hospitals. From home births, to school-based childhood immunization programs, to sex education for teens, to chronic disease management in adults, to hospice care, the nurse works with clients and the wide variety of community health organizations to provide wellness and illness care. Research has shown that community-based programs can have substantial positive impact on self-care and well-being (see, for example, Farrell, Wicks, & Martin, 2004). A wide variety of initiatives focused on care provided in the community for children is found at the American Academy of Pediatrics website.

Discharge Planning

Discharge planning is the process of preparing a client to leave one level of care for another within or outside the current health care agency. Usually, discharge planning refers to the client leaving the hospital for home. However, discharges occur among many other settings. Within a facility it can occur from one unit to another. For example, a client with a stroke may move from a medical unit to a rehabilitation unit, or a client with trauma may move from the emergency department to an intensive care unit. Clients may move from a hospital to a long-term care agency, from a rehabilitation center to home, or from a home health care setting to a hospital, and so on.

Each agency generally has its own policies and procedures related to discharge. Many agencies have case managers or discharge planners, a health or social services professional who coordinates the transition and acts as a link between the discharging agency and the receiving facility. Often, a nurse assumes this responsibility of providing continuity of care.

Discharge planning needs to begin when a client is admitted to an agency, especially in hospitals where stays are considerably shortened. Effective discharge planning involves ongoing assessment to obtain comprehensive information about the client's ongoing needs and nursing care plans to ensure the client's and caregivers' needs are met. In some situations discharge planning necessitates health team conferences and family conferences. At a health team conference, health care professionals focus on ways to individualize care for the client. At a family conference, both health professionals and the family discuss family issues related to the client. Both types of conferences give the client, family, and health care professionals the opportunity to mutually plan care and set goals.

Preparing Clients to Go Home

Nurses preparing to send clients home from the hospital need to assess their clients' personal and health data; abilities to perform the activities of daily living; any physical, cognitive, or other functional limitations; caregivers' responses and abilities; adequacy of financial resources; community supports; hazards or barriers that the home environment presents; and need for health care assistance in the home. Box 7–8 outlines details about each of these parameters.

The data establish nursing activities that are required before the client is discharged. These activities most often include (a) teaching the client to cope with continuing self-care at home and (b) a home care referral.

Home Health Care Teaching

Clients need help to understand their situation, to make health care decisions, and to learn new health behaviors. Because of today's shortened hospital stays, it is often unrealistic to teach clients everything they need to know. Referral to a home health agency for follow-up teaching may be necessary. Essential information before discharge includes information about medications, dietary and activity restrictions, signs of complications that need to be reported to the primary care provider, follow-up appointments and telephone numbers, and where supplies can be obtained. Clients or caregivers also need to demonstrate safe performance of any necessary treatments. Information needs to be provided verbally and in writing. Details about effective teaching strategies are provided in Chapter 27. ∞ Reinforcement of acute care discharge information will often fall in the domain of the community-oriented nurse. Client issues related to health literacy, language barriers, and access to resources to carry out the provided health care instruction are major concerns to community nurses.

Referrals

The referral process is a systematic problem-solving approach that helps clients to use resources that meet their health care needs. The process involves knowledge of community resources and an ability to solve problems, set priorities, coordinate, and collaborate. Home care referrals are often made before discharge for the following clients:

- Elders
- Children with complex conditions
- Frail persons who live alone
- Those who lack or have a limited support system
- Those who have a caregiver whose health is failing
- Those whose home presents barriers to their safety (e.g., stairs)

Referrals need to present as much information as possible about the client and the hospitalization to the agency. Most agencies have well-established protocols and detailed referral forms. The assessment parameters in Box 7–8 can also be used

---

BOX 7–8 **Discharge Planning: Home Assessment Parameters**

PERSONAL AND HEALTH DATA
Age; sex; height and weight; cultural beliefs and practices; medical history; current health status; prognosis; surgery

ABILITIES TO PERFORM ACTIVITIES OF DAILY LIVING
Abilities for dressing; eating; toileting; bathing (tub, shower, sponge); ambulating (with or without aids such as a cane, crutches, walker, wheelchair); transferring (from bed to chair, in and out of bath, in and out of car); meal preparation; transportation; shopping

DISABILITIES/LIMITATIONS
Sensory losses (auditory, visual); motor losses (paralysis, amputation); communication disorder; mental confusion or depression; incontinence

CAREGIVERS' RESPONSES/ABILITIES
Principal caregiver's relationship to client; thoughts and feelings about client's discharge; expectations for recovery; health and coping abilities; comfort with performing needed care

FINANCIAL RESOURCES
Financial resources and needs (note equipment, supplies, medications, special foods required)

COMMUNITY SUPPORTS
Family members, friends, neighbors, volunteers; resources such as Medicaid; food stamps; nutrition services; health centers; community health nurses; day programs; legal assistance; home care; respite care

HOME HAZARD APPRAISAL
Safety precautions (stairs with or without handrails; lighting in rooms, hallways, stairways; night-lights in hallways or bathroom; grab bars near toilet and tub; firmly attached carpets and rugs); self-care barriers (lack of running water, lack of wheelchair access to bathroom or home, lack of space for required equipment, lack of elevator) (A detailed home hazard appraisal is provided in Chapter 8. ∞)

NEED FOR HEALTH CARE ASSISTANCE
Home-delivered meals; special dietary needs; volunteers for telephone reassurance, friendly visiting, transportation, shopping; assistance with bathing; assistance with housekeeping; assistance with wound care, ostomies, tubes, intravenous medications

as a guide. The nurse caring for the hospital client is responsible for confirming and documenting that the relevant referrals have been made. In order to identify and recommend referrals, the nurse must already be familiar with the resources that are available in the community. Using this knowledge, plus information regarding the client's previous awareness and choice of community resources, hospital nurses play a key role in maintaining effective continuity of health care.

To ensure appropriate reimbursement to the home health agency, the primary care provider must provide a written order for a home care referral and subsequent home visits. Clients must meet specific criteria to have Medicare or other third-party payers reimburse them for home care services. Chapter 8 ∞ provides details about home health nursing.

LIFESPAN CONSIDERATIONS Health Care Delivery

CHILDREN

The Search Institute has identified evidence-based assets characteristic of healthy communities and of different age groups of children. These assets are both external and internal to the individual, and if promoted in communities, will contribute to the healthy development of children and families and the positive life of the community. The impact of these assets has been studied in children from birth through adolescence, and many communities across the United States are using them to structure programs for children and youth. Among the assets are such things as family support, family values of equality and social justice, involvement of children and youth with adults and community organizations, constructive use of young people's time, and engagement in learning. The institute also has five action strategies for transforming communities for the betterment of youth, which involve engaging adults, mobilizing youth, activating organizations, expanding programs, and influencing policy.

ELDERS

Due to the changes caused by aging and the increase of chronic illnesses in elders, various levels of health care delivery are often required. Clients may go back and forth between these levels as their needs fluctuate. At various times and situations, they might need care from hospitals, home care, extended care facilities, ambulatory care, and assisted living. Maintaining communications and providing continuity of care during these changes are essential.

Caregivers of elders are often older themselves and may have health problems of their own. Attention should be given to signs of emotional and physical fatigue and other problems that might arise for them. Community health nurses have the opportunity to do ongoing assessments of this as they see clients and caregivers in their home environment. They can then provide support and resources as needed.

CRITICAL THINKING CHECKPOINT

Nurses are, and should be, taking an active role in influencing the direction of health care. Recognizing that there are finite limits to the amount of money and health care providers available, desirable outcomes often compete for resources. Consider a clinical situation such as the so-called "drive-through (or 24-hour) mastectomies" in which clients are moved through the acute care (hospital) system extremely quickly compared to previously. *Nursing's Agenda for Health Care Reform* (ANA, 1991) stated that there should be (a) increased access to care via primary health care provided in community-based settings, (b) an emphasis on consumer self-care and decision making, and (c) cost-effective care provided in the most appropriate setting.

1. How does this clinical example reflect or not reflect the agenda?
2. Which of the three agenda items listed above do you consider the most important and why?
3. How might different community-based frameworks manage the clinical example?
4. How would the nurse use collaboration with insurance payers, women, or surgeons to resolve any concerns with the clinical example?

See Critical Thinking Possibilities in Appendix A. ∞

CHAPTER 7 REVIEW

CHAPTER HIGHLIGHTS

- Health care costs, access to health care, and the quality of health care are major areas of concern about the current health care system.
- A community is a collection of people who share some attribute of their lives.
- For community assessment, eight subsystems proposed by Anderson and McFarlane (2004) can be used: physical environment, education, safety and transportation, politics and

government, health and social services, communication, economics, and recreation.
- *Nursing's Agenda for Health Care Reform* by the ANA (1991) and *Healthy People 2010* by the USDHHS (2000) have set forth recommendations for health care reform. These focus on

accessibility of health care services, health promotion and disease prevention, and steps to consider how health care costs can be reduced.

- Consumers support an increased emphasis on health care measures that promote wellness.
- Community-based health care, akin to primary health care, provides health-related services in places where people spend their time—in homes, in shelters, in long-term care residences, at work, in schools, in senior citizen centers, and so on.
- Approaches are emerging to address community-based care. These include an integrated health care system, community initiatives, community coalitions, managed care, case management, and outreach programs using lay health workers.
- Numerous community settings have been established. More recent ones include nurse-managed community nursing centers, parish nursing, and telehealth projects.
- Community-based nursing directs nursing care toward specific individuals. It is not confined to one practice setting; it extends beyond institutional boundaries involving a network of nursing

services: nursing wellness centers, ambulatory care, long-term care, home health, and hospice care.

- To practice in community health care systems, nurses need knowledge and competencies such as determinants of a healthy community, primary and secondary preventive strategies, health-promotion strategies, collaborative and interdisciplinary teamwork, determinants of an accessible and cost-effective health care system, a decision-making process that involves consumers, and information management. Education in public health policy and strategies to influence and effect change are essential.
- Collaboration among health care providers is key to maintaining continuity of care as clients move through the health care system.
- A major responsibility of the nurse is to ensure continuity of care as clients move from one level of care to another.
- Continuity of care involves (a) discharge planning that begins when clients are admitted to an agency, (b) cooperation with the client and support persons, and (c) interdisciplinary collaboration.
- Nurses need to ensure that clients have essential information and skills to manage self-care before being discharged to their homes. In some situations referral to a home health agency is necessary.

TEST YOUR KNOWLEDGE

1. *Nursing's Agenda for Health Care Reform* submitted by the American Nurses' Association (ANA, 1991) included which of the following?
   1. Primary health care should be based in acute care hospitals.
   2. A minimum standard of health care for all persons should be paid for completely with public funds.
   3. Case management should be focused on clients with enduring health care needs.
   4. Essential services should be initiated simultaneously to avoid gaps.

2. A category of the Pew Commission *Competencies for Future Practitioners* emphasized the need for providers to become skilled in which of the following?
   1. Use of technology
   2. Budgetary and financial management strategies
   3. Traditional clinical approaches
   4. Making decisions for incompetent clients

3. Which of the following is characteristic of nursing care provided in community-based health?
   1. Clients are primarily those with identified illnesses.
   2. Clients are individuals in groups according to their geographic commonalities.
   3. Care is paid for by the community as a whole rather than by individuals.
   4. All clients are case managed.

4. When performing collaborative health care, the nurse must implement which of the following?

   1. Assume a leadership role in directing the health care team
   2. Rely on the expertise of other health care team members
   3. Be physically present for the implementation of all aspects of the care plan
   4. Delegate decision-making authority to each health care provider

5. The nurse concludes that effective discharge planning (hospital to home) has been conducted when the client states which of the following?
   1. "As soon as I get home, the nurse will come out, look at where I live, and see what kind of care I will need."
   2. "All I need are my medications and a ride home. Then I'm all ready for discharge."
   3. "When I visit my doctor in 10 days, they will show me how to change my bandages."
   4. "I have the phone numbers of the home care nurse and the therapist who will visit me at home tomorrow."

6. A large disaster in a community resulted in the destruction of many family homes and many individuals were injured. The assistance of community health nurses and home health nurses are needed. The home health nurse is most likely to perform which of the following?
   1. Provide for a safe water supply
   2. Monitor for communicable diseases
   3. Establish communication and support systems
   4. Assess and treat individual clients

See Answers to Test Your Knowledge in Appendix A.

EXPLORE MEDIALINK www.prenhall.com/berman

DVD-ROM
- Audio Glossary
- NCLEX Review

COMPANION WEBSITE
- Additional NCLEX Review
- Case Studies:
   The Amish
   Community Health Nursing
- Application Activities:
   Community Nursing Standards
   Government Services
- Link to Resources

READINGS AND REFERENCES

SUGGESTED READINGS

Brudenell, I. (2003). Parish nursing: Nurturing body, mind, spirit, and community. *Public Health Nursing, 20*(2), 85–94.
Parish nursing focuses on health promotion and disease prevention within a faith community. The authors recount a descriptive study that was conducted to determine how faith communities form parish nursing programs and what their effect is.

Huttlinger, K., Schaller-Ayers, J. M., Kenny, B., & Ayers, J. W. (2004). Research and collaboration in rural community health. *Online Journal of Rural Nursing and Health Care, 4* (1). Retrieved June 11, 2006, from http://www.rno.org/journal/issues/Vol-4/issue-1/Kulig_article.htm
Developing collaborative projects that involve community health nurses, researchers, health providers, community groups, and individuals is one way to increase an awareness of critical health needs. This paper describes a community, collaborative effort to bring a Remote Area Medical (RAM) event to southwestern Virginia and northeastern Tennessee. It also presents a description of the information gathered from the attendees of the RAM event that was used by local community health care agencies and politicians to leverage state and national officials for increased health care services for this area of Appalachia.

RELATED RESEARCH

Campbell, R., Sefl, T., Wasco, S. M., & Ahrens, C. E. (2004). Doing community research without a community: Creating safe space for rape survivors. *American Journal of Community Psychology, 33*, 253–261.

Cooper, L. A., Roter, D. L., Johnson, R. L., Ford, D. E., Steinwachs, D. M., & Powe, N. R. (2003). Patient-centered communication, ratings of care, and concordance of patient and physician race. *Annals of Internal Medicine, 13*, 907–915.

REFERENCES

American Nurses Association. (1991). *Nursing's agenda for health care reform.* Kansas City, MO: Author.

American Nurses Association. (1992). *House of delegates report: 1992 convention, Las Vegas, Nevada* (pp. 104–120). Kansas City, MO: Author.

American Public Health Association. (1996). *The definition and role of public health nursing: A Statement of APHA Public Health Nursing Section.* Washington, DC: Author.

Anderson, E. T., & McFarlane, J. (2004). *Community as partner: Theory and practice in nursing* (4th ed.). Philadelphia: Lippincott Williams & Wilkins.

Barnes, D., Eribes, C., Juarbe, T., Nelson, M., Proctor, S., Sawyer, L., et al. (1995). Primary health care and primary care: A confusion of philosophies. *Nursing Outlook, 43*(1), 7–16.

deTornyay, R. (1992). Reconsidering nursing education: The report of the Pew Health Professions Commission. *Journal of Nursing Education, 31*, 296–301.

Farrell, K., Wicks, M. N., & Martin, J. C. (2004). Chronic disease self management improved with enhanced self efficacy. *Clinical Nursing Research, 13*, 289–308.

Grumbach, K., Miller, J., Mertz, E., & Finocchio, L. (2004). How much public health in public health nursing practice? *Public Health Nursing, 21*, 266–276.

Institute of Medicine. (1994). *Defining primary care: An interim report.* Washington, DC: National Academy Press.

National Center for Health Statistics. (2005). *Health: United States, 2005.* Hyattsville, MD: Author.

Quad Council. (2003). *Quad Council PHN competencies.* Retrieved June 11, 2006, from http://www.achne.org/Documents/Final_PHN_Competencies.pdf

Smith, S. D. (Ed.). (2003). *Parish nursing: A handbook for the new millennium.* Binghamton, NY: Haworth Press.

U.S. Department of Health and Human Services. (2000). *Healthy people 2010: Understanding and improving health* (2nd ed.). Washington, DC: U.S. Government Printing Office.

World Health Organization. (1978). *Primary health care: Report of the international conference on primary health care.* Geneva: Author.

SELECTED BIBLIOGRAPHY

Abrams, S. E. (2004). From function to competency in public health nursing, 1931–2003. *Public Health Nursing, 21*, 507–510.

Allan, J., Barwick, T. A., Cashman, S., Cawley, J. F., Day, C., Douglass, C. W., et al. (2004). Clinical prevention and population health: Curriculum framework for health professions. *American Journal of Preventive Medicine, 27*, 471–476.

Allender, J. A., & Spradley, B. W. (2004). *Community health nursing: Promoting and protecting the public's health.* Philadelphia: Lippincott Williams & Wilkins.

Brudenell, I. (2003). Parish nursing: Nurturing body, mind, spirit, and community. *Public Health Nursing, 20*, 85–94.

Clark, M. J. (2003). *Community health nursing: Caring for populations* (4th ed.). Upper Saddle River, NJ: Prentice Hall.

Clark, N., & Buell, A. (2004). Community assessment: An innovative approach. *Nurse Educator, 29*, 203–207.

Davis, R., Cook, D., & Cohen, L. (2005). A community resilience approach to reducing ethnic and racial disparities in health. *American Journal of Public Health, 95*, 2168–2173.

Gesler, W. M., Dougherty, M., Arcury, T. A., Skelly, A. H., & Nash, S. (2003). The importance of obtaining information from assessment of community service providers for a disease prevention program. *Journal of Multicultural Nursing & Health, 9*(2), 14–21.

Kraus, M., Morgan, C., & Matteson, P. (2003). "Razoo Health": A community-based nursing education initiative. *Journal of Nursing Education, 42*, 304–310.

Mainous, A. G., Koopman, R. J., Gill, J. M., Baker, R., & Pearson, W. S. (2004). Relationship between continuity of care and diabetes control: Evidence from the Third National Health and Nutrition Examination Survey. *American Journal of Public Health, 94*, 66–70.

Maurer, F. A., & Smith, C. M. (2004). *Community/public health nursing practice: Health for families and populations.* St. Louis, MO: Elsevier.

Pew Health Professions Commission. (1991). *Healthy America: Practitioners for 2005. An agenda for action for U.S. health professional schools.* San Francisco: Author.

Porche, D. J. (2003). *Public and community health nursing practice: A population-based approach.* Thousand Oaks, CA: Sage.

Stanhope, M., & Lancaster, J. (2003). *Community and public health nursing* (6th ed.). St. Louis, MO: Elsevier.

Weisman, G. D., Kovach, D., & Cashin, S. E. (2004). Differences in dementia services and settings across place types and regions. *American Journal of Alzheimer's Disease and Other Dementias, 19*, 291–308.

Home Care

LEARNING OUTCOMES

After completing this chapter, you will be able to:

1. Define home health care.

2. Compare the characteristics of home health nursing to those of institutional nursing care.

3. Describe the types of home health agencies, including reimbursement and referral sources.

4. Describe the roles of the home health nurse.

5. Identify the essential aspects of the home visit.

6. Discuss the safety and infection control dimensions applicable to the home care setting.

7. Identify ways the nurse can recognize and minimize caregiver role strain.

KEY TERMS

caregiver role strain, *137*

durable medical equipment
   (DME) company, *134*

home care, *132*

home health care nursing, *132*

hospice nursing, *132*

registry, *133*

visiting nursing, *132*

MediaLink   Hospice Nursing Application

Historically, home care consisted primarily of nurses providing private duty care in clients' homes and care of the ill by their own family members. However, the delivery of professional nursing services in home settings has increased in frequency, scope, and complexity in the past two decades. **Home care** today involves a wide range of health care professionals providing services in the home setting to people recovering from an acute illness or injury, or who are disabled, or who have a chronic condition. A number of factors have contributed to this trend, among them rising health care costs, an aging population, and a growing emphasis on managing chronic illness and stress, preventing illness, and enhancing the quality of life. In the not-too-distant past, home health care occurred at the end of the client care continuum—that is, after discharge from an acute care facility. Today the trend is changing to use of home health care services to avoid hospitalization.

Because home health nurses must function independently in a variety of home settings and situations, employers generally prefer that the nurse be prepared at the baccalaureate level or above. The American Nurses Credentialing Center (ANCC) provides certification for home health nursing at both the generalist and advanced practice levels. Advanced practice certification requires a master's degree in nursing and recognizes the need for home health clinical specialists who can provide direct care, manage client care, and engage in consulting, education, administration, and research activities.

HOME HEALTH NURSING

The delivery of nursing services in the home has been called a variety of terms, including *home health care nursing* and *visiting nursing*. For an example of how the terms are used interchangeably, see the website for the Visiting Nurses Associations of America and note that their description of what a visiting nurse does is listed under the section entitled Home Health. **Home health care nursing** or **visiting nursing** includes the nursing services and products provided to clients in their homes that are needed to maintain, restore, or promote their physical, psychologic, and social well-being. The focus of home health care nursing is individuals and their families. This differs somewhat from the focus of community health nursing, which focuses on individuals, families, and aggregate groups (see Chapter 7). ∞

Hospice nursing, support and care of the dying person and family, is often considered a subspecialty of home health nursing because hospice services are frequently delivered to terminally ill clients in their residence. See Chapter 43 ∞ for further information about hospice care.

Home nursing care is one of the growing sectors of the health care system. Expenditures for home health are significantly influenced by increasing or decreasing Medicare payment policies, but they increase approximately 10% each year. Medicare payments for hospice services provided by home care agencies doubled between 2000 and 2003 (Smith, Cowan, Sensing, & Catlin, 2005). Factors that have contributed to the growth of home health care include (1) the increase in the older population, who are frequent recipients of home care; (2) third-party payers who favor home care to control costs; (3) the ability of agencies and institutions to successfully deliver high-technology services in the home; and (4) consumers who prefer to receive care in the home rather than in an institution. A common misperception by the general public is that home health nursing is only custodial in its scope of practice. However, health promotion is one of the intentions for the home health nurse in order to promote client self-care. Home care nurses are actively engaged in providing support and education for family caregivers as well as clients.

Unique Aspects of Home Health Nursing

Home care nurses must function independently in a variety of unfamiliar home settings and situations. Because the home is the family's territory, power and control issues in delivering nursing care differ from those in the hospital. For example, entry into a home is granted, not assumed; the nurse must therefore establish trust and rapport with the client and family. Due to the limited time for visits and the possibly lengthy interval between visits, this process does not always occur as quickly as it might when nursing within an acute care facility.

Health care that is provided in the home is often given with other family members present. Families may feel freer to question advice, to ignore directions, to do things differently, and to set their own priorities and schedules. Home care nurses implement every step of the nursing process, using critical-thinking skills in designing, implementing, and evaluating the plan of care.

Home health nurses have identified significant advantages in caring for individuals and families in the home. The home setting is intimate; this intimacy fosters familiarity, sharing, connections, and caring between clients, families, and their nurse. Behaviors are more natural, cultural beliefs and practices are more visible, and multigenerational interactions tend to be displayed. Nurses often get to know the client and family well as they may care for clients over weeks or months.

Home health nurses have also identified issues that negatively affect care in the home. More than any other care providers, these nurses have firsthand knowledge and experience about the burden of caregiving and the role of family dynamics in health care practices. In the interest of cutting health care costs, policy makers, third-party payers, and medical providers are placing increasingly complex responsibilities on clients' families and significant other(s). Family caregiving demands may go on for months or years, placing the caregivers themselves (many of whom are elders) at risk for physiological and psychosocial problems. Additionally, nurses enter homes where the living conditions and support systems may be inadequate.

Nurses caring for clients in rural home settings have challenges different from those in urban or suburban environments. These include the need for flexibility since clients may live far distances from the nurse and require care in the evening or at night, creativity and the ability to practice independently since fewer resources (including other nurses) are available, and the ability to work in an environment over which there is little nurse control (Boucher, 2005). Thus, those nurses who require a high degree of certainty, structure, and consistency are less likely to be successful in rural home health locations.

Practice of Home Health Nursing

The home health nurse will practice a variety of roles when caring for clients. Direct hands-on care for complex health conditions occurring in clients from birth to death is becoming common in home settings. Home health nurses routinely perform physical assessments, change wound dressings, insert and maintain intravenous access for various therapies, establish and monitor indwelling urinary catheters, monitor exercise or nutritional therapies, and in short do many nursing functions formerly thought of as being confined to acute care facilities.

Home health nurses serve as health educators to the client, caregivers, and families. They clarify misconceptions about the course of the illness, the treatment plan, and medications and potential interactions with over-the-counter drugs. They also educate the client and family on how to access the health care system appropriately. Indirect care is provided by the home health nurse to the client each time the nurse consults with other health care providers about ways to improve nursing care for the client. This consultation about client care issues often manifests itself in multidisciplinary care conferences where the role of the home health nurse is as client advocate.

THE HOME HEALTH CARE SYSTEM

The need for home health care may be identified by any person involved with the client. Clients are referred to a home health agency or private duty nursing agency. Individuals with extremely complex needs, beyond those that direct nursing care alone can provide, may benefit from the services of an agency with direct connections to a medical equipment company. Payment for home health is accomplished through private pay, third-party reimbursement, or a combination of sources.

Referral Process

Clients may be referred to home health care providers by a physician, nurse, social worker, therapist (e.g., physical therapist), discharge planner, or family member. Families often initiate the process by approaching one of these referral sources or by directly contacting the home health agency to make inquiries. Home care cannot begin, however, without a physician's order and a physician-approved treatment plan. This is a legal and reimbursement requirement.

After an initial set of physician's orders is obtained, a nursing evaluation visit is scheduled to enroll the client and identify the client's needs. The initial visit, often referred to as "opening the case," should include the client and the immediate family involved with the client's care. At this visit, the nurse develops a plan of care, which must be reviewed, approved, authorized, and signed by the attending physician before home health agency providers can continue with services.

Home Health Agencies

Home health agencies offer coordinated professional, skilled, and paraprofessional services. Because clients often require the services of several professionals, case coordination (case management) is essential. This responsibility generally rests with the registered nurse. Depending on the agency, additional providers may include nurse practitioners, practical nurses, nursing assistants, home health care aides, physical therapists, occupational therapists, respiratory therapists, speech therapists, social workers, dietitians, and a pastoral care minister or chaplain. In addition, it is not unusual for home health agencies to offer the services of specialized nurses such as wound-ostomy-continence nurses or diabetes educators. The care plan implemented by the home health agency may require services once or twice a day, up to 7 days a week. The minimum time of each period of care, or visit, is usually 1 hour.

There are several different types of home health agencies which include the following:

- Official or public agencies are operated by state or local governments and financed primarily by tax funds.
- Voluntary or private not-for-profit agencies are supported by donations, endowments, charities such as the United Way, and third-party reimbursement.
- Private, proprietary agencies are for-profit organizations and are governed by either individual owners or national corporations. Some of these agencies participate in third-party reimbursement; others rely on "private-pay" sources.
- Institution-based agencies operate under a parent organization, such as a hospital, funded by the same sources as the parent.

Regardless of the type of agency, all home health agencies must meet specific standards for licensing, certification, and accreditation.

Private Duty Agencies

This type of agency may be referred to as a **registry** which contracts with individual practitioners (e.g., nurses, home health aides) to care for the client in the home. The client may require care coverage from the agency for 4 to 24 hours a day. However, the agency is not focused uniquely on providing personnel for home care assignments but also supplies staff to hospitals, clinics, and other care settings. Thus, it does not afford the coordinated focus of a home care agency. Private duty care is expensive. Commercial insurance generally provides limited reimbursement. Otherwise, the client must pay privately.

Durable Medical Equipment Companies

A **durable medical equipment (DME) company** provides health care equipment for the client at home. The types of equipment can range from hospital beds and bedside commodes to ventilators and apnea monitors. Because of the cost associated with medical equipment, the nurse needs to ensure that clients have either Medicare/Medicaid or a DME benefit within their commercial insurance, or that they are able to pay privately. Before billing Medicare for any DME, it is wise to consult the list of equipment for which Medicare will reimburse the client. Most DME companies today seek accreditation from the Joint Commission on Accreditation of Healthcare Organizations (JCAHO) to ensure compliance with quality standards for equipment and services.

Reimbursement

Health care agencies in the United States receive reimbursement for services they provide from various sources: Medicare and Medicaid, private insurance companies, and private pay. The Medicare and Medicaid programs have strict guidelines governing reimbursement for home health care (Centers for Medicare & Medicaid Services, 2004). For example, the client must (a) need reasonable and necessary home care including skilled care; (b) be homebound, that is, confined to the home except for occasional outings for medical treatment, for a trip to the barber, or for a drive; and require the use of supportive devices, special transportation, or the escort of another person; (c) have a plan of care that includes all of Medicare's criteria; and (d) need nursing care on an intermittent basis (Caruso, Scala-Foley, Archer, & Reinhard, 2004). The agency too must meet specific conditions.

Payers other than Medicare or Medicaid, such as Blue Cross, Blue Shield, and HealthNet, typically negotiate reimbursement rates for home health care services. Not-for-profit agencies, like the Visiting Nurses Associations (VNAs), are reimbursed by public and private insurance plus charitable donations to the agency.

All health care agencies need to adhere to established guidelines and provide care within the predetermined reimbursement levels. Treatment plans (developed by the home health agency providers and authorized by the physician) are used by the reimbursement source. Only interventions identified on the treatment plan are paid for. Periodically the reimbursement source may request the home health provider's notes to substantiate what is being done in the home. This is a major reason why accurate documentation is critical.

ROLES OF THE HOME HEALTH NURSE

Historically, nurses who provided direct services in the home were strong generalists who focused on long-term preventive, educational, and rehabilitative outcomes. Today many home health nurses possess high-technology skills that were formerly used only in acute care settings. For example, nurses provide a variety of intravenous therapies in the home setting and monitor clients who are dependent on technologically complex medical equipment, such as ventilators and central intravenous lines. These nurses collaborate with physicians and other health care professionals in providing care. They play a key role in facilitating an effective plan of care as clients move among hospitals, home, school, work, and other care settings such as clinics or long-term care.

Major roles of the home health nurse are those of advocate, caregiver (provider of direct care), educator, and case manager or coordinator.

Advocate

Advocacy begins on the first visit. The nurse explores and supports the client's choices in health care; all viable options are considered. Advocacy includes having discussions about the client's rights, advance medical directives, living wills, and durable power of attorney for health care. It also usually involves assistance to access community resources, to make informed decisions, to recognize and cope with necessary changes in lifestyle, to negotiate medical insurance, and to understand ways to effectively use the complex medical system. Advocacy can be a particular challenge when family members' or other caregivers' views differ from those of the client. In the event of conflict, the nurse, being the client's primary advocate, ensures that the client's rights and desires are upheld.

Caregiver

The home health nurse's major role as caregiver is to assess and diagnose the client's actual and potential health problems, plan care, and evaluate the client's outcomes. Direct personal care activities such as bathing, changing linens, feeding, and light housekeeping activities to maintain a clean and safe home environment are usually provided by a family member or a home health aide arranged by the nurse. The home health nurse, however, will provide direct care for specific procedures and treatments such as ostomy care, wound care, intravenous therapy, and so on according to agency policies and practices (see Figure 8-1 ■). Much of the home health nurse's time is spent teaching others to provide required care.

Figure 8-1 ■ Home care nurses perform skilled direct care such as changing dressings.

Educator

The educator role of the home health nurse focuses on teaching illness care, the prevention of problems, and the promotion of optimal wellness or well-being to the client, the family, and other related persons. A common example is that of guiding the health and development of newborns. Some clients of all ages have acute illnesses that will resolve, while others have chronic conditions that will last the lifetime. The nurse's teaching and learning methods will vary based on the need of these clients. The nurse may also be involved in teaching others with whom the client interacts such as the schoolteachers of special-needs children. Education is ongoing and can be considered the crux of home care practice; its goal is to help clients learn to manage as independently as possible. All home health nurses need to be skilled in teaching and learning principles and strategies that facilitate learning. (See Chapter 27 ∞ for detailed information.)

Case Manager or Coordinator

The home health nurse coordinates the activities of all other home health team members involved in the client's treatment plan. Coordination can occur individually, in person or by telephone, with a specific team member such as the dietitian or respiratory therapist, or during a team conference where each team member provides information about the client's health status. The nurse is the main contact to report any changes in the client's condition and to bring about a revision in the plan of care as needed. Documentation of care coordination is a legal and reimbursement requirement and must be recorded on the client's medical record.

PERSPECTIVES OF HOME CARE CLIENTS

Home care clients include a diverse population that encompasses all ages, a variety of health problems, and families of different structures and cultural backgrounds. Home care clients have a wide range of health problems that include disabilities, perinatal problems, mental illnesses, and acute and chronic illnesses. The nurse should not assume that the client understands the various personnel and their roles in providing home health care. In one study, older women receiving home care were unclear regarding what they could expect of the nurse and how best to use home care services (Porter & Ganong, 2005).

Although the person receiving care is considered the primary client in home care, the client's family can be considered secondary clients because often they are associated with caregiving and have a major impact on the client's wellness status. The home health nurse will encounter many different family structures ranging from single families to extended families and dwellings that house multiple families. In the home setting, family members may include not only persons related by birth and marriage, but also friends, other significant individuals, and animals.

Various cultural influences also affect the client's health care beliefs and practices. The home health nurse needs to be culturally sensitive; that is, to become aware of the client's culture and form a nursing care plan with the client that incorporates his or her culture. See Chapter 18 ∞ for detailed information about making cultural assessments and providing culturally competent care.

SELECTED DIMENSIONS OF HOME HEALTH NURSING

Selected dimensions of home health care include assessing the home for safety features, infection control, and caregiver support.

Client Safety

Hazards in the home are major causes of falls, fire, poisoning, and other accidents, such as those caused by improper use of household equipment (e.g., tools and cooking utensils). The appraisal of such hazards and suggestions for remedies is an essential nursing function. See the Home Care Assessment box for a home hazard appraisal and Chapter 32 ∞ for a discussion of potential hazards and preventive actions for individuals of all ages.

HOME CARE ASSESSMENT   Home Hazard Appraisal for Adults

CLIENT AND ENVIRONMENT

- *Walkways and stairways (inside and outside):* Note uneven sidewalks or paths, broken or loose steps, absence of handrails or placement on only one side of stairways, insecure handrails, congested hallways or other traffic areas, and adequacy of lighting at night.
- *Floors:* Note uneven and highly polished or slippery floors and any unanchored rugs or mats.
- *Furniture:* Note hazardous placement of furniture with sharp corners. Note chairs or stools that are too low to get into and out of or that provide inadequate support.
- *Bathroom(s):* Note presence of grab bars around tubs and toilets, nonslip surfaces in tubs and shower stalls, handheld showerhead, adequacy of night lighting, need for raised toilet seat or bath chair in tub or shower, ease of access to shelves, and water temperature regulated at a maximum of 49°C (120°F).

- *Kitchen:* Note pilot lights (gas stove) in need of repair, inaccessible storage areas, and hazardous furniture.
- *Bedrooms:* Note adequacy of lighting, in particular the availability of night-lights and accessibility of light switches; ease of access to commode, urinal, or bedpan; and need for hospital bed or bed rails.
- *Electrical:* Note unanchored or frayed electrical cords and outlets that are overloaded or near water.
- *Fire protection:* Note presence or absence of smoke detectors, fire extinguisher, and fire escape plan, and improper storage of combustibles (e.g., gasoline) or corrosives (e.g., rust remover).
- *Toxic substances:* Note improperly labeled cleaning solutions.
- *Communication devices:* Note presence of method to call for help, such as a telephone or intercom in the bedroom and elsewhere (e.g., kitchen), and access to emergency telephone numbers.
- *Medications:* Note medications kept beyond date of expiration, adequacy of lighting for medication cabinet or storage, and method of disposal of sharp objects such as needles used for injections.

Figure 8-2 ■ MedicAlert emblems.
(Reproduced with permission: 2003. All rights reserved. MedicAlert® is a Federally Registered Trademark and Service Mark.)

Obviously home health nurses cannot expect to change a family's living space and lifestyle. However, they can express their concern and react appropriately when a situation suggests that an injury is imminent. Nurses must document information they provide and the family's response to instruction, and make ongoing assessments about the family's use of safety precautions.

Other aspects of client safety relate to emergency situations. The home health nurse can assist the client and caregivers as follows:

■ Post a list of all emergency telephone numbers (ambulance, fire, police, primary care provider) at each telephone.

■ Post a list of all the client's medications and potential side effects in a central location, such as on the refrigerator.

■ Help the client and family apply for a medical alert system such as a bracelet or necklace (see Figure 8-2 ■). Information on the MedicAlert System can be obtained by contacting MedicAlert Foundation International.

■ Enroll the client in a program that places all the client's vital medical information in one place for emergency per-

sonnel to have in the event of a life-threatening situation. The program can be obtained through a pharmacy, a primary care provider's office, the VNA, or other community support groups. The kit contains a plastic vial, a medical information form, a decal, and an instruction sheet. The information form is filled out, rolled, and placed in the vial. The vial is placed in the refrigerator, and emergency personnel are trained to routinely check there. The decal is placed on the refrigerator as a signal that the vial is inside.

■ Recommend the client enroll in an emergency response system. These systems provide a small device with a help button that attaches to a wrist or neck chain. The home base station can require the client to send a signal daily that indicates that he or she is OK. If the signal is not sent or if the portable device is activated, the system automatically calls the client and then dials a previously established list of emergency contacts. This system is particularly useful for clients who are alone because if they should fall, for instance, and be unable to reach a telephone, they might be left helpless for extended periods of time.

Nurse Safety

Some less desirable living locations pose additional personal safety concerns for the nurse. Many home health agencies have contracts with security firms to escort nurses needing to see clients in potentially unsafe neighborhoods. The nurse should avoid taking any personal belongings during these visits and have a preestablished mechanism to signal for help. Home health agencies provide training for nurses in ways to decrease personal risk. Little has been published on this important subject. See the accompanying Research Note for one example.

Infection Control

The goal of infection control in the home is to protect clients, caregivers, and the general community from the transmission of disease. This is particularly important for clients who are immunocompromised, who have infectious or communicable dis-

---

RESEARCH NOTE   Do Nurses Making Home Visits Worry About Their Own Safety?

The researchers in this study surveyed 83 rehabilitation nurses who performed home visits. A common theme in the responses was concern for personal safety. These concerns were broken down by community and home-based issues. Community issues related to poor communication systems, delayed notification of dangerous situations, weather conditions predisposing to automobile hazards, and difficulty in locating clients' homes due to unfamiliar and possibly dangerous neighborhoods. Home issues included poor sanitation, inadequate housing (e.g., heat, water), uncontrolled pets, and lifestyle (e.g., substance abuse, violence).

Based on these findings, the authors proposed specific guidelines for the nurses, consisting of actions to take to prevent or cope with issues that might arise. Examples were ensuring that cell phones functioned properly; having cars properly serviced, especially for hot or freezing weather; contacting family members for driving directions or meeting the nurse at a central location and guiding the nurse to the

home; carrying a signal device such as a whistle or alarm; carrying cleaning supplies such as gloves, drapes, water, and paper towels; advising the family regarding cancellation of visits; and reporting to agencies if violence or abuse is detected.

IMPLICATIONS

Although safety issues for any nurse visiting the client's home will vary somewhat based on the location and client characteristics, nurses must be prepared with strategies to prevent and cope with issues if they arise. All home care nurses should be thoroughly trained by the agency and know both public and private resources for assistance. The nurse also has a role in educating and assisting clients to avoid and correct unsafe situations.

From "Safety Concerns for Rehabilitation Nurses in Home Care," by B. Brillhart, B. Kruse, and L. Heard, 2004, *Rehabilitation Nursing, 29*, pp. 227–229.

eases, or who have draining wounds, drainage tubes, or other invasive access devices. The nurse's major role in infection control is health teaching. Clients and caregivers need to learn about effective hand washing, use of gloves, handling of linens, disposal of wastes and soiled dressings, and the practice of infection control (standard precautions). Infection control can present a challenge to the home health nurse, especially if the home care facilities are not conducive to basic aseptic requirements such as running water for hand washing.

An important aspect of infection control involves handling the home health nurse's equipment and supplies. Supplies may include materials for hand cleansing; assessment equipment such as stethoscope, blood pressure cuff and monitor, thermometer, and tape measure; infection control items such as gowns, goggles, masks, gloves, and blood spill kit; and antimicrobial cleaning agents.

The same organizations that accredit hospitals evaluate home health nurses' practice. Deficiencies in the use of appropriate infection control practices are common findings during these evaluations (Sturkey, Linker, Keith, & Comeau, 2005). Although some modifications in technique may be indicated in the home setting, such as the use of clean rather than sterile technique in caring for chronic wounds, all the basic principles still apply. Nurses need to follow agency protocol about aseptic practice in the home.

Caregiver Support

Caregiving may be directed to individuals of any age and varies from short term to long term according to the physical or mental disabilities of the care receivers. For example, some children who have permanent disabilities and adults who experience progressive deterioration such as those with Alzheimer's disease or multiple sclerosis require care on a permanent basis. Others who are recovering from a surgical procedure require care only on a temporary basis. Most caregivers have close relationships with the care receiver, that is, a spouse/partner, parent, child, friend, or other significant relationship. Many caregiving relationships, therefore, represent changes from the caring and caregiving intrinsic to all close relationships to an extraordinary and unequal burden for the caregiver. Caregivers may experience **caregiver role strain** when they have physical, emotional, social, and financial burdens that can seriously jeopardize their own health and well-being.

The home health nurse needs to recognize signs of caregiver role strain and suggest ways to minimize or alleviate this problem. Signs of caregiver overload include the following:

■ Difficulty performing routine tasks for the client
■ Reports of declining physical energy and insufficient time for caregiving
■ Concern that caregiving responsibilities interfere with other roles such as those of parent, spouse, worker, friend
■ Anxiety about ability to meet future care needs of client
■ Feelings of anger and depression
■ Dramatic change in the home environment's appearance

The nurse needs to encourage caregivers to express their feelings and at the same time convey understanding about the difficulties associated with caregiving and acknowledge the caregivers' competence. The nurse can obtain a realistic appraisal of the situation by asking a caregiver to describe a typical day and daily or weekly leisure and social activities. It is also helpful to identify activities for which assistance is desired. These activities may include client care needs such as hygiene, mobility, feeding, or treatments; house cleaning; laundry; shopping; house repairs; yard work; transportation; doctor's or hairdresser's appointments; or respite.

Activities that are commonly done by nurses and aides, such as changing an occupied bed and transferring a client from bed to chair, may be overwhelming to a caregiver who has not performed them before. Demonstrating them in the home and allowing caregivers to perform them with the nurse's supervision increases their confidence and increases the likelihood of them asking for assistance in other situations.

When activities for which assistance is required are identified, the nurse and caregiver need to identify possible sources of help. Both volunteer and agency sources need to be explored. Volunteer sources of help may include family members (cousins, siblings), neighbors, friends, church associates, or caregiver support groups in the community. Other sources include, for example, a home health aide for light housekeeping and grocery shopping, Meals on Wheels, day care, transportation, and counseling and social services. Families with a chronically ill member may benefit from a weekend respite—a program some hospitals provide in which the client is admitted to a skilled unit for observation and care, enabling the caregiver a break from ongoing health care needs.

Caregivers need to be reminded of the importance of caring for themselves by getting adequate rest, eating nutritious meals, asking for help, delegating household chores, and making time for leisure activities or simply some time alone. Family members other than the caregiver also may need help to learn ways to support the caregiver. The nurse may discuss the importance to the caregiver of regular phone calls, cards, letters, and visits; offer encouragement to take day trips or a vacation; listen without giving advice; acknowledge the burden of caregiving and the need to feel appreciated; and so on.

A particular challenge exists when the nurse is in a position to be a caregiver to a family member. Although the nurse's clinical expertise and familiarity with the client and setting can be especially useful, negotiating the professional distancing that is sometimes needed when providing care to clients can be difficult with family. The nurse may feel obligated to provide care, even when this is over and above regular employment responsibilities. The nurse must have the opportunity to step back and experience the role and emotions of being a family member—not only those of being a nurse.

THE PRACTICE OF NURSING IN THE HOME

The home health nurse assesses the health care demands of the client and family and the home and community environment. This process actually begins when the nurse contacts the client for the initial home visit and reviews documents received from the referral agency. The goal of the initial visit is to obtain a comprehensive clinical picture of the client's needs.

Most agencies have a packet that includes forms for consent to treatment; physical, psychosocial, and spiritual assessment; medications; pain assessment; family data; financial assessment including insurance verification; client's bill of rights; care plan; and daily visit notes. During the initial home visit, the home health nurse obtains a health history from the client (see Figure 8-3 ■), examines the client, observes the relationship of the client and caregiver, and assesses the home and community environment. Parameters of assessment of the home environment include client and caregiver mobility, client ability to perform self-care, the cleanliness of the environment, the availability of caregiver support, safety, food preparation, financial supports, and the emotional status of the client and caregiver.

Following this initial client examination, the nurse determines whether further consults and support personnel are needed. For example, would the client benefit from a dietary consult or Meals on Wheels? Is a home health aide needed to assist with activities of daily living and homemaker tasks? Is a social worker needed to help with financial resources or future care needs such as placement in a nursing home? What additional supplies does the client need?

Before completing the initial interview, the nurse also discusses what the client and family can expect from home care, what other health care providers may be needed to help the client achieve independence, and the frequency of home visits.

Establishing Health Issues

As in other care environments, the nurse identifies both actual and potential client problems. One of the most common examples of health issues that nurses address with clients in home care settings is lack of knowledge related to health conditions and self-care. Because client education is considered a skill re-

Figure 8-3 ■ Interviewing the home care client.

BOX 8–1 Medicare's Required Data for the Nursing Plan of Care

1. All pertinent diagnoses
2. A notation of the beneficiary's mental status
3. Types of services, supplies, and equipment ordered
4. Frequency of visits to be made
5. Client's prognosis
6. Client's rehabilitation potential
7. Client's functional limitations
8. Activities permitted
9. Client's nutritional requirements
10. Client's medications and treatments
11. Safety measures to protect against injuries
12. Discharge plans
13. Any other items the home health agency or physician wishes to include

Note: From *Medicare Home Health Agency Manual* (*HCFA Publication* 11 PB 98-955200), by Centers for Medicare & Medicaid Services 2001. Retrieved June 12, 2006, from http://new.cms.hhs.gov/manuals/downloads/pub_11.zip

---

imbursed by Medicare and other commercial insurance carriers, it is important for the nurse to include knowledge deficits within the plan of care.

Planning and Delivering Care

The nurse needs to encourage and permit clients to make their own health management decisions. Alternatives may need to be suggested for some decisions if the nurse identifies potential harm from a chosen course of action.

Strategies to meet goals generally include teaching the client and family techniques of care and identifying appropriate resources to assist the client and family in maintaining self-sufficiency. Box 8–1 lists Medicare's required data for the nursing plan of care.

To implement the plan, the home health nurse performs nursing interventions, including teaching; coordinates and uses referrals and resources; provides and monitors all levels of technical care; collaborates with other disciplines and providers; identifies clinical problems and solutions from research and other health literature; supervises ancillary personnel; and advocates for the client's right to self-determination. Technical skills commonly performed by home health nurses include blood pressure measurement; body fluid collection (blood, urine, stool, sputum); wound care; respiratory care; and all types of intravenous therapy, enteral nutrition, urinary catheterization, enterostomal care, and renal dialysis (see Figure 8-4 ■).

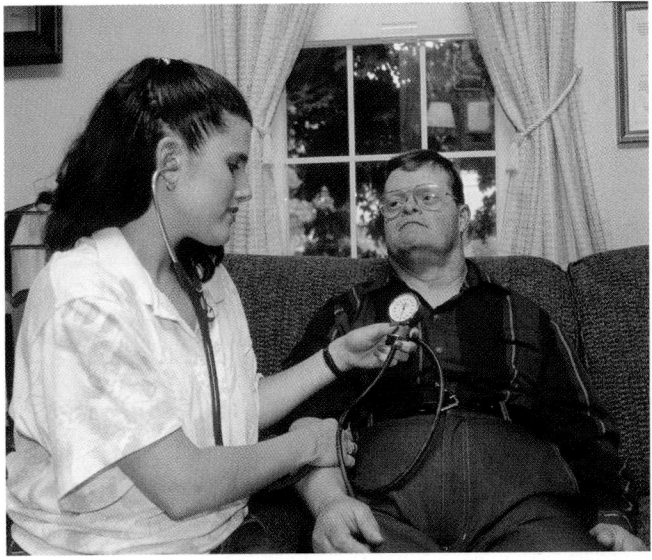

Figure 8-4 ■ The nurse monitors the client's response to treatments and therapy.

Figure 8-5 ■ Determining the success of the care plan includes comparing assessment findings to previous values. Weighing this tube-fed baby provides critical data about her progress.

A large part of the nurse's role involves teaching the client and caregiver the necessary skills for self-care—for example, administering insulin injections, measuring blood glucose, and administering medications. Medication instruction about dosage, frequency of administration, and possible side effects is of particular concern for many clients. (See Chapter 35 ∞ for more information.) Clients who are receiving high-technology interventions are often anxious about their ability to manage such sophisticated equipment. The home health nurse is challenged to alleviate the client's fears and to provide thorough instruction, demonstration, and periodic evaluation of the client and family's performance of such skills. Members of the home care team specially trained in the skill, such as intravenous nurses and respiratory therapists, generally make periodic visits to service the equipment and to monitor the client's skills.

Even though the client and family may become independent in self-care skills, the home health nurse still has the ultimate responsibility to ensure the client is receiving the prescribed therapy at the appropriate timed intervals. Ongoing communication with the primary care provider about the client's progress is critical, and the nurse must make ongoing assessments to ensure that all aspects of the care are being followed.

On subsequent home visits, the nurse observes the same parameters assessed on the initial home visit and relates findings to the expected outcomes or goals (see Figure 8-5 ■). The nurse can also teach caregivers parameters of evaluation so that they can obtain professional intervention if needed. Documentation of care given and the client's progress toward goal achievement at each visit is essential. Notes must also reflect plans for sub-sequent visits and when the client may be sufficiently prepared for self-care and discharge from the agency.

THE FUTURE OF HOME HEALTH CARE

What is the future for home health care? More studies are needed to determine the practicality, safety, effectiveness, cost, and satisfaction with home care—especially new models of "hospital-at-home" care. Trends in the home health care industry include:

1. Ethics committees to handle ethical issues that arise in the home. These committees may be necessary for agencies to receive accreditation.
2. Third-party reimbursement for community clinical nurse specialists and psychiatric nurse specialists. These advanced practice nurses can provide education, support, counseling, and therapy for clients and their families.
3. Third-party reimbursement for social workers. Social workers can assist clients and their families in the home with financial and household problems, freeing the nurse to focus on nursing care.
4. Nurse pain specialists to assess and manage pain in the home, thus avoiding costly hospitalizations and procedures.
5. Pet care for clients who may become too ill to care for them. Clients can make arrangements for the care of a pet if they are hospitalized or die.
6. Electronic home visits. A computerized system can obtain information, such as blood pressure readings, allowing case managers to review a client's progress from off-site.

MediaLink Home Care of a Diabetic Client Application

LIFESPAN CONSIDERATIONS   Home Care

CHILDREN

One goal of *Healthy People 2010* is to reduce the number of children with disabilities living in care facilities from over 24,000 in 1997 to 0 by 2010 (U.S. Department of Health and Human Services, 2000). Ideally, all children with disabilities would live in a secure, "permanent" family environment. Such an environment is one that supports family strengths, connects families to their community, and fosters ongoing, secure relationships. At times, children with disabilities may need to be placed in adoptive or medical foster homes. Home health nurses can strengthen family functioning by:

- Providing information, advice, and instruction on care of the child.
- Identifying natural support systems (e.g., extended family, neighbors, friends).
- Helping families find community resources to meet their needs (e.g., respite care, technical and equipment services).
- Assisting families with alternative placement options as needed (e.g., medical foster care).
- Advocating for families with other health care providers and policy makers.

ELDERS

Clients who have been hospitalized are often discharged after short stays and may still be acutely ill. This becomes a challenge for home health nurses in planning and implementing care. Special areas of concern for elders in this situation include the following:

- Healing time is slower due to changes that normally occur in aging, such as impaired circulation and alteration in immune response.
- Changes in medications or lingering traces of anesthesia may alter cognitive status, even though it is usually temporary.
- Weakness and fatigue create safety issues, such as risk for falling.
- Chronic diseases already present may have been complicated by other conditions acquired while hospitalized.
- Assessment should be initiated while the client is in the hospital to determine the need for assistive devices or environmental changes when the client returns home. Some examples of these devices are walkers, raised toilet seats, safety bars in the bathroom, and better lighting. Good planning eases the transition to home care for the client and caregiver.

In the future, although the number of elders will increase, fewer family caregivers may be available. However, elders appreciate receiving care from family members (Crist, 2005), and nurses should facilitate this when possible.

CRITICAL THINKING CHECKPOINT

Mr. Madden is a 67-year-old African American male with a 20-year history of hypertension and diabetes mellitus. He has recently undergone amputation of three toes due to poor circulation.

Because he is progressing well and his diabetes is under control, he is being discharged from the acute care setting to go home. He has been referred to the hospital-based home health agency, which will assign a nurse to change his foot dressings, administer IV antibiotics, and monitor his blood glucose levels.

1. When delivering care in the home environment, how will the nurse's role be similar to and different from that of the nurse's role in the acute care environment?

2. What rights does the client have when being cared for at home that may not be afforded him while institutionalized?
3. What factors could negatively affect the care of Mr. Madden in his own home?
4. Speculate about personal and financial savings derived by clients being cared for at home rather than in a hospital or other institution.

See Critical Thinking Possibilities in Appendix A. ∞

CHAPTER 8 REVIEW

CHAPTER HIGHLIGHTS

- Home health care is an alternative to acute and subacute health care facilities. The trend has changed from using home health care after hospitalization to using it to avoid hospitalization.
- Hospice nursing, often considered a subspecialty of home nursing, supports terminally ill clients and their families during the last stages of life and bereavement.
- Home health agencies offer skilled professional and paraprofessional services. Because clients often require the services of several professionals simultaneously, case coordination is essential.

- There are several types of home health agencies: official or public agencies, voluntary or private not-for-profit agencies, private proprietary agencies, and institution-based agencies. All home health agencies must meet specific standards for licensing, certification, and accreditation.
- Private duty agencies provide professional nursing and home health aide care for 4 to 24 hours per day.

- Health care agencies in the United States receive reimbursement for services they provide from various sources: Medicare and Medicaid, private insurance companies, and private pay. The Medicare and Medicaid programs have strict guidelines.
- Referrals for home health services may be made by the client's physician, a nurse, a social worker, a therapist, a discharge planner, or a family member. Home care requires, however, a physician's order and an approved treatment plan.
- Major roles of the home health nurse are those of advocate, caregiver, educator, and case manager.
- The home health nurse assesses the care needs of clients in their home; plans, implements, and supervises that care; teaches clients and their families self-care; and mobilizes the resources of

hospitals, primary care providers, and community agencies in meeting the needs of the clients and their families.
- Home care clients include a diverse population that encompasses all ages, a variety of health problems, and families of different structures and cultural backgrounds. The home health nurse needs to be culturally sensitive, that is, become aware of the client's culture, and form a nursing care plan with the client that incorporates the client's culture.
- Important dimensions of home health nursing include the home visit in which the nurse assesses the client and they make plans for care; client and nurse safety; infection control; and caregiver support.

TEST YOUR KNOWLEDGE

1. Care in the home is an alternative to hospital placement. Which of the following is one major difference associated with in-home care?
   1. Does not focus on curative and lifesaving approaches
   2. Is less able to manage complex symptoms
   3. Facilitates extensive involvement of significant others/family
   4. Permits use of pain medication regimens not allowed in the hospital

2. If a primary care provider prescribed the following, which could be delegated to the home health aide?
   1. Feeding and bathing the client
   2. Teaching the client about medications
   3. Assessing wound healing progress
   4. Adjusting oxygen flow

3. After the nurse instructed a client about the rationale for sitting with feet elevated to enhance venous return, the client refuses to perform the activity. Which statement by the nurse would be most useful?
   1. "If you won't cooperate, I can't help you."
   2. "Tell me the reasons you won't put your feet up."

3. "It is essential that you do this."
   4. "I'll notify your doctor that you are unable to keep your feet up."

4. A home health nurse is providing care for a client who has paralysis on one side and whose spouse provides most of the care. Which of the following may be a sign of caregiver role strain?
   1. The caregiver loses weight and has insomnia.
   2. The caregiver asks other family and friends for help.
   3. The caregiver asks the nurse what other ways he or she can help the client.
   4. The caregiver seems sad whenever the client's prognosis is discussed.

5. A client is scheduled to be discharged from the hospital. The discharge planner at the hospital should acquire which of the following first before home nursing care can be initiated?
   1. Insurance coverage
   2. An in-home caregiver
   3. A curable health problem
   4. A physician's authorization

See Answers to Test Your Knowledge in Appendix A.

EXPLORE MEDIALINK www.prenhall.com/berman

DVD-ROM
- Audio Glossary
- NCLEX Review

COMPANION WEBSITE
- Additional NCLEX Review
- Case Study: Home Care Nursing
- Application Activities:
    Hospice Nursing
    Duties of the Home Health Assistant
    Home Care of a Diabetic Client
- Links to Resources

READINGS AND REFERENCES

SUGGESTED READINGS
Bedard, M., Koivuranta, A., & Stuckey, A. (2004). Health impact on caregivers of providing informal care to a cognitively impaired older adult: Rural versus urban settings. *Canadian Journal of Rural Medicine, 9*(1), 15–34. *This article reports a study of informal caregiving for cognitively impaired Canadian elders in urban versus rural settings. The authors concluded that rural caregivers overall had more specialized needs in the promotion of healthy behaviors and care management of cognitively impaired elders.*
Ervin, N., Scrivener, K., & Simmons, T. (2004). Using the linkage model for integrating

evidence into home care nursing practice. *Home Health Care Nurse, 22*, 606–611. *The heart failure patient population of a home care agency shows improved outcomes following implementation of an evidence-based practice model by the agency.*

RELATED RESEARCH
Castleman, J., & Gailor, N. (2004). Informal caregiving burden: An overlooked aspect of the lives and health of women transitioning from welfare to employment? *Public Health Nursing, 21*, 24–31.
Grant, J. S., Glandon, G. L., Elliott, T. R., Giger, J. N., & Weaver, M. (2004). Caregiving problems

and feelings experienced by family caregivers of stroke survivors the first month after discharge. *International Journal of Rehabilitation Research, 27*, 105–111.
Langa, K., Valenstein, M., Fendrick, A., Kabeto, M., & Vijan, S. (2004). Extent and cost of informal caregiving for older Americans with symptoms of depression. *American Journal of Psychiatry, 161*, 857–863.
Taft, S. H., Pierce, C. A., & Gallo, C. L. (2005). From hospital to home and back again: A study in hospital admissions and deaths for home care patients. *Home Health Care Management and Practice, 17*, 467–480.

REFERENCES

Boucher, M. A. (2005). Making it: Qualities needed for rural home care nursing. *Home Healthcare Nurse, 23,* 103–108.

Brillhart, B., Kruse, B., & Heard, L. (2004). Safety concerns for rehabilitation nurses in home care. *Rehabilitation Nursing, 29,* 227–229.

Caruso, J. T., Scala-Foley, M. A., Archer, D., & Reinhard, S. C. (2004). Making sense of Medicare: A Medicare house call. *American Journal of Nursing, 104*(7), 71–72.

Centers for Medicare & Medicaid Services. (2001). *Medicare home health agency manual* (HCFA Publication No. 11, PB 98-955200). Retrieved June 12, 2006, from http://www.cms.hhs.gov/manuals/downloads/pub_11.zip

Centers for Medicare & Medicaid Services. (2004). *Medicare and home health care* (CMS Publication 10969). Baltimore: U.S. Department of Health & Human Services.

Crist, J. D. (2005). The meaning for elders of receiving family care. *Journal of Advanced Nursing, 49,* 485–493.

Porter, E. J., & Ganong, L. H. (2005). Older widows' speculations and expectancies concerning professional home-care providers. *Nursing Ethics, 12,* 507–521.

Smith, C., Cowan, C., Sensing, A., & Catlin, A. (2005). Health spending growth slows in 2003. *Health Affairs, 24,* 185–194.

Sturkey, E. N., Linker, S., Keith, D. D., & Comeau, E. (2005). Improving wound care outcomes in the home setting. *Journal of Nursing Care Quality, 20,* 349–355.

U.S. Department of Health and Human Services. (2000). *Healthy people 2010: Understanding and improving health* (2nd ed.). Washington, DC: U.S. Government Printing Office.

SELECTED BIBLIOGRAPHY

American Nurses Association. (1999). *Scope and standards of home health nursing practice.* Washington, DC: American Nurses Publishing.

Bradley, P. J. (2003). Family caregiver assessment: Essential for effective home health care. *Journal of Gerontological Nursing, 29*(2), 29–36.

Byrne, M. (2003). Culture-derived strategies of a pediatric home-care nursing specialty team. *International Nursing Review, 50*(1), 34–43.

Hartung, S. Q. (2005). Choosing home health as a specialty and successfully transitioning into practice. *Home Health Care Management and Practice, 17,* 70–87.

Hogue, E. (2003). Five crucial legal issues for home care providers. *Remington Report, 11*(1), 22–24.

Joint Commission on Accreditation of Healthcare Organizations. (2004). *2004–2005 Comprehensive accreditation manual for home care.* Oakbrook Terrace, IL: Author.

Keller, S., Hunter, D., & Shortt, S. (2004). The impact of hospital restructuring on home care nursing. *Canadian Journal of Nursing Leadership, 17*(2), 82–89.

Reinhart, E. (2005). *Infection control in home care.* Boston: Jones & Bartlett.

Schumacher, K., & Marren, J. (2004). Home care nursing for older adults: State of the science. *Nursing Clinics of North America, 39,* 443–471.

Nursing Informatics

LEARNING OUTCOMES

After completing this chapter, you will be able to:

1. Define the common components of desktop computers.

2. Recognize the uses of word processing, database, spreadsheet, and communications software in nursing.

3. Describe the uses of computers in nursing education.

4. Discuss the advantages of and concerns about computerized client documentation systems.

5. Identify computer applications used in client assessment and care.

6. List ways computers may be used by nurse administrators in the areas of human resources, facilities management, finance, quality assurance, and accreditation.

7. Identify the role of computers in each step of the research process.

Computers have become a part of everyday life for many people, including nurses. Computers are used for educating nursing students and clients; assessing, documenting, and testing clients' health conditions; managing medical records; communicating among health care providers and with clients; and conducting nursing research. All nurses must have a basic level of computer literacy in order to perform their jobs.

GENERAL CONCEPTS

Informatics refers to the science of computer information systems. **Nursing informatics** is the science of using computer information systems in the practice of nursing. It is defined by the American Nurses Association (ANA, 2001) as "A specialty that integrates nursing science, computer science, and information science to manage and communicate data, information, and knowledge in nursing practice... to support patients, nurses, and other providers in their decision-making in all roles and settings" (p. 46).

This is a relatively young science—the first Nursing Information Systems conference was held in the United States in 1977. Nurses have taken significant strides since then to design and adapt computer processes to enhance client care, education, administration and management, and nursing research. Advanced practice in nursing informatics is a growing specialty. The first ANA certification examination in nursing informatics was given in October 1995.

The terminology used to describe the parts and functions of computer systems can be confusing. New terms emerge daily and it is a challenge to keep up with them. This section describes the most common computer hardware and software nurses may come across in the work setting.

Computer Hardware

Hardware, the physical parts of the computer, allows the user to enter data into the computer, performs the actions of the computer's processing, and produces the computer output. Microcomputers, faster and smaller versions of the old supercomputer or mainframe, are individual systems referred to as desktop or **personal computers (PCs).** These include portable laptop, notebook, tablet, or handheld computers. The basic components of computer hardware include the central processing unit and one or more types of data input and output devices.

Central Processing Unit

The **central processing unit (CPU)** is in the box that contains the computer hardware necessary to process and store data. Also located with the CPU are the power supply, disk drives, chips, and connections for all the other computer hardware, referred to as **peripherals.** The speed of the computer is determined by three components: the CPU processor (measured in gigahertz), the amount of RAM (explained shortly), and the speed of data location or transfer rate of the disk drives (seek time). For example, at the time of this writing, a reasonably fast desktop computer would have a processing speed of more than 2.8 GHz, at least 256 MB of RAM, and a hard drive average seek time of less than 4 milliseconds. By the time you read this, standards will have changed.

Computer Memory and Storage

In order for data to be kept for later retrieval, the computer must store the information in an electronic form. Computer information is measured in bytes (usually 1 byte is one letter, digit, or character), kilobytes (1,000 bytes = 1 KB), megabytes (1 million bytes = 1 MB), or gigabytes (1 billion bytes = 1 GB).

While the computer is turned on, data and instructions for the computer are loaded into **random-access memory (RAM).** Storage in RAM is temporary and is lost when the computer is turned off. To save their work, computer users store data on magnetic hard disks or drives and "floppy" diskettes. Data can also be stored and retrieved from high-capacity disks (e.g., Zip disks), compact disks (CDs), magnetic tape, smartcards, and small, portable keychain-sized devices referred to as flash, thumb, or memory stick drives.

Input Devices

There are several ways to get information into a computer. The most common method is to use a keyboard. The mouse is a pointing device with buttons used to choose items or initiate an action. Some computer screens respond to touch from a finger, lightpen, or wand. Increasingly, print or cursive handwriting can be displayed directly on the computer screen or translated into typeface for storage, such as with a tablet computer or personal digital assistant (PDA). Many computers also have a microphone and can respond to voice commands. Other electronic devices used for entering data into a computer are scanners and analog-to-digital converters. Scanners allow data to be copied into the computer from a paper version or other "hardcopy" text or graphics. Analog signals such as those from biometric devices such as cardiac monitors can convert data to digital signals that can be stored by the computer.

CLINICAL ALERT

Personal digital assistants (PDAs) are handheld computers that can interface with PCs, networks, or phone systems. Nurses increasingly use them as calendar/date books, address books, drug and disease database storage devices, and data entry and retrieval devices. ■

Output Devices

The results of computer data entry or processing are usually displayed first on the computer screen or monitor and then through a printer. Both monitors and printers display text and graphics. Computer data can also be output to audio and video displays. For example, the popular free program Acrobat Reader (Adobe Systems) has a built-in function to read aloud portable document format (pdf) files—although the voice is very mechanical-sounding. Music, motion, and voice can also be presented in high fidelity.

Communications Devices

Sometimes computer data need to be sent long distances or directly to one or more other computers. The term **online** refers to a computer being connected to other computers in a **network.** The network is often coordinated by one computer, the network server. PCs linked directly to other nearby PCs and servers by wires or wireless communications devices constitute a **local-area network (LAN).** Distant locations can be linked through a **wide-area network (WAN),** virtual network, or private network. These larger distances can be covered by sending the data through standard telephone wires or a high-speed data connection (e.g., cable, digital subscriber line [DSL], or integrated services digital network [ISDN] line). The technology for network connections and devices changes rapidly.

Computer Software

Computer programs, also called applications or software, instruct the hardware to perform certain tasks. The most commonly used software programs are word processors, databases, spreadsheets, utilities such as communications, and presentation graphics programs.

Word Processing

The ability to save and manipulate words is probably the most used computer application. The word processing program has numerous options to permit the user to specify the typeface, spacing, and page layout. Documents can be automatically checked for spelling and grammar. Documents can also be individualized by merging them with name and address lists and can include pictures, tables and charts, and graphical designs.

Databases

Database programs are used to manage detailed information. Within a database file are individual records that represent the person, product, or area information. The record contains fields that are characteristics of the record. For example, a hospital client database has a record for each client that contains separate fields for age, gender, primary care provider's name, diagnosis, and so on. The pharmacy also has a database that lists each medication it has in stock (a record) and the strength, quantity, location, price, and manufacturer for each (the fields). The most common personal database is an electronic address book. The user enters data into the blank spaces which can then be retrieved in a variety of formats for viewing or printing (Figure 9-1 ■). The power of database programs is their ability to quickly search extremely large numbers of records and fields for commonalities, and then help the user generate detailed and complex reports.

Spreadsheets

Electronic **spreadsheets** are programs that manipulate words and numbers. The data are arranged in cells formatted into columns and rows. The program can perform many complicated manipulations on the data using formulas and directions that are entered or built into the software. Spreadsheets are used extensively for managing budgets but are also useful for working with staffing, scheduling, invoicing, research, and other analyses.

Communications

Communications devices require software to guide the computer in connecting to a remote device and knowing what data to send or receive. Communications programs use one or more standard protocols depending on the form of communication,

Figure 9-1 ■ An electronic address book is a type of database. After the details are entered into the computer for each contact person or organization, they can be retrieved, sorted, and displayed in many formats different from the one into which they were entered.

Microsoft product screen shot reprinted with permission from Microsoft Corporation.

such as fax or file transfer, in order to communicate effectively with the distant site.

An important type of communications software is electronic mail (e-mail). E-mail has become a standard method of communication worldwide.

Presentation Graphics Programs

Due in part to advances in color printing and computer display hardware, software programs to create charts, graphs, tables, pictures, videos, audio, and other nontext files have become increasingly popular. Many integrated software packages include graphics programs that can easily exchange materials with word processing and spreadsheet programs. Users can create so-called slide shows for use in teaching or research presentations.

Computer Systems

The concept of a computer system—not in the sense of one machine but of a network of computers, users, programs, and procedures in an organization—implies that there is identifiable input, processing, output, and feedback. The two most common types of computer systems used by nurses are management information systems and hospital information systems.

Management Information Systems

A **management information system (MIS)** is designed to facilitate the organization and application of data used to manage an organization or department. The system provides analyses used for strategic planning, decision making, and evaluation of management activities. All levels of management benefit from the ability to access the data.

Hospital Information Systems

A **hospital information system (HIS)** is an MIS that focuses on the types of data needed to manage client care activities and health care organizations. As with any system, the goal is to provide people with the data they need to determine appropriate actions and control them. Typically an HIS will have subsystems in the areas of admissions, medical records (Figure 9-2 ■), clinical laboratory, pharmacy, order entry, and finance. The personnel in these areas record the data needed to allow management of billing, quality assurance, scheduling, and inventory both within their own areas and across the institution. Increasingly, accrediting organizations mandate the use of an HIS and require that reports be submitted using computerized formats. Eventually, integrated HISs will form the center of all record keeping and analysis for interdisciplinary health care.

Often the "language" used in HISs varies from vendor to vendor. The National Library of Medicine (NLM) has created the Unified Medical Language System (UMLS) to facilitate the development of computer systems that recognize the language of health. UMLS Knowledge Sources (databases) and associated software programs are available to system developers of electronic information systems. A metathesaurus database contains multilingual terms and concepts which are then categorized in the UMLS Semantic Network.

The Health Insurance Portability and Accountability Act of 1996 (HIPAA) established legal requirements for the protection, security, and appropriate sharing of client personal health information (referred to as protected health information or PHI). Because PHI is now stored electronically, HIPAA regulations have mandated strict control over access and communication of

Figure 9-2 ■ Client list screen. This is the screen that the user sees when logging into an HIS application. It is the "home base" and displays alerts and notifications regarding new orders and new results. It also gives access to other areas of the chart such as documents or results.
(Courtesy of Sutter Health.)

HIS data (Rossel, 2003). Each health care agency in which nurses work will orient them to the specific technological controls in place.

World Wide Web and the Internet

The **Internet** is a worldwide network that connects other networks. Connections among networks and PCs via the Internet allow for almost instantaneous transmission among distant sites and can include text, audio, and video data. The **World Wide Web (WWW)** refers to the complex links among webpages or websites, accessed through "addresses" called universal resource locators (URLs). URLs begin with the designation http://, often followed by www. URLs end with a designation that denotes the type of site. For example, .com is for commercial sites, .org for organizations, .edu for educational institutions, and .gov for government sites.

Tens of thousands of health-related websites exist, many new ones appearing and others becoming "dead links" daily. No standardized controls exist to ensure that the information provided is current or accurate. Nurses should evaluate health websites as they access them and assist clients in doing the same. Tools for doing this include (as of this publication) *Evaluating Internet Resources* from the State University of New York at Albany and *Criteria for Assessing the Quality of Health Information on the Internet—Policy Paper* from the Health Information Technology Institute of Mitretek Systems Health Summit Working Group (Box 9–1).

The complexity and breadth of computer applications are expanding exponentially. Computer access is rapidly increasing while the cost tends to decrease over time. Technology is evolving in the areas of virtual reality, remote access, task automation, robotics, and bioengineering. Simultaneously, however, concerns regarding privacy, access by persons with disabilities and in underdeveloped countries, piracy, intellectual property debates (who owns Web content), destructive programs (computer viruses), and ergonomic injuries continue to arise.

COMPUTERS IN NURSING EDUCATION

Just as computers have become standard instructional tools in the primary and secondary school systems, they are used extensively in all aspects of nursing education. Nursing programs require computerized libraries, faculty members use technological teaching strategies in the classroom and for outside assignments as well as demonstrating and using applications in clinical rotations, and academic record keeping is facilitated by database programs.

Teaching and Learning

Computers enhance academics for both students and faculty in at least four ways. These include access to literature, computer-assisted instruction, classroom technologies, and strategies for learning at a distance.

Literature Access and Retrieval

In our information age, it is a challenge to keep abreast of the information on any subject. Computers have significantly improved our abilities in this area by presenting catalogs and text of materials in a way that can be searched systematically. Previously, users needed to leaf through multiple collections of printed indexes, one keyword or topic at a time. Now continuously updated cumulative indexes of related materials can be searched electronically in a fraction of the time. The searcher can specify the recency, language, document type, and other characteristics of the citation for desired materials. Once a list of search matches is displayed on the computer screen, users can select all or certain citations and either print them or store them on their own local computers. Box 9–2 lists commonly used bibliographic systems and databases.

In addition to searching lists of documents, actual complete publications and materials are available in computerized formats. These include medical textbooks, the full text of journals, drug references, digitized x-rays or scans, and graphics including clip art. Through the Internet and the World Wide Web, both classic and the most current information can be found on any topic. Users can access statistics from the Centers for Disease Control and Prevention, census data, and the National Library of Medicine.

BOX 9–1 Criteria for Evaluating Internet Health Information

- *Credibility:* includes the source, currency, relevance/utility, and editorial review process for the information.
- *Content:* must be accurate and complete, and an appropriate disclaimer provided.
- *Disclosure:* includes informing the user of the purpose of the site, as well as any profiling or collection of information associated with using the site.
- *Links:* evaluated according to selection, architecture, content, and back linkages.
- *Design:* encompasses accessibility, logical organization (navigability), and internal search capability.
- *Interactivity:* includes feedback mechanisms and means for exchange of information among users.
- *Caveats:* clarification of whether site function is to market products and services or is a primary information content provider.

BOX 9–2 Common Health-Related Bibliographic Systems and Databases

Acquired Immune Deficiency Syndrome information onLINE (AIDSLINE)
CANCER LITerature (CANCER LIT)
Cumulative Index to Nursing and Allied Health Literature (CINAHL)
Educational Resources Information Center (ERIC)
Medical Literature Analysis and Retrieval System (MEDLARS)
Mental Measurements Yearbook
Psychological Abstracts (PsychINFO)

Computer-Assisted Instruction

Nursing has enjoyed the computer revolution in the form of computer-assisted instruction (CAI). Dozens of software programs help nursing students and nurses learn and demonstrate learning. These have been created by individuals, educational institutions, technology companies, or print publishers. Programs cover topics from drug dosage calculations to ethical decision making and are classified according to format: tutorial, drill and practice, simulation, or testing. CAI can contain diagrams, graphics, animation, video, and audio and may be accessed on CD-ROMs or on the Internet. All forms of CAI allow almost instant access to any section of the program and can be designed to branch to different sections depending on the user's responses.

Tutorials on electrocardiogram (ECG, EKG) interpretation, drug interactions, and legal aspects of nursing are examples of these programs. Course syllabi that contain worksheets or activities students can complete on the computer may be distributed on disk, through the college network, or via the Internet. Students who become familiar with CAI will also find that they have an easier time adjusting to the software programs many employers require them to complete for annual competency testing mandated by accrediting bodies in certain areas (e.g., bloodborne pathogens and fire safety). Completion of CAI programs may also be an acceptable means of demonstrating continuing education activities required for license renewal.

Classroom Technology

Most new educational buildings are wired to accommodate technology. This includes adequate electric outlets for students to plug in laptop computers and wiring (or wireless technology) for network or Internet access. For the faculty, projectors and liquid crystal display (LCD) panels that allow computer screens to be displayed to the entire classroom are becoming standard. These enhancements allow faculty to use the full text, video, and audio capabilities of computers instead of overhead transparencies, slides, or writing on the board.

Distance Learning

There are several different models of **distance learning.** In one model, the student receives course materials, communicates with the faculty and other students, and submits assignments completely through the mail, phone or fax, e-mail, website, and electronic "dropbox" (a server folder accessible from the Internet). This may be referred to as an asynchronous mode because the persons involved are not interacting at the same "real" time. Another model of distance education involves groups of students in classrooms at different sites participating in a class session through two-way audio and video transmission. Computers are used to code and decode the sounds and visuals for transmission. Students who are not at the site where the faculty member is located can also communicate via voice-activated microphones or response pads. These pads have buttons that permit the students to indicate that they wish to ask a question or even to respond to multiple-choice test questions.

Synchronous distance learning can be accomplished through use of chat and instant messaging. Another computerized delivery of knowledge is through e-books—an entire textbook is available on a computer or PDA and can be annotated and searched. PDAs can also contain reference materials such as drug handbooks for instant, up-to-date information. As computer technology becomes more cost-effective and increases its transmission quality, it is anticipated that more schools will use distance learning strategies to reach students around the globe.

CLINICAL ALERT

Distance education courses held entirely on computer are called online courses, whereas part computer and part classroom-based courses are often referred to as Web-enhanced or hybrid courses. Course management software (such as Blackboard or Moodle) provides an organizing framework for delivery of the Internet content of distance courses. ■

Testing

The computer is ideal for conducting certain types of learning evaluations. Surveys can be completed online, including anonymous questionnaires. For testing, large banks of potential items can be written and the computer can generate different exams for each student depending on the selection criteria designated by the faculty. In addition, the students' answers can be scored electronically and the overall exam results analyzed quickly. In 1994, the National Council Licensure Examination for RNs in the United States (NCLEX-RN) moved from paper-and-pencil tests to computer tests. Applicants can complete the computerized exam in less than 5 hours compared to 2 days for the written exam, test results are available in about half the time, and exams can be taken at the applicant's convenience as opposed to two scheduled sessions each year. The computer determines if the applicant passed the examination by using a scoring algorithm that ensures all required competencies have been evaluated fairly.

Student and Course Record Management

Computers are also very useful for maintaining results of students' grades or attendance using spreadsheets. Often faculty are able to scan student exam answer sheets directly into a gradebook on the computer. The program can then calculate percentages, sort student scores in order, and print results for both students and faculty. Grades from multiple exams plus scores on essays or other projects are calculated into final grades.

Students are frequently asked to evaluate faculty and courses using machine-readable forms. These data are also scanned into the computer so that cumulative results can be calculated and stored. That is an example of what is called **data warehousing—** the accumulation of large amounts of data that are stored over time and can be examined for output in different types of reports (charts and tables).

Most schools now have all student records on computer. From application through graduation, the registrar's office keeps track of names, addresses, courses taken, grades, and all other pertinent student data. Students may be able to sign up for classes, check their tuition bills, and see their transcripts on computer terminals on campus or from anywhere that has a computer with Internet access.

COMPUTERS IN NURSING PRACTICE

Many activities of the registered nurse involve collecting, recording, and using data. Computers are well suited to assist the nurse in these functions. Specifically, the nurse records client information in computer records, accesses other departments' information on the client from centralized computers, uses computers to manage client scheduling, and uses programs for unique applications such as home health nursing and case management.

Documentation of Client Status and Medical Record Keeping

How might a computer assist individual nurses with their daily activities? In the typical 8-hour day of a nurse providing direct client care, as much as one-third of the time may be spent recording in the client's record. Additional time is spent trying to access data about the client that may be somewhere in the medical record or elsewhere in the health care agency. Nurses need access to standardized forms, policies, and procedures. Also, nurses need to be able to gather broader client information such as length of stay for specific diagnoses. Computers can assist with each of these.

Bedside Data Entry

There are several different types of computerized bedside data entry systems. These allow recording of client assessments, medication administration (Figure 9-3 ■), progress notes, care plan updating, client acuity, and accrued charges. The terminal can be fixed or handheld, and hardwired to the central system or cordless with the ability to transmit the data to distant sites, such as from the client's home to the agency office. A slightly

RESEARCH NOTE
Does Point-of-Care Nursing Documentation Make a Difference?

This article reports on five research studies aimed at determining whether or not bedside electronic charting made a difference in quality of documentation and nurses' satisfaction. The studies were very diverse, ranging from a pilot examination of functionality, usefulness, and acceptability to a large chart review of compliance with accreditation charting standards. In each case, results indicated that electronic charting improved compliance with documentation standards. Time spent charting was decreased and nurse satisfaction increased. The authors recognized that these were early studies and resistance to change may influence reproducibility of the magnitude of the results in larger institutions.

IMPLICATIONS

Novel approaches to charting that reduce the time and effort of recording will likely be of broad interest to nurses. Anything that allows more time to be spent with clients and enhances the ease of documentation—especially the more routine and standard reports required—is a positive move. However, it is far too early to have complete confidence that satisfaction with electronic bedside charting will be maintained over time as the novelty wears off. Institutions are spending many dollars on new computer charting systems. At the minimum, the cost is well spent even if only for the consistency of charting and the ability to mine the data for outcomes assessment and quality improvement. However, much more research on the effects of online charting is needed.

Note: From "The Times They Are a Changing: Effects of Online Nursing Documentation Systems," by C. Langowski, 2005, Quality Management in Health Care, 14, pp. 121–125.

Figure 9-3 ■ This screen shows a MAR (medication administration record) for several regularly scheduled medications. The worksheet displays the next time the medications are scheduled to be administered.

(Courtesy of Sutter Health.)

different type of bedside terminal is the point-of-care or point-of-service computer. In this case the terminal is located near, but not necessarily at, the client.

Computer-Based Client Records

Electronic medical records (EMRs) or **computer-based patient records (CPRs)** permit electronic client data retrieval by caregivers, administrators, accreditors, and other persons who require the data. The Computer-Based Patient Record Institute, established in 1992, identified four ways the EMR could improve health care: (a) constant availability of client health information across the life span, (b) ability to monitor quality, (c) access to warehoused (stored) data, and (d) ability for clients to share in knowledge and activities influencing their own health.

Because of the way computers provide access to the EMR, providers easily retrieve specific data such as trends in vital signs (Figure 9-4 ■), immunization records, and current problems. The system can be designed to warn providers about conflicting medications or client parameters that indicate dangerous conditions (Figure 9-5 ■). Sophisticated systems allow replay of audio, graphic, or video data for comparison with current status. All text is legible and can be searched for keywords.

There are several areas of concern with EMRs. Maintaining privacy and security of data is a significant issue (Olson, 2003). One way that computers can protect data is by user authentication via passwords or biometric identifiers (e.g., fingerprint or retinal scans)—only those persons who have a legitimate need to access the data receive the password. Addi-

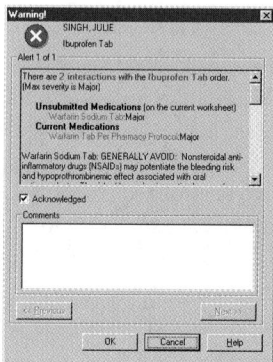

Figure 9-5 ■ One of the strengths of an electronic medical record is its ability to alert the clinician to potential drug interactions using warnings like the one displayed.
(Courtesy of Sutter Health.)

tional policies and procedures for protecting the confidentiality of EMRs are evolving as the use of computer systems becomes more widespread.

Following several previous reports, the ANA developed a position statement on privacy, confidentiality of medical records, and the nurse's role (see Box 9–3). One role of the **nurse informaticist,** an expert who combines computer, information, and nursing science, is to develop policies and procedures that promote effective and secure use of computerized records by nurses and other health care professionals.

Currently, there are no national standards for EMRs: not for the specific data that should be included nor for how the record

Figure 9-4 ■ This screen displays the client's vital signs. They can be entered by the nurse (or anyone with the security rights to do so) at the bedside, and they can then be displayed wherever needed.

(Courtesy of Sutter Health.)

BOX 9-3   ANA Position Statement on Privacy

THE ROLE OF NURSING IN PRIVACY AND CONFIDENTIALITY RELATED TO ACCESS TO ELECTRONIC DATA 1999 AMERICAN NURSES ASSOCIATION HOUSE OF DELEGATES

PRIVACY AND CONFIDENTIALITY

EXECUTIVE SUMMARY: Advances in technology have led to the development of computerized medical databases and telehealth systems and have raised serious concerns about patient privacy and the confidentiality of health care information. Threats to confidentiality of medical records and health care information affect the kinds of care that patients seek and potentially undermine the relationship of trust between health professionals and patients that is essential to quality health care. Nurses play a critical role in preserving patient privacy and confidentiality and should participate in the ongoing debate about and development of Federal laws designed to ensure patient privacy/confidentiality.

In keeping with the nursing profession's commitment to patient advocacy and the trust that is essential to the preservation of the high quality of care patients have come to expect from registered nurses, the American Nurses Association supports the following principles with respect to patient privacy and confidentiality:

- A patient's right to privacy with respect to individually identifiable health information, including genetic information, should be established statutorily. Individuals should retain the right to decide to whom, and under what circumstances, their individually identifiable health information will be disclosed. Confidentiality protections should extend not only to health records, but also to all other individually identifiable health information, including genetic information, clinical research records, and mental health therapy notes.
- Use and disclosure of individually identifiable health information should be limited.

- A patient should have the right to access his or her own health information and the right to supplement such information so that they are able to make informed health care decisions, to correct erroneous information, and to address discrepancies that they perceive.
- Patients should receive written, easily understood notification of how their health records are used and when their individually identifiable health information is disclosed to third parties.
- The use or disclosure of individually identifiable health information absent an individual's informed consent should be prohibited. Exceptions should be permitted only if a person's life is endangered, if there is a threat to the public, or if there is a compelling law enforcement need. In the case of such exceptions, information should be limited to the minimum amount necessary.
- Appropriate safeguards should be developed and required for the use, disclosure and storage of personal health information.
- Legislative or regulatory protections on individually identifiable health information should not unnecessarily impede public health efforts or clinical, medical, nursing, or quality of care research.
- Strong and enforceable remedies for violations of privacy protections should be established, and health care professionals who report violations should be protected from retaliation.
- Federal legislation should provide a floor for the protection of individual privacy and confidentiality rights, not a ceiling. Federal legislation should not preempt any other federal or state law or regulation that offers greater protection.

Note: Reprinted with permission from American Nurses Association, *Position Statement: Privacy and Confidentiality,* © 1999 American Nurses Association, Silver Spring, MD 20910.

---

should be organized. HIPAA regulations (also see Chapter 7 ∞) are playing a key role in establishing these. Nurses need to be involved in the design, implementation, and evaluation of EMRs to maximize their use and effectiveness.

Data Standardization and Classifications

There are many reasons why nursing would benefit from standard classifications of terms used to describe and measure clinical, disease, procedure, and outcomes data. One reason is that for nursing to be recognized for the value it adds to client well-being requires research-based findings showing client improvement by accepted standards. This necessitates agreement to use common, consistent, clear, and rule-based standards.

Standards for clinical data such as laboratory test results and their documentation in the EMR have been proposed by the American National Standards Institute Healthcare Informatics Standards Planning Panel, the American Society for Testing and Materials, the European Technical Committee for Standardization, the International Standards Organization, and the Workgroup for Electronic Data Interchange. Disease classification standards are in use in a variety of forms. The most common are the World Health Organization's *International Classification of Diseases* (ICD-9 and ICD-10), the World Organization of National Colleges *International Classification of Primary Care* (ICPC), and the American Psychiatric Association's *Diagnostic and Statistical Manual of Mental Disorders* (DSM).

Nursing classifications or taxonomies have been developed. The Nursing Minimum Data Set (NMDS) contains 16 elements of nursing data, along with their definitions, in three categories: nursing care, client demographics, and service. The NMDS can be used for data collection and documentation and allows sharing of information regarding the quality, cost, and effectiveness of nursing. In the United States, five classification systems are used: the North American Nursing Diagnosis Association (NANDA) taxonomy, the Omaha System, the Home Health Care Classification (HHCC), the Nursing Intervention Classification (NIC), and the Nursing Outcomes Classification (NOC). In addition, the International Council of Nurses has proposed an International Classification for Nursing Practice, a common language for describing nursing problems (or diagnoses), interventions, and outcomes. It may take years to determine which standards will allow optimal access to and manipulation of computerized records, and who will be the determining body.

Tracking Client Status

Once an EMR has been established, the nurse can retrieve and display a client's physiological parameters across time (see Figure 9-6 ■). In addition to the rather straightforward viewing of trends in vital signs, for example, the nurse can also track more global client progress. Standardized nursing care plans, care maps, critical pathways, or other prewritten treatment protocols can be stored in the computer and easily placed in the

Figure 9-6 ■ Lab results are displayed in a Trend view graph.
(Courtesy of Sutter Health.)

EMR electronically. Then the nurse and other health care personnel can examine progress toward and variance from the expected plan directly on the computer.

Electronic Access to Client Data

Besides computers designed for record keeping, other computers are used extensively in health care to assess and monitor clients' conditions. The data accumulated from various electronic devices can be part of the EMR and also stored for research purposes. Electronic records take up much less space than paper records and may be stored more securely. Copies can be made easily onto different electronic media (e.g., magnetic tape, microfiche) that tend to be more compact and durable than paper. Data can also be transmitted to a consulting specialist in another location.

Client Monitoring and Computerized Diagnostics

Nursing has benefited greatly from the myriad of client monitors. In everyday practice, nurses use digital or tympanic thermometers, digital scales, pulse oximetry, ECG/telemetry/hemodynamic monitoring, apnea monitors, fetal heart monitors, blood glucose analyzers, ventilators, and intravenous (IV) pumps. Although most of these monitors are applied externally, implanted electronic monitors are also proving to have great value. For example, a surgically placed wireless sensor can measure the pressure inside a bulging weakened blood vessel (aneurysm) and warn of potential rupture. These instruments can be used in any care setting, from intensive care to the home. Most keep a record of the most recent values. Some can transmit their data to a more sophisticated computer or print out a pa-

per record. Some have digital displays that "talk" to the user, giving instructions or results. Most also have error detection or alarms that indicate either that the instrument is malfunctioning or that the assessed value is outside predetermined parameters. These devices, with their minute but powerful computer chips, make it possible to extend the nurse's observations and provide valid and reliable data.

In various specialty areas of health care, clients undergo diagnostic procedures in which computers play a major role. Computerized axial tomography (CAT) scans, magnetic resonance imaging (MRI), and positron emission tomography (PET) scans use computers extensively to perform tests and analyze the findings. Blood gas analyzers, pulmonary function test machines, and intracranial pressure monitors all use computer processing. All of these can be linked directly to store data in the EMR (see Figure 9-7 ■). There are many more examples of ways that computers assist us in monitoring and diagnosing client conditions.

Telemedicine/Telehealth

One of the most exciting areas being developed in computer-assisted health care is telemedicine. **Telemedicine** uses technology to transmit electronic data about clients to persons at distant locations. In one example, two-way audiovisual communication allows an international expert to examine and consult on a client's case from thousands of miles away. X-rays, scans, stored computer data, and almost anything imaginable can be "sent" using computers. Another example is the ability for a few providers to provide primary health care to people living in remote areas using the kinds of monitors described previously plus telephone, fax, and other relatively simple equipment in the client's home.

Figure 9-7 ■ This screen displays a summary view of all available results for a particular client. The information is always reported from most summarized to most detailed so that the user gets an overview first and can then "drill down" to see the details.
(Courtesy of Sutter Health.)

Concerns regarding telehealth relate to legal and ethical issues. Who has responsibility for the client when a teleconsult is used? Does the care provider need to be licensed in the state or province where the client's primary care is given? The National Council of State Boards of Nursing has declared that the applicable regulations are those for where the client resides and not where the provider is located. This is also one of the reasons for the initiation of the Mutual Recognition Compact that boards of nursing are promulgating to facilitate nurses licensure in several states. How is the client's privacy protected? For example, if a provider in state A was teleconsulting with providers in states B, C, and D, which state privacy laws should take precedence over others? What if they conflict? HIPAA and several other projects are under way to answer these questions and to determine the most effective designs for telehealth programs.

Practice Management

Beyond direct client care, computers also assist nurses in many ways in the management of their work. In hospitals, data terminals are commonly used to order supplies, tests, meals, and services from other departments. Tracking of these orders allows the nursing service to determine the most frequent or most costly items used by a particular nursing unit. This information may lead to decisions to modify a budget, provide different staffing, move supplies to a different location, or make other changes for more efficient and higher quality care.

Computers are used extensively for scheduling. Client appointments can be easily entered or changed. Special notes or tags can be applied to the appointment as a reminder to the

provider to perform particular services. The schedule for a single day can be printed so that all personnel have a copy. Staffing patterns must also be coordinated. Special requests for days off or continuing education classes can be entered, and the schedule can be viewed for a day, week, month, or year.

Each practice needs to keep track of procedures health care workers perform, client diagnoses, and time spent with clients so that billing can be accurate. With managed care, information tracking is also aimed at determining trends in health problems and the need for providers with specific skills. The use of computerized databases filled with unique codes for each medication, medical and nursing diagnosis, treatment, and supply allows for accurate and timely management of these data.

Specific Applications of Computers in Nursing Practice

As previously described, numerous systems are in use for collecting and classifying the various types of data used in nursing practice. Some of these systems have been found particularly useful in specific settings.

Community and Home Health

Computer networks are being used in innovative ways in home settings. A computer placed in a high-risk client's or family's home allows them to access information on a variety of topics, search the Internet, or e-mail a health care provider with questions or concerns. Clients can also record data about their health status that can be transmitted to the health care provider at the central network computer. Examples that have been successful using this approach include monitoring women at risk for preterm labor, persons with AIDS, and Alzheimer's clients. Home alert systems that allow the client to signal the base station in an emergency are also widely used.

Nurses who visit clients in their homes are using notebook computer systems to record assessments and transmit data to the main office. Similar systems have been developed for nursing students in community health courses to communicate with their faculty.

Case Management

Case managers must be able to track a group of clients—the caseload. Software programs allow the case manager to enter client data and integrate this with predesigned care-tracking templates. In addition, the case manager must keep abreast of the latest regulations affecting eligibility for health care benefits, the reporting requirements of the payer agencies, and detailed facts about the variety of service providers the client may need to access. All of these data can be placed in integrated computer software programs. Finally, the case manager must document quality; that is, demonstrate client outcomes related to dollars spent.

COMPUTERS IN NURSING ADMINISTRATION

As indicated in the section of this chapter on computers in nursing practice, the volume of data that nurses need to have available and the additional volume of data generated by nurses can and must be managed electronically. Nursing administrators require these data to develop strategic plans for the organization.

Human Resources

All employers must maintain a database, computerized or not, on each employee. In addition to the usual demographic and salary data, the database for licensed or certified health care personnel has unique fields for areas such as life support certification, health requirements (e.g., tuberculosis testing, hepatitis immunization, rubella titers), and performance appraisals. Administrators can use this human resources database to communicate with employees, examine staffing patterns, and create budget projections.

Medical Records Management

Costs are inherent in and reflected by medical records. It is expensive to keep records, but it is even more expensive not to be able to access what is in them. Therefore, nurses require computer programs that allow client records to be searched for trends such as the most common presenting diagnoses, number of cases by diagnosis-related groups, most expensive cases, length of stay or total number of days the case was open, and client outcomes. Nurse informaticists can assist administrators with the design and implementation of systems that allow for such searches to be generated, analyzed, printed, and distributed.

Facilities Management

Many aspects of managing buildings and non-nursing services can be facilitated by computer. Heating, air conditioning, ventilation, and alarm systems are computer controlled. Security devices such as readers that scan identification cards, bar codes, or magnetic strips permit only authorized personnel to enter client or private areas. Computers also manage and report inventory, tracking everything from pillowcases to syringes.

Budget and Finance

Advantages of computerized billing are that claims are transmitted much more quickly and have a greater likelihood of being complete and accurate compared to handwritten documents. If this is the case, claims will be paid sooner and the agency will have better control over its financial status. Computers can also effect cost savings by reducing the clerical services time needed for accounts payable and receivable. In cases where nursing can directly bill and be reimbursed by payers, the same benefits of computerized accounting apply.

The budget itself is generally a spreadsheet program. This software allows tracking as well as forecasting and planning. In uncertain times, the ability to perform "what if" calculations is especially valuable.

Quality Assurance and Utilization Reviews

Both internal and external stakeholders in health care organizations need to know that the services and activities of the organization have positive results. Once standards, pathways, key indicators, and other vital data have been identified and described, computers can facilitate the accumulation of data for individuals and groups of clients and analysis of the data. Quality is considered a process and not an end point. Applying this perspective, computerized systems are ideal for taking a snapshot view of the institution's quality indices at any time.

Utilization review consists of examining trends and proposing advantageous disposition of resources (specifically, length of stay). For example, might clients who have had a fractured hip repaired have equivalent outcomes at lesser cost if transferred from the hospital to a skilled nursing facility sooner? Studies can be conducted with computer analyses to answer such questions.

Accreditation

The Joint Commission on Accreditation of Healthcare Organizations (JCAHO) has mandated that hospitals have online mechanisms to monitor quality indicators, so as to reduce the difficulty and time involved in the accreditation process. Health care agencies must maintain databases of policies and procedures, standards of care, and employee accomplishment of JCAHO requirements such as continuing education and in-service trainings. JCAHO has also required a move to computer systems that assess outcomes rather than processes.

Another aspect of accreditation review is demonstrating adequate staffing for the number and acuity of clients. Each agency, whether hospital, outpatient, or home care, must use a method of determining the number of hours of nursing care required for its current clients. This method can consider the severity of the clients' illnesses, length of time needed to perform certain procedures, training and expertise of the nursing staff, and any other parameters desired.

COMPUTERS IN NURSING RESEARCH

Computers are invaluable assistants in the conduct of both quantitative and qualitative nursing research. In each step of the research process, computers facilitate generation, refinement, analysis, and output of data. Computer resources are an important component of the planning phase of any research project: The size of the computer and its storage capacity must be adequate for the amount of data that will be collected, and the proper software programs must be in place to manage and analyze the data. Computerized word processing is also an integral component in the publication and dissemination of research.

Problem Identification

The first step of the research process is to identify and describe the problem of interest. The computer can be useful in locating current literature about the problem and related concepts. Perhaps, unknown to the researcher, a solution to the problem has already been found and reported. A search of existing documents, and e-mail to colleagues, may help define the problem.

Literature Review

An exhaustive review of the literature can be time consuming. Without computer access to online or CD-ROM bibliographic databases, the researcher must wade through huge volumes of publications. The software programs that facilitate searches contain thesauruses so that the most appropriate terms can be selected. If the researcher determines that little has been published on the topic of interest, closely related terms and topics must also be searched. It is not unusual for a researcher to collect more than 100 pertinent research or theoretical references during the literature review. The increase in availability of full-text journal articles online has made the electronic literature search process even more productive.

Research Design

The design of a research study, including the choice of specific research method, is always driven by the research question. At the design stage the investigator determines whether the study will use a qualitative or quantitative approach, what instruments will be used to collect data, and the types of analyses that will be carried out on the data to answer the research questions. Computers may be used during this step to search the literature for instruments that have already been established or to design and test instruments that need to be developed for the particular study. In addition, the investigator would not likely select an instrument or design that requires extensive computer or mathematical analysis if such resources are not available.

Data Collection and Analysis

Once the types of data to be collected have been determined, the investigator will create forms on the computer for collecting the data. These may include the informed consent document, a tool to collect demographic data, and recording forms for research variables. If possible, computer-readable forms are created so that the data can be scanned into the computer or the participant can key responses directly into the computer (e.g., an online survey). This eliminates the errors that may occur if the researcher must enter the data into the computer manually.

It is particularly important that all variables that will be computer analyzed are identified in a way that the computer can recognize and manipulate. This may mean determining how to code the data for optimal manipulation. For example, will age be recorded in specific years or by categories such as 1–10, 11–15, 16–20, and so on? Software programs can assist with the analysis and coding of qualitative data. Such programs as N6 (formerly Nud*ist, an acronym for Non-numerical Unstructured Data with powerful processes of Indexing Searching and Theorizing) and Ethnograph assist the researcher in finding and coding sections of text and organizing coded material.

When the variables have been coded, other programs can be used to calculate descriptive and analytic statistics. Calculations that formerly were extremely time consuming and complex can now be done by computer programs quickly and accurately. Commonly used software programs for quantitative data analysis include SPSS (Statistical Package for the Social Sciences), SAS (Statistical Analysis System), SysSTAT, and MYSTAT. These programs perform analyses and display output in tables, charts, lists, and other easily read formats.

Research Dissemination

Research is of limited value if the findings are not widely dispersed to the practitioners who can use the findings to improve their practice. Computer word processing programs are used to author the final reports of research and to send the reports to various readerships. Many journals now require that manuscripts submitted for publication include both hardcopy and electronic versions. As noted earlier in this chapter, the number of electronic journals is increasing. With the rapid growth of e-mail, authors can also send an article or data to interested persons instantaneously. Computers speed completion of a research project and the availability of the findings to the public.

Computers are frequently used to present research at meetings. Using computer projectors to display screens of data and findings also allows the researcher to highlight, modify, and manipulate content in an instant. In the future, we will see computer conferencing where researchers collaborate on a study from distant locations and can examine and analyze the data simultaneously on screen.

Research Grants

Funds are available from a variety of resources to support the conduct of nursing research. The budget in a grant application may include a request to purchase computers or software needed to carry out the proposed study. Funds may also be requested to pay

MediaLink Informatics Certification Exam Application

people to enter data into the computer and to run the statistical analyses.

Information about available grant funding is most easily found online. The U.S. federal government makes all of the grant applications for nursing projects available only by downloading them from Internet sites. Forms to be completed are computer generated and often must be submitted to the funding agency in electronic format.

LIFESPAN CONSIDERATIONS   Computer Use

CHILDREN AND ADULTS

Computer programs, both CD and Internet-based, are available for children and adults to learn everything from foreign language to algebra.

There are many issues of concern related to frequent and extended use of computers by all ages. In particular, repetitive motion injuries (especially of the hand) can occur with extensive typing and use of the computer mouse, eye strain can occur from computer monitor viewing, and musculoskeletal damage is related to inadequate ergonomic arrangement of desk chairs, surface height, and monitor placement. Students and adults who use computers daily should be thoroughly evaluated and instructed in the prevention of these conditions.

Parents need to be reminded of potential risks to children from Internet contact with strangers and adult-only websites. They also need to monitor schoolchildren's use of computers to ensure they are not being sidetracked from homework into computer games and messaging.

All persons should be wary to protect their financial and personal information when conducting business via computer.

ELDERS

Computer classes are being taught to increasing numbers of elders. Use of the computer provides them with an avenue of communication and exposure to a vast amount of health care information. Although nurses have little control over what Internet sites will be accessed, it is important to teach clients and the general public to evaluate information from the site and to be aware that misinformation can also be presented. Important guidelines that increase the validity of a site are as follows:

- The article or information lists the author and credentials and/or the institution from which the information came.
- A date is listed that states when information was updated.
- If health care information is presented, a disclaimer should be included. The disclaimer presents limitations of the information and should say that it is not medical advice.

Computer-assisted programs can be very effective teaching aids for elders. They may provide audio and visual instruction and may even be interactive. They are useful for teaching about medical conditions and medications and for providing information about procedures and surgeries to be performed.

CRITICAL THINKING CHECKPOINT

As a nurse working for a home care agency in a small, rural town, you would like your clients to receive up-to-date and accurate health information and care. High-speed computer access is available in your office, and many of the residents have computers in their homes since it provides a low-cost way of communicating with friends and relatives who are far away (for example, using e-mail and sending digitized photos).

1. You have a difficult clinical case and want to investigate possible interventions. What are some of the ways computers could assist in this endeavor?
2. You decide that sending photos of the client would be useful to your colleagues in providing input. Since time is an issue, you determine that sending them electronically would be most expeditious. The client agrees to the photos but is worried about privacy in sending them through the computer. How would you handle this?
3. A client shares with you a website that states it can guarantee a cure to the client's illness. How would you respond?
4. You are considering enrolling in an advanced degree program that is offered online. What would be some of the advantages and disadvantages of such a program?

See Critical Thinking Possibilities in Appendix A.

CHAPTER 9 **REVIEW**

CHAPTER HIGHLIGHTS

- Computer hardware consists of the central processing unit, memory, the keyboard and other input devices, and the monitor and other output devices.
- Common computer software programs used in nursing are word processors, databases, spreadsheets, communications, computer-assisted instruction, and presentation graphics.
- A hospital information system (HIS) organizes data from various areas in the hospital such as admissions, medical records, clinical laboratory, pharmacy, and finance.
- Concerns regarding privacy and confidentiality of health records have arisen as electronic databases and communications have proliferated.
- Computers are used extensively to locate and access data through online databases and Internet searching. Many nursing journals are electronic.
- Computer-assisted instruction programs include tutorial, drill and practice, and simulations. Programs are also available that simulate the national licensure examination in the United States.
- In distance learning, the faculty and student may be located far apart and communicate via computer, phone, fax, and video technologies.
- Bedside entry of nursing data is becoming more prevalent. Studies on whether these systems save nursing time have conflicting results.
- Electronic medical records (EMRs) enable longitudinal data to be collected on a client and made available to all health care providers who require it. Such data warehousing also enables research to be conducted on quality of care, client outcomes, and a variety of other parameters. However, no national standards exist for the structure or contents of these records.
- Nurses need to participate in the creation of taxonomies and classifications of electronic data. Existing models include the World Health Organization's *International Classification of Diseases* (ICD-9 and ICD-10), the World Organization of National Colleges'

International Classification of Primary Care (ICPC), the American Psychiatric Association's *Diagnostic and Statistical Manual of Mental Disorders* (DSM), the North American Nursing Diagnosis Association (NANDA) taxonomy, the Omaha System, the Home Health Care Classification (HHCC), the Nursing Intervention Classification (NIC), the Nursing Outcomes Classification (NOC), the International Council of Nurses' International Classification for Nursing Practice, and the Nursing Minimum Data Set (NMDS).

- Computer monitoring and diagnosing of client conditions is widespread. Examples include digital or tympanic thermometers, digital scales, pulse oximetry, ECG/telemetry/hemodynamic monitoring, apnea monitors, fetal heart monitors, blood glucose analyzers, ventilators, IV pumps, CAT scans, and MRI.
- Telehealth, the conduction of the health care profession using electronic means of communication, is a growing area that generates both excitement and concerns.
- Data terminals in health care settings allow placing of order requests and retrieval of client data and accounts. Appointments can be scheduled on computer.
- Computers are used by home health nurses to record client data and to communicate with the central office. Clients can also have computers in the home that allow them to monitor their own health status and send information about their condition to the nurse.
- Specialized computer software programs enable case managers to track clients' needs, resources, and health care outcomes.
- Computers are used in nursing administration to manage personnel, human resources, facilities, budgets, quality assurance, utilization review, staffing and scheduling, and accreditation.
- Each step of the nursing research process makes use of computer technology. In particular, computers are used to access literature, analyze data, and report findings.

TEST YOUR KNOWLEDGE

1. A textbook publisher wishes to store large amounts of data in a computer format that cannot be changed by other people. Which of the following would best serve this purpose?
   1. CD-ROM
   2. RAM
   3. Floppy diskette
   4. Network

2. The challenge most associated with the utilization of an electronic client record system is which of the following?
   1. Cost
   2. Accuracy
   3. Privacy
   4. Curability

3. One disadvantage associated with electronic (e.g., Internet-based) courses includes which of the following?
   1. They take longer.
   2. Interpersonal communication is not possible.
   3. Everyone has to "log on" at the same time.
   4. It is harder to establish a sense of community.

4. Which of the following is the primary advantage of using computers while conducting nursing research?
   1. Locating potential participants
   2. Designing the steps of the research plan
   3. Analyzing the quantitative data
   4. Disseminating the research findings

5. A client insists that the practitioner use a treatment method discovered on an Internet website. Which of the following is the most appropriate nursing response?
   1. "The treatment must be examined to see if it is appropriate."
   2. "Most website treatments have not been studied or researched."
   3. "The person establishing the website is the only one who can use it on clients."
   4. "Websites are like advertising; they are biased and may not be legitimate."

See Answers to Test Your Knowledge in Appendix A.

EXPLORE MEDIALINK www.prenhall.com/berman

DVD-ROM
- Audio Glossary
- NCLEX Review
- End of Unit Concept Map Activity

COMPANION WEBSITE
- Additional NCLEX Review
- Case Study:
  Computerizing Clinical Documentation
- Application Activities:
  Confidentiality Laws
  Working on the Hospital Informatics Committee
  Informatics Certification Exam
- Links to Resources

READINGS AND REFERENCES

SUGGESTED READINGS

Bartholomew, K., & Curtis, K. (2004). High tech, high touch, why wait? *Nursing Management, 35*, 48, 50–54.
This article describes a variety of technological advances intended to assist the nurse in accurate and timely provision of care. It discusses concerns about why nurses have not moved more quickly to adopt them.

RELATED RESEARCH

Anthony, D. (2004). Using a computer to perform statistical analysis. *Nurse Researcher, 11*, 7–27.

Chang, B. L. (2004). Nursing Informatics, Internet intervention for community elders, process and feasibility. *Western Journal of Nursing Research, 26*, 461–466.

Jiang, W., Chen, W., & Chen, Y. (2004). Important computer competencies for the nursing profession. *Journal of Nursing Research, 12*, 213–225.

REFERENCES

American Nurses Association. (1999). *Position statement: Privacy and confidentiality.* Retrieved June 14, 2006, from http://www.nursingworld.org/readroom/position/ethics/etprivcy.htm

American Nurses Association. (2001). *Scope and standards of nursing informatics practice.* Washington, DC: American Nurses Publishing.

Computer-Based Patient Record Institute. (1992). *Newsletters and membership brochures.* Chicago: Author.

Health Summit Working Group. (1999). *Criteria for assessing the quality of health information on the Internet: Policy paper.* McLean, VA: Mitretek Systems. Retrieved March 5, 2006, from http://hitiweb.mitretek.org/docs/policy.html

Langowski, C. (2005). The times they are a changing: Effects of online nursing documentation systems. *Quality Management in Health Care, 14*, 121–125.

Olson, L. (2003). Privacy and confidentiality in an electronic age. *Chart, 100*, 9.

Rossel, C. L. (2003). HIPAA: An informatics system perspective. *Chart, 100*, 11.

SELECTED BIBLIOGRAPHY

Bond, C. S. (2004). Web users' information retrieval methods and skills. *Online Information Review, 28*, 254–259.

Bowles, K. H. (2004). Sharpen decision making with computerized support tools. *Nursing Management, 35*, 19–20.

Burke, L., & Weill, B. (2004). *Information technology for the health professions* (2nd ed.). Upper Saddle River, NJ: Prentice Hall.

Burt, C. W., & Jing, E. (2005). Use of computerized clinical support systems in medical settings: United States, 2001-03. *Advance Data from Vital and Health Statistics,* No. 353 (PHS) 2005-1250. Hyattsville, MD: National Center for Health Statistics. Retrieved June 14, 2006, http://www.cdc.gov/nchs/data/ad/ad353.pdf

Chastain, A. R. (2003). Nursing informatics: Past, present and future. *Tennessee Nurse, 66*(1), 8–10.

Couvillon, J. S. (2006). *Nursing informatics: Practical issues for today's nurse.* Sudbury, MA: Jones & Bartlett.

Dickerson, S. S., Boehmke, M., Ogle, C., & Brown, J. K. (2005). Out of necessity: Oncology nurses' experiences integrating the Internet into practice. *Oncology Nursing Forum, 32*, 355–362.

Hunt, E. C., Sproat, S. B., & Kitzmiller, R. R. (2004). *The nursing informatics implementation guide.* New York: Springer-Verlag.

Joos, I., Nelson, R., Whitman, N., & Smith, M. (2005). *Introduction to computers for healthcare professionals* (4th ed.). Sudbury, MA: Jones & Bartlett.

Mascara, C. M., Czar, P., & Hebda, T. (2004). *Internet resource guide for nurses & health care professionals* (3rd ed.). Upper Saddle River, NJ: Prentice-Hall.

Montgomery, K. S., & Fitzpatrick, J. J. (Eds.). (2005). *Internet for nursing research.* New York: Springer.

Saba, V. K., & McCormick, K. A. (Eds.). (2006). *Essentials of nursing informatics* (4th ed.). New York: McGraw-Hill.

Seaver, M. (2005). A helping handheld computer: Technology at the point of care. *2005 Pathways to Success*, 46–50. Retrieved June 14, 2006, from at http://www2.nursingspectrum.com/CE/Self-Study_modules/course.html?ID=202

Simpson, R. L. (2004). Information technology. Measuring change: How technology increases nursing's diversity. *Nursing Management, 35*, 12, 14.

Tanner, A., Pierce, S., & Pravikoff, D. (2004). Moving the nursing information agenda forward. *CIN, Computers Informatics Nursing, 22*, 300–302.

Thede, L. Q. (2003). *Informatics and nursing: Opportunities and challenges.* Philadelphia: Lippincott Williams & Wilkins.

UNIT 3

The Nursing Process

The nursing process is a systematic, client-centered method for structuring the delivery of nursing care. The nursing process entails gathering and analyzing data in order to identify client strengths and potential or actual health problems, and developing and continually reviewing a plan of nursing interventions to achieve mutually agreed outcomes. At every stage of the process, the nurse works closely with the client to individualize care and build a relationship of mutual regard and trust.

CHAPTER
10

Critical Thinking and the Nursing Process

LEARNING OUTCOMES

After completing this chapter, you will be able to:

1. Discuss the skills and attitudes of critical thinking.

2. Describe the significance of developing critical-thinking abilities in order to practice safe, effective, and professional nursing care.

3. Discuss the relationships among the nursing process, critical thinking, the problem-solving process, and the decision-making process.

4. Explore ways of demonstrating critical thinking.

Although **critical thinking** has many definitions, one of the most useful for nursing is from the National League for Nursing (2000): "Critical thinking in nursing practice is a discipline specific, reflective reasoning process that guides a nurse in generating, implementing, and evaluating approaches for dealing with client care and professional concerns" (p. 2). Nurses are expected to use critical thinking to solve client problems and make better decisions. Thus, critical thinking, problem solving, and decision making are interrelated processes, with creativity enhancing the result.

CRITICAL THINKING

Critical thinking is essential to safe, competent, skillful nursing practice. The amount of knowledge that nurses must use and the continuing rapid growth of this knowledge prevent nurses from being effective practitioners if they attempt to function with only the information acquired in school or outlined in books. Decisions that nurses must make about client care and about the distribution of limited resources force them to think and act in areas where there are neither clear answers nor standard procedures and where conflicting forces turn decision making into a complex process. Nurses therefore need to embrace the attitudes that promote critical thinking and master critical-thinking skills in order to process and evaluate both previously learned and new information. Box 10–1 lists some reasons supporting the importance of critical thinking.

Nurses use critical-thinking skills in a variety of ways:

- *Nurses use knowledge from other subjects and fields.* Because nurses deal holistically with human responses, they must draw meaningful information from other subject areas (i.e., make interdisciplinary connections) in order to understand the meaning of client data and to plan effective interventions. Nursing students take courses in the biologic and social sciences and in the humanities so that they can acquire a strong foundation on which to build their nursing knowledge and skill. For example, the nurse might use knowledge from nutrition, physiology, and physics to promote wound healing and prevent further injury to a client with a pressure ulcer.
- *Nurses deal with change in stressful environments.* Nurses work in rapidly changing situations. Treatments, medications, and technology change constantly, and a client's condition may change from minute to minute. Routine actions may therefore not be adequate to deal with the situation at hand. Familiarity with the routine for giving medications, for example, does not help the nurse deal with a client who is frightened of injections or with

one who does not wish to take a medication. When unexpected situations arise, critical thinking enables the nurse to recognize important cues, respond quickly, and adapt interventions to meet specific client needs.

- *Nurses make important decisions.* During the course of a workday, nurses make vital decisions of many kinds. These decisions often determine the well-being of clients and even their very survival, so it is important that the decisions be sound. Nurses use critical thinking to collect and interpret the information needed to make decisions. Nurses must use good judgment, for example, to decide which observations must be reported to the primary care provider immediately and which can be noted in the client record for the primary care provider to address later, during a routine visit with the client.

Creativity is a major component of critical thinking. When nurses incorporate creativity into their thinking, they are able to find unique solutions to unique problems. **Creativity** is thinking that results in the development of new ideas and products. Creativity in problem solving and decision making is the ability to develop and implement new and better solutions.

Creativity is required when the nurse encounters a new situation or a client situation in which traditional interventions are

---

BOX 10–1 Top 10 Reasons to Improve Thinking

10. Things aren't what they used to be or what they will be.
9. Patients are sicker, with multiple problems.
8. More consumer involvement (patients and families).
7. Nurses must be able to move from one setting to another.
6. Rapid change and information explosion requires us to develop new learning and workplace skills.
5. Consumers and payers demand to see evidence of benefits, efficiency, and results.
4. Today's progress often creates new problems that can't be solved by old ways of thinking.
3. Redesigning care delivery and nursing curricula is useless if students and nurses don't have the thinking skills required to deal with today's world.
2. It can be done—it doesn't have to be that difficult.
1. **Your ability to focus your thinking to get the results you need can make the difference between whether you succeed or fail in this fast-paced world.**

Note: Reprinted from *Critical Thinking in Nursing: A Practical Approach* 3rd ed., R. Alfaro-LeFevre, Copyright 2004, with permission from Elsevier.

not effective. For example, a pediatric home health nurse is caring for a 9-year-old girl who has ineffective respirations following abdominal surgery. The primary care provider has ordered incentive spirometry (a treatment device that promotes alveolar expansion). The child is frightened by the equipment and tires quickly during the treatments. The nurse offers her a bottle of blow bubbles and a blowing wand. She is delighted with blowing bubbles. The nurse knows that the respiratory effort in blowing bubbles will promote alveolar expansion and suggests that she blow bubbles between incentive spirometry treatments.

Creative thinkers must have knowledge of the problem. They must have assessed the present problem and be knowledgeable about the underlying facts and principles that apply. For example, in the previous situation, the nurse knows the anatomy and physiology of respiratory function and is aware of the purpose of incentive spirometry. The nurse also understands pediatric growth and development. In trying to assist the child, the nurse builds on this knowledge and comes up with a creative solution. Using creativity, nurses

- Generate many ideas rapidly.
- Are generally flexible and natural; that is, they are able to change viewpoints or directions in thinking rapidly and easily.
- Create original solutions to problems.
- Tend to be independent and self-confident, even when under pressure.
- Demonstrate individuality.

SKILLS IN CRITICAL THINKING

Complex mental processes such as analysis, problem solving, and decision making require the use of cognitive critical-thinking skills. These skills include critical analysis, inductive and deductive reasoning, making valid inferences, differentiating facts from opinions, evaluating the credibility of information sources, clarifying concepts, and recognizing assumptions.

Critical analysis is the application of a set of questions to a particular situation or idea to determine essential information and ideas and discard superfluous information and ideas. The questions are not sequential steps; rather, they are a set of criteria for judging an idea. Not all questions will need to be applied to every situation, but one should be aware of all the questions in order to choose those questions appropriate to a given situation. Socrates (born about 470 BC) was a Greek philosopher who developed the Socratic method of posing a question and seeking an answer. Box 10–2 lists Socratic questions to use in critical analysis. **Socratic questioning** is a technique one can use to look beneath the surface, recognize and examine assumptions, search for inconsistencies, examine multiple points of view, and differentiate what one knows from what one merely believes. Nurses should employ Socratic questioning when listening to an end-of-shift report, reviewing a history or progress notes, planning care, or discussing a client's care with colleagues.

Two other critical-thinking skills are inductive and deductive reasoning. In **inductive reasoning,** generalizations are formed from a set of facts or observations. When viewed together, certain bits of information suggest a particular interpretation. In-

---

BOX 10–2 Socratic Questions

QUESTIONS ABOUT THE QUESTION (OR PROBLEM)
- Is this question clear, understandable, and correctly identified?
- Is this question important?
- Could this question be broken down into smaller parts?
- How might _____ state this question?

QUESTIONS ABOUT ASSUMPTIONS
- You seem to be assuming _____; is that so?
- What could you assume instead? Why?
- Does this assumption always hold true?

QUESTIONS ABOUT POINT OF VIEW
- You seem to be using the perspective of _____. Why?
- What would someone who disagrees with your perspective say?
- Can you see this any other way?

QUESTIONS ABOUT EVIDENCE AND REASONS
- What evidence do you have for that?
- Is there any reason to doubt that evidence?
- How do you know?
- What would change your mind?

QUESTIONS ABOUT IMPLICATIONS AND CONSEQUENCES
- What effect would that have?
- What is the probability that will actually happen?
- What are the alternatives?
- What are the implications of that?

---

ductive reasoning moves from specific examples (premises) to a generalized conclusion—for example, after touching several hot flames (premise), we conclude that *all* flames are hot. A nurse who observes a client who has dry skin, poor turgor, sunken eyes, and dark amber urine and who is otherwise determined to be dehydrated (premise) concludes that the presence of those signs indicate that other clients are dehydrated.

Deductive reasoning, by contrast, is reasoning from the general premise to the specific conclusion. If you begin with the premise that the sum of the angles in any triangle is always 180 degrees, you can then conclude that the sum of the angles in the triangle you happen to have is also 180 degrees. A nurse might start with a premise that all children love peanut butter sandwiches. If the client is a child, then the child will love peanut butter sandwiches. This is an example in which the premise is not always valid and, thus, the conclusion also may not be valid. Nurses use critical thinking to help analyze situations and establish which premises are valid.

In critical thinking, the nurse also differentiates statements of fact, inference, judgment, and opinion. Table 10–1 shows how these may be applied to a client. Evaluating the credibility of information sources is an important step in critical thinking. Unfortunately, we cannot always believe what we read or are told. The nurse may need to ascertain the accuracy of information by checking other documents or with other informants.

To comprehend a client situation clearly, the nurse and the client must agree on the meaning of terms. For example, if the client says to the nurse "I think I have a tumor," the nurse needs to clarify what this word means to the client—the medical def-

TABLE 10-1	**Differentiating Types of Statements**	
STATEMENT	**DESCRIPTION**	**EXAMPLE**
Facts	Can be verified through investigation	Blood pressure is affected by blood volume.
Inferences	Conclusions drawn from the facts, going beyond facts to make a statement about something not currently known	If blood volume is decreased (e.g., in hemorrhagic shock), the blood pressure will drop.
Judgments	Evaluation of facts or information that reflect values or other criteria; a type of opinion	It is harmful to the client's health if the blood pressure drops too low.
Opinions	Beliefs formed over time and include judgments that may fit facts or be in error	Nursing intervention can assist in maintaining the client's blood pressure within normal limits.

inition of tumor (a solid mass) or the common lay meaning of cancer—before responding.

Persons also live their lives under certain assumptions. Some people view humans as having a basically generous nature whereas others believe that the human tendency is to act in their own best interest. The nurse may believe that life should be considered worth living no matter what the condition whereas the client believes that quality of life is more important than quantity of life. If they recognize that they make choices based on these assumptions, they can still work together toward an acceptable plan of care. Difficulty arises when people do not take the time to consider what assumptions underlie their beliefs and actions.

ATTITUDES THAT FOSTER CRITICAL THINKING

Certain attitudes are crucial to critical thinking. These attitudes are based on the assumption that a rational person is motivated to develop, learn, and grow. A critical thinker works to develop the following attitudes or traits: independence, fair-mindedness, insight, intellectual humility, intellectual courage, integrity, perseverance, confidence, and curiosity.

Independence

Critical thinking requires that individuals think for themselves. People acquire many beliefs as children, not necessarily based on reason but in order to have an explanation they comprehend. As they mature and acquire knowledge and experience, critical thinkers examine their beliefs in the light of new evidence. Critical thinkers consider seriously a wide range of ideas, learn from them, and then make their own judgments about them. Nurses are open-minded about considering different methods of performing technical skills—not just the single way they may have been taught in school. They are not easily swayed by the opinions of others but take responsibility for their own views (Catalano, 2003).

Fair-Mindedness

Critical thinkers are fair-minded, assessing all viewpoints with the same standards and not basing their judgments on personal or group bias or prejudice (Catalano, 2003). Fair-mindedness helps one to consider opposing points of view and to try to understand new ideas fully before rejecting or accepting them. Critical thinkers strive to be open to the possibility that new ev-

idence could change their minds. The nurse listens to opinions of all the members of a family, young and old.

Insight into Egocentricity

Critical thinkers are open to the possibility that their personal biases or social pressures and customs could unduly affect their thinking. They actively try to examine their own biases and bring them to awareness each time they think or make a decision. For example, a nurse spends extensive time trying to teach a client how to prevent a future recurrence of some problem but is mystified when the client appears uninterested and does not follow the nurse's advice. The nurse's egocentric tendency to assume that all clients are motivated and interested in preventive care (just because the nurse is) resulted in an inaccurate assessment of the client's desire to learn; both the nurse's and the client's time was wasted. Had the nurse assessed the client's background and beliefs about the problem and collected sufficient evidence, the nurse might have identified a problem more relevant to the client's priorities and, thus, developed a better care plan.

Intellectual Humility

Intellectual humility means having an awareness of the limits of one's own knowledge. Critical thinkers are willing to admit what they do not know; they are willing to seek new information and to rethink their conclusions in light of new knowledge. They never assume that what everybody believes to be right will always be right, because new evidence may emerge. A hospital nurse might be unable to imagine how the elderly wife will care for her husband who has recently had a stroke. However, the nurse also recognizes that it is not really possible to know what the couple can achieve.

Intellectual Courage to Challenge the Status Quo and Rituals

With an attitude of courage, one is willing to consider and examine fairly one's own ideas or views, especially those to which one may have a strongly negative reaction. This type of courage comes from recognizing that beliefs are sometimes false or misleading. Values and beliefs are not always acquired rationally. Rational beliefs are those that have been examined and found to be supported by solid reasons and data. After such examination, it is inevitable that some beliefs previously held to be true will be found to contain questionable elements and that some truth will emerge from ideas considered dangerous or false. Courage is needed to be true to new thinking in such cases, especially if social penalties for nonconformity are severe. As an example, previously many nurses believed that allowing family members to observe an emergency (such as cardiopulmonary resuscitation) would be psychologically harmful to the family and that members would get in the health care team's way. Others felt that blanket exclusion of family members was unnecessary and extremely stressful for some of them. As a result, nurses initiated research that has demonstrated that family presence can be accomplished without detrimental effects to the nurse, the client, or the family.

Integrity

Intellectual integrity requires that individuals apply the same rigorous standards of proof to their own knowledge and beliefs as they apply to the knowledge and beliefs of others. Critical thinkers question their own knowledge and beliefs as quickly and thoroughly as they challenge those of another. They are readily able to admit and evaluate inconsistencies within their own beliefs and between their own beliefs and those of another. A nurse might believe that wound care always requires sterile technique. Reading a new article on the use and outcomes of clean technique for some wounds leads the critically thinking nurse to reconsider.

Perseverance

Nurses who are critical thinkers show perseverance in finding effective solutions to client and nursing problems. This determination enables them to clarify concepts and sort out related issues, in spite of difficulties and frustrations. Confusion and frustration are uncomfortable, but critical thinkers resist the temptation to find a quick and easy answer. Important questions tend to be complex and confusing and therefore often require a great deal of thought and research to arrive at an answer. The nurse needs to continue to address the issue until it is resolved. For example, the nurses on a unit have tried to establish a policy for selected clients to leave the hospital on a pass rather than have to be discharged and readmitted in the same day. The need for involvement of nursing, medical, administrative, and accounting staff gradually generates solutions to obstacles. The development of the policy moves forward, although very slowly.

Confidence

Critical thinkers believe that well-reasoned thinking will lead to trustworthy conclusions. Therefore, they cultivate an attitude of confidence in the reasoning process and examine emotion-laden arguments using the standards for evaluating thought, by asking questions such as these: Is that argument fair? Is it based on sufficient evidence? Consider nurses attempting to determine the best way to allocate holiday time off for staff. Should they go by seniority, use random selection (lottery), give preference to those who have children, use "first-come, first-served," or use another method?

The critical thinker develops skill in both inductive reasoning and deductive reasoning. As the nurse gains greater awareness of the thinking process and more experience in improving

TABLE 10–2	**Universal Intellectual Standards**
STANDARD	**SAMPLE QUESTION**
Clarity	What is an example of this?
Accuracy	How can I find out if that is true?
Relevance	How does that help me with the issue?
Logicalness	Does that follow from the evidence?
Breadth	Do I need to consider another point of view?
Precision	Can I be more specific?
Significance	Which of these facts is most important?
Completeness	Have I missed any important aspects?
Fairness	Am I considering the thinking of others?
Depth	What makes this a difficult problem?

Note: From *A Guide for Educators to Critical Thinking Competency Standards* by R. Paul & L. Elder, Foundation for Critical Thinking, 2005. Adapted with permission. www.criticalthinking.org.

such thinking, confidence in the process will grow. This nurse will not be afraid of disagreement and indeed will be concerned when others agree too quickly. Such a nurse can serve as a role model to colleagues, inspiring and encouraging them to think critically as well.

Curiosity

The mind of a critical thinker is filled with questions: Why do we believe this? What causes that? Does it have to be this way? Could something else work? What would happen if we did it another way? Who says that is so? The curious nurse may value tradition but is not afraid to examine traditions to be sure they are still valid. The nurse may, for example, apply these questions to the issue of moving responsibility for a procedure such as the drawing of arterial blood samples among the nursing, respiratory therapy, or laboratory department staff.

STANDARDS OF CRITICAL THINKING

How can one know whether one's thinking is critical thinking? Paul and Elder (2005) proposed that thinkers can use universal standards, shown in Table 10–2. Explicitly stating the standards for critical thinking promotes the reliability and validity of the thinking and thus makes appropriate action more likely. Forneris (2004), building on the work of many modern educational theorists, described core attributes of critical thinking: reflection, context, dialogue, and time. Reflection involves determining what data are relevant and making connections between that data and the decisions reached. Context is an essential consideration in nursing since care must always be individualized, taking knowledge and applying it to real people. Dialogue, which need not involve other persons, refers to the process of serving as both teacher and student in learning from situations, questioning, making connections, and determining motivation. Finally, the attribute of time emphasizes the value of using past learning in current situations that then guide future actions.

APPLYING CRITICAL THINKING TO NURSING PRACTICE

Nurses function effectively some part of every day without thinking critically. Many small decisions are based primarily on habit with minimal thinking involved; examples include selecting what uniform to wear, choosing which route to take to work, and deciding what to eat for lunch. Psychomotor skills in nursing often involve minimal thinking, such as operating a familiar piece of equipment. However, the higher order skills of critical thinking are put into play as soon as a new idea is encountered or a less-than-routine decision must be made.

The **nursing process** is a systematic, rational method of planning and providing individualized nursing care. The phases of the nursing process—assessing, diagnosing, planning, implementing, and evaluating—are discussed in detail in the chapters that follow. The phases of the nursing process and application to a clinical example of critical thinking are shown in Table 10–3. This demonstrates the use of critical thinking with individual clients. In addition, a nurse employs critical thinking when setting priorities for the day. When analyzing a situation and planning strategies for conflict resolution or change, the nurse manager uses critical-thinking attitudes and skills. The nurse clinician and nurse manager seek awareness of their thinking as they are thinking, as they apply standards for thinking, and as their thinking progresses.

Nurses use critical thinking in nursing practice primarily when solving problems and making decisions. These two processes are described in more detail.

Problem Solving

In **problem solving,** the nurse obtains information that clarifies the nature of the problem and suggests possible solutions. The nurse then carefully evaluates the possible solutions and chooses the best one to implement. The situation is carefully monitored over time to ensure its initial and continued effectiveness. The nurse does not discard the other solutions but holds them in reserve in the event that the first solution is not effective. The nurse may also encounter a similar problem in a different client situation where an alternative solution is determined to be the most effective. Therefore, problem solving for one situation contributes to the nurse's body of knowledge for problem solving in similar situations. Commonly used approaches to problem solving include trial and error, intuition, the research process, and the scientific/modified scientific method.

Trial and Error

One way to solve problems is through trial and error, in which a number of approaches are tried until a solution is found. However, without considering alternatives systematically, one cannot know why the solution works. Trial-and-error methods in nursing care can be dangerous because the client might suffer

TABLE 10–3 Phases of the Nursing Process and Clinical Examples of Critical Thinking

NURSING PROCESS	CLINICAL APPLICATION
Assessing	*Data*: A 45-year-old male Latino complains of severe headache; 20 lb overweight; blood pressure 180/95 mm Hg. States he has been taking high blood pressure pills only when he has a headache. Is self-employed as a gardener; lives with wife, mother-in-law, and four children.
	Given these data, a critical thinker is aware that more data must be obtained about the client's cultural health values and reasons for stated behavior. Failure to think critically and to obtain additional data leads to inaccurate goals, diagnosis, and interventions.
Goal setting	*Goal:* To increase compliance with medication regimen in order to relieve headaches and prevent a cerebrovascular accident (CVA). Thinking critically, a nurse will try to determine the client's goals and to agree to mutual goals.
Diagnosing	A critical thinker will defer identifying the client's diagnosis until more data are obtained and the client's priorities are known. This prevents a premature diagnosis based on insufficient data.
Diagnosing	As a critical thinker, the nurse is aware that the client's point of view may differ from the nurse's.
	Although the nurse may support the Western medical belief system that puts high priority on preventing disease, the critical thinker is also aware that the client may hold diverse views of health and illness, therapy, and preventive measures.
Diagnosing	The critical thinker recognizes that the client's erratic use of the prescribed medication may have multiple causes (e.g., troublesome side effects, or belief that illness is due to God's will and is not preventable) and will not infer a diagnosis with etiology until more data are obtained. Failure to think critically can lead to interpretations that are irrelevant, inadequate, and superficial (e.g., an erroneous interpretation that the client's problem is lack of sufficient knowledge).
Diagnosing	The critical thinker makes assumptions in accordance with a broad, unbiased database and mutually set client goals. The critical thinker avoids making unverified assumptions, such as that an increase in knowledge will increase this client's compliance or that this client is motivated to prevent a CVA.
Planning	The critical thinker uses concepts about motivation, change theory, and multicultural nursing to understand the client's behavior and motivation to change. Failure to think critically can lead to exclusive reliance on a simplistic concept, such as "knowledge creates change."
Planning Implementing	The critical thinker considers the implications and consequences of selected nursing strategies before implementing plans of care. Plans of care, including goals and outcomes, are based on ongoing assessment of the client's cultural values, beliefs, and needs. Failure to think critically may lead to ineffective interventions, such as client teaching that focuses only on resolving a knowledge deficit about the prescribed medication. The critical thinker recognizes that a knowledge deficit may or may not be one of several problems.
Evaluating	The critical thinker bases evaluation of client outcomes and the effectiveness of nursing interventions on well-developed, measurable criteria and considers rationally whether outcomes have been validated. Failure to think critically may lead to client noncompliance and an inference that the client did not learn effectively and needs further instruction.

REAL WORLD PRACTICE

When you hear the words, "critical thinking" many things enter your mind. It is more than just having the knowledge or psychomotor skill to do a task. In client care, it is the ability to recognize deviations from normal, the ability to prioritize, manage those deviations, and justify your actions. Traditionally, technical skills were considered the only measure of competency. That is no longer true.

The key to critical thinking is to use strategies that focus on your thought process to make decisions. Using critical thinking skills in the nursing process, you need to *assess*, identifying any risk factors; *diagnose*, including analyzing data, predicting any potential problems, and diagnosing any actual problems; *plan* your client care; and *implement* appropriate interventions; reassess, and finally *evaluate* each problem, determining if the interventions are effective to the desired outcome.

Ask yourself the following questions: What are the potential problems for this client and why? What would you do about these problems if they should occur? How would you prioritize and why? Critical thinking ability is developed over time through many experiences.

With the complexity of client care today and increasing all the time, the need to use critical thinking is crucial in the nursing world. The key area for development of new graduates is urgency and problem management. Both require coaching, mentoring and time for the development of critical thinking skills.

—*Jan Knudsen MSN, RN,*
Saint Elizabeth Regional Medical Center
Lincoln, NE

harm if an approach is inappropriate. However, nurses often use trial and error in the home setting where, due to logistics, equipment, and client lifestyle, hospital procedures cannot work as effectively (e.g., there may be no pole from which to hang an IV bag or no electricity to plug in a device).

Intuition

Intuition is the understanding or learning of things without the conscious use of reasoning. It is also known as sixth sense, hunch, instinct, feeling, or suspicion. As a problem-solving approach, intuition is viewed by some people as a form of guessing and, as such, an inappropriate basis for nursing decisions. However, others view intuition as an essential and legitimate aspect of clinical judgment acquired through knowledge and experience. The nurse must first have the knowledge base necessary to practice in the clinical area and then use that knowledge in clinical practice. Clinical experience allows the nurse to recognize cues and patterns and begin to reach correct conclusions.

Experience is important in improving intuition because the rapidity of the judgment depends on the nurse having seen similar client situations many times before. Sometimes nurses use the words "I had a feeling" to describe the critical-thinking element of considering evidence. These nurses are able to judge quickly which evidence is most important and to act on that limited evidence. Nurses in critical care often pay closer attention than usual to a client when they sense that the client's condition could change suddenly.

Although the intuitive method of problem solving is gaining recognition as part of nursing practice, it is not recommended for novices or students, however, because they usually lack the knowledge base and clinical experience on which to make a valid judgment.

Research Process and Scientific/ Modified Scientific Method

The research process, discussed in Chapter 2, is a formalized, logical, systematic approach to solving problems. The classic scientific method is most useful when the researcher is working in a controlled situation. Health professionals, often working with people in uncontrolled situations, require a modified approach to the scientific method for solving problems. For example, unlike experiments with animals, the effects of diet on health are complicated by a person's genetic variations, lifestyle, and personal preferences.

Table 10–4 compares the research process or scientific method with the modified scientific method. Critical thinking is important in all problem-solving processes as the nurse evaluates potential solutions to a given problem and makes a decision to select the most appropriate solution for that situation.

Decision Making

Decision making is a critical-thinking process for choosing the best actions to meet a desired goal. Decisions must be made whenever several mutually exclusive choices are available or when there is an option to act or not. For example, the individual who wishes to become a nurse in the United States has several possible courses of action: a diploma program, an associate degree program, or a baccalaureate program. Prospective students must choose. Therefore, they must evaluate the different types of programs, as well as personal circumstances, to make a decision appropriate to their situations.

Nurses make decisions in the course of solving problems. Decision making, however, is also used in situations that do not involve problem solving. Nurses make value decisions (e.g., to keep client information confidential), time management decisions (e.g., taking clean linens to the client's room at the same time as the medication in order to save steps), scheduling decisions (e.g., to bathe the client before visiting hours), and priority decisions (e.g., which interventions are most urgent and which can be delegated).

Nurses must make decisions and assist clients to make decisions. When faced with several client needs at the same time, the nurse must prioritize and decide which client to assist first. The nurse may (a) look at advantages and disadvantages of each option, (b) apply Maslow's hierarchy of needs, (c) consider which tasks can be delegated to others, or (d) use another priority-setting framework. When a client is trying to make a decision about what course of treatment to follow, the nurse may need to provide information or resources the client can use in making a decision. Nurses must make decisions in their own personal and professional lives. For example, the nurse must decide whether to work in a hospital or community setting, whether to join a professional association, and whether to carry professional liability insurance.

TABLE 10–4 **Comparison between the Research Process and the Modified Scientific Method**	
RESEARCH PROCESS (SCIENTIFIC METHOD)	**MODIFIED SCIENTIFIC METHOD**
State a research question or problem.	Define the problem.
Define the purpose of or the rationale for the study.	
Review related literature.	Gather information.
Formulate hypotheses and defining variables.	Analyze the information.
Select a method to test hypotheses.	Develop solutions.
Select a population, sample, and setting.	
Conduct a pilot study.	Make a decision.
Collect the data.	Implement the decision.
Analyze the data.	Evaluate the decision.
Communicate conclusions and implications.	

Here are sequential steps to the decision-making process:

1. *Identify the purpose.* The nurse identifies why a decision is needed and what needs to be determined.
2. *Set the criteria.* When the nurse sets the criteria for decision making, three questions must be answered: What is the desired outcome, what needs to be preserved, and what needs to be avoided? For example, for a client with pain, the criteria would be as follows:
   a. What is the desired outcome? Relief of pain.
   b. What needs to be preserved? Physical functioning, cognitive functioning, psychologic functioning.
   c. What needs to be avoided? Central nervous system depression, respiratory depression, nausea.
3. *Weight the criteria.* In this step, the decision maker sets priorities or ranks activities or services from least important to most important as they relate to the specific situation. Because the weighting is specific to the situation, an activity may be ranked as most important in one situation and of less importance in another situation. For example, the nurse avoids medication that can cause sedation of a client with a head injury, but for a client with terminal cancer, pain relief may be more important than avoiding the sedative side effects of the pain medication.
4. *Seek alternatives.* The decision maker identifies possible ways to meet the criteria. In clinical situations, the alternatives may be selected from a range of nursing interventions or client care strategies. Pain may be treated with oral or injectable medications, as needed (prn) or on a schedule, or without pharmacologic intervention at all, instead using complementary alternative modalities (CAM).
5. *Examine alternatives.* The nurse analyzes the alternatives to ensure that there is an objective rationale in relation to the established criteria for choosing one strategy over another. For pain that results from a procedure (such as removal of a foreign object), CAM may not be strong enough relief, and oral medication may be effective but act too slowly, so an intravenous narcotic might be the better choice.
6. *Project.* The nurse applies creative thinking and skepticism to determine what might go wrong as a result of a decision and develops plans to prevent, minimize, or overcome any problems. If the intravenous narcotic is se-

TABLE 10–5 **Comparison between the Nursing Process and the Decision-Making Process**	
NURSING PROCESS	**DECISION-MAKING PROCESS***
Assess	Identify the purpose.
Diagnose	
Plan	Set the criteria.
	Weight the criteria.
	Seek alternatives.
	Examine alternatives.
	Project.
Implement	Implement.
Evaluate	Evaluate the outcome.

*The decision-making process parallels the nursing process but is also used during each phase of the process.

lected, what safety procedures need to be in place—for example, a narcotic antidote and supplemental oxygen?
7. *Implement.* The decision plan is placed into action. The pain treatment is begun.
8. *Evaluate the outcome.* As with all nursing care, in evaluating, the nurse determines the effectiveness of the plan and whether the initial purpose was achieved. How does the client rate the level of pain following the procedure?

The decision-making process and the nursing process share similarities, and the nurse uses decision making in all phases of the nursing process. Table 10–5 compares these processes. It is essential that the nurse use critical thinking in each step or phase of these processes so that decisions and care are well considered and delivered with the highest possible quality.

DEVELOPING CRITICAL-THINKING ATTITUDES AND SKILLS

After gaining an idea of what it means to think critically, solve problems, and make decisions, nurses need to become aware of their own thinking style and abilities. Acquiring critical-thinking skills and a critical attitude then becomes a matter of practice. Critical thinking is not an "either-or" phenomenon; people develop and use it more or less effectively along a continuum. Some people make better evaluations than others do,

---

RESEARCH NOTE **Are Education, Experience, and Critical-Thinking Ability Related to Clinical Decision Making?**

This pilot study investigated the premise that there would be relationships between the education and experience of critical care nurses and their ability to make consistent clinical decisions. Critical-thinking ability, as measured by skills and dispositions tests, was also expected to correlate with decision making. Fifty-four nurses with a BSN or MSN working in adult critical care units in teaching hospitals were included in the study. Results showed that, overall, the more complex the clinical situation, the less consistent the nurses were in their decisions. Intuition, as a decision-making strategy, was most related to consistent decisions. No correlation was found between education or total years of experience and consistency in decision making. There was an association between years of experience in critical care and decision consistency.

IMPLICATIONS

This study reinforces that decision making and critical thinking are complex when applied in real clinical situations. That the results showed greater consistency in decisions when intuition was used and when the nurse had more years of critical care nursing experience (not just overall nursing experience) suggests that there is a type of nurse thinking in that clinical specialty that does not necessarily evolve with more global exposure to client care. It also suggests that the method of thinking used by nurses who choose critical care practice may be an inherent characteristic.

Note: From "Critical Thinking and Clinical Decision Making in Critical Care Nursing: A Pilot Study," by F. D. Hicks, S. L. Merritt, & A. S. Elstein, 2003, *Heart & Lung, 32,* pp. 169–180.

---

some people believe information from nearly any source, and still others seldom believe anything without carefully evaluating the credibility of the information. Critical thinking is not easy. Solving problems and making decisions is risky. Sometimes the outcome is not what was desired. With effort, however, everyone can achieve some level of critical thinking to become an effective problem solver and decision maker.

Self-Assessment

The nurse should consider some of the attitudes discussed earlier that facilitate critical thinking, such as curiosity, fair-mindedness, humility, courage, and perseverance. A nurse might benefit from a rigorous personal assessment to determine which attitudes he or she already possesses and which need to be cultivated. This could also be done with a partner or as a group. The nurse first determines which attitudes are held strongly and form a base for thinking and which are held minimally or not at all. The nurse also needs to reflect on situations where he or she made decisions that were later regretted, and analyzes thinking processes and attitudes or asks a trusted colleague to assess them. Identifying weak or vulnerable skills and attitudes is also important.

Reflection, at every step of critical thinking and nursing care, helps examine the ways in which the nurse gathers and analyzes data, makes decisions, and determines the effectiveness of interventions. Reflection requires the nurse to pause in order to consider his or her beliefs, knowledge, values, and abilities in the particular situation at hand. The purpose of this reflection is to determine if the current course of action is the best one and to improve future actions. Figure 10-1 ■, the Mind Map for Critical Thinking in Nursing, is a visual depiction of the interactive loops of concepts used in critical thinking. Note that the action of reflection appears as part of three of the steps shown: the starting points, processes, and outcomes.

Tolerating Dissonance and Ambiguity

The nurse needs to take deliberate efforts to cultivate critical-thinking attitudes. For example, to develop fair-mindedness,

one could deliberately seek out information that is in opposition to one's own views; this provides practice in understanding and learning to be open to other viewpoints. It is a human tendency to seek out information that corresponds to one's previously held beliefs and to ignore evidence that may contradict cherished ideas. This perspective is true for both the nurse and the client. Elders may have great difficulty accepting the pervasiveness of technology or that people don't stay in the hospital as long as they did in the 1970s or that having a diagnosis of cancer doesn't always mean that one is going to die. On the other hand, elders have a wealth of knowledge and experience and often know better than the health care provider knows what will work well and be acceptable to them. Nurses should increase their tolerance for ideas that contradict previously held beliefs, and they should practice suspending judgment.

Suspending judgment means tolerating ambiguity for a time. If an issue is complex, it may not be resolved quickly or neatly, and judgment should be postponed. For a while, the nurse will need to say, "I don't know" and be comfortable with that answer until more is known. Although postponing judgment may not be feasible in emergency situations where fast action is required, it is usually feasible in other situations.

Seeking Situations Where Good Thinking Is Practiced

Nurses will find it valuable to attend conferences in clinical or educational settings that support open examination of all sides of issues and respect for opposing viewpoints. Cultivating a questioning attitude, using either Socratic questioning or another technique, is vital. Nurses need to review the standards for evaluating thinking and apply them to their own thinking. If nurses are aware of their own thinking—while they are doing the thinking—they can detect thinking errors.

Creating Environments that Support Critical Thinking

A nurse cannot develop or maintain critical-thinking attitudes in a vacuum. Nurses in leadership positions must be particularly

Figure 10-1 ■ Mind Map for Critical Thinking in Nursing

Note: Duphorne, P. & Giddens, J. (2004) Critical Thinking in Nursing Resource funded by intramural grant of College of Nursing, University of New Mexico.

aware of the climate for thinking that they establish, and they must actively create a stimulating environment that encourages differences of opinion and fair examination of ideas and options. Nurses must embrace exploration of the perspectives of persons from different ages, cultures, religions, socioeconomic levels, and family structures. As leaders, nurses should encourage colleagues to examine evidence carefully before they come to conclusions, and to avoid "group think," the tendency to defer unthinkingly to the will of the group.

LIFESPAN CONSIDERATIONS   **Health Care Decisions**

CHILDREN

Parents most often make decisions about the health care of children. Growing children can participate in those decisions in age-appropriate ways. As described by Piaget, the ability of children to reason and critically think about themselves and their situation develops gradually (see Chapter 20). ∞ At each stage, nurses should be aware of the ways children think and sensitive to how they can be involved in health care decisions:

■ Infants progress from reflexive behavior to simple, repetitive behavior and then to imitative behaviors, learning the concepts of cause and effect and object permanence. Though not involved in making decisions, they need to be comforted and secure as care is given.

■ Toddlers and preschoolers are very egocentric and engage in magical thinking. They cannot reason out the implications of care, but need explanations in language they can understand. Play therapy and use of dolls and toys can help them adjust to care, and they can sometimes be given options (e.g., do you want your dressing changed before breakfast or after?).

■ School-age children tend to be concrete thinkers. They benefit from simple, direct explanations; hands-on exploration of equipment and materials; and helping the care provider as appropriate during procedures. Involving these children in care can increase cooperation and decrease anxiety.

■ Adolescents are increasingly able to think abstractly and may make many of their own health care decisions. They should be actively consulted as a part of the family system.

ELDERS

It is important to include all adult clients in decision making and planning nursing care, but it is especially difficult to do this when working with elders who have impaired cognitive abilities such as Alzheimer's disease. The nurse should allow them as much control and input as possible, keeping things simple and direct so they understand. Elders

continued on page 172

LIFESPAN CONSIDERATIONS   Health Care Decisions—*continued*

with impairments are usually unable to perform multiple tasks or even to think of more than one step at a time. The nurse must have patience and be willing to calmly repeat instructions if necessary. Presenting and discussing issues in basic terms helps to maintain respect and dignity

and allows elders to participate in their own care for as long as possible. If the elder is unable to perform self-care activities such as bathing or health-related activities such as a dressing change, the nurse seeks appropriate alternative methods for assisting the elder with these.

CRITICAL THINKING CHECKPOINT

Mr. W. is a 53-year-old recently retired engineer with a history of irritable bowel syndrome that causes frequent diarrhea and rectal bleeding. His wife is a schoolteacher. It is mid-December when he comes to your clinic complaining about "not feeling good." You conclude he is having a reoccurrence of his intestinal problem.

1. What questions would you ask yourself to check this assumption?
2. How would you demonstrate that you are using the critical-thinking attitude of "confidence in reasoning"?

3. Socrates might ask you about the consequences of your conclusion by posing the question "What are the implications of your thinking?" How would you answer? Consider the implications if you are correct and if you are incorrect in your assumption.
4. Critical thinkers look for subtle cues. Which cues in this situation require follow-up?

See Critical Thinking Possibilities in Appendix A.

CHAPTER 10 **REVIEW**

CHAPTER HIGHLIGHTS

- Nurses need critical-thinking skills and attitudes to be safe, competent, skillful practitioners.
- Critical thinking is a process that guides a nurse in generating, implementing, and evaluating approaches for dealing with client care and professional concepts (NLN, 2000).
- Nurses use critical thinking as they apply knowledge from other subjects and fields to nursing practice, deal with change in stressful environments, and make important decisions related to client care. When nurses incorporate creativity into their thinking, they are able to find unique solutions to unique problems.
- Creativity enhances critical thinking. Creative nurses generate many ideas rapidly, are flexible and natural, create original solutions to problems, tend to be independent and self-confident, and demonstrate individuality.
- Critical-thinking skills include the ability to do critical analysis, perform inductive and deductive reasoning, make valid inferences, differentiate facts from opinions, evaluate the credibility of information sources, clarify concepts, and recognize assumptions.
- Critical thinkers have certain attitudes: independence, fair-mindedness, insight, intellectual humility, intellectual courage to challenge the status quo and rituals, integrity, perseverance, confidence, and curiosity.

- Critical thinking consists of high-level cognitive processes that include problem solving and decision making. There are several problem-solving methods: trial and error, intuition, the nursing process, the scientific method, and the modified scientific method. Nurses use the scientific method or research process when they participate in nursing and health research.
- The nursing process and critical thinking are interrelated and interdependent, but they are not identical. Both involve problem solving, decision making, and creativity.
- Nurses must make decisions in both their personal and professional lives. The steps of the decision-making process include identifying the purpose of the decision, setting the criteria, weighting the criteria, seeking alternatives, examining alternatives, projecting, implementing, and evaluating the action.
- Everyone has at least some level of critical-thinking skill, and that skill can be developed with practice. Some guidelines to enhance critical-thinking skills and attitudes include performing a self-assessment, tolerating dissonance and ambiguity, seeking situations where good thinking is productive, and creating environments that support critical thinking.

TEST YOUR KNOWLEDGE

1. A client with diarrhea also has a physician's order for a bulk laxative daily. The nurse, not realizing that bulk laxatives can help solidify certain types of diarrhea, concludes "The physician does not know the client has diarrhea." This statement is an example of:
   1. A fact.
   2. An inference.
   3. A judgment.
   4. An opinion.

2. A client reports feeling hungry, but does not eat when food is served. Using critical-thinking skills, the nurse should perform which of the following?
   1. Assess why the client is not ingesting the food provided.
   2. Continue to leave the food at the beside until the client is hungry enough to eat.
   3. Notify the primary care provider that tube feeding may be indicated soon.
   4. Believe the client is not really hungry.

3. Although one nurse feels the manager prepared the holiday work schedule unfairly, the manager states that it is the same type of schedule used in the past and other nurses have no problems with it. The nurse continues to feel uncomfortable about how the schedule was created. Which response indicates the nurse is displaying an attitude of critical thinking?

1. Accepting the preferences of the other nurses since there are several of them
2. Recognizing that the nurse must have reached a false conclusion
3. Considering going to a higher authority than the manager for an explanation
4. Continuing to query the manager until the nurse understands the explanation

4. The client who is short of breath benefits from the head of the bed being elevated. Because this position can result in skin breakdown in the sacral area, the nurse decides to study the amount of sacral pressure occurring in other positions. This decision is an example of which of the following?

1. The scientific method
2. The trial-and-error method
3. Intuition
4. The nursing process

5. In the decision-making process, the nurse sets and weights the criteria, examines alternatives, and performs which of the following before implementing the plan?

1. Reexamines the purpose for making the decision
2. Consults the client and family members to determine their view of the criteria
3. Identifies and considers various means for reaching the outcomes
4. Determines the logical course of action should intervening problems arise

See Answers to Test Your Knowledge in Appendix A.

EXPLORE MEDIALINK www.prenhall.com/berman

DVD-ROM
- Audio Glossary
- NCLEX Review
- Video: Thinking Critically

COMPANION WEBSITE
- Additional NCLEX Review
- Case Study: Examining an Increase in Pressure Ulcers
- Application Activity: Practicing Critical Thinking
- Links to Resources

READINGS AND REFERENCES

SUGGESTED READINGS
Edwards, S. (2003). Professional issues. Critical thinking at the bedside: A practical perspective. *British Journal of Nursing, 12,* 1142–1149. *This article provides a comprehensive review of critical thinking from theoretical and practical perspectives. The many models from the literature are often complex and difficult to interpret in relation to clinical practice situations. If theory cannot be integrated into practice, then its value to nursing should be questioned. The task now is to formalize and cement the connections between the two concepts at the bedside.*

Oermann, M. H. (2004). Using active learning in lecture: Best of "both worlds." *International Journal of Nursing Education Scholarship, 1*(1), Article 1. *The lecture mode of content delivery has sometimes been viewed negatively. This well-known author in teaching and critical thinking explores another approach: integrating active learning within lecture, gaining the benefits of both methods. This article examines benefits of an integrated approach to teaching and presents strategies for active learning intended for use with lecture.*

RELATED RESEARCH
Gurney, D. (2004). Triage decisions. Exercises in critical thinking at triage: Prioritizing patients with similar acuities. *Journal of Emergency Nursing, 30,* 514–516.

Hoffman, K., & Elwin, C. (2004). The relationship between critical thinking and confidence in decision-making. *Australian Journal of Advanced Nursing, 22*(1), 8–12.

REFERENCES
Alfaro-LeFevre, R. (2004). *Critical thinking in nursing: A practical approach* (3rd ed.). Philadelphia: W. B. Saunders.

Catalano, J. T. (2003). *Nursing now! Today's issues, tomorrow's trends* (3rd ed.). Philadelphia: F. A. Davis.

Forneris, S. G. (2004). Exploring the attributes of critical thinking: A conceptual basis. *International Journal of Nursing Education Scholarship, 1* (1), Article 9, 1–19. Retrieved June 18, 2006, from http://www.bepress.comlijnes/vol1/iss1/art9

Hicks, F. D., Merritt, S. L., & Elstein, A. S. (2003). Critical thinking and clinical decision making in critical care nursing: A pilot study. *Heart & Lung, 32,* 169–180.

National League for Nursing. (2000). *Think tank on critical thinking*. New York: Author.

Paul, R., & Elder, L. (2005). *A guide for educators to critical thinking competency standards.* Dillon Beach, CA: Foundation for Critical Thinking.

SELECTED BIBLIOGRAPHY
Allen, G. D., Rubenfield, M. G., & Scheffer, B. K. (2004). Reliability assessment of critical thinking. *Journal of Professional Nursing, 20*(1), 15–22.

Benner, P. E., Hooper-Kyriakidis, P. L., & Stannard, D. (1999). *Clinical wisdom and interventions in critical care: A thinking-in-action approach.* Philadelphia: W. B. Saunders.

Elder, L., & Paul, R. (2003). *A miniature guide for students and faculty to the foundations of analytic thinking: How to take thinking apart and what to look for when you do.* Dillon Beach, CA: Foundation for Critical Thinking.

Hood, L. J., & Leddy, S. K. (2003). *Leddy & Pepper's conceptual bases of nursing practice* (5th ed.). Philadelphia: Lippincott Williams & Wilkins.

Jackson, M., Ignatavicius, D. D., & Case, B. (2006). *Conversations in critical thinking and clinical judgment.* Boston: Jones & Bartlett.

Moore, B. N., & Parker, R. (2007). *Critical thinking* (8th ed.). Boston: McGraw-Hill.

Rubenfeld, M. G., & Scheffer, B. (2006). *Critical thinking TACTICS for nurses.* Boston: Jones & Bartlett.

Staib, S. (2003). Teaching and measuring critical thinking. *Journal of Nursing Education, 42,* 498–507.

Wilkinson, J. M. (2007). *Nursing process and critical thinking* (4th ed.). Upper Saddle River, NJ: Prentice Hall Health.

CHAPTER
11

Assessing

LEARNING OUTCOMES

After completing this chapter, you will be able to:

1. Describe the phases of the nursing process.

2. Identify major characteristics of the nursing process.

3. Identify the purpose of assessing.

4. Identify the four major activities associated with the assessing phase.

5. Differentiate objective and subjective data and primary and secondary data.

6. Identify three methods of data collection, and give examples of how each is useful.

7. Compare directive and nondirective approaches to interviewing.

8. Compare closed and open-ended questions, providing examples and listing advantages and disadvantages of each.

9. Describe important aspects of the interview setting.

10. Contrast various frameworks used for nursing assessment.

Hall originated the term *nursing process* in 1955, and Johnson (1959), Orlando (1961), and Wiedenbach (1963) were among the first to use it to refer to a series of phases describing the practice of nursing. Since then, various nurses have described the process of nursing and organized the phases in different ways.

The purpose of the nursing process is to identify a client's health status and actual or potential health care problems or needs, to establish plans to meet the identified needs, and to deliver specific nursing interventions to meet those needs. The client may be an individual, a family, or a group.

OVERVIEW OF THE NURSING PROCESS

The use of the nursing process in clinical practice gained additional legitimacy in 1973 when the phases were included in the American Nurses Association (ANA) *Standards of Nursing Practice.* The Standards of Practice within the most current *Scope and Standards of Nursing Practice* (see Box 1–1 on page 14 ∞) include the five phases of the nursing process: assessment, diagnosis, planning, implementation, and evaluation (ANA, 2004). Most states have since revised their nurse practice acts to reflect the nursing process. See Figure 11-1 ■ for an illustration of the nursing process in action.

Phases of the Nursing Process

Although nurse theorists may use different terms to describe the phases of the nursing process, the activities of the nurse using the process are similar. For example, *diagnosing* may also be called *analysis,* and *implementing* may be called *intervention* or *intervening.*

An overview of the five-phase nursing process is shown in Table 11–1 on page 178. Each of the five phases is discussed in depth in this and subsequent chapters of this unit. The phases of the nursing process are not separate entities but overlapping, continuing subprocesses (see Figure 11-2 ■ on page 179). For example, assessing, which may be considered the first phase of the nursing process, is also carried out during the implementing and evaluating phases. For instance, while actually administering medications (implementing), the nurse continuously notes the client's skin color, level of consciousness, and so on.

Each phase of the nursing process affects the others; they are closely interrelated. For example, if inadequate data are obtained during assessing, the nursing diagnoses will be incomplete or incorrect; inaccuracy will also be reflected in the planning, implementing, and evaluating phases.

Characteristics of the Nursing Process

The nursing process has distinctive characteristics that enable the nurse to respond to the changing health status of the client. These characteristics include its cyclic and dynamic nature, client centeredness, focus on problem solving and decision making, interpersonal and collaborative style, universal applicability, and use of critical thinking.

- Data from each phase provide input into the next phase. Findings from evaluation feed back into assessment. Hence, the nursing process is a regularly repeated event or sequence of events (a cycle) that is continuously changing (dynamic) rather than staying the same (static).

- The nursing process is client centered. The nurse organizes the plan of care according to client problems rather than nursing goals. In the assessment phase, the nurse collects data to determine the client's habits, routines, and needs, enabling the nurse to incorporate client routines into the care plan as much as possible.

- The nursing process is an adaptation of problem solving (see Chapter 10 ∞) and systems theory (see Chapter 24 ∞). It can be viewed as parallel to but separate from the process used by physicians (the medical model). Both processes (a) begin with data gathering and analysis, (b) base action (intervention or treatment) on a problem statement (nursing diagnosis or medical diagnosis), and (c) include an evaluative component. However, the medical model focuses on physiological systems and the disease process, whereas the nursing process is directed toward a client's responses to disease and illness.

- Decision making is involved in every phase of the nursing process. Nurses can be highly creative in determining when and how to use data to make decisions. They are not bound by standard responses and may apply their repertoire of skills and knowledge to assist clients. This facilitates the individualization of the nurse's plan of care.

- The nursing process is interpersonal and collaborative. It requires the nurse to communicate directly and consistently with clients and families to meet their needs. It also requires that nurses collaborate, as members of the health care team, in a joint effort to provide quality client care.

The Nursing Process in Action

The nursing process is a systematic, rational method of planning and providing nursing care. Its purpose is to identify a client's health care status, and actual or potential health problems, to establish plans to meet the identified needs, and to deliver specific nursing interventions to address those needs. The nursing process is cyclical; that is, its components follow a logical sequence, but more than one component may be involved at one time. At the end of the first cycle, care may be terminated if goals are achieved, or the cycle may continue with reassessment, or the plan of care may be modified.

ASSESSING

ASSESSING
- Collect data
- Organize data
- Validate data
- Document data

DIAGNOSING

DIAGNOSING
- Analyze data
- Identify health problems, risks, and strengths
- Formulate diagnostic statements

PLANNING

PLANNING
- Prioritize problems/diagnoses
- Formulate goals/desired outcomes
- Select nursing interventions
- Write nursing interventions

IMPLEMENTING

IMPLEMENTING
- Reassess the client
- Determine the nurse's need for assistance
- Implement the nursing interventions
- Supervise delegated care
- Document nursing activities

EVALUATING

EVALUATING
- Collect data related to outcomes
- Compare data with outcomes
- Relate nursing actions to client goals/outcomes
- Draw conclusions about problem status
- Continue, modify, or terminate the client's care plan

Figure 11-1 ■ The nursing process in action.

Amanda Aquilini, a 28-year-old married attorney, was admitted to the hospital with an elevated temperature, a productive cough, and rapid, labored respirations. In taking a nursing history, Nurse Mary Medina, RN, finds that Amanda has had a "chest cold" for two weeks, and has been experiencing shortness of breath upon exertion. Yesterday she developed an elevated temperature and began to experience "pain" in her "lungs."

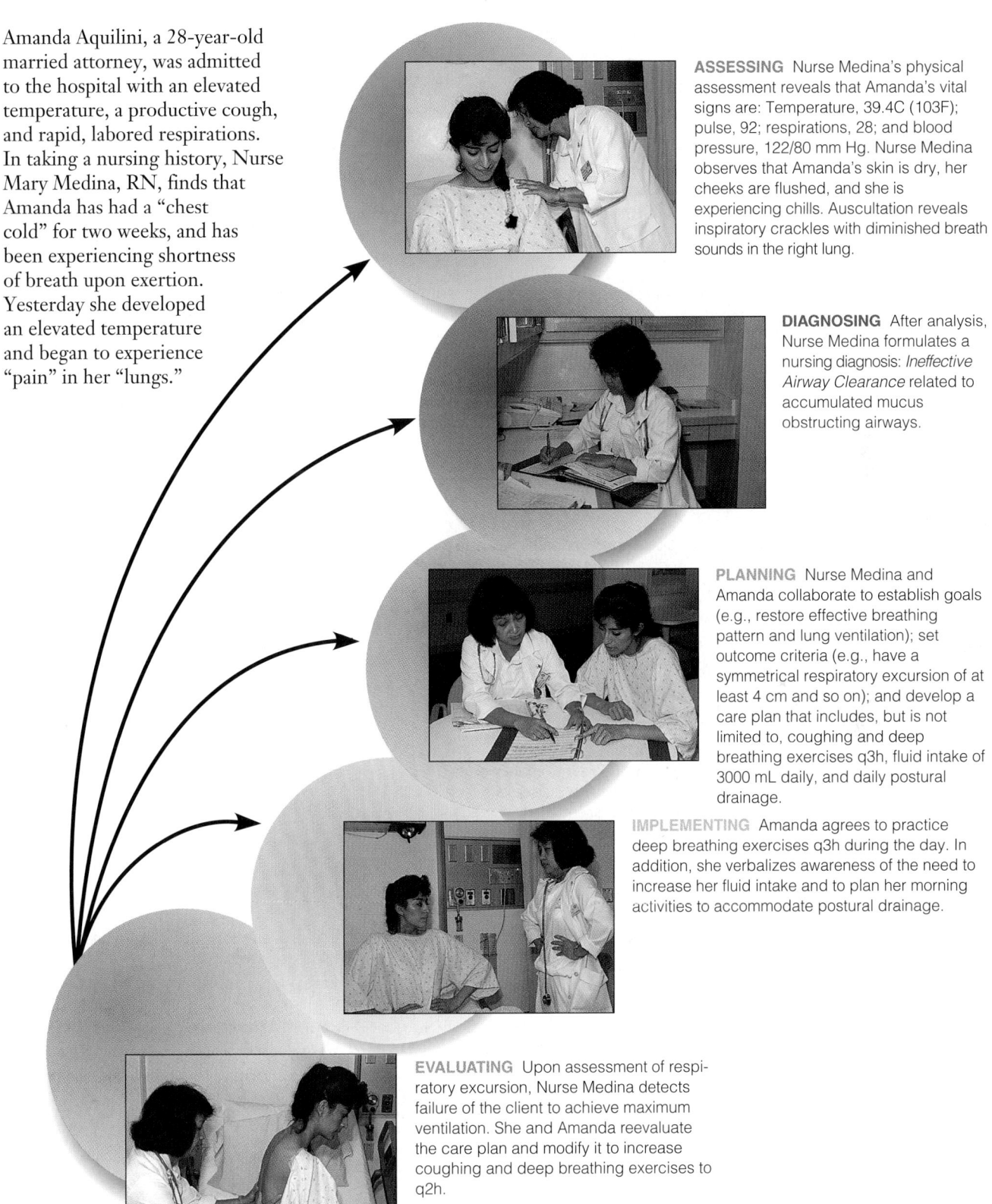

ASSESSING Nurse Medina's physical assessment reveals that Amanda's vital signs are: Temperature, 39.4C (103F); pulse, 92; respirations, 28; and blood pressure, 122/80 mm Hg. Nurse Medina observes that Amanda's skin is dry, her cheeks are flushed, and she is experiencing chills. Auscultation reveals inspiratory crackles with diminished breath sounds in the right lung.

DIAGNOSING After analysis, Nurse Medina formulates a nursing diagnosis: *Ineffective Airway Clearance* related to accumulated mucus obstructing airways.

PLANNING Nurse Medina and Amanda collaborate to establish goals (e.g., restore effective breathing pattern and lung ventilation); set outcome criteria (e.g., have a symmetrical respiratory excursion of at least 4 cm and so on); and develop a care plan that includes, but is not limited to, coughing and deep breathing exercises q3h, fluid intake of 3000 mL daily, and daily postural drainage.

IMPLEMENTING Amanda agrees to practice deep breathing exercises q3h during the day. In addition, she verbalizes awareness of the need to increase her fluid intake and to plan her morning activities to accommodate postural drainage.

EVALUATING Upon assessment of respiratory excursion, Nurse Medina detects failure of the client to achieve maximum ventilation. She and Amanda reevaluate the care plan and modify it to increase coughing and deep breathing exercises to q2h.

Figure 11-1 ■ *continued*

TABLE 11–1 Overview of the Nursing Process

PHASE AND DESCRIPTION	PURPOSE	ACTIVITIES
Assessing Collecting, organizing, validating, and documenting client data	To establish a database about the client's response to health concerns or illness and the ability to manage health care needs	Establish a database: ■ Obtain a nursing health history. ■ Conduct a physical assessment. ■ Review client records. ■ Review nursing literature. ■ Consult support persons. ■ Consult health professionals. Update data as needed. Organize data. Validate data. Communicate/document data.
Diagnosing Analyzing and synthesizing data	To identify client strengths and health problems that can be prevented or resolved by collaborative and independent nursing interventions To develop a list of nursing and collaborative problems	Interpret and analyze data. ■ Compare data against standards. ■ Cluster or group data (generate tentative hypotheses). ■ Identify gaps and inconsistencies. Determine client's strengths, risks, diagnoses, and problems. Formulate nursing diagnoses and collaborative problem statements. Document nursing diagnoses on the care plan.
Planning Determining how to prevent, reduce, or resolve the identified priority client problems; how to support client strengths; and how to implement nursing interventions in an organized, individualized, and goal-directed manner	To develop an individualized care plan that specifies client goals/desired outcomes, and related nursing interventions	Set priorities and goals/outcomes in collaboration with client. Write goals/desired outcomes. Select nursing strategies/interventions. Consult other health professionals. Write nursing interventions and nursing care plan. Communicate care plan to relevant health care providers.
Implementing Carrying out (or delegating) and documenting the planned nursing interventions	To assist the client to meet desired goals/outcomes; promote wellness; prevent illness and disease; restore health; and facilitate coping with altered functioning	Reassess the client to update the database. Determine the nurse's need for assistance. Perform planned nursing interventions. Communicate what nursing actions were implemented. ■ Document care and client responses to care. ■ Give verbal reports as necessary.
Evaluating Measuring the degree to which goals/outcomes have been achieved and identifying factors that positively or negatively influence goal achievement	To determine whether to continue, modify, or terminate the plan of care	Collaborate with client and collect data related to desired outcomes. Judge whether goals/outcomes have been achieved. Relate nursing actions to client outcomes. Make decisions about problem status. Review and modify the care plan as indicated or terminate nursing care. Document achievement of outcomes and modification of the care plan.

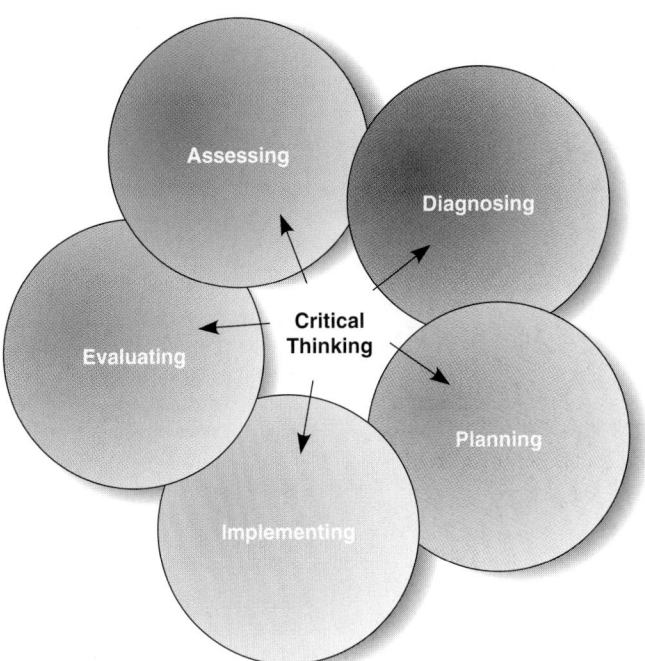

Figure 11-2 ■ The five overlapping phases of the nursing process. Each phase depends on the accuracy of the other phases. Each phase involves critical thinking.

- The universally applicable characteristic of the nursing process means that it is used as a framework for nursing care in all types of health care settings, with clients of all age groups.
- Nurses must use a variety of critical-thinking skills to carry out the nursing process. Table 11–2 provides examples of critical thinking in the nursing process.

ASSESSING

Assessing is the systematic and continuous collection, organization, validation, and documentation of **data** (information). In effect, assessing is a continuous process carried out during all phases of the nursing process. For example, in the evaluation phase, assessment is done to determine the outcomes of the nursing strategies and to evaluate goal achievement. All phases of the nursing process depend on the accurate and complete collection of data. There are four different types of assessments: initial assessment, problem-focused assessment, emergency assessment, and time-lapsed reassessment (see Table 11–3). Assessments vary according to their purpose, timing, time available, and client status.

Nursing assessments focus on a client's responses to a health problem. A nursing assessment should include the client's perceived needs, health problems, related experience, health practices, values, and lifestyles. To be most useful, the data collected should be relevant to a particular health problem. Therefore, nurses should think critically about what to assess. The Joint Commission on Accreditation of Healthcare Organizations (2005) requires that each client have an initial assessment consisting of a history and physical performed and documented within 24 hours of admission as an inpatient.

TABLE 11–2 Examples of Critical Thinking in the Nursing Process

NURSING PROCESS PHASE	CRITICAL-THINKING ACTIVITIES
Assessing	Making reliable observations
	Distinguishing relevant from irrelevant data
	Distinguishing important from unimportant data
	Validating data
	Organizing data
	Categorizing data according to a framework
	Recognizing assumptions
	Identifying gaps in the data
Diagnosing	Finding patterns and relationships among cues
	Making inferences
	Suspending judgment when lacking data
	Stating the problem
	Examining assumptions
	Comparing patterns with norms
	Identifying factors contributing to the problem
Planning	Forming valid generalizations
	Transferring knowledge from one situation to another
	Developing evaluative criteria
	Hypothesizing
	Making interdisciplinary connections
	Prioritizing client problems
	Generalizing principles from other sciences
Implementing	Applying knowledge to perform interventions
	Testing hypotheses
Evaluating	Deciding whether hypotheses are correct
	Making criterion-based evaluations

Note: From *Nursing Process & Critical Thinking,* 4th ed. (pp. 66–69), by J. M. Wilkinson, 2007, Upper Saddle River, NJ: Pearson Prentice Hall. Adapted with permission.

The assessment process involves four closely related activities: collecting data, organizing data, validating data, and documenting data (see Figure 11-3 ■).

COLLECTING DATA

Data collection is the process of gathering information about a client's health status. It must be both systematic and continuous to prevent the omission of significant data and reflect a client's changing health status.

A **database** is all the information about a client; it includes the nursing health history (see Box 11–1), physical assessment, primary care provider's history and physical examination, results of laboratory and diagnostic tests, and material contributed by other health personnel.

Client data should include past history as well as current problems. For example, a history of an allergic reaction to penicillin is

TABLE 11–3 Types of Assessment

TYPE	TIME PERFORMED	PURPOSE	EXAMPLE
Initial assessment	Performed within specified time after admission to a health care agency	To establish a complete database for problem identification, reference, and future comparison	Nursing admission assessment
Problem-focused assessment	Ongoing process integrated with nursing care	To determine the status of a specific problem identified in an earlier assessment	Hourly assessment of client's fluid intake and urinary output in an ICU
			Assessment of client's ability to perform self-care while assisting a client to bathe
Emergency assessment	During any physiologic or psychologic crisis of the client	To identify life-threatening problems	Rapid assessment of a person's airway, breathing status, and circulation during a cardiac arrest
		To identify new or overlooked problems	Assessment of suicidal tendencies or potential for violence
Time-lapsed reassessment	Several months after initial assessment	To compare the client's current status to baseline data previously obtained	Reassessment of a client's functional health patterns in a home care or outpatient setting or, in a hospital, at shift change

a vital piece of historical data. Past surgical procedures, folk healing practices, and chronic diseases are also examples of historical data. Current data relate to present circumstances, such as pain, nausea, sleep patterns, and religious practices. To collect data accurately, both the client and nurse must actively participate. Data

Figure 11-3 ■ Assessing. The assessment process involves four closely related activities.

can be of subjective or objective and constant or variable types, and from a primary or secondary source.

Types of Data

Subjective data, also referred to as **symptoms** or covert data, are apparent only to the person affected and can be described or verified only by that person. Itching, pain, and feelings of worry are examples of subjective data. Subjective data include the client's sensations, feelings, values, beliefs, attitudes, and perception of personal health status and life situation.

Objective data, also referred to as **signs** or overt data, are detectable by an observer or can be measured or tested against an accepted standard. They can be seen, heard, felt, or smelled, and they are obtained by observation or physical examination. For example, a discoloration of the skin or a blood pressure reading is objective data. During the physical examination, the nurse obtains objective data to validate subjective data and to complete the assessment phase of the nursing process.

Constant data is information that does not change over time such as race or blood type. Variable data can change quickly, frequently, or rarely and include such data as blood pressure, age, and level of pain.

A complete database provides a baseline for comparing the client's responses to nursing and medical interventions. Examples of subjective and objective data are shown in Table 11–4.

Sources of Data

Sources of data are primary or secondary. The client is the primary source of data. Family members or other support persons, other health professionals, records and reports, laboratory and diagnostic analyses, and relevant literature are secondary or indirect sources. In fact, all sources other than the client are con-

BOX 11–1 Components of a Nursing Health History

BIOGRAPHIC DATA
Client's name, address, age, sex, marital status, occupation, religious preference, health care financing, and usual source of medical care.

CHIEF COMPLAINT OR REASON FOR VISIT
The answer given to the question "What is troubling you?" or "Can you tell me the reason you came to the hospital or clinic today?" The chief complaint should be recorded in the client's own words.

HISTORY OF PRESENT ILLNESS
- When the symptoms started
- Whether the onset of symptoms was sudden or gradual
- How often the problem occurs
- Exact location of the distress
- Character of the complaint (e.g., intensity of pain or quality of sputum, emesis, or discharge)
- Activity in which the client was involved when the problem occurred
- Phenomena or symptoms associated with the chief complaint
- Factors that aggravate or alleviate the problem

PAST HISTORY
- *Childhood illnesses,* such as chickenpox, mumps, measles, rubella (German measles), rubeola (red measles), streptococcal infections, scarlet fever, rheumatic fever, and other significant illnesses
- *Childhood immunizations* and the date of the last tetanus shot
- *Allergies* to drugs, animals, insects, or other environmental agents, the type of reaction that occurs, and how the reaction is treated
- *Accidents and injuries:* how, when, and where the incident occurred, type of injury, treatment received, and any complications
- *Hospitalization for serious illnesses:* reasons for the hospitalization, dates, surgery performed, course of recovery, and any complications
- *Medications:* all currently used prescription and over-the-counter medications, such as aspirin, nasal spray, vitamins, or laxatives

FAMILY HISTORY OF ILLNESS
To ascertain risk factors for certain diseases, the ages of siblings, parents, and grandparents and their current state of health or, if they are deceased, the cause of death are obtained. Particular attention should be given to disorders such as heart disease, cancer, diabetes, hypertension, obesity, allergies, arthritis, tuberculosis, bleeding, alcoholism, and any mental health disorders.

LIFESTYLE
- *Personal habits:* the amount, frequency, and duration of substance use (tobacco, alcohol, coffee, cola, tea, and illicit or recreational drugs)
- *Diet:* description of a typical diet on a normal day or any special diet, number of meals and snacks per day, who cooks and shops for food, ethnically distinct food patterns, and allergies
- *Sleep/rest patterns:* usual daily sleep/wake times, difficulties sleeping, and remedies used for difficulties
- *Activities of daily living (ADLs):* any difficulties experienced in the basic activities of eating, grooming, dressing, elimination, and locomotion

- *Instrumental activities of daily living:* any difficulties experienced in food preparation, shopping, transportation, housekeeping, laundry, and ability to use the telephone, handle finances, and manage medications
- *Recreation/hobbies:* exercise activity and tolerance, hobbies and other interests, and vacations

SOCIAL DATA
- *Family relationships/friendships:* The client's support system in times of stress (who helps in time of need?), what effect the client's illness has on the family, and whether any family problems are affecting the client. See also the discussion of family assessment in Chapter 24. ∞
- *Ethnic affiliation:* Health customs and beliefs; cultural practices that may affect health care and recovery. See also detailed ethnic/cultural assessment guide in Chapter 18. ∞
- *Educational history:* Data about the client's highest level of education attained and any past difficulties with learning.
- *Occupational history:* Current employment status, the number of days missed from work because of illness, any history of accidents on the job, any occupational hazards with a potential for future disease or accident, the client's need to change jobs because of past illness, the employment status of spouses or partners and the way child care is handled, and the client's overall satisfaction with the work.
- *Economic status:* Information about how the client is paying for medical care (including what kind of medical and hospitalization coverage the client has), and whether the client's illness presents financial concerns.
- *Home and neighborhood conditions:* Home safety measures and adjustments in physical facilities that may be required to help the client manage a physical disability, activity intolerance, and activities of daily living; the availability of neighborhood and community services to meet the client's needs.

PSYCHOLOGIC DATA
- *Major stressors* experienced and the client's perception of them
- *Usual coping pattern* with a serious problem or a high level of stress
- *Communication style:* ability to verbalize appropriate emotion; nonverbal communication—such as eye movements, gestures, use of touch, and posture; interactions with support persons; and the congruence of nonverbal behavior and verbal expression

PATTERNS OF HEALTH CARE
All health care resources the client is currently using and has used in the past. These include the primary care provider, specialists (e.g., ophthalmologist or gynecologist), dentist, folk practitioners (e.g., herbalist or curandero), health clinic, or health center; whether the client considers the care being provided adequate; and whether access to health care is a problem.

---

sidered secondary sources. All data from secondary sources should be validated if possible.

Client

The best source of data is usually the client, unless the client is too ill, young, or confused to communicate clearly. The

client can provide subjective data that no one else can offer. Most often, primary data refers to statements made by the client but also include those objective data that can be directly obtained by the nurse from the client such as gender. Some clients cannot or do not wish to provide accurate data. These include young children, and clients who are confused, afraid,

TABLE 11-4	**Examples of Subjective and Objective Data**

SUBJECTIVE	OBJECTIVE
"I feel weak all over when I exert myself."	Blood pressure 90/50 * Apical pulse 104 Skin pale and diaphoretic
Client states he has a cramping pain in his abdomen. States, "I feel sick to my stomach."	Vomited 100 mL green-tinged fluid Abdomen firm and slightly distended Active bowel sounds auscultated in all four quadrants
"I'm short of breath." Wife states: "He doesn't seem so sad today." (This is subjective and secondary source data.) "I would like to see the chaplain before surgery."	Lung sounds clear bilaterally; diminished in right lower lobe Client cried during interview Holding open Bible Has small silver cross on bedside table

* Blood pressure obtained using an external cuff and manometer may be considered secondary or indirect data since it does not directly measure the pressure within the arteries.

embarrassed, or distrustful, or do not speak the nurse's language (D'Amico & Barbarito, 2007).

Support People

Family members, friends, and caregivers who know the client well often can supplement or verify information provided by the client. They might convey information about the client's response to illness, the stresses the client was experiencing before the illness, family attitudes on illness and health, and the client's home environment.

Support people are an especially important source of data for a client who is very young, unconscious, or confused. In some cases—a client who is physically or emotionally abused, for example—the person giving information may wish to remain anonymous. Before eliciting data from support people, the nurse should ensure that the client, if mentally able, accepts such input. The nurse should also indicate on the nursing history that the data were obtained from a support person.

Information supplied by family members, significant others, or other health professionals is considered subjective if it is not based on fact. If the client's daughter says, "Dad is very confused today," that is secondary subjective data because it is an interpretation of the client's behavior by the daughter. The nurse should attempt to verify the reported confusion by interviewing the client directly. However, if the daughter says, "Dad said he thought it was the year 1941 today," that may be considered secondary objective data since the daughter heard her father state this directly.

Client Records

Client records include information documented by various health care professionals. Client records also contain data regarding the client's occupation, religion, and marital status. By reviewing such records before interviewing the client, the nurse can avoid asking questions for which answers have already been supplied. Repeated questioning can be stressful and annoying to clients and cause concern about the lack of communication among health professionals. Types of client records include medical records, records of therapies, and laboratory records.

Medical records (e.g., medical history, physical examination, operative report, progress notes, and consultations done by primary care providers) are often a source of a client's present and past health and illness patterns. These records can provide nurses with information about the client's coping behaviors, health practices, previous illnesses, and allergies.

Records of therapies provided by other health professionals, such as social workers, nutritionists, dietitians, or physical therapists, help the nurse obtain relevant data not expressed by the client. For example, a social agency's report on a client's living conditions or a home health care agency's report on a client's coping at home can also be helpful to the nurse conducting an assessment.

Laboratory records also provide pertinent health information. For example, the determination of blood glucose level allows health professionals to monitor the administration of oral hypoglycemic medications. Any laboratory data about a client must be compared to the agency or performing laboratory's norms for that particular test and for the client's age, sex, and other significant client data. Diagnostic studies commonly ordered are discussed in Chapter 34. ∞

The nurse must always consider the information in client records in light of the present situation. For example, if the most recent medical record is 10 years old, the client's health practices and coping behaviors are likely to have changed. Older clients may have numerous previous records. These are very useful and contribute to a full understanding of the health history, especially if the client's memory is impaired.

Health Care Professionals

Because assessment is an ongoing process, verbal reports from other health care professionals serve as other potential sources of information about a client's health. Nurses, social workers, primary care providers, and physiotherapists, for example, may have information from either previous or current contact with the client. Sharing of information among professionals is especially important to ensure continuity of care when clients are transferred to and from home and health care agencies.

Literature

The review of nursing and related literature, such as professional journals and reference texts, can provide additional information for the database. A literature review includes but is not limited to the following information:

- Standards or norms against which to compare findings (e.g., height and weight tables, normal developmental tasks for an age group)
- Cultural and social health practices
- Spiritual beliefs
- Assessment data needed for specific client conditions
- Nursing interventions and evaluation criteria relevant to a client's health problems
- Information about medical diagnoses, treatment, and prognoses
- Current methodologies and research findings

Data Collection Methods

The principal methods used to collect data are observing, interviewing, and examining. Observation occurs whenever the nurse is in contact with the client or support persons. Interviewing is used mainly while taking the nursing health history. Examining is the major method used in the physical health assessment.

In reality, the nurse uses all three methods simultaneously when assessing clients. For example, during the client interview the nurse observes, listens, asks questions, and mentally retains information to explore in the physical examination.

Observing

To *observe* is to gather data by using the senses. Observation is a conscious, deliberate skill that is developed through effort and with an organized approach. Although nurses observe mainly through sight, most of the senses are engaged during careful observations. Examples of client data observed through the senses are shown in Table 11–5.

TABLE 11–5 Using the Senses to Observe Client Data

SENSE	EXAMPLE OF CLIENT DATA
Vision	Overall appearance (e.g., body size, general weight, posture, grooming); signs of distress or discomfort; facial and body gestures; skin color and lesions; abnormalities of movement; nonverbal demeanor (e.g., signs of anger or anxiety); religious or cultural artifacts (e.g., books, icons, candles, beads)
Smell	Body or breath odors
Hearing	Lung and heart sounds; bowel sounds; ability to communicate; language spoken; ability to initiate conversation; ability to respond when spoken to; orientation to time, person, and place; thoughts and feelings about self, others, and health status
Touch	Skin temperature and moisture; muscle strength (e.g., hand grip); pulse rate, rhythm, and volume; palpatory lesions (e.g., lumps, masses, nodules)

Observation has two aspects: (a) noticing the data and (b) selecting, organizing, and interpreting the data. A nurse who observes that a client's face is flushed must relate that observation to findings such as body temperature, activity, environmental temperature, and blood pressure. Errors can occur in selecting, organizing, and interpreting data. For example, a nurse might not notice certain signs, either because they are unexpected or because they do not conform to preconceptions about a client's illness. Nurses often need to focus on specific data in order not to be overwhelmed by a multitude of data. Observing, therefore, involves distinguishing data in a meaningful manner. For example, nurses caring for newborns learn to ignore the usual sounds of machines in the nursery but respond quickly to an infant's cry or movement.

The experienced nurse is often able to attend to an intervention (e.g., give a bed bath or monitor an intravenous infusion) and at the same time make important observations (e.g., note a change in respiratory status or skin color). The beginning student must learn to make observations and complete tasks simultaneously.

Nursing observations must be organized so that nothing significant is missed. Most nurses develop a particular sequence for observing events, usually focusing on the client first. For example, a nurse walks into a client's room and observes, in the following order:

1. Clinical signs of client distress (e.g., pallor or flushing, labored breathing, and behavior indicating pain or emotional distress)
2. Threats to the client's safety, real or anticipated (e.g., a lowered side rail)
3. The presence and functioning of associated equipment (e.g., intravenous equipment and oxygen)
4. The immediate environment, including the people in it

Interviewing

An **interview** is a planned communication or a conversation with a purpose, for example, to get or give information, identify problems of mutual concern, evaluate change, teach, provide support, or provide counseling or therapy. One example of the interview is the nursing health history, which is a part of the nursing admission assessment.

There are two approaches to interviewing: directive and nondirective. The **directive interview** is highly structured and elicits specific information. The nurse establishes the purpose of the interview and controls the interview, at least at the outset. The client responds to questions but may have limited opportunity to ask questions or discuss concerns. Nurses frequently use directive interviews to gather and to give information when time is limited (e.g., in an emergency situation).

During a **nondirective interview,** or rapport-building interview, by contrast, the nurse allows the client to control the purpose, subject matter, and pacing. **Rapport** is an understanding between two or more people.

A combination of directive and nondirective approaches is usually appropriate during the information-gathering interview. The nurse begins by determining areas of concern for the client. If, for example, a client expresses worry about surgery,

MediaLink

Anatomical Landmarks Animation

REAL WORLD PRACTICE

One of the most vulnerable times in a person's life may be hospitalization. When a person is hospitalized, he or she loses control over even the most basic decisions in his or her daily life, possibly for the first time in his or her life. Some coping mechanisms to deal with this sense of loss may be anger, or micro managing the few things over which the person does have control. The client may present this by being anxious, demanding or needy. Also, sometimes a person is just lonely and missing his or her familiar surroundings, family and pets, or daily routines.

The most important contact with my clients is at the beginning of my shift. I gather pertinent information, assess their needs and concerns, and inform them of what the plan of care will be for the next 12 hours. I have found that if a person is feeling anxious, demanding, or needy, I can minimize these behaviors by taking a little extra time at the beginning of my shift to address any issues he or she has or to just listen. Knowing that they are being heard and that I am concerned about their needs usually helps ease their anxiety. I also always ask about their level of pain. If this does not help I ask for assistance and feedback from my co-workers, because we've all been in this situation!

— *Toni Stamps BSN, RN,*
University Medical Center, Tucson, AZ

the nurse pauses to explore the client's worry and to provide support. Simply noting the worry, without dealing with it, can leave the impression that the nurse does not care about the client's concerns or dismisses them as unimportant.

TYPES OF INTERVIEW QUESTIONS. Questions are often classified as closed or open ended, and neutral or leading. **Closed questions**, used in the directive interview, are restrictive and generally require only "yes" or "no" or short factual answers giving specific information. Closed questions often begin with "when," "where," "who," "what," "do (did, does)," or "is (are, was)." Examples of closed questions are "What medication did you take?" "Are you having pain now? Show me where it is." "How old are you?" "When did you fall?" The highly stressed person and the person who has difficulty communicating will find closed questions easier to answer than open-ended questions.

Open-ended questions, associated with the nondirective interview, invite clients to discover and explore, elaborate, clarify, or illustrate their thoughts or feelings. An open-ended question specifies only the broad topic to be discussed, and invites answers longer than one or two words. Such questions give clients the freedom to divulge only the information that they are ready to disclose. The open-ended question is useful at the beginning of an interview or to change topics and to elicit attitudes.

Open-ended questions may begin with "what" or "how." Examples of open-ended questions are "How have you been feeling lately?" "What brought you to the hospital?" "How did you feel in that situation?" "Would you describe more about how you relate to your child?" "What would you like to talk about today?"

The type of question a nurse chooses depends on the needs of the client at the time. Nurses often find it necessary to use a combination of closed and open-ended questions throughout an interview to accomplish the goals of the interview and obtain needed information. See Box 11–2 for advantages and disadvantages of open-ended and closed questions.

A **neutral question** is a question the client can answer without direction or pressure from the nurse, is open ended, and is used in nondirective interviews. Examples are "How do you feel about that?" "Why do you think you had the operation?" A **leading question**, by contrast, is usually closed, used in a directive interview, and thus directs the client's answer. Examples are "You're stressed about surgery tomorrow, aren't you?" "You will take your medicine, won't you?" The leading question gives the client less opportunity to decide whether the answer is true or not. Leading questions create problems if the client, in an effort to please the nurse, gives inaccurate responses. This can result in inaccurate data.

PLANNING THE INTERVIEW AND SETTING. Before beginning an interview, the nurse reviews available information, for example, the operative report, information about the current illness, or literature about the client's health problem. The nurse also reviews the agency's data collection form to identify which data must be collected and which data are within the nurse's discretion to collect based on the specific client. If a form is not available, most nurses prepare an interview guide to help them remember areas of information and determine what questions to ask. The guide includes a list of topics and subtopics rather than a series of questions.

Both nurses and clients are made comfortable in order to encourage an effective interview by balancing several factors. Each interview is influenced by time, place, seating arrangement or distance, and language.

Time. Nurses need to plan interviews with clients when the client is physically comfortable and free of pain, and when interruptions by friends, family, and other health professionals are minimal. Nurses should schedule interviews with clients in their homes at a time selected by the client.

Place. A well-lighted, well-ventilated room that is relatively free of noise, movements, and distractions encourages communication. In addition, a place where others cannot overhear or see the client is desirable.

Seating Arrangement. Standing and looking down at a client who is in bed or in a chair, the nurse risks intimidating the client. When a client is in bed, the nurse can sit at a 45-degree angle to the bed. This position is less formal than sitting behind a table or standing at the foot of the bed. During an initial admission interview, a client may feel less confronted if there is an overbed table between the client and the nurse. Sitting on a client's bed hems the client in and makes staring difficult to avoid.

A seating arrangement with the nurse behind a desk and the client seated across creates a formal setting that suggests a business meeting between a superior and a subordinate. In contrast, a seating arrangement in which the parties sit on two chairs placed at right angles to a desk or table or a few feet apart, with

---

BOX 11–2 **Selected Advantages and Disadvantages of Open-Ended and Closed Questions**

OPEN-ENDED QUESTIONS

Advantages
1. They let the interviewee do the talking.
2. The interviewer is able to listen and observe.
3. They are easy to answer and nonthreatening.
4. They reveal what the interviewee thinks is important.
5. They may reveal the interviewee's lack of information, misunderstanding of words, frame of reference, prejudices, or stereotypes.
6. They can provide information the interviewer may not ask for.
7. They can reveal the interviewee's degree of feeling about an issue.
8. They can convey interest and trust because of the freedom they provide.

Disadvantages
1. They take more time.
2. Only brief answers may be given.
3. Valuable information may be withheld.
4. They often elicit more information than necessary.
5. Responses are difficult to document and require skill in recording.
6. The interviewer requires skill in controlling an open-ended interview.
7. Responses require psychologic insight and sensitivity from the interviewer.

CLOSED QUESTIONS

Advantages
1. Questions and answers can be controlled more effectively.
2. They require less effort from the interviewee.
3. They may be less threatening, since they do not require explanations or justifications.
4. They take less time.
5. Information can be asked for sooner than it would be volunteered.
6. Responses are easily documented.
7. Questions are easy to use and can be handled by unskilled interviewers.

Disadvantages
1. They may provide too little information and require follow-up questions.
2. They may not reveal how the interviewee feels.
3. They do not allow the interviewee to volunteer possibly valuable information.
4. They may inhibit communication and convey lack of interest by the interviewer.
5. The interviewer may dominate the interview with questions.

Note: From *Interviewing: Principles and Practices*, 11th ed. By C. J. Stewart and W. B. Cash, Jr., 2006, McGraw-Hill. Reprinted with permission from The McGraw-Hill Companies.

---

no table between, creates a less formal atmosphere, and the nurse and client tend to feel on equal terms. In groups, a horseshoe or circular chair arrangement can avoid a superior or head-of-the-table position.

Distance. The distance between the interviewer and interviewee should be neither too small nor too great, because people feel uncomfortable when talking to someone who is too close or too far away. Proxemics is the study of use of space. As a species, humans are highly territorial but we are rarely aware of it unless our space is somehow violated. Most people feel comfortable maintaining a distance of 2 to 3 feet during an interview. Some clients require more or less personal space, depending on their cultural and personal needs. See Box 11–3. For additional information, see Chapter 18. ∞

BOX 11–3 **Personal Space Variables**

- Accepted distance between individuals in conversation varies with ethnicity. It is about 8 to 12 inches in Arab countries, 18 inches in the United States, 24 inches in Britain, and 36 inches in Japan.
- Men of all cultures usually require more space than women.
- Anxiety increases the need for space.
- Direct eye contact increases the need for space.
- Physical contact is used only if it has a therapeutic purpose. Touch, even a simple hand on the shoulder, can be misinterpreted—especially between persons of opposite gender.

Language. Failure to communicate in language the client can understand is a form of discrimination. The nurse must convert complicated medical terminology into common English usage, and interpreters or translators are needed if the client and the nurse do not speak the same language or dialect (a variation in a language spoken in a particular geographic region). Translating medical terminology is a specialized skill because not all persons fluent in the conversational form of the language are familiar with anatomic or other health terms. Interpreters, however, may make judgments about precise wording but also about subtle meanings that require additional explanation or clarification according to the specific language and ethnicity. They may edit the original source to make the meaning clearer or more culturally appropriate.

If giving written documents to clients, the nurse must determine that the client can read in his or her native language. Live translation is preferred since the client can then ask questions for clarification. Nurses must be cautious when asking family members, client visitors, or agency nonprofessional staff to assist with translation. Issues of confidentiality or gender mismatch can interfere with effective communication. Services such as AT&T Language Line are available 24 hours a day in about 140 languages, for a fee paid by the health care provider. Many large agencies possess their own on-call translator services for the languages or dialects commonly spoken in their area.

Even among clients who speak English, there may be differences in understanding terminology. Clients from different parts of the country may have strong accents, or clients less well educated and teen clients may ascribe different meanings to words. For example, "cool" may imply something good to one client and something not warm to another. The nurse must always confirm accurate understandings.

STAGES OF AN INTERVIEW. An interview has three major stages: the opening or introduction, the body or development, and the closing.

The Opening. The opening can be the most important part of the interview because what is said and done at that time sets the tone for the remainder of the interview. The purposes of the opening are to establish rapport and orient the interviewee.

Establishing rapport is a process of creating goodwill and trust. It can begin with a greeting ("Good morning, Mr. Johnson") or a self-introduction ("Good morning. I'm Becky James, a nursing student") accompanied by nonverbal gestures such as a smile, a handshake, and a friendly manner. The nurse must be careful not to overdo this stage; too much superficial talk can arouse anxiety about what is to follow and may appear insincere.

In orientation, the nurse explains the purpose and nature of the interview, for example, what information is needed, how long it will take, and what is expected of the client. The nurse tells the client how the information will be used and usually states that the client has the right not to provide data.

The following is an example of an interview introduction:

Step 1—Establish Rapport

Nurse: Hello, Ms. Goodwin, I'm Ms. Fellows. I'm a nursing student, and I'll be assisting with your care here today.
Client: Hi. Are you a student from the college?
Nurse: Yes, I'm in my final year. Are you familiar with the campus?
Client: Oh, yes! I'm an avid football fan. My nephew graduated in 2004, and I often attend football games with him.
Nurse: That's great! Sounds like fun.
Client: Yes, I enjoy it very much.

Step 2—Orientation

Nurse: May I sit down with you here for about 10 minutes to talk about how I can help you while you're here?
Client: All right. What do you want to know?
Nurse: Well, to plan your care after your operation, I'd like to get some information about your usual daily activities and what you expect here in the hospital. I'll take notes while we talk to get the important points and have them available to the other staff who will also look after you.
Client: OK. That's all right with me.
Nurse: If there is anything you don't want to talk about, please feel free to say so. Everything you tell me will be confidential and only be shared with others who have the legal right to know it.
Client: Sure, that will be fine.

The Body. In the body of the interview, the client communicates what he or she thinks, feels, knows, and perceives in response to questions from the nurse. Effective development of the interview demands that the nurse use communication techniques that make both parties feel comfortable and serve the purpose of the interview (see Chapter 24 ∞). For communicating during an interview, see Practice Guidelines.

PRACTICE GUIDELINES
Communication during an Interview

- Listen attentively, using all your senses, and speak slowly and clearly.
- Use language the client understands, and clarify points that are not understood.
- Plan questions to follow a logical sequence.
- Ask only one question at a time. Multiple questions limit the client to one choice and may confuse the client.
- Acknowledge the client's right to look at things the way they appear to him or her and not the way they appear to the nurse or someone else.
- Do not impose your own values on the client.
- Avoid using personal examples, such as saying, "If I were you. . . ."
- Nonverbally convey respect, concern, interest, and acceptance.
- Be aware of the client's and your own body language.
- Be conscious of the client's and your own voice inflection, tone, and affect.
- Sit down to talk with the client (be at an even level).
- Use and accept silence to help the client search for more thoughts or to organize them.
- Use eye contact and be calm, unhurried, and sympathetic.

The Closing. The nurse terminates the interview when the needed information has been obtained. In some cases, however, a client terminates it, for example, when deciding not to give any more information or when unable to offer more information for some other reason—fatigue, for example. The closing is important for maintaining the rapport and trust and for facilitating future interactions. The following techniques are commonly used to close an interview:

1. Offer to answer questions: "Do you have any questions?" "I would be glad to answer any questions you have." Be sure to allow time for the person to answer, or the offer will be regarded as insincere.
2. Conclude by saying "Well, that's all I need to know for now" or "Well, those are all the questions I have for now." Preceding a remark with the word "well" generally signals that the end of the interaction is near.
3. Thank the client. "Thank you for your time and help. The questions you have answered will be helpful in planning your nursing care." You may also shake the client's hand.
4. Express concern for the person's welfare and future: "Take care of yourself." "I hope all goes well for you."
5. Plan for the next meeting, if there is to be one, or state what will happen next. Include the day, time, place, topic, and purpose: "Let's get together again here on the fifteenth at 9:00 a.m. to see how you are managing then." Or "Ms. Goodwin, I will be responsible for giving you care three mornings per week while you are here. I will be in to see you each Monday, Tuesday, and Wednesday between eight o'clock and noon. At those times, we can adjust your care as needed."
6. Provide a summary to verify accuracy and agreement. Summarizing serves several purposes: It helps to terminate the in-

terview, it reassures the client that the nurse has listened, it checks the accuracy of the nurse's perceptions, it clears the way for new ideas, and it helps the client to note progress and a forward direction. "Let's review what we have just covered in this interview." Summaries are particularly helpful for clients who are anxious or who have difficulty staying with the topic. "Well, it seems to me that you are especially worried about your hospitalization and chest pain because your father died of a heart attack five years ago. Is that correct? . . . I'll discuss this with you again tomorrow, and we'll decide what plans need to be made to help you."

Examining

The physical examination or physical assessment is a systematic data collection method that uses observation (i.e., the senses of sight, hearing, smell, and touch) to detect health problems. To conduct the examination the nurse uses techniques of inspection, auscultation, palpation, and percussion (see Chapter 30 ∞).

The physical examination is carried out systematically. It may be organized according to the examiner's preference, in a head-to-toe approach or a body systems approach. Usually, the nurse first records a general impression about the client's overall appearance and health status, for example, age, body size, mental and nutritional status, speech, and behavior. Then the nurse takes such measurements as vital signs, height, and weight. The **cephalocaudal** or head-to-toe approach begins the examination at the head; progresses to the neck, thorax, abdomen, and extremities; and ends at the toes. The nurse using a body systems approach investigates each system individually, that is, the respiratory system, the circulatory system, the nervous system, and so on. During the physical examination, the nurse assesses all body parts and compares findings on each side of the body (e.g., lungs). These techniques are discussed in detail in Chapters 29 and 30. ∞

Instead of giving a complete examination, the nurse may focus on a specific problem area noted from the nursing assessment, such as the inability to urinate. On occasion, the nurse may find it necessary to resolve a client complaint or problem (e.g., shortness of breath) before completing the examination. Alternatively, the nurse may perform a screening examination. A **screening examination,** also called a **review of systems,** is a brief review of essential functioning of various body parts or systems. An example of a screening examination is the nursing admission assessment form shown in Figure 11-4 ■. Data obtained from this examination are measured against norms or standards, such as ideal height and weight standards or norms for body temperature or blood pressure levels.

ORGANIZING DATA

The nurse uses a written (or computerized) format that organizes the assessment data systematically. This is often referred to as a nursing health history, nursing assessment, or nursing database form. The format may be modified according to the client's physical status such as one focused on musculoskeletal data for orthopedic clients.

Conceptual Models/Frameworks

Most schools of nursing and health care agencies have developed their own structured assessment format. Many of these are based on selected nursing models or frameworks (see Chapter 3 ∞). Three examples are Gordon's functional health pattern framework, Orem's self-care model, and Roy's adaptation model.

Gordon (2006) provides a framework of 11 functional health patterns (see Box 11–4 on page 190). Gordon uses the word *pattern* to signify a sequence of recurring behavior. The nurse collects data about dysfunctional as well as functional behavior. Thus, by using Gordon's framework to organize data, nurses are able to discern emerging patterns.

Orem (2001) delineates eight universal self-care requisites of humans (see Box 11–5 on page 190). Roy and Andrews (1998) outline the data to be collected according to the Roy adaptation model and classify observable behavior into four categories: physiologic, self-concept, role function, and interdependence (see Box 11–6 on page 190).

Figure 11-4 is a concise data collection tool that is organized according to body systems and specific nursing concerns (e.g., screening for falls and allergies); it does not use one particular nursing model. In Box 11–7 on page 191, the data for the case study client Amanda Aquilini from Figure 11-4 are shown after being organized according to the 11 functional health patterns. Note how the categories in the box differ from those in Figure 11-4. As a rule, the nurse organizes the data using the same model on which the data collection tool is based. However, different models are provided here to demonstrate differences in organizing frameworks, and to show that the nurse is not limited to the exact framework provided by the data collection tool.

Wellness Models

Nurses use wellness models to assist clients to identify health risks and to explore lifestyle habits and health behaviors, beliefs, values, and attitudes that influence levels of wellness. Such models generally include the following:

- Health history
- Physical fitness evaluation
- Nutritional assessment
- Life-stress analysis
- Lifestyle and health habits
- Health beliefs
- Sexual health
- Spiritual health
- Relationships
- Health risk appraisal

See Chapter 17 ∞ for details.

Nonnursing Models

Frameworks and models from other disciplines may also be helpful for organizing data. These frameworks are narrower than the model required in nursing; therefore, the nurse usually needs to combine these with other approaches to obtain a complete history.

ADMISSION DATA

Date _4-16-07_ Time _3:15p.m_ Primary Language _English_

Arrived Via: ☐ Wheelchair   ☐ Stretcher   ☑ Ambulatory

From: ☐ Admitting   ☐ ER   ☑ Home   ☐ Nursing Home   ☐ Other

Admitting M.D. _R. Katz_   Time Notified _5 p.m._

ORIENTATION TO UNIT

	YES	NO		YES	NO
Arm Band Correct	☒	☐	Visiting Hours	☒	☐
Allergy Band	☒	☐	Smoking Policy	☒	☐
Telephone	☒	☐	TV, Lights, Bed Controls,		
Electrical Policy	☒	☐	Call Lights, Side Rails	☒	☐
Educational Mat©l	☒	☐	Nurses Station	☒	☐
(TV Brochure)	☒	☐			

Family M.D. _R. Katz_

Weight _125 lb._ Height _5ft. 2in._   BP:R _—_ L _122/80_

Temp. _103F_   Pulse _92, weak_   Resp _28, shallow_

Source Providing Information ☑ Patient   ☐ Other _____

Unable to Obtain History ☐ _____

Reason for Admission (Onset, Duration, Pt.'s Perception) ("Chest cold" X2 weeks S.O.B on exertion. "Lung pain, fever," "Dr. says I have pneumonia.")

ALLERGIES & REACTIONS

Drugs _Penicillin_

Food/Other _____

Signs & Symptoms _rash, nausea_

Blood Reaction ☐ Yes ☑ No   Dyes/Shellfish ☐ Yes ☑ No

MEDICATIONS

Current Meds	Dose/Freq.	Last Dose
Synthroid	0.1 mg. daily	4-16, 8 a.m.

Disposition of Meds: ☒ Home   ☐ Pharmacy   ☐ Safe   *At Bedside

MEDICAL HISTORY

☑ No Major Problems   ☐ Gastro _____
☐ Cardiac _____   ☐ Arthritis _____
☐ Hyper/Hypotension _____   ☐ Stroke _____
☐ Diabetes _____   ☐ Seizures _____
☐ Cancer _____   ☐ Glaucoma _____
☐ Respiratory _____   ☑ Other _Childbirth-2000_

Surgery/Procedures	Date
Appendectomy	1985
Partial thyroidectomy	2000

SPECIAL ASSISTIVE DEVICES

☐ Wheelchair   ☐ Contacts   ☐ Venous   ☐ Dentures
☐ Braces   ☐ Hearing Aid   Access   ☐ Partial
☐ Cane/Crutches ☐ Prosthesis   Device   ☐ Upper
☐ Walker   ☐ Glasses   ☐ Epidural Catheter ☐ Lower
☐ Other _None_

VALUABLES

Patient informed Hospital not responsible for personal belongings.
Valuables Disposition: ☐ Patient ☐ Safe ☐ Given to _____
Patient/SO Signature _None_

PSYCHOSOCIAL HISTORY

Recent Stress _None_

Coping Mechanism _Not assessed because of fatigue_

Support System _Husband, coworkers, friends_

Calm: ☑ Yes ☐ No

Anxious: ☐ Yes ☐ No _Facial muscles tense; trembling_

Religion _Catholic. Would want Last Rites_

Tobacco Use: ☐ Yes ☑ No _____

Alcohol Use: ☐ Yes ☑ No _____

Drug Use: ☐ Yes ☑ No _____

NEUROLOGICAL

Oriented: ☑ Person ☑ Place ☑ Time ☐ Confused ☐ Sedated
☐ Alert ☐ Restless ☑ Lethargic ☐ Comatose

Pupils: ☑ Equal ☐ Unequal ☑ Reactive ☐ Sluggish
☐ Other _3mm._

Extremity Strength: ☑ Equal ☐ Unequal

Speech: ☑ Clear ☐ Slurred ☐ Other _____

MUSCULO-SKELETAL

Normal ROM of Extremities   ☑ Yes ☐ No

☑ Weakness ☐ Paralysis ☐ Contractures ☐ Joint Swelling ☑ Pain
☐ Other ↓ _related to fatigue_   _when coughing_

RESPIRATORY

Pattern: ☐ Even ☐ Uneven ☑ Shallow ☑ Dyspnea
☑ Other _diminished breath sounds_

Breathing Sounds: ☐ Clear ☑ Other _inspiratory crackles_

Secretions: ☐ None ☑ Other _pink, thick sputum_

Cough: ☐ None ☑ Productive ☐ Nonproductive

CARDIOVASCULAR

Pulses: Apical Rate _92-W_ ☑ Reg. ☐ Irregular ☐ Pacemaker
S = Strong W = Weak A = Absent D = Doppler

Radial R _92_ L _—_   Pedal R _—_ L _—_

Edema: ☑ Absent ☐ Present   Site _____

Perfusion: ☐ Warm ☐ Dry ☑ Diaphoretic ☐ Cool (Hot)

GASTROINTESTINAL

Oral Mucosa ☐ Normal ☑ Other _pale and dry_

Bowel Sounds: ☑ Normal ☐ Other _Abd. soft_

Wt. Change: ☐ ☑ N/V Stool Frequency/Character _1/day; soft_

Last B/M _4-15-07_   ☐ Ostomy (type) _____

Equip. _____

GENITOURINARY

Urine: Last Voided _This morning_

☐ Normal ☐ Anuria ☐ Hematuria ☐ Dysuri ☐ Incontinent

☒ Other ↓ _amount & frequency since ill_

☐ Catheter (type) _____   Other _____

LMP _4-1-07_   ☐ Vaginal/Penile Discharge

Other _____

SELF CARE

Need Assist with: ☐ Ambulating ☐ Elimination
☐ Meals ☒ Hygiene ☐ Dressing
While fatigued

Amanda Aquilini [F. age 28]
#4637651

✸ NORTH BROWARD HOSPITAL DISTRICT
NURSING ADMINISTRATION ASSESSMENT

Figure 11-4 ■ Assessment for Amanda Aquilini.

NUTRITION

General Appearance: ☑ Well Nourished ☐ Emaciated
☐ Other _____
Appetite: ☐ Good ☐ Fair ☑ Poor -x2 days
Diet _Liquid_ Meal Pattern _3/day_
☐ Feeds Self ☐ Assist ☐ Total Feed

SKIN ASSESSMENT

Color: ☐ Normal ☐ Flushed ☑ Pale ☐ Dusky ☐ Cyanotic
☐ Jaundiced ☑ Other _Cheeks flushed, hot_
General Description _Surgical scars:_
RLQ abdomen; anterior neck
_____
_____
_____
Note Cultures Obtained _____
_____
_____

PRESSURE SORE ™AT RISKʃ SCREENING CRITERIA

OVERALL SKIN CONDITION
Grade
- 0 Turgor (elasticity adequate, skin warm and moist)
- ✓ 1 Poor turgor, skin cold & dry
- 2 Areas mottled, red or denuded
- 3 Existing skin ulcer/lesions

BOWEL AND BLADDER CONTROL
Grade
- ✓ 0 Always able to ask for bedpan
- 1 Incontinence of urine
- 2 Incontinence of feces
- 3 Totally incontinent Confined to bed

REHABILITATIVE STATE
Grade
- 0 Fully ambulatory
- ✓ 1 Ambulated with assistance
- 2 Chair to bed ambulation only
- 3 Confined to bed
- 4 Immobile in bed

NUTRITIONAL STATE
Grade
- 0 Eats all
- ✓ 1 Eats very little
- 2 Refuses food often
- 3 Tube feeding
- 4 Intravenous feeding

MENTAL STATE
Grade
- ✓ 0 Alert and clear
- 1 Confused
- 2 Disoriented/senile
- 3 Stuporous
- 4 Unconcious

CHRONIC DISEASE STATUS (i.e. COPD, ASCVD. Peripheral Vascular Disease, Diabetes, or Renal Disease, Cancer, Motor or Sensory Deficits, Elderly, Other)
Grade
- ✓ 0 Absent
- 1 One Present
- 2 Two Present
- 3 Three or more Present

TOTAL _____ Refer to Skin Care Protocol

FALLS SCREENING

If one or more of the following are checked institute fall precautions/plan of care
☐ History of Falls ☐ Unsteady Gait ☐ Confusion/Disorientation ☐ Dizziness
If two or more of the following are checked institute fall precautions/plan of care
☐ Age over 80 ☐ Utilizes cane, walker, w/c ☐ Sleeplessness
☐ Impaired vision ☐ Urgency/frequency in elimination
☐ Multiple Diagnoses ☐ Impaired hearing
☐ Inability to understand or follow directions ☐ Medication/Sedative /Diuretic etc.

EDUCATION/DISCHARGE PLANNING

1. What do you know about your present illness? _"Dr. says I have pneumonia." "I will have an I.V."_
2. What information do you want or need about your illness? _____
3. Would you like family/SO involved in your care? _Husband, Michael_
4. How long do you expect to be in the hospital? _"1-2 days"_
5. What concerns do you have about leaving the hospital? ____

CHECK APPROPRIATE BOX

Will patient need post discharge assistance with ADLs/physical functioning? ☐ Yes ☑ No ☐ Unknown
Does patient have family capable of and willing to provide assistance post discharge?
☑ Yes ☐ No ☐ Unknown ☐ No family
Is assistance needed beyond that which family can provide?
☐ Yes ☑ No ☐ Unknown
Previous admission in the last six months?
☐ Yes ☑ No ☐ Unknown
Patient lives with _Husband and 1 child_
Planned discharge to _Home_
Comments: _Fatigue and anxiety may have interfered with learning. Re-teach anything covered at admission, later._

Social Services Notified ☐ Yes ☑ No

NARRATIVE NOTES

S--c/o sharp chest pain when coughing and dyspnea on exertion. States unable to carry out regular daily exercise for past week. Coughing relieved "if I sit up and sit still." Nausea associated with coughing. Having occasional "chills." Occasionally becomes frightened, stating, "I can't breathe." Well groomed but "too tired to put on make-up." O--Chest expansion < 3cm, no nasal flaring or use of accessory muscles. Breath sounds and insp. crackles in Ⓡ upper and lower chest. Assesses own supports as "good" (eg, relationship c̄ husband). Is "worried" about daughter. States husband will be out of town until tomorrow. Left 3-year-old daughter with neighbor. Concerned too about her work (is attorney). "I'll never get caught up." Had water at noon—no food today. Agrees to save urine for 24 hr. specimen. IV D₅W LR 1000 mL started in Ⓡ arm, 100 mL/hr. Slow capillary refill. Keeping head of bed↑ to facilitate breathing.

NURSE SIGNATURE/TITLE	DATE	TIME
Mary Medina, RN	4-16-07	3:30pm
NURSE SIGNATURE/TITLE	DATE	TIME

**✬ NORTH BROWARD HOSPITAL DISTRICT
NURSING ADMINISTRATION ASSESSMENT**

Figure 11-4 ■ continued

BOX 11—4   Gordon's Typology of 11 Functional Health Patterns

- *Health-perception/health-management pattern.* Describes the client's perceived pattern of health and well-being and how health is managed.
- *Nutritional-metabolic pattern.* Describes the client's pattern of food and fluid consumption relative to metabolic need and pattern indicators of local nutrient supply.
- *Elimination pattern.* Describes the patterns of excretory function (bowel, bladder, and skin).
- *Activity-exercise pattern.* Describes the pattern of exercise, activity, leisure, and recreation.
- *Sleep-rest pattern.* Describes patterns of sleep, rest, and relaxation.
- *Cognitive-perceptual pattern.* Describes sensory-perceptual and cognitive patterns.

- *Self-perception/self-concept pattern.* Describes the client's self-concept pattern and perceptions of self (e.g., self-conception/worth, comfort, body image, feeling state).
- *Role-relationship pattern.* Describes the client's pattern of role participation and relationships.
- *Sexuality-reproductive pattern.* Describes the client's patterns of satisfaction and dissatisfaction with sexuality pattern; describes reproductive patterns.
- *Coping/stress-tolerance pattern.* Describes the client's general coping pattern and the effectiveness of the pattern in terms of stress tolerance.
- *Value-belief pattern.* Describes the patterns of values, beliefs (including spiritual), and goals that guide the client's choices or decisions.

Note: From *Manual of Nursing Diagnosis,* 11th ed. (pp. 2–5), by M. Gordon, 2006, Boston: Jones & Bartlett. Reprinted with permission.

Body Systems Model

The body systems model focuses on abnormalities of the following anatomic systems:

- Integumentary system
- Respiratory system
- Cardiovascular system
- Nervous system
- Musculoskeletal system
- Gastrointestinal system
- Genitourinary system
- Reproductive system
- Immune system

Maslow's Hierarchy of Needs

Maslow's hierarchy of needs clusters data pertaining to the following:

- Physiologic needs (survival needs)
- Safety and security needs
- Love and belonging needs
- Self-esteem needs
- Self-actualization needs

See Chapter 16 ∞ for details.

Developmental Theories

Several physical, psychosocial, cognitive, and moral developmental theories may be used by the nurse in specific situations. Examples include the following:

BOX 11—5   Orem's Self-Care Model

UNIVERSAL SELF-CARE REQUISITES

1. The maintenance of a sufficient intake of air.
2. The maintenance of a sufficient intake of water.
3. The maintenance of a sufficient intake of food.
4. The provision of care associated with elimination processes and excrement.
5. The maintenance of a balance between activity and rest.
6. The maintenance of a balance between solitude and social interaction.
7. The prevention of hazards to human life, human functioning, and human well-being.
8. The promotion of human functioning and development within social groups in accord with human potential, known human limitations, and human desire to be normal. (Normalcy is used in the sense of that which is essentially human and that which is in accord with the genetic and constitutional characteristics and the talents of individuals.)

Note: Adapted from *Nursing: Concepts of Practice,* 6th ed. D. E. Orem, p. 225, Copyright 2001, with permission from Elsevier.

BOX 11—6   Roy's Adaptation Model

ADAPTIVE MODES

1. Physiologic needs
   - Activity and rest
   - Nutrition
   - Elimination
   - Fluid and electrolytes
   - Oxygenation
   - Protection
   - Regulation: temperature
   - Regulation: the senses
   - Regulation: endocrine system
2. Self-concept
   - Physical self
   - Personal self
3. Role function
4. Interdependence

Note: Adapted from *The Roy Adaptation Model: The Definitive Statement,* 2nd ed., by C. Roy and H. A. Andrews, 1999, Upper Saddle River, NJ: Prentice-Hall.

BOX 11–7 Data for Amanda Aquilini, Organized According to Functional Health Patterns

HEALTH PERCEPTION/HEALTH MANAGEMENT
- Aware/understands medical diagnosis
- Gives thorough history of illnesses and surgeries
- Complies with Synthroid regimen
- Relates progression of illness in detail
- Expects to have antibiotic therapy and "go home in a day or two"
- States usual eating pattern "3 meals a day"

NUTRITIONAL/METABOLIC
- 158 cm (5 ft, 2 in) tall; weighs 56 kg (125 lb)
- Usual eating pattern "3 meals a day"
- "No appetite" since having "cold"
- Has not eaten today; last fluids at noon
- Nauseated
- Oral temperature 39.4°C (103°F)
- Decreased skin turgor

ELIMINATION
- Usually no problem
- Decreased urinary frequency and amount × 2 days
- Last bowel movement yesterday, formed, states was "normal"

ACTIVITY/EXERCISE
- No musculoskeletal impairment
- Difficulty sleeping because of cough
- "Can't breathe lying down"
- States "I feel weak"
- Short of breath on exertion
- Exercises daily

COGNITIVE/PERCEPTUAL
- No sensory deficits
- Pupils 3 mm, equal, brisk reaction
- Oriented to time, place, and person
- Responsive, but fatigued
- Responds appropriately to verbal and physical stimuli
- Recent and remote memory intact
- States "short of breath" on exertion
- Reports "pain in lungs," especially when coughing
- Experiencing chills
- Reports nausea

ROLES/RELATIONSHIPS
- Lives with husband and 3-year-old daughter
- Husband out of town; will be back tomorrow afternoon
- Child with neighbor until husband returns
- States "good" relationships with friends and co-workers
- Working mother, attorney

SELF-PERCEPTION/SELF-CONCEPT
- Expresses "concern" and "worry" over leaving daughter with neighbors until husband returns
- Well-groomed, says, "Too tired to put on makeup"

COPING/STRESS
- Anxious: "I can't breathe"
- Facial muscles tense; trembling
- Expresses concerns about work: "I'll never get caught up"

VALUE/BELIEF
- Catholic
- No special practices desired except anointing of the sick
- Middle-class, professional orientation
- No wish to see chaplain or priest at present

MEDICATION/HISTORY
- Synthroid 0.1 mg per day
- Client has history of appendectomy, partial thyroidectomy

NURSING PHYSICAL ASSESSMENT
- 28 years old
- Height 158 cm (5 ft, 2 in); weight 56 kg (125 lb)
- TPR 39.4°C, 92, 28
- Radial pulses weak, regular
- Blood pressure 122/80 sitting
- Skin hot and pale, cheeks flushed
- Mucous membranes dry and pale
- Respirations shallow; chest expansion < 3 cm
- Cough productive of small amounts of pale pink sputum
- Inspiratory crackles auscultated throughout right upper and lower chest
- Diminished breath sounds on right side
- Abdomen soft, not distended
- Old surgical scars: anterior neck, RLQ abdomen
- Diaphoretic

- Havighurst's age periods and developmental tasks
- Freud's five stages of development
- Erikson's eight stages of development
- Piaget's phases of cognitive development
- Kohlberg's stages of moral development

See Chapter 20 ∞ for additional information.

VALIDATING DATA

The information gathered during the assessment phase must be complete, factual, and accurate because the nursing diagnoses and interventions are based on this information. **Validation** is the act of "double-checking" or verifying data to confirm that it is accurate and factual. Validating data helps the nurse complete these tasks:

- Ensure that assessment information is complete.
- Ensure that objective and related subjective data agree.
- Obtain additional information that may have been overlooked.
- Differentiate between cues and inferences. **Cues** are subjective or objective data that can be directly observed by the nurse; that is, what the client says or what the nurse can see, hear, feel, smell, or measure. **Inferences** are the nurse's interpretation or conclusions made based on the cues (e.g., a nurse observes the cues that an incision is red, hot, and swollen; the nurse makes the inference that the incision is infected).

TABLE 11–6 Validating Assessment Data

GUIDELINES	EXAMPLE
Compare subjective and objective data to verify the client's statements with your observations.	Client's perceptions of "feeling hot" need to be compared with measurement of the body temperature.
Clarify any ambiguous or vague statements.	*Client:* "I've felt sick on and off for 6 weeks."
	Nurse: "Describe what your sickness is like. Tell me what you mean by 'on and off.'"
Be sure your data consist of cues and not inferences.	*Observation:* Dry skin and reduced tissue turgor
	Inference: Dehydration
	Action: Collect additional data that are needed to make the inference in the diagnosing phase. For example, determine the client's fluid intake, amount and appearance of urine, and blood pressure.
Double-check data that are extremely abnormal.	*Observation:* A resting pulse of 30 beats per minute or a blood pressure of 210/95
	Action: Repeat the measurement. Use another piece of equipment as needed to confirm abnormalities, or ask someone else to collect the same data.
Determine the presence of factors that may interfere with accurate measurement.	A crying infant will have an abnormal respiratory rate and will need quieting before accurate assessment can be made.
Use references (textbooks, journals, research reports) to explain phenomena.	A nurse considers tiny purple or bluish black swollen areas under the tongue of an elderly client to be abnormal until reading about physical changes of aging. Such varicosities are common.

■ Avoid jumping to conclusions and focusing in the wrong direction to identify problems.

Not all data require validation. For example, data such as height, weight, birth date, and most laboratory studies that can be measured with an accurate scale can be accepted as factual. As a rule, the nurse validates data when there are discrepancies between data obtained in the nursing interview (subjective data) and the physical examination (objective data), or when the client's statements differ at different times in the assessment. Guidelines for validating data are shown in Table 11–6.

To collect data accurately, nurses need to be aware of their own biases, values, and beliefs and to separate fact from inference, interpretation, and assumption (see Chapter 10 ∞). For example, a nurse seeing a man holding his arm to his chest might assume that he is experiencing chest pain, when in fact he has a painful hand.

To build an accurate database, nurses must validate assumptions regarding the client's physical or emotional behavior. In the previous example, the nurse should ask the client why he is holding his arm to his chest. The client's response may validate the

nurse's assumptions or prompt further questioning. Figure 11-4 indicates that the nurse auscultated Amanda Aquilini's heart and lungs to validate her statement that she had "lung pain" and "shortness of breath" on exertion. Failure to validate assumptions can lead to an inaccurate or incomplete nursing assessment and could compromise client safety.

DOCUMENTING DATA

To complete the assessment phase, the nurse records client data. Accurate documentation is essential and should include all data collected about the client's health status. Data are recorded in a factual manner and not interpreted by the nurse. For example, the nurse records the client's breakfast intake (objective data) as "coffee 240 mL, juice 120 mL, 1 egg, and 1 slice of toast," rather than as "appetite good" (a judgment). A judgment or conclusion such as "appetite good" or "normal appetite" may have different meanings for different people. To increase accuracy, the nurse records subjective data in the client's own words, using quotation marks. Restating in other words what someone says increases the chance of changing the original meaning (see Chapter 15 ∞).

LIFESPAN CONSIDERATIONS Assessment

CHILDREN

Consider this example: A 4-year-old girl is admitted following emergency surgery for a ruptured appendix. She is awake and alert, but refuses to talk. Her parents have had little sleep for over 24 hours and are extremely anxious.

■ Gathering assessment data in this situation requires the nurse to be sensitive to the parents' needs for rest and assurance; at the same time, the nurse must collect information to compile an adequate database for appropriate nursing care decisions. Assessment will be problem focused, monitoring the condition of the child as she recovers from surgery and being alert to potential problems.

■ The parents become the major source of subjective data, although the child should be encouraged to tell the nurse how she is feeling.

■ Objective data collected include vital signs; level of and response to pain (often called the fifth vital sign); bleeding or discharge from the incision; mobility; integrity of dressings, intravenous lines, catheters, nasogastric tubes, or other medical devices; and affect.

■ Since children are a part of families, assessment will include observation of family dynamics and questions that could lead to care of the family system.

CRITICAL THINKING CHECKPOINT

Eighty-two-year-old Ms. T. is in the hospital for hip replacement surgery.

1. What are the key areas of information to obtain regarding her past history?
2. Which physiological systems are the most important for data collection before her surgery?
3. What exactly would you say to her to determine if someone will be at home to assist her after discharge?
4. Which other sources of data might be appropriate to access in her case?

See Critical Thinking Possibilities in Appendix A.

CHAPTER 11 REVIEW

CHAPTER HIGHLIGHTS

- The nursing process is a systematic, rational method of planning and providing individualized nursing care for individuals, families, groups, and communities.
- The goals of the nursing process are to identify a client's actual or potential health care needs, to establish plans to meet the identified needs, and to deliver and evaluate specific nursing interventions to meet those needs.
- The nursing process can be used in all health care settings. It is cyclic and dynamic, client centered, interpersonal and collaborative, and universally applicable, and it focuses on problem solving and decision making.
- The nursing process is organized into five interrelated, interdependent phases: assessing, diagnosing, planning, implementing, and evaluating.
- Assessing involves collecting, organizing, validating, and recording data.
- Diagnosing is the process of making a clinical judgment (nursing diagnosis) about a client's potential or actual health problems.
- Planning involves setting priorities, writing goals/desired outcomes, and establishing a written plan for nursing interventions.
- Implementing is carrying out the nursing interventions. It incorporates all the activities performed to promote health, prevent complications, treat present problems, and facilitate the client's coping with chronic alterations in health status.
- Evaluating is the process of comparing client responses to preselected outcomes to determine whether goals have been met. It includes review and modification of the care plan.

- Assessment involves active participation by the client and nurse in obtaining subjective and objective data about the client's health status.
- The client is the primary source of data. Secondary sources are family, friends, health team members, the health record, and pertinent literature.
- Subjective data are the client's personal perceptions, often gathered during the nursing health history.
- Objective data (e.g., data observed and collected during the physical examination) are detectable by an observer.
- The primary methods of data collection are observing, interviewing, and examining.
- Observation is a conscious, deliberate skill involving use of the senses.
- The nurse uses a combination of directive and nondirective interviewing (including closed and open-ended questions) to obtain the nursing health history.
- Nursing models provide formats for collecting and organizing client data.
- The nursing assessment must be complete and accurate because nursing diagnoses and interventions are based on this information.
- Some data must be validated. Subjective data can be used to validate objective data, and vice versa. Primary and secondary data can also be used to validate each other.
- Data must be recorded in a factual manner, without interpretation or inferences.

TEST YOUR KNOWLEDGE

1. Which of the following behaviors is most representative of the *nursing diagnosis* phase of the nursing process?
   1. Identifying major problems or needs
   2. Organizing data in the client's family history
   3. Establishing short-term and long-term goals
   4. Administering an antibiotic

2. Which of the following behaviors would indicate that the nurse was utilizing the assessment phase of the nursing process to provide nursing care?
   1. Proposes hypotheses
   2. Generates desired outcomes
   3. Reviews results of laboratory tests
   4. Documents care

3. Which of the following elements is best categorized as secondary subjective data?
   1. The nurse measures a weight loss of 10 pounds since the last clinic visit.
   2. Spouse states the client has lost all appetite.
   3. The nurse palpates edema in lower extremities.
   4. Client states severe pain when walking up stairs.

4. The nurse wishes to determine the client's feelings about a recent diagnosis. Which interview question is most likely to elicit this information?
   1. "What did the doctor tell you about your diagnosis?"
   2. "Are you worried about how the diagnosis will affect you in the future?"
   3. "Tell me about your reactions to the diagnosis."
   4. "How is your family responding to the diagnosis?"

5. The use of a conceptual or theoretical framework for collecting and organizing assessment data ensures which of the following?
   1. Correlation of the data with other members of the health care team
   2. Demonstration of cost-effective care
   3. Utilization of creativity and intuition in creating a plan of care
   4. Collection of all necessary information for a thorough appraisal

See Answers to Test Your Knowledge in Appendix A. ∞

EXPLORE MEDIALINK www.prenhall.com/berman

DVD-ROM
- Audio Glossary
- NCLEX Review
- Animations:
    Anatomical Landmarks
    Introduction to Body Systems
    A & P Review:
        Anterior View
        Posterior View
        Body Cavity
        Lymphatic System
        Body Organization

COMPANION WEBSITE
- Additional NCLEX Review
- Case Study: Down's Syndrome Client
- Application Activity:
    Care of a Disorganized Elderly Client
- Links to Resources

READINGS AND REFERENCES

SUGGESTED READINGS
Shattell, M. (2004). Nurse-patient interaction: A review of the literature. *Journal of Clinical Nursing, 13*, 714–722.
This article reviews a theoretical model for developing nursing knowledge related to nurse–patient interaction, reviews the literature on nurse–patient interaction, and discusses areas for further research. Issues such as power, the social and cultural context, and interpersonal competence are important in the quality of nurse–patient interactions, and nurses need to take cognizance of these factors in their interactions with patients.

RELATED RESEARCH
Hendry, C., & Walker, A. (2004). Priority setting in clinical nursing practice: Literature review. *Journal of Advanced Nursing, 47*, 427–436.

REFERENCES
American Nurses Association. (1973). *Standards of nursing practice*. Kansas City, MO: Author.
American Nurses Association. (2004). *Nursing: Scope and standards of nursing practice*. Kansas City, MO: Author.

D'Amico, D., & Barbarito, C. (2007). *Health & physical assessment in nursing*. Upper Saddle River, NJ: Pearson Prentice Hall.
Gordon, M. (2006). *Manual of nursing diagnosis* (11th ed.). Boston: Jones & Bartlett.
Hall, L. (1955, June). Quality of nursing care. *Public Health News*. Newark, NJ: State Department of Health.
Johnson, D. E. (1959). A philosophy of nursing. *Nursing Outlook, 7*, 198–200.
Joint Commission on Accreditation of Healthcare Organizations. (2005). *2005 Comprehensive accreditation manual for hospitals*. Chicago: Author.
Orem, D. E. (2001). *Nursing: Concepts of practice* (6th ed.). St. Louis, MO: Mosby.
Orlando, I. (1961). *The dynamic nurse–patient relationship*. New York: Putnam.
Roy, C., & Andrews, H. A. (1998). *The Roy adaptation model* (2nd ed.). Upper Saddle River, NJ: Prentice Hall.
Stewart, C. J., & Cash, Jr., W. B. (2006). *Interviewing principles and practices* (11th ed.). New York: McGraw-Hill.

Wiedenbach, E. (1963). The helping art of nursing. *American Journal of Nursing, 63*(11), 54–57.
Wilkinson, J. M. (2007). *Nursing process & critical thinking* (4th ed.). Upper Saddle River, NJ: Prentice Hall.

SELECTED BIBLIOGRAPHY
Ackley, B. J., & Ladwig, G. B. (2003). *Nursing diagnosis handbook: A guide to planning care* (5th ed.). St. Louis, MO: Mosby.
Alfaro-LeFevre, R. A. (2005). *Applying the nursing process: Promoting collaborative care* (6th ed.). Philadelphia: Lippincott Williams & Wilkins.
Alfaro-LeFevre, R. A. (2005). *The nursing process made easy: Concept mapping and care planning for students*. Philadelphia: Lippincott Williams & Wilkins.
Gardner, P. (2003). *Nursing process in action*. Albany, NY: Delmar.
Olenek, K., Skowronski, T., & Schmaltz, D. (2003). Geriatric nursing assessment. *Journal of Gerontological Nursing, 29*, 5–9.

Diagnosing

LEARNING OUTCOMES

After completing this chapter, you will be able to:

1. Differentiate various types of nursing diagnoses.

2. Identify the components of a nursing diagnosis.

3. Compare nursing diagnoses, medical diagnoses, and collaborative problems.

4. Identify basic steps in the diagnostic process.

5. Describe various formats for writing nursing diagnoses.

6. Describe the characteristics of a nursing diagnosis.

7. List guidelines for writing a nursing diagnosis statement.

8. Describe the evolution of the nursing diagnosis movement, including work currently in progress.

9. List advantages of a taxonomy of nursing diagnoses.

Diagnosing is the second phase of the nursing process. In this phase, nurses use critical-thinking skills to interpret assessment data and identify client strengths and problems. Diagnosing is a pivotal step in the nursing process. Activities preceding this phase are directed toward formulating the nursing diagnoses; the care-planning activities following this phase are based on the nursing diagnoses (see Figure 12-1■).

The identification and development of nursing diagnoses began formally in 1973, when two faculty members of Saint Louis University, Kristine Gebbie and Mary Ann Lavin, perceived a need to identify nurses' roles in an ambulatory care setting. The First National Conference to identify nursing diagnoses was sponsored by the Saint Louis University School of Nursing and Allied Health Professions in 1973. Subsequent national conferences occurred in 1975, in 1980, and every 2 years thereafter.

International recognition came with the First Canadian Conference in Toronto in 1977 and the International Nursing Conference in May 1987 in Calgary, Alberta, Canada. In 1982, the conference group accepted the name North American Nursing Diagnosis Association (NANDA), recognizing the participation and contributions of nurses in the United States and Canada.

The purpose of NANDA is to define, refine, and promote a taxonomy of nursing diagnostic terminology of general use to professional nurses. A **taxonomy** is a classification system or set of categories arranged based on a single principle or set of principles. The members of NANDA include staff nurses, clinical specialists, faculty, directors of nursing, deans, theorists, and researchers. The group has currently approved more than 170 nursing diagnosis labels for clinical use and testing. In 2000, Taxonomy I was revised and is now referred to as Taxonomy II (see the list in Appendix C on page 1530). ∞

NANDA NURSING DIAGNOSES

To use the concept of nursing diagnoses effectively in generating and completing a nursing care plan, the nurse must be familiar with the definitions of terms used, the types, and the components of nursing diagnoses.

Definitions

The term *diagnosing* refers to the reasoning process, whereas the term **diagnosis** is a statement or conclusion regarding the nature of a phenomenon. The standardized NANDA names for the diagnoses are called **diagnostic labels;** and the client's problem statement, consisting of the diagnostic label plus **etiology** (causal relationship between a problem and its related or risk factors), is called a **nursing diagnosis.**

In 1990, NANDA adopted an official working definition of nursing diagnosis: ". . . a clinical judgment about individual, family, or community responses to actual and potential health problems/life processes. A nursing diagnosis provides the basis for selection of nursing interventions to achieve outcomes for which the nurse is accountable" (as cited in NANDA International, 2005, p. 277). This definition implies the following:

- Professional nurses (registered nurses) are responsible for making nursing diagnoses, even though other nursing personnel may contribute data to the process of diagnosing and may implement specified nursing care. The American Nurses Association *Nursing: Scope and Standards of Practice* (2004) state that nurses are accountable for this phase of the nursing process. The Joint Commission on Accreditation of Healthcare Organizations (JCAHO) requires evidence of nursing diagnoses in clients' medical records as well (JCAHO, 2005).

- The domain of nursing diagnosis includes only those health states that nurses are educated and licensed to treat. For example, generalist nurses are not educated to diagnose or treat diseases such as diabetes mellitus; this task is defined legally as within the practice of medicine. Yet nurses can diagnose and treat *Deficient Knowledge, Ineffective Coping,* or *Imbalanced Nutrition,* all of which are

Figure 12-1 ■ Diagnosing. The pivotal second phase of the nursing process.

the human responses to the medical diagnosis of diabetes mellitus.

- A nursing diagnosis is a judgment made only after thorough, systematic data collection.
- Nursing diagnoses describe a continuum of health states: deviations from health, presence of risk factors, and areas of enhanced personal growth.

Types of Nursing Diagnoses

The five types of nursing diagnoses are actual, risk, wellness, possible, and syndrome.

1. An *actual diagnosis* is a client problem that is present at the time of the nursing assessment. Examples are *Ineffective Breathing Pattern* and *Anxiety*. An actual nursing diagnosis is based on the presence of associated signs and symptoms.
2. A **risk nursing diagnosis** is a clinical judgment that a problem does not exist, but the presence of **risk factors** indicates that a problem is likely to develop unless nurses intervene. For example, all people admitted to a hospital have some possibility of acquiring an infection; however, a client with diabetes or a compromised immune system is at higher risk than others. Therefore, the nurse would appropriately use the label *Risk for Infection* to describe the client's health status.
3. A **wellness diagnosis** "Describes human responses to levels of wellness in an individual, family or community that have a readiness for enhancement" (NANDA International, 2005, p. 277). Examples of wellness diagnoses would be *Readiness for Enhanced Spiritual Well-Being* or *Readiness for Enhanced Family Coping*.
4. A **possible nursing diagnosis** is one in which evidence about a health problem is incomplete or unclear. A possible diagnosis requires more data either to support or to refute it. For example, an elderly widow who lives alone is admitted to the hospital. The nurse notices that she has no visitors and is pleased with attention and conversation from the nursing staff. Until more data are collected, the nurse may write a nursing diagnosis of *Possible Social Isolation* related to unknown etiology.
5. A **syndrome diagnosis** is a diagnosis that is associated with a cluster of other diagnoses (Carpenito-Moyet, 2006). Currently six syndrome diagnoses are on the NANDA International list. *Risk for Disuse Syndrome*, for example, may be experienced by long-term bedridden clients. Clusters of diagnoses associated with this syndrome include *Impaired Physical Mobility, Risk for Impaired Tissue Integrity, Risk for Activity Intolerance, Risk for Constipation, Risk for Infection, Risk for Injury, Risk for Powerlessness, Impaired Gas Exchange*, and so on.

Components of a NANDA Nursing Diagnosis

A nursing diagnosis has three components: (1) the problem and its definition, (2) the etiology, and (3) the defining characteristics. Each component serves a specific purpose.

Problem (Diagnostic Label) and Definition

The problem statement, or diagnostic label, describes the client's health problem or response for which nursing therapy is given. It describes the client's health status clearly and concisely in a few words. The purpose of the diagnostic label is to direct the formation of client goals and desired outcomes. It may also suggest some nursing interventions.

To be clinically useful, diagnostic labels need to be specific; when the word *Specify* follows a NANDA label, the nurse states the area in which the problem occurs, for example, *Deficient Knowledge (Medications)* or *Deficient Knowledge (Dietary Adjustments)*.

Qualifiers are words that have been added to some NANDA labels to give additional meaning to the diagnostic statement; for example:

- *Deficient* (inadequate in amount, quality, or degree; not sufficient; incomplete)
- *Impaired* (made worse, weakened, damaged, reduced, deteriorated)
- *Decreased* (lesser in size, amount, or degree)
- *Ineffective* (not producing the desired effect)
- *Compromised* (to make vulnerable to threat)

Each diagnostic label approved by NANDA carries a definition that clarifies its meaning. For example, the definition of the diagnostic label *Activity Intolerance* is shown in Table 12–1.

Etiology (Related Factors and Risk Factors)

The etiology component of a nursing diagnosis identifies one or more probable causes of the health problem, gives direction to the required nursing therapy, and enables the nurse to individualize the client's care. As shown in Table 12–1, the probable

TABLE 12–1 **Components of a Nursing Diagnosis**		
DIAGNOSIS AND DEFINITION	**RELATED FACTORS**	**DEFINING CHARACTERISTICS**
Activity Intolerance: Insufficient physiological or psychological energy to endure or complete required or desired daily activities	Bedrest or immobility Generalized weakness Imbalance between oxygen supply/demand Sedentary lifestyle	Verbal report of fatigue or weakness Abnormal heart rate or blood pressure response to activity Electrocardiographic changes reflecting arrhythmias or ischemia Exertional discomfort or dyspnea

Note: From Definitions and Classification, 2003–2004, by NANDA International, 2003, Philadelphia, PA. Adapted with permission.

TABLE 12–2   Examples of Nursing Diagnoses with Different Etiologies

DIAGNOSTIC LABEL (PROBLEM)	CLIENT	ETIOLOGY
Constipation	Al Martinez	Long-term laxative use
	Jerry Wong	Inactivity and insufficient fluid intake
Anxiety	Tanya Brown	Threat to physiologic integrity: possible cancer diagnosis
	Caitlin Shea	Effects of aging (reduced hearing, vision, mobility)

causes of *Activity Intolerance* include sedentary lifestyle, generalized weakness, and so on. Differentiating among possible causes in the nursing diagnosis is essential because each may require different nursing interventions. Table 12–2 provides examples of problems that have different etiologies and therefore require different interventions.

Defining Characteristics

Defining characteristics are the cluster of signs and symptoms that indicate the presence of a particular diagnostic label. For actual nursing diagnoses, the defining characteristics are the client's signs and symptoms. For risk nursing diagnoses, no subjective and objective signs are present. Thus, the factors that cause the client to be more vulnerable to the problem form the etiology of a risk nursing diagnosis.

The NANDA lists of defining characteristics are still being developed and refined. Characteristics are listed separately according to whether they are subjective or objective in nature.

Differentiating Nursing Diagnoses from Medical Diagnoses

A nursing diagnosis is a statement of nursing judgment and refers to a condition that nurses, by virtue of their education, experience, and expertise, are licensed to treat. A medical diagnosis is made by a physician and refers to a condition that only a physician can treat. Medical diagnoses refer to disease processes—specific pathophysiologic responses that are fairly uniform from one client to another. In contrast, nursing diagnoses describe the human response, a client's physical, sociocultural, psychologic, and spiritual responses to an illness or a health problem. See how these responses vary among individuals:

Seventy-year-old Mary Cain and 20-year-old Kristi Vidan both have rheumatoid arthritis. Their disease processes are much the same. X-ray studies show that in both clients, the extent of inflammation and the number of joints involved are similar, and both clients experience almost constant pain. Ms. Cain views her condition as part of the aging process and is responding with acceptance. Ms. Vidan, however, is responding with anger and hostil-

ity because she views her disease as a threat to her personal identity, role performance, and self-esteem.

A client's medical diagnosis remains the same for as long as the disease process is present, but nursing diagnoses change as the client's responses change. Ms. Vidan's response to her illness may change over time to become more similar to that of Ms. Cain.

Nurses have responsibilities related to both medical and nursing diagnoses. Nursing diagnoses relate to the nurse's **independent functions,** that is, the areas of health care that are unique to nursing and separate and distinct from medical management.

It is possible that the nurse cannot prescribe all the care for a nursing diagnosis, but the nurse can prescribe most of the interventions needed for prevention or resolution. For example, most clients with a nursing diagnosis of *Pain* have medical orders for analgesics, but many independent nursing interventions can also alleviate pain (e.g., guided imagery or teaching a client to "splint" an incision). With regard to medical diagnoses, nurses are obligated to carry out physician-prescribed therapies and treatments, that is, **dependent functions.** See Chapter 13 ∞ for a discussion of independent and dependent nursing interventions.

Differentiating Nursing Diagnoses from Collaborative Problems

A collaborative problem is a type of potential problem that nurses manage using both independent and physician-prescribed interventions. Independent nursing interventions for a collaborative problem focus mainly on monitoring the client's condition and preventing development of the potential complication. Definitive treatment of the condition requires both medical and nursing interventions.

Collaborative problems are present when a particular disease or treatment is present; that is, each disease or treatment has specific complications that are always associated with it. For example, a statement of collaborative problems is "Potential complication of pneumonia: atelectasis, respiratory failure, pleural effusion, pericarditis, and meningitis."

Nursing diagnoses, by contrast, involve human responses, which vary greatly from one person to the next. Therefore, the same set of nursing diagnoses cannot be expected to occur with all persons who have a particular disease or condition; moreover, a single nursing diagnosis may occur as a response to any number of diseases. For example, all postpartum clients have similar collaborative problems, such as "Potential complication of childbearing: postpartum hemorrhage," but not all new mothers have the same nursing diagnoses. Some might experience *Impaired Parenting* (delayed bonding), but most will not; some might have *Deficient Knowledge* whereas others will not. Thus, the nurse uses nursing diagnoses rather than collaborative problems whenever possible, since nursing diagnoses are more individualized to a specific client and emphasize human responses to which the nurse can independently take action. Table 12–3 provides a comparison of nursing diagnoses, medical problems, and collaborative problems.

TABLE 12–3	**Comparison of Nursing Diagnoses, Medical Diagnoses, and Collaborative Problems**		
	NURSING DIAGNOSES	**MEDICAL DIAGNOSES**	**COLLABORATIVE PROBLEMS**
Example	*Activity Intolerance* related to decreased cardiac output	Myocardial infarction	Potential complication of myocardial infarction: congestive heart failure
Description	Describe human responses to disease process or health problem; consist of a one-, two-, or three-part statement, usually including problem and etiology	Describe disease and pathology; do not consider other human responses; usually consist of not more than three words	Involve human responses—mainly physiologic complications of disease, tests, or treatments; consist of a two-part statement of situation/pathophysiology and the potential complication
Orientation and responsibility for diagnosing	Oriented to the individual; nurses responsible for diagnosing	Oriented to pathology; physician responsible for diagnosing; diagnosis not within the scope of nursing practice	Oriented to pathophysiology; nurses responsible for diagnosing
Nursing focus	Treat and prevent	Implement medical orders for treatment and monitor status of condition	Prevent and monitor for onset or status of condition
Nursing actions	Independent	Dependent (primarily)	Some independent actions, but primarily for monitoring and preventing
Duration	Can change frequently	Remains the same while disease is present	Present when disease or situation is present
Classification system	Classification system is developed and being used but is not universally accepted	Well-developed classification system accepted by the medical profession	No universally accepted classification system

THE DIAGNOSTIC PROCESS

The diagnostic process uses the critical-thinking skills of analysis and synthesis. Critical thinking is a cognitive process during which a person reviews data and considers explanations before forming an opinion. Analysis is the separation into components, that is, the breaking down of the whole into its parts (deductive reasoning). Synthesis is the opposite, that is, the putting together of parts into the whole (inductive reasoning). See Chapter 10 ∞ to review the concepts of deductive and inductive reasoning.

The diagnostic process is used continuously by most nurses. An experienced nurse may enter a client's room and immediately observe significant data and draw conclusions about the client. As a result of attaining knowledge, skill, and expertise in the practice setting, the expert nurse may seem to perform these mental processes automatically. Novice nurses, however, need guidelines to understand and formulate nursing diagnoses. The diagnostic process has three steps:

- Analyzing data
- Identifying health problems, risks, and strengths
- Formulating diagnostic statements

Analyzing Data

In the diagnostic process, analyzing involves the following steps:

1. Compare data against standards (identify significant cues).
2. Cluster cues (generate tentative hypotheses).
3. Identify gaps and inconsistencies.

For experienced nurses, these activities occur continuously rather than sequentially.

Comparing Data with Standards

Nurses draw on knowledge and experience to compare client data to standards and norms and identify significant and relevant cues. A **standard** or **norm** is a generally accepted measure, rule, model, or pattern. The nurse uses a wide range of standards, such as growth and development patterns, normal vital signs, and laboratory values. A cue is considered significant if it does any of the following:

- Points to negative or positive change in a client's health status or pattern. For example, the client states: "I have recently experienced shortness of breath while climbing stairs" or "I have not smoked for 3 months."
- Varies from norms of the client population. The client's pattern may fit within cultural norms but vary from norms of the general society. The client may consider a pattern—for example, eating very small meals and having little appetite—to be normal. This pattern, however, may not be healthy and may require further exploration.
- Indicates a developmental delay. To identify significant cues, the nurse must be aware of the normal patterns and changes that occur as the person grows and develops. For example, by age 9 months an infant is usually able to sit alone without support. The infant who has not accomplished this task needs further assessment for possible developmental delays.

TABLE 12-4 Comparing Cues to Standards and Norms

TYPE OF CUE	CLIENT CUES	STANDARD/NORM
Deviation from population norms	Height is 158 cm (5 ft, 2 in). Woman with small frame. Weighs 109 kg (240 lb).	Height and weight tables indicate that the "ideal" weight for a woman 158 cm (5 ft, 2 in) with a small frame is 49–53 kg (108–121 lb).
Developmental delay	Child is 17 months old. Parents state child has not yet attempted to speak. Child laughs aloud and makes cooing sounds.	Children usually speak their first word by 10 to 12 months of age.
Changes in client's usual health status	States, "I'm just not hungry these days." Ate only 15% of food on breakfast tray. Has lost 13 kg (30 lb) in past 3 months.	Client usually eats three balanced meals per day. Adults typically maintain stable weight.
Dysfunctional behavior	Amy's mother reports that Amy has not left her room for 2 days. Amy is age 16. Amy has stopped attending school and has withdrawn from social contact.	Adolescents usually like to be with their peers; social group very important. Functional behavior includes school attendance.
Changes in client's usual behavior	Mrs. Stuart reports that lately her husband angers easily. "Yesterday he even yelled at the dog." "He just seems so tense."	Mr. Stuart is usually relaxed and easygoing. He is friendly and kind to animals.

Table 12–4 lists specific examples of client cues and norms to which they may be compared.

Clustering Cues

Data clustering or grouping cues is a process of determining the relatedness of facts and determining whether any patterns are present, whether the data represent isolated incidents, and whether the data are significant. This is the beginning of synthesis.

The nurse may cluster data inductively (as in Table 12–5) by combining data from different assessment areas to form a pattern. Or the nurse may begin with a framework, such as Gordon's functional health patterns, and organize the subjective and objective data into the appropriate categories (see Box 11–4, page 190). The latter is a deductive approach to data clustering (see Chapter 10). ∞

Experienced nurses may cluster data as they collect and interpret it, as evidenced in remarks or thoughts such as "I'm getting a sense of . . . " or "This cue doesn't fit the picture." The novice nurse does not have the knowledge base or the clinical experience that aids in recognizing cues. Thus, the novice must take careful assessment notes, search data for abnormal cues, and use textbook resources for comparing the client's cues with the defining characteristics and etiologic factors of the accepted nursing diagnoses.

Data clustering involves making inferences about the data. The nurse interprets the possible meaning of the cues, and labels the cue clusters with tentative diagnostic hypotheses. Data clustering or grouping for Amanda Aquilini is illustrated in Table 12–5, in which data are clustered according to standardized diagnosis labels.

Identifying Gaps and Inconsistencies in Data

Skillful assessment minimizes gaps and inconsistencies in data. However, data analysis should include a final check to ensure that data are complete and correct.

Inconsistencies are conflicting data. Possible sources of conflicting data include measurement error, expectations, and inconsistent or unreliable reports. For example, a nurse may learn from the nursing history that the client reports not having seen a doctor in 15 years, yet during the physical health examination he states, "My doctor takes my blood pressure every year." All inconsistencies must be clarified before a valid pattern can be established. See "Validating Data" in Chapter 11. ∞

Identifying Health Problems, Risks, and Strengths

After data are analyzed, the nurse and client can together identify strengths and problems. This is primarily a decision-making process (see Chapter 10 ∞).

Determining Problems and Risks

After grouping and clustering the data, the nurse and client together identify problems that support tentative actual, risk, and possible diagnoses. In addition the nurse must determine whether the client's problem is a nursing diagnosis, medical diagnosis, or collaborative problem. See Figure 12-2 ■ and Table 12-3.

Significant cues and data clusters for Amanda Aquilini that were extracted from Figure 11-4 on page 188 and Box 11–7 on page 191 are shown in Table 12–5. In this example, the nurse and client identified eight tentative problems: *Imbalanced Nutrition: Less than Body Requirements; Deficient Fluid Volume; Disturbed Sleep Pattern; Activity Intolerance; Acute Pain (Chest); Interrupted Family Processes; Anxiety;* and *Ineffective Airway Clearance.*

Note that some data may indicate a possible problem but when clustered with other data, the possible problem disappears. For example, the following data for Amanda Aquilini, "Decreased urinary frequency and amount × 2 days," suggests a possible urinary elimination problem. However, when these

TABLE 12–5 Formulating Nursing Diagnoses for Amanda Aquilini

FUNCTIONAL HEALTH PATTERN	CLIENT CUE CLUSTERS	INFERENCES (TENTATIVE IDENTIFICATION OF PROBLEMS)	FORMULATING DIAGNOSTIC STATEMENTS
Health perception/ health management			No problem *Strength:* Shows healthy lifestyle, understanding of and compliance with treatment regimens
Nutritional/ metabolic (includes hydration)	"No appetite" since having "cold" Has not eaten today; last fluids at noon today Nauseated × 2 days	*Imbalanced Nutrition: Less than Body Requirements*	*Imbalanced Nutrition: Less than Body Requirements* related to decreased appetite and nausea and increased metabolism (secondary to disease process) *Strength:* Normal weight for height
	Last fluids at noon today Oral temp 39.4C (103F) Skin hot and pale, cheeks flushed Mucous membranes dry Poor skin turgor *Cues from elimination pattern:* Decreased urinary frequency and amount × 2 days	*Deficient Fluid Volume*	*Deficient Fluid Volume* related to intake insufficient to replace fluid loss secondary to fever, diaphoresis, anorexia
Elimination	Decreased urinary frequency and amount × 2 days	Cues consist of elimination data but are actually symptoms of a fluid volume problem in the nutritional/metabolic functional health pattern	No elimination problem
Activity/exercise	Difficulty sleeping because of cough "Can't breathe lying down"	*Disturbed Sleep Pattern*	*Disturbed Sleep Pattern* related to cough, pain, orthopnea, fever, and diaphoresis
	States "I feel weak" Short of breath on exertion *Cues from cognitive/perceptual pattern:* Responsive but fatigued "I can think OK, just weak" *Cues from cardiovascular pattern:* Radial pulses weak, regular Pulse rate 92	*Activity Intolerance*	*Activity Intolerance* related to general weakness, imbalance between oxygen supply/demand *Strength:* No musculo-skeletal impairment, normal energy level is satisfactory, exercises regularly
Cognitive/ perceptual	Reports pain in chest, especially when coughing	*Acute Pain*	*Acute Pain (Chest)* related to cough secondary to pneumonia *Strength:* No cognitive or sensory deficits
	Responsive but fatigued "I can think OK, just weak"	These are cognitive/perceptual data, but they reflect symptoms of problems in the activity/exercise pattern	
Roles/ relationships	Husband out of town; will be back tomorrow afternoon Child with neighbor until husband returns	*Interrupted Family Processes* related to mother's illness and temporary unavailability of father to provide child care	*Risk for Interrupted Family Processes* related to mother's illness and temporary unavailability of father to provide child care *Strength:* Neighbors available and willing to help
Self-perception/ self-concept	Expresses "concern" and "worry" over leaving daughter with neighbors until husband returns	Cues also related to a problem in the coping/stress pattern Cue is a symptom of a problem in the coping/stress pattern	No self-perception/self-concept problem
Coping/stress	Anxious: "I can't breathe" Facial muscles tense; trembling Expresses concerns about work: "I'll never get caught up"	*Anxiety* related to difficulty breathing, inability to work, and child care	*Anxiety* related to difficulty breathing and concerns over work and parenting roles

continued

TABLE 12–5 **Formulating Nursing Diagnoses for Amanda Aquilini (continued)**			
FUNCTIONAL HEALTH PATTERN	**CLIENT CUE CLUSTERS**	**INFERENCES (TENTATIVE IDENTIFICATION OF PROBLEMS)**	**FORMULATING DIAGNOSTIC STATEMENTS**
Coping/stress (continued)	*Cues from role/relationship pattern:* Husband out of town; will be back tomorrow afternoon Child with neighbor until husband returns *Cues from self-perception/self-concept patterns:* Expresses "concern" and "worry" over leaving daughter with neighbors		
Medication/history Physical assessment	No significant cues	No problem	No problem
■ Cardiovascular	Radial pulses weak, regular Pulse rate 92	Cues are symptoms only; symptoms of exercise/rest and oxygenation problems	No cardiovascular problem
■ Oxygenation	Skin hot, pale, and moist Respirations shallow; chest expansion, 3 cm Cough productive of small amounts of thick pale pink sputum Inspiratory crackles auscultated throughout right upper and lower lungs Diminished breath sounds on right side Mucous membranes pale, dry	*Ineffective Airway Clearance* related to disease process	*Ineffective Airway Clearance* related to viscous secretions and shallow chest expansion secondary to pain, fluid volume deficit, and fatigue
■ Skin	Old surgical scars, anterior neck, RLQ abdomen	No problem now	Old problems; resolved

data are considered along with data associated with *Deficient Fluid Volume,* the nurse eliminates urinary elimination as a problem.

Determining Strengths

At this stage, the nurse and client also establish the client's strengths, resources, and abilities to cope. Most people have a clearer perception of their problems or weaknesses than of their strengths and assets, which they often take for granted. By taking an inventory of strengths, the client can develop a more well-rounded self-concept and self-image. Strengths can be an aid to mobilizing health and regenerative processes.

A client's strength might be weight that is within the normal range for age and height, thus enabling the client to cope better with surgery. In another instance, a client's strengths might be absence of allergies and being a nonsmoker.

A client's strengths can be found in the nursing assessment record (health, home life, education, recreation, exercise, work, family and friends, religious beliefs, and sense of humor, for example), the health examination, and the client's records. See Table 12–5 for the strengths identified for Amanda Aquilini.

Formulating Diagnostic Statements

Most nursing diagnoses are written as two-part or three-part statements, but there are variations of these.

Basic Two-Part Statements

The basic two-part statement includes the following:

1. *Problem (P):* statement of the client's response (NANDA label)

2. *Etiology (E):* factors contributing to or probable causes of the responses

The two parts are joined by the words *related to* rather than *due to.* The phrase *due to* implies that one part causes or is responsible for the other part. By contrast, the phrase *related to* merely implies a relationship. Some examples of two-part nursing diagnoses are shown in Box 12–1.

For NANDA labels that contain the word *Specify,* the nurse must add words to indicate the problem more specifically. The format is still a two-part statement. For example, *Noncompliance (Specify)* would be *Noncompliance (Diabetic Diet)* related to denial of having disease. For ease in alphabetizing, many NANDA lists are arranged with qualifying words after the main word (e.g., *Infection, Risk for*). Avoid writing diagnostic statements in that manner; instead, write them as they would be stated in normal conversation (e.g., *Risk for Infection*).

Basic Three-Part Statements

The basic three-part nursing diagnosis statement is called the **PES format** and includes the following:

1. *Problem (P):* statement of the client's response (NANDA label)
2. *Etiology (E):* factors contributing to or probable causes of the response
3. *Signs and symptoms (S):* defining characteristics manifested by the client

Actual nursing diagnoses can be documented by using the three-part statement (see Box 12–2) because the signs and symptoms have been identified. This format cannot be used for

Figure 12-2 ■ Decision tree for differentiating among nursing diagnoses, collaborative problems, and medical diagnoses.

risk diagnoses because the client does not have signs and symptoms of the diagnosis.

The PES format is especially recommended for beginning diagnosticians because the signs and symptoms validate why the diagnosis was chosen and make the problem statement more descriptive. The PES format can create very long problem statements, sometimes making the problem and etiology unclear. To minimize long problem statements, the nurse can record the signs and symptoms in the nursing notes instead of on the care plan. Another possibility, recommended for students, is to list the signs and symptoms on the care plan below the nursing diagnosis, grouping the subjective (S) and objective (O) data. The

signs and symptoms are easily accessible, and the problem and etiology stand out clearly. For example:

Noncompliance (Diabetic Diet) related to unresolved anger about diagnosis as manifested by

S— "I forget to take my pills."
"I can't live without sugar in my food."
O— Weight 98 kg (215 lb) [gain of 4.5 kg (10 lb)]
Blood pressure 190/100

One-Part Statements

Some diagnostic statements, such as wellness diagnoses and syndrome nursing diagnoses, consist of a NANDA label only. As the diagnostic labels are refined, they tend to become more specific, so that nursing interventions can be derived from the label itself. Therefore, an etiology may not be needed. For example, adding an etiology to the label *Rape-Trauma Syndrome* does not make the label any more descriptive or useful.

NANDA has specified that any new wellness diagnoses will be developed as one-part statements beginning with the words *Readiness for Enhanced* followed by the desired higher level wellness (for example, *Readiness for Enhanced Parenting*).

BOX 12—1	**Basic Two-Part Diagnostic Statement**	
Problem	*Related to*	*Etiology*
Constipation	related to	prolonged laxative use
Severe Anxiety	related to	threat to physiologic integrity: possible cancer diagnosis

BOX 12—2	**Basic Three-Part Diagnostic Statement**			
Problem	*Related to*	*Etiology*	*As Manifested by*	*Signs and Symptoms*
Situational Low Self-Esteem	related to (r/t)	feelings of rejection by husband	as manifested by (a.m.b.)	hypersensitivity to criticism; states "I don't know if I can manage by myself" and rejects positive feedback

Currently the NANDA list includes several wellness diagnoses. Some of these are *Spiritual Well-Being, Effective Breastfeeding, Health-Seeking Behaviors,* and *Anticipatory Grieving.* These are usually accepted as one-part statements but may be made more explicit by adding a descriptor, for example, *Health-Seeking Behaviors (Low-Fat Diet).*

Variations of Basic Formats

Variations of the basic one-, two-, and three-part statements include the following:

1. Writing *unknown etiology* when the defining characteristics are present but the nurse does not know the cause or contributing factors. One example is *Noncompliance (Medication Regimen)* related to unknown etiology.
2. Using the phrase *complex factors* when there are too many etiologic factors or when they are too complex to state in a brief phrase. The actual causes of chronic low self-esteem, for instance, may be long term and complex, as in the following nursing diagnosis: *Chronic Low Self-Esteem* related to complex factors.
3. Using the word *possible* to describe either the problem or the etiology. When the nurse believes more data are needed about the client's problem or the etiology, the word *possible* is inserted. Examples are *Possible Low Self-Esteem* related to loss of job and rejection by family; *Altered Thought Processes* possibly related to unfamiliar surroundings.
4. Using *secondary to* to divide the etiology into two parts, thereby making the statement more descriptive and useful. The part following *secondary to* is often a pathophysiologic or disease process or a medical diagnosis, as in *Risk for Impaired Skin Integrity* related to decreased peripheral circulation secondary to diabetes.
5. Adding a second part to the general response or NANDA label to make it more precise. For example, the diagnosis *Impaired Skin Integrity* does not indicate the location of the problem. To make this label more specific, the nurse can add a descriptor as follows: *Impaired Skin Integrity (Left Lateral Ankle)* related to decreased peripheral circulation.

Collaborative Problems

Carpenito-Moyet (2006) has suggested that all collaborative (multidisciplinary) problems begin with the diagnostic label *Potential Complication* (PC). Nurses should include in the diagnostic statement both the possible complication they are monitoring and the disease or treatment that is present to produce it. For example, if the client has a head injury and could develop increased intracranial pressure, the nurse should write the following:

Potential Complication of Head Injury:
Increased intracranial pressure

When monitoring for a group of complications associated with a disease or pathology, the nurse states the disease and follows it with a list of the complications:

Potential Complication of Pregnancy-Induced Hypertension:
seizures, fetal distress, pulmonary edema, hepatic/renal failure, premature labor, CNS hemorrhage

In some situations, an etiology might be helpful in suggesting interventions. Nurses should write the etiology when (a) it clarifies the problem statement, (b) it can be concisely stated, and (c) it helps to suggest nursing actions. See the examples in Box 12–3.

Evaluating the Quality of the Diagnostic Statement

In addition to using the correct format, nurses must consider the content of their diagnostic statements. The statements should, for example, be accurate, concise, descriptive, and specific. The nurse must always validate the diagnostic statements with the client and compare the client's signs and symptoms to the NANDA defining characteristics. For risk problems, the nurse compares the client's risk factors to NANDA risk factors. After writing nursing diagnoses, the nurse checks them against the criteria in Table 12–6.

Avoiding Errors in Diagnostic Reasoning

Some error is inherent in any human undertaking, and diagnosis is no exception. However, it is important that nurses make nursing diagnoses with a high level of accuracy. Nurses can avoid some common errors of reasoning by recognizing them and applying the appropriate critical-thinking skills. Error can occur at any point in the diagnostic process: data collection, data interpretation, and data clustering.

The following suggestions help to minimize diagnostic error:

- *Verify.* Hypothesize possible explanations of the data, but realize that all diagnoses are only tentative until they are verified. Begin and end the diagnostic process by talking with the client and family. When collecting data, ask them what their health problems are and what they believe the causes to be. At the end of the process, ask them to confirm the accuracy and relevance of your diagnoses.
- *Build a good knowledge base and acquire clinical experience.* Nurses must apply knowledge from many different

BOX 12–3 **Collaborative Problems**			
Disease/Situation	*Complication*	*Related to*	*Etiology*
Potential complication of childbirth:	hemorrhage	related to	uterine atony
			retained placental fragments
			bladder distention
Potential complication of diuretic therapy:	arrhythmia	related to	low serum potassium

TABLE 12–6 Guidelines for Writing a Nursing Diagnostic Statement

GUIDELINE	CORRECT STATEMENT	INCORRECT OR AMBIGUOUS STATEMENT
1. State in terms of a problem, not a need.	*Deficient Fluid Volume* (problem) related to fever	*Fluid Replacement* (need) related to fever
2. Word the statement so that it is legally advisable.	*Impaired Skin Integrity* related to immobility (legally acceptable)	*Impaired Skin Integrity* related to improper positioning (implies legal liability)
3. Use nonjudgmental statements.	*Spiritual Distress* related to inability to attend church services secondary to immobility (nonjudgmental)	*Spiritual Distress* related to strict rules necessitating church attendance (judgmental)
4. Make sure that both elements of the statement do not say the same thing.	*Risk for Impaired Skin Integrity* related to immobility	*Impaired Skin Integrity* related to ulceration of sacral area (response and probable cause are the same)
5. Be sure that cause and effect are correctly stated (i.e., the etiology causes the problem or puts the client at risk for the problem).	*Pain: Severe Headache* related to fear of addiction to narcotics	*Pain* related to severe headache
6. Word the diagnosis specifically and precisely to provide direction for planning nursing intervention.	*Impaired Oral Mucous Membrane* related to decreased salivation secondary to radiation of neck (specific)	*Impaired Oral Mucous Membrane* related to noxious agent (vague)
7. Use nursing terminology rather than medical terminology to describe the client's response.	*Risk for Ineffective Airway Clearance* related to accumulation of secretions in lungs (nursing terminology)	*Risk for Pneumonia* (medical terminology)
8. Use nursing terminology rather than medical terminology to describe the probable cause of the client's response.	*Risk for Ineffective Airway Clearance* related to accumulation of secretions in lungs (nursing terminology)	*Risk for Ineffective Airway Clearance* related to emphysema (medical terminology)

areas to recognize significant cues and patterns and generate hypotheses about the data. To name only a few, principles from chemistry, anatomy, and pharmacology each help the nurse understand client data in a different way.

■ *Have a working knowledge of what is normal.* Nurses need to know the population norms for vital signs, laboratory tests, speech development, breath sounds, and so on. In addition, nurses must determine what is usual for a particular person, taking into account age, physical makeup, lifestyle, culture, and the person's own perception of what his or her normal status is. For example, normal blood pressure for adults is in the range of 110/60 to 140/80. However, a nurse might obtain a reading of 90/50 that is perfectly normal for a particular client. The nurse should compare actual findings to the client's baseline when possible.

■ *Consult resources.* Both novices and experienced nurses should consult appropriate resources whenever in doubt about a diagnosis. Professional literature, nursing colleagues, and other professionals are all appropriate resources. The nurse should use a nursing diagnosis handbook to determine whether the client's signs and symptoms truly fit the NANDA label chosen.

■ *Base diagnoses on patterns—that is, on behavior over time—rather than on an isolated incident.* For example, even though Amanda Aquilini is concerned today about needing to leave her child with a neighbor, it is likely that this concern will be resolved without intervention by the next day. Therefore, the admitting nurse should not diagnose *Interrupted Family Processes.*

■ *Improve critical-thinking skills.* These skills help the nurse to be aware of and avoid errors in thinking, such as overgeneralizing, stereotyping, and making unwarranted assumptions. See Chapter 10. ∞

ONGOING DEVELOPMENT OF NURSING DIAGNOSES

The first taxonomy of nursing diagnoses was alphabetical. This ordering was considered unscientific by some, and a hierarchic structure was sought. In 1982, NANDA accepted the "nine patterns of unitary man" (based on the nursing models of Sr. Calista Roy and Martha Rogers—see Chapter 3 ∞) as an organizing principle. In 1984, NANDA renamed the "patterns of unitary man" as "human response patterns" based more on the work of Marjorie Gordon (Kim, McFarland, & McLane, 1984), as listed in Box 12–4.

Having undergone refinements, revisions, and acceptance of new diagnoses, the taxonomy is now called Taxonomy II (NANDA International, 2005). Taxonomy II has three levels: domains, classes, and nursing diagnoses (Figure 12-3 ■). The di-

BOX 12–4 Human Response Patterns

1. *Exchanging:* mutual giving and receiving
2. *Communicating:* sending messages
3. *Relating:* establishing bonds
4. *Valuing:* assigning relative worth
5. *Choosing:* selection of alternatives
6. *Moving:* activity
7. *Perceiving:* reception of information
8. *Knowing:* meaning associated with information
9. *Feeling:* subjective awareness of information

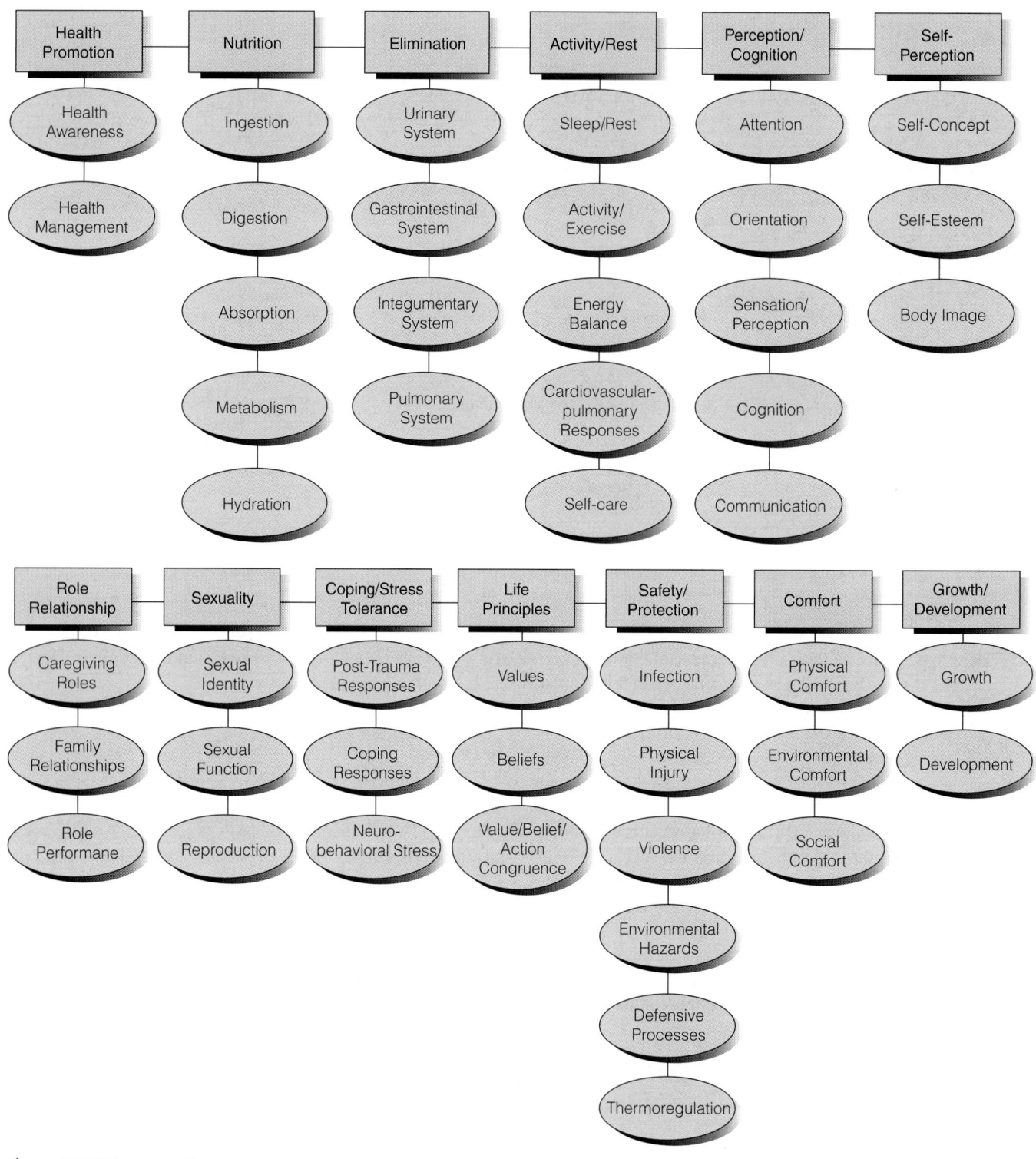

Figure 12-3 ■ Taxonomy II.

Source: From *Definitions and Classifications,* 2003–2004 by NANDA International, 2003, Philadelphia, PA. Adapted with permission

agnoses are no longer grouped by Gordon's patterns but coded according to seven axes: diagnostic concept, time, unit of care, age, health status, descriptor, and topology. In addition, diagnoses are now listed alphabetically by concept, not by first word.

Review and refinement of diagnostic labels continue as new and modified labels are discussed at each biannual conference. Nurses submit diagnoses to the Diagnostic Review Committee, which reviews and "stages" the diagnosis according to how well developed and supported it is. The NANDA board of directors gives final approval for incorporation of the diagnosis into the official list of labels. Diagnoses on the NANDA list are not finished products but are approved for clinical use and further study. Many on the list have been studied only minimally.

In 1997, NANDA changed the name of its official journal from *Nursing Diagnosis* to *Nursing Diagnosis: The International Journal of Nursing Language and Classification.* The subtitle emphasizes that nursing diagnosis is part of a larger, developing system of standardized nursing language. This system includes classifications of nursing interventions (NIC) and nursing outcomes (NOC) that are being developed by other research groups and linked to the NANDA diagnos-tic labels. NIC and NOC are discussed in greater detail in Chapter 13. ∞

Research groups are examining what nurses do from these three different perspectives (diagnoses, interventions, and outcomes) to clarify and communicate the role nurses play in the health care system. A standardized language will also enable nurses to implement a Nursing Minimum Data Set needed for computerized client records.

RESEARCH NOTE   What New Nursing Diagnoses Are Being Researched?

The *International Journal of Nursing Terminologies and Classifications* is a public forum for the publication of work currently conducted worldwide on the development of nursing diagnoses, outcomes, and interventions. In the paper by Lamont, the author reviewed published literature with the goal of establishing *discomfort* as a separate nursing diagnosis from *pain.* However, his review failed to provide clear evidence for this discrimination. He suggests that research be conducted to attempt to determine if pain and discomfort can be usefully separated.

Lopes and Higa conducted interviews with 148 women who had complaints of urinary incontinence. Over half the women (57%) described incontinence with characteristics of both urge and stress incontinence. They suggest that this should lead to a new nursing diagnosis of mixed urinary incontinence so that clients are not treated for urge or stress incontinence when they truly require a plan related to both types.

IMPLICATIONS

Many nursing diagnoses are being studied in a variety of settings. This is important work to determine the reliability and validity of existing diagnoses, identify gaps in the current list, and establish usefulness of the diagnoses in everyday practice. Nurses should be familiar with the direction of this work as it progresses.

Note: From "Discomfort as a Potential Nursing Diagnosis: A Concept Analysis and Literature Review," by S. C. Lamont, 2003, *International Journal of Nursing Terminologies and Classifications, 14*(4 Suppl), p. 5, and "Mixed Incontinence in Women: A New Nursing Diagnosis," by M. H. B. Lopes and R. Higa, 2003, *International Journal of Nursing Terminologies and Classifications, 14*(4 Suppl), p. 49.

LIFESPAN CONSIDERATIONS   Diagnosing

CHILDREN

Many developmental issues in pediatrics are not considered problems or illnesses, yet can benefit from nursing intervention. When applied to children and families, nursing diagnoses may reflect a condition or state of health. For example, parents of a newborn infant may be excited to learn all they can about infant care and child growth and development. Assessment of the family system might lead the nurse to conclude that the family is ready and able, even eager, to take on the new roles and responsibilities of being parents. An appropriate diagnosis for such a family could be *Readiness for Enhanced Family Processes,* and nursing care could be directed to educating and providing encouragement and support to the parents.

ELDERS

Elders tend to have multiple problems with complex physical and psychosocial needs when they are ill. If the nurse has done a thor-ough, accurate assessment, nursing diagnoses can be selected to cover all problems and, at the same time, prioritize the special needs. For example, if a client is admitted with severe congestive heart failure, prompt attention will be focused on *Decreased Cardiac Output* and *Excess Fluid Volume,* with interventions selected to improve these areas quickly. As these conditions improve, then other nursing diagnoses, such as *Activity Intolerance* and *Deficient Knowledge* related to a new medication regimen, might require more attention. They are all part of the same medical problem of congestive heart failure, but each nursing diagnosis has specific expected outcomes and nursing interventions. The client's strengths should be an essential consideration in all phases of the nursing process.

CRITICAL THINKING CHECKPOINT

Mr. H. has recently been diagnosed with lung cancer. Someone has written the nursing diagnosis of *Anxiety* on his care plan.

1. What data/defining characteristics would support this nursing diagnosis?
2. Which related factors might exist in his situation?
3. Which other nursing diagnoses might you expect to find in Mr. H.'s case?

4. Another nursing diagnosis on the care plan reads "Lung cancer related to smoking." Is this diagnosis written in an acceptable format? If not, why not?

See Critical Thinking Possibilities in Appendix A. ∞

CHAPTER 12 **REVIEW**

CHAPTER HIGHLIGHTS

- The purpose of the North American Nursing Diagnosis Association is to define, refine, and promote a taxonomy of nursing diagnostic terminology.
- Diagnosis is a reasoning process that uses critical thinking.
- Professional standards of care hold that registered nurses are responsible for making nursing diagnoses, even though others may contribute data or implement care.
- A nursing diagnosis is a clinical judgment about the client's responses to actual and potential health problems or life processes.
- A nursing diagnosis provides the basis for selecting independent nursing interventions to achieve outcomes for which the nurse is accountable.
- There are various types of nursing diagnoses: actual, risk, wellness, possible, and syndrome.
- A nursing diagnosis has three components: the problem (and its definition), the etiology, and the defining characteristics. Each component serves a specific purpose.
- Nursing diagnoses differ from medical diagnoses and collaborative problems in orientation, duration, and nursing focus.
- A collaborative problem is a type of potential problem that nurses manage using both independent and physician-prescribed interventions.
- The three phases of the diagnostic process are data analysis; identification of the client's health problems, health risks, and strengths; and formulation of diagnostic statements.
- In data analysis and processing, the nurse compares data against standards to identify significant cues, clusters the data, and identifies gaps and inconsistencies.
- Significant cues are those that (a) point to change in a client's health status or pattern, (b) vary from norms of the client population, or (c) indicate a developmental delay.
- It is important to identify client strengths as well as problems.
- The basic format for a nursing diagnostic statement is *"Problem related to etiology."* However, there are several variations on this format.
- The development of a taxonomy of nursing diagnosis labels is an ongoing process.
- The organizing principles for the NANDA Taxonomy II are the seven axes: diagnostic concept, time, unit of care, age, potentiality, descriptor, and topology.
- Work is progressing on a unified standardized nursing language that includes NANDA nursing diagnoses, a nursing interventions classification, and a nursing outcomes classification.

TEST YOUR KNOWLEDGE

1. The nurse is conducting the diagnosing phase (nursing diagnosis) for a client with a seizure disorder. Which of the following elements exists between data analysis and formulating the diagnostic statement?
   1. Assess the client's needs
   2. Delineate the client's problems and strengths
   3. Determine which interventions are most likely to succeed
   4. Estimate the cost of several different approaches

2. In the diagnostic statement "Excess fluid volume related to decreased venous return as manifested by lower extremity edema (swelling)," the etiology of the problem is which of the following?
   1. Excess fluid volume
   2. Decreased venous return
   3. Edema
   4. Unknown

3. Which of the following nursing diagnoses contains the proper components?
   1. Risk for caregiver role strain related to unpredictable illness course
   2. Risk for falls related to tendency to collapse when having difficulty breathing
   3. Decreased communication related to stroke
   4. Sleep deprivation secondary to fatigue and a noisy environment

4. One of the primary advantages of using a three-part diagnostic statement such as the problem-etiology-signs/symptoms (PES) format includes which of the following?
   1. Decreases the cost of health care
   2. Improves communication between nurse and client
   3. Helps the nurse focus on health and wellness elements
   4. Standardizes organization of client data

5. A collaborative (multidisciplinary) problem is indicated instead of a nursing or medical diagnosis:
   1. If both medical and nursing interventions are required to treat the problem
   2. When independent nursing actions can be utilized to treat the problem
   3. In cases where nursing interventions are the primary actions required to treat the problem
   4. When no medical diagnosis (disease) can be determined

See Answers to Test Your Knowledge in Appendix A. ∞

EXPLORE MEDIALINK www.prenhall.com/berman

DVD-ROM
- Audio Glossary
- NCLEX Review

COMPANION WEBSITE
- Additional NCLEX Review
- Case Study:
  Selecting Nursing Diagnoses for Client with Pneumonia
- Application Activity:
  Resources for a Chronically Ill Child
- Links to Resources

READINGS AND REFERENCES

SUGGESTED READINGS

Kelly, J. H., Weber, J., & Sprengel, A. (2005). Taxonomy of nursing practice: Adding an administrative domain. *International Journal of Nursing Terminologies and Classifications, 16*(3/4), 74–80.
In this article, the authors propose the addition of a fifth domain, Administrative, to the Taxonomy of Nursing Practice, and to introduce the related concept of organization nursing diagnoses. The current taxonomy does not include diagnoses that relate to the management/leadership roles of nurses.

RELATED RESEARCH

Junttila, K., Salanterä, S., & Hupli, M. (2005). Perioperative nurses' attitudes toward the use of nursing diagnoses in documentation. *Journal of Advanced Nursing, 52,* 271–280.
Keenan, G., Falan, S., Heath, C., & Treder, M. (2003). Establishing competency in the use of North American Nursing Diagnosis Association, nursing outcomes classification, and nursing interventions classification terminology. *Journal of Nursing Measurement, 11,* 183–198.

REFERENCES

American Nurses Association. (2004). *Nursing: Scope and standards of practice.* Kansas City, MO: Author.
Carpenito-Moyet, L. J. (2006). *Nursing diagnosis: Application to clinical practice* (11th ed.). Philadelphia: Lippincott Williams & Wilkins.
Joint Commission on Accreditation of Healthcare Organizations. (2005). *Accreditation manual for hospitals.* Chicago: Author.

Kim, M. J., McFarland, G. K., & McLane, A. M. (Eds.). (1984). *Classification of nursing diagnoses: Proceedings of the fifth national conference.* St. Louis, MO: Mosby.
Lamont, S. C. (2003). Discomfort as a potential nursing diagnosis: A concept analysis and literature review. *International Journal of Nursing Terminologies and Classifications, 14*(4 Suppl), 5.
Lopes, M. H. B., & Higa, R. (2003). Mixed incontinence in women: A new nursing diagnosis. *International Journal of Nursing Terminologies and Classifications, 14*(4 Suppl), 49.
NANDA International. (2005). *NANDA nursing diagnoses: Definitions and classification 2005–2006.* Philadelphia: Author.

SELECTED BIBLIOGRAPHY

Ackley, B. J., & Ladwig, G. B. (2006). *Nursing diagnosis handbook: A guide to planning care* (7th ed.). St. Louis, MO: Elsevier Health Sciences.
Alfaro-LeFevre, R. A. (2005). *Applying the nursing process: Promoting collaborative care* (6th ed.). Philadelphia: Lippincott Williams & Wilkins.
Alfaro-LeFevre, R. A. (2005). *The nursing process made easy: Concept mapping and care planning for students.* Philadelphia: Lippincott Williams & Wilkins.
Doenges, M. E., & Moorhouse, M. F. (2003). *Application of nursing process and nursing diagnosis: An interactive text for diagnostic reasoning* (4th ed.). Philadelphia: F.A. Davis.

Doenges, M. E., Moorhouse, M. F., & Geissler-Murr, A. C. (2005). *Nursing diagnosis manual: Planning, individualizing, and documenting client care.* Philadelphia: F. A. Davis.
Gardner, P. (2003). *Nursing process in action.* Albany, NY: Delmar.
Gordon, M. (1982). Historical perspective: The National Group for Classification of Nursing Diagnoses. In M. J. Kim & D. A. Moritz (Eds.), *Classification of nursing diagnoses: Proceedings of the fourth national conference.* New York: McGraw-Hill.
Gordon, M. (2006). *Manual of nursing diagnosis* (11th ed.). St. Louis, MO: Mosby.
Johnson, M., Bulechek, G. B., Butcher, H., Dochterman, J., Moorhead, S., Maas, M., et al. (Eds.). (2005). *NANDA, NOC and NIC linkages: Nursing diagnoses, outcomes, and interventions* (2nd ed.). St. Louis, MO: Elsevier Health Sciences.
Ladwig, G. B., & Ackley, B. J. (2005). *Mosby's guide to nursing diagnosis.* St. Louis, MO: Elsevier Health Sciences.
Seaback, W. (2005). *Nursing process: Concept & application* (2nd ed.). Albany, NY: Delmar.
Wilkinson, J. M. (2005). *Nursing diagnosis handbook: With NIC interventions and NOC outcomes* (8th ed.). Upper Saddle River, NJ: Prentice Hall.
Wilkinson, J. M. (2007). *Nursing process & critical thinking* (4th ed.). Upper Saddle River, NJ: Prentice Hall.

CHAPTER 13

Planning

LEARNING OUTCOMES

After completing this chapter, you will be able to:

1. Compare and contrast initial planning, ongoing planning, and discharge planning.

2. Identify activities that occur in the planning process.

3. Explain how standards of care and preprinted care plans can be individualized and used in creating a comprehensive nursing care plan.

4. Identify essential guidelines for writing nursing care plans.

5. Identify factors that the nurse must consider when setting priorities.

6. State the purposes of establishing client goals/desired outcomes.

7. Discuss the Nursing Outcomes Classification, including an explanation of how to use the outcomes and indicators in care planning.

8. Describe the relationship of goals/desired outcomes to the nursing diagnoses.

9. Identify guidelines for writing goals/desired outcomes.

10. Describe the process of selecting and choosing nursing interventions.

11. Discuss the Nursing Interventions Classification, including an explanation of how to use the interventions and activities in care planning.

Planning is a deliberative, systematic phase of the nursing process that involves decision making and problem solving. In planning, the nurse refers to the client's assessment data and diagnostic statements for direction in formulating client goals and designing the nursing interventions required to prevent, reduce, or eliminate the client's health problems (see Figure 13-1 ■). A **nursing intervention** is "any treatment, based upon clinical judgment and knowledge, that a nurse performs to enhance patient/client outcomes" (Dochterman & Bulechek, 2004, p. xxiii). The end product of the planning phase is a client care plan.

Although planning is basically the nurse's responsibility, input from the client and support persons is essential if a plan is to be effective. Nurses do not plan for the client, but encourage the client to participate actively to the extent possible. In a home setting, the client's support people and caregivers are the ones who implement the plan of care; thus, its effectiveness depends largely on them.

TYPES OF PLANNING

Planning begins with the first client contact and continues until the nurse–client relationship ends, usually when the client is

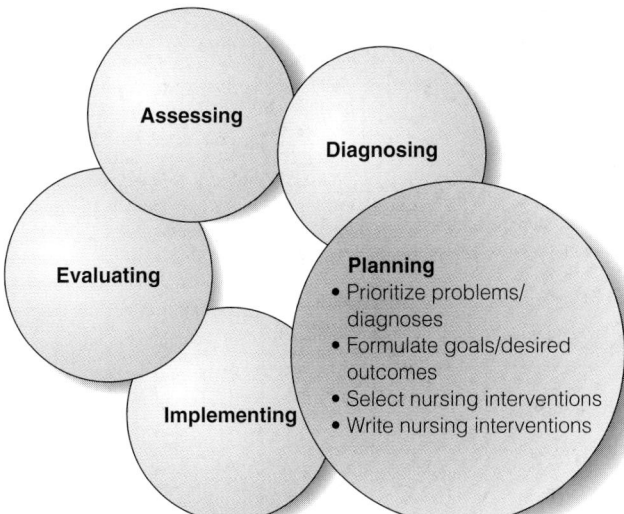

Figure 13-1 ■ Planning. The third phase of the nursing process, in which the nurse and client develop client goals/desired outcomes and nursing interventions to prevent, reduce, or alleviate the client's health problems.

discharged from the health care agency. All planning is multidisciplinary (involves all health care providers interacting with the client) and includes the client and family to the fullest extent possible in every step.

Initial Planning

The nurse who performs the admission assessment usually develops the initial comprehensive plan of care. This nurse has the benefit of the client's body language as well as some intuitive kinds of information that are not available solely from the written database. Planning should be initiated as soon as possible after the initial assessment, especially because of the trend toward shorter hospital stays.

Ongoing Planning

Ongoing planning is done by all nurses who work with the client. As nurses obtain new information and evaluate the client's responses to care, they can individualize the initial care plan further. Ongoing planning also occurs at the beginning of a shift as the nurse plans the care to be given that day. Using ongoing assessment data, the nurse carries out daily planning for the following purposes:

1. To determine whether the client's health status has changed
2. To set priorities for the client's care during the shift
3. To decide which problems to focus on during the shift
4. To coordinate the nurse's activities so that more than one problem can be addressed at each client contact

Discharge Planning

Discharge planning, the process of anticipating and planning for needs after discharge, is a crucial part of comprehensive health care and should be addressed in each client's care plan. Because the average stay of clients in acute care hospitals has become shorter, people are sometimes discharged still needing care. Although many clients are discharged to other agencies (e.g., long-term care facilities), such care is increasingly being delivered in the home. Effective discharge planning begins at first client contact and involves comprehensive and ongoing assessment to obtain information about the client's ongoing needs. For details about discharge planning, see "Continuity of Care" in Chapter 7. ∞

DEVELOPING NURSING CARE PLANS

The end product of the planning phase of the nursing process is a formal or informal plan of care. An **informal nursing care plan** is a strategy for action that exists in the nurse's mind. For example, the nurse may think, "Mrs. Phan is very tired. I will need to reinforce her teaching after she is rested." A **formal nursing care plan** is a written or computerized guide that organizes information about the client's care. The most obvious benefit of a formal written care plan is that it provides for continuity of care.

A **standardized care plan** is a formal plan that specifies the nursing care for groups of clients with common needs (e.g., all clients with myocardial infarction). An **individualized care plan** is tailored to meet the unique needs of a specific client—needs that are not addressed by the standardized plan. It is important that all caregivers work toward the same outcomes and, if available, use approaches shown to be effective with a particular client. Nurses also use the formal care plan for direction about what needs to be documented in client progress notes and as a guide for delegating and assigning staff to care for clients. When nurses use the client's nursing diagnoses to develop goals and nursing interventions, the result is a holistic, individualized plan of care that will meet the client's unique needs.

Care plans include the actions nurses must take to address the client's nursing diagnoses and produce the desired outcomes. The nurse begins the plan when the client is admitted to the agency and constantly updates it throughout the client's stay in response to changes in the client's condition and evaluations of goal achievement. During the planning phase, the nurse must (a) decide which of the client's problems need individualized plans and which problems can be addressed by standardized plans and routine care, and (b) write individualized desired outcomes and nursing interventions for client problems that require nursing attention beyond preplanned, routine care.

The complete plan of care for a client is made up of several different documents that (a) describe the routine care needed to meet basic needs (e.g., bathing, nutrition), (b) address the client's nursing diagnoses and collaborative problems, and (c) specify nursing responsibilities in carrying out the medical plan of care (e.g., keeping the client from eating or drinking before surgery; scheduling a laboratory test). A complete plan of care integrates dependent and independent nursing functions into a meaningful whole and provides a central source of client information. Figure 13-2 ■ illustrates the various documents that may be included in a nursing care plan.

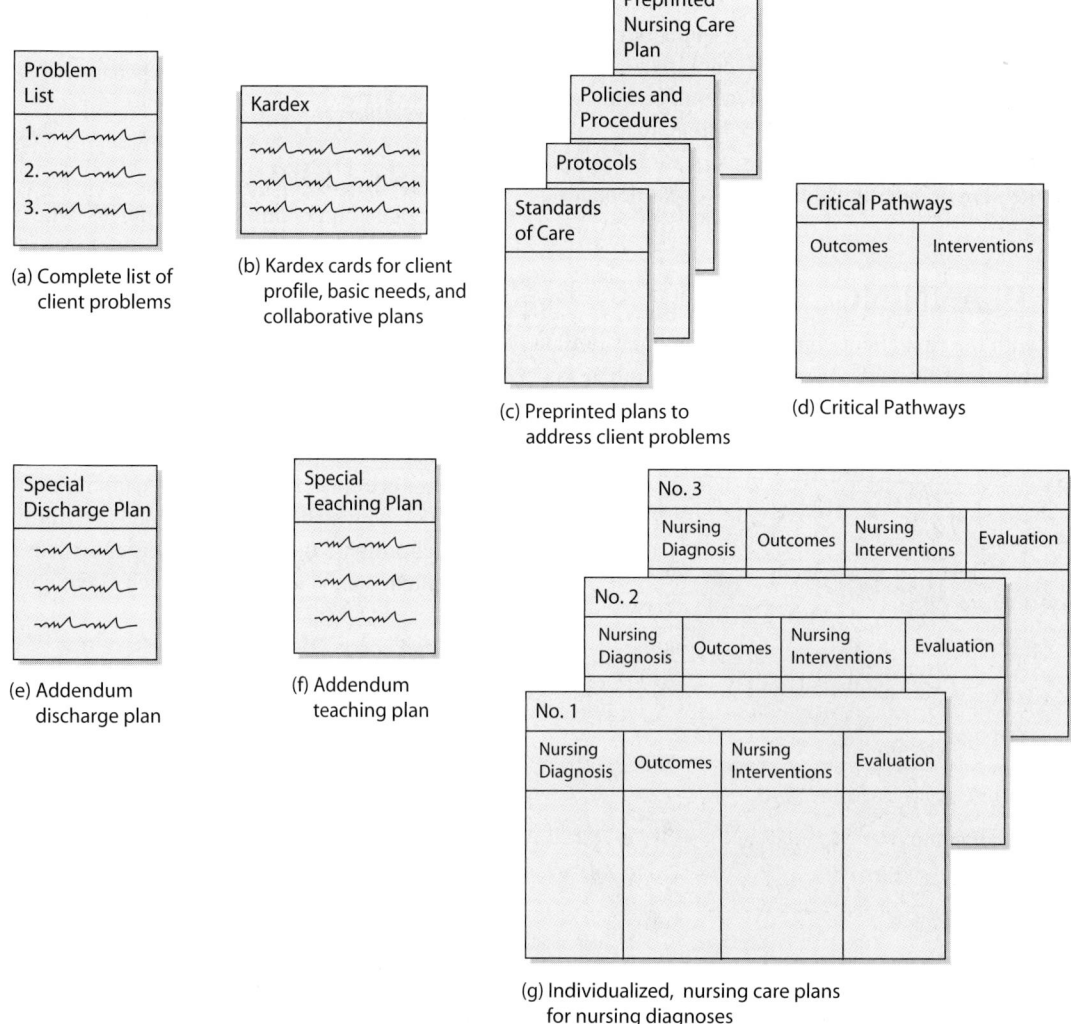

Figure 13-2 ■ Documents that may be included in a complete client care plan.

(*Note:* From *Nursing Process & Critical Thinking,* 4th ed. (p. 452), by J. M. Wilkinson, 2007, Upper Saddle River, NJ: Prentice Hall. Adapted with permission.)

Standardized Approaches to Care Planning

Most health care agencies have devised a variety of preprinted, standardized plans for providing essential nursing care to specified groups of clients who have certain needs in common (e.g., all clients with pneumonia). Standards of care, standardized care plans, protocols, policies, and procedures are developed and accepted by the nursing staff in order to (a) ensure that minimally acceptable standards are met and (b) promote efficient use of nurses' time by removing the need to author common activities that are done over and over for many of the clients on a nursing unit.

Standards of care describe nursing actions for clients with similar medical conditions rather than individuals, and they describe achievable rather than ideal nursing care. They define the interventions for which nurses are held accountable; they do not contain medical interventions. Standards of care are usually agency records and not part of the client's care plan, but they may be referred to in the plan (e.g., a nurse might write "See unit standards of care for cardiac catheterization"). Standards of care may or may not be organized according to problems or nursing diagnoses. They are written from the perspective of the nurse's responsibilities. Figure 13-3 ■ shows unit standards of care for the client with thrombophlebitis.

Standardized care plans are preprinted guides for the nursing care of a client who has a need that arises frequently in the agency (e.g., a specific nursing diagnosis or all nursing diagnoses associated with a particular medical condition). They are written from the perspective of what care the client can expect. They should not be confused with standards of care. Although the two have some similarities, they have important differences. Figure 13-4 ■ shows a standardized care plan for *Deficient Fluid Volume*. Standardized care plans:

- Are kept with the client's individualized care plan on the nursing unit. When the client is discharged, they become part of the permanent medical record.
- Provide detailed interventions and contain additions or deletions from the standards of care of the agency.
- Typically are written in the nursing process format:
  Problem → Goals/Desired Outcomes → Nursing Interventions → Evaluation
- Frequently include checklists, blank lines, or empty spaces to allow the nurse to individualize goals and nursing interventions.

STANDARDS OF CARE: Patient with Thrombophlebitis

Goal: 1. To monitor for early signs and symptoms of compromised respiratory status.
2. To report any abnormal signs and/or symptoms promptly to the medical staff.
3. To initiate appropriate nursing actions when signs and/or symptoms of compromised respiratory status occur.
4. To institute protocol for emergency intervention should the client develop cardiopulmonary dysfunction.

SUPPORTIVE DATA: The purpose of these standards of care is to prevent, monitor, report, and record the client's response to a diagnosis of thrombophlebitis. Thrombophlebitis places the client at risk for pulmonary embolism. The hemodynamic consequences of embolic obstruction to pulmonary blood flow involve increased pulmonary vascular resistance, increased right ventricular workload, decreased cardiac output, and development of shock and pulmonary arrest.

CLINICAL MANIFESTATIONS: Nursing assessments performed q3–4h should monitor for the following signs/symptoms:

- Dyspnea
- Sudden substernal pain
- Rapid/weak pulse
- Syncope
- Anxiety
- Fever
- Cough/hemoptysis
- Accelerated respiratory rate
- Pleuritic type chest pain
- Cyanosis

PREVENTIVE NURSING MEASURES:

- Encourage increased fluid intake to prevent dehydration.
- Maintain anticoagulant intravenous therapy as prescribed (See Protocol for Anticoagulant Administration).
- Maintain prescribed bedrest.
- Prevent venous stasis from improperly fitting elastic stockings; check q3–4h.
- Encourage dorsiflexion exercises of the lower extremities while on bedrest.

INDIVIDUALIZED PLANS/ADDITIONAL NURSING/MEDICAL ORDERS

Do not massage lower extremities.
Intake and output q8h.

Initiated by: _S. Ibarra, RN_   Date: _4-9-07_

Figure 13-3 ■ Standards of care for thrombophlebitis.

(*Note:* From *Nursing Process & Critical Thinking*, 4th ed. (p. 461), by J. M. Wilkinson, 2007, Upper Saddle River, NJ: Prentice Hall. Reprinted with permission.)

Etiology	Desired Outcomes	Nursing Interventions (Identify Frequency)
✓ Decreased oral intake	✓ Urinary output > 30 mL/hr	✓ Monitor intake and output q _1_ h
✓ Nausea	✓ Urine specific gravity 1.005–1.025	✓ Weigh daily
__ Depression	✓ Serum Na⁺ within normal limits	✓ Monitor serum electrolyte levels X 1 or until normal
✓ Fatigue, weakness		✓ Assess skin turgor and mucous membranes q _8 h_
__ Difficulty swallowing	✓ Mucous membranes moist	✓ Monitor temperature q _4 h_
__ Other:_____	✓ Skin turgor elastic	✓ Administer prescribed IV therapy (Monitor according to protocol for Intravenous Therapy) 1000 mL D₅ LR at 100 mL/hr
✓ Excess fluid loss	✓ No weight loss	✓ Offer 8 oz. oral liquids q _1_ h
✓ Fever or increased metabolic rate	✓ 8-hour intake = _400 mL oral_	Type _clear, cold_
✓ Diaphoresis	Other:	✓ Instruct client regarding amount, type, and schedule of fluid intake.
✓ Vomiting		✓ Assess understanding of type of fluid loss; teach accordingly
__ Diarrhea		✓ Mouth care prn with _mouthwash_
__ Burns		✓ Institute measures to reduce fever (e.g., lower room temperature, remove bed covers, offer cold liquids.)
__ Other_____		Other Nursing Orders:_____
		Monitor urine specific gravity
Defining Characteristics		_q shift_
✓ Insufficient intake		_____
✓ Negative balance of intake and output		_____
✓ Dry mucous membranes		_____
✓ Poor skin turgor		_____
__ Concentrated urine		_____
__ Hypernatremia		
✓ Rapid, weak pulse		
__ Falling B/P		
__ Weight loss		

Plan initiated by: _M. Medina RN_ Date _4-15-07_

Plan/outcomes evaluated_____ Date_____

Plan/outcomes evaluated_____ Date_____

Client: _Amanda Aquilini_

Figure 13-4 ■ A standardized care plan for the nursing diagnosis of *Deficient Fluid Volume.*

The use of standardized care plans is supported by the Joint Commission on Accreditation of Healthcare Organizations standards for nursing care, which no longer require a handwritten care plan for every client.

Like standards of care and standardized care plans, **protocols** are preprinted to indicate the actions commonly required for a particular group of clients. For example, an agency may have a protocol for admitting a client to the intensive care unit or for caring for a client receiving continuous epidural analgesia. Protocols may include both the physician's orders and nursing interventions. Depending on the agency, protocols may or may not be included in the client's permanent record.

Policies and **procedures** are developed to govern the handling of frequently occurring situations. For example, a hospital may have a policy specifying the number of visitors a client may have. Some policies and procedures are similar to protocols and specify what is to be done, for example, in the case of cardiac arrest. If a policy covers a situation pertinent to client care, it is usually noted on the care plan (e.g., "Make Social Service referral according to Policy Manual"). Policies are institutional records and do not become a part of the care plan or permanent record.

A **standing order** is a written document about policies, rules, regulations, or orders regarding client care. Standing orders give nurses the authority to carry out specific actions under certain circumstances, often when a physician is not immediately available. In a hospital critical care unit, a common example is the administration of emergency antiarrhythmic medications when a client's cardiac monitoring pattern changes. In a home care setting, a physician may write a standing order for the nurse to obtain blood tests for a client who has been on a certain therapy for a prescribed amount of time.

Regardless of whether care plans are handwritten, computerized, or standardized, nursing care must be individualized to fit the unique needs of each client. In practice, a care plan usually consists of both preprinted and nurse-created sections. The nurse uses standardized care plans for predictable, commonly occurring problems, and creates an individual plan for unusual problems or problems needing special attention. For example, a standardized care plan for all "clients with a medical diagnosis of pneumonia" would probably include a nursing diagnosis of *Deficient Fluid Volume* and direct the nurse to assess the client's hydration status. On a respiratory or medical unit this would be a common nursing diagnosis; therefore, Amanda Aquilini's nurse was able to obtain a standardized plan directing care commonly needed by clients with *Deficient Fluid Volume* (see Figure 13-4). However, the nursing diagnosis *Risk for Interrupted Family Processes* would not be common to all clients with pneumonia; it is specific to Amanda. Therefore, the goals and nursing interventions for that diagnosis would need to be created by the nurse.

Formats for Nursing Care Plans

Although formats differ from agency to agency, the care plan is often organized into four columns or categories: (a) nursing diagnoses, (b) goals/desired outcomes, (c) nursing interventions, and (d) evaluation. Some agencies use a three-column plan in which evaluation is done in the goals column or in the nurses' notes; others have a five-column plan that adds a column for assessment data preceding the nursing diagnosis column.

Student Care Plans

Because student care plans are a learning activity as well as a plan of care, they may be more lengthy and detailed than care plans used by working nurses. To help students learn to write care plans, educators may require that more of the plan be handwritten. They may also modify the three-, four-, or five-column plan by adding a column for "Rationale" after the nursing interventions column. A **rationale** is the scientific principle given as the reason for selecting a particular nursing intervention. Students may also be required to cite supporting literature for their stated rationale. Another method of organizing and representing care plan information is the use of a concept map. For an example of a Nursing Care Plan, see pages 224–225.

A **concept map** is a visual tool in which ideas or data are enclosed in circles or boxes of some shape and relationships between these are indicated by connecting lines or arrows. Concept maps are creative endeavors. They can take many different forms and encompass various categories of data, according to the creator's interpretation of the client or health condition. The concept map for Amanda Aquilini in this chapter is another way of depicting her nursing care plan and includes unique boxes that enclose assessment, nursing diagnosis, outcomes, and interventions. The arrows represent the flow of the phases of the nursing process. (See Concept Map on page 229.) Concept maps other than care plans are often used to depict complex relationships among ideas, processes, actions, and so on. Some are referred to as mind maps (see Chapter 10 ∞). Students are often asked to complete pathophysiology flow sheets or concept maps as a method of learning and demonstrating the linkages among disease processes, laboratory data, medications, signs and symptoms, risk factors, and other relevant data (Figure 13-5 ■).

Computerized Care Plans

Computers are increasingly being used to create and store nursing care plans. The computer can generate both standardized and individualized care plans. Nurses access the client's stored care plan from a centrally located terminal at the nurses' station or from terminals in client rooms. For an individualized plan, the nurse chooses the appropriate diagnoses from a menu suggested by the computer. The computer then lists possible goals and nursing interventions for those diagnoses; the nurse chooses those appropriate for the client and types in any additional goals and interventions or nursing actions not listed on the menu. The nurse can read the plan on the computer screen or print out an updated working copy.

Multidisciplinary (Collaborative) Care Plans

A **multidisciplinary care plan** is a standardized plan that outlines the care required for clients with common, predictable—usually medical—conditions. Such plans, also referred to as **collaborative care plans** and **critical pathways,** sequence the care

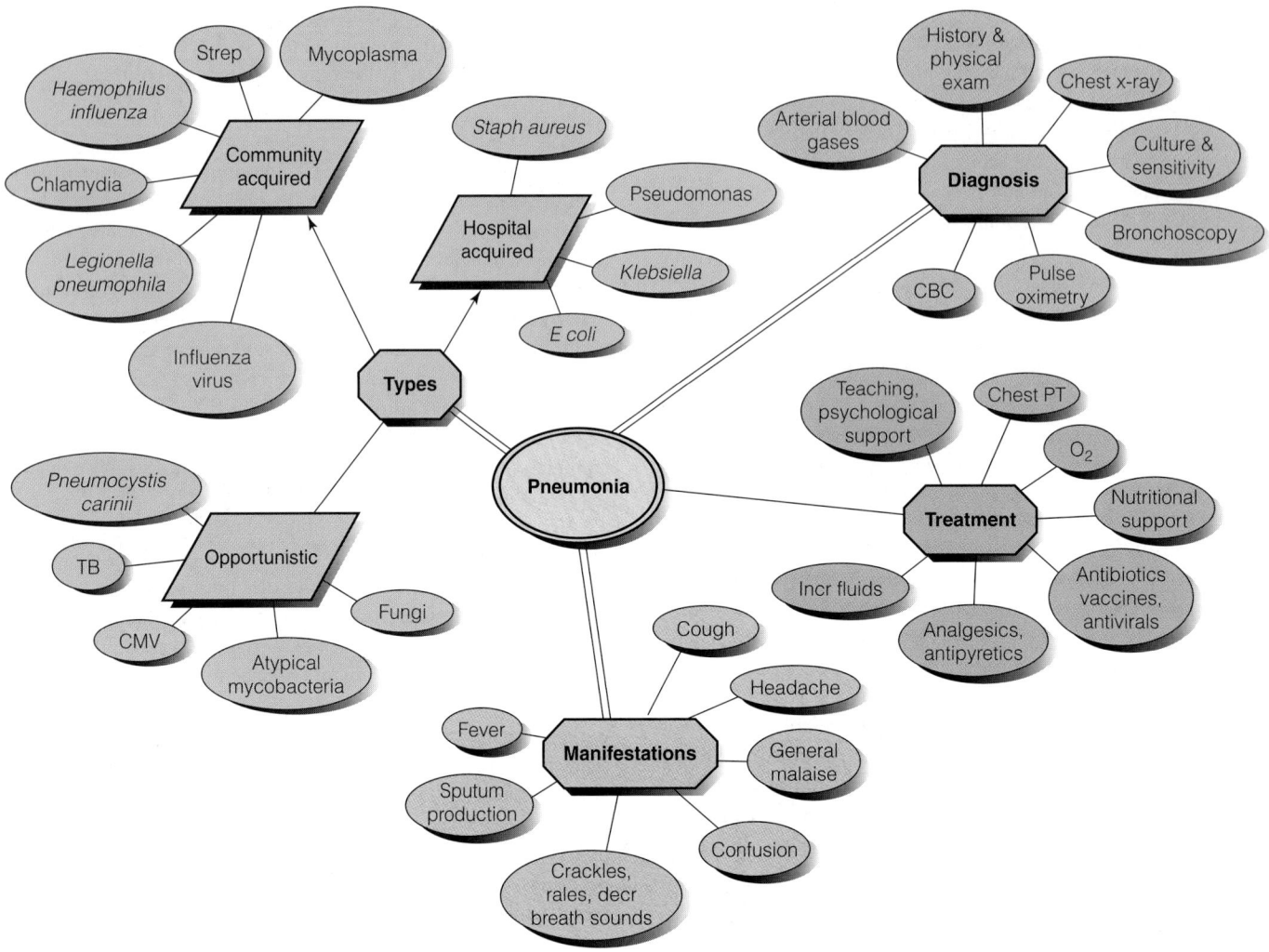

Figure 13-5 ■ A sample pathophysiology concept map.

that must be given on each day during the projected length of stay for the specific type of condition. Like the traditional nursing care plan, a multidisciplinary care plan can specify outcomes and nursing interventions to address client problems (including nursing diagnoses). However, it includes medical treatments to be performed by other health care providers as well.

The plan is usually organized with a column for each day, listing the interventions that should be carried out and the client outcomes that should be achieved on that day. There are as many columns on the multidisciplinary care plan as the preset number of days allowed for the client's diagnosis-related group (DRG). For further information, see Chapter 6 ∞ . Multidisciplinary care plans do not include detailed nursing activities. They should be drawn from but do not replace standards of care and standardized care plans.

Guidelines for Writing Nursing Care Plans

The nurse should use the following guidelines when writing nursing care plans:

1. *Date and sign the plan.* The date the plan is written is essential for evaluation, review, and future planning. The nurse's signature demonstrates accountability to the client and to the nursing profession, since the effectiveness of nursing actions can be evaluated.

2. *Use category headings:* "Nursing Diagnoses," "Goals/ Desired Outcomes," "Nursing Interventions," and "Evaluation." Include a date for the evaluation of each goal.

3. *Use standardized/approved medical or English symbols and key words rather than complete sentences to communicate your ideas unless the agency policy dictates otherwise.* For example, write "Turn and reposition q2h" rather than "Turn and reposition the client every two hours." Or, write "Clean wound c̄ H₂O₂ bid" rather than "Clean the client's wound with hydrogen peroxide twice a day, morning and evening." See Table 15–4 ∞ on page 259 for a list of standard medical abbreviations.

4. *Be specific.* Because nurses are now working shifts of different lengths, some working 12-hour shifts and some working 8-hour shifts, it is even more important to be specific about expected timing of an intervention. If the intervention reads "change incisional dressing q shift," it could mean either twice in 24 hours, or three times in 24 hours, depending on the shift time. This miscommunication becomes even more serious when medications are ordered to

be given "q shift." Writing down specific times during the 24-hour period will help clarify.

5. *Refer to procedure books or other sources of information rather than including all the steps on a written plan.* For example, write "See unit procedure book for tracheostomy care," or attach a standard nursing plan about such procedures as radiation-implantation care and preoperative or postoperative care.

6. *Tailor the plan to the unique characteristics of the client by ensuring that the client's choices, such as preferences about the times of care and the methods used, are included.* This reinforces the client's individuality and sense of control. For example, the written nursing intervention "Provide prune juice at breakfast rather than other juice" indicates that the client was given a choice of beverages.

7. *Ensure that the nursing plan incorporates preventive and health maintenance aspects as well as restorative ones.* For example, carrying out the intervention "Provide active-assistance ROM (range-of-motion) exercises to affected limbs q2h" prevents joint contractures and maintains muscle strength and joint mobility.

8. *Ensure that the plan contains interventions for ongoing assessment of the client* (e.g., "Inspect incision q8h").

9. *Include collaborative and coordination activities in the plan.* For example, the nurse may write interventions to ask a nutritionist or physical therapist about specific aspects of the client's care.

10. *Include plans for the client's discharge and home care needs.* The nurse begins discharge planning as soon as the client has been admitted. It is often necessary to consult and make arrangements with the community health nurse, social worker, and specific agencies that supply client information and needed equipment. Add teaching and discharge plans as addenda if they are lengthy and complex.

THE PLANNING PROCESS

In the process of developing client care plans, the nurse engages in the following activities:

- Setting priorities
- Establishing client goals/desired outcomes
- Selecting nursing interventions
- Writing individualized nursing interventions on care plans

Setting Priorities

Priority setting is the process of establishing a preferential sequence for addressing nursing diagnoses and interventions. The nurse and client begin planning by deciding which nursing diagnosis requires attention first, which second, and so on. Instead of rank-ordering diagnoses, nurses can group them as having high, medium, or low priority. Life-threatening problems, such as loss of respiratory or cardiac function, are designated as high priority. Health-threatening problems, such as acute illness and decreased coping ability, are assigned medium priority because they may result in delayed development or cause destructive physical or emotional changes. A low-priority problem is one

that arises from normal developmental needs or that requires only minimal nursing support.

Nurses frequently use Maslow's hierarchy of needs when setting priorities (see Figure 16-3 on page 274). In Maslow's hierarchy, physiologic needs such as air, food, and water are basic to life and receive higher priority than the need for security or activity. Growth needs, such as self-esteem, are not perceived as "basic" in this framework. Thus, nursing diagnoses such as *Ineffective Airway Clearance* and *Impaired Gas Exchange* would take priority over nursing diagnoses such as *Anxiety* or *Ineffective Coping*.

It is not necessary to resolve all high-priority diagnoses before addressing others. The nurse may partially address a high-priority diagnosis and then deal with a diagnosis of lesser priority. Furthermore, because the client may have several problems, the nurse often deals with more than one diagnosis at a time. Table 13–1 lists the priorities assigned to Amanda Aquilini's nursing diagnoses, which were identified in Chapter 12. ∞

Priorities change as the client's responses, problems, and therapies change. The nurse must consider a variety of factors when assigning priorities, including the following:

1. *Client's health values and beliefs:* Values concerning health may be more important to the nurse than to the client. For example, a client may believe being home for the children to be more urgent than a health problem. When there is such a difference of opinion, the client and nurse should discuss it openly to resolve any conflict. However, in a life-threatening situation the nurse usually must take the initiative.

2. *Client's priorities:* Involving the client in prioritizing and care planning enhances cooperation. Sometimes, however, the client's perception of what is important conflicts with the nurse's knowledge of potential problems or complications. For example, an elderly client may not regard turning and repositioning in bed as important, preferring to be undisturbed. The nurse, however, aware of the potential complications of prolonged bed rest (e.g., muscle weakness and pressure sores), needs to inform the client and carry out these necessary interventions.

3. *Resources available to the nurse and client:* If money, equipment, or personnel are scarce in a health care agency, then a problem may be given a lower priority than usual. Nurses in a home setting, for example, do not have the resources of a hospital. If the necessary resources are not available, the solution of that problem might need to be postponed, or the client may need a referral. Client resources, such as finances or coping ability, may also influence the setting of priorities. For example, a client who is unemployed may defer dental treatment; a client whose husband is terminally ill and dependent on her may feel unable to cope with nutritional guidance directed toward losing weight.

4. *Urgency of the health problem:* Regardless of the framework used, life-threatening situations require that the nurse assign them high priority. For example, in Table 13–1, although Amanda Aquilini is anxious about child care, her *Ineffective Airway Clearance* has higher priority. Situations

TABLE 13–1 Assigning Priorities to Nursing Diagnoses for Amanda Aquilini

NURSING DIAGNOSIS	PRIORITY	RATIONALE
Ineffective Airway Clearance related to (1) viscous secretions secondary to *Deficient Fluid Volume* and (2) shallow chest expansion secondary to pain and fatigue	High priority	Loss of respiratory functioning is a life-threatening problem. The nurse's primary concern must be to promote Amanda's oxygenation by addressing the etiologies of this problem.
Deficient Fluid Volume: intake insufficient to replace fluid loss related to fever and diaphoresis	High priority	Severe *Deficient Fluid Volume* is life threatening. Although not that severe for Amanda, it is a high-priority problem because it is also a contributing factor for *Ineffective Airway Clearance.* Collaborative efforts to improve her hydration have already begun (intravenous fluids). The nurse must immediately and continuously assess and promote Amanda's hydration.
Anxiety related to (1) difficulty breathing and (2) concerns over work and parenting roles	Medium priority	Although Amanda is concerned about work and parenting roles, these are not a threat to life. Also, treatment of her high-priority problem, *Ineffective Airway Clearance,* will relieve one of the etiologies of this problem (dyspnea). Meanwhile, the nurse must provide symptomatic relief of Amanda's anxiety during periods of dyspnea because extreme anxiety could further compromise her oxygenation by causing her to breathe ineffectively and increase the rate at which she uses oxygen.
Risk for Interrupted Family Processes related to mother's illness and potential temporary unavailability of father to provide child care	Low priority	Amanda's child is currently being cared for. If Amanda's husband returns as planned, this problem will not develop into an actual problem. No interventions are needed at present, except for continued assessment and reassurance.
Impaired Nutrition: Less than Body Requirements related to decreased appetite, nausea, and increased metabolism secondary to disease process	Low priority	This problem is not currently health threatening, but it could be if it were to persist. It will almost certainly resolve in a day or two as the medical problem is treated. If the medical problem does not resolve quickly, this will change to a medium priority.
Bathing/Hygiene Self-Care Deficit, related to weakness secondary to ineffective airway clearance and sleep pattern disturbance	Low priority	This problem is caused by the other higher priority problems; therefore, it will resolve as they resolve. Meanwhile, the nurse merely needs to assist Amanda with bathing and so on to support and conserve her energy until she is strong enough to resume her own care.
Sleep Pattern Disturbance related to cough, pain, orthopnea, fever, and diaphoresis	Low priority	Lack of sleep is health threatening. But for the moment (until night), the nurse does not need to address this problem. *Sleep Pattern Disturbance* does contribute to Amanda's *Ineffective Airway Clearance,* but it is not the main cause. Therefore, measures to promote sleep will be low priority until evening. After the nurse has attended to Amanda's oxygenation and hydration needs, this problem priority will change.
Acute Pain (Chest) related to cough secondary to pneumonia	Not on care plan	The nurse did not write *Pain* as a problem on the care plan because *Pain* is to be addressed as the etiology of *Sleep Pattern Disturbance* and *Ineffective Airway Clearance.* The pain etiologies (cough and pneumonia) will be treated by medications (collaborative interventions). Independent nursing actions would address the problem rather than the etiology and would be the same as the nursing actions for *Ineffective Airway Clearance.*

that affect the integrity of the client, that is, those that could have a negative or destructive effect on the client, also have high priority. Such health problems as drug abuse and radical alteration of self-concept due to amputation can be destructive both to the individual and to the family.

5. *Medical treatment plan:* The priorities for treating health problems must be congruent with treatment by other health professionals. For example, a high priority for the client might be to become ambulatory; however, if the primary care provider's therapeutic regimen calls for extended bed rest, then ambulation must assume a lower priority in the

nursing care plan. The nurse can provide or teach exercises to facilitate ambulation later, provided the client's health permits. The nursing diagnosis related to ambulation is not ignored; it is merely deferred.

Establishing Client Goals/ Desired Outcomes

After establishing priorities, the nurse and client set goals for each nursing diagnosis (see Figure 13-6 ■). On a care plan, the **goals/desired outcomes** describe, in terms of observable client re-

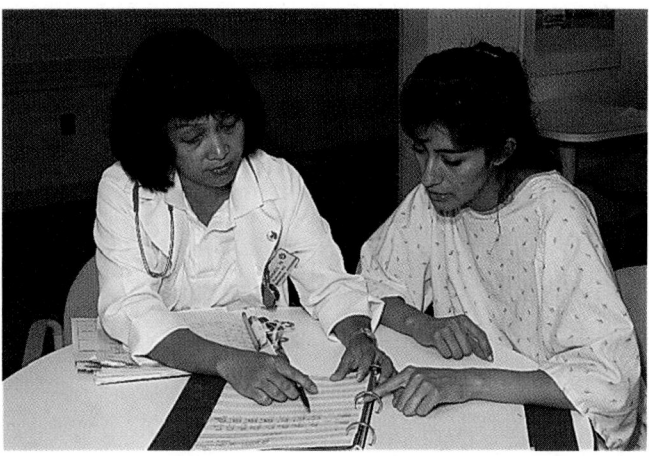

Figure 13-6 ■ Nurse Medina and Amanda collaborate to set goals and outcome criteria and develop a care plan.

sponses, what the nurse hopes to achieve by implementing the nursing interventions. The terms *goal* and *desired outcome* are used interchangeably in this text, except when discussing and using standardized language. Some references also use the terms *expected outcome, predicted outcome, outcome criterion,* and *objective.*

Some nursing literature differentiates the terms by defining goals as broad statements about the client's status and desired outcomes as the more specific, observable criteria used to evaluate whether the goals have been met. For example:

Goal (broad):   Improved nutritional status.
Desired outcome (specific): Gain 5 lb by April 25.

When goals are stated broadly, as in this example, the care plan must include both goals and desired outcomes. They are sometimes combined into one statement linked by the words "as evidenced by," as follows:

> Improved nutritional status as evidenced by weight gain of 5 lb by April 25.

Writing the broad, general goal first may help students to think of the specific outcomes that are needed, but the broad goal is just a starting point for planning. It is the specific, observable outcomes that must be written on the care plan and used to evaluate client progress. Table 13–2 shows both broad goals and specific outcomes.

The Nursing Outcomes Classification

Standardized or common nursing language is required in all phases of the nursing process if nursing data are to be included in computerized databases that are analyzed and used in nursing practice. Nurse leaders and researchers have been working since 1991 to develop a taxonomy, the **Nursing Outcomes Classification (NOC),** for describing client outcomes that respond to nursing interventions. In the taxonomy, over 330 outcomes belong to one of seven domains (e.g., physiologic health or family health) and a class within the domain (e.g., nutrition under physiologic health or family well-being under family health). Each NOC outcome is assigned a four-digit identifier, indicated in this text by square brackets, and a definition. Table 13–3 shows a NOC outcome associated with movement.

A NOC outcome is similar to a goal in traditional language. It is "An individual, family, or community state, behavior, or perception that is measured along a continuum in response to a nursing intervention(s)" (Moorhead, Johnson, & Maas, 2004, p. xix). The NOC outcomes are broadly stated and conceptual. To be measured, an outcome must be made more specific by identifying the indicators that apply to a particular client. An **indicator** is "a more concrete individual, family, or community state, behavior, or perception that serves as a cue for measuring an outcome" (Moorhead et al., p. xix) and is similar to desired outcomes in traditional language. Indicators are also stated in neutral terms, but each outcome includes a five-point scale (a measure) that is used to rate the client's status on each indicator. (See Appendix C ∞). When using the NOC taxonomy to write a desired outcome on a care plan, the nurse writes the label, the indicators that apply to the particular client, and the location on the measuring scale that is desired for each indicator. For example, using the NOC outcome in Table 13–3 for the client diagnosed in Table 13–2, the individualized desired outcomes would read as follows:

Mobility Level:

Transfer performance (5, completely independent)
Ambulation: walking (4, independent with assistive device)

Stated in traditional language, that goal would read: "Client will have improved mobility, as evidenced by ability to transfer independently and walk with assistive device (walker)."

TABLE 13–2 Deriving Desired Outcomes from Nursing Diagnoses

NURSING DIAGNOSIS	OPPOSITE HEALTHY RESPONSES (GOALS)	DESIRED OUTCOMES THE CLIENT WILL:
Impaired Physical Mobility: inability to bear weight on left leg, related to inflammation of knee joint	Improved mobility Ability to bear weight on left leg	Ambulate with crutches by end of the week. Stand without assistance by end of the month.
Ineffective Airway Clearance related to poor cough effort, secondary to incision pain and fear of damaging sutures	Effective airway clearance	Have lungs clear to auscultation during entire postoperative period. Have no skin pallor or cyanosis by 12 hours postoperation. Within 24 hours after surgery, demonstrate good cough effort.

TABLE 13–3 **Example of a Standardized Client Outcome (NOC)**					
Domain I: Functional Health Class C: Mobility Outcome: Mobility [0208] Definition: Ability to move purposefully in own environment independently with or without assistive device					
Mobility overall rating	Severely Compromised	Substantially Compromised	Moderately Compromised	Mildly Compromised	Not Compromised
Indicators					
Balance	1	2	3	4	5
Coordination	1	2	3	4	5
Body positioning performance	1	2	3	4	5
Muscle movement	1	2	3	4	5
Joint movement	1	2	3	4	5
Transfer performance	1	2	3	4	5
Gait	1	2	3	4	5
Walking	1	2	3	4	5
Running	1	2	3	4	5
Jumping	1	2	3	4	5
Moves with ease	1	2	3	4	5

Note: From *Nursing Outcomes and Classification (NOC),* (p. 203), by M. Johnson, M. Maas, and S. Moorehead, Eds., St. Louis, MO: Mosby. Reprinted with permission.

Purpose of Desired Goals/Outcomes

Desired outcomes/goals serve the following purposes:

1. Provide direction for planning nursing interventions. Ideas for interventions come more easily if the desired outcomes state clearly and specifically what the nurse hopes to achieve.
2. Serve as criteria for evaluating client progress. Although developed in the planning step of the nursing process, desired outcomes serve as the criteria for judging the effectiveness of nursing interventions and client progress in the evaluation step (see Chapter 14). ∞
3. Enable the client and nurse to determine when the problem has been resolved.
4. Help motivate the client and nurse by providing a sense of achievement. As goals are met, both client and nurse can see that their efforts have been worthwhile. This provides motivation to continue following the plan, especially when difficult lifestyle changes need to be made.

Long-Term and Short-Term Goals

Goals may be short term or long term. A short-term goal might be "Client will raise right arm to shoulder height by Friday." In the same context, a long-term goal might be "Client will regain full use of right arm in 6 weeks." Short-term goals are useful (a) for clients who require health care for a short time and (b) for those who are frustrated by long-term goals that seem difficult to attain and who need the satisfaction of achieving a short-term goal. In an acute care setting, much of the nurse's time is spent on the client's immediate needs, so most goals are short term. However, clients in acute care settings also need long-term goals to guide planning for their discharge to long-term agencies or home care, especially in a managed care environment. Long-term goals are often used for clients who live at home and have chronic health problems and for clients in nursing homes, extended care facilities, and rehabilitation centers.

Relationship of Desired Goals/ Outcomes to Nursing Diagnoses

Goals are derived from the client's nursing diagnoses—primarily from the diagnostic label. The diagnostic label contains the unhealthy response; it states what should change. For example, if the nursing diagnosis is *Risk for Deficient Fluid Volume* related to diarrhea and inadequate intake secondary to nausea, the essential goal statement might be

> The client will reestablish fluid balance, as evidenced by urinary and stool output in balance with fluid intake, normal skin turgor, and moist mucous membranes.

In this example, a general goal (fluid balance) is stated as the opposite of the problem (*Deficient Fluid Volume*) and then followed by a list of observable desired outcomes. If achieved, the outcomes would be evidence that the problem, *Deficient Fluid Volume,* has been prevented.

For every nursing diagnosis, the nurse must write the desired outcome or outcomes that, when achieved, directly demonstrates resolution of the problem. When developing goals/ desired outcomes, ask the following questions:

1. What is the client's problem?
2. What is the opposite, healthy response?
3. How will the client look or behave if the healthy response is achieved? (What will I be able to see, hear, measure, palpate, smell, or otherwise observe with my senses?)
4. What must the client do and how well must the client do it to demonstrate problem resolution or to demonstrate the capability of resolving the problem?

Components of Goal/ Desired Outcome Statements

Goal/desired outcome statements should usually have the following four components:

1. *Subject.* The subject, a noun, is the client, any part of the client, or some attribute of the client, such as the client's pulse or urinary output. The subject is often omitted in goals; it is assumed that the subject is the client unless indicated otherwise.

2. *Verb.* The verb specifies an action the client is to perform, for example, what the client is to do, learn, or experience. Verbs that denote directly observable behaviors, such as *administer, show,* or *walk,* must be used. See Box 13–1 for some examples.

3. *Conditions or modifiers.* Conditions or modifiers may be added to the verb to explain the circumstances under which the behavior is to be performed. They explain what, where, when, or how. For example:
Walks with the help of a cane (how).
After attending two group diabetes classes, lists signs and symptoms of diabetes (when).
When at home, maintains weight at existing level (where).
Discusses *food pyramid and recommended daily servings* (what).
Conditions need not be included if the criterion of performance clearly indicates what is expected.

4. *Criterion of desired performance.* The criterion indicates the standard by which a performance is evaluated or the level

at which the client will perform the specified behavior. These criteria may specify time or speed, accuracy, distance, and quality. To establish a time-achievement criterion, the nurse needs to ask "How long?" To establish an accuracy criterion, the nurse asks "How well?" Similarly, the nurse asks "How far?" and "What is the expected standard?" to establish distance and quality criteria, respectively. Examples are:
Weighs 75 kg *by April* (time).
Lists *five out of six* signs of diabetes (accuracy).
Walks *one block per day* (time and distance).
Administers insulin *using aseptic technique* (quality).

Table 13–4 illustrates the format that should be used to write outcomes. Table 13–5 lists desired outcomes that were developed for Amanda Aquilini.

Guidelines for Writing Goals/ Desired Outcomes

The following guidelines can help nurses write useful goals and desired outcomes:

1. Write goals and outcomes in terms of client responses, not nurse activities. Beginning each goal statement with *the client will* may help focus the goal on client behaviors and responses. Avoid statements that start with *enable, facilitate, allow, let, permit,* or similar verbs followed by the word *client.* These verbs indicate what the nurse hopes to accomplish, not what the client will do.
Correct: Client will drink 100 mL of water per hour (client behavior).
Incorrect: Maintain client hydration (nursing action).

2. Be sure that desired outcomes are realistic for the client's capabilities, limitations, and designated time span, if it is indicated. Limitations refers to finances, equipment, family support, social services, physical and mental condition, and time. For example, the outcome "Measures insulin accurately" may be unrealistic for a client who has poor vision due to cataracts.

3. Ensure that the goals and desired outcomes are compatible with the therapies of other professionals. For example, the outcome "Will increase the time spent out of bed by 15 minutes each day" is not compatible with a primary care provider's prescribed therapy of bed rest.

BOX 13–1 Examples of Action Verbs

Apply	Drink	Select
Assemble	Explain	Share
Breathe	Help	Sit
Choose	Identify	Sleep
Compare	Inject	State
Define	List	Talk
Demonstrate	Move	Transfer
Describe	Name	Turn
Differentiate	Prepare	Verbalize
Discuss	Report	

TABLE 13–4 Components of Goals/Desired Outcomes

SUBJECT	VERB	CONDITIONS/MODIFIERS	CRITERION OF DESIRED PERFORMANCE
Client	drinks	2500 mL of fluid	daily (time)
Client	administers	correct insulin dose	using aseptic technique (quality standard)
Client	lists	three hazards of smoking (after reading literature)	(accuracy indicated by "three hazards")
Client	recalls	five symptoms of diabetes before discharge	(accuracy indicated by "five symptoms")
Client	walks	the length of the hall without a cane	by date of discharge (time)
Client's ankle	measures	less than 10 inches in circumference	in 48 hours (time)
Client	performs	leg ROM exercises as taught	every 8 hours (time)
Client	identifies	foods high in salt from a prepared list	before discharge (time)
Client	states	the purposes of his medications	before discharge (time)

4. Make sure that each goal is derived from only one nursing diagnosis. For example, the goal "The client will increase the amount of nutrients ingested and show progress in the ability to feed self" is derived from two nursing diagnoses: *Feeding Self-Care Deficit* and *Impaired Nutrition: Less than Body Requirements*. Keeping the goal statement related to only one diagnosis facilitates evaluation of care by ensuring that planned nursing interventions are clearly related to the diagnosis.

5. Use observable, measurable terms for outcomes. Avoid words that are vague and require interpretation or judgment by the observer. For example, phrases such as *increase daily exercise* and *improve knowledge of nutrition* can mean different things to different people. If used in outcomes, these phrases can lead to disagreements about whether the outcome was met. These phrases may be suitable for a broad client goal but are not sufficiently clear and specific to guide the nurse when evaluating client responses.

6. Make sure the client considers the goals/desired outcomes important and values them. Some outcomes, such as those for problems related to self-esteem, parenting, and communication, involve choices that are best made by the client or in collaboration with the client.

Some clients may know what they wish to accomplish with regard to their health problem; others may not know all the outcome

TABLE 13–5 **Desired Outcomes for Amanda Aquilini**	
NURSING DIAGNOSIS*	**GOAL STATEMENTS [NOC]/DESIRED OUTCOMES**
Ineffective Airway Clearance related to viscous secretions and shallow chest expansion secondary to fluid volume deficit, pain, and fatigue	Respiratory Status: Gas exchange [0402], as evidenced by ■ Absence of pallor and cyanosis (skin and mucous membranes) ■ Use of correct breathing/coughing technique after instruction ■ Productive cough ■ Symmetric chest excursion of at least 4 cm Within 48–72 hours: ■ Lungs clear to auscultation ■ Respirations 12–22/min, pulse <100 beats/min ■ Inhales normal volume of air on incentive spirometer
Deficient Fluid Volume: intake insufficient to replace fluid loss related to vomiting, fever, and diaphoresis	Fluid balance [0601], as evidenced by ■ Urine output greater than 30 mL/h ■ Urine specific gravity 1.005–1.025 ■ Good skin turgor ■ Moist mucous membranes ■ Stating the need for oral fluid intake
Anxiety related to difficulty breathing and concerns about work and parenting roles	Anxiety control [1402], as evidenced by ■ Listening to and following instructions for correct breathing and coughing technique, even during periods of dyspnea ■ Verbalizing understanding of condition, diagnostic tests, and treatments (by end of day) ■ Decrease in reports of fear and anxiety; none within 12 h ■ Voice steady, not shaky ■ Respiratory rate of 12–22/min ■ Freely expressing concerns and possible solutions about work and parenting roles
Risk for Interrupted Family Processes related to mother's illness and temporary unavailability of father to provide child care	Family coping [2600], as evidenced by ■ Report of satisfactory child care arrangements having been made ■ Client and husband communicating effectively and working together to solve problems ■ Family members expressing feelings and providing mutual support
Imbalanced Nutrition: Less than Body Requirements related to decreased appetite, nausea, and increased metabolism secondary to disease process	Nutritional status: Nutrient intake [1009], as evidenced by ■ Eating at least 85% of each meal ■ Maintaining present weight ■ Verbalizing importance of adequate nutrition ■ Verbalizing improved appetite
Bathing/Hygiene Self-Care Deficit related to activity intolerance secondary to airway clearance and sleep pattern disturbance	Self-care: Activities of daily living [0300], as evidenced by ■ Ambulates to bathroom without dyspnea, fatigue, ineffective or shortness of breath ■ Within 24 hours, bathes with assistance in bed; within 48 hours, bathes with assistance at sink; within 72 hours, bathes in shower without dyspnea ■ Reports satisfaction and comfort with hygiene needs
Disturbed Sleep Pattern related to cough, pain, orthopnea, and diaphoresis	Sleep [0004], as evidenced by ■ Observed sleeping at night rounds ■ Reports feeling rested ■ Does not experience orthopnea

* The nursing diagnoses are listed in priority order.

possibilities. The nurse must actively listen to the client to determine personal values, goals, and desired outcomes in relation to current health concerns. Clients are usually motivated and expend the necessary energy to reach goals they consider important.

See the Nursing Care Plan on pages 227–228 for three of Amanda Aquilini's nursing diagnoses.

Selecting Nursing Interventions and Activities

Nursing interventions and activities are the actions that a nurse performs to achieve client goals. The specific interventions chosen should focus on eliminating or reducing the etiology of the nursing diagnosis, which is the second clause of the diagnostic statement.

When it is not possible to change the etiologic factors, the nurse chooses interventions to treat the signs and symptoms or the defining characteristics in NANDA terminology. Examples of this situation would be *Pain* related to surgical incision and *Anxiety* related to unknown etiology.

Interventions for risk nursing diagnoses should focus on measures to reduce the client's risk factors, which are also found in the second clause.

Correct identification of the etiology during the diagnosing phase provides the framework for choosing successful nursing interventions. For example, the diagnostic label *Activity Intolerance* may have several etiologies: pain, weakness, sedentary lifestyle, anxiety, or cardiac arrhythmias. Interventions will vary according to the cause of the problem.

Types of Nursing Interventions

Nursing interventions are identified and written during the planning step of the nursing process; however, they are actually performed during the implementing step. Nursing interventions include both direct and indirect care, as well as nurse-initiated, physician-initiated, and other provider-initiated treatments. Direct care is an intervention performed through interaction with the client. Indirect care is an intervention performed away from but on behalf of the client such as interdisciplinary collaboration or management of the care environment.

Independent interventions are those activities that nurses are licensed to initiate on the basis of their knowledge and skills. They include physical care, ongoing assessment, emotional support and comfort, teaching, counseling, environmental management, and making referrals to other health care professionals. Recall from Chapter 12 ∞ that nursing diagnoses are client problems that can be treated primarily by independent nursing interventions. In performing an autonomous activity, the nurse determines that the client requires certain nursing interventions, either carries these out or delegates them to other nursing personnel, and is accountable or answerable for the decision and the actions. An example of an independent action is planning and providing special mouth care for a client after diagnosing *Impaired Oral Mucous Membranes.*

Dependent interventions are activities carried out under the physician's orders or supervision, or according to specified routines. Physicians' orders commonly direct the nurse to provide medications, intravenous therapy, diagnostic tests, treatments, diet, and activity. The nurse is responsible for assessing the need for, explaining, and administering the medical orders. Nursing interventions may be written to individualize the medical order based on the client's status. For example, for a medical order of "Progressive ambulation, as tolerated," a nurse might write the following:

1. Dangle for 5 min, 12 h postop.
2. Stand at bedside 24 h postop; observe for pallor, dizziness, and weakness.
3. Check pulse before and after ambulating. Do not progress if pulse > 110.

Collaborative interventions are actions the nurse carries out in collaboration with other health team members, such as physical therapists, social workers, dietitians, and physicians. Collaborative nursing activities reflect the overlapping responsibilities of, and collegial relationships between, health personnel. For example, the physician might order physical therapy to teach the client crutch-walking. The nurse would be responsible for informing the physical therapy department and for coordinating the client's care to include the physical therapy sessions. When the client returns to the nursing unit, the nurse would assist with crutch-walking and collaborate with the physical therapist to evaluate the client's progress.

The amount of time the nurse spends in an independent versus a collaborative or dependent role varies according to the clinical area, type of institution, and specific position of the nurse.

Considering the Consequences of Each Intervention

Usually several possible interventions can be identified for each nursing goal. The nurse's task is to choose those that are most likely to achieve the desired client outcomes. The nurse begins by considering the risks and benefits of each intervention. An intervention may have more than one consequence. For example, "Provide accurate information" could result in the following client behaviors:

- Increased anxiety
- Decreased anxiety
- Wish to talk with the primary care provider
- Desire to leave the hospital
- Relaxation

Determining the consequences of each intervention requires nursing knowledge and experience. For example, the nurse's experience may suggest that providing information the night before the client's surgery may increase the client's worry and tension, whereas maintaining the usual rituals before sleep is more effective. The nurse might then consider providing information several days before surgery.

Criteria for Choosing Nursing Interventions

After considering the consequences of the alternative nursing interventions, the nurse chooses one or more that are likely to be most effective. Although the nurse bases this decision on knowledge and experience, the client's input is important.

The following criteria can help the nurse choose the best nursing interventions. The plan must be

- Safe and appropriate for the individual's age, health, and condition.
- Achievable with the resources available. For example, a home care nurse might wish to include an intervention for an elderly client to "Check blood glucose daily"; but in order for that to occur, either the client must have intact sight, cognition, and memory to carry this out independently, or daily visits from a home care nurse must be available and affordable.
- Congruent with the client's values, beliefs, and culture.
- Congruent with other therapies (e.g., if the client is not permitted food, the strategy of an evening snack must be deferred until health permits).
- Based on nursing knowledge and experience or knowledge from relevant sciences (i.e., based on a rationale). For examples of rationales, refer to the Nursing Care Plan for Amanda Aquilini on pages 227–228.
- Within established standards of care as determined by state laws, professional associations (American Nurses Association), and the policies of the institution. Many agencies have policies to guide the activities of health professionals and to safeguard clients. Rules for visiting hours and procedures to follow when a client has cardiac arrest are examples. If a policy does not benefit clients, nurses have a responsibility to bring this to the attention of the appropriate people.

Writing Individualized Nursing Interventions

After choosing the appropriate nursing interventions, the nurse writes them on the care plan. See examples of nursing interventions for Amanda Aquilini in the Nursing Care Plan on pages 227–228.

Nursing interventions on the care plan are dated when they are written and reviewed regularly at intervals that depend on the individual's needs. In an intensive care unit, for example, the plan of care will be continually monitored and revised. In a community clinic, weekly or biweekly reviews may be indicated.

The format of written interventions is similar to that of outcomes: verb, conditions, and modifiers, plus time element. The action verb starts the intervention and must be precise. For example, "Explain (to the client) the actions of insulin" is a more precise statement than "Teach (the client) about insulin." "Measure and record ankle circumference daily at 0900 h" is more precise than "Assess edema of left ankle daily." Sometimes a modifier for the verb can make the nursing intervention more precise. For example, "Apply spiral bandage firmly to left lower leg" is more precise than "Apply spiral bandage to left leg."

The time element answers when, how long, or how often the nursing action is to occur. Examples are "Assist client with tub bath at 0700 daily" and "Administer analgesic 30 minutes prior to physical therapy."

In some settings, the intervention (and other segments of the nursing care plan) is signed. The signature of the nurse prescribing the intervention shows the nurse's accountability and has legal significance.

Relationship of Nursing Interventions to Problem Status

Depending on the type of client problem, the nurse writes interventions for observation, prevention, treatment, and health promotion.

Observations include assessments made to determine whether a complication is developing, as well as observation of the client's responses to nursing and other therapies. The nurse should write observations for both real problems and those for which the client is at risk. Some examples are "Auscultate lungs q8h," "Observe for redness over sacrum q2h," and "Record intake and output hourly."

Prevention interventions prescribe the care needed to avoid complications or reduce risk factors. They are needed mainly for potential nursing diagnoses and collaborative problems. Examples are "Turn, cough, and deep breathe q2h" (prevents respiratory complications) and "Keep bed rails raised and bed in low position" (minimizes chances of client falling out of bed).

Treatments include teaching, referrals, physical care, and other care needed for an actual nursing diagnosis. Some interventions may accomplish either prevention or treatment functions, depending on the status of the problem. In the preceding examples, "Turn, cough, and deep breathe q2h" can also be intended to treat an existing respiratory problem.

Health promotion interventions are appropriate when the client has no health problems or when the nurse makes a wellness nursing diagnosis. Such nursing interventions focus on helping the client identify areas for improvement that will lead to a higher level of wellness and actualize the client's overall health potential. Examples are "Discuss the importance of daily exercise" and "Explore infant stimulation techniques."

Delegating Implementation

Delegating is another activity that occurs during the planning phase of the nursing process. While choosing and writing nursing interventions on the client's care plan, the nurse must also determine who should actually perform the activity. The American Nurses Association defines delegation as "the transfer of responsibility for the performance of an activity from one person to another while retaining accountability for the outcome." This differs from **assignment,** which is a "downward or lateral transfer of both the responsibility *and accountability* [emphasis added] of an activity from one individual to another" (ANA, 1997, Attachment I, #5–6). The ability to delegate client care and assign tasks is a vital skill for registered nurses because many health care institutions use assistive personnel (e.g., licensed practical nurses and unlicensed nursing assistants). To delegate appropriately, the nurse must match the needs of the client and family with the skills and knowledge of the available caregivers. This requires knowing the background, experience, knowledge, skills, and strengths of each person, and understanding which tasks are and are not within their legal scope of practice.

The nurse has two responsibilities in delegating and assigning: (1) appropriate delegation of duties (that is, giving people duties within their scope of practice) and (2) adequate supervision of personnel to whom work is delegated or assigned. The RN can delegate certain tasks to an unlicensed person but cannot assign responsibility for total nursing care. The RN is responsible for seeing that delegated tasks are carried out properly. Assistive personnel may perform tasks such as mea-suring intake and output, but the RN is still responsible for analyzing data, planning care, and evaluating outcomes. Because there are no universal standards for the training of unlicensed personnel, nurses often must assume responsibility for supplementing the training those staff members have received (see also Chapter 28). ∞

THE NURSING INTERVENTIONS CLASSIFICATION

In addition to the efforts of NANDA to standardize the language for describing problems that require nursing care and to create a taxonomy of standardized client outcome labels, nurse researchers also recognized the need for a standardized language to describe the interventions that nurses perform. A taxonomy of nursing interventions referred to as the **Nursing Interventions**

Classification (NIC) taxonomy, developed by the Iowa Intervention Project, was first published in 1992 and has been updated every 4 years after then. This taxonomy consists of three levels: (a) level 1, domains; (b) level 2, classes; and (c) level 3, interventions. Table 13–6 shows the seven domains and 30 classes of interventions within the taxonomy.

More than 514 interventions (level 3) have been developed. Similar to NANDA diagnoses, each broadly stated intervention includes a label (name), a definition, and a list of activities that outline the key actions of nurses in carrying out the intervention. For example, the level 3 intervention Touch is one of several interventions developed within the Behavioral domain and its class entitled Coping Assistance (see Box 13–2).

All NIC interventions have been linked to NANDA nursing diagnostic labels. The nurse can look up a client's nursing diagnosis to see which nursing interventions are suggested. However, each nursing diagnosis contains suggestions for several interventions, so nurses need to select the appropriate interventions based on their judgment and knowledge of the client. For example, the nursing diagnostic label *Disturbed Sleep Pattern* has 10 NIC interventions listed for problem resolution and 18 additional optional interventions (see Box 13–3).

BOX 13–2 Example of a NIC Nursing Intervention Label

INTERVENTION: TOUCH [5460]
DEFINITION: Providing comfort and communication through purposeful tactile contact
ACTIVITIES:
- Observe cultural taboos about touch.
- Give a reassuring hug, as appropriate.
- Put arm around patient's shoulders, as appropriate.
- Hold patient's hand to provide emotional support.
- Apply gentle pressure at wrist, hand, or shoulder of seriously ill patient.
- Rub back in synchrony with patient's breathing, as appropriate.
- Stroke body part in slow, rhythmical fashion, as appropriate.
- Massage around painful area, as appropriate.
- Elicit from parents common actions used to soothe and calm their child.
- Hold infant or child firmly and snugly.

- Encourage parents to touch newborn or ill child.
- Surround premature infant with blanket rolls (nesting).
- Swaddle infant snugly in a blanket to keep arms and legs close to the body.
- Place infant on mother's body immediately after birth.
- Encourage mother to hold, touch, and examine the infant while umbilical cord is being severed.
- Encourage parents to hold infant.
- Encourage parents to massage infant.
- Demonstrate quieting techniques for infants.
- Provide appropriate pacifier for nonnutritional sucking in newborns.
- Provide oral stimulation exercises before tube feedings in premature infants.

Note: From *Nursing Interventions Classification (NIC)* 4th ed. (p. 738), by J. C. Dochterman and G. M. Bulechek, Eds., 2004, St. Louis, MO: Mosby. Reprinted with permission.

BOX 13–3 Examples of NIC Interventions Linked to the NANDA Nursing Diagnosis of Disturbed Sleep Pattern

DISTURBED SLEEP PATTERN
Definition: Time limited disruption of sleep (natural, periodic suspension of consciousness) amount and quality

SUGGESTED NURSING INTERVENTIONS FOR PROBLEM RESOLUTION

Dementia Management	Medication Prescribing
Environmental Management	Security Enhancement
Environmental Management: Comfort	Simple Relaxation Therapy
Medication Administration	Sleep Enhancement
Medication Management	Touch

ADDITIONAL OPTIONAL INTERVENTIONS

Anxiety Reduction	Meditation
Autogenic Training	Music Therapy
Bathing	Nutrition Management
Calming Technique	Pain Management
Coping Enhancement	Positioning
Energy Management	Progressive Muscle Relaxation
Exercise Promotion	Self-Care Assistance: Toileting
Exercise Therapy: Ambulation	Simple Massage
Kangaroo Care	Urinary Incontinence Care: Enuresis

Note: From *Nursing Interventions Classification (NIC)* 4th ed. (p. 877), by J. C. Dochterman and G. M. Bulechek, Eds., 2004, St. Louis, MO: Mosby. Reprinted with permission.

TABLE 13–6 NIC Taxonomy

LEVEL 1: DOMAINS	LEVEL 2: CLASSES (LETTERED FOR CROSS-REFERENCING)
Domain 1 *Physiological: Basic* Care that supports physical functioning	A. Activity and Exercise Management: Interventions to organize or assist with physical activity and energy conservation and expenditure B. Elimination Management: Interventions to establish and maintain regular bowel and urinary elimination patterns and manage complications due to altered patterns C. Immobility Management: Interventions to manage restricted body movement and the sequelae D. Nutrition Support: Interventions to modify or maintain nutritional status E. Physical Comfort Promotion: Interventions to promote comfort using physical techniques F. Self-Care Facilitation: Interventions to provide or assist with routine activities of daily living
Domain 2 *Physiological: Complex* Care that supports homeostatic regulation	G. Electrolyte and Acid–Base Management: Interventions to regulate electrolyte/acid–base balance and prevent complications H. Drug Management: Interventions to facilitate desired effects of pharmacological agents I. Neurologic Management: Interventions to optimize neurologic functions J. Perioperative Care: Interventions to provide care before, during, and immediately after surgery K. Respiratory Management: Interventions to promote airway patency and gas exchange L. Skin/Wound Management: Interventions to maintain or restore tissue integrity M. Thermoregulation: Interventions to maintain body temperature within a normal range N. Tissue Perfusion Management: Interventions to optimize circulation of blood and fluids to the tissue
Domain 3 *Behavioral* Care that supports psychosocial functioning and facilitates lifestyle changes	O. Behavior Therapy: Interventions to reinforce or promote desirable behaviors or alter undesirable behaviors P. Cognitive Therapy: Interventions to reinforce or promote desirable cognitive functioning or alter undesirable cognitive functioning Q. Communication Enhancement: Interventions to facilitate delivering and receiving verbal and nonverbal messages R. Coping Assistance: Interventions to assist another to build on own strengths, to adapt to a change in function, or to achieve a higher level of function S. Patient Education: Interventions to facilitate learning T. Psychological Comfort Promotion: Interventions to promote comforts using psychological techniques
Domain 4 *Safety* Care that supports protection against harm	U. Crisis Management: Interventions to provide immediate short-term help in both psychological and physiological crises V. Risk Management: Interventions to initiate risk-reduction activities and continue monitoring risks over time
Domain 5 *Family* Care that supports the family unit	W. Childbearing Care: Interventions to assist in understanding and coping with the psychological and physiological changes during the childbearing period Z. Childrearing Care: Interventions to assist in child rearing X. Lifespan Care: Interventions to facilitate family unit functioning and promote the health and welfare of family members throughout the lifespan
Domain 6 *Health System* Care that supports effective use of the health care delivery system *Domain 7* *Community* Care that supports the health of the community	Y. Health System Mediation: Interventions to facilitate the interface between patient/family and the health care system a. Health System Management: Interventions to provide and enhance support services for the delivery of care b. Information Management: Interventions to facilitate communication among health care providers c. Community Health Promotion: Interventions that promote the health of the whole community d. Community Risk Management: Interventions that assist in detecting or preventing health risks to the whole community

Note: From *Nursing Interventions Classification (NIC)*, 4th ed. (pp. 112–113), by J. C. Dochterman and G. M. Bulechek, Eds., 2004, St. Louis, MO: Mosby. Reprinted with permission.

When planning and documenting care in an agency that uses the NIC taxonomy, the nurse chooses the broad intervention label (e.g., Touch). Not all activities suggested for the intervention would be needed for every client, so the nurse chooses the activities appropriate for the client and individualizes them to fit the supplies, equipment, and other resources available in the agency. When writing individualized nursing interventions on a care plan, the nurse should record customized activities rather than the broad intervention labels.

The NIC taxonomy provides many benefits to nurse practitioners, nurse educators, nurse administrators, and the nursing profession as a whole (see Box 13–4).

LIFESPAN CONSIDERATIONS   Nursing Care Plan

ELDERS

When a client is in an extended care facility or a long-term care facility, interventions and medications often remain the same day after day. It is important to review the care plan on a regular basis, because changes in the condition of elders may be subtle and go unnoticed. This applies to both changes of improvement or deterioration. Either one should receive attention so that appropriate revisions can be made in expected outcomes and interventions. Outcomes need to be realistic with consideration given to the client's physical condition, emotional condition, support systems, and mental status. Outcomes often have to be stated and expected to be completed in very small steps. For instance, a client who has had a cerebrovascular accident may spend weeks learning to brush her own teeth or dress herself. When these small steps are successfully completed, it gives the client a sense of accomplishment and motivation to continue working toward increasing self-care. This particular example also demonstrates the need to work collaboratively with other departments, such as physical and occupational therapy, to develop the nursing care plan.

NURSING CARE PLAN   Amanda Aquilini

NURSING DIAGNOSIS: Ineffective Airway Clearance Related to Viscous Secretions and Shallow Chest Expansion Secondary to Deficient Fluid Volume, Pain, and Fatigue

DESIRED OUTCOMES*/ INDICATORS	NURSING INTERVENTIONS	RATIONALE
Respiratory Status: Gas exchange [0402], as evidenced by ■ Absence of pallor and cyanosis (skin and mucous membranes) ■ Use of correct breathing/coughing technique after instruction ■ Productive cough ■ Symmetric chest excursion of at least 4 cm	Monitor respiratory status q4h: rate, depth, effort, skin color, mucous membranes, amount and color of sputum. Monitor results of blood gases, chest x-ray studies, and incentive spirometer volume as available. Monitor level of consciousness. Auscultate lungs q4h. Vital signs q4h (TPR, BP, pulse oximetry).	To identify progress toward or deviations from goal. *Ineffective Airway Clearance* leads to poor oxygenation, as evidenced by pallor, cyanosis, lethargy, and drowsiness. Inadequate oxygenation causes increased pulse rate. Respiratory rate may be decreased by narcotic analgesics. Shallow breathing further compromises oxygenation.
Within 48–72 hours ■ Lungs clear to auscultation ■ Respirations 12–22/min; pulse, 100 beats/min ■ Inhales normal volume of air on incentive spirometer	Instruct in breathing and coughing techniques. Remind to perform, and assist q3h. Administer prescribed expectorant; schedule for maximum effectiveness. Maintain Fowler's or semi-Fowler's position. Administer prescribed analgesics. Notify physician if pain not relieved.	To enable client to cough up secretions. May need encouragement and support because of fatigue and pain. Helps loosen secretions so they can be coughed up and expelled. Gravity allows for fuller lung expansion by decreasing pressure of abdomen on diaphragm. Controls pleuritic pain by blocking pain pathways and altering perception of pain, enabling client to increase thoracic expansion. Unrelieved pain may signal impending complication.

* The NOC # for desired outcomes are listed in brackets following the appropriate outcome. Outcomes, interventions, and activities selected are only a sample of those suggested by NOC and NIC and should be further individualized for each client.

continued

NURSING CARE PLAN **Amanda Aquilini** *continued*

DESIRED OUTCOMES*/ INDICATORS	NURSING INTERVENTIONS	RATIONALE
	Administer oxygen by nasal cannula as prescribed. Provide portable oxygen if client goes off unit (e.g., for x-ray examination).	Supplemental oxygen makes more oxygen available to the cells, even though less air is being moved by the client, thereby reducing the work of breathing.
	Assist with postural drainage daily at 0930.	Gravity facilitates movement of secretions upward through the respiratory passage.
	Administer prescribed antibiotic to maintain constant blood level. Observe for rash and GI or other side effects.	Resolves infection by bacteriostatic or bactericidal effect, depending on type of antibiotic used. Constant level required to prevent pathogens from multiplying. Allergies to antibiotics are common.

NURSING DIAGNOSIS: Deficient Fluid Volume: Intake insufficient to replace fluid loss (See standardized care plan for Deficient Fluid Volume, Figure 13-4).

NURSING DIAGNOSIS: Anxiety related to difficulty breathing and concern about work and parenting roles.

DESIRED OUTCOMES*/ INDICATORS	NURSING INTERVENTIONS	RATIONALE
Anxiety control [1402], as evidenced by ■ Listening to and following instructions for correct breathing and coughing technique, even during periods of dyspnea ■ Verbalizing understanding of condition, diagnostic tests, and treatments (by end of day) ■ Decrease in reports of fear and anxiety ■ Voice steady, not shaky ■ Respiratory rate of 12–22/min ■ Freely expressing concerns and possible solutions about work and parenting roles Explore alternatives as needed. Note whether husband returns as scheduled. If not, institute care plan for actual *Interrupted Family Processes*	When client is dyspneic, stay with her; reassure her you will stay. Remain calm; appear confident. Encourage slow, deep breathing. When client is dyspneic, give brief explanations of treatments and procedures. When acute episode is over, give detailed information about nature of condition, treatments, and tests. As client can tolerate, encourage to express and expand on her concerns about her child and her work.	Presence of a competent caregiver reduces fear of being unable to breathe. Control of anxiety will help client to maintain effective breathing pattern. Reassures client the nurse can help her. Focusing on breathing may help client feel in control and decrease anxiety. Anxiety and pain interfere with learning. Knowing what to expect reduces anxiety. Awareness of source of anxiety enables client to gain control over it. Husband's continued absence would constitute a defining characteristic for this nursing diagnosis.

APPLYING CRITICAL THINKING

1. What assumptions does the nurse make when deciding that using a standardized care plan for *Deficient Fluid Volume* is appropriate for this client?
2. Identify an outcome in the care plan and its nursing intervention that contribute to discharge care planning. What evidence supports your choice?
3. Consider how the nurse shares the development of the care plan and outcomes with the client.
4. Not every intervention has a time frame or interval specified. It may be implied. Under what circumstances is this acceptable practice?
5. In Table 13–1, *Ineffective Airway Clearance* is Amanda's highest priority nursing diagnosis. Under what conditions might this diagnosis be of only moderate priority in Amanda's case?

See Critical Thinking Possibilities in Appendix A.

* The NOC # for desired outcomes is listed in brackets following the appropriate outcome. Outcomes, interventions, and activities selected are only a sample of those suggested by NOC and NIC and should be further individualized for each client.

CONCEPT MAP   Ineffective Airway Clearance (Gas Exchange)

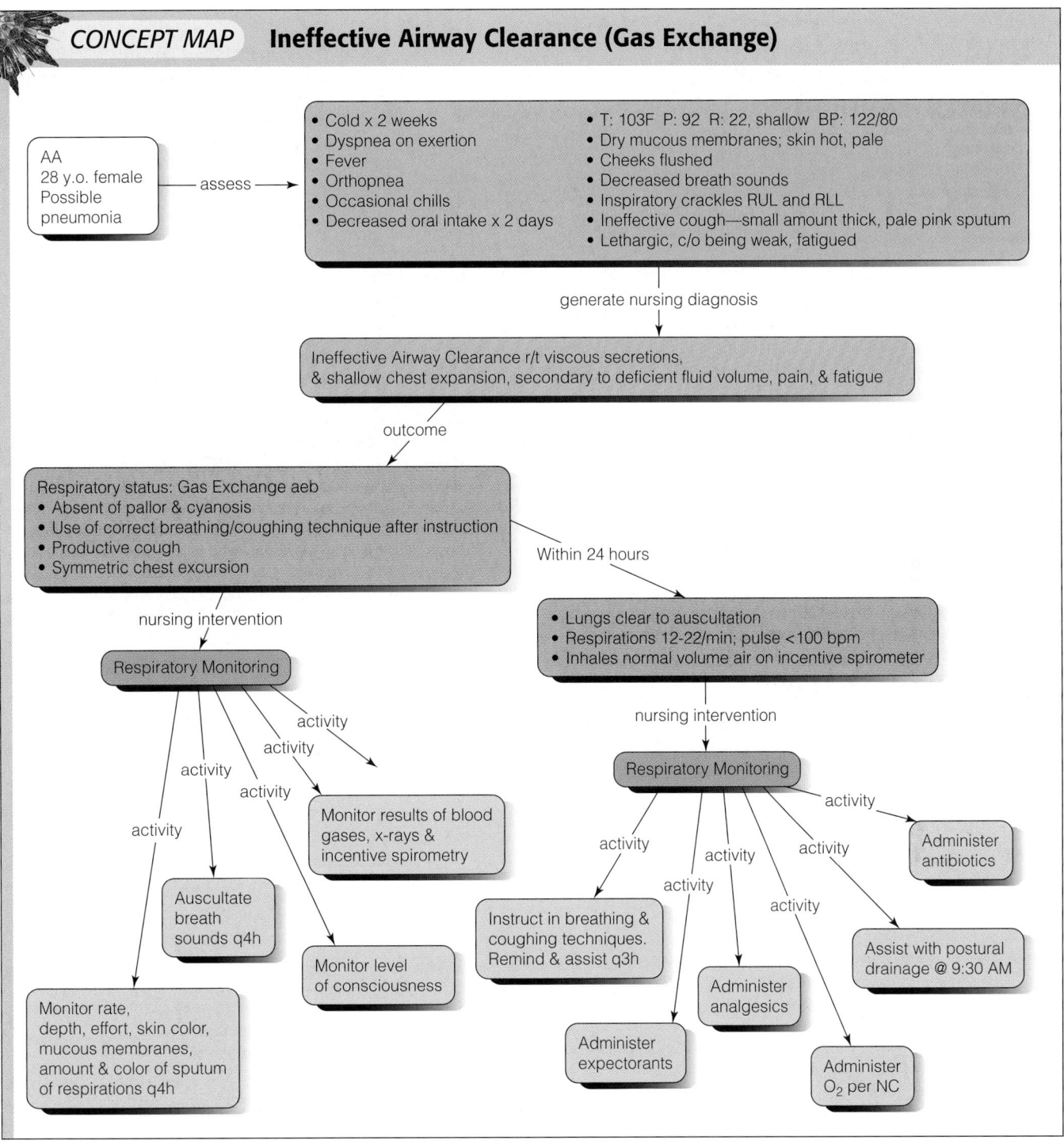

AA
28 y.o. female
Possible
pneumonia

→ assess →

- Cold x 2 weeks
- Dyspnea on exertion
- Fever
- Orthopnea
- Occasional chills
- Decreased oral intake x 2 days

- T: 103F P: 92 R: 22, shallow BP: 122/80
- Dry mucous membranes; skin hot, pale
- Cheeks flushed
- Decreased breath sounds
- Inspiratory crackles RUL and RLL
- Ineffective cough—small amount thick, pale pink sputum
- Lethargic, c/o being weak, fatigued

generate nursing diagnosis

Ineffective Airway Clearance r/t viscous secretions,
& shallow chest expansion, secondary to deficient fluid volume, pain, & fatigue

outcome

Respiratory status: Gas Exchange aeb
- Absent of pallor & cyanosis
- Use of correct breathing/coughing technique after instruction
- Productive cough
- Symmetric chest excursion

Within 24 hours

- Lungs clear to auscultation
- Respirations 12-22/min; pulse <100 bpm
- Inhales normal volume air on incentive spirometer

nursing intervention

Respiratory Monitoring

activity

Monitor results of blood gases, x-rays & incentive spirometry

Auscultate breath sounds q4h

Monitor level of consciousness

Monitor rate, depth, effort, skin color, mucous membranes, amount & color of sputum of respirations q4h

nursing intervention

Respiratory Monitoring

activity

Administer antibiotics

Instruct in breathing & coughing techniques. Remind & assist q3h

Administer expectorants

Administer analgesics

Administer O₂ per NC

Assist with postural drainage @ 9:30 AM

CHAPTER 13 **REVIEW**

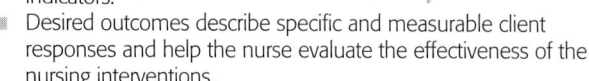

CHAPTER HIGHLIGHTS

- Planning is the process of designing nursing activities required to prevent, reduce, or eliminate a client's health problems.
- Planning involves the nurse, the client, support persons, and other caregivers.
- Shorter acute care hospitalization necessitates careful discharge planning.
- Standardized care plans should be adapted and used with individualized plans to meet individual client needs.
- The nursing care plan provides direction for individualized care of the client.
- The planning process includes setting diagnostic priorities, establishing client goals/desired outcomes, selecting nursing interventions, and writing individualized nursing interventions on the care plan.
- The nurse consults with other nurses or health professionals to verify information, implement changes, or obtain additional knowledge to aid in client goals.
- Nursing diagnoses are assigned high, medium, and low priorities in consultation with the client, if health permits.
- Client goals/desired outcomes are used to plan nursing interventions that will achieve anticipated changes in the client.
- A taxonomy of nursing outcome statements, the Nursing Outcomes Classification (NOC) has been developed to describe measurable states, behaviors, or perceptions that respond to

nursing interventions. Each has a definition, a measuring scale, and indicators.
- Desired outcomes describe specific and measurable client responses and help the nurse evaluate the effectiveness of the nursing interventions.
- Client goals/desired outcomes are derived from the first clause of the nursing diagnosis.
- Goal statements and desired outcomes are written in terms of the client's behavior.
- Nursing interventions are focused on the etiology or second clause of the nursing diagnosis.
- Independent nursing interventions are those the nurse is licensed to prescribe or delegate.
- Projecting the consequences of each nursing strategy requires nursing knowledge and experience.
- A taxonomy of nursing interventions referred to as the Nursing Interventions Classification (NIC) taxonomy has been developed. These interventions have been linked to the NANDA nursing diagnostic labels. Similar to NANDA diagnoses, each broadly stated intervention includes a label (name), a definition, and a list of activities that outline the key actions of nurses in carrying out the intervention.

TEST YOUR KNOWLEDGE

1. After being admitted directly to the surgery unit a 75-year-old client who had elective surgery to replace an arthritic hip, was discharged from the postanesthesia recovery unit. The client has been on the orthopedic floor several hours. Which of the following types of planning will be *least* useful during the first shift on the orthopedic unit?
   1. Initial
   2. Ongoing
   3. Discharge
   4. Strategic

2. The client with a fractured pelvis requests that family members be allowed to stay overnight in the hospital room. Before determining whether or not this request can be honored, the nurse should consult which of the following?
   1. Hospital policies
   2. Standardized care plans
   3. Orthopedic protocols
   4. Standards of care

3. The nurse assesses a postoperative client with an abdominal wound and finds the client drowsy when not aroused. The client's pain is ranked 2 on a scale of 0 to 10, vital signs are within preoperative range, extremities are warm with good pulses but very dry skin. The client declines oral fluids due to nausea, and reports no bowel movement in the past 2 days.

Hip dressing is dry with drains intact. Which of the following elements is most likely to be considered of high priority for a change in the current care plan?
   1. Pain
   2. Nausea
   3. Constipation
   4. Potential for wound infection

4. The nurse selects the nursing diagnosis of *Risk for Impaired Skin Integrity* related to immobility, dry skin, and surgical incision. Which of the following represents a properly stated outcome/goal? The client will:
   1. Turn in bed q2h.
   2. Report the importance of applying lotion to skin daily.
   3. Have intact skin during hospitalization.
   4. Use a pressure-reducing mattress.

5. The care plan includes a nursing intervention "4/2/07 Measure client's fluid intake and output. F. Jenkins, RN." What element of a proper nursing intervention has been omitted?
   1. Action verb
   2. Content
   3. Time
   4. None

See Answers to Test Your Knowledge in Appendix A.

EXPLORE MEDIALINK   www.prenhall.com/berman

DVD-ROM
- Audio Glossary
- NCLEX Review

COMPANION WEBSITE
- Additional NCLEX Review
- Case Study: Client Struck by a Car
- Application Activity: Client with Peptic Ulcers

READINGS AND REFERENCES

SUGGESTED READINGS

NIC/NOC letter—published twice a year, available online at http://www.nursing.uiowa.edu/centers/cncce/nicnocnews.htm

Hendry, C., & Walker, A. (2004). Priority setting in clinical nursing practice: Literature review. *Journal of Advanced Nursing, 47*, 427–436. *This article describes a review of the literature on clinical decision making, problem solving or planning, and setting priorities. Factors found in the literature that influenced setting of priorities included expertise of the nurse, client's condition, resources, organization of the unit, models of care, nurse–client relationship, and nurses' priority-setting strategy.*

RELATED RESEARCH

Allen, G. D., Rubenfield, M. G., & Scheffer, B. K. (2004). Reliability assessment of critical thinking. *Journal of Professional Nursing, 20*(1), 15–22.

Benner, P. (2004). Designing formal classification systems to better articulate knowledge, skills, and meanings in nursing practice. *American Journal of Critical Care, 13*, 426–430.

Hinck, S. M., Webb, P., Simms-Giddens, S., Helton, C., Hope, K., Utley, R., et al. (2006). Student learning with concept mapping of care plans in community-based education. *Journal of Professional Nursing, 22*, 23–29.

REFERENCES

American Nurses Association. (1997). *The American Nurses Association position statement on registered nurse utilization of unlicensed personnel.* Kansas City, MO: Author. Retrieved April 14, 2006, from http://www.nursingworld.org/readroom/position/uap/uapuse.htm

Dochterman, J. C., & Bulechek, G. M. (Eds.). (2004). *Nursing interventions classification (NIC)* (4th ed.). St. Louis, MO: Mosby.

Moorhead, S., Johnson, M., & Maas, M. (Eds.). (2004). *Nursing outcomes classification (NOC)* (3rd ed.). St. Louis, MO: Mosby.

Wilkinson, J. M. (2007). *Nursing process & critical thinking* (4th ed.). Upper Saddle River, NJ: Prentice Hall Health.

SELECTED BIBLIOGRAPHY

Alfaro-LeFevre, R. A. (2005). *Applying the nursing process: Promoting collaborative care* (6th ed.). Philadelphia: Lippincott Williams & Wilkins.

Alfaro-LeFevre, R. A. (2005). T*he nursing process made easy: Concept mapping and care planning for students.* Philadelphia: Lippincott Williams & Wilkins.

Doenges, M. E., & Moorhouse, M. F. (2003). *Application of nursing process and nursing diagnosis: An interactive text for diagnostic reasoning* (4th ed.). Philadelphia: F. A. Davis.

Gardner, P. (2003). *Nursing process in action.* Albany, NY: Delmar.

Johnson, M., Bulechek, G. B., Butcher, H., Dochterman, J., Moorhead, S., Maas, M., et al. (Eds.). (2005). *NANDA, NOC, and NIC linkages: Nursing diagnoses, outcomes, and interventions* (2nd ed.). St. Louis, MO: Elsevier Health Sciences.

Martinez de Castillo, S. L. (2003). *Strategies, techniques, & approaches to thinking: Case studies in clinical nursing* (2nd ed.). St. Louis, MO: Saunders.

Seaback, W. (2005). *Nursing process: Concept & application* (2nd ed.). Albany, NY: Delmar.

Wilkinson, J. M. (2005). *Nursing diagnosis handbook: With NIC interventions and NOC outcomes* (8th ed.). Upper Saddle River, NJ: Prentice Hall.

CHAPTER 14

Implementing and Evaluating

LEARNING OUTCOMES

After completing this chapter, you will be able to:

1. Explain how implementing relates to other phases of the nursing process.

2. Describe three categories of skills used to implement nursing interventions.

3. Discuss the five activities of the implementing phase.

4. Identify guidelines for implementing nursing interventions.

5. Explain how evaluating relates to other phases of the nursing process.

6. Describe five components of the evaluation process.

7. Describe the steps involved in reviewing and modifying the client's care plan.

8. Differentiate quality improvement from quality assurance.

9. Name the two components of an evaluation statement.

10. Describe three components of quality evaluation: structure, process, and outcomes.

The nursing process is action oriented, client centered, and outcome directed. After developing a plan of care based on the assessing and diagnosing phases, the nurse implements the interventions and evaluates the desired outcomes. On the basis of this evaluation, the plan of care is either continued, modified, or terminated. As in all phases of the nursing process, clients and support persons are encouraged to participate as much as possible.

IMPLEMENTING

In the nursing process, implementing is the action phase in which the nurse performs the nursing interventions. Using NIC terminology, **implementing** consists of doing and documenting the activities that are the specific nursing actions needed to carry out the interventions. The nurse performs or delegates the nursing activities for the interventions that were developed in the planning step and then concludes the implementing step by recording nursing activities and the resulting client responses.

Although the nurse may act on the client's behalf (e.g., referring the client to a community health nurse for home care), professional standards support client and family participation, as in all phases of the nursing process. The degree of participation depends on the client's health status. For example, an unconscious man is unable to participate in his care and therefore needs to have care given to him. By contrast, an ambulatory client may require very little care from the nurse and carry out health care activities independently.

Relationship of Implementing to Other Nursing Process Phases

The first three nursing process phases—assessing, diagnosing, and planning—provide the basis for the nursing actions performed during the implementing step. In turn, the implementing phase provides the actual nursing activities and client responses that are examined in the final phase, the evaluating phase. Using data acquired during assessment, the nurse can individualize the care given in the implementing phase, tailoring the interventions to fit a specific client rather than applying them routinely to categories of clients (e.g., all clients with pneumonia).

While implementing nursing care, the nurse continues to reassess the client at every contact, gathering data about the client's responses to the nursing activities and about any new problems that may develop. A nursing activity on the client's care plan for the NIC intervention *Airway Management* might read "Auscultate breath sounds q4h." When performing this activity, the nurse is both carrying out the intervention (implementing) and performing an assessment. Some routine nursing activities are, themselves, assessments. For example, while bathing an elderly client, the nurse observes a reddened area on the client's sacrum. Or, when emptying a urinary catheter bag, the nurse measures 200 mL of offensive smelling, brown urine.

Implementing Skills

To implement the care plan successfully, nurses need cognitive, interpersonal, and technical skills. These skills are distinct from one another; in practice, however, nurses use them in various combinations and with different emphasis, depending on the activity. For instance, when inserting a urinary catheter the nurse needs cognitive knowledge of the principles and steps of the procedure, interpersonal skills to inform and reassure the client, and technical skill in draping the client and manipulating the equipment.

The **cognitive skills** (intellectual skills) include problem solving, decision making, critical thinking, and creativity. They are crucial to safe, intelligent nursing care (see Chapter 10). ∞

Interpersonal skills are all of the activities, verbal and nonverbal, people use when interacting directly with one another. The effectiveness of a nursing action often depends largely on the nurse's ability to communicate with others. The nurse uses therapeutic communication to understand the client and in turn be understood. A nurse also needs to work effectively with others as a member of the health care team.

Interpersonal skills are necessary for all nursing activities: caring, comforting, advocating, referring, counseling, and supporting are just a few. Interpersonal skills include conveying knowledge, attitudes, feelings, interest, and appreciation of the client's cultural values and lifestyle. Before nurses can be highly skilled in interpersonal relations, they must have self-awareness and sensitivity to others (see Chapters 25 and 39). ∞

Technical skills are purposeful "hands-on" skills such as manipulating equipment, giving injections, bandaging, moving, lifting, and repositioning clients. These skills are also called tasks, procedures, or psychomotor skills. The term *psychomotor* refers to physical actions that are controlled by the mind, not reflexive.

Technical skills require knowledge and, frequently, manual dexterity. The number of technical skills expected of a nurse has greatly increased in recent years because of the pervasive use of technology, especially in acute care hospitals.

Process of Implementing

The process of implementing (see Figure 14-1 ■) normally includes the following:

- Reassessing the client
- Determining the nurse's need for assistance
- Implementing the nursing interventions
- Supervising the delegated care
- Documenting nursing activities

Reassessing the Client

Just before implementing an intervention, the nurse must reassess the client to make sure the intervention is still needed. Even though an order is written on the care plan, the client's condition may have changed. For example, a client has a nursing diagnosis of *Disturbed Sleep Pattern* related to anxiety and unfamiliar surroundings. During rounds, the nurse discovers that she is sleeping and therefore defers the back massage that had been planned as a relaxation strategy.

New data may indicate a need to change the priorities of care or the nursing activities. For example, a nurse begins to teach a client who has diabetes, how to give himself insulin injections. Shortly after beginning the teaching, the nurse realizes that he is not concentrating on the lesson. Subsequent discussion reveals that he is worried about his eyesight and fears he is going blind. Realizing that the client's level of stress is interfering with his learning, the nurse ends the lesson and arranges for a primary care provider to examine the client's eyes. The nurse also provides supportive communication to help alleviate the client's stress.

Figure 14-1 ■ Implementing. The fourth phase of the nursing process, in which the nurse implements the nursing interventions and documents the care provided.

Determining the Nurse's Need for Assistance

When implementing some nursing interventions, the nurse may require assistance for one or more of the following reasons:

- The nurse is unable to implement the nursing activity safely or efficiently alone (e.g., ambulating an unsteady obese client).
- Assistance would reduce stress on the client (e.g., turning a person who experiences acute pain when moved).
- The nurse lacks the knowledge or skills to implement a particular nursing activity (e.g., a nurse who is not familiar with a particular model of traction equipment needs assistance the first time it is applied).

Implementing the Nursing Interventions

It is important to explain to the client what interventions will be done, what sensations to expect, what the client is expected to do, and what the expected outcome is. For many nursing activities it is also important to ensure the client's privacy, for example by closing doors, pulling curtains, or draping the client. The number and kind of direct nursing interventions are almost unlimited. Nurses also coordinate client care. This activity involves scheduling client contacts with other departments (e.g., laboratory and x-ray technicians, physical and respiratory therapists) and serving as a liaison among the members of the health care team.

When implementing interventions, nurses should follow these guidelines:

- Base nursing interventions on scientific knowledge, nursing research, and professional standards of care (evidence-based practice) when these exist. The nurse must be aware of the scientific rationale, as well as possible side effects or complications, of all interventions. For example, a client prefers to take an oral medication after meals; however, this medication is not absorbed well in the presence of food. Therefore, the nurse will need to explain why this preference cannot be honored.
- Clearly understand the interventions to be implemented and question any that are not understood. The nurse is responsible for intelligent implementation of medical and nursing plans of care. This requires knowledge of each intervention, its purpose in the client's plan of care, any contraindications (e.g., allergies), and changes in the client's condition that may affect the order.
- Adapt activities to the individual client. A client's beliefs, values, age, health status, and environment are factors that can affect the success of a nursing action. For example, the nurse determines that a client chokes when swallowing pills, so consults with the physician to change the order to a liquid form of the medication. Or, the nurse recognizes that many Asian persons prefer to drink hot water rather than ice water and, after confirming it with a specific client, supplies this at the bedside.
- Implement safe care. For example, when changing a sterile dressing, the nurse practices sterile technique to prevent infection; when giving a medication, the nurse administers the correct dosage by the ordered route.

- Provide teaching, support, and comfort. See Chapter 27 ∞ for details on client teaching and Box 27–3 for examples of verbs used in writing learning outcomes. The nurse should always explain the purpose of interventions, what the client will experience, and how the client can participate. The client must have sufficient knowledge to agree to the plan of care and to be able to assume responsibility for as much self-care as possible. These independent nursing activities enhance the effectiveness of nursing care plans (see Figure 14-2 ■).

- Be holistic. The nurse must always view the client as a whole and consider the client's responses in that context. For example, whenever possible, the nurse honors the client's expressed preference that interventions be planned for times that fit with the client's usual schedule of visitors, work, sleep, or eating.

- Respect the dignity of the client and enhance the client's self-esteem. Providing privacy and encouraging clients to make their own decisions are ways of respecting dignity and enhancing self-esteem.

- Encourage clients to participate actively in implementing the nursing interventions. Active participation enhances the client's sense of independence and control. However, clients vary in the degree of participation they desire. Some want total involvement in their care, whereas others prefer little involvement. The amount of desired involvement may be related to the severity of the illness; the client's culture; or the client's fear, understanding of the illness, and understanding of the intervention.

Supervising Delegated Care

If care has been delegated to other health care personnel, the nurse responsible for the client's overall care must ensure that the activities have been implemented according to the care plan. Other caregivers may be required to communicate their activities to the nurse by documenting them on the client record, reporting verbally, or filling out a written form. The nurse validates and responds to any adverse findings or client responses. This may involve modifying the nursing care plan.

Figure 14-2 ■ Amanda agrees to practice deep-breathing exercises q3h during the day. In addition, she verbalizes awareness of the need to increase her fluid intake.

Documenting Nursing Activities

After carrying out the nursing activities, the nurse completes the implementing phase by recording the interventions and client responses in the nursing progress notes. These are a part of the agency's permanent record for the client. Nursing care must not be recorded in advance because the nurse may determine on reassessment of the client that the intervention should not or cannot be implemented. For example, a nurse is authorized to inject 10 mg of morphine sulfate subcutaneously to a client, but the nurse finds that the client's respiratory rate is 4 breaths per minute. This finding contraindicates the administration of morphine (a respiratory depressant). The nurse withholds the morphine and reports the client's respiratory rate to the nurse in charge and/or physician.

The nurse may record routine or recurring activities (e.g., mouth care) in the client record at the end of a shift. In the meantime, the nurse maintains a personal record of these interventions on a worksheet. In some instances, it is important to record a nursing intervention immediately after it is implemented. This is particularly true of the administration of medications and treatments because recorded data about a client must be up to date, accurate, and available to other nurses and health care professionals. Immediate recording helps safeguard the client, for example, from receiving a duplicate dose of medication.

Nursing activities are communicated verbally as well as in writing. When a client's health is changing rapidly, the charge nurse and/or the physician may want to be kept up to date with verbal reports. Nurses also report client status at a change of shift and on a client's discharge to another unit or health agency in person, via a voice recording, or in writing. For information on documenting and reporting, see Chapter 15. ∞

EVALUATING

To evaluate is to judge or to appraise. Evaluating is the fifth and last phase of the nursing process. In this context, **evaluating** is a planned, ongoing, purposeful activity in which clients and health care professionals determine (a) the client's progress toward achievement of goals/outcomes and (b) the effectiveness of the nursing care plan. Evaluation is an important aspect of the nursing process because conclusions drawn from the evaluation determine whether the nursing interventions should be terminated, continued, or changed.

Evaluation is continuous. Evaluation done while or immediately after implementing a nursing order enables the nurse to make on-the-spot modifications in an intervention. Evaluation performed at specified intervals (e.g., once a week for the home care client) shows the extent of progress toward goal achievement and enables the nurse to correct any deficiencies and modify the care plan as needed. Evaluation continues until the client achieves the health goals or is discharged from nursing care. Evaluation at discharge includes the status of goal achievement and the client's self-care abilities with regard to follow-up care. Most agencies have a special discharge record for this evaluation.

Through evaluating, nurses demonstrate responsibility and accountability for their actions, indicate interest in the results of the nursing activities, and demonstrate a desire not to perpetuate ineffective actions but to adopt more effective ones.

Relationship of Evaluating to Other Nursing Process Phases

Successful evaluation depends on the effectiveness of the steps that precede it. Assessment data must be accurate and complete so that the nurse can formulate appropriate nursing diagnoses and desired outcomes. The desired outcomes must be stated concretely in behavioral terms if they are to be useful for evaluating client responses. And finally, without the implementing phase in which the plan is put into action, there would be nothing to evaluate.

The evaluating and assessing phases overlap. As previously stated, assessment (data collection) is ongoing and continuous at every client contact. However, data are collected for different purposes at different points in the nursing process. During the assessment phase the nurse collects data for the purpose of making diagnoses. During the evaluation step the nurse collects data for the purpose of comparing it to preselected goals and judging the effectiveness of the nursing care. The act of assessing (data collection) is the same; the differences lie in (a) when the data are collected and (b) how the data are used.

Process of Evaluating Client Responses

Before evaluation, the nurse identifies the desired outcomes (indicators) that will be used to measure client goal achievement. (This is done in the planning step.) Desired outcomes serve two purposes: They establish the kind of evaluative data that need to be collected and provide a standard against which the data are judged. For example, given the following expected outcomes, any nurse caring for the client would know what data to collect:

- Daily fluid intake will not be less than 2500 mL.
- Urinary output will balance with fluid intake.
- Residual urine will be less than 100 mL.

The evaluation process has five components (see Figure 14-3 ■):

- Collecting data related to the desired outcomes (NOC indicators)
- Comparing the data with outcomes
- Relating nursing activities to outcomes
- Drawing conclusions about problem status
- Continuing, modifying, or terminating the nursing care plan

Collecting Data

Using the clearly stated, precise, and measurable desired outcomes as a guide, the nurse collects data so that conclusions can be drawn about whether goals have been met. It is usually necessary to collect both objective and subjective data.

Some data may require interpretation. Examples of objective data requiring interpretation are the degree of tissue turgor of a dehydrated client or the degree of restlessness of a client with pain. Examples of subjective data needing interpretation include complaints of nausea or pain by the client. When interpreting subjective data, the nurse must rely upon either (a) the client's statements (e.g., "My pain is worse now than it was after breakfast") or (b) objective indicators of the subjective data,

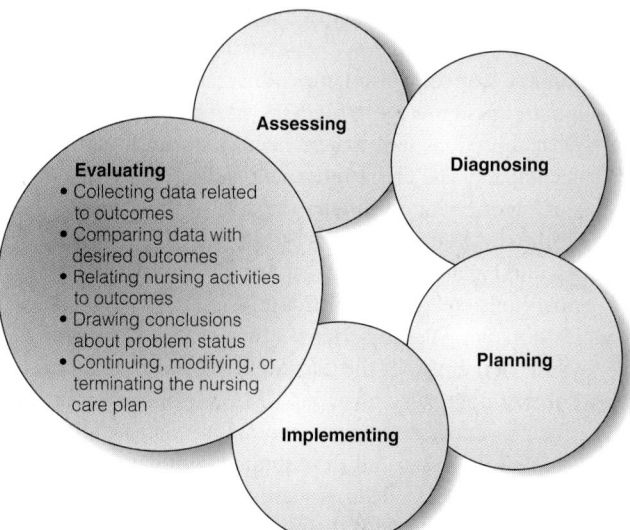

Figure 14-3 ■ Evaluating. The final phase of the nursing process, in which the nurse determines the client's progress toward goal achievement and the effectiveness of the nursing care plan. The plan may be continued, modified, or terminated.

even though these indicators may require further interpretation (e.g., decreased restlessness, decreased pulse and respiratory rates, and relaxed facial muscles as indicators of pain relief). Data must be recorded concisely and accurately to facilitate the next part of the evaluating process.

Comparing Data with Outcomes

If the first two parts of the evaluation process have been carried out effectively, it is relatively simple to determine whether a desired outcome has been met. Both the nurse and client play an active role in comparing the client's actual responses with the desired outcomes. Did the client drink 3000 mL of fluid in 24 hours? Did the client walk unassisted the specified distance per day? When determining whether a goal has been achieved, the nurse can draw one of three possible conclusions:

1. The goal was met; that is, the client response is the same as the desired outcome.
2. The goal was partially met; that is, either a short-term goal was achieved but the long-term goal was not, or the desired outcome was only partially attained.
3. The goal was not met.

After determining whether a goal has been met, the nurse writes an evaluative statement (either on the care plan or in the nurse's notes). An **evaluation statement** consists of two parts: a conclusion and supporting data. The conclusion is a statement that the goal/desired outcome was met, partially met, or not met. The supporting data are the list of client responses that support the conclusion, for example:

Goal met: Oral intake 300 mL more than output; skin turgor resilient; mucous membranes moist.

See the Nursing Care Plan at the end of the chapter for evaluation statements for Amanda Aquilini. Data in the Evaluation Statements column on this table represent Ms. Aquilini's responses to care as observed by the night nurse on the morning after her admission to the unit. In practice, care plans usually do not have a column for evaluation statements; rather, these are recorded in the nurse's notes. If NOC indicators are being used with the outcomes, scores on the scales after intervention would be compared with those measured at baseline to determine improvement. See Table 13–3 on ∞ page 220 for an example of the NOC rating scales used for indicators of mobility. The column explaining rationale for continuing or modifying the plan is included in a student care plan.

Relating Nursing Activities to Outcomes

The fourth aspect of the evaluating process is determining whether the nursing activities had any relation to the outcomes. It should never be assumed that a nursing activity was the cause of or the only factor in meeting, partially meeting, or not meeting a goal.

For example, a client was obese and needed to lose 14 kg (30 lb). When the nurse and client drew up a care plan, one goal was "Lose 1.4 kg (3 lb) in 4 weeks." A nursing strategy in the care plan was "Explain how to plan and prepare a 1200-calorie diet." Four weeks later, the client weighed herself and had lost 1.8 kg (4 lb). The goal had been met—in fact, exceeded. It is easy to assume that the nursing strategy was highly effective. However, it is important to collect more data before drawing that conclusion. On questioning the client, the nurse might find any of the following: (a) The client planned a 1200-calorie diet and prepared and ate the food; (b) the client planned a 1200-calorie diet but did not prepare the correct food; (c) the client did not understand how to plan a 1200-calorie diet, so she did not bother with it.

If the first possibility is found to be true, the nurse can safely judge that the nursing strategy "Explain how to plan and prepare a 1200-calorie diet" was effective in helping the client lose weight. However, if the nurse learns that either the second or third possibility actually happened, then it must be assumed that the nursing strategy did not affect the outcome. The next step for the nurse is to collect data about what the client actually did to lose weight. It is important to establish the relationship (or lack thereof) of the nursing actions to the client responses.

Drawing Conclusions about Problem Status

The nurse uses the judgments about goal achievement to determine whether the care plan was effective in resolving, reducing, or preventing client problems. When goals have been met, the nurse can draw one of the following conclusions about the status of the client's problem:

- The actual problem stated in the nursing diagnosis has been resolved, or the potential problem is being prevented and the risk factors no longer exist. In these instances, the nurse documents that the goals have been met and discontinues the care for the problem.
- The potential problem stated in the nursing diagnosis is being prevented, but the risk factors are still present. In this case, the nurse keeps the problem on the care plan.
- The actual problem still exists even though some goals are being met. For example, a desired outcome on a client's care plan is "Will drink 3000 mL of fluid daily."

Even though the data may show this outcome has been achieved, other data (dry oral mucous membranes) may indicate that there is *Deficient Fluid Volume*. Therefore, the nursing interventions must be continued even though this one goal was met.

When goals have been partially met or when goals have not been met, two conclusions may be drawn:

- The care plan may need to be revised, since the problem is only partially resolved. The revisions may need to occur during assessing, diagnosing, or planning phases, as well as implementing.

OR

- The care plan does not need revision, because the client merely needs more time to achieve the previously established goal(s). To make this decision, the nurse must assess why the goals are being only partially achieved, including whether the evaluation was conducted too soon (see Figure 14-4 ■).

Continuing, Modifying, and Terminating the Nursing Care Plan

After drawing conclusions about the status of the client's problems, the nurse modifies the care plan as indicated. Depending on the agency, modifications may be made by drawing a line through portions of the care plan, or marking portions using a highlighting pen, or writing "Discontinued" (dc'd), "goal met," or "problem resolved" and the date.

Whether or not goals were met, a number of decisions need to be made about continuing, modifying, or terminating nursing care for each problem. See Table 14–1 for a checklist to use when reviewing a care plan. Although the checklist uses a closed-ended yes/no format, its only intent is to identify areas that require the nurse's further examination.

Before making modifications, the nurse must determine if the plan as a whole was not completely effective. This requires

Figure 14-4 ■ Upon assessment of respiratory excursion, Nurse Medina detects failure of the client to achieve maximum ventilation. She and Amanda reevaluate the care plan and modify it to increase coughing and deep-breathing exercises to q2h.

TABLE 14–1 Evaluation Checklist

ASSESSING	DIAGNOSING	PLANNING	IMPLEMENTING
____ Are data complete, accurate, and validated? ____ Do new data require changes in the care plan?	____ Are nursing diagnoses relevant and accurate? ____ Are nursing diagnoses supported by the data? ____ Has problem status changed (i.e., potential, actual, risk)? ____ Are the diagnoses stated clearly and in correct format? ____ Have any nursing diagnoses been resolved?	**Desired Outcomes** ____ Do new nursing diagnoses require new goals? ____ Are goals realistic? ____ Was enough time allowed for goal achievement? ____ Do the goals address all aspects of the problem? ____ Does the client still concur with the goals? ____ Have client priorities changed? **Nursing Interventions** ____ Do nursing interventions need to be written for new nursing diagnoses or new goals? ____ Do the nursing interventions seem to be related to the stated goals? ____ Is there a rationale to justify each nursing order? ____ Are the nursing interventions clear, specific, and detailed? ____ Are new resources available? ____ Do the nursing interventions address all aspects of the client's goals? ____ Were the nursing interventions actually carried out?	____ Was client input obtained at each step of the nursing process? ____ Were goals and nursing interventions acceptable to the client? ____ Did the caregivers have the knowledge and skill to perform the interventions correctly? ____ Were explanations given to the client prior to implementing?

a review of the entire care plan and a critique of each step of the nursing process involved in its development.

ASSESSING. An incomplete or incorrect database influences all subsequent steps of the nursing process and care plan. If data are incomplete, the nurse needs to reassess the client and record the new data. In some instances, new data may indicate the need for new nursing diagnoses, new goals, and new nursing interventions.

DIAGNOSING. If the database was incomplete, new diagnostic statements may be required. If the database was complete, the nurse needs to analyze whether the problems were identified correctly and whether the nursing diagnoses were relevant to that database. After making judgments about problem status, the nurse revises or adds new diagnoses as needed to reflect the most recent client data.

PLANNING: DESIRED OUTCOMES. If a nursing diagnosis was inaccurate, obviously the goal statement will need revision. If the nursing diagnosis was appropriate, the nurse then checks if the goals were realistic and attainable. Unrealistic goals require correction. The nurse should also determine whether priorities have changed and whether the client still agrees with the priorities. For example, the amount of time delineated for a specific amount

of weight loss was possibly too short and should be extended. Goals must also be written for any new nursing diagnoses.

PLANNING: NURSING INTERVENTIONS. The nurse investigates whether the nursing interventions were related to goal achievement and whether the best nursing interventions were selected. Even when diagnoses and goals were appropriate, the nursing interventions selected may not have been the best ones to achieve the goal. New nursing interventions may reflect changes in the amount of nursing care the client needs, scheduling changes, or rearrangement of nursing activities to group similar activities or to permit longer rest or activity periods for the client. For example, for a client who wishes to stop smoking, there are many potential interventions. If medication was prescribed but the client is still smoking, possibly a behavioral intervention such as group counseling needs to be added. If new nursing diagnoses have been written, then new nursing interventions will also be necessary.

IMPLEMENTING. Even if all sections of the care plan appear to be satisfactory, the manner in which the plan was implemented may have interfered with goal achievement. Before selecting new interventions, the nurse should check whether they were carried out. Other personnel may not have carried them out, either because the interventions were unclear or because they were unreasonable in terms of external constraints such as money, staff, time, and equipment.

After making the necessary modifications to the care plan, the nurse implements the modified plan and begins the nursing process cycle again. Refer to the Nursing Care Plan at the end of this chapter to see how the plan for Amanda Aquilini was modified after evaluation of goal achievement and review of the nursing process. A line has been drawn through portions the nurse wished to delete; additions to the care plan are shown in italics.

Evaluating the Quality of Nursing Care

In addition to evaluating goal achievement for individual clients, nurses are also involved in evaluating and modifying the overall quality of care given to groups of clients. This is an essential part of professional accountability. In each of the processes described as follows, nurses and all other health care providers work together as an interdisciplinary team focused on improving client care. The activities both use and contribute to evidence-based practice.

Quality Assurance

A **quality-assurance (QA) program** is an ongoing, systematic process designed to evaluate and promote excellence in the health care provided to clients. Quality assurance frequently refers to evaluation of the level of care provided in a health care agency, but it may be limited to the evaluation of the performance of one nurse or more broadly involve the evaluation of the quality of the care in an agency, or even in a country.

Quality assurance requires evaluation of three components of care: structure, process, and outcome. Each type of evaluation requires different criteria and methods, and each has a different focus.

Structure evaluation focuses on the setting in which care is given. It answers this question: What effect does the setting have on the quality of care? Structural standards describe desirable environmental and organizational characteristics that influence care, such as equipment and staffing.

Process evaluation focuses on how the care was given. It answers questions such as these: Is the care relevant to the client's needs? Is the care appropriate, complete, and timely? Process standards focus on the manner in which the nurse uses the nursing process. Some examples of process criteria are "Checks client's identification band before giving medication" and "Performs and records chest assessment, including auscultation, once per shift."

Outcome evaluation focuses on demonstrable changes in the client's health status as a result of nursing care. Outcome criteria are written in terms of client responses or health status, just as they are for evaluation within the nursing process. For example, "How many clients undergoing hip repairs develop pneumonia?" or "How many clients who have a colostomy experience an infection that delays discharge?"

Quality Improvement

There are currently strong national efforts at evaluating and improving the quality of health care based on internal assessment by health care providers and increasing awareness by the public that medical errors are not uncommon and can be lethal. The Quality of Health Care in America Committee of the Institute of Medicine issued a landmark report: *To Err Is Human: Building a Safer Health System* in 2000. The entire report is available at the National Academies Press website. The emphases of the report are increasing knowledge related to medical errors and establishing systems for enhancing safe care. Since the report was issued, improved attention to these issues has come from a variety of sources. However, the complexity of the health care system (including methods of reimbursement), difficulties with leadership, and fear of threats to autonomy have limited progress (Leape & Berwick, 2005).

CLINICAL ALERT

Bad systems—and not bad people—lead to most errors. ■

The Center for Quality Improvement and Patient Safety (CQuIPS) within the Agency for Healthcare Research and Quality (2004) has as its mission to "improve[s] the quality and safety of all Americans through strategic partnerships. Specifically, CQuIPS:

1. Conducts and supports user-driven research on patient safety and health care quality measurement, reporting, and improvement.

RESEARCH NOTE   **How Is Quality Improvement Being Conducted in Nursing Homes?**

The purpose of this study, conducted in 35 nursing homes managed by the Veterans Administration, was to examine the association between quality improvement (QI) and client outcomes. Over 1,000 of the nursing staff completed surveys on the culture of the setting, satisfaction, and specific information regarding implementation of pressure ulcer prevention guidelines. There were differences among the nursing homes in their implementation of QI practices, and QI appeared to be associated with employee satisfaction and the perception of providing better care. However, the results were inconclusive in terms of demonstrating an effect of QI on quality of care.

IMPLICATIONS

The results demonstrated the need for continued study before QI is widely promoted as a means for improving nursing home quality. The relationship between use of QI and satisfaction of the nursing staff is an optimistic sign. Quality improvement, as well as other interventions to improve care, is unlikely to be successfully implemented in nursing homes that are not suitably predisposed to making the necessary changes in how care is delivered.

Note: From "Quality Improvement Implementation in the Nursing Home," by D. R. Berlowitz, G. J. Young, E. C. Hickey, D. Saliba, B. S. Mittman, E. Czarnowski, et al., 2003, *Health Services Research, 38* (1 Part 1), pp. 65–83.

2. Develops and disseminates reports and information on health care quality measurement, reporting, and improvement.
3. Collaborates with stakeholders across the health care system to implement evidence-based practices, accelerating and amplifying improvements in quality and safety for patients.
4. Assesses our own practices to ensure continuous learning and improvement for the Center and its members."

In addition, the mission of the Joint Commission on Accreditation of Healthcare Organizations (JCAHO, 2005a) is: "To continuously improve the safety and quality of care provided to the public through the provision of health care accreditation and related services that support performance improvement in health care organizations." JCAHO has put great emphasis on the importance of what are called "sentinel events." Although each agency must define sentinel events for itself, the definition must be consistent with that given by JCAHO (2005b):

■ A **sentinel event** is an unexpected occurrence involving death or serious physical or psychological injury, or the risk thereof. Serious injury specifically includes loss of limb or function. The phrase, "or the risk thereof" includes any process variation for which a recurrence would carry a significant chance of a serious adverse outcome.

■ Such events are called "sentinel" because they signal the need for immediate investigation and response.

The organization must respond to the sentinel event by assessing the cause, identifying a plan for intervention, and evaluating the results of the plan. Often, assessment involves a root cause analysis. **Root cause analysis** is a process for identifying the factors that bring about deviations in practices that lead to the event. It focuses primarily on systems and processes, not individual performance. It begins with examination of the single event but with the goal of determining which organizational improvements are needed to decrease the likelihood of such events occurring again.

Unlike quality assurance, **quality improvement (QI)** follows client care rather than organizational structure, focuses on process rather than individuals, and uses a systematic approach with the intention of *improving* the quality of care rather than *ensuring* the quality of care. QI studies often focus on identifying and correcting a system's problems, such as duplication of services in a hospital. QI is also known as continuous quality improvement (CQI), total quality management (TQM), performance improvement (PI), or persistent quality improvement (PQI).

Nursing Audit

An **audit** means the examination or review of records. A **retrospective audit** is the evaluation of a client's record after discharge from an agency. *Retrospective* means "relating to past events." A **concurrent audit** is the evaluation of a client's health care while the client is still receiving care from the agency. These evaluations use interviewing, direct observation of nursing care, and review of clinical records to determine whether specific evaluative criteria have been met.

Another type of evaluation of care is the *peer review*. In nurse peer review, nurses functioning in the same capacity, that is, peers, appraise the quality of care or practice performed by other equally qualified nurses. The peer review is based on preestablished standards or criteria.

There are two types of peer reviews: individual and nursing audits. The individual peer review focuses on the performance of an individual nurse. The nursing audit focuses on evaluating nursing care through the review of records. The success of these audits depends on accurate documentation.

LIFESPAN CONSIDERATIONS Evaluating

Evaluation of goals, selected outcomes, and interventions needs to be continuous, with ongoing assessment and reassessment of the situation. Priority needs can change quickly and must be reprioritized when problems occur. Infants and young children are vulnerable to rapid change in their condition due to their small body size, disproportionate size of organs, and immaturity of body systems. Also, they may not be able to verbalize how they are feeling. Older adults may have conditions that impair communication, such as aphasia from a cerebrovascular accident, dementia, multiple sclerosis, or other neurological conditions. In such cases, the nurse needs to be even more astute in performing nonverbal assessments, being alert to potential problems, and detecting changes in the client's condition. If evaluations are done often and thoroughly, changes can be made quickly to intervene more effectively and improve outcomes. Constant assessment, communication, and interpersonal skills are as essential in the evaluation phase as they are in the initial assessment.

NURSING CARE PLAN For Amanda Aquilini Modified Following Implementation and Evaluation

NURSING DIAGNOSIS: Ineffective Airway Clearance related to viscous secretions and shallow chest expansion secondary to deficient fluid volume, pain, and fatigue.

DESIRED OUTCOMES*/ INDICATORS	EVALUATION STATEMENTS	NURSING INTERVENTIONS**	EXPLANATION FOR CONTINUING OR MODIFYING NURSING INTERVENTIONS
Respiratory status: gas exchange [0402], as evidenced by			
■ Absence of pallor and cyanosis (skin and mucous membranes)	Partially met. Skin and mucous membranes not cyanotic, but still pale.	Monitor respiratory status q4h; rate, depth, effort, skin color, mucous membranes, amount and color of sputum.	Retain nursing interventions to continue to identify progress. Goal status indicates problem not resolved.
■ Use of correct breathing/coughing technique after instruction	Partially met. Uses correct technique when pain well controlled by narcotic analgesics.	Monitor results of blood gases, chest x-ray studies, pulse oximetry, and incentive spirometer volume as available.	
■ Productive cough	Met. Cough productive of moderate amounts of thick, yellow, pink-tinged sputum.	Monitor level of consciousness.	
		Auscultate lungs q4h.	
■ Symmetric chest excursion of at least 4 cm	Not met. Chest excursion = 3 cm.	Vital signs q4h (TPR, BP, pulse oximetry).	
■ Lungs clear to auscultation within 48–72 h	Not met. Scattered inspiratory crackles auscultated throughout right anterior and posterior chest.	Instruct in breathing and coughing techniques. Remind to perform and assist q3h. *Support and encourage. (4/17/07, JW)*	Does not need to be reinstructed as client demonstrates correct techniques. May still need support and encouragement because of fatigue and pain of breathing.
		Administer prescribed expectorant; schedule for maximum effectiveness.	
■ Respirations 12–22/min, pulse <100 beats/min	Partially met. Respirations 26/min, pulse 96.	Maintain Fowler's or semi-Fowler's position.	
■ Inhaling normal volume of air on incentive spirometer	Not met. Tidal volume only 350 mL *(Evaluated 4/17/07, JW)*	Administer prescribed analgesics. Notify primary care provider if pain not relieved.	
		Administer oxygen by nasal cannula as prescribed. Provide portable oxygen if client goes off unit (e.g., for x-ray examination).	
		Assist with postural drainage daily at 0930. *On 4/17 teach to continue prn at home. (4/17/07, JW)*	As soon as client is hydrated and fever is controlled, she will probably be discharged to self-care at home.
		Administer prescribed antibiotic to maintain constant blood level. Observe for rash and GI or other side effects.	

continued on page 242

NURSING CARE PLAN For Amanda Aquilini Modified Following Implementation and Evaluation—continued

NURSING DIAGNOSIS: Ineffective Airway Clearance related to viscous secretions and shallow chest expansion secondary to deficient fluid volume, pain, and fatigue.

DESIRED OUTCOMES*/ INDICATORS	EVALUATION STATEMENTS	NURSING INTERVENTIONS**	EXPLANATION FOR CONTINUING OR MODIFYING NURSING INTERVENTIONS
Anxiety control [1402], as evidenced by			
■ Listening to and following instructions for correct breathing and coughing technique, even during periods of dyspnea	Met. Performed coughing techniques as instructed during periods of dyspnea.	When client is dyspneic, stay with her; reassure her you will stay.	
■ Verbalizing understanding of condition, diagnostic tests, and treatments (by end of day)	Met. See nurse's notes for 3–11 shift. Stated, "I know I need to try to breathe deeply even when it hurts." Demonstrated correct use of incentive spirometer and stated understanding of the need to use it. Understands IV is for hydration and antibiotics. *(Evaluated 4/17/07, JW)*	Remain calm, appear confident. Encourage slow, deep breathing. When client is dyspneic, give brief explanations of treatments and procedures.	
■ Decrease in reports of fear and anxiety	Met. Stated, "I know I can get enough air, but it still hurts to breathe."		
■ Voice steady, not shaky	Met. Speaks in steady voice.		
■ Respiratory rate of 12–22 min	Not met. Rate 26–36/min.	~~When acute episode is over, give detailed information about nature of condition, treatments, and tests.~~ *Reassess whether client needs any information on condition, treatments, or tests. (4/17/07, JW).*	Detailed information has been given. Because client shows understanding, there is no need to repeat information.
■ Freely expresses concerns and possible solutions about work and parenting roles	Partially met. Discussed only briefly on 3–11 shift. Not done on 11–7 shift because of client's need to rest. *(Evaluated 4/17/07, JW)*	As client can tolerate, encourage to express and expand on her concerns about her child and her work. Explore alternatives as needed. Note whether husband returns as scheduled. If he does not, institute care plan for actual *Interrupted Family Process. (Do on 4/17, day shift) (4/17/07, JW)*	It is important that this assessment be made right away, so child care can be arranged if needed.

*The NOC # for desired outcomes is listed in brackets following the appropriate outcome. Outcomes are only a sample of those suggested by NOC and should be further individualized for each client.

**In this care plan, a line has been drawn through portions the nurse wished to delete; additions to the care plan are shown in italics.

APPLYING CRITICAL THINKING

NURSING CARE PLAN **Amanda Aquilini** (continued)

1. From reviewing Amanda Aquilini's nursing care plan, what general conclusions can you make about the desired outcomes for *Ineffective Airway Clearance* and *Anxiety*?
2. Despite some of the outcomes being only partially met or not met, no new interventions were written for several outcomes. What reasons might there be for this?
3. For the nursing diagnosis of *Anxiety,* most of the outcomes are fully met. Would you delete this diagnosis from the care plan at this time? Why or why not?
4. Since the Evaluation Statements column is generally not used on written care plans, where would auditors or persons conducting quality assessments find these data?

See Critical Thinking Possibilities in Appendix A.

CHAPTER 14 **REVIEW**

CHAPTER HIGHLIGHTS

- Implementing is putting planned nursing interventions into action.
- Reassessing occurs simultaneously with the implementing phase of the nursing process.
- Successful implementing and evaluating depend in part on the quality of the preceding phases of assessing, diagnosing, and planning.
- Cognitive, interpersonal, and technical skills are used to implement nursing strategies.
- Before implementing an order, the nurse reassesses the client to be sure that the order is still appropriate.
- The nurse must determine whether assistance is needed to perform a nursing intervention knowledgeably, safely, and comfortably for the client.
- The implementing phase terminates with the documentation of the nursing activities and client responses.
- After the care plan has been implemented, the nurse evaluates the client's health status and the effectiveness of the care plan in achieving client goals.

- The desired outcomes formulated during the planning phase serve as criteria for evaluating client progress and improved health status.
- The desired outcomes determine the data that must be collected to evaluate the client's health status.
- Reexamining the client care plan is a process of making decisions about problem status and critiquing each phase of the nursing process.
- Professional standards of care hold that nurses are responsible and accountable for implementing and evaluating the plan of care.
- Quality assurance evaluation includes consideration of the structures, processes, and outcomes of nursing care.
- Quality improvement is a philosophy and process internal to the institution, and does not rely on inspections by an external agency.

TEST YOUR KNOWLEDGE

1. When initiating the implementation phase of the nursing process, the nurse performs which of the following steps first?
   1. Carrying out nursing interventions
   2. Determining the need for assistance
   3. Reassessing the client
   4. Documenting interventions

2. Under what circumstances is it considered acceptable practice for the nurse to document a nursing activity *before* it is carried out?
   1. When the activity is routine (e.g., raising the bed rails)
   2. When the activity occurs at regular intervals (e.g., turning the client in bed)
   3. When the activity is to be carried out immediately (e.g., a stat medication)
   4. It is never acceptable

3. Which of the following is the primary purpose of the evaluating phase of the care-planning process to determine whether:
   1. Desired outcomes have been met.
   2. Nursing activities were carried out.
   3. Nursing activities were effective.
   4. Client's condition has changed.

4. The client has a high-priority nursing diagnosis of *Risk for Impaired Skin Integrity* related to the need for several weeks of imposed bed rest. The nurse evaluates the client after 1 week and finds the skin integrity is not impaired. When the care plan is reviewed, the nurse should perform which of the following?
   1. Delete the diagnosis since the problem has not occurred.
   2. Keep the diagnosis since the risk factors are still present.
   3. Modify the nursing diagnosis to *Impaired Mobility*.
   4. Demote the nursing diagnosis to a lower priority.

5. If the nurse planned to evaluate the length of time clients must wait for a nurse to respond to the client need reported over the intercom system on each shift, which of the following processes does this reflect?
   1. Structure evaluation
   2. Process evaluation
   3. Outcome evaluation
   4. Audit

See Answers to Test Your Knowledge in Appendix A.

EXPLORE MEDIALINK www.prenhall.com/berman

DVD-ROM
- Audio Glossary
- NCLEX Review

COMPANION WEBSITE
- Additional NCLEX Review
- Case Study: Treating a Client for Pain
- Application Activity:
  Analyzing Effective Quality Assurance
- Links to Resources

READINGS AND REFERENCES

SUGGESTED READINGS

Dochterman, J., Titler, M., Wang, J., Reed, D., Pettit, D., Mathew-Wilson, M., et al. (2005). Describing use of nursing interventions for three groups of patients. *Journal of Nursing Scholarship, 37*, 57–66.
This article describes the nursing interventions implemented most frequently during an acute hospital stay for clients with heart failure, hip fractures, or fall risk by use of the Nursing Interventions Classification (NIC).

QI project cuts patients' chronic pain dramatically: Facility earns Codman Award from JCAHO. (2003). *Healthcare Benchmarks and Quality Improvement, 10*(8), 94–96.
A quality improvement project at a Michigan long-term care facility resulted in a decrease in the prevalence of chronic pain among its residents from 33% to 18%. The reduction is even more significant given that the assessment of an individual's pain is a highly complex procedure, particularly among the elderly, who may experience cognitive or communication difficulties. For this work, the facility earned the Ernest A. Codman Award, which recognizes excellence in the use of outcomes measurement by health care organizations to achieve improvements in the quality and safety of health care from the Joint Commission on Accreditation of Healthcare Organizations.

RELATED RESEARCH

Cavendish, R., Konecny, L., Mitzeliotis, C., Russo, D., Luise, B., Lanza, M., et al. (2003). Spiritual care activities of nurses using nursing interventions classification (NIC) labels. *International Journal of Nursing Terminologies and Classifications, 14*, 13–24.

Wallace, T., O' Connell, S., & Frisch, S. R. (2005). Community psychiatric practice: What do nurses do when they take to the streets? An analysis of psychiatric and mental health nursing interventions in the community. *Community Mental Health Journal, 41*, 481–496.

REFERENCES

Agency for Healthcare Research and Quality. (2004). *Mission statement: Center for Quality Improvement and Patient Safety.* Rockville, MD. Retrieved April 16, 2006, from http://www.ahrq.gov/about/cquips/cquipsmiss.htm

Berlowitz, D. R., Young, G. J., Hickey, E. C., Saliba, D., Mittman, B. S., Czarnowski, E., et al. (2003). Quality improvement implementation in the nursing home. *Health Services Research, 38*(1 Part 1), 65–83.

Dochterman, J., & Bulechek, G. B. (Eds.). (2004). *Nursing interventions classification (NIC)* (4th ed.). St. Louis, MO: Mosby.

Joint Commission on Accreditation of Healthcare Organizations. (2005a). *Mission statement.* Retrieved April 16, 2006, from http://www.jointcommission.org/AboutUs/joint_commission_facts.htm

Joint Commission on Accreditation of Healthcare Organizations. (2005b). *Sentinel event policy and procedures.* Retrieved April 16, 2006, from http://www.jointcommission.org/SentinelEvents/

Kohn, L. T., Corrigan, J. M., & Donaldson, M. S. (Eds.). (2000). *To err is human: Building a safer health system.* Washington, DC: Committee on Quality of Health Care in America, Institute of Medicine National Academy Press. Retrieved June 21, 2006, from http://books.nap.edu/books/0309068371/html/index.html

Leape, L. L., & Berwick, D. M. (2005). Five years after To Err Is Human: What have we learned? *Journal of the American Medical Association, 293*, 2384–2390.

Moorhead, S., Johnson, M., & Maas, M. (Eds.). (2004). *Nursing outcomes classification (NOC)* (3rd ed). St. Louis, MO: Mosby.

NANDA International. (2005). *NANDA nursing diagnoses: Definitions and classification 2005–2006.* Philadelphia: Author.

SELECTED BIBLIOGRAPHY

Alfaro-LeFevre. R. A. (2005). *Applying the nursing process: Promoting collaborative care* (6th ed.). Philadelphia: Lippincott Williams & Wilkins.

American Nurses Association. (1999). *Nursing quality indicators: Guide for implementation.* Washington, DC: Author.

American Nurses Association. (2000). *Nursing quality indicators beyond acute care: Literature review.* Washington, DC: Author.

Burkhart, L., Konicek, D., Moorhead, S., & Androwich, I. (2005). Mapping parish nurse documentation into the Nursing Interventions Classification: A research method. *CIN: Computers Informatics Nursing, 23*, 220–229.

Johnson, M., Bulechek, G. B., Butcher, H., Dochterman, J., Moorhead, S., Maas, M., et al. (Eds.). (2005). *NANDA, NOC and NIC linkages: Nursing diagnoses, outcomes, and intervention* (2nd ed.). St. Louis, MO: Elsevier Health Sciences.

von Krogh, G., Dale, C., & Naden, D. (2005). A framework for integrating NANDA, NIC, and NOC terminology in electronic patient records. *Journal of Nursing Scholarship, 37*, 275–281.

Wilkinson, J. M. (2005). *Nursing diagnosis handbook: With NIC interventions and NOC outcomes* (8th ed.). Upper Saddle River, NJ: Prentice Hall.

Wilkinson, J. M. (2007). *Nursing process & critical thinking* (4th ed.). Upper Saddle River, NJ: Prentice Hall.

Documenting and Reporting

CHAPTER 15

LEARNING OUTCOMES

After completing this chapter, you will be able to:

1. List the measures used to maintain the confidentiality of client records.

2. Discuss reasons for keeping client records.

3. Compare and contrast different documentation methods: source-oriented and problem-oriented medical records, PIE, focus charting, charting by exception, computerized records, and the case management model.

4. Explain how various forms in the client record (e.g., flow sheets, progress notes, care plans, critical pathways, Kardexes, discharge/transfer forms) are used to document steps of the nursing process (assessment, diagnosis, planning, implementation, and evaluation).

5. Compare and contrast the documentation needed for clients in acute care, home health care, and long-term care settings.

6. Identify and discuss guidelines for effective recording that meets legal and ethical standards.

7. Identify essential guidelines for reporting client data.

8. Identify prohibited abbreviations, acronyms, and symbols that cannot be used in any form of clinical documentation.

Effective communication among health professionals is vital to the quality of client care. Generally, health personnel communicate through discussion, reports, and records. A **discussion** is an informal oral consideration of a subject by two or more health care personnel to identify a problem or establish strategies to resolve a problem. A **report** is oral, written, or computer-based communication intended to convey information to others. For instance, nurses always report on clients at the end of a hospital work shift. A **record** is written or computer based. The process of making an entry on a client record is called **recording, charting,** or **documenting.**

A clinical record, also called a **chart** or **client record,** is a formal, legal document that provides evidence of a client's care. Although health care organizations use different systems and forms for documentation, all client records have similar information.

Each health care organization has policies about recording and reporting client data, and each nurse is accountable for practicing according to these standards. Agencies also indicate which nursing assessments and interventions can be recorded by RNs and which can be charted by unlicensed personnel. In addition, the Joint Commission on Accreditation of Healthcare Organizations (JCAHO) requires client record documentation to be timely, complete, accurate, confidential, and specific to the client.

ETHICAL AND LEGAL CONSIDERATIONS

The American Nurses Association code of ethics (2001) states that ". . . the nurse has a duty to maintain confidentiality of all patient information" (p. 12). The client's record is also protected legally as a private record of the client's care. Access to the record is restricted to health professionals involved in giving care to the client. The institution or agency is the rightful owner of the client's record. This does not, however, exclude the client's rights to the same records.

Changes in the laws regarding client privacy became the official standard on April 14, 2003. The new HIPAA regulations maintain privacy and confidentiality of protected health information (PHI). HIPAA refers to the Health Insurance Portability and Accountability Act of 1996. PHI is identifiable health information that is transmitted or maintained in any form or medium, including verbal discussions, electronic communications with or about clients, and written communications (Clark, 2003, p. 7).

CLINICAL ALERT

Take safety measures before faxing confidential information. A fax cover sheet should contain instruction that the faxed material is to be given only to the named recipient. Consent is needed from the client to fax information. Make sure that personally identifiable information (e.g., client name, social security number) has been removed. Finally, check that the fax number is correct, check the number on the display of the machine after dialing, and check a third time before pressing the "send" button. ■

For purposes of education and research, most agencies allow student and graduate health professionals access to client records. The records are used in client conferences, clinics, rounds, client studies, and written papers. The student or graduate is bound by a strict ethical code and legal responsibility to hold all information in confidence. It is the responsibility of the student or health professional to protect the client's privacy by not using a name or any statements in the notations that would identify the client.

Ensuring Confidentiality of Computer Records

Because of the increased use of computerized client records, health care agencies have developed policies and procedures to ensure the privacy and confidentiality of client information stored in computers. In addition, the Security Rule of HIPAA became mandatory in 2005. This rule governs the security of electronic protected health information (Gallagher, 2004). The following are some suggestions for ensuring the confidentiality and security of computerized records:

1. A personal password is required to enter and sign off computer files. Do not share this password with anyone, including other health team members.
2. After logging on, never leave a computer terminal unattended.
3. Do not leave client information displayed on the monitor where others may see it.
4. Shred all unneeded computer-generated worksheets.
5. Know the facility's policy and procedure for correcting an entry error.
6. Follow agency procedures for documenting sensitive material, such as a diagnosis of AIDS.
7. Information technology (IT) personnel must install a firewall to protect the server from unauthorized access.

PURPOSES OF CLIENT RECORDS

Client records are kept for a number of purposes.

Communication

The record serves as the vehicle by which different health professionals who interact with a client communicate with each other. This prevents fragmentation, repetition, and delays in client care.

Planning Client Care

Each health professional uses data from the client's record to plan care for that client. A primary care provider, for example, may order a specific antibiotic after establishing that the client's temperature is steadily rising and that laboratory tests reveal the presence of a certain microorganism. Nurses use baseline and ongoing data to evaluate the effectiveness of the nursing care plan.

Auditing Health Agencies

An audit is a review of client records for quality-assurance purposes (see Chapter 14 ∞). Accrediting agencies such as JCAHO may review client records to determine if a particular health agency is meeting its stated standards.

Research

The information contained in a record can be a valuable source of data for research. The treatment plans for a number of clients with the same health problems can yield information helpful in treating other clients.

Education

Students in health disciplines often use client records as educational tools. A record can frequently provide a comprehensive view of the client, the illness, effective treatment strategies, and factors that affect the outcome of the illness.

Reimbursement

Documentation also helps a facility receive reimbursement from the federal government. For a facility to obtain payment through Medicare, the client's clinical record must contain the correct diagnosis-related group (DRG) codes and reveal that the appropriate care has been given.

Codable diagnoses, such as DRGs, are supported by accurate, thorough recording by nurses. This not only facilitates reimbursement from the federal government, but also facilitates reimbursement from insurance companies and other third-party payers. If additional care, treatment, or length of stay becomes necessary for the client's welfare, thorough charting will help justify these needs.

Legal Documentation

The client's record is a legal document and is usually admissible in court as evidence. In some jurisdictions, however, the record is considered inadmissible as evidence when the client objects, because information the client gives to the physician is confidential.

Health Care Analysis

Information from records may assist health care planners to identify agency needs, such as overutilized and underutilized hospital services. Records can be used to establish the costs of various services and to identify those services that cost the agency money and those that generate revenue.

DOCUMENTATION SYSTEMS

A number of documentation systems are in current use: the source-oriented record; the problem-oriented medical record; the problems, interventions, evaluation (PIE) model; focus charting; charting by exception (CBE); computerized documentation; and case management.

Source-Oriented Record

The traditional client record is a **source-oriented record.** Each person or department makes notations in a separate section or sections of the client's chart. For example, the admissions department has an admission sheet; the physician has a physician's order sheet, a physician's history sheet, and progress notes; nurses use the nurses' notes; and other departments or personnel have their own records. In this type of record, information about a particular problem is distributed throughout the record. For example, if a client had left hemiplegia (paralysis of the left side of the body), data about this problem might be found in the physician's history sheet, on the physician's order sheet, in the nurses' notes, in the physical therapist's record, and in the social service record. Table 15–1 lists the components of a source-oriented record.

Narrative charting is a traditional part of the source-oriented record. It consists of written notes that include routine care, normal findings, and client problems. There is no right or wrong order to the information, although chronological order is frequently used. Few institutions use only narrative charting today. Narrative recording is being replaced by other systems, such as charting by exception and focus charting. However, narrative charting is expedient in emergency situations (see Figure 15-1 ■ on page 249). Many agencies combine narrative charting with another system. For example, an agency using a charting-by-exception system (discussed later) may use narrative charting when describing abnormal findings. When using narrative charting, it is important to organize the information in a clear, coherent manner. Using the nursing process as a framework is one way to do this. See Box 15–1 on page 249.

Source-oriented records are convenient because care providers from each discipline can easily locate the forms on which to record data and it is easy to trace the information specific to one's discipline. The disadvantage is that information about a particular client problem is scattered throughout the chart, so it is difficult to find chronological information on a client's problems and progress. This can lead to decreased communication among the health team, an incomplete picture of the client's care, and a lack of coordination of care, (Lippincott, Williams, & Wilkins, 2003, 2007).

TABLE 15-1	Components of the Source-Oriented Record	

FORM	INFORMATION
Admission (face) sheet	Legal name, birth date, age, gender
	Social Security number
	Address
	Marital status; closest relatives or person to notify in case of emergency
	Date, time, and admitting diagnosis
	Food or drug allergies
	Name of admitting (attending) physician
	Insurance information
	Any assigned diagnosis-related group (DRG)
Initial nursing assessment	Findings from the initial nursing history and physical health assessment
Graphic record	Body temperature, pulse rate, respiratory rate, blood pressure, daily weight, and special measurements such as fluid intake and output and oxygen saturation
Daily care record	Activity, diet, bathing, and elimination records
Special flow sheets	Examples: fluid balance record, skin assessment
Medication record	Name, dosage, route, time, date of regularly administered medications
	Name or initials of person administering the medication
Nurses' notes	Pertinent assessment of client
	Specific nursing care including teaching and client's responses
	Client's complaints and how client is coping
Medical history and physical examination	Past and family medical history, present medical problems, differential or current diagnoses, findings of physical examination by the primary care provider
Physician's order sheet	Medical orders for medications, treatments, and so on
Physician's progress notes	Medical observations, treatments, client progress, and so on
Consultation records	Reports by medical and clinical specialists
Diagnostic reports	Examples: laboratory reports, x-ray reports, CT scan reports
Consultation reports	Physical therapy, respiratory therapy
Client discharge plan and referral summary	Started on admission and completed on discharge; includes nursing problems, general information, and referral data

Problem-Oriented Medical Record

In the **problem-oriented medical record (POMR),** or **problem-oriented record (POR),** established by Lawrence Weed in the 1960s, the data are arranged according to the problems the client has rather than the source of the information. Members of the health care team contribute to the problem list, plan of care, and progress notes. Plans for each active or potential problem are drawn up, and progress notes are recorded for each problem.

The advantage of POMR is that (a) it encourages collaboration and (b) the problem list in the front of the chart alerts caregivers to the client's needs and makes it easier to track the status of each problem. Its disadvantages are that (a) caregivers differ in their ability to use the required charting format, (b) it takes constant vigilance to maintain an up-to-date problem list, and (c) it is somewhat inefficient because assessments and interventions that apply to more than one problem must be repeated.

The POMR has four basic components:

- Database
- Problem list
- Plan of care
- Progress notes

In addition, flow sheets and discharge notes are added to the record as needed.

Database

The database consists of all information known about the client when the client first enters the health care agency. It includes the nursing assessment, the physician's history, social and family data, and the results of the physical examination and baseline diagnostic tests. Data are constantly updated as the client's health status changes.

Problem List

The problem list (see Figure 15-2 ■) is derived from the database. It is usually kept at the front of the chart and serves as an index to the numbered entries in the progress notes. Problems are listed in the order in which they are identified, and the list is continually updated as new problems are identified and others resolved. All caregivers may contribute to the problem list, which includes the client's physiologic, psychologic, social, cultural, spiritual, developmental, and environmental needs. Primary care providers write problems as medical diagnoses, surgical procedures, or symptoms; nurses write problems as nursing diagnoses.

As the client's condition changes or more data are obtained, it may be necessary to "redefine" problems. Figure 15-2 illustrates how this has been done for Problems 1B, 1C, and 2. When a problem is resolved, a line is drawn through it and the number is not used again for that client.

NURSING NOTES

Date	Time	
6/6/07	1400	Passive ROM exercises provided for R arm and leg.
		Active assistive exercises to L arm and leg. Has scratch
		marks on L and R forearms. States, "My skin on my back
		and arms has been itchy for a week." Rash not evident.
		No previous history of pruritus. Is allergic to elastoplast
		but has not been in contact. Dr. J. Wong notified.
		———————————————————— T. Ritchie, RN
	1430	Applied calamine lotion to back and arms. Incontinent
		of urine. Is restless. ——————— T. Ritchie, RN

Figure 15-1 ■ An example of narrative notes.

Plan of Care

The initial list of orders or plan of care is made with reference to the active problems. Care plans are generated by the person who lists the problems. Physicians write physician's orders or medical care plans; nurses write nursing orders or nursing care plans. The written plan in the record is listed under each problem in the progress notes and is not isolated as a separate list of orders.

BOX 15–1   Example of Organizing Narrative Charting

Situation: Client is postop day # 2 after abdominal surgery.
   Questions to ask yourself:
- What assessment data are relevant?
- What nursing interventions have I completed?
- What is my evaluation of the result of the interventions and/or what is the client's response to the interventions?

EXAMPLE
1000 Diminished breath sounds in all lung fields with crackles in LLL. Not using incentive spirometer (IS). Stated he's "not sure how to use it." Temperature 99.6. Instructed how to use IS. Discussed the importance of deep breathing and coughing after surgery. Administered analgesic for c/o abdominal pain rating of 5/10. After pain relief (1/10), able to demonstrate correct use of IS. ———
——————————————————————— S. Martin, RN

1400 Using IS each hour. Lungs less diminished with fewer LLL crackles. Temp 99. ——————————— S. Martin, RN

Progress Notes

A **progress note** in the POMR is a chart entry made by all health professionals involved in a client's care; they all use the same type of sheet for notes. Progress notes are numbered to correspond to the problems on the problem list and may be lettered for the type of data. For example, the SOAP format is frequently used. **SOAP** is an acronym for subjective data, objective data, assessment, and planning.

S—*Subjective data* consist of information obtained from what the client says. It describes the client's perceptions of and experience with the problem (see Chapter 11 ∞). When possible, the nurse quotes the client's words; otherwise, they are summarized. Subjective data are included only when it is important and relevant to the problem.
O—*Objective data* consist of information that is measured or observed by use of the senses (e.g., vital signs, laboratory and x-ray results).
A—*Assessment* is the interpretation or conclusions drawn about the subjective and objective data. During the initial assessment, the problem list is created from the database, so the "A" entry should be a statement of the problem. In all subsequent SOAP notes for that problem, the "A" should describe the client's condition and level of progress rather than merely restating the diagnosis or problem.
P—The *plan* is the plan of care designed to resolve the stated problem. The initial plan is written by the person who enters the problem into the record. All subsequent plans, including revisions, are entered into the progress notes.

No.	Date Entered	Date Inactive	Client Problem
#1	3/9/07		CVA resulting in Rt hemiplegia and left-sided weakness
#1A	3/9/07		Self-care deficit (hygiene, toileting, grooming, feeding)
#1B	3/9/07		Impaired physical mobility (unable to turn and position self) *Redefined 2/7/08*
#1C	3/9/07		Total urinary incontinence *Redefined 1/17/08*
#1D	3/9/07		Progressive dysphasia
#2	3/9/07		Constipation r/t immobility *Redefined 6/10/07*
#3	3/9/07		History of depression
#4	3/9/07		Essential hypertension
~~#5~~	~~6/6/07~~	~~7/11/07~~	~~Pruritus~~
#2	6/10/07		Risk for constipation r/t insufficient fiber intake
#1C	1/17/08		Urge urinary incontinence at night
#1B	2/7/08		*Impaired physical mobility (needs 2-person assistance to transfer and walk)*

Figure 15-2 ■ A client's problem list in the POMR. Note that problems 1B, 1C, and 2 were redefined on the dates indicated and listed subsequently.

Over the years, the SOAP format has been modified. The acronyms *SOAPIE* and *SOAPIER* refer to formats that add interventions, evaluation, and revision.

    I—*Interventions* refer to the specific interventions that have actually been performed by the caregiver.
    E—*Evaluation* includes client responses to nursing interventions and medical treatments. This is primarily reassessment data.
    R—*Revision* reflects care plan modifications suggested by the evaluation. Changes may be made in desired outcomes, interventions, or target dates.

Newer versions of this format eliminate the subjective and objective data and start with *assessment,* which combines the subjective and objective data. The acronym then becomes *AP, APIE,* or *APIER.* See Figure 15-3 ■.

PIE

The **PIE** documentation model groups information into three categories. PIE is an acronym for problems, interventions, and

evaluation of nursing care. This system consists of a client care assessment flow sheet and progress notes. The **flow sheet** uses specific assessment criteria in a particular format, such as human needs or functional health patterns. The time parameters for a flow sheet can vary from minutes to months. In a hospital intensive care unit, for example, a client's blood pressure may be monitored by the minute, whereas in an ambulatory clinic a client's blood glucose level may be recorded once a month.

    After the assessment, the nurse establishes and records specific problems on the progress notes, often using North American Nursing Diagnosis Association (NANDA) diagnoses to word the problem. If there is no approved nursing diagnosis for a problem, the nurse develops a problem statement using NANDA's three-part format: client's response, contributing or probable causes of the response, and characteristics manifested by the client (see Chapter 12 ∞). The *problem statement* is labeled "P" and referred to by number (e.g., P #5). The *interventions* employed to manage the problem are labeled "I" and numbered according to the problem (e.g., I #5). The

SOAP Format	SOAPIER Format	APIE Format
6/6/07 #5 Generalized pruritus	6/6/07 #5 Generalized pruritus	6/6/07 A— Generalized pruritus r/t unknown cause
1400 S— "My skin is itchy on my back and arms, and it's been like this for a week."	1400 S— "My skin is itchy on my back and arms, and it's been like this for a week."	1400 States, "My skin is itchy on my back and arms, and it's been like this for a week." Skin appears clear.
O— Skin appears clear—no rash or irritation noted. Marks where client has scratched noted on left and right forearms. Allergic to elastoplast but has not been in contact. No previous history of pruritus.	O— Skin appears clear—no rash or irritation noted. Marks where client has scratched noted on left and right forearms. Allergic to elastoplast but has not been in contact. No previous history of pruritus.	No rash or irritations noted. Marks where client has scratched noted on left and right forearms. Allergic to elastoplast but has not been in contact. No previous history of pruritus.
A— Altered comfort (pruritus): cause unknown.	A— Altered comfort (pruritus): cause unknown.	P— Instruct to not scratch skin.
P— Instructed not to scratch skin.	P— Instruct to not scratch skin.	— Apply calamine lotion as necessary.
— Applied calamine lotion to back and arms at 1430 h.	— Apply calamine lotion as necessary.	— Cut nails to avoid scratches.
— Cut fingernails.	— Cut nails to avoid scratches.	— Assess further to determine whether recurrence associated with specific drugs or foods.
— Assess further to determine whether recurrence associated with specific drugs or foods.	— Assess further to determine whether recurrence associated with specific drugs or foods.	— Refer to physician and pharmacist for assessment.
— Refer to physician and pharmacist for assessment.	— Refer to physician and pharmacist for assessment.	I — Instructed not to scratch skin. Applied calamine lotion to back and arms at 1430 h. Assisted to cut fingernails. Notified physician and pharmacist of problem.
T. Ritchie, RN	I — Instructed not to scratch skin. Applied calamine lotion to back and arms at 1430 h. Assisted to cut fingernails. Notified physician and pharmacist of problem.	E— States, "I'm still itchy. That lotion didn't help."
	1600 E— States, "I'm still itchy. That lotion didn't help."	T. Ritchie, RN
	R— Remove calamine lotion and apply hydrocortisone cream as ordered.	
	T. Ritchie, RN	

Figure 15-3 ■ Examples of nursing progress notes using SOAP, SOAPIER, and APIE formats.

evaluation of the effectiveness of the interventions is also labeled and numbered according to the problem (e.g., E #5).

The PIE system eliminates the traditional care plan and incorporates an ongoing care plan into the progress notes. Therefore, the nurse does not have to create and update a separate plan. A disadvantage is that the nurse must review all the nursing notes before giving care to determine which problems are current and which interventions were effective.

Focus Charting

Focus charting is intended to make the client and client concerns and strengths the focus of care. Three columns for recording are usually used: date and time, focus, and progress notes. The *focus* may be a condition, a nursing diagnosis, a behavior, a sign or symptom, an acute change in the client's condition, or a client strength. The progress notes are organized into (D) data, (A) ac-

tion, and (R) response, referred to as DAR. The *data* category reflects the assessment phase of the nursing process and consists of observations of client status and behaviors, including data from flow sheets (e.g., vital signs, pupil reactivity). The nurse records both subjective and objective data in this section.

The *action* category reflects planning and implementation and includes immediate and future nursing actions. It may also include any changes to the plan of care. The *response category* reflects the evaluation phase of the nursing process and describes the client's response to any nursing and medical care.

The focus charting system provides a holistic perspective of the client and the client's needs. It also provides a nursing process framework for the progress notes (DAR). The three components do not need to be recorded in order and each note does not need to have all three categories. Flow sheets and checklists are frequently used on the client's chart to record routine nursing tasks and assessment data.

Date/Hour	Focus	Progress Notes
2/11/07 0900	Pain	**D:** Guarding abdominal incision. Facial grimacing. Rates pain at "8" on scale of 0–10.
		A: Administered morphine sulfate 4 mg IV.
0930		**R:** Rates pain at "1." States willing to ambulate.

Charting by Exception

Charting by exception (CBE) is a documentation system in which only abnormal or significant findings or exceptions to norms are recorded. CBE incorporates three key elements (Guido, 2005):

1. Flow sheets. Examples of flow sheets include a graphic record (Figure 15-4 ■), fluid balance record, daily nursing

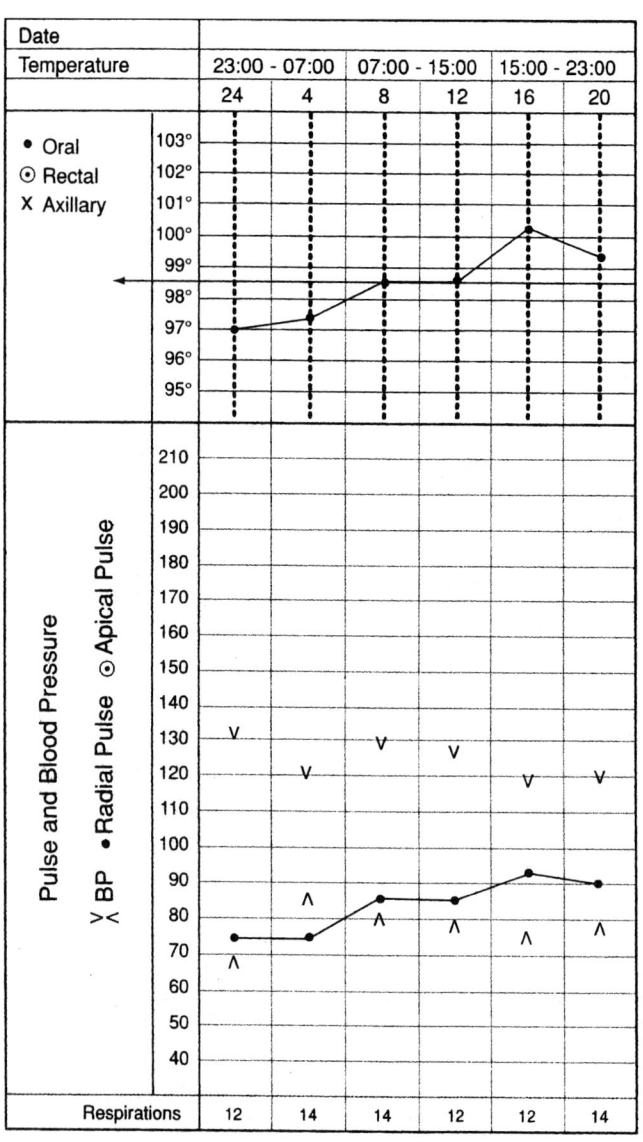

Figure 15-4 ■ Sample vital signs graphic record.

assessments record (Figure 15-5 ■), client teaching record, client discharge record, and skin assessment record (Figure 15-6 ■).

2. Standards of nursing care. Documentation by reference to the agency's printed standards of nursing practice eliminates much of the repetitive charting of routine care. An agency using CBE must develop its own specific standards of nursing practice that identify the minimum criteria for client care regardless of clinical area. Some units may also have unit-specific standards unique to their type of client. For example, "The nurse must ensure that the unconscious client has oral care at least q4h." Documentation of care according to these specified standards involves only a check mark in the routine standards box on the graphic record. If all of the standards are not implemented, an asterisk on the flow sheet is made with reference to the nurses' notes. All exceptions to the standards are fully described in narrative form on the nurses' notes.

3. Bedside access to chart forms. In the CBE system, all flow sheets are kept at the client's bedside to allow immediate recording and to eliminate the need to transcribe data from the nurse's worksheet to the permanent record.

The advantage to this system is the elimination of lengthy, repetitive notes and it makes client changes in condition more obvious. Inherent in CBE is the presumption that the nurse did assess the client and determined what responses were normal and abnormal. Many nurses believe in the saying "not charted, not done" and subsequently may feel uncomfortable with the CBE documentation system. Sullivan (2004) suggests writing N/A on flow sheets where the items are not applicable and to not leave blank spaces. This would then avoid the possible misinterpretation that the assessment or intervention was not done by the nurse.

Computerized Documentation

Computerized clinical record systems are being developed as a way to manage the huge volume of information required in contemporary health care. Nurses use computers to store the client's database, add new data, create and revise care plans, and document client progress (see Figure 15-7 ■). Some institutions have a computer terminal at each client's bedside, or nurses carry a small handheld terminal, enabling the nurse to document care immediately after it is given.

Multiple flow sheets are not needed in computerized record systems because information can be easily retrieved in a variety of formats. For example, the nurse can obtain results of a client's blood test, a schedule of all clients on the unit who are to have surgery during the day, a suggested list of interventions for a nursing diagnosis, a graphic chart of a client's vital signs, or a printout of all progress notes for a client. Many systems can generate a work list for the shift, with a list of all treatments, procedures, and medications needed by the client.

Computers make care planning and documentation relatively easy. To record nursing actions and client responses, the nurse either chooses from standardized lists of terms or types narrative information into the computer. Automated speech-

Medical-Surgical
NURSING ASSESSMENT RECORD

| Date: 9/12/2007 | 0700–1900 | Initials: NS | Signature: Nancy Smith RN |

Assessment Parameters	Time: 0800 Notes	Time: 1000 Notes	Time: Notes
NEUROMUSCULAR: Alert & oriented to person, place, & time. Behavior appropriate to situation. PERL. MAE with symmetry of strength and no muscle weakness. Ambulates independently and performs self-care. Speech clear. Hears normal conversation. Swallows without difficulty. No c/o numbness or tingling, blurred vision, dizziness, or headache.	☑	☑	☐
CARDIOVASCULAR: Regular apical pulse with no extra sounds. Nail beds pink. Pedal pulses present. No edema. No c/o chest pain.	☑	☑	☐
RESPIRATORY: Respirations regular and unlabored. Breath sounds clear in all fields. No cough or sputum production. No c/o dyspnea.	✳ Coarse crackles at bases—clears with coughing. Encouraged C + DB	➞	☐
GASTROINTESTINAL: Abdomen soft, non-tender. No distention. Bowel sounds present in all 4 quadrants. No nausea or vomiting. Continent. Soft, brown BMs every 1–2 days.	✳ Bowel sounds absent. N/G Tube draining mod. amt lt. brownish fluid	➞	☐
URINARY: Urine clear and yellow to amber. Continent. No c/o discomfort with voiding.	☑	☑	☐

KEY: ✓ = Assessment matches normal assessment parameters
       ★ = Abnormal finding
       → = No change in abnormal finding since last assessment

Figure 15-5 ■ Sample of a daily nursing assessment form used in CBE.

recognition technology now allows nurses to enter data by voice for conversion to written documentation. Again, according to HIPAA, if the spoken word is used to create PHI, the nurse must be alert and aware of others who might hear the dictation.

The computerization of clinical records has made it possible to transmit information from one care setting to another. The Nursing Minimum Data Set (NMDS) is an effort to establish standards for collecting standardized, essential nursing data for inclusion in computer databases. Selected pros and cons of computer documentation are shown in Box 15–2.

Case Management

The case management model emphasizes quality, cost-effective care delivered within an established length of stay. This model uses a multidisciplinary approach to planning and documenting client care, using *critical pathways.* These forms identify the outcomes that certain groups of clients are expected to achieve on each day of care, along with the interventions necessary for each day. See Figure 15-8 ■ and Chapter 6 for more information about critical pathways. ∞

SKIN ASSESSMENT FLOW CHART

Date: _____ Assessed by: _____

Number each skin injury/wound on the diagram. Complete information for each skin injury/wound.

Stage 1:   Nonblanchable erythema of intact skin
Stage 2:   Superficial skin break, shallow crater/blister
Stage 3:   Deep tissue involvement/cavity not through fascia
Stage 4:   Full thickness skin loss with extensive
             destruction of tissue, tissue necrosis, or damage
             to muscle, bone, or supporting structures

Injury/Wound Types:

Stasis ulcer   Bruise
Pressure ulcer   Skin tear
Arterial ulcer   Rash
Surgical wound   Hematoma
Laceration   Other: specify

Photographs on admission, weekly, and on discharge (note due dates on Kardex).

Site #	Injury/Wound Type (specify)	Stage	Length Width cm	Depth cm	Tunneling Yes/No	Color	Drainage Amt/Type	Odor	Culture Date	Treatments & Comments

Figure 15-6 ■ Sample skin assessment flow sheet.

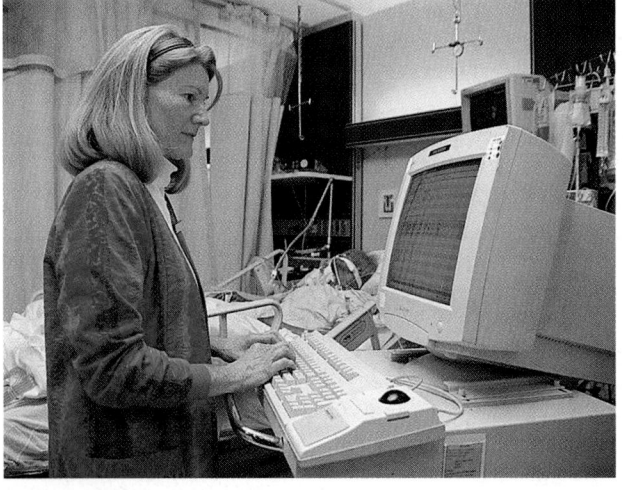

Figure 15-7 ■ A bedside computer.

Along with critical pathways, the case management model incorporates graphics and flow sheets. Progress notes typically use some type of charting by exception. For example, if goals are met, no further charting is required. A goal that is not met is called a **variance.** A variance is a deviation to what is planned on the critical pathway—unexpected occurrences that affect the planned care or the client's responses to care. When a variance occurs, the nurse writes a note documenting the unexpected event, the cause, and actions taken to correct the situation or justify the actions taken. See Table 15–2 for an example of how a variance might be documented.

The case management model promotes collaboration and teamwork among caregivers, helps to decrease length of stay, and makes efficient use of time. Because care is goal focused, the quality may improve. However, critical pathways work best for clients with one or two diagnoses and few individualized needs. Clients with multiple diagnoses (e.g., a client with a hip fracture, pneumonia, diabetes, and pressure sore) or those with an unpredictable course of symptoms (e.g., a neurological client with seizures) are difficult to document on a critical path.

BOX 15–2 Selected Pros and Cons of Computer Documentation

PROS
- Computer records can facilitate a focus on client outcomes.
- Bedside terminals can synthesize information from monitoring equipment.
- It allows nurses to use their time more efficiently.
- The system links various sources of client information.
- Client information, requests, and results are sent and received quickly.
- Links to monitors improve accuracy of documentation.
- Bedside terminals eliminate the need to take notes on a worksheet before recording.
- Bedside terminals permit the nurse to check an order immediately before administering a treatment or medication.
- Information is legible.
- The system incorporates and reinforces standards of care.
- Standard terminology improves communication.

CONS
- Client's privacy may be infringed on if security measures are not used.
- Breakdowns make information temporarily unavailable.
- The system is expensive.
- Extended training periods may be required when a new or updated system is installed.

CRITICAL PATHWAY: TOTAL HIP REPLACEMENT

	DOS/Day 1	Days 2–3
Pain Management	Outcome: • Verbalizes comfort or tolerance of pain Circle: V NV Variance:	Outcome: • Verbalizes comfort with pain control measures Circle: V NV Variance:
Respiratory	Outcomes: • Breath sounds clear to auscultation • Achieves 50% of volume goal on incentive spirometer Circle: V NV Variance:	Outcomes: • Breath sounds clear to auscultation • Achieves 100% of volume goal on incentive spirometer Circle: V NV Variance:
Key: V = Variance	NV = No Variance	
Signature:	Initials:	
Signature:	Initials:	

Figure 15-8 ■ Excerpt from a critical pathway documentation form.

health problems and risks, nursing model, or type of health care setting (e.g., labor and delivery, pediatrics, mental health). The nurse generally records ongoing assessments or reassessments on flow sheets or on nursing progress notes.

DOCUMENTING NURSING ACTIVITIES

The client record should describe the client's ongoing status and reflect the full range of the nursing process. Regardless of the records system used in an agency, nurses document evidence of the nursing process on a variety of forms throughout the clinical record (Table 15–3).

Admission Nursing Assessment

A comprehensive admission assessment, also referred to as an initial database, nursing history, or nursing assessment, is completed when the client is admitted to the nursing unit. As discussed in Chapter 11 ∞, these forms can be organized according to health patterns, body systems, functional abilities,

Nursing Care Plans

According to Smith and Dougherty (2001), JCAHO requires that the clinical record include evidence of client assessments, nursing diagnoses and/or client needs, nursing interventions, client outcomes, and evidence of a current nursing care plan. Depending on the records system being used, the nursing care plan may be separate from the client's chart, recorded in progress notes and other forms in the client record, or incorporated into a multidisciplinary plan of care.

There are two types of nursing care plans: traditional and standardized. The *traditional care plan* is written for each client. The form varies from agency to agency according to the needs of the client and the department. Most forms have three columns: one for nursing diagnoses, a second for expected outcomes, and a

TABLE 15–2 Example of Variance Documentation (Critical Pathway)

A client has had a below-the-knee amputation. On the third postoperative day he has a temperature of 38.8C (102F). Lung sounds are clear and he is not coughing. The nurse notices redness and skin breakdown over the client's sacrum. The critical pathway outcomes specified for Day 3 are "Oral temperature 37.7C (100F)" and "Skin intact over bony prominences." The nurse should chart the following variances:

DATE/TIME	VARIANCE	CAUSE	ACTION TAKEN/PLANS
4/16/07 0900	Elevated temperature (102F)	Possible sepsis	4/16—Blood cultures ×3 per order. Monitor temp. q1h. Monitor I&O, hydration, and mental status.
4/16/07 1130	Impaired skin integrity: Stage 1 redness, 2-inch circular area on sacrum	Client does not move about in bed unless reminded	4/16—Positioned on L side. Turn side-to-side q2h while awake. On every client contact, remind client to move about in bed. Apply Duoderm after bath.

TABLE 15–3 Documentation for the Nursing Process

STEP*	DOCUMENTATION FORMS
Assessment	Initial assessment form, various flow sheets
Nursing diagnosis	Nursing care plan, critical pathway, progress notes, problem list
Planning	Nursing care plan, critical pathway
Implementing	Progress notes, flow sheets
Evaluating	Progress notes

*All steps are recorded on discharge/referral summaries.

third for nursing interventions. See Chapter 13 ∞ for additional information.

Standardized care plans were developed to save documentation time. These plans may be based on an institution's standards of practice, thereby helping to provide a high quality of nursing care. For further information, see Chapter 13 ∞. Standardized plans must be individualized by the nurse in order to adequately address individual client needs.

Kardexes

The **Kardex** is a widely used, concise method of organizing and recording data about a client, making information quickly accessible to all health professionals. The system consists of a series of cards kept in a portable index file or on computer-generated forms. The card for a particular client can be quickly accessed to reveal specific data. The Kardex may or may not become a part of the client's permanent record. In some organizations it is a temporary worksheet written in pencil for ease in recording frequent changes in details of a client's care. The information on Kardexes may be organized into sections, for example:

- Pertinent information about the client, such as name, room number, age, admission date, physician's name, diagnosis, and type of surgery and date
- Allergies
- List of medications, with the date of order and the times of administration for each
- List of intravenous fluids, with dates of infusions
- List of daily treatments and procedures, such as irrigations, dressing changes, postural drainage, or measurement of vital signs
- List of diagnostic procedures ordered, such as x-ray or laboratory tests
- Specific data on how the client's physical needs are to be met, such as type of diet, assistance needed with feeding, elimination devices, activity, hygienic needs, and safety precautions (e.g., one-person assist)
- A problem list, stated goals, and a list of nursing approaches to meet the goals and relieve the problems

Although much of the information on the Kardex may be recorded by the nurse in charge or a delegate (e.g., the nursing

unit clerk), any nurse who cares for the client plays a key role in initiating the record and keeping the data current. Whether the Kardex is a written paper or computerized, it is important to have a place on it to record date and initials of the person reviewing or revising it. It is a quick visual guide to ensure that information is current and updated on a regular basis.

Flow Sheets

A flow sheet enables nurses to record nursing data quickly and concisely and provides an easy-to-read record of the client's condition over time.

Graphic Record

This record typically indicates body temperature, pulse, respiratory rate, blood pressure, weight, and, in some agencies, other significant clinical data such as admission or postoperative day, bowel movements, appetite, and activity.

Intake and Output Record

All routes of fluid intake and all routes of fluid loss or output are measured and recorded on this form. See Chapter 52 ∞ for more information.

Medication Administration Record

Medication flow sheets usually include designated areas for the date of the medication order, the expiration date, the medication name and dose, the frequency of administration and route, and the nurse's signature. Some records also include a place to document the client's allergies (see Chapter 35 ∞).

Skin Assessment Record

A skin or wound assessment is often recorded on a flow sheet such as the one shown in Figure 15-6. These records may include categories related to stage of skin injury, drainage, odor, culture information, and treatments.

Progress Notes

Progress notes made by nurses provide information about the progress a client is making toward achieving desired outcomes. Therefore, in addition to assessment and reassessment data, progress notes include information about client problems and nursing interventions. The format used depends on the documentation system in place in the institution. Various kinds of nursing progress notes are discussed in the "Documentation Systems" section earlier in this chapter.

Nursing Discharge/ Referral Summaries

A discharge note and referral summary are completed when the client is being discharged and transferred to another institution or to a home setting where a visit by a community health nurse is required. See the discussion of discharge planning in Chapter 7 ∞, and the assessment parameters suggested when preparing clients to go home. Many institutions provide forms for these summaries. Some records combine the discharge plan, including instructions for care, and the final progress note. Many are designed with checklists to facilitate data recording.

If the discharge plan is given directly to the client and family, it is imperative that instructions be written in terms that can be readily understood. For example, medications, treatments, and activities should be written in layman's terms, and use of medical abbreviations (such as t.i.d.) should be avoided.

If a client is transferred within the facility or from a long-term facility to a hospital, a report needs to accompany the client to ensure continuity of care in the new area. It should include all components of the discharge instructions, but also describe the condition of the client before the transfer. Any teaching or client instruction that has been done should also be described and recorded.

If the client is being transferred to another institution or to a home setting where a visit by a home health nurse is required, the discharge note takes the form of a referral summary. Regardless of format, discharge and referral summaries usually include some or all of the following:

- Description of client's physical, mental, and emotional status at discharge or transfer
- Resolved health problems
- Unresolved continuing health problems and continuing care needs; may include a review-of-systems checklist that considers integumentary, respiratory, cardiovascular, neurological, musculoskeletal, gastrointestinal, elimination, and reproductive problems
- Treatments that are to be continued (e.g., wound care, oxygen therapy)
- Current medications
- Restrictions that relate to (a) activity such as lifting, stair climbing, walking, driving, work, (b) diet, and (c) bathing such as sponge bath, tub, or shower
- Functional/self-care abilities in terms of vision, hearing, speech, mobility with or without aids, meal preparation and eating, preparing and administering medications, and so on
- Comfort level
- Support networks including family, significant others, religious adviser, community self-help groups, home care and other community agencies available, and so on
- Client education provided in relation to disease process, activities and exercise, special diet, medications, specialized care or treatments, follow-up appointments, and so on
- Discharge destination (e.g., home, nursing home) and mode of discharge (e.g., walking, wheelchair, ambulance)
- Referral services (e.g., social worker, home health nurse)

LONG-TERM CARE DOCUMENTATION

Long-term facilities usually provide two types of care: skilled or intermediate. Clients needing skilled care require more extensive nursing care and specialized nursing skills. In contrast, an intermediate care focus is needed for clients who usually have chronic illnesses and may only need assistance with activities of daily living (such as bathing and dressing).

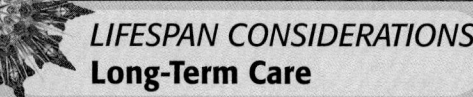

LIFESPAN CONSIDERATIONS
Long-Term Care

ELDERS

Elders in long-term care facilities tend to have chronic conditions and generally experience subtle small changes in their condition. However, when problems do occur, such as a hip fracture, CVA, or pneumonia, they are serious and require prompt attention. This points out the importance of keeping Kardexes and charting in long-term facilities current and up to date in the event that the client needs to be transferred for more skilled care and further treatment. A thorough transfer summary will facilitate communication and promote continuity of care in these situations.

Requirements for documentation in long-term care settings are based on professional standards, federal and state regulations, and the policies of the health care agency. Laws influencing the kind and frequency of documentation required are the Health Care Financing Administration and the Omnibus Budget Reconciliation Act (OBRA) of 1987. The OBRA law, for example, requires that (a) a comprehensive assessment (the Minimum Data Set [MDS] for Resident Assessment and Care Screening) be performed within 4 days of a client's admission to a long-term care facility, (b) a formulated plan of care must be completed within 7 days of admission, and (c) the assessment and care screening process must be reviewed every 3 months.

Documentation must also comply with requirements set by Medicare and Medicaid. These requirements vary with the level of service provided and other factors. For example, Medicare provides little reimbursement for services provided in long-term care facilities except for services that require skilled care such as chemotherapy, tube feedings, ventilators, and so on. For such Medicare clients, the nurse must provide daily documentation to verify the need for service and reimbursement.

Nurses need to familiarize themselves with regulations influencing the kind and frequency of documentation required in long-term care facilities. Usually the nurse completes a nursing care *summary* at least once a week for clients requiring skilled care and every 2 weeks for those requiring intermediate care. Summaries should address the following:

- Specific problems noted in the care plan
- Mental status
- Activities of daily living
- Hydration and nutrition status
- Safety measures needed
- Medications
- Treatments
- Preventive measures
- Behavioral modification assessments, if pertinent (if client is taking psychotropic medications or demonstrates behavioral problems)

See the Practice Guidelines for documentation in long-term care facilities.

PRACTICE GUIDELINES Long-Term Care Documentation

- Complete the assessment and screening forms (MDS) and plan of care within the time period specified by regulatory bodies.
- Keep a record of any visits and of phone calls from family, friends, and others regarding the client.
- Write nursing summaries and progress notes that comply with the frequency and standards required by regulatory bodies.
- Review and revise the plan of care every 3 months or whenever the client's health status changes.
- Document and report any change in the client's condition to the primary care provider and the client's family within 24 hours.
- Document all measures implemented in response to a change in the client's condition.
- Make sure that progress notes address the client's progress in relation to the goals or outcomes defined in the plan of care.

PRACTICE GUIDELINES Home Health Care Documentation

- Complete a comprehensive nursing assessment and develop a plan of care to meet Medicare and other third-party payer requirements. Some agencies use the certification and plan of treatment form as the client's official plan of care.
- Write a progress note at each client visit, noting any changes in the client condition; nursing interventions performed (including education and instructional brochures and materials provided to the client and home caregiver); client responses to nursing care; and vital signs as indicated.
- Provide a monthly progress nursing summary to the attending physician and to the reimburser to confirm the need to continue services.
- Keep a copy of the care plan in the client's home and update it as the client's condition changes.
- Report changes in the plan of care to the physician and document that these were reported. Medicare and Medicaid will reimburse only for the skilled services provided that are reported to the physician.
- Encourage the client or home caregiver to record data when appropriate.
- Write a discharge summary for the physician to approve the discharge and to notify the reimbursers that services have been discontinued. Include all services provided, the client's health status at discharge, outcomes achieved, and recommendations for further care.

HOME CARE DOCUMENTATION

In 1985 the Health Care Financing Administration, a branch of the U.S. Department of Health and Human Services, mandated that home health care agencies standardize their documentation methods to meet requirements for Medicare and Medicaid and other third-party disbursements. Two records are required: (a) a home health certification and plan of treatment form and (b) a medical update and patient information form. The nurse assigned to the home care client usually completes the forms, which must be signed by both the nurse and the attending physician. See the Practice Guidelines for home health care documentation.

Some home health agencies provide nurses with laptop or handheld computers to make records available in multiple locations. With the use of a modem, the nurse can add new client information to records at the agency without traveling to the office.

GENERAL GUIDELINES FOR RECORDING

Because the client's record is a legal document and may be used to provide evidence in court, many factors are considered in recording. Health care personnel must not only maintain the confidentiality of the client's record but also meet legal standards in the process of recording.

Date and Time

Document the date and time of each recording. This is essential not only for legal reasons but also for client safety. Record the time in the conventional manner (e.g., 9:00 AM or 3:15 PM) or according to the 24-hour clock (military clock), which avoids confusion about whether a time was AM or PM (see Figure 15-9 ■).

Timing

Follow the agency's policy about the frequency of documenting, and adjust the frequency as a client's condition indicates;

for example, a client whose blood pressure is changing requires more frequent documentation than a client whose blood pressure is constant. As a rule, documenting should be done as soon as possible after an assessment or intervention. No recording should be done *before* providing nursing care.

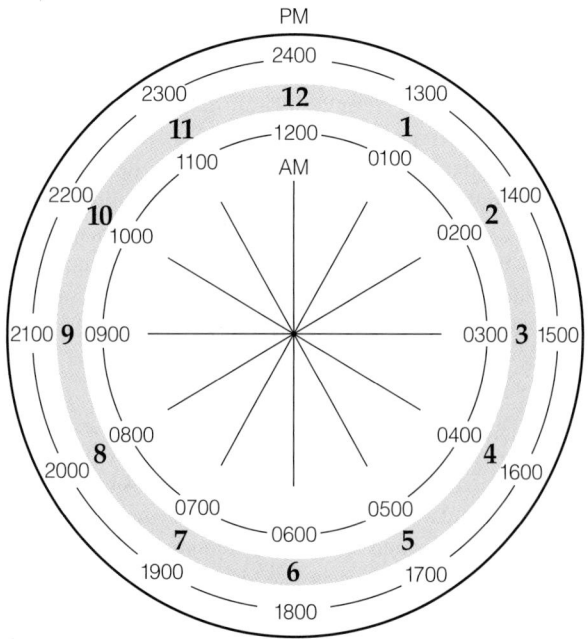

Figure 15-9 ■ The 24-hour clock.

Legibility

All entries must be legible and easy to read to prevent interpretation errors. Hand printing or easily understood handwriting is usually permissible. Follow the agency's policies about handwritten recording.

Permanence

All entries on the client's record are made in dark ink so that the record is permanent and changes can be identified. Dark ink reproduces well on microfilm and in duplication processes. Follow the agency's policies about the type of pen and ink used for recording.

Accepted Terminology

Use only commonly accepted abbreviations, symbols, and terms that are specified by the agency. Many abbreviations are standard and used universally; others are used only in certain geographic areas. Many health care facilities supply an approved list of abbreviations and symbols to prevent confusion. When in doubt about whether to use an abbreviation, write the term out in full until certain about the abbreviation. Table 15–4 lists some common abbreviations (except those used for medications, which are described in Chapter 35 ∞).

In 2004, JCAHO developed National Patient Safety Goals (NPSGs) to reduce communication errors. These goals are required to be implemented by all organizations accredited by JCAHO. As a result, the accredited organizations must develop a "Do Not Use" list of abbreviations, acronyms, and symbols. This list must include those banned by JCAHO (see Table 15–5).

Correct Spelling

Correct spelling is essential for accuracy in recording. If unsure how to spell a word, look it up in a dictionary or other resource book. Two decidedly different medications may have similar spellings; for example, Fosamax and Flomax.

TABLE 15–4 Commonly Used Abbreviations*

ABBREVIATION	TERM	ABBREVIATION	TERM
Abd	Abdomen	mL (ml)	Milliliter
ABO	The main blood group system	mod	Moderate
ac	Before meals	neg	Negative
ADL	Activities of daily living	Ø	None
ad lib	As desired	#	Number or pounds
Adm	Admitted or admission	NPO (NBM)	Nothing by mouth
AM	Morning	NS (N/S)	Normal saline
amb	Ambulatory	O$_2$	Oxygen
amt	Amount	OD	Right eye or overdose
approx	Approximately	OOB	Out of bed
bid	Twice daily	OS	Left eye
BM (bm)	Bowel movement	pc	After meals
BP	Blood pressure	PE (PX)	Physical examination
BRP	Bathroom privileges	per	By or through
c̄	With	PM	Afternoon
C	Celsius (centigrade)	po	By mouth
CBC	Complete blood count	postop	Postoperatively
c/o	Complains of	preop	Preoperatively
DAT	Diet as tolerated	prep	Preparation
drsg	Dressing	prn	When necessary
Dx	Diagnosis	qid	Four times a day
ECG (EKG)	Electrocardiogram	(R)	Right
F	Fahrenheit	s̄	Without
fld	Fluid	stat	At once, immediately
GI	Gastrointestinal	tid	Three times a day
gtt	Drop	TO	Telephone order
h (hr)	Hour	TPR	Temperature, pulse, respirations
H$_2$0	Water		
I&O	Intake and output	VO	Verbal order
IV	Intravenous	VS	Vital signs
LMP	Last menstrual period	WNL	Within normal limits
(L)	Left	wt	Weight
meds	Medications		

*Institutions may elect to include some of these abbreviations on their "Do Not Use" list. Check the agency's policy.

TABLE 15–5   "Do Not Use" List

ABBREVIATION	POTENTIAL PROBLEM	PREFERRED TERM
The Minimum Required List required by JCAHO		
U (for unit)	Mistaken as zero, four, or cc	Write "unit"
IU (for international unit)	Mistaken as IV (intravenous) or 10 (ten)	Write "international unit"
Q.D., Q.O.D. (Latin abbreviation for once daily and every other day)	Mistaken for each other. The period after the Q can be mistaken for an "I" and the "O" can be mistaken for "I".	Write "daily" and "every other day"
Trailing zero (X.0 mg) [Note: prohibited only for medication-related notations]; Lack of leading zero (.X mg)	Decimal point is missed.	Never write a zero by itself after a decimal point (X mg), and always use a zero before a decimal point (0.X mg)
MS MSO$_4$ MgSO$_4$	Confused for one another. Can mean morphine sulfate or magnesium sulfate.	Write "morphine sulfate" or "magnesium sulfate"
In addition to the "minimum required list" above, the following should be considered when expanding the "Do Not Use" list.		
μg (for microgram)	Mistaken for mg (milligrams) resulting in one thousand-fold dosing overdose.	Write "mcg"
H.S. (for half-strength or Latin abbreviation for bedtime)	Mistaken for either half-strength or hour of sleep (at bedtime). q.H.S. mistaken for every hour. All can result in a dosing error.	Write out "half-strength" or "at bedtime"
T.I.W. (for three times a week)	Mistaken for three times a day or twice weekly resulting in an overdose.	Write "3 times weekly" or "three times weekly"
S.C. or S.Q. (for subcutaneous)	Mistaken as SL for sublingual, or "5 every."	Write "Sub-Q," "subQ," or "subcutaneously"
D/C (for discharge)	Interpreted as discontinue whatever medications follow (typically discharge meds).	Write "discharge"
c.c. (for cubic centimeter)	Mistaken for U (units) when poorly written.	Write "ml" or "milliliters"
A.S., A.D., A.U. (Latin abbreviation for left, right, or both ears)	Mistaken for OS, OD, and OU, etc.	Write "left ear," "right ear" or "both ears"

Note: © Joint Commission Resources: *2006 National Patient Safety Goals—FAQs.* Oakbrook Terrace, IL: Joint Commission on Accreditation of Healthcare Organizations, 2006. Reprinted with permission.

CLINICAL ALERT

Incorrect spelling gives a negative impression to the reader and, thereby, decreases the nurse's credibility. ■

Signature

Each recording on the nursing notes is signed by the nurse making it. The signature includes the name and title; for example, "Susan J. Green, RN" or "SJ Green, RN." Some agencies have a signature sheet and after signing this signature sheet, nurses can use their initials. With computerized charting, each nurse has his or her own code, which allows the documentation to be identified.

The following title abbreviations are often used, but nurses need to follow agency policy about how to sign their names.

RN	registered nurse
LVN	licensed vocational nurse
LPN	licensed practical nurse
NA	nursing assistant
NS	nursing student
PCA	patient care associate
SN	student nurse

Accuracy

The client's name and identifying information should be stamped or written on each page of the clinical record. Before making any entry, check that it is the correct chart. Do not identify charts by room number only; check the client's name. Special care is needed when caring for clients with the same last name.

Notations on records must be accurate and correct. Accurate notations consist of facts or observations rather than opinions or interpretations. It is more accurate, for example, to write that the client "refused medication" (fact) than to write that the client "was uncooperative" (opinion); to write that a client "was crying" (observation) is preferable to noting that the client "was depressed" (interpretation). Similarly, when a client expresses worry about the diagnosis or problem, this should be quoted directly on the record:

"Stated: 'I'm worried about my leg.'" When describing something, avoid general words, such as *large, good,* or *normal,* which can be interpreted differently. For example, chart specific data such as "2 cm × 3 cm bruise" rather than "large bruise."

When a recording mistake is made, draw a line through it and write the words *mistaken entry* above or next to the original entry, with your initials or name (depending on agency policy). Do not erase, blot out, or use correction fluid. The original entry must remain visible. When using computerized charting, the nurse needs to be aware of the agency's policy and process for correcting documentation mistakes. (See Figure 15-10 ■ for an example.)

Write on every line but never between lines. If a blank appears in a notation, draw a line through the blank space so that no additional information can be recorded at any other time or by any other person, and sign the notation.

> **CLINICAL ALERT**
>
> Avoid writing the word *error* when a recording mistake has been made. Some believe that the word error is a "red flag" for juries and can lead to the assumption that a clinical error has caused a client injury. ■

Sequence

Document events in the order in which they occur; for example, record assessments, then the nursing interventions, and then the client's responses. Update or delete problems as needed.

Appropriateness

Record only information that pertains to the client's health problems and care. Any other personal information that the client conveys is inappropriate for the record. Recording irrelevant information may be considered an invasion of the client's privacy and/or libelous. A client's disclosure that she was addicted to heroin 15 years ago, for example, would *not* be recorded on the client's medical record unless it had a direct bearing on the client's health problem.

Completeness

Not all data that a nurse obtains about a client can be recorded. However, the information that is recorded needs to be complete and helpful to the client and health care professionals.

Nurses' notes need to reflect the nursing process. Record all assessments, dependent and independent nursing interventions, client problems, client comments and responses to interventions and tests, progress toward goals, and communication with other members of the health team.

Care that is *omitted* because of the client's condition or refusal of treatment must also be recorded. Document what was omitted, why it was omitted, and who was notified.

> **CLINICAL ALERT**
>
> Do not assume that the person reading your charting will know that a common intervention (e.g., turning) has occurred because you believe it to be an "obvious" component of care. ■

Conciseness

Recordings need to be brief as well as complete to save time in communication. The client's name and the word *client* are omitted. For example, write "Perspiring profusely. Respirations shallow, 28/min." End each thought or sentence with a period.

Legal Prudence

Accurate, complete documentation should give legal protection to the nurse, the client's other caregivers, the health care facility, and the client. Admissible in court as a legal document, the clinical record provides proof of the quality of care given to a client. Documentation is usually viewed by juries and attorneys as the best evidence of what really happened to the client.

> **CLINICAL ALERT**
>
> Complete charting, for example, by using the steps of the nursing process as a framework, is the best defense against malpractice. ■

For the best legal protection, the nurse should not only adhere to professional standards of nursing care but also follow agency policy and procedures for intervention and documentation in all situations—especially high-risk situations. For example:

> 1100—c/o of feeling dizzy. Raised top two side rails and instructed to stay in bed and ring call bell if requiring assistance. 1130—found lying on floor beside the bed. Stated, "I climbed out of bed all by myself." When asked about pain, replied, "I feel fine but a little dizzy." Helped into bed. BP 100/60 P90 R24. Dr. RJ Naden notified.
> — *RG Woo RN*

Date	Time	Progress Notes
9/12/2007	0800	~~Breath sounds diminished throughout all lung fields. C/O "shortness of breath".~~ N. Smith, RN.
9/12/2007	0805	Mistaken entry above, wrong client --N. Smith, RN.

Figure 15-10 ■ Correcting a charting error.

PRACTICE GUIDELINES   Documentation

DO

- Chart a change in a client's condition *and* show that follow-up actions were taken.
- Read the nurses' notes prior to care to determine if there has been a change in the client's condition.
- Be timely. A late entry is better than no entry; however, the longer the period of time between actual care and charting, the greater the suspicion.
- Use objective, specific, and factual descriptions.
- Correct charting errors.
- Chart all teaching.
- Record the client's actual words by putting quotes around the words.
- Chart the client's response to interventions.
- Review your notes—are they clear and do they reflect what you want to say?

DON'T

- Leave a blank space for a colleague to chart later.
- Chart in advance of the event (e.g., procedure, medication).
- Use vague terms (e.g., "appears to be comfortable," "had a good night").
- Chart for someone else.
- Use "patient" or "client" as it is their chart.
- Alter a record even if requested by a superior or a physician.
- Record assumptions or words reflecting bias (e.g., "complainer," "disagreeable").

RESEARCH NOTE   Does Nursing Documentation Reflect Individualized Client Care?

Using qualitative metasynthesis, the researchers reviewed and analyzed qualitative research reports focusing on the documentation of nursing care published between 1996 and 2003. The aim of this study was to increase understanding of the content of documenting nursing care and to show how ethical principles relating to individualized care are visible in the documentation. Ethical care includes the value of respecting clients and, therefore, documenting what the clients believe to be important in their care.

Three different themes emerged. One of the themes reflected the demands of the organization. That is, the organizations wanted the documentation to show measurable results of nursing care that could subsequently affect financial implications. The second theme reflected nurses' attitudes and duties. Nurses did not consider documentation to be important and viewed it negatively or with indifference. The third theme reflected clients' involvement in their care. It became clear that the client's views were seldom referred to in the documentation. Nurses mainly documented physical functions of the client.

IMPLICATIONS

This study reflected the small amount of documentation given to clients' wishes and needs. The researchers point out that the more structured the documentation system (i.e., computerized charting), the more the focus will be on nursing tasks rather than individualizing nursing care for the health of the client. Although nurses advocate the need for individualized client care, it is not visible in the nursing documentation. Is it time to clearly define the purpose of documentation? Who is the documentation for—the organization, the nurse, or the client?

Note: From "Documentation of Individualized Patient Care: A Qualitative Metasynthesis," by O. Karkkainen, T. Bondas, and K. Eriksson, 2005, *Nursing Ethics, 12*(2), pp. 123–132. Copyright © Sage Publications Ltd, 2005. Reproduced with permission of Sage Publications, London.

REPORTING

The purpose of reporting is to communicate specific information to a person or group of people. A report, whether oral or written, should be concise, including pertinent information but no extraneous detail. In addition to change-of-shift reports and telephone reports, reporting can also include the sharing of information or ideas with colleagues and other health professionals about some aspect of a client's care. Examples include the care plan conference and nursing rounds.

Change-of-Shift Reports

A **change-of-shift report** is given to all nurses on the next shift. Its purpose is to provide continuity of care for clients by providing the new caregivers a quick summary of client needs and details of care to be given.

Change-of-shift reports may be written or given orally, either in a face-to-face exchange or by audiotape recording. The face-to-face report permits the listener to ask questions during the report; written and tape-recorded reports are often briefer and less time consuming. Reports are sometimes given at the bedside, and clients as well as nurses may participate in the exchange of information. Box 15–3 lists key elements of a change-of-shift report. Box 15–4 provides a sample change-of-shift report.

CLINICAL ALERT

Be aware of where the shift report takes place in order to maintain client confidentiality. An area that is private and free from interruption is best. ■

Telephone Reports

Health professionals frequently report about a client by telephone. Nurses inform primary care providers about a change in a client's

---

BOX 15–3 Key Elements of a Change-of-Shift Report

- Follow a particular order (e.g., follow room numbers in a hospital).
- Provide basic identifying information for each client (e.g., name, room number, bed designation).
- For new clients, provide the reason for admission or medical diagnosis (or diagnoses), surgery (date), diagnostic tests, and therapies in past 24 hours.
- Include significant changes in client's condition and present information in order (i.e., assessment, nursing diagnoses, interventions, outcomes, and evaluation). For example, "Mr. Ronald Oakes said he had an aching pain in his left calf at 1400 hours. Inspection revealed no other signs. Calf pain is related to altered blood circulation. Rest and elevation of his legs on a footstool for 30 minutes provided relief."
- Provide exact information, such as "Ms. Jessie Jones received morphine 6 mg IV at 1500 hours," not "Ms. Jessie Jones received some morphine during the evening."
- Report clients' need for special emotional support. For example, a client who has just learned that his biopsy results revealed malignancy

and who is now scheduled for a laryngectomy needs time to discuss his feelings before preoperative teaching is begun.
- Include current nurse-prescribed and primary care provider-prescribed orders.
- Provide a summary of newly admitted clients, including diagnosis, age, general condition, plan of therapy, and significant information about the client's support people.
- Report on clients who have been transferred or discharged from the unit.
- Clearly state priorities of care and care that is due after the shift begins. For example, in a 7 AM report the nurse might say, "Mr. Li's vital signs are due at 0730, and his IV bag will need to be replaced by 0800." Give this information at the end of that client's report, because memory is best for the first and last information given.
- Be concise. Don't elaborate on background data or routine care (e.g., do not report "Vital signs at 0800 and 1150" when that is the unit standard). Do not report coming and going of visitors unless there is a problem or concern, or visitors are involved in teaching and care. Social support and visits are the norm.

BOX 15–4 Sample Change-of-Shift Report

ROOM 201—C.W.

Admitted last night for pneumonia
Allergic to penicillin
DNR
IV of D5/0.45 NS infusing at 100 mL/hour in (L) forearm
Need sputum specimen for C&S
Temp 102.4. Tylenol given at 0600
Lung sounds diminished in lower lobes

ROOM 202—G. H.

Admitted for (L) total knee arthroplasty. POD # 3
Has discharge orders to go to rehab today
Dressing clean, dry, and intact
Regular diet. Taking fluids well.
Had BM yesterday
Pain rating of 4/10—last medicated with Percocet at 0400

---

condition; a radiologist reports the results of an x-ray study; a nurse may report to a nurse on another unit about a transferred client.

The nurse receiving a telephone report should document the date and time, the name of the person giving the information, and the subject of the information received, and sign the notation. For example:

6/6/03 1035 GL Messina, laboratory technician, reported by telephone that Mrs. Sara Ames's hematocrit was 39/100 mL. ———————————— *B. Ireland RN*

The person receiving the information should repeat it back to the sender to ensure accuracy.

When giving a telephone report to a primary care provider, it is important that the nurse be concise and accurate. Begin with name and relationship to the client (e.g., "This is Jana

Gomez, RN; I'm calling about your client, Dorothy Mendes. I'm her nurse on the 7 PM to 7 AM shift").

Telephone reports usually include the client's name and medical diagnosis, changes in nursing assessment, vital signs related to baseline vital signs, significant laboratory data, and related nursing interventions. The nurse should have the client's chart ready to give the primary care provider any further information.

After reporting, the nurse should document the date, time, and content of the call. For example:

1200-Admitted from ED. c/o burning upper right quadrant abdominal pain. Rates pain at 6/10. BP 115/80, P100, R15. Demerol 100 mg given IM per order. 1300-BP 100/40, P115, R30. Pain unchanged. Color pale and diaphoretic. Reported by telephone to Dr. Burns at 1305.
———————————— *TG Jones RN*

Telephone Orders

Physicians often order a therapy (e.g., a medication) for a client by telephone. Most agencies have specific policies about telephone orders. Many agencies allow only registered nurses to take telephone orders.

While the primary care provider gives the order, *write* the complete order down and *read* it back to the primary care provider to ensure accuracy. Question the primary care provider about any order that is ambiguous, unusual (e.g., an abnormally high dosage of a medication), or contraindicated by the client's condition. Then transcribe the order onto the physician's order sheet, indicating it as a verbal order (VO) or telephone order (TO). See Box 15–5 for selected guidelines.

Once the order is transcribed on the physician's order sheet, the order must be countersigned by the primary care provider within a time period described by agency policy. Many acute care hospitals require that this be done within 24 hours.

BOX 15—5 Guidelines for Telephone and Verbal Orders

1. Know the state nursing board's position on who can give and accept verbal and phone orders.
2. Know the agency's policy regarding phone orders (e.g., colleague listens on extension and cosigns order sheet).
3. Ask the prescriber to speak slowly and clearly.
4. Ask the prescriber to spell out the medication if you are not familiar with it.
5. Question the drug, dosage, or changes if they seem inappropriate for this client.
6. Write the order down or enter into a computer.
7. Read the order back to the prescriber. Use words instead of abbreviations (i.e., three times a day for tid).
8. Write the order on the physician's order sheet. Record date and time and indicate it was a telephone order (TO). Sign name and credentials.
9. When writing a dosage always put a number before a decimal (i.e., 0.3 mL) but never after a decimal (i.e., 6 mg).
10. Write out units (i.e., 15 units of insulin, not 15 u of insulin).
11. Transcribe the order.
12. Follow agency protocol about the prescriber's protocol for signing telephone orders (i.e., within 24 hours).

    Other:
- Never follow a voice-mail order. Call the prescriber for a client order. Write it down and read it back for confirmation.

Note: Adapted from "JCAHO Says Watch Your P's and Q's," by editors of *Nursing 2004*, 2004, *Nursing, 34*(3), p. 55; and "FAQs for the 2006 National Patient Safety Goals—" by Joint Commission on Accreditation of Healthcare Organizations, 2006. Retrieved April 30, 2006, from http://www.jointcommission.org/NR/rdonlyres/7C116D6D-AE82-449E-BA45-1DE49D2A0A34/0/06_npsg_faq.pdf

Care Plan Conference

A care plan conference is a meeting of a group of nurses to discuss possible solutions to certain problems of a client, such as inability to cope with an event or lack of progress toward goal attainment. The care plan conference allows each nurse an opportunity to offer an opinion about possible solutions to the problem. Other health professionals may be invited to attend the conference to offer their expertise; for example, a social worker may discuss the family problems of a severely burned child, or a dietitian may discuss the dietary problems of a client who has diabetes.

Care plan conferences are most effective when there is a climate of respect—that is, nonjudgmental acceptance of others even though their values, opinions, and beliefs may seem different. Nurses need to accept and respect each person's contributions, listening with an open mind to what others are saying even when there is disagreement.

Nursing Rounds

Nursing rounds are procedures in which two or more nurses visit selected clients at each client's bedside to:

- Obtain information that will help plan nursing care.
- Provide clients the opportunity to discuss their care.
- Evaluate the nursing care the client has received.

During rounds, the nurse assigned to the client provides a brief summary of the client's nursing needs and the interventions being implemented. Nursing rounds offer advantages to both clients and nurses: Clients can participate in the discussions, and nurses can see the client and the equipment being used. To facilitate client participation in nursing rounds, nurses need to use terms that the client can understand. Medical terminology excludes the client from discussion.

CRITICAL THINKING CHECKPOINT

Mr. Anderson, an 80-year-old male, was admitted for back pain. He has a past medical history of hypertension. He told the admitting nurse that he has lost interest in many of his normal activities because of the constant pain.

You read the following documentation entry by a previous nurse:

> 8—Client is a complainer. I listened to him for 15 minutes with no success. BP 210/90 and 180/70. P 72, R 18.
> 12—Refused lunch
> 2—Client fell out of bed

1. What guidelines were *not* used in this documentation?
2. The nursing diagnosis for Mr. Anderson is *Acute Pain.* What would you expect to document?
3. Using the following pieces of data for Mr. Anderson, sort them into a SOAP note:
   a. "I didn't sleep last night"
   b. positioned on side with pillows behind back
   c. continues to need narcotic medication to progress toward goal of pain relief
   d. states pain is 8 out of 10
   e. "I feel better" (after interventions)
   f. last medicated 5 hours previously
   g. heating pad applied to lower back
   h. BP 210/90, P 72, R 18.
   i. Add to plan of care to offer analgesic around the clock q 4 hours versus prn
   j. 6/6/03 #1 Pain
   k. "sharp, stabbing pain in lower back that radiates to left leg"
   l. medicated with ordered analgesic
4. Use the same pieces of data and sort them into a DAR note.

See Critical Thinking Possibilities in Appendix A.

CHAPTER 15 **REVIEW**

CHAPTER HIGHLIGHTS

- Client records are legal documents that provide evidence of a client's care.
- The nurse has a legal and ethical duty to maintain confidentiality of the client's record; this includes special measures to protect client information stored in computers.
- Client records are kept for a number of purposes, including communication, planning client care, auditing health agencies, research, education, reimbursement, legal documentation, and health care analysis.
- In source-oriented clinical records, each health care professional group provides its own record. Recording is oriented around the source of the information.
- In problem-oriented clinical records, recording is organized around client problems.
- Examples of documentation systems include PIE, focus charting, charting by exception (CBE), computerized documentation, and case management.
- Computers make care planning and documentation relatively easy. The use of computer terminals at the bedside allows immediate documentation of nursing actions.
- The case management model emphasizes quality, cost-effective care delivered within an established length of stay.

- The Kardex is used to organize client data, making information quick to access for health professionals.
- Nursing progress notes provide information about the progress the client is making toward desired outcomes. The format for the progress note depends on the documentation system at the facility.
- Long-term documentation varies depending on the level of care provided and requirements set by Medicare and Medicaid.
- Home health agencies must standardize their documentation methods to meet requirements for Medicare and Medicaid and other third-party disbursements.
- Legal guidelines for the process of recording in a client record include documenting date and time, legible entries, using dark ink, using correct terminology and spelling, accuracy, appropriateness, completeness, conciseness, and including an appropriate signature.
- The purpose of reporting is to communicate specific information for the goal of improving quality of care. Examples include change-of-shift reports, telephone reports, telephone orders, care plan conferences, and nursing rounds.

TEST YOUR KNOWLEDGE

1. Which of the following actions by a nurse ensures confidentiality of a client's computer record?
1. The nurse logs on to the client's file and leaves the computer to answer the client's call light.
2. The nurse shares her computer password.
3. The nurse closes a client's computer file and logs off.
4. The nurse leaves client computer worksheets at the computer workstation.

2. The case management model using critical pathways would be appropriate for a client with which diagnosis?
1. Myocardial infarction (heart attack)
2. Diabetes, hypertension
3. Myocardial infarction, diabetes, hypertension
4. Diabetes, hypertension, an infected foot ulcer, senile dementia

3. After making a documentation error, which action should the nurse take?
1. Use correcting liquid to cover the mistake and make a new entry.
2. Draw a line through it and write *error* above the entry.
3. Draw a line through it and write *mistaken entry* above it.
4. Draw a line through the mistake and write *mistaken entry* with initials above it.

4. Which charting entry would be the most defensible in court?
1. Client fell out of bed
2. Client drunk on admission

3. Large bruise on left thigh
4. Notified Dr. Jones of BP of 90/40

5. The client has NKA. He has BRP and he receives his pain pill prn. His nutrition is DAT. Interpret the commonly used abbreviations.
1. NKA:_____
2. BRP:_____
3. prn:_____
4. DAT:_____

6. During the first day a nurse is caring for a client who has been in the hospital for 2 days, the nurse thinks that the client's blood pressure (B/P) seems high. What is the next step?
1. Ask the client about past blood pressure ranges.
2. Review the graphic record on the client's record.
3. Examine the medication record for antihypertensive medications.
4. Review the progress notes included in the client's record.

7. A student nurse observes the change-of-shift report. Which of the following behaviors by the reporting nurse represent effective nursing practice? Select all that apply.
1. Provides the medical diagnosis or reason for admission
2. States the time the client last received pain medication
3. Speaks loudly when giving report
4. States priorities of care that are due shortly after the report
5. Reports on number of visitors for each client

8. Which charting entries are written correctly? Select all that apply.
   1. MS 5 gr given IV for c/o abdominal pain
   2. Lanoxin 0.25 mg given orally per Dr. Smith's stat order
   3. KCl 15cc's given orally for K+ level of 2.9
   4. regular insulin 10.0 u given SQ for capillary blood glucose of 180
   5. Ambien 5 mg given orally at bedtime per request

9. A 74-year-old female is brought to the E.D. c/o right hip pain. The right leg is shorter than the left and is externally rotated. During inspection, the nurse observes what appears to be cigarette burns on the client's inner thighs. Which of the following is the most appropriate documentation?

   1. Six round skin lesions partially healed, on the inner thighs bilaterally
   2. Several burned areas on both of the client's inner thighs
   3. Multiple lesions on inner thighs possibly related to elder abuse
   4. Several lesions on inner thighs similar to cigarette burns

10. Which of the following charting rules will keep the nurse legally safe? Select all that apply.
    1. Use military time.
    2. Document worries or concerns expressed by the client.
    3. Perform most of the charting at the end of the shift.
    4. Record only information that pertains to the client's health problems.

See Answers to Test Your Knowledge in Appendix A.

EXPLORE MEDIALINK www.prenhall.com/berman

DVD-ROM
- Audio Glossary
- NCLEX Review
- End of Unit Concept Map Activity

COMPANION WEBSITE
- Additional NCLEX Review
- Case Study:
  Client with Delirium Tremens
- Application Activities:
  Establishing a Documentation System
  HIPAA and Client Privacy
- Links to Resources

READINGS AND REFERENCES

SUGGESTED READINGS

Austin, S. (2006). "Ladies & gentlemen of the jury, I present . . . the nursing documentation." *Nursing, 36*(1), 56–62.
The author, a nurse attorney, reviews documentation guidelines to help prevent liability. Of particular interest are the scenarios included in the article. They are based on actual cases and reflect common allegations of professional negligence.

Kirkley, D., & Stein, M. (2004). Nurses and clinical technology: Sources of resistance and strategies for acceptance. *Nursing Economics, 22*(4), 216–222.
The authors conducted an electronic roundtable followed up by phone interviews with nurse leaders in the United States and United Kingdom with the focus to identify barriers to the process of introducing online clinical documentation. They found that the resistance had less to do with computer experience and more to do with cultural

factors. One identified cultural factor was lack of time as nurses resist the idea of one more thing being added to their workload. The other identified cultural factor was loyalty to the historic mode of paper documentation. Finally, the article finishes with ideas that can be used as part of a change management program to ease the process of introducing and using computer information systems.*

RELATED RESEARCH

Ammenwerth, E., Mansmann, U., Iller, C., & Eichstadter, R. (2003). Factors affecting and affected by user acceptance of computer-based nursing documentation: Results of a two-year study. *Journal of the American Medical Informatics Association, 10*(1), 69–84.

Bjorvell, C., Wredling, R., & Thorell-Ekstrand, I. (2003). Prerequisites and consequences of nursing documentation in patient records as perceived by a group of registered nurses. *Journal of Clinical Nursing, 12*(2), 206–214.

REFERENCES

American Nurses Association. (2001). *Code of ethics for nurses with interpretive statements.* Washington, DC: Author.

Clark, A. P. (2003). What's all the HIPAA hype? *Nurse Practitioner Supplement: the 2004 Sourcebook for Advanced Practice Nurses,* 6–11.

Editors of Nursing 2004. (2004). JCAHO says watch your p's and q's. *Nursing, 34*(3), 55.

Gallagher, P. M. (2004). Maintain privacy with electronic charting. *Nursing Management, 35*(2), 16–17.

Guido, G. W. (2005). *Legal and ethical issues in nursing* (4th ed). Upper Saddle River, NJ: Prentice Hall.

Joint Commission on Accreditation of Healthcare Organizations. (2006). *2006 National Patient Safety Goals—FAQs.* Retrieved April 30, 2006, from http://www.jointcommission.org/NR/rdonlyres/7C116D6D-AE82-449E-BA45-1DE49D2A0A34/0/06_npsg_faq.pdf

Lippincott Williams & Wilkins. (2003). *Complete guide to documentation.* Philadelphia: Author.

Lippincott Williams & Wilkins. (2007). *Chart smart* (2nd ed.). Philadelphia: Author.

Smith, C. M., & Dougherty, M. (2001). Practice brief: Requirements for the acute care record. *Journal of AHIMA, 72*(3), 56A–56G.

Sullivan, G. H. (2004). Legally speaking: Does your charting measure up? *RN, 67*(3), 61–65.

SELECTED BIBLIOGRAPHY

Feeg, V. D. (2003). What's this HIPAA stuff . . . and does it affect me? *Pediatric Nursing, 29*(2), 93, 133.

Fernandez, R. D., & Spragley, F. (2004). Focus on streamlined documentation. *Nursing Management, 35*(10), 25–29.

Hamilton, A. V., Coyle, G. A., & Heinen, M. G. (2004). Applied technology rounds out e-documentation. *Nursing Management, 35*(9), 44–47.

Hendrix, L. (2004). Paging pointers: Here's how to make the most of your calls to health care providers. *Nursing, 34*(5), 32hn4–32hn6.

Kirkley, D., & Stein, M. (2004). Nurses and clinical technology: Sources of resistance and strategies for acceptance. *Nursing Economics, 22*(4), 216–222.

Kroll, M. (2003). What were you thinking? Charting rules to keep you legally safe. *Journal of Gerontological Nursing, 29*(3), 15–16.

Maddox, P. J. (2003). HIPAA: Update on rule revisions and compliance requirements. *Medsurg Nursing, 12*(1), 59–63.

Miller, J., & Glusko, J. (2003). Standing up to the scrutiny of medical malpractice. *Nursing Management, 34*(10), 20–22.

Murphy, E. K. (2003). Charting by exception. *AORN Journal, 78*(5), 821–823.

Smith, L. S. (2003). Chart smart: Handling documentation errors. *Nursing, 33*(10), 73.

Smith, L. S. (2004). Documenting refusal of treatment. *Nursing, 34*(4), 79.

UNIT 4

Health Beliefs and Practices

As increasingly knowledgeable health care consumers, clients expect and deserve quality care. While assisting the client—whether an individual, family, or entire community—quality nursing care seeks to emphasize illness prevention and health promotion. Nurses recognize that a client's state of health and wellness encompasses many dimensions, including social, spiritual, cultural, sexual, and environmental, as well as physical and psychological. Each client encounter affords the nurse an opportunity to influence and encourage both traditional and innovative health-seeking behaviors.

CHAPTER 16

Health Promotion

LEARNING OUTCOMES

After completing this chapter, you will be able to:

1. Explain the relationship of individuality and holism to nursing practice.

2. Give four main characteristics of homeostatic mechanisms.

3. Identify theoretical frameworks used in individual health promotion.

4. Identify Maslow's characteristics of the self-actualized person.

5. Describe how the *Healthy People 2010* leading health indicators can help improve the health of a community.

6. Differentiate health promotion from health protection or illness prevention.

7. Identify various types and sites of health promotion programs.

8. Discuss the Health Promotion Model.

9. Explain the stages of health behavior change.

10. Discuss the nurse's role in health promotion.

11. Assess the health of individuals.

12. Develop, implement, and evaluate plans for health promotion.

Health promotion is an important component of nursing practice. It is a way of thinking that revolves around a philosophy of wholeness, wellness, and well-being. In the past two decades, the public has become increasingly aware of and interested in health promotion. Many people are aware of the relationship between lifestyle and illness and are developing health-promoting habits, such as getting adequate exercise, rest, and relaxation; maintaining good nutrition; and controlling the use of tobacco, alcohol, and other drugs.

Assessing and planning health care of the individual client is enhanced when the nurse understands the concepts of individuality, holism, homeostasis, and human needs. The beliefs and values of each person and the support he or she receives come in large part from the family and are reinforced by the community. The reverse is also true—the health of a community is affected by the beliefs, attitudes, and behaviors of the individuals in the community.

INDIVIDUAL HEALTH

Dimensions of individuality include the person's total character, self-identity, and perceptions. The person's total character encompasses behaviors, emotional state, attitudes, values, motives, abilities, habits, and appearances. The person's self-identity encompasses perception of self as a separate and distinct entity alone and in interactions with others. The person's perceptions encompass the way the person interprets the environment or situation, directly affecting how he or she thinks, feels, and acts in any given situation.

Concept of Individuality

To help clients attain, maintain, or regain an optimal level of health, nurses need to understand clients as individuals. Each individual is a unique being who is different from every other human being, with a different combination of genetics, life experiences, and environmental interactions.

When providing care, nurses need to focus on the client within both a total care and an individualized care context. In the total care context, the nurse considers all the principles and areas that apply when taking care of any client of that age and condition. In the individualized care context, the nurse becomes acquainted with the client as an individual, using the total care principles that apply to this person at this time. For example, a nurse who is advising the mother of a preschooler understands that the child's desire to explore his or her world is a developmental stage that all preschoolers experience. However, the preschooler diagnosed with attention deficit/hyperactivity disorder may have an increased risk of accidents and injuries when interacting with the environment, due to his or her impulsivity and poor self-control.

Concept of Holism

Nurses are concerned with the individual as a whole, complete, or holistic person, not as an assembly of parts and processes. When applied in nursing, the concept of **holism** emphasizes that nurses must keep the whole person in mind and strive to understand how one area of concern relates to the whole person. The nurse must also consider the relationship of the individual to the external environment and to others. For example, in helping a man who is grieving over the death of his spouse, the nurse explores the impact of the loss on the whole person (i.e., on the man's appetite, rest and sleep pattern, energy level, sense of well-being, mood, usual activities, family relationships, and relationships with others). Nursing interventions are directed toward restoring overall harmony, so they depend on the man's sense of purpose and meaning of his life. For additional information about holistic practices, see Chapter 19. ∞

Concept of Homeostasis

The concept of **homeostasis** was first introduced by Cannon (1939) to describe the relative constancy of the internal processes of the body, such as blood oxygen and carbon dioxide levels, blood pressure, body temperature, blood glucose, and fluid and electrolyte balance. To Cannon, the word *homeostasis* did not imply something stagnant, set, or immobile; it meant a condition that might vary but remained relatively constant. Cannon viewed the human being as separate from the external environment and constantly endeavoring to maintain physiologic **equilibrium,** or balance, through adaptation to that environment.

Homeostasis, then, is the tendency of the body to maintain a state of balance or equilibrium while continually changing.

Physiologic Homeostasis

Physiologic homeostasis means that the internal environment of the body is relatively stable and constant. All cells of the body require a relatively constant environment to function; thus the body's internal environment must be maintained within narrow limits. Homeostatic mechanisms have four main characteristics:

1. They are self-regulating.
2. They are compensatory.
3. They tend to be regulated by negative feedback systems.
4. They may require several feedback mechanisms to correct only one physiologic imbalance.

Self-regulation means that homeostatic mechanisms come into play automatically in the healthy person. However, if a person is ill, or if a respiratory organ such as a lung is injured, the homeostatic mechanisms may not be able to respond to the stimulus as they would normally. Homeostatic mechanisms are **compensatory** (counterbalancing) because they tend to counteract conditions that are abnormal for the person. An example is a sudden drop in air temperature. The compensatory mechanisms are that the peripheral blood vessels constrict, thereby diverting most of the blood internally, and increased muscular activity and shivering occur to create heat. Through these mechanisms the body temperature remains stable despite the cold.

Homeostasis occurs within the physiologic **system,** a set of interacting identifiable parts or components. The fundamental components of a system are matter, energy, and communication. Without any one of these, a system does not exist. The individual is a human system with matter (the body), energy (chemical or thermal), and communication (e.g., the nervous system). The **boundary** of a system, such as the skin in the human system, is a real or imaginary line that differentiates one system from another system or a system from its environment.

There are two general types of systems: closed and open. A **closed system** does not exchange energy, matter, or information with its environment; it receives no input from the environment and gives no output to the environment. An example of a closed system is a chemical reaction that takes place in a test tube. In reality, outside the laboratory, no closed systems exist. In an **open system,** energy, matter, and information move into and out of the system through the system boundary. All living systems, such as plants, animals, people, families, and communities, are open systems, since their survival depends on a continuous exchange of energy. They are, therefore, in a constant state of change.

An open system depends on the quality and quantity of its input, output, and feedback. **Input** consists of information, material, or energy that enters the system. After the input is absorbed by the system, it is processed in a way useful to the system. This transformation is called **throughput.** For example, food is input to the digestive system; it is digested (throughput) so that it can be used by the body. **Output** from a system is energy, matter, or information given out by the system as a result of its processes. Output from the digestive system includes caloric energy, nutrients, urine, and feces.

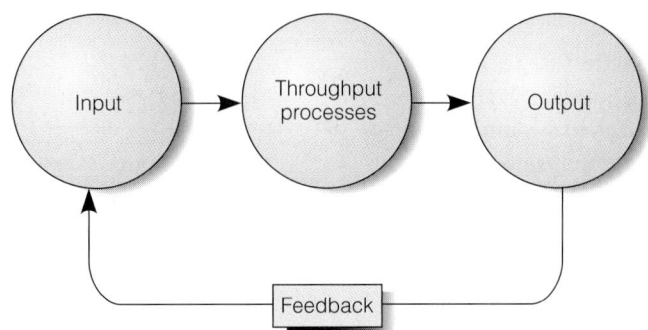

Figure 16-1 ■ An open system with a feedback mechanism.

Feedback is the mechanism by which some of the output of a system is returned to the system as input. Feedback enables a system to regulate itself by redirecting the output back into the system, thus forming a feedback loop (see Figure 16-1 ■). This input influences the behavior of the system and its future output. **Negative feedback** inhibits change; **positive feedback** stimulates change. Most biologic systems are controlled by negative feedback to bring the system back to stability. This type of feedback system senses and counteracts any deviations from normal. The deviations may be greater or less than the normal level or range. For example, an increase in the production of parathyroid hormone is stimulated by a drop in blood calcium, but when additional parathyroid hormone raises the level of blood calcium, the hormone's production is then inhibited (see Figure 16-2 ■). With hypoxia (shortage of oxygen), the concentration of red blood cells increases and the heart rate becomes faster to transport the blood and available oxygen around the body adequately. People interact with the environment by adjusting themselves to it or adjusting it to themselves. This premise directs the nurse to look at environmental factors influencing the system and to plan nursing interventions to help the client maintain homeostasis. For example, the individual who is experiencing severe anxiety may be taught a variety of stress management techniques.

Psychologic Homeostasis

The term **psychologic homeostasis** refers to emotional or psychologic balance or a state of mental well-being. It is maintained by a variety of mechanisms. Each person has certain psychologic needs, such as the need for love, security, and self-esteem, which must be met to maintain psychologic homeostasis. When one or more of these needs is not met or is threatened, certain coping mechanisms are activated to protect the person and provide psychologic homeostasis.

Psychologic homeostasis is acquired or learned through the experience of living and interacting with others. In addition, societal norms and culture influence behavior. Some prerequisites for a person to develop psychologic homeostasis can be summarized as follows:

■ A stable physical environment in which the person feels safe and secure. For example, the basic needs for food, shelter, and clothing must be met consistently from birth onward.

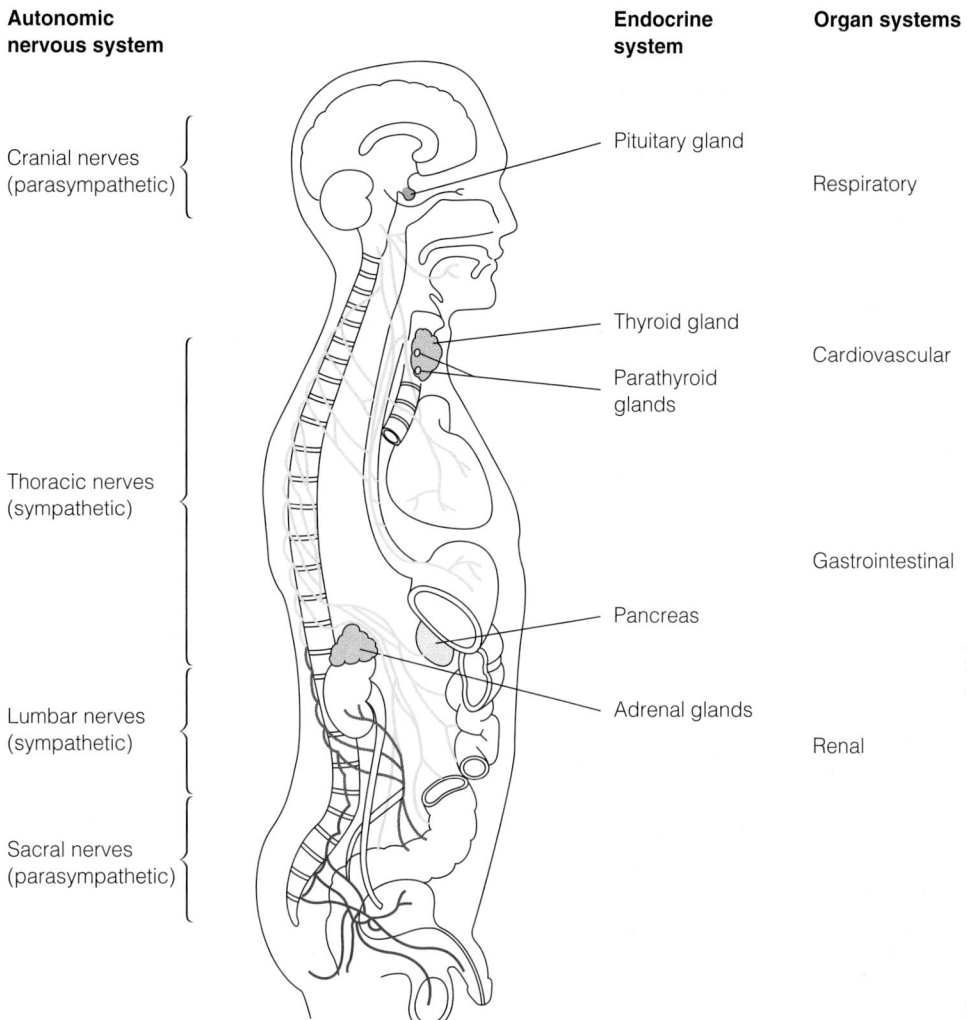

Figure 16-2 ■ The homeostatic regulators of the body: autonomic nervous system, endocrine system, and specific organ systems.

- A stable psychologic environment from infancy onward, so that feelings of trust and love develop. Growing children and adolescents also need kind but firm and consistent discipline, encouragement, and support to be their own unique selves.
- A social environment that includes adults who are healthy role models. Children learn the customs and values of society from these individuals.
- A life experience that provides satisfactions. Throughout life, people encounter many frustrations. People deal with these better if enough satisfying experiences have occurred to counterbalance the frustrating ones.

Assessing the Health of Individuals

A thorough assessment of the individual's health status is basic to health promotion. Components of this assessment are the health history and physical examination, physical fitness assessment, lifestyle assessment, health risk appraisal, health beliefs review, and life-stress review. Details about these assessments are discussed in Chapters 11 and 30. ∞

APPLYING THEORETICAL FRAMEWORKS

A variety of theoretical frameworks provide the nurse with a holistic overview of health promotion for the individual and families across the life span. Two major theoretical frameworks that nurses use in promoting the health of the individual are needs theories and developmental stage theories.

Needs Theories

In needs theories, human needs are ranked on an ascending scale according to how essential the needs are for survival. Abraham Maslow (1970), perhaps the most renowned needs theorist, ranks human needs on five levels (see Figure 16-3 ■ and Box 16–1). The five levels in ascending order are as follows:

- *Physiologic needs.* Needs such as air, food, water, shelter, rest, sleep, activity, and temperature maintenance are crucial for survival.
- *Safety and security needs.* The need for safety has both physical and psychologic aspects. The person needs to

Maslow's hierarchy of needs   Maslow's hierarchy of needs, as adapted by Kalish

Figure 16-3 ■ Maslow's needs.

(From *Psychology of Human Behavior,* 5th ed. by Kalish, copyright 1983. Reprinted with permission of Wadsworth, a division of Thomson Learning: www.thomsonrights.com. Fax 800-730-2215.)

feel safe, both in the physical environment and in relationships.

■ *Love and belonging needs.* The third level of needs includes giving and receiving affection, attaining a place in a group, and maintaining the feeling of belonging.

■ *Self-esteem needs.* The individual needs both self-esteem (i.e., feelings of independence, competence, and self-respect) and esteem from others (i.e., recognition, respect, and appreciation).

■ *Self-actualization.* When the need for self-esteem is satisfied, the individual strives for self-actualization, the innate need to develop one's maximum potential and realize one's abilities and qualities.

Kalish's Hierarchy of Needs

Richard Kalish (1983) adapted Maslow's hierarchy of needs into six levels rather than five. He suggests an additional category between the physiologic needs and the safety and security needs. This category, referred to as *stimulation needs,* includes sex, activity, exploration, manipulation, and novelty (see Figure 16-3). Kalish emphasizes that children need to explore and manipulate their environments to achieve optimal growth and development. He notes that adults, too, often seek novel adventures or stimulating experiences before considering their safety or security needs.

Characteristics of Basic Needs

All people have the same basic needs; however, each person's needs and reactions to those needs are influenced by the culture with which the person identifies. For example, professional achievement, independent functioning, and privacy may be important in one culture or subculture and unimportant in another.

■ People meet their own needs relative to their own priorities. For example, a poor mother might give up her share of food so that her child might have sufficient food to live.
■ Although basic needs generally must be met, some needs can be deferred. An example is the need for independence, which an ill person can defer until well.
■ Failure to meet needs results in one or more homeostatic imbalances, which can eventually result in illness.
■ A need can make itself felt by either external or internal stimuli. An example is the need for food. A person may experience hunger as a result of physiologic processes (internal stimulation) or as a result of seeing a beautiful cake (external stimulation).

- A person who perceives a need can respond in several ways to meet it. The choice of response is largely a result of learned experiences, lifestyle, and the values of the culture. For example, many people's food choices at mealtimes and snack times are based on past experiences, lifestyle, and culture.
- Needs are interrelated. Some needs cannot be met unless related needs are also met. The need for hydration can be influenced by the need for elimination of urine. Likewise, the need for security can be markedly altered if the need for oxygen is threatened by a respiratory obstruction.

Needs can be satisfied in healthy and unhealthy ways. Ways of meeting basic needs are considered healthy when they are not harmful to others or to self, conform to the individual's sociocultural values, and are within the law. Conversely, unhealthy behavior may be harmful to others or to self, does not conform to the individual's sociocultural values, or is not within the law. People who satisfy their basic needs appropriately are healthier, happier, and more effective than those whose needs are frustrated.

Knowledge of the theoretical bases of human needs assists nurses in responding therapeutically to a client's behaviors and in understanding themselves and their own responses to needs. Human needs serve as a framework for assessing behaviors, assigning priorities to desired outcomes, and planning nursing interventions. For example, an adult with poor self-esteem would have difficulty accomplishing self-actualization. Therefore, nursing interventions would focus on increasing the client's self-esteem.

Developmental Stage Theories

Developmental stage theories categorize a person's behaviors or tasks into approximate age ranges or in terms that describe the features of an age group. The age ranges of the stages do not take into account individual differences; however, the categories do describe characteristics associated with the majority of individuals at periods when distinctive developmental changes occur and with the specific tasks that must be accomplished. See Chapter 20 ∞ for further information about developmental stages.

Developmental stage theories allow nurses to describe typical behaviors of an individual within a certain age group, explain the significance of those behaviors, predict behaviors that might occur in a given situation, and provide a rationale to control behavioral manifestations. Individuals can be compared with a representative group of people at the same point in time or compared at different points in time. The nurse's knowledge of developmental stage theories can be used in parental and client education, counseling, and anticipatory guidance.

HEALTHY PEOPLE 2010

The vision of health promotion was initially expressed in 1979 with the surgeon general's report *Healthy People,* which emphasized health promotion and disease prevention. *Healthy People 2000* followed in 1990 and provided a framework for national health promotion, health protection, and preventive service

strategy. The current *Healthy People 2010: Understanding and Improving Health* (U.S. Department of Health and Human Services [USDHHS], 2000) presents a comprehensive 10-year strategy for promoting health and preventing illness, disability, and premature death. The two major goals of *Healthy People 2010* reflect the nation's changing demographics:

- "Increase quality and years of healthy life" indicates the aging or "graying" of the population.
- "Eliminate health disparities" reflects the diversity of the population.

To support these goals, *Healthy People 2010* is organized into 28 focus areas to improve health (see Box 16–2). *Healthy People 2010* also establishes a set of leading health indicators that reflect the major public health concerns in the United States at the beginning of the 21st century (see Box 16–3). Each indicator relates to a number of the health objectives. It is expected that these indicators will help develop action plans to improve the health of both individuals and communities.

The foundation for *Healthy People 2010* is the belief that individual health is closely linked to community health and the reverse. For example, community health is affected by the beliefs, attitudes, and behaviors of the individuals who live in

---

BOX 16–2 The 28 Focus Areas in *Healthy People 2010*

- Access to quality health services
- Arthritis, osteoporosis, and chronic back conditions
- Cancer
- Chronic kidney disease
- Diabetes
- Disability and secondary conditions
- Educational and community-based programs
- Environmental health
- Family planning
- Food safety
- Health communication
- Heart disease and stroke
- HIV
- Immunization and infectious diseases
- Injury and violence prevention
- Maternal, infant, and child health
- Medical product safety
- Mental health and mental disorders
- Nutrition and overweight
- Occupational safety and health
- Oral health
- Physical activity and fitness
- Public health infrastructure
- Respiratory diseases
- Sexually transmitted diseases
- Substance abuse
- Tobacco use
- Vision and hearing

Note: U.S. Department of Health and Human Services.

BOX 16–3 **The Leading Health Indicators in *Healthy People 2010***

■ Physical Activity
  ● Regular physical activity throughout life is important for maintaining a healthy body, enhancing psychological well-being, and preventing premature death (p. 26).
■ Overweight and Obesity
  ● Overweight and obesity are major contributors to many preventable causes of death. On average, higher body weights are associated with higher death rates. The number of overweight children, adolescents, and adults has risen over the past four decades (p. 28).
■ Tobacco Use
  ● Cigarette smoking is the single most preventable cause of disease and death in the United States (p. 30).
■ Substance Abuse
  ● Alcohol and illicit drug use are associated with many of this country's most serious problems, including violence, injury, and HIV infection (p. 32).
■ Responsible Sexual Behavior
  ● Unintended pregnancies and sexually transmitted diseases (STDs), including infection with the human immunodeficiency virus that causes AIDS, can result from unprotected sexual behaviors (p. 34).
■ Mental Health
  ● Approximately 20% of the U.S. population is affected by mental illness during a given year; no one is immune. Of all mental ill-

ness, depression is the most common disorder. Major depression is the leading cause of disability and is the cause of more than two-thirds of suicides each year (p. 36).
■ Injury and Violence
  ● More than 400 Americans die each day from injuries due primarily to motor vehicle crashes, firearms, poisonings, suffocation, falls, fires, and drowning (p. 38).
■ Environmental Quality
  ● An estimated 25% of preventable illnesses worldwide can be attributed to poor environmental quality. Two indicators of air quality are ozone (outdoor) and environmental tobacco smoke (indoor) (p. 40).
■ Immunization
  ● Vaccines are among the greatest public health achievements of the 20th century. Immunizations can prevent disability and death from infectious diseases for individuals and can help control the spread of infections within communities (p. 42).
■ Access to Health Care
  ● Strong predictors of access to quality health care include having health insurance, a higher income level, and a regular primary care provider or other source of ongoing health care. Use of clinical preventive services, such as early prenatal care, can serve as indicators of access to quality health care services (p. 44).

Note: U.S. Department of Health and Human Services.

---

the community. Thus, the vision for *Healthy People 2010* is "Healthy People in Healthy Communities" (USDHHS, 2000, p. 3). As a result, partnerships are important to improve individual and community health. Businesses, local government, and civic, professional, and religious organizations can all participate. Examples include sponsoring a health fair, establishing fitness programs, beginning community recycling, and printing immunization schedules.

DEFINING HEALTH PROMOTION

Considerable differences appear in the literature regarding the use of the terms *health promotion, primary prevention, health protection,* and *illness prevention.* Edelman and Mandle (2006) state that "prevention, in a narrow sense, means avoiding the development of disease in the future, and, in the broader sense, consists of all interventions to limit progression of a disease" (p. 13). The levels of prevention occur at various points of a course of disease progression. Leavell and Clark (1965) defined three levels of prevention: primary, secondary, and tertiary. Five steps describe these levels: **Primary prevention** focuses on (a) health promotion and (b) protection against specific health problems (e.g., immunization against hepatitis B). The purpose of primary prevention is to decrease the risk or exposure of the individual or community to disease. **Secondary prevention** focuses on (a) early identification of health problems and (b) prompt intervention to alleviate health problems. Its goal is to identify individuals in an early stage of a disease process and to limit future disability. **Tertiary prevention** focuses on restoration and rehabilitation with the goal of returning the individual to an

optimal level of functioning. Table 16–1 provides examples of activities for each level of prevention. The three levels of prevention may overlap in practice. For example, a client may have experienced a heart attack, and a goal of secondary prevention is to limit disability. The teaching (e.g., lifestyle changes) for the client's rehabilitation will be similar to health education activities in primary prevention.

Pender, Murdaugh, and Parsons (2006) consider health promotion to be different from disease prevention or health protection. They define **health promotion** as "behavior motivated by the desire to increase well-being and actualize human health potential," and **disease prevention** or **health protection** as "behavior motivated by a desire to actively avoid illness, detect it early, or maintain functioning within the constraints of illness" (p. 7). The individual's underlying motivation for the behavior is the major difference. Box 16–4 provides an overview of the differences between health promotion and health protection.

The difficulty in separating the terms *health promotion* and *disease prevention/health protection* lies in the fact that an activity may be carried out for numerous reasons. For example, a 40-year-old male may begin a program of walking 3 miles each day. If the goal of his program were to "decrease the risk of cardiovascular disease," then the activity would be considered disease prevention or health protection. By contrast, if the motivation for his walking regimen were to "increase his overall health and feeling of well-being," then the activity would be considered a health promotion behavior. It is most helpful to think of health promotion and health protection as being complementary processes because both affect quality of health.

TABLE 16–1 Levels of Prevention

LEVEL AND DESCRIPTION	EXAMPLES
Primary prevention Generalized health promotion and specific protection against disease. It precedes disease or dysfunction and is applied to generally healthy individuals or groups.	■ Health education about injury and poisoning prevention, standards of nutrition and of growth and development for each stage of life, exercise requirements, stress management, protection against occupational hazards, and so on ■ Immunizations ■ Risk assessments for specific disease ■ Family planning services ■ Environmental sanitation and provision of adequate housing, recreation, and work conditions
Secondary prevention Emphasizes early detection of disease, prompt intervention, and health maintenance for individuals experiencing health problems. Includes prevention of complications and disabilities.	■ Screening surveys and procedures of any type (e.g., Denver Developmental Screening Test, hypertension screening) ■ Encouraging regular medical and dental checkups ■ Teaching self-examination for breast and testicular cancer ■ Assessing the growth and development of children ■ Nursing assessments and care provided in home, hospital, or other agency to prevent complications (e.g., maintaining skin integrity; turning, positioning, and exercising clients; ensuring adequate rest, food, and fluid intake; promoting fecal and urinary elimination; administering medical therapies such as medications; and so on)
Tertiary prevention Begins after an illness, when a defect or disability is fixed, stabilized, or determined to be irreversible. Its focus is to help rehabilitate individuals and restore them to an optimum level of functioning within the constraints of the disability.	■ Referring a client who has had a colostomy to a support group ■ Teaching a client who has diabetes to identify and prevent complications ■ Referring a client with a spinal cord injury to a rehabilitation center to receive training that will maximize use of remaining abilities

Health promotion can be offered to all clients regardless of their health and illness status or age. For example, weight-control measures can benefit both overweight clients without disease and clients with cardiac or joint disease. Age-specific health promotion activities are discussed in Chapters 21, 22, and 23 ∞ . See Lifespan Considerations for examples of health promotion topics.

SITES FOR HEALTH PROMOTION ACTIVITIES

Health promotion programs are found in many settings. Programs and activities may be offered to individuals and families in the home or in the community setting and at schools, hospitals, or worksites. Some individuals may feel more comfortable having a nurse, diet counselor, or fitness expert come to their home for teaching and follow-up on individual needs. This type

BOX 16–4 Differences between Health Promotion and Health Protection

Health Promotion	Health Protection
Not disease oriented	Illness or injury specific
Motivated by personal, positive "approach" to wellness	Motivated by "avoidance" of illness
Seeks to expand positive potential for health	Seeks to thwart the occurrence of insults to health and well-being

Note: From *Health Promotion in Nursing Practice,* 5th ed. (p. 8), by N. J. Pender, C. L. Murdaugh, and M. A. Parsons, 2006, Upper Saddle River, NJ: Prentice Hall. Reprinted with permission.

of program, however, is not cost-effective for most individuals. Many people prefer the group approach, find it more motivating, and enjoy the socializing and support. Most programs offered in the community are group oriented.

Community programs are frequently offered by cities and towns. The type of program depends on the current concerns and the expertise of the sponsoring department or group. Program offerings may include health promotion, specific protection, and screening for early detection of disease. The local health department may offer a townwide immunization program because immunization provides one of the most cost-effective means of protecting infants and children. Other examples include the fire department disseminating fire prevention information, or the police offering a bicycle safety program for children or a safe-driving campaign for young adults.

Hospitals began the emphasis on health promotion and prevention by focusing on the health of their employees. Because of the stress involved in caring for the sick and the various shifts that nurses and other health care workers must work, the lifestyles and health habits of health care employees were given priority.

Programs offered by health care organizations initially began with a specific focus on prevention. Examples include infection control, fire prevention and fire drills, limiting exposure to x-rays, and the prevention of back injuries. Gradually, issues related to the health and lifestyle of the employee were addressed with programs on topics such as smoking cessation, exercise and fitness, stress reduction, and time management. Increasingly, hospitals have offered a variety of these programs and others (e.g., women's health) to the community as well as to their employees. Such community activities enhance the public image of

---

LIFESPAN CONSIDERATIONS **Health Promotion Topics**

INFANTS

Infant-parent attachment/bonding
Breastfeeding
Sleep patterns
Playful activity to stimulate development
Immunizations
Safety promotion and injury control

CHILDREN

Nutrition
Dental checkups
Rest and exercise
Immunizations
Safety promotion and injury control

ADOLESCENTS

Communicating with the teen
Hormonal changes
Nutrition
Exercise and rest
Peer group influences
Self-concept and body image

Sexuality
Safety promotion and accident prevention

ELDERS

Adequate sleep
Appropriate use of alcohol
Dental/oral health
Drug management
Exercise
Foot health
Health screening recommendations
Hearing aid use
Immunizations
Medication instruction
Mental health
Nutrition
Physical fitness
Preventive health services
Safety precautions
Smoking cessation
Weight control

---

the hospital, increase the health of the surrounding population, and generate some additional income.

School health promotion programs may serve as a foundation for children of all ages to gain basic knowledge about personal hygiene and issues in the health sciences. Because school is the focus of a child's life for so many years, the school provides a cost-effective and convenient setting for health-focused programs. The school nurse may teach programs about basic nutrition, dental care, activity and play, drug and alcohol abuse, domestic violence, child abuse, and issues related to sexuality and pregnancy. Classroom teachers may include health-related topics in their lesson plans, for example, the way the normal heart functions or the need for clean air and water in the environment.

Worksite programs for health promotion have developed out of the need for businesses to control the rising cost of health care and employee absenteeism. Many industries feel that both employers and employees benefit from healthy lifestyles and behaviors. The convenience of the worksite setting makes these programs particularly attractive to many adults who would otherwise not be aware of them or motivated to attend them. Health promotion programs may be held in the company cafeteria so that employees can watch a film or attend a discussion group during their lunch break. Worksite programs may include programs that address air quality standards for the office, classroom, or plant; programs aimed at specific populations, such as injury prevention for the machine worker or back-saver programs for the individual involved in heavy lifting; programs to screen for high blood pressure; or health enhancement programs, such as fitness information and relaxation techniques. Benefits to the worker may include an increased feeling of well-being, fitness, weight control, and decreased stress. Benefits to the employer may include an increase in employee motivation and productivity, an increase in employee morale, a decrease in

absenteeism, and a lower rate of employee turnover, all of which may decrease business and health care costs.

Older adults who have retired often have more time for health promotion activities than they did before retirement. The nurse can inform elders of available community resources such as walking groups. Nurses can address the need for health protection and health promotion through teaching classes at retirement communities and other community resource centers for elders.

HEALTH PROMOTION MODEL

The initial version of the Health Promotion Model (HPM) appeared in the nursing literature in the early 1980s and focused on health-promoting behaviors rather than health protection or illness prevention behaviors. The initial model has been replaced by the Health Promotion Model (Revised) as shown in Figure 16-4 ■. The HPM is a competence- or approach-oriented model in which the motivational source for behavior change is based on the individual's subjective value of the change—that is, how the client perceives the benefits of changing the given health behavior. The HPM does not include "fear" or "threat" as a motivating source for changing health behavior (Pender et al., 2006, p. 48). The assumptions of the HPM are stated in Box 16–5. The variables in the revised HPM and their interrelationships are described next.

Individual Characteristics and Experiences

The importance of an individual's unique personal factors or characteristics and experiences will depend on the target behavior for health promotion. There is flexibility in the HPM to select those characteristics that are relevant to the particular health behavior. Personal factors are categorized as biological (e.g., age,

Individual Characteristics and Experiences — Behavior-Specific Cognitions and Affect — Behavioral Outcome

Figure 16-4 ■ The Health Promotion Model (revised).

(*Note:* From *Health Promotion in Nursing Practice,* 5th ed. (p. 50), by N. J. Pender, C. L. Murdaugh, and M. A. Parsons, 2006, Upper Saddle River, NJ: Prentice Hall. Reprinted with permission.)

BOX 16–5 Assumptions of the Health Promotion Model

- Persons seek to create conditions of living through which they can express their unique human health potential.
- Persons have the capacity for reflective self-awareness, including assessment of their own competencies.
- Persons value growth in directions viewed as positive and attempt to achieve a personally acceptable balance between change and stability.
- Individuals seek to actively regulate their own behavior.
- Individuals in all their biopsychosocial complexity interact with the environment, progressively transforming the environment and being transformed over time.
- Health professionals constitute a part of the interpersonal environment, which exerts influence on persons throughout their life span.
- Self-initiated reconfiguration of person–environment interactive patterns is essential to behavior change.

Note: From *Health Promotion in Nursing Practice,* 5th ed. (pp. 120–122), by N. J. Pender, C. L. Murdaugh, and M. A. Parsons, 2006, Upper Saddle River, NJ: Prentice Hall. Reprinted with permission.

strength, balance), psychological (e.g., self-esteem, self-motivation), and sociocultural (e.g., race, ethnicity, education, socioeconomic status). Some personal factors can influence health behaviors whereas others, such as age, cannot be changed. Prior related behavior includes previous experience, knowledge, and skill in health-promoting actions. Individuals who made a habit of a previous health-promoting behavior and received a positive benefit as a result will engage in future health-promoting behaviors. In contrast, a person with a history of barriers to achieving the behavior remembers the "hurdles," which creates a negative effect. The nurse can assist by focusing on the positive benefits of the behavior, teaching how to overcome the hurdles and providing positive feedback for the client's successes.

Nursing interventions usually focus on factors that can be modified. It is just as important, however, to also focus on factors that cannot be changed, such as family history. For instance, if a woman has a strong family history of breast cancer, she may neglect self-care practices such as performing breast self-exams and having regular mammograms. She may do this out of fear of finding a lump, or just feeling that with her family history, it is inevitable that she will have breast cancer. Nurses should recognize this and direct more support and information to this group of women, reinforcing the idea that even with a strong family history, early detection and treatment are especially important and offer more hope for a cure. Helping to transform that fear into hope for early detection can make a difference in health attitudes and behaviors.

Behavior-Specific Cognitions and Affect

This set of variables is considered to be of major motivational significance for acquiring and maintaining health-promoting behaviors. Behavior-specific cognitions constitute a critical "core" for intervention because they can be modified through nursing interventions. They include the following:

- *Perceived benefits of action.* Anticipated benefits or outcomes (e.g., physical fitness, stress reduction) affect the person's plan to participate in health-promoting behaviors and may facilitate continued practice. Prior positive experience with the behavior or observations of others engaged in the behavior is a motivational factor.
- *Perceived barriers to action.* A person's perceptions about available time, inconvenience, expense, and difficulty performing the activity may act as barriers (imagined or real). Perceived barriers to action affect health-promoting behaviors by decreasing the individual's commitment to a plan of action.
- *Perceived self-efficacy.* This concept refers to the conviction that a person can successfully carry out the behavior necessary to achieve a desired outcome, such as maintaining an exercise program to lose weight. Often people who have serious doubts about their capabilities decrease their efforts and give up, whereas those with a strong sense of efficacy exert greater effort to master problems or challenges.
- *Activity-related affect.* The subjective feelings that occur before, during, and following an activity can influence whether a person will repeat the behavior again or maintain the behavior. What is the individual's reaction to the thought of the behavior? Is it perceived as fun, enjoyable, or unpleasant? A behavior associated with a positive affect or emotional response is likely to be repeated, and behaviors associated with a negative affect are usually avoided.
- *Interpersonal influences.* Interpersonal influences are a person's perceptions concerning the behaviors, beliefs, or attitudes of others. Family, peers, and health professionals are sources of interpersonal influences that can influence a person's health-promoting behaviors. Interpersonal influences include expectations of significant others, social support (e.g., emotional encouragement), and learning through observing others or modeling.
- *Situational influences.* Situational influences are direct and indirect influences on health-promoting behaviors and include perceptions of available options, demand characteristics, and the aesthetic features of the environment. An example of an individual's perception of available options can include easy access to healthy alternatives such as

vending machines and restaurants that provide healthful menu options. Demand characteristics can directly affect healthy behaviors through policies such as a company regulation that demands safety equipment to be worn or that establishes a "no smoking" environment. Individuals are more apt to perform health promotion behaviors if they are comfortable in the environment versus feeling alienated. Environments that are considered safe as well as interesting are also desirable aesthetic features that facilitate health promotion behaviors.

Commitment to a Plan of Action

Commitment to a plan of action involves two processes: commitment and identifying specific strategies for carrying out and reinforcing the behavior. Strategies are important because commitment alone often results in "good intentions" and not actual performance of the behavior.

Immediate Competing Demands and Preferences

Competing demands are those behaviors over which an individual has a low level of control. For example, an unexpected work or family responsibility may compete with a planned visit to the health club, and not responding to this responsibility may cause a more negative outcome than missing the exercise routine. Competing preferences are behaviors over which an individual has a high level of control; however, this control depends on the individual's ability to be self-regulating or to not "give in." For example, a person who chooses a high-fat food over a low-fat food because it tastes better has "given in" to an urge based on a competing preference.

Behavioral Outcome

Health-promoting behavior, the outcome of the Health Promotion Model, is directed toward attaining positive health outcomes for the client. Health-promoting behaviors should result in improved health, enhanced functional ability, and better quality of life at all stages of development (Pender et al., 2006, p. 57).

STAGES OF HEALTH BEHAVIOR CHANGE

Health behavior change is a cyclic phenomenon in which people progress through several stages. In the first stage, the person does not think seriously about changing a behavior; by the time the person reaches the final stage, he or she is successfully maintaining the change in behavior. Several behavior change models have been proposed. The Transtheoretical Model (TTM), proposed by Prochaska, Redding, and Evers (2002) is discussed here. As shown in Figure 16-5 ■, the stages are (a) precontemplation, (b) contemplation, (c) preparation, (d) action, (e) maintenance, and (f) termination. If the person does not succeed in changing behavior, relapse occurs.

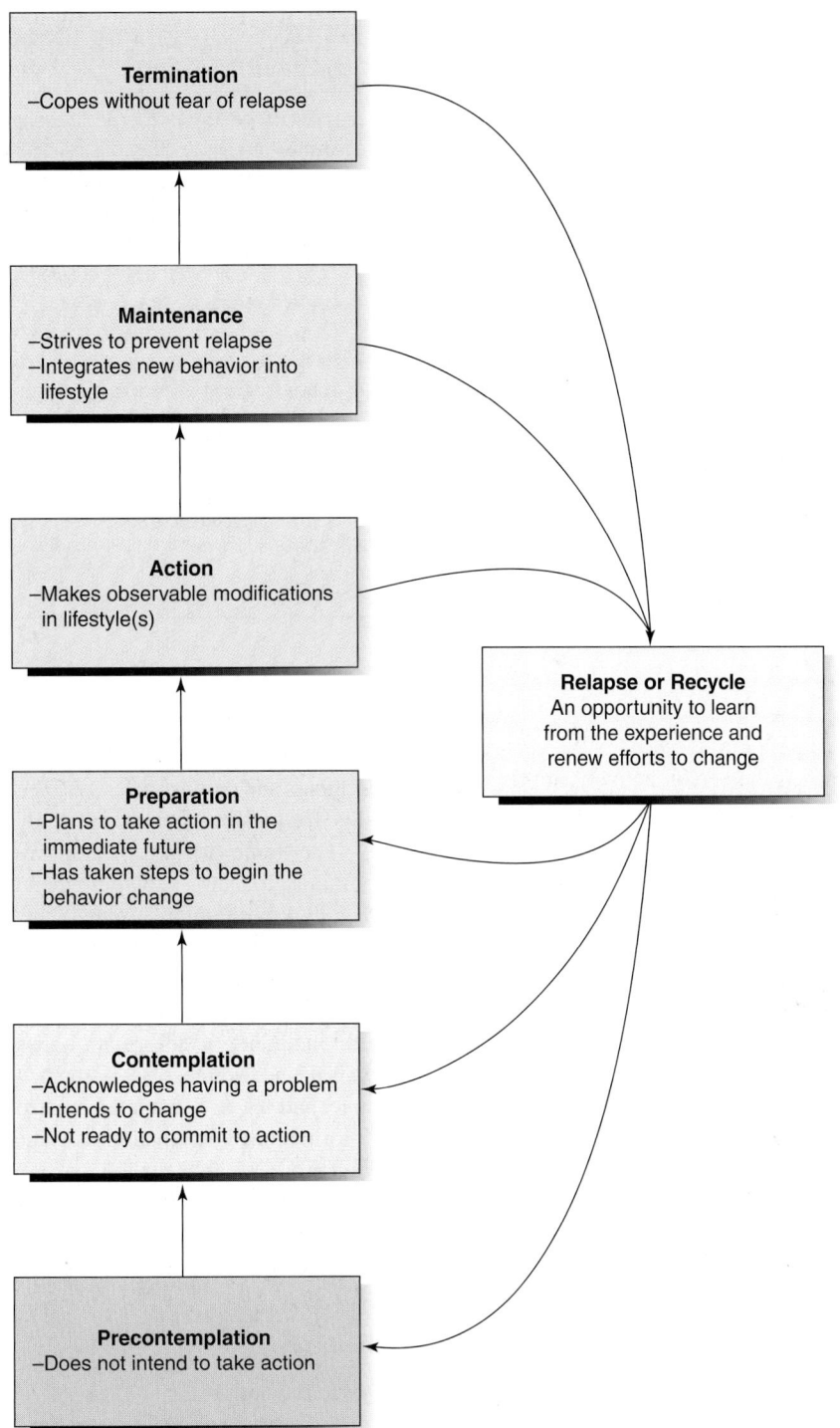

Figure 16-5 ■ The stages of change are rarely linear. It is more common for people to recycle several times through the stages. The person who takes action and has a relapse (recycles through some or all of the stages again) is more apt to be successful the next time than the individual who never takes action.

(Diagram based on content from *Changing for Good* by James O. Prochaska, John C. Norcross, and Carlo C. DiClemente. Copyright 1994 by James O. Prochaska, John C. Norcross, and Carlo C. DiClemente. Reprinted by permission of HarperCollins Publishers, Inc.; and "The Transtheoretical Model and Stages of Change" by James O. Prochaska, Colleen A. Redding, and Kerry E. Evers in *Health Behaviors and Health Education: Theory, Research, and Practice* (3rd ed.), 2002, by Karen Glanz, Barbara K. Rimer, and Frances Marcus Lewis, Eds.)

Precontemplation Stage

In the **precontemplation stage,** the person does not think about changing his or her behavior in the next 6 months. They may be uninformed or underinformed about the consequences of the risk behavior(s). The person who has tried changing previously and was unsuccessful may now see the behavior as his or her "fate" or believe that change is hopeless. Individuals in this stage tend to avoid reading, talking, or thinking about their high-risk behaviors (Prochaska et al., 2002, p. 100).

Contemplation Stage

During the **contemplation stage,** the person acknowledges having a problem, seriously considers changing a specific behavior, actively gathers information, and verbalizes plans to change the behavior in the near future (e.g., next 6 months). The person, however, may not be ready to commit to action. Some people may stay in the contemplative stage for months or years before taking action. When contemplators begin the transition to the preparation stage, their thinking is clearly marked by two changes: focusing on the solution rather than the problem and thinking more about the future than the past (Prochaska, Norcross, & DiClemente, 1994, p. 43).

Preparation Stage

The **preparation stage** occurs when the person intends to take action in the immediate future (e.g., within the next month). Some people in this stage may have already started making small behavioral changes, such as buying a self-help book. At this stage, the person makes the final specific plans to accomplish the change.

Action Stage

The **action stage** occurs when the person actively implements behavioral and cognitive strategies of the action plan to interrupt previous health risk behaviors and adopt new ones. This stage requires the greatest commitment of time and energy.

Maintenance Stage

During the **maintenance stage,** the person strives to prevent relapse by integrating newly adopted behaviors into his or her lifestyle. This stage lasts until the person no longer experiences temptation to return to previous unhealthy behaviors. Without a strong commitment to maintenance, there will be a relapse, usually to the precontemplation or contemplation stage (Prochaska et al., 1994, p. 45).

Termination Stage

The **termination stage** is the ultimate goal where the individual has complete confidence that the problem is no longer a temptation or threat. It is as if they never acquired the habit in the first place (Prochaska et al., 2002, p. 102). Experts debate whether some behaviors can be terminated versus requiring continual maintenance.

These six stages are cyclical; people generally move through one stage before progressing to the next. However, at any point a person may relapse or recycle to any previous stage. In fact, the average successful self-changer recycles through the stages several times before making it to the top and exiting the cycle (Prochaska et al., 1994, pp. 47–48). The majority of individuals who relapse return to the contemplation stage. During this time they can think about what they learned and plan for the next action attempt. Box 16–6 suggests a method to assess your stage of change for a health behavior.

BOX 16–6 Assessing Stages of Behavior Change

Stages of change for positive health behaviors may be assessed with the following true-false questions:

1. I currently do not (specify exact behavior, e.g., exercise 30 minutes three times a week, eat two to four servings of fruit daily) and do not intend to start in the next 6 months. (Precontemplation)
2. I currently do not (specify behavior), but I am thinking about starting to do so in the next 6 months. (Contemplation)
3. I have tried several times to (specify behavior), but I am seriously thinking of trying again in the next month. (Planning)
4. I have (specify behavior) regularly for less than 6 months. (Action)
5. I have (specify behavior) regularly for more than 6 months. (Maintenance)

Note: From "A Transtheoretical Model of Behaviors and Change," by J. O. Prochaska, C. A. Redding, & K. E. Evers. In K. Glanz, B. K. Rimer, & F. M. Lewis (Eds.), *Health Behavior and Health Education: Theory, Research and Practice.* Copyright © 2002 Jossey-Bass. Reprinted with permission of John Wiley & Sons, Inc.

THE NURSE'S ROLE IN HEALTH PROMOTION

Individuals and communities who seek to increase their responsibility for personal health and self-care require health education. The trend toward health promotion has created the opportunity for nurses to strengthen the profession's influence on health promotion, disseminate information that promotes an educated public, and assist individuals and communities to change long-standing health behaviors.

A variety of programs can be used for the promotion of health, including (a) information dissemination, (b) health risk appraisal and wellness assessment, (c) lifestyle and behavior change, and (d) environmental control programs.

Information dissemination is the most basic type of health promotion program. This method makes use of a variety of media to offer information to the public about the risk of particular lifestyle choices and personal behavior, as well as the benefits of changing that behavior and improving the quality of life. Billboards, posters, brochures, newspaper features, books, and health fairs all offer opportunities for the dissemination of health promotion information. Alcohol and drug abuse, driving under the influence of alcohol, hypertension, and the need for immunizations are some of the topics frequently discussed. Information dissemination is a useful strategy for raising the level of knowledge and awareness of individuals and groups about health habits.

When planning information dissemination, it is important to consider factors such as cultural factors and different age groups. Knowing the best place and method to distribute information will increase the effectiveness. For example, older African Americans usually have strong ties to their churches for social support as well as religious practices. Knowing this, the church can often be the appropriate place to hold health fairs or even small group discussions on various health topics. It provides a stepping stone for providing information and suggesting resources for special needs—all done in a comfortable, nonthreatening environment for persons in that age group and culture.

It is just as critical to know where people get "misinformation." Sending multiple mailings has become a marketing ploy for advertising "miracle" vitamins, herbs, and food supplements. These are heavily directed toward elders who may choose this route of purchasing items if they have transportation problems.

Health risk appraisal and wellness assessment programs are used to apprise individuals of the risk factors that are inherent in their lives in order to motivate them to reduce specific risks and develop positive health habits. Wellness assessment programs are focused on more positive methods of enhancement, in contrast to the risk factor approach used in the health appraisal. A variety of tools are available to facilitate these assessments. Some of these tools are computer based and can therefore be offered to educational institutions and industries at a reasonable cost.

Lifestyle and behavior change programs require the participation of the individual and are geared toward enhancing the quality of life and extending the life span. Individuals generally consider lifestyle changes after they have been informed of the need to change their health behavior and have become aware of the potential benefits of the process. Many programs are available to the public, both on a group and individual basis, some of which address stress management, nutrition awareness, weight control, smoking cessation, and exercise.

Environmental control programs have been developed in response to the continuing increase of contaminants of human origin that have been introduced into our environment. The amounts of contaminants that are already present in the air, food, and water will affect the health of our descendants for several generations. The most common concerns of community groups are toxic and nuclear wastes, nuclear power plants, air and water pollution, and herbicide and pesticide use.

Health promotion activities, such as the variety of programs previously discussed, involve collaborative relationships with both clients and primary care provider. The role of the nurse is to work *with* people, not *for* them—that is, to act as a facilitator of the process of assessing, evaluating, and understanding health. The nurse may act as advocate, consultant, teacher, or coordinator of services. For examples of the nurse's role in health promotion, see Box 16–7.

In these roles, the nurse may work with individuals of all age groups and diverse family units or concentrate on a specific population, such as new parents, school-age children, or older adults. In any case, the nursing process is a basic tool for the nurse in a health promotion role. Although the process is the same, the nurse emphasizes teaching the client (who can be either an individual or a family unit) self-care responsibility. Adult clients decide the goals, determine the health promotion plans, and take responsibility for the success of the plans.

THE NURSING PROCESS AND HEALTH PROMOTION

A thorough assessment of the individual's health status is basic to health promotion. As nurses move toward greater autonomy

---

BOX 16–7 The Nurse's Role in Health Promotion

- Model healthy lifestyle behaviors and attitudes.
- Facilitate client involvement in the assessment, implementation, and evaluation of health goals.
- Teach clients self-care strategies to enhance fitness, improve nutrition, manage stress, and enhance relationships.
- Assist individuals, families, and communities to increase their levels of health.
- Educate clients to be effective health care consumers.
- Assist clients, families, and communities to develop and choose health-promoting options.
- Guide clients' development in effective problem solving and decision making.
- Reinforce clients' personal and family health-promoting behaviors.
- Advocate in the community for changes that promote a healthy environment.

---

in providing client care, expanded assessment skills are essential to provide the meaningful data needed for health planning.

NURSING MANAGEMENT

Assessing

Components of this assessment are the health history and physical examination, physical fitness assessment, lifestyle assessment, spiritual assessment, social support systems review, health risk assessment, health beliefs review, and life-stress review.

Health History and Physical Examination

The health history and physical examination discussed in Chapter 30 ∞ provide a means for detecting any existing problems. The age of the individual must be considered when collecting data. For example, an environmental safety assessment and immunization history must be appropriate to the person's age. A nutritional assessment is an important part of the health history. The nurse must consider both age and body build of the client when gathering information on dietary patterns. See Chapter 47 ∞ for more information about nutritional assessment.

Physical Fitness Assessment

During an evaluation of physical fitness, the nurse assesses several components of the body's physical functioning: muscle endurance, flexibility, body composition, and cardiorespiratory endurance. Specific guidelines for obtaining measurements and the optimal values for men, women, and children can be found in physical fitness texts (see Table 16–2). Elders need to be monitored carefully for fatigue during strength and endurance tests.

A common test for muscular endurance is performing sit-ups with knees bent (bent-knee sit-ups) for one minute. The number of sit-ups performed during that time is compared to standardized charts.

TABLE 16–2 Physical Fitness Values

TEST	AGE	DESIRED OUTCOMES	UNDESIRED OUTCOMES
Sit-ups	36 to 45 years	Men: 42 or more Women: 39 or more	21 or less 12 or less
	Over 46 years	Men: 38 or more Women: 24 or more	18 or less 11 or less
Trunk flexion		Men: 11 to 15 inches Women: 12 to 16 inches	Below −6 inches Below −4 inches
Skin folds		Men: 21 mm Women: 30 mm	Marked deviations above or below desired ratings
Step test		Men: recovery pulse rate 124 Women: recovery pulse rate 140 (95th percentile rankings)	Men: recovery pulse rate 178 Women: recovery pulse rate 184 (10th percentile rankings)

Note: From *Health Promotion in Nursing Practice,* 5th ed. (pp. 98–100) by N. J. Pender, C. L. Murdaugh, and M. A. Parsons, 2006, Upper Saddle River, NJ: Prentice Hall. Reprinted with permission.

Flexibility of the joints and muscles greatly increases an individual's ability to move about with ease and comfort. Trunk flexion is one test used to measure the client's ability to stretch the back and thigh muscles. In this test the client sits on an examining table or the floor with the legs fully extended, the feet placed flat against a box, and the arms and hands stretched forward as far as possible, and holds for a count of three. The distance the client can reach beyond the near edge of the box is measured in inches or, if the client is unable to reach the box, the distance between the fingertips and the box is measured and recorded as a negative number.

Body composition indicates the ratio of body fat to muscle and is estimated through skinfold measurements. Skinfold measurements are obtained by grasping the skinfold (skin layers and subcutaneous fat) between the thumb and forefinger and measuring the skinfold at subcutaneous sites (chest, midaxillary, triceps, subscapula, abdomen, suprailiac, and thigh) with special calipers. Generally three measurements are taken at each site and the average values summed. The technique for measuring skin folds is described in Chapter 47 ∞ . One test for cardiorespiratory endurance is the step test. Individuals step up and down on a 16- to 17-inch step for 3 minutes at a prescribed rate (e.g., 22 to 24 steps per minute). After the test, the client sits in a chair while the nurse assesses the apical or carotid pulse rate from 5 to 20 seconds into recovery.

Lifestyle Assessment

Lifestyle assessment focuses on the personal lifestyle and habits of the client as they affect health. Categories of lifestyle generally assessed are physical activity, nutritional practices, stress management, and such habits as smoking, alcohol consumption, and drug use. Other categories may be included. Several tools are available to assess lifestyle. The goals of lifestyle assessment tools are to provide the following:

1. An opportunity for clients to assess the impact of their present lifestyle on their health
2. A basis for decisions related to desired behavior and lifestyle change

Spiritual Health Assessment

Spiritual health is the ability to develop one's inner nature to its fullest potential, including the ability to discover and articulate one's basic purpose in life, to learn how to experience love, joy, peace, and fulfillment, and how to help ourselves and others achieve their fullest potential (Pender et al., 2006, p. 108). Spiritual beliefs can affect a person's interpretation of events in his or her life and, therefore, an assessment of spiritual well-being is a part of evaluating the person's overall health. See Chapter 41 ∞ , Spirituality, for more information.

Social Support Systems Review

Understanding the social context in which a person lives and works is important in health promotion. Individuals and groups, through interpersonal relationships, can provide comfort, assistance, encouragement, and information. Social support fosters successful coping and promotes satisfying and effective living.

Social support systems contribute to health by creating an environment that encourages healthy behaviors, promotes self-esteem and wellness, and provides feedback that the person's actions will lead to desirable outcomes. Examples of social support systems include family, peer support groups (including computer-based support groups), community-organized religious support systems (e.g., churches), and self-help groups (e.g., Mended Hearts, Weight Watchers). The Culturally Competent Care feature addresses aspects of social support within the context of culture.

According to Pender et al. (2002), the nurse begins a social support system review by asking the client to do these tasks:

- List individuals who provide personal support.
- Indicate the relationship of each person (e.g., family member, fellow worker or colleague, social acquaintance).
- Identify which individuals have been a source of support for 5 or more years.

This assessment allows the nurse and client to discuss and evaluate the adequacy of the client's support system together and, if necessary, plan options for enhancing the support system.

CULTURALLY COMPETENT CARE
Cultural Aspects of Social Support

It is important to understand how various subgroups of American society may define social support.

- In the African American community, the family and church have been major providers of social support.
- Hispanic-Latino Americans and Asian Americans view the family as being a major social support system.
- Asian Americans respect older adults and use shame and harmony in giving and receiving support.
- Native Americans live in social networks that foster mutual assistance and support.

Note: From *Health Promotion in Nursing Practice,* 5th ed. (pp. 239–240), by N. J. Pender, C. L. Murdaugh, and M. A. Parsons, 2006, Upper Saddle River, NJ: Prentice Hall. Reprinted with permission.

Health Risk Assessment

A **health risk assessment (HRA)** is an assessment and educational tool that indicates a client's risk for disease or injury during the next 10 years by comparing the client's risk with the mortality risk of the corresponding age, sex, and racial group. The client's general health, lifestyle behaviors, and demographic data are compared to data from a large national sample. Individual risk reports are based on statistics for the population group that matches the individual's surveyed characteristics. The HRA includes a summary of the person's health risks and lifestyle behaviors with educational suggestions on how to reduce the risk.

Many HRA instruments are available today in paper-and-pencil as well as computerized forms. Recently, HRAs have begun to reflect a broader approach to health as companies use the HRA as a means to begin a health promotion and risk reduction program. Occupational health nurses can identify risk factors and subsequently plan interventions aimed to decrease illness, absenteeism, and disability.

HRAs are helpful for assessing individual and group health risks. They are not, however, substitutes for medical care and are not appropriate for all individuals. For example, people with chronic illnesses such as cancer or heart disease may not obtain accurate risk assessments. Certain populations (e.g., very young, elderly, some sociocultural groups) may not be fully represented in the population databases and, therefore, the HRA may not project an accurate risk assessment.

Health Beliefs Review

Clients' health beliefs need to be clarified, particularly those beliefs that determine how they perceive control of their own health care status. Locus of control is a measurable concept that can be used to predict which people are most likely to change their behavior (see Chapter 17 ∞). Several instruments are available that assess a person's health-belief measures. Assessment of clients' health beliefs provides the nurse with an indication of how much the clients believe they can influence or control health through personal behaviors. Several cultures have a strong belief in fate: "Whatever will be, will be." If people hold this belief, they do not feel that they can do anything to change the course of their disease. An example is doing diabetic teaching, which often requires many lifestyle changes in diet, exercise, and close control of glucose to prevent complications. If the person believes he or she has no control of the outcome, it is difficult to provide motivations to make the necessary changes. Being aware of these differences can provide a better indication of readiness and motivation on the part of the client to engage in healthy behaviors. See the Lifespan Considerations for factors that might indicate a need for additional information or resources for elders.

MediaLink Health Belief Model Application

LIFESPAN CONSIDERATIONS   Factors Affecting Health Promotion and Illness Prevention

CHILDREN

Childhood obesity is becoming a serious health problem. Data collected by the Centers for Disease Control and Prevention (CDC) show that nearly 16% of American children are overweight, up from 6.5% in 1980 (National Center for Health Statistics, 2004). Obesity and overweight in children contributes to long-term health problems such as heart disease and diabetes mellitus.

Although specific causes of obesity and appropriate management to reduce weight will vary from child to child, healthy eating habits and adequate exercise patterns form the basis for healthy growth and prevention of overweight in children. It is the responsibility of parents and caregivers to provide children with healthy food choices and an environment that makes eating a pleasure. It is the responsibility of children to decide how much and what foods to eat. Adults must be role models for their children, eating well and exercising regularly themselves.

ELDERS

In elders, health promotion and illness prevention are important, but often the focus is on learning to adapt to and live with increasing changes and limitations. Maximizing strengths continues to be of prime importance in maintaining optimal function and quality of life. Factors to be aware of that might indicate a need for additional information or resources include these:

- An increase in physical limitations
- Presence of one or more chronic illnesses
- Change in cognitive status
- Difficulty in accessing health care services due to transportation problems
- Poor support system
- Need for environmental modifications for safety and to maintain independence
- Attitude of hopelessness and depression, which decreases the motivation to use resources or learn new information

Life Stress Review

There is abundant literature about the impact of stress on mental and physical well-being. A variety of stress-related instruments have been found in the literature. For example, Holmes and Rahe (1967, p. 213) developed a Life-Change Index, a tool that assigns numerical values to life events (see Box 16–8). Studies have shown that a high score is associated with the increased possibility of illness in an individual.

Validating Assessment Data

Following the collection of assessment data, the nurse and client need to review, validate, and summarize the information. This step is carried out jointly by the nurse and the client. During this process, the nurse verbally reviews the current practices and attitudes of the client. This allows validation of the information by the client and may increase awareness of the need to change behavior. The nurse and client need to consider the following:

- Any existing health problems
- The client's perceived degree of control over health status
- Key health beliefs
- Level of physical fitness and nutritional status
- Illnesses for which the client is at risk
- Current positive health practices
- Spirituality
- Sources of life stress and ability to handle stress

- Social support systems
- Information needed to enhance health care practices

Diagnosing

Nursing diagnoses accepted by the North American Nursing Diagnosis Association (NANDA) have generally focused on impaired or imbalanced health patterns or problems. The definition, however, of the NANDA **wellness diagnoses** states: "Describes human responses to levels of wellness in an individual, family, or community that have a readiness for enhancement" (2005, p. 277).

Wellness diagnoses can be applied at all levels of prevention but are particularly useful for healthy clients who require teaching for health promotion, disease prevention, and personal growth. When the nurse and client conclude that the client has positive function in a certain pattern area, such as adequate nutrition or effective coping, the nurse can use this information to help the client reach a higher level of functioning.

A wellness diagnosis is preceded by the modifier "readiness for enhanced". The following examples are included in the NANDA taxonomy:

- *Readiness for Enhanced Spiritual Well-being*
- *Readiness for Enhanced Coping*
- *Readiness for Enhanced Nutrition*
- *Readiness for Enhanced Knowledge (Specify)*

BOX 16–8 Life-Change Index

Life Event	Impact Score	Life Event	Impact Score
Death of spouse	100	Begin or end school	26
Divorce	73	Change in living conditions	25
Marital separation	65	Revisions of personal habits	24
Jail term	63	Trouble with boss	23
Death of close family member	63	Change in work hours or conditions	20
Personal injury or illness	53	Change in residence	20
Marriage	50	Change in schools	20
Fired at work	47	Change in recreations	19
Marital reconciliation	45	Change in church activities	19
Retirement	45	Change in social activities	19
Change in health of family member	44	Mortgage or loan less than $20,000	17
Pregnancy	40	Change in sleeping habits	16
Sex difficulties	39	Change in number of family get-togethers	15
Gain of a new family member	39	Change in eating habits	15
Business readjustment	39	Vacation	13
Change in financial state	38	Christmas approaching	11
Death of a close friend	37	Minor violation of the law	11
Change to a different line of work	36		
Change in number of arguments with spouse	35		
Mortgage over $20,000	31		
Foreclosure of mortgage or loan	30		
Change in responsibilities at work	29		
Son or daughter leaving home	29		
Trouble with in-laws	29		
Outstanding personal achievement	28		
Spouse begins or stops work	26		

Life-Change Units	Likelihood of Illness in Near Future
300+	About 80%
150–299	About 50%
Less than 150	About 30%

The higher your life-change score, the harder you have to work to get yourself back into a state of good health.

Note: Reprinted from *Journal of Psychosomatic Research, 11* (8), Holmes, T. H., and Rahe, T. H., "Social Readjustment Rating Scale," p. 213, copyright 1967, with permission from Elsevier.

- *Readiness for Enhanced Parenting*
- *Readiness for Enhanced Self-concept*
- *Readiness for Enhanced Immunization Status*
- *Readiness for Enhanced Self-Care*

Wellness diagnoses provide a clear focus for planning interventions without indicating that a problem exists.

Planning

Health promotion plans need to be developed according to the needs, desires, and priorities of the client. The client decides on health promotion goals, the activities or interventions to achieve those goals, the frequency and duration of the activities, and the method of evaluation. During the planning process the nurse acts as a resource person rather than as an advisor or counselor. The nurse provides information when asked, emphasizes the importance of small steps to behavioral change, and reviews the client's goals and plans to make sure they are realistic, measurable, and acceptable to the client.

Steps in Planning

Pender et al. (2006, pp. 127–141) outline several steps in the process of developing a joint health promotion-prevention plan

(see Box 16–9). These steps actively involve both the nurse and the client:

1. *Review and summarize data from assessment.* The nurse shares with the client a summary of the data collected from the various assessments (e.g., physical health and fitness, nutrition, sources of stress, spirituality, health practices).
2. *Reinforce strengths and competencies of the client.* The nurse and the client come to consensus about areas in which the client is doing well and areas that need further development.
3. *Identify health goals and related behavior-change options.* The client selects two or three top priority personal health goals, prioritizes them, and reviews behavior-change options.
4. *Identify behavioral or health outcomes.* For each of the selected goals or areas in step 1, the nurse and client determine what specific behavioral changes are needed to bring about the desired outcome. For example, to reduce the risk of cardiovascular disease, the client may need to stop smoking, lose weight, and increase activity level.
5. *Develop a behavior-change plan.* A constructive program of change is based on client "ownership" of those behavior changes selected for implementation within everyday life (Pender et al., 2006, p. 134). Clients may need to be assisted

---

BOX 16–9	**Example of an Individual Health Promotion-Prevention Plan**

Designed for: James Moore
Home Address: 714 George
Home Telephone Number: 222-3333
Occupation (if employed): Building services supervisor
Work Telephone Number: 445-6666
Cultural Identification: African American
Birth Date: 3/14/59   Date of Initial Plan: 1/15/2007

Client strengths	Satisfactory peer relationships, spiritual strength, adequate sleep pattern
Major risk factors	Elevated cholesterol, mild obesity, sedentary lifestyle, moderate life change, multiple daily hassles, few reported uplifts
Nursing diagnoses	Deficient Diversional Activity
(derived from assessment	Imbalanced Nutrition: More than Body Requirements
of functional health patterns)	Caregiver Role Strain (elderly mother)
Medical diagnoses (if any)	Mild hypertension
Age-specific screening recommendations	Blood pressure, cholesterol, fecal occult blood, malignant skin lesions, depression
Desired behavioral and health outcomes	Become a regular exerciser (3×/week), lower my blood pressure, weigh 165 lb

Personal Health Goals (1 = highest priority)	Selected Behaviors to Accomplish Goals	Stage of Change	Strategies/Interventions for Change
1. Achieve desired body weight	Begin a progressive walking program	Planning	Counterconditioning Reinforcement management Client contracting
	Decrease caloric intake while maintaining good nutrition	Action (eating 2 fruits and 2 vegetables daily; using low-fat dairy products for last 2 months)	Stimulus control Cognitive restructuring
2. Decrease risk for hypertension-related disorders	Change from high- to low-sodium snacks	Contemplation	Consciousness raising Learning facilitation
3. Learn to manage stress effectively	Attend relaxation classes and use home relaxation tapes	Contemplation	Consciousness raising Self-reevaluation Simple relaxation therapy
4. Increase leisure-time activities	Join a local bowling league	Contemplation	Support system enhancement

Note: From *Health Promotion in Nursing Practice,* 5th ed. (pp. 129–130), by N. J. Pender, C. L. Murdaugh, and M. A. Parsons, 2006, Upper Saddle River, NJ: Prentice Hall. Reprinted with permission.

in examining value-behavior inconsistencies and in selecting behavioral options that are most appealing and that they are most willing to try. The client's priorities will reflect personal values, activity preferences, and expectations for success.

6. *Reiterate benefits of change.* The positive benefits will probably need to be reiterated by both the nurse and the client even though the client is committed to the change. The health-related and non-health-related benefits should be kept before the client as central motivating factors.

7. *Address environmental and interpersonal facilitators and barriers to change.* Environmental and interpersonal factors that support positive change should be used to reinforce the client's efforts to change lifestyle. All people experience barriers, some of which can be anticipated and planned for, thereby making the change more likely to occur.

8. *Determine a time frame for implementation.* By developing a time frame, the appropriate knowledge and skills can be developed before a new behavior is implemented. The time frame may be several weeks or months. Scheduling short-term goals and rewards can offer encouragement to achieve long-term objectives. Clients may need help to be realistic and to deal with one behavior at a time.

9. *Formalize commitment to behavior-change plan.* Commitments to changing behaviors have usually been verbal. Increasingly, a formal, written behavioral contract is being used to motivate the client to follow through with selected actions (see Chapter 27 ∞). Motivation to follow through is provided by a positive reinforcement or re-ward stated in the contract. Contracting is based on the belief that all people have the potential for growth and the right of self-determination, even though their choices may be different from the norm.

Exploring Available Resources

Another essential aspect of planning is identifying support resources available to the client. These may be community resources such as a fitness program at a local gymnasium, or educational programs such as stress management, breast self-examination, nutrition, smoking cessation, and health lectures.

Implementing

Implementing is the "doing" part of behavior change. Self-responsibility is emphasized for implementing the plan. Depending on the client's needs, the nursing interventions may include supporting, counseling, facilitating, teaching, consulting, enhancing the behavior change, and modeling.

Providing and Facilitating Support

A major nursing role is to support the client. A vital component of lifestyle change is ongoing support that focuses on the desired behavior change and is provided in a nonjudgmental manner. Support can be offered by the nurse on an individual basis or in a group setting. The nurse can also facilitate the development of support networks for the client, such as family members and friends.

RESEARCH NOTE   Adolescents and Their Control of Tobacco Use

Studies show that, in 2003, approximately 3.6 million U.S. children between 12 and 17 years of age (14.4% of that population) used tobacco products. This use increases in older adolescents and young adults, with individuals aged 18 to 25 years having the highest rate of tobacco use (48.8%) of all Americans (Substance Abuse and Mental Health Services Administration, 2004). In its 2003 study of youth risk behaviors, the Centers for Disease Control and Prevention (CDC) found that 27.5% of all adolescents currently use tobacco (Grunbaum et al., 2004). Smoking cigarettes is the most common type of tobacco use.

Johnson et al. (2004) used a grounded theory approach to study how adolescents perceived their smoking, how it fit into a "typical" adolescent framework of experimentation and establishing independence, and how adolescents attempted to control their amount of cigarette use. The researchers found that adolescents go through a process of determining if smoking is a problem, "crossing the line" to unacceptable tobacco use, using strategies to regain control once the "line" has been crossed, and then "reconstructing" the line either where it was originally (e.g., no smoking or very limited cigarette use) or at a higher level of use.

Most adolescents expressed a desire to maintain control of their smoking and not become "addicted." They used strategies such as not buying cigarettes, rationing smokes, limiting the situations in which they would smoke, cutting out "unnecessary" cigarettes, delaying smoking, and "half-butting" (taking a few puffs and saving the butt for later) to limit their use. Replacing smoking with other activities was also used to gain control, for example, substituting chewing gum, getting help from friends or family to limit or stop use, using transitions such as moving to a new school to get a "fresh start," and making efforts to "quit" completely.

The authors conclude that the way adolescents manage their cigarette use, including their active efforts to maintain control over it, may be a part of the typical adolescent process of establishing independence, and adolescents do not intend or desire to become addicted to nicotine. Many adolescents who limited smoking went on to quit completely.

IMPLICATIONS

A "harm reduction" approach in which smokers are encouraged to limit their cigarette use validates the adolescent's propensity to establish self-control and may be more effective than a conventional smoking cessation program alone when working with adolescent smokers.

Note: From "Crossing the Line: Adolescents' Experiences of Controlling Their Tobacco Use" by J. L. Johnson, C. Kalaw, C. Y. Lovato, L. Baillie, and N. A. Chambers. 2004, *Qualitative Health Research, 14*(9), 1276–1291; "Youth risk behavior surveillance—United States, 2003" by J. A. Grunbaum, L. Kann, S. Kinchen, J. Ross, J. Hawkings, R. Lowry, et al., May 21, 2004, *MMWR Surveillance Summaries, 53 (No. SS-2); 1–96;* and "Results from the 2003 National Survey on Drug Use and Health: National Findings" by Substance Abuse and Mental Health Services Administration. 2004, *Office of Applied Studies, NSDUH Series H-25, DHHS Publication No. SMA 04-3964. Rockville, MD.*

INDIVIDUAL COUNSELING SESSIONS. Counseling sessions may be routinely scheduled as part of the plan or may be provided if the client encounters difficulty in carrying out interventions or meets insurmountable barriers to change. In a counseling relationship, the nurse and client share ideas. In this sharing relationship, the nurse acts as a facilitator, promoting the client's decision-making in regard to the health promotion plan.

TELEPHONE OR COMPUTER COUNSELING. Regular telephone sessions or computer interaction may be provided to the client to help in answering questions, reviewing goals and strategies, and reinforcing progress. The client may find that scheduling a weekly interaction is helpful or may wish to initiate a call if a problem occurs. The client is asked, "Is your plan working?" If the plan is not working, the nurse asks, "What would you like to do?" The client may wish to continue or may wish to change the plan to a more realistic one. Telephone or computer support is efficient for the busy client who may not have the time for regular, in-person sessions.

GROUP SUPPORT. Group sessions provide an opportunity for participants to learn the experiences of others in changing behavior. Group contact gives individuals a renewed commitment to their goals. Groups can be scheduled at monthly or less frequent intervals for over a year.

FACILITATING SOCIAL SUPPORT. Social networks, such as family and friends, can facilitate or impede the efforts directed toward health promotion and prevention. The nurse's role is to assist the client to assess, modify, and develop the social support necessary to achieve the desired change. To provide the necessary support, families must communicate effectively, be aware of and support each other's needs and goals, and provide help and assistance to one another to achieve those goals. The client may wish the nurse to meet with the family or significant others and help enlist their understanding and support.

PROVIDING HEALTH EDUCATION. Health education programs on a variety of topics discussed earlier can be provided to groups, individuals, or communities. Group programs need to be planned carefully before they are implemented. The decision to establish a health promotion program must be based on the health needs of the people; also, specific health promotion goals must be set. After the program is implemented, outcomes must be evaluated.

ENHANCING BEHAVIOR CHANGE. Whether people will make and maintain changes to improve health or prevent disease depends on many interrelated factors. To help clients succeed in implementing behavior changes, the nurse needs to understand the stages of change and effective interventions that focus on progressing the individual through the stages of change. Guidelines for assisting the client toward behavior change are offered in the Practice Guidelines. Figure 16-6 ■ provides suggested strategies to assist clients depending on their stage of change. As Saarmann, Daugherty, and Riegel (2000) point out, the nursing goal is not necessarily to change behavior but to advance the client to the next stage of change (p. 285).

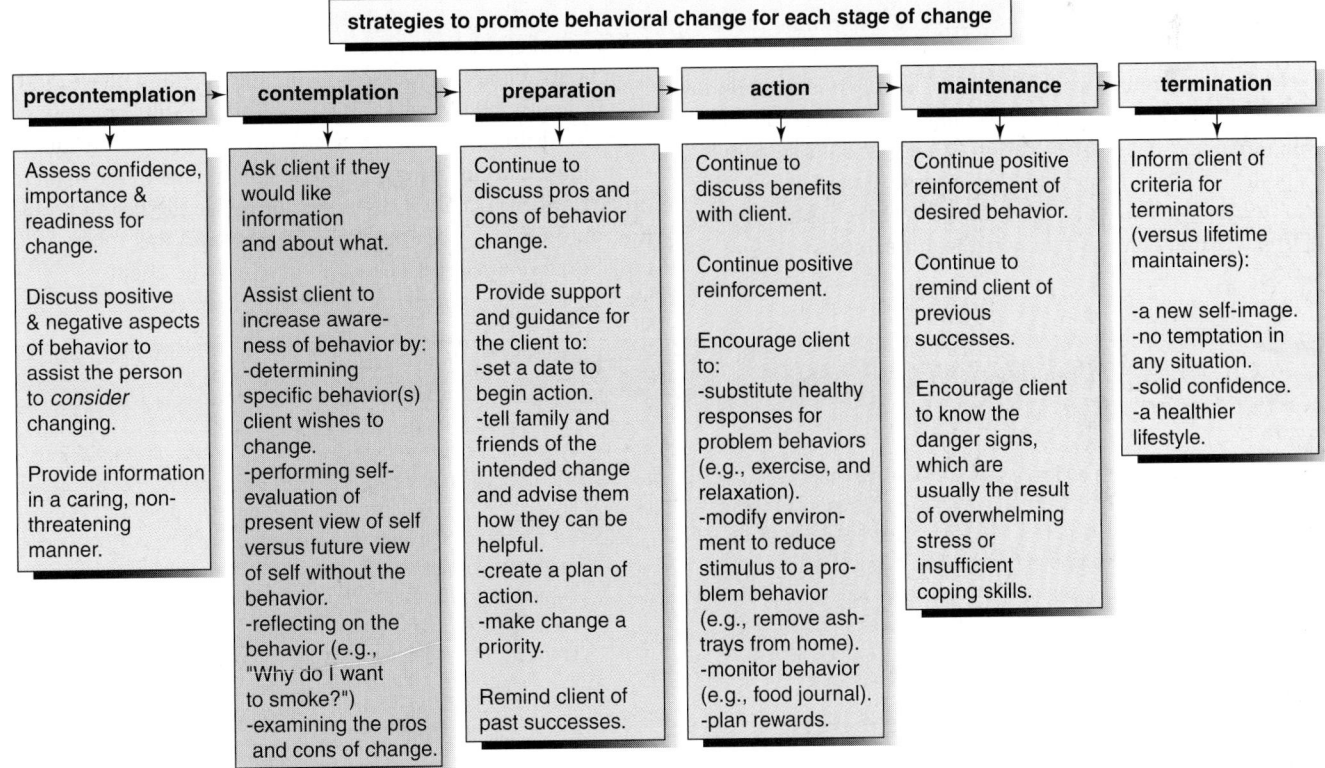

Figure 16-6 ■ Strategies to promote behavioral change for each stage of change.

PRACTICE GUIDELINES   Enhancing Behavior Change

ESTABLISH RAPPORT

■ Provide privacy and a perception of a collaborative, equal-power relationship.

■ If time allows, ask the client to describe a "typical" day. Usually the problematic behavior is described; however, even if it is not, the listening will strengthen rapport and the personal information may be helpful in understanding the client's current situation.

SET AGENDA

■ Allow the client to identify concerns. If there are multiple concerns (e.g., smoking, exercise, diet, stress), it is best to focus on one specific behavior at a time. Ask the client which behavior he or she feels most ready to *think* about changing.

ASSESS IMPORTANCE, CONFIDENCE, AND READINESS

■ A client's readiness to change is often influenced by his or her perception of importance and confidence.

■ Importance refers to the personal value of change. Questions that obtain this information can include: "How do you feel at the moment about [state the change]?" "How important is it to you to [state the change]?" "On a scale of 1 to 10, with 1 being not important and 10 very important, what number would you give yourself?"

■ Confidence relates to mastering the skills needed to achieve the behavior and the situations in which behavior change will be challenging to the client. A potential question to use to assess confidence is "If you decided right now to change, how confident would you feel about succeeding?"

EXCHANGE INFORMATION AND REDUCE RESISTANCE

■ These two tasks are performed throughout the various stages of behavior change.

■ Ask clients if they would like information and about what.

■ Present information in a neutral tone of voice, and avoid using the word "you" too much. Referring to other people (versus "you") and what happens to them makes the information less threatening to the client.

■ After presenting the information, ask for the client's interpretation of the information.

■ Three *traps* that increase resistance and *strategies to avoid the traps* include:

• Taking control away. *Instead,* emphasize personal choice and control.

• Misjudging importance, confidence, or readiness. Often this results in talking about action before the client is ready. It is important to *reexamine* the client's feelings about importance and confidence as they influence readiness to make a specific change.

• Meeting force with force. Instead of attacking or defending through argument, sit back and use reflective listening. Try to understand how the client is feeling. The resistance usually subsides and the discussion can move in a different direction.

Note: From *Health Behavior Change: A Guide for Practitioners,* by S. Rollnick, P. Mason, and C. Butler. Copyright © 1999, with permission from Elsevier.

MODELING. Through observing a model, the client acquires ideas for behavior and coping strategies that can be used with specific problems. The client is not expected to mimic the sequence of actions or behavior patterns of the model. The nurse and client should mutually select models with whom the client can identify, since the cultural and ethnic backgrounds and age of the nurse and client often differ. Models should be people the client respects. Nurses should also serve as models of wellness. To model effectively, nurses need to have a philosophy and lifestyle that demonstrate good health habits.

Evaluating

Evaluation takes place on an ongoing basis, both during the attainment of short-term goals and after the completion of long-term goals. Goals are written during the planning phase, and a date is determined for attaining the specific results or behaviors that are desired to promote health or prevent illness. During evaluation, the client may decide to continue with the plan, reorder priorities, change strategies, or revise the health protection promotion contract. Evaluation of the plan is a collaborative effort between the nurse and the client.

CRITICAL THINKING CHECKPOINT

Mr. W., a 50-year-old professional man, has pneumonia and is currently being treated with antibiotics. He smokes two packs of cigarettes a day. Since this bout of pneumonia he voices concern about his smoking and wonders if he should try to quit again. He states, "I've tried everything and nothing works. The longest I last is about one month." He admits to being 30 pounds overweight and states that his wife and he have started walking for 30 minutes every evening. His wife has also started making low-fat meals. He is concerned that if he quits smoking he will gain more weight.

1. What information/knowledge is important for the nurse to remember when assisting a client to advance to the next stage of change?

2. Each contact between a nurse and a client is an opportunity for health promotion. Based on the knowledge or key concepts listed above, what question(s) would you ask Mr. W.?

3. Mr. W. is in which stage of change relating to his cigarette smoking? What strategies could you, the nurse, consider?

See Critical Thinking Possibilities in Appendix A.

CHAPTER 16 **REVIEW**

CHAPTER HIGHLIGHTS

- Nursing involves viewing the client as an individual and in a holistic way.
- To ensure holistic health care, the nurse considers all components of health (health promotion, health maintenance, health education and illness prevention, and restorative-rehabilitative care) and recognizes that disturbance in one part of a person affects the whole being.
- Homeostasis is the tendency of the body to maintain a state of relative balance or constancy in response to a changing internal and external environment.
- Physiologic homeostasis is maintained by coordinated functioning of the autonomic nervous, endocrine, respiratory, cardiovascular, renal, and gastrointestinal systems.
- Homeostatic mechanisms regulate hormone secretion, fluid and electrolyte levels, the functions of body viscera, and metabolic processes that provide energy for the body.
- Psychologic homeostasis, or emotional well-being, is acquired or learned through the experience of living and interacting with others.
- Although each individual has unique characteristics, certain needs are common to all people.
- Maslow's hierarchy of human needs consists of five categories: physiologic (survival) needs, safety needs, love and belonging needs, self-esteem needs, and self-actualization needs.
- People vary in how they rank their needs at any given moment.
- *Healthy People 2010* (USDHHS, 2000) presents a comprehensive 10-year strategy for promoting health and preventing illness of both individuals and communities.
- Health promotion is defined as client behavior directed toward developing well-being and actualizing human health potential. Health protection is client behavior geared toward preventing illness, detecting it early, or maintaining function.
- The Health Promotion Model (Pender et al., 2006) is a competence- or approach-oriented model that depicts the multidimensional nature of persons interacting with their interpersonal and physical environments as they pursue health. The major motivational variables that can be modified through nursing interventions include perceived benefits of action, perceived barriers to action, perceived self-efficacy, activity-related affect, interpersonal influences, and situational influences.
- Prochaska et al. (1994, 2002) propose a six-stage model for health behavior change. The stages are (a) precontemplation,

(b) contemplation, (c) preparation, (d) action, (e) maintenance, and (f) termination. If the person is not successful in changing behavior, relapse occurs. However, at any point in these stages, people may move to any previous stage. An understanding of these stages enables the nurse to provide appropriate nursing interventions.

- The nurse's role in health promotion is to act as a facilitator of the process of assessing, evaluating, and understanding health. It is the opportunity for nurses to strengthen the profession's influence on health promotion, disseminate information that promotes an educated public, and assist individuals and communities to change long-standing adverse health behaviors.
- A complete and accurate assessment of the individual's health status is basic to health promotion. Lifestyle assessment tools give clients the opportunity to assess the impact of their present lifestyle behaviors on their health and to make decisions about specific lifestyle changes. Health risk appraisals provide the data that may influence the individual to adopt healthier life behaviors. Assessments or reviews of a client's spiritual health, social support, health beliefs, and life stress are also important because they impact a person's health.
- Organizing assessment data from individual and family assessments enables the nurse to make wellness diagnoses that identify client strengths, recognize self-care abilities, and enhance health promotion goals to help the client reach a higher level of functioning.
- Health promotion plans need to be developed according to the needs, desires, and priorities of the client.
- The nurse acts as a resource person, provides ongoing support, and supplies additional information and education in a nonjudgmental manner to help individuals change their lifestyles or health behaviors.
- As role models for their clients, nurses should have a philosophy and lifestyle that demonstrate good health habits.
- During the evaluation phase of the health promotion process, the nurse assists clients in determining whether they will continue with the plan, reorder priorities, or revise the plan.

TEST YOUR KNOWLEDGE

1. A nurse and a primary care provider inform a client that chemotherapy is recommended for the diagnosis of cancer. Which of the following nursing actions is most representative of the concept of holism?
   1. Offer to come to the client's home to provide needed physical care.
   2. Contact the client's spiritual adviser.
   3. Inquire how this will affect other aspects of the client's life.
   4. Provide the client with information about how to join a support group.

2. When a father prepares to leave for work in the morning, his 3-year-old son starts to cry and scream. The father picks him up and delays leaving for a while. The child's behavior most reflects which part of a system?
   1. Input
   2. Throughput

   3. Output
   4. Feedback

3. While hospitalized, a client is very worried about business activities. The client spends a great deal of time on the phone and with colleagues instead of resting. Which of the following principles of need therapy applies?
   1. His higher level need cannot be met unless the lower level physiologic need is met.
   2. His lower level physiologic needs are being deferred while higher needs are addressed.
   3. The higher need takes precedence and the lower need no longer must be met.
   4. It is necessary for someone else to meet his higher level needs so he can focus on the lower level need.

4. Which of the following statements best represents the contemplation stage of the stages of behavior change?
1. "I currently do not need to exercise and do not intend to start in the next 6 months."
2. "I have tried several times to exercise 30 minutes three times a week but am seriously thinking of trying again in the next month."
3. "I currently do not exercise 30 minutes three times a week, but I am thinking about starting to do so within the next 6 months."
4. "I have exercised 30 minutes three times a week regularly for more than 6 months."

5. A client who is 46 pounds overweight tells you, "I was just born to be fat. I don't have the willpower." Although weight loss occurred while attending two previous programs that "guaranteed" weight loss, the weight returned along with extra pounds after each program. According to the Health Promotion Model, the nurse is most likely to focus on which of the following behavior-specific cognitions and affects variable for this client?
1. Perceived barriers to action
2. Perceived self-efficacy
3. Interpersonal influences
4. Situational influences

6. Which of the following individuals would have an increased possibility of illness in the near future?
1. A 25-year-old man who recently married his high school sweetheart
2. A 35-year-old man who was fired from his job
3. A 40-year-old woman who started a nursing program
4. A 50-year-old woman whose husband died a month ago

7. The nurse who is assisting a client in the action stage of change would use which of the following strategies?

1. Reinforce the importance of providing rewards for positive behavior.
2. Ask the client if he or she would like information.
3. Guide the client to create a plan of action.
4. Remind the client of previous successes.

8. If a client fails to follow the information or teaching provided, how should the nurse respond?
1. Give up, as the client doesn't want to change.
2. Develop a tough approach.
3. Reteach the information, as the nurse is the expert.
4. Reassess the client's importance given to the behavior and readiness to change it.

9. A client is admitted for heart failure. The nurse assesses that the client's BP is below normal range and the apical pulse is 110. The nurse knows that the increase in the client's pulse illustrates which aspect of the client's homeostatic mechanism?
1. Compensation
2. Decompensation
3. Self-regulation
4. Equilibrium

10. Using Maslow's framework, which statement characterizes the highest level of need?
1. "Nurse, my pain is severe . . . is it time for my shot?"
2. "I felt welcomed when I first joined the group and I look forward to the monthly meetings."
3. "I'm very proud of receiving the Employee of the Month award."
4. "There have been home break-ins with burglary in our neighborhood. We are thinking of moving."

See Answers to Test Your Knowledge in Appendix A.

EXPLORE MEDIALINK www.prenhall.com/berman

DVD-ROM
- Audio Glossary
- NCLEX Review

COMPANION WEBSITE
- Additional NCLEX Review
- Case Study: Health Promotion Program
- Care Plan Activity: Health Promotion, Health Fair, and Nursing Students
- Application Activity
    Health Belief Model
- Links to Resources

READINGS AND REFERENCES

SUGGESTED READINGS
Daniels, J. (2006). Obesity: America's epidemic. *American Journal of Nursing, 106*(1), 40–49.
One of the goals of Healthy People 2010 is to reduce the percentage of obese adults to 15% and develop measures to prevent excess weight and obesity. This article explores the rising incidence of obesity in the United States, the reasons so many people fail to lose or maintain a weight loss, and the potential for nurses to help clients make lifestyle changes.
Haber, D. (2003). *Health promotion and aging. Practical applications for health professionals* (3rd ed.). New York: Springer.
This book is easy to read and includes humor (e.g., the 10-calorie diet). It is focused on

current research findings and practical applications which include health-promoting tools, illustrations, checklists, and tips. It is a basic, comprehensive review of health promotion topics and interventions when working with older adults.
MacPherson, S. L., Joseph, D., & Sullivan, E. (2004). The benefits of peer support with diabetes. *Nursing Forum, 39*(4), 5–12.
The authors describe a project to see if peer coaching assists a person with diabetes to make the correct diet and activity choices. The project involved a program aimed at helping people change behaviors using the Transtheoretical Model described in the chapter. The authors use an example of a

typical client in the program and how she moved between the stages of change. Once she was in the action stage, the authors described how the peer support moved the client to the maintenance stage. This article helps the reader understand the importance of assessing a client's stage of change and the relevance of peer support in health promotion.

RELATED RESEARCH
Berg, J. A. (2003). Mexican American women's willingness to promote health. *Journal of Multicultural Nursing & Health, 9*(2), 34–43.
Chalmers, K., Sequire, M., & Brown, J. (2003). Health promotion and tobacco control:

Student nurses' perspectives. *Journal of Nursing Education, 42*(3), 106–112.

Kim, S., Koniak-Griffin, D., Flaskerud, J. H., & Guarnero, P. A. (2004). The impact of lay health advisors on cardiovascular health promotion: Using a community-based participatory approach. *Journal of Cardiovascular Nursing, 19*(3), 192–199.

Padula, C. A., & McNatt, M. (2004). Older married couples and health promotion: Joint decision-making process for long-term spouses. *Journal of Gerontological Nursing, 30*(8), 38–46.

Stuifbergen, A. K., Becker, H., Timmerman, G. M., & Kullberg, V. (2003). The use of individualized goal setting to facilitate behavior change in women with multiple sclerosis. *Journal of Neuroscience Nursing, 35*(2), 94–106.

Yarcheski, A., Mahon, N. E., Yarcheski, T. J., & Cannella, B. L. (2004). A meta-analysis of predictors of positive health practices. *Journal of Nursing Scholarship, 36*(2), 102–108.

Yoon, S. L., & Horne, C. H. (2004). Perceived health promotion practice by older women. *Journal of Gerontological Nursing, 30*(7), 9–15.

REFERENCES

Cannon, W. B. (1939). *The wisdom of the body* (2nd ed.). New York: Norton.

Edelman, C. L., & Mandle, C. L. (2006). *Health promotion throughout the lifespan* (6th ed.). St. Louis, MO: Mosby.

Grunbaum, J. A., Kann, L., Kinchen, S., Ross, J., Hawkings, J., Lowry, R., et al. (2004, May 21). Youth risk behavior surveillance—United States, 2003. *MMWR Surveillance Summaries, 53* (No. SS-2), 1–96.

Holmes, T. H., & Rahe, T. H. (1967). The social readjustment rating scale. *Journal of Psychosomatic Research, 11*(8), 213–218.

Johnson, J. L., Kalaw, C., Lovato, C. Y., Baillie, L., & Chambers, N. A. (2004). Crossing the line:

Adolescents' experiences of controlling their tobacco use. *Qualitative Health Research, 14*(9), 1276–1291.

Kalish, R. A. (1983). *The psychology of human behavior* (5th ed.). Monterey, CA: Brooks/Cole.

Leavell, H. R., & Clark, E. G. (1965). *Preventive medicine for the doctor in the community* (3rd ed.). New York: McGraw-Hill.

Maslow, A. H. (1968). *Toward a psychology of being* (2nd ed.). New York: John Wiley & Sons.

Maslow, A. H. (1970). *Motivation and personality* (2nd ed.). New York: Harper & Row.

National Center for Health Statistics. (2004). *Health, United States, 2004. With chartbook on trends in the health of Americans.* Hyattsville, MD: Author.

North American Nursing Diagnosis Association. (2007). *Nursing diagnoses: Definitions & classification 2007–2008.* Philadelphia: Author.

Pender, N. J., Murdaugh, C. L., & Parsons, M. A. (2002). *Health promotion in nursing practice* (4th ed.). Upper Saddle River, NJ: Prentice Hall.

Pender, N. J., Murdaugh, C. L., & Parsons, M. A. (2006). *Health promotion in nursing practice* (5th ed.). Upper Saddle River, NJ: Prentice Hall.

Prochaska, J. O., Norcross, J. C., & DiClemente, C. C. (1994). *Changing for good: A revolutionary six-stage program for overcoming bad habits and moving your life positively forward.* New York: Avon Books/Harper Collins.

Prochaska, J. O., Redding, C. A., & Evers, K. E. (2002). The transtheoretical model and stages of change. In *Health behavior and health education: Theory, research, and practice* (3rd ed., pp. 99–120). San Francisco: Jossey-Bass.

Rollnick, S., Mason, P., & Butler, C. (1999). *Health behavior change. A guide for practitioners.* Edinburgh: Churchill Livingstone.

Saarmann, L., Daugherty, J., & Riegel, B. (2000). Patient teaching to promote behavioral change. *Nursing Outlook, 48*(6), 281–287.

Substance Abuse and Mental Health Services Administration. (2004). *Results from the 2003 national survey on drug use and health: National findings (Office of Applied Studies, NSDUH Series H-25,* DHHS Publications No. SMA 04-3964). Rockville, MD. U.S. Department of Health and Human Services, Substance Abuse and Mental Health Services Administration, Office of Applied Studies.

U.S. Department of Health and Human Services. (2000). *Healthy people 2010: Understanding and improving health* (2nd ed.). Washington, DC: U.S. Government Printing Office.

U.S. Surgeon General. (1979). *Healthy people: The surgeon general's report on health promotion and disease prevention* (DHHS Pub. No. 79-55071). Washington, DC: U.S. Government Printing Office.

SELECTED BIBLIOGRAPHY

Anspaugh, D. J., Hamrick, M. H., & Rosato, F. D. (2003). *Wellness: Concepts and applications* (5th ed.). New York: McGraw-Hill.

Gunderson, A. J., & Tomkowiak, J. M. (2004). Dynamic health promotion for the geriatric population. *Rehabilitation Nursing, 29*(2), 45–48.

Laverack, G. (2004). *Health promotion practice: Power & empowerment.* Thousand Oaks, CA: Sage Publications.

Murray, R. B., & Zentner, J. P. (2001). *Health promotion strategies through the life span* (7th ed.). Upper Saddle River, NJ: Prentice Hall.

Schenk, S., & Hartley, K. (2002). Nurse coach: Healthcare resource for this millennium. *Nursing Forum, 37*(3), 14–20.

CHAPTER 17

Health, Wellness, and Illness

LEARNING OUTCOMES

After completing this chapter, you will be able to:

1. Differentiate health, wellness, and well-being.

2. Describe five dimensions of wellness.

3. Compare various models of health outlined in this chapter.

4. Identify factors affecting health status, beliefs, and practices.

5. Describe factors affecting health care adherence.

6. Differentiate illness from disease and acute illness from chronic illness.

7. Identify Parsons' four aspects of the sick role.

8. Explain Suchman's stages of illness.

9. Describe effects of illness on individuals' and family members' roles and functions.

Nurses' understanding of health and wellness largely determines the scope and nature of nursing practice. Clients' health beliefs also influence their health practices. Some people think of health and wellness (or well-being) as the same thing or, at the very least, as accompanying one another. However, health may not always accompany well-being: A person who has a terminal illness may have a sense of well-being; conversely, another person may lack a sense of well-being yet be in a state of good health. For many years the concept of disease was the yardstick by which health was measured. In the late 19th century the "how" of disease (pathogenesis) was the major concern of health professionals. The 20th century focused on finding cures for diseases. Currently health care providers are increasing their emphasis on promoting health and wellness in individuals, families, and communities.

CONCEPTS OF HEALTH, WELLNESS, AND WELL-BEING

Health, wellness, and well-being have many definitions and interpretations. The nurse should be familiar with the most common aspects of the concepts and consider how they may be individualized with specific clients.

Health

Traditionally **health** was defined in terms of the presence or absence of disease. Nightingale defined health as a state of being well and using every power the individual possesses to the fullest extent (Nightingale, 1860/1969). The World Health Organization (WHO) takes a more holistic view of health. Its constitution defines health as "a state of complete physical, mental, and social well-being, and not merely the absence of disease or infirmity" (WHO, 1948). This definition

- Reflects concern for the individual as a total person functioning physically, psychologically, and socially. Mental processes determine people's relationship with their physical and social surroundings, their attitudes about life, and their interaction with others.
- Places health in the context of environment. People's lives, and therefore their health, are affected by everything they interact with—not only environmental influences such as climate and the availability of food, shelter, clean air, and water to drink, but also other people, including family, lovers, employers, co-workers, friends, and associates.

Health has also been defined in terms of role and performance. Talcott Parsons (1951), an eminent American sociologist and creator of the concept "sick role," conceptualized health as the ability to maintain normal roles.

In 1953, the (United States) President's Commission on Health Needs of the Nation made the following statement about health: "Health is not a condition; it is an adjustment. It is not a state but a process. The process adapts the individual not only to our physical but also our social environments" (President's Commission, 1953, p. 4). This definition emphasizes health as an adaptive process rather than a state.

In 1980, the American Nurses Association (ANA) defined health in its social policy statement as "a dynamic state of being in which the developmental and behavioral potential of an individual is realized to the fullest extent possible" (ANA, 1980, p. 5). In this definition, health is more than a state or the absence of disease; it includes striving toward optimal functioning. In 2004, the ANA also stated that health was "An experience that is often expressed in terms of wellness and illness, and may occur in the presence or absence of disease or injury" (2004, p. 48).

Personal Definitions of Health

Health is a highly individual perception. Consider the following examples of individuals who would probably say they are healthy even though they have physical impairments that some would consider an illness:

- A 15-year-old with diabetes takes injectable insulin each morning. He plays on the school soccer team and is editor of the high school newspaper.
- A 32-year-old is paralyzed from the waist down and needs a wheelchair for mobility. He is taking accounting at a nearby college and uses a specially designed automobile for transportation.
- A 72-year-old takes antihypertensive medications to treat high blood pressure. She bowls once a week, is a member of the neighborhood golf club, makes handicrafts for a local charity, and travels 2 months each year.

Many people define and describe health as the following:

- Being free from symptoms of disease and pain as much as possible
- Being able to be active and to do what they want or must
- Being in good spirits most of the time

These characteristics indicate that health is not something that a person achieves suddenly at a specific time. It is an ongoing

Figure 17-1 ■ Satisfaction with work enhances a sense of well-being and contributes to wellness.

process—a way of life—through which a person develops and encourages every aspect of the body, mind, and feelings to interrelate harmoniously as much as possible (see Figure 17-1 ■).

Many factors affect individual definitions of health. Definitions vary according to an individual's previous experiences, expectations of self, age, and sociocultural influences.

Nurses should be aware of their own personal definitions of health and appreciate that other people have their own individual definitions as well. A person's definition of health influences behavior related to health and illness. By understanding clients' perceptions of health and illness, nurses can provide more meaningful assistance to help them regain or attain a state of health. For aid in developing a personal definition of health, see Box 17–1.

Wellness and Well-Being

Wellness is a state of well-being. Basic aspects of wellness include self-responsibility; an ultimate goal; a dynamic, growing process; daily decision making in the areas of nutrition, stress management, physical fitness, preventive health care, and emotional health; and, most importantly, the whole being of the individual.

Anspaugh, Hamrick, and Rosato (2006) propose seven components of wellness (see Figure 17-2 ■). To realize optimal health and wellness, people must deal with the factors within each component:

The following questions can help nurses develop a personal definition of health.

■ Is a person more than a biophysiologic system?
■ Is health more than the absence of disease symptoms?
■ Is health the ability of an individual to perform work?
■ Is health the ability of an individual to adapt to the environment?
■ Is health a condition of a person's actualization?
■ Is health a state or a process?
■ Is health the effective functioning of self-care activities?
■ Is health static or changing?
■ Are health and wellness the same?
■ Are disease and illness different?
■ Are there levels of health?
■ Are wellness, health, and illness separate entities or points along a continuum?
■ Is health socially determined?
■ How do you rate your health and why?

■ *Physical.* The ability to carry out daily tasks, achieve fitness (e.g., pulmonary, cardiovascular, gastrointestinal), maintain adequate nutrition and proper body fat, avoid abusing drugs and alcohol or using tobacco products, and generally practice positive lifestyle habits.

REAL WORLD PRACTICE

Health, wellness, and illness are terms commonly used to indicate or measure the well-being of an individual. However, personal interpretation of these terms indicates that the definitions are highly subjective and can vary from client to client. Consider John, a 26-year-old paraplegic. His permanent condition may lead some to believe that a state of illness exists, or that a state of wellness is not experienced. However, John is gainfully employed, participates in various extracurricular activities, perceives himself as healthy, and enjoys a state of well-being. Variations in the definitions of health, wellness, and illness set the state for situations in which illness and wellness can co-exist. Consider Mary, an 84-year-old woman who is blind and has advanced rheumatoid arthritis, hypertension, and diabetes. She recognizes the limitations imposed by the diagnoses, but adheres to her health care plan and enjoys an active and fulfilling lifestyle. Conversely, Anita, a 75-year-old woman with the same diagnoses as Mary, considers herself ill and does not perceive herself as having the potential to experience wellness.

The client's perception of health, wellness, and illness must be considered in order to provide individualized, quality health care. Challenges may arise when the client's interpretation of these terms varies significantly from those of the health care professional. While it is important to value our own definitions, the views of the client must be kept in focus. Wellness may not necessarily co-exist with health; and the presence of illness does not negate the opportunity to experience wellness. Individualized interpretation of these terms sets the foundation for the provision of quality health care that best meets the needs of our clients.

—Carol Olff, MSN, RN, CCRN,
Clinical Coordinator, Neuro ICU
John Muir Health, Walnut Creek, CA

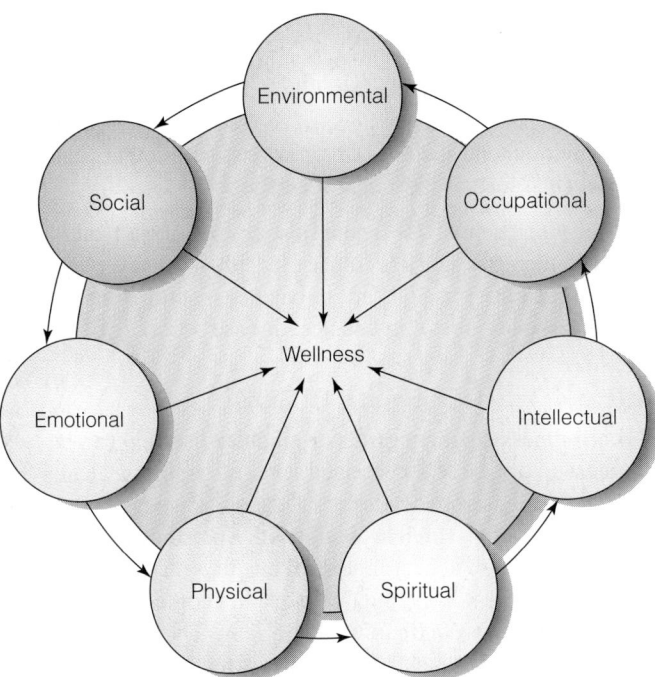

Figure 17-2 ■ The seven components of wellness.
(From *Wellness: Concepts and Applications,* 6th ed. (p. 4), by D. J. Anspaugh, M. H. Hamrick, and F. D. Rosato, copyright 2006. Reproduced with permission of the McGraw-Hill Companies.)

- *Social.* The ability to interact successfully with people and within the environment of which each person is a part, to develop and maintain intimacy with significant others, and to develop respect and tolerance for those with different opinions and beliefs.
- *Emotional.* The ability to manage stress and to express emotions appropriately. Emotional wellness involves the ability to recognize, accept, and express feelings and to accept one's limitations.
- *Intellectual.* The ability to learn and use information effectively for personal, family, and career development. Intellectual wellness involves striving for continued growth and learning to deal with new challenges effectively.
- *Spiritual.* The belief in some force (nature, science, religion, or a higher power) that serves to unite human beings and provide meaning and purpose to life. It includes a person's own morals, values, and ethics.
- *Occupational.* The ability to achieve a balance between work and leisure time. A person's beliefs about education, employment, and home influence personal satisfaction and relationships with others.
- *Environmental.* The ability to promote health measures that improve the standard of living and quality of life in the community. This includes influences such as food, water, and air.

The seven components overlap to some extent, and factors in one component often directly affect factors in another. For example, a person who learns to control daily stress levels from a physiologic perspective is also helping to maintain the emotional stamina needed to cope with a crisis. Wellness involves working on all aspects of the model.

"**Well-being** is a subjective perception of vitality and feeling well . . . can be described objectively, experienced, and measured . . . and can be plotted on a continuum" (Hood & Leddy, 2003, p. 264). It is a component of health.

MODELS OF HEALTH AND WELLNESS

Because health is such a complex concept, various researchers have developed models or paradigms to explain health and in some instances its relationship to illness or injury. Models can be helpful in assisting health professionals to meet the health and wellness needs of individuals. Nurses need to clarify their understanding of health, wellness, and illness for the following reasons:

- Nurses' definitions of health largely determine the scope and nature of nursing practice. For example, when health is defined narrowly as a physiologic phenomenon, nurses confine themselves to assisting clients to regain normal physiologic functioning. When health is defined more broadly, the scope of nursing practice enlarges correspondingly.
- People's health beliefs influence their health practices. A nurse's health values and practices may differ from those of a client. Nurses need to ensure that a plan of care developed for an individual relates to the client's conception of health rather than the nurse's belief system. Otherwise the client may fail to respond to the health care regimen.

Models of health include the clinical model, the role performance model, the adaptive model, the eudemonistic model, the agent-host-environment model, and health-illness continua.

Clinical Model

The narrowest interpretation of health occurs in the clinical model. People are viewed as physiologic systems with related functions, and health is identified by the absence of signs and symptoms of disease or injury. It is considered the state of not being "sick." In this model the opposite of health is disease or injury.

Many medical practitioners use the clinical model in their focus on the relief of signs and symptoms of disease and elimination of malfunction and pain. When these signs and symptoms are no longer present, the medical practitioner considers the individual's health restored.

Role Performance Model

Health is defined in terms of the individual's ability to fulfill societal roles, that is, to perform his or her work. People usually fulfill several roles (e.g., mother, daughter, friend), and certain individuals may consider nonwork roles paramount in their lives. According to this model, people who can fulfill their roles are healthy even if they have clinical illness. For example, a man who works all day at his job as expected is healthy even though an x-ray of his lung indicates a tumor. It is assumed in this model that sickness is the inability to perform one's work role.

Adaptive Model

In the adaptive model, health is a creative process; disease is a failure in adaptation, or maladaptation. The aim of treatment is to restore the ability of the person to adapt, that is, to cope. According to this model, extreme good health is flexible adaptation to the environment and interaction with the environment to maximum advantage. Sister Callista Roy's adaptation model of nursing (Roy, 1999) views the person as an adaptive system (see Chapter 3 ∞). The focus of this model is stability, although there is also an element of growth and change.

Eudemonistic Model

The eudemonistic model incorporates a comprehensive view of health. Health is seen as a condition of actualization or realization of a person's potential. Actualization is the apex of the fully developed personality, described by Abraham Maslow (see Chapter 16 ∞). In this model the highest aspiration of people is fulfillment and complete development, which is actualization. Illness, in this model, is a condition that prevents self-actualization.

Pender includes stabilizing and actualizing tendencies in her definition of health: "Health is the actualization of inherent and acquired human potential through goal-directed behavior, competent self-care, and satisfying relationships with others while adjustments are made as needed to maintain structural integrity and harmony with relevant environments" (Pender, Murdaugh, & Parsons, 2006, p. 23).

Agent-Host-Environment Model

The agent-host-environment model of health and illness, also called the ecologic model, originated in the community health work of Leavell and Clark (1965) and has been expanded into a general theory of the multiple causes of disease. The model is used primarily in predicting illness rather than in promoting wellness, although identification of risk factors that result from the interactions of agent, host, and environment are helpful in promoting and maintaining health. The model has three dynamic interactive elements (see Figure 17-3 ■):

1. *Agent.* Any environmental factor or stressor (biologic, chemical, mechanical, physical, or psychosocial) that by its presence or absence (e.g., lack of essential nutrients) can lead to illness or disease.
2. *Host.* Person(s) who may or may not be at risk of acquiring a disease. Family history, age, and lifestyle habits influence the host's reaction.

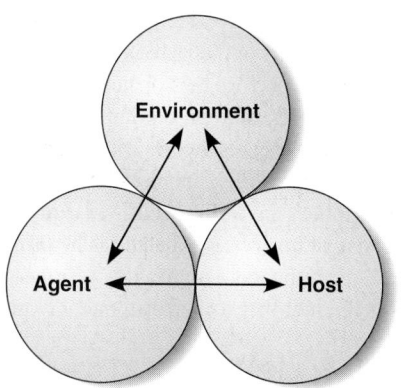

Figure 17-3 ■ The agent-host-environment triangle.

3. *Environment.* All factors external to the host that may or may not predispose the person to the development of disease. Physical environment includes climate, living conditions, sound (noise) levels, and economic level. Social environment includes interactions with others and life events, such as the death of a spouse.

Because each of the agent-host-environment factors constantly interacts with the others, health is an ever-changing state. When the variables are in balance, health is maintained; when variables are not in balance, disease occurs.

Health-Illness Continua

Health-illness continua (grids or graduated scales) can be used to measure a person's perceived level of wellness. Health and illness or disease can be viewed as the opposite ends of a health continuum. From a high level of health a person's condition can move through good health, normal health, poor health, and extremely poor health, eventually to death. People move back and forth within this continuum day by day. There is no distinct boundary across which people move from health to illness or from illness back to health. How people perceive themselves and how others see them in terms of health and illness will also affect their placement on the continuum. The ranges in which people can be thought of as healthy or ill are considerable.

Dunn's High-Level Wellness Grid

Dunn (1959) described a health grid in which a health axis and an environmental axis intersect. The grid demonstrates the interaction of the environment with the illness-wellness continuum (see Figure 17-4 ■). The health axis extends from peak wellness to death, and the environmental axis extends from very favorable to very unfavorable. The intersection of the two axes forms four quadrants of health and wellness:

1. *High-level wellness in a favorable environment.* An example is a person who implements healthy lifestyle behaviors and has the biopsychosocial, spiritual, and economic resources to support this lifestyle.
2. *Emergent high-level wellness in an unfavorable environment.* An example is a woman who has the knowledge to implement healthy lifestyle practices but does not implement adequate self-care practices because of family responsibilities, job demands, or other factors.
3. *Protected poor health in a favorable environment.* An example is an ill person (e.g., one with multiple fractures or severe hypertension) whose needs are met by the health care system and who has access to appropriate medications, diet, and health care instruction.
4. *Poor health in an unfavorable environment.* An example is a young child who is starving in a drought-stricken country.

Family wellness enhances wellness in individuals. In a well family that offers trust, love, and support, the individual does not have to expend energy to meet basic needs and can move forward on the wellness continuum. By providing effective sanitation and safe water, disposing of sewage safely, and preserving beauty and wildlife, the community enhances both family

Very favorable environment

Environmental

Protected poor health
(in favorable environment,
i.e., through social and
cultural institutions)

High-level wellness
(in favorable environment)

Death ●– – – Health – – – – – Axis – – – ● Peak wellness

Axis

Poor health
(in unfavorable
environment)

Emergent high-level wellness
(in unfavorable environment)

Very unfavorable environment

Figure 17-4 ■ Dunn's health grid: its axes and quadrants.

(From "High-Level Wellness for Man and Society," by H. L. Dunn, 1959, *American Journal of Public Health, 49*, p. 786–792. Reprinted with permission of American Public Health Association.)

and individual wellness. Environmental wellness is related to the premise that humans must be at peace with and guard the environment. Societal wellness is significant because the status of the larger, social group affects the status of smaller groups. Dunn believes that social wellness must be considered on a worldwide basis.

Travis's Illness-Wellness Continuum

The illness-wellness continuum (Figure 17-5 ■) developed by Travis ranges from high-level wellness to premature death (Travis & Ryan, 2001). The model illustrates two arrows pointing in opposite directions and joined at a neutral point. Movement to the right of the neutral point indicates increasing levels of health and well-being for an individual. This is achieved in

three steps: (a) awareness, (b) education, and (c) growth. In contrast, movement to the left of the neutral point indicates progressively decreasing levels of health. Travis and Ryan believe it is possible to be physically ill and at the same time oriented toward wellness, or be physically healthy and at the same time function from an illness mentality.

The model also compares the traditional treatment model with the wellness model. The former can help an individual move from the left only to the neutral point, where symptoms of the illness are alleviated. For example, a man who takes an antihypertensive medication to reduce blood pressure and relieve any associated symptoms moves to the neutral point. However, wellness-oriented measures such as reducing weight or ceasing to smoke are needed to move the person beyond the neutral point to a higher level of

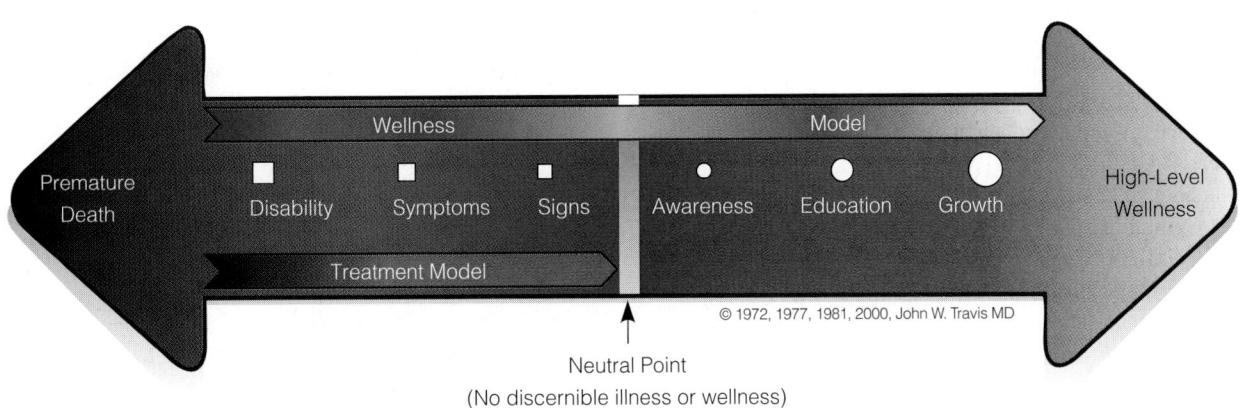

Figure 17-5 ■ Illness-wellness continuum.

(Reprinted with permission, *Wellness Workbook,* Travis & Ryan, Ten Speed Press, Berkeley, CA. © 1981, 1988 by John W. Travis, MD. www.thewellspring.com.)

wellness. Note that wellness interventions can be initiated at any point on the continuum. Thus, the wellness model and the treatment model can work together.

The 4+ Model of Wellness

A newer model, the 4+ model of wellness (Baldwin & Conger, 2001), consists of the four domains of the inner self—physical, spiritual, emotional, and intellectual—plus the elements of the outer systems (environment, culture, nutrition, safety, and many other elements). The nurse assesses the inner self for strengths and excesses, sources of nurturing and of depletion, and the interactions between the inner self and the outer systems. This model is useful when working with individuals, families, or communities.

VARIABLES INFLUENCING HEALTH STATUS, BELIEFS, AND PRACTICES

Many variables influence a person's health status, beliefs, and behaviors or practices. These factors may or may not be under conscious control. People can usually control their health behaviors and can choose healthy or unhealthy activities. In contrast, people have little or no choice over their genetic makeup, age, sex, culture, and sometimes their geographic environments. Box 17–2 differentiates health status, beliefs, and behaviors or practices.

Internal Variables

Internal variables include biologic, psychologic, and cognitive dimensions. They are often described as nonmodifiable variables because, for the most part, they cannot be changed. However, when internal variables are linked to health problems, the nurse must be even more diligent about working with the client to influence external variables (such as exercise and diet) that may assist in health promotion and prevention of illness. Regular health exams and appropriate screening for early detection of health problems become even more important.

Biologic Dimension

Genetic makeup, gender, age, and developmental level all significantly influence a person's health.

Genetic makeup influences biologic characteristics, innate temperament, activity level, and intellectual potential. It has been related to susceptibility to specific disease, such as diabetes and breast cancer. In some cases, genetic predisposition for health or illness is enhanced when parents are from the same ethnic genetic pool. For example, people of African heritage have a higher incidence of sickle-cell anemia and hypertension than the general population but may be less susceptible to malaria.

Gender influences the distribution of disease. Certain acquired and genetic diseases are more common in one sex than in the other. Disorders more common among females include osteoporosis and autoimmune disease such as rheumatoid arthritis. Those more common among males are stomach ulcers, abdominal hernias, and respiratory diseases.

Age is also a significant factor. The distribution of disease varies with age. For example, arteriosclerotic heart disease is

---

BOX 17–2 Health Status, Beliefs, and Behaviors

- **Health status.** State of health of an individual at a given time. A report of health status may include anxiety, depression, or acute illness and thus describe the individual's problem in general. Health status can also describe such specifics as pulse rate and body temperature.
- **Health beliefs.** Concepts about health that an individual believes are true. Such beliefs may or may not be founded on fact. Some of these are influenced by culture, such as the "hot-cold" system of some Hispanic Americans. In this system, health is viewed as a balance of hot and cold qualities within a person. Citrus fruits and some fowl are considered cold foods, and meats and bread are hot foods. In this context hot and cold do not denote temperature or spiciness but innate qualities of the food. For example, a fever is said to be caused by an excess of hot foods. Another example of a culturally related health belief is the belief that health and illness are closely associated with the amount and quality of blood in the body. For example, some Southerners say that "high blood," meaning too much blood in the body, causes headaches and dizziness. For additional information about cultural views of health and illness, see Chapter 18. ∞
- **Health behaviors.** The actions people take to understand their health state, maintain an optimal state of health, prevent illness and injury, and reach their maximum physical and mental potential. Behaviors such as eating wisely, exercising, paying attention to signs of illness, following treatment advice, avoiding known health hazards such as smoking, taking time for rest and relaxation, and managing one's time effectively are all examples.

  Health behavior is intended to prevent illness or disease or to provide for early detection of disease. Nurses preparing a plan of care with an individual need to consider the person's health beliefs before they suggest a change in health behaviors.

---

common in middle-aged males but occurs infrequently in younger people; such communicable diseases as whooping cough and measles are common in children but rare in elders, who have acquired immunity to them.

Developmental level has a major impact on health status. Consider these examples:

- Infants lack physiologic and psychologic maturity so their defenses against disease are lower during the first years of life.
- Toddlers who are learning to walk are more prone to falls and injury.
- Adolescents who need to conform to peers are more prone to risk-taking behavior and subsequent injury.
- Declining physical and sensory-perceptual abilities limit the ability of elders to respond to environmental hazards and stressors.

Psychologic Dimension

Psychologic (emotional) factors influencing health include mind-body interactions and self-concept.

Mind-body interactions can affect health status positively or negatively. Emotional responses to stress affect body function. For example, a student who is extremely anxious before a test may experience urinary frequency and diarrhea. A person worried about the outcome of surgery or about the behavior of a teenager may chain-smoke. Prolonged emotional distress may increase susceptibility to organic disease or precipitate it. Emotional distress may influence the immune system through central nervous system and endocrine alterations. Alterations in the immune system are related to the incidence of infections, cancer, and autoimmune diseases.

Increasing attention is being given to the mind's ability to direct the body's functioning. Relaxation, meditation, and biofeedback techniques are gaining wider recognition by individuals and health care professionals. For example, women often use relaxation techniques to decrease pain during childbirth. Other people may learn biofeedback skills to reduce hypertension.

Emotional reactions also occur in response to body conditions. For example, a person diagnosed with a terminal illness may experience fear and depression. *Self-concept* is how a person feels about self (self-esteem) and perceives the physical self (body image), needs, roles, and abilities. Self-concept affects how people view and handle situations. Such attitudes can affect health practices, responses to stress and illness, and the times when treatment is sought. An example is the anorexic woman who deprives herself of needed nutrients because she believes she is too fat even though she is well below an acceptable weight level. Self-concept is discussed in detail in Chapter 39 ∞ . Self-perceptions are also associated with a person's definition of health. For example, a 75-year-old man who can no longer move large objects as he was accustomed to do may need to examine and redefine his concept of health in view of his age and abilities.

Cognitive Dimension

Cognitive or intellectual factors influencing health include lifestyle choices and spiritual and religious beliefs.

Lifestyle refers to a person's general way of living, including living conditions and individual patterns of behavior that are influenced by sociocultural factors and personal characteristics. In brief, lifestyle is often considered as behavior and activities over which people have control. Lifestyle choices may have positive or negative effects on health. Practices that have potentially negative effects on health are often referred to as **risk factors.** For example, overeating, getting insufficient exercise, and being overweight are closely related to the incidence of heart disease, arteriosclerosis, diabetes, and hypertension. Excessive use of tobacco is clearly implicated in lung cancer, emphysema, and cardiovascular diseases. See Box 17–3 for examples of healthy lifestyle choices.

Spiritual and religious beliefs can significantly affect health behavior. For example, Jehovah's Witnesses oppose blood transfusions; some fundamentalists believe that a serious illness is a punishment from God; some religious groups are strict vegetarians; and religious Jews perform circumcision on the eighth day of a male baby's life. The influence of spirituality and religion is discussed further in Chapter 41. ∞

External Variables

External variables affecting health include the physical environment, standards of living, family and cultural beliefs, and social support networks.

BOX 17–3 Examples of Healthy Lifestyle Choices

- Regular exercise
- Weight control
- Avoidance of saturated fats
- Alcohol and tobacco avoidance
- Seat belt use
- Bike helmet use
- Immunization updates
- Regular dental checkups
- Regular health maintenance visits for screening examinations or tests

---

Environment

People are becoming increasingly aware of their environment and how it affects their health and level of wellness. Geographic location determines climate, and climate affects health. For instance, malaria and malaria-related conditions occur more frequently in tropical rather than temperate climates. Pollution of the water, air, and soil affects the health of cells. Pollution can occur naturally (e.g., lightning-caused fires produce smoke, which pollutes the air). Other substances in the environment, such as asbestos, are considered carcinogenic (i.e., they cause cancer). Tobacco is "hazardous to one's health," with rates of cancer higher among both smokers and those who live or work near smokers.

Another environmental hazard is radiation. The improper use of x-rays, for example, can harm many of the body's organs. Another common source of radiation is the sun's ultraviolet rays. Light-skinned people are more susceptible to the harmful effects of the sun than are dark-skinned people.

The main component of acid rain is sulfur dioxide, produced by ore smelters and related industries. The other components are nitrogen oxides. These emissions are thought by scientists to damage forests, lakes, and rivers.

Another environmental hazard that is receiving more attention is an increase in the "greenhouse effect." The glass roof of a greenhouse permits the sun's radiation to penetrate, but the resulting heat does not escape back through the glass. Carbon dioxide in the earth's atmosphere acts like the glass roof of a greenhouse, and as carbon dioxide levels increase due to industrial and automobile emissions, the surface temperature of the earth may also be increasing.

Other sources of environmental contamination are pesticides and chemicals used to control weeds and plant diseases. These contaminants can be found in some animals and plants that are subsequently ingested by people. In excessive levels, they are harmful to health.

Standards of Living

An individual's standard of living (reflecting occupation, income, and education) is related to health, morbidity, and mortality. Hygiene, food habits, and the propensity to seek health care advice and follow health regimens vary among high-income and low-income groups.

Low-income families often define health in terms of work; if people can work they are healthy. They tend to be fatalistic and believe that illness is not preventable. Because their present problems are so great and all efforts are exerted toward survival, an orientation to the future may be lacking.

The environmental conditions of poverty-stricken areas also have a bearing on overall health. Slum neighborhoods are overcrowded and in a state of deterioration. Sanitation services tend to be inadequate. Many streets are strewn with garbage, and rodents are common. Fires and crime are constant threats. Recreational facilities are almost nonexistent, forcing children to play in streets and alleys.

Occupational roles also predispose people to certain illnesses. For instance, some industrial workers may be exposed to carcinogenic agents. More affluent people may fulfill stressful social or occupational roles that predispose them to stress-related diseases. Such roles may also encourage overeating or social use of drugs or alcohol.

Family and Cultural Beliefs

The family passes on patterns of daily living and lifestyles to offspring. For example, a man who was abused as a child may physically abuse his own children. Physical or emotional abuse may cause long-term health problems. Emotional health depends on a social environment that is free of excessive tension and does not isolate the person from others. A climate of open communication, sharing, and love fosters the fulfillment of the person's optimum potential.

Culture and social interactions also influence how a person perceives, experiences, and copes with health and illness. Each culture has ideas about health, and these are often transmitted from parents to children. Heritage and cultural influences on health are discussed in detail in Chapter 18. ∞

People of certain cultures may perceive home remedies or tribal health customs as superior to and more dependable than the health care practices of North American society. For example, a person of Asian origin may prefer to use herbal remedies and acupuncture to treat pain rather than analgesic medications. Cultural rules, values, and beliefs give people a sense of being stable and able to predict outcomes. The challenging of old beliefs and values by second-generation cultural groups may give rise to conflict, instability, and insecurity, in turn contributing to illness.

Social Support Networks

Having a support network (family, friends, or a confidant) and job satisfaction helps people avoid illness. Support people also help the person confirm that illness exists. People with inadequate support networks sometimes allow themselves to become increasingly ill before confirming the illness and seeking therapy. Support people also provide the stimulus for an ill person to become well again.

HEALTH BELIEF MODELS

Several theories or models of health beliefs and behaviors have been developed to help determine whether an individual is likely to participate in disease prevention and health promotion activities. These models can be useful tools in developing programs for helping people change to healthier lifestyles and develop a more positive attitude toward preventive health measures (see also Chapter 16). ∞

Health Locus of Control Model

Locus of control (LOC) is a concept from social learning theory that nurses can use to determine whether clients are likely to take action regarding health, that is, whether clients believe that their health status is under their own or others' control. People who believe that they have a major influence on their own health status—that health is largely self-determined—are called *internals*. People who exercise internal control are more likely than others to take the initiative on their own health care, be more knowledgeable about their health, and adhere to prescribed health care regimens such as taking medication, making and keeping appointments with primary care providers, maintaining diets, and giving up smoking. By contrast, people who believe their health is largely controlled by outside forces (e.g., chance or powerful others) are referred to as *externals*.

Research has shown that locus of control plays a role in clients' choices about health behaviors. In some cases, externals demonstrate better adherence to medical regimens; in others, internals have better adherence. For example, Leong, Molassiotis, and Marsh (2004) found externals adhered better to weight loss regimens whereas internals adhered better to exercise programs.

RESEARCH NOTE   How Can Nurses Help Prevent Childhood Obesity?

The prevalence rate of obesity among children in the United States has been rising in recent years. Crawford and colleagues' (2004) pilot study aimed to improve the self-efficacy of staff counseling clients enrolled in the Women, Infants, and Children (WIC) program about childhood obesity. The study compared a sample of 51 WIC employees split into an intervention group that received educational sessions to help them identify ways to make changes in eating habits, activity information, and pedometers to promote the 10,000-steps-per-day program, and a control group. The intervention group was more likely to make healthy food choices when supported by the environment, to make positive changes in counseling parents about their children's weight issues, and to feel more confident in encouraging the WIC clients to be physically active with their own children.

IMPLICATIONS

Evidence suggests that overweight children have at least one associated biochemical or cardiovascular risk factor. The need for effective programs to help control America's growing waistline among our youngest citizens is becoming imperative. Chronic health issues such as obesity require the establishment of long-term supportive relationships between the nurse and the client. Nurses can contribute and encourage lifestyle alterations to improve client health by modeling behaviors, providing educational materials, and counseling.

Note: From "Walking the Talk: Fit WIC Wellness Programs Improve Self-Efficacy in Pediatric Obesity Prevention Counseling," by P. B. Crawford, W. Gosliner, P. Strode, S. E. Samuels, L. Craypo, C. Burnett, et al., 2004, American Journal of Public Health, 94, pp. 1480–1485.

Locus of control is a measurable concept that can be used to predict which people are most likely to change their behavior. Many measurement instruments are available to assess LOC. One widely used example is the Multidimensional Health Locus of Control (MHLC) Scale (Wallston, Wallston, & DeVellis, 1978), most recently expanded to Form C (Wallston, Stein, & Smith, 1994). Nurses can use LOC results to plan internal reinforcement training if necessary in order to improve client efforts toward better health.

Rosenstock's and Becker's Health Belief Models

In the 1950s Rosenstock (1974) proposed a health belief model intended to predict which individuals would or would not use preventive measures such as screening for early detection of cancer. Becker (1974) modified the health belief model to include these components: individual perceptions, modifying factors, and variables likely to affect initiating action. The health belief model (see Figure 17-6 ■) is based on motivational theory. Rosenstock (1974) assumed that good health is an objective common to all people. Becker added "positive health motivation" as a consideration.

Individual Perceptions

Individual perceptions include the following:

- *Perceived susceptibility.* A family history of a certain disorder, such as diabetes or heart disease, may make the individual feel at high risk.

- *Perceived seriousness.* In the perception of the individual, does the illness cause death or have serious consequences? For example, concern about the spread of acquired immune deficiency syndrome (AIDS) reflects the general public's perception of the seriousness of this illness.

- *Perceived threat.* According to Becker (1974), perceived susceptibility and perceived seriousness combine to determine the total perceived threat of an illness to a specific individual. For example, a person who perceives that many individuals in the community have AIDS may not necessarily perceive a threat of the disease; if the person is a drug addict or a homosexual, however, the perceived threat of illness is likely to increase because the susceptibility is combined with seriousness.

Modifying Factors

Factors that modify a person's perceptions include the following:

- *Demographic variables.* Demographic variables include age, gender, race, and ethnicity. An infant, for example, does not perceive the importance of a healthy diet; an adolescent may perceive peer approval as more important than family approval and as a consequence may participate in hazardous activities or adopt unhealthy eating and sleeping patterns.

- *Sociopsychologic variables.* Social pressure or influence from peers or other reference groups (e.g., self-help or vocational groups) may encourage preventive health behaviors even when individual motivation is low. Expectations

Figure 17–6 ■ The health belief model.

(From "Selected Psychosocial Models and Correlates of Individual Health-Related Behaviors," by M. H. Becker, et al., 1977, *Medical Care, 15*(5 Suppl), pp. 27–46. Reprinted with permission.)

of others may motivate people, for example, not to drive an automobile after drinking alcohol.

- *Structural variables.* Knowledge about the target disease and prior contact with it are structural variables that are presumed to influence preventive behavior. Becker (1974) found higher adherence rates with prescribed treatments among mothers whose children had frequent ear infections and occurrences of asthma.
- *Cues to action.* Cues can be either internal or external. Internal cues include feelings of fatigue, uncomfortable symptoms, or thoughts about the condition of an ill person who is close. External cues are listed in Figure 17–6.

Likelihood of Action

The likelihood of a person's taking recommended preventive health action depends on the perceived benefits of the action minus the perceived barriers to the action.

- *Perceived benefits of the action.* Examples include that in order to prevent lung cancer one refrains from smoking, and to maintain weight, one eats nutritious foods and avoids snacking.
- *Perceived barriers to action.* Examples include cost, inconvenience, unpleasantness, and lifestyle changes.

Nurses play a major role in helping clients implement healthy behaviors. They help clients monitor health, they supply anticipatory guidance, and they impart knowledge about health. Nurses can also reduce barriers to action (e.g., by minimizing inconvenience or discomfort) and can support positive actions.

Pender et al. (2006) have modified this health belief model to develop a health promotion model. According to Pender, the Health Belief Model explains health-protecting or preventive behaviors but does not emphasize health-promoting behaviors. See Pender's Health Promotion Model in Chapter 16. ∞

In addition to applying these models, the nurse uses other resources to evaluate options in planning interventions to maximize wellness. Two very useful documents developed by federal agencies are the *Guide to Community Preventive Services* from the Centers for Disease Control and Prevention and the third edition of the *Guide to Clinical Preventive Services* from the U.S. Public Health Service. A major emphasis in both sets of documents is providing evidence-based recommendations for practices and policies aimed at improving health. Both documents are updated as the data become available and can be retrieved from their respective websites.

BOX 17–4   Factors Influencing Adherence

- Client motivation to become well
- Degree of lifestyle change necessary
- Perceived severity of the health care problem
- Value placed on reducing the threat of illness
- Difficulty in understanding and performing specific behaviors
- Degree of inconvenience of the illness itself or of the regimens
- Beliefs that the prescribed therapy or regimen will or will not help
- Complexity, side effects, and duration of the proposed therapy
- Specific cultural heritage that may make adherence difficult
- Degree of satisfaction and quality and type of relationship with the health care providers
- Overall cost of prescribed therapy

HEALTH CARE ADHERENCE

Adherence is the extent to which an individual's behavior (for example, taking medications, following diets, or making lifestyle changes) coincides with medical or health advice. Degree of adherence may range from disregarding every aspect of the recommendations to following the total therapeutic plan. There are many reasons why some people adhere and others do not (see Box 17–4).

To enhance adherence, nurses need to ensure that the client is able to perform the prescribed therapy, understands the necessary instructions, is a willing participant in establishing goals of therapy, and values the planned outcomes of behavior changes. Examples of questions to be included in assessment are found in the Assessment Interview box.

When a nurse identifies nonadherence, it is important to take the following steps:

- *Establish why the client is not following the regimen.* Depending on the reason, the nurse can provide information, correct misconceptions, attempt to decrease expense, or suggest counseling if psychologic problems are interfering with adherence. It is also essential that the nurse reevaluate the suitability of the health advice provided. In situations where the client's cultural beliefs or age conflict with planned therapies, the nurse needs to consider ways to repattern and restructure care that will preserve and accommodate the client's practices. See "Providing Cultural Care" in Chapter 18. ∞
- *Demonstrate caring.* Show sincere concern about the client's problems and decisions and at the same time ac-

---

ASSESSMENT INTERVIEW   Determining the Risk for Medication Nonadherence

- Are you having side effects from any of your medications?
- Do you think your medications are helping?
- Do you have "tools" to remind you to take your medication? Examples could be an alarm or environmental cues (e.g., 6:00 news).
- Is there someone at home who helps you with your medications?
- How many times per day are your medications prescribed?

- How many pills do you take every day?
- Are there any special storage requirements for your medications?
- How much do your medication requirements interfere with your lifestyle?
- How well are you able to follow special dosing requirements?
- How many doses of your medications have you missed over the last 3 days?

cept the client's right to a course of action. For example, a nurse might tell a client who is not taking his heart medication, "I can appreciate how you feel about this, but I am very concerned about your heart."

- *Encourage healthy behaviors through positive reinforcement.* If the man who is not taking his heart medication is walking every day, the nurse might say, "You are really doing well with your walking."
- *Use aids to reinforce teaching.* For instance, the nurse can leave pamphlets for the client to read later or make a "pill calendar," a paper with the date and number of pills to be taken.
- *Establish a therapeutic relationship of freedom, mutual understanding, and mutual responsibility with the client and support persons.* By providing knowledge, skills, and information, the nurse gives clients control over their health and establishes a cooperative relationship, which results in greater adherence.

CLINICAL ALERT

Chronic illness often requires complicated treatment regimens for lengthy periods that may include significant adverse reactions and be very costly. Thus, clients with chronic illnesses may be at increased risk for treatment nonadherence. ■

Aspects influencing clients of varying ages are found in the Lifespan Considerations box.

ILLNESS AND DISEASE

Illness is a highly personal state in which the person's physical, emotional, intellectual, social, developmental, or spiritual functioning is thought to be diminished. It is not synonymous with disease and may or may not be related to disease. An individual could have a disease, for example, a growth in the stomach, and not feel ill. Similarly a person can feel ill, that is, feel uncomfortable, and yet have no discernible disease. Illness is highly subjective; only the individual person can say he or she is ill.

Disease can be described as an alteration in body functions resulting in a reduction of capacities or a shortening of the normal life span. Traditionally intervention by primary care providers has the goal of eliminating or ameliorating disease processes. Primitive people thought "forces" or spirits caused disease. Later this belief was replaced by the single-causation theory. Today multiple factors are considered to interact in causing disease and determining an individual's response to treatment.

The causation of a disease is called its **etiology.** A description of the etiology of a disease includes the identification of all causal factors that act together to bring about the particular disease. For example, the tubercle bacillus is designated as the biologic agent of tuberculosis. However, other etiologic factors, such as age, nutritional status, and even occupation, are involved in the development of tuberculosis and influence the course of infection. There are many diseases for which the cause is unknown (e.g., multiple sclerosis).

LIFESPAN CONSIDERATIONS   Medication Nonadherence

CHILDREN

Microbial resistance to antibiotics has increased significantly in recent years, making it critical that antibiotics given to children are necessary, administered correctly by parents in the home, and taken as prescribed. Providers, parents, and children must work together in order to increase the adherence rate in taking antibiotics.

Adherence is influenced by

- attitudes toward medications; some parents may think that when their child is feeling better, the medication is no longer necessary.
- past experience; children may remember a bad experience with taking a medication and resist parents' efforts to give an antibiotic.
- cost of medication; generic drugs are less costly than brand-name drugs, and can be equally effective.
- cultural issues; providers must work with families who have language or cultural differences to make sure they understand the family's needs and communicate the provider's recommendations.
- number of doses necessary; adherence improves if there are fewer doses per day, and fewer days that the antibiotic will be taken.
- taste and palatability; pharmaceutical companies continue to develop liquid medication that will be more acceptable to young children.

ADOLESCENTS

Several causes of nonadherence are specific to teenagers. It is important for the nurse to consider these when working with adolescents, because they

- don't consider the consequences of their actions.
- are in the early stages of problem solving.
- assert independence by rejecting adult values.
- conform to their peers and don't like being "different."
- focus on self-concept and body image.
- live in the "here and now."
- may regress developmentally at times of stress or illness.
- may be unable to distinguish benefits from disadvantages.

ELDERS

Issues that influence adherence in elders include the following:

- Lifestyle choices and individual responsibility for health maintenance
- Availability of home and community-based services to maximize independence
- Alternative/complementary therapies
- Housing and home modifications to accommodate the physical aspects of aging
- Affordable and accessible transportation
- Preventive nursing and medical care
- Available mental health services
- The caregiving crisis that overburdens some family and informal caregivers
- Forgetfulness
- Dementia
- Feeling that they have lived their life and it is time for life to end

Nurses have traditionally taken a holistic view of people and base their practice on the multiple-causation theory of health problems.

There are many ways to classify illness and disease; one of the most common is as acute or chronic. **Acute illness** is typically characterized by severe symptoms of relatively short duration. The symptoms often appear abruptly and subside quickly and, depending on the cause, may or may not require intervention by health care professionals. Some acute illnesses are serious (for example, appendicitis may require surgical intervention), but many acute illnesses, such as colds, subside without medical intervention or with the help of over-the-counter medications. Following an acute illness, most people return to their normal level of wellness.

A **chronic illness** is one that lasts for an extended period, usually 6 months or longer, and often for the person's life. Chronic illnesses usually have a slow onset and often have periods of **remission,** when the symptoms disappear, and **exacerbation,** when the symptoms reappear.

Examples of chronic illnesses are arthritis, heart and lung diseases, and diabetes mellitus. Nurses are involved in caring for chronically ill individuals of all ages in all types of settings—homes, nursing homes, hospitals, clinics, and other institutions. Care needs to be focused on promoting the highest level possible of independence, sense of control, and wellness. Clients often need to modify their activities of daily living, social relationships, and perception of self and body image. In addition, many must learn how to live with increasing physical limitations and discomfort.

Illness Behaviors

When people become ill, they behave in certain ways that sociologists refer to as illness behavior. **Illness behavior,** a coping mechanism, involves ways individuals describe, monitor, and interpret their symptoms, take remedial actions, and use the health care system. How people behave when they are ill is highly individualized and affected by many variables, such as age, sex, occupation, socioeconomic status, religion, ethnic origin, psychologic stability, personality, education, and modes of coping.

Parsons (1979) described four aspects of the sick role:

1. Clients are not held responsible for their condition.
2. Clients are excused from certain social roles and tasks.
3. Clients are obliged to try to get well as quickly as possible.
4. Clients or their families are obliged to seek competent help.

Suchman (1979) described five stages of illness: symptoms, sick role, medical care contact, dependent client role, and recovery or rehabilitation. Not all clients progress through each stage. For example, the client who experiences a sudden heart attack is taken to the emergency department and immediately enters stages 3 and 4, medical care contact and dependent client role.

Other clients may progress through only the first two stages and then recover. Details of Suchman's five stages follow.

Stage 1 Symptom Experiences

At this stage the person comes to believe something is wrong. Either someone significant mentions that the person looks unwell, or the person experiences some symptoms such as pain, rash, cough, fever, or bleeding. Stage 1 has three aspects:

- The physical experience of symptoms
- The cognitive aspect (the interpretation of the symptoms in terms that have some meaning to the person)
- The emotional response (e.g., fear or anxiety)

During this stage, the unwell person usually consults others about the symptoms or feelings, validating with a spouse or support people that the symptoms are real. At this stage the sick person may try home remedies. If self-management is ineffective, the individual enters the next stage.

Stage 2 Assumption of the Sick Role

The individual now accepts the sick role and seeks confirmation from family and friends. Often people continue with self-treatment and delay contact with health care professionals as long as possible. During this stage people may be excused from normal duties and role expectations. Emotional responses such as withdrawal, anxiety, fear, and depression are not uncommon depending on the severity of the illness, perceived degree of disability, and anticipated duration of the illness. When symptoms of illness persist or increase, the person is motivated to seek professional help.

Stage 3 Medical Care Contact

Sick people seek the advice of a health professional either on their own initiative or at the urging of significant others. When people seek professional advice they are really asking for three types of information:

- Validation of real illness
- Explanation of the symptoms in understandable terms
- Reassurance that they will be all right or prediction of what the outcome will be

The health professional may determine that the client does not have an illness or that an illness is present and may even be life threatening. The client may accept or deny the diagnosis. If the diagnosis is accepted, the client usually follows the prescribed treatment plan. If the diagnosis is not accepted, the client may seek the advice of other health care professionals or quasi-practitioners who will provide a diagnosis that fits the client's perceptions.

Stage 4 Dependent Client Role

After accepting the illness and seeking treatment, the client becomes dependent on the professional for help. People vary greatly in the degree of ease with which they can give up their independence, particularly in relation to life and death. Role obligations—such as those of wage earner, father, mother, student, baseball team member, or choir member—complicate the decision to give up independence.

Most people accept their dependence on the primary care provider, although they retain varying degrees of control over their own lives. For example, some people request precise information about their disease, their treatment, and the cost of treatment, and they delay the decision to accept treatment until they have all this information. Others prefer that the primary care provider proceed with treatment and do not request additional information.

For some clients illness may meet dependence needs that have never been met and thus provide satisfaction. Other people have minimal dependence needs and do everything possible to return to independent functioning. A few may even try to maintain independence to the detriment of their recovery.

Stage 5 Recovery or Rehabilitation

During this stage the client is expected to relinquish the dependent role and resume former roles and responsibilities. For people with acute illness, the time as an ill person is generally short and recovery is usually rapid. Thus most find it relatively easy to return to their former lifestyles. People who have long-term illnesses and must adjust their lifestyles may find recovery more difficult. For clients with a permanent disability, this final stage may require therapy to learn how to make major adjustments in functioning.

Effects of Illness

Illness brings about changes in both the involved individual and in the family. The changes vary depending on the nature, severity, and duration of the illness, attitudes associated with the illness by the client and others, the financial demands, the lifestyle changes incurred, adjustments to usual roles, and so on.

Impact on the Client

Ill clients may experience behavioral and emotional changes, changes in self-concept and body image, and lifestyle changes. Behavioral and emotional changes associated with short-term illness are generally mild and short lived. The individual, for example, may become irritable and lack the energy or desire to interact in the usual fashion with family members or friends. More acute responses are likely with severe, life-threatening, chronic, or disabling illness. Anxiety, fear, anger, withdrawal, denial, a sense of hopelessness, and feelings of powerlessness are all common responses to severe or disabling illness. For example, a client experiencing a heart attack fears for his life and the financial burden it may place on his family. Another client informed about a diagnosis of cancer or AIDS or crippling neurologic disease may, over time, experience episodes of denial, anger, fear, and hopelessness.

Certain illnesses can also change the client's body image or physical appearance, especially if there is severe scarring or loss of a limb or special sense organ. The client's self-esteem and self-concept may also be affected. Many factors can play a part in low self-esteem and a disturbance in self-concept: loss of body parts and function, pain, disfigurement, dependence on others, unemployment, financial problems, inability to participate in social functions, strained relationships with others, and spiritual distress. Nurses need to help clients express their thoughts and feelings, and to provide care that helps the client effectively cope with change.

Ill individuals are also vulnerable to loss of autonomy, the state of being independent and self-directed without outside control. Family interactions may change so that clients may no longer be involved in making family decisions or even decisions about their own health care. Nurses need to support clients' right to self-determination and autonomy as much as possible by providing them with sufficient information to participate in decision-making processes and to maintain a feeling of being in control.

Illness also often necessitates a change in lifestyle. In addition to participating in treatments and taking medications, the ill person may need to change diet, activity and exercise, and rest and sleep patterns.

Nurses can help clients adjust their lifestyles by these means:

- Providing explanations about necessary adjustments
- Making arrangements wherever possible to accommodate the client's lifestyle
- Encouraging other health professionals to become aware of the person's lifestyle practices and to support healthy aspects of that lifestyle
- Reinforcing desirable changes in practices with a view to making them a permanent part of the client's lifestyle

Impact on the Family

A person's illness affects not only the person who is ill but also the family or significant others. The kind of effect and its extent depend chiefly on three factors: (a) the member of the family who is ill, (b) the seriousness and length of the illness, and (c) the cultural and social customs the family follows.

The changes that can occur in the family include the following:

- Role changes
- Task reassignments and increased demands on time
- Increased stress due to anxiety about the outcome of the illness for the client and conflict about unaccustomed responsibilities
- Financial problems
- Loneliness as a result of separation and pending loss
- Change in social customs

See Chapter 24 for further information about the effects of illness on the family. ∞

MediaLink Health Promotion Activities in a Senior Citizen Residence Care Plan Activity

CRITICAL THINKING CHECKPOINT

Jerry and Joe have both suffered heart attacks. Jerry, upon advice from his physician, started exercising, changed his dietary intake, entered stress reduction classes, and returned to work 6 weeks after his heart attack. He has a positive outlook, is doing well, and talks about being "well." Joe also changed his dietary habits and started exercising. However, Joe has been unable to quit smoking even though he wants to and has been advised to do so. Joe is frequently despondent, is very fearful of having another heart attack, has not yet returned to work, and frequently talks about being "ill."

1. How does Jerry's psychologic dimension of health status differ from Joe's?

2. Both Jerry and Joe have heart disease. Jerry considers himself "well" whereas Joe considers himself "ill." Explain this phenomenon based on the health locus of control model.

3. What external factors may have influenced Jerry's decision to implement positive health behaviors?

4. What factors may have prevented Joe from developing the same positive outlook and actions that Jerry was able to take in regard to his illness?

5. What nursing interventions would be most beneficial to Joe concerning his smoking problem?

See Critical Thinking Possibilities in Appendix A.

CHAPTER 17 **REVIEW**

CHAPTER HIGHLIGHTS

- Nurses need to clarify their understanding of health because their definitions of health largely determine the scope and nature of nursing practice. Likewise, people's health beliefs influence their health practices.
- The perspective from which health is viewed has changed; instead of absence of disease, health has come to mean a high level of wellness or the fulfillment of one's maximum potential for physical, psychosocial, and spiritual functioning.
- Wellness is an active, seven-dimensional process of becoming aware of and making choices toward a higher level of well-being. The seven dimensions of wellness are the physical, social, emotional, intellectual, spiritual, occupational, and environmental dimensions.
- Well-being is considered a subjective perception of balance, harmony, and vitality. It is a state rather than a process.
- Most people describe health as freedom from symptoms of disease, the ability to be active, and a state of being in good spirits.
- Definitions of health and ability are culturally determined.
- Because notions of health are highly individual, the nurse must determine a client's perception of health in order to provide meaningful assistance. This involves well-developed communication skills. Nurses need to be aware of their own personal definitions of health.
- Various models have been developed to explain health: clinical, role performance, adaptive, and eudemonistic models and Leavell and Clark's agent-host-environment model, Dunn's high-level wellness grid, and Travis's illness-wellness continuum.
- The health status of a person is affected by many internal and external variables over which the person has varying degrees of control.
- Internal variables include biologic, psychologic, and cognitive dimensions. The biologic dimension includes genetic makeup, sex, age, and developmental level. The psychologic dimension includes mind-body interactions and self-concept. The cognitive dimension includes lifestyle choices and spiritual and religious beliefs.
- External variables influencing health are physical environment, standards of living, family and cultural beliefs, and social support networks.

- Health belief and behavior models have been developed to help determine whether an individual is likely to participate in disease prevention and health promotion activities. Two of these are the locus of control model and Rosenstock's and Becker's health belief models.
- A person's decision to implement health behaviors or to take action to improve health depends on such factors as the importance of health to the person, perceived threat of a particular disease or severity of the health care problems, perceived benefits of preventive or therapeutic actions, inconvenience and unpleasantness involved, degree of lifestyle change necessary, cultural ramifications, and cost.
- Nurses can enhance health care adherence by identifying the reasons for nonadherence if it occurs, demonstrating caring, using positive reinforcement to encourage healthy behaviors, using aids to reinforce teaching, and establishing a therapeutic relationship of freedom, mutual understanding, and mutual responsibility with the client and support persons.
- Illness is usually associated with disease but may occur independently of it. Illness is a highly personal state in which the person feels unhealthy or ill. Disease alters body functions and results in a reduction of capacities or a shortened life span.
- Various theorists have described stages and aspects of illness. Parsons describes four aspects of the sick role. Suchman outlines five stages of illness: symptom experience, assumption of the sick role, medical care contact, dependent client role, and recovery or rehabilitation.
- An individual's usual pattern of behavior changes with illness and hospitalization, which disrupt a person's privacy, autonomy, lifestyle, roles, and finances.
- Nurses need to be aware that the illness of one member of a family affects all other members.

TEST YOUR KNOWLEDGE

1. Which one of the following is an example of the emotional component of wellness?
   1. The client chooses health foods.
   2. A new father decides to take parenting classes.
   3. A client expresses frustration with her partner's substance abuse.
   4. A widow with no family decides to join a bowling league.

2. Which one of the following individuals appears to have "taken on" the sick role?
   1. An obese client states, "I deserve to have a heart attack."
   2. A mother is ill and says, "I won't be able to make your lunch today."
   3. A man with low back pain misses several physical therapy appointments.
   4. An elder states, "My horoscope says I will be well again."

3. Because a client recently diagnosed with diabetes mellitus is confident that blood sugar control can be improved with diet and exercise alone, and recently checked out a video on the management of diabetes at the HMO education center, the client's actions are most representative of which one of the following models:
   1. Health belief model
   2. Clinical model
   3. Role performance model
   4. Agent-host-environment model

4. Because a client with human immunodeficiency virus (HIV) is scheduled to begin several medications to manage the infection, the nurse will need to provide client education. Which of the following client characteristics is most likely to predict adherence with the treatment program? Mark all that apply.
   1. Educational level
   2. A trusting relationship with the health care provider
   3. An expectation that the medications will be helpful
   4. Being able to take the medications twice daily instead of four times daily
   5. Gender

5. Which one of the following might be the BEST way to measure adherence to a prescribed medication regime?
   1. Direct observation of medication administration
   2. Evidence of illness complications or exacerbations
   3. Monitoring laboratory values of elements influenced by the medication
   4. Questioning the client about his or her medication routine

See Answers to Test Your Knowledge in Appendix A.

EXPLORE MEDIALINK www.prenhall.com/berman

DVD-ROM
- Audio Glossary
- NCLEX Review

COMPANION WEBSITE
- Additional NCLEX Review
- Care Plan: Health Care Promotion in a Senior Citizen Residence
- Case Study: Nonadherent Diabetic Client
- Application Activity: Multidisciplinary Care and Resources
- Links to Resources

READINGS AND REFERENCES

SUGGESTED READINGS

Wardle, J., Haase, A., Steptoe, A., Nillapun, M., Jonwutiwes, K., & Bellisle, F. (2004). Gender difference in food choice: The contribution of health beliefs and dieting. *Annals of Behavioral Medicine, 27*(2), 107–116. *This study examined food choice behaviors in a large sample of young adults from 23 countries and tests two possible explanatory mechanisms for women's greater likelihood of dieting and women's greater beliefs in the importance of healthy diets. Health beliefs were found to explain 40% of the variation in dietary selections.*

RELATED RESEARCH

Cheadle, A., Senter, S., Procello, A., Pearson, D., Nelson, G.D., Greenwald, H.P., et al. (2005). The California Wellness Foundation's Health Improvement Initiative: Evaluation findings and lessons learned. *American Journal of Health Promotion, 19,* 286–296.

Javors, J., & Bramble, J. (2003). Uncontrolled chronic disease: Patient non-compliance or clinical mismanagement? *Disease Management, 6,* 169–178.

REFERENCES

American Nurses Association. (1980). *Nursing: A social policy statement.* Kansas City, MO: Author.

American Nurses Association. (2003). *Nursing: A social policy statement* (2nd ed.). Kansas City, MO: Author.

American Nurses Association. (2004). *Nursing: Scope and standards of practice.* Washington, DC: Author.

Anspaugh, D. J., Hamrick, M., & Rosato, F. D. (2006). *Wellness: Concepts and applications* (6th ed.). New York: McGraw-Hill.

Baldwin, J. H., & Conger, C. O. (2001). Health promotion and wellness. In K. S. Lundy & S. Janes (Eds.), *Community health nursing: Caring for the public's health* (pp. 286–307). Boston: Jones & Bartlett.

Becker, M. H. (Ed.). (1974). *The health belief model and personal health behavior.* Thorofare, NJ: Charles B. Slack.

Crawford, P. B., Gosliner, W., Strode, P., Samuels, S. E., Craypo, L., Burnett, C., et al. (2004). Walking the talk: Fit WIC wellness programs improve self-efficacy in pediatric obesity prevention counseling. *American Journal of Public Health, 94,* 1480–1485.

Dunn, H. L. (1959). High-level wellness for man and society. *American Journal of Public Health, 49,* 786–792.

Hood, L., & Leddy, S. K. (2003). *Leddy & Pepper's conceptual bases of professional nursing* (5th ed.). Philadelphia: Lippincott Williams & Wilkins.

Leavell, H. R., & Clark, E. G. (1965). *Preventive medicine for the doctor in his community* (3rd ed.). New York: McGraw-Hill.

Leong, J., Molassiotis, A., & Marsh, H. (2004). Adherence to health recommendations after a cardiac rehabilitation programme in post-myocardial infarction patients: The role of health beliefs, locus of control and psychological status. *Clinical Effectiveness in Nursing, 8*(1), 26–38.

Nightingale, F. (1969). *Notes on nursing: What it is, and what it is not.* New York: Dover Books. (Original work published 1860)

Parsons, T. (1951). *The social system.* Glencoe, IL: Free Press.

Parsons, T. (1979). Definitions of health and illness in the light of American values and social structure. In E. G. Jaco (Ed.), *Patients, physicians, and illness* (3rd ed.). New York: Free Press.

Pender, N. J., Murdaugh, C. L., & Parsons, M. J. (2006). *Health promotion in nursing practice* (5th ed.). Upper Saddle River, NJ: Prentice Hall.

President's Commission on Health Needs of the Nation. (1953). *Building Americans' health* (Vol. 2). Washington, DC: U.S. Government Printing Office.

Rosenstock, I. M. (1974). Historical origins of the health belief model. In M. H. Becker (Ed.), *The health belief model and personal health behavior.* Thorofare, NJ: Charles B. Slack.

Roy, C. (1999).*The Roy adaptation model* (2nd ed.). Upper Saddle River, NJ: Prentice Hall.

Suchman, E. A. (1979). Stages of illness and medical care. In E. G. Jaco (Ed.), *Patients, physicians, and illness* (3rd ed.). New York: Free Press.

Travis, J. W., & Ryan, R. S. (2001). *Simply well.* Berkeley, CA: Ten Speed Press.

Wallston, K. A., Stein, M. J., & Smith, C. A. (1994). Form C of the MHLC scales: A condition-specific measure of locus of control. *Journal of Personality Assessment, 63,* 534–553.

Wallston, K. A., Wallston, B. S., & DeVellis, R. (1978, Spring). Development of the Multidimensional Locus of Control (MHLC) scales. *Health Education Monographs, 6,* 160–170.

World Health Organization. (1948). *Preamble to the constitution of the World Health Organization as adopted by the International Health Conference.* New York, 19–22 June 1946; signed on 22 July 1946 by the representatives of 61 States (Official Records of the World Health Organization, no. 2, p. 100) and entered into force on 7 April 1948.

SELECTED BIBLIOGRAPHY

Briss, P. A., Brownson, R. C., Fielding, J. E., & Zaza, S. (2004). Developing and using the Guide to Community Preventive Services: Lessons learned about evidence-based public health. *Annual Review of Public Health, 25,* 281–302.

Coughlin, S. S., Uhler, R. J., Richards, T., & Wilson, K. M. (2003). Breast and cervical cancer screening practices among Hispanic and non-Hispanic women residing near the United States–Mexico border, 1999–2000. *Family & Community Health, 26*(2), 130–139.

Cross, M. (2004). CDC begins to provide resources for workplace wellness programs. *Managed Care, 13*(6), 54–55.

Goode, M., Wales, S., & Crisp, J. (2004). The role of specialist nurses in improving treatment adherence in children with a chronic illness. *Australian Journal of Advanced Nursing, 21*(4), 41–45.

Rosina, R., Crisp, J., & Steinbeck, K. (2003). Treatment adherence of youth and young adults with and without a chronic illness. *Nursing & Health Sciences, 5*(2), 139–147.

Toth, E., Mahumdar, S., Guirguis, L., Lawanczuk, R., Lee, T., & Johnson, J. (2003). Compliance with clinical practice guideline for type 2 diabetes in rural patients: Treatment gaps and opportunities for improvement. *Pharmacotherapy, 23,* 659–665.

Wu, A. M., Tang, C. S., & Kwok, T. C. (2004). Self-efficacy, health locus of control, and psychological distress in elderly Chinese women with chronic illnesses. *Aging & Mental Health, 8*(1), 21–28.

Culture and Heritage

LEARNING OUTCOMES

After completing this chapter, you will be able to:

1. Describe the role of federal agencies, initiatives, and laws on provision of cultural health care.

2. Discuss the components of culturally focused nursing, heritage consistency, and health traditions.

3. Describe examples of the different health views of culturally diverse people.

4. Differentiate biomedical care from folk healing.

5. Identify factors related to communication with culturally diverse clients and colleagues.

6. Recognize the core practice competencies of culturally competent nursing care.

7. Identify methods of heritage assessment.

8. Plan culturally sensitive, appropriate, and competent nursing interventions.

KEY TERMS

acculturation, *314*	**ethnic,** *315*	**race,** *314*
assimilation, *314*	**ethnocentrism,** *315*	**religion,** *315*
bicultural, *314*	**folk medicine,** *318*	**scientific health belief,** *318*
biomedical health belief, *318*	**heritage,** *312*	**socialization,** *316*
culturally appropriate, *313*	**heritage consistency,** *315*	**stereotyping,** *315*
culturally competent, *313*	**heritage inconsistency,** *315*	**subculture,** *314*
culturally sensitive, *313*	**holistic health belief,** *318*	**traditional,** *315*
culture, *312*	**interpreter,** *320*	**transcultural nursing,** *313*
culture shock, *315*	**magico-religious health**	**translator,** *320*
discrimination, *315*	**belief,** *317*	**xenophobia,** *315*
diversity, *314*	**prejudice,** *315*	

To provide quality care, nurses must become informed about and be sensitive to the culturally diverse subjective meanings of health, illness, caring, and healing practices. **Culture** can be defined as the nonphysical traits, such as values, beliefs, attitudes, and customs, that are shared by a group of people and passed from one generation to the next (Spector, 2004). Culture is also the "thoughts, communications, actions, customs, beliefs, values, and institutions of racial, ethnic, religious, or social groups" (Office of Minority Health [OMH], 2001, p. 131). Culture defines how health is perceived, how health care information is received, how rights and protections are exercised, what is considered to be a health problem, how symptoms and concerns about the health problem are expressed, who should provide treatment and how, and what kind of treatment should be given.

Nurses must be aware that, although people from a given group share certain beliefs, values, and experiences, often there is also widespread intragroup diversity. Major differences within groups may be due to such factors as age, gender, level of education, socioeconomic status, and area of origin in the home country (rural or urban). Such factors influence the client's beliefs about health and illness, practices, help-seeking behaviors, and expectations of nurses. For these reasons, effort must be made and care taken to avoid stereotyping people from a specific group.

The United States has been called a "melting pot" of peoples. However, the term *cultural mosaic* may be a more accurate description of the way in which many people of different cultures maintain the cultural values, beliefs, traditions, and practices of their **heritage** (things passed down from previous generations) for many generations. In addition to the indigenous peoples (Native Americans and Native Alaskans), much diversity is seen in the long-term resident populations and immigrant groups in North America.

CLINICAL ALERT

Culture and language are vital factors in how nursing care is delivered and received, and the diverse cultural needs of clients are expected to be met. ■

NATIONAL AGENCIES AND TRENDS

The demographic changes in the overall population of the United States and the influence of immigration on health services are major reasons for the immense need for culturally focused nursing care. The efforts described in the following list are evidence of increased emphasis on providing culturally appropriate health care.

- The U.S. Department of Health and Human Services US (DHHS) houses the Office of Minority Health "to improve and protect the health of racial and ethnic minority populations through the development of health policies and programs that will eliminate health disparities (n.d.)." In collaboration with other organizations, it developed the *National Standards for Culturally and Linguistically Appropriate Services in Health Care* (CLAS). Culture and language have a considerable impact on how clients access and respond to health care services.

- The Centers for Disease Control and Prevention (CDC) also has an Office of Minority Health to "promote health and quality of life by preventing and controlling the disproportionate burden of disease, injury and disability among racial and ethnic minority populations (n.d.)."

- The purpose of the National Center on Minority Health and Health Disparities (NCMHD) in the National Institutes of Health "is to promote minority health and to lead, coordinate, support, and assess the NIH effort to reduce and ultimately eliminate health disparities (n.d.)."

- The nursing profession plays a major role in REACH: Racial and Ethnic Approaches to Community Health, which strives to eliminate racial and ethnic disparities (inequalities) in infant mortality; in screening and management of breast and cervical cancer, cardiovascular diseases, diabetes, and HIV infections/AIDS; and in child and adult immunizations.

- One of the major goals of *Healthy People 2010* is to eliminate health disparities by gender, race or ethnicity, education, income, disability, geographic location, and sexual orientation (details of *Healthy People 2010* are discussed in Chapter 16 ∞). To achieve these goals, the Health Resources and Services Administration (HRSA) aims to increase the number of underrepresented racial and ethnic groups entering the nursing profession (Public Health Foundation, 2001).

- Current nursing practice has been largely influenced by the *National Healthcare Disparities Report*, which is a comprehensive overview of disparities in health care among racial, ethnic, and socioeconomic groups in the general U.S. population and among priority populations (Agency for Healthcare Research and Quality, 2005). This report indicates that, although the quality of health care has improved and differences in access and quality between whites and minorities have decreased overall, the quality and access disparity for Hispanics has widened.

Demographic Changes

Statistics of the ethnicity of the population can be complicated to interpret. The U.S. Census Bureau (2005a) revealed that in 2004, 98.5% of Americans identified themselves as belonging to a single race. Of the total, 80.4% identify themselves as white, 12.7% as black or African American, 4.2% as Asian, and 1% as American Indian or Alaska Native. Those Americans who indicated they were of Hispanic or Latino origin (which is different from race) were 14.1% of the total American population. Census Bureau projections (2004) are that the U.S. population overall will continue to increase by approximately 27 million persons each decade, and that by 2050, Hispanics will increase by 70 million to represent 24% of the total while White non-Hispanics will decrease from 69% to 50% of the total.

Nurses are predominantly White, and in percentage disproportionate to the demographic profile of the United States. Table 18–1 compares the percentages of American Indian, Asian/Pacific Islander, black non-Hispanic, Hispanic, and White non-Hispanic nurses in 2004 (US DHHS, 2004).

Immigration

According to the U.S. Census Bureau (2005b), the foreign-born population in the United States numbered 34.2 million in 2004, which corresponds to 12% of the total U.S. population. This is a 2.3% increase from 2003. Of these, 53% were born in Latin America (Central and South America), 25% in Asia, 14% in Europe, and the remaining 8% in other regions of the world. Second-generation Americans who were born in the United States but have one or both parents born in a foreign country accounted for 11% of the total U.S. population (30.4 million).

TABLE 18–1 Percentages of American Indian, Asian/Pacific Islander, Black Non-Hispanic, Hispanic, and White Non-Hispanic Nurses in 2004

POPULATION	PERCENT
American Indian/Alaska Native	0.4
Asian/Pacific Islander and other	3.3
Black non-Hispanic	4.6
Hispanic	1.8
White non-Hispanic	88.4
Two or more races	1.5

Note: From "The Registered Nurse Population: Preliminary Findings from the National Sample Survey of Registered Nurses, March 2004," by U.S. Department of Health and Human Services Health Resources and Service Administration Bureau of Health Professions. Retrieved April 21, 2006, from http://bhpr.hrsa.gov/healthworkforce/reports/rnpopulation/preliminaryfindings.htm

LIFESPAN CONSIDERATIONS
International Adoption

CHILDREN

International adoption of children by families in the United States is increasing, with over 150,000 children adopted in the past 14 years. These children present many challenges, and the care given by pediatric health providers can strongly influence the success with which they are assimilated into their new families. Understanding and assessing adopted children's potential issues early and intervening appropriately can lead to stronger family bonds. Children who arrive in the United States should be evaluated within 10 to 14 days for the following:

- Immunization history (blood titers may be appropriate)
- Infectious disease, parasites, general health (CBC, thyroid, liver function, and other blood work)
- Tuberculosis exposure (PPD)
- Developmental history and status, including speech, language, motor, and social development
- Vision and hearing
- Dental health

Note: Adapted from "International adoption: A health and developmental prospective," by P. Mason & C. Narad, 2005, *Seminars in Speech and Language, 26*(1), 1–9.

CULTURAL NURSING CARE

Responsibility for cultural health care is shared among "individuals, professional associations, regulatory bodies, health services delivery and accreditation organizations, educational institutions, and governments" (Canadian Nurses Association, 2004, p. 1). Professional nursing care is culturally sensitive, culturally appropriate, and culturally competent. This type of nursing is critical to meeting the complex nursing care needs of a given person, family, and community. It is the provision of nursing care across cultural boundaries and takes into account the context in which the client lives as well as the situations in which the client's health problems arise.

- **Culturally sensitive** implies that nurses possess some basic knowledge of and constructive attitudes toward the health traditions observed among the diverse cultural groups found in the setting in which they are practicing.
- **Culturally appropriate** implies that nurses apply the underlying background knowledge that must be possessed to provide a given client with the best possible health care.
- **Culturally competent** implies that, within the delivered care, nurses understand and attend to the total context of the client's situation and use a complex combination of knowledge, attitudes, and skills.

The term "transcultural nursing" has been promulgated by nurse Madeleine Leininger since the 1950s. **Transcultural nursing** focuses on providing care within the differences and similarities of the beliefs, values, and patterns of cultures (Leininger & McFarland, 2005). Leininger created the theory of culture care diversity and universality. Her transcultural research has involved international studies that have served the nursing profession by providing a framework to understand the needs of immigrants and multicultural populations in the United States and around the world.

Countless conflicts in the health care delivery arenas are predicated on cultural misunderstandings. Although many of these misunderstandings are related to universal situations, such as verbal and nonverbal language misunderstandings, the conventions of courtesy, sequencing of interactions, phasing of interactions, objectivity, and so forth, many cultural misunderstandings are unique to the delivery of nursing care. Cultural nursing care is essential and demands that nurses be able to assess and interpret a given client's health beliefs and practices and cultural needs. Cultural nursing care alters the perspective of nursing care delivery because it enables the nurse to understand, from a cultural perspective, the manifestations of the client's health care beliefs and practices.

CONCEPTS RELATED TO CULTURAL NURSING CARE

All groups of people face issues in adapting to their environment: providing nutrition and shelter, caring for and educating children, dividing labor, developing social organization, controlling disease, and maintaining health. Humans adapt to varying environments by developing cultural solutions to meet these needs. Culture is a universal experience, but no two cultures are exactly alike. Cultural patterns are learned, and it is important for nurses to note that members of a particular group may not share identical cultural experiences. Thus, each member of a cultural group will be somewhat different from his or her own cultural counterparts. For example, third-generation Japanese Americans (Sansei) will differ in cultural understandings from first-generation Japanese (Issei).

Subculture

Large cultural groups often have cultural subgroups or subsystems. A **subculture** is usually composed of people who have a distinct identity and yet are related to a larger cultural group. A subcultural group generally shares ethnic origin or physical characteristics with the larger cultural group. Examples of cultural subgroups include occupational groups (e.g., nurses), societal groups (e.g., feminists), and ethnic groups (e.g., Cajuns, who are descendants of French Acadians—17th-century settlers in Canadian Nova Scotia, New Brunswick, and Prince Edward Island).

Bicultural

Bicultural is used to describe a person who has dual patterns of identification and crosses two cultures, lifestyles, and sets of values (Spector, 2004). For example, a young man whose father is Cherokee and whose mother is European American may honor his traditional Cherokee heritage while also being influenced by his mother's cultural values. Another example exists in large areas of Canada where both British and French influences are strong.

Diversity

Diversity refers to the fact or state of being different. Many factors account for diversity: race, gender, sexual orientation, culture, ethnicity, socioeconomic status, educational attainment, religious affiliation, and so on. Diversity therefore occurs not only between cultural groups but also within a cultural group.

Acculturation

While becoming participants in the dominant culture, members of a nondominant cultural group are always identified as members of the culture from which they originate. People immigrating to the United States from any country will be associated with their native countries for many years, if not for all of their lives. The involuntary process of **acculturation** occurs when people adapt to or borrow traits from another culture. The member of the nondominant cultural group is often forced to learn the new culture to survive. Acculturation can also be defined as the changes of one's cultural patterns to those of the host society (Spector, 2004).

Assimilation

Assimilation is the process by which an individual develops a new cultural identity. Assimilation means becoming like the members of the dominant culture. The process of assimilation encompasses various aspects, such as behavioral, marital, identification, and civic. The underlying assumption is that the person from a given cultural group loses his or her original cultural identity to acquire the new one. In fact, because this is a conscious effort, it is not always possible, and the process may cause severe stress and anxiety. Assimilation can also be described as a collection of subprocesses: a process of inclusion through which a person gradually ceases to conform to any standard of life that differs from the dominant group standards and, at the same time, a process through which the person learns to conform to all the dominant group standards. The process of assimilation is considered complete when the foreigner is fully merged into the dominant cultural group (McLemore & Romo, 2005).

The concepts of assimilation and acculturation are complex and sensitive. The dominant society may expect that all immigrants are in the process of acculturation and assimilation and that the world view that we have as nurses is commonly shared by our clients. Because we live in a society with many cultures, however, many variations of health beliefs and practices exist.

Race

Race is the classification of people according to shared biologic characteristics, genetic markers, or features. People of the same race have common characteristics such as skin color, bone structure, facial features, hair texture, and blood type. Different ethnic groups can belong to the same race, and different cultures can be found within one ethnic group. For example, the terms *Caucasian* and *European American* describe the race of White people whose origins are in Europe. Whereas British Americans are a subgroup of European Americans, Scottish Americans (an ethnic subgroup of British Americans) may share different cultural practices than other British Americans. It is important to understand that not all people of the same race have the same culture. Culture should not be confused with either race or ethnic group. The U.S. Census in 2004 used the following categories as possible for race identification: White; Black; American Indian, Eskimo, or Aleut; Asian or Pacific Islander; and other. People of Hispanic or Latino origin can be of any race.

Prejudice

Prejudice is a negative belief or preference that is generalized about a group and that leads to "prejudgment." Prejudice occurs because either the person making the judgment does not understand the particular person or his or her heritage, or the person making the judgment generalizes an experience of one individual from a culture to all members of that group. It may also be referred to as racism. A related concept is **xenophobia**—the fear or dislike of people different from one's self.

Stereotyping

Stereotyping is assuming that all members of a culture or ethnic group are alike. For example, a nurse may assume that all Italians verbally express pain loudly or that all Chinese people like rice. Stereotyping may be based on generalizations founded in research, or it may be unrelated to reality. For example, research indicates that most Italians are likely to express pain verbally; however, a specific Italian client may not do so. Stereotyping that is unrelated to reality is frequently an outcome of racism or discrimination. Nurses need to realize that not all people of a specific group have the same health beliefs, practices, and values. It is therefore essential to identify a specific client's beliefs, needs, and values rather than assuming they are the same as those attributable to the larger group.

Ethnocentrism

Ethnocentrism is the belief that one's own culture or way of life is better than that of others. Ethnocentric individuals tend to view the world from their own cultural perspective and may have difficulty recognizing that others view the same world differently. Other viewpoints are considered not only different, but wrong or of lesser importance.

Discrimination

Discrimination, the differential treatment of individuals or groups based on categories such as race, ethnicity, gender, social class, or exceptionality, occurs when a person acts on prejudice and denies other persons one or more of their fundamental rights.

Culture Shock

Culture shock is a disorder that occurs in response to transition from one cultural setting to another. A person's former behavior patterns are ineffective in such a setting, and basic cues for social behavior are absent (Spector, 2004). This phenomenon may occur when one moves from one geographic location to another or when a person immigrates to a new country. It may occur when a person is admitted into a hospital and has to adapt to a foreign situation. Expressions of culture shock may range from

confusion and anxiety, to silence and immobility, to agitation, rage, or fury.

HERITAGE CONSISTENCY

Heritage consistency, a concept developed by Zitzow and Estes (1981), relates to the observance of beliefs and practices of a person's traditional cultural system (Spector, 2004). The concept has been expanded in an attempt to study the degree to which a person's lifestyle reflects his or her traditional culture, whether European, Asian, African, or Hispanic. The values indicating heritage consistency exist on a continuum, and a person can possess characteristics of both heritage consistency (**traditional**), that is, observance of the beliefs and practices of one's traditional cultural belief system; and **heritage inconsistency,** the observance of the beliefs and practices of one's acculturated (or modern) belief system. The model of heritage consistency has four overlapping components: culture, ethnicity, religion, and socialization.

Culture

Culture is a complex whole in which each part is related to every other part. It is learned, and the capacity to learn culture is genetic, but the subject matter is not genetic and must be learned by each person in his or her family and social community. Culture also depends on an underlying social matrix, including knowledge, belief, art, law, morals, and custom. Nursing involves the identification of cultural traits and the integration of such cultural elements in the delivery of care (Turton, 2003).

Ethnicity

Cultural background is a fundamental component of one's **ethnic** background or ethnicity, a group within the social system that claims to possess variable traits such as a common religion or language.

There are at least 106 groups in the United States that meet many of the characteristics of an ethnic group. People from every country in the world have immigrated to this country. Among the foreign-born peoples of the United States, the largest numbers of Latin American immigrants have come from Cuba, El Salvador, and Mexico; African immigrants from Egypt, Ghana, and Nigeria; Asian immigrants from China, India, and the Philippines; and European immigrants from the British Isles, Germany, and the former Soviet Union. The percent of the total numbers coming from a specific area have remained relatively constant during the past 15 years for some groups (e.g., Europe and the Caribbean), while others have experienced greater increases (e.g., Africa) (U.S. Census Bureau, 2005b).

Religion

The third major component of a person's heritage is religion. Although the word has many definitions, **religion** may be considered a system of beliefs, practices, and ethical values about divine or superhuman power or powers worshiped as the creator(s) and ruler(s) of the universe. The practice of religion is revealed in numerous cults, sects, denominations, and churches. Ethnicity and religion are clearly related, and one's religion

Figure 18-1 ■ Celebrations of the passage to adulthood are often based on culture or religion: for example, the Jewish bar mitzvah at age 13 and the Mexican quinceañera or "sweet fifteen" party.

quite often is determined by one's ethnic group (Figure 18-1 ■). Religion gives a person a frame of reference and a perspective with which to organize information. Religious teachings about health help to present a meaningful philosophy and system of practices within a system of social controls having specific values, norms, and ethics. Illness is sometimes seen as the punishment for the violation of religious codes and morals. It is not possible to isolate the aspects of culture, religion, and ethnicity that shape a person's worldview. Each is part of the other, and all three are united within the person. See Chapter 41 ∞ for more information on spirituality.

Socialization

Socialization is the process of being raised within a culture and acquiring the characteristics of that group. Education—be it elementary school, high school, college, or nursing—is a form of socialization. For many people who have been socialized within the boundaries of a traditional culture or a nonmodern culture (usually associated with the East or third world nations), modern "American," or Western, first world culture becomes a second cultural identity. Those who immigrate here from non-Western or nonmodern countries may find socialization into the American culture to be an extremely difficult and painful process. As time passes, many people experience biculturalism and divided loyalties. In addition, many people who have been socialized in cultures wherein traditional health care resources are used may prefer to use this type of care even when residing within a cultural setting with modern health care resources available.

SELECTED PARAMETERS FOR CULTURAL NURSING CARE

This section outlines selected phenomena of significance to nursing. Information about cultural aspects of death and dying are found in Chapter 43 and about pain management in Chapter 46. ∞

HEALTH Traditions Model

The HEALTH traditions model (Spector, 2004) is predicated on the concept of holistic health and describes what people do from a traditional perspective to maintain, protect, and restore health. Imagine health as a complex, interrelated, threefold phenomenon, that is, the balance of all aspects of the person—the body, mind, and spirit.

- The body includes all physical aspects, such as genetic inheritance, body chemistry, gender, age, nutrition, and physical condition.
- The mind includes cognitive processes, such as thoughts, memories, and knowledge of such emotional processes as feelings, defenses, and self-esteem.
- The spiritual facet includes both positive and negative learned spiritual practices and teachings, dreams, symbols, stories, protecting forces, and metaphysical or native forces.

These aspects are in constant flux and change over time, yet each is completely related to the others and also related to the context of the person. The context includes the person's family, culture, work, community, history, and environment (Spector, 2004).

The HEALTH traditions model, Table 18–2, consists of nine interrelated facets, represented by the following:

1. *Traditional methods of maintaining HEALTH*—physical, mental, and spiritual—include following a proper diet and wearing proper clothing, concentrating and using the mind, and practicing one's religion.
2. *Traditional methods of protecting HEALTH*—physical, mental, and spiritual—include wearing protective objects, such as amulets, avoiding people who may cause trouble, and placing religious objects in the home.

TABLE 18–2 **The Nine Interrelated Facets of Health (Physical, Mental, and Spiritual) and Personal Methods of Maintaining Health, Protecting Health, and Restoring Health**			
	PHYSICAL	**MENTAL**	**SPIRITUAL**
MAINTAIN HEALTH	Proper clothing Proper diet Exercise/rest	Concentration Social and family support systems Hobbies	Religious worship Prayer Meditation

PROTECT HEALTH	Special foods and food
	  combination
	Symbolic clothing
		Avoid certain people who can
		  cause illness
		Family activities
			Religious customs
			Superstitions
			Wearing amulets and other
			  symbolic objects to prevent
			  the "Evil Eye" or defray other
			  sources of harm

RESTORE HEALTH	Homeopathic remedies Liniments Herbal teas Special foods Massage Acupuncture/moxibustion	Relaxation Exorcism Curanderos and other traditional healers Nerve teas	Religious rituals, special prayers Meditation Traditional healings Exorcism

Note: From *Cultural Diversity in Health and Illness,* 6th ed. (p. 76) by R. E. Spector, 2004, Upper Saddle River, NJ: Prentice Hall.

3. *Traditional methods of restoring HEALTH*—physical, mental, and spiritual—include the use of herbal remedies, exorcism, and healing rituals.

Symbolic Examples

Figure 18-2 ■ depicts symbolic, HEALTH-related images that may be used to maintain, protect, or restore physical, mental, or spiritual HEALTH by people of different heritages.

1. Thousand-year-old eggs, from China, represent traditional foods that may be eaten daily to maintain physical HEALTH.
2. The enjoyment of nature, the natural environment, may be a universal way of maintaining mental HEALTH.

Figure 18-2 ■ Symbols of the HEALTH traditions model and themes.
(From *Cultural Diversity in Health and Illness,* 6th ed., by R. E. Spector, 2004, p. 73, Upper Saddle River, NJ: Prentice Hall.)

3. The Islamic prayer, from East Jerusalem, represents prayer, a way of maintaining spiritual HEALTH.
4. Red string, from the Tomb of Rachel in Bethlehem, Israel, may be worn to protect physical HEALTH.
5. The eye, from Cuba, represents the plethora of eye-related objects that may be worn or hung in the home to protect the mental HEALTH of people by shielding them from the envy and bad wishes of others.
6. The thunderbird, from the Hopi nation, may be worn for spiritual protection and good luck.
7. The herbal remedy, from Africa, represents aromatic plants that may be used by people from all ethnocultural traditional backgrounds as one method of restoring physical HEALTH.
8. Tiger balm, from Singapore, represents substances that are used in massage therapy as a way of restoring mental HEALTH.
9. Rosary beads, from Italy, symbolize prayer and meditation methods used in the spiritual restoration of HEALTH.

There are an infinite number of examples one could present. A major aspect of conducting the heritage assessment of a client is to determine what items are used by a specific person and its meaning to the person.

Health Beliefs and Practices

Three views of health beliefs include magico-religious, scientific, and holistic. In the **magico-religious health belief** view, health and illness are controlled by supernatural forces. The client may believe that illness is the result of "being bad" or opposing God's will. Getting well is also viewed as dependent on God's will. The client may make statements such as "If it is God's will, I will recover" or "What did I do wrong to be punished with cancer?" Some cultures believe that magic can cause illness. A sorcerer or witch may put a spell or hex on the client. Some people view illness as possession by an evil spirit. Although these beliefs are not supported by empirical evidence, clients who believe that such things can cause illness may in fact become ill as a result. Such illnesses may require magical treatments in addition to scientific treatments. For example, a man who experiences gastric distress, headaches, and hypertension after being told that a spell has been placed on him may recover only if the spell is removed by the culture's healer.

The **scientific** or **biomedical health belief** is based on the belief that life and life processes are controlled by physical and biochemical processes that can be manipulated by humans. The client with this view will believe that illness is caused by germs, viruses, bacteria, or a breakdown of the human machine, the body. This client will expect a pill, or treatment, or surgery to cure health problems.

The **holistic health belief** holds that the forces of nature must be maintained in balance or harmony. Human life is one aspect of nature that must be in harmony with the rest of nature. When the natural balance or harmony is disturbed, illness results. The medicine wheel is an ancient symbol used by Native Americans of North and South America to express many concepts. For health and wellness, the medicine wheel teaches the four aspects of the individual's nature: the physical, the mental, the emotional, and the spiritual. The four dimensions must be in balance to be healthy. The medicine wheel can also be used to express the individual's relationship with the environment as a dimension of wellness.

The concept of yin and yang in the Chinese culture and the hot–cold theory of illness in many Spanish cultures are examples of holistic health beliefs. When a Chinese client has a yin illness or a "cold" illness such as cancer, the treatment may include a yang or "hot" food (e.g., hot tea).

What is considered hot or cold varies considerably across cultures. In many cultures, the mother who has just delivered a baby should be offered warm or hot foods and kept warm with blankets because childbirth is seen as a "cold" condition. Conventional scientific thought recommends cooling the body to reduce a fever. The primary care provider may order liquids for the client and cool compresses to be applied to the forehead, the axillae, or the groin. Many cultures believe that the best way to treat a fever is to increase elimination of toxins through sweat baths (Fontaine, 2005). Clients from these cultures may want to cover up with several blankets, take hot baths, and drink hot beverages. The nurse must keep in mind that a treatment strategy that is consistent with the client's beliefs may have a better chance of being successful. For example, the Latino client who avoids "hot" foods when experiencing a stomach disturbance may be eating foods consistent with the bland diet that is normally prescribed by primary care providers.

Sociocultural forces, such as politics, economics, geography, religion, and the predominant health care system, influence the client's health status and health care behavior. For example, people who have limited access to scientific health care may turn to folk medicine or folk healing. **Folk medicine** is defined as those beliefs and practices relating to illness prevention and healing that derive from cultural traditions rather than from modern medicine's scientific base. Many persons have special teas or "cures" (such as chicken soup) used by older family members to prevent or treat colds, fevers, indigestion, and other common health problems. Why do individuals use nontraditional healing methods? Folk medicine is thought to be more humanistic than biomedical health care. The consultation and treatment takes place in the community of the recipient, frequently in the home of the healer. It may be less expensive than scientific or biomedical care. The healer often prepares the treatments, for example, herbs to be ingested, poultices to be applied, or charms or amulets to be worn. A frequent component of treatment is some ritual practice on the part of the healer or the client to cause healing to occur. Because folk healing is more culturally based, it is often more comfortable and less frightening for the client.

CLINICAL ALERT

Treatments once considered to be folk treatments, including acupuncture, therapeutic touch, and massage, are now being investigated for their therapeutic effect. The National Center for Complementary and Alternative Medicine at the National Institutes of Health provides up-to-date information on this line of research. ■

It is important for the nurse to obtain information about folk or family healing practices that may have been used before or while the client used Western medical treatment. Often clients are reluctant to disclose the use of home remedies with health care professionals for fear of being laughed at or rebuked. However, a study on complementary and alternative medicine (CAM) use among adults in 2002 indicated that 62% of adults in the United States had used some form of CAM therapy during the previous 12 months when the definition of CAM therapy included prayer specifically for health reasons (Barnes, Powell-Griner, McFann, & Nahin, 2004). When prayer was excluded, 36% of adults reported using CAM healing practices. The increased use of alternative healing practices in the United States represents an opportunity for nurses to inform clients about what the nursing profession offers in this regard (see Chapter 19). ∞

Family Patterns

The family is the basic unit of society. Cultural values can determine communication within the family group, the norm for family size, and the roles of specific family members. In some families, the man is considered the provider and decision maker. The woman may need to consult her husband before making decisions about her medical treatment or the treatment of her children. Some families are matriarchal; that is, the mother or grandmother is viewed as the leader of the family and is usually the decision maker. The nurse needs to identify who has the "authority" to make decisions in a client's family. If the decision maker is someone other than the client, the nurse needs to include that person in health care discussions.

The value placed on children and elders within a society is culturally derived. In some cultures, children are not disciplined by spanking or other forms of physical punishment. Rather, children are allowed to interact with their environment while caregivers provide subtle direction to prevent harm or injury. In other cultures, elders are considered the holders of the culture's wisdom and are therefore highly respected. Responsibility for caring for older relatives is determined by cultural practices. In many cultures, older relatives who cannot live independently live with a married son or daughter and family.

Cultural gender-role behavior may also affect nurse–client interactions. In some countries, men dominate and women have little status. Men from these countries may not accept instruction from a female nurse or primary care provider but will be receptive to the same instruction given by a male primary care provider or nurse. Some cultures have a prevailing concept of machismo, or male superiority. The positive aspects of machismo require that the adult man provide for and protect his family, including extended family members. The woman is expected to maintain the home and raise the children.

Cultural family values may also dictate the extent of the family's involvement in the hospitalized client's care. In some cultures, only the nuclear and the extended family will want to visit for long periods and participate in care. In other cultures, the entire community may want to visit and participate in the client's care. This can cause concern on nursing units with strict visiting policies. The nurse should evaluate the positive benefits of family participation in the client's care and modify visiting policies as appropriate.

Cultures that value the needs of the extended family as much as those of the individual may believe that personal and family information must stay within the family. Some cultural groups are very reluctant to disclose family information to outsiders, including health care professionals. This attitude can present difficulties for health care professionals who require knowledge of family interaction patterns to help clients with emotional problems.

Naming systems in many cultures differ from those in North America. In some cultures (e.g., Japanese and Vietnamese), the family name comes first and the given name second. One or two names may be added between the family and given names. Other nomenclature may be used to delineate gender, child, or adult status. For example, in traditional Japanese culture, adults address other adults by their surname followed by *san,* meaning *Mr., Mrs.,* or *Miss.* An example is Maurakami san. The children are referred to by their first names followed by *kun* for boys and *chan* for girls. Sikhs and Hindus traditionally have three names. Hindus have a personal name, a complimentary name, and then a family name. Sikhs have a personal name, then the title *Singh* for men and *Kaur* for women, and lastly the family name. Names by marriage also vary. In Central America, a woman who marries retains her father's name and takes her husband's. For example, if Louisa Viccario marries Carlos Gonzales she becomes Louisa Viccario de Gonzales. The connecting *de* means "belonging to." Their son is Pedro Gonzales Viccario. Nurses need to become familiar with appropriate ways to address clients.

Communication Style

Communication and culture are closely interconnected. Through communication, the culture is transmitted from one generation to the next, and knowledge about the culture is trans-

mitted within the group and to those outside the group. Communicating effectively with clients of various ethnic and cultural backgrounds is critical to providing culturally competent nursing care. There are cultural variations in both verbal and nonverbal communication.

Verbal Communication

The most obvious cultural difference is in verbal communication: vocabulary, grammatical structure, voice qualities, intonation, rhythm, speed, pronunciation, and silence. In North America, the dominant language is English; however, immigrant groups who speak English still encounter language differences because English words can have different meanings in different English-speaking cultures. For example, in the United States, a *boot* is a type of footwear that comes to the ankle or higher; in England, a boot can also be the trunk of a car. Spanish is spoken by people in several regions of the world: Spain, South America, Central America, Mexico, the Caribbean, and the Philippines, for example. It is the second most commonly spoken language in the United States. Nevertheless, each cultural group that speaks Spanish may use different vocabulary, apply rules of grammar differently, and use different pronunciation, so that often two people of different Latino cultures, speaking Spanish together, may not completely understand each other.

Initiating verbal communication may be influenced by cultural values. The busy nurse may want to complete nursing admission assessments quickly. The client, however, may be offended when the nurse immediately asks personal questions. In some cultures, social courtesies should be established before business or personal topics are discussed. Discussing general topics can convey that the nurse is interested and has time for the client. This enables the nurse to develop a rapport with the client before progressing to discussion that is more personal.

Verbal communication becomes even more difficult when an interaction involves people who speak different languages. Both clients and health professionals experience frustration when they are unable to communicate verbally with each other. Techniques for therapeutic communication with persons who have limited English are shown in the accompanying Practice Guidelines.

PRACTICE GUIDELINES

Verbal Communication with Clients Who Have Limited Knowledge of English

- Avoid slang words, medical terminology, and abbreviations.
- Augment spoken conversation with gestures or pictures to increase the client's understanding.
- Speak slowly, in a respectful manner, and at a normal volume. Speaking loudly does not help the client understand and may be offensive.
- Frequently validate the client's understanding of what is being communicated. Do not automatically interpret a client's smiling and nodding to mean that the client understands; the client may only be trying to please the nurse and not understand what is being said.

For the client whose language is not the same as that of the health care provider, an intermediary may be necessary. A **translator** converts written material (such as client education pamphlets) from one language into another. An **interpreter** is "an individual who mediates spoken or signed communication between people speaking different languages without adding, omitting, or distorting meaning or editorializing. The objective of the professional interpreter is for the complete transfer of the thought behind the utterance in one language into an utterance in a second language" (California Healthcare Interpreters Association, 2002, p. 70). Thus, a true interpreter has demonstrated ethical and interpreting skills and the knowledge and expertise required to function in a health care situation. In some states, mandates require hospitals to have certified interpreters available for clients who require them. Many institutions that are located in culturally diverse communities have translators available on staff or maintain a list of employees who are fluent in other languages. Embassies, consulates, ethnic churches (e.g., Russian Orthodox, Greek Orthodox), ethnic clubs (e.g., Polish American Club, Italian American Club), or telephone companies may also be able to provide interpreters. However, asking a family member or other nonprofessional to interpret can create difficulties. Cultural rules often dictate who can discuss what with whom. The first program in the United States to provide a master's degree in Health Interpreting and Health Applied Linguistics (HIHAL) has been established at the University of North Texas Health Science Center at Fort Worth, School of Public Health. Guidelines for using an interpreter are shown in the Practice Guidelines.

Nurses and other health care providers must remember that clients for whom English is a second language may lose command of their English when they are in stressful situations. Clients who have used English comfortably for years in social and business communication may forget and revert back to their primary language when they are ill or distressed. It is important for the nurse to assure the client that this is normal and to promote behaviors to facilitate verbal communication.

CLINICAL ALERT

Nurses who speak a second language may be asked to interpret for others. Nursing schools and health care institutions may not permit nursing students to interpret for consent for a procedure because limited knowledge about the procedure may lead the student to give inaccurate information. Check the institution's policy before agreeing to interpret for institutional staff and physicians. ■

Nonverbal Communication

To communicate effectively with culturally diverse clients, the nurse needs to be aware of two aspects of nonverbal communication behaviors: what nonverbal behaviors mean to the client and what specific nonverbal behaviors mean in the client's culture. Before assigning meaning to nonverbal behavior, the nurse must consider the possibility that the behavior may have a different meaning for the client and the family. To provide safe and

PRACTICE GUIDELINES
Using an Interpreter

- Avoid asking a member of the client's family, especially a child or spouse, to act as interpreter. The client, not wishing family members to know about his or her problem, may not provide complete or accurate information.
- Be aware of gender and age differences; it is preferable to use an interpreter of the same gender as the client to avoid embarrassment and faulty translation of sexual matters.
- Avoid an interpreter who is politically or socially incompatible with the client. For example, a Bosnian Serb may not be the best interpreter for a Muslim, even if he speaks the language.
- Address the questions to the client, not to the interpreter.
- Ask the interpreter to translate as closely as possible the words used by the nurse.
- Speak slowly and distinctly. Do not use metaphors, for example, "Does it swell like a grapefruit?" or "Is the pain stabbing like a knife?"
- Observe the facial expressions and body language that the client assumes when listening and talking to the interpreter.
- Become aware of the individual expressions and colloquial words used in specific regions and acknowledge them when using interpreting services.

effective care, nurses who work with specific cultural groups should learn more about cultural behavior and communication patterns within these cultures.

Nonverbal communication can include the use of silence, touch, eye movement, facial expressions, and body posture. Some cultures are quite comfortable with long periods of silence, whereas others consider it appropriate to speak before the other person has finished talking. Many people value silence and view it as essential to understanding a person's needs or use silence to preserve privacy. Some cultures view silence as a sign of respect, whereas to other people silence may indicate agreement.

Touching involves learned behaviors that can have both positive and negative meanings. In the American culture, a firm handshake is a recognized form of greeting that conveys character and strength. In some European cultures, greetings may include a kiss on one or both cheeks. In some societies, touch is considered magical and because of the belief that the soul can leave the body on physical contact, casual touching is forbidden. In some Asian cultures (e.g., people from India, Sri Lanka, Thailand, and Laos), only certain elders are permitted to touch the head of others, and children are never patted on the head. Nurses should therefore touch a client's head only with permission.

Cultures dictate what forms of touch are appropriate for individuals of the same and opposite gender. In many cultures, for example, a kiss is not appropriate for a public greeting between persons of the opposite sex, even those who are family members; however, a kiss on the cheek is acceptable as a greeting among individuals of the same sex. The nurse should watch interaction among clients and families for cues to the appropriate degree of touch in that culture. The nurse can also assess the client's response to touch when providing nursing care, for example, by noting the client's reaction to the physical examination or the bath.

Facial expression can also vary between cultures. Italian, Jewish, African American, and Spanish-speaking persons are more likely to smile readily and use facial expression to communicate feelings, whereas Irish, English, and Northern European people tend to have less facial expression and are less open in their response, especially to strangers (Spector, 2004). Facial expressions can also convey a meaning opposite to what is felt or understood.

Eye movement during communication has cultural foundations. In Western cultures, direct eye contact is regarded as important and generally shows that the other is attentive and listening. It conveys self-confidence, openness, interest, and honesty. Lack of eye contact may be interpreted as secretiveness, shyness, guilt, lack of interest, or even a sign of mental illness. However, other cultures may view eye contact as impolite or an invasion of privacy. In the Hmong culture, continuous direct eye contact is considered rude, but intermittent eye contact is acceptable. The nurse should not misinterpret the character of the client who avoids eye contact.

Body posture and hand gestures are also culturally learned. For example, the V sign means victory in some cultures, but it is an offensive gesture in other cultures. Tapping the index finger on one's temple may mean someone is intelligent in the United States but crazy in Holland.

Communication is an essential part of establishing a relationship with a client and his or her family. It is also important for developing effective working relationships with health care colleagues. To enhance their practice, nurses can observe the communication patterns of clients and colleagues and be aware of their own communication behaviors.

Space Orientation

Space is a relative concept that includes the individual, the body, the surrounding environment, and objects within that environment. The relationship between the individual's own body and objects and persons within space is learned and is influenced by culture. For example, in nomadic societies, space is not owned; it is occupied temporarily until the tribe moves on. In Western societies people tend to be more territorial, as reflected in phrases such as "This is my space" or "Get out of my space." In Western cultures, spatial distances are defined as the intimate zone, the personal zone, and the social and public zones. The size of these areas may vary with the specific culture. Nurses move through all three zones as they provide care for clients. The nurse needs to be aware of the client's response to movement toward the client. The client may physically withdraw or back away if the nurse is perceived as being too close. The nurse will need to explain to the client why there is a need to be close. To assess the lungs with a stethoscope, for example, the nurse needs to move into the client's intimate space. The nurse should first explain the procedure and await permission to continue.

Clients who reside in long-term care facilities, or who are hospitalized for an extended time, may want to personalize their space. They may want to arrange their room differently or control the placement of objects on their bedside cabinet or overbed table. The nurse should be responsive to clients' needs to have some control over their space. When there are no medical contraindications, clients should be permitted and encouraged to have objects of personal significance. Having personal and cultural items in one's environment can increase self-esteem by promoting not only one's individuality but also one's cultural identity. Of course, the nurse should caution the client about responsibility for loss of personal items.

Time Orientation

Time orientation refers to an individual's focus on the past, the present, or the future. Most cultures include all three time orientations, but one orientation is more likely to dominate. The American focus on time tends to be directed to the future, emphasizing time and schedules. Nursing students know what times they must be in class or clinical. They know what courses they will take in future semesters. European Americans often plan for next week, their vacation, or their retirement. Other cultures may have a different concept of time. For example, the Navajo Indians do not have a word for "late" and a Navajo mother may not become upset if her child does not achieve a specific developmental milestone, such as walking or toileting, on schedule.

The culture of nursing and health care values time. Appointments are scheduled, and treatments are prescribed with time parameters (e.g., changing a dressing once a day). Medication orders include how often the medicine is to be taken and when (e.g., digoxin 0.25 mg, once a day, in the morning). Nurses need to be aware of the meaning of time for clients. When caring for clients who are "present oriented," it is important to avoid fixed schedules. The nurse can offer a time range for activities and treatments. For example, instead of telling the client to take digoxin every day at 10:00 AM, the nurse might tell the client to take it every day in the morning or every day after getting out of bed.

Nutritional Patterns

Most cultures have staple foods that are plentiful or readily accessible in the environment. For example, the staple food of Asians is rice; of Italians, pasta; and of Eastern Europeans, wheat. Even clients who have been in the United States or Canada for several generations often continue to eat the foods of their cultural homeland.

The way food is prepared and served is also related to cultural practices. For example, in the United States a traditional food served for the Thanksgiving holiday is stuffed turkey; however, in different regions of the country the contents of the stuffing may vary. In Southern states, the stuffing may be made of cornbread; in New England, of seasoned bread and chestnuts.

The way in which staple foods are prepared also varies. For example, some Asian cultures prefer steamed rice; others prefer boiled rice. Southern Asians from India prepare unleavened bread from wheat flour rather than the leavened bread of European Americans.

Food-related cultural behaviors can include whether to breast-feed or bottle-feed infants, and when to introduce solid foods to them. Food can also be considered part of the remedy for illness. Foods classified as "hot" foods or foods that are hot in temperature may be used to treat illnesses that are classified as "cold" illnesses. For example, corn meal (a "hot" food) may be used to treat arthritis (a "cold" illness). Each culture group defines what it considers to be hot and cold entities.

Religious practice associated with specific cultures also affects diet. Some Roman Catholics avoid meat on certain days, such as Ash Wednesday and Good Friday, and some Protestant faiths prohibit meat, tea, coffee, or alcohol. Both Orthodox Judaism and Islam prohibit the ingestion of pork or pork products. Orthodox Jews observe kosher customs, eating certain foods only if they have been inspected by a rabbi and prepared according to dietary laws. For example, the eating of milk products and meat products at the same meal is prohibited. Some Buddhists, Hindus, and Sikhs are strict vegetarians. The nurse must be sensitive to such religious dietary practices.

PROVIDING CULTURAL NURSING CARE

All phases of the nursing process are affected by the client's and the nurse's cultural values, beliefs, and behaviors. As the client's culture and the nurse's culture come together in the nurse–client relationship, a unique cultural environment is created that can improve or impair the client's outcome. Self-awareness of personal biases can enable nurses to develop modifying behaviors or (if they are unable to do so) to remove themselves from situations where care may be compromised. Nurses can become more aware of their own culture through values clarification (see Chapter 5 ∞). The nurse must also consider the cultural values dominant in the health care setting because those, too, may influence the client's outcome.

Campinha-Bacote's model of cultural competence (2003) is also of special relevance to understand the core practice competences of culturally appropriate nursing care. This model is based on a framework that integrates transcultural nursing, medical anthropology, and multicultural counseling. In this model, nurses are encouraged to integrate into their practice the following five constructs: (a) cultural awareness, (b) cultural knowledge, (c) cultural skills, (d) cultural encounters, and (e) cultural desires. According to this model, nurses need to have a desire to become culturally competent and sensitive, as well as actively look for opportunities and experiences that are cross-cultural. Box 18–1 lists texts authored by nurses that may be helpful in developing cultural knowledge.

 NURSING MANAGEMENT

Assessing

The Assessment Interview on page 323 depicts the questions to ask when conducting a heritage assessment. The tool is a way of interviewing and facilitating communication with clients and their families. It is designed to enhance the process in order to determine if clients are identifying with their traditional cultural heritage (heritage consistent) or if they have acculturated into

---

BOX 18–1 Selected Nurse Authored Texts

Andrews, J. D. (2005). *Cultural, ethnic and religious reference manual for health care providers* (3rd ed.). Winston-Salem, NC: Jamarda Resources.

Campinha-Bacote, J. (2003). *The process of cultural competence in the delivery of healthcare services* (3rd ed.). Cincinnati, OH: Transcultural C.A.R.E. Associates.

D'Avanzo, C., & Geissler, E. M. (2003). *Pocket guide to cultural health assessment* (3rd ed.). St. Louis, MO: Mosby.

Giger, J. N., & Davidhizar, R. E. (2004). *Transcultural nursing* (4th ed.). St. Louis, MO: Mosby Year Book.

Kavanaugh, K. H., & Knowlden, V. (2004). *Many voices: Toward caring culture in healthcare and healing.* Madison: University of Wisconsin Press.

Leininger, M. M., & McFarland, M. R. (2005). *Culture care diversity & universality: A worldwide nursing theory* (2nd ed.). Boston: Jones & Bartlett.

Lipson, J. G., & Dibble, S. L. (Eds.). (2005). *Culture & clinical care.* San Francisco: UCSF Nursing Press.

Munoz, C. C., & Luckman, J. (2004). *Transcultural communication in nursing* (2nd ed.). Clifton Park, NY: Thomson Delmar.

Purnell, L., & Paulanka, B. (2004). *A guide to culturally competent healthcare.* Philadelphia: F.A. Davis.

Spector, R. E. (2004). *Cultural diversity in health and illness* (6th ed.). Upper Saddle River, NJ: Pearson Education.

---

the dominant culture of the modern society they reside in (heritage inconsistent). The tool may be used in any setting and both facilitates conversation and helps in the planning of cultural care. Once a conversation begins and the person describes aspects of cultural heritage, it becomes possible to develop an understanding of the person's unique health and illness beliefs, practices, and cultural needs.

Examples of Heritage Consistency

The following factors and examples indicative of heritage consistency can be explored to determine the depth to which a person identifies with his or her traditional heritage, that is, the cultural beliefs and practices of his or her family heritage:

1. The person's childhood development occurred in the person's country of origin or in an immigrant neighborhood of like ethnic group in the United States. For example, the person was raised in a specific ethnic neighborhood, such as an Italian, African American, Hispanic, or Jewish one, in a given part of a city and was exposed only to the culture, language, foods, and customs of that particular group.

2. Extended family members encouraged participation in traditional religious and cultural activities. For example, the parents sent the person to religious (parochial) school, and most social activities were church related.

3. The individual engages in frequent visits to the country of origin or returns to the "old neighborhood" in the United States. The desire to return to the old country or to the old

ASSESSMENT INTERVIEW   Heritage Assessment Tool

This set of questions is to be used to describe a given client's—or your own—ethnic, cultural, and religious background. In performing a *heritage assessment* it is helpful to determine how deeply a given person identifies with his or her traditional heritage. This tool is most useful in setting the stage for assessing and understanding a person's traditional health and illness beliefs and practices and in helping to determine the community resources that will be appropriate to target for support when necessary. The greater the number of positive responses, the greater the degree to which the person may identify with his or her traditional heritage. The one exception to positive answers is the question about whether a person's name was changed.

1. Where was your mother born? _____
2. Where was your father born? _____
3. Where were your grandparents born? _____
   a. Your mother's mother? _____
   b. Your mother's father? _____
   c. Your father's mother? _____
   d. Your father's father? _____
4. How many brothers _____ and sisters _____ do you have?
5. What setting did you grow up in? Urban _____ Rural _____
6. What country did your parents grow up in?
   Father _____
   Mother _____
7. How old were you when you came to the United States?
   _____
8. How old were your parents when they came to the United States?
   Mother _____
   Father _____
9. When you were growing up, who lived with you?
   _____
10. Have you maintained contact with
    a. Aunts, uncles, cousins?   (1) Yes _____   (2) No _____
    b. Brothers and sisters?   (1) Yes _____   (2) No _____
    c. Parents?   (1) Yes _____   (2) No _____
    d. Your own children?   (1) Yes _____   (2) No _____
11. Did most of your aunts, uncles, cousins live near your home?
    (1) Yes _____ (2) No _____
12. Approximately how often did you visit family members who lived outside of your home?
    (1) Daily _____ (2) Weekly _____ (3) Monthly _____
    (4) Once a year or less _____ (5) Never _____
13. Was your original family name changed?
    (1) Yes _____ (2) No _____

14. What is your religious preference?
    (1) Catholic _____ (2) Jewish _____
    (3) Protestant _____ Denomination _____
    (4) Other _____ (5) None _____
15. Is your spouse the same religion as you?
    (1) Yes _____ (2) No _____
16. Is your spouse the same ethnic background as you?
    (1) Yes _____ (2) No _____
17. What kind of school did you go to?
    (1) Public _____ (2) Private _____ (3) Parochial _____
18. As an adult, do you live in a neighborhood where the neighbors are the same religion and ethnic background as yourself?
    (1) Yes _____ (2) No _____
19. Do you belong to a religious institution?
    (1) Yes _____ (2) No _____
20. Would you describe yourself as an active member?
    (1) Yes _____ (2) No _____
21. How often do you attend your religious institution?
    (1) More than once a week _____ (2) Weekly _____
    (3) Monthly _____
    (4) Special holidays only _____ (5) Never _____
22. Do you practice your religion in your home?
    (1) Yes _____ (2) No _____ (if yes, please specify)
    (3) Praying _____ (4) Bible reading _____ (5) Diet _____
    (6) Celebrating religious holidays _____
23. Do you prepare foods special to your ethnic background?
    (1) Yes _____ (2) No _____
24. Do you participate in ethnic activities?
    (1) Yes _____ (2) No _____ (if yes, please specify)
    (3) Singing _____ (4) Holiday celebrations _____
    (5) Dancing _____ (6) Festivals _____
    (7) Costumes _____ (8) Other _____
25. Are your friends from the same religious background as you?
    (1) Yes _____ (2) No _____
26. Are your friends from the same ethnic background as you?
    (1) Yes _____ (2) No _____
27. What is your native language? _____
28. Do you speak this language?
    (1) Prefer _____ (2) Occasionally _____ (3) Rarely _____
29. Do you read your native language?
    (1) Yes _____ (2) No _____

Note: From *Cultural Diversity in Health & Illness,* 6th ed. (pp. 321–323), by R. E. Spector, 2004, Upper Saddle River, NJ: Prentice Hall.

neighborhood is prevalent in many people; however, many people, for various reasons, cannot return. The people who left to escape religious persecution or whose families were killed during World War II, during the Holocaust, in the killing fields of Cambodia, or in other recent massacres may not want to return to their homelands. Other reasons why people may not return to their native country include political conditions in the homeland or lack of relatives or friends in that land.

4. The individual's family home is within the ethnic community of which he or she is a member. As adults, persons elect to live with their families in the ethnic neighborhood wherein the people are from a similar heritage.
5. The individual participates in ethnic cultural events, such as religious festivals or national holidays, sometimes with singing, dancing, and costumes. For example, the person is active in social and cultural groups and participates in family festivities.

RESEARCH NOTE **What are the Knowledge, Skills, and Attitudes Required of Nursing Students to Provide Culturally Competent Care for Native American Groups?**

This study investigated the perceptions, beliefs, and practices of associate degree nursing students related to providing culturally competent health care for Native Americans, particularly the Cherokee tribe. A total of 28 participants answered an open-ended survey addressing three major issues: (a) type of knowledge, (b) skills, and (c) attitudes/beliefs nursing students should acquire to provide culturally competent health for this population.

Regarding knowledge, participants indicated that in their academic preparation nursing students should learn the cultural factors of Native Americans, their spiritual and religious beliefs, their dietary habits, health conditions, and risk factors. The participants also recognized that nursing students should do a self-analysis of the prejudices and preconceived beliefs they may have regarding this population. Regarding skills, participants indicated that nursing students need to learn basic nursing skills and communication skills when working with this particular group. Regarding attitudes and beliefs, the respondents indicated that nursing students should de-velop an open-minded, nonjudgmental, and caring attitude, as well as respect for diversity.

IMPLICATIONS

This research provides the nursing profession with a better understanding of the training needs of nursing students. The development of a solid knowledge base of a cultural group, the acquisition of skills for the delivery of nursing care, the development of effective communication patterns, and the nurturing of a genuine appreciation for diversity ought to be major goals in the nursing curriculum. Although this research is centered on Native American populations, the findings of this study can be applicable when working with other cultural groups. Recognizing the variations within cultural groups is also important when providing health care for underrepresented populations.

Note: From "Knowledge, Skills, and Attitudes of Nursing Students Regarding Culturally Congruent Care of Native Americans" by D. R. Wittig, 2004, *Journal of Transcultural Nursing, 15*(1), pp. 54–61.

---

6. The individual was raised in an extended family setting. For example, when the person was growing up, grandparents or aunts and uncles may have been living in the same house or close by. The person's social frame of reference was the family.

7. The individual maintains regular contact with the extended family. For example, the person maintains close ties with family members of the same generation, the surviving members of the older generation, and members of the younger generation.

8. The individual's name has not been Americanized. For example, the person has restored the family name to its original if it had been changed by immigration authorities at the time the family immigrated or if the family changed the name at a later time in an attempt to assimilate to the dominant culture more fully.

9. The individual was educated in a parochial (nonpublic) school with a religious or ethnic philosophy similar to the family's background. The person's education plays an enormous role in socialization, and the major purpose of education is to socialize a given person into the dominant culture. Children learn English and the customs and norms of American life in the schools. In the parochial or private schools, they not only learn English but also are socialized in the culture and norms of the particular religious or ethnic group that is sponsoring the school.

10. The individual engages in social activities primarily with others of the same religious or ethnic background. For example, the major portion of the person's personal time is spent attending meetings and events sponsored by those with whom he or she identifies.

11. The individual has knowledge of the culture and language of origin. For example, the person has been socialized in the traditional ways of the family and expresses this as a central theme of life.

12. The individual expresses pride in his or her heritage. For example, the person may identify him- or herself as ethnic American and display flags, wear clothing, or participate in ethnic activities to a great extent.

Conveying Cultural Sensitivity

The process of heritage and health traditions assessment is important. How and when questions are asked requires sensitivity and clinical judgment. The timing and phrasing of questions need to be adapted to the individual. Timing is important in introducing questions. Sensitivity is needed in phrasing questions. Trust must be established before clients can be expected to volunteer and share sensitive information. The nurse therefore needs to spend time with clients, introduce some social conversation, and convey a genuine desire to understand their values and beliefs.

Before a heritage assessment begins, determine what language the client speaks and the client's degree of fluency in the English language. It is also important to learn about the client's communications patterns and space orientation. This is accomplished by observing both verbal and nonverbal communication. For example, does the client do the speaking or defer to another? What nonverbal communication behaviors does the client exhibit (e.g., touching, eye contact)? What significance do these behaviors have for the nurse–client interaction? What is the client's proximity to other people and objects within the environment? How does the client react to the nurse's movement toward the client? What cultural objects within the environment have importance for health promotion or health maintenance?

It is vital for nurses to be culturally sensitive and to convey this sensitivity to clients, support people, and other health care personnel. Some ways to do so follow:

- Always address clients, support people, and other health care personnel by their last names (e.g., Mrs. Aylia, Dr. Rush) until they give you permission to use other names. In some cultures, the more formal style of address is a sign of respect, whereas the informal use of first names may be considered disrespect. It is important to ask people how they wish to be addressed.

- When meeting a person for the first time, introduce yourself by your full name, and then explain your role (e.g., "My name is Alicia Bernett and I am a student nurse at Nightingale School of Nursing"). This helps establish a relationship and provides an opportunity for clients, others, and nurses to learn the pronunciation of one another's names and their roles.
- Be authentic with people, and be honest about the knowledge you lack about their culture. When you do not understand a person's actions, politely and respectfully seek information.
- Use language that is culturally sensitive; for example, say "gay," "lesbian," or "bisexual" rather than "homosexual"; do not use "man" or "mankind" when referring to a woman. Ask if the person prefers to be referred to as an "Hispanic" or "Latino"; as an "African American" or "Black."
- Find out what the client thinks about his or her health problems, illness, and treatments. Assess whether this information is congruent with the dominant health care culture. If the beliefs and practices are incongruent, establish whether this will have a negative effect on the client's health.
- Do not make any assumptions about the client, and always ask about anything you do not understand.
- Show respect for the client's values, beliefs, and practices, even if they differ from your own or from those of the dominant culture. If you do not agree with them, it is important to respect the client's right to hold these beliefs.
- Show respect for the client's support people. In some cultures, men in the family make decisions affecting the client, while in other cultures women make the decisions.
- Make a concerted effort to obtain the client's trust, but do not be surprised if it develops slowly or not at all. The heritage assessment takes time and usually needs to extend over several meetings.

Diagnosing

The nursing diagnoses developed by NANDA are focused on nursing care provided in the United States and Canada and are based on Western cultural beliefs. It is essential to expand the understanding of the nursing practice to include cultural beliefs of the Eastern culture. Nurses must provide appropriate care to clients of any culture. This is accomplished through developing cultural sensitivity and considering how a client's culture influences his or her responses to health conditions, much as the nurse considers how a client's age or gender influences a nursing diagnosis, plan, and delivery of nursing care.

Planning

Cultural competence in nursing involves delivering care that integrates the mind, the body, the spirit, and the cultural values of the individual (Fontaine, 2005). A potential outcome is that the client can "promote, maintain, and/or regain mutually desired and obtainable levels of health within the realities of their life circumstances" (Kagawa-Singer & Kassim-Lakha, 2003, p. 580). There are several steps involved in the process that lead to the development of cultural competency. The knowledge and skills necessary to incorporate cultural care into standard nursing require the acquisition of a broad base of knowledge about different heritages and social structures. It is an ongoing process and the skills and knowledge base grow over time. As one's knowledge base grows, the ability to convey cultural sensitivity also grows (see Box 18–2).

The following are examples of the necessary steps:

1. Become aware of one's own cultural heritage. Where were your parents and grandparents born? What are examples of their traditional health and illness beliefs and practices? Do they value stoic behavior in relation to pain, or is it permissible to state that you are in pain? Are the rights of the individual valued over and above the rights of the family? Only by knowing one's own culture

---

BOX 18–2 Health-Related Practices of Asian, African American, and Hispanic Peoples

ASIAN
- Coining and cupping are traditional medical practices, not forms of abuse.
- Fevers are treated by wrapping the ill person in warm blankets and having him or her drink warm liquids.
- Do not provide ice water unless requested. May prefer hot liquids, such as tea.
- Rich tradition of herbal remedies. Health care providers should be sure to discuss the use of home or herbal remedies to avoid potential drug interactions.
- Instruct on the use of Western medication because traditional Chinese medicine is taken differently. Explain the importance of taking pills as prescribed, even after symptoms have disappeared.

AFRICAN AMERICAN
- Menstruation is believed to rid the body of dirty and excess blood. With too little flow, they may fear bad blood is staying in the body; too much flow can weaken the body. Influences views of birth control.

- Have rich tradition of herbal remedies. Health care providers should be sure to discuss the use of home or herbal remedies to avoid potential drug interactions.
- May avoid dairy products due to high incidence of lactose intolerance. Check for family history.
- Focus on present time may interfere with use of preventive medicine and follow-up care.

HISPANIC
- Certain foods or medications upset hot–cold body balance. Try offering alternative foods or liquids for medications.
- Do not provide ice water unless requested.
- Respect postpartum prescriptions for rest.
- Sponge baths may be preferred after giving birth.
- Allow family members to spend as much time with the client as possible and provide nontechnical care.
- Strong beliefs in fate and external control over events may lead to fewer adherences to medical regimens.

(values, practices, and beliefs) can a person be ready to learn about another's.

2. Become aware of the client's heritage and health traditions as described by the client. It is important to avoid assuming that all people of one ethnic background have the same cultural beliefs and values. When the nurse has knowledge of the client's culture, mutual respect between client and nurse is more likely to develop.

3. Become aware of adaptations the client made to live in a North American culture. During this part of the interview, a nurse can also identify the client's preferences in health practices, diet, hygiene, and so on.

4. Form a nursing plan with the client that incorporates his or her cultural beliefs regarding the maintenance, protection, and restoration of health. In this way, cultural values, practices, and beliefs can be incorporated with the necessary nursing care.

Many research studies have documented the need for culturally focused care planning. Two examples follow:

■ A study sponsored by the Agency for Healthcare Research and Quality demonstrated that regular home visits by a nurse–health advocate team can substantially improve the maternal and infant health of economically challenged and minority populations. Positive outcomes of nurse-led home visits were demonstrated in terms of better maternal documentation of infant immunizations, more developmentally appropriate parenting expectations, and higher infant developmental scores (Norr et al., 2003).

■ The study "Determinants of Physical Activity and Low-Fat Diet Among Low Income African American and Hispanic Middle School Students" demonstrated that school-based approaches, in which the school nurse or parish nurse helps build appropriate family roles, reduce health problems associated with low physical activity and high-fat diets (Frenn et al., 2005).

Implementing

The implementation of cultural nursing care includes (a) cultural preservation and maintenance and (b) cultural accommodation and negotiation. Cultural preservation may involve the use of cultural health care practices, such as giving herbal tea, chicken soup, or "hot foods" to the ill client. Accommodation of the client's viewpoint and negotiating appropriate care requires expert communication skills, such as responding empathetically, validating information, and effectively summarizing content. Negotiation is a collaborative process. It acknowledges that the nurse–client relationship is reciprocal and that different views exist of health, illness, and treatment. The nurse attempts to bridge the gap between the nurse's scientific and the client's cultural perspectives. During the negotiation process, the client's views are explored and acknowledged. Relevant scientific information is then provided. If the client's views reveal that certain behaviors would not affect the client's condition adversely, then they are incorporated in planning care. If the client's views can lead to harmful behavior or outcomes, then an attempt is made to shift the client's perspectives to the scientific view.

Negotiation occurs when cultural treatment practices conflict with those of the health care system. It must be determined precisely how the client is managing the illness, what practices could be harmful, and which practices can be safely combined with Western medicine. For example, reducing dosages of an antihypertensive medication or replacing insulin therapy with herbal measures may be detrimental. Some herbal remedies are synergistic with Western medicines and others are antagonistic; therefore, it is necessary to fully inform the client about the possible outcomes. Consider these examples of potential conflicts between cultural beliefs or practices and the dominant American health care system:

■ Native American women value large body size and may be resistant to weight control.

■ The decision to circumcise male infants is often made based on cultural and family beliefs and can occasionally conflict with medical advice.

■ An Hispanic or Asian client may be unable to obtain hospice care if the family will not permit the client to be informed of the diagnosis or prognosis.

■ Members of the Jehovah's Witness faith do not accept blood transfusions even in life-threatening situations.

■ Orthodox Sikhs do not cut their hair. This can conflict with the need to shave the skin for medical procedures.

When a client chooses to follow only cultural practices and declines all prescribed medical or nursing interventions, the nurse and client must adjust the client goals. Monitoring the client's condition to identify changes in health and to recognize impending crises before they become irreversible may be all that is realistically achievable. At a time of crisis, the opportunity may arise to renegotiate care.

Providing cultural nursing care is challenging. It requires discovery of the meaning of the client's behavior, flexibility, creativity, and knowledge to adapt nursing interventions. An effort must be made to learn from each experience. This knowl-

---

CULTURALLY COMPETENT CARE
Families

■ Include cultural assessment of the client and family as part of overall assessment.

■ Learn the rituals, customs, and practices of the major cultural groups with whom you come into contact. Learn to appreciate the richness of diversity and consider it an asset rather than a hindrance in your practice.

■ Don't make assumptions about beliefs or practices.

■ Ask about the client's use of cultural or alternative approaches to healing.

■ Identify your personal biases, attitudes, prejudices, and stereotypes.

■ Recognize that it is the client's (or family's) right to make their own health care choices. Explain in detail the client's condition and the treatment plan if the client is willing for you to do this.

■ Convey respect and cooperate with traditional helpers and caregivers.

edge will improve the delivery of culture-specific care to future clients. The accompanying box offers suggestions for providing such care to clients and families.

Evaluating

Evaluating nursing care of clients that incorporates the concepts of heritage and ethnicity is performed in the same way as with any client. Client outcomes are compared with the goals and expected outcomes established following comprehensive assessment that includes sensitivity to cultural diversity. However, if the outcomes are not achieved, and the client and nurse are from different cultures, the nurse should be especially careful to consider whether the client's belief system has been adequately included as an influencing factor.

CRITICAL THINKING CHECKPOINT

Rachel was born to a Jewish couple and lists her religion as Jewish. Her father died when she was 10 years old and her mother remarried 3 years later. Rachel was legally adopted by her Italian stepfather, who was a devout Catholic. Although the family participated in Catholic–Italian traditions, Rachel's mother taught her many Jewish traditions as well, so that her heritage would be preserved. Rachel is now 58 years old, practices traditions from both her Jewish and Italian upbringing, and is dying of cancer. You are the nurse caring for Rachel during her final days.

1. Differentiate between Rachel's culture, ethnicity, and race.

2. How might Rachel's mixed cultural background pose a dilemma for you as her nurse or for her family?
3. How might Rachel's culture affect her approach to death and the care of her body following her death?
4. Of what benefit would a cultural assessment be to Rachel or her family since she is dying?
5. How could nurses' race, culture, or religion influence their care of clients who are racially or culturally different?

See Critical Thinking Possibilities in Appendix A.

CHAPTER 18 **REVIEW**

CHAPTER HIGHLIGHTS

- The Office of Minority Health is a major resource for nursing students when working with racial, ethnic, and cultural groups.
- *The National Standards for Culturally and Linguistically Appropriate Services in Health Care* (CLAS) should be understood by nurses and applied their professional practice.
- *Healthy People 2010* calls for nursing to contribute to eliminating health disparities by gender, race or ethnicity, education, income, disability, geographic location, and sexual orientation.
- Racial and Ethnic Approaches to Community Health (REACH 2010) is an initiative that motivates nurses and other health professionals to center their academic and research efforts on infant mortality, deficits in breast and cervical cancer screening/management, cardiovascular diseases, diabetes, HIV infections/AIDS, and child and adult immunizations.
- People in the United States come from a variety of backgrounds, and many retain at least some of their traditional values, including health beliefs and practices.

- People may live within their traditional heritage or they may embrace both their original ethnocultural traditional heritage(s) and the modern culture of the United States.
- An individual's heritage and cultural background can influence health beliefs and practices.
- Through acculturation, most groups in the United States modify some of their traditional cultural characteristics.
- Personal characteristics also modify an individual's cultural values, beliefs, and practices.
- Health beliefs and practices, family patterns, communication style, space and time orientation, and nutritional patterns may influence the relationship between the nurse and the client who have different cultural backgrounds.
- When assessing a client, the nurse considers the client's cultural values, beliefs, and practices related to health and health care.

TEST YOUR KNOWLEDGE

1. The major factor contributing to the increased emphasis on the need for proficiency in cultural nursing practice in the United States includes which of the following?
   1. An increasing birth rate
   2. Limited access to health care services
   3. Demographic changes
   4. A decreasing rate of immigration

2. Which of the following behaviors is most indicative of culturally *sensitive* nursing practice?
   1. Helps client recognize the need to adapt health practices to fit commonly accepted practices

   2. Discusses the meaning of the medical regime to the client
   3. Informs client that lack of adherence to medical regime may be detrimental
   4. Asks a person from the same culture to explain the relevance of the intervention

3. In initiating care for a client of a different culture than the nurse, which of the following would be an appropriate statement?
   1. "Since, in your culture, people don't drink ice water, I will bring you hot tea."
   2. "Do you have any books I could read about people of your culture?"

3. "Please let me know if I do anything that is not acceptable in your culture."
4. "You will need to set aside your usual customs and practices while you are in the hospital."

4. Which of the following behaviors is most representative of a *culturally competent* nurse?
1. Helps clients of Native-American heritage identify ways to relate more to their culture
2. Helps parents of Latino heritage recognize that their children need to speak English
3. Interprets and validates beliefs of a client with African American heritage
4. Asks a nurse of Japanese heritage to teach others dosage calculations since Asians are good at math

5. Students ask the nurse to explain the differences between culture and race. Which of the following is the best response?
1. Culture is limited to a shared language or religion.
2. Race describes common characteristics within a specific heritage group.
3. Culture is socially oriented and race addresses shared physical traits.
4. Culture is the degree by which one's lifestyle matches one's heritage.

See Answers to Test Your Knowledge in Appendix A.

EXPLORE MEDIALINK www.prenhall.com/berman

DVD-ROM
- Audio Glossary
- NCLEX Review

COMPANION WEBSITE
- Additional NCLEX Review
- Care Plan Activity: Client in the ICU
- Case Study: Conveying Cultural Sensitivity
- Application Activity: Chinese Childbearing Beliefs
- Links to Resources

READINGS AND REFERENCES

SUGGESTED READINGS
Cook, C. (2003). The many faces of diversity: Overview and summary. *Online Journal of Issues in Nursing, 8*(1). Retrieved June 25, 2006, from http://nursingworld.org/ojin/topic20/tpc20ntr.htm
This citation is the introduction to the remaining articles in the issue dedicated to cultural diversity. It describes the discussions that follow regarding health and health care disparities, cultural competence, race consciousness, and diversity and health policy.
Green-Hernandez, C., Quinn, A. A., Denman-Vitale, S., Falkenstern, S. K., & Judge-Ellis, T. (2004). Making nursing care culturally competent. *Holistic Nursing Practice, 18*(4), 215–218.
Nursing practice traditionally is client centered, using holistic modalities that recognize the importance of cultural competence. The delivery of comprehensive and quality primary care can be more complex for those clinicians who work with clients from diverse cultures. The authors suggest that clients need to have at least some knowledge about the culture, including common beliefs and practices, of all diverse clients.
Muñoz, C., & Hilgenberg, C. (2005). Ethnopharmacology: Understanding how ethnicity can affect drug response is essential to providing culturally competent care. *American Journal of Nursing, 105*(8), 40–49.
Studies have shown that clients of some genetic or cultural backgrounds respond to certain medications differently from those with other backgrounds. This article describes the known variations in response to psychotropic and antihypertensive medications according to culture.
Rawlings-Anderson, K. (2004). Assessing the cultural and religious needs of older people. *Nursing Older People, 16*(8), 29–33.
In this article, the author focuses on the general need for assessment of culture and its impact on health care of the population 65 and older. Recommendations for specific questions to ask during history taking and assessment are included.

RELATED RESEARCH
Pinquart, M., & Sörenson, S. (2005). Ethnic differences in stressors, resources, and psychological outcomes of family caregiving: A meta-analysis. *Gerontologist, 45,* 90–106.
Rhee, H. (2005). Racial/ethnic differences in adolescents' physical symptoms. *Journal of Pediatric Nursing Nursing Care of Children and Families, 20,* 153–162.
Yeo, S. (2004). Language barriers and access to care. *Annual Review of Nursing Research, 22,* 59–73.

REFERENCES
Agency for Healthcare Research and Quality. (2005). *2005 national healthcare quality and disparities report.* Rockville, MD: Author.
Barnes, P. M., Powell-Griner, E., McFann, K., & Nahin, R. L. (2004). Complementary and alternative medicine use among adults: United States, 2002. *Advance Data from Vital and Health Statistics,* no. 343. Hyattsville, MD: U.S. Department of Health and Human Services, CDC, National Center for Health Statistics. Retrieved April 22, 2006, from http://www.cdc.gov/nchs/data/ad/ad343.pdf
California Healthcare Interpreters Association. (2002). *California standards for healthcare interpreters: Ethical principles, protocols, and guidance on roles and interventions.* Los Angeles: Author.
Campinha-Bacote, J. (2003). *The process of cultural competence in the delivery of healthcare services* (3rd ed.). Cincinnati, OH: Transcultural C.A.R.E. Associates.
Canadian Nurses Association. (2004). *Position statement: Promoting culturally competent care.* Retrieved April 22, 2006, from http://cna-aiic.ca/CNA/documents/pdf/publications/PS73_Promoting_Culturally_Competent_CareMarch_2004_e.pdf
Centers for Disease Control and Prevention. (n.d.). *Mission.* Retrieved June 25, 2006, from http://www.cdc.gov/omh/AboutUs/aboutUs.htm
Fontaine, K. L. (2005). *Complementary and alternative therapies for nursing practice* (2nd ed.). Upper Saddle River, NJ: Pearson Prentice Hall.
Frenn, M., Malin, S., Villarruel, A., Slaikeu, K., McCarthy, S., Freeman, J., et al. (2005). Determinants of physical activity and low-fat diet among low income African American and Hispanic middle school students. *Public Health Nursing, 22,* 89–97.
Kagawa-Singer, M., & Kassim-Lakha, S. (2003). A strategy to reduce cross-cultural miscommunication and increase the likelihood of improving health outcomes. *Academic Medicine, 78,* 577–587.
Leininger, M. M., & McFarland, M. R. (2005). *Culture care diversity & universality: A worldwide nursing theory* (2nd ed.). Boston: Jones & Bartlett.
Mason, P., & Narad, C. (2005). International adoption: A health and developmental prospective. *Seminars in Speech and Language 26*(1),1–9.
McLemore, S. D., & Romo, H. D. (2005). *Racial and ethnic relations in America* (7th ed.). Boston: Allyn & Bacon.
National Center on Minority Health and Health Disparities. (n.d.) *Mission.* Retrieved June 25, 2006, from http://ncmhd.nih.gov/about_ncmhd/mission.asp
Norr, K. F., Crittenden, K. S., Lehrer, E. L., Reyes, O., Boyd, C. B., Nacion, K. W. et al. (2003). Maternal and infant outcomes at one year for a nurse-health advocate home visiting program serving African Americans and Mexican Americans. *Public Health Nursing, 20,* 190–203.
Office of Minority Health. (2001). *National standards for culturally and linguistically appropriate services in health care.* Washington, DC: U. S. Department of Health and Human Services.
Public Health Foundation. (2001). *The key ingredient of the National Prevention Agenda: Workforce development—A companion*

document to *Healthy People 2010*. Retrieved April 22, 2006, from ftp://ftp.hrsa.gov/bhpr/nationalcenter/hp2010.pdf

Spector, R. E. (2004). *Cultural diversity in health and illness* (6th ed.). Upper Saddle River, NJ: Pearson Prentice Hall.

Turton, P. (2003). Education for integration: A view from the bridge! *Complementary Therapies in Nursing and Midwifery, 9*(1), 20–22.

U.S. Department of Health and Human Services Health Resources and Service Administration Bureau of Health Professions. (2004). *The registered nurse population: Preliminary findings from the National Sample Survey of Registered Nurses, March 2004.* Retrieved April 21, 2006, from http://bhpr.hrsa.gov/healthworkforce/reports/rnpopulation/preliminaryfindings.htm

U. S. Bureau of Labor Statistics. (2004). *Table 3c. The 10 occupations with the largest job growth, 2002–12.* Retrieved April 22, 2006, from http://www.bls.gov/news.release/ecopro.t05.htm

U.S. Census Bureau. (2001). *Profiles of general demographic characteristics 2000.* Washington, DC: U.S. Department of Commerce.

U.S. Census Bureau. (2004). *U.S. interim projections by age, sex, race, and Hispanic origin.* Retrieved April 22, 2006, from http://www.census.gov/ipc/www/usinterimproj

U.S. Census Bureau. (2005a). *Annual estimates of the population by sex, race and Hispanic or Latino origin for the United States: April 1, 2000 to July 1, 2004* (NC-EST2004-03). Retrieved April 22, 2006, from http://www.census.gov/popest/national/asrh/NC-EST2004-srh.html

U.S. Census Bureau. (2005b). *Foreign born population tops 34 million.* Retrieved April 22, 2006, from http://www.census.gov/Press-Release/www/releases/archives/foreignborn_population/003969.html

U.S. Department of Health and Human Services Office of Minority Health, (n.d.) *Mission.* Retrieved June 25, 2006, from http://www.omhrc.gov/templates/browse.aspx?lvl=1&lvlID=7

Wittig, D. R. (2004). Knowledge, skills, and attitudes of nursing students regarding culturally congruent care of Native Americans. *Journal of Transcultural Nursing, 15(1)*, 54–61.

Zitzow, D., & Estes, G. (1981). The heritage consistency continuum in counseling Native American students. In *Contemporary American Indian issues in higher education.* Los Angeles: American Indian Studies Center, University of California.

SELECTED BIBLIOGRAPHY

Alexander, R. (2006). Diversity, cultural competence, and the nursing student. *Imprint, 53*(2), 43–45.

Andrews, J. D. (2005). *Cultural, ethnic and religious reference manual for health care providers* (3rd ed.). Winston-Salem, NC: Jamarda Resources.

Betancourt, J. R., Green, A. R., Carrillo, J. E., & Park, E. R. (2005). Cultural competence and health care disparities: Key perspectives and trends. *Health Affairs, 24,* 499–505.

Buerhaus, P. I., Staiger, D. O., & Auerbach, D. I. (2004). New signs of a strengthening U.S. nurse labor market? *Health Affairs, 23,* 526–533.

Campinha-Bacote, J. (2003). Many faces: Addressing diversity in health care. *Online Journal of Issues in Nursing,* 8(1), Manuscript 2. Retrieved April 22, 2006, from http://www.nursingworld.org/ojin/topic20/tpc202.htm

Campinha-Bacote, J. (2003). *The process of cultural competence in the delivery of healthcare services* (3rd ed.). Cincinnati, OH: Transcultural C.A.R.E. Associates.

Collins, C. C., Decker, S. I., & Esquibel, K. A. (2004). Definitions of health: Comparison of Hispanic and African-American elders. *Journal of Multicultural Nursing & Health, 10*(3), 13–18.

Dennis, B. P., & Small, E. B. (2003). Incorporating cultural diversity in nursing care: An action plan. *ABNF Journal, 14,* 17–26.

Galanti, G. A. (2004). *Caring for patients from different cultures* (3rd ed.). Philadelphia: University of Pennsylvania Press.

Giger, J. N., & Davidhizar, R. E. (2004). *Transcultural nursing: Assessment and intervention* (4th ed.). St. Louis, MO: Mosby.

Giorgianni, S. J. (Ed.). (2004). Diversity in healthcare delivery. *Pfizer Journal. VIII*(2), 4–14.

Hascup, V. A. (2004). Transcultural nursing. *Advance for Nurses, 2*(15), 28–29.

Jeffreys, M. (2006). Cultural competence in clinical practice. *Imprint, 53*(2), 37–41.

Jones, M. E., Cason, C. L., & Bond, M. L. (2004). Cultural attitudes, knowledge, and skills of a health workforce. *Journal of Transcultural Nursing, 15,* 283–290.

Lipson, J. G., & Dibble, S. L. (Eds.). (2005). *Culture and clinical care.* San Francisco: UCSF Nursing Press.

Sensor, C. S. (2006). Culturally competent care in the workplace. *Imprint, 53*(2), 46–51.

Shen, Z. (2004). Cultural competence models in nursing: A selected annotated bibliography. *Journal of Transcultural Nursing, 15,* 317–322.

Vivian, C., & Dundes, L. (2004). The crossroads of culture and health among the Roma (Gypsies). *Journal of Nursing Scholarship, 36,* 86–91.

Waters, V. L. (2004). Cultivate corporate culture and diversity. *Nursing Management, 35*(1), 36–37.

Complementary and Alternative Healing Modalities

LEARNING OUTCOMES

After completing this chapter, you will be able to:

1. Describe concepts basic to alternative practices.

2. Give examples of healing environments.

3. Develop a self-care plan using alternative practices.

4. Explain how herbs are similar to many prescription drugs.

5. Discuss how naturopathic medicine may be the model health care system of the future.

6. Identify the role of manual healing methods in health and illness.

7. Describe the goals that yoga, meditation, hypnotherapy, guided imagery, qigong, and t'ai chi have in common.

8. Explain the theory underlying bioelectromagnetics and infrared photoenergy therapy.

9. Compare the various types of detoxification.

10. Discuss uses of animals, prayer, and humor as treatment modalities.

KEY TERMS

acupressure, *337*	**curanderismo,** *334*	**meditation,** *338*
acupuncture, *337*	**detoxification,** *342*	**music therapy,** *341*
allopathic medicine, *331*	**energy,** *332*	**naturopathic**
alternative medicine, *331*	**faith,** *340*	** medicine,** *335*
animal-assisted therapy, *342*	**guided imagery,** *339*	**Pilates,** *340*
aromatherapy, *334*	**herbal medicine,** *334*	**prayer,** *340*
Ayurveda, *332*	**holism,** *331*	**qi,** *333*
balance, *332*	**homeopathy,** *335*	**qigong,** *340*
bioelectromagnetics, *341*	**horticultural therapy,** *343*	**reflexology,** *337*
biofeedback, *340*	**humanist,** *331*	**spirituality,** *332*
biomedicine, *331*	**hypnotherapy,** *339*	**t'ai chi,** *340*
chiropractic, *336*	**imagery,** *339*	**traditional Chinese**
complementary medicine, *331*	**infrared photoenergy**	** medicine,** *333*
conventional medicine, *331*	** therapy,** *342*	**yoga,** *338*

Most of nursing education in the United States, Canada, Europe, and Australia has been under the umbrella of biomedicine. Thus, nurses from these parts of the world are familiar and comfortable with biomedical beliefs, theories, practices, strengths, and limitations. Fewer nurses have studied alternative medical theories and practices and as a result may lack information or even harbor misinformation about these healing practices. In this chapter the terms **conventional medicine, biomedicine, and allopathic medicine** are used to describe Western medical practices. The terms **alternative medicine** or **complementary medicine** are used to describe as many as 1,800 other therapies practiced all over the world. Many of these have been handed down over thousands of years, both orally and as written records. They are based on the medical systems of ancient people, including Egyptians, Chinese, Asian Indians, Greeks, and Native Americans. Other therapies, such as bioelectromagnetics and chiropractic, evolved in the United States over the past two centuries. Still others, such as some of the mind-body and bioelectromagnetic approaches, are on the frontier of scientific knowledge and understanding.

CLINICAL ALERT

What constitutes traditional, alternative, complementary, or holistic to one person may be considered mainstream to another. Do not assume anything about the client's belief system—be sure to assess. ■

The conventional medical community cannot ignore complementary and alternative therapies. The public interest is extensive and growing. One has only to look at the proliferation of popular health books, health food stores, and clinics offering healing therapies to realize this. In 1998, the National Institutes of Health established the National Center for Complementary and Alternative Medicine to provide research, educational grants, and dissemination of information to the public. In March 2000, President Clinton ordered the establishment of the White House Commission on Complementary and Alternative Medicine Policy whose mission it is to make legislative and administrative recommendations for the integration of conventional and alternative medicine.

BASIC CONCEPTS

Several concepts are common to most alternative practices. These are holism, humanism, balance, spirituality, energy, and healing environments.

Holism

Although they represent diverse approaches, alternative therapies share certain attributes. They are based on the paradigm of whole systems and the belief that people are more than physical bodies with fixable and replaceable parts. Combined mental, emotional, spiritual, relationship, and environmental components, referred to as **holism,** are considered to play crucial and equal roles in a person's state of health. Interventions are individualized within the entire context of the person's life. The focus of the American Holistic Nurses Association (AHNA) is to enhance the healing of the whole person from birth to death.

Humanism

The **humanist** perspective includes propositions such as the following: the mind and body are indivisible, people have the power to solve their own problems, people are responsible for the patterns of their lives, and well-being is a combination of personal satisfaction and contributions to the larger community. Nursing is in a unique position to take a leadership role in integrating alternative healing methods into Western health care systems. We have historically used our hands, heart, and head in more natural and traditional healing interactions. As nurses, by virtue of our education and relationships with clients, we can help consumers assert their right to choose their own healing journey and the quality of their life and death experiences (Fontaine, 2005).

Balance

In terms of optimal wellness, the concept of **balance** consists of mental, physical, emotional, spiritual, and environmental components. Not only does each component have to be balanced, equilibrium is needed among the components. *Physical* aspects include optimal functioning of all body systems. *Emotional* aspects include the ability to feel and express the entire range of human emotions. *Mental* aspects include feelings of self-worth, a positive identity, a sense of accomplishment, and the ability to appreciate and create. *Spiritual* aspects involve moral values, a meaningful purpose in life, and a feeling of connectedness to others and a divine source. *Environmental* aspects include physical, biologic, economic, social, and political conditions. Being in balance is a learned skill and one that must be practiced regularly to engage in the process of healthful living. This concept of balance appears throughout the various alternative therapies.

Spirituality

Spiritual healing techniques and spiritually based health care systems are among the most ancient healing practices. Spirit is the liveliness, richness, and beauty of one's life. It is who we are and how we are in the world. **Spirituality** (see Chapter 41 ∞) includes the drive to become all that one can be, and is bound to intuition, creativity, and motivation. It is the dimension that involves relationship with oneself, with others, and with a higher power. Spirituality is that which gives people meaning and purpose in their lives. It involves finding significant meaning in the entirety of life, including illness and death.

Energy

The concept of energy has been recognized for centuries, and in most cultures. **Energy** is viewed as the force that integrates the body, mind, and spirit; it is that which connects everything.

Chinese Taoist scholars believed that energy was the basic building material of the universe. Albert Einstein and other physicists proved that matter and energy are the same and that energy is not only the raw material of the cosmos but the glue that holds it together. Modern scientists now look at the universe in terms of forces of tiny particles of matter. Their experimental findings are similar to the intuitive observation of China's ancient scholars. Everything in the world—animate and inanimate—is made of energy. People are beings of energy, living in a universe composed of energy.

Two terms common in various healing practices and related to energy and balance are grounding and centering. *Grounding,* as its name suggests, relates to one's connection with the ground and, in a broader sense, to one's whole contact with reality. Being grounded suggests stability, security, independence, having a solid foundation, and living in the present rather than escaping into dreams. *Centering* refers to the process of bringing oneself to the center or middle. When people are centered, they are fully connected to the part of their bodies where all their energies meet. Centering is the process of focusing one's mind on the center of energy allowing one to operate intuitively, with awareness, and to channel energy throughout the body.

Healing Environments

Nursing has always focused on creating healing environments for those who have been entrusted to our care. We create healing environments when we use our hands, heart, and mind to provide holistic nursing care. We create healing environments when we empower others by providing the knowledge, skills, and support that allow them to tap into their inner wisdom and make healthy decisions for themselves. Healing environments are a synthesis of the medical-curing approach and the nursing-healing approach. We need a healthy balance between technology and compassion. We create healing environments when we take the time to be with clients in deeply caring ways. It is when we stop, become still, and enter the other's subjective world that we are able to be wholly present for that person (Fontaine, 2005).

We must also create healing environments for ourselves. Working with people can be draining work. As nurses, we need to learn how to restore our energy and replenish ourselves. You might compare your ability to care for others to a well of fresh, healing water. If the well is never dipped into, the water becomes stagnant and brackish. If the water is constantly drawn out and given away, with no source of replenishment, the well will soon run dry. What happens to nurses who don't sincerely care for others or take the time to replenish themselves? It soon becomes obvious by their behavior that they are stagnant or depleted; they are less patient, less tolerant, more irritable, and unhappy. Their state of "burnout" contaminates all aspects of their professional and personal lives. Box 19–1 lists methods that can be useful to nurses working to foster their own health and well-being.

HEALING MODALITIES

Ethnocentrism, the assumption that one's own cultural or ethnic group is superior to others, has often prevented Western health care practitioners from learning new ways to promote health and prevent chronic illness. With consumer demand for a broader range of options, we must open our minds to the idea that other cultures and countries have valid ways of preventing and curing diseases. Although the information may be new to us, many of these traditions are hundreds or even thousands of years old and have long been part of the medical mainstream in other cultures. This information could be useful for Western countries. The nurse should inquire about healing modalities the client may have used previously (see Assessment Interview).

Systematized Health Care Practices

There are a number of health care practices that have been systematized throughout the centuries and throughout the world. These typically include an entire set of values, attitudes, and beliefs that generate a philosophy of life, not simply a group of remedies.

Ayurveda

The Indian system of medicine, **Ayurveda,** is at least 2,500 years old. Illness is viewed as a state of imbalance among the body's systems. Ayurveda emphasizes the interdependence of the health of the individual and the quality of societal life. Mentally healthy people have good memory, comprehension, intelligence, and rea-

BOX 19–1   Self-Healing Methods for Nurses

- *Clarify values and beliefs.*   Identify those things that are important, meaningful, and valuable to you, and assess whether your actions are consistent with your beliefs. For example, do you value time spent with your children and time reading or listening to music?
- *Set realistic goals.*   Identify long-term goals and then short-term goals that will help you meet the long-term goals. For example, a long-term goal might be to experience an increase in emotional and physical comfort. A short-term goal might be to take a 30-minute walk each evening.
- *Challenge the belief that others always come first.*   Overinvolvement with clients leads to overwork and overly solicitous helping that neglects the client's responsibilities, autonomy, and resources. It leaves little time for fulfillment of personal needs. Identify behaviors that indicate overinvolvement, such as saying yes much too often, a tendency to avoid conflict whenever possible, feeling selfish when not responding to someone else's needs, and always listening to others who need emotional support but seldom asking anyone to pay attention to your emotional needs. Assess whether you need to adjust your perspective and behavior. Learn to ask for what you need, acknowledge that you are doing the best you can, and affirm that you can meet your own needs as well as care for others.

- *Learn to manage stress.*   Stress management requires the following:
  - Acknowledge the mind–body connection, that is, the relationship among thoughts, feelings, behaviors, and the physiologic response to stress.
  - Monitor stress warning signals and invoke the relaxation response on a regular basis such as once a day for 20 minutes or twice a day for 10 minutes. "Mini-relaxations" (e.g., taking several deep breaths and thinking about something pleasant such as your favorite pet) throughout the day can also be used to counter the tension and anxiety associated with stress.
  - Develop the skill of personal presence (physically "being there" and psychologically "being with" a client or other person). To be available to others in this way requires practicing the skill of being present to yourself. Avoid allowing yourself to be hurried, distracted, or fragmented. Focus full attention on the activity you are doing at the moment.
  - *Maintain and enhance physical health.*   Eat healthy, balanced meals, exercise regularly, and obtain adequate rest.
  - *Develop a support network.*   Fellow nurses can often provide perspectives and insights to help cope with commonly shared experiences.

Note: From "Awakening the Healer Within," by C. L. Wells-Federman, 1996, *Holistic Nursing Practice, 10,* pp. 13–29. Adapted with permission.

ASSESSMENT INTERVIEW
Complementary and Alternative Therapies

- Tell me about your use of teas, herbs, vitamins, or other natural products to improve your health.
- What traditional or folk remedies are used in your family?
- Do you meditate, pray, or use relaxation techniques, music, or yoga for healing purposes?
- What alternative therapies have you used (acupuncture, touch therapies, magnets, hypnosis, etc.)?

soning ability. Emotionally healthy people experience evenly balanced emotional states and a sense of well-being or happiness. Physically healthy people have abundant energy with proper functioning of the senses, digestion, and elimination. From a spiritual perspective, healthy people have a sense of aliveness and richness of life, are developing in the direction of their full potential, and are in good relationships with themselves, other people, and the larger cosmos. Environmentally healthy individuals have minimal economic, social, and political stress.

Specific lifestyle interventions are a major preventive and therapeutic approach in Ayurveda. Each person is prescribed an individualized diet and exercise program depending on dosha (body) type and the nature of the underlying dosha imbalance. Herbal preparations are added to the diet for preventive or regenerative purposes as well as for the treatment of specific disorders. Yoga, breathing exercises, and meditative techniques are also prescribed by the practitioner. This ancient system has adapted to modern science and technology, including biomedical science and quantum physics.

Traditional Chinese Medicine

Traditional Chinese medicine (TCM) has developed over 3,000 years and is based on the premise that the body's vital energy or **qi** (pronounced *chee*) circulates through pathways or meridians and can be accessed and manipulated through specific anatomical points along the surface of the body. Disease is described as an imbalance or interruption in the flow of qi. In TCM the mind, body, spirit, and emotions are never separated. Thus, the heart is not just a blood pump; it also influences one's capacity for joy, one's sense of purpose in life, and one's connectedness with others. The kidneys filter fluids, but they also manage one's capacity for fear, one's will and motivation, and one's faith in life. The lungs breathe in air and breathe out waste products, but they also regulate one's capacity to grieve, as well as one's acknowledgment of self and others. The liver cleanses the body, and it also influences one's feeling of anger as well as that of vision and creativity. The stomach has a part in digestion of food and influences one's ability to be thoughtful, kind, and nurturing as well. These are just a few of the mind–body connections that TCM practitioners recognize.

Practitioners are trained to use a variety of ancient and modern therapeutic methods, including acupuncture, acupressure, herbal medicine, massage, heat therapy, qigong, t'ai chi, and nutritional lifestyle counseling.

Native American Healing

Spirituality and medicine are inseparable in Native American healing. Medicine women and men see themselves as channels through which the Great Power helps others achieve well-being in mind, body, and spirit. The only healer is the One who created all things. Medicine people consider that they have certain knowledge to put things together to help the sick person heal and that knowledge has to be dispensed in a certain way, often through ritual or ceremony. The healer enters into the healing relationship with love and compassion. The two individuals experience a joining or merging as this process unfolds. This merger symbolizes the cementing together of people and the Divine Spirit. Healers use medicine objects to assist them and ceremony treatments such as the sweat lodge, singing, pipe ceremony, sun dance, and vision quest. Other treatments include smudging, drumming and chanting, healing touch, acupressure, and herbs.

Health is viewed as a balance or harmony of mind and body. The goal is to be in harmony with all things, which means first being in harmony with oneself. It is believed that most illness begins in the head and people must get rid of ideas that predispose illness. If the mind is negative, the body will be drained, making it more vulnerable. When people open up to the universe, learn what is good for them, and find ways to be happier, they can begin to work toward a longer and healthier life.

Curanderismo

Curanderismo (pronounced *koo rahn dare ees mo*) is a cultural healing tradition found in Latin America and among many Latinos in the United States. Although it is a traditional healing system, it utilizes Western biomedical beliefs, treatment, and practices. Three levels of care are practiced among curanderos (men) and curanderas (women): the material level, the spiritual level, and the mental level. Healers have the gift for working at only one of these levels. The majority of healers work at the material level, and most combine spiritual healing, herbal medicine, and first-aid techniques.

Botanical Healing

Botanical (plant) healings are used by 80% of the world's population. These include herbs, aromatherapy, homeopathy, and naturopathy.

Herbal Medicine

Before pharmaceutical companies existed, there was **herbal medicine.** In many parts of the world, treating illness with herbs is still the only medicine available. Even though only a tiny fraction of plants have been studied for medicinal benefits, conventional primary care providers use plant-derived products regularly. Thirty percent of all prescription drugs sold in the United States are derived from plants. Examples of herbal remedies that have been synthesized into modern drugs are reserpine from the Indian snakeroot plant, digoxin from foxglove, quinine from Peruvian bark, aspirin from willow tree bark, morphine from opium poppy, cocaine from coca leaves, and atropine from deadly nightshade. Recently, researchers discovered paclitaxel (Taxol), found in Pacific yew bark, which is currently being used in the treatment of breast and ovarian cancer.

Not all plant life is beneficial. Most plant-related poisonings are due to accidental consumption of toxic ornamental plants

PRACTICE GUIDELINES

Cautions and Contraindications for Popular Herbal Preparations

- Feverfew, garlic, ginger, and ginkgo may increase the anticoagulant effects of aspirin and anticoagulant medications.
- Echinacea may reduce the effectiveness of immunosuppressants. It has not been found effective in treating colds in children ages 2 to 11 (Taylor et al., 2003).
- Garlic may cause a need for an increased dose of antihypertensives.
- Ginseng may interact with caffeine and cause irritability. It may decrease the effectiveness of glaucoma medications.
- Milk thistle reduces the effectiveness of oral contraceptives.
- St. John's wort may potentiate antidepressant medications, causing severe agitation, nausea, confusion, and possible cardiac problems.
- Saw palmetto may give false low prostate-specific antigen (PSA) levels, thereby delaying diagnosis of prostate cancer.
- Valerian may increase the sedative effects of antianxiety medication.

such as jade, holly, and poinsettia. The vast majority of herbal medicines present no danger if taken appropriately. Some can, however, cause serious side effects if taken in excess or, for some, if taken over a prolonged period of time. Herbs can also interact with drugs, and caution should be used when combining herbs with prescription and over-the-counter (OTC) medications (see Practice Guidelines). Pregnant and breast-feeding women should be cautioned not to take herbs internally except for mild herb teas.

Although herbs can be quite effective, it is important to caution people about becoming overdependent on them. If they have a life-threatening illness such as asthma, experience chest pain, or notice symptoms that persist for longer than a few days, they should seek medical attention. For example, while it may be healthy to take echinacea if they feel a cold coming on, any serious ailment should be diagnosed by a health care practitioner before undertaking an herbal cure. Conventional medicine is best used in crisis situations, and herbs are best used in noncrisis situations.

Nurses must be open to exploring and discussing their clients' uses of and questions regarding herbal medicine. This clinical screening allows for evaluation of herbal intake against known and potential adverse interactions with prescriptions and OTC medications. See Practice Guidelines for some cautions and contraindications.

Aromatherapy

Aromatherapy is the therapeutic use of essential oils of plants in which the odor or fragrance plays an important part. It is an offshoot of herbal medicine with the basis of action the same as that of modern pharmacology. The chemicals found in the essential oils are absorbed into the body, resulting in physiologic or psychologic benefit. Essential oils are extracted from plants and are massaged into the skin, inhaled, placed in baths, used as compresses, or mixed into ointments. Different oils may calm, stimulate, improve sleep, change eating habits, or boost the immune system.

Essential oils, other than lavender or tea tree oil, are quite potent and can irritate the skin, so they should be diluted with a carrier oil before being used on the skin. Carrier oils such as sunflower oil, grapeseed oil and soy oil contain vitamins, proteins, and minerals that provide added nutrients to the body. Essential oils should not be ingested, because even modest amounts can be fatal. Pregnant women and persons with epilepsy should consult a knowledgeable health care practitioner or qualified aromatherapist prior to the use of essential oils. Some oils can trigger bronchial spasms, so persons with asthma should consult their primary health care provider before using oils. Table 19–1 describes helpful oils you can encourage people to have available at home.

Homeopathy

Homeopathy is a self-healing system, assisted by small doses of remedies or medicines, which is useful in a variety of acute and chronic disorders. It was developed by Samuel Hahnemann, a German physician and chemist. He proposed the use of the *law of similars*, which claims that a natural substance that produces a given symptom in a healthy person, cures it in a sick person. If taken in large amounts, these natural compounds will produce symptoms of disease. In the doses used by homeopaths, however, these remedies stimulate a person's self-healing capacity.

Natural healing compounds are prepared through a process of serial dilution. The compound is first dissolved in a water-alcohol mixture called the "mother tincture." One drop of the tincture is then mixed with 10 drops of water-alcohol, and this process is repeated hundreds or thousands of times depending on the potency being prepared. The remedies are diluted beyond the point at which any molecules of the substance can theoretically still be found in the solution. The homeopathic belief is that the more the substance is diluted, the more potent it becomes as a remedy.

It is not presently understood how homeopathic remedies work. A number of theories are proposed. A remedy may be like a hologram. No matter how many times a substance is diluted, a smaller but complete essence of the substance remains. Modern chaos theory supports the observation that major changes occur in living organisms when body substances are activated only slightly. The basic assumption of chaos theory is that minute changes can have huge effects. Advances in quantum physics have led some scientists to suggest that electromagnetic energy in the remedies interacts with the body on some level. Researchers in physical chemistry have proposed the memory of water theory in which the structure of the water-alcohol solutions is altered during the process of dilution and retains its new structure even after the substance is no longer present. It seems likely that remedies work through a bioenergetic or subatomic mechanism that we are not as yet capable of understanding.

Naturopathy

Naturopathic medicine is not only a system of medicine but also a way of life with emphasis on client responsibility, client education, health maintenance, and disease prevention. It may be the model health system of the future with the movement toward healthy lifestyles, healthy diets, and preventive health care.

The education of naturopathic physicians is extensive and similar to conventional medical education. Four years of medical school follow a college degree in a biologic science. Naturopathic medicine holds the same view of human physiology, body functions, and disease processes as conventional medicine. Naturopathic physicians do not provide emergency care nor do they perform major surgery. They rarely prescribe drugs and they treat clients in private practice and outpatient clinics, not in hospitals.

The goal of treatment is the restoration of health and normal body function, rather than the application of a particular therapy. Virtually every complementary and alternative medicine (CAM) therapy is utilized, most of which are described in this chapter. Physicians mix and match different approaches, customizing treatment for each person. The least invasive intervention to support the body's natural healing processes is a primary consideration. These interventions include dietetics, therapeutic nutrition, herbs (European, Native American, and Chinese), physical therapy, spinal manipulation, acupuncture, lifestyle counseling, stress management, exercise therapy, homeopathy, and hydrotherapy.

Nutritional Therapy

Nutritional therapy consists of the consumption of specific types of diets (see Chapter 47 ∞) or supplements, including vitamins, minerals, amino acids, herbs and other botanicals, and miscellaneous substances such as enzymes and fish oils for the

TABLE 19–1	**Helpful Oils to Have at Home**
OIL	**USE**
Chamomile	Soothes muscle aches, sprains, swollen joints; GI antispasmodic; rub on abdomen for colic, indigestion, gas; decreases anxiety, stress-related headaches; decreases insomnia; can be used with children
Eucalyptus	Feels cool to skin and warm to muscles; decreases fever; relieves pain; anti-inflammatory; antiseptic, antiviral, and expectorant to respiratory system in steam inhalation; boosts immune system
Ginger	Helps ward off colds; calms upset stomach, decreases nausea; soothes sprains, muscle spasms
Jasmine	Uplifting and stimulating, antidepressant; massage abdomen and lower back for menstrual cramps
Lavender	Calming, sedative for insomnia; massage around temples for headache; inhale to speed recovery from colds, flu; massage chest to decrease congestion; heals burns
Tea Tree	First-aid kit in a bottle; antifungal, good for athlete's foot; soothes insect bites, stings, cuts, wounds; in bath for yeast infection; drops on handkerchief for coughs, congestion

purpose of preventing or treating illness. Supplements are not considered medications. The Dietary Supplement Health and Education Act of 1994 requires that the companies selling these products determine their safety but they are not required to publicize this information or to inform the Food and Drug Administration of reports of adverse reactions.

There are three major concerns for clients' use of nutritional supplements: efficacy, consistency, and safety. Often, research conducted to determine the effectiveness of supplements has been flawed in design or produced conflicting results. Nurses should assist clients in gathering reliable information about supplements such as information available from the National Institutes of Health Office of Dietary Supplements website. Supplements are manufactured by many different companies and often contain a variety of substances in varying amounts. The specific amount of a substance needed to produce the desired effect may not be known and there is no guarantee that each dose (pill, capsule, tablet, or liquid) contains a consistent amount of the substance. There are no legal definitions of the words *standardized, certified,* or *verified* for supplements. As mentioned in the discussion of herbs, not all supplements are harmless. Some supplements cause adverse effects such as diarrhea or high blood pressure while others become dangerous when taken in combination with certain medications (see Practice Guidelines). Another safety concern with supplements is that they may contain contamination with dangerous substances such as mold, bacteria, pesticides, and metals (Rolfes, Pinna, & Whitney, 2006). Nurses must assess clients for use of dietary supplements and include teaching about the known benefits and risks of supplements in the care planning.

Manual Healing Methods

Some manual healing methods come from ancient times, and some have been developed in the latter half of the twentieth century. These healing practices include chiropractic, massage, acupuncture/acupressure/reflexology, and hand-mediated biofield therapies.

Chiropractic

Chiropractic is the third largest independent health profession in the Western world after conventional medicine and dentistry. Chiropractic practitioners believe that health is a state of balance, especially of the nervous and musculoskeletal systems. When the spine is fully aligned, nerve energy flows freely to every cell and organ in the body. This free flow of energy nurtures the innate ability of the body to work effectively and coordinate normal body functions. Although chiropractic embraces a multifactorial explanation of disease, the chiropractic treatment of choice is spinal adjustment. The biomechanical explanation states that range of motion is improved when fibrous adhesions within joints are broken or small tags from the joint capsule are released through manipulation. The neurophysiologic explanation proposes that mechanoreceptors in the joint are stimulated through manipulation, resulting in a relaxation of the paraspinal muscles.

Three primary clinical goals guide chiropractic intervention. The first clinical goal is to reduce or eliminate pain. The second goal is to correct the spinal dysfunction, thereby restoring biomechanical balance to reestablish shock absorption, leverage, and range of motion. In addition, muscles and ligaments are strengthened by spinal rehabilitative exercises to increase resistance to further injury. The third clinical goal is preventive maintenance to ensure the problem does not recur.

Orthogonal chiropractors focus on the cervical spine using a precision instrument. This instrument delivers a mechanical impulse which allows the doctor to adjust spinal misalignment with a high degree of precision combined with minimal physical pressure.

As holistic practitioners, chiropractors work with many facets of clients' lifestyles. Exercise programs are designed, rehabilitation measures are planned, correct posture and lifting techniques are explained, and activities of daily living are assessed and improved.

Massage

It is believed that massage aids the ability of the body to heal itself and is aimed at achieving or increasing health and wellbeing. In the United States, massage is considered an alternative or complementary treatment compared to many areas of the world where massage is an integral part of health systems.

Strong, sustained touch in massage can have an even greater effect than other forms of touch. A skilled massage therapist not only stretches and loosens muscle and connective tissue, but also greatly improves blood flow and the movement of lymph fluid throughout the body (Figure 19-1 ■). Massage speeds the removal of metabolic waste products resulting from exercise or inactivity, allowing more oxygen and nutrients to reach the cells and tissues. The release of muscular tension also helps to unblock and balance the overall flow of life energy throughout the body.

On the physical level, massage relieves muscle tension, reduces muscle spasms, improves joint flexibility and range of motion, improves posture, lowers blood pressure, slows heart rate, promotes deeper and easier breathing, and improves the

Figure 19-1 ■ Massage over the shoulders and back.

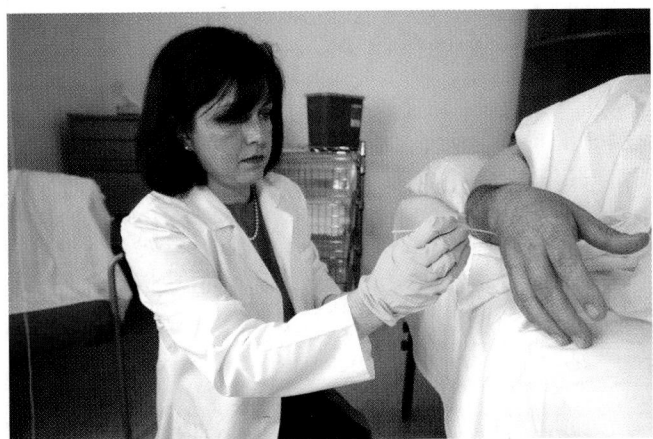

Figure 19-2 ■ Acupuncture involves the insertion of thin, sterile needles.

(Yoav Levy/Phototake NYC.)

health of the skin. On the mental level, massage induces a relaxed state of alertness, reduces mental stress, and increases the capacity for clearer thinking. On the emotional level, massage satisfies the need for caring and nurturing touch, increases feelings of well-being, decreases mild depression, enhances self-image, reduces levels of anxiety, and increases awareness of mind–body connection (Fontaine, 2005). For back massage techniques see Skill 46-1 in Chapter 46. ∞

Acupuncture/Acupressure/Reflexology

Acupuncture and **acupressure** are techniques of applying pressure or stimulation to specific points on the body, known as acupuncture points, to relieve pain, cure certain illnesses, and promote wellness. Acupuncture uses needles (see Figure 19-2 ■), whereas acupres-

sure uses finger pressure. **Reflexology** is a form of acupressure most commonly performed on the feet but the hands or ears may also be manipulated. See Figure 19-3 ■ for the foot reflex areas.

Acupuncture, acupressure, and reflexology are treatments rooted in the traditional Eastern philosophy that qi, or life energy, flows through the body along pathways known as *meridians*. As vital energy flows through the meridians, it forms tiny whirlpools close to the skin's surface at places called acupuncture points. These points function somewhat like gates to moderate the flow of qi.

When the flow of energy becomes blocked or congested, people experience discomfort or pain on a physical level, may feel frustrated or irritable on an emotional level, and may experience a sense of vulnerability or lack of purpose in life on a spiritual level. The goal of care in wellness acupuncture is to recognize and manage the disruption before illness or disease occurs. Practitioners bring balance to the body's energies, which promotes optimal health and well-being, and facilitates people's own healing capacity (Stibich & Wissow, 2006).

A number of clinical trials have studied the effectiveness of acupuncture for symptoms of osteoarthritis (Novey, 2002), most reporting decreased pain, increased function, and general improvement. Likewise, studies have demonstrated significant improvement in pain in people with fibromyalgia syndrome (Singh et al., 2006).

Research has demonstrated that acupuncture improves memory, orientation, and activities of daily living for individuals with certain types of dementia (Yu, Zhang, Liu, Meng, & Han, 2006). Another disorder responding to acupuncture includes chronic low back pain (Brinkhaus et al., 2006).

Hand-Mediated Biofield Therapies

The three most prominent therapies using the hands to alter the biofield, or energy field, are therapeutic touch (TT), healing

Figure 19-3 ■ Foot reflex areas.

RESEARCH NOTE Can Massage Help Renal Clients' Sleep Disturbances?

It is common for persons living with end-stage renal disease (ESRD) to report occurrences of sleep disturbances. Due to this recurring problem, the purpose of this study was to test the effectiveness of acupoints massage for clients with ESRD experiencing sleep disturbances and diminished quality of life. Ninety-eight participants were recruited for this double-blind, randomized control trial. Participants were randomized into the treatment group (receiving acupressure per protocol plus usual care), placebo group (receiving sham acupressure plus usual care), or control group (usual care).

Results of the study indicated significant differences between the acupressure and control groups in subjective sleep quality, sleep duration, habitual sleep efficiency, and sleep sufficiency. The sham acupres-

sure group did report improvements in subjective sleep quality but not as great compared with the participants in the acupressure group.

IMPLICATIONS

Nurses caring for persons living with ESRD may use the data from this study in addressing sleep problems with nonpharmacological interventions. Acupoints massage can be considered a rapid and effective intervention in promoting an enhanced quality of life for persons with ESRD.

Note: From "Acupoints massage in improving the quality of sleep and quality of life in patients with end-stage renal disease," by S. L. Tsay, J. R. Rong, and P. F. Lin, 2003, *Journal of Advanced Nursing, 42*(2), pp. 134–142. Contributed by Dolores Huffman, PhD, RN, Associate Professor of Nursing, Purdue University Calumet.

touch (HT), and Reiki. All three approaches could be simply defined as the use of the hands on or near the body with the intention to help or to heal. The goals are to accelerate the person's own healing process and to facilitate healing at all levels of body, mind, emotions, and spirit. All three are forms of treatment and are not designed to diagnose physical conditions. Nor are they meant to replace conventional surgery, medicine, or drugs in treating organic disease.

Hand-mediated biofield therapies of TT and HT have been pioneered by nurses and are easily learned by nurses. You can use TT, HT, and Reiki in almost any clinical setting, including hospitals, nursing homes, home health care, hospice, and private practice. These therapies are helpful for people with a variety of medical and nursing diagnoses. The National League for Nurses and the American Nurses Association support TT. Energy-field disturbance, defined as a state in which a disruption of the flow of energy surrounding a person's being results in a disharmony of the body, mind, or spirit, is listed as a nursing diagnosis by the North American Nursing Diagnosis Association (NANDA, 2005).

Mind–Body Therapies

In mind–body therapies, individuals focus on realigning or creating balance in mental processes to bring about healing. These therapies include yoga, meditation, hypnotherapy, guided imagery, biofeedback, qigong, t'ai chi, and Pilates.

Yoga

Yoga has been practiced for thousands of years in India, where it is a way of life that includes ethical models for behavior and mental and physical exercises aimed at producing spiritual enlightenment. It is a method for life that can complement and enhance any system of religion, or it can be practiced completely apart from religion. The Western approach to yoga tends to be more fitness oriented with the goal of managing stress, learning to relax, and increasing vitality and well-being. A typical yoga session lasts 20 minutes to an hour. Some people spend 30 minutes doing the poses and another 30 minutes doing breathing practices and meditations. Others spend the majority of the time doing poses and end with a short meditation or relaxation procedure. Even for those who are inactive and out of shape, sick, or weak, sets of

easy exercises can help to loosen the joints and stimulate circulation. If practiced regularly, these simple exercises alone make a great difference in people's health and well-being.

Beginning research indicates people with diabetes who practice yoga may increase the release of insulin from the pancreas (Manjunatha, Vempati, Ghosh, & Bijlani, 2005). Other research demonstrates that yoga as a lifestyle intervention reduces oxidative stress which is increased in a variety of chronic degenerative diseases (Yadav, Ray, Vempati, & Bijlani, 2005). People with exercise-induced bronchoconstriction experience a significant improvement after 40 days of 90 minutes of yoga in the morning and 60 minutes in the evening (Jaber, 2002).

Meditation

Meditation is a general term for a wide range of practices that involve relaxing the body and easing the mind. Meditation is a process that anyone can use to calm themselves, cope with stress, and, for those with spiritual inclinations, feel as one with God or the universe. Meditation can be practiced individually or in groups and is easy to learn. It requires no change in belief system and is compatible with most religious practices.

If practiced regularly, such as 20 minutes twice a day, meditation produces widespread positive effects on physical and psychologic functioning. The autonomic nervous system responds with a decrease in heart rate, lower blood pressure, decreased respiratory rate and oxygen consumption, and a lower arousal threshold. People who meditate say that they have clearer minds and sharper thoughts. Meditation's residual effects—improved stress-coping abilities—are a protection against daily stress and anxiety. All other self-healing methods are improved with the practice of meditation.

The following are guidelines for meditation:

1. Create a special time and place for meditation. Ideally, choose the early morning or evening, and wait at least 2 hours after eating so that complete energy is devoted to meditation rather than to digestive demands. A quiet, comfortable place, devoid of distractions, is helpful.
2. Sit either cross-legged on the floor or upright in a straight-backed chair, keeping the spine straight and the body relaxed. Avoid a lying position; this increases the tendency to fall asleep.

BOX 19–2 Guidelines for Progressive Relaxation

- Sit comfortably in a chair, with your feet flat on the ground.
- Tense and tighten your right fist. Focus on the feeling of tension as you do so.
- Allow the muscles in your right fist to relax. Contrast the difference in feeling from tension to relaxation.
- Repeat the preceding two steps for the left fist.
- Now tense and relax both your left and right fists.
- Focus on and relish the feeling of relaxation.
- Now tighten the muscles in both fists and both arms. Feel the tension, fully relax the muscles, and again focus on the sensation of relaxation.
- Progressively tighten and relax each muscle group in the body: toes, ankles, knees, buttocks and groin, stomach and lower back muscles, chest and upper back muscles, shoulders, forehead, jaw muscles.
- Couple deep breathing with progressive relaxation. While relaxing your muscles, inhale deeply, send the breath to the fist (or other muscle group), and exhale.

The entire exercise should last a minimum of 10 minutes.

3. Support the palms on the thighs, and close the eyes.
4. Follow deep-breathing or progressive relaxation exercises (see Box 19–2).
5. Focus attention completely on either breathing or a chosen mental image. If using a mantra, repeat the word or phrase either aloud or silently while exhaling. When distracting thoughts appear, allow them to drift into and out of your mind without giving them undue attention; then refocus on your breathing or your mantra.
6. Practice this process daily for 10- to 20-minute periods.

Hypnotherapy

Hypnotherapy is the application of hypnosis in a wide variety of medical and psychologic disorders. Hypnosis is a trance state or an altered state of consciousness in which an individual's concentration is focused and distraction is minimized. People in trances are aware of what is going on around them but choose not to focus on it and can return to normal awareness whenever they choose. Hypnosis is not a surrender of control; it is only an advanced form of relaxation. Hypnotherapy can be used to help people gain self-control, improve self-esteem, and become more autonomous. In some medical facilities, hypnosis is routinely used with a variety of conditions, usually in conjunction with other forms of medical, surgical, psychiatric, or psychologic treatment. It can be used with nonmedical clients as well, in working through problems of living or situations of performance anxiety, and in changing bad habits. Depending on the complexity and seriousness of the complaint, treatment typically runs from two to ten sessions.

Guided Imagery

Imagery is a two-way communication between the conscious and unconscious mind and involves the whole body and all of its senses. Most of us image frequently throughout the day. Worry is the most common form of imagery that affects our health. In our imagination we react to current stressors and anticipated dangers. Our bodies become aroused and tense and we activate the fight-or-flight mechanism. **Guided imagery** is a state of focused attention, much like hypnosis, that encourages changes in attitudes, behavior, and physiologic reactions. Guided imagery can help us learn how to stop troublesome thoughts and focus on images that help us relax and decrease the negative impact of stressors.

In guided imagery, the images may be created by the therapist based on the needs and desires of the client. Clients can also create the images as a way to understand the meaning of symptoms or to access inner resources. Imagery stimulates changes in many body functions such as heart rate, blood pressure, respiratory patterns, brain wave rhythms and patterns, electrical characteristics of the skin, local blood flow and temperature, gastrointestinal motility and secretions, sexual arousal, and levels of various hormones and neurotransmitters.

The American Holistic Nurses Association and an organization called Beyond Ordinary Nursing offer a nurses' certificate program in imagery. The program consists of 110 hours of in-depth, hands-on training to provide nurses with experience in relaxation and therapeutic imagery skills. These skills are used to promote healing; decrease pain and symptoms; minimize side effects; manage chronic illness; prepare for procedures, surgery, or childbirth; and access inner wisdom and resources. Table 19–2 describes several types of imagery.

TABLE 19–2 Types of Imagery

TYPE	DESCRIPTION	EXAMPLE
Feeling state	Move from a feeling state of tension to one of peace	May imagine self at a beach or floating gently on the water
End-state	Imagine self in the situation wished for	See self as strong and healthy
Energetic	Imagine free flowing energy	Feel self pulling up energy from the earth through the soles of the feet
Cellular	Imagine events at cellular level	Imagine natural killer cells surrounding and attacking cancer cells
Physiologic	Involves entire body	Imagine all blood vessels relaxed and wider in order to lower blood pressure
Psychologic	Involves perception of self	Imagine a dialogue with a person with whom one is in conflict in an effort to find a new solution to the problem
Spiritual	Make contact with God or the Divine	Imagine being held in the hands of God where you are perfectly safe

Biofeedback

Biofeedback is a method for learned control of physiologic responses of the body. It is a relaxation technique that uses electronic equipment to amplify the electrochemical energy produced by body responses. Normally out of conscious awareness, biofeedback provides perceptible information that individuals can use to gain voluntary control over various physiologic processes such as blood flow in the hands, sweat gland activity, insomnia, muscle spasms, hyperventilation, gastrointestinal symptoms, and incontinence.

Qigong and T'ai Chi

A number of therapies focus on movement, body awareness, and breathing and their purpose is to maintain health as well as to correct specific problems. **Qigong** (pronounced *chee goong*) is a Chinese discipline consisting of breathing and mental exercises combined with body movements. **T'ai chi** (pronounced *teye chee*) arose out of qigong and is a discipline that combines physical fitness, meditation, and self-defense. Both disciplines consist of soft, slow, continuous movements that are circular in nature. The softness of movements develops energy without nervousness. The slowness of movements requires attentive control that quiets the mind and develops one's powers of awareness and concentration. The continuous circular nature of the movements develops strength and endurance.

Almost anyone can participate in movement-oriented therapies. They can be learned by the young and old, by people physically challenged or physically fit, and by those in good health and those recovering from long-term injury or illness. In China, 80-, 90-, and 100-year-old people get up every morning before dawn and go out to the parks to practice qigong or t'ai chi, even in the middle of winter. These Eastern practices can be done alone, in pairs, or in large groups.

Pilates

Pilates (pronounced *pih lah tes*) is a method of physical movement and exercise designed to stretch, strengthen, and balance the body, in particular the core or center including the abdominal region. It is based in principles of yoga, Zen meditation, and ancient Greek and Roman physical regimens. Pilates exercises were developed by Joseph Pilates, a German national in England at the outbreak of World War I, who was interned in a "camp" for enemy aliens. While there he devised his system of exercises to strengthen his frail asthmatic body, which he then taught to his fellow inmates. Exercises, coupled with focused breathing patterns, are done on the floor or with simple types of equipment. Benefits include increased lung capacity, improved flexibility and joint health, muscular coordination, increased bone density, and better posture and balance. Pilates can help rehabilitate back, knee, hip, shoulder, and stress injuries, and relieve muscle aches.

CLINICAL ALERT

Although meditation, biofeedback, and imagery are different techniques, all three involve the process of physical resting and rhythmic breathing. ■

Spiritual Therapy

Health care sciences have begun to demonstrate that spirituality, faith, and religious commitment may play a role in promoting health and reducing illness. For more information about spirituality, see Chapter 41. ∞

Faith and Prayer

Faith refers to our beliefs and expectations about life, ourselves, and others. In a religious context, faith refers to a belief in a Supreme Being who listens and responds to people and who cares about their well-being. In a spiritual context, faith is thought of as the power to accept the nature of life as it is and live in the present moment. It is a sense of letting go of the need to control while trusting and waiting for the moment when answers come.

Prayer is most often defined simply as a form of communication and fellowship with the Deity or Creator. It is also defined as an "active process of appealing to a higher spiritual power, specifically for health reasons" when used within CAM (Barnes, Powell-Griner, McFann, & Nahin, 2004). The universality of prayer is evidenced in all cultures having some form of prayer. Prayer has been and continues to be used in times of difficulty and illness even in the most secular societies. Ninety percent of Americans believe in prayer, 72% to 82% have prayed for personal healing, and 87% have prayed for the healing of others (Taylor, 2003). In *directed prayer,* the praying person asks for a specific outcome, such as for the cancer to go away or for the baby to be born healthy. In contrast, in *nondirected prayer,* no specific outcome is asked. The praying person simply asks for the best thing to occur in a given situation.

Prayer can also be described according to form. *Colloquial prayer* is an informal talk with God, as if one were talking to a good friend. *Intercessory prayer* is asking God for things for oneself or others. The focus is on what God can provide. Intercessory prayer for others may be called "distant" prayer, if the person being prayed for is remote from the person who is praying. This form of prayer is of interest to researchers, but at the present time scientific evidence is not conclusive. *Ritual prayer* is the use of formal prayers or rituals such as prayers from a prayer book or the Jewish siddur, or the Catholic practice of saying the rosary. *Meditative prayer,* also known as contemplative prayer, is similar to meditation and is a process of focusing the mind on an aspect of God for a period of time. Prayer is a self-care strategy that provides comfort, increases hope, and promotes healing and psychologic well-being (Dijoseph & Cavendish, 2005; Hampton & Weinert, 2006).

Miscellaneous Therapies

There are some therapies that do not fit into any of the above categories. These include music therapy, humor and laughter, bioelectromagnetics, detoxifying therapies, and animal-assisted therapy.

Music Therapy

Health is about balance or harmony of body, mind, and spirit. In a state of optimal health, all frequencies are in harmony, like a

Figure 19-4 ■ Listening to music can provide a variety of therapeutic benefits.

finely tuned piano. In fact, music is often used in healing, from the ancient sounds of the drum, rattle, bone flute, and other primitive instruments to the use of current music as a prescription for health.

Music therapy can be used in a variety of practice settings. Quiet, soothing music without words is often used to induce relaxation (see Figure 19-4 ■). Music recordings are often used to relax and distract clients in operative settings, intensive care units, birthing rooms, rehabilitation and physical therapy units, and sleep induction units.

CLINICAL ALERT

CAM modalities may be combined, for example, listening to music while being massaged with essential oils. ■

Humor and Laughter

Health care professionals recently have focused on the positive effects of humor and laughter on health and disease, although Florence Nightingale wrote about the therapeutic effects of laughing in 1860. Humor involves the ability to discover, express, or appreciate the comical or bizarre, to be amused by one's own imperfections or the whimsical aspects of life, and to see the funny side of an otherwise serious situation. Humor in nursing is defined as helping the client "to perceive, appreciate, and express what is funny, amusing, or ludicrous in order to establish relationships, relieve tension, release anger, facilitate learning, or cope with painful feelings" (Dochterman & Bulechek, 2004, p. 422). Elaboration of these functions of humor in nursing situations follows:

- *Establishing relationships.* Humor decreases the social distance between persons and assists in putting persons at ease. When tension is decreased, people can focus on the message and on other people rather than on their own feelings. Use of humor helps the nurse establish rapport with clients, an important factor in achieving success in nursing interventions.
- *Relieving tension and anxiety.* The effective use of humor relieves the tension of emotionally charged events. The personal nature of humor, for example, helps clients deal with the impersonal nature of wearing a hospital gown and numbered ID band and with embarrassing questions and uncomfortable tests. People can also use humor prophylactically to decrease stress.
- *Releasing anger and aggression.* Humor helps individuals act out impulses or feelings in a safe and nonthreatening manner. It dissipates feelings of anger and aggression by focusing on the comic elements of a situation.
- *Facilitating learning.* Many lectures and presentations begin with a joke or cartoon. Humor not only reduces the presenter's anxiety but also gains the audience's attention. People learn more when humor is used and anxiety levels are reduced. People also recall more information when they associate information with a joke. Use of humor in instruction, however, needs to be carefully planned so that it will contribute to learning.
- *Coping with painful feelings.* People may use humor to blunt the immediate effect of situations that are too painful, such as the effect of a threatening diagnosis or treatment. Humor diminishes anxiety and fear and reduces tension, thus enabling the person to confront and deal with the situation (Christie & Moore, 2005).

Humor also has physiologic benefits that involve alternating states of stimulation and relaxation. Laughter stimulates increases in respiratory rate, heart rate, muscular tension, and oxygen exchange. A state of relaxation follows laughter, during which heart rate, blood pressure, respiration, and muscle tension decrease. Humor stimulates the production of catecholamines and hormones. It also releases endorphins, thereby increasing pain tolerance.

Humor brings out and integrates people's positive emotions: hope, faith, will to live, festivity, purpose, and determination. It therefore has healing properties. To use humor effectively, nurses need to be aware of their own feelings as well as the feelings of others and cultural variations in what people consider humorous.

Many health care settings are now interested in providing humor as a caring skill and have recognized that "laughter is the best medicine." "Humor" rooms are being created for clients and staff that are supplied with items such as games, funny audiotapes and videotapes, humorous books, and collections of cartoons.

Bioelectromagnetics

Bioelectromagnetics is the emerging science that studies how living organisms interact with electromagnetic fields. It works on the principle that every animal, plant, and mineral has an electromagnetic field that enables organic beings and inorganic objects, such as crystals, to communicate and interact as part of a single, unified energy system. Magnetic fields are able to penetrate the body and affect the functioning of cells, tissues, organs, and systems. These therapies work best in combination with other healing modalities and are considered to be adjunct treatments to conventional medicine. Magnets are used to relieve joint pain and headaches, to speed up healing of wounds by increasing blood flow, and to improve bone repair (Wolsko et al., 2004).

Contraindications for magnetic therapy include pregnancy, pacemakers, implanted defibrillators, aneurysm clips in the brain, cochlear implants, or other implanted electrical devices. They should not be used by people on anticoagulants, those with an actively bleeding or open wound, or those with a freshly torn muscle.

Infrared Photoenergy Therapy

Infrared photoenergy therapy is a safe and effective treatment to improve sensory impairment associated with peripheral neuropathy. The treatments are given with the Anodyne Therapy System three to five times a week for 2 weeks. It is believed that the treatment works by increasing energy inside cells, as well as by improving circulation. Research demonstrates improved sensation in the feet, less pain, and improved balance (Leonard, Farooqi, & Myers, 2004).

Detoxifying Therapies

Many cultures and religions, past and present, have rituals of purification. In Western cultures, some people are currently fascinated with the concept of **detoxification,** the belief that physical impurities and toxins must be cleared from the body to achieve better health.

The use of water as a healing treatment is known as *hydrotherapy.* The use of hot and cold moisture in the form of solid, liquid, or gas makes use of the body's response to heat and cold. Hydrotherapy is used to decrease pain, decrease fever, reduce swelling, reduce cramps, induce sleep, and improve physical and mental tone. It must be used with great care in the very young or old who have poor heat regulation and also with people experiencing a prolonged illness or fatigue.

Colonics, or colon therapy, is based on the idea that high-fat, Western diets lead to an accumulation of a thick, gluelike substance in the colon, which in turn produces toxins that lead to disease. Colonics is the procedure for washing the inner wall of the colon by filling it with water or herbal solutions and then draining it. Colon cleansing is a controversial method of detoxification, and there tends to be no middle group in the beliefs about the usefulness of colonics. Contraindications include people in a weakened state and those having ulcerative colitis, diverticulitis, Crohn's disease, severe hemorrhoids, or tumors of the large intestine or rectum.

Chelation therapy is the introduction of chemicals into the bloodstream that bind with heavy metals in the body. Ethylene diamine tetraacetic acid (EDTA) is a synthetic amino acid that readily binds to lead. The U.S. Federal Drug Administration has approved EDTA for the treatment of lead poisoning, hypercalcemia, and ventricular fibrillation secondary to digitalis toxicity.

Animal-Assisted Therapy

Animal-assisted therapy is the use of specifically selected animals as a treatment modality in health and human service settings. It has been shown to be a successful intervention for people with a variety of physical or psychologic conditions. Throwing an object for a dog to retrieve or brushing the animal increases upper extremity range of motion. Reaching for the object the dog has retrieved improves coordination. Ambulating with a dog improves mobility. Recalling the animal's name helps with memory. Using simple commands to the animal increases language production. Attending to the animal and the situation increases attention and concentration. Therapeutic horseback riding, or hippotherapy, is the use of the rhythmic movement of the horse to increase sensory processing and improve posture, balance, and mobility in people with movement dysfunctions.

Resident animals live at long-term health care facilities. Species include fish, birds, hamsters, gerbils, guinea pigs, rabbits, cats, and dogs. Some staff report that full-time pets become

REAL WORLD PRACTICE

Pet Therapy is gaining popularity as a form of pain management throughout the nation. Pet therapy can reduce pain level, and in some cases decrease the blood pressure and heart rates of hospitalized clients. Many clients leave beloved pets at home when they are hospitalized, and become quite sad without this companionship during a stressful time. The use of specially trained and certified pets in visitations, such as those who have been certified by the International Delta Society (IDS), can help to ease a client's discomfort and anxiety. One example of the great work a pet therapy dog provided, involves a child whose siblings were killed in a house fire. This child suffered extensive injuries and permanent disabilities. During the initial hospitalization and rehabilitation a pet therapy dog provided loving comfort through multiple visits to this child.

The child began to verbalize more and became much more cooperative with her required rehabilitation exercises. This very special dog became friends with a child who had suffered great loss. The dog's always affectionate and happy demeanor provided comfort in a way that only a very special pet can.

Another example of pet therapy involved an IDS certified cat. Not too many cats are pet therapy trained. However one very special cat is a routine visitor to all client care units in a hospital on a weekly basis. This totally calm cat has proven himself to be a super pain management tool. A client in Critical Care had been suffering from intractable pain, unrelieved by any of the medications or other interventions employed. The client had been crying and restless all morning. When the cat was brought by his handler into the room to visit, the client began to smile and talk to him. The cat lay down on the bed, allowing the client to pet him. While purring loudly, he fell asleep as the client stroked the cat's fur for over an hour. When it was time for the cat to leave, the client remained calm, denied any pain, and then slept the entire night!

—*Pat Larson, RN,*
La Porte Hospital, Indiana

so perceptive that they actually gravitate to the rooms of people who are the most isolated or depressed. Those residents who have regular visits are more receptive to treatment, have a greater incentive to recover, and have an increased will to live (*Animals in Residential Facilities*, 2003). The contributions companion animals (personal pets) make to the emotional well-being of people include providing unconditional love and opportunities for affection; achievement of trust, responsibility, and empathy toward others; a reason to get up in the morning; and a source of reassurance.

Horticultural Therapy

Horticultural therapy, also called gardening or a healing garden, is an adjunct therapy to occupational and physical therapy. People may view nature, visit a healing garden or a wander garden, or actually participate in gardening. When it is a communal activity, gardening decreases social isolation by fostering interactions with others. Horticultural therapy stimulates the five senses, provides leisure activities, improves motor function, provides a sense of achievement, and improves self-esteem (Detweiler & Warf, 2005; Milligan, Gatrell, & Bingley, 2004).

LIFESPAN CONSIDERATIONS   Examples of CAM Use

There are many examples of CAM use among different age groups. Following are a few illustrating alternative therapy in children and elders.

PEDIATRICS

Mask making can be used as a therapeutic tool when working with children who are chronically or terminally ill. Chronic or terminal illnesses strain the emotional and spiritual integrity of children and families. As a form of art therapy, mask making helps children cope with their illness by "making special," or moving their understanding of the illness and its effects beyond the ordinary, often into the spiritual realm. The process of making the mask can help the child confront the illness, express his or her emotions, develop meaning, and, ultimately, gain a sense of control in an overwhelming situation.

Masks can be made from materials found in the health care setting—gauze, plastic cups for dispensing medication, plastic covers from IV ports, gloves, and tubing. They can be hung from doors, put on walls, or made into mobiles. Children can be very creative in making masks. After a child's death, the mask can be a way parents and others remember the child. "For me, there is no technology to date that addresses the uniqueness of the individual or the healing of the human spirit in the way art does" (Driessnack, 2004, p. 214).

ELDERS

The practice of t'ai chi has been found to have the following benefits:

- T'ai chi improves the balance of older adults and reduces the risk of falls (Hakim, Newton, Segal, & DuCette, 2004). This is especially important for people with osteoporosis. Those who have better postural control and increased flexibility reduce their risk of falls and risk of hip fractures, which are a major contributor to dysfunction and death in elderly women.

- Older adults with moderate sleep complaints improved self-rated sleep quality through a 6-month, low- to moderate-intensity t'ai chi program. T'ai chi appears to be effective as a nonpharmacological approach to sleep enhancement for sleep-disturbed elderly individuals (Li et al., 2004).

- A randomized study found that older adults who performed t'ai chi had an increase in varicella zoster virus–specific cell-mediated immunity and thus decreased risk for herpes zoster. This is the first study to demonstrate that a behavioral intervention can influence a virus-specific response (Irwin et al., 2003).

- The first prospective and randomized study showed that a programmed t'ai chi exercise intervention is beneficial for retarding bone loss in weight-bearing bones in early postmenopausal women (Chan et al., 2004).

CRITICAL THINKING CHECKPOINT

Tim Le is a 68-year-old accountant who has been diagnosed with gastric cancer. He lost a great deal of weight before the diagnosis and during treatment with chemotherapy and radiation. He is now admitted to the hospital with pain and weakness preventing him from working or performing many activities of daily living. His wife, Susan Carter, stays with him the majority of the day. His elderly parents visit often and bring him homemade food and drink. They do not speak English. In the process of placing bathing items in Tim's bedside stand, the nurse notes several plastic bags of a tea-like product in the drawer.

1. What aspects of this case suggest that it would be appropriate for the nurse to discuss the use of alternative therapies with the client or family?

2. Which alternative therapies might be most useful for this client and are in keeping with the principle of "do no harm"?

3. How should the nurse respond to finding the bags in the client's drawer? What options should be considered and what are the likely results of each?

4. How might the nurse's own belief system influence his or her interactions with the client and family regarding CAM?

See Critical Thinking Possibilities in Appendix A. ∞

CHAPTER 19 **REVIEW**

CHAPTER HIGHLIGHTS

- The concepts common to most alternative practices include holism, humanism, balance, spirituality, energy, and healing environments.
- We create healing environments when we provide holistic nursing care, take time to be with clients in deeply caring ways, and balance technology and compassion.
- If we do not create healing environments for ourselves, we are in danger of nursing "burnout."
- Ancient health care practices typically include an entire set of values, attitudes, and beliefs that generate a philosophy of life, not simply a group of remedies. Biomedicine is reductionistic rather than holistic.

- Thirty percent of all prescription drugs sold in the United States are derived from plants.
- Although many botanical and nutritional supplements can be helpful in certain conditions, their effectiveness and safety are not all well studied.
- Mind–body therapies such as yoga, meditation, hypnotherapy, guided imagery, biofeedback, qigong, t'ai chi, and Pilates all focus on realigning or creating balance in mental and physical processes to bring about healing.

TEST YOUR KNOWLEDGE

1. A client asks the nurse the differences between traditional therapies and alternative therapies. Which of the following is the best response?
   1. Alternative therapies cost less than traditional therapies.
   2. Alternative therapies are used if traditional therapies are ineffective.
   3. Alternative therapies can be as effective as traditional therapies for some conditions.
   4. Alternative therapies utilize products from nature but traditional therapies do not.

2. Before meeting with a client with a terminal illness, a new graduate nurse reviews information on spirituality. Which of the following is the *best* explanation of spirituality?
   1. That which gives people purpose and meaning in their lives
   2. A formalized religious dogma
   3. A nondenominational community service
   4. People being responsible for their life patterns

3. In which of the following ways do nurses create healing environments?
   1. Use technology to prevent hospital-acquired infections
   2. Empower clients to make healthy decisions for themselves
   3. Place aquariums in day rooms of nursing homes
   4. Ensure that physicians' orders are carried out

4. A client asks the nurse to state one of the primary principles associated with naturopathy. Which of the following is the best response?
   1. A higher being guides the learning needed to treat disease
   2. Focuses on enviornmental causes when treating illnesses
   3. Focuses on early detection and treatment of disease
   4. Is a way of life to maintain health and prevent disease

5. From the perspective of traditional Chinese medicine (TCM), which is the best definition of disease?
   1. Imbalance or disruption in food digestion
   2. Imbalance or interruption in the flow of qi
   3. Imbalance or disruption in key social relationships
   4. Imbalance or disruption in thoughts or emotions

See Answers to Test Your Knowledge in Appendix A.

EXPLORE MEDIALINK www.prenhall.com/berman

DVD-ROM
- Audio Glossary
- NCLEX Review
- End of Unit Concept Map Activity

COMPANION WEBSITE
- Additional NCLEX Review
- Care Plan Activity: Lyme Disease
- Case Study: Complementary Alternative Medicine
- Application Activity: Support for Alternative Therapies
- Links to Resources

READINGS AND REFERENCES

SUGGESTED READINGS
Fontaine, K. L. (2005). *Complementary & alternative therapies for nursing practice* (2nd ed.). Upper Saddle River, NJ: Prentice Hall. *This practical guide covers the principles, techniques, research, and health promotion methods and healing practices of specific illnesses and symptoms. It discusses over 40 alternative therapies.*

RELATED RESEARCH
Arais, D. C. (2004). Alternative medicines' popularity prompts concern: Use of alternative and complementary remedies on the rise. *Nation's Health, 34*(6). Retrieved March 6, 2005, from www.medscape.com/viewarticle/484309?src=search
Larden, C. N., Palmer, M. L., & Janssen, P. (2004). Efficacy of therapeutic touch in treating

pregnant inpatients who have a chemical dependency. *Journal of Holistic Nursing, 22*, 320–332.
Weze, C., Leathard, H. L., Grange, J., Tiplady, P., & Stevens, G. (2005). Evaluation of healing by gentle touch. *Public Health, 119*(1), 3–10.

REFERENCES

Animals in residential facilities: Guidelines and resources for success. (2003). Renton, WA: Delta Society.

Barnes, P. M., Powell-Griner, E., McFann, K., & Nahin, R. L. (2004). Complementary and alternative medicine use among adults, United States, 2002. *Advance Data from Vital and Health Statistics,* no. 343. Hyattsville, MD: Anderson National Center for Health Statistics.

Brinkhaus, B., Witt, C. M., Jena, S., Linde, K., Streng, A., Wagenpfeil, S., et al. (2006). Acupuncture in patients with chronic low back pain. *Archives of Internal Medicine, 166,* 450–457.

Chan, K., Qin, L., Lau, M., Woo, J., Au, S., Choy, W., et al. (2004). A randomized, prospective study of the effects of Tai Chi Chun exercise on bone mineral density in postmenopausal women. *Archives of Physical Medicine and Rehabilitation, 85,* 717–722.

Christie, W., & Moore, C. (2005). The impact of humor on patients with cancer. *Clinical Journal of Oncology Nursing, 9,* 211–218.

Detweiler, M. B., & Warf, C. (2005). Dementia wander garden aids post cerebrovascular stroke restorative therapy. *Alternative Therapies in Health and Medicine, 11*(4), 54–58.

Dijoseph, J., & Cavendish, R. (2005). Expanding the dialogue on prayer relevant to holistic care. *Holistic Nursing Practice, 19,* 147–154.

Dochterman, J., & Bulechek, G. B. (Eds.). (2004). *Nursing interventions classification (NIC)* (4th ed.). St. Louis, MO: Mosby.

Driessnack, M. (2004). Remember me: Mask making with chronically and terminally ill children. *Holistic Nursing Practice, 18,* 211–214.

Fontaine, K. L. (2005). *Complementary & alternative therapies for nursing practice* (2nd ed.). Upper Saddle River, NJ: Prentice Hall.

Hakim, R. M., Newton, R. A., Segal, J., & DuCette, J. P. (2004). A group intervention to reduce fall risk factors in community dwelling older adults. *Physical and Occupational Therapy in Geriatrics, 22*(1), 1–20.

Hampton, J. S., & Weinert, C. (2006). An exploration of spirituality in rural women with chronic illness. *Holistic Nursing Practice, 20*(1), 27–33.

Irwin, M. R., Pike, J. L., Cole, J. C., & Oxman, M. N. (2003). Effects of a behavioral intervention, tai chi chih, on varicella-zoster virus specific immunity and health functioning in older adults. *Psychosomatic Medicine, 65,* 824–830.

Jaber, R. (2002). Respiratory and allergic diseases. *Primary Care, 29,* 231–261.

Leonard, D. R., Farooqi, M. H., & Myers, S. (2004). Restoration of sensation, reduced pain, and improved balance in subjects with diabetic peripheral neuropathy. *Diabetes Care, 27*(1), 168–172.

Li, F., Fisher, K. J., Harmer, P., Irbe, D., Tearse, R. G., & Weimer, C. (2004). Tai chi and self rated quality of sleep and daytime sleepiness in older adults: A randomized controlled trial. *Journal of the American Geriatrics Society, 52,* 892–900.

Manjunatha, S., Vempati, R. P., Ghosh, D., & Bijlani, R. L. (2005). An investigation into the acute and long-term effects of selected yogic postures on fasting and postprandial glycemia and insulinemia in healthy young subjects. *Indian Journal of Physiology and Pharmacology, 49,* 319–324.

Milligan, C., Gatrell, A., & Bingley, A. (2004). Cultivating health. *Social Science & Medicine, 58,* 1781–1793.

Nightingale, F. (1969). *Notes on nursing: What it is, and what it is not.* New York: Dover. (Original work published 1860)

Novey, D. W. (2002). Osteoarthritis. *Primary Care, 29,* 263–277.

Rolfes, S. R., Pinna, K., & Whitney, E. (2006). *Understanding normal and clinical nutrition* (7th ed.). Belmont, CA: Thomson.

Singh, B. B., Wu, W. S., Hwang, S. H., Khorsan, R., Der-Martirosian, C., Vinjamury, S. P., et al. (2006). Effectiveness of acupuncture in the treatment of fibromyalgia. *Alternative Therapies in Health and Medicine, 12*(2), 34–41.

Stibich, M., & Wissow, L. (2006). Meaning shift: Findings from wellness acupuncture. *Alternative Therapies in Health and Medicine, 12*(2), 42–48.

Taylor, E. J. (2003). Prayer's clinical issues and implications. *Holistic Nursing Practice, 17,* 179–188.

Taylor, J. A., Weber, W., Standish, L., Quinn, H., Goesling, J., McGann, M., et al. (2003). Efficacy and safety of Echinacea in treating upper respiratory tract infections in children. *Journal of the American Medical Association, 290,* 2824–2830.

Tsay, S. L., Rong, J. R., & Lin, P. F. (2003). Acupoints massage in improving the quality of sleep and quality of life in patients with end-stage renal disease. *Journal of Advanced Nursing, 42*(2), 134–142.

Wells-Federman, C. L. (1996). Awakening the healer within. *Holistic Nursing Practice, 10,* 13–29.

Wolsko, P. M., Eisenberg, D. M., Simon, L. S., Davis, R. B., Walleczek, J., Mayo Smith, M., et al.

(2004). Double blind placebo controlled trial of static magnets for the treatment of osteoarthritis of the knee: Results of a pilot study. *Alternative Therapies in Health and Medicine, 10*(2), 36–43.

Yadav, R. K., Ray, R. B., Vempati, R., & Bijlani, R. L. (2005). Effect of a comprehensive yoga-based lifestyle modification program on lipid peroxidation. *Indian Journal of Physiology and Pharmacology, 49,* 358–362.

Yu, J., Zhang, X., Liu, C., Meng, Y., & Han, J. (2006). Effect of acupuncture treatment on vascular dementia. *Neurological Research, 28,* 97–103.

SELECTED BIBLIOGRAPHY

Benson, H., Dusek, J. A., Sherwood, J. B., Lam, P., Bethea, C. F., Carpenter, W., et al. (2006). The Study of Therapeutic Effects of Intercessory Prayer (STEP) in cardiac bypass patients: A multicenter randomized trial of uncertainty and certainty of receiving intercessory prayer. *American Heart Journal, 151,* 934–942.

Bulkeley, K. (2003). *Dreams of healing.* New York: Paulist Press.

Denison, B. (2004). Touch the pain away. *Holistic Nursing Practice, 18*(3), 142–151.

Dossey, B. M., Keegan, L., & Guzzetta, C. (2004). *Pocket guide for holistic nursing.* Boston: Jones & Bartlett.

Lenarz, M. (2003). *The chiropractic way.* New York: Bantam Books.

Moore, T. (2005). Best practice guidelines: An invitation to reflect on therapeutic touch practice. *Journal of Nursing Care Quality, 20*(1), 90–94.

NANDA International. (2005). NANDA *nursing diagnoses: Definitions and classification 2005–2006.* Philadelphia: Author.

National Center for Complementary and Alternative Medicine. (2004). *Expanding horizons of health care: Strategic plan 2005–2009.* Washington, DC: U.S. Department of Health and Human Services.

Ornish, D. (2004). *Dr. Dean Ornish's program for reversing heart disease* (rev. ed.). New York: Ballantine Books.

Potter, P. (2003). What are the distinctions between Reiki and therapeutic touch? *Clinical Journal of Oncology Nursing, 7*(1), 1–3.

Wardell, D. W., & Weymouth, K. F. (2004). Review of studies of healing touch. *Journal of Nursing Scholarship, 36,* 147–154.

UNIT
5

Life Span Development

Along the intriguing journey from infancy through old age, human beings encounter new and often challenging life changes. An understanding and appreciation of how people develop at various stages of life influences much of nursing practice. The nurse's ability to consider the impact of prevailing life span issues as well as the needs of the individual promotes care that is appropriate, meaningful, and more likely to achieve desired outcomes.

CHAPTER 20

Concepts of Growth and Development

LEARNING OUTCOMES

After completing this chapter, you will be able to:

1. Differentiate between the terms *growth* and *development*.

2. Describe essential principles related to growth and development.

3. List factors that influence growth and development.

4. Explain the concept of temperament.

5. Describe the stages of growth and development according to various theorists.

6. Describe characteristics and implications of Freud's five stages of development.

7. Identify Erikson's eight stages of development.

8. Identify developmental tasks associated with Havighurst's six age periods.

9. Compare Peck's and Gould's stages of adult development.

10. Explain Piaget's theory of cognitive development.

11. Compare Kohlberg's and Gilligan's theories of moral development.

12. Compare Fowler's and Westerhoff's stages of spiritual development.

The terms *growth* and *development* both refer to dynamic processes. Often used interchangeably, these terms have different meanings. **Growth** is physical change and increase in size. It can be measured quantitatively. Indicators of growth include height, weight, bone size, and dentition. The pattern of physiologic growth is similar for all people. However, growth rates vary during different stages of growth and development. The growth rate is rapid during the prenatal, neonatal, infancy, and adolescent stages and slows during childhood. Physical growth is minimal during adulthood.

Development is an increase in the complexity of function and skill progression. It is the capacity and skill of a person to adapt to the environment. Development is the behavioral aspect of growth (e.g., a person develops the ability to walk, to talk, and to run).

Growth and development are independent, interrelated processes. For example, an infant's muscles, bones, and nervous system must grow to a certain point before the infant is able to sit up or walk. Growth generally takes place during the first 20 years of life; development takes place during that time and also continues after that point. Principles of growth and development are shown in Box 20–1.

FACTORS INFLUENCING GROWTH AND DEVELOPMENT

Many factors can influence growth and development. Knowledge of these factors helps the nurse to intervene to promote positive growth and development of the individual.

BOX 20–1 Principles of Growth and Development

- Growth and development are continuous, orderly, sequential processes influenced by maturational, environmental, and genetic factors.
- All humans follow the same pattern of growth and development.
- The sequence of each stage is predictable, although the time of onset, the length of the stage, and the effects of each stage vary with the person.
- Learning can either help or hinder the maturational process, depending on what is learned.
- Each developmental stage has its own characteristics. For example, Piaget suggested that in the sensorimotor stage (birth to 2 years) children learn to coordinate simple motor tasks.
- Growth and development occur in a cephalocaudal direction, that is, starting at the head and moving to the trunk, the legs, and the feet (see Figure 20-1■). This pattern is particularly obvious at birth, when the head of the infant is disproportionately large.
- Growth and development occur in a proximodistal direction, that is, from the center of the body outward (Figure 20-1). For example, infants can roll over before they can grasp an object with the thumb and second finger.
- Development proceeds from simple to complex, or from single acts to integrated acts. To accomplish the integrated act of drinking and swallowing from a cup, for example, the child must first learn a series of single acts: eye-hand coordination, grasping, hand-mouth coordination, controlled tipping of the cup, and then mouth, lip, and tongue movements to drink and swallow.
- Development becomes increasingly differentiated. Differentiated development begins with a generalized response and progresses to a skilled specific response. For example, an infant's initial response

Figure 20-1 ■ Cephalocaudal and proximodistal growth.

to a stimulus involves the total body; a 5-year-old child can respond more specifically with laughter or fear.
- Certain stages of growth and development are more critical than others. It is known, for example, that the first 10 to 12 weeks after conception are critical. The incidence of congenital anomalies as a result of exposure to certain viruses, chemicals, or drugs is greater during this stage than others.
- The pace of growth and development is uneven. It is known that growth is greater during infancy than during childhood. Asynchronous development is demonstrated by rapid growth of the head during infancy and the extremities at puberty.

Genetic

The genetic inheritance of an individual is established at conception. It remains unchanged throughout life and determines such characteristics as gender, physical characteristics (e.g., eye color, potential height), and, to some extent, temperament.

Temperament

Temperament (i.e., the way individuals respond to their external and internal environment) sets the stage for the interactive dynamics of growth and development. Temperament may persist throughout the life span, though caution must be taken not to irrevocably "label" or categorize infants and children.

Family

The purpose of a family is to provide support and safety for the child. The family is the major constant in a child's life. Families are involved in their children's physical and psychologic well-being and development (Ball & Bindler, 2006). Children are socialized through family dynamics. The parents set expected behaviors and model appropriate behavior.

Nutrition

Adequate nutrition is an essential component of growth and development. For example, poorly nourished children are more likely to have infections than are well-nourished children. In addition, poorly nourished children may not attain their full height potential.

Environment

A few environmental factors that can influence growth and development include living conditions of the child (e.g., homelessness), socioeconomic status (e.g., poor versus financial stability), climate, and community (e.g., provides developmental support versus exposes the child to hazards).

Health

Illness or injury can affect growth and development. Being hospitalized is stressful for a child and can affect coping mechanisms of the child. Prolonged or chronic illness may affect normal developmental processes.

Culture

Cultural customs can influence a child's growth and development. Nutritional practices may influence the rate of growth for infants. Child-rearing practices may influence development. For example, the Native American practice of carrying infants on boards often delays walking (Ball & Bindler, 2006, p. 146).

STAGES OF GROWTH AND DEVELOPMENT

The rate of a person's growth and development is highly individual; however, the sequence of growth and development is predictable. Stages of growth usually correspond to certain developmental changes (see Table 20–1).

Growth and development are commonly thought of as having five major components: biophysical, psychosocial, cognitive, moral, and spiritual. A discussion of some of the major theories relating to these components follows.

GROWTH AND DEVELOPMENT THEORIES

Researchers have advanced several theories about the various stages and aspects of growth and development, particularly with regard to infant and child development.

Biophysical Theory (Gesell, 1880–1961)

Biophysical development theories describe the development of the physical body—how it grows and changes. These changes are compared against established norms. Arnold Gesell is often identified as the "father of child development" in the United States. His theory states that development is directed by genetics. He conducted extensive research at Yale University in the 1920s and 1930s, asserting that child development is a maturational process based on an in-born "timetable." Although children benefit from experience, they will achieve maturational milestones such as rolling over, sitting, and walking at specific times. Gesell's most important work is found in *An Atlas of Infant Behavior* (Gesell, 1934), but his research documented a fixed sequence of developmental milestones of children from infancy through adolescence (Ball, 1977). Between 1930 and 1960, Gesell's books were read by many parents as guides to bringing up children (Gesell, 2006).

Psychosocial Theories

Psychosocial development refers to the development of personality. **Personality,** a complex concept that is difficult to define, can be considered as the outward (interpersonal) expression of the inner (intrapersonal) self. It encompasses a person's temperament, feelings, character traits, independence, self-esteem, self-concept, behavior, ability to interact with others, and ability to adapt to life changes.

Many theorists attempt to account for psychosocial development in humans. Many of these theories explain the development of a person's personality and the causes of behavior.

Freud (1856–1939)

Sigmund Freud introduced a number of concepts about development that are still used today. The concepts of the unconscious mind, defense mechanisms, and the id, ego, and superego are Freud's. The **unconscious mind** is the part of a person's mental life that the person is unaware of. This concept of the unconscious is one of Freud's major contributions to the field of psychiatry. The **id** resides in the unconscious and, operating on the pleasure principle, seeks immediate pleasure and gratification. The **ego,** the realistic part of the person, balances the gratification demands of the id with the limitations of social and physical circumstances. The methods the ego uses to fulfill the needs of the id in a socially acceptable manner are called de-

TABLE 20–1 Stages of Growth and Development

STAGE	AGE	SIGNIFICANT CHARACTERISTICS	NURSING IMPLICATIONS
Neonatal	Birth to 28 days	Behavior is largely reflexive and develops to more purposeful behavior.	Assist parents to identify and meet unmet needs.
Infancy	1 month to 1 year	Physical growth is rapid.	Control the infant's environment so that physical and psychologic needs are met.
Toddlerhood	1 to 3 years	Motor development permits increased physical autonomy. Psychosocial skills increase.	Safety and risk-taking strategies must be balanced to permit growth.
Preschool	3 to 6 years	The preschooler's world is expanding. New experiences and the preschooler's social role are tried during play. Physical growth is slower.	Provide opportunities for play and social activity.
School age	6 to 12 years	Stage includes the preadolescent period (10 to 12 years). Peer group increasingly influences behavior. Physical, cognitive, and social development increases, and communication skills improve.	Allow time and energy for the school-age child to pursue hobbies and school activities. Recognize and support child's achievement.
Adolescence	12 to 20 years	Self-concept changes with biologic development. Values are tested. Physical growth accelerates. Stress increases, especially in face of conflicts.	Assist adolescents to develop coping behaviors. Help adolescents develop strategies for resolving conflicts.
Young adulthood	20 to 40 years	A personal lifestyle develops. Person establishes a relationship with a significant other and a commitment to something.	Accept adult's chosen lifestyle and assist with necessary adjustments relating to health. Recognize the person's commitments. Support change as necessary for health.
Middle adulthood	40 to 65 years	Lifestyle changes due to other changes; for example, children leave home, occupational goals change.	Assist clients to plan for anticipated changes in life, to recognize the risk factors related to health, and to focus on strengths rather than weaknesses.
Older adulthood			
Young-old	65 to 74 years	Adaptation to retirement and changing physical abilities is often necessary. Chronic illness may develop.	Assist clients to keep physically and socially active and to maintain peer group interactions.
Middle-old	75 to 84 years	Adaptation to decline in speed of movement, reaction time, and increasing dependence on others may be necessary.	Assist clients to cope with loss (e.g., hearing, sensory abilities and eyesight, death of loved one). Provide necessary safety measures.
Old-old	85 and over	Increasing physical problems may develop.	Assist clients with self-care as required, and with maintaining as much independence as possible.

fense mechanisms or adaptive mechanisms. **Defense mechanisms,** or **adaptive mechanisms** as they are more commonly called today, are the result of conflicts between the id's impulses and the anxiety created by the conflicts due to social and environmental restrictions. The third aspect of the personality, according to Freud, is the superego. The **superego** contains the conscience and the ego ideal. The conscience consists of society's "do not's," usually as a result of parental and cultural expectations. The ego ideal comprises the standards of perfection toward which the individual strives. Freud proposed that the underlying motivation to human development is a dynamic, psychic energy, which he called **libido.**

According to Freud's theory of psychosexual development, the personality develops in five overlapping stages from birth to adulthood. The libido changes its location of emphasis within the body from one stage to another. Therefore, a particular body area has special significance to a client at a particular stage. The first three stages (oral, anal, and phallic) are called *pregenital stages.* The culminating stage is the *genital stage.* Table 20–2 indicates characteristics for each stage.

Freudian theory asserts that the individual must meet the needs of each stage in order to move successfully to the next developmental stage. For example, during an infant's oral stage, nurses can assist an infant's development by making feeding a pleasurable experience. This provides comfort and security for the infant. Freud also emphasized the importance of infant-parent interaction. Therefore, the nurse as a caregiver should provide a warm, caring atmosphere for an infant and assist parents to do so when the infant returns to their care.

If the person does not achieve a satisfactory progression at one stage, the personality becomes fixated at that stage. **Fixation** is immobilization or the inability of the personality to proceed to the next stage because of anxiety. For example, making toilet training a positive experience during the anal stage enhances the

TABLE 20-2 Freud's Five Stages of Development

STAGE	AGE	CHARACTERISTICS	IMPLICATIONS
Oral	Birth to 1 1/2 year	Mouth is the center of pleasure (major source of gratification and exploration). Security is primary need. Major conflict: weaning	Feeding produces pleasure and sense of comfort and safety. Feeding should be pleasurable and provided when required.
Anal	1 1/2 to 3 years	Anus and bladder are the sources of pleasure (sensual satisfaction, self-control). Major conflict: toilet training	Controlling and expelling feces provide pleasure and sense of control. Toilet training should be a pleasurable experience.
Phallic	4 to 6 years	The child's genitals are the center of pleasure. Masturbation offers pleasure. Other activities can include fantasy, experimentation with peers, and questioning of adults about sexual topics. Major conflict: the Oedipus or Electra complex, which resolves when the child identifies with parent of same sex. (The Oedipus complex refers to the male child's attraction for his mother and hostile attitudes toward his father. The Electra complex refers to the female's attraction for her father and hostile attitudes toward her mother.)	The child identifies with the parent of the opposite sex and later takes on a love relationship outside the family. Encourage identity.
Latency	6 years to puberty	Energy is directed to physical and intellectual activities. Sexual impulses tend to be repressed. Develop relationships between peers of the same sex.	Encourage child with physical and intellectual pursuits. Encourage sports and other activities with same-sex peers.
Genital	Puberty and after	Energy is directed toward full sexual maturity and function and development of skills needed to cope with the environment.	Encourage separation from parents, achievement of independence, and decision making.

Note: From *Health Promotion Strategies Through the Life Span,* 7th ed. (p. 238), by R. B. Murray and J. P. Zentner, 2001, Upper Saddle River, NJ: Merrill/Prentice Hall. Adapted with permission.

child's feeling of self-control. If, however, the toilet training was a negative experience, the resulting conflict or stress can delay or prolong progression through a stage or cause a person to regress to a previous stage. Ideally, an individual progresses through each stage with balance between the id, ego, and superego.

Erikson (1902–1996)

Erik H. Erikson (1963, 1964) adapted and expanded Freud's theory of development to include the entire life span, believing that people continue to develop throughout life. He described eight stages of development (see Table 20–3).

Erikson's theory proposes that life is a sequence of **developmental stages** or levels of achievement. Each stage signals a task that must be accomplished. The resolution of the task can be complete, partial, or unsuccessful. Erikson believed that the more success an individual has at each developmental stage, the healthier the personality of the individual. Failure to complete any developmental stage influences the person's ability to progress to the next level. These developmental stages can be viewed as a series of crises. Successful resolution of these crises supports healthy ego development. Failure to resolve the crises damages the ego.

Erikson's eight stages reflect both positive and negative aspects of the critical life periods. The resolution of the conflicts at each stage enables the person to function effectively in society. Each phase has its own developmental task, and the individual must find a balance between, for example, trust versus mistrust (stage 1) or integrity versus despair (stage 8). See Figure 20-2 ■ and 20-3 ■.

When using Erikson's developmental framework, nurses should be aware of indicators of positive and negative resolution of each developmental stage. According to Erikson, the environment is highly influential in development. Nurses can enhance a client's development by being aware of the individual's developmental stage and assisting with the development of coping skills related to stressors experienced at that specific level. Nurses can strengthen a client's positive resolution of a developmental task by providing the individual with appropriate opportunities and encouragement. For example, a 10-year-old child (industry versus inferiority) can be encouraged to be

Figure 20-2 ■ Trust is established when the infant's basic needs are met.

TABLE 20–3 Erikson's Eight Stages of Development

STAGE	AGE	CENTRAL TASK	INDICATORS OF POSITIVE RESOLUTION	INDICATORS OF NEGATIVE RESOLUTION
Infancy	Birth to 18 months	Trust versus mistrust	Learning to trust others	Mistrust, withdrawal, estrangement
Early childhood	18 months to 3 years	Autonomy versus shame and doubt	Self-control without loss of self-esteem Ability to cooperate and to express oneself	Compulsive self-restraint or compliance Willfulness and defiance
Late childhood	3 to 5 years	Initiative versus guilt	Learning the degree to which assertiveness and purpose influence the environment Beginning ability to evaluate one's own behavior	Lack of self-confidence Pessimism, fear of wrongdoing Overcontrol and overrestriction of own activity
School age	6 to 12 years	Industry versus inferiority	Beginning to create, develop, and manipulate Developing sense of competence and perseverance	Loss of hope, sense of being mediocre Withdrawal from school and peers
Adolescence	12 to 20 years	Identity versus role confusion	Coherent sense of self Plans to actualize one's abilities	Feelings of confusion, indecisiveness, and possible antisocial behavior
Young adulthood	18 to 25 years	Intimacy versus isolation	Intimate relationship with another person Commitment to work and relationships	Impersonal relationships Avoidance of relationship, career, or lifestyle commitments
Adulthood	25 to 65 years	Generativity versus stagnation	Creativity, productivity, concern for others	Self-indulgence, self-concern, lack of interests and commitments
Maturity	65 years to death	Integrity versus despair	Acceptance of worth and uniqueness of one's own life Acceptance of death	Sense of loss, contempt for others

Note: "Figure of Erickson's Stages of Personality Development," from Childhood and Society by Erik H. Erikson. Copyright 1950, © 1963 by W. W. Norton & Company Inc., renewed © 1978, 1991 by Erik H. Erikson. Used by permission of W. W. Norton & Company, Inc.

creative, to finish schoolwork, and to learn how to accomplish these tasks within the limitations imposed by health status.

Erikson emphasized that people must change and adapt their behavior to maintain control over their lives. In his view, no stage in personality development can be bypassed, but people can become fixated at one stage or regress to a previous stage under anxious or stressful conditions. For example, a middle-aged woman who has never satisfactorily accomplished the task of resolving identity versus role confusion might regress to an earlier stage when stressed by an illness with which she cannot cope.

Havighurst (1900–1991)

Robert Havighurst believed that learning is basic to life and that people continue to learn throughout life. He described growth and development as occurring during six stages, each associated with six to ten tasks to be learned (see Table 20–4).

Havighurst promoted the concept of developmental tasks in the 1950s. A **developmental task** is "a task which arises at or about a certain period in the life of an individual, successful achievement of which leads to his happiness and to success with later tasks, while failure leads to unhappiness in the individual, disapproval by society, and difficulty with later tasks" (Havighurst, 1972, p. 2).

Havighurst's developmental tasks provide a framework that the nurse can use to evaluate a person's general accomplishments. However, some nurses find that the broad categories limit its usefulness as a tool in assessing specific accomplishments, particularly those of infancy and childhood. In a multicultural society, the definition of success of tasks may vary with values and belief systems as well (e.g., not all individuals may wish to marry or bear children), making these tasks less relevant for some.

Chess and Thomas

Early research on temperament, conducted in the 1950s by Stella Chess and Alexander Thomas, identified nine temperamental qualities seen in children's behavior (see Table 20–5). The "goodness of fit" between children's temperamental qualities and the demands of their environment contributes to positive interaction and positive growth and development (Rothbart, 2004). Goodness of fit refers to whether parents' expectations of their child's behavior are consistent with the child's temperament type. When parents understand a child's temperament characteristics, they are better able to shape the environment to meet the child's needs (Ball & Bindler, 2006, p. 143).

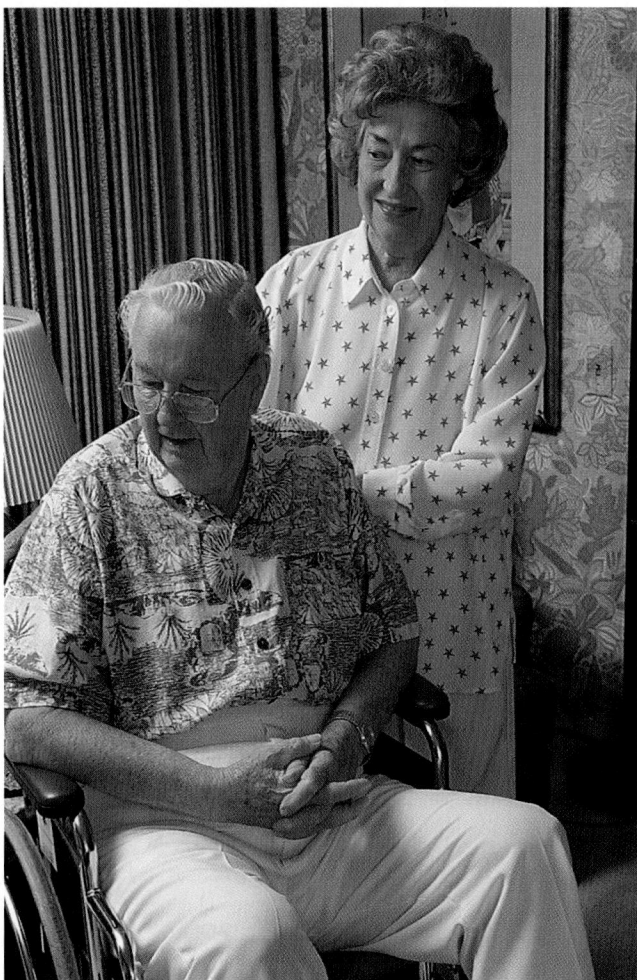

Figure 20-3 ■ Assistive devices help maintain independence and self-esteem, which also helps the older adult's ego integrity to adapt and cope with the reality of aging.

Vygotsky (1896–1934)

Lev Vygotsky, referred to as a "social constructivist," explored the concept of cognitive development within a social, historical, and cultural context, arguing that adults guide children to learn and that development depends on the use of language, play, and extensive social interaction. These ideas have been used in treatment of children with learning disorders, autism, mental handicaps, and other disabilities (Edwards, 2002). These ideas also support the benefit of adult social learning opportunities via group interaction and observation. Vygotsky truly supported social learning and reinforcement through work, group discussion, and other means.

Peck

Theories and models about adult development are relatively recent compared with theories of infant and child development. Research into adult development has been stimulated by a number of factors, including increased longevity and healthier old age. In the past, development was viewed as complete by the time of physical maturity, and aging was considered a decline following maturity. The emphasis was on the negative aspects rather than the positive aspects of aging. However, Robert Peck (1968) believes that although physical capabilities and func-

tions decrease with old age, mental and social capacities tend to increase in the latter part of life.

Peck proposes three developmental tasks during old age, in contrast to Erikson's one (integrity versus despair):

1. *Ego differentiation versus work-role preoccupation.* An adult's identity and feelings of worth are highly dependent on that person's work role. On retirement, people may experience feelings of worthlessness unless they derive their sense of identity from a number of roles so that one such role can replace the work role or occupation as a source of self-esteem. For example, a man who likes to garden or golf can obtain ego rewards from those activities, replacing rewards formerly obtained from his occupation.
2. *Body transcendence versus body preoccupation.* This task calls for the individual to adjust to decreasing physical capacities and at the same time maintain feelings of well-being. Preoccupation with declining body functions reduces happiness and satisfaction with life.
3. *Ego transcendence versus ego preoccupation.* Ego transcendence is the acceptance without fear of one's death as inevitable. This acceptance includes being actively involved in one's own future beyond death. Ego preoccupation, by contrast, results in holding onto life and a preoccupation with self-gratification.

Gould

Roger Gould is another theorist who has studied adult development. He believes that transformation is a central theme during adulthood: "Adults continue to change over the period of time considered to be adulthood and developmental phases may be found during the adult span of life" (Gould, 1972, p. 33). According to Gould, the 20s is the time when a person assumes new roles; in the 30s, role confusion often occurs; in the 40s the person becomes aware of time limitations in relation to accomplishing life's goals; and in the 50s, the acceptance of each stage as a natural progression of life marks the path to adult maturity. Gould's study of 524 men and women led him to describe seven stages of adult development:

■ *Stage 1 (ages 16–18).* Individuals consider themselves part of the family rather than individuals and want to separate from their parents.
■ *Stage 2 (ages 18–22).* Although the individuals have established autonomy, they feel it is in jeopardy; they feel they could be pulled back into their families.
■ *Stage 3 (ages 22–28).* Individuals feel established as adults and autonomous from their families. They see themselves as well-defined but still feel the need to prove themselves to their parents. They see this as the time for growing and building for the future (see Figure 20-4 ■).
■ *Stage 4 (ages 29–34).* Marriage and careers are well established. Individuals question what life is all about and wish to be accepted as they are, no longer finding it necessary to prove themselves.
■ *Stage 5 (ages 35–43).* This is a period of self-reflection. Individuals question values and life itself. They see time as finite, with little time left to shape the lives of adolescent children.

TABLE 20–4 Havighurst's Age Periods and Developmental Tasks

Infancy and Early Childhood
1. Learning to walk
2. Learning to take solid foods
3. Learning to talk
4. Learning to control the elimination of body wastes
5. Learning sex differences and sexual modesty
6. Achieving psychologic stability
7. Forming simple concepts of social and physical reality
8. Learning to relate emotionally to parents, siblings, and other people
9. Learning to distinguish right from wrong and developing a conscience

Middle Childhood
1. Learning physical skills necessary for ordinary games
2. Building wholesome attitudes toward oneself as a growing organism
3. Learning to get along with age-mates
4. Learning an appropriate masculine or feminine social role
5. Developing fundamental skills in reading, writing, and calculating
6. Developing concepts necessary for everyday living
7. Developing conscience, morality, and a scale of values
8. Achieving personal independence
9. Developing attitudes toward social groups and institutions

Adolescence
1. Achieving new and more mature relations with age-mates of both sexes
2. Achieving a masculine or feminine social role
3. Accepting one's physique and using the body effectively
4. Achieving emotional independence from parents and other adults
5. Achieving assurance of economic independence

6. Selecting and preparing for an occupation
7. Preparing for marriage and family life
8. Developing intellectual skills and concepts necessary for civic competence
9. Desiring and achieving socially responsible behavior
10. Acquiring a set of values and an ethical system as a guide to behavior

Early Adulthood
1. Selecting a mate
2. Learning to live with a partner
3. Starting a family
4. Rearing children
5. Managing a home
6. Getting started in an occupation
7. Taking on civic responsibility
8. Finding a congenial social group

Middle Age
1. Achieving adult civic and social responsibility
2. Establishing and maintaining an economic standard of living
3. Assisting teenage children to become responsible and happy adults
4. Developing adult leisure-time activities
5. Relating oneself to one's spouse as a person
6. Accepting and adjusting to the physiologic changes of middle age
7. Adjusting to aging parents

Later Maturity
1. Adjusting to decreasing physical strength and health
2. Adjusting to retirement and reduced income
3. Adjusting to death of a spouse
4. Establishing an explicit affiliation with one's age group
5. Meeting social and civil obligations
6. Establishing satisfactory physical living arrangements

Note: From Robert J. Havighurst, Developmental Tasks and Education, 3rd ed. Published by Allyn and Bacon, Boston, MA. Copyright © 1972 by Pearson Education. Reprinted by permission of the publisher.

■ *Stage 6 (ages 43–50).* Personalities are seen as set. Time is accepted as finite. Individuals are interested in social activities with friends and spouse and desire both sympathy and affection from spouse.

■ *Stage 7 (ages 50–60).* This is a period of transformation, with a realization of mortality and a concern for health. There is an increase in warmth and a decrease in negativism. The spouse is seen as a valuable companion (Gould, 1972, pp. 525–527).

TABLE 20–5 Characteristics of Temperament

CHARACTERISTIC	EXAMPLES OF BEHAVIOR STYLE
Activity level	Active, restless, always on the move versus quiet, inactive
Sensitivity	Apparently oblivious to stimuli versus reacts to minimal stimuli
Intensity	Minimal reaction to stimuli versus reacts strongly and intensely
Adaptability	Responds smoothly to unexpected events versus resists change
Distractibility	Focuses on tasks versus easily distracted by minimal stimuli
Approach/ withdrawal	Jumps right into activities versus hesitant to engage, slow to warm up
Mood	Cheerful, happy versus serious, somber
Persistence	Sticks to tasks versus easily gives up
Regularity	Demonstrates patterns of behavior versus random activity

Figure 20-4 ■ Young adults develop meaningful relationships and begin considering a home and family for themselves.

CONCEPT MAP   **Overview of Growth and Development Psychosocial Theories and Theorists**

Cognitive Theory (Piaget, 1896–1980)

Cognitive development refers to the manner in which people learn to think, reason, and use language. It involves a person's intelligence, perceptual ability, and ability to process information. Cognitive development represents a progression of mental abilities from illogical to logical thinking, from simple to complex problem solving, and from understanding concrete ideas to understanding abstract concepts.

The most widely known cognitive theorist is Jean Piaget. His theory of cognitive development has contributed to other theories, such as Kohlberg's theory of moral development and Fowler's theory of the development of faith, both discussed in this chapter.

According to Piaget (1966), cognitive development is an orderly, sequential process in which a variety of new experiences (stimuli) must exist before intellectual abilities can develop. Piaget's cognitive developmental process is divided into five major phases: the sensorimotor phase, the preconceptual phase, the

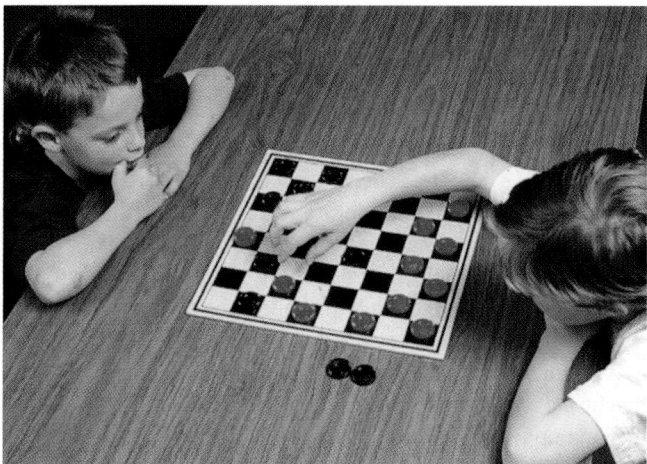

Figure 20-5 ■ School-age (7 to 11 years) children can understand cause-and-effect and concrete relationships or problems.

intuitive thought phase, the concrete operations phase (see Figure 20-5 ■), and the formal operations phase.

A person develops through each of these phases; each phase has its own unique characteristics (see Table 20–6). In each phase, the person uses three primary abilities: assimilation, accommodation, and adaptation. **Assimilation** is the process through which humans encounter and react to new situations by using the mechanisms they already possess. In this way, people acquire knowledge and skills as well as insights into the world around them. **Accommodation** is a process of change whereby cognitive processes mature sufficiently to allow the person to solve problems that were unsolvable before. This adjustment is possible chiefly because new knowledge has been assimilated. **Adaptation,** or coping behavior, is the ability to handle the demands made by the environment.

Nurses can employ Piaget's theory of cognitive development when developing teaching strategies. For example, a nurse can

expect a toddler to be egocentric and literal; therefore, explanations to the toddler should focus on the needs of the toddler rather than on the needs of others. A 13-year-old can be expected to use rational thinking and to reason; therefore, when explaining the need for a medication a nurse can outline the consequences of taking and not taking the medication, enabling the adolescent to make a rational decision. Nurses must remember, however, that the range of normal cognitive development is broad, despite the ages arbitrarily associated with each level. When teaching adults, nurses may become aware that some adults are more comfortable with concrete thought and slower to acquire and apply new information than are other adults.

Behaviorism (Skinner, 1904–1990)

Behaviorist theory states that learning takes place when an individual's reaction to a stimulus is either positively or negatively reinforced. The more rapid, consistent, and positive the reinforcement is, the more likely a behavior is to be learned and retained.

B.F. Skinner believed that organisms learn as they respond to or "operate on" their environment. His research led to the term "operant conditioning," in which he maintained that rewarded or reinforced behavior will be repeated; behavior that is punished will be suppressed. Most of his work was with laboratory animals.

Social Learning (Bandura, 1925–present)

Social learning theory is based on the principle that individuals learn by observing and thinking about the behavior of others. Social learning theorists contend that this process may not always lead to change in the individual's behavior; in contrast, behaviorist theory says that learning will result in a permanent change in behavior. Social learning theory can be seen as spanning both behaviorist and cognitive learning theories.

TABLE 20–6 Piaget's Phases of Cognitive Development

PHASES AND STAGES	AGE	SIGNIFICANT BEHAVIOR
Sensorimotor phase	Birth to 2 years	
Stage 1 Use of reflexes	Birth to 1 month	Most action is reflexive.
Stage 2 Primary circular reaction	1 to 4 months	Perception of events is centered on the body. Objects are extension of self.
Stage 3 Secondary circular reaction	4 to 8 months	Acknowledges the external environment. Actively makes changes in the environment.
Stage 4 Coordination of secondary schemata	8 to 12 months	Can distinguish a goal from a means of attaining it.
Stage 5 Tertiary circular reaction	12 to 18 months	Tries and discovers new goals and ways to attain goals. Rituals are important.
Stage 6 Inventions of new means	18 to 24 months	Interprets the environment by mental image. Uses make-believe and pretend play.
Preconceptual phase	2 to 4 years	Uses an egocentric approach to accommodate the demands of an environment. Everything is significant and relates to "me." Explores the environment. Language development is rapid. Associates words with objects.
Intuitive thought phase	4 to 7 years	Egocentric thinking diminishes. Thinks of one idea at a time. Includes others in the environment. Words express thoughts.
Concrete operations phase	7 to 11 years	Solves concrete problems. Begins to understand relationships such as size. Understands right and left. Cognizant of viewpoints.
Formal operations phase	11 to 15 years	Uses rational thinking. Reasoning is deductive and futuristic.

Note: Adapted from *The Origin of Intelligence*, by J. Piaget, 1966, Copyright © 1966. International Universities Press, Inc. Reprinted with permission.

In contrast to Skinner's "operant conditioning," Alfred Bandura believes that learning occurs through imitation and practice and requires more awareness, self-motivation, and self-regulation of the individual. In Bandura's "social learning theory," the individual actively interacts with the environment to learn new skills and behaviors.

Ecologic Theory (Bronfenbrenner—1917–present)

Bronfenbrenner established the ecologic theory of development. He views the child as interacting with the environment at different levels, or systems. Urie Bronfenbrenner believes each child brings a unique set of genes—and specific attributes such as age,

gender, health, and other characteristics—to his or her interactions with the environment. The child interacts in many settings at different levels or systems (Ball & Bindler, 2006, p. 141).

There are five levels or systems in the ecologic theory. The microsystem includes close relationships the child has on a daily basis (e.g., home, school, friends). The mesosystem level includes relationships of microsystems with one another. For example, two common microsystems for children are home and school. The exosystem includes those settings that may influence the child but with which the child does not have daily contact (e.g., parent's job, local school board). The macrosystem level includes attitudes and beliefs of the child's culture. And the chronosystem involves the time period in which the child is growing up as it influences views of health and illness.

CONCEPT MAP Overview of Growth and Development Theories and Theorists

Moral Theories

Moral development, a complex process not fully understood, involves learning what ought to be and what ought not to be done. It is more than imprinting parents' rules and virtues or values on children. The term **moral** means "relating to right and wrong." The terms *morality, moral behavior*, and *moral development* need to be distinguished from each other. **Morality** refers to the requirements necessary for people to live together in society; **moral behavior** is the way a person perceives those requirements and responds to them; **moral development** is the pattern of change in moral behavior with age (see Chapter 5 ∞).

Kohlberg (1927–1987)

Lawrence Kohlberg's theory specifically addresses moral development in children and adults (Kohlberg, 1981, 1984). The morality of an individual's decision was not Kohlberg's concern; rather, he focused on the reasons an individual makes a decision. According to Kohlberg, moral development progresses through three levels and six stages. Levels and stages are not always linked to a certain developmental stage, because some people progress to a higher level of moral development than others.

At Kohlberg's first level, called the *premoral* or *preconventional level*, children are responsive to cultural rules and labels of good and bad, right and wrong. However, children interpret these in terms of the physical consequences of their actions, that is, punishment or reward. At the second level, the *conventional level*, the individual is concerned about maintaining the expectations of the family, group, or nation and sees this as right. The emphasis at this level is conformity and loyalty to one's own expectations as well as society's. Level three is called the *postconventional, autonomous*, or *principled level*. At this level, people make an effort to define valid values and principles without regard to outside authority or to the expectations of others (see Table 20–7).

TABLE 20–7 Kohlberg's Stages of Moral Development

LEVEL	STAGE	AVERAGE AGE
I. Preconventional Person is responsive to cultural rules of labels of good and bad, right or wrong. Externally established rules determine right or wrong actions. Person reasons in terms of punishment, reward, or exchange of favors. **Egocentric focus**	1. Punishment and Obedient Orientation Fear of punishment, not respect for authority, is the reason for decisions, behavior, and conformity.	Toddler to 7 years
	2. Instrumental Relativist Orientation Conformity is based on egocentricity and narcissistic needs. There is no feeling of justice, loyalty, or gratitude. "I'll do something if I get something for it or because it pleases you."	Preschooler through school age
II. Conventional Person is concerned with maintaining expectations and rules of the family, group, nation, or society. A sense of guilt has developed and affects behavior. The person values conformity, loyalty, and active maintenance of social order and control. Conformity means good behavior or what pleases or helps another and is approved. **Societal focus**	3. Interpersonal Concordance Orientation Decisions and behavior are based on concerns about others' reactions; the person wants others' approval or a reward. An empathic response, based on understanding of how another person feels, is a determinant for decisions and behavior. ("I can put myself in your shoes.")	School age through adulthood (Most American women are in this stage)
	4. Law-and-Order Orientation The person wants established rules from authorities, and the reason for decisions and behavior is that social and sexual rules and traditions demand the response. ("I'll do something because it's the law and my duty.")	Adolescence and adulthood (Most men are in this stage)
III. Postconventional The person lives autonomously and defines moral values and principles that are distinct from personal identification with group values. He or she lives according to principles that are universally agreed on and that the person considers appropriate for life. **Universal focus**	5. Social Contract Legalistic Orientation The social rules are not the sole basis for decisions and behavior because the person believes a higher moral principle applies such as equality, justice, or due process.	Middle-age or older adult. Only 20% or less of Americans achieve this stage.
	6. Universal Ethical Principle Orientation Decisions and behaviors are based on internalized rules, on conscience rather than social laws, and on self-chosen ethical and abstract principles that are universal, comprehensive, and consistent.	Middle-age or older adult. Few people attain or maintain this stage. Examples of this stage are seen in times of crisis or extreme situations.

Note: From *Health Promotion Strategies Through the Life Span,* 7th ed. (pp. 252–253), by R. B. Murray and J. P. Zentner, 2001, Upper Saddle River, NJ: Merrill/Prentice Hall. Adapted with permission.

RESEARCH NOTE What Predicts Conscience in Preschoolers?

Forman and his colleagues (2004) hypothesized that toddlers who show the ability and eagerness to imitate their caregivers are likely to demonstrate a conscience as preschoolers. In a longitudinal study, they examined children at 14 months of age (n=108), and again at 22 months (n=106), 33 months (n=104), and 45 months (n=101).

At the first two ages, interactions between the mother and child were observed to see how the toddler imitated the mother's behavior. Mothers demonstrated three tasks—cleaning a table, having a tea party, and feeding a teddy bear—and the toddler was given the opportunity to imitate. The researchers looked specifically at how much help the mother gave the child, how well the child imitated the mother, how responsive the child was to the mother, and the child's affect during the interaction.

At the latter two ages, preschool-age children were studied for internalized conduct and guilt, two parameters of conscience. The children were presented with three situations. In one situation, toys were verbally forbidden but easily available. In the second situation, the only way to get a reward was to cheat at a game. In the third situation, the child was given a toy that "broke"; after being gently chastised, the child was observed for signs of guilt (i.e., gaze avoidance and bodily tension).

Findings from the study confirmed a strong relationship between imitation among toddlers and conscience as a preschooler. Toddlers who most avidly and successfully imitated mothers' behavior also demonstrated strong internalized conduct (i.e., resisted forbidden toys or cheating) and guilt (i.e., became tense and avoided eye contact). Although the relationship was correlational rather than causative, and other factors (such as temperament, parenting styles, and experience) may influence the development of conscience, it is evident that imitation can be an important predictor.

IMPLICATIONS

Nurses often work with parents around parenting issues. This research supports interventions that encourage parents to allow children to practice or imitate healthful behaviors, even at very early ages. Such practice could strengthen family relationships, teach values, and enhance positive social functioning.

Note: From "Toddlers' Responsive Imitation Predicts Preschool-age Conscience," by D.R. Forman, N. Aksan, & G. Kochanska, *Psychological Science*, 2004, pp. 699–704. Copyright © 2004 Blackwell Publishing. Reprinted with permission.

Gilligan

After more than 10 years of research with women subjects, Carol Gilligan (1982) reported that women often consider the dilemmas Kohlberg used in his research to be irrelevant. Women scored consistently lower on Kohlberg's scale of moral development in spite of the fact that they approached moral dilemmas with considerable sophistication. Gilligan believes that most frameworks for research in moral development do not include the concepts of caring and responsibility.

Gilligan found that moral development proceeds through three levels and two transitions, with each level representing a more complex understanding of the relationship of self and others and each transition resulting in a crucial reevaluation of the conflict between selfishness and responsibility (Murray & Zentner, 2001, p. 251).

■ *Stage 1: caring for oneself.* In this first stage of development, the person is concerned only with caring for the self. The individual feels isolated, alone, and unconnected to others. There is no concern or conflict with the needs of others because the self is the most important. The focus of this stage is survival. The transition of this stage occurs when the individual begins to view this approach as selfishness and moves toward responsibility. The person begins to realize a need for relationships and connections with other people.

■ *Stage 2: caring for others.* During this stage, the individual recognizes the selfishness of earlier behavior and begins to understand the need for caring relationships with others. Caring relationships bring with them responsibility. The definition of responsibility includes self-sacrifice, where "good" is considered to be "caring for others." The individual now approaches relationships with a focus of not hurting others. This approach causes the individual to be more responsive and submissive to others' needs, excluding any thoughts of meeting one's

own needs. A transition from goodness to truth occurs when the individual recognizes that this approach can cause difficulties with relationships because of the lack of balance between caring for oneself and caring for others. The woman makes decisions on personal intentions and consequences of actions rather than on how she thinks others will react (Murray & Zentner, 2001, p. 253).

■ *Stage 3: caring for self and others.* During this last stage, a person sees the need for a balance between caring for others and caring for the self. The concept of responsibility now includes responsibility for the self and for other people. Care remains the focus on which decisions are made. However, the person recognizes the interconnections between the self and others and realizes that if one's own needs are not met, other people may also suffer.

Gilligan (1982) believes women often see morality in the integrity of relationships and caring, so that the moral problems they encounter are different from those of men. Men tend to consider what is right to be what is just, whereas for women what is right is taking responsibility for others as a self-chosen decision (p. 140). The ethic of justice, or fairness, is based on the idea of equality: Everyone should receive the same treatment. This is the development path usually followed by men and widely accepted by moral theorists. By contrast, the ethic of care is based on the premise of nonviolence: No one should be harmed. This is the path typically followed by women but given little attention in the literature of moral theory.

In the development of maturity, according to Gilligan (1982), both viewpoints blend "in the realization that just as inequality adversely affects both perspectives in an unequal relationship, so too violence is destructive for everyone involved" (p. 174). The blending of these two perspectives could give rise to a new view of human development and a better understanding of human relations.

TABLE 20–8 Fowler's Stages of Spiritual Development

STAGE	AGE	DESCRIPTION
0. Undifferentiated	0 to 3 years	Infant unable to formulate concepts about self or the environment
1. Intuitive-projective	4 to 6 years	A combination of images and beliefs given by trusted others, mixed with the child's own experience and imagination
2. Mythic-literal	7 to 12 years	Private world of fantasy and wonder; symbols refer to something specific; dramatic stories and myths used to communicate spiritual meanings
3. Synthetic-conventional	Adolescent or adult	World and ultimate environment structured by the expectations and judgments of others; interpersonal focus
4. Individuating-reflexive	After 18 years	Constructing one's own explicit system; high degree of self-consciousness
5. Paradoxical-consolidative	After 30 years	Awareness of truth from a variety of viewpoints
6. Universalizing	Maybe never	Becoming an incarnation of the principles of love and justice

Note: From *Life Maps: Conversations in the Journey of Faith,* by J. Fowler and S. Keen, 1985, Waco, TX: Word Books; and *How to Help Your Child Have a Spiritual Life: A Parents' Guide to Inner Development,* by A. Hollander, 1980, New York: A and W Publishers. Adapted with permission.

Spiritual Theories

The spiritual component of growth and development refers to individuals' understanding of their relationship with the universe and their perceptions about the direction and meaning of life.

Fowler

James Fowler describes the development of faith as a force that gives meaning to a person's life. He uses the term *faith* as a form of knowing, a way of being in relation to "an ultimate environment." To Fowler, "faith is a relational phenomenon; it is an active 'mode-of-being-in-relation' to another or others in which we invest commitment, belief, love, risk and hope" (Fowler & Keen, 1985, p. 18). Fowler's stages in the development of faith are given in Table 20–8.

Fowler's theory and developmental stages were influenced by the work of Piaget, Kohlberg, and Erikson. Fowler believes

that the development of faith is an interactive process between the person and the environment (Fowler, Streib, & Keller, 2004). In each of Fowler's stages, new patterns of thought, values, and beliefs are added to those already held by the individual; therefore the stages must follow in sequence. Faith stages, according to Fowler, are separate from the cognitive stages of Piaget: They evolve from a combination of knowledge and values.

Westerhoff

Westerhoff describes faith as a way of being and behaving that evolves from an experienced faith guided by parents and others during a person's infancy and childhood to an owned faith that is internalized in adulthood and serves as a directive for personal action (see Table 20–9). For the client who is ill, faith—whether in a higher authority (e.g., God, Allah, Jehovah), in the client's own self, in the health care team, or in a combination of all—provides strength and trust.

TABLE 20–9 Westerhoff's Four Stages of Faith

STAGE	AGE	BEHAVIOR
Experienced faith	Infancy/early adolescence	Experiences faith through interaction with others who are living a particular faith tradition.
Affiliative faith	Late adolescence	Actively participates in activities that characterize a particular faith tradition; experiences awe and wonderment; feels a sense of belonging.
Searching faith	Young adulthood	Through a process of questioning and doubting own faith, acquires a cognitive as well as an affective faith.
Owned faith	Middle adulthood/old age	Puts faith into personal and social action and is willing to stand up for what the individual believes even against the nurturing community.

Note: From *Will Our Children Have Faith?* By John Westerhoff. Reprinted with permission from the author.

CONCEPT MAP **Overview of Growth and Development Moral and Spiritual Theories and Theorists**

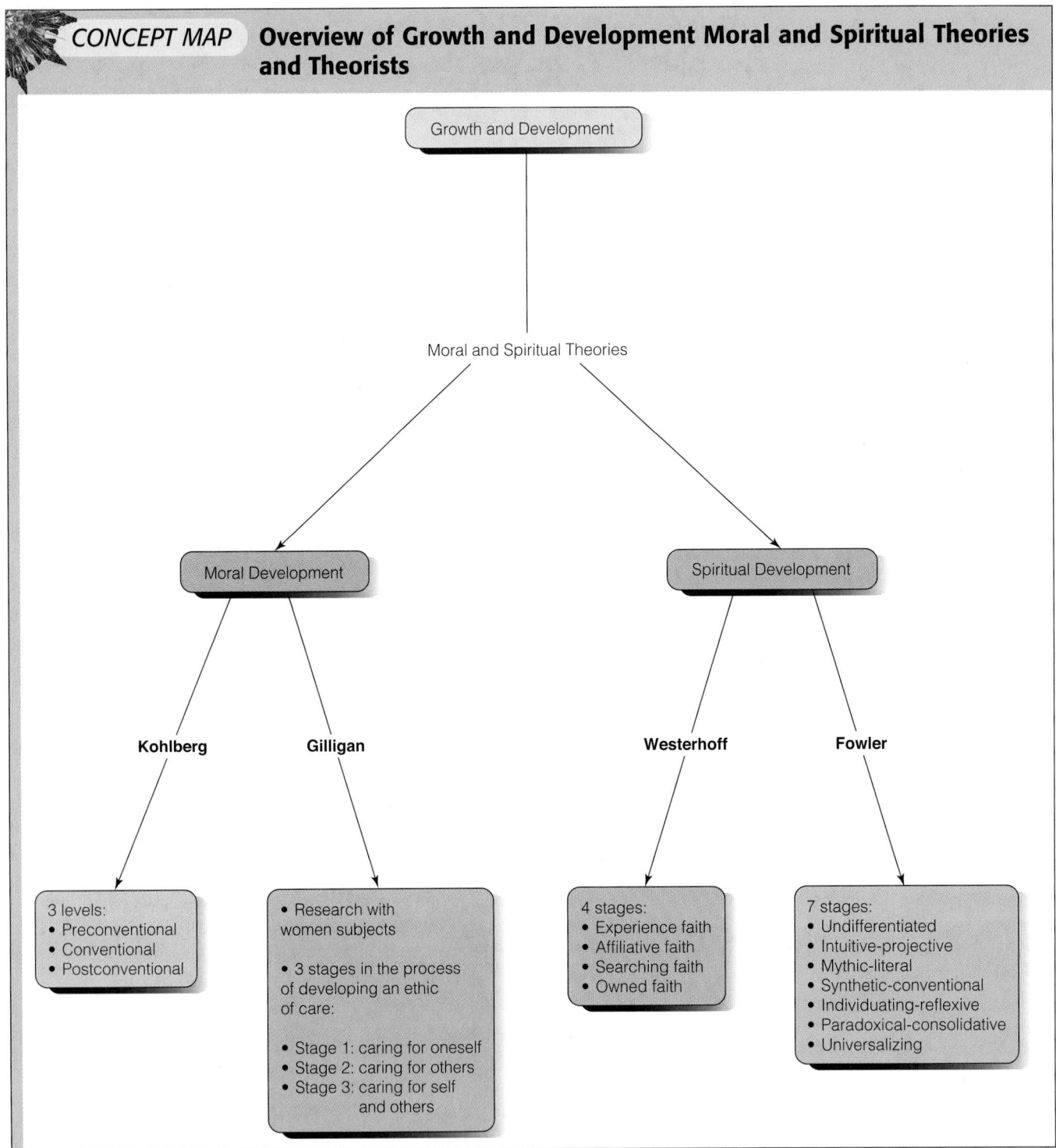

APPLYING GROWTH AND DEVELOPMENT CONCEPTS TO NURSING PRACTICE

Different theories explain one or more aspects of an individual's growth and development. Typically, theorists examine only one aspect of an individual's development, such as the cognitive, moral, or physical aspects. The area chosen for examination usually reflects the researcher's academic discipline and personal interest. The theorists may also limit the population that is studied to a particular part of the life span, such as infancy, childhood, or adulthood.

Although such theories can be useful, they have limitations. First, the theory chosen may explain only one aspect of the growth and development process. Yet a person does not develop in fragmented sections but rather as a whole human being. Thus the nurse may find it necessary to apply several theories for an adequate understanding of the growth and development of a client.

Another limitation of some theories is the suggestion that certain tasks are performed at a specific age. In most cases, the child or adult does accomplish the task at the time specified by the guidelines. In other cases, however, the nurse may find that an individual does not accomplish the task or meet the milestone at the exact time suggested by the theory. Such individual differences are not easily defined or categorized by a single theory. Human development is a complex synthesis of physiologic, cognitive, psychologic, moral, and spiritual development. Nurses should expect individual variations and take these into consideration when applying these theories about growth and development. In so doing, they will be better able to understand a client's development and plan effective nursing interventions.

In nursing, developmental theories can be useful in guiding assessment, explaining behavior, and providing a direction for nursing interventions. An understanding of a child's intellectual ability helps a nurse to anticipate and explain certain reactions, responses, and needs. Nurses can then encourage client behavior that is appropriate for that particular developmental stage.

Theories are also useful in planning a nursing intervention. For instance, choosing the appropriate toy for a 3-year-old boy requires some knowledge of the physical and cognitive development of the child, as well as a sensitivity for individual preferences.

In adult care, knowledge about the physical, cognitive, and psychologic aspects of the aging process is a fundamental as-

pect of administering sensitive nursing care. For example, nurses can use their familiarity with the theories of development to help clients understand and anticipate the psychosocial changes that take place after retirement or the physical limitations that come with aging.

CRITICAL THINKING CHECKPOINT

Chloe, a shy, quiet 13-year-old, and her mother arrive at your clinic for a sports physical prior to school. You ask Chloe if she wants her mother in the room for the exam. Her mother responds before Chloe can answer, saying, "Of course I'll come with you. I want to hear all about how you are growing."

1. According to Erikson, at what stage of development is Chloe?
2. How do you expect Chloe might respond to her mother's comment?
3. According to temperamental theory and based on your observations, what temperamental style is Chloe most likely displaying?

See Critical Thinking Possibilities in Appendix A.

CHAPTER 20 **REVIEW**

CHAPTER HIGHLIGHTS

- The terms *growth* and *development* represent independent, interrelated, and dynamic processes.
- Growth is physical change and increase in size. The pattern of physiologic growth is similar for all people.
- Development is an increase in the complexity of function and skill progression. It is the capacity and skill of the individual to adapt to the environment.
- The rate of a person's growth and development is highly individual, but the sequence of growth and development is predictable.
- Genetics and environment are the primary factors influencing growth and development.
- Temperament, the way in which individuals respond to their internal and external environment, influences interactive dynamics of growth and development.
- Components of growth and development are generally categorized as physiologic, psychosocial, cognitive, moral, and spiritual.
- Robert Havighurst believed that learning is basic to life and that people continue to learn throughout life. His theory describes six age periods with developmental tasks for each period.
- Psychosocial development refers to the development of personality. Psychosocial theorists include Freud, Erickson, Peck, and Gould.
- Cognitive development refers to the manner in which people learn to think, reason, and use language. The most widely known cognitive theorist is Piaget.

- Behaviorist learning theory emphasizes stimulus-response and either positive or negative reinforcement as the basis for learning and behavior change.
- Social learning theory states that learning can occur by observation. Role modeling and learning from watching role models are a part of social learning theory. Attention and cognitive function, in which the individual thinks about the behavior of self and others, as well as the expected rewards and punishments for certain behaviors, are important to social learning.
- Moral development, a complex process not fully understood, involves learning what ought to be and what ought not to be done. Kohlberg's theory focuses on the reasons an individual makes a decision.
- The spiritual component of growth and development refers to individuals' understanding of their relationship with the universe and their perceptions about the direction and meaning of life. Fowler and Westerhoff are two theorists who describe stages of spiritual development or faith.
- In nursing, developmental theories can be useful in guiding assessment, explaining behavior, and providing a direction for nursing interventions.

TEST YOUR KNOWLEDGE

1. The parents of a 5-month-old infant and a 3-year-old child ask the nurse about the sequence and timing of developmental milestones. Which of the following is the most appropriate response?

1. "This infant should reach the milestones at the same time as your older child."
2. "The infant may reach the milestones in a different order than your older child."

3. "The sequence of reaching each milestone should follow the same pattern but may be at a different rate."
4. "There are no predictable patterns. Try to enjoy the uniqueness of each child."

2. The nurse knows that the study of growth and development is exploration of the:
   1. Physical changes of the growing child.
   2. Increasing complexity of function and skill progression of the growing child.
   3. Environmental factors such as family, religion, and culture of the growing child.
   4. Physical developments and the increasing level and progression of function and skill of the growing child.

3. The nurse examines a 2-year-old child recently hospitalized with pneumonia. Which patterns of behavior are most likely to be exhibited by the child?
   1. Lies quietly while the nurse listens to the lungs
   2. Asks many questions about what the nurse is doing and hearing
   3. The child fusses, cries, and pushes the nurse away during assessment of the breath sounds
   4. Enjoys playing "nurse" with the stethoscope, and listens to self and others' breath sounds

4. A 14-year-old is scheduled to have surgical repair of a spinal curvature (scoliosis). The adolescent will be hospitalized for about two weeks. What nursing intervention will be most helpful during the hospital stay?
   1. Have peers visit frequently during the day.
   2. Instruct parents to room-in with her.
   3. Encourage her to go to the recreation room.
   4. Encourage her to arrange for her teachers to provide her with homework.

5. A 65-year-old man who recently retired from 40 years of work as an independent contractor, is scheduled for a physical examination. The nurse should be concerned about which of the following comments?
   1. "My wife and I are planning to drive to Nebraska in June to visit our grandkids."
   2. "Every day, when I wake up, it's hard to find a reason to get out of bed."
   3. "I often take ibuprofen for the pain in my knees."
   4. "People still call me for advice on building projects. I may never get to retire!"

6. An eleven-year-old child is scheduled for a yearly physical examination. The accompanying parent expresses concern because the child "seems all wrapped up in the soccer teammates and other peers leaving, very little time for the family." Using Havighurst's developmental tasks, what would be the nurse's *best* response?
   1. "This is somewhat unusual. Are there problems that we need to discuss?"
   2. "Although this is normal for 11-year-olds, this transition can be difficult for families."
   3. "Become involved in her life and insist that she set aside time for the family."
   4. "This is normal development. You need to let her grow up."

7. A nurse decides that a review of which of the following theorists would be helpful before teaching a preschool class (4–5-year-olds) about how to brush their teeth?
   1. Fowler
   2. Erikson
   3. Gould
   4. Peck

8. A 5-year-old boy arrives for the preadmission work-up for a surgical procedure. When the nurse brings in the intravenous (IV) control pump the child states: I am afraid that it "will bite me because I have been bad." Using knowledge of Piaget, Erikson, and Fowler, which of the following is the best nursing action?
   1. Reassure the child by providing opportunies for touching and exploring the machine, as well as explaining how it works.
   2. Understand that his imagination is out of control. Tell him that his fears are unfounded and that he needs to be a "big boy."
   3. Recognize that he is too young to understand and that he needs to be quickly distracted.
   4. Acknowledge his need for fantasy by reassuring him that if he is a "good boy" the bad machine will not bite him.

See Answers to Test Your Knowledge in Appendix A.

EXPLORE MEDIALINK www.prenhall.com/berman

DVD-ROM
- Audio Glossary
- NCLEX Review

COMPANION WEBSITE
- Additional NCLEX Review
- Case Study: Treating a Six-Year-Old Client
- Care Plan Activity: Child with Developmental Problems
- Application Activity: Discharging a Young Client
- Links to Resources

READINGS AND REFERENCES

SUGGESTED READINGS

Berk, L. E. (2004). *Development through the lifespan* (3rd ed.). Boston: Allyn & Bacon. *This text examines physical, cognitive, emotional, and social development from the prenatal period to the end of life. Introductory chapters discuss theory and research in human development as well as biological and environmental foundations of development.*

Paludi, M. A. (2002). *Human development in multicultural contexts. A book of readings.* Upper Saddle River, NJ: Prentice Hall. *The author focuses on the ways in which culture influences development. Each chapter includes two parts. The first is an overview of cultural influences for the specific life stages from infancy to adulthood. The second consists of readings that present multicultural studies pertaining to the specific stages of development.*

RELATED RESEARCH

Bauer, J. J., & McAdams, D. P. (2004). Personal growth in adults' stories of life transitions. *Journal of Personality, 72*(3), 573–602.

Chang, F., & Burns, B. M. (2005). Attention in preschoolers: Associations with effortful control and motivation. *Child Development, 76*(1), 247–263.

Cook, J. T., Frank, D. A., Berkowitz, C., Black, M.M., Casey, P.H., Cutts, D.B., et al. (2004). Food insecurity is associated with adverse health outcomes among human infants and toddlers. *Journal of Nutrition, 134*(6), 1432–1438.

Manners, J., Durkin, K., & Nesdale, A. (2004). Promoting advanced ego development among adults. *Journal of Adult Development, 11*(1), 19–28.

Oman, R. F., Vesely, S., Aspy, C. B., McLeroy, K. R., Rodine, S., & Marshall, L. (2004). The potential protective effect of youth assets on adolescent alcohol and drug use. *American Journal of Public Health, 94*(8), 1425–1430.

REFERENCES

Ball, R. S. (1977). The Gesell developmental schedules: Arnold Gesell (1880–1961). *Journal of Abnormal Child Psychology, 5*(3), 233–239.

Ball, J. W., & Bindler, R. C. (2006). *Child health nursing.* Upper Saddle River, NJ: Pearson Education.

Edwards, M. E. (2002). Attachment, mastery, and interdependence: A model of parenting processes. *Family Process, 41*(3), 389–404.

Erikson, E. H. (1963). *Childhood and society* (2nd ed.). New York: Norton.

Erikson, E. H. (1964). *Insight and responsibility: Lectures on the ethical implications of psychoanalytic insight.* New York: Norton.

Forman, D. R., Aksan, N., & Kochanska, G. (2004). Toddler's responsive imitation predicts preschool-age conscience. *Psychological Science, 15*(10), 699–704.

Fowler, J., & Keen, S. (1985). *Life maps: Conversations in the journey of faith.* Waco, TX: Word Books.

Fowler, J. W., Streib, H., & Keller, B. (2004). *Manual for faith development research* (3rd ed.). Bielefeld, Atlanta, Research Center for Biographical Studies in Contemporary Religion; Center for Research in Faith and Moral Development, Emory University.

Gesell, A. (1934). *An atlas of infant behavior: A systematic delineation of the forms and early growth of human behavior patterns.* New Haven, CT: Yale University Press.

Gesell, A. (2006). *Britannica student encyclopedia.* Retrieved May 14, 2006, from http://www.britannica.com/ebi/article-927-4541

Gilligan, C. (1982). *In a different voice: Psychological theory and women's development.* Cambridge, MA: Harvard University Press.

Gould, R. L. (1972). The phases of adult life: A study in developmental psychology. *American Journal of Psychiatry, 129*, 33–43.

Havighurst, R. J. (1972). *Developmental tasks and education* (3rd ed.). Boston: Allyn & Bacon.

Hollander, A. (1980). *How to help your child have a spiritual life: A parent's guide to inner development.* New York: A and W Publishers.

Kohlberg, L. (1981). *Essays on moral development: Vol. 1. The philosophy of moral development.* San Francisco: Harper & Row.

Kohlberg, L. (1984). *Essays on moral development: Vol. 2. The psychology of moral development.* San Francisco: Harper & Row.

Murray, R. B., & Zentner, J. P. (2001). *Health promotion strategies through the life span* (7th ed.). Upper Saddle River, NJ: Prentice Hall.

Peck, R. (1968). Psychological developments in the second half of life. In B. L. Neugarten (Ed.), *Middle age and aging.* Chicago: University of Chicago Press.

Piaget, J. (1966). *Origins of intelligence in children.* New York: Norton.

Rothbart, M. K. (2004). Commentary: Differentiated measures of temperament and multiple pathways to childhood disorders. *Journal of Clinical Child and Adolescent Psychology, 33*(1), 82–87.

Westerhoff, J. (1976). *Will our children have faith?* New York: Seabury Press.

SELECTED BIBLIOGRAPHY

Armstrong, T. D., & Crowther, M. R. (2002). Spirituality among older African Americans. *Journal of Adult Development, 9*(1), 3–12.

Erikson, E. H. (1985). *The life cycle completed: A review.* New York: Norton.

Fowler, J. W. (1982). *Stages of faith.* San Francisco: Harper Collins.

Freud, S. (1923). *The ego and the id.* London: Hogarth Press.

Freud, S. (1961). *The ego and the id and other works* (Vol. 19). J. Strachey, Trans. London: Hogarth Press and the Institute of Psychoanalysis.

Mitchell, K. (2002). Women's morality: A test of Carol Gilligan's theory. *Journal of Social Distress and the Homeless, 11*(1), 81–110.

Polan, E., & Taylor, D. (2003). *Journey across the life span. Human development and health promotion* (2nd ed.). Philadelphia: F. A. Davis.

Stuart-Hamilton, I. (2000). *The psychology of ageing. An introduction* (3rd ed.). London and Philadelphia: Jessica Kingsley Publishers.

CHAPTER 21

Promoting Health from Conception through Adolescence

LEARNING OUTCOMES

After completing this chapter, you will be able to:

1. Identify tasks characteristic of different stages of development from infancy through adolescence.

2. Describe usual physical development from infancy through adolescence.

3. Trace psychosocial development according to Erikson from infancy through adolescence.

4. Explain cognitive development according to Piaget from infancy through adolescence.

5. Describe moral development according to Kohlberg from childhood through adolescence.

6. Describe spiritual development according to Fowler throughout childhood and adolescence.

7. Identify assessment activities and expected characteristics from birth through late childhood.

8. Identify essential activities of health promotion and protection to meet the needs of infants, toddlers, preschoolers, school-age children, and adolescents.

A knowledge of growth and development is essential for nurses if they are to identify developmental needs and problems. This chapter applies the concepts of growth and development introduced in Chapter 20 ∞ to the prenatal period and to the neonate, infant, toddler, preschooler, school-age child, and adolescent. Each developmental stage includes physical, psychosocial, cognitive, moral, and spiritual aspects. Health assessment and promotion of health and wellness are emphasized.

CONCEPTION AND PRENATAL DEVELOPMENT

Prenatal or intrauterine development lasts approximately 9 calendar months (10 lunar months) or 38 to 40 weeks, depending on the method of calculation. (A lunar month is 28 days.) If the time is calculated from the day of conception, this stage of life is 38 weeks or 9 1/2 lunar months. If the time is calculated from the first day of the last menstrual period, its average length is 10 lunar months or 40 weeks.

Traditionally, pregnancy has been divided into three periods called **trimesters,** each of which lasts about 3 months. Each trimester includes certain landmarks for developmental changes in the mother and the fetus. The two phases of intrauterine life can also be considered in trimestral terms. The embryonic phase is the first trimester, and the fetal phase includes the second and third trimesters.

The **embryonic phase** is the period during which the fertilized ovum develops into an organism with most of the features of the human. This period is considered to encompass the first 8 weeks of pregnancy.

Within the first 3 weeks of life, the embryonic tissues differentiate into three layers—the **ectoderm** (outer layer), **mesoderm** (middle layer), and **endoderm** or **entoderm** (inner layer). The ectoderm and endoderm are formed in the second week; the mesoderm forms in the third week. From the beginning of the third week through the eighth week after conception, these layers form the basic structure of all of the body's complex organs and systems. For example, the ectoderm forms the brain and spinal cord, the mesoderm forms the heart, and the endoderm forms the bladder and urethra (Pillitteri, 2003).

Three other events occur concurrently during the first 3 weeks:

1. The embryo is implanted in the endometrium of the uterus.
2. The fetal membranes differentiate into the chorion, precursor to the placenta, and the amnion, precursor to the amniotic sac.
3. Placental function starts. The **placenta** is a flat, disc-shaped organ that is highly vascular. It normally forms in the upper segment of the endometrium of the uterus. Its function is to facilitate nutrients and gas exchange between the embryo or fetus and the mother.

The **fetal phase** of development is characterized by a period of rapid growth in the size of the fetus. Both genetic and environmental factors affect its growth.

At the end of the second trimester, or 6 lunar months, the fetus resembles a small baby. Because very little fat is present beneath the skin, the skin appears wrinkled, red, and transparent. Underlying vessels are visible. A protective covering called **vernix caseosa** begins to develop over the skin. This is a white, cheeselike substance that adheres to the skin and can become one-eighth inch thick by birth. **Lanugo,** a fine downy hair, also covers the body. At about 5 months, fetal movement can be felt by the mother, and the first fetal heartbeat may be heard.

At the end of the third trimester (9 1/2 lunar months), the fetus has developed to approximately 50 cm (20 in.) and 3.2 to 3.4 kg (7.0 to 7.5 lb). The lanugo has disappeared, and the skin is a more normal color and appears less wrinkled. A large amount of subcutaneous fat makes the baby look more rotund. The baby gains most of its weight during the last 2 months in utero. Box 21–1 lists maternal factors that can lead to a higher risk of a low-birth-weight baby.

MediaLink

Oogenesis and Cell Division Animations

> ## BOX 21–1   Maternal Factors that Contribute to a Higher Risk of Low-Birth-Weight Babies
>
> - Underweight before pregnancy
> - Less than 21 pounds gained during pregnancy
> - Inadequate prenatal care
> - Age of 16 years or younger or 35 years or older
> - Low socioeconomic level
> - Poor nutrition during pregnancy
> - Smoking cigarettes during pregnancy
> - Use of addictive drugs or alcohol during pregnancy
> - History of abortion
> - Complications during pregnancy, poor health status, exposure to infections
> - High stress levels, including physical or emotional abuse
>
> *Note:* From *Health Promotion Strategies Through the Life Span,* 7th ed. (p. 309), by R. B. Murray and J. P. Zentner, 2001. Reprinted by permission.

Health Promotion

During the intrauterine stage of development, the embryo or fetus relies on the maternal blood flow through the placenta to meet its basic survival needs. The health of the mother is essential for proper growth and development.

Oxygen

To meet the fetal demands for oxygen, the pregnant mother gradually increases her normal blood flow by about one-third, peaking at about 8 months. Respiratory rate and cardiac output increase significantly during this period. Initially the heart of the embryo lies outside its body. It is then repositioned in the chest early in the second trimester. Fetal circulation travels from the placenta through two umbilical arteries, which carry deoxygenated blood away from the fetus. By 20 weeks the fetal heartbeat is audible through a fetoscope; the heartbeat is audible as early as the 10th week if a Doppler stethoscope with ultrasound is used.

Nutrition and Fluids

The fetus obtains nourishment from the placental circulation and by swallowing amniotic fluid. Nutritional needs are met when the mother eats a well-balanced diet containing sufficient calories and nutrients to meet both her needs and those of the fetus.

Adequate folic acid, one of the B vitamins, is important in order to prevent neural tube defects (e.g., spina bifida) in the fetus. One of the objectives of *Healthy People 2010* is to increase consumption of folic acid at the beginning and throughout pregnancies to prevent neural tube defects (U.S. Department of Health and Human Services [USDHHS], 2000). Neural tube defects occur in the first few weeks of fetal development. As a result, it is recommended that all women capable of becoming pregnant consume 400 micrograms of folic acid daily. The nurse should teach the client about folic-rich foods (e.g., green leafy vegetables, oranges, dried beans) and suggest she take a vitamin supplement that contains folic acid.

Rest and Activity

The fetus sleeps most of the time and develops a pattern of sleep and wakefulness that usually persists after birth. Fetal activity can be felt by the mother at about the fifth lunar month of pregnancy.

Elimination

Fetal feces are formed in the intestines from swallowed amniotic fluid throughout pregnancy, but are normally not excreted until after birth. Inadequate oxygenation of the fetus during the third trimester can result in relaxation of the anal sphincter and passage of feces into the amniotic fluid. Urine normally is excreted into the amniotic fluid when the kidneys mature (16 to 20 weeks).

Temperature Maintenance

Amniotic fluid usually provides a safe and comfortable temperature for the fetus. Significant changes in maternal temperature can alter the temperature of the amniotic fluid and the fetus. Significant temperature increases due to illness, hot whirlpool baths, or saunas may result in birth defects. In the last weeks of gestation, the fetus develops subcutaneous fatty tissue stores that will help maintain body temperature at birth.

Safety

As stated earlier, the body systems form during the embryonic period. As a result, the embryo is particularly vulnerable to damage from a **teratogen,** which is anything that adversely affects normal cellular development in the embryo or fetus (Venes, 2005). It is important for the nurse to inquire about possible pregnancy when giving medications that are known teratogens and to also ask when the woman is scheduled for tests that involve radiography (x-ray).

Smoking, alcohol, and drugs can affect the environment for the fetus. Smoking has been associated with preterm labor, spontaneous abortion, low-birth-weight infants, sudden infant death syndrome, and learning disorders (Albrecht et al. 2004; Anderson, Johnson, & Batal, 2005). Maternal, neonatal, and infant mortality are significantly increased with maternal use of drugs and/or alcohol (Wolfe, Davis, Guydish, & Delucchi, 2005). Fetal alcohol syndrome (FAS), a result of impaired mitochondrial development, leads to microcephaly, mental retardation, learning disorders, and other central nervous system defects (Kvigne et al. 2004). All women of childbearing age should be educated about the risk of FAS and, if seeking to become pregnant, encouraged to abstain from alcohol. Adolescents who engage in risky behaviors such as drinking and unprotected sex are at significant risk for pregnancy and FAS.

NEONATES AND INFANTS (BIRTH TO 1 YEAR)

Babies are considered neonates from birth to the end of the first month. Infants are babies from 1 month to 1 year of age.

Physical Development

A neonate's basic task is adjustment to the environment outside the uterus, which requires breathing, sleeping, sucking, eating, swallowing, digesting, and eliminating. Because newborns are so vulnerable, the first 3 months of life have been called by some as the "fourth trimester" (Karp, 2003). Infants continue to grow and develop rapidly during the first year, learning more skills as they interact with their world. Infants undergo significant physiologic change in weight, length, head growth, vision, and motor development. Some of these changes can be assessed using standardized growth charts based on growth of groups of American children (Centers for Disease Control [CDC], 2000). The World Health Organization's global Child Growth Standards are available to assess optimal growth given adequate nutrition, feeding practices, environment, and health care for children around the world (WHO Multicentre Growth Reference Study Group, 2006).

Weight

At birth, most babies weigh from 2.7 to 3.8 kg (6.0 to 8.5 lb). Just after birth, most infants lose 5% to 10% of their birth weight because of fluid loss. This weight loss is normal, and infants usually regain that weight in about 1 week. After several days, babies usually gain weight at the rate of 150 to 210 g (5 to 7 oz) weekly for 6 months. By 5 months of age, infants usually reach twice their birth weight, and by age 12 months, three times their birth weight.

Length

The average length of a European American newborn in the United States is about 50 cm (20 in.). Female babies on the average are smaller than male babies. Babies from different ethnic groups may vary by height, weight, and head circumference, so ethnicity must be considered when determining what is "normal" for any particular infant.

Two recumbent lengths are the crown-to-rump length (the sitting length) and the head-to-heel length (from the top of the head to the base of the heels). (See Figure 21-1 ■). Normally the crown-to-rump length is approximately the same as the head circumference. By 6 months infants gain another 13.75 cm (5.5 in.) of height. By 12 months they add another 7.5 cm (3 in.). The rate of increase in height is largely influenced by the baby's size at birth and by nutrition.

Figure 21-1 ■ Measuring an infant head to heel, from the top of the head to the base of the heels.

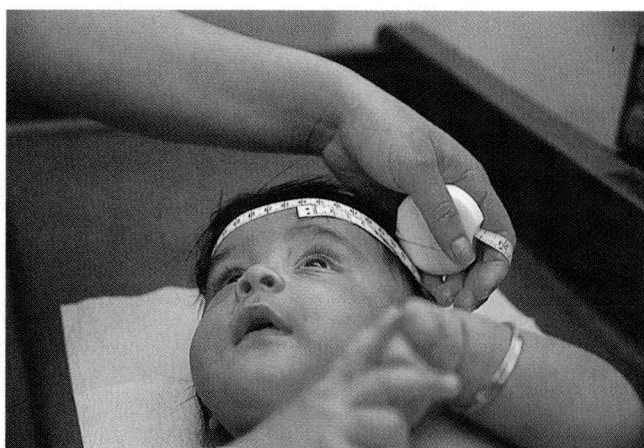

Figure 21-2 ■ An infant's head circumference is measured around the skull, above the eyebrows and around the occiput.

Head and Chest Circumference

Assessment of head circumference is of particular importance in infants and children to determine the growth rate of the skull and the brain. An infant's head should be measured at every visit to the primary care provider or nurse until the child is 2 years old (see Figure 21-2 ■). Normal head circumference (**normocephaly**) is often related to chest circumference. At birth the average infant's head circumference is 35 cm (14 in.) and generally varies only 1 or 2 cm (0.5 in.). The chest circumference of the newborn is usually less than the head circumference by about 2.5 cm (1 in.). As the infant grows, the chest circumference becomes larger than the head circumference. At about 9 or 10 months the head and chest circumferences are about the same, and after 1 year of age the chest circumference is larger.

Head Molding

The heads of many newborn babies are misshapen because of the molding of the head that occurs during vaginal deliveries. Molding of the head occurs due to fontanels and sutures in the skull. **Fontanels** are unossified membranous gaps in the bone structure of the skull. **Sutures** are junction lines of the skull bones that override to provide flexibility for molding of the head. Within a week, a newborn's head usually regains its symmetry, which is reassuring to the parents. The larger anterior fontanel (4 to 6 cm in diameter and diamond shaped) can increase in size for several months after birth. After 6 months the size gradually decreases until closure occurs between 9 and 18 months. The posterior fontanel between the parietal bones and the occipital bone closes between 2 and 3 months after birth (see Figure 21-3 ■).

Vision

The newborn can follow large moving objects and blinks in response to bright light and sound. The pupils of the newborn respond slowly, and the eyes cannot focus on close objects. By 1 month the infant can focus his or her gaze on objects and follow moving ones. At 4 months the infant recognizes a parent's smile, although social smiles may appear as early as 2 months. The 4-month-old has almost complete color vision and follows objects through a 180-degree arc. A 5-month-old infant reaches for

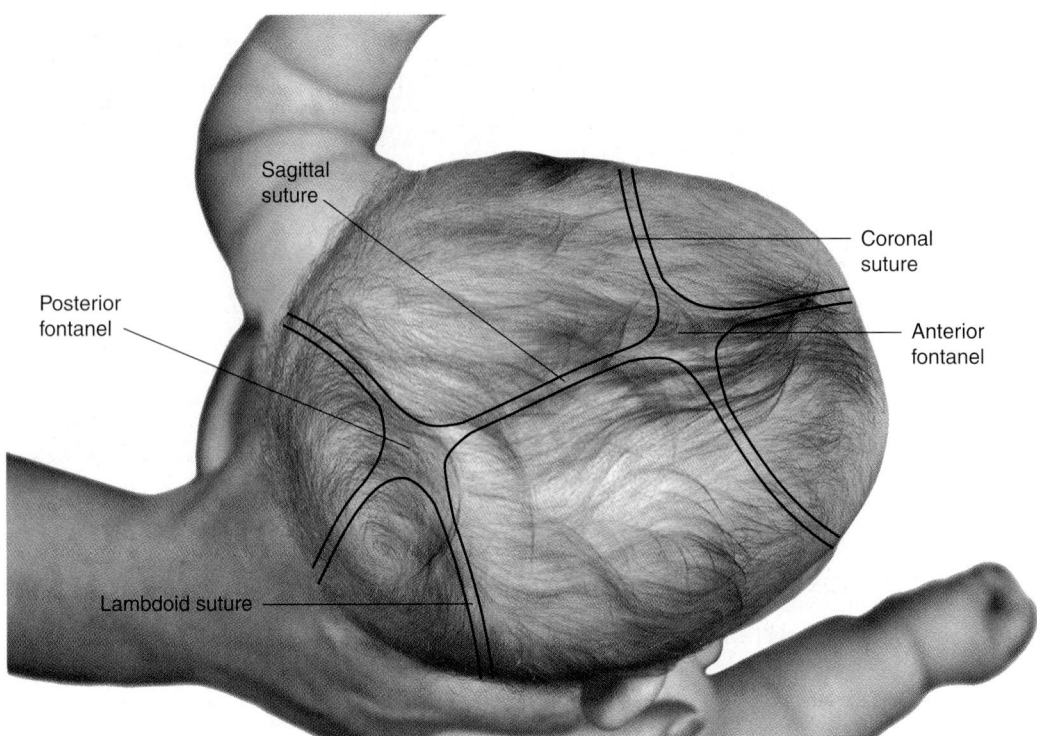

Figure 21-3 ■ The bones of the skull, showing the fontanels and suture lines.

objects. Between 6 and 10 months the infant can fix on an object and follow it in all directions. By 12 months depth perception has fully developed, and the infant will consistently be able to recognize where a change in level occurs, such as at the edge of the bed.

Hearing

Newborns with intact hearing will react with a startle to a loud noise, a reaction called the *Moro reflex* . Within a few days, they are able to distinguish different sounds. For example, they can tell the difference between their mother's voice and that of another woman. By 2 to 3 months they will actively coo, smile, or gurgle to sounds and voices. Between 3 and 6 months the infant will look for sounds, pausing an activity to listen and responding with distress or pleasure to angry or happy voices. Between 6 and 9 months individual words begin to take on meaning and the infant may look at named objects or people. The 9- to 12-month-old infant understands many words (e.g., "no," "hot," "dog"), uses gestures (e.g., waves "bye-bye"), may articulate one or two words with a specific reference (e.g., "mama," "dada"), and, by 1 year of age, responds to simple commands.

Smell and Taste

The senses of smell and taste are functional shortly after birth. Newborns prefer sweet tastes and tend to decrease their sucking in response to liquids with a salty content. They are able to recognize the smell of their mother's milk and respond to this smell by turning toward the mother.

Touch

The sense of touch is well developed at birth. Skin-to-skin touching is important for an infant's development. The infant responds positively to the warmth, love, and security it perceives

when touched, held, and cuddled. The newborn is sensitive to temperature extremes and has poor self-regulation of body temperature. In response to pain, young babies react diffusely and cannot isolate the discomfort. The pain of an open safety pin in the buttock, for example, is not isolated in the buttock.

Reflexes

Reflexes of the newborn are unconscious, involuntary responses of the nervous system to external and internal stimuli. Reflexes normally present at birth are the rooting, sucking, Moro, palmar grasp, plantar, tonic neck, stepping, and Babinski reflexes (see Box 21–2). Infant reflexes disappear during the first year of life in an ordered sequence, a process that allows the infant to develop voluntary movements. In addition, the abilities to yawn, stretch, sneeze, burp, and hiccup are all present at birth.

Motor Development

Motor development is the development of the baby's abilities to move and to control the body. Initially, body movement is uncoordinated. At 1 month of age the infant lifts the head momentarily when prone, turns the head when prone, and has a head lag when pulled to a sitting position. Head lag should be minimal by 4 months of age. After 6 months infants may sit without support (see Figure 21-4 ■). At 9 months they can reach, grasp a rattle, and transfer it from hand to hand. At 12 months they can turn the pages of a book, put objects into a container, walk with some assistance, and help to dress themselves.

Psychosocial Development

According to Erikson (1963), the central crisis at this stage is trust versus mistrust. Resolution of this stage determines how

BOX 21–2 Infant Reflexes

- *Sucking reflex:* A feeding reflex that occurs when the infant's lips are touched. The reflex persists throughout infancy.
- *Rooting reflex:* A feeding reflex elicited by touching the baby's cheek, causing the baby's head to turn to the side that was touched. The reflex usually disappears after 4 months.
- *Moro reflex:* Often assessed to estimate the maturity of the central nervous system. A loud noise, a sudden change in position, or an abrupt jarring of the crib elicits this reflex. The infant reacts by extending both arms and legs outward with the fingers spread, then suddenly retracting the limbs. Often the infant cries at the same time. This reflex disappears after 4 months.
- *Palmar grasp reflex:* Occurs when a small object is placed against the palm of the hand, causing the fingers to curl around it. This reflex disappears after 3 to 6 months.
- *Plantar reflex:* Similar to the palmar grasp reflex; an object placed just beneath the toes causes them to curl around it. This reflex disappears after 8 to 10 months.
- *Tonic neck reflex (TNR) or fencing reflex:* A postural reflex. When a baby who is lying on its back turns its head to the right side, for example, the left side of the body shows a flexing of the left arm and the left leg. This reflex disappears after 4 to 6 months.
- *Stepping reflex (walking or dancing reflex):* Can be elicited by holding the baby upright so that the feet touch a flat surface. The legs then move up and down as if the baby were walking. This reflex usually disappears at about 2 months.
- *Babinski reflex:* When the sole of the foot is stroked, the big toe rises and the other toes fan out. A newborn baby has a positive Babinski. After age 1, the infant exhibits a negative Babinski; that is, the toes curl downward. A positive Babinski after age 1 can indicate possible upper motor neuron damage.

Figure 21-4 ■ An infant sits without support at 6 months of age.

the person approaches subsequent developmental stages. During the first year of life, infants depend on the parents for all their physiologic and psychologic needs. Fulfillment of these needs is required for the infant to develop a basic sense of trust. Parents can enhance this sense of trust by (a) being sensitive to the infant's needs and meeting these needs promptly and skillfully; (b) responding consistently to an infant's needs; and (c) providing a predictable environment in which routines are established. Mothering or nurturing behavior, such as consistent care, handling, stroking, and cuddling, is essential for healthy psychosocial development. By 8 months, most infants exhibit attachment to their parents and may show displeasure when left with strangers.

The newborn reacts socially to caregivers by paying attention to the face or voice and by cuddling when held. The baby is able to interact with the environment by responding to various stimuli such as touch and sound. Table 21–1 provides examples of motor and social development.

Infants have no understanding of waiting and no time frame by which to measure waiting. Crying is their initial reaction to stress, and the major way they communicate stress. Infants learn gradually to tolerate stress. According to Freud, infants have an

TABLE 21–1 Examples of Motor and Social Development in Infancy

AGE	MOTOR DEVELOPMENT	SOCIAL DEVELOPMENT
Newborn	Turns head from side to side when in a prone position. Grasps by reflex when object is placed in palm of hand.	Displays displeasure by crying and satisfaction by soft vocalizations. Attends to adult face and voice by eye contact and quieting.
4 months	Rolls over. Sits with support, holds head steady when sitting.	Babbles, laughs, and increased response to verbal play.
6 months	Lifts chest and shoulders off table when prone, bearing weight on hands. Manipulates small objects.	Starts to imitate sounds. Vocalizes one-syllable sounds: "ma ma," "da da"
9 months	Creeps and crawls. Uses pincer grasp with thumb and forefinger.	Complies with simple verbal commands. Displays fear of being left alone (e.g., going to bed). Waves "bye-bye"
12 months	Walks alone with help. Uses spoon to feed self.	Clings to mother in unfamiliar situations. Demonstrates emotions such as anger and affection

oral focus, many of their activities and pleasures are mouth-centered, and they reduce tension by sucking and chewing on objects. Nurses and parents can reduce the stress of an infant by maintaining the infant's routine as much as possible and providing a consistent, predictable environment.

Cognitive Development

According to Piaget (1966), cognitive development is a result of interaction between an individual and the environment. Piaget referred to the initial period of cognitive development as the sensorimotor phase. This phase has six stages, three of which take place during the first year. From 4 to 8 months infants begin to have perceptual recognition. By 6 months they respond to new stimuli, and they remember certain objects and look for them for a short time. By 12 months infants have a concept of both space and time. They experiment to reach a goal, such as a toy on a chair.

An infant's cognitive development also proceeds from reflexive ability of the newborn to using one or two actions to attain a goal by the age of 1 year.

Moral Development

Infants associate right and wrong with pleasure and pain. What gives them pleasure is right, since they are too young to reason otherwise. When infants receive abundant positive responses from the parent such as smiles, caresses, and voice tones of approval in these early months, they learn that certain behaviors are wrong or good and that pain or pleasure is the consequence. In later months and years, children can tell easily and quickly by changes in parental facial expressions and voice tones that their behavior is either approved or disapproved.

Health Risks

A number of health problems of neonates and infants require interventions from health care personnel. Safety concerns are of particular importance.

Failure to Thrive

Failure to thrive is a unique syndrome in which an infant falls below the fifth percentile for weight and height on a standard growth chart or is falling in percentiles on a growth chart (Pillitteri, 2003, p. 1700). The two categories for this syndrome are organic causes (e.g., cardiac disease) and inorganic causes, which usually involve the parent-child relationship. Infants deprived of mothering, especially from months 3 to 15, will not learn to form significant relationships or to trust others. Touch, cuddling, and visual and auditory stimulation are all critical for the infant. It is through these mechanisms that the baby comes to know self and the environment. Infants who fail to establish a loving, responsive relationship with a caregiver often fail to develop normally. Infants with inorganic failure to thrive show delayed development without any physical cause. They are often malnourished and fail to gain weight and grow normally.

Infant Colic

Colic is acute abdominal pain caused by periodic contractions of the intestines. It occurs in infants as young as 2 weeks of age and for most infants disappears by 3 months of age. Although the direct cause is not known, colic tends to occur in babies with sensitive temperaments. Factors such as swallowing air, feeding too rapidly, allergies, taking excessive amounts of carbohydrates, infant emotional distress, and anxiety of the caregiver may be associated with colic.

To help relieve the colic, the nurse can assess the infant during feeding and suggest possible changes. Suggestions may include cuddling the infant, swaddling, rocking, and finding the position that provides the infant with the most comfort (e.g., wearing the baby in a front pack, placing the infant in a swinging or vibrating chair) (Karp, 2003, Schmitt, 2004).

Crying

Crying is often of great concern. When an infant's crying lasts up to 10 to 12 hours a day it is described as colicky (see the preceding section). A crying or fussy period lasting 1 to 2 hours a day is usually considered normal for infants.

Child Abuse

Reports of child abuse have increased in recent years, and the stress of having a baby with colic or excessive crying can put some parents at risk for child abuse. It can take various forms including physical abuse, physical neglect, sexual abuse, and emotional abuse and neglect. **Shaken baby syndrome (SBS)** is violent shaking of the infant, causing a whiplash. The shaking, combined with impact, often against a soft surface (e.g., mattress), can lead to severe brain injury in infants. Cerebral damage, subdural hematoma, neurologic defects, blindness, and spinal cord damage can result. These injuries often occur without external evidence of head injury. Subdural and retinal hemorrhages accompanied by the absence of external signs of trauma are hallmarks of the syndrome (Geddes, 2004). Nurses should teach parents about the dangers in shaking infants and the need to call their primary care provider if they feel they could harm their baby.

Sudden Infant Death Syndrome

The sudden and unexpected death of an infant may be a case of **sudden infant death syndrome (SIDS).** A postmortem examination usually fails to reveal a cause. The highest incidence of SIDS occurs in the second to fourth month of life, and boys are more susceptible than girls. Research has shown that sleeping on the back, not prone, greatly decreases the risk of SIDS. The back is preferred because infants may roll onto their stomach from a side-lying position (see Figure 21-5 ■). *Healthy People 2010* includes an objective to increase the percentage of healthy full-term infants who are put down to sleep on their backs (USDHHS, 2000).

Health Assessment and Promotion

Health assessment occurs immediately at birth and continues for the promotion of wellness.

Apgar Scoring

Newborn babies can be assessed immediately by the **Apgar scoring system.** This provides a numeric indicator of the baby's physiologic capacities to adapt to extrauterine life. Each of five

Identifying Child Abuse Video   MediaLink

SIDS Video   MediaLink

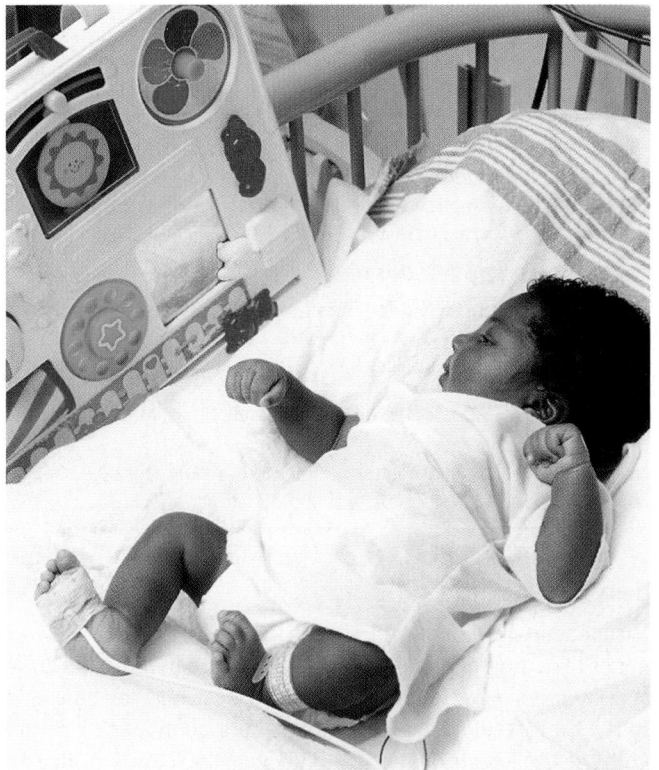

Figure 21-5 ■ Place infant on back for sleeping. Note the infant's tonic neck reflex.

signs is assigned a maximum score of 2, so that the maximum score achievable is 10. A score under 7 suggests that the baby is having difficulty, and a score under 4 indicates that the baby's condition is critical. Apgar scoring is usually carried out 60 seconds after birth and is repeated in 5 minutes. Those with very low scores require special resuscitative measures and care. See Table 21–2.

Developmental Screening Tests

Development can be assessed by observing the infant's behavior and by using standardized tests such as the **Denver Developmental Screening Test (DDST-II).** The DDST-II is used to screen children from birth to 6 years of age. The test is intended to estimate the abilities of a child compared to those of an average group of children of the same age. Four main areas of development are screened: personal-social, fine-motor adaptive, language, and gross motor.

Ongoing Nursing Assessments

During ongoing assessments, the nurse examines and observes the infant, taking into account variations that occur with developmental age and activity. For example, the pulse of the baby at birth is affected by the child's activity, rising up to 170 when the infant is crying and falling to as low as 70 during sleep.

In addition, the nurse actively listens to the caregiver for possible problems or areas of concern and reviews with the parent the expected behavior or characteristics for the particular age group. It is important for the caregiver to know that certain behaviors, responses, and activities of the infant are normal and expected. It is also important to discuss the many individual differences that can, quite normally, occur.

The assessment interview is also a time to be supportive of the parent's role, to assess the attachment of the mother to the infant, and to observe the interactions between the infant and parent. Assessment guidelines for the infant are shown in the Developmental Assessment Guidelines.

The first month of life is critical for physical adjustments to extrauterine life and for the psychosocial adjustment of the parents. From 1 month to 1 year, infants experience rapid change, with advances in physical growth and psychosocial development. For a summary of health and wellness promotion, see Box 21–3.

TODDLERS (1 TO 3 YEARS)

Toddlers develop from having no voluntary control to being able to walk and speak. They also learn to control their bladder and bowels, and they acquire a wide variety of information about their environment.

Physical Development

Two-year-old children lose the baby look. Toddlers are usually chubby, with relatively short legs and a large head. The face appears small when compared to the skull, but as the toddler grows, the face seems to grow from under the skull and appears better proportioned. Toddlers have a pronounced lumbar lordosis and a protruding abdomen. The abdominal muscles develop gradually with growth, and the abdomen flattens.

Weight

Two-year-olds can be expected to weigh approximately four times their birth weight. The weight gain is about 2 kg (5 lb) between ages 1 and 2 years and about 1 to 2 kg (2 to 5 lb) between 2 and 3 years. The 3-year-old weighs about 13.6 kg (30 lb).

TABLE 21–2	**Apgar Scoring System to Assess the Newborn**		
		SCORE	
SIGN	**0**	**1**	**2**
1. Heart rate	Absent	Slow (below 100 per minute)	Above 100 per minute
2. Respirations	Absent	Slow, irregular	Regular rate, crying
3. Muscle tone	Flaccid	Some flexion of extremities	Active movements
4. Reflex irritability	None	Grimace	Cries
5. Color	Body pale cyanotic	Body pink (for African American babies, pink mucous membranes), extremities blue	Body completely pink, pink mucous membranes in African American babies

DEVELOPMENTAL ASSESSMENT GUIDELINES   The Infant

In these five developmental areas, does the infant do the following?

PHYSICAL DEVELOPMENT

- Demonstrate physical growth (weight, length, head and chest circumference) within the normal range.
- Manifest appropriately sized fontanels for age.
- Exhibit vital signs within normal range for age.
- Display ability to habituate to stimuli and to calm self.

MOTOR DEVELOPMENT

- Perform gross and fine motor milestones within the normal range for age.
- Exhibit reflexes appropriate for age.
- Display symmetric movements.
- Exhibit no hyper- or hypotonia.

SENSORY DEVELOPMENT

- Follow a moving object within normal range for age.
- Respond to sounds, such as talking or clapping hands.
- Coo, babble, laugh, vocalize, and imitate sounds as expected for age.

PSYCHOSOCIAL DEVELOPMENT

- Interact appropriately with parent through body movements and vocalizations.

DEVELOPMENT IN ACTIVITIES OF DAILY LIVING

- Eat and drink appropriate amounts of breast milk, formula, and/or solid foods.
- Exhibit an elimination pattern within normal range for age.
- Exhibit a rest and sleep pattern appropriate for age.

Height

A toddler's height can be measured as height or length. Height is measured while the toddler stands, and length is measured while the toddler is in a recumbent position. Although the measurements differ slightly, nurses must specify which measurement is used to avoid confusion. Between ages 1 and 2 years, the average growth in height is 10 to 12 cm (4 to 5 in.), and between 2 and 3 years it slows to 6 to 8 cm (2 1/2 to 3 1/2 in.).

Head Circumference

The head circumference of the toddler increases about 2.5 cm (1 in.) on average each year. By 24 months the head is 80% of the average adult size and the brain is 70% of its adult size.

Sensory Abilities

Visual acuity is fairly well established at 1 year; average estimates of acuity for the toddler are 20/70 at 18 months and 20/40 at 2 years of age. Accommodation to near and far objects is fairly well developed by 18 months and continues to mature with age. At 3 years of age, the toddler can look away from a toy prior to reaching out and picking it up. This ability requires the integration of visual and neuromuscular mechanisms.

The senses of hearing, taste, smell, and touch become increasingly developed and associated with each other. Hearing in the 3-year-old is at adult levels. The taste buds of the toddler are sensitive to the natural flavors of food, and the 3-year-old prefers familiar odors and tastes. Touch is a very important sense, and a distressed toddler is often soothed by tactile sensations.

BOX 21–3   Health Promotion Guidelines for Infants

HEALTH EXAMINATIONS

- Screening of newborns for hearing loss; follow-up at 3 months and early intervention by 6 months if appropriate
- At 2 weeks and at 2, 4, 6, and 12 months

PROTECTIVE MEASURES

- Immunizations: diphtheria, tetanus, acellular pertussis (DTaP), inactivated poliovirus vaccine (IPV), pneumococcal, measles-mumps-rubella (MMR), *Haemophilus influenzae* type B (HIB), hepatitis B (HepB), varicella and influenza vaccines as recommended
- Fluoride supplements if there is inadequate water fluoridation (less than 0.7 part per million)
- Screening for tuberculosis
- Screening for phenylketonuria (PKU) and other metabolic conditions
- Prompt attention for illnesses
- Appropriate skin hygiene and clothing

INFANT SAFETY

- Importance of supervision
- Car seat, crib, playpen, bath, and home environment safety measures
- Feeding measures (e.g., avoid propping bottle)
- Provide toys with no small parts or sharp edges

- Eliminate toxins in the environment (e.g., chemicals, radon, lead, mercury)
- Use smoke and carbon monoxide (CO) detectors in home

NUTRITION

- Breast-feeding to age 12 months
- Breast-feeding and bottle-feeding techniques
- Formula preparation
- Feeding schedule
- Introduction of solid foods
- Need for iron supplements at 4 to 6 months

ELIMINATION

- Characteristics and frequency of stool and urine elimination
- Diarrhea and its effects

REST/SLEEP

- Establish routine for sleep and rest patterns

SENSORY STIMULATION

- Touch: holding, cuddling, rocking
- Vision: colorful, moving toys
- Hearing: soothing voice tones, music, singing
- Play: toys appropriate for development

Motor Abilities

Fine muscle coordination and gross motor skills improve during toddlerhood. At the age of 18 months babies can pick up raisins or cereal pieces and place them in a receptacle. They can also hold a spoon and a cup and can walk upstairs with assistance. They will probably crawl down the stairs.

At 2 years, toddlers can hold a spoon and put it into the mouth correctly. They are able to run, their gait is steady, and they can balance on one foot and ride a tricycle (Figure 21-6 ■). By 3 years most children are toilet trained, although they still may have the occasional accident when playing or during the night.

Psychosocial Development

According to Freud, the ages of 2 and 3 years represent the anal phase of development, when the rectum and anus are the specially significant areas of the body. Erikson viewed the period from 18 months to 3 years as the time when the central developmental task is autonomy versus shame and doubt.

Toddlers begin to develop their sense of autonomy by asserting themselves with the frequent use of the word "no." They are often frustrated by restraints to their behavior and between ages 1 and 3 may have temper tantrums. However, with the guidance of their caregivers they slowly gain control over their emotions.

Figure 21-6 ■ A toddler has enough gross and fine motor ability to jump and kick a ball.

BOX 21-4 Fostering the Toddler's Psychosocial Development

- Provide toys suitable for the toddler, including some toys challenging enough to motivate but not so difficult that the toddler will fail. (Failure will intensify feelings of self-doubt and shame.)
- Make positive suggestions rather than commands. Avoid an emotional climate of negativism, blame, and punishment.
- Give the toddler choices, all of which are safe; however, limit number to two or three.
- When toddler has a temper tantrum, make sure the child is safe, and then leave.
- Help the toddler to develop inner control by setting and enforcing consistent, reasonable limits.
- Praise the toddler's accomplishments; give random and spontaneous feedback for positive behavior.

Parents need to have a great deal of patience coupled with an understanding of the importance of this developmental milestone. To be effective, caregivers need to give the child some measure of control and at the same time be consistent in setting limits so that the child learns the results of misbehavior. The nurse can also assist the parents and caregivers in promoting the toddler's development by suggesting the activities summarized in Box 21–4.

Self-concept is made up of body image development, feelings about self, adaptive and defensive mechanisms, reactions from others, and one's perceptions of these reactions, attitudes, values, and many of life's experiences (Starr, 2004). Children learn to develop a sense of self-concept through their immediate social environment, in which their parents play a significant role. If the children's social interactions with their parents are negative (e.g., constant disapproval regarding eating, toilet training, or other behavior), the children may begin to see themselves as bad. This perception is the basis of a negative self-concept. Parents need to give toddlers positive input so that they can develop a positive and healthy self-concept. With a healthy sense of self-esteem and security, the toddler is able to deal with periodic failures later in life without damage to self-esteem.

Although toddlers like to explore the environment, they always need to have a significant person nearby. Parents need to know that young children experience acute **separation anxiety,** the fear and frustration that come with parental absences. Abandonment is their greatest fear. At this age, the child may have difficulty accepting a baby-sitter or strongly resist being left by the parents at a day-care center. For example, toddlers may become highly anxious when separated from their parents and admitted to a hospital. **Regression** or reverting to an earlier development stage may be indicated by bed-wetting or using baby talk. Nurses can assist parents by helping them understand that this behavior is normal and indicates that these toddlers are trying to establish their position in the family.

Experience with separation helps the child cope with parental absences. Children need room for exploration and interaction with other children and adults. At the same time, they need to know that the parental bond of a loving and close relationship remains secure.

Toddlers assert their independence by saying "no" or by dawdling. During the toddler stage, receptive and expressive language skills are developing quickly. Children can understand words and follow directions long before they can actually form them into sentences.

Cognitive Development

According to Piaget, the toddler completes the fifth and sixth stages of the sensorimotor phase and starts the preconceptual phase at about 2 years of age. In the fifth stage, the toddler solves problems by a trial-and-error process. By stage 6, toddlers can solve problems mentally. For example, when given a new toy the toddler will not immediately handle the toy to see how it works, but will instead look at it carefully to think about how it works.

During Piaget's preconceptual phase, toddlers develop considerable cognitive and intellectual skills. They learn about the sequence of time. They have some symbolic thought; for example, a chair may represent a place of safety, and a blanket may symbolize comfort. Concepts start to form in late toddlerhood. A concept develops when the child learns words to represent classes of objects or thoughts. An example of a concrete concept is *table*, representing a number of articles of furniture that are all different but all tables.

Moral Development

According to Kohlberg, the first level of moral development is the preconventional when children respond to punishment and reward. During the second year of life, children begin to know that some activities elicit affection and approval. They also recognize that certain rituals, such as repeating phrases from prayers, also elicit approval. This provides children with feelings of security. By 2 years of age, toddlers are learning what attitudes their parents hold about moral matters.

Spiritual Development

According to Fowler (1981), the toddler's stage of spiritual development is undifferentiated. Toddlers may be aware of some religious practices, but they are primarily involved in learning knowledge and emotional reactions rather than establishing spiritual beliefs. A toddler may repeat short prayers at bedtime, conforming to a ritual, because praise and affection result. This parental or caregiver response enhances the toddler's sense of security.

Health Risks

Toddlers experience significant health problems due to injuries, visual problems, dental caries, and respiratory and ear infections.

Injuries

Injuries are the leading cause of mortality of toddlers. They are curious and like to feel and taste everything. The most common causes of fatal injuries are automobile crashes, drowning, burns, poisoning, and falls. Parents or other caregivers need to take the appropriate preventive measures to guard against these health threats (Figure 21-7 ■).

Figure 21-7 ■ Keep medicines and other poisonous materials locked away.

Visual Problems

During this period, the toddler should be screened for amblyopia. **Amblyopia** (reduced visual acuity in one eye) is usually the result of **strabismus** (cross-eye) but can be caused by refractive errors (e.g., myopia) or opacities in the lens. Initially the child with amblyopia has straight eyes, but the condition can lead to deviation of the "lazy" eye and loss of vision.

Dental Caries

Dental caries occur frequently during the toddler period, resulting from the interaction between the tooth surface, the *Streptococcus mutans* bacterium, and carbohydrates, especially sugar, in the diet. Prolonged exposure of teeth to carbohydrates (use of the bottle during naps and at bedtime) can cause caries.

Respiratory Tract and Ear Infections

Respiratory and middle ear infections are common during toddlerhood; their incidence increases with exposure to other children (as in day-care centers or preschools), with use of a bottle during naps or at bedtime, or if bottles are propped for feedings. Respiratory infections contribute significantly to visits to the pediatric primary care provider in the toddler years.

Health Assessment and Promotion

Growth and development in the toddler and preschool years provide the basis for a child's future health and well-being. It is essential that nurses do accurate and timely assessments to promote health and detect problems early, thus allowing for early interventions. Providing health education, information about growth and development, and anticipatory guidance to parents is also an important nursing role. Assessment activities for the

MediaLink ● Drowning Video

DEVELOPMENTAL ASSESSMENT GUIDELINES The Toddler

In these four developmental areas, does the toddler do the following?

PHYSICAL DEVELOPMENT

- Demonstrate physical growth (weight, height, and head circumference) within normal range.
- Manifest vital signs within normal range for age.
- Exhibit vision and hearing abilities within normal range.

MOTOR DEVELOPMENT

- Perform gross and fine motor milestones within the normal range for age. For example, by 3 years of age is the toddler able to do the following?
  - Walk up steps without assistance.
  - Balance on one foot, jump, and walk on toes.
  - Copy a circle.
  - Build a bridge from blocks.
  - Ride a tricycle.

PSYCHOSOCIAL DEVELOPMENT

- Perform psychosocial developmental milestones for age. For example, by 3 years of age is the toddler able to do the following?
  - Express likes and dislikes.
  - Display curiosity and ask questions.
  - Accept separation from mother for short periods of time.
  - Begin to play and communicate with children and others outside the immediate family.
  - Understand words such as *up, down, cold,* and *hungry.*
  - Speak in sentences of three to four words.
  - Imitate religious rituals of the family.

DEVELOPMENT IN ACTIVITIES OF DAILY LIVING

- Feed self.
- Eat and drink a variety of foods.
- Begin to develop bowel and bladder control.
- Exhibit a sleep pattern appropriate for age.
- Dress self.

---

toddler are similar to those for the infant in terms of measuring weight, length (height), and vital signs (see the Developmental Assessment Guidelines).

Promoting health and wellness includes such areas as accident prevention, toilet training, and good dental hygiene. For a summary of health promotion for toddlers, see Box 21–5.

PRESCHOOLERS (4 AND 5 YEARS)

During the preschool period physical growth slows, but control of the body and coordination increase greatly. Preschoolers' worlds gets larger as they meet relatives, friends, and neighbors.

Physical Development

By the time children are 4 or 5 years old, they appear taller and thinner than toddlers because children tend to grow more in height than in weight. The preschooler's brain almost reaches its adult size by 5 years. The extremities of the body grow more quickly than the body trunk, making the child's body appear somewhat out of proportion. The posture of preschoolers gradually changes as the pelvis is straightened and the abdominal muscles become stronger. Thus the preschooler appears slender with erect posture.

Weight

Weight gain in preschool children is generally slow. By 5 years they have added only another 3 to 5 kg (7 to 12 lb) to their 3-year-old weight, increasing it to somewhere between 18 and 20 kg (40 and 45 lb).

Height

Preschool children grow about 5 to 6.25 cm (2.0 to 2.5 in.) each year. Thus by 4 years of age they double the birth length and measure about 102 cm (41 in.).

BOX 21–5 Health Promotion Guidelines for Toddlers

HEALTH EXAMINATIONS
- At 15 and 18 months and then as recommended by the primary care provider
- Dental visit starting at age 3 or earlier

PROTECTIVE MEASURES
- Immunizations: continuing DTaP, IPV series, pneumococcal, MMR, *Haemophilus influenzae* type B, hepatitis B, hepatitis A, and influenza vaccines as recommended
- Screenings for tuberculosis and lead poisoning
- Fluoride supplements if there is inadequate water fluoridation (less than 0.7 part per million)

TODDLER SAFETY
- Importance of constant supervision and teaching child to obey commands
- Home environment safety measures (e.g., lock medicine cabinet)
- Outdoor safety measures (e.g., close supervision near water)
- Appropriate toys

- Eliminate toxins in environment (e.g., pesticides, herbicides, mercury, lead, arsenic in playground materials)
- Use smoke and carbon monoxide (CO) detectors in home

NUTRITION
- Importance of nutritious meals and snacks
- Teaching simple mealtime manners
- Dental care

ELIMINATION
- Toilet training techniques

REST/SLEEP
- Dealing with sleep disturbances

PLAY
- Providing adequate space and a variety of activities
- Toys that allow "acting on" behaviors and provide motor and sensory stimulation

Vision

Preschool children are generally **hyperopic** (farsighted), that is, unable to focus on near objects. As the eye grows in length, it becomes **emmetropic** (it refracts light normally). If the eyes become too long, the child becomes **myopic** (nearsighted), that is, unable to focus on objects that are far away. In severe cases of hyperopia or myopia, glasses may be prescribed. By the end of the preschool years, visual ability has improved; normal vision for the 5-year-old is approximately 20/30. The Snellen E chart can be used to assess the preschooler's vision.

Hearing and Taste

The hearing of the preschool child has reached optimal levels, and the ability to listen (attend to and comprehend what is said) has matured since the toddler age. As for the sense of taste, preschoolers show their preferences by asking for something "yummy," and may refuse something they consider "yucky." At about age 3, children may display food "jags," refusing to eat some foods or only eating a few particular foods. It is important that parents not engage the child in a "battle of wills" over food. If parents provide healthful foods in an environment that is pleasant and comfortable for eating, the child will eat what is needed.

Motor Abilities

By 5 years of age, children are able to wash their hands and face and brush their teeth (see Figure 21-8 ■). They are self-conscious about exposing their bodies and go to the bathroom without telling others. Typically, preschool children run with increasing skill each year. By 5 years of age, they run skillfully and can jump three steps. Preschoolers can balance on their toes and dress themselves without assistance.

Psychosocial Development

Erikson wrote that the major developmental crisis of the preschooler is initiative versus guilt. Preschoolers must solve problems in accordance with their consciences. Their personalities continue to develop. Erikson viewed the success of this milestone as determining the individual's self-concept. According to

Figure 21-8 ■ A preschooler brushing her teeth.

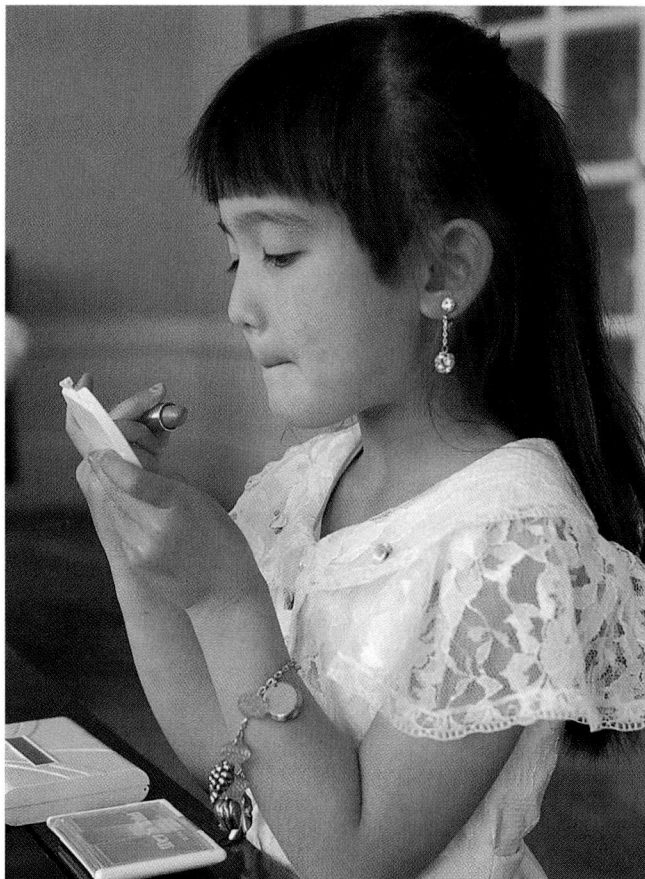

Figure 21-9 ■ Preschoolers often identify with the parent of the same sex and like to mimic behavior.

Erikson, preschoolers must learn what they can do. As a result, preschoolers imitate behavior, and their imaginations and creativity become lively.

Parents can enhance the self-concept of the preschooler by providing opportunities for new achievements where the child can learn, repeat, and master. For example, a child obtains a two-wheel bike with safety wheels and quickly learns coordination, balance, use of the brakes, and bicycle safety. Mastery of these tasks provides the child with a sense of accomplishment. The child is soon ready for the new challenge of mastering the two-wheeler.

The self-concept of the preschooler is also based on gender identification. Preschoolers are aware of the two sexes and identify with the correct one. They often imitate sexual stereotypes and usually begin by identifying with the parent of the same sex. They may mimic the parent's behavior, attitudes, and appearance (see Figure 21-9 ■). Parents need to be aware that preschoolers are curious about their own bodies and sexual functions, as well as those of others, and will often ask questions. Parents should answer questions calmly and frankly, using words and concepts the child understands. Children do not have the social, emotional, or moral context that adults do, so a simple answer may be more than adequate. When parents overreact to a child's question, refuse to answer, or punish or shame the child, the child can become confused.

Freud theorized that the preschooler is in the phallic stage of development. The biologic focus of the child during this stage is the genital area, and masturbation is common. The phase of close emotional relationships with both parents changes to the phase Freud referred to as the Electra or Oedipus complex. At this time, the child focuses feelings of love chiefly on the parent of the opposite sex, and the parent of the same sex may receive some hostile feelings. The child begins to develop sexual interests and becomes interested in clothes and hair styles.

During the preschool years, four adaptive mechanisms are learned: identification, introjection, imagination, and repression. **Identification** occurs when the child perceives the self as similar to another person and behaves like that person. For example, a boy may internalize the attitudes and gender behavior of his father. **Introjection** is similar to identification. It is the assimilation of the attributes of others. When preschoolers observe their parents, they assimilate many of their values and attitudes. **Imagination** is an important part of preschoolers' lives, helping children make sense of the world and giving them a sense of control and mastery. The preschooler has an active imagination and fantasizes in play; for example, a chair becomes a beautiful throne to a girl, and she is the ruler of all she sees. **Repression** is removing experiences, thoughts, and impulses from awareness. The preschooler generally represses thoughts related to the Oedipus or Electra complex.

Preschool children gradually emerge as social beings. At the age of 3 or 4, they learn to play with a small number of their peers. They gradually learn to play with more people as they grow older. Preschoolers participate more in the family than they did previously. In associations with neighbors, family guests, and baby-sitters, too, they learn about social relationships.

In their speech, children of 4 years are often dogmatic; they tend to believe that what they know is right. Four-year-olds love nonsense words such as "jump-jump" and can string them together much to an adult's exasperation. At 4, children are aggressive in their speech and capable of long conversations, often mixing fact and fiction. By 5 years of age, speaking skills are well developed. Children use words purposefully and ask questions to acquire information. They do not merely practice speaking as 3- and 4-year-olds do, but speak as a means of social interaction. Exaggeration is common among 4- and 5-year-olds.

Preschoolers also become increasingly aware of themselves. They play with their bodies largely out of curiosity. They know where the body begins and ends as well as the correct names for the different parts. By 5 years of age, they are able to draw a person including all the features. Preschoolers also learn about their feelings; they know the words *cry*, *sad*, *laugh*, and the feelings related to them. They also begin to learn how to control their feelings and behavior. The preschooler uses the same types of coping mechanisms in response to stress as the toddler does, although protest behavior (kicking, screaming) is less likely to occur in the older preschooler. Preschoolers usually have greater ability to verbalize stress.

Preschoolers need to feel that they are loved and that they are an important part of the family. The child who has to compete with siblings for parental attention will often display jealousy. Parents and caregivers should be aware that preschoolers need time to adjust to a new baby and may need additional attention or special activities to help them through this adjustment period.

Preschoolers with older siblings may also experience sibling rivalry. Siblings may fight and argue and become aggressive because of their daily proximity or competition for parental attention. Parents who can plan some special time or activity for each child will help that child to feel loved and may decrease the sibling rivalry.

Guidance and discipline are important parts of the parental role during the preschool years. As children seek independence from adults, they often test limits by refusing to cooperate and by repeatedly ignoring parental requests. These power struggles can sometimes be avoided by encouraging children to be responsible for their own behavior as much as possible and by setting reasonable expectations and consistent limits. When conflict does occur, parents can employ mutual discussion and compromise.

Cognitive Development

The preschooler's cognitive development, according to Piaget, is the phase of intuitive thought. Children are still egocentric, but egocentrism gradually subsides as they experience their expanding world. Preschoolers learn through trial and error, and they think of only one idea at a time. They do not understand relationships such as those between mother and father or sister and brother. Children start to understand that words are associated with objects in late toddlerhood or the early preschool years. Preschoolers become concerned about death as something inevitable, but they do not explain it. They also associate death with others rather than themselves.

Most children at the age of 5 years can count pennies; however, the opportunity to spend money usually does not occur until they attend school. Reading skills also start to develop at this age. Young children like fairy tales and books about animals and other children.

Moral Development

Preschoolers are capable of prosocial behavior, that is, any action that a person takes to benefit someone else. The term *prosocial* is synonymous with *kind* and connotes sharing, helping, protecting, giving aid, befriending, showing affection, and giving encouragement.

At this stage of development, preschoolers do not have a fully formed conscience; however, they do develop some internal controls. Moral behavior is largely learned by modeling, initially after parents and later significant others. The preschooler usually behaves well in social settings.

Children who perceive their parents as strict may become resentful or overly obedient. Preschoolers usually control their behavior because they want love and approval from their parents. Moral behavior to a preschooler may mean taking turns at play or sharing. Nurses can assist parents by discussing moral development and encouraging parents to give preschoolers recognition for actions such as sharing. It is also important for parents to answer preschoolers' "why" questions and discuss values with them.

Spiritual Development

Many preschoolers enroll in Sunday school or faith-oriented classes. The preschooler usually enjoys the social interaction of these classes. According to Fowler, children from the ages of 4 to 6 years are at the intuitive-projective stage of spiritual development. Faith at this stage is primarily a result of the teaching of significant others, such as parents and teachers. Children learn to imitate religious behavior, for example, bowing the head in prayer, although they don't understand the meaning of the behavior. Preschoolers require simple explanations, such as those in picture books, of spiritual matters. Children at this age use their imaginations to envision such ideas as angels or the devil.

Health Risks

Preschoolers often have health problems similar to those they had in toddlerhood. Respiratory tract problems and communicable diseases frequently occur as the preschooler interacts with other children at nursery schools and day care. Accidents and dental caries continue to be problems during this age. Congenital abnormalities such as cardiac disorders and hernias are often corrected at this age.

Health Assessment and Promotion

During assessment, the preschooler can often participate in answering questions with assistance from parents or caregivers. For instance, children who attend preschool can describe the typical lunch and how much of it they usually eat. Preschoolers can also describe the types of activities they enjoy. Guidelines for the preschooler are shown in the Developmental Assessment Guidelines.

Promoting health and wellness includes such areas as accident prevention, dental health, good nutrition, cognitive stimulation, and sufficient sleep. For a summary of health promotion, see Box 21–6.

BOX 21–6 Health Promotion Guidelines for Preschoolers

HEALTH EXAMINATIONS
- Every 1 to 2 years

PROTECTIVE MEASURES
- Immunizations: continuing DTaP, IPV series, MMR, hepatitis, pneumococcal, influenza, and other immunizations as recommended
- Screenings for tuberculosis
- Vision and hearing screening
- Regular dental screenings and fluoride treatment

PRESCHOOLER SAFETY
- Educating child about simple safety rules (e.g., crossing the street)
- Teaching child to play safely (e.g., bicycle and playground safety)
- Educating to prevent poisoning; exposure to toxic materials

NUTRITION
- Importance of nutritious meals and snacks

ELIMINATION
- Teaching proper hygiene (e.g., washing hands after using bathroom)

REST/SLEEP
- Dealing with sleep disturbances (e.g., night terrors, sleepwalking)

PLAY
- Providing times for group play activities
- Teaching child simple games that require cooperation and interaction
- Providing toys and dress-ups for role-playing

SCHOOL-AGE CHILDREN (6 TO 12 YEARS)

The school-age period starts when children are about 6 years of age, when the deciduous teeth are shed. This period includes the preadolescent (prepuberty) period. It ends at about 12 years,

---

DEVELOPMENTAL ASSESSMENT GUIDELINES The Preschooler

In these four developmental areas, does the preschooler do the following?

PHYSICAL DEVELOPMENT
- Demonstrate physical growth (weight, height) within normal range.
- Manifest vital signs within normal range for age.
- Exhibit vision and hearing abilities within normal range.

MOTOR DEVELOPMENT
- Perform gross and fine motor milestones within the normal range for age. For example, by 5 years of age is the preschooler able to do the following?
  - Jump rope and skip.
  - Climb playground equipment.
  - Ride a bicycle with training wheels.
  - Print letters and numbers.

PSYCHOSOCIAL DEVELOPMENT
- Perform psychosocial developmental milestones for age. For example, by 5 years of age is the preschooler able to do the following?
  - Separate easily from parents.
  - Display imagination and creativity.
  - Enjoy playing with peers in cooperative activities.
  - Understand right from wrong and respond to others' expectations of behavior.
  - Identify four colors.
  - Exhibit increasing vocabulary using complete sentences and all parts of speech.
  - Cooperate in doing simple chores (e.g., putting away toys).
  - Demonstrate awareness of sexual differences.

DEVELOPMENT IN ACTIVITIES OF DAILY LIVING
- Demonstrate development of toilet training.
- Perform simple hygiene measures.
- Dress and undress self.
- Engage in bedtime rituals and demonstrate ability to put self to sleep.

with the onset of puberty. Puberty is the age when the reproductive organs become functional and secondary sex characteristics develop. Because the average age of onset of puberty is 10 for girls and 12 for boys, some people define the school-age years as 6 to 10 for girls and 6 to 12 for boys. Skills learned during this stage are particularly important in relation to work later in life and willingness to try new tasks. In general, the period from 6 to 12 years is one of significant growth.

Physical Development

The school-age child gains weight rapidly and thus appears less thin than previously. Individual differences due to both genetic and environmental factors are obvious at this time.

Weight

At 6 years boys tend to weigh about 21 kg (46 lb), about 1 kg (2 lb) more than girls. The weight gain of schoolchildren from 6 to 12 years of age averages about 3.2 kg (7 lb) per year, but the major weight gains occur from age 10 to 12 for boys and from 9 to 12 for girls. By 12 years of age boys and girls weigh on the average 40 to 42 kg (88 to 95 lb); girls are usually heavier.

Height

At 6 years both boys and girls are about the same height, 115 cm (46 in.). They are about 150 cm (60 in.) by 12 years. Before puberty, children of both sexes have a growth spurt, girls between 10 and 12 years and boys between 12 and 14 years. Thus girls may be taller than boys at 12 years.

The extremities tend to grow more quickly than the trunk; thus school-age children's bodies appear somewhat ill proportioned. By 6 years of age the thoracic curvature starts to develop and the lordosis disappears. Full adult posture is not assumed, however, until after the complete development of the skeletal musculature during the adolescent period.

Vision

The depth and distance perception of children 6 to 8 years of age is accurate. By age 6 children have full binocular vision. The eye muscles are well developed and coordinated, and both eyes can focus on one object at the same time. Because the shape of the eye changes during growth, the farsightedness of the preschool years gradually changes to 20/20 vision during the school-age years; 20/20 vision is usually well established between 9 and 11 years of age.

Hearing and Touch

Auditory perception is fully developed in school-age children, who are able to identify fine differences in voices, both in sound and in pitch. At this stage, children also have a well-developed sense of touch and are able to locate points of heat and cold on all body surfaces. They are also able to identify an unseen object, such as a pencil or a book, simply by touch. This ability is called **stereognosis.**

Prepubertal Changes

Little change takes place in the reproductive and endocrine systems until the prepuberty period. During prepuberty, at about ages 9 to 13, endocrine functions slowly increase. This change in endocrine function can result in increased perspiration and more active sebaceous glands. Girls may have a sticky vaginal discharge (leukorrhea) prior to puberty.

Motor Abilities

During the middle years (6 to 10), children perfect their muscular skills and coordination. By 9 years most children are becoming skilled in games of interest, such as football or baseball. These skills are often associated with school, and many of them are learned there. By 9 years most children have sufficient fine motor control for such activities as drawing, building models, or playing musical instruments.

Psychosocial Development

According to Erikson, the central task of school-age children is industry versus inferiority. At this time children begin to create and develop a sense of competence and perseverance. School-age children are motivated by activities that provide a sense of worth. They concentrate on mastering skills that will help them function in the adult world. Although children of this age work hard to succeed, they are always faced with the possibility of failure, which can lead to a sense of inferiority. If children have been successful in previous stages, they are motivated to be industrious and to cooperate with others toward a common goal.

Freud described the period from 6 through 12 years of age as the latency stage. During this time the focus is on physical and intellectual activities, while sexual tendencies seem to be repressed.

In school, children have the restraints of the school system imposed on their behavior, and they learn to develop internal controls. Children tend to compare their skills with those of their peers in a number of areas, including motor development, social development, and language. This comparison assists in the development of self-concept.

As school-age children grow older, they learn to play in groups. The typical 6- and 7-year-old is a member of a peer group that is usually informal and transitory with the leadership changing from time to time. During this period of socialization with others, children gradually become less self-centered and more cooperative within a group. Peers can have a greater influence than the family. During middle to late childhood, children may join a more formalized group of peers, which is often structured around common interests. These groups may consist of children of the same gender later in the school-age period.

Self-concept continues to mature in this period. Children recognize similarities and differences between themselves and others. School-age children compare themselves with others. Children who are successful and receive recognition for their efforts feel competent and in control of themselves and of their environment. Conversely, children who feel unaccepted by peers or constantly receive negative feedback and little recognition may experience feelings of inferiority and worthlessness.

Although the focus of interest for this age group has moved to school, peers, and other activities, the home remains the crucial place for the child's development of high self-esteem.

MediaLink Teen with Lymphocytic Leukemia Care Plan Activity

Figure 21-10 ■ Expanding cognitive skills enable school-age children to interact cooperatively in activities of an increasingly complex nature, as shown by the children playing this board game.

Cognitive Development

According to Piaget, the ages 7 to 11 years mark the phase of concrete operations. During this stage the child changes from egocentric interactions to cooperative interactions (see Figure 21-10 ■). School-age children also develop an increased understanding of concepts that are associated with specific objects, for example, environmental conservation or wildlife preservation. Children at this time develop logical reasoning from intuitive reasoning. For example, they learn to add and subtract to obtain an answer to a problem. Children also learn about cause-and-effect relationships at this age; for example, they know that a stone will not float because it is heavier than water.

Money is a concept that gains meaning for children when they start school. By the time they are 7 or 8 years old, children usually know the value of most coins. The concept of time is also learned at this age. By 6 years of age children enter school; the schedule in school helps them learn time periods. However, it is not until 9 or 10 years of age that children are able to understand the long periods of time in the past. Knowing the time of day and the day of the week are relatively easy for children because they relate time to routine activities. For example, a girl may go to school Monday through Friday, play on Saturday, go to Sunday school on Sunday morning, and go out with her father Sunday afternoon. Children are beginning to read a clock by the time they are 6 years old; they can learn to read both digital and numerical clocks.

Reading skills are usually well developed later in childhood, and what a child reads is largely influenced by the family. By 9 years of age most children are self-motivated. They compete with themselves, and they like to plan in advance. By 12 years they are motivated by inner drive rather than by competition with peers. They like to talk, to discuss different subjects, and to debate.

Moral Development

Some school-age children are at Kohlberg's stage 1 of the preconventional level (punishment and obedience); that is, they act to avoid being punished. Some school-age children, however, are at stage 2 (instrumental-relativist orientation). These children do things to benefit themselves. Fairness, that is, everyone getting a fair share or chance, becomes important. Later in childhood, most children progress to the conventional level. This level has two stages: Stage 3 is the "good boy-nice girl" stage, and stage 4 is the law and order orientation. Children usually reach the conventional level between the ages of 10 and 13. The child shifts from the concrete interests of individuals to the interests of groups. The motivation for moral action at this stage is to live up to what significant others think of the child.

Spiritual Development

According to Fowler, the school-age child is at stage 2 in spiritual development, the mythic-literal stage. Children learn to distinguish fantasy from fact. Spiritual facts are those beliefs that are accepted by a religious group, whereas fantasy is thoughts and images formed in the child's mind. Parents and the minister, rabbi, or priest help the child distinguish fact from fantasy. These people still influence the child more than peers in spiritual matters.

When children do not understand such events as the creation of the world, they use fantasy to explain them. The school-age child needs to have concepts such as prayer presented in concrete terms. For example, the child thinks of God as having human qualities, such as a kind old man or a person who punishes when behavior does not meet his standards.

School-age children may ask many questions about God and religion in these years and will generally believe that God is good and always present to help. Just before puberty, children become aware that their prayers are not always answered and become disappointed. At this age, some children reject religion, whereas others continue to accept it. This decision is largely influenced by the parents. If a child continues religious training, the child is ready to apply reason rather than blind belief in most situations.

Health Risks

School-age children continue to have as many communicable diseases, dental caries, and accidents as preschoolers (see Figure 21-11 ■). Another health concern is the increasing number of overweight children. Being overweight is the most common nutritional problem among children and contributes to the increasing incidence of hypertension and type 2 diabetes in children (Strock et al., 2005). Obesity in childhood can lead to obesity and increased risk for diabetes, hypertension, and cardiovascular disease among adults.

Health Assessment and Promotion

During the assessment interview the nurse responds to questions from the parent or other caregiver, gives appropriate feedback, and lends encouragement and support. The nurse also demonstrates interest in the child and enthusiasm for the child's strengths. Guidelines for the school-age child are shown in the Developmental Assessment Guidelines.

Figure 21-11 ■ Teach children never to touch guns without a parent present.

Promoting health and wellness includes dental hygiene and regular dental examinations, safety measures to prevent accidents, promoting a healthy diet and physical fitness, supporting autonomy and self-esteem, and hygiene measures to prevent infections. Box 21–7 provides health promotion guidelines for this age group.

BOX 21–7 Health Promotion Guidelines for School-Age Children

HEALTH EXAMINATIONS
- Annual physical examination or as recommended

PROTECTIVE MEASURES
- Immunizations as recommended (e.g., MMR, meningococcal, tetanus-diphtheria, adult preparation [Td])
- Screening for tuberculosis
- Periodic vision, speech, and hearing screenings
- Regular dental screenings and fluoride treatment
- Providing accurate information about sexual issues (e.g., reproduction, AIDS)

SCHOOL-AGE CHILD SAFETY
- Using proper equipment when participating in sports and other physical activities (e.g., helmets, pads)
- Encouraging child to take responsibility for own safety (e.g., participating in bicycle and water safety courses)

NUTRITION
- Importance of child not skipping meals and eating a balanced diet
- Experiences with food that may lead to obesity

ELIMINATION
- Utilizing positive approaches for elimination problems (e.g., enuresis)

PLAY AND SOCIAL INTERACTIONS
- Providing opportunities for a variety of organized group activities
- Accepting realistic expectations of child's abilities
- Acting as role models in acceptance of other persons who may be different
- Providing a home environment that limits TV viewing and video games and encourages completion of homework and healthy exercise

---

DEVELOPMENTAL ASSESSMENT GUIDELINES   The School-Age Child

In these four developmental areas, does the school-age child do the following?

PHYSICAL DEVELOPMENT
- Demonstrate physical growth (weight, height) within normal range.
- Manifest vital signs within normal range for age.
- Exhibit vision and hearing abilities within normal range.
- Demonstrate male or female prepubertal changes within normal range.

MOTOR DEVELOPMENT
- Possess coordinated motor skills for age. For example, by 12 years of age, is the child able to do the following?
  - Do tricks on a bike, climb a tree, shinny up a rope.
  - Throw and catch a small ball.
  - Play a musical instrument.

PSYCHOSOCIAL DEVELOPMENT
- Perform psychosocial developmental milestones for age. For example, by 12 years of age is the child able to do the following?
  - Make friends of the same sex and establish a peer group.

- Become less dependent on family and venture away from them.
- Interact well with parents.
- Control strong and impulsive feelings.
- Articulate an understanding of right and wrong.
- Participate in organized competitions.
- Read, print, and manipulate numbers and letters easily.
- Express positive feelings about school and school activities.
- Exhibit a concept of money and make change for small amounts of money.
- Express self in a logical manner and talk through problems.
- Enjoy riddles and read and understand comics.
- Invest in a hobby or collection.
- Like to help others.
- Think of self as likable and healthy.

DEVELOPMENT IN ACTIVITIES OF DAILY LIVING
- Demonstrate concern for personal cleanliness and appearance.
- Express need for privacy.

ADOLESCENTS (12 TO 18 YEARS)

Adolescence is the period during which the person becomes physically and psychologically mature and acquires a personal identity. At the end of this critical period in development, the person should be ready to enter adulthood and assume its responsibilities. The length of adolescence is culturally determined to some extent. In North America, adolescence is longer than in some cultures, extending to 18 or 20 years of age.

Puberty is the first stage of adolescence in which sexual organs begin to grow and mature. **Menarche** (onset of menstruation) occurs in girls. **Ejaculation** (expulsion of semen) occurs in boys. For girls, puberty normally starts between 10 and 14 years; for boys, between 12 and 16 years. The adolescent period is often subdivided into three stages: early adolescence lasts from ages 12 to 13; middle adolescence extends from 14 to 16 years; and late adolescence extends from 17 to 18 or 20 years. Late adolescence is a more stable stage than the other two. In the late period, adolescents are involved mostly with planning their future and economic independence.

Physical Development

During puberty, growth is markedly accelerated compared to the slow, steady growth of the child. This period, marked by sudden and dramatic physical changes, is referred to as the **adolescent growth spurt.** In boys, the growth spurt usually begins between ages 12 and 16; in girls, it begins earlier, usually between ages 10 and 14. Because the growth spurt begins earlier in girls, many girls surpass boys in height at this time.

Physical Growth

Physical growth continues throughout adolescence. Growth is fastest for boys at about 14 years, and the maximum height is often reached at about 18 or 19 years. Some men add another 1 or 2 cm to their height during their 20s as the vertebral column gradually continues to grow. During the period of 10 to 18 years of age, the average American male doubles his weight, gaining about 32 kg (72 lb), and grows about 41 cm (16 in.). The fastest rate of growth in girls occurs at about age 12; they reach their maximum height at about 15 to 16 years. During ages 10 to 18, the average American female gains about 25 kg (55 lb) and grows about 24 cm (9 in.).

Physical growth during adolescence is greatly influenced by a number of factors, such as heredity, nutrition, medical care, illness, physical and emotional environment, family size, and culture. Generally, people in the United States have grown taller in recent years. This increase in average height is thought to be due to many of the preceding factors.

Growth is noted first in the musculoskeletal system. This growth follows a sequential pattern: The head, hands, and feet are the first to grow to adult status. Next, the extremities reach their adult size. Because the extremities grow before the trunk, the adolescent looks leggy, awkward, and uncoordinated. After the trunk grows to full size, the shoulders, chest, and hips grow. Skull and facial bones also change proportions: The forehead becomes more prominent, and the jawbones develop.

Glandular Changes

The eccrine and apocrine glands increase their secretions and become fully functional during puberty. The **eccrine glands,** found over most of the body, produce sweat. The **apocrine glands** develop in the axillae, in the anal and genital areas, in the external auditory canals, and around the umbilicus and the areola of the breasts. Apocrine sweat is released onto the skin in response to emotional stimuli only. **Sebaceous glands** also become active under the influence of androgens in both males and females. The sebaceous glands, which secrete sebum, become most active on the face, neck, shoulder, upper back, and chest and are often the cause of an increased incidence of acne.

Sexual Characteristics

During puberty, both primary and secondary sex characteristics develop. **Primary sexual characteristics** relate to the organs necessary for reproduction, such as the testes, penis, ovaries, vagina, and uterus. **Secondary sexual characteristics** differentiate the male from the female but do not relate directly to reproduction. Examples are pubic hair growth, breast development, and voice changes.

The first noticeable sign that puberty has begun in males is the appearance of pubic hair and the enlargement of the scrotum and testes. The milestone of male puberty is considered to be the first ejaculation, which commonly occurs at about 14 years of age. Fertility follows several months later. Sexual maturity is achieved by age 18.

Often the first noticeable sign of puberty in females is the appearance of the breast bud (thelarche), although the appearance of hair along the labia may precede this. The milestone of female puberty is the menarche, which occurs about 1 1/2 to 2 years after the breast bud appears. At first, menstrual periods are scanty and irregular and may occur without ovulation. Ovulation is usually established 1 to 2 years after menarche; ovulation, and pregnancy, however, can occur early in menarche or as an immediate precursor to a girl's first menstruation. Female internal reproductive organs reach adult size about age 18 to 20.

Psychosocial Development

According to Erikson (1963), the psychosocial task of the adolescent is the establishment of identity. The danger of this stage is role confusion. The inability to settle on an occupational identity commonly disturbs the adolescent. Less commonly, doubts about sexual identity arise. Because of the adolescent's dramatic body changes, the development of a stable identity is difficult. Erikson says that adolescents help one another through this identity crisis by forming cliques and a separate youth culture. These cliques often exclude all those who are "different" in skin color, cultural background, aspects of dress, gestures, and tastes.

Adolescents are usually concerned about their body, their appearance, and their physical abilities. Hair styling, skin care, and clothes become very important. In-groupers of an adolescent clique can be excessively clannish and cruel in excluding out-groupers; this intolerance is a temporary defense against identity confusion (Erikson, 1963, p. 236).

In their search for a new identity, adolescents have to reprocess many of the previous stages of development. The task of developing trust in self and others is again encountered when adolescents look for ideal persons whom they can trust and with whom they can prove trustworthy. Development of autonomy is restaged in their search for ways to express the right to choose freely. The search for an occupational role that allows expression of an autonomous, freely chosen direction is one example. Free choice and autonomy present conflicts to the adolescent. Conflict arises between behaving well in the eyes of the parents and behaving in a manner that may expose them to the ridicule of peers. The sense of initiative is also restaged. The adolescent has unlimited imagination and ambition and aspires to great accomplishments. The sense of industry is reenacted when the adolescent chooses a career. The extent to which these tasks are successfully achieved earlier influences the adolescent's ability to develop a healthy self-concept and self-identity.

The adolescent needs to establish a self-concept that accepts both personal strengths and weaknesses. Many adolescents experience temporary difficulty in developing a positive self-image. This is due to dramatic changes in body structure and function as well as greater expectations to assume responsibilities. Many adolescents experience temporary difficulty in developing a positive self-image. Adolescents who are accepted, loved, and valued by family and peers generally tend to gain confidence and feel good about themselves. Teenagers with physical disabilities or illnesses are particularly vulnerable to peer rejection. Nurses and educators can promote peer understanding and acceptance by discussing within the peer group the problems an individual with a particular disability or condition might face. Establishing groups of peers who have similar problems can provide an opportunity for the individual to develop close relationships with others and feel valued and accepted.

Although sexual identification begins at about 3 or 4 years of age, it is a significant part of adolescence. Establishing a sense of sexual identity and clarifying one's sexual orientation occurs during late adolescence. Adolescents explore sexual images, fantasies, ideas, and roles. Experimenting with dress, language, and social interactions (e.g., dances, dating, youth activities, workplace) help them define who they are. Adult role models (e.g., parents, movie stars, music idols) can influence greatly the way adolescents think and behave, helping teens to decide which aspects of masculinity or femininity to adopt or reject. Later, adolescents begin to establish intimacy with a partner or partners. This intimacy lays the groundwork for the commitments of adulthood. Sexual experimentation is not part of true intimacy, but once intimacy is achieved, sexual activity is often included. Homosexual youth may experience a great deal of confusion during this process, since homosexuality is not openly accepted in all groups and their questions about self and identity may go unanswered.

Many adolescents are sexually active and may engage in masturbation as well as heterosexual and homosexual activity. The 2003 Youth Risk Behavior Surveillance reported that 46.7% of high school students had had sexual intercourse during their lifetime; 34% were currently sexually active (had had sexual intercourse in the 3 months prior to the survey); and 37% of sexually active students had not used a condom at their last sexual intercourse (Grunbaum et al., 2004). Although the pregnancy rate for teenagers 15 to 19 years of age dropped to 84.5/1,000 women between 1990 and 2000 (Ventura, Abrna, Moshe, Hanshaw, et al., 2004), nearly 5% of all high school aged girls had been pregnant, and over 7% of girls had had sex before they were 13 years old (Grunbaum et al., 2004). These behaviors increase the risk for sexually transmitted diseases

---

RESEARCH NOTE   What Effect Would Mandated Parental Notification Have on Adolescent Contraceptive Use?

Jones and her colleagues (2005) surveyed 1,526 adolescent girls younger than 18 years who were seeking reproductive health services to determine what effect notifying their parents would have on their choices about contraception and sexual activity.

Sixty percent of the sample stated that their parents were aware of the adolescent's visit to the clinic, and many parents had encouraged their daughters to seek reproductive health care services at the clinic. Characteristics of the girls who were most likely to have parents aware of their clinic visit included: younger than 15 years, non-Hispanic blacks, used a hormonal method of contraception, had made two or more clinic visits for prescription contraceptives in the past year, and lived with their mothers.

Of those who had not told their parents of their visit to the clinic, 25% stated they did not want their parents to know they were sexually active. Another 22% said they were responsible for their own health care and made decisions independently.

When asked what contraceptive or sexual activity choices they would make if parental notification were required, respondents indicated several strategies. Fifty-nine percent said they would continue to access care in the clinic; most of these were girls whose parents were

already aware of their visit. Over 45% said they would use over-the-counter (OTC) methods such as condoms. Seven percent said they would stop having sex, but only 1% listed this as their only option.

Teenagers whose parents were not aware of their clinic visit said they would be less likely to continue to visit the clinic and more likely to use OTC methods. Overall, nearly 20% of the sample said they would engage in risky sexual behavior (including no protection or withdrawal) if parental notification were mandated, and 5% indicated they would not seek care for STDs.

IMPLICATIONS

This research suggests that, although the parents of many adolescent girls are aware of their daughters' reproductive health care, mandating providers to notify parents could lead to increased risky sexual behavior and subsequent increases in adolescent pregnancy and sexually transmitted disease.

Note: From "Adolescents' Reports of Parental Knowledge of Adolescents' Use of Sexual Health Services and Their Reactions to Mandated Parental Notification for Prescription Contraception," by R. K. Jones, A. Purcell, S. Singh, L. B. Finder, 2005, *Journal of the American Medical Association 293*(3), pp. 340–348. Reprinted with permission.

(STDs) and pregnancy. Almost 4 million of the new cases of STDs each year occur in adolescents, and about 1 million teenagers become pregnant each year (USDHHS, 2000).

At about the age of 15 years, many adolescents gradually draw away from the family and gain independence. This need for independence combined with the need for family support sometimes creates conflict within the adolescent and between the adolescent and the family. The young person may appear hostile or depressed at times during this painful process. At this age, adolescents prefer to be with their peers rather than their parents and may seek advice from adults other than their parents. Parents sometimes are bewildered by this stage of development; instead of reducing controls, they increase them, causing the adolescent to rebel.

Adolescents also have to resolve their ambivalent feelings toward the parent of the opposite sex. As part of the resolution, adolescents may develop brief crushes on adults outside the family—teachers or neighbors, for example. Adolescents sometimes adopt some of the attributes of the adults with whom they are infatuated. This modeling can be helpful in the maturing process.

Some of the discord in the family at this time is due to the generation gap. The values of the adolescent may differ from those of the parents. This difference may be difficult for the parents to understand and to accept. Adolescents still need guidance from their parents, although they appear to neither want it nor need it. However, adolescents need to know that their parents care about them and that their parents still want to help them. Restrictions and guidance need to be presented in a manner that makes adolescents feel loved. They need consistency in guidance and fewer restrictions than previously. They should have the independence they can handle yet know that their parents will assist them when they need help.

During adolescence, **peer groups** assume great importance (see Figure 21-12 ■). The peer group has a number of functions. It provides a sense of belonging, pride, social learning, and sexual roles. Most peer groups have well-defined, sex-specific modes of acceptable behavior. In adolescence, the peer groups change with age. They start as single-sex groups, evolve to mixed groups, and finally narrow to couples who share activities.

Not all adolescents, however, are heterosexual. For homosexuals, adolescence is a difficult time. Because peer acceptance is crucial to self-acceptance, lesbian and gay adolescents usually conform to the heterosexual codes and behaviors of their peer groups even though these do not feel natural or correct. Conforming may exact a great personal cost. Adolescents who choose to be openly gay or lesbian face not only the ostracism of their peers but also the misunderstanding and hostility of parents, teachers, and other important adults.

Cognitive Development

Cognitive abilities mature during adolescence. Between the ages of 11 and 15, the adolescent begins Piaget's formal operations stage of cognitive development. The main feature of this stage is that people can think beyond the present and beyond the world of reality. Adolescents are highly imaginative and idealistic. They consider things that do not exist but that might be and

Figure 21-12 ■ Adolescent peer group relationships enhance a sense of belonging, self-esteem, and self-identity.

consider ways things could be or ought to be. This type of thinking requires logic, organization, and consistency. In social interactions, adolescents often practice this increasing ability to think abstractly, and parents may misunderstand their child's intent, seeing the teen as arguing or being contrary, which can lead to unnecessary confusion and conflict.

The adolescent becomes more informed about the world and environment. Adolescents use new information to solve everyday problems and can communicate with adults on most subjects. The adolescent's capacity to absorb and use knowledge is great. Adolescents usually select their own areas for learning; they explore interests from which they may evolve a career plan. Study habits and learning skills developed in adolescence are used throughout life.

Moral Development

According to Kohlberg, the young adolescent is usually at the conventional level of moral development. Most still accept the Golden Rule and want to abide by social order and existing laws. Adolescents examine their values, standards, and morals. They may discard the values they have adopted from parents in favor of values they consider more suitable.

When adolescents move into the postconventional or principled level, they start to question the rules and laws of society. Right thinking and right action become a matter of personal values and opinions, which may conflict with societal laws. Adolescents consider the possibility of rationally changing the law and emphasize individual rights. Not all adolescents or even adults proceed to this postconventional level. See the discussion about Kohlberg's stages of moral development in Chapter 20. ∞

Spiritual Development

According to Fowler, the adolescent or young adult reaches the synthetic-conventional stage of spiritual development. As adolescents encounter different groups in society, they are exposed to a wide variety of opinions, beliefs, and behaviors regarding religious matters. The adolescent may reconcile the differences in one of the following ways:

- Deciding any differences are wrong
- Compartmentalizing the differences (For example, a friend may not be able to go to dances on Friday evenings because of religious observances, but the friend can share activities on other days.)
- Obtaining advice from a significant other, such as a parent or a minister

Often the adolescent believes that various religious beliefs and practices have more similarities than differences. At this stage, the adolescent's focus is on interpersonal rather than conceptual matters.

Nursing activities relative to this stage of spiritual development include

- Presenting an open, accepting attitude to adolescents' questions and statements regarding spiritual matters and their implications for health.
- Arranging for adolescents to see a member of their religious faith if so desired, or to talk with members of their church peer group for support.
- Providing a comfortable environment in which adolescents can practice the rituals of their faith.

Health Risks

Adolescents face many health risks as they negotiate the intricate process of becoming young adults. Principal among these are consequences of risky behavior, such as injury related to accidents, sexually transmitted disease, and teen pregnancy. Psychologic and emotional challenges of adolescence may lead to psychologic problems. Also, the developing brain is susceptible to addiction; and the first manifestation of schizophrenia may appear in late adolescence (Toga, Thompson, & Sowell, 2006). In late adolescence, with communal living, as in college dormitories, adolescents are at increased risk for infectious diseases such as measles and pneumococcal meningitis.

The 2003 Youth Risk Behavior Surveillance reported the following health-risk behaviors for youth and young adults (Grun-

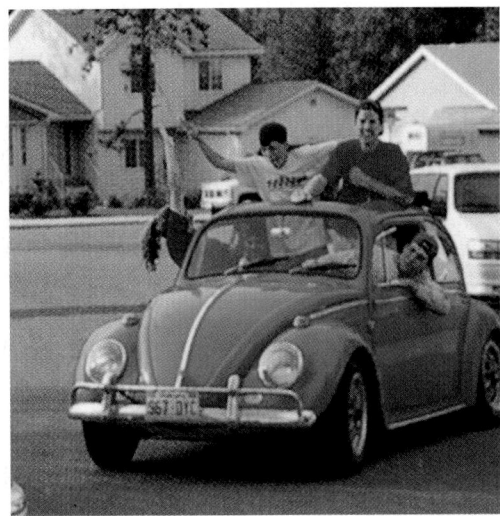

Figure 21-13 ■ To prevent motor vehicle crashes, insist on driver's education classes and enforce rules about safe driving.

baum et al., 2004): 70.8% of all deaths in the 10 to 24 age group resulted from four causes:

- Motor vehicle crashes (see Figure 21-13 ■)
- Other unintentional injuries (e.g., falls, drowning, poisoning)
- Homicides
- Suicide

During the month prior to the survey, high school students engaged in the following risk behaviors:

- 18.2% never wore a seat belt
- 30% had ridden with a driver who had been drinking alcohol
- 17% had carried a weapon
- 44.9% had drunk alcohol
- 22.4% had used marijuana
- 8.5% had attempted suicide at sometime in the previous 12 months

Suicide in adolescents has declined in recent years, but continues to be a significant problem. Older adolescents, males, and

---

DEVELOPMENTAL ASSESSMENT GUIDELINES   **The Adolescent**

In these three developmental areas, does the adolescent do the following?

PHYSICAL DEVELOPMENT

- Exhibit physical growth (weight, height) within normal range for age and sex.
- Demonstrate male or female sexual development consistent with standards.
- Manifest vital signs within normal range for age and sex.
- Exhibit vision and hearing abilities within normal range.

PSYCHOSOCIAL DEVELOPMENT

- Interact well with parents, teachers, peers, siblings, and persons in authority.

- Like self.
- Think and plan for the future, such as college or a career.
- Choose a lifestyle and interests that fit own identity.
- Determine own beliefs and values.
- Begin to establish a sense of identity in the family.
- Seek help from appropriate persons about problems.

DEVELOPMENT IN ACTIVITIES OF DAILY LIVING

- Demonstrate knowledge of physical development, menstruation, reproduction, and birth control.
- Exhibit healthy lifestyle practices in nutrition, exercise, recreation, sleep patterns, and personal habits.
- Demonstrate concern for personal cleanliness and appearance.

non-Hispanic American Indians and Alaskan Natives have the highest rates of suicides among adolescents (National Adolescent Health Information Center, 2004). Suicide in adolescents may be reported as an accidental death. Motor vehicle accidents, drug and alcohol overdoses, firearm accidents, and even homicides can be disguised suicides. Psychologic, social, and physiologic stressors are apparent causes for the rising number of suicides; recent research indicates that use of antidepressant drugs in children is associated with a slight increase of suicide risk (Hammad, Laughren, & Racoosin, 2006). Other adolescent health problems are cardiovascular disease, depression, tooth decay, gingivitis, malalignment of teeth, neglect, and abuse.

Eating Disorders

The highest nutrient and energy demands occur during the growth spurt in adolescence. The addition of sports and other physical activities increases these demands. However, the desire to "fit in" often leads to unhealthy dietary practices (Edelman &

Mandle, 2006, p. 508). As discussed in Chapter 47, ∞ common problems related to nutrition and self-esteem among adolescents include obesity, anorexia nervosa, and bulimia. Nurses need to help adolescents create a wellness plan that addresses body image, diet, weight concerns, and exercise.

Health Assessment and Promotion

Guidelines for growth and development of the adolescent are shown in the Developmental Assessment Guidelines.

Adolescents are usually self-directed in meeting their health needs. Because of maturation changes, however, they need teaching and guidance in a number of health care areas.

Promoting health and wellness includes screening for tobacco, alcohol, and drug use; screening for sexual practices; checking blood pressure, height, and weight; and ensuring that immunizations are current. For a summary of health promotion, see Box 21–8.

BOX 21–8   Health Promotion Guidelines for Adolescents

HEALTH EXAMINATIONS
- As recommended by the primary care provider

PROTECTIVE MEASURES
- Immunizations as recommended, such as adult tetanus-diphtheria vaccine, MMR, pneumococcal, and hepatitis B vaccine
- Screening for tuberculosis
- Periodic vision and hearing screenings
- Regular dental assessments
- Obtaining and providing accurate information about sexual issues

ADOLESCENT SAFETY
- Adolescent's taking responsibility for using motor vehicles safely (e.g., completing a driver's education course, wearing seat belt and helmet)
- Making certain that proper precautions are taken during all athletic activities (e.g., medical supervision, proper equipment)
- Parents' keeping lines of communication open and being alert to signs of substance abuse and emotional disturbances in the adolescent

NUTRITION AND EXERCISE
- Importance of healthy snacks and appropriate patterns of food intake and exercise
- Factors that may lead to nutritional problems (e.g., obesity, anorexia nervosa, bulimia)
- Balancing sedentary activities with regular exercise

SOCIAL INTERACTIONS
- Encouraging and facilitating adolescent success in school
- Encouraging adolescent to establish relationships that promote discussion of feelings, concerns, and fears
- Parents' encouraging adolescent peer group activities that promote appropriate moral and spiritual values
- Parents' acting as role models for appropriate social interactions
- Parents' providing a comfortable home environment for appropriate adolescent peer group activities
- Parents' expecting adolescents to participate in and contribute to family activities

---

CRITICAL THINKING CHECKPOINT

Sean Malloy, 3 years old, is admitted to the emergency department with a fractured humerus and dislocated shoulder. He is accompanied by his mother. As you assess Sean you notice he is very quiet, crying almost silently. He cringes when you approach but does not protest when you touch him. He has multiple bruises, in various stages of healing, on his torso and buttocks. His mother says he "fell out of his bunk bed" and he is "always getting into trouble."

1. According to Erikson, Sean is at what stage of development?
2. What behavior does Sean exhibit that causes you most concern? What behavior would you expect of a 3-year-old child?
3. Knowing that accidents are a major cause of morbidity and mortality in toddlers, what information do you have that makes you suspect Sean's injuries are not accidental?
4. Nurses are mandated reporters for suspected child abuse. Given this scenario, how you would approach Sean's mother?

See Critical Thinking Possibilities in Appendix A.

CHAPTER 21 **REVIEW**

CHAPTER HIGHLIGHTS

- Prenatal or intrauterine development lasts about 9 calendar months.
- The embryonic phase is the 8-week period during which the fertilized ovum develops into an organism with most of the features of the human.
- The infant's weight, length, head and chest circumferences, fontanel size and status, vision, hearing, smell and taste, touch, reflexes, and motor development are important indicators to the newborn's growth and health.
- Infants from birth to 12 months reveal marked growth in size and stature with appropriate nutrition and care: Birth weight doubles by about 5 months and triples by 12 months.
- During infancy, motor development is notable: At 1 month infants can lift their heads momentarily when prone, at 6 months they can sit unsupported, and at 12 months they can walk with help.
- Fulfillment of the infant's physiologic and psychologic needs is required to develop a basic sense of trust. Parents can enhance this sense of trust by responding consistently to an infant's needs, providing a predictable environment in which routines are established, and being sensitive to the infant's needs and meeting those needs skillfully and promptly.
- Cognitive development, for the infant, is a result of interaction between an individual and the environment. The infant needs a variety of sensory and motor stimuli.
- The toddler group, ages 12 months to 3 years, is, according to Erikson, developing a sense of autonomy. Voluntary control increases and they learn to walk and speak. They also learn to control their bladders and bowels, and they acquire all kinds of information about their environment.
- During the preschool years, ages 4 to 5, physical growth slows, but control of the body and coordination increase greatly. The preschooler's world gets larger as they meet relatives, friends, and neighbors. They are engaged in Erikson's task of initiative versus guilt and shame.

- The school-age period starts when children are about 6 years of age, when deciduous teeth are shed. In general, this period from 6 to 12 years is one of significant change. Skills learned during this stage are particularly important in relation to work later in life and willingness to try new tasks.
- During psychosocial development, school-age children face Erikson's conflict of industry versus inferiority.
- School-age children begin to understand relationships and change from being egocentric to having cooperative interactions; according to Piaget, they are in the concrete operations phase of cognitive development.
- Most school-age children progress to the conventional level of moral development and to the mythic-literal stage of spiritual development.
- Rapid growth in height, development of secondary sexual characteristics, sexual maturity, and increasing independence from the family are major landmarks of adolescence.
- Peer groups assume great importance during adolescence; they provide a sense of belonging, pride, social learning, and sexual roles.
- Adolescents are at Fowler's synthetic-conventional stage of spiritual development.
- Adolescents between the ages of 11 and 15 begin the formal operations stage of cognitive development; they are able to think logically, rationally, and futuristically and can conceptualize things as they could be rather than as they are.
- The adolescent is at Kohlberg's conventional level of moral development, and some proceed to the postconventional or principled level.
- The four leading causes of adolescent death are motor vehicle crashes, homicide, suicide, and other unintentional injuries.

TEST YOUR KNOWLEDGE

1. The parent of an 8-month-old girl who has been admitted to the hospital with pneumonia is worried about the infant having sudden death syndrome (SIDS). The parent stated that "My sister's baby died at the age of 2 months and all he had was a little cold." The nurse's best response includes which of the following?
   1. "You don't need to worry. Your daughter is too old for SIDS."
   2. "Girls are less likely to have SIDS than boys are."
   3. "We don't know what causes SIDS, so I would try not to worry about it."
   4. "You must be very anxious; let's talk about SIDS and what you are thinking."

2. Four-year-old Angie whose grandmother recently died, tells the nurse, "My grandma has wings just like angels. She flew to heaven yesterday and tomorrow she'll be back." The nurse's best response includes which of the following?
   1. "She's not coming back, honey."
   2. "It is normal for a little one to make believe."
   3. "You must miss your grandma a lot."
   4. "When people get old they die."

3. Because near-drowning is one of the leading causes of vegetative state in young children, nurses need to teach parents to:

1. Supervise children at all times when near any source of water.
2. Enroll children in swimming classes at an early age to ensure water safety.
3. Make bathroom doors and toilets easily accessible and appropriate for a toddler's size.
4. Allow unsupervised play only in "kiddy pools" designated for young children.

4. Which of the following statements most accurately describes physical development during the school-age years?
   1. Child's weight almost triples.
   2. Child begins shedding deciduous teeth.
   3. Few physical changes occur during middle childhood.
   4. Fat gradually increases, which contributes to child's heavier appearance.

5. Females experience an increase in weight and fat deposition during puberty. Nursing actions most appropriate to this age group include which of the following?
   1. Give reassurance that these changes are normal.
   2. Suggest dietary measures to control weight gain.
   3. Recommend increased exercise to control weight gain.
   4. Encourage low-fat diet to prevent fat deposition.

6. A night shift nurse notices that a postpartum (after delivery of a baby) client is crying and rubbing her baby's head. The mother states, "Look how lopsided my little Sam's head is. It is all my fault. My mom told me that I should have laid down more instead of sitting. Now, Sam's head is all smashed and funny looking." The nurse's best response is:
    1. "Do you mean to tell me that your mother told you that? Are you serious?"
    2. "The head is soft and changed shapes as it moved through the birth canal."
    3. "I will provide you with materials to read that will clear that up for you."
    4. "There is no need to cry. His head will return to normal in a few days."

7. During a physical examination a 24-month-old child clings to the parent and cries every time the nurse attempts to touch her. From knowledge of psychosocial development, the nurse knows that this:
    1. Is normal toddler development
    2. Child needs further psychological evaluation
    3. Child is manipulative and should be taken from the parent to be examined
    4. Is normal behavior for a 12-month-old, but this child is too old for this action and is showing signs of regression

8. After falling off playground equipment, a 5-year-old is brought to the emergency department with a broken arm. The parents ask for ways to keep her occupied while wearing the cast. The nurse should tell them which of the following?
    1. "You will need to talk to the primary care provider about this."
    2. "Let her watch television or do puzzles and other quiet games."
    3. "Activities that do not involve the use of the arm or risk damage to the cast are okay."
    4. "She can ride a bike, jump rope, or play with friends if you watch her closely."

9. According to Piaget's theory of cognitive development, the movement from intuitive reasoning to logical reasoning in school-age children is called the concrete operations phase. Which of the following is an example of this phase?
    1. A science-fair project comparing how fast different objects fall from a set height
    2. Feeling responsible for wishing that a sibling would go away, and now that sibling is ill and hospitalized
    3. Understanding how geometric figures might fit into a futuristic and idealistic world
    4. Learning to ride a bike

10. Parents ask the nurse how they will know that their daughter has reached puberty. The best response includes which of the following?
    1. "The first noticeable sign of puberty in females is appearance of the breast bud."
    2. "The growth spurt usually begins between ages 10 and 14."
    3. "The apocrine glands, found over most of the body, begin to produce sweat."
    4. "The adolescent will display significant mood swings."

See Answers to Test Your Knowledge in Appendix A.

EXPLORE MEDIALINK www.prenhall.com/berman

DVD-ROM
- Audio Glossary
- NCLEX Review
- Animations:
    Oogenesis
    Cell Division
    Conception
    Embryonic Heart Formation and Circulation
    Formation of Placenta
    Sperm Production
    Adolescent Ear
- Videos:
    Identifying Child Abuse
    Drowning
    SIDS

COMPANION WEBSITE
- Additional NCLEX Review
- Case Study: Motor and Social Development in Infancy
- Care Plan Activity: Teen with Lymphocytic Leukemia
- Application Activities:
    Safety Tips for Children
    Playground Bullies
- Links to Resources

READINGS AND REFERENCES

SUGGESTED READINGS
Society for Adolescent Medicine. (2003). *Health guide for America's teens.* Germantown, WI: Securitec Publications.
Written for teenagers, this pamphlet emphasizes health promotion and discusses a wide range of topics, including development, self-care, psychosocial (e.g., relationships, suicide), and physical issues and changes. Adolescents are encouraged to consult their primary care provider with additional questions; several resources are listed.

Stewart, S. H., Conrod, P. J., Marlatt, G. A., Comeau, M. N., Thush, C., & Krank, M. (2005). New developments in prevention and early intervention for alcohol abuse in youths. *Alcoholism, Clinical and Experimental Research, 29* (2), 278–286.
A symposium held at the 2004 Annual Meeting of the Research Society on Alcoholism in Vancouver, British Columbia, Canada, is summarized. Participants presented new developments in alcohol intervention with adolescents that focus on addressing factors that motivate teens to drink and misuse alcohol. Techniques for approaching teenagers are outlined, including traditional cognitive behavioral approaches combined with "expectancy challenge and motivational interviewing."

RELATED RESEARCH

Berger, L. M. (2005). Income, family characteristics, and physical violence toward children. *Child Abuse and Neglect, 29* (2), 107–133.

Jones, R. K., Purcell, A., Singh, S., & Finer, L. B. (2005). Adolescents' reports of parental knowledge of adolescents' use of sexual health services and their reactions to mandated parental notification for prescription contraception. *Journal of the American Medical Association, 293*(3), 340–348.

Malloy, M. H., & Freeman, D. H. (2004). Age at death, season, and day of death as indicators of the effect of the back to sleep program on sudden infant death syndrome in the United States, 1992–1999. *Archives of Pediatric and Adolescent Medicine, 158*(4), 359–365.

REFERENCES

Albrecht, S. A., Maloni, J. A., Thomas, K. K., Jones, R., Halleran, J., & Osborne, J. (2004). Smoking cessation counseling for pregnant women who smoke: Scientific basis for practice for AWHONN's SUCCESS project. *Journal of Obstetric, Gynecologic & Neonatal Nursing, 33*(3), 298–305.

Anderson, M. E., Johnson, D.C., & Batal, H. A. (2005). Sudden infant death syndrome and prenatal maternal smoking: Rising attributed risk in the back to sleep era. *BMC Medicine, 3*(1), 4.

Centers for Disease Control. (2000). *2000 growth charts: United States.* Retrieved April 26, 2006, from http://www.cdc.gov/growthcharts

Edelman, C. L., & Mandle, C. L. (2006). Health promotion throughout the life span (6th ed.). St. Louis, MO: Mosby.

Erikson, E. H. (1963). *Childhood and society* (2nd ed.). New York: Norton.

Fowler, J. W. (1981). *Stages of faith: The psychology of human development and the quest for meaning.* New York: Harper & Row.

Geddes, J. F. (2004). The evidence base for shaken baby syndrome. *BMJ, 328,* 719–720.

Grunbaum, J. A., Kann, L., Kinchen, S. A., Ross, J., Hawkins, J., Lowry, R., et al. (2004). Youth risk behavior surveillance—United States, 2003.

Morbidity and Mortality Weekly Report, 53(SS-2), 1–96.

Hammad, T. A., Laughren, T., & Racoosin, J. (2006). Suicidality in pediatric patients treated with antidepressant drugs. *Archives of General Psychiatry, 63*(3), 246–248.

Karp, H. (2003). *The happiest baby on the block.* New York: Bantam Books.

Kvigne, V. L., Leonardson, G. R., Neff-Smith, M., Brock, E., Borzelleca, J., & Welty, T. K. (2004). Characteristics of children who have full or incomplete fetal alcohol syndrome. *Journal of Pediatrics, 145*(5), 635–640.

Murray, R. B., & Zentner, J. P. (2001). *Health promotion strategies through the life span* (7th ed.). Upper Saddle River, NJ: Prentice Hall.

National Adolescent Health Information Center. (2004). Fact sheet on suicide: Adolescents & young adults. San Francisco: Author, University of California, San Francisco.

Piaget, J. (1966). *Origins of intelligence in children.* New York: Norton.

Pillitteri, A. (2003). *Maternal & child health nursing: Care of the childbearing & childrearing family* (4th ed.). Philadelphia: Lippincott Williams & Wilkins.

Schmitt, B. D. (2004). *Pediatric telephone protocols: Office version* (10th ed.). Elk Grove Village, IL: American Academy of Pediatrics.

Starr, N. B. (2004). Self-perception. In C. E. Burns et al., *Pediatric primary care: A handbook for nurse practitioners.* Philadelphia: W. B. Saunders.

Strock, G. A., Cottrell, E. R., Abang, A. E., Buschbacher, R. M., & Hannon, T. S. (2005). Childhood obesity: A simple equation with complex variables. *Journal of Long Term Effects of Medical Implants, 15*(1), 15–32.

Toga, A. W., Thompson, P. M., & Sowell, E. R. (2006). Mapping brain maturation. *Trends in Neurosciences, 29(3),* 148–159.

U.S. Department of Health and Human Services. (2000). *Healthy people 2010: Objectives for improving health. Part B: Focus area 16. Maternal, infant, and child health. Understanding and improving health* (2nd ed.) [Electronic version]. Washington, DC: Author. Retrieved March 14, 2005, from

http://www.healthypeople.gov/document/html/volume2/16mich.htm

Venes, D. (Ed.). (2005). *Taber's cyclopedic medical dictionary* (20th ed.). Philadelphia: F. A. Davis.

Ventura, J. J., Abrna, J. C., Mosher, W. D., Hanshaw, S. (2004). Estimated Pregnancy rates for the United States, 1990–2000: An update. *National Vital Statistics Report, 52*(23), 1–10. Center's for Disease Control. USDHHS.

Wolfe, E. L., Davis, T., Guydish, J., & Delucchi, K. L. (2005). Mortality risk associated with perinatal drug and alcohol use in California. *Journal of Perinatology, 25*(2), 93–100.

WHO Multicentre Growth Reference Study Group. (2006). WHO Child Growth Standards based on length/height, weight and age. *Acta Pædiatrica,* Suppl. 450, 76–85.

SELECTED BIBLIOGRAPHY

Burns, C. E., Dunn, A. M., Brady, M. A., Starr, N. B., & Blosser, C. G. (2004). *Pediatric primary care: A handbook for nurse practitioners* (3rd ed.). Philadelphia: W. B. Saunders.

Doswell, W. M., Portis, S., Jemison, T., Kaufmann, J., Braxter, B., & Green, L. (2004). The NIA Group. Building a sense of purpose in preadolescent African American girls: A novel approach to nursing leadership in community health. *Nursing Leadership Forum, 8*(3), 95–100.

Dubowitz, L. M. S., & Dubowitz, V. (1977). *Gestational age of the newborn.* Menlo Park, CA: Addison-Wesley.

Edelman, C. L., & Mandle, C. L. (2006). *Health promotion throughout the lifespan* (6th ed.). St. Louis, MO: Mosby.

Elkins, M., & Cavendish, R. (2004). Developing a plan for pediatric spiritual care. *Holistic Nursing Practice, 18*(4), 179–184.

Mattson, S. (2000). Providing culturally competent care strategies and approaches for perinatal clients. *AWHONN Lifelines, 4*(5), 37–39.

McKinney, E. S. (2005). *Maternal-child nursing* (2nd ed.). Philadelphia: W. B. Saunders.

Roberts, K. S. (2003). Providing culturally sensitive care to the childbearing Islamic family: Part II. *Advances in Neonatal Care, 3*(5), 250–255.

Simpson, K. R., & Creehan, P. A. (2001). *AWHONN'S perinatal nursing* (2nd ed.). Philadelphia: Lippincott.

CHAPTER 22

Promoting Health in Young and Middle-Aged Adults

LEARNING OUTCOMES

After completing this chapter, you will be able to:

1. Compare and contrast the following generational groups: Baby boomers, Generation X and Generation Y.

2. Describe the usual physical development occurring during young and middle adulthood.

3. Identify characteristic tasks of development during young and middle adulthood.

4. Explain changes in cognitive development throughout adulthood.

5. Describe moral development according to Kohlberg throughout adulthood.

6. Describe spiritual development according to Fowler throughout adulthood.

7. Identify selected health problems associated with young and middle-aged adults.

8. Identify developmental assessment guidelines for young and middle-aged adults.

9. List examples of health promotion topics for young and middle adulthood.

The adult phase of development encompasses the years from the end of adolescence to death. Because the developmental tasks of young adults differ from those of older adults, adulthood is often divided into three phases: young adulthood, middle adulthood, and late adulthood. In this book, young adults are defined as people 20 to 40 years old, and middle-aged adults as 40 to 65.

It is important to remember that the adult age span includes three very different generations: the **Baby Boomers** (born in years 1945–1964), **Generation X** (birth years 1965–1978), and **Generation Y** or the Millennials (birth years 1979–2000). Each cohort has shared specific life events and has its own world view, making them quite diverse in some ways. At this point, it is unclear if these generational differences will prompt new developmental theories, or if the differences are in "generational personalities" and values. Baby Boomers are characterized by an individualistic outlook, tend toward a "workaholic" orientation, want to be respected at work, but feel role overload (Hill, 2004; Hu, Herrick, & Hodgin, 2004; Sanots & Cox, 2000). Generation Xers were frequently raised in two-worker households where long hours at work were common. They may now be less impressed with corporate values, are more skeptical, resist authority, but enjoy challenges and opportunities to creatively problem solve. Finally, Generation Y (or Millennials) have come of age in an increasingly multicultural America, are technologically sophisticated (and dependent), and enjoy public affirmation of their efforts.

This chapter applies the concepts of growth and development introduced in Chapter 21 to the young adult and middle-aged adult. Each developmental stage includes physical, psychosocial, cognitive, moral, and spiritual aspects. Also included are health problems and health assessment and promotion guidelines.

YOUNG ADULTS (20 TO 40 YEARS)

The age at which a person is considered an adult depends on how adulthood is described in the social context of the individual, and this defining age is changing. Legally, a person in the United States can vote at 18 years. The legal age for alcohol consumption outside the home varies among states from 18 to 21 years. Another criterion of adulthood is financial independence, which is also highly variable. Some adolescents support themselves as early as 16 years of age, usually because of family circumstances. By contrast, some adults are financially dependent on their families for many years, for example, during prolonged periods of education.

Adulthood may also be indicated by moving away from home and establishing one's own living arrangements. Yet this independence also varies greatly. Some adolescents leave home because of family problems. In recent years, however, "**Boomerang Kids**" have evolved, as young adults have moved back into their parents' homes after an initial period of independent living. In

---

RESEARCH NOTE · **What Workforce Differences Exist Between Nursing Staff of Different Generations?**

Difficulties in understanding differences in work habits and communication styles of those in another age group are now common in the workplace. This descriptive research study examined the generational profiles of two groups (the Silent Generation (born in years 1925–1942) and Baby Boomers versus Generation X and Generation Y) regarding communication styles and significance of tasks to help nurse managers maximize their department's effectiveness.

One of the authors developed a survey tool to examine the generational profiles of staff members of two departments (medical-surgical and critical care) and the communication styles of the participants. The survey consisted of 22 questions asking about the characteristics of the respondent's generation, the significance of tasks, and their communication styles.

There were no statistically significant differences between the generational groups in the area of communication styles and significance of tasks. Other findings were consistent with generational profiles revealed in other studies. For example:

- The Silent Generation and Baby Boomer group identified themselves as principled, idealistic, experts, caring, savvy, and diverse. However, they viewed computers as frightening and complicated.
- Generations X and Y perceived themselves as idealistic. They wanted freedom and flexibility plus immediate feedback in terms of job completion and performance.

IMPLICATIONS

Nurse managers need to understand each generation's different values and expectations. Knowing this information will help the nurse manager to facilitate a positive work environment. It can also mean that different orientations, training, opportunities for advancement, benefits, and perks may need to be implemented.

Note: From J. Hu, C. Herrick, and K. A. Hodgin, "Managing the Multigenerational Nursing Team," *Health Care Manager*, 23(4), pp. 334–341. Copyright © 2004 Lippincott, Williams & Wilkins. Reprinted with permission.

2003, 13% of young men (ages 24–34 years) and 7% of young women were living with one or both of their parents (Fields, 2004). The factors contributing to this trend include high housing costs, high divorce rates, high unemployment rates, and the problems resulting from substance abuse and maladaptive behaviors. Some young people who are employed full-time receive only minimum wage and are unable to earn enough money to be self-supporting.

Young adults are typically busy people who face many challenges. They are expected to assume new roles at work, in the home, and in the community, and to develop interests, values, and attitudes related to these roles.

Physical Development

People in their early 20s are in their prime physical years. The human body is at its most efficient functioning at about age 25 years. The musculoskeletal system is well developed and coordinated. This is the period when athletic endeavors reach their peak. All other systems of the body (e.g., cardiovascular, visual, auditory, and reproductive) are also functioning at peak efficiency. Emerging adults, however, tend to be high-risk takers (Nelson & Barry, 2005), placing their high-functioning bodies at substantial risk of serious injury.

Although physical changes are minimal during this stage, weight and muscle mass may change as a result of diet and exercise. Health outcomes in older adulthood may have their genesis in younger adult behaviors (Hartman-Stein & Potkanowicz, 2003). In addition, extensive physical and psychosocial changes occur in pregnant and lactating women. These changes are discussed in maternal/child textbooks.

Psychosocial Development

In contrast to the minimal physical changes, psychosocial development of the young adult is great. Box 22–1 reviews this psychosocial development according to the theories of Freud, Erikson, and Havighurst. The basic developmental task is establishing **intimacy** or very close friendship. Establishing a firm sense of self, and then reaching to others to develop loving, intimate relationships is key. Choice of a lifelong partner and considerations of childbearing depend upon successful negotiation of intimacy.

Young adults face a number of new experiences and changes in lifestyle as they progress toward maturity. They make choices about education and employment, about whether to marry or remain single, about starting a home, and about rearing children. Social responsibilities include forming new friendships and assuming some community activities.

Many young adults have experienced the stressors of divorce of their parents, and being raised in blended families or stepfamilies. As children of divorce, feelings of being "caught" between two divorced parents may be heavy burdens as they move into young adulthood (Afifi, 2003). Common problems among young adults raised in blended families include concerns about adequate financial resources, difficulty deciding how much personal information to share with others, and worries about loy-

---

> **BOX 22–1** **Psychosocial Development: Young Adult**
>
> The young adult
> - Is in the genital stage in which energy is directed toward attaining a mature sexual relationship, according to Freud's theory.
> - Is in the intimacy versus isolation phase of Erikson's stages of development.
> - Has the following developmental tasks, according to Havighurst:
>   - Selecting a mate
>   - Learning to live with a partner
>   - Starting a family
>   - Rearing children
>   - Managing a home
>   - Getting started in an occupation
>   - Taking on civic responsibility
>   - Finding a congenial social group
> - Has the following characteristics, according to Nelson and Barry (2005):
>   - Separation from parents
>   - Exploration of new identities for self
>   - Personal discovery and self-discovery
>   - High-risk behavior

---

alty and disloyalty to others (Afifi, 2003). These added concerns have obvious implications for the development of intimate relationships in young adults.

Occupational choice and education are largely inseparable. Education influences occupational opportunities; conversely, an occupation, once chosen, can determine the education needed and sought. Education enhances employment opportunities and usually ensures economic survival. As the role of women has changed, many women now choose to assume active careers and civic roles in society in addition to their roles as mother and/or wife. Some women work out of necessity, rather than choice (Figure 22-1 ■).

Remaining single is becoming the lifestyle of more and more young adults. Many people choose to remain single, perhaps to pursue an education and then to have the freedom to pursue their chosen vocation. Some unmarried individuals choose to live with another person of the opposite or same sex and share living arrangements and certain expenses. Some people who are gay or lesbian commit themselves legally to a partner as in marriage, and do not consider themselves to be "single."

Although nontraditional lifestyles are becoming more acceptable in society, attitudes toward these various lifestyles can contribute social pressures that lead to stress responses. The multiple roles of adulthood (citizen, worker, taxpayer, homeowner, wife/husband, daughter/son, brother/sister, parent, friend, and so on) may also create stress as a result of role conflict.

Cognitive Development

Young adults are able to use formal operations, characterized by the ability to think abstractly and employ logic. For example, young adults are able to generate hypotheses about what will happen, given a set of circumstances, and do not have to engage

Figure 22-1 ■ Many young women combine active careers with motherhood.

in trial-and-error behavior. Most adults identify strongly with the values and norms of their social group and will act in ways that are consistent with those norms (Pfaffenberger, 2005).

Recently, researchers in the field of psychology have suggested that Piaget's formal operational stage is not the last stage of human development. Some have proposed a concept of post-formal thought. *Postformal thought* includes creativity, intuition, and the ability to consider information in relationship to other ideas (Murray & Zentner, 2001). Postformal thinkers possess an understanding of the temporary or relative nature of knowledge. They are able to comprehend and balance arguments created by both logic and emotion. Few adults reach these stage (only about 10%), but these adults are marked by greater tolerance and the skills of noticing and resolving complex problems (Pfaffenberger, 2005). Meditation and other insight-oriented practices facilitate becoming a postformal thinker.

Moral Development

Young adults who have mastered the previous stages of Kohlberg's theory of moral development enter the postconventional level. At this time, the person is able to separate self from the expectations and rules of others and to define morality in terms of personal principles. When individuals perceive a conflict with society's rules or laws, they judge according to their own principles. For example, a person may intentionally break the law and join a protest group to stop hunters from killing wild animals, believing that the principle of wildlife conservation justifies the protest action. This type of reasoning is called *principled reasoning.* See also Gilligan's ethic of care in Chapter 21. ∞ Gilligan argues that as individuals approach young adulthood, men and women tend to define moral problems somewhat differently. Men often use an "ethic of justice" and define moral problems in terms of rules and rights. Women, by contrast, often define moral problems in terms of obligation to care and to avoid hurt.

Spiritual Development

According to Fowler, the individual enters the individuating-reflective period sometime after 18 years of age. During this period, the individual focuses on reality. A 27-year-old adult may ask philosophical questions regarding spirituality and may be self-conscious about spiritual matters. The religious teaching that the young adult had as a child may now be accepted or redefined. Cavendish, Luise, Bauer, et al. (2001) demonstrated that young adults may depend on spirituality and seek guidance from a Higher Power, but do so privately.

Health Risks

Young adulthood is generally a healthy time of life. Health risks that do occur and are common in this age group include injuries, suicide, substance abuse, hypertension, sexually transmitted infection (STI), abuse of women, and certain malignancies. Some of the problems such as injuries, substance abuse, and STIs are related to behaviors that could possibly be prevented through appropriate education and other primary prevention strategies.

Injuries

Healthy People 2010 (U.S. Department of Health and Human Services [USDHHS], 2000) reports that leading causes of death differ among the various population groups. For example, unintentional injuries (primarily motor vehicle crashes) are the fifth leading cause of death for the total population but the leading cause of death for people 1 to 44 years of age. Education about safety precautions and injury prevention is a major role of the nurse in promoting the health of young adults. For a further discussion of safety education for young adults, see Chapter 30. ∞

Suicide

Suicide is the third leading cause of death among adolescents and the leading cause of death among young adults in the United States (Edelman & Mandle, 2006, pp. 515, 540). Many suicides may actually be mistaken for accidental death (motor vehicle crashes, combining alcohol and barbiturates, or discharging a gun while cleaning it). Suicide may result from problems with close relationships such as those with marriage partners or parents, or from depression related to perceived occupational, academic, or financial failure. In general, suicide results from the young adult's inability to cope with the pressures, responsibilities, and expectations of adulthood.

The nurse's role in the prevention of suicide includes identifying behaviors that may indicate potential problems: depression; a variety of physical complaints, including weight loss, sleep disturbances, and digestive disorders; and decreased interest in social and work roles along with an increase in isolation. A young adult identified as at risk for suicide should be referred to a mental health specialist or a crisis center. A suicide threat should never be ignored. Nurses can also reduce the incidence of suicide by participating in educational programs that provide information about the early signs of suicide.

Hypertension

Hypertension is a major problem for young African American adults, particularly men. Many of the causes for this higher incidence of hypertension are unknown. In addition to biologic inheritance, contributing factors may include smoking, obesity, a high-sodium diet, and high stress levels. Hypertension is a major risk factor in the development of chronic heart disease or stroke (cerebrovascular accidents). Blood pressure measurements are usually advised at least every 2 years for young adults to screen for hypertension.

Substance Abuse

Substance abuse is a major threat to the health of young adults. Alcohol, marijuana, amphetamines, and cocaine, for example, can bring about feelings of well-being that may be highly valued by people with adjustment problems. Prolonged use can lead to physical and psychologic dependency and subsequent health problems. Addiction, or physical and psychologic dependence on a substance, is related to properties of the substance, the individual user, and the social network of the individual (Mathre, 2004). For example, drug abuse during pregnancy can lead to fetal damage. Prolonged use of alcohol can lead to such diseases as cirrhosis of the liver and cancer of the esophagus.

Nursing strategies related to drug abuse include teaching about the complications of their use, changing individual attitudes toward drug abuse, and counseling regarding problems that lead to drug abuse. In addition, assessment of the young adult for substance abuse may help the nurse identify a problem early on, and assist the young adult client to access intervention services.

Smoking is another type of drug abuse that can lead to diseases such as lung cancer and cardiovascular disease. The nurse's role regarding smoking is to (a) serve as a role model by not smoking; (b) provide educational information regarding the dangers of smoking; (c) help make smoking socially unacceptable, for example, by posting No Smoking signs in client lounges and offices; and (d) suggest resources such as hypnosis, lifestyle training, and behavior modification to clients who desire to stop smoking. Nurses can also promote health related to tobacco by being aware of marketing efforts that target young adults (Ling & Glantz, 2002). The tobacco industry has developed very effective campaigns to encourage smoking among young adults by advertising and sponsoring entertainment events. Nurses can help young adults recognize and resist these marketing efforts.

Sexually Transmitted Infection

STIs such as genital herpes, AIDS, syphilis, and gonorrhea are common infections in young adults. Chlamydia is the most prevalent STI, and in fact is the most prevalent infectious disease in the United States (Centers for Disease Control and Prevention, 2004). Other STIs, such as gonorrhea, are becoming resistant to multiple antibiotics, and therefore cause an increased risk for future health. Nursing functions are largely educational. The use of condoms greatly reduces the transfer of infectious microorganisms from one partner to another. Knowl-edge about the symptoms of these diseases can help the client obtain early treatment. In dealing with clients with an STI, the nurse must be nonjudgmental and accepting of the client's lifestyle and treat any information obtained as confidential (see Chapter 38). ∞

Eating Disorders

Many young adults also battle with obesity. According to *Healthy People 2010*, 23% of adults age 20 and older are obese (USDHHS, 2000). The nurse needs to assess nutritional concerns, and discuss diet and exercise patterns with the client for the subsequent development of an individualized wellness plan. Other areas of nutritional needs for young women include meeting calcium requirements and proper nutrition during the childbearing years (see Chapter 47 ∞).

Violence

Violence has spread throughout the United States and claims lives or threatens the well-being of all ages of people. The youth are perpetrators and victims of violence. For example, *Healthy People 2010* (USDHHS, 2000) reports that homicide is the second leading cause of death for young persons 15 to 24 years of age and the leading cause of death for African Americans in this age group. The elderly, females, and children continue to be targets of both physical and sexual assaults.

Abuse of Women

The problem of battering or abuse of women affects families at all socioeconomic levels. Stresses that predispose families to abuse may include financial problems, separation from family and community support, and physical as well as social isolation. It is essential that nurses make assessment for domestic violence part of their routine (Landenburger & Campbell, 2003). A nurse who works with women should explicitly ask if they are frightened or hurt by someone they know. The nurse should become familiar with community resources, such as adult protective services, shelters, Partners Anonymous, advocacy programs, victim assistance programs, and hotlines (Landenburger & Campbell, 2003).

Malignancies

Testicular cancer is the most common neoplasm in men aged 20 to 34 (USDHHS, 2004). Monthly testicular self-examination, a means of early identification of malignancy, used to be recommended for all men. More recent recommendations from the American Cancer Society (ACS, 2005) are that men should have a testicular exam as part of a yearly physical exam. Men who have risk factors for testicular cancer should discuss monthly testicular self-examination with their primary care provider. For additional information, see Chapter 40. ∞

Of all cancers among women, cancer of the breast is a leading cause of death. Breast cancer is rare under the age of 25, but the risk increases after the age of 30 (ACS, 2005). Strong evidence exists that yearly mammography for all women over the age of 40 decreases mortality from breast cancer, and should be encouraged (U.S. Preventive Services Task Force, 2003). An annual breast exam performed by a primary care provider is also recommended (ACS, 2005), but breast self-exam is no longer recommended for all women. The American Cancer Society recommends that young women who choose to do breast self-exam have their technique validated by a health care practitioner at a yearly physical exam. For detailed information, see Chapter 38. ∞ The earlier a breast lump is discovered, the greater the effectiveness of treatment.

Young adult women should also be screened for cervical cancer by having a routine **Papanicolaou (Pap) test**. A Pap test is done by obtaining and examining cells from the uterine cervical os. The cells are obtained during a pelvic examination. For more information on the vaginal exam, see Chapter 30. ∞ The nurse should also screen for high-risk factors for cervical cancer: sexual activity at an early age, multiple sexual partners, or a history of syphilis, herpes genitalis, or *Trichomonas vaginitis*. Many young adults are reluctant to have these examinations and screenings. Therefore, it is important for nurses to explain the purpose of the test and to encourage all young women to begin this preventive measure by age 21 (ACS, 2005). See cancer screening guidelines in Chapter 30. ∞

Health Assessment and Promotion

Assessment guidelines for the growth and development of the young adult are shown in the accompanying Developmental Assessment Guidelines.

Young adults are usually interested in meeting their health needs. However, because of the many stresses and changes that occur throughout this 20-year period, the nurse needs to offer teaching and guidance in several health care areas. The nurse may wish to discuss some or all of the health promotion topics outlined in Box 22–2. These topics are discussed in detail in subsequent chapters throughout the book.

MIDDLE-AGED ADULTS (40 TO 65 YEARS)

The middle years, from 40 to 65, have been called the years of stability and consolidation. For most people, it is a time when children have grown and moved away or are moving away from

home. Thus partners generally have more time for and with each other and time to pursue interests they may have deferred for years (see Figure 22-2 ■).

BOX 22–2 Health Promotion Guidelines for Young Adults

HEALTH TESTS AND SCREENINGS
- Routine physical examination (every 1 to 3 years for females; every 5 years for males)
- Immunizations as recommended, such as tetanus-diphtheria boosters every 10 years, meningococcal vaccine if not given in early adolescence (Bilukha & Rosenstein, 2005), and hepatitis B vaccine
- Regular dental assessments (every 6 months)
- Periodic vision and hearing screenings
- Professional breast examination every 1 to 3 years
- Papanicolaou smear annually within 3 years of onset of sexual activity
- Testicular examination every year
- Screening for cardiovascular disease (e.g., cholesterol test every 5 years if results are normal; blood pressure to detect hypertension; baseline electrocardiogram at age 35)
- Tuberculosis skin test every 2 years
- Smoking: history and counseling, if needed

SAFETY
- Motor vehicle safety reinforcement (e.g., using designated drivers when drinking, maintaining brakes and tires)
- Sun protection measures
- Workplace safety measures
- Water safety reinforcement (e.g., no diving in shallow water)

NUTRITION AND EXERCISE
- Importance of adequate iron intake in diet
- Nutritional and exercise factors that may lead to cardiovascular disease (e.g., obesity, cholesterol and fat intake, lack of vigorous exercise)

SOCIAL INTERACTIONS
- Encouraging personal relationships that promote discussion of feelings, concerns, and fears
- Setting short- and long-term goals for work and career choices

---

DEVELOPMENTAL ASSESSMENT GUIDELINES   The Young Adult

In these three developmental areas, does the young adult do the following?

PHYSICAL DEVELOPMENT
- Exhibit weight within normal range for age and sex.
- Manifest vital signs (e.g., blood pressure) within normal range for age and sex.
- Demonstrate visual and hearing abilities within normal range.
- Exhibit appropriate knowledge (e.g., about sexually transmitted infections) and attitudes about sexuality.

PSYCHOSOCIAL DEVELOPMENT
- Feel independent from parents.
- Have a realistic self-concept.

- Like self and direction life is going.
- Interact well with family.
- Cope with the stresses of change and growth.
- Have well-established bonds with significant others, such as marriage partner or close friends.
- Have a meaningful social life.
- Demonstrate emotional, social, and economic responsibility for own life.
- Have a set of values that guide behavior.

DEVELOPMENT IN ACTIVITIES OF DAILY LIVING
- Have a healthy lifestyle.

Figure 22-2 ■ Middle-aged adults have time to pursue interests that may have been put aside for child care.

Maturity is the state of maximal function and integration, or the state of being fully developed. Many other characteristics are generally recognized as representative of maturity. Mature individuals are guided by an underlying philosophy of life. They take many perspectives into account and are tolerant of the views of others. A comprehensive philosophy allows a person to make sense out of life and thus helps that person maintain a sense of purpose and hope in the face of human tragedies. Mature persons are open to new experiences and continued growth; they can tolerate ambiguity, are flexible, and can adapt to change. In addition, mature people have the quality of self-acceptance; they are able to be reflective and insightful about life and to see themselves as others see them. Mature persons also assume responsibility for themselves and expect others to do the same. They confront the tasks of life in a realistic and mature manner, make decisions, and accept responsibility for those decisions.

Physical Development

A number of changes that start when young adults are in their mid-20s become noticeable as the fifth decade approaches. At 40, most adults can function as effectively as they did in their 20s. However, during ages 40 to 65 many physical changes take place. These are summarized in Table 22–1.

Both men and women experience decreasing hormonal production during the middle years. The **menopause** refers to the so-called change of life in women, when menstruation ceases. It is said to have occurred when a woman has not had a menstrual period for 12 months. The menopause usually occurs sometime between ages 40 and 55. The average is about 47 years. At this time, ovarian activity declines until ovulation ceases. Common symptoms, related to a decline in estrogen, are hot flashes, chilliness, a tendency of the breasts to become smaller and less dense, and a decrease in metabolic rate that may lead to weight gain. Insomnia and headaches may also occur. Psychologically, the menopause can be an anxiety-producing time, especially if the ability to bear children is an integral part of the woman's self-concept. For other women, menopause may produce few symptoms, physically or psychologically (Banister, 2000).

Sexual arousal in both men and women takes longer after midlife than in younger adulthood. In men there is no change comparable to the menopause in women, although the term **climacteric** (andropause) has been used to denote the change in sexual response in men. Androgen levels decrease very slowly; however, men can father children even in late life. Some men may have difficulties achieving sexual arousal for psychologic reasons, such as anxiety. See Chapter 40 for further details about sexual health. ∞

Psychosocial Development

Before the mid-1990s, the developmental tasks of middle-aged adults received little attention (Lachman, 2004). Havighurst outlined seven tasks for this age group (see Box 22–3). Erikson

TABLE 22–1	**Physical Changes of the Middle-Aged Adult**
CATEGORY	**DESCRIPTION**
Appearance	Hair begins to thin, and gray hair appears. Skin turgor and moisture decrease, subcutaneous fat decreases, and wrinkling occurs. Fatty tissue is redistributed, resulting in fat deposits in the abdominal area.
Musculoskeletal system	Skeletal muscle bulk decreases at about age 60. Thinning of the intervertebral discs causes a decrease in height of about 1 inch. Calcium loss from bone tissue is more common among postmenopausal women. Muscle growth continues in proportion to use.
Cardiovascular system	Blood vessels lose elasticity and become thicker.
Sensory perception	Visual acuity declines, often by the late 40s, especially for near vision (presbyopia). Auditory acuity for high-frequency sounds also decreases (presbycusis), particularly in men. Taste sensations also diminish.
Metabolism	Metabolism slows, and may result in weight gain.
Gastrointestinal system	Gradual decrease in tone of large intestine may predispose the individual to constipation.
Urinary system	Nephron units are lost during this time, and glomerular filtration rate decreases.
Sexuality	Hormonal changes take place in both men and women.

BOX 22–3 *Psychosocial Development: Middle-Aged Adult*

The middle-aged adult

- Is in the generativity versus stagnation phase of Erikson's stages of development.
- According to Havighurst, has the following developmental tasks:
  - Achieving adult civic and social responsibility
  - Establishing and maintaining an economic standard of living
  - Assisting teenage children to become responsible and happy adults
  - Developing adult leisure-time activities
  - Relating oneself to one's spouse as a person
  - Accepting and adjusting to the physiologic changes of middle age
  - Adjusting to aging parents
  - Balances the needs of multiple constituencies (children, parents, work, etc.).
  - Has work as a central theme.
- According to Slater (2003), has the additional developmental tasks of:
  - Inclusivity versus exclusivity
  - Pride versus embarrassment (in children, work, or creativity)
  - Responsibility versus ambivalence (making choices about commitments)
  - Career productivity versus inadequacy
  - Parenthood versus self-absorption
  - Being needed versus alienation
  - Honesty versus denial (with oneself)

(1963, p. 266) viewed the developmental choice of the middle-aged adult as generativity versus stagnation. **Generativity** is defined as the concern for establishing and guiding the next generation. In other words, the concern about providing for the welfare of humankind is equal to the concern of providing for self. People in their 20s and 30s tend to be self- and family-centered. In middle age, the individual is "linked to the welfare of others" (Lachman, 2004, p. 306). Marriage partners have more time for companionship and recreation, thus marriage may be more satisfying in the middle years of life. Partners have time to work together in volunteer activities, and time for one partner to go out for lunch and for the other to go fishing. Generative middle-aged persons are able to feel a sense of comfort in their lifestyle and receive gratification from charitable endeavors.

Erikson wrote that people who are unable to expand their interests at this time and who do not assume the responsibilities of middle age suffer a sense of boredom and impoverishment, that is, stagnation. These people have difficulty accepting their aging bodies and become withdrawn and isolated. They are preoccupied with self and unable to give to others. Some may regress to younger patterns of behavior, for example, adolescent behavior.

The middle-aged person looks older and may also feel older (Banister, 2000). People usually accept the fact that they are aging; however, some try to defy the years by changing their dress and even their actions. A new freedom to be independent and follow one's individual interests arises. Prior to this period, the marriage partner or lover and other persons were crucial to a definition of self. Now the middle-aged person does not make comparisons with others, often no longer fears aging or death, relaxes the sense of competitiveness, and enjoys the independence and freedom of middle age. Other people's opinions become less important, and the earlier habit of trying to please everyone is overcome. The person establishes ethical and moral standards that are independent of the standards of others. The focus shifts from inner self and being to others and doing. Religious and philosophical concerns become important.

The "midlife crisis" is a popular idea, and one that is the source of many jokes and humorous anecdotes. This crisis occurs when individuals recognize that they have reached the halfway mark of life. The universality of midlife crisis is disputed by some who suggest that some midlifers may experience a crisis that promotes further development, while some may have consistently functioned in a crisis mode from early life (Lachman, 2004). Midlifers begin to recognize that time is at a premium and that life is finite. Youthfulness and physical strength can no longer be taken for granted.

Cognitive Development

The middle-aged adult's cognitive and intellectual abilities change very little. Cognitive processes include reaction time, memory, perception, learning, problem solving, and creativity. Reaction time during the middle years stays much the same or diminishes during the later part of the middle years. Memory and problem solving are maintained through middle adulthood. Learning continues and can be enhanced by increased motivation at this time in life.

Genetic, environmental, and personality factors in early and middle adulthood account for the large difference in the ways in which individuals maintain mental abilities (Edelman & Mandle, 2006, p. 557). The experiences of the professional, social, and personal life of middle-aged persons will be reflected in their cognitive performance. Thus, approaches to problem solving and task completion will vary considerably in a middle-aged group.

Moral Development

According to Kohlberg, the adult can move beyond the conventional level to the postconventional level (see Chapter 21 ∞). Kohlberg believed that extensive experience of personal moral choice and responsibility is required before people can reach the postconventional level. Kohlberg found that few of his subjects achieved the highest level of moral reasoning. To move from stage 4, a law and order orientation, to stage 5, a social contract orientation, requires that the individual move to a stage in which rights of others take precedence. Recent research demonstrates that moral development continues through adulthood, and that few individuals attain stage 5 before age 40 (Dawson, 2002).

Spiritual Development

Not all adults progress through Fowler's stages to the fifth, called the paradoxical-consolidative stage. At this stage, the individual can view "truth" from a number of viewpoints.

MediaLink Developmental Phases of Adulthood Case Study

Fowler's fifth stage corresponds to Kohlberg's fifth stage of moral development. Fowler believes that only some individuals after the age of 30 years reach this stage.

In middle age, people tend to be less dogmatic about religious beliefs, and religion often offers more comfort to the middle-aged person than it did previously. People in this age group often rely on spiritual beliefs to help them deal with illness, death, and tragedy.

Health Problems

Many middle-aged adults remain healthy; however, the risk of developing a health problem is greater than that of the young adult. Leading causes of death in this age group include motor vehicle and occupational injuries, chronic disease such as cancer, and cardiovascular disease. Lifestyle patterns in combination with aging, family history, and developmental stressors (e.g., menopause, climacteric) and situational stressors (e.g., divorce) are often related to health problems that do arise. For example, smoking and excessive alcohol consumption place an individual at greater risk of developing chronic respiratory problems, lung cancer, and liver disease. Overeating can result in obesity, diabetes mellitus, atherosclerosis, and its associated risk for hypertension and coronary artery disease. Many diseases of older age may be decreased by health conscious decisions made, and acted upon, in midlife (Hartman-Stein & Potkanowicz, 2003). The nurse can play an important role in teaching middle-aged clients about preventive health care to avoid or minimize the risk of such health problems.

Injuries

Changing physiologic factors, as well as concern over personal and work-related responsibilities, may contribute to the injury rate of middle-aged people. Motor vehicle crashes are the most common cause of unintentional death in this age group. Decreased reaction times and visual acuity may make the middle-aged adult prone to injury. Other unintentional causes of death for middle-aged adults include falls, fires, burns, poisonings, and drownings. Work-related injuries continue to be a significant safety hazard during the middle years.

Cancer

Cancer accounts for considerable mortality and morbidity in both men and women. It is the second leading cause of death among people between the ages of 25 and 64 in the United States. The patterns of cancer types and incidences for men and women have changed during the past several decades. Men have a high incidence of cancer of the lung and bladder. In women, breast cancer is highest in incidence, followed by cancer of the colon and rectum, uterus, and lung. The incidence of lung cancer is increasing in women.

Screening guidelines for early detection of cancer are constantly evolving as new data are analyzed. The American Cancer Society has a helpful website.

Cardiovascular Disease

Coronary heart disease (CHD) is the leading cause of death in the United States for the middle-aged adult. Several factors contribute to risk of CHD. These include smoking, obesity, hypertension, hyperlipidemia, diabetes mellitus, sedentary lifestyle, a family history of myocardial infarction or sudden death in a father less than 55 years old or in a mother less than 65 years old, and the individual's age. A newly recognized cluster of risk factors that often occur together, termed *metabolic syndrome*, increases the risk for CHD. This syndrome includes the following risk factors: excessive abdominal fat, hypertension, high lipid levels and insulin resistance (Edelman & Mandle, 2006 p. 526).

Men over 45 years of age and women over 55 years of age are at greater risk of developing CHD than younger adults. Physical inactivity places individuals at greater risk of developing CHD, and midlife adults should be helped to incorporate some physical activity in activities of daily living.

Obesity

Middle-aged adults who gain weight may not be aware of some common facts about this age period. Decreased metabolic activity and decreased physical activity mean a decrease in caloric need. The nurse's role in nutritional health promotion is to counsel clients to prevent obesity by reducing caloric intake and participating in regular exercise. Clients should also be educated that being overweight is a risk factor for many chronic diseases such as diabetes and hypertension and for problems of mobility such as arthritis. Recent changes in the Food Pyramid propagated by the U.S. Department of Agriculture now encourage nutrient intake based on physical activity, age, and gender. Clients may be directed to the Food Pyramid website to design a customized, healthy diet plan for themselves. Clients should seek medical advice before considering any major changes in their diets.

Alcoholism

The excessive use of alcohol can result in unemployment, disrupted homes, injuries, and diseases. It is estimated that 4 million people in the United States are dependent on alcohol and can be considered alcoholics. Alcohol use may exacerbate other health problems, and is a leading cause of hospitalization (Bostwick & Seaman, 2004). Nurses can help clients by providing information about the dangers of excessive alcohol use, by helping the individual clarify values about health, and by referring the client who abuses alcohol to special groups such as Alcoholics Anonymous.

Mental Health Alterations

Developmental stressors, such as the menopause, the climacteric, aging, and impending retirement, and situational stressors, such as divorce, unemployment, and death of a spouse, can precipitate increased anxiety and depression in middle-aged adults. Clients may benefit from support groups or individual therapy to help them cope with specific crises.

Health Assessment and Promotion

Assessment guidelines for the growth and development of the middle-aged adult are shown in the accompanying Developmental Assessment Guidelines. Middle-aged adults usually take care of their health needs and are interested in maintaining health and preventing the acceleration of the aging process (Acton & Malathum, 2000).

The nurse may choose to discuss some or all of the health promotion topics with the middle-aged adult client (see Box 22–4). These topics are discussed in detail in subsequent chapters throughout the book.

DEVELOPMENTAL ASSESSMENT GUIDELINES The Middle-Aged Adult

In these three developmental areas, does the middle-aged adult do the following?

PHYSICAL DEVELOPMENT

- Exhibit weight within normal range for age and sex.
- Manifest vital signs (e.g., blood pressure) within normal range for age and sex.
- Manifest visual and hearing abilities within normal range.
- Exhibit appropriate knowledge and attitudes about sexuality (e.g., about menopause).
- Verbalize any changes in eating, elimination, or exercise.

PSYCHOSOCIAL DEVELOPMENT

- Accept aging body.
- Feel comfortable and respect self.

- Enjoy new freedom to be independent.
- Accept changes in family roles (e.g., having teenage children and aging parents).
- Interact effectively and share companionable activities with life partner.
- Expand and renew previous interests.
- Pursue charitable and altruistic activities.
- Have a meaningful philosophy of life.

DEVELOPMENT IN ACTIVITIES OF DAILY LIVING

- Follow preventive health practice.

BOX 22–4 Health Promotion Guidelines for Middle-Aged Adults

HEALTH TESTS AND SCREENING

- Physical examination (every 3 to 5 years until age 40, then annually)
- Immunizations as recommended, such as a tetanus booster every 10 years, and current recommendations for influenza vaccine
- Regular dental assessments (e.g., every 6 months)
- Tonometry for signs of glaucoma and other eye diseases every 2 to 3 years or annually if indicated
- Breast examination annually by primary care provider
- Testicular examination annually by primary care provider
- Screenings for cardiovascular disease (e.g., blood pressure measurement; electrocardiogram and cholesterol test as directed by the primary care provider)
- Screenings for colorectal, breast, cervical, uterine, and prostate cancer (see cancer screening guidelines in Chapter 30) ∞
- Screening for tuberculosis every 2 years
- Smoking: history and counseling, if needed

SAFETY

- Motor vehicle safety reinforcement, especially when driving at night
- Workplace safety measures
- Home safety measures: keeping hallways and stairways lighted and uncluttered, using smoke detectors, using nonskid mats and handrails in the bathrooms

NUTRITION AND EXERCISE

- Importance of adequate protein, calcium, and vitamin D in diet
- Nutritional and exercise factors that may lead to cardiovascular disease (e.g., obesity, cholesterol and fat intake, lack of vigorous exercise)
- An exercise program that emphasizes skill and coordination

SOCIAL INTERACTIONS

- The possibility of a midlife crisis: encourage discussion of feelings, concerns, and fears
- Providing time to expand and review previous interests
- Retirement planning (financial and possible diversional activities), with partner if appropriate

---

CRITICAL THINKING CHECKPOINT

Mark Jones, a 22-year-old construction worker, comes into the health center for a "physical." He states that the last time he saw a health care provider was during high school, and he is only here today because his employer required that he be examined prior to returning to work. Mr. Jones has been off the job for 2 weeks following an accident in which he fell off a ladder, sustaining multiple contusions and a concussion. He mentions that he and "his buddies" have enjoyed his 2 weeks off from work, and have used the time to "drink beer and chase women."

1. What questions would you ask Mr. Jones about his usual health promotion activities?

2. How would you ask Mr. Jones about his risk for sexually transmitted infections?
3. What health conditions are young adults at risk for, and how would you explain these to Mr. Jones?
4. What health screening activities would you suggest to Mr. Jones? How would you explain the rationale to him?
5. How would you assess Mr. Jones's psychosocial development?

See Critical Thinking Possibilities in Appendix A. ∞

CHAPTER 22 **REVIEW**

CHAPTER HIGHLIGHTS

▥ Three distinct generations are included in adulthood: Baby Boomers, Generation Xers, and Generation Ys. Each has its own world view.

▥ Physical growth and development peaks in the middle 20s, and then becomes decremental.

▥ Emerging and young adults develop a self-identity and prepare for intimate relationships with others.

▥ Moral development continues throughout adulthood.

▥ Spirituality may be important to young adults, but is considered a private matter.

▥ Health risks for young adults are primarily related to lifestyle and behavior.

▥ Midlife adults begin to notice physical changes associated with aging.

▥ The developmental issue for midlife adults is generativity.

▥ Adults in midlife must balance the needs of many, including their own parents and children.

▥ Health decisions made by midlife adults may affect their health in later life.

▥ A variety of health threats, including cancer and heart disease, begin to affect persons in their middle age.

▥ Physical activity, healthy nutrition choices, and routine care by a health provider are important throughout the adult years.

TEST YOUR KNOWLEDGE

1. Because a 45-year-old woman is worried that she still has regular menstrual periods, she asks about menopause. Which of the following answers by the nurse is most appropriate?
   1. Regular menses in a 45-year-old woman should be promptly evaluated by a gynecologist.
   2. Although you continue to have menstrual periods, you are unlikely to become pregnant.
   3. It is common for women to experience menopause in their late 40s.
   4. Many women dread menopause because it is an unpleasant experience.

2. A nurse is planning a teaching session on a wellness topic. Which adult generation group would be most likely to be skeptical about health teaching by the nurse?
   1. Baby Boomer
   2. Generation X
   3. Generation Y
   4. Millennial

3. The routine physical examination of a female client between the ages of 25 and 64 is most likely to reveal that the client has which of the following types of cancer?
   1. Cervical cancer
   2. Lymphoma
   3. Lung cancer
   4. Colon cancer

4. The nurse is planning an educational program on sexually transmitted infections (STIs) for young adults. Which of the following topics should be given priority?
   1. Syphilis
   2. HIV
   3. Gonorrhea
   4. Chlamydia

5. Which statement about moral development in adults is the most correct?
   1. Moral development is completed during adolescence.
   2. Moral development continues throughout adulthood.
   3. Moral development is highly individualized.
   4. Moral development correlates to spiritual development.

6. If the nurse were assessing the status of a middle-aged client's psychosocial development, which of the following should be the focus?
   1. Selecting a life partner
   2. Balancing the needs of others
   3. Reviewing one's life course
   4. Establishing a sense of self

7. The nurse is developing a health promotion teaching plan for a community group of middle-aged adults. Information about which immunizations should be included?
   1. Pneumococcal, meningococcal
   2. Pertussis, influenza, meningococcal
   3. Influenza, pneumococcal
   4. Meningococcal, pertussis

8. When planning a screening program for cardiovascular disease in the middle-aged adult, the nurse has limited funds and must address which of the following most significant elements? Select all that apply.
   1. Blood pressure measurement
   2. Electrocardiogram
   3. Cholesterol measurement
   4. Sexual performance
   5. Activity level

9. A woman comes into the emergency department with multiple bruises about the face and head. The nurse suspects that domestic violence may be related to the injuries. What is the most appropriate action for the nurse to take at this time?
   1. Ask the woman if she is afraid of someone at home who is hurting her.
   2. Refer the woman to a shelter for battered women.
   3. Call a social worker to assess the woman for domestic violence.
   4. Document the concern in the chart, but do nothing else.

10. The nurse is completing a health history on a 24-year-old male. Which activity is the best indicator of appropriate psychosocial development?
    1. Creating a scrapbook of his life experiences
    2. Joining the board of directors for three charities
    3. Decorating his new apartment
    4. Attending seminars on choosing a career

See Test Your Knowledge Answers in Appendix A .

EXPLORE MEDIALINK www.prenhall.com/berman

DVD-ROM
- Audio Glossary
- NCLEX Review

COMPANION WEBSITE
- Case Study: Developmental Phases of Adulthood
- Care Plan Activity: Parenting Responsibilities
- Application Activity: College Student with Manic Depression
- Links to Resources

READINGS AND REFERENCES

SUGGESTED READINGS

Brown, C. G. (2004). Testicular cancer: An overview. *Urologic Nursing, 24*(2), 83–93. *The author points out that testicular cancer (TC) is the most common malignancy in males between 15 and 35, the second most common cancer in men from 35 to 39, and the third most common from 15 to 19 years of age. The incidence is rising in the United States and Canada. This article provides a review of the epidemiology, risk factors, early detection, signs and symptoms, diagnosis, treatment, and the nurse's role in educating men.*

Ehrenreich, B. (2002). *Nickled and dimed: On (not) getting by in America*. New York: Owl Books. *An insightful look into daily life for many adults, it will help nurses understand the decisions many face when it comes to health promotion and everyday needs.*

Glanz, K., Rimer, B. K., & Lewis, F. M. (2002). *Health behavior and health education: Theory, research, and practice* (3rd ed.). San Francisco: Jossey-Bass. *The editors of this text have done a wonderful job of explaining why people make the decisions they make about health. They also offer suggestions on how to be a more effective health educator.*

Swearingen, S., & Liberman, A. (2004). Nursing generations: An expanded look at the emergence of conflict and its resolution. *Health Care Manager, 23*(1), 54–65. *The authors point out that the coexistence of three generations in nursing is leading to intergenerational conflict. This conflict is exacerbating the nursing shortage because Generation X individuals are either not pursuing nursing or maintaining their nursing careers. The article, using cohort and conflict theories, examines and suggests the impact of generational diversity on the future of nursing.*

RELATED RESEARCH

Callahan, S. T., & Cooper, W. O. (2005). Uninsurance and health care access among young adults in the United States. *Pediatrics, 116*(1), 88–95.

Jack, S. M., Bouck, L. M. S., Beynon, C. E., Ciliska, D. K., & Mitchell, M. J. L. (2005). Marketing a hard-to-swallow message. Recommendations for the design of media campaigns to increase awareness about the risks of binge drinking. *Canadian Journal of Public Health, 96*(3), 189–193.

Morrone, M., & Rathbun, A. (2003). Health education and food safety behavior in the university setting. *Journal of Environmental Health, 65*(7), 9–15.

Schmidt, M. I., Duncan, B. B., Bang, H., Pankow, J. S., Ballantyne, C. M., Golden, S.H., et al. (2005). Identifying individuals at high risk for diabetes: The atherosclerosis risk in communities study. *Diabetes Care, 28*(8), 2013–2018.

Thornton, E. W., Sykes, K. S., & Tang, W. K. (2004). Health benefits of tai chi exercise: Improved balance and blood pressure in middle-aged women. *Health Promotion International, 19*(1), 33–36.

Tucker, J. S., Klein, D. J., & Elliott, M. N. (2004). Social control of health behaviors: A comparison of young, middle-aged, and older adults. *Journal of Gerontology, 59B*(4), 147–150.

REFERENCES

Acton, G. J., & Malathum, P. (2000). Basic need status and health-promoting self-care behaviors in adults. *Western Journal of Nursing Research 22*(7), 796–811.

Afifi, T. D. (2003). "Feeling caught" in stepfamilies: Managing boundary turbulence through appropriate communication privacy rules. *Journal of Social and Personal Relationships, 20*, 729–755.

American Cancer Society. (2005). *Cancer facts and figures, 2005*. Retrieved June 6, 2006, from http://www.cancer.org/docroot/STT/content/STT_1x_Cancer_Facts__Figures_2005.asp

Banister, E. M. (2000). Women's midlife confusion: "Why am I feeling this way?" *Issues in Mental Health Nursing, 21*, 745–764.

Bilukha, O. O., & Rosenstein, N. (2005). Prevention and control of meningococcal disease. Recommendations of the Advisory Committee on Immunization Practices (ACIP). *Morbidity and Mortality Weekly Report, 54* (RR-7), 1–21.

Bostwick, J. M., & Seaman, J. S. (2004). Hospitalized patients and alcohol: Who is being missed? *General Hospital Psychiatry, 26*(1), 59–62.

Cavendish, R., Luise, B. K., Bauer, M., et al. (2001). Recognizing opportunities for spiritual enhancement in young adults. *Nursing Diagnosis, 12*(3), 77–92.

Centers for Disease Control and Prevention. (2004). *Trends in reportable sexually transmitted diseases in the United States, 2003*. Atlanta, GA: Author.

Dawson, T. L. (2002). New tools, new insights: Kohlberg's moral judgement stages revisited. *International Journal of Behavioral development, 26*(2), 154–166.

Edelman, C. L., & Mandle, C. L. (2006). *Health promotion throughout the life span* (6th ed.). St. Louis, MO: Mosby.

Erikson, E. H. (1963). *Childhood and society* (2nd ed.). New York: Norton.

Fields, J. (2004). America's families and living arrangements: 2003. *Current population reports* (U.S. Census Bureau Report No. P20–553). Washington, DC: Author.

Hartman-Stein, P. E., & Potkanowicz, E. S. (2003). Behavioral determinants of healthy aging: Good news for the baby boomer generation. *Online Journal of Issues in Nursing, 8*(2), Manuscript #5. Retrieved June 6, 2006, from http://www.nursingworld.org/ojin/topic21/tpc21_5.htm

Hill, K. S. (2004). Defy the decades with multigenerational teams. *Nursing Management, 35*(1), 32–35.

Hu, J., Herrick, C., & Hodgin, K. A. (2004). Managing the multigenerational nursing team. *Health Care Manager, 22*, 334–341.

Lachman, M. E. (2004). Development in midlife. *Annual Review of Psychology, 55*, 305–31.

Landenburger, K. M., & Campbell, J. C. (2003). Violence and human abuse. In M. Stanhope & J. Lancaster (Eds.), *Community and public health nursing* (6th ed., pp. 874–901). St. Louis, MO: Mosby.

Ling, P. M., & Glantz, S. A. (2002). Why and how the tobacco industry sells cigarettes to young adults: Evidence from industry documents. *American Journal of Public Health, 92*, 908–916.

Mathre, M. L. (2004). Alcohol, tobacco, and other drug problems in the community. In M. Stanhope & J. Lancaster (Eds.), *Community and public health nursing* (6th ed., pp. 848–873). St. Louis, MO: Mosby.

Murray, R. B., & Zentner, J. P. (2001). *Health promotion strategies through the life span* (7th ed.). Upper Saddle River, NJ: Prentice Hall.

Nelson, L. J., & Barry, C. M. (2005). Distinguishing features of emerging adulthood: The role of self-classification as an adult. *Journal of Adolescent Research, 20*, 242–262.

Paludi, M. A. (2002). *Human development in multicultural contexts. A book of readings*. Upper Saddle River, NJ: Prentice Hall.

Pfaffenberger, A. H. (2005). Optimal adult development: An inquiry into the dynamics of growth. *Journal of Humanistic Psychology, 45*(3), 279–301.

Polan, E., & Taylor, D. (2003). *Journey across the life span. Human development and health promotion* (2nd ed.). Philadelphia: F. A. Davis.

Sanots, S. R., & Cox, K. (2000). Workplace adjustment and intergenerational differences between Matures, Boomers, and Xers. *Nursing Economics, 18*(1), 7–13.

Slater, C. L. (2003). Generativity versus stagnation: An elaboration of Erikson's adult stage of human development. *Journal of Adult Development, 10*, 53–65.

U.S. Department of Health and Human Services (USDHHS). (2000). *Healthy people 2010* (2nd. ed.). Washington, DC: Government Printing Office.

U.S. Department of Health and Human Services. (2004). *Summary health statistics for U. S.*

adults: *National Health Interview Survey, 2002.* DHHS Publication No. (PHS) 2004-1550. Hyattsville, MD: Author.

U. S. Preventive Services Task Force. (2003). *Guide to clinical preventive services, 3rd edition: Periodic updates.* Rockville, MD: Agency for Health Care Research and Quality. Retrieved June 6, 2006, from http://www.ahrq.gov/clinic/gcpspu.htm

U. S. Preventive Services Task Force. (2004). *Screening for testicular cancer: Recommendation statement.* Rockville, MD: Agency for Health Care Research and Quality. Retrieved June 6, 2006, from http://www.ahrq.gov/clinic/uspstf/uspstest.htm

SELECTED BIBLIOGRAPHY

Erikson, E. H. (1982). *The life cycle completed: A review.* New York: Norton.

Fowler, J. W. (1981). *Stages of faith: The psychology of human development and the quest for meaning.* New York: Harper & Row.

Freud, S. (1922). *The ego and the id.* London: Hogarth Press.

Gilligan, C. (1982). *In a different voice: Psychological theory and women's development.* Cambridge, MA: Harvard University Press.

Havighurst, R. J. (1972). *Developmental tasks and education* (3rd ed.). New York: Longman.

Kohlberg, L. (1971). *Recent research in moral development.* New York: Holt, Rinehart & Winston.

Kohlberg, L. (1981). *The psychology of moral development: Moral stages and the idea of justice.* San Francisco: Harper & Row.

Kohlberg, L. (1984). *The psychology of moral development: The nature and validity of moral stages.* San Francisco: Harper & Row.

Maslow, A. H. (1970). *Motivation and personality.* New York: Harper & Row.

Piaget, J. (1966). *Origins of intelligence in children.* New York: Norton.

Sheehy, G. (1995). *New passages. Mapping your life across time.* New York: Ballantine Books.

Stevenson, J. S. (1977). *Issues and crises during middlescence.* New York: Appleton-Century-Crofts.

Promoting Health in Elders

LEARNING OUTCOMES

After completing this chapter, you will be able to:

1. Identify the different categories of elders as they range from 65 to 100 years of age.

2. Describe the demographic, socioeconomic, ethnicity, and health characteristics of elders in the United States.

3. Describe ageism and its contribution to the development of negative stereotypes about elders.

4. Compare and contrast gerontology and geriatrics.

5. Describe the development of gerontological nursing and the roles of the gerontological nurse.

6. Describe the different care settings for elders.

7. List the common biologic theories of aging.

8. Describe the usual physical changes that occur during older adulthood.

9. List the common psychosocial theories about aging.

10. Describe developmental tasks of the older adult.

11. Describe psychosocial changes that the older adult adjusts to during the aging process.

12. Explain changes in cognitive abilities while aging.

13. Compare and contrast Kohlberg's and Gilligan's theories of moral reasoning in elders.

14. Describe spirituality and aging.

15. Describe selected health problems associated with elders.

16. List examples of health promotion topics for older adulthood.

The United States is experiencing a "graying of America" as the elder population steadily grows. By the mid-21st century, elders are projected to outnumber young people (Mauk, 2006, p. 30).

CHARACTERISTICS OF ELDERS IN THE UNITED STATES

Elders represent an increasingly diverse population in the United States. A review of the major characteristics of the elder population includes demographic, socioeconomic, ethnicity, and health characteristics.

Demographic

At one time, all individuals over the age of 65 were considered old. With advancements in disease control, living conditions, and health technology, people are living longer. A 65-year-old American woman may expect to live another 19 years, and a 65-year-old American man may expect to reach the age of 81 (Federal Interagency Forum on Age-Related Statistics [FIFAS], 2004). People 85 years and older are the fastest growing of all age groups in the country, numbering 4.6 million in 2002, but projected to reach 9.6 million by the year 2030 (U.S. Department of Health and Human Services [USDHHS], 2003). The elderly are as heterogeneous as any other age group that spans 40 years or more. As a result, the categories of elders have expanded from one to four with each one having a distinct set of interests and health care needs. See Box 23–1.

Socioeconomic

Socioeconomic characteristics such as gender, marital status, education, income, and living arrangements vary among the young-old and old-old groups (Miller, 2004). Women outnumber men. For example, the young-old and old-old groups have nearly 2 million more women than men (Mauk, 2006, p. 31).

Women have a longer life expectancy than men. In addition, women are more likely than men to be widowed and there are higher remarriage rates for older men.

The level of education can affect the socioeconomic status of the elder. Higher education is usually associated with higher incomes. According to Miller (2004), educational levels for older adults are gradually increasing as indicated by the increasing percentage rates of people 65 years and older who have completed high school. However, there is significant variation among racial and ethnic groups. Usually, older adults have lower incomes than younger adults, and people 85 years and older have the lowest median income (Miller, 2004, p. 14).

Living arrangements of elders are linked not only to income, but also to health status. Most live in a variety of community settings with only 4.3% living in nursing homes (FIFAS, 2004). Older people who live alone are more likely to live in poverty than people in the same age category who are married (Mauk, 2006). Older women are twice as likely to be living alone. Living arrangements vary by race and ethnicity (see Table 23–1). The rate of living alone increases as age increases.

Ethnicity

The growing population of elders consists of increasing numbers of minority elders. When projecting to 2050, the higher proportion of the elder white population will continue. However, the nonwhite elder population is expected to increase with elder Hispanics being the fastest growing subpopulation group (Meiner & Lueckenotte, 2006). These numbers emphasize the importance of nurses being culturally sensitive and competent. See Table 23–2 for a comparison of the elder population growth.

BOX 23–1 Categorizing the Aging Population

- Young-old: 65 to 75 years
- Old: 75 to 85 years
- Old-old: 85 to 100 years
- Elite old: Over 100 years

Note: From C. Eliopoulos, *Gerontological Nursing*, 6th ed. Copyright © Lippincott Williams & Wilkins, 2005. Reprinted with permission.

TABLE 23–1 Common Living Arrangements of Elders by Gender, Race, and Ethnicity

WHO	LIVING ARRANGEMENT
Asian female	Live with relatives other than a spouse
Non-Hispanic white female	Live alone
Black female	Live alone
Black male	Live alone
Asian male	Live with relatives other than a spouse

Note: K. L. Mauk, *Gerontological Nursing* 2006: Jones and Bartlett Publishers, Sudbury, MA. www.jbpub.com. Reprinted with permission.

TABLE 23–2 **Comparison of Elderly Population for 2003 Census and Projected Elderly Population for 2050 Census Ethnicity**

ETHNICITY	2003 CENSUS	2050 PROJECTION
White	83%	61%
Black	8%	12%
Asian	3%	8%
Hispanic	6%	18%

Note: K. L. Mauk, *Gerontological Nursing* 2006: Jones and Bartlett Publishers, Sudbury, MA. www.jbpub.com. Reprinted with permission.

Health

Chronic health problems and disabilities increase as age increases. However, disease is *not* a normal outcome of aging. The vast majority (73%) of older Americans rated their health as good, very good, or excellent (National Center for Health Statistics [NCHS], 2003), even though most have chronic health conditions, and 20% report a disability (FIFAS, 2004). Nurses need to be aware that promoting health and wellness and assessing and promoting functional abilities for activities of daily living continue to be valid and important for 65-year-old clients who have 16 to 19 more years to enjoy life. In fact, the goals of *Healthy People 2010* include focus areas relevant to elders. See Box 23–2.

ATTITUDES TOWARD AGING

Because elder numbers are increasing, nurses will be caring for older adults at some point. It is important for nurses to be aware of their own values and attitudes toward aging and the elderly, and examine whether myths or stereotypes influence those attitudes.

BOX 23–2 **Focus Areas in *Healthy People 2010* That Are Relevant to Elders**

- Access to quality health services
- Arthritis, osteoporosis, and chronic back conditions
- Cancer
- Chronic kidney disease
- Diabetes
- Disability and secondary conditions
- Educational and community-based programs
- Food safety
- Health communication
- Heart disease and stroke
- Immunization and infectious diseases
- Injury and violence prevention
- Mental health and mental conditions
- Nutrition and obesity
- Oral health
- Physical activity and fitness
- Respiratory diseases
- Substance abuse
- Tobacco use
- Vision and hearing

Note: U.S. Department of Health and Human Services.

Ageism

American society values youth. See the Culturally Competent Care box to see how different cultures view elders. **Ageism** is a term to describe the deep and profound prejudice in American society

CULTURALLY COMPETENT CARE
How Different Cultures View Elders

CHINESE
- Traditional Chinese values place the family and society over the individual. Many American-born Chinese may not be as traditional but still hold values of respect for elders and authority.
- The oldest son has obligations toward the family and is expected to respect and care for parents.
- The tradition of "filial piety" is the value of total respect for the family, especially the elders. This respect for elders was advocated by Confucius, the famous Chinese philosopher and many Chinese and Chinese-American families choose to follow these ancient principles.

NATIVE AMERICAN
- Traditionally, elders are respected for their wisdom, experience, and knowledge.
- Elders, regardless of tribe, assume significant roles as teachers and caretakers of the young.

VIETNAMESE
- Elders are given high respect in Vietnamese society. They are considered the carriers of tradition, knowledge, and wisdom. Age is considered an asset, not a liability.
- Elderly grandparents and parents stay with the family for support and care.
- Elders may prepare meals and care for grandchildren if both the husband and wife work.
- In Vietnam, elders are the leaders and decision-makers in the family and often sought for advice. When these elders move to the U.S., they can become socially and culturally isolated for many reasons (e.g., lack of English, age, lack of training for work). In contrast, the younger family members become more Americanized and may behave in ways their elders do not approve. This can create tension in families where elders feel ignored and not respected.

BLACK/AFRICAN AMERICAN
- Elders are respected, obeyed and considered a source of wisdom.
- To survive to old age is often considered an accomplishment reflecting personal strength, resourcefulness, and faith.

HISPANIC/LATINO
- Elders are held in high esteem.
- Old age is viewed as a positive time in the life of the elder.
- Care for elders is provided by the extended family. It is expected that children will care for their elderly parents.

KOREAN
- Traditional Koreans value filial piety and respect for elders.
- In Korean culture, children are taught to respect elders whether they are right or wrong.
- There is the expectation that the children will take care of their parents in old age.
- Two important family holidays that are celebrated with feasts include the 60th birthday and the 70th birthday.

MediaLink

Cultural Diversity Video

against older adults (Meiner & Lueckenotte, 2006, p. 13). It is a discrimination based solely on age. Unfortunately, this negative attitude toward aging or elders exists among some health care professionals (Ebersole, Hess, Touhy, & Jett, 2005; Mauk, 2006). This attitude is another reason for nurses to self-reflect personal beliefs and values toward elders.

Myths and Stereotypes

Ageism contributes to the development of negative stereotypes about older adults. Stereotypes occur when younger people do not understand or identify with elders as unique human beings. Instead, they generalize undesirable characteristics (e.g., senile, old-fashioned, unproductive, inflexible) to all elders. Many negative attitudes about aging are based on myths and incorrect information. See Table 23–3. As a result, it is important for nurses to provide accurate information about aging. This has been found to be an effective intervention for reducing negative stereotypes and improving attitudes about aging (Miller, 2004, p. 11).

GERONTOLOGICAL NURSING

The growth of the elder population is characterized by unique and diverse individuals who may require a variety of health care professionals to meet their health care needs. **Gerontology** is a term used to define the study of aging and older adults. Gerontology is multidisciplinary and is a specialized area within various disciplines such as nursing, psychology, and social work. **Geriatrics** is associated with the medical care (e.g., diseases and disabilities) of the elderly.

Development

Gerontological nursing involves advocating for the health of older persons at all levels of prevention (Mauk, 2006, p. 9). In the 1960s, gerontological nursing became a subspecialty of nursing. In the 1980s, gerontological nursing leaders stated that most practicing nurses did not have sufficient knowledge about gerontology. This prompted discussion of how to prepare nurses for gerontological nursing. Since the late 1990s, the nursing profession has recognized the importance of preparing all practicing nurses with basic gerontological knowledge. As a result, schools of nursing provide classes or courses about nursing care of the elderly. Practicing gerontological nurses can obtain gerontological nursing certification through the American Nurses Association. Advanced practice in gerontological nursing requires a master's degree in nursing, of which there are two options: the gerontological clinical nurse specialist and the gerontological nurse practitioner.

Roles

The gerontological nurse has many roles: provider of care, teacher, manager, advocate, and research consumer. As provider of care, the nurse gives direct care to older adults in a variety of settings. The teaching of gerontological nurses often focuses on modifiable risk factors (e.g., healthy diet, physical activity, stress management). Gerontological nurse managers balance the concerns of the elder, family, and nurses and other interdisciplinary team members. As an advocate, the gerontological nurse empowers elders by helping them remain independent and strengthen their autonomy and decision making. Being a research consumer requires nurses to read the latest professional literature for evidence-based practice to improve the quality of nursing care for the elderly.

CARE SETTINGS FOR ELDERS

Gerontological nurses practice in many settings. Older adults are the primary users of health care services from acute care facilities to rehabilitation, long-term care, and the community (Stanley, Blair, & Beare, 2005). No matter the setting, older adults require health assessment and promotion.

TABLE 23–3 **Myths and Realities of Aging**	
MYTH	**REALITY**
People consider themselves to be old at 65.	People feel old based on their health and functional ability, rather than their chronological age.
In today's society, families no longer care for older people.	In the United States, 80% of the care of older adults is provided by their families.
As people grow older, it is natural for them to want to withdraw from society.	Because older people are unique individuals, each of them responds differently to society.
By age 70, an individual's psychologic growth is complete.	People never lose their capacity for psychologic growth.
In old age, there is an inevitable decline in all intellectual abilities.	A few areas of cognitive ability decline in older adulthood, but other areas show improvement.
Older adults cannot learn complex new skills.	Older adults are capable of learning new things, but the speed with which they process information slows with age.
Older people decrease the level of their sexual activity because they are less able to perform sexually.	If sexual activity in older people declines, it is because of social reasons (e.g., loss of partner) or risk factors, such as diseases and adverse medication effects.
Most old people are depressed and should be allowed to withdraw from society.	About one-third of older people exhibit depressive symptoms; however, depression is a very treatable condition at any age.

Note: From C. A. Miller, *Nursing for Wellness in Older Adults,* 4th ed. Copyright © Lippincott, Williams & Wilkins, 2004. Reprinted with permission.

Acute Care Facilities

Elders are the majority of clients cared for in acute care. For example, people who are 65 and older use the emergency department (ED) at a higher rate than any other age group (Capezuti & Harrington, 2004). Nearly half of the clients who die in hospitals spend part or all of their last 3 days in critical care (Seery, 2004).

Nurses in an acute care setting focus on protecting the health of the older adult, with the goal of the older adult returning to his or her prior level of independence. Examples include:

- Preventing nosocomial infections (e.g., urinary tract infections, pneumonia).
- Preventing therapy-related problems (e.g., confusion, sleeplessness, dehydration, decreased nutrition).
- Treating the health problem that resulted in the older adult's admission plus assessing for potential undiagnosed health problems (e.g., depression, drug and/or alcohol abuse).
- Preventing complications (e.g., decubitus ulcer).

Elders often perceive that being in the hospital could change their ability to be autonomous and independent. As a result, nurses need to assess the elder's stage or perception of need for control and autonomy during hospitalization and his or her fears and hopes about being discharged from the hospital setting.

Long-Term Care Facilities

The objective of long-term care is to provide a place of safety and care to attain optimal wellness and independence for each individual (Stanley et al., 2005, p. 94). In the long-term care setting, the individual is referred to as a resident. Long-term care includes many different levels of care. These may include assisted living, intermediate care, skilled care, and Alzheimer's units. Elders who do not feel safe living alone or require additional help with activities of daily living (ADLs) may desire **assisted living.** They usually have their own apartment. The assisted living facility provides meals, weekly activities, and a pleasant environment to socialize with other residents. Some assisted living units are part of a larger facility. When residents require additional assistance, they may enter intermediate care. Residents of intermediate care are no longer able to live independently. This level of care provides 24-hour direct nursing contact (Mauk, 2006).

Skilled care units or skilled nursing facilities (SNFs) are for elders who require a higher level of nursing care because the acuity level of the client requires a greater nurse-to-client ratio. Gerontological nurses working in SNFs often care for clients with tube feedings, IVs, chronic wounds, and ventilators.

Many long-term care facilities offer specialized units for clients with **Alzheimer's disease** (AD), which involves progressive dementia, memory loss, and inability to care for themselves. The gerontological nurses working in Alzheimer's units have specialized knowledge and help family members understand and cope with the disease process affecting their loved one.

Hospice

Gerontological nurses may also work in hospice and care for dying persons and their families. The majority of hospice clients are elders. Hospice requires a great deal of patience, expertise, understanding, interdisciplinary communication,

MediaLink

Nursing Issues and the Elderly Video

RESEARCH NOTE — How Do Elders Manage Personal Integrity During Hospitalization?

For this grounded theory research study the researcher collected in-depth interviews of five older adults ranging from 77 to 85 years of age. These elders, who lived independently in the community prior to hospitalization, were admitted for medical reasons related to a chronic underlying health problem. The researcher also interviewed family members of each elder and an RN who provided nursing care for each elder. In addition to the interviews, the researcher observed each elder for at least 2 hours each day.

The research findings resulted in a theory entitled Managing Personal Integrity. Jacelon, the researcher, defines personal integrity as a dynamic, intrinsic quality of the self with the properties of health, dignity, and autonomy. The findings indicated that each property was a focus of the elders during their hospitalization.

Hospital routine was strange and different for the elder. All of their prior routines were taken away and they felt a loss of control. According to this research, the elder progressed through three stages of independence and autonomy. First, they willingly gave up their autonomy and sense of control when they were admitted to the hospital because they wanted to get better. They focused primarily on their health. As they started to improve, the elders wanted to increase their autonomy and sense of control, focusing on their dignity. For example, they accomplished more by themselves and took more responsibility for self-care. They also participated more in the plan of care by asking questions about their medications and tests. Before dis-

charge, with the reasons for the hospitalization resolving, the elders felt more of a sense of control and began to reassert their autonomy. They took more responsibility for both their activities of daily living and their health by preparing for discharge and resuming independent functioning at home.

IMPLICATIONS

This study reflects the importance of autonomy to the elder. According to Jacelon, autonomy has two components: independence (the physical ability to act) and control (the ability to make decisions on one's own behalf). As nurses work with more and more elders in the acute care hospital setting, it is important to remember the stages of independence and autonomy experienced by elders during the different phases of hospitalization as reflected in this study. Strategies to enhance an increased sense of control and autonomy by the elder include providing adequate information in a timely manner, allowing participation in the scheduling of activities, explaining any changes in the plan of care, and viewing hospitalized elders as individuals who wish to regain their autonomy and dignity.

Note: From "Older Adults and Autonomy in Acute Care: Increasing Patients' Independence and Control During Hospitalization," by C. S. Jacelon, 2004, *Journal of Gerontological Nursing, 30*.(11), pp. 29–36. Copyright © 2004 SLACK, Inc. Reprinted with permission.

REAL WORLD PRACTICE

Some of my earliest memories are playing with the nurse kit my grandmother bought for me. I have always wanted to be a nurse. The nursing profession is so integrated into who I am; I would truly be lost without it.

The geriatric population is growing so rapidly the health care industry is having difficulty keeping up with the demands. Working with the elderly whether in a long-term care facility, home care, or transitioning them from one to the other is a specialty in which the nurse uses all of the knowledge gained throughout nursing school. This population has complex needs that need to be addressed by competent, caring professionals who have the knowledge, evidence base, and creativity to solve them. Many co-morbid chronic illnesses, multiple medications, dealing with the normal changes that happen as we age, and the abnormal findings that often pop up are just some of the problems geriatric nurses are faced with daily. To keep the client in the setting where they want to live, or the challenge of needing to change settings to meet a client's needs are dilemmas the nurse frequently faces. Providing basic assessments, seeing the client as a whole, and providing the care that is needed and deserved are a few things geriatric nurses do best to solve or make these transitions easier.

The rewards for the efforts made every day are expressed in the faces of our clients whether it is from doing the best we can for the clients, putting kindness and laughter into their day, solving a health-related problem, treating them as they would like to be treated, or holding their hand as they die in peace. These are small acts dedicated nurses do every day that make a world of difference in the lives of the clients we touch.

—*Constance Lemley, MSN, RN*
LaPorte Hospital, LaPorte, IN

and compassion skills on the part of gerontology nurses (Mauk, 2006, p. 23).

Rehabilitation

Rehabilitation may be found in several settings: acute care hospital, subacute or transitional care, and long-term care facilities. Many elders benefit from a rehabilitation program where the goal is to maintain physical independence (e.g., after orthopedic surgery, stroke, or amputation). The nurse is an important member of the interdisciplinary rehabilitation team. The role of the nurse is often as a health care coordinator, manager, and counselor for elders and their families (Stanley et al., 2005). For example, nurses monitor the client's health care, assist with ADLs, and facilitate the client's adjustment and coping with the disability.

Community

Gerontological nurses provide nursing care in many types of community settings. Nurses often assess the elder's needs and then try to match the need with a community resource. A few of

the different community areas for gerontological nurses to practice include:

- *Home health care.* Home care is designed for those who are homebound due to severity of illness or disability (Mauk, 2006). Research has shown that home health for older adults prevents hospital readmissions (Stanley et al., 2005).
- *Nurse-run clinics.* The clinics focus on managing chronic illness. Nurses follow up with either telephone contacts or home visits within a week after discharge from a hospital. Again, this often helps decrease hospital readmissions.
- *Adult day care.* The older adult may receive **adult day care** where the focus is on social activities or health care where the level of nursing care can vary (e.g., bathing, medication administration, wound dressing). Some adult day-care centers provide both social and health care. Family members who care for older parents but may need to work during the day or need some respite from the continual care often use these services. This is an alternative to institutionalizing the older adult.

PHYSIOLOGICAL AGING

In the past half-century, scientists have proposed numerous theories of why people age. More recently, as both the absolute number and the population percentage of elders increase, there is renewed scientific interest in why people age, how people age, and what factors affect the physical, psychologic, and functional status of older persons. There are nearly 40 different theories of aging in the biologic, psychologic, and social sciences, and many in gerontological nursing. Clearly, there are more questions as to how people age than there are answers. At this point, it is helpful to distinguish between normal or usual aging (the typical aging course, with concomitant diseases and disabilities) and successful aging (the aging course without disease). Unfortunately, it is extremely difficult to know one from the other, as 80% of older adults have one chronic health condition, and 50% have two (Centers for Disease Control and Prevention [CDC], 2004). The most promising theories for explaining physical aging include genetics (Kirkwood & Austad, 2000), oxidative stress (Finkel & Holbrook, 2000), and cellular changes (DePinto, 2000). These theories may be generally grouped into (a) theories that hypothesize aging as a consequence of accumulated damage to informational molecules, and (b) theories that hypothesize aging as a consequence of regulation by specific genes (Kane, Ouslander, & Abrass, 2004). Table 23–4 describes the various biologic theories of aging.

As the person ages, a number of physical changes occur; some are visible, some are not. In general, lean body mass is reduced, fat tissue increases, and bone mass decreases. Extracellular fluid remains constant; however, intracellular fluid decreases and leads to reduced total body fluid. Thus, elders are at risk for developing dehydration (Eliopoulos, 2005). Table 23–5 provides a summary of the normal physical changes associated with aging.

TABLE 23–4 **Common Biologic Theories of Aging**

THEORY TYPE	HYPOTHESES
Wear-and-tear theories	Proposes that humans, like automobiles, have vital parts that run down with time, leading to aging and death. Proposes that the faster an organism lives, the quicker it dies. Proposes that cells wear out through exposure to internal and external stressors, including trauma, chemicals, and buildup of natural wastes.
Endocrine theory	Proposes that events occurring in the hypothalamus and pituitary are responsible for changes in hormone production and response that result in the organism's decline.
Free-radical theory	Proposes that unstable free radicals (groups of atoms) result from the oxidation of organic materials, such as carbohydrates and proteins. These radicals cause biochemical changes in the cells, and the cells cannot regenerate themselves.
Genetic theories	Proposes that the organism is genetically programmed for a predetermined number of cell divisions, after which the cells/organism dies. Proposes that when damage to the protein synthesis occurs, faulty proteins will be synthesized and will gradually accumulate, causing a progressive decline in the organism.
Cross-linking theories	Proposes that the irreversible aging of proteins such as collagen is responsible for the ultimate failure of tissues and organs. Proposes that as cells age, chemical reactions create strong bonds, or cross-linkages, between proteins. These bonds cause loss of elasticity, stiffness, and eventual loss of function.
Immunological theories	Proposes that the immune system becomes less effective with age, resulting in reduced resistance to infectious disease and viruses. Proposes that a decrease in immune function may result in an increase in autoimmune responses, causing the body to produce antibodies that attack itself.

Integument

Obvious changes occur in the integumentary system (skin, hair, nails) with age. The skin becomes drier, less elastic, and more fragile, making the older person more susceptible to skin tears and shearing injuries. The hair loses color, the fingernails and toenails become thickened and brittle, and in women over 60, facial hair increases.

Responses to these changes vary among individuals and cultures. For example, one person may feel distinguished with gray hair, whereas another may feel embarrassed or depressed, interpreting gray hair as a sign of losing one's youth.

These integumentary changes accompany progressive losses of subcutaneous fat and muscle tissue, muscle atrophy, and loss of elastic fiber, resulting in a "double" chin, sagging of eyelids and earlobes, and wrinkling of skin, especially in areas exposed to sun. Bony prominences may become visible. In older women, the breasts become less firm and may sag. Loss of subcutaneous fat also decreases elders' tolerance of cold.

Health promotion teaching about skin care for elders can include the following:

- Maintaining healthy skin
  - Ensure optimal nutrition.
  - Maintain adequate hydration.
  - Prevent skin dryness by using emollient lotions after bathing or showering, when the skin is still moist.
  - Avoid skin products that contain perfume or alcohol.
  - Assess the frequency of bathing/showering.
- Avoiding sun damage
  - Use sun-screening lotions with sun protection factor (SPF) of 15 or higher.
  - Wear wide-brimmed hats, sun visors, and sunglasses when exposed to the sun.

- Observe for any skin changes (e.g., new lesions, change in mole size or color) and seek medical evaluation.
- Preventing skin injury
  - Do not use strong detergent to launder clothes.
  - Avoid rough texture in clothing.
  - Avoid highly starched linens.
  - Use soft washcloths, towels, and bed linens.

Neuromusculoskeletal

With aging comes gradual reduction in the speed and power of skeletal or voluntary muscle contractions and sustained muscular effort. Exercise can strengthen weakened muscles, and up to about age 50 the skeletal muscles can increase in bulk and density. After that time there is a steady decrease in muscle fibers (**sarcopenia**), even in elderly master athletes (Taylor et al., 2004), ultimately leading to the typical wasted appearance of the very old person. The mechanism of age-related sarcopenia appears to be related to denervation of the muscle. Thus elders often complain about their lack of strength and how quickly they tire. Activities can still be carried out, but at a slower pace, and with greater expenditure of energy (Taylor et al., 2004). Often balance is impaired with age, and is related to loss of muscle strength. Muscle endurance diminishes with age, resulting in muscle fatigue after short periods of exercise for the elder. There is substantial evidence, however, that the muscles that do remain in the older adult can be strengthened through exercise and training, with resulting improvements in functional status.

The person's reaction time slows with age. Reaction time can be delayed further by decreased muscle tone as a result of diminished physical activity. Elders compensate for this reaction difference by being exceptionally cautious, for instance, in their driving habits, which exasperates some impatient younger drivers.

TABLE 23–5 Normal Physical Changes Associated with Aging

PHYSICAL CHANGES	RATIONALE
Integumentary	
Increased skin dryness	Decrease in sebaceous gland activity and tissue fluid
Increased skin pallor	Decreased vascularity
Increased skin fragility	Reduced thickness and vascularity of the dermis; loss of subcutaneous fat
Progressive wrinkling and sagging of the skin	Loss of skin elasticity, increased dryness, and decreased subcutaneous fat
Brown "age spots" (lentigo senilis) on exposed body parts (e.g., face, hands, arms)	Clustering of melanocytes (pigment-producing cells)
Decreased perspiration	Reduced number and function of sweat glands
Thinning and graying of scalp, pubic, and axillary hair	Progressive loss of pigment cells from the hair bulbs
Slower nail growth and increased thickening with ridges	Increased calcium deposition
Neuromuscular	
Decreased speed and power of skeletal muscle contractions	Decrease in muscle fibers
Slowed reaction time	Diminished conduction speed of nerve fibers and decreased muscle tone
Loss of height (stature)	Atrophy of intervertebral discs, increased flexion at hips and knees
Loss of bone mass	Bone reabsorption outpaces bone reformation
Joint stiffness	Drying and loss of elasticity in joint cartilage
Impaired balance	Decreased muscle strength, reaction time, and coordination, change in center of gravity
Greater difficulty in complex learning and abstraction	Fewer cells in cerebral cortex
Sensory/Perceptual	
Loss of visual acuity	Degeneration leading to lens opacity (cataracts), thickening, and inelasticity (presbyopia)
Increased sensitivity to glare and decreased ability to adjust to darkness	Changes in the ciliary muscles; rigid pupil sphincter; decrease in pupil size
Partial or complete glossy white circle around the periphery of the cornea (arcus senilis)	Fatty deposits
Progressive loss of hearing (presbycusis)	Changes in the structures and nerve tissues in the inner ear; thickening of the eardrum
Decreased sense of taste, especially the sweet sensations at the tip of the tongue	Decreased number of taste buds in the tongue because of tongue atrophy
Decreased sense of smell	Atrophy of the olfactory bulb at the base of the brain (responsible for smell perception)
Increased threshold for sensations of pain, touch, and temperature	Possible nerve conduction and neuron changes
Pulmonary	
Decreased ability to expel foreign or accumulated matter	Decreased elasticity and ciliary activity
Decreased lung expansion, less effective exhalation, reduced vital capacity, and increased residual volume	Weakened thoracic muscles; calcification of costal cartilage, making the rib cage more rigid with increased anterior-posterior diameter; dilation from inelasticity of alveoli
Difficult, short, heavy, rapid breathing (dyspnea) following intense exercise	Diminished delivery and diffusion of oxygen to the tissues to repay the normal oxygen debt because of exertion or changes in both respiratory and vascular tissues
Cardiovascular	
Reduced cardiac output and stroke volume, particularly during increased activity or unusual demands; may result in shortness of breath on exertion and pooling of blood in the extremities	Increased rigidity and thickness of heart valves (hence decreased filling/emptying abilities); decreased contractile strength
Reduced elasticity and increased rigidity of arteries	Increased calcium deposits in the muscular layer
Increase in diastolic and systolic blood pressure	Inelasticity of systemic arteries and increased peripheral resistance
Orthostatic hypertension	Reduced sensitivity of the blood pressure–regulating baroreceptors

TABLE 23–5 **Normal Physical Changes Associated with Aging—continued**	
PHYSICAL CHANGES	**RATIONALE**
Gastrointestinal	
Delayed swallowing time	Alterations in the swallowing mechanism
Increased tendency for indigestion	Gradual decrease in digestive enzymes, reduction in gastric pH, and slower absorption rate
Increased tendency for constipation	Decreased muscle tone of the intestines; decreased peristalsis; decreased free body fluid
Urinary	
Reduced filtering ability of the kidney and impaired renal function	Decreased number of functioning nephrons (basic functional units of the kidney) and arteriosclerotic changes in blood flow
Less effective concentration of urine	Decreased tubular function
Urinary urgency and urinary frequency	Enlarged prostate gland in men; weakened muscles supporting the bladder or weakness of the urinary sphincter in women
Tendency for nocturnal frequency and retention of residual urine	Decreased bladder capacity and tone
Genitals	
Prostate enlargement (benign) in men	Exact mechanism is unclear; possible endocrine changes
Multiple changes in women (shrinkage and atrophy of the vulva, cervix, uterus, fallopian tubes, and ovaries; reduction in secretions; and changes in vaginal flora)	Diminished secretion of female hormones and more alkaline vaginal pH
Increased time to sexual arousal	Changes in blood supply to penis, clitoris
Decreased firmness of erection, increased refractory period (men)	Changes in blood supply
Decreased vaginal lubrication and elasticity (women)	Loss of estrogen effects
Immunological	
Decreased immune response; lowered resistance to infections	T cells less responsive to antigens; B cells produce fewer antibodies
Poor response to immunization	Immune system changes may precipitate insulin resistance
Decreased stress response	
Endocrine	
Increased insulin resistance	Unclear mechanism
Decreased thyroid function	

Loss in overall stature occurs with age. This can be exaggerated by muscular weakness resulting in a stooping posture and **kyphosis** (humpback of the upper spine). Imbalance in the rates of absorption and formation of bone tissue occurs with aging, so that older adults have more porous and fragile bones than do younger adults, making elders prone to serious fractures. **Osteoporosis,** a pathologic decrease in bone density that is more common in older than younger adults, may lead to spontaneous (i.e., without a fall or other trauma to the bone) fractures that are called **pathologic fractures.** Osteoporosis occurs more frequently in people with insufficient intake of dietary calcium, in women after menopause, in Caucasians and Asians, and in individuals who are immobilized or physically inactive. Often considered a woman's disease, it is important to remember that osteoporosis affects men also (Curry & Hogstel, 2002).

Joints and their supporting structures change with age, including decreased elasticity, strength, and hydration of the tendons and ligaments, making movement stiffer and more restricted. Stiffness is aggravated by inactivity; for example, if a person sits too long, the joints become stiff, and the person has difficulty standing and walking. These changes may be compounded by osteoarthritis. A continual program of physical activity and proper nutrition will slow bone density loss and decrease muscle atrophy and stiffness (see Figure 23-1 ■).

As indicated, these age-related changes may affect the mobility and safety of the elder. For example, decreased muscle strength, decreased balance, and osteoporosis put the elder at risk for falls and fractures. For health promotion, the nurse assesses

Figure 23-1 ■ A regular program of exercise is important for maintenance of joint mobility and muscle tone and can promote socialization.

the musculoskeletal functioning of the elder and identifies any risk factors that may contribute to falls or the ability of the elder to perform ADLs. Health promotion interventions often include providing information about the risk factors for osteoporosis and the importance of adequate intake of calcium and vitamin D.

Sensory/Perceptual

Each of the five senses becomes less efficient in older adulthood. Changes in vision associated with aging include the obvious changes around the eye, such as the shrunken appearance of the eyes due to loss of orbital fat, the slowed blink reflex, and the looseness of the eyelids, particularly the lower lid, due to poorer muscle tone. Other changes result in loss of visual acuity, less power of adaptation to darkness and dim light, a decrease in accommodation to near and far objects, loss of peripheral vision, atrophy of lacrimal glands resulting in dry eyes, and difficulty in discriminating similar colors, especially blues, greens, and purples.

Presbyopia, the inability to focus or accommodate due to a loss of flexibility of the lens, causes a decrease in near vision. This generally starts around age 40. Visual acuity lessens gradually after age 50 and more rapidly after age 70 (Tabloski, 2006).

By the age of 80, nearly all elders have some lens opacity (**cataracts**) that reduces visual acuity and causes glare to be a problem. In addition to cataracts, three other conditions result in visual impairment and blindness in the elderly: age-related macular degeneration (ARMD), glaucoma, and diabetic retinopathy (Tabloski, 2006). It is important for the nurse to promote health by informing elders to schedule routine eye examinations to maintain and protect their vision. Also, wearing sunglasses will help avoid the damaging effect of ultraviolet light.

The loss of hearing ability related to aging, called **presbycusis,** affects people over age 65. Gradual loss of hearing is more common among men than women, perhaps because men are more frequently in noisy work environments. Hearing loss is greater in the higher frequencies than the lower. Thus older adults with hearing loss usually hear speakers with low, distinct voices best. Hard consonants (e.g., *k, d, t*) and long vowel sounds (e.g., *ay, ee*) are more easily recognized, and sibilant sounds (*s, th, f*) are the most difficult to hear. Elders may have more difficulty compensating for hearing loss than the young, who pay closer attention to the lip movements of the speaker.

If family members notice communication problems or social withdrawal of the elder, the nurse should provide health promotion teaching by suggesting that the elder be referred for hearing screening. Also, the elder's ears should be checked for impacted earwax. If hearing has diminished, assistive listening devices are available and the nurse can provide information to the elder and family. To help avoid increased hearing loss, inform the elder to use ear protection devices when working in or around activities that give off loud noise.

Older people have a poorer sense of taste and smell and are less stimulated by food than the young. It is common for the sense of smell to decline more than the sense of taste. These changes significantly affect appetite in the elder, contributing to poor nutrition. Decreased or absent sense of smell and taste also

add to the health hazard of increased salt usage and safety issues (e.g., being unable to smell a gas leak). It is important for the nurse to teach the elder and family about the safety issues involved with a decreased sense of taste and smell and what strategies can be implemented to promote the elder's safety (e.g., dating and labeling foods, using smoke alarms).

Loss of skin receptors takes place gradually, producing an increased threshold for sensations of pain, touch, and temperature. The older person may not be able to distinguish hot from cold or the intensity of heat. Stimuli causing severe pain in a younger person may cause only minor sensation or pressure in elders. This places the older adult at higher risk for burns and other injuries. Again, it is important for the nurse to teach about the involved safety risks and subsequent interventions (e.g., setting the temperature of the water heater to 110°F to prevent scalding).

Pulmonary

Respiratory efficiency is reduced with age. Tidal volume (the amount of air moved in and out during normal respiration) remains the same, but the older adult has a decreased vital capacity. This means the older adult is unable to compensate for increased oxygen need by significantly increasing the amount of air inspired. **Dyspnea** (difficult breathing) occurs frequently with increased activity, such as running for a bus or carrying heavy parcels upstairs. A greater volume of residual air is left in the lungs after expiration, and the capacity to cough efficiently decreases because of weaker expiratory muscles. Mucous secretions tend to collect more readily in the respiratory tree. Thus susceptibility to respiratory infections increases in elders.

Health promotion teaching includes information about the following:

- Cessation of smoking, if appropriate
- Preventing respiratory infections by washing hands
- Ensuring the influenza and pneumonia vaccinations are up to date

Cardiovascular

The working capacity of the heart diminishes with age. This is particularly evident when increased demands are made on the heart, such as during periods of exercise or emotional stress. The heart rate at normal rest may decrease with age. However, the heart rate of the older person is slower to respond to stress and slower to return to normal after periods of physical activity.

Changes in the arteries occur concurrently. Reduced arterial elasticity may result in diminished blood supply to, for instance, the legs and the brain, resulting in pain on exertion in the calf muscles and dizziness, respectively. In addition, there may be a delay in the circulatory adjustments required when a person quickly stands up from a lying or sitting position. The delay results in an abrupt drop in systolic blood pressure known as *orthostatic hypotension.*

For blood pressure measurements, it is not unusual to have a slight increase in the systolic pressure while the diastolic pressure remains the same. For many years, isolated systolic hypertension was considered to be "normal" in elders, and was frequently not treated. Newer evidence indicates that a systolic pressure of greater than 140 mm Hg is as problematic in older adults as in younger ones, and should be as aggressively treated (Joint National Committee on Prevention, Detection, Evaluation, and Treatment of High Blood Pressure [JNC 7], 2003). A significant increase in blood pressure is more likely the result of other factors such as diet, weight, or stress rather than age (Polan & Taylor, 2003, p. 231).

Health promotion activities involve detecting and reducing risks for cardiovascular disease. To detect risks, the elder should have his or her blood pressure checked annually. The elder should be aware of his or her cholesterol level and have it rechecked at appropriate intervals, depending on the results of the blood test (e.g., the higher the level, the more frequently it should be rechecked). To reduce risks of cardiovascular disease, the nurse should inform the elder about the importance of the following: smoking cessation (if applicable), maintaining ideal body weight, exercising daily, avoiding foods high in sodium and fat and eating fruits and vegetables, and discussing the use of low-dose aspirin therapy with the elder's primary provider (Miller, 2004).

Gastrointestinal

Age-related changes in the gastrointestinal system include:

- Periodontal disease, which can lead to tooth loss. With age, tooth enamel becomes harder and more brittle, making teeth more susceptible to fractures. The root of the tooth shrinks and the gingival retracts. The bones that support the teeth decrease in density and height, all leading to tooth loss (Eliopoulos, 2005, p. 55).
- Reduced saliva which may lead to xerostomia (dry mouth) and make the oral mucosa of the elder more susceptible to infection.
- Decreased esophageal motility slowing the esophageal emptying process.
- Decreased stomach motility and emptying time. Also, a higher pH of the stomach contributes to increased incidence of gastric irritation in the elderly.
- Decreased production of intrinsic factor leading to pernicious anemia.
- Decreased intestinal absorption, motility, and blood flow.

Health promotion teaching for elders includes effective oral hygiene and preventive dental care (e.g., semiannual teeth cleaning). Nutrition is important including appropriate diet, as needed by the elder, and sufficient fluid intake. Maintenance of a regular bowel routine is helpful, and screening for colorectal cancer is important (e.g., annual fecal occult blood test, sigmoidoscopy every 5 years, and colonoscopy every 10 years) (Meiner & Lueckenotte, 2006, p. 563).

Urinary

The excretory function of the kidney diminishes with age, but usually not significantly below normal levels unless a disease process intervenes. The kidney's filtering abilities may also be impaired; thus waste products may be filtered and excreted more slowly. For this reason, the nurse should be aware of whether medications that are administered are excreted via the kidney or liver. Drugs that are metabolized predominantly in the kidney may accumulate in the older adult, and the nurse needs to watch for signs of toxicity.

More noticeable changes are those related to the bladder. Complaints of urinary urgency and urinary frequency are common. The capacity of the bladder and its ability to completely empty diminish with age. Many elders need to arise during the night to void (nocturia) and may experience retention of residual urine, predisposing the elderly adult to bladder infections.

Although elders are susceptible to urinary incontinence (UI) because of changes in the kidney and bladder, UI is *never* normal. The nurse must promptly investigate UI, particularly when of new onset. Urinary incontinence has many ill effects on older adults, including social isolation, falls, and skin breakdown.

The nurse can teach the following health promotion activities for good urinary function in the elder:

- Drink sufficient fluids daily (e.g., 8 to 10 glasses of non-caffeinated liquid).
- Drink fluids even if you do not feel thirsty. (The thirst mechanism in elders is diminished.)
- Avoid foods that can irritate the bladder (e.g., sugar, caffeine, alcohol, chocolate, artificial sweeteners, and spicy and acidic foods).
- Practice pelvic muscle exercises to stop or control stress incontinence.

The nurse should explain that incontinence is not a normal change related to aging.

Genitals

Degenerative changes in the gonads are gradual in men. Production of testosterone continues, and the testes can produce sperm well into old age although there is a gradual decrease in the number of sperm produced. In women the degenerative changes in the ovaries are noticed by the cessation of menses in middle age during the menopause.

Changes in the gonads of older women result from diminished secretion of the ovarian hormones. Some changes, such as the shrinking of the uterus and ovaries, go unnoticed. Other changes are obvious. The breasts atrophy, and lubricating vaginal secretions are reduced. Reduced natural lubrication may be the cause of painful intercourse, which may be addressed through the use of lubricating jellies.

The elder man will notice several age-related changes in his sexual response and performance, but it is important for both the client and nurse to know that sexual response and performance should be present in the older adult. For both men and women, the major age-related change in sexual response is timing: it takes longer to become sexually aroused, longer to complete intercourse, and longer before sexual arousal can occur again (Butler & Lewis, 2003). In general, the elder man's libido may decrease, but not disappear. If an elder man reports a loss in sexual interest, the nurse should be as concerned as when a younger man reports a loss of interest in sexual activity. Elder men achieve an erection that is less firm than in younger men, but still capable of penetration. Ejaculation may take longer to occur, and the older man may have difficulty anticipating or delaying ejaculation.

Elder women also experience changes in their sexual responses. It takes longer for the elder woman to become sexually aroused and produce vaginal lubrication, and the labia and uterus do not fully elevate, making penetration slightly more difficult (Butler & Lewis, 2003). The clitoris remains an important part of orgasm, but may become irritated more easily because the clitoral hood is less protective than in younger women. During orgasm, the uterus will contract less frequently, but the contractions remain vigorous, and orgasm is as intense as in younger women.

The nurse needs excellent communication skills when providing health education about sexual function in the elderly. A survey of elders found that they prefer that the health care professional use open, respectful, nonjudgmental, and plain English when discussing sexuality (Miller, 2004, p. 488). Elders are fully capable of enjoying sexual activity. If they experience problems with sexual function, they should seek professional advice from their primary care provider or other appropriate health care professional.

PSYCHOSOCIAL AGING

A number of theories have attempted to explain psychosocial aging. These theories focus on behavior and attitude changes during the aging process. One of the earliest, **disengagement theory,** developed in the early 1960s by Cumming and Henry, proposed that aging involves mutual withdrawal (disengagement) between the older person and others in the elderly person's environment. It has been widely criticized for the assumptions that disengagement is appropriate for the older adult. According to Havighurst's **activity theory,** the best way to age is to stay active physically and mentally, and according to Atchley's **continuity theory,** people maintain their values, habits, and behavior in old age. A person who is accustomed to having people around will continue to do so, and the person who prefers not to be involved with others is more likely to disengage. This theory accounts for the great variety of behavior seen in elderly people.

According to Erikson, the developmental task at this time is ego integrity versus despair. People who attain ego integrity view life with a sense of wholeness and derive satisfaction from past accomplishments. They view death as an acceptable completion of life. People who develop integrity accept "one's one and only life cycle" (Erikson, 1963, p. 263). By contrast, people who despair often believe they have made poor choices during life and wish they could live life over.

Acknowledging that the "young-old" and "old-old" differ not only in physical characteristics but also in psychosocial responses, many people have difficulty with Erikson's singular developmental task. Peck (1968) proposed the following three developmental tasks of the elder in contrast to Erikson's task of ego integrity versus despair:

1. Ego differentiation versus work-role preoccupation
2. Body transcendence versus body preoccupation
3. Ego transcendence versus ego preoccupation

For details about these tasks see Chapter 20. ∞ See Box 23–3 for further developmental tasks of the older adult.

BOX 23–3 **Developmental Tasks of the Elder**

65 TO 75 YEARS
- Adjusting to decreasing physical strength and health
- Adjusting to retirement and lower and fixed income
- Adjusting to the death of parents, spouses, and friends
- Adjusting to new relationships with adult children
- Adjusting to leisure time
- Adjusting to slower physical and cognitive responses
- Keeping active and involved
- Making satisfying living arrangements as aging progresses

75 YEARS AND OLDER
- Adapting to living alone
- Safeguarding physical and mental health
- Adjusting to the possibility of moving into a nursing home
- Remaining in touch with other family members
- Finding meaning in life
- Adjusting to one's own death

Note: From *Health Promotion Strategies Through the Life Span,* 7th ed., by R. B. Murray & J. P. Zentner, 2001, Upper Saddle River, NJ: Prentice Hall.

Retirement

A majority of the people in the United States over age 65 are unemployed (FIFAS, 2004). However, many who are healthy continue to work on a full- or part-time basis. Work offers these people a better income, a sense of self-worth, and the chance to continue long-established routines. It is important to remember that setting the retirement age at 65 is arbitrary and has no relationship to the abilities of the worker. Also, some elders need to work for economic reasons. Retirement usually causes income to decrease by 35% or more (Meiner & Lueckenotte, 2006, p. 143). Elders may find that their retirement income has not kept up with inflation. They may also realize that they need to continue working to meet medical and insurance costs.

Retirement can be a time when projects or recreational activities deferred for a long time can be pursued, or it can be a difficult time of adjustment. Either way, retirement requires a process of adaptation (see Figure 23-2 ■). Retired people are no longer gov-

Figure 23-2 ■ Many elders find creative outlets during retirement.

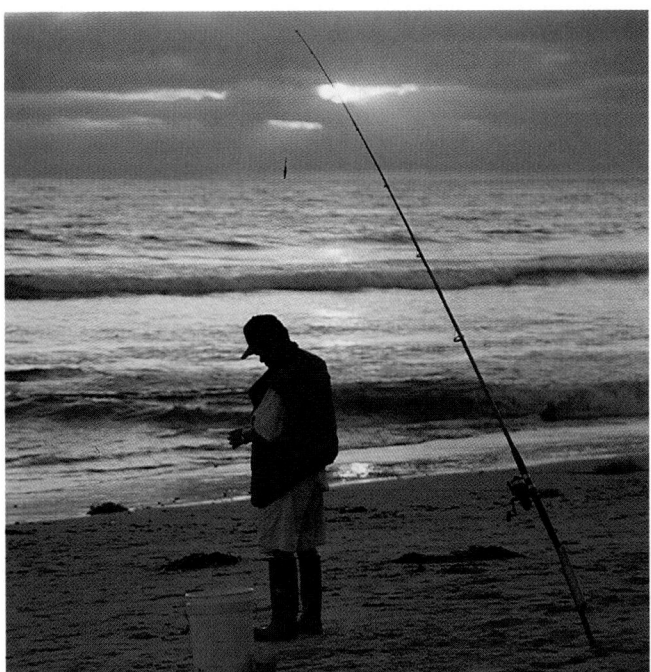

Figure 23-3 ■ Retirement provides time for enjoying hobbies.

erned by an alarm clock and can get up when they please. The enjoyment of staying up later is another luxury. Few elders, however, spend much time resting or sleeping. Being accustomed to activity most of their lives, most elders find many outlets, including jobs, community projects, travel, volunteer services, intellectual or recreational pursuits, or hobbies (Figure 23-3 ■).

The lifestyle of later years is to a large degree formulated in youth. This fact was recognized by the poet Robert Browning: "Grow old along with me! / The best is yet to be, / The last of life, for which the first was made." People who attempt suddenly to refocus and enrich their lives at retirement usually have difficulty. Those who learned early in life to live well-balanced and fulfilling lives are generally more successful in retirement. The woman who has been concerned only with the accomplishments of her children or the man who has been concerned only with the paycheck and his job status can be left with a feeling of emptiness when children leave and the job no longer exists. The later years can foster a sense of integrity and continuity, or they can be years of despair.

Economic Change

The financial needs of elders vary considerably (FIFAS, 2004). Though most need less money for clothing, entertainment, and work, and although some own their homes outright, costs continue to rise, making it difficult for some to manage. Food and medical costs alone are often a financial burden. Adequate financial resources enable the older person to remain independent.

Problems with income are often related to low retirement benefits, lack of pension plans for many workers, and the increased length of the retirement years. Older members of minority groups often have greater financial problems than older whites (FIFAS, 2004). Older women of all ages usually have lower incomes than men, and the oldest women may be the poorest.

Nurses should be aware of the costs of health care. For example, while assisting a client to plan a diet, the nurse must consider which foods the client can afford to buy. The nurse or the client can request the physician to order lower priced medications, or assist the older client to apply for medication assistance programs operated by pharmaceutical companies. In addition, the supplies used in a client's care should be as economical as possible.

Grandparenting

Grandparents traditionally provide gifts, money, and other forms of support (e.g., baby-sitting) for younger family members. They also provide a sense of continuity, family heritage, rituals, and folklore (Ebersole, Hess, Touhy, & Jett, 2005). However, the rate of grandparents being the primary caregiver for their grandchildren is increasing. The major reasons for grandparents raising grandchildren include substance abuse, incarceration, teen pregnancy, emotional problems, and parental death (Butler & Zakari, 2005).

While loving their grandchildren, the grandparents often experience stress, anxiety, financial hardships, and potential deteriorating health. For example, they must cope with their own chronic health problems while caring for their grandchildren. It is important for nurses to assess and help maintain the health of the grandparents.

Relocation

During late adulthood, many people experience relocation. A variety of factors may lead to this decision. The house or apartment may be too large or too expensive. The work involved in maintaining the house may become burdensome or impossible for the aged person or couple. Some elders with decreased mobility want living arrangements that are all on one floor or need more accessible bathroom facilities.

Making the decision to move is stressful. Moving to an apartment may mean leaving the comfort of the family home and the neighbors and friends of several decades. Some elders need to move nearer to their children for general support and supervision. For many, this decision is difficult and stressful. For others, relocation is voluntary. The person may be seeking a more moderate climate with better recreational facilities geared to a more leisurely lifestyle. Adjustment will be much easier for the elder making a voluntary move.

More living choices and options are available for the older adult today. Depending on their needs, examples include:

- *Assisted living.* This is a facility that meets the needs of the older person (e.g., wide doorways, grab bars in the bathroom, a call light). Various degrees of personal care assistance may be provided.
- *Adult day care.* The older adult who lives at home can attend a day-care center that provides health and social services to the older person. While the older adult is at day care, the caregiver has a respite from the daily care.
- *Adult foster care and group homes.* These programs offer services to individuals who can care for themselves but require some form of supervision for safety purposes.

Some elders, however, must relocate to long-term care facilities or nursing homes. The decision to enter a nursing home is frequently made when elders can no longer care for themselves, often because of problems of mobility and memory impairment. The facilities in nursing homes differ in many ways and offer varying degrees of independence to the residents. All provide meals but vary in giving other services, such as assistance with hygiene and dressing, physical therapy or exercise, recreational activities, transportation services, and medical and nursing supervision.

Nurses in hospitals should find out whether a client is being discharged to a nursing home or to a private home. Nursing homes require appropriate information to provide for continuity of care. Clients returning home, however, may require the assistance of a home care nurse.

Maintaining Independence and Self-Esteem

Most American elders thrive on independence. It is important to them to be able to look after themselves even if they have to struggle to do so. Although it may be difficult for younger family members to watch an older person completing tasks in a slow, determined way, elders need this sense of accomplishment. Children might notice that the aging father or mother with failing vision cannot keep the kitchen as clean as before. The aging parent may be slower and less meticulous in carpentry tasks or gardening. To maintain the elder's sense of self-respect, nurses and family members need to encourage them to do as much as possible for themselves, provided that safety is maintained. Many young people, including nurses, mistakenly think that they are helpful to elders when they take over for them and do the job much faster and more efficiently.

Nurses need to acknowledge the elder's ability to think, reason, and make decisions. Most elders are willing to listen to suggestions and advice, but they do not want to be ordered around. The nurse can support a decision by an elder even if eventually the decision is reversed because of failing health.

Elders appreciate the same thoughtfulness, consideration, and acceptance of their abilities as younger people do. They are not "wrinkled babies," and certainly do not represent a homogeneous group. There is as much diversity among older adults as there is in any other population group, and the nurse should be just as wary of stereotyping elders as with stereotyping any other group. The values and standards held by older people need to be accepted, whether they are related to ethical, religious, or household matters. For example, the nurse should respect an older person's decision to hang the laundry outside rather than to use a dryer, or to cook on a conventional stove rather than in a microwave oven.

Facing Death and Grieving

Well-adjusted aging couples usually thrive on companionship. Many couples rely increasingly on their partners for this company and may have few outside friends. Great bonds of affection and closeness can develop during this period of aging together and nurturing each other. When a mate dies, the remaining part-ner inevitably experiences feelings of loss, emptiness, and loneliness. Many are capable of living alone and can manage to do so; however, reliance on younger family members may increase as age advances and ill health occurs. Some widows and widowers remarry, particularly the latter because most widowers are less inclined than widows to maintain a household.

More women than men face bereavement and solitude because women usually live longer (FIFAS, 2004). Elders are often reminded of the brevity of life by the death of friends. It is a time when they review their life with happiness or regret. Feelings of serenity or guilt and inadequacy can arise. Independence established prior to loss of a partner makes this adjustment period easier. A person who has some meaningful friendships, economic security, ongoing interests in the community, private hobbies, and a peaceful philosophy of life copes more easily with bereavement. Successful relationships with children and grandchildren are also of inestimable value. See Chapter 43 ∞ for a discussion about facing death.

Nurses help clients who are alone a great deal to adjust to their living arrangements or lifestyle so that they have more companionship. Moving to a retirement home that has other people in similar circumstances and organized social activities is one example. Many communities provide social centers for the elders, for example, drop-in centers or community centers that offer day trips for seniors. Nurses refer clients to services and encourage them to obtain companionship.

COGNITIVE ABILITIES AND AGING

Piaget's phases of cognitive development end with the formal operations phase. However, considerable research on cognitive abilities and aging is currently being conducted. Intellectual capacity includes perception, cognitive agility, memory, and learning.

Perception

Perception, or the ability to interpret the environment, depends on the acuteness of the senses. If the aging person's senses are impaired, the ability to perceive the environment and react appropriately is diminished. Changes in the nervous system may also affect perceptual capacity.

Changes in the cognitive structures occur as a person ages. The brain loses mass with aging. In addition, blood flow to the brain decreases, the meninges thicken, and brain metabolism slows. As yet, little is known about the effect of these physical changes on the cognitive functioning of the older adult. Lifelong mental activity, particularly verbal activity, helps the elder retain a high level of cognitive function and helps maintain long-term memory.

Cognitive Ability

In elders, changes in cognitive abilities are more often a difference in speed than in ability. Overall the older adult maintains intelligence, problem solving, judgment, creativity, and other well-practiced cognitive skills. Intellectual loss generally reflects a disease process such as atherosclerosis, which causes the blood vessels to narrow and diminishes perfusion of nutrients to the brain. Most elders do not experience cognitive impairments, with only

15% of older men and 11% of older women manifesting moderate or severe memory impairment (FIFAS, 2004). It is important to note, however, that memory impairment is more prevalent in persons over age 85 than persons between the ages of 65 and 69. Cognitive impairment that interferes with normal life is not considered part of normal aging. A decline in intellectual abilities that interferes with social or occupational functions should always be regarded as abnormal. Family members should be advised to seek prompt medical evaluation.

Memory

Memory is also a component of intellectual capacity that involves the following steps:

1. Momentary perception of stimuli from the environment referred to as **sensory memory.**
2. Storage in **short-term memory** (information held in the brain for immediate use or what one has in mind at a given moment). An example of this type of memory is when you call information for a telephone number and remember the number only for the brief time needed to dial the number. Short-term memory also deals with activities or the recent past of minutes to a few hours that is often referred to as **recent memory.**
3. Encoding in which the information leaves short-term memory and enters **long-term memory,** the repository for information stored for periods longer than 72 hours and usually weeks and years. Memories of childhood friends, teachers, and events are stored in long-term memory. Older people who remember the flowers in their wedding bouquet or the names of the boys on their dance card are drawing from long-term memory.

In elders, retrieval of information from long-term memory can be slower, especially if the information is not frequently used. Most age-related differences, however, occur in short-term memory. Older adults tend to forget the recent past. This forgetfulness can be improved by the use of memory aids, making notes or lists, and placing objects in consistent locations.

Learning

Older people need additional time for learning, largely because of the problem of retrieving information. Motivation is also important. Older adults have more difficulty than younger ones in learning information they do not consider meaningful; therefore, the nurse should be particularly careful to discover what is meaningful to the older adult before attempting client education. See Chapter 27. ∞

MORAL REASONING

Much of the theoretical and empirical work related to moral development in elders was conducted in the 1980s, and few current studies can be found. According to Kohlberg (1984), moral development is completed in the early adult years. Kohlberg hypothesized that an older person at the preconventional level obeys rules to avoid pain and the displeasure of others. At stage 1, a person defines good and bad in relation to self, whereas older people at stage 2 may act to meet another's needs as well as their own. Elders at the conventional level follow society's rules of conduct in response to the expectations of others. Pratt, Diessner, Pratt, Hunsberger, and Pancer (1996) found that moral reasoning does not decline in old age.

Gilligan (1982), however, challenged Kohlberg's stages as not being applicable to women. She developed a theory of moral reasoning based on the concept of caring. She believed that women base moral judgments on connectedness to others and the value of relationships, while Kohlberg based his stages on concepts of justice, objectivity, and preservation of rights. Subsequent research has demonstrated that men and women do make moral decisions differently, and represent Kohlberg (men) and Gilligan (women) along gender lines. Older adults, however, begin to make moral decisions that are consistent with *both* Kohlberg and Gilligan (Pinch & Parsons, 1997). Older men consider relationships, as well as justice, in moral decisions, and older women add justice to the factors they consider in moral situations.

The value and belief patterns that are important to elders may be different from those held by younger people because they developed during a time that was very different from today. In addition, a large number of today's elders are either foreign-born or first-generation citizens. Cultural background, life experiences, gender, religion, and socioeconomic status all influence one's values. The nurse must identify and consider the specific values of the older client when nursing care is planned.

SPIRITUALITY AND AGING

Elders can contemplate new religious and philosophical views and try to understand ideas missed previously or interpreted differently. The older person may derive a sense of worth by sharing experiences or views. In contrast, the older adult who has not matured spiritually may feel impoverishment or despair as the drive for economic and professional success lessens.

Many elders take their faith and religious practice very seriously, and display a high level of spirituality. It would be a mistake, however, to assume that religiosity increases with age. Today's elders grew up in a time when religion was much more important than it is for younger people today. The participation of older adults in religious organizations, therefore, is more likely to be a continuation of lifelong habits than a correlate of aging (McFadden, 1996). Many older people have strong religious convictions and continue to attend religious meetings or services. Involvement in religion often helps the older adult to resolve issues related to the meaning of life, to adversity, or to good fortune. Religion may also be an important coping resource, leading to enhanced well-being. The "old-old" person who cannot attend formal services often continues religious participation in a more private manner. Assisting the older person to participate in religious and spiritual practices is an important nursing responsibility.

HEALTH PROBLEMS

Health problems that older adults may experience include injuries, chronic disabling disease such as hypertension and arthritis, drug abuse and misuse, alcoholism, dementia, and abuse. Leading causes of death in people ages 65 and over are heart disease, cancer, cerebrovascular disease (stroke), lower respiratory disease, pneumonia/influenza, and diabetes mellitus (FIFAS, 2004).

Injuries

Injury prevention is a major concern for older people. *Healthy People 2010* (USDHHS, 2000) reports that falls account for 87% of all fractures among adults 65 years and older (pp. 13–15). Because vision is limited, reflexes are slowed, and bones are brittle, caution is required in climbing stairs, driving a car, and even walking. Driving, particularly night driving, requires caution because accommodation of the eye to light is impaired and peripheral vision is diminished. Older persons need to learn to turn the head before changing lanes and should not rely on side vision, for example, when crossing a street. Driving in fog or other hazardous conditions should be avoided.

Fires are a hazard for the elder with a failing memory. Elders may forget that the iron or stove is left on or may not extinguish a cigarette completely. Because of reduced sensitivity to pain and heat, care must be taken to prevent burns when the person bathes or uses heating devices.

Many elders suffer and die each year from hypothermia. **Hypothermia** is a body temperature below normal. A lowered metabolism and loss of normal insulation from thinning subcutaneous tissue decrease the older client's ability to retain heat. The elder who spends time outdoors in cold weather, or who does not turn on the heat in the home is at significant risk for hypothermia.

Nurses can help elders make the home environment safe by identifying and correcting specific hazards; for example, installing handrails on staircases. The nurse teaches the importance of taking only prescribed medications and contacting a health professional at the first indication of intolerance to them.

Persons with Alzheimer's disease or other types of dementia experience increasing safety needs as their condition deteriorates. Judgment becomes impaired as the disease progresses, and some environmental modification is needed to help the older adult remain safe. Some of these are keeping poisons and medications out of reach (preferably locked up), taking knobs off kitchen stoves to prevent burns and fires, and putting special locks on doors for persons who tend to wander. Attention should be given to these potential problems whether the client lives at home or is in a health facility.

Guidelines for injury prevention for the older adult are detailed in Chapter 32. ∞

Chronic Disabling Illness

Many older adults function well within the community without impairments; others are afflicted with one or more chronic illnesses that may seriously impair their functioning. Examples of these are arthritis, osteoporosis, heart disease, stroke, obstructive lung disease, hearing and visual alterations, and cognitive dysfunctions. In addition, acute illnesses such as pneumonia, fractures, trauma from falls, motor vehicle crashes, or other incidents may create chronic health problems. Chronic illness brings many changes to the client and the family members. The client, for ex-

---

RESEARCH NOTE   How Do You Take Away the Car Keys?

The issue of older drivers is a troublesome one. Driving is an important aspect of autonomy, and cherished by many older adults; yet there are concerns for the safety of the older driver as well as for others on the road. Nurses may be asked to assist family members to convince an elder to stop driving.

The researchers studied interventions used to stop cognitively impaired elders from driving. Older adults with mild cognitive impairment, family members of such adults, and professionals in elder care (n = 216) were interviewed about the decision to stop an elder from driving, and the ways used to enforce the decision. The data were qualitatively analyzed using a grounded theory methodology. There was more agreement than disagreement among those interviewed. Unsafe behaviors that the participants identified included getting lost easily, being less aware of other drivers and pedestrians, and forgetting how to use equipment, such as brakes, in the car. Themes related to an increased likelihood that cognitively impaired elders continued to drive included a desire to drive, availability of a car, lack of alternative transportation, and the willingness of someone to ride with the impaired elder and "co-pilot." Strategies to keep the impaired older adult from driving fell into two main categories: those that included the elder in the decision-making process, and those that were imposed by professionals or significant others. Involving the elder in the decision making is an important nursing goal, but a restriction may need to be imposed for safety reasons. Factors that facilitate a successful intervention include a strong relationship between the elder,

primary care provider, and family members, and the obviousness of the driving impairment including "near misses."

Participants in the study identified the following strategies that family members can initiate, with coaching by the primary care provider:

- Begin to discuss the possibility of giving up driving before safety is a concern.
- Observe the older adult's driving abilities, and point out specific driving errors in a nonjudgmental way.
- Acknowledge that giving up driving is a loss for the older adult.
- Develop a feasible plan for alternative transportation.
- Point out the possibility of harming someone, or of possible legal action and financial repercussions.
- Have the older adult tested for driving safety. State and local agencies may be helpful in identifying sites that will specifically test for driving safety in relation to cognitive impairment.

IMPLICATIONS

Both the autonomy of the older adult and the safety of the older adult and others are nursing concerns. Anticipatory guidance may help ease the transition from independent mobility to collaborative mobility with alternative transportation.

Note: Reprinted from *Geriatric Nursing,* vol. 26, by K. Jett, R. M. Tappen, and M. Rosselli, "Imposed Versus Involved: Different Strategies to Effect Driving Cessation in Cognitively Impaired Older Adults," pp. 111–116. Copyright 2005, with permission from Elsevier.

ample, may need increasing help with the activities of daily living such as ambulation, feeding, hygiene, and so on; health care expenses often escalate and may become an economic concern; family roles may need to be altered; and family members may need to change their lifestyle to meet caregiving needs.

Drug Use and Misuse

The average elder in the United States takes four to five prescription drugs and two over-the-counter OTC medicines every day. Episodes of acute illness may require additional medications. Clients may purchase OTC drugs to remedy common discomforts related to aging, such as constipation, sleep disturbance, and joint pain. Over the last few years, the use of vitamins, food supplements, and herbal remedies has increased. These agents fall under the category of OTC drugs and are often not reported by clients as part of their medicine regimen. An accurate assessment should include a listing of all these agents. Many of these agents have not had adequate testing for effectiveness, side effects, or interactions with other medications.

The complexities involved in the self-administration of medication may lead to a variety of misuse situations, including taking too much or too little medication, combining alcohol and medication, combining prescribed medications with OTC drugs, taking medications at the wrong time, or taking someone else's medication. Other potential misuse situations occur when more than one primary care provider prescribes medications and the client fails to tell each primary care provider what has been previously prescribed.

Additionally, the pharmacodynamics of drugs are altered in older adults. The variations in absorption, distribution, metabolism, and excretion of drugs are related to physiologic changes associated with aging. These variations are discussed in Chapter 35. ∞

Most elders living independently in the community take their medications with no supervision. Therefore, education about medications is important for safe medication-taking behaviors (Miller, 2004). The following strategies, taught by the nurse, can promote safe medication use by the elder:

- Write a list of all the medications you are taking, including over-the-counter drugs and herbal supplements. Include any medication allergies on the list. Keep the list current and carry it in your purse or billfold.
- Know the reason you are taking each medication. Ask your primary care practitioner the reason for any new medication.
- Consider using a "pill organizer" system to help you remember to take your medications. This is helpful if you have many medications to take each day.
- Ask your pharmacist for easy-to-open containers if you have difficulty opening the medications.
- If possible, obtain all medications from the same pharmacy. This allows the pharmacist to monitor for drug duplications and interactions.

Alcoholism

There are two types of older alcoholics: those who began drinking alcohol in their youth and those who began excessive alcohol use later in life to help them cope with the changes and problems of their older years. Many late-onset alcoholics are widowers.

Chronic drinking has major effects on all body systems, causes progressive liver and kidney damage, damages the stomach and related organs, and slows mental response, frequently leading to injuries and death. Alcohol interacts with various drugs, altering the normal effect of the medication on the body. Some medications have an increased effect when taken with alcohol (e.g., anticoagulants and narcotics), whereas the action of other medications (e.g., antibiotics) is inhibited. For the older adult who has a chronic illness and takes many medications, the combination of drugs and alcohol can lead to serious drug overdose.

Clients who are alcoholics should not be stereotyped or prejudged by the nurse. Rather, they should be accepted, listened to, and offered help. The nurse should assess the number and type of alcoholic beverages consumed as well as the pattern and frequency of consumption. It is important that the nurse discuss any medications the client is taking and review the side effects and interaction effects of alcohol and medication. The role of the nurse is to act as a client advocate and facilitate the treatment of the drinking problem in addition to the prevention of possible complications.

Dementia

Dementia is a progressive loss of cognitive function. It is critical that dementia be differentiated from delirium, an acute and reversible syndrome. Both may be characterized by changes in memory, judgment, language, mathematic calculation, abstract reasoning, and problem-solving ability. The most common causes of delirium are infection, medications, and dehydration. The most common type of dementia is Alzheimer's disease (AD), although there are other dementias. The cause of Alzheimer's disease is unknown, and the course is slow and insidious. Alzheimer's disease affects about 3 million people in the United States. Unless a prevention or cure is found, 14 million Americans will have Alzheimer's disease by the year 2050 (Agency on Aging, 2004).

The symptoms of AD may vary somewhat from client to client. The most prominent symptoms are cognitive dysfunctions, including decline in memory, learning, attention, judgment, orientation, and language skills. The symptoms are progressive and exhibit a steady decline in cognitive and physical abilities, lasting between 7 and 15 years and ending in death. In the last stage, the client requires total assistance, is unable to communicate, is incontinent, and may be unable to walk. There is no cure or specific treatment for AD. Several drugs have been developed, but none has been shown consistently to reverse the progression of the disease.

It is estimated that about 1 million people with AD are cared for in the home. The burden of care is frequently on women—wives and daughters—who are themselves aging. AD is devastating for the families and caregivers of its victims. The caregivers may experience physical and emotional exhaustion while they render continuous care. Caregiving is complicated when the client no longer recognizes family members or close

MediaLink

Alzheimer's Disease Video

DRUG CAPSULE **Parasympathomimetic or** **donepezil (Aricept)**
Cholinesterase Inhibitor

THE CLIENT WITH ALZHEIMER'S DISEASE (AD)

Cholinesterase inhibitors improve cholinergic function by inhibiting acetylcholinesterase; thus, increasing the amount of acetylcholine in the brain.

In normal brain function, acetylcholine is an essential neurotransmitter and plays an important role in cognitive function, including memory storage and retrieval (Abrams, 2004, p. 298).

Cholinesterase inhibitors do not alter Alzheimer's disease but may stabilize the elder at the current level of dementia and/or lessen symptoms for a short period of time (e.g., average of 6 months).

NURSING RESPONSIBILITIES

■ Assess cognitive ability of the client.
■ Monitor heart rate as bradycardia may occur.

CLIENT AND FAMILY TEACHING

■ Explain that donepezil may cause dizziness and the client may want to take the medication in the evening before going to bed.
■ Teach that the medication can be taken with or without food.

■ Emphasize the importance of taking the medication every day. A missed dose should be skipped, and the client should return to the regular schedule the next day.
■ Explain that the medication is started at a lower dose with a gradual increase in dosage. Higher doses may not increase the effects but may increase the side effects (gastrointestinal disturbance, sleep disturbance, and sedation).

Note: Prior to administering any medication, review all aspects with a current drug handbook or other reliable source.

---

friends. The nurse's responsibility is to provide supportive nursing care, accurate information, and referral assistance, if placement in a nursing care facility becomes necessary. Respite services may also be very helpful to the caregiver. It is important for the nurse to do an ongoing assessment of both the client and the caregiver, because changes will occur as the client's condition deteriorates.

Elder Mistreatment

Approximately 1 million to 2 million Americans over the age of 65 have been abused, neglected, or exploited (National Research Council Panel to Review Risk and Prevalence of Elder Abuse and Neglect, 2003). Elder mistreatment may affect either sex; however, the victims most often are women over 75 years of age, physically or mentally impaired, and dependent for care on the abuser. The abuse may involve physical, psychologic, or emotional abuse; sexual abuse; financial abuse; violation of human or civil rights; and active or passive neglect.

When elder mistreatment involves physical neglect, victims may suffer from dehydration, malnutrition, and oversedation. The victim may be deprived of necessary articles, such as glasses, hearing aids, or walkers. Psychologically, the person may suffer verbal assaults, threats, humiliation, or harassment. Abuse may also include failure to provide appropriate medications or medical treatment, isolation, unreasonable confinement, lack of privacy, an unsafe environment, and involuntary servitude. Some are financially exploited by relatives who steal from them or misuse their property or funds. Others are beaten and even raped by family members. Most victims experience two or more forms of abuse.

Elder abuse or neglect may occur in private homes, senior citizens' homes, nursing homes, hospitals, and long-term care facilities. Many of the abusers are either sons or daughters; others include spouses, relatives (grandchildren, siblings, nieces, and nephews), and in some instances health care providers.

Elders at home may fail to report abuse or neglect for many reasons. They may be ashamed to admit that their children have mistreated them or fear retaliation if they seek help. They may fear being sent to an institution. They frequently lack financial resources or lack the mental capacity to be aware of abuse or neglect and to report the situation. Examples of crimes are assault and financial abuse of an older person who is physically or mentally incompetent and has no trustworthy friend or relative to help. In some instances, nurses can intervene by educating caregivers about the needs of elders and available resources to provide increased home support. They should also report the situation to the appropriate person in the health care agency.

Nurses should be familiar with the laws of their particular state regarding the reporting of suspected or known abuse. The legally competent adult cannot be forced, however, to leave the abusive situation and in many cases may decide to stay. If the client is not legally competent, court proceedings to attain guardianship can be initiated.

HEALTH ASSESSMENT AND PROMOTION

Assessment guidelines for the development of the older adult are shown in the accompanying Developmental Assessment Guidelines. Assessment activities include measurement of weight, height, and vital signs; observation of the skin for hydration status or presence of lesions; examination of visual acuity using the Snellen chart; examination of hearing acuity using the Weber and Rinne tests (see Chapter 30 ∞); and questions about the following:

■ Usual dietary pattern
■ Any problems with bowel or urinary elimination
■ Activity/exercise and sleep/rest patterns
■ Family and social activities and interests
■ Any problems with reading, writing, or problem solving
■ Adjustment to retirement or loss of partner

Health care professionals should also be alert for these signs:

- Symptoms of depression
- Risk factors for suicide
- Signs of abnormal bereavement
- Changes in cognitive function
- Medications that increase risk of falls
- Signs of physical abuse or neglect
- Skin lesions (malignant and peripheral)

- Tooth decay, gingivitis, loose teeth
- Peripheral arterial disease

Older persons are usually concerned about their health and interested in information and behavioral strategies directed toward improving it. The nurse may wish to discuss some or all of the health promotion topics outlined in Box 23–4. These topics are discussed in detail in subsequent chapters throughout the book.

BOX 23–4 Health Promotion Guidelines for Elders

HEALTH TESTS AND SCREENING
- Total cholesterol and high-density lipid protein measurement every 3 to 5 years until age 75
- Aspirin, 81 mg, daily, if in high-risk group
- Diabetes mellitus screen every 3 years, if in high-risk group
- Smoking cessation
- Screening mammogram every 1 to 2 years (women)
- Clinical breast exam annually (women)
- Pap smear annually if there is a history of abnormal smears or previous hysterectomy for malignancy (United States Preventive Services Task Force, 2003)
  - Older women who have regular, normal Pap smears or hysterectomy for nonmalignant causes do NOT need Pap smears beyond the age of 65 (United States Preventive Services Task Force, 2003).
- Annual digital rectal exam
- Annual prostate-specific antigen (PSA)
- Annual fecal occult blood test (FOBT)
- Sigmoidoscopy every 5 years; colonoscopy every 10 years
- Visual acuity screen annually
- Hearing screen annually
- Depression screen periodically
- Family violence screen periodically
- Height and weight measurements annually
- Sexually transmitted disease testing, if in high-risk group
- Annual flu vaccine if over 65 or in high-risk group
- Pneumococcal vaccine at 65 and every 10 years thereafter
- Td vaccine every 10 years

SAFETY
- Home safety measures to prevent falls, fire, burns, scalds, and electrocution
- Working smoke detectors and carbon monoxide detectors in the home
- Motor vehicle safety reinforcement, especially when driving at night
- Elder driver skills evaluation (some states require for license renewal)
- Precautions to prevent pedestrian accidents

NUTRITION AND EXERCISE
- Importance of a well-balanced diet with fewer calories to accommodate lower metabolic rate and decreased physical activity
- Importance of sufficient amounts of vitamin D and calcium to prevent osteoporosis
- Nutritional and exercise factors that may lead to cardiovascular disease (e.g., obesity, cholesterol and fat intake, lack of exercise)
- Importance of 30 minutes of moderate physical activity daily; 20 minutes of vigorous physical activity 3 times per week

ELIMINATION
- Importance of adequate roughage in the diet, adequate exercise, and at least six 8-ounce glasses of fluid daily to prevent constipation

SOCIAL INTERACTIONS
- Encouraging intellectual and recreational pursuits
- Encouraging personal relationships that promote discussion of feelings, concerns, and fears
- Assessment of risk factors for maltreatment
- Availability of social community centers and programs for seniors

---

DEVELOPMENTAL ASSESSMENT GUIDELINES   The Elder

In these three developmental areas, does the elder do the following?

PHYSICAL DEVELOPMENT
- Adjust to physiologic changes (e.g., appearance, sensory/perceptual, musculoskeletal, neurologic, cardiovascular).
- Adapt lifestyle to diminishing energy and ability.
- Maintain vital signs (especially blood pressure) within normal range for age and sex.

PSYCHOSOCIAL DEVELOPMENT
- Manage retirement years in a satisfying manner.
- Participate in social and leisure activities.
- Have a social network of friends and support persons.

- View life as worthwhile.
- Have high self-esteem.
- Gain support from value system and/or spiritual philosophy.
- Accept and adjust to the death of significant others.

DEVELOPMENT IN ACTIVITIES OF DAILY LIVING
- Exhibit healthy practices in nutrition, exercise, recreation, sleep patterns, and personal habits.
- Have the ability to care for self or to secure appropriate help with activities of daily living.
- Have satisfactory living arrangements and income to meet changing needs.

CRITICAL THINKING CHECKPOINT

Alice Green, a 78-year-old female, has had a bone density scan as part of a regular physical exam and has been told that she has severe osteoporosis. Her physician has ordered a new experimental medication that is supposed to maintain bone mass in clients with osteoporosis. She lives alone in her own home and is able to perform activities of daily living independently.

1. How would you define osteoporosis to Mrs. Green?
2. What risk factors related to osteoporosis should be included in an assessment of Mrs. Green?

3. Which of the risk factors are modifiable or can be altered by a change in lifestyle?
4. What medication teaching is essential when a client is taking medications to increase or maintain bone mass in osteoporosis?
5. What preventive measures should be taught to decrease risks of fractures and to maintain bone mass?

See Critical Thinking Possibilities in Appendix A.

CHAPTER 23 REVIEW

CHAPTER HIGHLIGHTS

- The elder population is steadily growing and projected to outnumber young people by the middle of the 21st century.
- Elders are categorized into young-old (65 to 75 years), old (75 to 85 years), old-old (85 to 100 years), and elite old (over 100 years).
- Elders represent a diverse population in the United States. For example, women outnumber men, elder Hispanics are the fastest growing subpopulation group, and the majority of elders rate their health as good even though most have chronic health conditions.
- It is important for nurses to be aware of their own values and attitudes toward aging and the elderly, to avoid ageism, and to examine whether myths or stereotypes influence their personal attitudes and beliefs about the elderly.
- The gerontological nurse has many roles: provider of care, teacher, manager, advocate, and research consumer.
- Elders are primary users of health care services in different types of care settings, including acute care, rehabilitation, long-term care, and the community. No matter the setting, the elder requires health assessment and health promotion.
- Several theories have been proposed to account for the biologic aging process: wear-and-tear, free-radical, genetic, cross-linking, and immunity theories.
- Elders experience many physical changes associated with aging. All body systems undergo change: integumentary, neuromuscular, sensory/perceptual, pulmonary, cardiovascular, gastrointestinal, and genitourinary.
- Psychosocial theories about aging include the disengagement, activity, and continuity theories.

- The elder has to adjust to possible psychosocial changes, including retirement (which necessitates financial and social adjustments), grandparenting, relocation, increasing dependence on others, and coping with losses and death.
- The cognitive abilities of the healthy elder undergo some changes in perception, cognitive agility, memory, and learning.
- In the realm of moral reasoning, most elders begin to blend concepts of justice and caring relationships into their moral decision making.
- Many elders take their faith and religious practice seriously and display a high level of spirituality.
- Health problems of elders include injuries, chronic disabling disease, drug use and misuse, alcoholism, dementia, and elder mistreatment.
- Health promotion information for all adults needs to include positive health practices that can promote health and wellness. These include (a) recommended physical, visual, hearing, and dental assessments; (b) screenings for cardiovascular disease and tuberculosis; (c) breast and testicular self-examinations; (d) immunizations; (e) Papanicolaou smears for some older women; (f) safety precautions to prevent injuries; (g) the importance of appropriate nutrition and exercise; and (h) the importance of measures to prevent constipation.

TEST YOUR KNOWLEDGE

1. The nurse provides care for an elder whose husband died 8 months ago. Which of the following behaviors indicates that the client is experiencing ineffective coping?
   1. She always shows the nurse photographs of her family.
   2. She no longer has her hair done at the beauty shop.
   3. She visits the cemetery and her husband's grave every 2 weeks.
   4. She is Catholic and goes to mass on a regular daily basis.

2. A nurse in a long-term care facility is caring for several elders with noticeable hearing losses. The best way to communicate with the clients includes which of the following?
   1. Speak slowly using the proper volume and as few words as possible.

2. Write the information using large lettering.
3. Speak in a low and distinct voice tone.
4. Have the client increase the volume in the hearing aid.

3. The nurse notices that an 85-year-old man at an adult day-care center frequently tells stories about when he was younger and how he came from New York City on the "orphan trains" and was adopted by a Swedish family in Nebraska. His stories are told in a very positive manner. How would the nurse assess his behavior?
   1. Would refer him for a geriatric psychiatric evaluation.
   2. Would consider this a normal response for his developmental level.

3. Would converse with him, but distract him and change the conversation.
4. Would perceive a need to involve him in more social activities.

4. A 70-year-old woman with Alzheimer's disease becomes agitated every evening, pacing and insisting on leaving to go "home." Which of the following is/are most appropriate nursing intervention(s) to assist this client? Select all that apply.
   1. Take her to her room, turn the lights out, and leave her alone.
   2. Allow her to pace and inform her that she is at home.
   3. Turn on the television and encourage her to watch it with you.
   4. Touch her in a gentle way.

5. While being admitted to a rehabilitation unit, an 82-year-old woman mentions to the nurse that she "has trouble holding her water" and adds "if I could have that tube back in me like I had in the hospital, I wouldn't have so many accidents." What is the best response to this client?
   1. "Don't worry, the staff will bring plenty of pads to keep you dry."
   2. "I'll put the tube back in you so you will stay dry."
   3. "Tell me more about your 'leaking' problem."
   4. "Just call the staff and we'll help you to the bathroom in time."

6. The nurse notices that when an 80-year-old man rises from a seated position, the client uses both arms to push himself up, and also "rocks" back and forth before finally standing. What is the most appropriate intervention for this client?
   1. Suggest a referral to physical therapy for strengthening exercises.
   2. Suggest a waist restraint to remind the client not to stand by himself.
   3. Praise the client for his attempts to remain independent.
   4. Assist the client to rise by grasping both his shoulders and pulling forward.

7. A healthy 78-year-old woman who is considering marriage to a healthy 79-year-old neighbor tells the nurse she wonders if they will be able to have sexual intercourse. Which of the following is the most appropriate response?
   1. Sexual activity may be too demanding for the cardiac systems.
   2. Older women maintain sexual function, but most older men are impotent.
   3. Most older people are not interested in sexual activity.
   4. Older men and older women may have slower responses to sexual stimulation.

8. The client informs the nurse that he has difficulty clearly seeing the words in the newspaper unless he places the newspaper an arm's length away. The nurse documents this age-related change as
   1. Presbycusis.
   2. Xerostomia.
   3. Presbyopia.
   4. Presbyesophagus.

9. The nurse integrates the theories of psychosocial aging into nursing care of elders by applying which of the following principles? Elders:
   1. Experience physical changes at a predictable rate.
   2. Are as individual as younger adults.
   3. Are best supported in long-term facilities.
   4. Cause an economic drain on society.

10. The nursing student is planning care for an elder client who had a total knee replacement yesterday evening. Which of the following interventions would be *most* appropriate?
   1. Ask the client how much of his bath he can perform.
   2. Ask the client about his thoughts regarding discharge from the hospital.
   3. Tell the client that he needs to decide when he wants his medications.
   4. Tell the client that he needs to rest and that he (the nursing student) will bathe him today.

See Answers to Test Your Knowledge in Appendix A.

EXPLORE MEDIALINK www.prenhall.com/berman

DVD-ROM
- Audio Glossary
- NCLEX Review
- Videos:
  - The Study of Aging
  - Cultural Diversity
  - Nursing Issues and the Elderly
  - Immune System
  - Respiratory System
  - Cardiovascular System
  - Gastrointestinal Sytem

Geritourinary and Renal System
Nutrition and Aging
Alzheimer's Disease
Mistreatment and Abuse of the Elderly

COMPANION WEBSITE
- Additional NCLEX Review
- Case Study: Home Health and Elderly Siblings
- Care Plan Activity: Elderly Client with Nose Bleed
- Application Activity: Gerontology as a Nusing Speciality
- Links to Resources

READINGS AND REFERENCES

SUGGESTED READINGS
Arnold, E. (2004). Sorting out the 3 D's: Delirium, dementia, depression. *Nursing, 34*(6), 36–42. *This helpful article differentiates the sometimes overlapping signs and symptoms of delirium, dementia, and depression.*

Knowing these differences helps the nurse provide appropriate nursing interventions.
Baier, F. (2006). The Medicare prescription drug benefit: Understanding the benefits and the gaps in this new coverage. *American Journal of Nursing, 106*(6), 66–72.

This article reviews the reasons for the implementation of Medicare Part D and outlines basic provision of this new drug benefit. In addition, three nurses discuss their experiences with Medicare Part D.

Edwards, H., & Chapman, H. (2004). Contemplating, caring, coping, conversing. A model for promoting mental wellness in later life. *Journal of Gerontological Nursing, 30*(5), 16–21.
This article reviews barriers to communications for the older adult, followed by a conceptual model for promoting mental wellness for older adults (contemplating, caring, coping, and conversing).

Gray-Vickrey, P. (2004). Combating elder abuse. *Nursing, 34*(10), 47–51.
The author provides clear information as to what to look for, what to ask, and how to respond if the nurse suspects an older adult is a victim of violence, abuse, or neglect.

RELATED RESEARCH

Resnick, B. (2003). Health promotion practices of older adults: Model testing. *Public Health Nursing, 2*(1), 2–12.

Schneider, J. K., Mercer, G. T., Herning, M., Smith, C. A., & Prysak, M. D. (2004). Promoting exercise behavior in older adults: Using a cognitive behavioral intervention. *Journal of Gerontological Nursing, 30*(4), 45–53.

Schneider, J. K., Eveker, A., Bronder, D. R., Meiner, S. E., & Binder, E. F. (2003). Exercise training program for older adults. Incentives and disincentives for participation. *Journal of Gerontological Nursing, 29*(9), 21–31.

Wagnild, G. (2003). Resilience and successful aging: Comparison among low and high income older adults. *Journal of Gerontological Nursing, 29*(12), 42–49.

Wikstrom, B. M. (2004). Older adults and the arts. The importance of aesthetic forms of expression in later life. *Journal of Gerontological Nursing, 30*(9), 30–36.

REFERENCES

Abrams, A. C. (2004). *Clinical drug therapy* (7th ed.). Philadelphia: Lippincott Williams & Wilkins.

Agency on Aging. (2004). *Alzheimer's resource room: Professionals and Providers.* Retrieved June 11, 2006, from http://www.aoa.gov/ALZ/Public/alzprof/alz_prof.asp

Butler, F. R., & Zakari, N. (2005). Grandparents parenting grandchildren: Assessing health status, parental stress, and social supports. *Journal of Gerontological Nursing, 31*(3), 43–54.

Butler, R. N., & Lewis, M. I. (2003). Sexuality and aging. In W. R. Hazzard, J. P. Blass, J. B. Halter, J. G. Ouslander, & M. E. Tinetti (Eds.), *Principles of geriatric medicine and gerontology* (5th ed) (pp. 1277–1282). New York: McGraw-Hill.

Capezuti, E., & Harrington, C. (2004). Older adults in the ED. *American Journal of Nursing, 104*(5), 73.

Centers for Disease Control and Prevention (CDC). (2004). *Healthy aging: Preventing disease and improving quality of life among older Americans.* Retrieved June 11, 2006, from http://www.cdc.gov/nccdphp/aag/aag_aging.htm#2

Curry, L., & Hogstel, M. (2002). Osteoporosis: Education and awareness can make a difference. *American Journal of Nursing, 102*(1), 26–33.

De Pinto, R. A. (2000). The age of cancer. *Nature, 408*(9), 248–255.

Ebersole, P., Hess, P., Touhy, T., & Jett, K. (2005). *Gerontological nursing & healthy aging* (2nd ed.). Philadelphia: Elsevier Mosby.

Eliopoulos, C. (2005). *Gerontological nursing* (6th ed.). Philadelphia: Lippincott.

Erikson, E. H. (1963). *Childhood and society* (2nd ed.). New York: Norton.

Federal Interagency Forum on Aging-Related Statistics (FIFAS). (2004). *Older Americans 2004: Key indicators of well-being.* Washington, DC: U.S. Government Printing Office.

Finkel, T., & Holbrook, N. J. (2000). Oxidants, oxidative stress and the biology of aging. *Nature, 408*(9), 239–247.

Gilligan, C. (1982). *In a different voice: Psychological theory and women's development.* Cambridge, MA: Harvard University Press.

Havighurst, R. J. (1972). *Developmental tasks and education* (3rd ed.). New York: Longman.

Jacelon, C. S. (2004). Older adults and autonomy in acute care. Increasing patients' independence and control during hospitalization. *Journal of Gerontological Nursing, 30*(11), 29–36.

Jett, K., Tappen, R. M., & Rosselli, M. (2005). Imposed versus involved: Different strategies to effect driving cessation in cognitively impaired older adults. *Geriatric Nursing, 26*(2), 111–116.

Joint National Committee on Prevention, Detection, Evaluation, and Treatment of High Blood Pressure [JNC 7]. (2003). *Seventh report* (NIH Publication No. 03–5233). Rockville, MD: Author.

Kane, R. L., Ouslander, J. G., & Abrass, I. B. (2004). *Essentials of clinical geriatrics* (5th ed). New York: McGraw-Hill Medical Publishing Division.

Kirkwood, T. B. L., & Austad, S. N. (2000). Why do we age? *Nature, 408*(9), 233–238.

Kohlberg, L. (1984). *The psychology of moral development: The nature and validity of moral stages.* San Francisco: Harper & Row.

Mauk, K. L. (2006). *Gerontological nursing: Competencies for care.* Boston: Jones & Bartlett.

McFadden, S. H. (1996). Religion and spirituality. In J. E. Birren (Ed.), *Encyclopedia of gerontology: Age, aging, and the aged* (pp. 387–397). San Diego: Academic Press.

Meiner, S. E., & Lueckenotte, A. G. (2006). *Gerontologic nursing* (3rd ed.). Philadelphia: Mosby Elsevier.

Miller, C. A. (2004). *Nursing for wellness in older adults: Theory and practice* (4th ed.). Philadelphia: Lippincott Williams & Wilkins.

Murray, R. B., & Zentner, J. P. (2001). *Health promotion strategies through the life span* (7th ed.). Upper Saddle River, NJ: Prentice Hall.

National Center for Health Statistics. (2003). *Health, United States, 2003.* Hyattsville, MD: Author.

National Research Council Panel to Review Risk and Prevalence of Elder Abuse and Neglect. (2003). *Elder mistreatment: Abuse, neglect, and exploitation in an aging America.* Washington, DC: Author.

Peck, R. (1968). Psychological development in the second half of life. In B. L. Neugarten (Ed.), *Middle age and aging.* Chicago: University of Chicago Press.

Pinch, W. J. E., & Parsons, M. E. (1997). Moral orientation of elderly persons: Considering ethical dilemmas in health care. *Nursing Ethics, 4*(5), 380–393.

Polan, E., & Taylor, D. (2003). *Journey across the life span. Human development and health promotion* (2nd ed.). Philadelphia: F. A. Davis.

Pratt, M. W., Diessner, R., Pratt, A., Hunsberger, B., & Pancer, S. M. (1996). Moral and social reasoning and perspective taking in later life: A

longitudinal study. *Psychology and Aging, 11*(1), 66–73.

Purnell, L. D., & Paulanka, B. J. (2003). *Transcultural health care: A culturally competent approach* (2nd ed.). Philadelphia: F. A. Davis.

Seery, D. H. (2004). Shifting gears: From cure to comfort. *RN, 67*(11), 52–57.

Stanley, M., Blair, K. A., & Beare, P. G. (2005). *Gerontological nursing: Promoting successful aging with older adults* (3rd ed.). Philadelphia: F. A. Davis.

Tabloski, P. A. (2006). *Gerontological nursing.* Upper Saddle River, NJ: Pearson Prentice Hall.

Taylor, A. H., Cable, N. T., Faulkner, G., Hillsdon, M., Narici, M., & Van Der Bij, A. K. (2004). Physical activity and older adults: A review of health benefits and the effectiveness of interventions. *Journal of Sports Science, 22*(8), 703–723.

U.S. Department of Health and Human Services. (2000). *Healthy people 2010: Understanding and improving health* (2nd ed.). *Goal 15: Injury and violence prevention.* Washington, DC: Author.

U.S. Department of Health and Human Services. (2003). *A profile of older Americans: 2003.* Washington, DC: Administration on Aging.

U.S. Department of Health and Human Services. (2005). *28 focus areas of healthy people 2010.* Retrieved June 11, 2006, from http://www.healthypeople.gov/lhi/touch_fact.htm

U.S. Preventive Services Task Force. *Screening for Cervical Cancer. Recommendations and Rationale.* AHRQ Publication No. 03-515A. January 2003. Agency for Healthcare Research and Quality, Rockville, MD. Retrieved June 30, 2006, from, http://www.ahrq.gov/clinic/3rduspstf/cervcan/cervcanrr.htm

SELECTED BIBLIOGRAPHY

Amella, E. J. (2004). Presentation of illness in older adults. *American Journal of Nursing, 104*(10), 40–51.

Atchley, R. C. (1989). A continuity theory of normal aging. *Gerontologist, 29,* 183–190.

Averill, J. B. (2005). Studies of rural elderly individuals: Merging critical ethnography with community-based action research. *Journal of Gerontological Nursing, 31*(12), 11–18.

Cataldo, J. K. (2003). Smoking and aging. Clinical implications part 1: Health and consequence. *Journal of Gerontological Nursing, 29*(3), 15–20.

Clark, M. J. (2003). *Community health nursing. Caring for populations* (4th ed.). Upper Saddle River, NJ: Prentice Hall.

Cumming, E., & Henry, W. E. (1961). *Growing old: The process of disengagement.* New York: Basic Books.

Danter, J. H. (2003). Put a realistic spin on geriatric assessment. *Nursing, 33*(12), 52–55.

Ebersole, P., Hess, P., & Luggen, A. S. (2004). *Toward healthy aging: Human needs and nursing response* (6th ed.). St. Louis, MO: Mosby.

Edelman, C. L., & Mandle, C. L. (2006). *Health promotion throughout the life span* (6th ed.). St. Louis, MO: Mosby Elsevier.

Erikson, E. H. (1982). *The life cycle completed: A review.* New York: Norton.

Fowler, J. W. (1981). *Stages of faith: The psychology of human development and the quest for meaning.* New York: Harper & Row.

Freud, S. (1923). *The ego and the id.* London: Hogarth Press.

Graf, C. (2006). Functional decline in hospitalized older adults. *American Journal of Nursing, 106*(1), 58–67.

Haber, D. (2003). *Health promotion and aging: Practical applications for health professionals* (3rd ed.). New York: Springer.

Havighurst, R. J. (1963). Successful aging. In R. H. Williams, C. Tibbitts, & W. Donohue (Eds.), *Processes of aging: Social and psychological perspectives* (Vol. 1, pp. 299–320). New York: Atherton.

Hetzel, L., & Smith, A. (2001). *The 65 years and over population: 2000. Census 2000 brief.* Washington, DC: U.S. Census Bureau.

Kohlberg, L. (1971). *Recent research in moral development.* New York: Holt, Rinehart & Winston.

Kohlberg, L. (1981). *The psychology of moral development: Moral stages and the idea of justice.* San Francisco: Harper & Row.

Mezey, M. D. (2001). *The encyclopedia of elder care.* New York: Springer.

Neugarten, B. (1974). Age groups in American society and the rise of the young-old. *Annals of the American Academy of Political and Social Science, 415,* 187–198.

Oeppen, J., & Vaupel, J. W. (2002). Broken limits to life expectancy. *Science, 296,* 1029–1031.

Paludi, M. A. (2002). *Human development in multicultural contexts. A book of readings.* Upper Saddle River, NJ: Prentice Hall.

Peck, R. (1955). Psychological developments in the second half of life. In J. Anderson (Ed.), *Psychological aspects of aging.* Washington, DC: American Psychological Association.

Piaget, J. (1966). *Origins of intelligence in children.* New York: Norton.

Ross-Kerr, J. C., Warren, S., Schalm, C., Smith, D. L., & Godkin, M. D. (2003). Adult day programs: Who needs them? *Journal of Gerontological Nursing, 29*(12), 11–17.

Sheehy, G. (1995). *New passages. Mapping your life across time.* New York: Ballantine Books.

Stotts, N. A., & Deitrich, C. E. (2004). The challenge to come: The care of older adults. *American Journal of Nursing, 104*(8), 40–47.

Substance Abuse and Mental Health Services Administration (SAMHSA). (2005, April 22). Substance abuse among older adults: 2002 and 2003 update. *NDSUH Report.* Retrieved June 11, 2006, from http://oas.samhsa.gov/2k5/olderadults/olderadults.htm

CHAPTER 24

Promoting Family Health

LEARNING OUTCOMES

After completing this chapter, you will be able to:

1. Describe the roles and functions of the family.

2. Describe different types of families.

3. Identify theoretical frameworks used in family health promotion.

4. Identify the components of a family health assessment.

5. Identify common risk factors regarding family health.

6. Develop nursing diagnoses, outcomes, and interventions pertaining to family functioning.

7. Develop outcome criteria for specific nursing diagnoses related to family functioning.

Nurses assess and plan health care for three types of clients: the individual, the family, and the community. The beliefs and values of each person and the support he or she receives come in large part from the family and are reinforced by the community. Thus an understanding of family dynamics and the context of the community assists the nurse in planning care. When a family is the client, the nurse determines the health status of the family and its individual members, the level of family functioning, family interaction patterns, and family strengths and weaknesses.

FAMILY HEALTH

The **family** is a basic unit of society. It consists of those individuals, male or female, youth or adult, legally or not legally related, genetically or not genetically related, who are considered by the others to represent their significant persons. In the nursing profession, interest in the family unit and its impact on the health, values, and productivity of individual family members is expressed by **family-centered nursing:** nursing that considers the health of the family as a unit in addition to the health of individual family members.

Functions of the Family

The economic resources needed by the family are secured by adult members. The family protects the physical health of its members by providing adequate nutrition and health care services. Nutritional and lifestyle practices of the family also directly affect the developing health attitudes and lifestyle practices of the children.

In addition to providing an environment conducive to physical growth and health, the family creates an atmosphere that influences the cognitive and the psychosocial growth of its members. Children and adults in healthy, functional families receive support, understanding, and encouragement as they progress through predictable developmental stages, as they move in or out of the family unit, and as they establish new family units. In families where members are physically and emotionally nurtured, individuals are challenged to achieve their potential in the family unit. As individual needs are met, family members are able to reach out to others in the family and the community, and to society.

Families from different cultures are an integral part of North America's rich heritage. Each family has values and beliefs that are unique to their culture of origin and that shape the family's structure, methods of interaction, health care practices, and coping mechanisms. These factors interact to influence the health of families. Families of a particular culture may cluster to form mutual support systems and to preserve their heritage; however, this practice may isolate them from the larger society (see Figure 24-1 ■).

Becoming acculturated is a slow, stressful process of learning the language and customs of a new country. Children in cultural clusters often have greater contact with the world around them than do adults; through school, children become more proficient in language and more comfortable with new customs and behaviors. Sometimes children create conflict in the family when they bring home new ideas and values. For more information about cultural aspects of health of individuals and families, see Chapter 18. ∞

Types of Families in Today's Society

Families consist of persons (structure) and their responsibilities within the family (roles). Government data are grouped by types of *households*: married couples with children, married couples without children, other family households (single-parent families), men living alone, women living alone, and other nonfamily households. A family structure of parents and their offspring is known as the **nuclear family.** The relatives of nuclear families, such as grandparents or aunts and uncles, compose the **extended family.** In some families, members of the extended family live with the nuclear family. Although members of the extended family may live in different areas, they may be a source of emotional or financial support for the family.

Some families live in houses, some in apartments; some live in urban areas, some in rural towns; and some are homeless. In

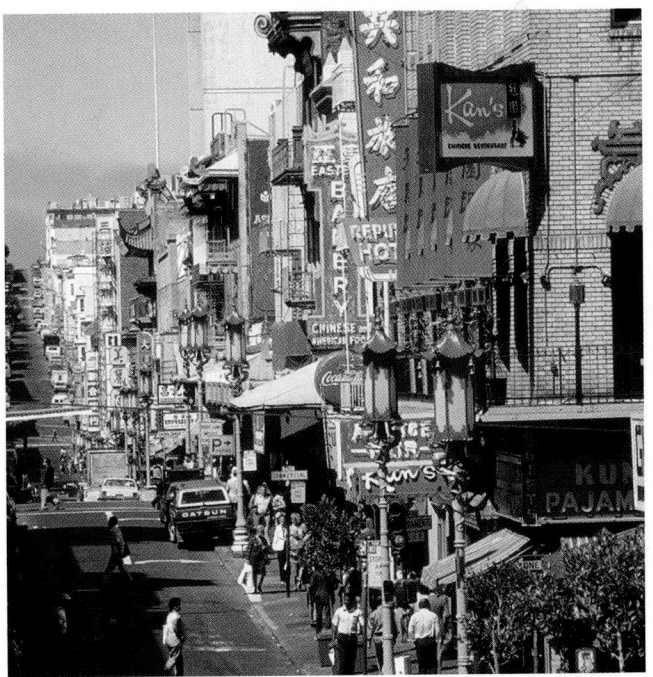

Figure 24-1 ■ Cultural separation.

cities, 40% of the homeless population may consist of families with children (U.S. Conference of Mayors, 2004).

Traditional Family

The traditional family is viewed as an autonomous unit in which both parents reside in the home with their children, the mother often assuming the nurturing role and the father providing the necessary economic resources. In today's society both males and females are less bound to traditional role patterns. For example, fathers are more likely to be involved with the household chores, their children, and family life (see Figure 24-2 ■). The U.S. Census Bureau reported 26.5 million fathers in married-couple families, 98,000 of whom were stay-at-home fathers (caring for 336,000 children) in 2004. This was the first time the number of stay-at-home parents was analyzed in the census. Of all the families with children, the percentage consisting of married couples declined between 1980 and 1996 and has remained constant since then at about 68% (Fields, 2003).

Two-Career Family

In two-career (or dual-career) families, both partners are employed. They may or may not have children. Two-career families have steadily increased since the 1960s because of increased career opportunities for women, a desire to increase their standard of living, and economic necessity. Finding good-quality, affordable child care is one of the greatest stresses faced by working parents.

Single-Parent Family

Of all types of households, about 9% (12 million) are single-parent families and the number continues to increase (Fields, 2003). Of these families, 10 million are headed by women and 2 million by men. There are many reasons for single parenthood, including death of a spouse, separation, divorce, birth of

Figure 24-2 ■ Role patterns within traditional families are changing.

a child to an unmarried woman, or adoption of a child by a single man or woman. The stresses of single parenthood are many: child care concerns, financial concerns, role overload and fatigue in managing daily tasks, and social isolation.

Adolescent Family

Birth rates among teenagers peaked in 1991 and have decreased progressively since then to 47.7 births per 1,000 women aged 15 to 19 in 2000 (Alan Guttmacher Institute, 2004). Rates are highest among black teens, followed by Hispanic and then white women. These young parents are often developmentally, physically, emotionally, and financially ill prepared to undertake the responsibility of parenthood. Adolescent pregnancies frequently interrupt or stop formal education. Children born to an adolescent are often at greater risk for health and social problems, and they have few role models to assist in breaking out of the cycle of poverty.

Foster Family

Children who can no longer live with their birth parents may require placement with a family that has agreed to include them temporarily. The legal agreement between the foster family and the court to care for the child includes the expectations of the foster parents and the financial compensation they will receive. A family (with or without their own children) may house more than one foster child at a time or different children over many years. Hopefully, at some time the fostered child can return to the birth parent(s) or be legally and permanently adopted by other parents.

Blended Family

Existing family units who join together to form new families are known as *blended, step,* or *reconstituted families.* There are no official statistics on the number of blended families, but a commonly accepted view is that about one of every three Americans is a member of a stepfamily. Family integration requires time and effort. Stresses occur as blended families get acquainted with each other, respect differences, and establish new patterns of behavior. When blended families with children form following the divorce or death of a parent, adjustment can be particularly challenged by the normal processes of grief and loss (see Chapter 43). ∞

Intragenerational Family

In some cultures, and as people live longer, more than two generations may live together. Children may continue to live with their parents even after having their own children, or the grandparents may move in with their grown children's families after some years of living apart. In other situations, a generation is skipped or missing; that is, grandparents live with and care for their grandchildren but the children's parents are not a part of this family. Many life events and choices can lead to this type of family.

Cohabiting Family

Cohabiting (or communal) families consist of unrelated individuals or families who live under one roof. Reasons for cohabiting may be a need for companionship, a desire to achieve a sense of family, testing a relationship or commitment, or sharing expenses and household management. Cohabiting families

REAL WORLD REFLECTION

THE STORY: "ALL THIS AND CALVIN KLEINS TOO"

This was my first shift in the Neonatal Intensive Care Unit (NICU). The infant I was caring for was born around 34 weeks gestation. She was being evaluated because she was small for her gestational age. The infant had a nasogastric tube and was being gavaged to meet the minimum daily intake, but also was doing well at bottle feeding. The nurse showed me how to check for residuals from the last feeding.

The infant had been hospitalized for about one month, and now she was ready for discharge the following day. While I was interested in the infant's medical condition, I was most interested in the mother's psychosocial status. She was very passive about holding her baby, and indicated that the infant's grandmother would be taking care of the baby when she came home because of her need to return to work. The mother didn't seem interested in participating in any teaching/learning before discharge. She did request a prescription for a specialized formula so she could obtain it from a public assistance program. I am sure that the special formula is expensive, but I also noticed that this young (probably late teens) mom was in full make-up, hair, and Calvin Klein jeans.

STUDENT REFLECTION

As the evening progressed the parents went home and the lights dimmed in the NICU. I continued assessing, feeding, changing, and comforting my clients. As I look back on this experience, I think most about my inclination to judge the parents and think that they are responsible for the infant's medical problems. As I talked with other nurses they stressed that even moms who do everything right can find their baby in the NICU for a short or extensive stay. I know that there are many risks in pregnancy and delivery, but looking at these tiny babies fighting to live made me want to blame someone.

I also assumed that all parents would want to be with their baby day in and out if they were in the NICU. While some parents do spend as much time as possible with their child, many of the infants are in the NICU for weeks or months making a parental vigil nearly impossible.

FACULTY REFLECTION

Jennifer did a great job on reflecting on how she felt while caring for this infant and mother. She recognized the feeling in herself of assigning blame for what she considered an injustice, and yet, she did not know where to direct that blame. As nurses we may verbally say to ourselves and others that we don't judge our clients. But often our nonverbal language is "screaming" something to the contrary. Until we recognize, name, and understand those feelings in ourselves, we cannot effectively deliver caring and compassionate care.

—Student: Jennifer Trucke
Faculty member: Deb Filer, PhD, RN
College of St. Catherine, St. Paul, MN

---

illustrate the flexibility and creativity of the family unit in adapting to individual challenges and changing societal needs.

Gay and Lesbian Family

Homosexual adults form gay and lesbian families based on the same goals of caring and commitment seen in heterosexual relationships. In addition, the structure of gay and lesbian families is as diverse as that of heterosexual families—including stepfamilies and single-parent families. Children raised in these family units develop sex role orientations and behaviors similar to children in the general population.

Legal issues for same-sex couples are significant and constantly changing. *Domestic partner* policies extend the same rights and privileges to the partner of a nonmarried employee of the same or opposite gender as would be offered to spouses. California Family Code Section 297–297.5 defines domestic partners as "two adults who have chosen to share one another's lives in an intimate and committed relationship of mutual caring." Numerous state and federal legislation has been introduced in the United States to either allow or prohibit same-sex marriages or civil unions. It can be a challenge for the nurse to keep current on how such legislation affects health care issues such as insurance coverage and the right to consent for health care.

Single Adults Living Alone

Individuals who live by themselves represent a significant portion of today's society. In younger adults 18 to 34 years of age, about 10% live alone with little variation between males and females. However, among adults 65 years and older, about 20% of men live alone while about 40% of women live alone (Fields, 2003). Singles include young self-supporting adults who have recently left the nuclear family as well as older adults living alone. Young adults typically move in and out of living situations and may have membership in family, nonfamily household, and living alone categories at several different times. Older adults may find themselves single through divorce, separation, or the death of a spouse but generally remain living alone for the remainder of their lives.

APPLYING THEORETICAL FRAMEWORKS TO FAMILIES

A variety of theoretical frameworks provide the nurse with a holistic overview of health promotion for families across the life span. Major theoretical frameworks that nurses use in promoting the health of families are systems theory and structural–functional theory.

Systems Theory

A **system** is a set of interacting identifiable parts or components. The basic concepts of general systems theory were proposed in the 1950s. One of its major proponents, Ludwig von Bertalanffy (1980) introduced systems theory as a universal theory that could be applied to many fields of study. Nurses are increasingly using systems theory to understand not only biologic systems but also

---

RESEARCH NOTE ◆ **Are Adolescent Mothers Able to Promote a Healthy Life for Their Families?**

Much of the research on families headed by adolescent mothers has focused on the negative health aspects of these family units. Yet family and community theory suggests that no unit, family, or community will continue to exist with only negative factors. Black and Ford-Gilboe conducted a study with 41 adolescent mothers to test the families' resilience and ability to promote healthy lifestyles. The young mothers were asked to provide verbal responses to items on three questionnaires designed to gather information on the mother's health-promoting lifestyle practices and demographic background. The results validated the theoretical relationships between increased family resilience and the teenage mother's ability to promote healthy lifestyles for herself and her children.

IMPLICATIONS

Nursing focuses on the complete individual by assessing for both positive and negative health behaviors and risks. In the past, families headed by young single mothers tended to be viewed only in negative terms. By conducting research to examine the positive strengths of these types of family units, nursing is helping to place these families in a more positive light.

Note: From "Adolescent Mothers: Resilience, Family Health, Work, and Health-Promoting Practices," by C. Black and M. Ford-Gilboe, 2004, *Journal of Advanced Nursing, 48*, pp. 351–360.

---

systems in families, communities, and nursing and health care. General systems theory provides a way of examining interrelationships and deriving principles.

Systems may be complex and the systems components are often studied as **subsystems.** For family systems, the subsystems would be individuals. Looking back up the hierarchy, the systems above other systems are referred to as **suprasystems**—the family is the suprasystem of the individual. See Figure 24-3 ■ for a hierarchy of the human system.

A system depends on the quality and quantity of its input, throughput, output, and feedback. **Input** consists of information, material, or energy that enters the system. After the input is absorbed by the system, it is processed in a way useful to the system. This transformation is called **throughput.** For example, food is input to the digestive system; it is digested (throughput) so that it can be used by the body. **Output** from a system is energy, matter, or information given out by the system as a result of its processes. Output from the digestive system includes caloric energy, nutrients, urine, and feces.

Feedback is the mechanism by which some of the output of a system is returned to the system as input. Feedback enables a system to regulate itself by redirecting the output of a system back into the system as input, thus forming a feedback loop (see Figure 24-4 ■). This input influences the behavior of the system and its future output. **Negative feedback** inhibits change; **positive feedback** stimulates change.

The biologic system can be subdivided into the neurologic, musculoskeletal, respiratory, circulatory, gastrointestinal, and urinary subsystems, among others. Each subsystem can in turn be subdivided. For example, the urinary system consists of the kidneys, the ureters, and the bladder; the circulatory system consists of the heart and the blood vessels; the neurologic system consists of the brain, the spinal cord, and the nerves. The biologic system can also be subdivided into categories of needs or functional health patterns or activities of daily living, such as nutrition and hydration, sleep/rest, activity/exercise, elimination, and so on.

The psychologic and social systems consist of subsystems that include thinking, feeling, and interaction patterns. Names of the psychologic and social subsystems vary considerably according to individual nurse theorists. For example, Dorothy Johnson (as cited in Wilkerson & Loveland-Cherry, 2004), who describes the human system in terms of behaviors, lists the psychologic subsystems of attachment—affiliative, dependence, achievement, and aggressive.

The interrelatedness of all the parts of a system is the basis for nursing's holistic view of the client. A tumor of the liver affects the whole individual, that is, the person may be nauseated, tired, anxious, and so on. A psychologic problem such as stress

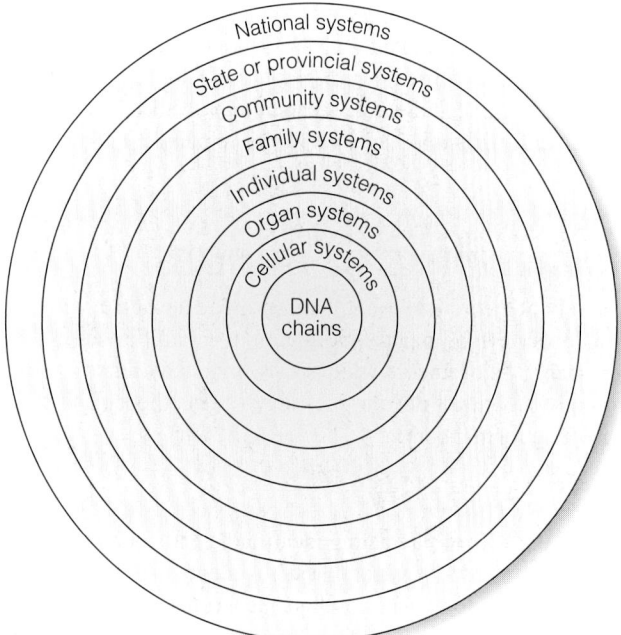

Figure 24-3 ■ A common system hierarchy.

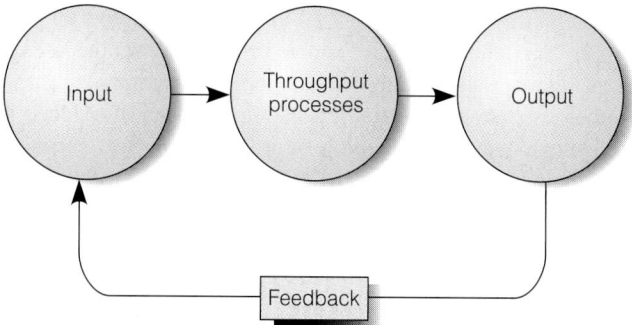

Figure 24-4 ■ A system with a feedback mechanism.

or anxiety may also manifest itself by physiologic symptoms, such as sleeplessness, nausea, or changes in cardiac function.

The family unit can also be viewed as a system. Its members are interdependent, working toward specific purposes and goals. Families, as open systems, are continually interacting with and influenced by other systems in the community. Boundaries regulate the input from other systems that interact with the family system; they also regulate output from the family system to the community or to society. Boundaries protect the family from the demands and influences of other systems. Families are likely to welcome input from without, encourage individual members to adapt beliefs and practices to meet the changing demands of society, seek out health care information, and use community resources.

Structural–Functional Theory

The structural–functional theory, as the name implies, focuses on family structure and function. The structural component of the theory addresses the membership of the family and the relationships among family members. Intrafamily relationships are complex because of the numerous relationships that exist within the family structure—mother–daughter, brother–sister, spouse–partner, and so on. These relationships are constantly evolving as children mature and leave the family nest and adults age and become more dependent on others to meet their daily needs.

The functional aspect of the theory examines the effects of intrafamily relationships on the family system, as well as their effects on other systems. Some of the main functions of the family include developing a sense of family purpose and affiliation, adding and socializing new members, and providing and distributing care and services to members. A healthy family organizes its members and resources in meeting family goals; it functions in harmony, working toward shared goals.

Nurses generally use a combination of theoretical frameworks in promoting the health of individuals and families. For example, the nurse may provide education for the mother of a toddler who is struggling to accomplish the developmental stage of autonomy described by Erikson (1963). Simultaneously, the nurse may provide guidance for the same family in its stressful transition period between developmental stages as their older school-age child becomes an adolescent.

 NURSING MANAGEMENT

Assessing

The purpose of family assessment is to determine the level of family functioning, clarify family interaction patterns, identify family strengths and weaknesses, and describe the health status of the family and its individual members. Also important are family living patterns, including communication, child rearing, coping strategies, and health practices. Family assessment gives an overview of the family process and helps the nurse identify areas that need further investigation. Nurses carry out a detailed assessment in specific target areas as they become more acquainted with the family and begin to understand family needs and strengths more fully. In planning interventions, nurses need

to focus not only on problems but also on family strengths and resources as part of the nursing care plan (see Box 24–1).

The assessment begins with a complete health history. The nurse focuses first on the family unit and then on the individuals in that family. The health history is one of the most effective ways of identifying existing or potential health problems. Employment of a genogram will aid the nurse to visualize how all family members are genetically related to each other and to grasp how patterns of chronic conditions are present within the family unit. Genograms are composed of visual representations of gender and lines of birth descent through the generations (Figure 24-5 ■). The history is followed by physical assessment of family members. If further evaluation is indicated, a referral is made to the appropriate health care professional.

The nurse should also develop an ecomap for family members individually and as a group to document the family unit's

---

BOX 24–1 **Family Assessment Guide**

FAMILY STRUCTURE
- Size and type: nuclear, extended, or other type of family
- Age and gender of family members

FAMILY ROLES AND FUNCTIONS
- Family members working outside the home; type of work and satisfaction with it
- Household roles and responsibilities and how tasks are distributed
- Ways child-rearing responsibilities are shared
- Major decision maker and methods of decision making
- Family members' satisfaction with roles, the way tasks are divided, and the way decisions are made

PHYSICAL HEALTH STATUS
- Current physical health status of each member
- Perceptions of own and other family members' health
- Preventive health practices (e.g., status of immunizations, oral hygiene practices, regularity of visual examinations)
- Routine health care, when and why primary care provider last seen

INTERACTION PATTERNS
- Ways of expressing affection, love, sorrow, anger, and so on
- Most significant family member in person's life
- Openness of communication with all family members

FAMILY VALUES
- Cultural and religious orientations; degree to which cultural practices are followed
- Use of leisure time and whether leisure time is shared with total family unit
- Family's view of education, teachers, and the school system
- Health values: how much emphasis is put on exercise, diet, preventive health care

COPING RESOURCES
- Degree of emotional support offered to one another
- Availability of support persons and affiliations outside the family (e.g., friends, church memberships)
- Sources of stress
- Methods of handling stressful situations and conflicting goals of family members
- Financial ability to meet current and future needs

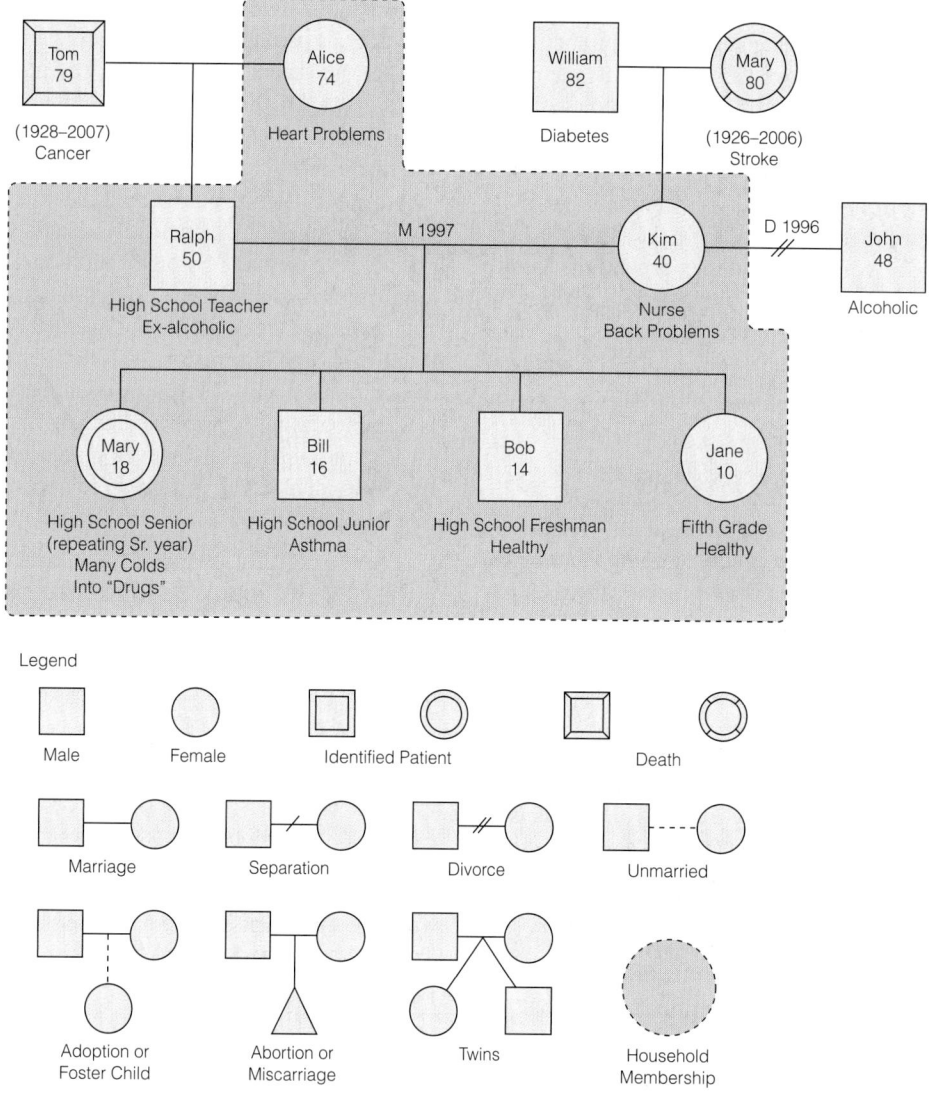

Figure 24-5 ■ Example of a family genogram with accompanying legend (symbols used in genograms).

energy expenditures within the community setting. Ecomaps provide a visualization of how the family unit interacts with the external community environment such as schools, religious commitments, occupational duties, and recreational pursuits (see Figure 24-6 ■). When the focus is on health, the appraisal includes information on lifestyle behaviors and health beliefs. The nurse uses data from the health appraisal to formulate a health profile. The health profile provides the data necessary to determine wellness or to establish a nursing diagnosis and to plan appropriate nursing interventions to promote optimal health through lifestyle modification.

Health Beliefs

To promote health, the nurse must understand the health beliefs of individuals and families. Health beliefs may reflect a lack of information or misinformation about health or disease. They may also include folklore and practices from different cultures. Because of the many advances in medicine and health care during the last few decades, clients may have outdated information about health, illness, treatment, and prevention. The nurse is fre-

quently in a position to give information or correct misconceptions. This function is an important component of the nursing care plan. For additional information on health beliefs, see Chapter 17. ∞

Family Communication Patterns

The effectiveness of family communication determines the family's ability to function as a cooperative, growth-producing unit. Messages are constantly being communicated among family members, both verbally and nonverbally. The information transmitted influences how members work together, fulfill their assigned roles in the family, incorporate family values, and develop skills to function in society. Intrafamily communication plays a significant role in the development of self-esteem, which is necessary for the growth of personality.

Families that communicate effectively transmit messages clearly. Members are free to express their feelings without fear of jeopardizing their standing in the family. Family members support one another and have the ability to listen, empathize, and reach out to one another in times of crisis. When the needs

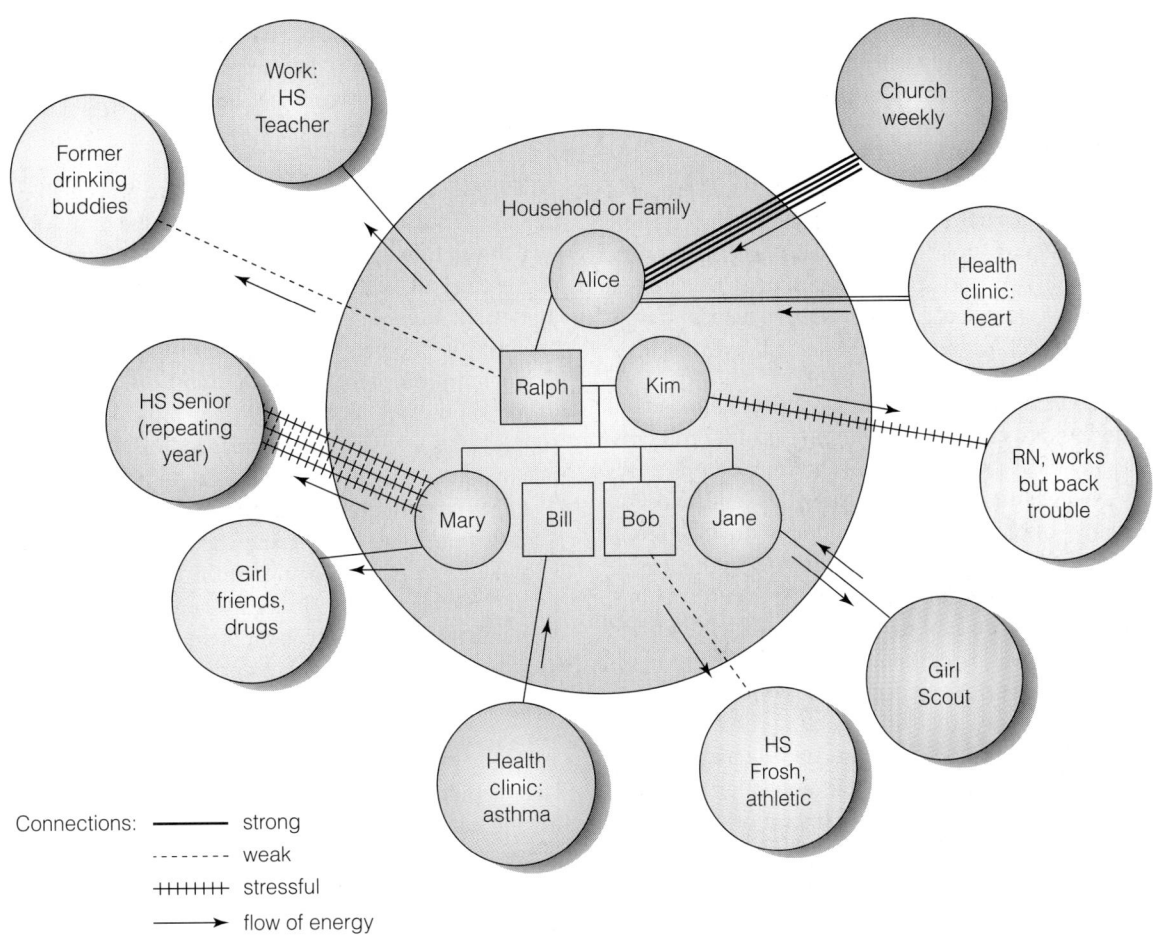

Connections:
———— strong
- - - - - weak
++++++ stressful
———→ flow of energy

Figure 24-6 ■ Example of a family ecomap. Many more components may be added to the map.

of family members are met, they are more able to reach out to meet the needs of others in society.

When patterns of communication among family members are dysfunctional, messages are often communicated unclearly. Verbal communication may be incongruent with nonverbal messages. Power struggles may be evidenced by hostility, anger, or silence. Members may be cautious in expressing their feelings because they cannot predict how others in the family will respond. When family communication is impaired, the growth of individual members is stunted. Members often turn to other systems to seek personal validation and gratification.

The nurse needs to observe intrafamily communication patterns closely. Nurses should pay special attention to who does the talking for the family, which members are silent, how disagreements are handled, and how well the members listen to one another and encourage the participation of others. Nonverbal communication is important because it gives valuable clues about what people are feeling.

Family Coping Mechanisms

Family coping mechanisms are the behaviors families use to deal with stress or changes imposed from either within or without. Coping mechanisms can be viewed as an active method of problem solving developed to meet life's challenges. The coping mechanisms families and individuals develop reflect their

individual resourcefulness. Families may use coping patterns rather consistently over time or may change their coping strategies when new demands are made on the family. The success of a family largely depends on how well it copes with the stresses it experiences.

Nurses working with families realize the importance of assessing coping mechanisms as a way of determining how families relate to stress. Also important are the resources available to the family. Internal resources, such as knowledge, skills, effective communication patterns, and a sense of mutuality and purpose within the family, assist in the problem-solving process. In addition, external support systems promote coping and adaptation. These external systems may be extended family, friends, religious affiliations, health care professionals, or social services. The development of social support systems is particularly valuable today because many families, due to stress, mobility, or poverty, are isolated from the resources that would traditionally have helped them cope.

FAMILY VIOLENCE. The incidence of family violence has increased in recent years. Statistics are not accurate, because many cases remain unreported. Family violence includes abuse between intimate partners, child abuse, and elder abuse, and may include physical, mental, and verbal abuse, as well as neglect. Early symptoms are evident in burns, cuts, fractures, and even death. Other manifestations often seen are depression, alcohol

MediaLink

Involving Families in NICU Settings Video

and substance abuse, and suicide attempts. Nurses should be alert to the symptoms of family violence and take appropriate measures to report it and obtain resources for the family.

Risk for Health Problems

Risk assessment helps the nurse identify individuals and groups at higher risk than the general population of developing specific health problems, such as stroke, diabetes, and lung cancer. The vulnerability of family units to health problems may be based on the maturity level of individual family members, heredity or genetic factors, sex or race, sociologic factors, and lifestyle practices.

MATURITY FACTORS. Families with members at both ends of the age continuum are at risk of developing health problems. Families entering childbearing and child-rearing phases experience many changes in roles, responsibilities, and expectations. The many, often conflicting, demands on the family cause stress and fatigue, which may impede growth of individual family members and the functioning of the group as a unit. Adolescent mothers, because of their developmental level and lack of knowledge about parenthood, and single-parent families, because of role overload experienced by the head of the household, are more likely to develop health problems. Many elderly persons feel a lack of purpose and decreased self-esteem. These feelings in turn reduce their motivation to engage in health-promoting behaviors, such as exercise or community and family involvement.

HEREDITARY FACTORS. Persons born into families with a history of certain diseases, such as diabetes or cardiovascular disease, are at greater risk of developing these conditions. A detailed family health history, including genetically transmitted disorders, is crucial to the identification of persons and families at risk. These data are used not only to monitor the health of individual family members but also to recommend modifications in health practices that potentially reduce the risk, minimize the consequences, or postpone the development of genetically related conditions.

GENDER OR RACE. Some family units or family members may be at risk of developing a disease by reason of gender or race. Males, for example, are at greater risk of having cardiovascular disease at an earlier age than females, and females are at greater risk of developing osteoporosis, particularly after menopause. Although it is sometimes difficult to separate genetic factors from cultural factors, certain risk factors seem to be related to race. Sickle-cell anemia, for example, is a hereditary disease limited to people of African descent, and Tay-Sachs is a neurodegenerative disease that occurs primarily in descendants of Eastern European Jews.

SOCIOLOGIC FACTORS. Poverty is a major problem that affects not only the family but also the community and society. Poverty is a real concern among the rising number of single-parent families. As the number of these families increases, poverty will affect a large number of growing children.

When ill, the poor are likely to put off seeking services until the illness reaches an advanced state and requires longer or more complex treatment. Although the health of the people of industrialized nations has improved significantly during the past century, this progress has not benefited all segments of society, particularly the poor.

LIFESTYLE FACTORS. Many diseases are preventable, the effects of some diseases can be minimized, or the onset of disease can be delayed through lifestyle modifications. Certain cancers, cardiovascular disease, adult-onset diabetes, and tooth decay are among the lifestyle diseases. The incidence of lung cancer, for example, would be greatly reduced if people stopped smoking. Good nutrition, dental hygiene, and use of fluoride—in the water supply, in toothpaste, as a topical application, or as supplements—have been shown to reduce dental decay or caries, one of America's most prevalent health problems.

Other important lifestyle considerations are exercise, stress management, and rest. Today health professionals have the knowledge to prevent or minimize the effects of some of the main causes of disease, disability, and death. The challenge is to disseminate information about prevention and to motivate families to make lifestyle changes prior to the onset of illness.

Diagnosing and Planning

Data gathered during a family assessment may lead to the following nursing diagnoses:

- *Interrupted Family Processes,* a change in family relationships
- *Readiness for Enhanced Family Coping,* effective management of adaptive tasks by family member involved with the client's health challenge, who now exhibits desire and readiness for enhanced health and growth in regard to self and in relation to the client
- *Disabled Family Coping,* behavior of significant person (family member or other primary person) that disables his/her capacities to effectively address tasks essential to either person's adaptation to the health challenge
- *Impaired Parenting,* inability of the primary caretaker to create, maintain, or regain an environment that promotes the optimum growth and development of the child
- *Impaired Home Maintenance,* inability to independently maintain a safe growth-promoting immediate environment
- *Caregiver Role Strain,* difficulty in performing family caregiver role

Examples of contributing factors for one selected diagnosis, desired outcomes to evaluate the achievement of client goals, and the effectiveness of nursing interventions are listed in Identifying Nursing Diagnoses, Outcomes, and Interventions.

Being sensitive to cultural differences is important in assessment and planning care. Knowing who makes most of the decisions in the family, especially in health care, helps the nurse know to whom to direct questions in order to obtain information and also to whom to give instructions. The extended family unit is found in many cultures and there may be a difference in health beliefs and health practices within the family. Older members of the family may use their traditional practices, while younger members may have had more exposure to modern practices.

IDENTIFYING NURSING DIAGNOSES, OUTCOMES, AND INTERVENTIONS
Clients with Disruption in Family Health

DATA CLUSTER Mr. & Mrs. G's 6-year-old son has just been diagnosed with acute leukemia. They also have a 9-year-old daughter and a 4-year-old son.

NURSING DIAGNOSIS/ DEFINITION	SAMPLE DESIRED OUTCOMES*/ DEFINITION	NOC INDICATORS	SELECTED INTERVENTIONS*/ DEFINITION	SAMPLE NIC ACTIVITIES
Interrupted Family Processes/Change in family relationships	Family Coping [2600]/*Family actions to manage stressors that tax family resources.*	Often demonstrated ▪ Involves family members in decision making ▪ Uses stress reduction strategies ▪ Arranges for respite care	Family Integrity Promotion [7100]/ *Promotion of family cohesion and unity* Normalization Promotion [7200]/ *Assisting parents and other family members of children with chronic illness or disabilities in providing normal life experiences for their children and families*	▪ Determine family understanding of illness ▪ Tell family members it is safe and acceptable to use typical expressions of affection ▪ Refer for family therapy, as indicated ▪ De-emphasize uniqueness of child's condition ▪ Involve siblings in care and activities of child as appropriate
	Psychosocial Adjustment: Life Change [1305]/ Adaptive *psychosocial response of an individual to a significant life change.*	Sometimes demonstrated ▪ Sets realistic goals ▪ Reports of feeling empowered	Family Process Maintenance [7130]/ *Minimization of family process disruption effects*	▪ Determine typical family processes ▪ Discuss strategies for normalizing family life with family members

*The NOC# for desired outcomes and the NIC# for nursing interventions are listed in brackets following the appropriate outcome or intervention. Outcomes, indicators, interventions, and activities are only a sample of those suggested by NOC and NIC and should be further individualized for each client.

Building a trusting relationship with these families is the first step toward planning more effective care by being able to talk to them about their beliefs and practices.

Nursing needs to focus on assisting the family to plan realistic goals/outcomes and strategies that enhance family functioning, such as improving communication skills, identifying and utilizing support systems, and developing and rehearsing parenting skills. Anticipatory guidance may assist well-functioning families in preparing for predictable developmental transitions that occur in the life of families.

The Family Experiencing a Health Crisis

Illness of a family member is a crisis that affects the entire family system. The family is disrupted as members abandon their usual activities and focus their energy on restoring family equilibrium. Roles and responsibilities previously assumed by the ill person are delegated to other family members, or those functions may remain undone for the duration of the illness. The family experiences anxiety because members are concerned about the sick person and the resolution of the illness. This anxiety is compounded by additional responsibilities when there is less time or motivation to complete the normal tasks of daily living. See Box 24–2 for some factors that determine the impact of illness on the family unit.

The family's ability to deal with the stress of illness depends on the members' coping skills. Families with good communication skills are better able to discuss how they feel about the illness and how it affects family functioning. They can plan for the future and are flexible in adapting these plans as the situation changes. An established social support network provides strength, encouragement, and services to the family during the

BOX 24–2 Factors Determining the Impact of Illness on the Family

- The nature of the illness, which can range from minor to life threatening
- The duration of the illness, which ranges from short term to long term
- The residual effects of the illness, including none to permanent disability
- The meaning of the illness to the family and its significance to family systems
- The financial impact of the illness, which is influenced by factors such as insurance and ability of the ill member to return to work
- The effect of the illness on future family functioning (for instance, previous patterns may be restored or new patterns may be established)

illness. During health crises, families need to realize that it is a strength, not a sign of weakness, to turn to others for support. Nurses can be part of the support system for families, or they can identify other sources of support in the community.

During a crisis, families are often drawn together by a common purpose. In this time of closeness, family members have the opportunity to reaffirm personal and family values and their commitment to one another. Indeed, illness may provide a unique opportunity for family growth.

The Nurse's Role with Families Experiencing Illness

Nurses committed to family-centered care involve both the ailing individual and the family in the nursing process. Through their interaction with families, nurses can give support and information. Nurses make sure that not only the individual but also each family member understands the disease, its management, and the effect of these two factors on family functioning. The nurse also assesses the family's readiness and ability to provide continued care and supervision at home when warranted. After carefully planned instruction and practice, families are given an opportunity to demonstrate their ability to provide care under the supportive guidance of the nurse. When the care indicated is beyond the capability of the family, nurses work with families to identify available resources that are socially and financially acceptable.

In helping families reintegrate the ill person into the home, nurses use data gathered during family assessment to identify family resources and deficits. By formulating mutually acceptable goals for reintegration, nurses help families cope with the realities of the illness and the changes it may have brought about, which may include new roles and functions of family members or the need to provide continued medical care to the ill or recovering person. Working together, nurses and families can create environments that restore or reorganize family functioning during illness and throughout the recovery process.

Death of a Family Member

The death of a family member often has a profound effect on the family. The structure of the family is altered, and this change may in turn affect how it functions as a unit. Individual members experience a sense of loss. They grieve for the lost person, and they grieve for the family that once was. Family disorganization may occur. However, as the family begins to recover, a new sense of normalcy develops, the family reintegrates its roles and functions, and it comes to grips with the reality of the situation. This painful blow takes time to heal.

After the death of a member, families may need counseling to deal with their feelings and to talk about the person who died. They may also want to talk about their fears and hopes for the future. At this time, families often derive comfort from their religious beliefs and their spiritual advisers. Support groups are also available for families experiencing the pain of death. It is often difficult for nurses to deal with grieving families because the nurses also feel the loss and feel inadequate in knowing what to say or do. By understanding the effect death has on families, nurses can help families resolve their grief and move ahead with life. (See Chapter 43 ∞ for a discussion of loss and grieving.)

Implementing and Evaluating

Nursing interventions are based on the medical diagnoses, nursing diagnoses, and selected goals or outcomes (see Identifying Nursing Diagnoses, Outcomes, and Interventions). In evaluating the success of the family care plan, the nurse assesses for the presence of the indicators identified for the chosen outcomes. If the indicators are present, it is likely that the outcome has been achieved. If the indicators or outcomes are partially or not met, all aspects of the family situation must be reexamined: Have the intervention activities been carried out? Are the indicators and outcomes appropriate? Is the nursing diagnosis proper? Has the medical condition or diagnosis changed?

Recognition of individual and family strengths helps to maintain wellness and also directs behavior in crises situations. If a plan of care has to be modified to be more effective, these strengths should be identified and utilized.

CRITICAL THINKING CHECKPOINT

Linda is a young mother of three children who has developed a severe arthritic condition that has affected her ability to work and adequately care for her family. Her illness has created a financial hardship for the family and has strained their roles. Linda and her husband have custody of their children from previous marriages as well as a daughter of their own. They are reluctant to seek assistance from outside sources because they fear interference from their ex-spouses with regard to their children.

1. What aspects of Linda's physical problem must the nurse be concerned about as they relate to the other issues occurring in Linda's life?
2. Explain why Linda's family is considered to be in a health crisis when only Linda is experiencing an illness.
3. What are the advantages or disadvantages of facing illness as a member of a family as opposed to individually?
4. Describe Linda's family from the perspective of general systems theory.

See Critical Thinking Possibilities in Appendix A. ∞

CHAPTER 24 **REVIEW**

CHAPTER HIGHLIGHTS

- The family is the basic unit of society.
- The family plays an important role in forming the health beliefs and practices of its members.
- Information on how family members are genetically related is gathered via a genogram, while an ecomap allows the nurse to see where the family's energy is being expended.
- Family-centered nursing addresses the health of the family as a unit, as well as the health of family members.
- In today's society, many types of families exist: traditional, two-career, single-parent, those headed by one or more adolescent parents, foster, blended, intragenerational, cohabiting, and gay and lesbian. In addition, many single adults live alone.
- The purpose of family assessment is to determine the level of family functioning, to clarify family interaction patterns, to identify family strengths and weaknesses, and to describe the health status of the family and its individual members.

- Families at risk for health problems may be considered on the basis of family maturity level, presence of hereditary factors, sex or race, lifestyle practices, and sociologic factors such as poverty.
- Nursing diagnoses that relate to family health needs and problems include *Interrupted Family Processes; Readiness for Enhanced Family Coping; Disabled Family Coping; Impaired Parenting; Impaired Home Maintenance;* and *Caregiver Role Strain.*
- Nurses must examine their own values about family, health, illness, and death to be effective in supporting families in crisis.
- A variety of nursing theoretical frameworks provide the nurse with a holistic overview of health promotion of families across the life span.

TEST YOUR KNOWLEDGE

1. Because a severely injured middle-aged client informed the nurse that he did not have any immediate family members, the nurse contacted extended family members. Which of the following is most representative of extended family members?
   1. Grandparents, aunts and uncles
   2. Parents and spouse
   3. Children who no longer live at home
   4. Roommates and close family friends

2. When a father prepares to leave for work in the morning, his 3-year-old son starts to cry and scream. The father picks him up and delays leaving for a while. The child's behavior most reflects which part of a system?
   1. Input
   2. Throughput
   3. Output
   4. Feedback

3. A nurse should instruct a client who identifies "the family" as two college roommates, a dog, and a cat to perform which of the following when completing a family health history form?
   1. Include all information about blood relatives and the animals and roommates that might influence his health.
   2. Include only information about genetic/hereditary and environmental illnesses of blood relatives.
   3. Leave the area blank since the client does not live with blood relatives.
   4. Use the client's own judgment in completing the area since the physical exam is more important than the history.

4. A visual representation of family members by gender, age, health status, and lines of relationships through the generations is referred to as a _____.

5. In order to assess the impact of illness on the family as a unit, it is **essential** that the nurse assess which of the following factors? (Choose all that apply.)
   1. The duration of the illness
   2. The meaning of the illness to the family and its significance to family systems
   3. The coping mechanisms used by other families with similar illnesses
   4. The financial impact of the illness (including factors such as insurance and ability of the ill member to work)
   5. The incidence of the illness in the community at large

6. An adult child brings a parent to an agency with signs and symptoms of potential fluid retention (e.g., high blood pressure, swollen feet) possibly related to excessive sodium intake. Further nursing assessment indicates inadequate food storage and preparation techniques in the home. Which of the following would be the most appropriate nursing diagnosis?
   1. *Readiness for enhanced family coping*
   2. *Disabled family coping*
   3. *Impaired parenting*
   4. *Caregiver role strain*

7. Prior to finalizing a family-oriented nursing care plan and implementing interventions, it is essential for the nurse to perform which of the following?
   1. Meet with all family members simultaneously
   2. Confirm that the family health insurance covers all the family members
   3. Establish a trusting relationship with the family as a group
   4. Complete a thorough history and physical examination of each family member

8. Nurses often utilize systems theory to assess family units. Which of the examples listed below illustrates a family unit that *does not* meet the criteria of a well-functioning system?
   1. The family members allow input from outside the family unit
   2. The family members are interdependent
   3. Each member's personal boundaries are well-defined
   4. The primary activities of each member focus on personal purposes

See Answers to Test Your Knowledge in Appendix A.

EXPLORE MEDIALINK www.prenhall.com/berman

DVD-ROM
- Audio Glossary
- NCLEX Review
- End of Unit Concept Map Activity
- Video: Involving Families in NICU Settings

COMPANION WEBSITE
- Additional NCLEX Review
- Case Study: Home Health and an Elderly Family
- Care Plan Activity: Client in the ICU and the Family
- Application Activity: Health Care Resources
- Links to Resources

READINGS AND REFERENCES

SUGGESTED READINGS
Willgerodt, M. A., & Killien, M. G. (2004). Family nursing research with Asian families. *Journal of Family Nursing, 10,* 149–172.
This article reviews nursing research conducted with Asian families over the past decade. The aim was to better understand what has been accomplished with Asian families and what still needs to be addressed by nursing for this group.
Wuest, J., Ford-Gilboe, M., Merritt-Gray, M., & Berman, H. (2003). Intrusion: The central problem for family health promotion among children and single mothers after leaving an abusive partner. *Qualitative Health Research, 13,* 597–622.
Mothers and their children who leave abusive partners/fathers are seen as having viewed a high-risk susceptibility to multiple problems. The authors discuss the complex nature of intrusion, demonstrating how health is socially determined, and the challenges of health promotion faced by the study families.

RELATED RESEARCH
Byrd, M., & Garwick, A. (2004). A feminist critique of research on interracial family identity: Implications for family health. *Journal of Family Nursing, 10,* 302–320.
Sgarbossa, D., & Ford-Gilboe, M. (2004). Mother's friendship quality, parental support, quality of life, and family health work in families led by adolescent mothers with preschool children. *Journal of Family Nursing, 10,* 232–261.

REFERENCES
Alan Guttmacher Institute. (2004). *U.S. teenage pregnancy statistics: Overall trends, trends by race and ethnicity and state-by-state information.* New York: Author.
Black, C., & Ford-Gilboe, M. (2004). Adolescent mothers: Resilience, family health work and health-promoting practices. *Journal of Advanced Nursing, 48,* 351–360.
Dochterman, J., & Bulechek, G. B. (Eds.). (2004). *Nursing interventions classification (NIC)* (4th ed.). St. Louis, MO: Mosby.

Erikson, E. (1963). *Childhood and society* (2nd ed.). New York: Norton.
Fields, J. (2003). *America's families and living arrangements: 2003.* Current Population Reports, P20–553. Washington, DC: U.S. Census Bureau.
Moorhead, S., Johnson, M., & Maas, M. (Eds.). (2004). *Nursing outcomes classification (NOC)* (3rd ed.). St. Louis, MO: Mosby.
NANDA International. (2007). NANDA *nursing diagnoses: Definitions and classification 2007–2008.* Philadelphia: Author.
U.S. Census Bureau. (2004). *"Stay-at-home" parents top 5 million.* Washington, DC: Author. Retrieved May 5, 2006, from http:// www.census.gov/Press-Release/www/ releases/archives/families_households/ 003118.html
U.S. Conference of Mayors. (2004). *A status report on hunger and homelessness in America's cities: 2004.* Retrieved May 5, 2006, from http://www.usmayors.org/uscm/

us_mayor_newspaper/documents/01_10_05/
hunger_survey.asp

von Bertalanffy, L. (1980). *General system theory* (revised from original 1969). New York: George Braziller.

Wilkerson, S. A., & Loveland-Cherry, C. J. (2004). Johnson's behavioral system model. In J. J. Fitzpatrick & A. L. Whall (Eds.), *Conceptual models of nursing: Analysis and application* (4th ed., pp. 83–103). Upper Saddle River, NJ: Prentice Hall Health.

SELECTED BIBLIOGRAPHY

American Nurses Association. (1998). *Culturally competent assessment for family violence.* Washington, DC: American Nurses Publishing.

Doane, G. H., & Varcoe, C. (2004). *Family nursing as relational inquiry*. Philadelphia: Lippincott Williams & Wilkins.

Friedman, M. M., Bowden, V. R., & Jones, E. G. (2003). *Family nursing: Research, theory and practice* (5th ed.). Upper Saddle River, NJ: Prentice Hall.

Locsin, R. C. (2003). Culture perspectives. The integration of family health, culture, and nursing: Prescriptions and practices. *Holistic Nursing Practice, 17*(1), 8–10.

Rigazio-DiGilio, S. A. (2005). *Community genograms: Using individual, family, and cultural narratives with clients.* New York: Teacher's College Press.

UNIT
6

Integral Aspects of Nursing

Caring and effective communication are essential elements of an optimal nurse–client relationship and of the leader–manager role. Nurses are attuned to all forms of communication, recognizing that gestures, expressions, and other kinds of body language often convey a message more powerfully and accurately than mere words. The nurse responds not only to the factual content of a message but also to the feelings expressed through verbal and nonverbal modes. Establishing client rapport facilitates a vital nursing role—the process of teaching, a structured form of communication designed to produce learning.

CHAPTER
25

Caring

LEARNING OUTCOMES
After completing this chapter, you will be able to:

1. Discuss the meaning of caring.

2. Identify nursing theories focusing on caring.

3. Analyze the importance of different types of knowledge in nursing.

4. Describe how nurses demonstrate caring in practice.

5. Evaluate the importance of self-care for the professional nurse.

6. Identify the value of reflective practice in nursing.

KEY TERMS

aesthetic knowing, *450*
caring , *445*
caring practice, *445*

empirical knowing, *449*
ethical knowing, *450*

personal knowing, *450*
reflection, *454*

In this age of technological competence and efficiency, the knowledge and skills embedded in caring practices are often overlooked. Phillips and Benner (1994) identified a "crisis in caring" across our society, especially involving members of the helping professions, such as nursing. Caring is central to all helping professions, and enables persons to create meaning in their lives. **Caring** means that people, relationships, and things matter.

PROFESSIONALIZATION OF CARING

Caring practice involves connection, mutual recognition, and involvement. Consider the following examples of caring, emerging from nursing situations:

- A client experiencing postoperative pain is given medication to control her symptoms, and then the nurse talks quietly and holds her hand for a few minutes as the pain resolves. The nurse's presence, in itself, provides comfort for the client.
- After the student nurse washes her hair and applies makeup, an immobilized elderly woman is helped to sit up in a wheelchair to greet her daughter and grandchildren. She is extremely grateful just to be able to sit up af-

ter weeks in bed. Her sense of dignity is enhanced by this personal care.

Just as clients benefit from caring practices, the nurses involved in these situations experience caring through knowing that they have made a difference in their clients' lives. Consider, for example, one nurse's feeling of satisfaction: "It is not something that can be defined but, you know, . . . the feeling that you've made a difference to an individual, and had I not been there at that time, that would never have occurred" (Pask, 2003, p. 169).

As nurses feel free to concentrate their attention upon the other, they can make a positive difference to clients. The ability to give focused attention to clients means leaving the egocentric self behind. Students of nursing can develop this ability by studying the meaning of caring in nursing.

Caring as "Helping the Other Grow"

Milton Mayeroff (1990), a noted philosopher, has proposed that to care for another person is to help him grow and actualize himself. Caring is a process that develops over time, resulting in a deepening and transformation of the relationship. Recognizing the other as having potential and the need to grow, the caregiver

REAL WORLD PRACTICE

As a nursing student I once cared for a client by the name of Mr. Johnson.* He was an older gentleman, who was very ill and noncommunicative. He was in the first room to the right past the nursing station. There were few personal belongings in his room, and I never observed visiting family or friends. The room was dark and all I could see and hear was Mr. Johnson's labored breathing through his tracheostomy and the cyclical clicking of the intravenous pump. Both his legs were immobilized and pinned from feet to the knees. Every time I would walk into his room I spoke to him. "Hi Mr. Johnson, it's Danene, your student nurse, I'm here to" . . . and I would tell him what I was there to do. When I would turn, bathe, clean his leg pins or suction his trach, I would tell him I hoped he slept well last night and what the weather was like that day. I would talk with him in a conversation as though he was returning a dialogue with me. Every now and then he would move or make a grunting sound and I began to understand what he needed. Over a couple of hours he "told" me what was okay for him and never spoke a word.

The next morning I walked into his room and introduced myself again. I could see the tension in his face fade as his cheeks relaxed. He knew I was there for him. Later that day when the floor

nurse came into the room, I was talking to Mr. Johnson as I usually did. She looked at me with disgust and said, "He can't hear you and he doesn't talk." I decided to continue my conversations with Mr. Johnson despite the floor nurse's disapproval. As my shift was ending one day, I told Mr. Johnson that I would be back in the morning bright and early. I held his hand and then gave it a little pat and said, "I'll see you in the morning—sleep well . . ."

The next morning I found Mr. Johnson's room empty. I was told Mr. Johnson had died in the early hours of the morning. To this day I will never know if Mr. Johnson actually heard or understood my words but if he did, he knew I was his advocate and someone he could count on. My interactions with Mr. Johnson and the floor nurse forever changed the way I practice nursing. I have relived this experience many times over and would never change a single thing.

— *Danene Shannon MS Ed, BSN, BA, RN,*
Professional Clinical Educator/Patient Education Specialist,
Advocate Lutheran General Hospital, Park Ridge, IL

*Name has been changed for client privacy.

does not impose direction, but allows the direction of the other person's growth to help determine how to respond.

Major ingredients of caring provide structure and further description of this process: (a) *knowing* means understanding the other's needs and how to respond to these needs; (b) *alternating rhythms* signifies moving back and forth between the immediate and long-term meanings of behavior, considering the past; (c) *patience* enables the other to grow in his own way and time; (d) *honesty* includes awareness and openness to one's own feelings and a genuineness in caring for the other; (e) *trust* involves letting go, to allow the other to grow in his own way and own time; (f) *humility* means acknowledging that there is always more to learn, and that learning may come from any source; (g) *hope* is belief in the possibilities of the other's growth; and (h) *courage* is the sense of going into the unknown, informed by insight from past experiences.

Mayeroff proposes that the caring process has benefits for the one giving care. By helping the other grow, the caregiver moves toward self-actualization. By caring and being cared for, each person "finds his place" in the world. Through serving others through caring, persons live the meaning of their own lives.

NURSING THEORIES ON CARING

Caring is a multidimensional concept. In a comprehensive review of the concept of caring, Morse, Solberg, Neander, Battorff, and Johnson (1990) identified different definitions of caring, which were summarized as the following five viewpoints:

- Caring as a moral imperative
- Caring as an affect
- Caring as a human trait
- Caring as an interpersonal relationship
- Caring as a therapeutic intervention

Nurse scholars have reviewed the literature, conducted research, and analyzed nurses' experiences, resulting in the development of theories and models of caring. These theories and models are grounded in humanism and the idea that caring is the basis for human science. Several nursing theorists focus on caring: Leininger, Ray, Roach, Boykin and Schoenhofer, Watson, Swanson, and Benner and Wrubel.

Culture Care Diversity and Universality (Leininger)

Based on studies in nursing and anthropology, Leininger noted that caring, as nurturing behavior, has been present throughout history and is one of the most critical factors in helping people maintain or regain health. Leininger proposes that "caring is the essence of nursing, and the distinct, dominant, central, and unifying focus of nursing" (Leininger, 2001, p. 35). Her theory of culture care diversity and universality is based on the assumption that nurses must understand different cultures in order to function effectively.

Transcultural nursing focuses on both the differences and similarities among persons in diverse cultures. While cultures have different ways of caring for others, there are also universal behaviors among all cultures of the world. In order to provide care that is congruent with cultural values, beliefs, and practices, the nurse must understand these differences and similarities. To understand the care desired by clients and "enter their broader worldview," the nurse requires knowledge of the culture and local language (Leininger, 2001, p. 58). When nursing care fails to be reasonably congruent with the client's beliefs, lifeways, and values, there may be signs of conflict, noncompliance, and stress.

Culturally congruent care is provided in three major ways: (a) by preserving the client's familiar lifeways, (b) by making accommodations in care that are satisfying to clients, and (c) by repatterning nursing care to help the client move toward wellness (Leininger, 2001). Leininger defines caring as "assisting, supporting, or enabling another individual or group with evident or anticipated needs to ameliorate or improve a human condition or lifeway, or to face death" (2001, p. 46).

Theory of Bureaucratic Caring (Ray)

Ray's theory of bureaucratic caring focuses on caring in organizations (e.g., hospitals) as cultures. The theory suggests that caring in nursing is contextual and is influenced by the organizational structure. In Ray's research, the meaning of caring varied in the emergency department, intensive care unit, oncology unit, and other areas of the hospital. For example, an intensive care unit had a dominant value of technological caring (i.e., monitors, ventilators, treatments, and pharmacotherapeutics), and an oncology unit had a value of a more intimate, spiritual caring (i.e., family focused, comforting, compassionate). Furthermore, the meaning of caring was further influenced by the role and position a person held. Staff nurses valued caring in terms of its relatedness to clients, while administrators valued caring as more system-related, such as safeguarding the economic well-being of the hospital (Coffman, 2006).

As depicted in Figure 25-1■, spiritual-ethical caring influences each of the aspects of the bureaucratic system (political, legal, economic, educational, physiologic, social-cultural, and technological). Each of these aspects is different, but they make up a whole bureaucratic system (e.g., a hospital). Nurses influence client care by making choices about each of these aspects (Ray, 2001). Nurses make these choices with the interest of the client at heart and use ethical principles as the foundation for the basis of professional decision making. According to Ray (2001), "Spiritual-ethical caring for nursing does not question whether or not to care in complex systems, but intimates how sincere deliberations and ultimately the facilitation of choices for the good of others can or should be accomplished" (p. 429).

Caring, the Human Mode of Being (Roach)

M. Simone Roach focuses on caring as a philosophical concept and proposes that caring is the human mode of being, or the "most common, authentic criterion of humanness" (Roach, 2002, p. 28). All persons are caring, and develop their caring abilities by being true to self, being real, and being who they truly are. Thus, caring is not unique to nursing.

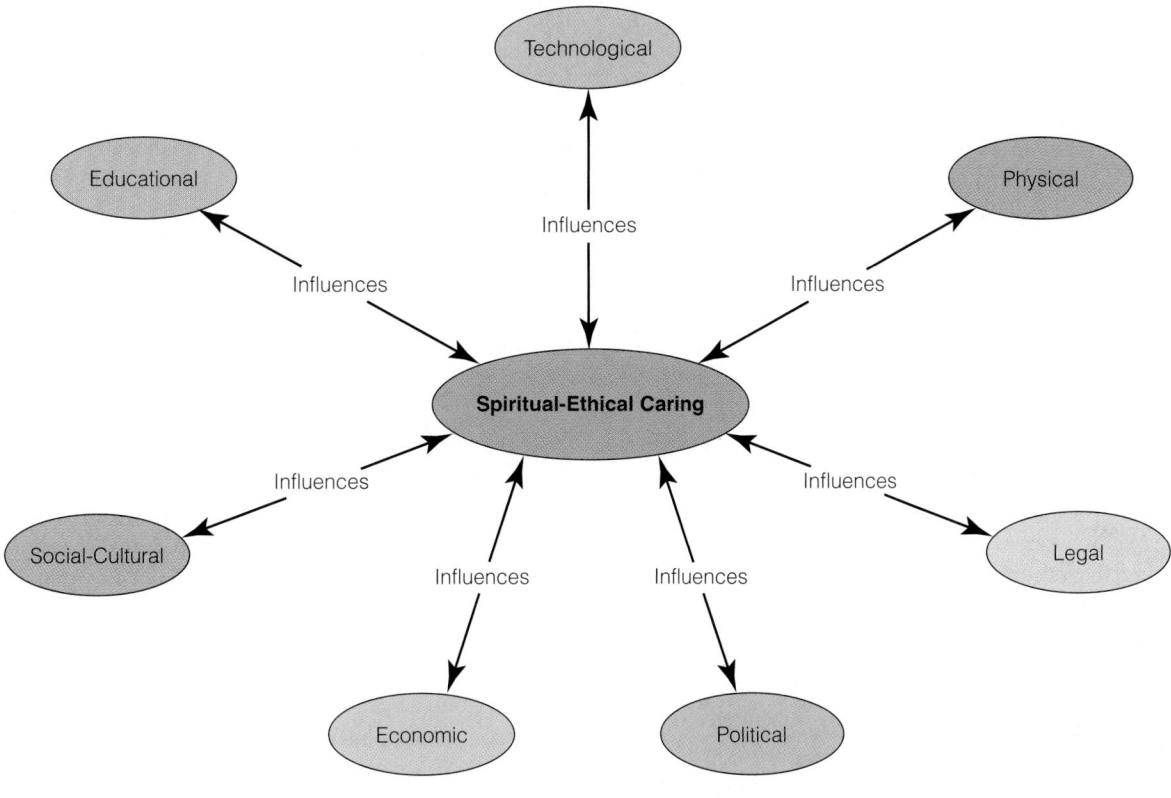

Figure 25-1 ■ Concept map reflecting the theory of bureaucratic caring.

Roach visualizes caring to be unique in nursing, however, because caring is the center of all attributes used to describe nursing. Roach defines these attributes as the six Cs of caring: compassion, competence, confidence, conscience, commitment, and comportment. See Box 25–1 for definitions of each characteristic. The six Cs are used as a broad framework, suggesting categories of behavior that describe professional caring. Each category reflects specific values and includes virtuous actions by which a nurse can demonstrate caring.

Nursing as Caring (Boykin and Schoenhofer)

Boykin and Schoenhofer suggest that the purpose of the discipline and profession of nursing is to know persons and nurture them as persons living in caring and growing in caring (Purnell, 2006). Respect for persons as caring individuals and respect for what matters to them are assumptions underlying the theory of nursing as caring. Similar to Roach's idea that all persons are caring, Boykin and Schoenhofer emphasize the importance of the nurse knowing self as a caring person. Maintaining this approach may be difficult in practice environments which may depersonalize the nurse and view nursing care only as tasks that need to be completed. However, caring is a lifetime process, lived moment to moment by the nurse, and constantly unfolding. Through knowing self as a caring person, the nurse can be authentic to self, freeing oneself to truly be with others. This

---

BOX 25–1 **The Six Cs of Caring in Nursing**

COMPASSION
Awareness of one's relationship to others, sharing their joys, sorrows, pain, and accomplishments. Participation in the experience of another.

COMPETENCE
Having the knowledge, judgment, skills, energy, experience, and motivation to respond adequately to others within the demands of professional responsibilities.

CONFIDENCE
The quality that fosters trusting relationships. Comfort with self, client, and family.

CONSCIENCE
Morals, ethics, and an informed sense of right and wrong. Awareness of personal responsibility.

COMMITMENT
Convergence between one's desires and obligations and the deliberate choice to act in accordance with them.

COMPORTMENT
Appropriate bearing, demeanor, dress, and language, that are in harmony with a caring presence. Presenting oneself as someone who respects others and demands respect.

Note: Adapted from *Caring, the Human Mode of Being,* 2nd ed. by M. S. Roach. Copyright © 2002 CHA Press. Reprinted with permission.

awareness of self allows the nurse to authentically care for others in nursing practice.

Caring in nursing is "an altruistic, active expression of love, and is the intentional and embodied recognition of value and connectedness" (Boykin & Schoenhofer, 2001, p. 393). From the perspective of the theory of nursing as caring, the nurse approaches each client as a caring person, whole and complete in the moment. The idea of wholeness includes the understanding that people are not perfect, but constantly growing and changing. By living nursing as caring, the nurse establishes a mutual relationship of trust and respect with the client. Through fully appreciating the life-world of others, the nurse energizes self and others to grow as caring persons.

Theory of Human Care (Watson)

Watson's theory of human care views caring as the essence and the moral ideal of nursing. Human care is the basis for nursing's role in society; indeed, nursing's contribution to society lies in its moral commitment to human care. Nursing as human care goes beyond the realm of ethics, as described by Watson (1999, p. 29):

> Human caring in nursing, therefore, is not just an emotion, concern, attitude, or benevolent desire. Caring is the moral ideal of nursing whereby the end is protection, enhancement, and preservation of human dignity. Human caring involves values, a will and a commitment to care, knowledge, caring action, and consequences. All of human caring is related to intersubjective human responses to health-illness conditions; a knowledge of health-illness, environmental-personal interactions; a knowledge of the nurse caring process; self-knowledge, knowledge of one's power and transaction limitations.

Assumptions of Watson's theory and nursing interventions related to human care, or her carative factors, are presented in Chapter 3. ∞

Watson emphasizes nursing's commitment to care of the whole person as well as a concern for the health of individuals and groups. The nurse and client are co-participants in the client's movement toward health and wholeness. This human connection is further described in Box 25–2. Watson labels this process transpersonal human caring through which the nurse enters into the experience of the client, and the client can enter

into the nurse's experience. By identifying with each other, the nurse and client gain self-knowledge and keep alive his or her common humanity, avoiding reducing the other to an object.

Watson emphasizes that the practice of nursing is both transpersonal and metaphysical. While the nurse maintains professional objectivity as a scientist, scholar, clinician, and moral agent, the nurse is also subjectively engaged in the interpersonal relationship with the client. Within the actual caring situation, each person (nurse and client) seeks a sense of harmony within the mind, body, and soul, thereby actualizing the real self. This transpersonal contact has the potential to touch the higher, spiritual sense of self, or the soul. Such contact, which touches the soul, has the power to generate the self-healing process.

Theory of Caring (Swanson)

Swanson defines caring as "a nurturing way of relating to a valued 'other,' toward whom one feels a personal sense of commitment and responsibility" (2001, p. 415). An assumption of her theory is that a client's well-being should be enhanced through the caring of a nurse who understands the common human responses to a specific health problem. The theory focuses on caring processes as nursing interventions. Swanson's theory was developed through interactions with parents at the time of pregnancy, miscarriage, and birth. The five caring processes and their subdimensions are described in Table 25–1. These processes pro-

BOX 25–2 Watson's Description of a Caring Transaction

The two individuals (the nurse and the client) in a caring transaction are both in a process of being and becoming. Both individuals bring with them to the relationship a unique life history and phenomenal field, and both are influenced and affected by the nature of the transaction, which in turn becomes part of the life history of each person. In this sense of a caring transaction, caring is a moral ideal, rather than an interpersonal technique and it entails a commitment of a particular end. The end is the protection, enhancement, and preservation of the person's humanity, which help to restore inner harmony and potential healing.

Note: J. Watson, *Nursing: Human Science and Human Care. A Theory of Nursing* 1999: Copyright Jones and Bartlett Publishers, Sudbury, MA. www.jbpub.com. Reprinted with permission.

TABLE 25–1 Caring Processes and Subdimensions from Swanson's Theory of Caring

PROCESS AND DEFINITION	SUBDIMENSIONS
Knowing Striving to understand an event as it has meaning in the life of the other	Avoiding assumptions Centering on the one cared Assessing thoroughly Seeing cues Engaging the self of both
Being With Being emotionally present to the other	Being there Conveying ability Sharing feelings Not burdening
Doing For Doing for the other as he/she would do for the self if it were at all possible	Comforting Anticipating Performing competently/skillfully Protecting Preserving dignity
Enabling Facilitating the other's passage through life transitions and unfamiliar events	Informing/explaining Supporting/allowing Focusing Generating alternatives/thinking it through Validating/giving feedback
Maintaining Belief Sustaining faith in the other's capacity to get through an event or transition and face a future with meaning	Believing in/holding in esteem Maintaining a hope-filled attitude Offering realistic optimism "Going the distance"

Note: From K. Swanson, "Empirical Development of a Middle Range Theory of Caring," *Nursing Research, 40*(3), pp. 162–163. Copyright © 1991 Lippincott, Williams & Wilkins. Reprinted with permission.

vide guidance to nurses who work with pregnant and postpartum clients. Further research will test the applicability of these caring dimensions to other client populations.

The Primacy of Caring (Benner and Wrubel)

As Benner and Wrubel listened to expert nurses' stories and analyzed their meanings, caring emerged as the essence of excellence in nursing. Nursing is described as a relationship in which caring is primary because it sets up the possibility of giving and receiving help (Benner & Wrubel, 1989). Caring practice requires attending to the particular client over time, determining what matters to the person, and using this knowledge in clinical judgments. As nurses gain expertise, they are more effective in focusing on what the client brings to the health care encounter. Caring facilitates the nurse's ability to problem solve and to implement individualized solutions.

Caring is interactive, in that the strengths and abilities of the person who is cared for are as important as the skills of the nurse. A caring relationship requires a certain amount of openness and capacity to respond to care on the part of the client. In caring practice, being with someone may be just as important as doing something for that person, if not more so. As the nurse gains expertise, he or she learns how to be with people, to respect who they are and where they are at, and to stop doing for them. Thus, caring practice involves client advocacy and provides the necessary conditions to help the client grow and develop (Gordon, Benner, & Noddings, 1996).

TYPES OF KNOWLEDGE IN NURSING

Nursing involves different types of knowledge that are integrated to guide nursing practice. Nurses require scientific competence (empirical knowledge), therapeutic use of self (personal knowing), moral/ethical awareness (ethical knowing), and creative action (aesthetic knowing). These four types of knowledge were identified by Carper (1978) from her observations of nurses' activities. An understanding of each type of knowledge is important for the student of nursing because only by integrating all ways of knowing can the nurse develop a professional practice. Figure 25-2 ■ illustrates the interconnection of these different types of knowledge.

Empirical Knowing: The Science of Nursing

Knowledge about the empirical world is systematically organized into laws and theories for the purpose of describing, explaining, and predicting phenomena of special concern to the discipline of nursing. **Empirical knowing** ranges from factual, observable phenomena (e.g., anatomy, physiology, chemistry) to theoretical analysis (e.g., developmental theory, adaptation theory).

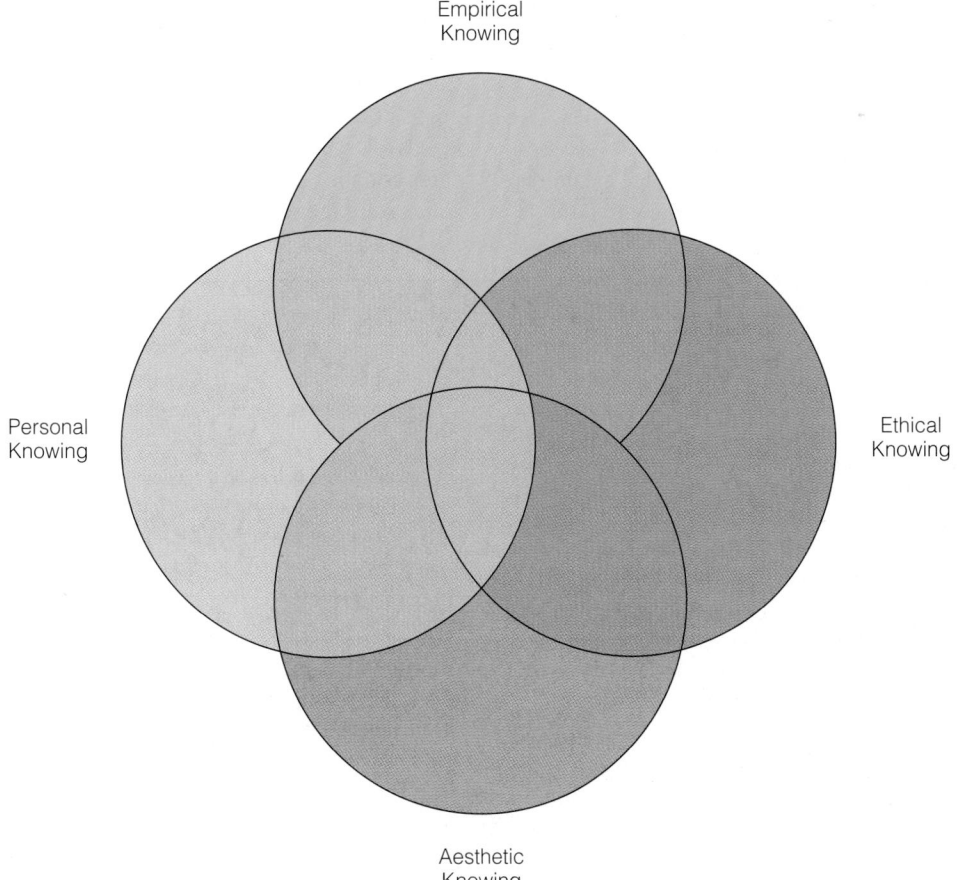

Figure 25-2 ■ The four ways of knowing.

Aesthetic Knowing: The Art of Nursing

Aesthetic knowing is the art of nursing and is expressed by the individual nurse through his or her creativity and style in meeting the needs of clients. The nurse uses aesthetic knowing to provide care that is both effective and satisfying. Empathy, compassion, holism, and sensitivity are important modes in the aesthetic pattern of knowing.

Personal Knowing: The Therapeutic Use of Self

Personal knowledge is concerned with the knowing, encountering, and actualizing of the concrete, individual self. Because nursing is an interpersonal process, the way in which nurses view their own selves and the client is of primary concern in any therapeutic relationship. **Personal knowing** promotes wholeness and integrity in the personal encounter, achieves engagement rather than detachment, and denies the manipulative or impersonal approach.

Ethical Knowing: The Moral Component

Goals of nursing include the conservation of life, alleviation of suffering, and promotion of health. **Ethical knowing** focuses on matters of obligation or what ought to be done, and goes beyond simply following the ethical codes of the discipline. Nursing care involves a series of deliberate actions or choices that are subject to the judgment of right or wrong. Occasionally, the principles and norms that guide choices may be in conflict. The more sensitive and knowledgeable the nurse is to these issues, the more "ethical" he or she will be.

Developing Ways of Knowing

The methods for developing each type of knowledge are unique (Chinn & Kramer, 2004). The methods that are required for de-veloping one pattern cannot be used to develop knowledge within another pattern. For example, personal knowing is developed through critical reflection on one's own actions and feelings in practice. Empirical knowing is gained from studying scientific models and theories and from making objective observations. Ethical knowing involves confronting and resolving conflicting values and beliefs. Aesthetic knowing arises from a deep appreciation of the uniqueness of each individual and the meanings that individual ascribes to a given situation. The nurse who practices effectively is able to integrate all types of knowledge to understand situations more holistically.

CARING ENCOUNTERS

How does a nurse demonstrate caring? Given similar situations, why is one nurse judged to be "caring" while another is said to be "uncaring"? Nurse theorists and researchers have studied this question and identified caring attributes and behaviors. Consider, for example, Roach's six Cs, Watson's carative factors (Chapter 3 ∞), and Swanson's structure of caring (Table 25–1). Because caring is contextual, a nursing approach used with a client in one situation may be ineffective in another. Caring responses are as varied as clients' needs, environmental resources, and nurses' imaginations. Caring encounters are influenced by the diversity of human responses, the nurse's workload, and the preferences of the nurse and client (Cooper, 2001). When clients perceive the encounter to be caring, their sense of dignity and self-worth is increased, and feelings of connectedness are expressed.

Knowing the Client

Caring attends to the totality of the client's experience. The nurse asks: Who is this person? What is his or her history? Needs? Desires? Dreams? Spiritual beliefs? Who loves and cares for this person at home? Where is home and what resources are there? What does this person need today, from me,

---

RESEARCH NOTE **Believing That I Make a Difference**

The development of the nurse's moral agency, or sense of what should be done in a nursing situation, is a critical concept for caring practitioners. The purpose of this analysis was to describe the nature of moral agency in nursing by revealing how and why nurses see value in the work they do. The researcher analyzed interviews that had been transcribed and coded to draw out analytical themes. The analysis was based on the philosophy of Iris Murdoch, who drew attention to how individuals examine their responses to events in their lives, and in so doing develop how they see the world and themselves in relation to others.

When asked what sustained them in their work, nurses in the study often pointed to moments when their personal presence made a difference in clients' lives. For example:

■ "When someone says you have really helped me, all the other things about it are invisible, it doesn't make any difference [speaking of the stress that she had to sustain]." (p. 166)
■ "After a while things become a little bit routine . . . And when I end up feeling like that something always seems to happen that makes you re-evaluate what you are doing, and that always tends to be

very patient focused. . . . it's where you get feedback from a patient and you realize, well no one else, unless they were in this position, could have actually achieved that." (p. 168)

When nurses achieved their expectations and desires to make a positive difference to their clients, the nurses saw value in their work that was affirming to them. There is, then, a positive connection between nurses' view of themselves and what they achieve for their clients.

IMPLICATIONS

Students and developing practitioners of nursing need guidance and support in order to feel free to concentrate their attention upon the client. By knowing the client, nurses learn how they can make a positive difference in that person's life. Nurses who perceive this difference are able to embrace the goals of nursing as their own goals, and to better recognize the good that they do.

Note: Reprinted with permission from Sage Publications Ltd., from E. Pask, "Moral Agency in Nursing: Seeing Value in the Work and Believing That I Make a Difference." Copyright © 2003 Sage Publications Ltd., 2003.

right now? Can he or she tell me what is needed? Personal knowledge of the client is a key in the caring relationship between nurse and client. The nurse aims to know who the client is, in his or her *uniqueness*. This knowledge is gained by observing and talking with the client and family, using listening and communication skills. The nurse cannot remain detached, but is actively engaged with the client.

Take, for example, an elderly man experiencing postoperative pain after removal of a cancerous prostate. The nurse assesses the client's pain, using an appropriate pain scale. The client's positioning, hygiene, amount of rest, and other physiological variables are assessed for their effect on pain. In addition, there are a multitude of other factors that affect the client's perception of pain. Is this surgery likely to cure the cancer, or is it primarily palliative? The meaning of the diagnosis and surgery to this client affects his pain experience. The nurse discovers that this man lost his wife to cancer 2 years ago. His daughter, at the bedside, is his primary support. The nurse discusses with his daughter how she can make her father more comfortable.

Knowing the client and family ultimately involves the nurse and client in a caring transaction. By attending broadly to personal, ethical, aesthetic, and empirical knowledge, the nurse understands events as they have meaning in the life of the client. The nurse's *knowing the client* ultimately increases the possibilities for therapeutic interventions to be perceived as relevant.

Nursing Presence

Caring in nursing always takes place in a relationship. Watson (2002) describes the transpersonal caring relationship, in which the nurse enters into the life space of another person. Establishment of a caring relationship depends on a moral commitment by the nurse and the nurse's ability to assess and realize another person's state of being. Mutuality within this relationship involves a partnership between the nurse and client.

Swanson's category *being with* (Table 25–1) provides a description of nursing presence. By being emotionally present to the client and family, the nurse conveys that they and their experiences matter. Being present is a way of sharing in the meanings, feelings, and lived experiences of the client. Physical presence is combined with the promise of availability, especially during a time of need. This may be as simple as responding promptly to a call bell on a hospital unit, or as complex as sitting with a parent who has just lost a child in a neonatal intensive care unit. In an account by the parent of a newborn with a serious heart defect, Schroeder (1998) described how a nurse periodically sat with her. "Her words and presence began to fill some of the emptiness inside me," (p. 19) she said. Quietly talking with the nurse helped this mother find meaning in her experience, as she "began to see that perhaps this experience wasn't just meaningless destruction, torture and death: regardless of outcome, we were all growing in ways denied ordinary people" (p. 20).

Covington (2003) defines caring presence as an "interpersonal, intersubjective human experience of connection within a nurse-client relationship that makes it safe for sharing oneself with another" (p. 312). The nurse brings conscious awareness (intentionality), and is open to opportunities for connection with the

client. Through this sharing, both client and nurse attempt to discover meaning in the experience of health and illness. A possible outcome is transformation and growth of both client and nurse.

Empowering the Client

Through knowing the client and engaging in a mutual relationship, the nurse is able to identify and build upon client/family strengths. This empowering relationship includes mutual respect, trust, and confidence in the other's abilities and motives. According to Swanson (1993), the caring behavior of *enabling* is defined as "facilitating the other's passage through life transitions and unfamiliar events" (p. 356). Enabling also includes coaching, informing, explaining, supporting, assisting, guiding, focusing, and validating. There are times when enabling involves substitutive care (doing for the client who is unable to do for oneself), but doing no more than is needed at the time. At other times, enabling involves providing an environment in which the client can function safely and effectively. The nurse should remain mindful of professional boundaries and responsibilities, to avoid enabling pathological choices by the client. The goal is always to facilitate growth and development.

Nurses both *advocate for* (verb) and are *advocates* (noun) for clients and families. Knowlden (1998) explored the meaning of caring in nursing and identified four dimensions of advocacy: (a) being a client advocate, (b) following through or following up, (c) providing resources, and (d) going above and beyond. A client in Knowlden's study described how his nurse was an advocate for him: "She keeps in touch with [my practitioner] to find out what's to be done. She gets through right away. They give us the run-around and get back 5 days later. . . She has been instrumental in getting the tube changed" (p. 37). Through advocacy, nurses are champions for their clients. They empower clients and families through activities that enhance well-being, understanding, and self-care.

Compassion

Universally, clients equate compassion with caring. The caring nurse is described as warm and empathic, compassionate and concerned. In order to demonstrate empathy, the nurse must be able to identify with the client, appreciating the pain and discomfort of illness, or imagining "walking in his shoes," in regard to some part of the client's life experience.

Roach (2002) defines compassion as "a way of living born out of an awareness of one's relationship to all living creatures" (p. 50). Like empathy, compassion involves participating in the client's experience, with sensitivity to the person's pain or discomfort, and a willingness to share in their experience. Compassion is given as part of the caring relationship, as the nurse shares the client's joys, sorrows, pain, and accomplishments. Compassion is a gift from the heart, rather than an advanced skill or technique.

Attention to spiritual needs is part of compassionate care, particularly in the face of death and bereavement. The nurse is aware that spiritual and religious beliefs are important coping mechanisms in dealing with issues of mortality (see Chapter 41 ∞). The nurse does not impose his or her own spiritual beliefs, but rather assists the client and family in drawing upon their own beliefs as spiritual resources.

Comfort is often associated with compassionate care, and many nursing interventions are carried out to provide comfort. For example, bathing, positioning, talking, touching, and listening are often performed to increase the client's comfort level. Just like pain or discomfort, comfort is subjective and is defined as "whatever the client says it is," based on the individual's perceptions. Despite this subjectivity, comfort care is often the basis for nursing in settings ranging from intensive care to hospice, and serves as a motivator for nursing interventions. Nurses are challenged to be creative and innovative, basing interventions on knowledge of the client's preferences, in order to provide comfort care.

Competence

The competent nurse employs the necessary knowledge, judgment, skills, and motivation to respond adequately to the client's needs. Just as competence without compassion is cold and inhumane, compassion without competence is meaningless and dangerous. The competent nurse, as described by Roach (2002), understands the client's condition, its treatment, and associated care. The nurse is able to provide the necessary care, while guiding the client and family through the process. The nurse's abilities to assess, plan, implement, and evaluate a plan of care are focused on meeting the client/family needs. Practice of these skills requires a high level of cognitive, affective, technical, and administrative skills.

MAINTAINING CARING PRACTICE

The concept of caring for self seems almost foreign to many nurses and students of nursing, because of the professional emphasis on meeting others' needs. Yet, as nurses take on multiple commitments to family, work, school, and community, they risk exhaustion, burnout, and stress. Obstacles to self-care may be professional, related to the demands of a particular work setting, or may be personal, such as poor health habits or unrealistic expectations of self (see Chapter 42 ∞ for more information on stress and coping). Despite these challenges, it is imperative that nurses attend to their own needs, because caring for self is central to caring for others.

Caring for Self

Mayeroff (1990) describes caring for self as helping oneself grow and actualize one's possibilities. Self-care, when defined as responding to one's own needs to grow, is the opposite of the self-complacency that often accompanies egocentricity. Caring for self means taking the time to nurture oneself. This involves initiating and maintaining behaviors that promote healthy living and well-being. Although different activities may be helpful to different people, some examples of these activities are the following:

- A balanced diet
- Regular exercise
- Adequate rest and sleep
- Recreational activities
- Meditation and prayer

Self-care focuses on care of the self in the deepest sense. Self-awareness and self-esteem are intimately connected to self-care. Each person is unique and possesses individual strengths and weaknesses. Self-care practices are intentionally created by the self and vigilantly maintained. This is a lifelong unfolding process, leading to wholeness that comes from and contributes to self-esteem. In its code of ethics, the American Holistic Nurses Association states that "the nurse has a responsibility to model healthy behaviors. Holistic nurses strive to achieve harmony in their own lives and to assist others who are striving to do the same" (American Holistic Nurses Association, 1992, p. 275). Individuals with high self-esteem can critically problem solve and tackle obstacles more effectively. Self-care practices build self-esteem, leading to feelings of comfort and accomplishment. The self-esteem questionnaire in Box 25–3 is

BOX 25–3 **Self-Esteem Questionnaire**		
Answer Yes or No to the following questions. Check the box appropriate for how you feel the majority of time.		
	Yes	No
Do you have a hard time nurturing yourself?		
Have you ever turned down an invitation to a party or function because of the way you felt about yourself?		
Do you get your sense of self-worth from the approval of others?		
Are you supportive of others but berate yourself?		
Whenever things go wrong in life do you blame yourself?		
Do you react to disappointment by blaming others?		
Do you begin each day with a negative attitude?		
Do you feel undeserving?		
Do you ever feel like an impostor and that soon your deficiencies will be exposed?		
Do you have an inner-critic who is disparaging or demeaning?		
Do you believe that being hard on yourself is the best motivation for change?		
Do your good points seem ordinary and your failings all-important?		
Do you feel unattractive?		
Have you ever felt your accomplishments are due to luck, but your failures due to incompetence or inadequacy?		
Have you ever felt that if you are not a total success, then you are a failure, and that there is no middle ground with no points for effort?		
Do you feel unappreciated?		
Do you feel lonely?		
Do you struggle with feelings of inferiority?		
Do other people's opinions count more to you than your own?		
Do you criticize yourself often?		
Do others criticize you often?		
Do you hesitate to do things because of what others might think?		
TOTALS		

Note: © 1998 Catherine A. Martin, The Positive Way, Used with permission. www.positive-way.com

a measure to assess self-esteem. The more "yes" answers on the tool, the more opportunity exists for improving self-esteem.

A Healthy Lifestyle

Everyone needs to pay attention to nutrition and exercise, and to avoid unhealthy lifestyle practices. Key words for a healthy lifestyle are *balance* and *moderation*. These lifestyle practices are supplemented by regular physical examinations and health screenings.

NUTRITION. Healthy eating is important for everyone. A nutritionally balanced eating plan provides more energy, builds endurance to carry out daily activities, and reduces the risk for certain health problems. Healthy eating means learning to make good choices in the foods eaten, preparing foods appropriately, and eating in moderation. It is important to select a variety of foods, to eat regular meals, and to eat the correct amount to maintain a healthy weight. Determining a healthy weight depends on several factors, including age, activity level, and the presence of weight-related medical problems such as high blood pressure. Dietary guidelines and standards for a healthy diet are included in Chapter 47. ∞

ACTIVITY AND EXERCISE. Exercise is recognized as a lifetime endeavor that is essential for energetic, active, and healthy living (see Figure 25-3 ■). The benefits of exercise have been linked to many physiologic and psychologic responses, from a reduced feeling of stress to an increased sense of well-being. Exercise strengthens the heart, lungs, and blood vessels to prevent heart disease, keeps the joints flexible, and helps many people deal with sad or unhappy feelings. For persons who are overweight, exercise has the added benefit of burning calories, resulting in weight loss or maintenance. Whatever the exercise, whether walking or working out in a gym, 20 minutes of exercise two to three times a week is recommended (Maville & Huerta, 2002).

Nurses participate in strenuous activities that call for specialized knowledge of body mechanics and movement techniques to prevent self-injuries. Self-care practices are based on competence and compliance with these specialized techniques and knowledge of how to use assistive devices such as hydraulic lifts, belts, and sliding boards. An in-depth discussion of these techniques is included in Chapter 32. ∞

Figure 25-3 ■ Regular activity and exercise is an effective self-care practice.

> ### BOX 25–4 Twelve Things You Would Love to Do
>
> We often put off doing the simple things that bring us joy and happiness. Make a list of 12 things you would love to do after reviewing the list on the left. Post your list where you can see it. Resolve to carry out one activity by a specified time. Enjoy!
>
> | *Some Ideas:* | *Your List:* |
> |---|---|
> | 1. Go out for ice cream | 1. _____ |
> | 2. Take a nap | 2. _____ |
> | 3. Dance a polka | 3. _____ |
> | 4. Make a campfire | 4. _____ |
> | 5. Roast marshmallows | 5. _____ |
> | 6. Ride a bike | 6. _____ |
> | 7. Shop for new shoes | 7. _____ |
> | 8. Watch your favorite movie | 8. _____ |
> | 9. Rearrange your furniture | 9. _____ |
> | 10. Take a ceramics class | 10. _____ |
> | 11. Read a mystery novel | 11. _____ |
> | 12. Walk in the park | 12. _____ |

RECREATION. Self-care also includes taking time to do the things that bring joy and stimulate creativity. Nurses need to reward themselves, to experience spontaneity, and even to take downtime or time to do nothing. Defending the right to this time may take courage and conviction in the face of others' demands. "Forbidden Joys, An Exercise" (see Box 25–4) is intended to help a person recapture a sense of joy and self-reward.

AVOIDING UNHEALTHY PATTERNS. Part of staying healthy is avoiding unhealthy life patterns. This means avoiding activities or thought patterns that contribute to negative health outcomes. Negative thinking can create a stress response, with all its physiological, mental, and emotional outcomes. It is not what happens, but how events are perceived, that determines an individual's reaction. Practices such as identifying negative feelings, refocusing on the positive, and using humor are helpful to avert the stress response by changing thought patterns. Using positive affirmations, as listed in Box 25–5, can lead to greater self-esteem and control self-doubt. It is also important to avoid destructive lifestyle choices such as smoking, abuse of alcohol or drugs, and misusing medications.

Mind–Body Therapies

The interconnectedness of the mind and body is the basis for the complementary therapies. Imagery, meditation, storytelling, music

---

> ### BOX 25–5 Positive Affirmations
>
> Begin the day with positive statements about how you want to think and act:
>
> I am a person of worth and goodness.
> I am happy to be alive.
> I am in the right place at the right time.
> I am prepared to do a good job today.
> I am surrounded by people that I love, who love me.
> I am doing what brings me joy.
> This is an opportunity to grow.

therapy, and yoga are complementary therapies that bring balance to thoughts and emotions. Practice of one or more mind–body therapies is an effective self-care strategy to help restore peace and balance. More in-depth information on different types of complementary therapies is included in Chapter 19. ∞

GUIDED IMAGERY. Imagery is a mind–body intervention that uses the power of the imagination as a therapeutic tool. Imagery is used to promote relaxation, decrease anxiety, and enhance psychologic or spiritual insight. Through forming mental images of an object, event, or situation, the individual can reframe negative responses into positive images, enhancing healing and emotional well-being.

MEDITATION. Through quieting the mind and focusing it on the present, meditation assists the individual in releasing fears, worries, and doubts. The technique involves both relaxation and focused attention. Guidelines for mindfulness meditation include choosing a quiet space, sitting comfortably, achieving progressive relaxation through deep breathing, and focusing attention on breathing or a mental image.

STORYTELLING. Telling stories is a natural component of everyday conversation that can be utilized as a powerful tool to communicate with others (Struthers, 2002). As expressions of human consciousness, stories help individuals move toward wholeness. Indigenous groups conducted storytelling sessions with the participants sitting in a talking circle, a shape that assists the intuition in discerning that things occur in the manner they are intended to happen.

MUSIC THERAPY. Using music as therapy includes listening, singing, rhythm, and body movement. Quiet, soothing music is often used to induce relaxation. Active rhythms can awaken feelings of power and control. Familiar music allows the listener to recall past events or feelings. Music can also serve as an effective distraction technique. Each person's likes and dislikes are taken into account in order to achieve the desired emotional response.

YOGA. The practice of yoga unites the body, mind, and spirit (see Figure 25-4 ■). Through daily practice of the various postures and breathing practices of yoga, an individual can achieve increased balance and flexibility, mental alertness, and calmness. The bending, stretching, and holding properties of the postures help to relax and tone the muscles and improve function of the internal organs. Breath control is designed to still the mind and enhance awareness.

Reflection on Practice

Critical thinking, self-analysis, and reflection are required in order to learn from one's experience. The student matures as a practitioner by thinking about how values and standards guide practical experience. **Reflection** is thinking from a critical point of view, analyzing why one acted in a certain way, and assessing the results of one's actions. In order to develop oneself as a caring practitioner, reflection on practice must be personal and meaningful.

Figure 25-4 ■ Yoga is a mind–body self-care strategy to help restore peace and balance.
(Russell Saur © Dorling Kindersley)

Reflective practice is a method of self-examination that involves thinking back over what happened in a nursing situation. It involves the whole person, including his or her emotions. Reflectivity includes becoming aware of how one feels about oneself and recognizing how one thinks and acts. This exploration of experiences leads to new understandings and appreciations. Through reflection, nurses can become more comfortable with an authentic way of being-in-the-world and can participate more fully in caring-healing relationships (Cumbie, 2001).

Using Four Ways of Knowing

Reflection provides a method to explore alternative forms of nursing knowledge, including empirical, aesthetic, personal, and ethical types. Johns suggests the following questions for exploration of different ways of knowing (2000, p. 47):

- *Empirical knowing:* What knowledge informed me in this situation? What additional information did I need? Was I prepared to deal with this situation?
- *Personal knowing:* What were my thoughts and emotions in this situation? Why did I feel the way I did? To what extent was I concerned for the person? To what extent was I preoccupied with self?
- *Aesthetic knowing:* What was I trying to achieve? Why did I respond as I did? What were the consequences for the client/family? How were others feeling and how did I know this?
- *Ethical knowing:* Did I act for the best? What standards were relevant in this situation? Was there conflict of values between different persons' perspectives?

Reflective practice requires discipline, action, openness, and trust. It is a form of self-evaluation. Reflective journaling, as a tool for learning, is usually shared with a mentor or teacher, who works in partnership with the student. A guideline, such as the one in Box 25–6, provides structure for the journaling process. Writing reflections in a journal provides a space for the student to look at and acknowledge the deeper self. Guidance from a mentor or teacher can help the student view a nursing situation from many different perspectives. It helps the student find

meaning in the event, understand and learn through it, and emerge at a higher level of understanding.

Box 25–7 provides an example of a beginning nursing student's experience. See how it compares to your own. Think about the questions and use them for your own reflection.

BOX 25–6 Guidelines for Reflective Journaling

Reflection is a window through which the student can view and focus on self, in ways that enable him or her to understand, confront, and work towards resolving the contradictions between actual and desirable practice. Reflection facilitates learning through everyday lived experiences. This guideline focuses on the concept of *being available*, which is the essence of effective holistic practice (Johns, 2000). The following outline can be used as a guide for journaling after each clinical experience:

1. Knowing what is desirable (ethical knowing)
   - What are your beliefs and values in relation to the situation?
   - Describe the contradictions between your values and the reality of the situation.
2. Knowing the person/family
   - What is the meaning of the health event to each person?
   - What are each person's values and needs?
   - What behaviors did you assess to reveal these meanings and needs?
   - How did your relationship (trust) with each person influence your knowing?
3. Concern for the person/family
   - Evaluate your level of concern for the person/family.
   - How easy or difficult was it to care about each person?
   - How did your personal reactions influence your concern?

4. The aesthetic response to the person (aesthetic knowing)
   - Assess the extent to which you were able to interpret the situation, envision what needed to be done, and respond appropriately to the person/family.
   - Were you able to expand on your ability to be available to the person and respond effectively?
5. Knowing and managing self's involvement with the person (personal knowing)
   - In what ways did you feel vulnerable in the situation?
   - How did you manage negative influences such as anxiety, stress, prejudice, loss of concern, preoccupation with self?
   - What did you feel you did well, or improved upon from previous experiences?
6. Creating and sustaining an environment where being available is possible
   - Were there environmental factors that constrained your availability to work with the client and family (norms, ways of relating, lack of resources, time, etc.)?

Note: From "*Becoming a Reflective Practitioner,*" by Chris Johns, 2000, pp. 69–70, Blackwell Science. Copyright © 2000 Blackwell Publishing. Reprinted with permission.

BOX 25–7 Nursing Student Reflection Checkpoint

Debbie started nursing school in September, and by October felt overwhelmed by the amount of reading and studying that was required. Her anxiety level began to rise, but at the same time, she became more aware of her feelings and reactions to situations. In her nursing courses she was studying nursing as caring, and in the clinical setting she focused on applying these ideas in her practice with clients. She was surprised how genuinely her clients responded to a kind word of encouragement, the attention of personal care, and her concern for their well-being. Her clients' responses boosted her confidence and motivated her to learn more about their conditions and needs.

Each week Debbie analyzed and described the clinical situations encountered in practice in a reflective journal. Through reflecting on her clinical experiences and feedback from her clinical instructor, she was able to identify her personal strengths and areas for growth. She began to think about how she could better organize her study schedule, plan time with her family, and provide the same level of caring for herself that she desired to give her clients.

1. Being in nursing school is often an overwhelming experience. Can you relate to Debbie's situation?
2. As you study caring in nursing, what ideas interest you most? How have you implemented these ideas in your own practice as a student nurse?
3. According to Carper's four ways of knowing, give examples of how you practiced each of these ways of knowing in your care of clients.
4. What value do you see in keeping a reflective journal? As you reflect on practice situations, have you written down your thoughts?
5. What changes can you make in your weekly schedule, to be more efficient with studying and also plan time for self-care?
6. What self-care activities would be most helpful to you right now? Changes in diet? Scheduled exercise or recreation? Meditation, yoga, or another mind–body therapy?
7. Do you have unhealthy patterns, such as smoking or negative thinking, that you need to work on? Develop an action plan to change these behaviors.

CRITICAL THINKING CHECKPOINT

After morning report, the nurse, Megan, approaches Robbie James, a 10-year-old boy lying quietly in his hospital bed. She introduces herself and writes her name on the white board in the room, so that when Robbie's mother arrives, she will know the name of Robbie's nurse. Megan's client assignment today consists of four acutely ill children of different ages. As Megan makes her initial rounds, she assesses the immediate needs of each child and begins to prioritize her nursing activities.

Megan has her own needs. She is tired from the night before when her own daughter was up late with coughing and fever. She is comfortable with her arrangements for child care, however, and is able to focus on her care of the clients on the pediatric unit.

When Megan returns with intravenous morphine, Robbie barely speaks, a pinched look of discomfort on his face. Using the FACES pain scale, Robbie has identified his pain as the "worst possible pain." This is his first day postop after surgery for a ruptured appendix, and he has a nasogastric (NG) tube in place, draining to wall suction. Megan administers the medication according to unit protocol and continues her assessment. She checks patency and placement of the NG tube and measures Robbie's vital signs.

Megan notes a "walking chart" on the wall beside Robbie's bed. The walking chart includes spaces to place a sticker each time Robbie walks in the hall. Robbie knows that after three stickers, he can choose a prize from the treasure box. Before Megan leaves the room, she suggests to Robbie, "When you feel better from this medicine, I'll help you walk, and we'll put another sticker on that chart!"

1. Describe which aspect of the nurse's approach relates to each of the following six Cs of caring in nursing as outlined by Roach: Compassion, Competence, Confidence, Conscience, Commitment, Comportment

2. In analyzing this case study and reflecting on the four ways of knowing (e.g., personal, empirical, aesthetic, and ethical), describe how each type of knowing prepared the nurse, Megan, for her caring approach.

3. In the theory of bureaucratic caring, Ray suggests that different aspects of the hospital system influence the choice making of the nurse. Describe how each of the following aspects influences the nurse's care:
   - Spiritual-ethical-caring
   - Physical
   - Technological
   - Social-cultural
   - Educational
   - Legal

See Critical Thinking Possibilities in Appendix A.

CHAPTER 25 **REVIEW**

CHAPTER HIGHLIGHTS

- Caring practice involves connection, mutual recognition, and involvement between nurse and client. Caring is central to nursing practice.
- To care for another person is to help the person grow and actualize him or herself. By helping the other grow, the caregiver moves toward self-actualization. Caring behaviors described by Mayeroff include knowing, alternating rhythms, patience, honesty, trust, humility, hope, and courage.
- Caring is a multidimensional concept, summarized by Morse et al. as five viewpoints: (a) moral imperative, (b) affect, (c) human trait, (d) interpersonal relationship, and (e) therapeutic intervention.
- Various theorists have focused on caring as the essence of nursing. Each theory develops different aspects of caring, describing how caring is unique in nursing.
- Nursing involves different types of knowledge that are integrated to guide nursing practice. Empirical knowing includes scientific competence, personal knowing focuses on the self, ethical knowing requires moral/ethical awareness, and aesthetic knowing is the creative art of nursing.
- Caring encounters are influenced by the diversity of human responses. Common caring patterns include knowing the client, nursing presence, empowering the client, compassion, and competence.
- Caring for self is central to caring for others. Nurse self-care includes a balanced diet, regular exercise, adequate rest and sleep, recreational activities, and mind–body therapies.
- The nurse matures as a practitioner by reflecting on practice. Through reflection, nurses can grow and participate more fully in caring-healing relationships.

TEST YOUR KNOWLEDGE

1. Which of the following examples illustrates the principle of knowing the client?
   1. The nurse provides a back rub to help the client relax, and then makes the bed with clean linen.
   2. The nurse listens as the client describes how he has been caring for his diabetes at home.
   3. The nurse administers a piggyback antibiotic for a client with pneumonia.
   4. The nurse collects a urine specimen to send to the lab, and explains to the client the reason for the test.

2. The nurse teaches a client with diabetes how to make decisions about insulin management after discharge. This teaching most clearly reflects which caring activity?
   1. Empowering the client
   2. Compassion
   3. Knowing the client
   4. Nursing presence

3. Mayeroff described allowing the other to grow in his own way and time. This behavior most clearly reflects which major ingredient of caring?
   1. Humility
   2. Knowing
   3. Patience
   4. Courage

4. Leininger's theory, culture care diversity and universality, would provide the best framework for assessing which of the following nursing situations?
   1. Because the Indonesian parents of an infant preferred to use hot/cold therapies to prevent seizures, they withheld the prescribed phenobarbital medication.
   2. Staff nurses on a hospital unit discuss how to reorganize client care to provide more continuity of staff with clients.
   3. Nurses in a community agency search for learning resources about intravenous therapy in the home setting.
   4. A nurse manager explores ways to assist new nursing graduates to develop clinical skills on the hospital unit.

5. In a reflective journal, a nursing student writes this statement about a comatose client on the hospice unit: "The Do-Not-Resuscitate order was not on the chart, and none of the nurses knew what measures should be taken if the client stopped breathing." This statement most clearly reflects which of the four ways of knowing?
   1. Empirical
   2. Personal
   3. Ethical
   4. Aesthetic

6. The nurse sits with the client and holds the client's hand as his pain decreases. This situation is an example of the following caring practice:
   1. Nursing presence.
   2. Assessment.
   3. Knowing the client.
   4. Empowering.

7. Which nursing theory is depicted by a model with spiritual-ethical caring in the center, surrounded by political, legal, economic, educational, physiologic, social-cultural, and technological systems?
   1. Nursing as caring
   2. Theory of bureaucratic caring
   3. Caring, the human mode of being
   4. Theory of human care

8. The nursing student reviews the pathophysiology of myocardial infarction, in preparation for the next day's clinical experience. This activity is an example of which type of knowledge development?
   1. Empirical knowing
   2. Aesthetic knowing
   3. Personal knowing
   4. Ethical knowing

9. Which mind–body therapy is described by the following activity: "The person sits quietly in a chair, breathing deeply and focusing on the mental image of a crystal"?
   1. Storytelling
   2. Yoga
   3. Music therapy
   4. Meditation

10. A 40-year-old client who comes to the clinic for a routine physical exam asks the nurse how much exercise is recommended for a healthy lifestyle. Which answer is most appropriate?
   1. 10 minutes daily
   2. 30 minutes daily
   3. 20 minutes two to three times a week
   4. 1 hour every other day

See Answers to Test Your Knowledge in Appendix A.

EXPLORE MEDIALINK www.prenhall.com/berman

DVD-ROM
▨ Audio Glossary
▨ NCLEX Review

COMPANION WEBSITE
▨ Additional NCLEX Review
▨ Case Study: Six C's of Caring in Nursing
▨ Care Plan Activity: Care of Client After Motor Vehicle Crash
▨ Application Activity: Watson's Theory of Human Caring
▨ Links to Resources

READINGS AND REFERENCES

SUGGESTED READINGS
Cooper, C. (2001). *The art of nursing*. Philadelphia: W. B. Saunders. *Rich narratives from practicing nurses paint a vivid picture of the artful practice of nursing.*

Scholarly sources are cited to support understanding of how nurses care for clients through advocacy, spiritual support, compassion, nurse presence, and self-care. Guided exercises and group discussion

activities help nursing students develop their own caring approaches.
Henry, L. G., & Henry, J. D. (2004). *The soul of the caring nurse.*

Stories & resources for revitalizing professional passion. Washington, D.C.: American Nurses Association.
This book reflects much of what is included in this chapter on caring. It consists of stories told by nurses. The book offers "a perspective on how nurses can and do practice caring in spite of the current system" (p. xvii). The last section of the book consists of strategies and resources for nurse self-care.

Miller, J., & Cutshall, S. (2001). *The art of being a healing presence: A guide for those in caring relationships.* Ft. Wayne, IN: Willowgreen.
As the title of this book implies, healing presence is an art, and there are universal principles that apply. Steps for being a healing presence begin with opening oneself, honoring self and other, and giving and receiving the gifts that come. Insights presented here will assist nurses in fulfilling professional as well as personal responsibilities.

Wendler, M. C. (2002). *The heart of nursing: Expressions of creative art in nursing.* Indianapolis, IN: Sigma Theta Tau International.
This diverse and extraordinary collection of nurses' artistic work includes photography, poetry, short stories, quilting, painting, and needlework. Produced by more than 50 nurse-artists, the contributions serve as examples of the beauty of human caring processes and relationships.

RELATED RESEARCH

Jackson, C. (2004). Healing ourselves, healing others. *Holistic Nursing Practice, 18*(3), 127–141.

Kapborg, I., & Bertero, C. (2003). The phenomenon of caring from the novice student nurse's perspective: A qualitative content analysis. *International Nursing Review, 50*, 183–192.

Ray, M., Turkel, M., & Marino, F. (2002). The transformative process for nursing in workforce redevelopment. *Nursing Administration Quarterly, 26*(2), 1–14.

Ruth-Sahd, L. (2003). Reflective practice: A critical analysis of data-based studies and implications for nursing education. *Journal of Nursing Education, 42*(11), 488–497.

Turkel, M. (2003). A journey into caring as experienced by nurse managers. *International Journal for Human Caring, 7*(1), 20–26.

Wiman, E., & Wikbland, K. (2004). Caring and uncaring encounters in nursing in an emergency department. *Journal of Clinical Nursing, 13*, 422–429.

REFERENCES

American Holistic Nurses Association. (1992). Code of ethics for holistic nurses. *Journal of Holistic Nursing, 10*(3), 275–276.

Benner, P., & Wrubel, J. (1989). *The primacy of caring: Stress and coping in health and illness.* Menlo Park, CA: Addison-Wesley.

Boykin, A., & Schoenhofer, S. (2001). Nursing as caring: An overview of a general theory of nursing. In M. Parker (Ed.), *Nursing theories and nursing practice* (pp. 391–402). Philadelphia: F. A. Davis.

Cameron, J. (2002). *The artist's way.* New York: Jeremy P. Tarcher/Putnam.

Carper, B. (1978). Fundamental patterns of knowing in nursing. *Advances in Nursing Science, 1*(1), 13–23.

Chinn, P., & Kramer, M. (2004). *Integrated knowledge development in nursing* (6th ed.). St. Louis, MO: Mosby.

Coffman, S. (2006). Marilyn Anne Ray: Theory of bureaucratic caring. In A. Tomey & M. Alligood (Eds.), *Nursing theorists and their work* (6th ed., pp. 116–139). St. Louis, MO: Mosby.

Cooper, C. (2001). *The art of nursing.* Philadelphia: W. B. Saunders.

Covington, H. (2003). Caring presence. *Journal of Holistic Nursing, 21*(3), 301–317.

Cumbie, S. (2001). The integration of mind-body-soul and the practice of humanistic nursing. *Holistic Nursing Practice, 15*(3), 56–62.

Gordon, S., Benner, P., & Noddings, N. (1996). *Caregiving.* Philadelphia: University of Pennsylvania Press.

Johns, C. (2000). *Becoming a reflective practitioner.* Oxford, England: Blackwell Science.

Knowlden, V. (1998). *The communication of caring in nursing.* Indianapolis, IN: Center Nursing Press.

Leininger, M. M. (2001). *Culture care diversity & universality: A theory of nursing.* Sudbury, MA: Jones & Bartlett.

Maville, J., & Huerta, C. (2002). *Health promotion in nursing.* Albany, NY: Delmar.

Mayeroff, M. (1990). *On caring.* New York: Harper Collins.

Morse, J., Solberg, S., Neander, W., Battorff, J., & Johnson, J. (1990). Concepts of caring and caring as a concept. *Advances in Nursing Science, 13*(1), 1–14.

Parker, M. (2006). *Nursing theories and nursing practice* (2nd ed.). Philadelphia: F. A. Davis.

Pask, E. (2003). Moral agency in nursing: Seeing value in the work and believing that I make a difference. *Nursing Ethics, 10*(2), 165–174.

Phillips, S., & Benner, P. (1994). *The crisis of care: Affirming and restoring caring practices in the helping professions.* Washington, DC: Georgetown University Press.

The Positive Way. (2006). Self-esteem questionnaire. Retrieved June 7, 2006, from http://www.positive-way.com/self-est1.htm

Purnell, M. (2006). Nursing as caring: A model for transforming practice. In A. Tomey & M. Alligood (Eds.), *Nursing theorists and their work* (6th ed.). St. Louis, MO: Mosby.

Ray, M. (2001). The theory of bureaucratic caring. In M. Parker (Ed.), *Nursing theories and nursing practice* (pp. 422–431). Philadelphia: F. A. Davis.

Roach, M. S. (2002). *Caring, the human mode of being* (2nd ed.). Ottawa, Ontario, Canada: CHA Press.

Schroeder, C. (1998). So this is what it's like: Struggling to survive in pediatric intensive care. *Advances in Nursing Science, 10*(4), 13–22.

Struthers, R. (2002). Storytelling as a healing tool. In M. Snyder & R. Lindquist (Eds.), *Complementary/alternative therapies in nursing* (4th ed., pp. 124–134). New York: Springer.

Swanson, K. (1991). Empirical development of a middle range theory of caring. *Nursing Research, 40*(3), 161–166.

Swanson, K. (1993). Nursing as informed caring for the well-being of others. *IMAGE: Journal of Nursing Scholarship, 25*(4), 352–357.

Swanson, K. (2001). A program of research on caring. In M. Parker (Ed.), *Nursing theories and nursing practice* (pp. 411–420). Philadelphia: F. A. Davis.

Watson, J. (1999). *Nursing: Human science and human care. A theory of nursing.* Boston: Jones & Bartlett.

Watson, J. (2002). Intentionality and caring-healing consciousness: A practice of transpersonal nursing. *Holistic Nursing Practice, 16*(4), 12–19.

SELECTED BIBLIOGRAPHY

Benner, P. (2002). *From novice to expert: Excellence and power in clinical nursing practice.* Upper Saddle River, NJ: Prentice Hall Health.

Canfield, J., Hansen, M. V., Mitchell-Autoio, N., & Thieman, L. (2001). *Chicken soup for the nurse's soul: 101 stories to celebrate, honor, and inspire the nursing profession.* Deerfield Beach, FL: Health Communications.

Chenevert, M. (2002). *Mosby's tour guide to nursing school: A student's road survival kit* (4th ed.). St. Louis, MO: Mosby.

Dowling, M. (2004). Exploring the relationship between caring, love and intimacy in nursing. *British Journal of Nursing, 13*(21), 1289–1292.

Fink, J. (2005). Burned out? Here's help. *Nursing, 35*(4), 53.

Freshwater, D. (2002). *Therapeutic nursing.* London: Sage Publications.

Gaydos, H. (2004). "Making special": A framework for understanding the art of holistic nursing. *Journal of Holistic Nursing, 22*(2), 152–163.

Godkin, J., & Godkin, L. (2004). Caring behaviors among nurses: Fostering a conversation of gestures. *Health Care Management Review, 29*(3), 258–267.

Graber, D., & Mitcham, M. (2004). Compassionate clinicians take patient care beyond the ordinary. *Holistic Nursing Practice, 18*(2), 87–94.

Hudacek, S. (2004). *Making a difference: Stories from the point of care,* (Vol. II). Indianapolis, IN: Sigma Theta Tau International.

Hunter, L. (2002). Being with women: A guiding concept for the care of laboring women. *Journal of Obstetric, Gynecologic, and Neonatal Nursing, 31*(31), 555–562.

Johns, C. (2002). *Guided reflection: Advancing practice.* Oxford, England: Blackwell Science.

Poirier, S., & Ayres, L. (2002). *Stories of family caregiving.* Indianapolis, IN: Center Nursing Publishing.

Snyder, M., & Lindquist, R. (2002). *Complementary/alternative therapies in nursing* (4th ed.). New York: Springer.

Tomey, A. M., & Alligood, M. (2006). *Nursing theorists and their work* (6th ed.). St. Louis, MO: Mosby.

Tutton, E., & Seers, K. (2003). An exploration of the concept of comfort. *Journal of Clinical Nursing, 12*, 689–696.

Watson, J., & Foster, R. (2003). The attending nurse caring model: Integrating theory, evidence and advanced caring-healing therapeutics for transforming professional practice. *Journal of Clinical Nursing, 12*(3), 360–365.

Wieck, K. L. (2003). *Stories for nurses. Acts of caring.* St. Louis: Mosby.

Wilkin, K. (2003). The meaning of caring in the practice of intensive care nursing. *British Journal of Nursing, 12*(20), 1178–1292.

Wilt, D., & Smucker, C. (2001). *Nursing the spirit: The art and science of applying spiritual care.* Washington, DC: American Nurses Association.

Communicating

LEARNING OUTCOMES

After completing this chapter, you will be able to:

1. Describe factors influencing the communication process.

2. Discuss nurse–client communication as a dynamic process.

3. Describe four phases of the helping relationship.

4. Identify features of effective groups.

5. Identify types of groups helpful in promoting health and comfort.

6. Discuss how nurses use communication skills in each phase of the nursing process.

7. State why effective communication is imperative among health professionals.

8. Differentiate major characteristics between assertive and nonassertive communication.

Communication is a critical skill for nursing. It is the process by which humans meet their survival needs, build relationships, and experience emotions. In nursing, communication is a dynamic process used to gather assessment data, to teach and persuade, and to express caring and comfort. It is an integral part of the helping relationship.

COMMUNICATING

The term *communication* has various meanings, depending on the context in which it is used. To some, communication is the interchange of information between two or more people; in other words, the exchange of ideas or thoughts. This kind of communication uses methods such as talking and listening or writing and reading. However, painting, dancing, and storytelling are also methods of communication. In addition, thoughts are conveyed to others not only by spoken or written words but also by gestures or body actions.

Communication may have a more personal connotation than the interchange of ideas or thoughts. It can be a transmission of feelings or a more personal and social interaction between people. Frequently, one member of a couple comments that the other is not communicating. Some teenagers complain about a generation gap—being unable to communicate with understanding or feeling to a parent or authority figure. Sometimes a nurse is said to be efficient but lacking in something called *bedside manner*. For the purpose of this text, **communication** is any means of exchanging information or feelings between two or more people. It is a basic component of human relationships, including nursing.

The intent of any communication is to elicit a response. Thus, communication is a process. It has two main purposes: to influence others and to obtain information. Communication can be described as helpful or unhelpful. The former encourages a sharing of information, thoughts, or feelings between two or more people. The latter hinders or blocks the transfer of information and feelings.

Nurses who communicate effectively are better able to collect assessment data, initiate interventions, evaluate outcomes of interventions, initiate change that promotes health, and prevent legal problems associated with nursing practice. The communication process is built on a trusting relationship with a client and support persons. Effective communication is essential for the establishment of a nurse–client relationship.

Communication can occur on an intrapersonal level within a single individual as well as on interpersonal and group levels. Intrapersonal communication is the communication that you have with yourself; another name is *self-talk*. Both the sender and the receiver of a message usually engage in self-talk. It involves thinking about the message before it is sent, while it is being sent, and after it is sent, and it occurs constantly. Consequently, intrapersonal communication can interfere with a person's ability to hear a message as the sender intended (see Figure 26-1 ■).

Figure 26-1 ■ Improving student nurse self-talk.

The Communication Process

Face-to-face communication involves a sender, a message, a receiver, and a response, or feedback (see Figure 26-2 ■). In its simplest form, communication is a two-way process involving the sending and the receiving of a message. Because the intent of communication is to elicit a response, the process is ongoing; the receiver of the message then becomes the sender of a response, and the original sender then becomes the receiver.

Sender

The *sender,* a person or group who wishes to convey a message to another, can be considered the *source-encoder.* This term suggests that the person or group sending the message must have an idea or reason for communicating (source) and must put the idea or feeling into a form that can be transmitted. **Encoding** involves the selection of specific signs or symbols (codes) to transmit the message, such as which language and words to use, how to arrange the words, and what tone of voice and gestures to use. For example, if the receiver speaks English, the sender usually selects English words. If the message is "Mr. Johnson, you have to wait another hour for your pain medication," the tone of voice selected and a shake of the head can reinforce it. The nurse must not only deal with dialects and foreign languages but also cope with two language levels—the layperson's and the health professional's.

Message

The second component of the communication process is the *message* itself—what is actually said or written, the body language that accompanies the words, and how the message is transmitted. The medium used to convey the message is the channel, and it can target any of the receiver's senses. It is important for the channel to be appropriate for the message and it should help make the intent of the message more clear.

Talking face to face with a person may be more effective in some instances than telephoning or writing a message. Recording messages on tape or communicating by radio or television may be more appropriate for larger audiences. Written communication is often appropriate for long explanations or for a communication that needs to be preserved. The nonverbal channel of touch is often highly effective (see Figure 26-3 ■).

Receiver

The *receiver,* the third component of the communication process, is the listener, who must listen, observe, and attend. This person is the *decoder,* who must perceive what the sender

Figure 26-3 ■ Appropriate forms of touch can communicate caring.

intended (interpretation). Perception uses all of the senses to receive verbal and nonverbal messages. To **decode** means to relate the message perceived to the receiver's storehouse of knowledge and experience and to sort out the meaning of the message. Whether the message is decoded accurately by the receiver, according to the sender's intent, depends largely on their similarities in knowledge and experience and sociocultural background. If the meaning of the decoded message matches the intent of the sender, then the communication has been effective. Ineffective communication occurs when the message sent is misinterpreted by the receiver. For example, Mr. Johnson may perceive the message accurately—"No pain medication for another hour." However, if experience has taught him that he can receive the pain medication early if a certain nurse is on duty, he will interpret the intent of the message differently.

Response

The fourth component of the communication process, the response, is the message that the receiver returns to the sender. It is also called **feedback.** Feedback can be either verbal, nonverbal, or both. Nonverbal examples are a nod of the head or a yawn. Either way, feedback allows the sender to correct or reword a message. In the case of Mr. Johnson, the receiver may appear irritated or say, "Well, the nurse on the other shift gives me my pain medication early if I need it." The sender then knows the message was interpreted accurately. However, now the original sender becomes the receiver, who is required to decode and respond.

Modes of Communication

Communication is generally carried out in two different modes: verbal and nonverbal. **Verbal communication** uses the spoken or written word; **nonverbal communication** uses other forms, such as gestures or facial expressions, and touch. Although both kinds of communication occur concurrently, the majority of communication is nonverbal. Learning about nonverbal communication is important for nurses in developing effective communication patterns and relationships with clients. Another

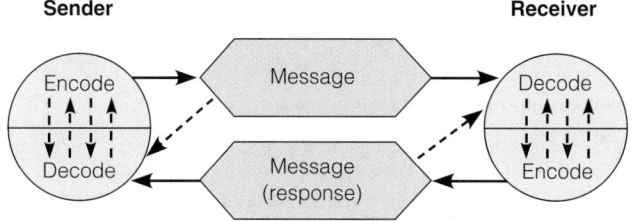

Sender   Receiver

Figure 26-2 ■ The communication process. The dashed arrows indicate intrapersonal communication (self-talk). The solid lines indicate interpersonal communication.

form of communication has evolved with technology—**electronic communication**. The most common form of electronic communication is e-mail where an individual can send a message, by computer, to another person or group of people. It is important for nurses to know when it is appropriate and not appropriate to use e-mail when communicating with clients.

Verbal Communication

Verbal communication is largely conscious because people choose the words they use. The words used vary among individuals according to culture, socioeconomic background, age, and education. As a result, countless possibilities exist for the way ideas are exchanged. An abundance of words can be used to form messages. In addition, a wide variety of feelings can be conveyed when people talk.

When choosing words to say or write, nurses need to consider pace and intonation, simplicity, clarity and brevity, timing and relevance, adaptability, credibility, and humor.

PACE AND INTONATION. The manner of speech, as in the pace or rhythm and intonation, will modify the feeling and impact of the message. The intonation can express enthusiasm, sadness, anger, or amusement. The pace of speech may indicate interest, anxiety, boredom, or fear. For example, speaking slowly and softly to an excited client may help calm the client.

SIMPLICITY. Simplicity includes the use of commonly understood words, brevity, and completeness. Many complex technical terms become natural to nurses. However, laypersons often misunderstand these terms. Words such as *vasoconstriction* or *cholecystectomy* are meaningful to the nurse and easy to use but are ill advised when communicating with clients. Nurses need to learn to select appropriate, understandable terms based on the age, knowledge, culture, and education of the client. For example, instead of saying to a client, "The nurses will be catheterizing you tomorrow for a urine analysis," it may be more appropriate and understandable to say, "Tomorrow we need to get a sample of your urine, so we will collect it by putting a small tube into your bladder." The latter statement is more likely to elicit a response from the client as to why it is needed and whether it will be uncomfortable, because the person understands the message being conveyed by the nurse.

CLARITY AND BREVITY. A message that is direct and simple will be more effective. Clarity is saying precisely what is meant, and brevity is using the fewest words necessary. The result is a message that is simple and clear. An aspect of this is congruence, or consistency, where the nurse's behavior or nonverbal communication matches the words spoken. When the nurse tells the client, "I am interested in hearing what you have to say," the nonverbal behavior would include the nurse facing the client, making eye contact, and leaning forward. The goal is to communicate clearly so that all aspects of a situation or circumstance are understood. To ensure clarity in communication, nurses also need to speak slowly and enunciate carefully.

TIMING AND RELEVANCE. Nurses need to be aware of both relevance and timing when communicating with clients. No matter how clearly or simply words are stated or written, the timing needs to be appropriate to ensure that words are heard. Moreover, the messages need to relate to the person or to the person's interests and concerns.

This involves sensitivity to the client's needs and concerns. For example, a client who is enmeshed in fear of cancer may not hear the nurse's explanations about the expected procedures before and after gallbladder surgery. In this situation it is better for the nurse first to encourage the client to express concerns, and then to deal with those concerns. The necessary explanations can be provided at another time when the client is able to listen.

Another problem in timing is asking several questions at once. For example, a nurse enters a client's room and says in one breath, "Good morning, Mrs. Brody. How are you this morning? Did you sleep well last night? Your husband is coming to see you before your surgery, isn't he?" The client no doubt wonders which question to answer first, if any. A related pattern of poor timing is to ask a question and then not wait for an answer before making another comment. On the other hand, research shows that by allowing the client to respond to the social talk or chat, the nurse develops a rapport with the client (Fenwick, Barclay, & Schmeid, 2001). This rapport can help facilitate effective therapeutic communication.

ADAPTABILITY. Spoken messages need to be altered in accordance with behavioral cues from the client. This adjustment is referred to as *adaptability*. What the nurse says and how it is said must be individualized and carefully considered. This requires astute assessment and sensitivity on the part of the nurse. For example, a nurse who usually smiles, appears cheerful, and greets his client with an enthusiastic "Hi, Mrs. Brown!" notices that the client is not smiling and appears distressed. It is important for the nurse to then modify his tone of speech and express concern in his facial expression while moving toward the client.

CREDIBILITY. *Credibility* means worthiness of belief, trustworthiness, and reliability. Credibility may be the most important criterion of effective communication. Nurses foster credibility by being consistent, dependable, and honest. The nurse needs to be knowledgeable about what is being discussed and to have accurate information. Nurses should convey confidence and certainty in what they are saying, while being able to acknowledge their limitations (e.g., "I don't know the answer to that, but I will find someone who does").

HUMOR. The use of humor can be a positive and powerful tool in the nurse–client relationship, but it must be used with care. Humor can be used to help clients adjust to difficult and painful situations. The physical act of laughter can be an emotional and physical release, reducing tension by providing a different perspective and promoting a sense of well-being.

When using humor, it is important to consider the client's perception of what is considered humorous. Timing is also important to consider. MacDonald (2004) states that while humor and laughter can help reduce stress and anxiety in the early and recovery stages of a crisis, it may be considered offensive or distracting at a peak crisis period (p. 23).

Nonverbal Communication

Nonverbal communication is sometimes called *body language.* It includes gestures, body movements, use of touch, and physical appearance, including adornment. Nonverbal communication often tells others more about what a person is feeling than what is actually said, because nonverbal behavior is controlled less consciously than verbal behavior (see Figure 26-4 ■). Nonverbal communication either reinforces or contradicts what is said verbally. For example, if a nurse says to a client, "I'd be happy to sit here and talk to you for a while," yet glances nervously at a watch every few seconds, the actions contradict the verbal message. The client is more likely to believe the nonverbal behavior, which conveys "I am very busy and need to leave."

Observing and interpreting the client's nonverbal behavior is an essential skill for nurses to develop. To observe nonverbal behavior efficiently requires a systematic assessment of the person's overall physical appearance, posture, gait, facial expres-

A

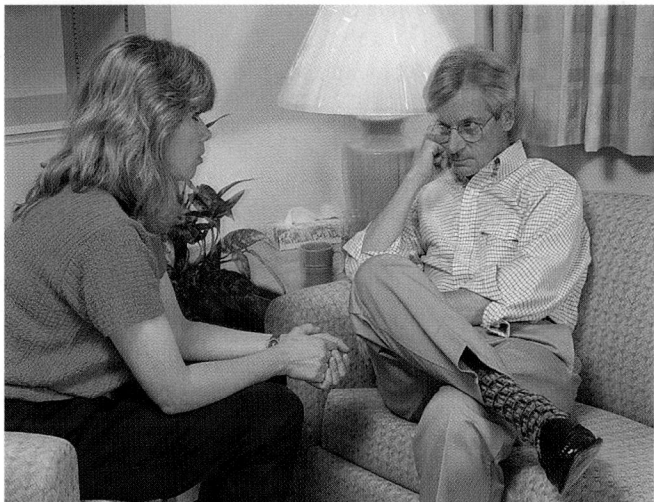

B

Figure 26-4 ■ Nonverbal communication sometimes conveys meaning more effectively than words. *A,* The postures of these women indicate openness to communication. *B,* The listener's posture suggests resistance to communication.

sions, and gestures. Whatever is observed, the nurse needs to exercise caution in interpretation, always clarifying any observation with the client.

Clients who have altered thought processes, such as in schizophrenia or dementia, may experience times when expressing themselves verbally is difficult or impossible. During these times, the nurse needs to be able to interpret the feeling or emotion that the client is expressing nonverbally. An attentive nurse who clarifies observations very often portrays caring and acceptance to the client. This can be a beginning for establishing a trusting relationship between the nurse and the client, even in clients who have difficulty communicating appropriately.

Transculturally, nonverbal communication varies widely. Even for behaviors such as smiling and handshaking, cultures differ. For example, to many Hispanics smiling and handshaking are an integral part of an interaction and essential to establishing trust. The same behavior might be perceived by a Russian as insolent and frivolous.

The nurse cannot always be sure of the correct interpretation of the feelings expressed nonverbally. The same feeling can be expressed nonverbally in more than one way, even within the same cultural group. For example, anger may be communicated by aggressive or excessive body motion, or it may be communicated by frozen stillness. In some cultures, a smile may be used to conceal anger. Therefore, the interpretation of such observations requires validation with the client. For example, the nurse might say, "You look like you have been crying. Is something upsetting you?"

PERSONAL APPEARANCE. Clothing and adornments can be sources of information about a person. Although choice of apparel is highly personal, it may convey social and financial status, culture, religion, group association, and self-concept. Charms and amulets may be worn for decorative or for health protection purposes. When the symbolic meaning of an object is unfamiliar the nurse can inquire about its significance, which may foster rapport with the client.

How a person dresses is often an indicator of how the person feels. Someone who is tired or ill may not have the energy or the desire to maintain their normal grooming. When a person known for immaculate grooming becomes lax about appearance, the nurse may suspect a loss of self-esteem or a physical illness. The nurse must validate these observed nonverbal data by asking the client. For acutely ill clients in hospital or home care settings, a change in grooming habits may signal that the client is feeling better. A man may request a shave, or a woman may request a shampoo and some makeup.

POSTURE AND GAIT. The ways people walk and carry themselves are often reliable indicators of self-concept, current mood, and health. Erect posture and an active, purposeful stride suggest a feeling of well-being. Slouched posture and a slow, shuffling gait suggest depression or physical discomfort. Tense posture and a rapid, determined gait suggest anxiety or anger. The posture of people when they are sitting or lying can also indicate feelings or mood. Again, the nurse clarifies the meaning of the observed behavior by describing to the client what the nurse sees and then asking what it means or whether the nurse's interpretation is correct. For example, "You look like it really hurts you to move. I'm wondering how your pain is and if you might need something to make you more comfortable?"

FACIAL EXPRESSION. No part of the body is as expressive as the face (see Figure 26-5 ■). Feelings of surprise, fear, anger, disgust, happiness, and sadness can be conveyed by facial expressions. Although the face may express the person's genuine emotions, it is also possible to control these muscles so the emotion expressed does not reflect what the person is feeling. When the message is not clear, it is important to get feedback to be sure of the intent of the expression. Many facial expressions convey a universal meaning. The smile expresses happiness. Contempt is conveyed by the mouth turned down, the head tilted back, and the eyes directed down the nose. No single expression can be interpreted accurately, however, without considering other reinforcing physical cues, the setting in which it occurs, the expression of others in the same setting, and the cultural background of the client.

Nurses need to be aware of their own expressions and what they are communicating to others. Clients are quick to notice the nurse's facial expression, particularly when the client feels unsure or uncomfortable. The client who questions the nurse about a feared diagnostic result will watch whether the nurse maintains eye contact or looks away when answering. The client who has had disfiguring surgery will examine the nurse's face for signs of disgust. It is impossible to control all facial expression, but the nurse must learn to control expressions of feelings such as fear or disgust in some circumstances.

Eye contact is another essential element of facial communication. In many cultures, mutual eye contact acknowledges recognition of the other person and a willingness to maintain communication. Often a person initiates contact with another person with a glance, capturing the person's attention prior to communicating. A person who feels weak or defenseless often averts the eyes or avoids eye contact; the communication received may be too embarrassing or too dominating.

GESTURES. Hand and body gestures may emphasize and clarify the spoken word, or they may occur without words to indicate a particular feeling or to give a sign. A father awaiting information about his daughter in surgery may wring his hands, tap his foot, pick at his nails, or pace back and forth. A gesture may more clearly indicate the size or shape of an object. A wave good-bye and the motioning of a visitor toward a chair are gestures that have relatively universal meanings. Some gestures, however, are culture specific. The Anglo American gesture meaning "shoo" or "go away" means "come here" or "come back" in some Asian cultures. In the Hmong culture it is considered rude to point at something with your toe.

For people with special communication problems, such as the deaf, the hands are invaluable in communication. Many people who are deaf learn sign language. Ill persons who are unable to reply verbally can similarly devise a communication system using the hands. The client may be able to raise an index finger once for "yes" and twice for "no." Other signals can often be devised by the client and the nurse to denote other meanings.

Electronic Communication

Computers are increasingly playing a big role in nursing practice. Many health care agencies are moving toward electronic medical records where nurses document their assessments and nursing care. Electronic mail (e-mail) can be used in health care facilities for many purposes: schedule and confirm appointments, report normal lab results, conduct client education, and follow up with discharged clients (Austin, 2006, p. 76).

E-MAIL. E-mail is the most common form of electronic communication. It is important for the nurse to know the advantages and disadvantages of e-mail and also other guidelines to ensure client confidentiality.

Advantages. E-mail has many positive advantages. It is a fast, efficient way to communicate and it is legible. It provides a record of the date and time of the message that was sent or received. Some health facilities provide information to their clients on how they can reach, via e-mail, specified staff members. This improves communication and continuity of client care. E-mail promises better access, and one research study indicated that half of Internet users would like to communicate with a doctor online (Delbanco & Sands, 2004).

Disadvantages. The disadvantage or negative aspect of e-mail is the risk to client confidentiality. The Health Insurance Portability and Accountability Act (HIPAA) requires organizations to apply "reasonable and appropriate safeguards" when e-mailing protected health information (PHI) (Anonymous, 2005). The health care agency needs to have an e-mail encryption system to ensure security. An agency may have their own system or outsource an encryption service.

Another disadvantage is one of socioeconomics. Not everyone has a computer. While there may be available access to a computer, not everyone has the necessary computer skills. E-mail may enhance communication with some clients but not all clients. Other forms of communication will be needed for clients who have limited abilities with speaking English, reading, writing, or using a computer.

When Not to Use E-mail. Austin (2006) lists the following situations when it is best to avoid using e-mail:

Figure 26-5 ■ The nurse's facial expression communicates warmth and caring.

LIFESPAN CONSIDERATIONS Communication

The ability to communicate is directly related to the development of thought processes, the presence of intact sensory and motor systems, and the extent and nature of an individual's opportunities to practice communication skills. As children grow, their communication abilities change markedly.

INFANTS

■ Infants communicate nonverbally, often in response to body feelings rather than in a conscious effort to be expressive.
■ Infants' perceptions are related to sensory stimuli, so a gentle voice is soothing, for example, while tension and anger around them creates distress.

TODDLERS AND PRESCHOOLERS

■ Toddlers and young children gain skills in both expressive (i.e., telling others what they feel, think, want, care about) and receptive (hearing and understanding what others are communicating to them) language.
■ Allow time for them to complete verbalizing their thoughts without interruption.
■ Provide a simple response to questions because they have short attention spans.
■ Drawing a picture can provide another way for the child to communicate.

SCHOOL-AGE CHILDREN

■ Talk to the child at his or her eye level to help decrease intimidation.
■ Include the child in the conversation when communicating with the parents.

ADOLESCENTS

■ Take time to build rapport with the adolescent.
■ Use active listening skills.
■ Project a nonjudgmental attitude and nonreactive behaviors, even when the adolescent says disturbing remarks.

Nurses can use the following communication techniques to work effectively with children and their families:

■ Play, the universal language, allows children to use other symbols, not just words, to express themselves.
■ Drawing, painting, and other art forms can be used by even nonverbal children.
■ Storytelling, in which the nurse and child take turns adding to a story or putting words to pictures, can help the child feel safer in expressing emotions and feelings.
■ Word games that pose hypothetical situations or put the child in control, such as "What if . . . ?" "If you could . . . ," "If a genie came and gave you a wish . . . ," can help a child feel more powerful or explore ideas about how to manage the illness.
■ Read books with a theme similar to the child's condition or problem, then discuss the meaning, characters, and feelings generated by the book. Movies or videos can also be used in this way.
■ Writing can be used by older children to reflect on their situation, develop meaning, and gain a sense of control.

In all interactions with children, it is important to give them opportunities to be expressive, listen openly, and respond honestly, using words and concepts they understand.

■ When the information is urgent and the client's health could be in jeopardy if he or she doesn't read it immediately.
■ Highly confidential information (e.g., HIV status, mental health, chemical dependency).
■ Abnormal lab data. If the information is confusing and could prompt many questions by the client, it is better to either see or telephone the person.

Other Guidelines. Agencies usually develop standards and guidelines for the use of e-mail in health care. It is important to know, per the agency's guidelines, what can be e-mailed to clients. Usually there is an e-mail consent form that the client signs. This form provides information about the risks of e-mail and authorizes the health agency to communicate with the client at a specified e-mail address.

Austin (2006) cautions the nurse to be sure to identify that the e-mail is "confidential" in the subject line. She advises including a disclaimer that the message is to be read only by the person to whom it is addressed and that no one else is authorized to read the message. Additionally, the disclaimer should state that if the e-mail is sent to anyone else by mistake, they should contact the sender.

Information sent to a client via e-mail is considered part of the client's medical record. Therefore, a copy of the e-mail needs to be put in the client's chart. E-mails, like other documentation in the client's record, may be used as evidence during litigation.

E-mail is another form of communication that can enhance effective relationships with clients. It is not, however, a substitute for effective verbal and nonverbal communication. Nurses need to use their professional judgment about what form of communication(s) will best meet their client's health needs.

Factors Influencing the Communication Process

Many factors influence the communication process. Some of these are development, gender, values and perceptions, personal space, territoriality, roles and relationships, environment, congruence, and attitudes.

Development

Language, psychosocial, and intellectual development move through stages across the life span. Knowledge of a client's developmental stage will allow the nurse to modify the message accordingly. The use of dolls and games with simple language may help explain a procedure to an 8-year-old. With adolescents who have developed more abstract thinking skills, a more detailed explanation can be given, whereas a well-educated, middle-aged business executive may wish to have detailed technical information provided. Older clients are apt to have had a wider range of experiences with the health care system, which may influence their response or understanding. With aging also come changes in vision and hearing acuity that can affect nurse–client interactions.

Gender

From an early age, females and males communicate differently. Girls tend to use language to seek confirmation, minimize differences, and establish intimacy. Boys use language to establish independence and negotiate status within a group. These differences can continue into adulthood so that the same communication may be interpreted differently by a man and a woman.

Values and Perceptions

Values are the standards that influence behavior, and *perceptions* are the personal view of an event. Because each person has unique personality traits, values, and life experiences, each will perceive and interpret messages and experiences differently. For example, if the nurse draws the curtains around a crying woman and leaves her alone, the woman may interpret this as "The nurse thinks that I will upset others and that I shouldn't cry" or "The nurse respects my need to be alone." It is important for the nurse to be aware of a client's values and to validate or correct perceptions to avoid creating barriers in the nurse–client relationship.

Personal Space

Personal space is the distance people prefer in interactions with others. **Proxemics** is the study of distance between people in their interactions. Middle-class North Americans use definite distances in various interpersonal relationships, along with specific voice tones and body language. Communication thus alters in accordance with four distances, each with a close and a far phase. Tamparo and Lindh (2000, p. 31) list the following examples:

1. *Intimate:* Touching to 1½ feet
2. *Personal:* 1½ to 4 feet
3. *Social:* 4 to 12 feet
4. *Public:* 12 to 15 feet

Intimate distance communication is characterized by body contact, heightened sensations of body heat and smell, and vocalizations that are low. Vision is intense, is restricted to a small body part, and may be distorted. Intimate distance is frequently used by nurses. Examples include cuddling a baby, touching the sightless client, positioning clients, observing an incision, and restraining a toddler for an injection. It is a natural protective instinct for people to maintain a certain amount of space immediately around them, and the amount varies with individuals and cultures. When someone who wants to communicate steps too close, the receiver automatically steps back a pace or two. In their therapeutic roles, nurses often are required to violate this personal space. However, it is important for them to be aware when this will occur and to forewarn the client. In many instances, the nurse can respect (not come as close as) a person's intimate distance. In other instances, the nurse may come within intimate distance to communicate warmth and caring.

Personal distance is less overwhelming than intimate distance. Voice tones are moderate, and body heat and smell are noticed less. Physical contact such as a handshake or touching a shoulder is possible. More of the person is perceived at a personal distance, so that nonverbal behaviors such as body stance or full facial expressions are seen with less distortion. Much communication be-

Figure 26-6 ■ Personal space influences communication in social and professional interactions. Encroachment into another individual's personal space creates tension.
(Photographer, Patrick Watson)

tween nurses and clients occurs at this distance. Examples occur when nurses are sitting with a client, giving medications, or establishing an intravenous infusion. Communication at a close personal distance can convey involvement by facilitating the sharing of thoughts and feelings. On the other hand, it can also create tension if the distance encroaches upon the other's personal space (Figure 26-6 ■). At the outer extreme of 4 feet, however, less involvement is conveyed. Bantering and some social conversations usually take place at this distance.

Social distance is characterized by a clear visual perception of the whole person. Body heat and odor are imperceptible, eye contact is increased, and vocalizations are loud enough to be overheard by others. Communication is therefore more formal and is limited to seeing and hearing. The person is protected and out of reach for touch or personal sharing of thoughts or feelings. Social distance allows more activity and movement back and forth. It is expedient in communicating with several people at the same time or within a short time. Examples occur when nurses make rounds or wave a greeting to someone. Social distance is important in accomplishing the business of the day. However, it is frequently misused. For example, the nurse who stands in the doorway and asks a client, "How are you today?" will receive a more noncommittal reply than the nurse who moves to a personal distance to make the same inquiry.

Public distance requires loud, clear vocalizations with careful enunciation. Although the faces and forms of people are seen at public distance, individuality is lost. Instead, the perception is of the group of people or the community.

Territoriality

Territoriality is a concept of the space and things that an individual considers as belonging to the self. Territories marked off by people may be visible to others. For example, clients in a hospital often consider their territory as bounded by the curtains around the bed unit or by the walls of a private room. This human tendency to claim territory must be recognized by all health care workers. Clients often feel the need to defend their territory when it is invaded by others; for example, when a visitor or nurse removes a chair to use at another bed, the visitor has inadvertently violated the territoriality of the client whose chair was removed. Nurses need to obtain permission from clients to remove, rearrange, or borrow objects in their hospital area.

Roles and Relationships

The roles and the relationships between sender and receiver affect the communication process. Roles such as nursing student and instructor, client and primary care provider, or parent and child affect the content and responses in the communication process. Choice of words, sentence structure, and tone of voice vary considerably from role to role. In addition, the specific relationship between the communicators is significant. The nurse who meets with a client for the first time communicates differently from the nurse who has previously developed a relationship with that client.

Environment

People usually communicate most effectively in a comfortable environment. Temperature extremes, excessive noise, and a poorly ventilated environment can all interfere with communication. Also, lack of privacy may interfere with a client's communication about matters the client considers private. For example, a client who is worried about the ability of his wife to care for him after discharge from the hospital may not wish to discuss this concern with a nurse within hearing of other clients in the room. Environmental distraction can impair and distort communication.

Congruence

In **congruent communication,** the verbal and nonverbal aspects of the message match. Clients more readily trust the nurse when they perceive the nurse's communication as congruent. This will also help to prevent miscommunication. Congruence between verbal expression and nonverbal expression is easily seen by the nurse and the client. Nurses are taught to assess clients, but clients are often just as adept at reading a nurse's expression or body language. If there is an incongruence, the body language or nonverbal communication is usually the one with the true meaning. For example, when teaching a client how to care for a colostomy, the nurse might say, "You won't have any problem with this." However, if the nurse looks worried or disgusted while saying this, the client is less likely to trust the nurse's words.

Interpersonal Attitudes

Attitudes convey beliefs, thoughts, and feelings about people and events. Attitudes are communicated convincingly and rapidly to others. Attitudes such as caring, warmth, respect, and acceptance facilitate communication, whereas condescension, lack of interest, and coldness inhibit communication.

Caring and *warmth* convey a feeling of emotional closeness, in contrast to an impersonal approach. Caring is more enduring and intense than warmth. It conveys deep and genuine concern for the person, whereas warmth conveys friendliness and consideration, shown by acts of smiling and attention to physical comforts (Brammer, 1988). Caring involves giving feelings, thoughts, skill, and knowledge. It requires psychologic energy and poses the risk of gaining little in return, yet by caring, people usually reap the benefits of greater communication and understanding.

Respect is an attitude that emphasizes the other person's worth and individuality. It conveys that the person's hopes and feelings are special and unique even though similar to others in many ways. People have a need to be different from—and at the same time similar to—others. Being too different can be isolating and threatening. A nurse conveys respect by listening open-mindedly to what the other person is saying, even if the nurse disagrees. Nurses can learn new ways of approaching situations when they conscientiously listen to another person's perspective.

Health care providers may unknowingly use speech that they believe shows caring but the client perceives as demeaning or patronizing. This frequently happens in settings that provide health care to older adults and/or individuals with obvious physical or mental disabilities (Williams, Kemper, & Hummert, 2004). **Elderspeak** is a speech style similar to babytalk, that gives the message of dependence and incompetence to older adults. It does not communicate respect. Many health care providers are not aware that they use elderspeak or that it can have negative meanings to the client. The characteristics of elderspeak include diminutives (inappropriate terms of endearment), inappropriate plural pronoun use, tag questions, and slow, loud speech (Williams et al., 2004, p. 22). See Table 26–1 for features of elderspeak and alternative strategies to use.

Acceptance emphasizes neither approval nor disapproval. The nurse willingly receives the client's honest feelings. An accepting attitude allows clients to express personal feelings freely and to be themselves. The nurse may need to restrict acceptance in situations where clients' behaviors are harmful to themselves or to others. Helping the client to find appropriate behaviors for feelings is often part of client teaching.

Therapeutic Communication

Therapeutic communication promotes understanding and can help establish a constructive relationship between the nurse and the client. Unlike the social relationship, where there may not be a specific purpose or direction, the therapeutic helping relationship is client and goal directed.

Nurses need to respond not only to the content of a client's verbal message but also to the feelings expressed. It is important to understand how the client views the situation and feels about it before responding. The content of the client's communication is the words or thoughts, as distinct from the feelings. Sometimes people can convey a thought in words while their emotions contradict the words; that is, words and feelings are incongruent. For example, a client says, "I am glad he has left me; he was very cruel." However, the nurse observes that the client has tears in her eyes as she says this. To respond to the client's *words,* the nurse might simply rephrase, saying, "You are pleased that he has left you." To respond to the client's *feelings,* the nurse would need to acknowledge the tears in the client's eyes, saying, for example, "You seem saddened by all this." Such a response helps the client to focus on her feelings. In some instances, the nurse may need to know more about the client and her resources for coping with these feelings.

Sometimes clients need time to deal with their feelings. Strong emotions are often draining. People usually need to deal

TABLE 26–1 **Features of Elderspeak and Alternative Strategies**	
ELDERSPEAK	**ALTERNATIVE STRATEGY**
Diminutives (inappropriately intimate terms of endearment, imply parent–child relationship). Examples: honey, sweetie, dearie, grandma	Refer to clients by their full name (i.e., Mrs. Robinson) or by their preferred name.
Inappropriate plural pronouns (substituting a collective pronoun, e.g., *we*, when referring to an independent older adult). Example: "Are *we* ready for *our* medicine?"	"Are *you* ready for *your* medicine?"
Tag questions (prompts the answer to the questions and implies the older adult can't act alone). Example: "You would rather wear the blue socks, *wouldn't you*?"	"Would you like to wear the blue socks?"
Shortened sentences, slow speech rate, and simple vocabulary (sounds like baby talk)	Use usual sentence structure, speech rate, and vocabulary.

Note: From "Enhancing Communication with Older Adults: Overcoming Elderspeak," by K. Williams, S. Kemper, & M. L. Hummert, 2004, *Journal of Gerontological Nursing.* Copyright © 2004 *SLACK,* Inc. Reprinted with permission.

with feelings before they can cope with other matters, such as learning new skills or planning for the future. This is most evident in hospitals when clients learn that they have a terminal illness. Some require hours, days, or even weeks before they are ready to start other tasks. Some need only time to themselves, others need someone to listen, others need assistance identifying and verbalizing feelings, and others need assistance making decisions about future courses of action.

Attentive Listening

Attentive listening is listening actively, using all the senses, as opposed to listening passively with just the ear. It is probably the most important technique in nursing and is basic to all other techniques. Attentive listening is an active process that requires energy and concentration. It involves paying attention to the total message, both verbal and nonverbal, and noting whether these communications are congruent. Attentive listening means absorbing both the content and the feeling the person is conveying, without selectivity. The listener does not select or listen solely to what the listener wants to hear; the nurse focuses not on the nurse's own needs but rather on the client's needs. Attentive listening conveys an attitude of caring and interest, thereby encouraging the client to talk (see Figure 26-7 ■).

Attentive listening also involves listening for key themes in the communication. The nurse must be careful not to react quickly to the message. The speaker should not be interrupted and the nurse (the responder) should take time to think about the message before responding. As a listener, the nurse also should ask questions either to obtain additional information or to clarify.

Nurses need to be aware of their own biases. A message that reflects different values or beliefs should not be discredited for that reason. According to Rondeau (1992), the message sender (i.e., the client) should decide when to close a conversation. When the nurse closes the conversation, the client may assume that the nurse considers the message unimportant.

In summary, attentive listening is a highly developed skill, but fortunately it can be learned with practice. A nurse can convey attentiveness in listening to clients in various ways. Common responses are nodding the head, uttering "uh huh" or "mmm," repeating the words that the client has used, or saying "I see what you mean." Each nurse has characteristic ways of responding, and the nurse must take care not to sound insincere or phony.

Physical Attending

Egan (1998) has outlined five specific ways to convey physical attending, which he defines as the manner of being present to

Figure 26-7 ■ The nurse conveys attentive listening through a posture of involvement.

REAL WORLD PRACTICE

After 20 years of nursing I have discovered that one of my greatest skills is the ability to listen. When you are dealing with those labeled "difficult," approach them with an open mind. Many times they just need to be heard, to feel as though someone cares and has taken the time to listen to them. Giving them three minutes of your undivided attention is often enough to diffuse their anger. More often than not, you will find the anger is justified, and you will be able to advocate for the clients and families more effectively.

—*Sherrie Hatch RN BSN CCRN,*
Clinical Resource Nurse, PICU, UC Davis Medical Center, Sacramento CA

BOX 26–1 Actions of Physical Attending

■ Face the other person squarely. This position says, "I am available to you." Moving to the side lessens the degree of involvement.

■ Adopt an open posture. The nondefensive position is one in which neither arms nor legs are crossed. It conveys that the person wishes to encourage the passage of communication, as the open door of a home or an office does.

■ Lean toward the person. People move naturally toward one another when they want to say or hear something—by moving to the front of a class, by moving a chair nearer a friend, or by leaning across a table with arms propped in front. The nurse conveys involvement by leaning forward, closer to the client.

■ Maintain good eye contact. Mutual eye contact, preferably at the same level, recognizes the other person and denotes willingness to maintain communication. Eye contact neither glares at nor stares down another but is natural.

■ Try to be relatively relaxed. Total relaxation is not feasible when the nurse is listening with intensity, but the nurse can show relaxation by taking time in responding, allowing pauses as needed, balancing periods of tension with relaxation, and using gestures that are natural.

These five attending postures need to be adapted to the specific needs of clients in a given situation. For example, leaning forward may not be appropriate at the beginning of an interview. It may be reserved until a closer relationship grows between the nurse and the client. The same applies to eye contact, which is generally uninterrupted when the communicators are very involved in the interaction.

another or being with another. Listening, in his frame of reference, is what a person does while attending. The five actions of physical attending, which convey a "posture of involvement," are described in Box 26–1.

Therapeutic communication techniques facilitate communication and focus on the client's concerns (see Table 26–2).

Barriers to Communication

Nurses need to recognize barriers or nontherapeutic responses to effective communication (see Table 26–3). Failure to listen, improperly decoding the client's intended message, and placing the nurse's needs above the client's needs are major barriers to communication.

TABLE 26–2 Therapeutic Communication Techniques

TECHNIQUE	DESCRIPTION	EXAMPLES
Using silence	Accepting pauses or silences that may extend for several seconds or minutes without interjecting any verbal response.	Sitting quietly (or walking with the client) and waiting attentively until the client is able to put thoughts and feelings into words.
Providing general leads	Using statements or questions that (a) encourage the client to verbalize, (b) choose a topic of conversation, and (c) facilitate continued verbalization.	"Can you tell me how it is for you?" "Perhaps you would like to talk about. . . ." "Would it help to discuss your feelings?" "Where would you like to begin?" "And then what?"
Being specific and tentative	Making statements that are specific rather than general, and tentative rather than absolute.	"Rate your pain on a scale of 0–10." (specific statement) "Are you in pain?" (general statement) "You seem unconcerned about your diabetes." (tentative statement) "You don't care about your diabetes and you never will." (absolute statement)
Using open-ended questions	Asking broad questions that lead or invite the client to explore (elaborate, clarify, describe, compare, or illustrate) thoughts or feelings. Open-ended questions specify only the topic to be discussed and invite answers that are longer than one or two words.	"I'd like to hear more about that." "Tell me about. . . . " "How have you been feeling lately?" "What brought you to the hospital?" "What is your opinion?" "You said you were frightened yesterday. How do you feel now?"
Using touch	Providing appropriate forms of touch to reinforce caring feelings. Because tactile contacts vary considerably among individuals, families, and cultures, the nurse must be sensitive to the differences in attitudes and practices of clients and self.	Putting an arm over the client's shoulder. Placing your hand over the client's hand.
Restating or paraphrasing	Actively listening for the client's basic message and then repeating those thoughts and/or feelings in similar words. This conveys that the nurse has listened and understood the client's basic message and also offers clients a clearer idea of what they have said.	*Client:* "I couldn't manage to eat any dinner last night—not even the dessert." *Nurse:* "You had difficulty eating yesterday." *Client:* "Yes, I was very upset after my family left." *Client:* "I have trouble talking to strangers." *Nurse:* "You find it difficult talking to people you do not know?"

continued

TABLE 26–2 Therapeutic Communication Techniques—*continued*

TECHNIQUE	DESCRIPTION	EXAMPLES
Seeking clarification	A method of making the client's broad overall meaning of the message more understandable. It is used when paraphrasing is difficult or when the communication is rambling or garbled. To clarify the message, the nurse can restate the basic message or confess confusion and ask the client to repeat or restate the message. Nurses can also clarify their own message with statements.	"I'm puzzled." "I'm not sure I understand that." "Would you please say that again?" "Would you tell me more?" "I meant this rather than that." "I'm sorry that wasn't very clear. Let me try to explain another way."
Perception checking or seeking consensual validation	A method similar to clarifying that verifies the meaning of specific words rather than the overall meaning of a message.	*Client:* "My husband never gives me any presents." *Nurse:* "You mean he has never given you a present for your birthday or Christmas?" *Client:* "Well—not never. He does get me something for my birthday and Christmas, but he never thinks of giving me anything at any other time."
Offering self	Suggesting one's presence, interest, or wish to understand the client without making any demands or attaching conditions that the client must comply with to receive the nurse's attention.	"I'll stay with you until your daughter arrives." "We can sit here quietly for a while; we don't need to talk unless you would like to." "I'll help you to dress to go home, if you like."
Giving information	Providing, in a simple and direct manner, specific factual information the client may or may not request. When information is not known, the nurse states this and indicates who has it or when the nurse will obtain it.	"Your surgery is scheduled for 11 AM tomorrow." "You will feel a pulling sensation when the tube is removed from your abdomen." "I do not know the answer to that, but I will find out from Mrs. King, the nurse in charge."
Acknowledging	Giving recognition, in a nonjudgmental way, of a change in behavior, an effort the client has made, or a contribution to a communication. Acknowledgment may be with or without understanding, verbal or nonverbal.	"You trimmed your beard and mustache and washed your hair." "I notice you keep squinting your eyes. Are you having difficulty seeing?" "You walked twice as far today with your walker."
Clarifying time or sequence	Helping the client clarify an event, situation, or happening in relationship to time.	*Client:* "I vomited this morning." *Nurse:* "Was that after breakfast?" *Client:* "I feel that I have been asleep for weeks." *Nurse:* "You had your operation Monday, and today is Tuesday."
Presenting reality	Helping the client to differentiate the real from the unreal.	"That telephone ring came from the program on television." "I see shadows from the window coverings." "Your magazine is here in the drawer. It has not been stolen."
Focusing	Helping the client expand on and develop a topic of importance. It is important for the nurse to wait until the client finishes stating the main concerns before attempting to focus. The focus may be an idea or a feeling; however, the nurse often emphasizes a feeling to help the client recognize an emotion disguised behind words.	*Client:* "My wife says she will look after me, but I don't think she can, what with the children to take care of, and they're always after her about something—clothes, homework, what's for dinner that night." *Nurse:* "Sounds like you are worried about how well she can manage."
Reflecting	Directing ideas, feelings, questions, or content back to clients to enable them to explore their own ideas and feelings about a situation.	*Client:* "What can I do?" *Nurse:* "What do you think would be helpful?" *Client:* "Do you think I should tell my husband?" *Nurse:* "You seem unsure about telling your husband."
Summarizing and planning	Stating the main points of a discussion to clarify the relevant points discussed. This technique is useful at the end of an interview or to review a health teaching session. It often acts as an introduction to future care planning.	"During the past half hour we have talked about. . . ." "Tomorrow afternoon we may explore this further." "In a few days I'll review what you have learned about the actions and effects of your insulin." "Tomorrow, I will look at your feeling journal."

TABLE 26–3 Barriers to Communication

TECHNIQUE	DESCRIPTION	EXAMPLES
Stereotyping	Offering generalized and oversimplified beliefs about groups of people that are based on experiences too limited to be valid. These responses categorize clients and negate their uniqueness as individuals.	"Two-year-olds are brats." "Women are complainers." "Men don't cry." "Most people don't have any pain after this type of surgery."
Agreeing and disagreeing	Akin to judgmental responses, agreeing and disagreeing imply that the client is either right or wrong and that the nurse is in a position to judge this. These responses deter clients from thinking through their position and may cause a client to become defensive.	*Client:* "I don't think Dr. Broad is a very good doctor. He doesn't seem interested in his patients." *Nurse:* "Dr. Broad is head of the department of surgery and is an excellent surgeon."
Being defensive	Attempting to protect a person or health care services from negative comments. These responses prevent the client from expressing true concerns. The nurse is saying, "You have no right to complain." Defensive responses protect the nurse from admitting weaknesses in the health care services, including personal weaknesses.	*Client:* "Those night nurses must just sit around and talk all night. They didn't answer my light for over an hour." *Nurse:* "I'll have you know we literally run around on nights. You're not the only client, you know."
Challenging	Giving a response that makes clients prove their statement or point of view. These responses indicate that the nurse is failing to consider the client's feelings, making the client feel it necessary to defend a position.	*Client:* "I felt nauseated after that red pill." *Nurse:* "Surely you don't think I gave you the wrong pill?" *Client:* "I feel as if I am dying." *Nurse:* "How can you feel that way when your pulse is 60?" *Client:* "I believe my husband doesn't love me." *Nurse:* "You can't say that; why, he visits you every day."
Probing	Asking for information chiefly out of curiosity rather than with the intent to assist the client. These responses are considered prying and violate the client's privacy. Asking "why" is often probing and places the client in a defensive position.	*Client:* "I was speeding along the street and didn't see the stop sign." *Nurse:* "Why were you speeding?" *Client:* "I didn't ask the doctor when he was here." *Nurse:* "Why didn't you?"
Testing	Asking questions that make the client admit to something. These responses permit the client only limited answers and often meet the nurse's need rather than the client's.	"Who do you think you are?" (forces people to admit their status is only that of client) "Do you think I am not busy?" (forces the client to admit that the nurse really is busy)
Rejecting	Refusing to discuss certain topics with the client. These responses often make clients feel that the nurse is rejecting not only their communication but also the clients themselves.	"I don't want to discuss that. Let's talk about. . . . " "Let's discuss other areas of interest to you rather than the two problems you keep mentioning." "I can't talk now. I'm on my way for coffee break."
Changing topics and subjects	Directing the communication into areas of self-interest rather than considering the client's concerns is often a self-protective response to a topic that causes anxiety. These responses imply that what the nurse considers important will be discussed and that clients should not discuss certain topics.	*Client:* "I'm separated from my wife. Do you think I should have sexual relations with another woman?" *Nurse:* "I see that you're 36 and that you like gardening. This sunshine is good for my roses. I have a beautiful rose garden."
Unwarranted reassurance	Using clichés or comforting statements of advice as a means to reassure the client. These responses block the fears, feelings, and other thoughts of the client.	"You'll feel better soon." "I'm sure everything will turn out all right." "Don't worry."
Passing judgment	Giving opinions and approving or disapproving responses, moralizing, or implying one's own values. These responses imply that the client must think as the nurse thinks, fostering client dependence.	"That's good (bad)." "You shouldn't do that." "That's not good enough." "What you did was wrong (right)."
Giving common advice	Telling the client what to do. These responses deny the client's right to be an equal partner. Note that giving expert rather than common advice is therapeutic.	*Client:* "Should I move from my home to a nursing home?" *Nurse:* "If I were you, I'd go to a nursing home, where you'll get your meals cooked for you."

THE HELPING RELATIONSHIP

Nurse–client relationships are referred to by some as *interpersonal relationships,* by others as *therapeutic relationships,* and by still others as **helping relationships.** Helping is a growth-facilitating process that strives to achieve two basic goals (Egan, 1998):

1. Help clients manage their problems in living more effectively and develop unused or underused opportunities more fully.
2. Help clients become better at helping themselves in their everyday lives.

A helping relationship may develop over weeks of working with a client, or within minutes. The keys to the helping relationship are (a) the development of trust and acceptance between the nurse and the client and (b) an underlying belief that the nurse cares about and wants to help the client.

The helping relationship is influenced by the personal and professional characteristics of the nurse and the client. Age, sex, appearance, diagnosis, education, values, ethnic and cultural background, personality, expectations, and setting can all affect the development of the nurse–client relationship. Consideration of all of these factors, combined with good communication skills and sincere interest in the client's welfare, will enable the nurse to create a helping relationship. Characteristics of helping relationships are named in Box 26–2.

Phases of the Helping Relationship

The helping relationship process can be described in terms of four sequential phases, each characterized by identifiable tasks and skills. The relationship must progress through the stages in succession because each builds on the one before. Nurses can identify the progress of a relationship by understanding these phases: preinteraction phase, introductory phase, working (maintaining) phase, and termination phase. Table 26–4 summarizes the tasks and skills required.

Preinteraction Phase

The preinteraction phase is similar to the planning stage before an interview. In most situations, the nurse has information about the client before the first face-to-face meeting. Such information may include the client's name, address, age, medical his-

tory, and/or social history. Planning for the initial visit may generate some anxious feelings in the nurse. If the nurse recognizes these feelings and identifies specific information to be discussed, positive outcomes can evolve.

Introductory Phase

The introductory phase, also referred to as the *orientation phase* or the *prehelping phase,* is important because it sets the tone for the rest of the relationship. During this initial encounter, the client and the nurse closely observe each other and form judgments about the other's behavior. The three stages of this introductory phase are opening the relationship, clarifying the problem, and structuring and formulating the contract (Brammer, 1988). Other important tasks of the introductory phase include getting to know each other and developing a degree of trust.

After introductions, the nurse may initially engage in some social interaction to put the client at ease. For example, the nurse and client may talk about what a nice day it is and what they would like to do if at home.

During the initial parts of the introductory phase, the client may display some resistive behaviors. *Resistive behaviors* are those that inhibit involvement, cooperation, or change. They may be due to difficulty in acknowledging the need for help and thus a dependent role, fear of exposing and facing feelings, anxiety about the discomfort involved in changing problem-causing behavior patterns, and fear or anxiety in response to the nurse's approach, which may, in the client's opinion, be inappropriate.

Resistive behaviors can be overcome by conveying a caring attitude, genuine interest in the client, and competence. These behaviors of the nurse also foster the development of trust in the relationship. Trust can be described as a reliance on someone without doubt or question, or the belief that the other person is capable of assisting in times of distress and in all likelihood will do so. To trust another person involves risk; clients become vulnerable when they share thoughts, feelings, and attitudes with the nurse. Trust, however, enables the client to express thoughts and feelings openly.

By the end of the introductory phase, clients should begin to

- Develop trust in the nurse.
- View the nurse as a competent professional capable of helping.
- View the nurse as honest, open, and concerned about their welfare.
- Believe the nurse will try to understand and respect their cultural values and beliefs.
- Believe the nurse will respect client confidentiality.
- Feel comfortable talking with the nurse about feelings and other sensitive issues.
- Understand the purpose of the relationship and the roles.
- Feel that they are active participants in developing a mutually agreeable plan of care.

Working Phase

During the working phase of a helping relationship, the nurse and the client begin to view each other as unique individuals. They begin to appreciate this uniqueness and care about each other. Caring is sharing deep and genuine concern about the

---

BOX 26–2 **Characteristics of a Helping Relationship**

A HELPING RELATIONSHIP
- Is an intellectual and emotional bond between the nurse and the client and is focused on the client.
- Respects the client as an individual, including
  • Maximizing the client's abilities to participate in decision making and treatments.
  • Considering ethnic and cultural aspects.
  • Considering family relationships and values.
- Respects client confidentiality.
- Focuses on the client's well-being.
- Is based on mutual trust, respect, and acceptance.

TABLE 26–4 Tasks and Skills for Each Phase of the Helping Relationship

PHASE	TASKS	SKILLS
Preinteraction Phase	The nurse reviews pertinent assessment data and knowledge, considers potential areas of concern, and develops plans for interaction.	Organized data gathering; recognizing limitations and seeking assistance as required.
Introductory Phase		
1. Opening the relationship	Both client and nurse identify each other by name. When the nurse initiates the relationship, it is important to explain the nurse's role to give the client an idea of what to expect. When the client initiates the relationship, the nurse needs to help the client express concerns and reasons for seeking help. Vague, open-ended questions, such as "What's on your mind today?" are helpful at this stage.	A relaxed, attending attitude to put the client at ease. It is not easy for all clients to receive help.
2. Clarifying the problem	Because the client initially may not see the problem clearly, the nurse's major task is to help clarify the problem.	Attentive listening, paraphrasing, clarifying, and other effective communication techniques discussed in this chapter. A common error at this stage is to ask too many questions of the client. Instead focus on priorities.
3. Structuring and formulating the contract (obligations to be met by both the nurse and client)	Nurse and client develop a degree of trust and verbally agree about (a) location, frequency, and length of meetings, (b) overall purpose of the relationship, (c) how confidential material will be handled, (d) tasks to be accomplished, and (e) duration and indications for termination of the relationship.	Communication skills listed above and ability to overcome resistive behaviors if they occur.
Working Phase	Nurse and client accomplish the tasks outlined in the introductory phase, enhance trust and rapport, and develop caring.	Listening and attending skills, empathy, respect, genuineness, concreteness, self-disclosure, and confrontation. Skills acquired by the client are nondefensive listening and self-understanding.
1. Exploring and understanding thoughts and feelings	The nurse assists the client to explore thoughts and feelings and acquires an understanding of the client. The client explores thoughts and feelings associated with problems, develops the skill of listening, and gains insight into personal behavior.	
2. Facilitating and taking action	The nurse plans programs within the client's capabilities and considers long- and short-term goals. The client needs to learn to take risks (i.e., accept that either failure or success may be the outcome). The nurse needs to reinforce successes and help the client recognize failures realistically.	Decision-making and goal-setting skills. Also, for the nurse: reinforcement skills; for the client: risk taking.
Termination Phase	Nurse and client accept feelings of loss. The client accepts the end of the relationship without feelings of anxiety or dependence.	For the nurse: summarizing skills; for the client: ability to handle problems independently.

welfare of another person. Once caring develops, the potential for empathy increases.

The working phase has two major stages: exploring and understanding thoughts and feelings, and facilitating and taking action. The nurse helps the client to explore thoughts, feelings, and actions and helps the client plan a program of action to meet preestablished goals.

EXPLORING AND UNDERSTANDING THOUGHTS AND FEELINGS. The nurse requires the following skills for this phase of the helping relationship:

- *Empathetic listening and responding.* Nurses must listen attentively and communicate (respond) in ways that indicate they have listened to what was said and understand how the client feels. The nurse responds to content or feelings or both, as appropriate. The nurse's nonverbal behaviors are also important. Nonverbal behaviors indicating empathy include moderate head nodding, a

steady gaze, moderate gesturing, and little activity or body movement. According to Egan (1998), **empathy** "can be seen as an intellectual process that involves understanding correctly another person's emotional state and point of view" and also as an emotional response experienced by the helper (p. 73). Empathetic listening focuses on a kind of "being with" clients to develop an understanding of them and their world. This understanding, however, must also be communicated effectively to the client—empathetic response. The end result of empathy is comforting and caring for the client and a helping, healing relationship.

- *Respect.* The nurse must show respect for the client's willingness to be available, desire to work with the client, and a manner that conveys the idea of taking the client's point of view seriously.

- *Genuineness.* Personal statements can be helpful in solidifying the rapport between the nurse and the client. The

---

BOX 26–3   **Components of Genuineness**

- The genuine helper does not take refuge in or overemphasize the role of counselor.
- The genuine person is spontaneous.
- The genuine person is nondefensive.
- The genuine person displays few discrepancies—that is, the person is consistent and does not think or feel one thing but say another.
- The genuine person is capable of deep self-disclosure (self-sharing) when it is appropriate.

---

nurse might offer such comments as "I recall when I was in (a similar situation), and I felt angry about being put down." Egan (1998) has outlined five behaviors that are components of genuineness (see Box 26–3). Nurses need to exercise caution when making references about themselves. These statements must be used with discretion. The extreme of matching each of the client's problems with a better story of the nurse's own is of little value to the client.

- *Concreteness.* The nurse must assist the client to be concrete and specific rather than to speak in generalities. When the client says, "I'm stupid and clumsy," the nurse narrows the topic to the specific by pointing out, "You tripped on the rug."
- *Confrontation.* The nurse points out discrepancies between thoughts, feelings, and actions that inhibit the client's self-understanding or exploration of specific areas. This is done empathetically, not judgmentally.

During this first stage of the working phase, the intensity of interaction increases, and feelings such as anger, shame, or self-consciousness may be expressed. If the nurse is skilled in this stage and if the client is willing to pursue self-exploration, the outcome is a beginning understanding on the part of the client about behavior and feelings.

FACILITATING TAKING ACTION. Ultimately the client must make decisions and take action to become more effective. The responsibility for action belongs to the client. The nurse, however, collaborates in these decisions, provides support, and may offer options or information.

Termination Phase

The termination phase of the relationship is often expected to be difficult and filled with ambivalence. However, if the previous phases have evolved effectively, the client generally has a positive outlook and feels able to handle problems independently. On the other hand, because caring attitudes have developed, it is natural to expect some feelings of loss, and each person needs to develop a way of saying good-bye.

Many methods can be used to terminate relationships. Summarizing or reviewing the process can produce a sense of accomplishment. This may include sharing reminiscences of how things were at the beginning of the relationship and comparing them to how they are now. It is also helpful for both the nurse and the client to express their feelings about termination openly and honestly. Thus termination discussions need to start in advance of the termination interview. This allows time for the client to adjust to independence. In some situations referrals are necessary, or it may be appropriate to offer an occasional standby meeting to give support as needed. Follow-up phone calls or e-mails are other interventions that ease the client's transition to independence.

Developing Helping Relationships

Whatever the practice setting, the nurse establishes some type of helping relationship in which mutual goals (outcomes) are set with the client or, if the client is unable to participate, with support persons. Although special training in counseling techniques is advantageous, there are many ways of helping clients that do not require special training.

- Listen actively.
- Help to identify what the person is feeling. Often clients who are troubled are unable to identify or to label their feelings and consequently have difficulty working them out or talking about them. Responses such as "You seem angry about taking orders from your boss" or "You sound as if you've been lonely since your wife died" can help clients recognize what they are feeling and talk about it.
- Put yourself in the other person's shoes (i.e., empathize). Communicate to the client in a way that shows an understanding of the client's feelings and the behavior and experience underlying these feelings.
- Be honest. In effective relationships nurses honestly recognize any lack of knowledge by saying "I don't know the answer to that right now"; openly discuss their own discomfort by saying, for example, "I feel uncomfortable about this discussion"; and admit tactfully that problems do exist, for instance, when a client says "I'm a mess, aren't I?"
- Be genuine and credible. Clients will sense whether the nurse is truly concerned.
- Use your ingenuity. There are always many courses of action to consider in handling problems. Whatever course is chosen needs to further the achievement of the client's goals (outcomes), be compatible with the client's value system, and offer the probability of success.
- Be aware of cultural differences that may affect meaning and understanding (see Chapter 18 ∞). To facilitate nurse–client interaction, recognize the language(s) and/or dialect(s) the client uses. Provide a bilingual interpreter as needed for clients limited in the English language.
- Maintain client confidentiality. To maintain the client's right to privacy, share information only with other health care professionals as needed for effective care and treatment.
- Know your role and your limitations. Every person has unique strengths and problems. When you feel unable to handle some problems, the client should be informed and referred to the appropriate health professional. Clarify functions and roles, specifically what is expected of the client, the nurse, and the primary care provider.

GROUP COMMUNICATION

People are born into a group (i.e., a family) and interact with others at all stages of life in various groups: peer groups, work groups, recreational groups, religious groups, and so on. A **group** is two or more people who have shared needs and goals, who take each other into account in their actions, and who thus are held together and set apart from others by virtue of their interactions. Groups exist to help people achieve goals (outcomes) that would be unattainable by individual effort alone. For example, groups can often solve problems more effectively than one person by pooling the ideas and expertise of several individuals; in addition, information can be disseminated to groups more quickly than to individuals.

Group Dynamics

The communication that takes place between members of any group is known as **group dynamics.** The manner of this communication will be determined by a number of interrelated factors and variables. Each member of the group will have an effect on the group dynamics, based on their motivation for participating, their similarity to other group members, the maturity of the group members in expressing their feelings, and the goal of the group.

The unique dynamics of each group will influence its maturation or group process, as well as the effectiveness of the group. Three main functions are required for any group to be effective. It must maintain a degree of group unity or cohesion. It needs to develop and modify its structure to improve its effectiveness. And it must accomplish its goals. The characteristics of an effectively functioning group are shown in Table 26–5.

Types of Health Care Groups

Much of a nurse's professional life is spent in a wide variety of groups, ranging from dyads (two-person groups) to large professional organizations. As a participant in a group, the nurse may be required to fulfill different roles: member or leader, teacher or learner, adviser or advisee, and so on.

Common types of health care groups include task groups, teaching groups, self-help groups, self-awareness/growth groups, therapy groups, and work-related social support groups. There are similarities and differences among the characteristics of these various types of groups and the nurse's role.

Task Groups

The task group is one of the most common types of work-related groups to which nurses belong. Examples are health care planning

TABLE 26–5   Comparative Features of Effective and Ineffective Groups

FACTOR	EFFECTIVE GROUPS	INEFFECTIVE GROUPS
Atmosphere	Comfortable and relaxed; a working atmosphere in which people demonstrate their interest and involvement.	Tense; lacks privacy or voluntary commitment to the group.
Purpose	Goals, tasks, and outcomes are clarified, understood, and modified so that members of the group can commit themselves to purposes through cooperation.	Purposes are unclear, misunderstood, or imposed.
Leadership and member participation	Leadership is democratic with a shift in leadership from time to time depending on knowledge or experience.	Authoritarian; leader may dominate the group, or the members may defer unduly. Member participation is unequal, with some members dominating.
Communication	Open; ideas and feelings are encouraged.	Closed; only idea production is encouraged. Feelings are ignored. Members may have "hidden agendas" (personal goals at cross-purposes with group goals).
Decision making	By the group, although various decision-making procedures appropriate to the situation may be instituted.	By the highest authority in the group, or one or two strong members of the group, with minimal involvement by members. Disagreements are ignored.
Cohesion	Facilitated through valuing other group members, open expression of feelings, trust, and support.	Leader claims full credit for achievements. Comments are critical and focus on personal characteristics.
Conflict tolerance	The reasons for disagreements or conflicts are carefully examined, and the group seeks to resolve them.	Fear of conflict prevents decisions and growth.
Power	Determined by the members' abilities and the information they possess. Power is shared.	Determined by position in the group. Obedience to authority is strong. The issue is who controls, based on individual emotional needs of members.
Problem solving	High; constructive criticism is frequent, frank, relatively comfortable, and oriented toward problem solving.	Low; criticism may be destructive, taking the form of either overt or covert personal attacks.
Creativity	Encouraged.	Discouraged.

committees, nursing service committees, nursing team meetings, nursing care conference groups, and hospital staff meetings. The focus of such groups is the completion of a specific task, and the format is defined at the outset by the leader and/or members. The methods vary according to the task to be performed.

The leader of a task group, usually called the chairperson, must be accepted by the members as an appropriate leader and therefore should be an expert in the area of task emphasis. The chairperson's role is to identify the specific task, clarify communication, and assist in expressing opinions and offering solutions. Committee members are generally selected in terms of their individual functional role and employment status, rather than in terms of their personal characteristics. Member participation is determined by the task. A target date for termination of the group is usually set in advance.

Teaching Groups

The major purpose of teaching groups is to impart information to the participants. Examples of teaching groups include continuing education and client health care groups. Numerous subjects are often handled via the group teaching format: childbirth techniques, birth control methods, effective parenting, nutrition, management of chronic illness such as diabetes, exercise for middle-aged and older adults, and instructions to family members about follow-up care for discharged clients. A nurse who leads a group in which the primary purpose is to teach or learn must be skilled in the teaching-learning process (see Chapter 27). ∞

Self-Help Groups

A self-help group is a small, voluntary organization composed of individuals who share a similar health, social, or daily living problem. One of the central beliefs of the self-help movement is that people who experience a particular social or health problem have an understanding of that condition which those without it do not.

Self-help groups are available for a range of problems (e.g., stillbirth, parenting, pregnant adolescents, divorce, drug abuse, cancer, menopause, mental illness, diabetes, AIDS, women's health, caregivers of elderly people, and grief). Alcoholics Anonymous was the first self-help group. Positive aspects of self-help groups are outlined in Box 26–4.

The major functions of the nurse's role in self-help groups include the following:

- Help clients form such groups by identifying key people who can act as facilitators.
- Share expertise with clients and help them gain appropriate knowledge and skills.
- Inform clients and support persons about existing self-help groups available to them.
- Participate as a member of a self-help group when this is appropriate. The nurse's role is that of a resource person, that is, of being "on tap, but not on top."
- Help out in times of crisis.

Self-Awareness/Growth Groups

The purpose of self-awareness/growth groups is to develop or use interpersonal strengths. The overall aim is to improve the

---

BOX 26–4 Positive Aspects of Self-Help Groups

- Members can experience almost instant kinship because the essence of the group is the idea that "you are not alone."
- Members can talk about their feelings and listen to the concerns of others, knowing they all share this experience.
- The group atmosphere is generally one of acceptance, support, encouragement, and caring.
- Many members act as role models for newer members and can inspire them to attempt tasks they might consider impossible.
- The group provides the opportunity for people to help as well as to be helped—a critical component in restoring self-esteem after significant losses.

---

person's functioning in the group to which they return, whether job, family, or community. From the beginning, broad goals are usually apparent, for example, to study communication patterns, group process, or problem solving. Because the focus of these groups is interpersonal concerns around current situations, the work of the group is oriented to reality testing with a here-and-now emphasis. Members are responsible for correcting inefficient patterns of relating and communicating with each other. They learn group process through participation and involvement and guided exercises.

Therapy Groups

Therapy groups work toward self-understanding, more satisfactory ways of relating or handling stress, and changing patterns of behavior toward health.

Members of the therapy group are referred to as clients or, in some settings, as patients. They are selected by health professionals after extensive selection interviews that consider the pattern of personalities, behaviors, needs, and identification of group therapy as the treatment of choice. Duration of therapy groups is not usually set. A termination date is usually mutually determined by the therapist and members.

Work-Related Social Support Groups

Many nurses, for example, hospice, emergency, and acute care nurses, experience high levels of vocational stress. Various types of group support can buffer such stress. Group members who know about the work of others can encourage and challenge members to be more creative and enthusiastic about their work and to achieve more. For example, a nurse may help another team member consider alternative strategies for intervention. Members also can share the joys of success and the frustration of failure through active listening without giving advice or making judgments. This type of social support is best given outside of the work environment.

COMMUNICATION AND THE NURSING PROCESS

Communication is an integral part of the nursing process. Nurses use communication skills in each phase of the nursing process. Communication is also important when caring for clients who have communication problems. Communication skills are even more important when the client has sensory, language, or cognitive deficits.

NURSING MANAGEMENT

Assessing

To assess the client's communication, the nurse determines communication impairments or barriers and communication style. Remember that culture may influence when and how a client speaks. Obviously, language varies according to age and development. With children, the nurse observes sounds, gestures, and vocabulary.

Impairments to Communication

Various barriers may alter a client's ability to send, receive, or comprehend messages. These include language deficits, sensory deficits, cognitive impairments, structural deficits, and paralysis. The nurse must assess each to determine their presence.

LANGUAGE DEFICITS. Determine the client's primary language for communicating and whether a fluent interpreter is required. Some clients who use English as a second language may have language skills that are inadequate to meet their needs.

SENSORY DEFICITS. The ability to hear, see, feel, and smell are important adjuncts to communication. Deafness can significantly alter the message the client receives; impaired vision alters the ability to observe nonverbal behavior, such as a smile or a gesture; inability to feel and smell can impair the client's capabilities to report injuries or detect the smoke from a fire. For clients with severe hearing impairments, follow these steps:

- Look for a Medic-Alert bracelet (or necklace or tag) indicating hearing loss.

- Determine whether the client wears a hearing aid and whether it is functioning.
- Observe whether the client is attempting to see your face to read lips.
- Observe whether the client is attempting to use hands to communicate with sign language.

COGNITIVE IMPAIRMENTS. Any disorder that impairs cognitive functioning (e.g., cerebrovascular disease, Alzheimer's disease, and brain tumors or injuries) may affect a client's ability to use and understand language. These clients may develop total loss of speech, impaired articulation, or the inability to find or name words. Certain medications such as sedatives, antidepressants, and neuroleptics may also impair speech, causing the client to use incomplete sentences or to slur words.

The nurse assesses whether these clients respond when asked a question and, if so, assesses the following: Is the client's speech fluent or hesitant? Does the client use words correctly? Can the client comprehend instructions as evidenced by following directions? Can the client repeat words or phrases? In addition, the nurse assesses the client's ability to understand written words: Can the client follow written directions? Can the client respond correctly by pointing to a written word? Can the client read aloud? Can the client recognize words or letters if unable to read whole sentences? The nurse uses large, clearly written words when trying to establish abilities in this area.

When the client is unconscious, the nurse looks for any indication that suggests comprehension of what is communicated (e.g., tries to arouse the client verbally and through touch). Ask a closed question like "Can you hear me?" and watch for a nonverbal response such as a nod of the head for yes or a shake for no; or ask for a hand squeeze or blink of the eye once for yes or twice for no.

STRUCTURAL DEFICITS. Structural deficits of the oral and nasal cavities and respiratory system can alter a person's ability to speak clearly and spontaneously. Examples include cleft

---

LIFESPAN CONSIDERATIONS   Communication with Elders

Older adults may have physical or cognitive problems that necessitate nursing interventions for improvement of communication skills. Some of the common ones are as follows:

- Sensory deficits, such as vision and hearing
- Cognitive impairment, as in dementia
- Neurological deficits from strokes or other neurological conditions, such as aphasia (expressive and/or receptive) and lack of movement
- Psychosocial problems, such as depression

Recognition of specific needs and obtaining appropriate resources for clients can greatly increase their socialization and quality of life. Interventions directed toward improving communication in clients with these special needs are as follows:

- Make sure that assistive devices, glasses, and hearing aids are being used and are in good working order.
- Make referrals to appropriate resources, such as speech therapy.
- Make use of communications aids, such as communication boards, computers, or pictures, when possible.

- Keep environmental distractions to a minimum.
- Speak in short, simple sentences, one subject at a time—reinforce or repeat what is said when necessary.
- Always face the person when speaking—coming up behind someone may be frightening.
- Include family and friends in conversation.
- Use reminiscing, either in individual conversations or in groups, to maintain memory connections and to enhance self-identity and self-esteem in the older adult.
- When verbal expression and nonverbal expression are incongruent, believe the nonverbal. Clarification of this and attentiveness to their feelings will help promote a feeling of caring and acceptance.
- Find out what has been important and has meaning to the person and try to maintain these things as much as possible. Even simple things such as bedtime rituals become important if they are lost in a hospital or extended care setting.

RESEARCH NOTE **Can Clients with Advanced Dementia Participate in a Social Conversation?**

The nursing literature provides general principles to use when communicating with clients with dementia. However, there is little research that documents the effectiveness of the principles or strategies. The purpose of this study by Perry, Galloway, Bottorff, and Nixon (2005) was to describe the communication strategies used by expert nurses in communicating with residents with advanced dementia and to assess the effectiveness of the strategies in supporting participation in social conversations.

The researchers used a descriptive study design. Two of the researchers led a weekly socialization group over a 10-week period for eight women with dementia. The socialization group sessions were audiotaped and transcribed verbatim. These data resulted in the formation of two taxonomies: one represented the nurses' communication and the other represented the participants' communication repertoire.

The research supported the use of a greater number of conversational strategies than what is often stated in the nursing literature. The findings also suggested that clients with advanced dementia are able to engage in social conversation beyond what was expected given their Mini-Mental State Examination (MMSE) score.

IMPLICATIONS

This study suggests that individuals with advanced dementia are able to participate in a conversation when nurses use a broad range of conversational strategies. Moreover, the use of socialization groups to allow clients with advanced dementia to interact with others is a cost-effective way of enhancing their quality of life.

Note: From "Nurse-Patient Communication in Dementia. Improving the Odds," by J. Perry, S. Galloway, J. Bottorff, and S. Nixon, 2005, *Journal of Gerontological Nursing*, Copyright © 2005 *SLACK*, Inc. Reprinted with permission.

MediaLink — Medical-Surgical Care Area Case Study

palate, artificial airways such as an endotracheal tube or tracheostomy, and laryngectomy (removal of the larynx). Extreme dyspnea (shortness of breath) can also impair speech patterns.

PARALYSIS. If verbal impairment is combined with paralysis of the upper extremities that impairs the client's ability to write, the nurse should determine whether the client can point, nod, shrug, blink, or squeeze a hand. Any of these could be used to devise a beginning communication system.

Style of Communication

In assessing communication style, the nurse considers both verbal and nonverbal communication. In addition to physical barriers, some psychologic illnesses (e.g., depression or psychosis) influence the ability to communicate. The client may demonstrate constant verbalization of the same words or phrases, a loose association of ideas, or flight of ideas.

VERBAL COMMUNICATION. When assessing verbal communication, the nurse focuses on three areas: the content of the message, the themes, and verbalized emotions. In addition, the nurse considers the following:

- Whether the communication pattern is slow, rapid, quiet, spontaneous, hesitant, evasive, and so on
- The vocabulary of the individual, particularly any changes from the vocabulary normally used (For example, a person who normally never swears may indicate increased stress or illness by an uncharacteristic use of profanity.)
- The presence of hostility, aggression, assertiveness, reticence, hesitance, anxiety, or loquaciousness (incessant verbalization) in communication
- Difficulties with verbal communication, such as slurring, stuttering, inability to pronounce a particular sound, lack of clarity in enunciation, inability to speak in sentences, loose association of ideas, flight of ideas, or the inability to find or name words or identify objects
- Refusal or inability to speak

NONVERBAL COMMUNICATION. Consider nonverbal communication in relation to the client's culture. Pay particular attention to facial expression, gestures, body movements, affect, tone of voice, posture, and eye contact.

Diagnosing

Impaired verbal communication may be used as a nursing diagnosis when "an individual experiences a decreased, delayed, or absent ability to receive, process, transmit, and use a system of symbols—anything that has meaning (i.e., transmits meaning)" (Wilkinson, 2005, p. 80). Communication problems may be *receptive* (e.g., difficulty hearing) or *expressive* (e.g., difficulty speaking).

Wilkinson (2005) points out that the *Impaired Verbal Communication* diagnosis may not be useful when an individual's communication problems are caused by a psychiatric illness or a coping problem. In those instances, the diagnoses of *Fear* or *Anxiety* may be more appropriate. Other nursing diagnoses (NANDA International, 2007) used for clients experiencing communication problems that involve impaired verbal communication as the *etiology* could include the following:

- *Anxiety* related to impaired verbal communication
- *Powerlessness* related to impaired verbal communication
- *Situational Low Self-Esteem* related to impaired verbal communication
- *Social Isolation* related to impaired verbal communication
- *Impaired Social Interaction* related to impaired verbal communication.

Planning

When a nursing diagnosis related to impaired verbal communication has been made, the nurse and client determine outcomes and begin planning ways to promote effective communication. The overall client outcome for persons with *Impaired Verbal Communication* is to reduce or resolve the factors impairing the communication. Specific nursing interventions will be planned from the stated etiology. Examples of outcome criteria to evaluate the effectiveness of nursing interventions and achievement of client goals follow.

The client:

- Communicates that needs are being met.
- Begins to establish a method of communication:
  - Signals yes/no to direct questions using vocalization or agreed-on physical cue (i.e., eye blink, hand squeeze).
  - Uses verbal or nonverbal techniques to indicate needs.
- Perceives the message accurately, as evidenced by appropriate verbal and/or nonverbal responses.
- Communicates effectively:
  - Using dominant language
  - Using translator/interpreter
  - Using sign language
  - Using word board or picture board
  - Using a computer
- Regains maximum communication abilities.
- Expresses minimum fear, anxiety, frustration, and depression.
- Uses resources appropriately.

Implementing

Nursing interventions to facilitate communication with clients who have problems with speech or language include manipulating the environment, providing support, employing measures to enhance communication, and educating the client and support person.

Manipulate the Environment

A quiet environment with limited distractions will make the most of the communication efforts of both the client and the nurse and increase the possibility of effective communication. Sufficient light will help in conveying nonverbal messages, which is especially important if visual or auditory acuity is impaired. Initially, the nurse needs to provide a calm, relaxed environment, which will help reduce any anxiety the client may have. Remember that any factor that affects communication can create feelings of frustration, anxiety, depression, or hostility in the client. Communication normally contributes to a client's sense of security and feelings that he or she is not alone, so communication problems may cause some clients to feel isolated and confused. To further reduce these emotions, the nurse should acknowledge and praise the client's attempts at communication.

Provide Support

The nurse should convey encouragement to the client and provide nonverbal reassurance, perhaps by touch if appropriate. If the nurse does not understand, it is critical to let the client know so that he or she can provide clarification with other words or through some other means of communication. When speaking with a client who will have difficulty understanding, the nurse should check frequently to determine what the client has heard and understood. Using open-ended questions will assist the nurse in obtaining accurate information about the effectiveness of communication. For example, Maria Perez, who has limited English skills, is being taught about diet related to her Crohn's disease. If the nurse asks, "Do you understand what to eat?"

Maria may nod her head yes. However, this does not give the nurse confirmation that the message given has been received. Rather the nurse needs to say, "What do you think will be good for you to eat when you go home?" The nurse's body language (e.g., gestures, posture, facial expression, and eye contact) should convey acceptance and approval.

Employ Measures to Enhance Communication

First determine how the client can best receive messages: by listening, by looking, through touch, or through an interpreter. Ways to help communication include keeping words simple and concrete and discussing topics of interest to the client. It is often helpful to use alternative communication strategies such as word boards, pictures, or paper and pencil.

Often interpreters can assist a client and nurse to communicate when the client lacks fluency in the dominant language. Some hospitals have a list of interpreters for various languages who can assist at the bedside. If the client's support person offers to interpret it is important to ask the client's permission, for the sake of confidentiality. Then instruct the person interpreting to translate as precisely as possible, without interpretation.

Educate the Client and Support Persons

Sometimes clients and support people can be prepared in advance for communication problems, for example, before an intubation or throat surgery. By explaining anticipated problems, the client is often less anxious when problems arise.

Evaluating

Evaluation is useful for both client and nurse communication.

Client Communication

To establish whether client outcomes have been met in relation to communication, the nurse must listen actively, observe nonverbal cues, and use therapeutic communication skills to determine that communication was effective. Examples of statements indicating outcome achievement include "Using picture board effectively to indicate needs" or "The client stated, 'I listened more closely to my daughter yesterday and found out how she feels about our divorce.'"

Nurse Communication

For nurses to evaluate the effectiveness of their own communication with clients, process recordings are frequently used. A **process recording** is a verbatim (word-for-word) account of a conversation. It can be taped or written and includes all verbal and nonverbal interactions of both the client and nurse.

One method of writing a process recording is to make two columns on a page. The first column lists what the nurse and the client said along with the associated nonverbal behavior. The second column contains an analysis about the nurse's responses. An example of a process recording is found in Table 26–6.

Once a process recording has been completed, it should be analyzed in terms of the content and meaning of the interaction based on communication theory. Each of the nurse's statements is interpreted in terms of the communication skill used, with the rationale for and effectiveness of its use. Any barriers to effective

MediaLink Treating an Immigrant Family Care Plan Activity

TABLE 26–6   Sample Process Recording

Mary Jane Adams, a nursing aide, reports to Irene Olsen, the staff nurse, that Sandra Barrett, the client in room 815, had finished only her orange juice when Ms. Adams collected the breakfast trays. Mrs. Barrett had been admitted 2 days earlier for diagnostic studies. Concerned about her client, Ms. Olsen walks down the corridor to room 815, knocks, and enters. Mrs. Barrett turns away from the window, tears in her eyes, as Ms. Olsen enters.

NURSE/CLIENT DIALOGUE	ANALYSIS
NURSE: Good morning, Mrs. Barrett.	Acknowledging.
CLIENT: Hello.	
NURSE: I understand you didn't eat your breakfast.	Making a specific statement but ignoring the nonverbal.
CLIENT: I wasn't hungry.	
NURSE: Is something wrong?	Asking a closed question that fails to facilitate exploration.
CLIENT: No. (Eyes fill with tears.)	
NURSE: You look sad, as if you're about to cry.	Giving feedback.
CLIENT: (Cries)	
NURSE: I'll sit here awhile with you. (Sits down.)	Offering self.
CLIENT: (Continues to cry.)	
NURSE: (After a 30-second pause) Sometimes it's hard to share the things you're concerned about with someone you don't know well. I'd like to be able to help.	Empathizing. Supporting. Offering self.
CLIENT: (Angrily) You can help me by telling me the truth.	
NURSE: (Leans forward and maintains eye contact.)	Actively listening and demonstrating interest.
CLIENT: Everyone beats around the bush when I ask them what's wrong with me. The nurse manager said, "What do you think is wrong?" That kind of put-off drives me up the wall!	
NURSE: You're angry because you're not getting any answers. It seems as if the staff knows something about your condition and they're keeping it from you.	Paraphrasing.
CLIENT: They all seem to be in cahoots. Nobody tells me anything. (Pause.) (Softly) If the news was good, they wouldn't beat around the bush.	
NURSE: I'm wondering if you're worried that because people haven't answered your question it means that you have a serious illness?	Paraphrasing.
CLIENT: Good news is always easy to give.	
NURSE: Yes, people do seem to be able to deliver good news easier and faster. I also know that we don't have any news—good or bad—to give you because none of the laboratory or x-ray results are back yet. I know that doesn't help answer your questions, but I hope it relieves you a bit from worrying that there is some bad news that's being withheld.	Giving information. Supporting.
CLIENT: Well, when my father-in-law had surgery for a bleeding ulcer, the x-ray and laboratory results were available immediately.	
NURSE: When there's a question of emergency surgery being needed, then test results are asked for immediately. Usually, though, it's preferable to wait for an accurate reading and a thorough written report.	Giving information.
CLIENT: Are you absolutely sure?	
NURSE: You don't sound convinced.	Acknowledging the implied.
CLIENT: Listen, I don't mean to give you a hard time. It's just that . . . it may not seem like an emergency to my doctor or the lab people, but it sure is to me. I can't stand not knowing. I don't know the results of the tests I had yesterday. I don't know how many more tests I have to have. Will I have to have surgery? When can I go home?	
NURSE: The problem you need help with now is finding out the answers to four questions: What are the results of yesterday's tests? Is your doctor considering any other tests for you and, if so, what are they? Is surgery being planned? And when can you go home? Let's try to figure out how you can get the answers to these questions.	Summarizing. Encouraging problem solving.
CLIENT: Well, I can't call my doctor on the phone. All his receptionist will do is take the message. And, anyway, I'm afraid that he'll be offended if he thinks I'm complaining about him. You won't tell him, will you?	

TABLE 26–6 **Sample Process Recording—*continued***

NURSE/CLIENT DIALOGUE	ANALYSIS
NURSE: No, not unless you and I decide together that it would be the best solution.	Encouraging collaboration.
CLIENT: I suppose I could try to forget about it and be patient, just like everyone tells me to.	
NURSE: You've tried that, but you're still worried, fearful, and angry. Let's think of some other possibilities.	Encouraging further exploration.
CLIENT: Maybe you could call his office for me! Since you're a nurse, they'll probably put your call right through.	
NURSE: So far there are three possible solutions—calling his office yourself, waiting until he comes to visit you later this afternoon, or having me call his office. Are there any other possible solutions that we haven't considered?	Focusing on solutions.
CLIENT: I can't think of any other.	
NURSE: Okay, then, which do you think would be best?	
CLIENT: I guess I'd feel better if you called his office. I just don't want him to think that I'm criticizing him.	
NURSE: You're concerned about what he might think of you because of this phone call. Let's discuss how I should handle the call and what I should say.	Demonstrating respect for the client. Paraphrasing. Encouraging collaboration and problem solving.

Note: From material by Carol Ren Kneisl, RN, MS, APRN, Orange Beach, AL. Adapted with permission.

---

communication can be identified with a possible alternative response noted. The outcome for nurses should be increased awareness and insight regarding their communication strengths, as well as identification of areas for future skills development.

COMMUNICATION AMONG HEALTH PROFESSIONALS

Effective communication among the health professions is as important as the promotion of therapeutic communication between the nurse and the client. For example, past studies show that more than 60% of medication errors are caused by mistakes in interpersonal communication (Maxfield, Grenny, McMillan, Patterson, & Switzler, 2005, p. 2).

A 2004 research study collected survey data from over 17,000 nurses, physicians, clinical-care staff, and administrators. This study explored their concerns of difficulty in communicating which may then cause errors and poor health outcomes. The findings resulted in a compelling report entitled *Silence Kills*. As Maxfield et al. (2005) reported, the study identified the categories of conversations that were especially difficult and, at the same time, especially essential for people in health care to master. How effective their conversations were related strongly to medical errors, client safety, quality of care, staff satisfaction, and turnover. The seven areas of concern were broken rules, mistakes, lack of support, incompetence, poor teamwork, disrespect, and micromanagement (p. 3). The report indicates, for example, that many of the health care workers observed colleagues taking dangerous shortcuts, showing poor clinical judgment, and exhibiting verbal abuse and/or intimidating behaviors. Despite their concerns, very few discussed their concerns with the co-worker. This silence strongly related to poorer health outcomes for clients.

On the other hand, the study also showed that those health care workers who were confident in their communication abilities to discuss their concerns with their co-workers were more satisfied and committed to staying in health care. Moreover, better client outcomes (i.e., fewer errors) were observed.

In response to the findings of this study, the American Association of Critical-Care Nurses (AACN) developed a set of national standards. One of their six standards for establishing and sustaining healthy work environments is skilled communication. Skilled communication states that nurses must be as proficient in communication skills as they are in clinical skills. See Box 26–5 which

---

BOX 26–5 **AACN Communication Standard for Establishing and Sustaining Healthy Work Environments**

Standard: Skilled Communication: Nurses must be as proficient in communication skills as they are in clinical skills.

CRITICAL ELEMENTS FOR THE NURSE

- Skilled communicators focus on finding solutions and achieving desirable outcomes.
- Skilled communicators seek to protect and advance collaborative relationships among colleagues.
- Skilled communicators invite and hear all relevant perspectives.
- Skilled communicators call upon goodwill and mutual respect to build consensus and arrive at common understanding.
- Skilled communicators demonstrate congruence between words and actions, holding others accountable for doing the same.
- Skilled communicators have access to appropriate communication technologies and are proficient in their use.

Note: From *AACN standards for establishing and sustaining healthy work environments: A journey to excellence* by American Association of Critical-Care Nurses, 2005. Aliso Viejo, CA. Adapted with permission. The six behaviors above have been identified as critical elements for the individual nurse to achieve skilled communication as part of creating a healthy work environment. Becasue communication involves at least two individuals and does not occur in a vacuum, the nurse should be congnizant that each healthcare organization shares reponsiblity in supporting skilled communication, and critical elements for the organization have also been identified.

RESEARCH NOTE   What Are Effects of Disruptive Behavior?

The goals of this study by Rosenstein and O'Daniel (2005) were to assess perceptions of the impact of disruptive behavior of both physicians and nurses and its effects on both providers and clinical outcomes. Disruptive behavior was defined as any inappropriate behavior, confrontation, or conflict, ranging from verbal abuse to physical and sexual harassment.

The researchers distributed surveys to over 1,500 RNs (72%), physicians (27%), and executive administrators (1%) in 50 hospitals across the country. The research revealed a high prevalence of disruptive behavior among nurses and physicians. This behavior affected nurse–physician relationships and also nurse–nurse and physician–physician relationships, indicating a problem within and across disciplines. All respondents reported that the disruptive behavior had a significant negative impact on their level of stress, frustration, concentration, collaboration, communication, and relationships. The research results also

showed a strong perception of an association between disruptive behavior and medical errors which affected client safety, quality of care, and satisfaction.

IMPLICATIONS

This study confirms that disruptive behavior is associated with decreased psychologic well-being of health care providers. This impacts job satisfaction and retention of nurses, which affects the current nursing shortage. Disruptive behavior also affects client safety and clinical outcomes. Health care organizations must develop strategies, policies, and an organizational culture that reinforces acceptable codes of behavior.

Note: From "Disruptive Behavior & Clinical Outcomes: Perceptions of Nurses & Physicians," by A. Rosenstein and M. O'Daniel, 2005, *American Journal of Nursing,* *105*(1), pp. 54–64.

---

lists the critical elements for skilled communication that preserves a nurse's professional integrity while ensuring a client's safety (AACN, 2005).

Nurse and Physician Communication

There are guidelines for written documentation and for nurses communicating with clients. However, few guidelines exist for the frequent verbal communication that occurs between nurses and doctors. This lack of guidelines or format may contribute to medical errors as a result of communication problems.

Communication Styles

A few authors describe differences between nurse and physician communication. For example, Lindeke and Sieckert (2005) state that nurses usually strive for consensus where physicians focus on ruling out alternatives. These differences can make collaboration more difficult. Beyea (2004) describes nurses' communication style as narrative and descriptive versus the physician's style being focused on a need or problem. One model, called the situational briefing model, addresses these differences and provides a framework for nurses when communicating with a physician. See Box 26–6 for more details on this communication framework.

BOX 26–6   Situational Briefing or SBAR (Situation, Background, Assessment, Recommendation) Model

A FRAMEWORK FOR NURSE–PHYSICIAN COMMUNICATION
Provide the following:

- Information about the client's current situation
- Background for the current clinical situation
- Assessment of the current problem
- Recommendation that addresses the client's need

Note: Reprinted from *AORN Journal,* vol. 790, S. Beyea, "Improving Verbal Communication in Clinical Care" pp. 1053–1057, Copyright 2004, with permission from AORN, Inc.

Assertive Communication

Assertive communication promotes client safety by minimizing miscommunication with colleagues. People who use assertive communication are honest, direct, and appropriate while being open to ideas and respecting the rights of others.

An important characteristic of assertive communication includes the use of "I" statements versus "you" statements. The "you" statement places blame and puts the listener in a defensive position. On the other hand, the "I" statement encourages discussion. For example, a nurse who states "I am concerned about . . ." to a physician will be gaining the attention of the doctor while also giving the message of the importance to work together for the benefit of the client. It is then important for the nurse to be clear, concise, organized, and fully informed when verbally presenting the client concern.

Nonassertive Communication

Two types of interpersonal behaviors are considered nonassertive: submissive and aggressive.

SUBMISSIVE. When people use a submissive communication style they allow their rights to be violated by others (Catalano, 2006). They meet the demands and requests of others without regard to their own feelings and needs as they believe their own feelings are not important. Some experts believe that people who use the submissive behaviors or communication style are insecure and try to maintain their self-esteem by avoiding conflict (e.g., negative criticism and disagreement from others).

AGGRESSIVE. There is a fine line between assertive and aggressive communication. Assertive communication is an open expression of ideas and opinions while respecting the rights, opinions, and ideas of others. Aggressive communication strongly asserts the person's legitimate rights and opinions with little regard or respect for the rights and opinions of others (Catalano, 2006, p. 278). Aggressive communication is often perceived as a personal attack by the other person because aggressive communication humiliates, dominates, controls, or embarrasses the other person. By lowering the other person's self-esteem, the person using aggressive communication may feel superior which helps increase his or her self-esteem. Cata-

lano (2006) states that aggressive communication can take several different forms, including screaming, sarcasm, rudeness, belittling jokes, and even direct personal insults (p. 278).

CRITICAL THINKING CHECKPOINT

You are the nursing student assigned to care for Mr. Manasovitz, a 45-year-old man who will be returning from the recovery room after undergoing the removal of a mass from his abdomen. While you are preparing his room for his return, the nurse and physician arrive to talk with Mrs. Manasovitz about her husband's surgery. The physician explains that the mass was malignant and invasive. Mr. Manasovitz is a candidate for chemotherapy, but his prognosis is guarded because of the extent of the tumor growth. Mrs. Manasovitz looks away, closes her eyes, and only nods her head "yes." As the physician leaves, the nurse approaches Mrs. Manasovitz, sits next to her, and puts her arm around Mrs. Manasovitz, who begins to cry. The nurse uses a soothing voice to tell Mrs. Manasovitz that it is okay to cry and assures her she will remain with her. The two of them sit in silence until Mrs. Manasovitz is

able to express her feelings. The nurse listens attentively. Later the nurse offers to get a cup of coffee for Mrs. Manasovitz and asks if there is anything she can do to assist Mrs. Manasovitz at this difficult time.

1. Interpret Mrs. Manasovitz's nonverbal behavior in response to the news about her husband's surgery.
2. Evaluate the nurse's response toward Mrs. Manasovitz based on the concepts of caring and comforting.
3. Why is it important for the nurse to effectively communicate with Mrs. Manasovitz at this time?
4. The nurse was described as listening attentively to Mrs. Manasovitz. Cite actions that portray attentive listening.

See Critical Thinking Possibilities in Appendix A. ∞

CHAPTER 26 **REVIEW**

CHAPTER HIGHLIGHTS

- Communication is a critical nursing skill used to gather assessment data for nursing diagnoses, to teach and persuade, and to express caring and comfort.
- Communication is a two-way interpersonal process involving the sender of the message and the receiver of the message. It also involves intrapersonal messages, or self-talk, which can affect the message, the interpretation of the message, and the response.
- Because the sender must encode the message and determine the appropriate channels for conveying it, and because the receiver must perceive the message, decode it, and then respond, the communication process includes four elements: sender, message, receiver, and feedback.
- Verbal communication is effective when the criteria of pace and intonation, simplicity, clarity and brevity, timing, relevance, adaptability, and credibility are met.
- Nonverbal communication often reveals more about a person's thoughts and feelings than verbal communication; it includes personal appearance, posture and gait, facial expressions, and gestures.
- When assessing verbal and nonverbal behaviors, the nurse needs to consider cultural influences and be aware that a single nonverbal expression can indicate any of a variety of feelings and that words can have various meanings.
- When communication is effective, verbal and nonverbal expressions are congruent.
- Electronic communication, particularly e-mail, is evolving into nursing practice. While e-mail provides positive advantages for improving communication and continuity of client care, the nurse needs to be aware of the risk to client confidentiality.
- Many factors influence the communication process: development, gender, values and perceptions, personal space (intimate, personal, social, and public distance), territoriality, roles and relationships, environment, congruence, and interpersonal attitudes.

- Many techniques facilitate therapeutic communication: using silence, providing general leads, being specific and tentative, using open-ended questions, using touch, restating or paraphrasing, seeking clarification, perception checking or seeking consensual validation, offering self, giving information, acknowledging, clarifying time or sequence, presenting reality, focusing, reflecting, summarizing, and planning.
- Techniques that inhibit communication include stereotyping, being defensive, challenging, testing, rejecting, changing topics and subjects, unwarranted reassurance, passing judgment, and giving common advice.
- The effective nurse–client relationship is a helping relationship that facilitates growth of the individual.
- Four phases of the helping relationship include the preinteraction phase, the introductory phase, the working phase, and the termination phase; each has a specific purpose or goal and requires specific skills of the nurse.
- Nurses interact with groups of clients and colleagues in a wide variety of settings. To use groups rationally and effectively, nurses must understand the features of effective groups.
- To help clients with communication problems the nurse manipulates the environment, provides support, employs measures to enhance communication, and educates the client and support persons.
- Process recordings are frequently made by nurses to evaluate their own communication. With them, nurses can analyze both the process and the content of the communication.
- Effective communication between health professionals is vital for client safety. A compelling research report entitled *Silence Kills* indicated that many health care workers observed concerning behaviors of their co-workers (e.g., poor clinical judgment,

dangerous shortcuts, disrespectful communication). However, they did not discuss their concerns with the co-worker. As a result, this silence strongly related to poorer health outcomes for clients.

■ Communication styles can differ between nurses and physicians. Nurses tend to be more narrative and descriptive and strive for consensus. Physicians focus on a need or problem and rule out alternatives. The situational briefing model is one approach to addressing these differences in communication style and approach.

■ Assertive communication promotes client safety by minimizing miscommunication with colleagues. An important characteristic of assertive communication is to use "I" statements.

■ Nonassertive communication includes two types of interpersonal behaviors: submissive and aggressive.

TEST YOUR KNOWLEDGE

1. A student nurse is caring for a 72-year-old client with Alzheimer's disease who is very confused. The most appropriate communication strategy should include which of the following?
   1. Written directions for bathing
   2. Speaking very loudly
   3. Gentle touch while providing ADLs
   4. Flat facial expression

2. Using the phases of the helping relationship as a framework, place the following descriptions in the correct sequence.
   1. After introductions, the nurse asks, "What plans do you have for the upcoming holiday weekend?"
   2. The nurse states, "It sounds like you are concerned about the possible complications of having diabetes. What would be the most helpful for you at this time?"
   3. The nurse reads in the medical history that the client was diagnosed with diabetes 1 week ago.
   4. The nurse states, "When we met, you knew very little about diabetes and now you are able to use your new information and apply it to your own personal situations."

3. The nurse who uses appropriate therapeutic listening skills will display which of the following behaviors? Select all that apply.
   1. Absorb both the content and the feeling the client is conveying.
   2. Presume an understanding of the client needs.
   3. Adopt an open professional posture.
   4. React quickly to the message.

4. A nurse tells a client who is struggling with cancer pain, "It is normal to feel frustrated about the discomfort." Which of the following is most representative of the skills associated with the working phase of the helping relationship?
   1. Respect
   2. Genuineness
   3. Concreteness
   4. Confrontation

5. A depressed client who has not bathed or dressed in clean clothes today is reading the lunch menu but is unable to make a decision. Which of the following would be the most appropriate nursing diagnosis for this client?
   1. *Anxiety*
   2. *Powerlessness*
   3. *Chronic Low Self-Esteem*
   4. *Social Isolation*

6. After being admitted for emergency surgery, an 80-year-old client has just returned to the room from PAR (post-anesthesia room). Which nursing interventions are most likely to facilitate effective communication with this client? Select all that apply.
   1. Ask the client, "Do you know where you are?"
   2. Ask the client or support person about visual or learning problems.
   3. Inform the client and support person(s) about events likely to occur during the next 2 hours.
   4. Provide the client with instructions about discharge.

7. The nurse is communicating with a well-oriented older adult client in a long-term care setting. Which statement best reflects respectful and caring communication?
   1. "Are we ready for our shower?"
   2. "It's time to go to the dining room, honey."
   3. "Are you comfortable, Mrs. Smith?"
   4. "You would rather wear the slacks, wouldn't you?"

8. The client made the following statement to the nurse, "My doctor just told me that he cannot save my leg and that I need to have an above-the-knee amputation." Which of the following responses by the nurse is most appropriate?
   1. "Dr. Jones is an excellent surgeon."
   2. "Are you in pain?"
   3. "If I were you, I'd get a second opinion."
   4. "Tell me more. . . ."

9. The nurse is communicating with a primary care provider about medical interventions prescribed for a client. Which of the following statements is most representative of a collaborative nurse-physician relationship?
   1. "That new medication you prescribed for Mr. Black is ineffective."
   2. "I am worried about Mr. Black's blood pressure. It is not decreasing even with the new antihypertensive medication."
   3. "Can we talk about Mr. Black?"
   4. "Excuse me doctor. I think we need to talk about Mr. Black's blood pressure."

10. The nurse asks the client, "What do you fear most about your surgery tomorrow?" This is an example of which of the following communication techniques?
   1. Providing general leads
   2. Seeking clarification
   3. Presenting reality
   4. Summarizing

See Answers to Test Your Knowledge in Appendix A. ∞

EXPLORE MEDIALINK www.prenhall.com/berman

DVD-ROM
- Audio Glossary
- NCLEX Review
- Videos
    Communication
    Communicating Effectively

COMPANION WEBSITE
- Additional NCLEX Review
- Case Study: Facilitating Communication
- Care Plan Activity: Treating an Immigrant Family
- Application Activity: Communication
    Resources
- Links to Resources

READINGS AND REFERENCES

SUGGESTED READINGS

Burke, M., Boal, J., & Mitchell, R. (2004). Communicating for better care. Improving nurse-physician communication. *American Journal of Nursing, 104*(12), 40–47. *The authors examine the current state of nurse-physician communication and present strategies for improving communication and collaboration.*

Maxfield, D., Grenny, J., McMillan, R., Patterson, K., & Switzler, A. (2005). *Silence kills. The seven crucial conversations for healthcare.* VitalSmarts, L.C. *The authors provide compelling information and anecdotal examples of the seven crucial conversations for health care: broken rules, mistakes, lack of support, incompetence, poor teamwork, disrespect, and micromanagement. These are the concerns that health care workers experience and yet have difficulty communicating. Moreover, they perceive that these concerns contribute to medical problems and errors. The report focuses on three of the seven crucial conversations (i.e., incompetence, poor teamwork, and disrespect) and describes the frequency and impact of people's concerns.*

Preston, P. (2005). Nonverbal communication: Do you really say what you mean? *Journal of Healthcare Management, 50*(2), 83–86. *This helpful article reinforces the role of nonverbal communication in professional image and communication. It includes helpful strategies to improve your ability to read nonverbal cues and to guide your own body language.*

RELATED RESEARCH

Jonas-Simpson, C. M., Mitchell, G. J., Fisher, A., Jones, G., & Linscott, J. (2006). The experience of being listened to: A qualitative study of older adults in long-term settings. *Journal of Gerontological Nursing, 32*(1), 46–53.

Stiles, A. S., & Raney, T. J. (2004). Relationships among personal space boundaries, peer acceptance, and peer reputation in adolescents. *Journal of Child and Adolescent Psychiatric Nursing, 16*(4), 29–40.

Utley-Smith, Q. (2004). Nursing competencies needed by new baccalaureate graduates. *Nursing Education Perspectives, 25*(4), 166–170.

Vazirani, S., Hays, R. D., Shapiro, M. F., & Cowan, M. (2005). Effect of a multidisciplinary intervention on communication and collaboration among physicians and nurses. *American Journal of Critical Care, 14*(1), 71–76.

REFERENCES

American Association of Critical-Care Nurses (AACN). (2005). *AACN standards for establishing and sustaining healthy work environment: A journey to excellence.* Aliso Viejo, CA: Author.

Anonymous. (2005). Meeting security regulations for e-mail. *Health Management Technology, 26*(10), 52–54.

Austin, S. (2006). E-mail: So fast, so convenient, so . . . risky? *Nursing, 36*(2), 76–77.

Beyea, S. C. (2004). Improving verbal communication in clinical care. *AORN Journal, 79*(5), 1053–1057.

Brammer, L. M. (1988). *The helping relationship: Process and skills* (4th ed.). Upper Saddle River, NJ: Prentice Hall.

Catalano, J. T. (2006). *Nursing now! Today's issues, tomorrow's trends* (4th ed.). Philadelphia: F. A. Davis.

Delbanco, T., & Sands, D. Z. (2004). Electrons in flight—E-mail between doctors and patients. *New England Journal of Medicine, 350*(17), 1705–1708.

Dochtermaun, J. M. & Bulachek, G. H. (2004). *Nursing Interventions Classification (NIC),* (4th ed.) St. Louis: Mosby.

Egan, G. (1998). *The skilled helper: A problem-management approach to helping* (6th ed.). Pacific Grove, CA: Brooks/Cole.

Fenwick, J., Barclay, L., & Schmeid, V. (2001). Chatting: An important clinical tool in facilitating mothering in neonatal nurseries. *Advances in Nursing Science, 24,* 34–49.

Lindeke, L. L., & Sieckert, A. M. (2005). Nurse-physician workplace collaboration. *Online Journal of Issues in Nursing, 10*(1), manuscript 4. Retrieved February 2, 2005, from http://www.nursingworld.org/ojin/topic26/tpc26_4.htm

MacDonald, C. M. (2004). A chuckle a day keeps the doctor away: Therapeutic humor & laughter. *Journal of Psychosocial Nursing & Mental Health Services, 42*(3), 18–25.

Maxfield, D., Grenny, J., McMillan, R., Patterson, K., & Switzler, A. (2005). *Silence kills. The seven crucial conversations for healthcare.* VitalSmarts, L.C.

Moorhead, S., Johnson, M., & Maas, M. (2004). *Nursing Outcomes Classification (NOC).* (3rd ed.). St. Louis: Mosby.

NANDA International. (2007). *NANDA nursing diagnosis: Definitions & classification 2007–2008.* Philadelphia: Author.

Perry, J., Galloway, S., Bottorff, J. L., & Nixon, S. (2005). Nurse-patient communication in dementia: Improving the odds. *Journal of Gerontological Nursing, 31*(4), 43–52.

Rondeau, K. V. (1992). Effective communication means really listening. *Canadian Journal of Medical Technology, 52*(2), 78–80.

Rosenstein, A. H., & O'Daniel, M. (2005). Disruptive behavior & clinical outcomes: Perceptions of nurses & physicians. *American Journal of Nursing, 105*(1), 54–64.

Tamparo, C. T., & Lindh, W. Q. (2000). *Therapeutic communications for health professionals* (2nd ed.). Albany, NY: Delmar: Thomson Learning.

Wilkinson, J. M. (2005). *Nursing diagnosis handbook with NIC interventions and NOC outcomes* (8th ed.). Upper Saddle River, NJ: Prentice Hall Health.

Williams, K., Kemper, S., & Hummert, M. L. (2004). Enhancing communication with older adults: Overcoming elderspeak. *Journal of Gerontological Nursing, 30*(10), 17–25.

SELECTED BIBLIOGRAPHY

Adubato, S. (2004). Making the communication connection. *Nursing Management, 35*(9), 33–35.

Arford, P. H. (2005). Nurse-physician communication: An organizational accountability. *Nursing Economics, 23*(2), 72–77.

Leonard, M., Frankel, A., Simmonds, T., & Vega, K. (2004). *Achieving safe and reliable healthcare: Strategies and solutions.* Chicago, IL: Health Administration Press.

Mathew, F. M. (2003). Laughter is the best medicine: The value of humour in current nursing practice. *Nursing Journal of India, 94*(7), 146–147.

Mikanowicz, C. K. (2005). *Strategies for developing communication between nurses and physicians.* Retrieved May 29, 2005, from http://www.nursece.com/onlinecourses/957.html

Slaven, A. (2003). Communication and the hearing-impaired patient. *Nursing Standard, 18*(1), 39–41.

Weeks, M. B. (2004). Nurse-physician communication—Discourse analysis. *Canadian Operating Room Nursing Journal, 22*(4), 33–37.

Weeks, M. B. (2005). Nurse-physician communication. *Canadian Operating Room Nursing Journal, 23*(1), 48–56.

CHAPTER 27

Teaching

Teaching client education is a major aspect of nursing practice and an important independent nursing function. In 1992, the American Hospital Association passed *A Patient's Bill of Rights* mandating client education as a right of all clients. State nurse practice acts include client teaching as a function of nursing, thereby making teaching a legal and professional responsibility. In addition, the Joint Commission on Accreditation of Healthcare Organizations (JCAHO) recently expanded its standards of client education by nurses to include "evidence that patients and their significant others understand what they have been taught. This requirement means that providers must consider the literacy level, educational background, language skills, and culture of every client during the education process" (Bastable, 2003, p. 5).

Client education is multifaceted, involving promoting, protecting, and maintaining health. It involves teaching about reducing health risk factors, increasing a person's level of wellness, and taking specific protective health measures. Box 27–1 lists specific areas of health teaching.

TEACHING

Teaching is a system of activities intended to produce learning. The teaching process is intentionally designed to produce specific learning.

The teaching–learning process involves dynamic interaction between teacher and learner. Each participant in the process communicates information, emotions, perceptions, and attitudes to the other. The teaching process and the nursing process are much alike (see Table 27–1).

Nurses teach a variety of learners in various settings. They teach clients and their families or significant others in the hospital, primary care clinics, urgent care, managed care, the home, and assisted living and long-term care facilities. Nurses teach large and small groups of learners in community health education programs.

Nurses also teach professional colleagues and other health care personnel in academic institutions such as vocational schools, colleges, and universities, and in health care facilities such as hospitals or nursing homes.

Teaching Clients and Their Families

Nurses may teach individual clients in one-to-one teaching episodes. For example, the nurse may teach about wound care while changing a client's dressing or may teach about diet, exercise, and other lifestyle behaviors that minimize the risk of a heart attack for a client who has a cardiac problem. The nurse may also be involved in teaching family members or other support people who are caring for the client. Nurses working in obstetric and pediatric areas teach parents and sometimes grandparents how to care for children.

Because of decreased length of hospital stays, time constraints on client education may occur. Nurses need to provide client education that will ensure the client's safe transition from one level of care to another and make appropriate plans for follow-up education in the client's home. Discharge plans must include information about what the client has been taught before transfer or

---

BOX 27–1   Areas for Client Education

PROMOTION OF HEALTH

- Increasing a person's level of wellness
- Growth and development topics
- Fertility control
- Hygiene
- Nutrition
- Exercise
- Stress management
- Lifestyle modification
- Resources within the community

PREVENTION OF ILLNESS/INJURY

- Health screening (e.g., blood glucose levels, blood pressure, blood cholesterol, Pap test, mammograms, vision, hearing, routine physical examinations)
- Reducing health risk factors (e.g., lowering cholesterol level)
- Specific protective health measures (e.g., immunizations, use of condoms, use of sunscreen, use of medication, umbilical cord care)
- First aid
- Safety (e.g., using seat belts, helmets, walkers)

RESTORATION OF HEALTH

- Information about tests, diagnosis, treatment, medications
- Self-care skills or skills needed to care for family member
- Resources within health care setting and community

ADAPTING TO ALTERED HEALTH AND FUNCTION

- Adaptations in lifestyle
- Problem-solving skills
- Adaptation to changing health status
- Strategies to deal with current problems (e.g., home IV skills, medications, diet, activity limits, prostheses)
- Strategies to deal with future problems (e.g., fear of pain with terminal cancer, future surgeries, or treatments)
- Information about treatments and likely outcomes
- Referrals to other health care facilities or services
- Facilitation of strong self-image
- Grief and bereavement counseling

TABLE 27–1	Comparison of the Teaching Process and the Nursing Process	
STEP	**TEACHING PROCESS**	**NURSING PROCESS**
1	Collect data; analyze client's learning strengths and deficits.	Collect data; analyze client's strengths and deficits.
2	Make educational diagnoses.	Make nursing diagnoses.
3	Prepare teaching plan: ■ Write learning outcomes. ■ Select content and time frame. ■ Select teaching strategies.	Plan nursing goals/desired outcomes and select interventions.
4	Implement teaching plan.	Implement nursing strategies.
5	Evaluate client learning based on achievement of learning outcomes.	Evaluate client outcomes based on achievement of goal criteria.

discharge and what remains for the client to learn to perform self-care in the home or other residence (see Chapter 7). ∞

Teaching in the Community

Nurses are often involved in community health education programs. Such teaching activities may be voluntary as part of the nurse's involvement in an organization such as the Red Cross or Planned Parenthood, or they may be compensated as part of the nurse's work role, such as school nurses. Community teaching activities may be aimed at large groups of people who have an interest in some aspect of health, such as nutrition classes, CPR or cardiac risk factor reduction classes, and bicycle or swimming safety programs. Community education programs can also be designed for small groups or individual learners, such as childbirth classes or family planning classes.

Teaching Health Personnel

Nurses are also involved in the instruction of professional colleagues through continuing education, in-service programs, and staff development. For example, experienced nurses may function as preceptors for new graduate nurses or for newly employed nurses. Nurses with specialized knowledge and experience share that knowledge and experience with nurses who are new to that practice area. Examples of such specialized courses include critical-care nursing, perioperative nursing, and quality improvement/quality assurance. In addition, nurses in nursing practice settings are often involved in the clinical instruction of nursing students.

Nurses are also involved in teaching other health professionals. Nurses may participate in the education of medical students or allied health students. In this capacity, the nurse educator clarifies the role of the nurse for other health professionals or how nurses can assist them in their care of the client.

LEARNING

Like all people, clients have a variety of learning needs. A **learning need** is a desire or a requirement to know something that is presently unknown to the learner. Learning needs include new knowledge or information but can also include a new or different skill or physical ability, or a new behavior or a need to change an old behavior. **Learning** is a change in human disposition or capability that persists and that cannot be solely accounted for by growth. Learning is represented by a change in behavior. See Client Teaching for attributes of learning.

An important aspect of learning is the individual's desire to learn and to act on the learning, referred to as **compliance.** In the health care context, compliance is the extent to which a person's behavior coincides with medical or health advice. Compliance is best illustrated when the person recognizes and accepts the need to learn, and then follows through with the appropriate behaviors that reflect the learning. For example, a person diagnosed as having diabetes willingly learns about the needed special diet and then plans and follows the learned diet. Many people, however, view the term *compliance* in a negative perspective because the term implies the learner is submissive and this is in conflict with the learner's right to determine his

REAL WORLD PRACTICE

Teachable moments occur every day and it is important to take advantage of them. When providing care for the client, it is easy to talk about the activity you are performing and why it is necessary. For example, while bathing a client, talk about skin care. When bringing a meal tray to the client, discuss the selections on the tray to help the client understand his or her particular diet. Whatever the activity, there is a teachable moment within it, if you recognize the opportunity.

—Joy Plamann, RN, BSN, BC,
St. Cloud Hospital, St. Cloud, MN

CLIENT TEACHING
Attributes of Learning

Learning is
■ An experience that occurs inside the learner.
■ The discovery of the personal meaning and relevance of ideas.
■ A consequence of experience.
■ A collaborative and cooperative process.
■ An evolutionary process that builds on past learning and experiences.
■ A process that is both intellectual and emotional.

or her own health care decisions rather than be told what to do by a health care professional. In addition, it is important not to label a client as noncompliant without obtaining further information. For example, the client intended to comply but was unable to do so because he could not afford the cost of the medications.

Another term seen in health care literature is **adherence,** which is commitment or attachment to a regimen. Bastable (2003) explains that both compliance and adherence refer to the "ability to maintain health-promoting regimens, which are determined largely by a health care provider" (p. 169).

Andragogy is the art and science of teaching adults, in contrast to **pedagogy,** the discipline concerned with helping children learn. **Geragogy** is the term used to describe the process involved in stimulating and helping elders to learn (Hayes, 2005; John, 1988).

Nurses can use the following andragogic concepts about adult learners as a guide for client teaching (Hayes, 2005; Knowles, 1984):

- As people mature, they move from dependence to independence.
- An adult's previous experiences can be used as a resource for learning.
- An adult's readiness to learn is often related to a developmental task or social role (i.e., perceive a need in their life situation).
- An adult is more oriented to learning when the material is useful immediately, not sometime in the future.

Learning Theories

Three main theoretical constructs are behaviorism, cognitivism, and humanism.

Behaviorism

Thorndike originally advanced behaviorism. His major contribution that applied to teaching is that learning should be based on the learner's behavior. In addition to Thorndike, major behaviorist theorists include Pavlov, Skinner, and Bandura.

In the behaviorist school of thought, an act is called a *response* when it can be traced to the effects of a stimulus. Behaviorists closely observe responses and then manipulate the environment to bring about the intended change. Thus, to modify a person's attitude and response, a behaviorist would either alter the stimulus condition in the environment or change what happens after a response occurs (Bastable, 2003, p. 45).

Skinner's and Pavlov's work focused on conditioning behavioral responses to a stimulus that causes the response or behavior. To increase the probability of a response, Skinner introduced the importance of **positive reinforcement** (e.g., a pleasant experience such as praise and encouragement) in fostering repetition of an action. Bandura, however, claims that most learning comes from observational learning and instruction rather than trial-and-error behavior. Bandura's research focuses on **imitation,** the process by which individuals copy or reproduce what they have observed, and **modeling,** the process by which a person learns by observing the behavior of others.

Nurses applying behavioristic theory will

- Provide sufficient practice time and both immediate and repeat testing and redemonstration.
- Provide opportunities for learners to solve problems by trial and error.
- Select teaching strategies that avoid distracting information and that evoke the desired response.
- Praise the learner for correct behavior and provide positive feedback at intervals throughout the learning experience.
- Provide role models of desired behavior.

Cognitivism

Cognitivism depicts learning as a complex cognitive activity. In other words, learning is largely a mental or intellectual or thinking process. The learner structures and processes information. Perceptions are selectively chosen by the individual, and personal characteristics have an impact on how a cue is perceived. Cognitivists also emphasize the importance of social, emotional, and physical contexts in which learning occurs, such as the teacher–learner relationship and the environment. Developmental readiness and individual readiness (expressed as motivation) are other key factors associated with cognitive approaches.

Major cognitive theorists include Piaget, Lewin, and Bloom. Piaget's five major phases of cognitive development include the sensorimotor phase, the preconceptual phase, the intuitive phase, the concrete operations phase, and the formal operations phase. Each phase is discussed in Chapter 20. ∞ According to Lewin, learning involves four different types of changes: change in cognitive structure, change in motivation, change in one's sense of belonging to the group, and gain in voluntary muscle control. His widely known theory of change has three basic stages: unfreezing, moving, and refreezing. These stages are discussed in detail in Chapter 28. ∞

Bloom (1956) identified three domains or areas of learning: cognitive, affective, and psychomotor. The **cognitive domain,** the "thinking" domain, includes six intellectual abilities and thinking processes beginning with knowing, comprehending, and applying to analysis, synthesis, and evaluation. The **affective domain,** known as the "feeling" domain, is divided into categories that specify the degree of a "person's depth of emotional response to tasks" (Bastable, 2003, p. 330). It includes feelings, emotions, interests, attitudes, and appreciations. The **psychomotor domain,** the "skill" domain, includes motor skills such as giving an injection.

Nurses should include each of Bloom's three domains in client teaching plans. For example, teaching a client how to self-administer insulin is in the psychomotor domain. But an important part of a teaching plan for a client with diabetes is to teach why insulin is needed and what to do when not feeling well; this is in the cognitive domain. Helping the client accept the chronic implications of diabetes and maintain self-esteem is in the affective domain.

Nurses applying cognitive theory will

- Provide a social, emotional, and physical environment conducive to learning.
- Encourage a positive teacher–learner relationship.

- Select multisensory teaching strategies since perception is influenced by the senses.
- Recognize that personal characteristics have an impact on how cues are perceived and develop appropriate teaching approaches to target different learning styles.
- Assess a person's developmental and individual readiness to learn and adapt teaching strategies to the learner's developmental level.
- Select behavioral objectives and teaching strategies that encompass the cognitive, affective, and psychomotor domains of learning.

Humanism

Humanistic learning theory focuses on both cognitive and affective qualities of the learner. Prominent members of this school of thought include Abraham Maslow and Carl Rogers. According to humanistic theory, learning is believed to be self-motivated, self-initiated, and self-evaluated. Each individual is viewed as a unique composite of biologic, psychologic, social, cultural, and spiritual factors. Learning focuses on self-development and achieving full potential; it is best when it is relevant to the learner. Autonomy and self-determination are important; the learner identifies the learning needs and takes the initiative to meet these needs. The learner is an active participant and takes responsibility for meeting individual learning needs.

Nurses applying humanistic theory will

- Convey empathy in the nurse–client relationship.
- Encourage the learner to establish goals and promote self-directed learning.
- Encourage active learning by serving as a facilitator, mentor, or resource for the learner.
- Use active learning strategies to assist the client's adoption of new behavior.
- Expose the learner to new relevant information and ask appropriate questions to encourage the learner to seek answers.

Using Learning Theories

Nurses using the **behaviorist theory** identify what is to be taught, and they immediately identify and reward correct responses. However, the theory is not easily applied to complex learning situations and limits the learner's role in the teaching process.

Uses of **cognitive theory** recognize the developmental level of the learner and acknowledge, the learner's motivation and environment. However, some or many of the motivational and environmental factors may be beyond the teacher's control.

Using **humanism,** the nurse focuses on the feelings and attitudes of learners, on the importance of the individual in identifying learning needs and in taking responsibility for them, and on the self-motivation of the learners to work toward self-reliance and independence.

Being aware of the focus and limitations of the various learning theories allows the nurse to use one or more of them when developing a teaching plan for a client. Knowing what is important (e.g., knowledge, motivation, feelings, attitudes) assists the nurse in choosing the appropriate learning theory or theories.

The nurse also needs to be aware of the different factors that can affect the client's learning.

Factors Affecting Learning

Many factors can facilitate or hinder learning by a client. The nurse should be aware of these factors, particularly when available teaching time is limited.

Motivation

Motivation to learn is the desire to learn. It greatly influences how quickly and how much a person learns. Motivation is generally greatest when a person recognizes a need and believes the need will be met through learning. It is not enough for the need to be identified and verbalized by the nurse; it must be experienced by the client. Often the nurse's task is to help the client personally work through the problem and identify the need. Sometimes clients or support people need help identifying information relevant to their situation before they can see a need. For instance, clients with heart disease may need to know the effects of smoking before they recognize the need to stop smoking. Or adolescents may need to know the consequences of an untreated sexually transmitted disease before they see the need for treatment.

Readiness

Readiness to learn is the demonstration of behaviors or cues that reflect the learner's motivation to learn at a specific time. Readiness reflects not only the desire or willingness to learn but also the ability to learn at a specific time. For example, a client may want to learn self-care during a dressing change, but if the client experiences pain or discomfort he or she may not be able to learn. The nurse can provide pain medication to make the client more comfortable and more able to learn. The nurse's role is often to encourage the development of readiness.

Active Involvement

When the learner is actively involved in the process of learning, learning becomes more meaningful. If the learner actively participates in planning and discussion, learning is faster and retention is better (Figure 27-1 ■). Active learning promotes critical thinking, enabling learners to problem solve more effectively. Clients who are actively involved in learning about their health care may be more able to apply the learning to their own situation. For example, clients who are actively involved in learning about their therapeutic diets may be more able to apply the principles being taught to their cultural food preferences and their usual eating habits. Passive learning, such as listening to a lecture or watching a film, does not foster optimal learning.

Relevance

The knowledge or skill to be learned must be personally relevant to the learner. Clients learn more easily if they can connect the new knowledge to that which they already know or have experienced. For example, if a client is diagnosed with hypertension, is overweight, and has symptoms of headaches and fatigue, he is more likely to understand the need to lose weight if he remembers having more energy when he weighed less. The

Figure 27-1 ■ Learning is facilitated when the client is interested and actively involved.

nurse needs to validate the relevance of learning with the client throughout the learning process.

Feedback

Feedback is information regarding a person's performance to a desired goal. It has to be meaningful to the learner. Feedback that accompanies the practice of psychomotor skills helps the person to learn those skills. Support of desired behavior through praise, positively worded corrections, and suggestions of alternative methods are ways of providing positive feedback. Negative feedback such as ridicule, anger, or sarcasm can lead people to withdraw from learning. Such feedback, viewed as a type of punishment, may cause the client to avoid the teacher in order to avoid punishment.

Nonjudgmental Support

People learn best when they believe they are accepted and will not be judged. The person who expects to be judged as a "poor" or "good" client will not learn as well as the person who feels no such threat. Once learners have succeeded in accomplishing a task or understanding a concept, they gain self-confidence in their ability to learn. This reduces their anxiety about failure and can motivate greater learning. Successful learners have increased confidence with which to accept failure.

Simple to Complex

Learning is facilitated by material that is logically organized and proceeds from the simple to the complex. Such organization enables the learner to comprehend new information, assimilate it with previous learning, and form new understandings. Of course, *simple* and *complex* are relative terms, depending on the level at which the person is learning. What is simple for one person may be complex for another.

Repetition

Repetition of key concepts and facts facilitates retention of newly learned material. Practice of psychomotor skills, particu-

larly with feedback from the nurse, improves performance of those skills and facilitates their transfer to another setting.

Timing

People retain information and psychomotor skills best when the time between learning and active use of the learning is short; the longer the time interval, the easier it is to forget the learning. For example, a client who is only shown literature and videotapes about administering insulin but is not permitted to administer his or her own insulin until discharge from the hospital is unlikely to remember what was learned. However, giving his or her own injections while in the hospital enhances the client's learning.

Environment

An optimal learning environment facilitates learning by reducing distraction and providing physical and psychologic comfort. It has adequate lighting that is free from glare, a comfortable room temperature, and good ventilation. Most students know what it is like to try to learn in a hot, stuffy room; the consequent drowsiness interferes with concentration. Noise can also distract the student and interfere with listening and thinking. To facilitate learning in a hospital setting, nurses should choose a time when no visitors are present and interruptions are unlikely.

Privacy is essential for some learning. For example, when a client is learning to change a colostomy bag, the presence of others can be embarrassing and thus interfere with learning. However, when a client is particularly anxious, having a support person present may give the client confidence.

Many factors inhibit learning. Some of the most common barriers to learning are described next and in Table 27–2.

Emotions

Emotions such as fear, anger, and depression can impede learning. A high level of anxiety resulting in agitation and the inability to focus or concentrate can also inhibit learning. Clients or families who are experiencing extreme emotional states may not hear spoken words or may retain only part of the communication. Emotional responses such as fear and anxiety decrease with information that relieves uncertainty. Medications may be prescribed for extremely distraught clients or families to reduce their anxiety and put them in an emotional state in which understanding or learning can occur.

Physiologic Events

Physiologic events such as a critical illness, pain, or sensory deficits inhibit learning. Because the client cannot concentrate and apply energy to learning, the learning itself is impaired. The nurse should try to reduce the physiologic barriers to learning as much as possible before teaching. For example, providing analgesics and rest before teaching is often helpful.

Cultural Aspects

There are also cultural barriers to learning, such as language or values. The client who does not understand the nurse's language may learn little. Western medicine may conflict with a client's cultural healing beliefs and practices. To be effective, nurses must be

TABLE 27–2	**Barriers to Learning**	
BARRIER	**EXPLANATION**	**NURSING IMPLICATIONS**
Acute illness	Client requires all resources and energy to cope with illness.	Defer teaching until client is less ill.
Pain	Pain decreases ability to concentrate.	Conduct pain assessment before teaching.
Prognosis	Client can be preoccupied with illness and unable to concentrate on new information.	Defer teaching to a better time.
Biorhythms	Mental and physical performances have a circadian rhythm.	Adapt time of teaching to suit client.
Emotion (e.g., anxiety, denial, depression, grief)	Emotions require energy and distract from learning.	Deal with emotions and possible misinformation first.
Language	Client may not be fluent in the nurse's language.	Obtain services of an interpreter or nurse with appropriate language skills.
Age		
■ Elders	Vision, hearing, and motor control can be impaired in elders.	Consider sensory and motor deficits and adapt in teaching plan.
■ Children	Children have a shorter attention span and vocabulary differences.	Plan shorter and more active learning episodes.
Culture/religion	There may be cultural or religious restrictions on certain types of knowledge, for example, birth control information.	Assess the client's cultural/religious needs when planning learning activities.
Physical disability	Visual, hearing, sensory, or motor impairments may interfere with a client's ability to learn.	Plan teaching activities appropriate to learner's physical abilities. For example, provide audio learning tools for the client who is blind, or large-print materials for the client whose vision is impaired.
Mental disability	Impaired cognitive ability may affect the client's capacity for learning.	Assess client's capacity for learning and plan teaching activities to complement the client's ability while planning more complex learning for the client's caregivers.

culturally sensitive and competent; otherwise the client may be partially or totally noncompliant with recommended treatments. Another impediment to learning is differing values held by the client and the health team. For example, if a client comes from a culture that views being overweight or "plump" as positive, the nurse negotiates with the client to determine an acceptable weight and they develop a plan together (Purnell & Paulanka, 2005).

Psychomotor Ability

It is important that the nurse be aware of a client's psychomotor skills when planning teaching. Psychomotor skills can be affected by health. For example, an older client who has severe osteoarthritis of the hands may not be able to wrap a bandage. The following physical abilities are important for learning psychomotor skills:

1. *Muscle strength.* For example, an older client who cannot rise from a chair because of insufficient leg and muscle strength cannot be expected to learn to lift herself out of a bathtub.
2. *Motor coordination.* Gross motor coordination is required for movements such as walking, and fine motor coordination is needed when using utensils such as a fork for eating. For example, a client who has advanced amyotrophic lateral sclerosis (ALS) involving the lower limbs will probably be unable to use a walker.
3. *Energy.* Energy is required for most psychomotor skills, and learning these skills uses more energy. People who are ill or elderly often have limited energy resources; learning and carrying out these skills must be timed for when the client's energy sources are at their peak.

4. *Sensory acuity.* Sight is used for most learning (i.e., walking with crutches, changing a dressing, drawing a medication into a syringe). Clients who have a visual impairment often need the assistance of a support person to carry out such tasks.

THE INTERNET AND HEALTH INFORMATION

The Internet has become a part of the lives of many Americans, allowing them to communicate and obtain information quickly. Internet technology has dramatically changed the activities of business, including health care. The term *e-health* is defined as "the application of Internet and other related technologies in the healthcare industry to improve the access, efficiency, effectiveness, and quality of clinical and business processes utilized by healthcare organizations, practitioners, patients, and consumers in an effort to improve the health status of patients" (Healthcare Information and Management Systems Society E-Health Special Interest Group, 2003, p. 4). E-health includes many aspects such as online appointment access, billing review, e-mail access between the client and health care provider, and online health information.

Online Health Information

The Pew Internet & American Life Project (2006) reports that 73% of American adults use the Internet. Using the Internet to locate health information is common. Health care online usage is growing twice as fast as any other online type of usage (Curran & Curran, 2005, p. 496). Eight out of 10 American Internet

---

RESEARCH NOTE Do College Students Use the Internet to Obtain Health Information?

Previous studies have found that a majority of college students use the Internet, with the most frequent activities for e-mail and instant messaging. The authors found little research data, however, about college students' use of the Internet for locating health information. This study examined college students' Internet use, health-seeking behaviors on the Internet, and attitudes toward use of the Internet for health information.

The researchers used an anonymous, cross-sectional survey that was completed by college students from two universities over a two-semester time frame. The questionnaire was administered two ways: either a paper survey or online. The 743 students who completed the survey were primarily women (58%), first-year (49%) or sophomore (25%), and white (78%).

The findings indicated the following:

- More than 98% of the college students in the study used the Internet, and 68% reported being very experienced with the Internet.
- Fifty-three percent reported that they would like to get health information on the Internet.
- Seventy-three percent reported getting health information from the Internet for themselves. Of this group, the majority (91%) re-

ported retrieving information from "some" to "a little." About 37% of this group, seeking health information, felt the information improved the way they took care of their health.

- The majority of the students used a variety of search engines to locate health information. However, 89% of the students did not always find the desired information.
- The top topics researched included fitness/exercise, diet and nutrition, and prescription drugs or medications.

IMPLICATIONS

The authors suggest that there is great potential for using the Internet for health education at colleges and universities. Campus health centers could use the Internet as a tool for health education. The results also suggest a need for training students how to search for and evaluate the health information.

Note: Journal of American College Health, 53(4), pp. 183–188, 2005. Reprinted with permission of Helen Dwight Reid Educational Foundation. Published by Heldref Publications, 1319 Eighteenth St., NW, Washington, DC 20036-1802. Copyright © 2005.

users have searched for information on at least one major health topic online. Certain groups of users are more likely to search the Internet for health information: women, adults younger than 65, college graduates, people with online experience, and those with broadband (high-speed) access (Pew Internet & American Life Project, 2005a, p. 1).

Access

The Pew Internet & American Life Project (2005b, p. 7) reported that there are three groups of adults in the United States: those who do not use the Internet, those with a modest connection, and those highly engaged with the Internet. Each group has its distinct characteristics.

Twenty-two percent of American adults have never used the Internet. They tend to have a high school or less education and to be over the age of 65. Forty percent of adults have a loose connection to the Internet. That is, they have access (usually dial-up) but do not use the Internet regularly. They are younger and more educated than the previous group. Thirty-three percent of American adults are highly engaged by using the Internet daily. They tend to have attended college and be under age 50; however, there are "pockets" of elders who are also highly engaged in Internet use.

Elders and Use of the Internet

The Kaiser Family Foundation (2005, pp. 3–10) conducted a survey research study that provided the first close look at how elders use the Internet for health information. Key findings of the report included:

- Only four in 10 elders age 65 and over have used a computer.
- Seventy percent of "Baby Boomers" (age 50–64) use the Internet. Thus, the number of elders using the Internet will increase over the next decade.

- There is a "digital divide" among elders. Those elders whose annual income is under $20,000, those who have a high school degree or less, those who are older (e.g., 75 and above), and elder women are less likely to use the Internet.
- One in five elders (65 and over) use the Internet for health information. These elders are more likely to use TV and books for their health information.
- Many elders do not trust the Internet as a source for health information except for the 50 to 64 age group who trust the Internet "a lot."
- Information on prescription drugs is the top reason for using the Internet for health information.
- Of those elders who have used the Internet for health information, about half say it helped them and the other half say it wasn't helpful.
- Most elders do not check the source of health information they find online.

Implications

The Internet is an important source of health information for many adult clients in the United States. Therefore, nurses need to know and be able to integrate this technology into the teaching plans for those clients who use the Internet. On the other hand, nurses also need to apply effective teaching strategies for those clients who do not use the Internet.

NURSE AS EDUCATOR

Being an educator or teacher is an important and primary role for the nurse. Clients and families have the right to health education in order to make informed decisions about their health. The nurse is in a position to promote healthy lifestyles through the application of health knowledge, the change process, learning theories, and the nursing and teaching process when teaching clients and their families.

NURSING MANAGEMENT

Assessing

A comprehensive assessment of learning needs incorporates data from the nursing history and physical assessment and addresses the client's support system. It also considers client characteristics that may influence the learning process: readiness to learn, motivation to learn, and reading and comprehension level, for example. Assessing a person's stage of change and any barriers to change is also important and often overlooked (see Chapter 16). ∞

The nurse's knowledge of common learning needs required by clients experiencing similar health problems is another source of information. Learning needs change as the client's health status changes, so nurses must constantly reassess them.

Nursing History

Several elements in the nursing history provide clues to learning needs. These elements include (a) age, (b) the client's understanding and perceptions of the health problem, (c) health beliefs and practices, (d) cultural factors, (e) economic factors, (f) learning style, and (g) the client's support systems. Examples of interview questions to elicit this information are shown in the accompanying Assessment Interview. Note the number of open-ended questions.

AGE. Age provides information on the person's developmental status that may indicate distinctive health teaching content

and teaching approaches. Simple questions to school-age children and adolescents will elicit information on what they know. Observing children at play provides information about their motor and intellectual development as well as relationships with other children. For older people, conversation and questioning may reveal slow recall or limited psychomotor skills, sensory deficits, and learning difficulties (see Lifespan Considerations).

CLIENTS' UNDERSTANDING OF HEALTH PROBLEM. Clients' perceptions of their current health problems and concerns may indicate deficient knowledge or misinformation. In addition, the effects of the problem on the client's usual activities can alert the nurse to other areas requiring instruction. For example, people who cannot manage self-care at home often need information about community resources and services.

HEALTH BELIEFS AND PRACTICES. A client's health beliefs and practices are important to consider in any teaching plan. The health belief model described in Chapter 17 ∞ provides a predictor of preventive health behavior. However, even if a nurse is convinced that a particular client's health beliefs should be changed, doing so may not be possible because so many factors are involved in a person's health beliefs.

CULTURAL FACTORS. Many cultural groups have their own folk beliefs and practices with a number of them related to diet, health, illness, and lifestyle. It is therefore important to discuss the client's cultural perspective on illness and therapy. The cultural practices and values held by clients will affect

---

ASSESSMENT INTERVIEW   Learning Needs and Characteristics

PRIMARY HEALTH PROBLEM

- Tell me what you know about your current health problem. What do you think caused it?
- What concerns do you have about it?
- How has the problem affected what you can or cannot do during your usual activities (e.g., work, recreation, shopping, housework)?
- What do you or did you do at home to relieve the problem? How helpful was it?
- How have the treatments you have started helped your problem?
- What, if any, difficulties have the treatments caused you (e.g., inconvenience, cost, discomfort)?
- Tell me about the tests (surgery, treatments) you are going to have.

HEALTH BELIEFS

- How would you describe your health generally?
- What things do you usually do to keep healthy?
- What health problems do you think you may be at risk for because of family history, age, diet, occupation, inadequate exercise, or other habits, such as smoking?
- What changes would you be willing to make to decrease your risk for these problems or to improve your health?

CULTURAL FACTORS

- What language do you use most often when speaking and writing?
- Do you seek the advice of another health practitioner?

- Do you use herbs or other medications or treatments commonly used in your cultural group?
- Does your current primary care provider know about these?
- What advice or treatments given previously by your primary care provider conflicted with values or beliefs you consider important?
- When a conflict arose, what did you do?

LEARNING STYLE

- Note the client's age and developmental level.
- What level of education have you received?
- Do you like to read?
- Where do you obtain health information (e.g., primary care provider, nurse, magazines, books, pharmacist, and so on)?
- How do you best learn new things?
  a. By reading about them
  b. By talking about them
  c. By watching a movie or demonstration
  d. By computer
  e. By listening to the teacher
  f. By first being shown how something works and then doing it
  g. On your own or in a group

CLIENT SUPPORT SYSTEM

- Would you like a family member or friend to help you learn about things you need to do to take care of yourself?
- Who do you think would be interested in learning with you?

LIFESPAN CONSIDERATIONS   Special Teaching Considerations

ELDERS

Elders often have chronic illnesses that require multiple treatments and/or medications. Health teaching will focus on the same areas as with other ages—health and wellness promotion and prevention of illness and accidents—but often the needs are greatest in learning to manage their lives in order to live with their chronic health conditions and to maintain optimal health and functioning. For older adults to be motivated to learn, the material must be practical and have meaning for them individually, especially if the information is new to them. Special considerations in teaching elders include the following:

- Health promotion is a priority need and should include these areas:
  - Exercise
  - Nutrition
  - Safety habits
  - Having regular health checkups
  - Understanding medications
- Set achievable goals—involve the client and family in doing this.
- If developing written materials:
  - Use large print (e.g., at least 14-point font) in bulleted format.
  - Use buff-colored paper (avoids the glare of white paper).
  - Present the information at a fifth- to sixth-grade reading level.
- Increase time for teaching and allow for rest periods as processing of information is slower.
  - Verbal presentation of material should be well organized. Ensure that there is minimal distraction.
- Repeat information if necessary.
- Use return demonstrations with psychomotor skills, such as teaching someone to learn to do insulin injections.
- Determine where clients obtain most of their health information (e.g., newspapers, magazines, television).
- Use examples that they can relate to in their daily lives.
- Be aware of sensory deficits, such as hearing and vision.
- Use the setting with which the individual is most comfortable—either a group or one-on-one setting.
- If noncompliance is a problem, investigate the cause. It could be due to lack of finances, transportation problems, poor access to medical care, and so on.

Elders come with a lifetime of experiences and learned knowledge of their own. Respect this and always have them use their strengths to work with any problems. Positive reinforcement and ongoing evaluation of what has been taught are important factors in effective health teaching with older adults.

CHILDREN

It has often been said that the parent is a child's first and most important teacher. Every interaction between a child and parent (or other adults and children) is a moment in which teaching and learning occurs, often unconsciously. Sometimes the results are ones parents desire and strive for; sometimes they are not what the parent would have wished.

In order to make parents more aware of the teaching they are doing, nurses can point out how the parent is using the concept of a "teaching loop" and how that "formal" teaching strategy can be applied more consciously to many parent–child interactions.

The teaching loop consists of four specific teaching behaviors that give children verbal instruction, role modeling, and positive feedback. These include:

- *Alerting:* Get children's attention by calling their name, touching them, or making a noise.
- *Instructing:* Give the child a short, specific instruction about what is to be done; modeling or demonstrating behavior can also be done (e.g., "Try it like this...").
- *Performing:* Give the child opportunity to practice the task, play with the toy, and explore the materials being used. Provide "enough" time, but with some structure or direction.
- *Reinforcing:* Give the child feedback; a positive or negative comment (e.g., "You poured the milk very well" or "No, that's not quite right; try turning it this way") that is specific to the task lets children know how they have done and encourages them to continue to learn.

Note: From *Gerontological Nursing: Promoting Successful Aging with Older Adults,* 3rd ed. (pp. 67–75) by M. Stanley, K. Blair, and P. G. Beare, 2005, Philadelphia: F. A. Davis; "Designing Written Medication Instructions: Effective Ways to Help Older Adults Self-Medicate" by K. Hayes, 2005, *Journal of Gerontological Nursing, 31*(5), 5–10. Adapted with permission; and "The Observation of Anglo-Mexican and Chinese-American Mothers Teaching Their Young Sons," by D. Steward and M. Steward, 1973, *Child Development, 44,* 329–337.

---

their learning needs. For example, the client may understand the health care information being taught but this learning may not be used if the client primarily believes in folk medical practices (see Chapter 18). ∞

ECONOMIC FACTORS. Economic factors can also affect a client's learning. For example, a client who cannot afford to obtain a new sterile syringe for each injection of insulin may find it difficult to learn to administer the insulin when the nurse teaches that a new syringe should be used each time.

LEARNING STYLE. Considerable research has been done on people's learning styles. The best way to learn varies with the individual. Some people are visual learners and learn best by watching. Other people do not visualize an activity well; they learn best by actually manipulating equipment and discovering how it works. Other people can learn well from reading things presented in an orderly fashion. Still other people learn best in groups where they can relate to other people. For some, stressing the thinking part of a skill and its logic will promote learning. For other people, stressing the feeling part or interpersonal aspect motivates and promotes learning.

A client's learning style may be based in his or her cultural background. For example, clients from cultures that have a strong oral tradition may prefer educational videos presented in their language (Munoz & Luckmann, 2005).

The nurse seldom has the time or skills to assess each learner, identify the person's particular learning style, and then adapt teaching accordingly. What the nurse can do, however, is ask clients how they have learned things best in the past or how they like to learn. Many people know what helps them learn, and the nurse can use this information in planning the teaching. Using a variety of teaching techniques and varying activities during teaching are good ways to match learners with learning styles. One technique will be most effective for some clients, whereas other techniques will be suited to clients with different learning styles.

CLIENT SUPPORT SYSTEM. The nurse explores the client's support system to determine the extent to which others may enhance learning and offer support. Family members or a close friend may help the client perform required skills at home and maintain required lifestyle changes.

Physical Examination

The general survey part of the physical examination provides useful clues to the client's learning needs, such as mental status, energy level, and nutritional status. Other parts of the physical examination reveal data about the client's physical capacity to learn and to perform self-care activities. For example, visual ability, hearing ability, and muscle coordination affect the selection of content and approaches to teaching.

Readiness to Learn

Clients who are ready to learn often behave differently from those who are not. A client who is ready may search out information, for instance, by asking questions, reading books or articles, talking to others, and generally showing interest. The person who is not ready to learn is more likely to avoid the subject or situation. In addition, the unready client may change the subject when it is brought up by the nurse. For example, the nurse might say, "I was wondering about a good time to show you how to change your dressing," and the client responds, "Oh, my wife will take care of everything."

The nurse assesses for these readiness characteristics:

- *Physical readiness.* Is the client able to focus on things other than physical status, or are pain, fatigue, and immobility using up all of the client's time and energy?
- *Emotional readiness.* Is the client emotionally ready to learn self-care activities? Clients who are extremely anxious, depressed, or grieving over their health status are not ready.
- *Cognitive readiness.* Can the client think clearly at this point? Are the effects of anesthesia and analgesia altering the client's level of consciousness?

Nurses can promote readiness to learn by providing physical and emotional support during the critical stage of recovery. As the client stabilizes physically and emotionally, the nurse can provide opportunities to learn.

Motivation

Motivation relates to whether the client wants to learn and is usually greatest when the client is ready, the learning need is recognized, and the information being offered is meaningful to the client. Assessment of motivation, however, may be difficult. Communication skills used by the nurse can obtain helpful information indicating a readiness for change such as "I'm really ready to lose weight this time." On the other hand, nonverbal behaviors such as disinterest, lack of attention, and missed appointments can indicate a decreased motivation to learn.

Nurses can increase a client's motivation in several ways:

- By relating the learning to something the client values and helping the client see the relevance of the learning
- By helping the client make the learning situation pleasant and nonthreatening

- By encouraging self-direction and independence
- By demonstrating a positive attitude about the client's ability to learn
- By offering continuing support and encouragement as the client attempts to learn (i.e., positive reinforcement)
- By creating a learning situation in which the client is likely to succeed (Succeeding in small tasks motivates the client to continue learning.)
- By assisting the client to identify the benefits of changing behavior

Health Literacy

A 1993 National Adult Literacy Study reported that the average reading ability of many American adults is at the fifth-grade level (Edmunds, 2005). A report from the Institute of Medicine (IOM, 2004) titled *Health Literacy: A Prescription to End Confusion* states that nearly half of all Americans — 90 million people—have difficulty understanding and acting upon health information (p. 1). Moreover, studies that assessed a variety of health-related materials found that the reading level exceeded the twelfth-grade level.

Health literacy is the ability to read, understand, and act on health information, including such tasks as comprehending prescription labels, interpreting appointment slips, completing health insurance forms, and following instructions for diagnostic tests (Redman, 2004, pp. 30–31). Limited health literacy skills are often greater among certain groups: older adults, people with limited education, poor people, minority populations, and people with limited English proficiency.

Low health literacy skills are associated with poor health outcomes and higher health care costs (IOM, 2004). For example, a client may not be able to read a prescription to know how many pills to take or may take the wrong number of pills (e.g., "once" means eleven in Spanish). Clients with low literacy skills have less information about health promotion and/or management of a disease process for themselves and their families because they are unable to read the educational materials. As a result, they have higher rates of hospitalization than people with adequate health literacy.

It is a challenge for the nurse to teach clients with low or no reading and writing skills. However, such teaching is vitally important because clients with low literacy skills need learning opportunities to improve their health practices.

CLINICAL ALERT

The majority of people at the lowest reading levels will report that they "read well." ∎

It is difficult, however, to assess a client's literacy skills because the shame and stigma associated with limited health literacy skills are major barriers. Clients may be too embarrassed to admit they cannot read. The following client behaviors may cause a nurse to suspect a literacy problem:

- Pattern of noncompliance
- Insisting that they already know the information
- Having a friend or family member read the document for them
- Pattern of excuses for not reading the instructions (e.g., glasses broken, stating will read later or when they get home)

BOX 27–2 Determining Readability Using Word Processing Programs

MICROSOFT WORD
- Click on "Tools"
- Click on "Options"
- Click on the tab "Spelling and Grammar"
- Select or check "Show readability statistics"
- Click "OK"

When finished with the document, click on "Spelling and Grammar" again. When Microsoft Word finishes checking the spelling and grammar, it will provide information about the reading level of the document.

COREL WORDPERFECT
- Click on "Tools"
- Click on "Grammatik"
- Click on "Options"
- Click on "Analysis"
- Click on "Readability"
- In the Readability dialog box, choose a comparison document

Information will then be provided about the reading level of the document.

Note: Instructions from *Microsoft Word for Windows, 2003* computer software and Corel *WordPerfect 12, 2004* computer software.

There are many formulas for assessing reading level of written material. Most word processing programs have a feature that will calculate the readability for you (see Box 27–2). Nurses involved in developing written health teaching materials should write for lower reading levels (see Client Teaching). The goal is to have the education materials at a fifth-or sixth-grade level (Aldridge, 2004). People with good reading skills are not offended by simple reading material and prefer easy-to-read information. Even the simplest written directions, however, won't be helpful for the client with low or no reading skills. See the Client Teaching box for suggestions on how to teach clients with low literacy levels.

CLIENT TEACHING Developing Written Teaching Aids

- Keep language level at or below the fifth-grade level.
- Use active, not passive, voice.
- Use easy, common words of one or two syllables (e.g., *use* instead of *utilize,* or *give* instead of *administer*).
- Use the second person (*you*) rather than the third person (*the client*).
- Use a large type size (14 to 16 point).
- Write short sentences.
- Avoid using all capital letters.
- Place priority information first and repeat more than once.
- Use bold for emphasis.
- Use simple pictures, drawings, or cartoons, if appropriate.
- Leave plenty of white space.
- Obtain feedback from nurses and clients.

CLIENT TEACHING Teaching Clients with Low Literacy Levels

- Use multiple teaching methods: Show pictures. Read important information. Lead a small group discussion. Role-play. Demonstrate a skill. Provide hands-on practice.
- Emphasize key points in simple terms and provide examples.
- Limit the amount of information in a single teaching session. Instead of one long session with a great deal of information, it is better to have more frequent sessions with a major point at each session.
- Associate new information with something the client already knows and/or associates with his or her job or lifestyle.
- Reinforce information through repetition.
- Involve the client in the teaching.
- Obtain feedback: Ask the client specific questions about the information presented or ask the client to repeat it in his or her own words.
- Avoid handouts with many pages and classroom lecture format with a large group.

RESEARCH NOTE Can Animated Cartoons Increase Knowledge of Educational Information?

Printed client information may not be helpful because of low English-language literacy levels. The researchers in this study compared the gain of knowledge about polio vaccination from information presented in two formats: printed pamphlet and videotape of animated cartoons. Both formats contained the same information. The participants were parents/caretakers of pediatric clinic clients. Ninety-six participants were in the treatment group who watched the videotape in the clinic waiting room in the midst of intense client traffic. The comparison group consisted of ninety-six participants who were given a written pamphlet to read. Both groups completed a pretest that included demographics and five questions related to understanding polio vaccine. After the two groups completed either reading the pamphlet or viewing the videotape, the participants completed a posttest which included the same five pretest questions and three additional questions.

There was no statistical difference between the two groups regarding demographic information or pretreatment knowledge. There was

a significant statistical difference between the two groups in post-test knowledge. Both groups scored higher on the post-test in comparison to the pretest. However, 30% of the participants in the videotape group answered all of the posttest questions correctly while none of the participants in the pamphlet group responded correctly to all the questions.

IMPLICATIONS

This study showed that animated cartoons can improve client knowledge independent of the level of literacy. The production cost of the videotape used in this study was $6,000 with a production time of 6 weeks. Printed material is less costly and can be developed quickly. However, if the client does not or cannot read the material, what is the ultimate cost to the client and the health care system?

Note: Health Education Research by M. Leiner, G. Handal, and D. Williams. Copyright 2004 by Oxford University Press Journals. Reproduced with permission of Oxford University Press Journals in the format Textbook via Copyright Clearance Center.

Diagnosing

Nursing diagnoses for clients with learning needs can be designated in two ways: as the client's primary concern or problem, or as the etiology of a nursing diagnosis associated with the client's response to health alterations or dysfunction (see Identifying Nursing Diagnoses, Outcomes, and Interventions).

Learning Need as the Diagnostic Label

The North American Nursing Diagnosis Association (NANDA) includes the following diagnostic labels appropriate to a client's learning needs when the learning need is the primary concern:

- *Deficient Knowledge:* absence or deficiency of cognitive information related to a specific topic (NANDA, 2005, p. 109)

    Whenever the diagnostic label *Deficient Knowledge* is used, either the client is seeking health information or the nurse has identified a learning need. The area of deficiency should always be included in the diagnosis. Following are examples using the NANDA label *Deficient Knowledge* as the primary concern:

- *Deficient Knowledge (Low-Calorie Diet)* related to inexperience with newly ordered therapy
- *Deficient Knowledge (Home Safety Hazards)* related to denial of declining health and living alone

    Wilkinson (2005) stresses that if *Deficient Knowledge* is used as the primary concern, one client goal must be "client will acquire knowledge about." The nurse needs to provide information that has the potential to change the client's behavior rather than focus on the behaviors caused by the client's lack of knowledge.

    A second nursing diagnostic label where a learning need may be the primary concern is

- *Health-Seeking Behavior:* active seeking (by a person in stable health) of ways to alter personal health habits and/or the environment in order to move toward a higher level of health (NANDA, 2005, p. 88)

    When this diagnostic label is used, the client is seeking health information; the client may or may not have an altered response or dysfunction at the time but may be seeking information to improve health or prevent illness. This diagnosis is especially appropriate for clients attending community health education programs. The following are examples using the NANDA label *Health-Seeking Behavior* as the primary concern:

- *Health-Seeking Behavior (Exercise and Activity)* related to desire to improve health behaviors and decrease risk of heart disease. This diagnosis may be appropriate for the client who has identified a personal health risk for a cardiac condition and wants to minimize that risk through exercise.
- *Health-Seeking Behavior (Home Safety Hazards)* related to desire to minimize risk of injury. This diagnosis may be appropriate for parents of a toddler who are seeking information to ensure that their home is safe for their child. The diagnosis might also be used when an adult child seeks information to ensure that the home of an elderly parent is free of risk factors for falls or other injuries common to the elderly.

A third nursing diagnostic label where a learning need may be the primary concern is

- *Noncompliance:* behavior of person and/or caregiver that fails to coincide with a health-promoting or therapeutic plan agreed on by the person (and/or family and/or community) and health-care professional. In the presence of an agreed-on, health-promoting or therapeutic plan, person's or caregiver's behavior is fully or partially nonadherent and may lead to clinically ineffective or partially ineffective outcomes (NANDA, 2005, p. 120).

The diagnostic label *Noncompliance* should be used with caution. In general, the diagnosis *Noncompliance* is associated with the *intent* to comply, but situational factors make it difficult (Wilkinson, 2005, p. 323). Factors that influence a client's compliance with health teaching include understanding or comprehension of the teaching, the experienced negative side effects of the treatment, financial inability to carry out the treatment plan, language barriers, or poor teaching on the part of the health care team. *Noncompliance* should *not* be used for a client who is unable to follow instructions (e.g., cognitive disability) or for a client who makes an informed decision to refuse or not follow the medical treatment (Wilkinson, 2005, p. 323).

CLINICAL ALERT

The term *noncompliance* is often perceived as a negative label. Be sure to state the etiology in neutral, nonjudgmental words. ■

Deficient Knowledge as the Etiology

Another way to deal with identified learning needs of clients is to write deficient knowledge as the etiology, or second part, of the diagnosis statement. Such nursing diagnoses are written in the following format:

- *Risk for (Specify)* related to deficient knowledge (specify).

    Examples include the following:

- *Risk for Impaired Parenting* related to deficient knowledge (skills in infant care and feeding)
- *Risk for Infection* related to deficient knowledge (sexually transmitted diseases and their prevention)
- *Anxiety* related to deficient knowledge (bone marrow aspiration)

Other nursing diagnoses in which a knowledge deficit can be the etiology follow:

- Risk for Injury
- Ineffective Breast-feeding
- Impaired Adjustment
- Ineffective Coping
- Ineffective Health Maintenance.

Note also that most NANDA-approved nursing diagnoses imply a teaching–learning need. For example, the nursing diagnosis *Constipation* suggests the need for a review of bowel hygiene practices including diet, hydration, and exercise/activity.

IDENTIFYING NURSING DIAGNOSES, OUTCOMES, AND INTERVENTIONS
Clients Requiring Teaching

DATA CLUSTER The nurse brings Mr. Steinberg the first dose of a medication ordered by his physician. The nurse asks whether anyone has explained what this medication is and why he is taking it. He says no.

NURSING DIAGNOSIS/ DEFINITION	SAMPLE DESIRED OUTCOME*/ DEFINITION	INDICATORS	SELECTED INTERVENTIONS*/ DEFINITION	SAMPLE NIC ACTIVITIES
Deficient Knowledge (Medication Information) related to lack of exposure to newly prescribed medication/*Absence or deficiency of cognitive information related to specific topic*	Knowledge: Medication [1808]/*Extent of understanding conveyed about the safe use of medication*	Substantial: ▪ Identification of correct medication name ▪ Description of action of medication ▪ Description of side effects of medication ▪ Description of medication precautions	Teaching, Prescribed Medication [5616]/ *Preparing a client to safely take prescribed medications and monitor for their effects*	▪ Inform the client of both the generic and brand names of the medication ▪ Instruct the client on the purpose and action of the medication ▪ Instruct the client on the dosage, route, and duration of the medication ▪ Instruct the client on specific precautions to observe when taking the medication (e.g., no driving) as appropriate

DATA CLUSTER George Evans is a 45-year-old man who has come to the clinic for his annual physical examination. He expresses concern about his family history of heart disease and requests information about activities to decrease his risk of heart disease.

Health-Seeking Behavior (Nutrition, Activity and Exercise Information) to reduce risk of heart disease/*Active seeking (by a person in stable health) of ways to alter personal health habits and/or the environment in order to move toward a higher level of health*	Adherence Behavior [1600]/*Self-initiated action taken to promote wellness, recovery, and rehabilitation*	Often demonstrated: ▪ Asks health-related questions when indicated ▪ Seeks health-related information from a variety of sources ▪ Uses strategies to eliminate unhealthy behavior	Self-Modification Assistance [4470]/ *Reinforcement of self-directed change initiated by the client to achieve personally important goals*	▪ Assist the client in identifying a specific goal for change ▪ Assist the client in identifying target behaviors that need to change to achieve the desired goal ▪ Appraise the client's present knowledge and skill level in relationship to the desired change ▪ Explore with the client potential barriers to change behavior

DATA CLUSTER Mildred Cumming is a 74-year-old widow with a history of hypertension. Her blood pressure is 150/96. She is on daily antihypertensive therapy. When asked if she is taking her medication as prescribed, she tells the nurse that she is taking her medication every other day because it is expensive and she cannot afford to take it every day.

Noncompliance (With Medication Plan) related to insufficient finances/*Behavior of person and/or caregiver that fails to coincide with a health-promoting or therapeutic plan agreed on by the person (and/or family and/or community) and health-care professional. In the presence of an agreed-on, health-promoting or therapeutic plan, person's or caregiver's behavior is fully or partially nonadherent and may lead to clinically ineffective or partially ineffective outcomes*	Compliance Behavior [1601]/ *Personal actions to promote wellness, recovery, and rehabilitation based on professional advice*	Consistently demonstrated: ▪ Discusses prescribed treatment regimen with health care professional ▪ Modifies treatment regimen as directed by a health care professional	Financial Resource Assistance [7380]/ *Assisting an individual/ family to secure and manage finances to meet health care needs*	▪ Determine if client is eligible for waiver programs ▪ Inform client of available resources and assist in accessing resources (e.g., medication assistance program)

*The NOC # for desired outcomes and the NIC # for nursing interventions are listed in brackets following the appropriate outcome or intervention. Outcomes, indicators, interventions, and activities selected are only a sample of those suggested by NOC and NIC and should be further individualized for each client.

Planning

Developing a teaching plan is accomplished in a series of steps. Involving the client at this time promotes the formation of a meaningful plan and stimulates client motivation. The client who helps develop the teaching plan is more likely to achieve the desired outcomes (see Client Teaching: Sample Teaching Plan for Wound Care).

CLINICAL ALERT

Knowing the client's stage of change helps determine which interventions will be useful to help the client change. ■

Determining Teaching Priorities

The client's learning needs must be ranked according to priority. The client and the nurse should do this together, with the client's priorities always being considered. Once a client's priorities have been addressed, the client is generally more motivated to concentrate on other identified learning needs. For example, a man who wants to know all about coronary artery disease may not be ready to learn how to change his lifestyle until he meets his own need to learn more about the disease. Nurses can also use theoretical frameworks, such as Maslow's hierarchy of needs, to establish priorities (see Chapter 8). ∞

Setting Learning Outcomes

Learning outcomes can be considered the same as desired outcomes for other nursing diagnoses. They are written in the same way. Like client outcomes, learning outcomes

■ State the client (learner) behavior or performance, not nurse behavior. For example, "Identify personal risk factors for heart disease" (client behavior), *not* "Teach the client about cardiac risk factors" (nurse behavior).

CLIENT TEACHING Sample Teaching Plan for Wound Care

Assessment of learner: A 24-year-old male college student suffered a 7-cm (2.5-inch) laceration on the left lower anterior leg during a hockey game. The laceration was cleaned, sutured, and bandaged. The client was given an appointment to return to the health clinic in 10 days for suture removal. Client states that he lives in the college dormitory and is able to do wound care if given instructions. Client is able to understand and read English. Assessed to be in the "preparation" and "action" stages of change.

Nursing Diagnosis: Deficient Knowledge (Care of Sutured Wound) related to no prior experience.
Long-Term Goal: Client's wound will heal completely without infection or other complications.
Intermediate Goal: At clinic appointment, client's wound will be healing without signs of infection, loss of function, or other complication.
Short-Term Goals: Client will (a) correctly list three signs and symptoms of wound infection and (b) correctly perform a return demonstration of wound cleansing and bandaging.

LEARNING OUTCOMES	CONTENT OUTLINE	TEACHING METHODS
Upon completion of the instructional session, The client will		
1. Describe normal wound healing.	I. Normal wound healing	Describe normal wound healing with the use of audiovisuals.
2. Describe signs and symptoms of wound infection.	II. Infection Signs and symptoms include wound warm to touch, misalignment of wound edges, and purulent wound drainage. Signs of systemic infection include fever and malaise.	Discuss the mechanism of wound infection. Use audiovisuals to demonstrate infected wound appearance. Provide handout describing signs and symptoms of wound infection.
3. Identify equipment needed for wound care.	III. Wound care equipment a. Cleansing solution as prescribed by physician (e.g., clear water, mild soap and water, or antimicrobial solution) b. Bandaging material: Telfa, gauze wrap, adhesive tape.	Demonstrate equipment needed for cleansing and bandaging wound. Provide handout listing equipment needed.
4. Demonstrate wound cleansing and bandaging.	IV. Demonstration of wound cleansing and bandaging on the client's wound or a mannequin.	Demonstrate wound cleansing and bandaging on the client's wound or a mannequin. Provide handout describing procedure for cleansing and bandaging wound.
5. Describe appropriate action if questions or complications arise.	V. Resources available for client questions include health clinic, emergency department.	Discuss available resources. Provide handout listing available resources and follow-up treatment plan.
6. Identify date, time, and location of follow-up appointment for suture removal.	VI. Follow-up treatment plan; where and when	Provide written instructions.

Evaluation: The client will:
1. Respond to questions regarding self-care of wound.
2. Return demonstration of wound cleansing and bandaging.
3. State contact person and telephone number to obtain assistance.
4. State date, time, and location of follow-up appointment.

BOX 27–3 Examples of Verbs for Writing Learning Outcomes

Cognitive Domain	Affective Domain	Psychomotor Domain
Compares	Accepts	Assembles
Describes	Attends	Calculates
Evaluates	Chooses	Changes
Explains	Discusses	Demonstrates
Identifies	Displays	Measures
Labels	Initiates	Moves
Lists	Joins	Organizes
Names	Participates	Shows
Plans	Shares	
Selects	Uses	
States		
Writes		

■ Reflect an observable, measurable activity. The performance may be visible (e.g., walking) or invisible (e.g., adding a column of figures). It is necessary, however, to be able to evaluate whether an unobservable activity has been mastered from some performance that represents the activity. For example, the performance of an outcome might be written: "Selects low-fat foods from a menu" (observable), *not* "understands low-fat diet" (unobservable). Examples of measurable verbs used for learning outcomes are shown in Box 27–3. Avoid using words such as *knows, understands, believes,* and *appreciates* because they are neither observable nor measurable.

■ May add conditions or modifiers as required to clarify what, where, when, or how the behavior will be performed. Examples are "Demonstrates four-point crutch gait *correctly*" (condition), "Administers own insulin *independently* (condition) as taught," or "States *three* (condition) factors that affect blood sugar level."

■ Include criteria specifying the time by which learning should have occurred. For example, "The client will state three things that affect blood sugar level *by end of second diabetic class.*"

Learning outcomes can reflect the learner's command of simple to complex concepts. For example, the learning outcome "The client will list cardiac risk factors" is a low-level knowledge outcome that simply requires the learner to identify all cardiac risk factors; it does not suggest application of the knowledge to the learner's own behaviors. The learning outcome "The client will list personal cardiac risk factors" requires that the learner not only know cardiac risk factors in general but also know his own behaviors that place him at risk for cardiac disease.

In writing learning outcomes, the nurse must be specific about what behaviors and knowledge (cognitive, psychomotor, and affective) learners must have to be able to positively influence their health state. In most cases, the learning needs are more complex than simple acquisition of knowledge and include the application of that knowledge to oneself (see Identifying Nursing Diagnoses, Outcomes, and Interventions on page 499).

Choosing Content

The content, or what is to be taught, is determined by learning outcomes. For instance, "Identify appropriate sites for insulin injection" means the nurse must include content about the body sites suitable for insulin injections. Nurses can select among many sources of information including books, nursing journals, Internet, and other nurses and primary care providers. Whatever sources the nurse chooses, content should be

■ Accurate.
■ Current.
■ Based on learning outcomes.
■ Adjusted for the learner's age, culture, and ability.
■ Consistent with information the nurse is teaching.
■ Selected with consideration of how much time and what resources are available for teaching.

Selecting Teaching Strategies

The method of teaching that the nurse chooses should be suited to the individual and to the material to be learned (Figure 27-2 ■). For example, the person who cannot read needs material presented in other ways; a discussion is usually not the best strategy for teaching how to give an injection; and a nurse using group discussion for teaching should be a competent group leader. As stated earlier, some people are visually oriented and learn best through seeing; others learn best through hearing and having the skill explained. Table 27–3 lists selected teaching strategies.

Organizing Learning Experiences

To save nurses time in constructing their own teaching guides, some health agencies have developed teaching guides for teaching sessions that nurses commonly give. These guides standardize content and teaching methods and make it easier for the nurse to plan and implement client teaching. Standardized teaching plans also ensure consistency of content for the learner, thereby decreasing the risk of confusion if different practices are taught. For example, when teaching infant bathing, the nurse

Figure 27-2 ■ Teaching materials and strategies should be suited to the client's age and learning abilities.

TABLE 27–3	**Selected Teaching Strategies**	
STRATEGY	**MAJOR TYPE OF LEARNING**	**CHARACTERISTICS**
Explanation or description (e.g., lecture)	Cognitive	Teacher controls content and pace. Learner is passive; therefore retains less information than when actively participating. Feedback is determined by teacher. May be given to individual or group.
One-to-one discussion	Affective, cognitive	Encourages participation by learner. Permits reinforcement and repetition at learner's level. Permits introduction of sensitive subjects.
Answering questions	Cognitive	Teacher controls most of content and pace. Teacher must understand question and what it means to learner. Learner may need to overcome cultural perception that asking questions is impolite and may embarrass the teacher. Can be used with individuals and groups. Teacher sometimes needs to confirm whether question has been answered by asking learner, for example, "Does that answer your question?"
Demonstration	Psychomotor	Often used with explanation. Can be used with individuals, small or large groups. Does not permit use of equipment by learner; learner is passive.
Discovery	Cognitive, affective	Teacher guides problem-solving situation. Learner is active participant; therefore, retention of information is high.
Group discussions	Affective, cognitive	Learner can obtain assistance from supportive group. Group members learn from one another. Teacher needs to keep the discussion focused and prevent monopolization by one or two learners.
Practice	Psychomotor	Allows repetition and immediate feedback. Permits hands-on experience.
Printed and audiovisual materials	Cognitive	Forms include books, pamphlets, films, programmed instruction, and computer learning. Learners can proceed at their own speed. Nurse can act as resource person, need not be present during learning. Potentially ineffective if reading level is too high. Teacher needs to select language of materials that meets learner needs if English is a second language (e.g., Spanish).
Role-playing	Affective, cognitive	Permits expression of attitudes, values, and emotions. Can assist in development of communication skills. Involves active participation by learner. Teacher must create supportive, safe environment for learners to minimize anxiety.
Modeling	Affective, psychomotor	Nurse sets example by attitude, psychomotor skill.
Computer-assisted learning programs	All types of learning	Learner is active. Learner controls pace. Provides immediate reinforcement and review. Use with individuals or groups.

on the unit should be consistent about which soaps are appropriate for the infant's bath and distinguish those that are not. Whether the nurse is implementing a plan devised by another or developing an individualized teaching plan, some guidelines can help the nurse sequence the learning experience:

- Start with something the learner is concerned about; for example, before learning how to administer insulin to himself,

an adolescent wants to know how to adjust his lifestyle and yet still play football.

CLINICAL ALERT

Leave a note pad and pen at the client's bedside and encourage him to write down his questions for the nurse or the primary care provider. ∎

- Discover what the learner knows, and then proceed to the unknown. This gives the learner confidence. Sometimes you will not know the client's knowledge or skill base and will need to elicit this information either by asking questions or by having the client fill out a form, such as a pretest.
- Address early on any area that is causing the client anxiety. A high level of anxiety can impair concentration in other areas. For example, a woman highly anxious about her fear of the needle breaking off into the skin may not be able to learn how to self-administer an insulin injection until her fear is resolved.
- Teach the basics before proceeding to the variations or adjustments (e.g., simple to complex). It is confusing to learners to have to consider possible adjustments and variations before they master the basic concepts. For example, when teaching a female client how to insert a retention catheter, it is best to teach the basic procedure before teaching any adjustments that might be needed if the catheter stops draining after insertion.
- Schedule time for review of content and questions the client(s) may have to clarify information.

CLINICAL ALERT

If the client has no questions, you can help introduce questions by saying, "A few frequently asked questions are." ■

Implementing

The nurse needs to be flexible in implementing any teaching plan because the plan may need revising. The client may tire sooner than anticipated or be faced with too much information too quickly, the client's needs may change, or external factors may intervene. For instance, the nurse and the client plan to change his dressing at 10 AM, but when the time comes, the client wants to observe the nurse once more before actually doing it himself.

In this case, the nurse alters the teaching plan and discusses any desired information, provides another demonstration, and defers teaching the psychomotor skill until the next day. It is also important for nurses to use teaching techniques that enhance learning and reduce or eliminate any barrier to learning such as pain or fatigue (see Table 27–2 earlier in this chapter).

CLINICAL ALERT

Many nurses find that they teach while performing nursing care (e.g., giving medication). Remember to document this informal teaching also. ■

Guidelines for Teaching

Knowledge alone is not enough to motivate a person to change a behavior. Do not assume that providing information will automatically result in clients changing their behavior. Learning what needs to be done to change behavior and acting on that knowledge are two different processes (Saarmann, Daugherty, & Riegel, 2000, p. 281). The stages of change, the person's willingness and perceived need to change, and barriers to change are important elements to reflect on when implementing a teaching plan (see Chapter 16 ∞). When a client is ready to change a health behavior and when implementing a teaching plan, the nurse may find the following guidelines helpful:

- Rapport between teacher and learner is essential. A relationship that is both accepting and constructive will best assist learning. Knowing the learner and the previously described factors that affect learning should be established before planning the teaching.
- The teacher who uses the client's previous learning in the present situation encourages the client and facilitates learning new skills. For instance, a person who already knows how to cook can use this knowledge when learning to prepare food for a special diet.
- The optimal time for each session depends largely on the learner. Whenever possible, ask the client for help to choose the best time, for example, when she feels most rested or when no other activities are scheduled. Look for "teachable moments" that may occur during normal routine care (Hohler, 2004). For example, if a client asks you why he needs a certain medication (e.g., Coumadin) it is an opportunity to explain the reason for the medication, signs to watch for, and if follow-up laboratory work is needed.
- The nurse teacher must be able to communicate clearly and concisely. The words used need to have the same meaning to the client as to the teacher. A client who is taught not to put water on an area of skin may think a wet washcloth is permissible for washing the area. In effect, the nurse needs to explain that no water or moisture should touch the area.
- Using a layperson's vocabulary enhances communication. Often nurses use terms and abbreviations that have meaning to other health professionals but make little sense to clients. Even words such as *urine* or *feces* may be unfamiliar to clients, and abbreviations such as ICU (intensive care unit) or PACU (post-anesthesia care unit) are often misunderstood.
- The pace of each teaching session also affects learning. Nurses should be sensitive to any signs that the pace is too fast or too slow. A client who appears confused or does not comprehend material when questioned may be finding the pace too fast. When the client appears bored and loses interest, the pace may be too slow, the learning period may be too long, or the client may be tired.
- An environment can detract from or assist learning; for example, noise or interruptions usually interfere with concentration, whereas a comfortable environment promotes learning. If possible, the client should be out of bed for learning activities. Most people associate their bed with rest and sleep, not with learning. Placing the client in a position and location associated with activity or learning may influence the amount of learning that takes place. For instance, a client who is shown a videotape while in bed may be more likely to become drowsy during instruction than a client who is sitting in a bedside chair.
- Teaching aids can foster learning and help focus a learner's attention. To ensure the transfer of learning, the nurse should use the type of supplies or equipment the client will eventually use. Before the teaching session, the nurse needs to assemble all

Figure 27-3 ■ Teaching activities may need to include hands-on client participation.

equipment and visual aids and ensure that all audiovisual equipment is functioning effectively. See Client Teaching for teaching tools for children.

- Teaching that involves a number of the learner's senses often enhances learning. For instance, when teaching about changing a surgical dressing, the nurse can tell the client about the procedure (hearing), show how to change the dressing (sight), and show how to manipulate the equipment (touch).
- Learning is more effective when the learners discover the content for themselves. Ways to increase learning include stimulating motivation and self-direction, for example, (a) by providing specific, realistic, achievable outcomes; (b) by giving feedback; and (c) by helping the learner derive satisfaction from learning. The nurse may also encourage self-directed independent learning by encouraging the client to explore sources of information required. If certain activities do not assist the learner to attain outcomes, these need to be reassessed; perhaps other activities can replace them. Explanation alone may not be able to teach a client to handle a syringe. Actually handling the syringe may be more effective (Figure 27-3 ■).
- Repetition reinforces learning. Summarizing content, rephrasing (using other words), and approaching the material from another point of view are ways of repeating and clarifying content. For instance, after discussing the kinds of foods that can be included in a diet, the nurse describes the foods again, but in the context of the three meals eaten during one day.
- It is helpful to employ "organizers" to introduce material to be learned. Advanced organizers provide a means of connecting unknown material to known material and generating logical

relationships. The following statement can be an advanced organizer: "You understand how urine flows down a catheter from the bladder. Now I will show you how to inject fluid so that it flows up the catheter into the bladder." The details that follow are then seen within a framework that adds meaning.

- The anticipated behavioral changes that indicate learning has taken place must always be within the context of the client's lifestyle and resources. It would be unreasonable to expect a woman to soak in a tub of hot water two times a day if she did not have a bathtub or had to heat water on a stove.

Special Teaching Strategies

One-on-one discussion is the most common method of teaching used by nurses. However, nurses can choose from a number of special teaching strategies: client contracting, group teaching, computer-assisted instruction, discovery/problem solving, and behavior modification. Any strategy the nurse selects must be appropriate for the learner and the learning objectives.

CLIENT CONTRACTING. Client contracting involves establishing a learning contract with a client that specifies certain outcomes and when they are to be met. Here is an example of a self-contract:

> I, Amy Martin, will exercise strenuously for 20 minutes three times per week for a period of 2 weeks and will then buy myself six yellow roses.
>
> Amy Martin   A. Ward, RN
>
> July 30, 2007

The contract, drawn up and signed by the client and the nurse, may specify the learning outcomes, the responsibilities of the client and the nurse, and the methods of follow-up and evaluation. The contract can be changed in two ways: if the client meets the contract outcomes and wants to negotiate new learning outcomes, and if the client decides that he or she is unable to meet the existing learning outcomes and wants to revise them (Rankin, Stallings, & London, 2005, pp. 207–209). The learning contract allows for freedom, mutual respect, and mutual responsibility.

GROUP TEACHING. Group instruction is economical, and it provides members with an opportunity to share with and learn from others. A small group allows for discussion in which everyone can participate. A large group often necessitates a lecture technique or use of films, videos, slides, or role-playing by teachers.

It is important that all members involved in group instruction have a common need (e.g., prenatal health or preoperative instruction). It is also important that sociocultural factors be considered in the formation of a group.

COMPUTER-ASSISTED INSTRUCTION (CAI). Computer-assisted instruction is popular. Initially, the primary use of computer educational methods was cognitive learning of facts. Now, however, computers can also be used to teach the following:

- Application of information (e.g., answering questions after reading the information about a health subject)
- Psychomotor skills (e.g., filling a syringe on the computer screen to the correct dosage line on the syringe)
- Complex problem-solving skills (e.g., responding to questions based on a client situation)

Computers can be used in a variety of ways:

- Individual health care professionals or clients using one computer
- Families or small groups of three to five clients gathered around one computer taking turns running the program and answering questions together
- Large groups with the computer display screen projected onto an overhead screen and a teacher or one learner using the keyboard
- Individuals or small groups at computers using programs through shared network platforms or through Internet websites.

Individuals using a computer are able to set the pace that meets their particular learning needs. Small groups are less able to do this, and large groups progress through the program at a pace that may be too slow for some learners and too fast for others. It is therefore helpful to group learners of similar needs and abilities together. Whether using the computer alone or in large groups, learners read and view informational material, answer questions, and receive immediate feedback. The correct answer is usually indicated by the use of colors, flashing signs, or written praise. When the learner selects an incorrect answer, the computer may respond with an explanation of why that was not the best answer and encouragement to try again. Many programs ask learners whether they want to review material on which the question and answer were based. Some computer programs feature simulated situations that allow learners to manipulate objects on the screen to learn psychomotor skills. When used to teach such skills, CAI must be followed up with practice on actual equipment supervised by the teacher.

Some clients may have a negative attitude about computers that could act as a barrier to learning. The nurse helps these clients by explaining how the computer can help meet their needs. Matching a computer program or website to the client's individual health circumstances may encourage computer use.

Providing a resource list of free available community sites for training and access may also help. For clients who use the Internet, it is important for the nurse to teach the client how to evaluate if the site is a relevant and credible source for health information.

Most media catalogs, professional journals, and health care libraries contain information about computer software programs available to the nurse for client education. The media specialist or librarian in a health care facility or college is an excellent resource to help the nurse locate appropriate computer programs. Computer educational material is also available for clients with different language needs, for clients with special visual needs, and for clients at different growth and development levels.

DISCOVERY/PROBLEM SOLVING. In using the discovery/problem-solving technique, the nurse presents some initial information and then asks the learners a question or presents a situation related to the information. The learner applies the new information to the situation and decides what to do. Learners can work alone or in groups. This technique is well suited to family learning. The teacher guides the learners through the thinking process necessary to reach the best solution to the question or the best action to take in the situation. This may also be referred to as *anticipatory problem solving*. For example, the nurse educator might present information on diabetes and glucose management. Then the nurse might ask the learners how they think their insulin and/or diet should be adjusted if their morning glucose was too low. In this way, clients learn what critical components they need to consider to reach the best solution to the problem.

BEHAVIOR MODIFICATION. The behavior modification system for changing behavior has as its basic assumptions (a) that human behaviors are learned and can be selectively strengthened, weakened, eliminated, or replaced; and (b) that a person's behavior is under conscious control. Under this system, desirable behavior is rewarded and undesirable behavior is ignored. The client's response is the key to behavior change. For example, clients trying to quit smoking are not criticized when they smoke, but they are praised or rewarded when they go without a cigarette for a certain period of time. For some people, a learning contract is combined with behavior modification, and includes the following pertinent features:

- Positive reinforcement (e.g., praise) is used.
- The client participates in the development of the learning plan.
- Undesirable behavior is ignored, not criticized.
- The expectation of the client and the nurse is that the task will be mastered (i.e., the behavior will change).

Transcultural Teaching

The nurse and clients of different cultural and ethnic backgrounds have additional barriers to overcome in the teaching–learning process. These barriers include language and communication problems, differing concepts of time, conflicting cultural healing practices, beliefs that may positively or negatively influence compliance with health teaching, and unique high-risk or high-frequency health problems that can be addressed with health-promotion instruction (see Chapter 13 ∞). Nurses should consider the following guidelines when teaching clients from various ethnic backgrounds:

- *Obtain teaching materials, pamphlets, and instructions in languages used by clients.* Nurses who are unable to read the foreign language material for themselves can have the translator read the material to them. The nurse can then evaluate the quality of the information and update it with the translator's help as needed.
- *Use visual aids, such as pictures, charts, or diagrams, to communicate meaning.* Audiovisual material may be helpful if the English is spoken clearly and slowly. Even if understanding the verbal message is a problem for the client, seeing a skill or procedure may be helpful. In some instances, a translator can be asked to clarify the video. Alternatively the video may be available in several languages, and the nurse can request the necessary version from the company.
- *Use concrete rather than abstract words.* Use simple language (short sentences, short words), and present only one idea at a time.
- *Allow time for questions.* This helps the client mentally separate one idea or skill from another.
- *Avoid the use of medical terminology or health care language,* such as "taking your vital signs" or "apical pulse." Rather, nurses should say they are going to take a blood pressure or listen to the client's heart.
- *If understanding another's pronunciation is a problem, validate brief information in writing.* For example, during assessments, write down numbers, words, or phrases and have the client read them to verify accuracy.
- *Use humor very cautiously.* Meaning can change in the translation process.
- *Do not use slang words or colloquialisms.* These may be interpreted literally.
- *Do not assume that a client who nods, uses eye contact, or smiles is indicating an understanding of what is being taught.* These responses may simply be the client's way of indicating respect. The client may feel that asking the nurse questions or stating a lack of understanding is inappropriate because it might embarrass the nurse or cause the nurse to "lose face.".
- *Invite and encourage questions during teaching.* Let clients know they are urged to ask questions and be involved in making information clearer. When asking questions to evaluate client understanding, avoid asking negative questions. These can be interpreted differently by people for whom English is a second language. "Do you understand how far you can bend your hip after surgery?" is better than the negative question "You don't understand how far you can bend your hip after surgery, do you?" With particularly difficult information or skills teaching, the nurse might say, "Most people have some trouble with this. May I please help you go through this one more time?" In some cultures, expressing a need is not appropriate, and expressing confusion or asking to be shown something again is considered rude.
- *When explaining procedures or functioning related to personal areas of the body, it may be appropriate to have a nurse of the same sex do the teaching.* Because of modesty concerns in

many cultures and beliefs about what is considered appropriate and inappropriate male–female interaction, it is wise to have a female nurse teach a female client about personal care, birth control, sexually transmitted diseases, and other potentially sensitive areas. If a translator is needed during explanation of procedures or teaching, the translator should also be female.
- *Include the family in planning and teaching. This promotes trust and mutual respect.* Identify the authoritative family member and incorporate that person into the planning and teaching to promote compliance and support of health teaching. In some cultures, the male head of household is the critical family member to include in health teaching; in other cultures, it is the eldest female member. See the Culturally Competent Care box.
- *Consider the client's time orientation.* The client may be more oriented to the present than the nurse. Cultures with a predominant orientation to the present include the Mexican American, Navajo Native American, Appalachian, Eskimo, and Filipino American cultures. Preventing future problems may be less significant for these clients than for others, so teaching prevention may be more difficult. For example, teaching a client why and when to take medications may be more difficult if the client is oriented to the present. In such instances, the nurse can emphasize preventing short-term problems rather than

---

CULTURALLY COMPETENT CARE
Examples of Cultures That Value Family Inclusion in Client Teaching

HISPANIC AMERICANS

- Because of the value of family, it is important for the nurse to direct teaching to include all interested family members. Hispanic families provide support to each other and decision-making is usually made by the male and elder figures in the family.
- Ensure adequate space when teaching to allow for all of the family members who may accompany the client seeking health information and care.

BLACK AMERICANS

- The family structure has traditionally been matriarchal.
- It is important to recognize the dominant role that black women have in decision making and to share health information with them.
- Grandmothers play a central role in the Black American family and are often involved in support and care of their grandchildren.

ASIAN/PACIFIC ISLANDERS

- Decision making is often a family matter. Therefore, it is important to include the family, especially the male authority figure, in the process of decision making for a situation.
- Respect is automatically given to health care professionals as they are viewed as knowledgeable.
- Asians often want to "save face" for themselves and others. As a result, they may agree to what is being said or nod their heads in agreement to avoid being considered offensive or disruptive by disagreeing with the nurse or doctor. They may need to be given permission to ask questions.

Note: From *Nurse as Educator: Principles of Teaching and Learning for Nursing Practice,* 2nd ed., by S. B. Bastable, 2003, Sudbury, MA: Jones and Bartlett.

long-term problems. Failure to keep clinic appointments or to arrive on time is common in clients who have a present-time orientation. The nurse can help by accommodating these clients when they arrive for their appointment.

Schedules may be very flexible in present-oriented societies, with sleeping and eating patterns varying greatly. Teaching clients to take medications at bedtime or with a meal does not necessarily mean that these activities will occur at the same time each day. For this reason, the nurse should assess the client's daily routine before teaching the client to pair a treatment or medication with an event the nurse assumes occurs at the same time every day. When teaching a client when to take medication, the nurse should determine whether a clock or watch is available to the client and whether the client can tell time.

■ *Identify cultural health practices and beliefs.* Noncompliance with health teaching may be related to conflict with folk medicine beliefs. Noncompliance may also be related to lack of understanding or fatalism, a belief system in which life events are held to be predestined or fixed in advance and the individual is powerless to change them. To encourage compliance, the nurse needs to learn the client's explanation of why the illness developed and how it might be treated (Munoz & Luckmann, 2005).

The nurse should treat the client's cultural healing beliefs with respect and try to identify whether any are in agreement or in conflict with what is being taught. The nurse can then focus on the ones in agreement to promote the integration of new learning with the familiar health practices. The goal is to arrive at a mutually agreeable plan: Decide which instructions must be followed for client safety and negotiate less crucial folk healing practices.

Evaluating

Evaluating is both an ongoing and a final process in which the client, the nurse, and often the support people determine what has been learned.

Evaluating Learning

The process of evaluating learning is the same as evaluating client achievement of desired outcomes for other nursing diagnoses. Learning is measured against the predetermined learning outcomes selected in the planning phase of the teaching process. Thus the outcomes serve not only to direct the teaching plan but also to provide outcome criteria for evaluation. For example, the outcome "Selects foods that are low in carbohydrates" can be evaluated by asking the client to name such foods or to select low-carbohydrate foods from a list.

The best method for evaluating depends on the type of learning. In *cognitive learning,* the client demonstrates acquisition of knowledge. Examples of the evaluation tools for cognitive learning include the following:

■ Direct observation of behavior (e.g., observing the client selecting the solution to a problem using the new knowledge)
■ Written measurements (e.g., tests)
■ Oral questioning (e.g., asking the client to restate information or correct verbal responses to questions)

■ Self-reports and self-monitoring. These can be useful during follow-up phone calls and home visits. Evaluating individual self-paced learning, as might occur with computer-assisted instruction, often incorporates self-monitoring.

The acquisition of *psychomotor skills* is best evaluated by observing how well the client carries out a procedure such as self-administration of insulin.

Affective learning is more difficult to evaluate. Whether attitudes or values have been learned may be inferred by listening to the client's responses to questions, noting how the client speaks about relevant subjects, and observing the client's behavior that expresses feelings and values. For example, have parents learned to value health sufficiently to have their children immunized? Do clients who state that they value health actually use condoms every time they have sex with a new partner?

Following evaluation, the nurse may find it necessary to modify or repeat the teaching plan if the objectives have not been met or have been met only partially. Follow-up teaching in the home or by phone may be needed for the client discharged from a health facility.

Behavior change does not always take place immediately after learning. Often individuals accept change intellectually first and then change their behavior only periodically (for example, a client who knows that she must lose weight, diets and exercises off and on). If the new behavior is to replace the old behavior, it must emerge gradually; otherwise, the old behavior may prevail. The nurse can assist clients with behavior change by allowing for client vacillation and by providing encouragement.

Evaluating Teaching

It is important for nurses to evaluate their own teaching and the content of the teaching program, just as they evaluate the effectiveness of nursing interventions for other nursing diagnoses. Evaluation should include a consideration of all factors—the timing, the teaching strategies, the amount of information, whether the teaching was helpful, and so on. The nurse may find, for example, that the client was overwhelmed with too much information, was bored, or was motivated to learn more.

Both the client and the nurse should evaluate the learning experience. The client may tell the nurse what was helpful, interesting, and so on. Feedback questionnaires and videotapes of the learning sessions can also be helpful.

The nurse should not feel ineffective as a teacher if the client forgets some of what is taught. Forgetting is normal and should be anticipated. Having the client write down information, repeating it during teaching, giving handouts on the information, and having the client be active in the learning process all promote retention.

Documenting

Documentation of the teaching process is essential because it provides a legal record that the teaching took place and communicates the teaching to other health professionals. If teaching is not documented, legally it did not occur.

It is also important to document the responses of the client and support people to teaching activities. What did the client or support person say or do to indicate that learning occurred? Has the client demonstrated mastery of a skill or the acquisition of knowledge? The nurse records this in the client's chart as evidence of learning. A sample documentation of charting follows:

6/8/2007 1130 Learning to use glucometer to check her own capillary blood glucose levels. Noted a slight hesitation with each step. Demonstrated correct technique. Stated that she is "feeling more comfortable" each time she does it but still "needs to stop and think about the process." Will continue to monitor client's progress. ————————————————————— S. Brown, RN

Many agencies have multiple-copy client teaching forms that include the medical and nursing diagnoses, the treatment plan, and the client education. After the teaching session is completed, the client and the nurse sign the form and a copy of the form is given to the client as a record of teaching and as reinforcement of the content taught. A second copy of the completed and signed form is placed in the client's chart. The parts of the teaching process that should be documented in the client's chart include the following:

- Diagnosed learning needs
- Learning outcomes
- Topics taught
- Client outcomes
- Need for additional teaching
- Resources provided

The written teaching plan that the nurse uses as a resource to guide future teaching sessions might also include these elements:

- Actual information and skills taught
- Teaching strategies used
- Time framework and content for each class
- Teaching outcomes and methods of evaluation

CRITICAL THINKING CHECKPOINT

Mrs. Yorty is a 59-year-old African American bank vice president who is heavily relied on by her boss and co-workers. Three days ago she was admitted to the hospital with complaints of shortness of breath and mild chest pain. A diagnostic evaluation indicates that she has significant coronary artery disease but has not yet suffered a heart attack. Her primary care provider has indicated that Mrs. Yorty will need to make significant lifestyle changes to reduce her heart attack risk. As her nurse, you have been requested to teach Mrs. Yorty about her disease process, diet, exercise, and stress reduction. As you begin teaching Mrs. Yorty, you note that she is very pleasant and frequently nods her head, but she also seems preoccupied and is readily distracted.

1. How would you evaluate Mrs. Yorty's readiness to learn?
2. Of what benefit would a learning needs assessment be since Mrs. Yorty is obviously a well-educated client?
3. You recognize that you have a great deal of information to deliver to Mrs. Yorty and you are concerned that you will not be able to teach it all. What can you do to help Mrs. Yorty and still accomplish the learning outcomes?
4. How will you know if your teaching is effective?
5. How might your teaching differ if you were teaching Mrs. Yorty at home rather than in a hospital or acute care setting?

See Critical Thinking Possibilities in Appendix A.

CHAPTER 27 **REVIEW**

CHAPTER HIGHLIGHTS

- Teaching clients and families about their health needs is a major role of the nurse. Nurses also teach colleagues, subordinates, nursing and other health care students, and groups in community education programs.
- Learning is represented by a change in behavior.
- Three main theories of learning are behaviorism, cognitivism, and humanism.
- Bloom identified three learning domains: cognitive, affective, and psychomotor.
- A number of factors affect learning, including motivation, readiness, active involvement, relevance, feedback, nonjudgmental support, repetition, timing, environment, emotions, physiologic events, psychomotor ability, and cultural aspects.
- Many adults in the United States use the Internet to access health information. The 22% of adults who have never used the Internet tend to have less education and to be over age 65. The current "Baby Boomers" (ages 50–64), however, use the Internet. As a result, it is projected that Internet use among elders will increase as the Baby Boomers age.

- Teaching, like the nursing process, consists of six activities: assessing the learner, diagnosing learning needs, developing a teaching plan, implementing the plan, evaluating learning outcomes and teaching effectiveness, and documenting instructional activities.
- Teaching strategies chosen by the nurse should be suited to the client and to the material to be learned.
- A teaching plan is a written plan consisting of learning outcomes, content to teach, and strategies to use in teaching the content. The plan must be revised when the client's needs change or the teaching strategies prove ineffective.
- Evaluating the teaching–learning process is both an ongoing and a final process in which the client, nurse, and support people determine what has been learned.
- Documentation of client teaching is essential to communicate the teaching to other health professionals and to provide a record for legal and accreditation purposes.

TEST YOUR KNOWLEDGE

1. Which of the following activities would be classified as the affective domain of Bloom's taxonomy?
   1. Teaching how to administer an injection
   2. Learning to accept the loss of a limb
   3. Learning to insert a catheter
   4. Teaching how to read

2. Which of the following is the best method of helping a newly diagnosed diabetic client to learn the dietary requirements associated with the disease?
   1. Provide a videotape that addresses the dietary requirements associated with the disease.
   2. Ask a nutritionist to visit the client to present information and handouts about the diabetic diet.
   3. Ask the client to make a list of her favorite foods and how to work them into her diet.
   4. Have the client attend a group meeting for diabetic clients to discuss their adaptation to this chronic health condition.

3. A nurse is scheduling a teaching situation. Which of the following clients is most ready to learn?
   1. A 45-year-old man whose doctor just informed him that he has cancer
   2. A 3-year-old child whose parents are reading a story book about going to the hospital
   3. A 60-year-old female who received medication 5 minutes ago for relief of abdominal pain
   4. A 70-year-old man, recovering from a stroke, who has returned from physical therapy

4. How can the nurse best assess a client's style of learning?
   1. Ask the client how he or she learns best.
   2. Use a variety of teaching strategies.
   3. Observe the client's interactions with others.
   4. Ask family members.

5. A 74-year-old client who takes multiple medications tells the nurse, "I have no idea what that little yellow pill is for." What is the best nursing diagnosis for this client?
   1. *Knowledge Deficit*
   2. *Health-Seeking Behavior*
   3. *Deficient Knowledge (Medication Information)*
   4. *Noncompliance*

6. A client is scheduled to have a diagnostic procedure. Which questions by the nurse will most likely produce a "teachable moment"? Select all that apply.

   1. "Have you ever had this procedure before?"
   2. "What are your concerns about this procedure?"
   3. "What would you like to know about the procedure?"
   4. "Are you prepared for this procedure?"

7. A client needs to learn to self-administer insulin injections. Which statements reflect possible low literacy skills? Select all that apply.
   1. "I will read the information later – I'm too tired right now."
   2. "I've watched my brother give his own shots. I know how to do it."
   3. "Just show my wife."
   4. "Do you have a video showing how I should give myself the shot?"

8. A primary care provider admitted a client experiencing hypertensive crisis because of the failure to ingest prescribed medications. To determine learning needs, which assessment would have the highest priority?
   1. Client's age
   2. Client's perception of the effects of hypertension
   3. Client's ability to purchase needed medications
   4. Client's support system

9. A client has a learning outcome of: Select foods that are low in fat content. Which of the following statements reflect that the client has met this learning outcome?
   1. "I understand the importance of maintaining a low-fat diet."
   2. "I feel better about myself now."
   3. "See how I revised my favorite recipe to be lower in fat."
   4. "Since changing my diet, my husband is also losing weight."

10. A client's learning outcome is: Client will verbalize medication name, purpose, and appropriate precautions. Which of the following documented statements reflect evidence of learning?
    1. Taught name, purpose, and precautions for the new cardiac medication; seemed to understand
    2. Written information about the medication provided and reviewed; correct responses were given to follow-up questions
    3. Written information read to client; stated he would read it when he got home
    4. Asked questions about the new cardiac medication; satisfied with the information

See Answers to Test Your Knowledge in Appendix A. ∞

EXPLORE MEDIALINK www.prenhall.com/berman

DVD-ROM
▥ Audio Glossary
▥ NCLEX Review

COMPANION WEBSITE
▥ Additional NCLEX Review
▥ Case Study: Planning a Rural Health Education Program
▥ Care Plan Activity: Discharge of Client with Cardiomyopathy
▥ Application Activity: Overseeing a Health Fair
▥ Links to Resources

READINGS AND REFERENCES

SUGGESTED READINGS

Wingard, R. (2005). Patient education and the nursing process: Meeting the patient's needs. *Nephrology Nursing Journal, 32*(2), 211–214. *This article clearly shows the integration of the nursing process and client teaching. The author uses anemia-related examples to highlight the key principles.*

RELATED RESEARCH

Hsu, J., Huang, J., Kinsman, J., Fireman, B., Miller, R., Selby, J., & Ortiz, E. A. (2005). Use of e-health services between 1999 and 2002: A growing digital divide. *Journal of the American Medical Informatics Association, 12*(2), 164 – 171.

Wilson, E. V., & Lankton, N. K. (2004). Modeling patients' acceptance of provider-delivered e-health. *Journal of the American Medical Informatics Association, 11*(4), 241–248.

REFERENCES

Aldridge, M. D. (2004). Writing and designing readable patient education materials. *Nephrology Nursing Journal, 31*(4), 373–377.

Bastable, S. (2003). *Nurse as educator: Principles of teaching and learning for nursing practice* (2nd ed.). Boston: Jones & Bartlett.

Bloom, B. S. (Ed.). (1956). *Taxonomy of education objectives. Book 1, Cognitive domain.* New York: Longman.

Brownson, K. (n.d.). *Improving patient education for poor readers.* Retrieved June 26, 2006 from http:// www.nursingspectrum.com/ce/ self-study_modules/syllabus.html?CCID=3121

Curran, M. A., & Curran, K. E. (2005). The e-health revolution: Competitive options for nurse practitioners as local providers. *Journal of the American Academy of Nurse Practitioners, 17*(12), 495–498.

Dochterman, J. M., & Bulechek, G. M. (2004). *Nursing interventions classification (NIC)* (4th ed.). St. Louis, MO: Mosby.

Edmunds, M. (2005). Health literacy a barrier to patient education. *Nurse Practitioner, 30*(3), 54.

Escoffery, C., Miner, K. R., Adame, D.D., Butler, S., McCormick, L., & Mendell, E. (2005). Internet use for health information among college students. *Journal of American College Health, 53*(4), 183–188.

Hayes, K. (2005). Designing written medication instructions: Effective ways to help older adults self-medicate. *Journal of Gerontological Nursing, 31*(5), 5–10.

Healthcare Information and Management Systems Society E-Health Special Interest Group (SIG). (2003). *HIMSS e-health SIG white paper.* Retrieved June 9, 2006, from http://www. himss.org/content/files/ehealth_whitepaper.pdf

Hohler, S. E. (2004). Tips for better patient teaching. *Nursing, 34*(7), 32hn7–32hn8.

Institute of Medicine. (2004). *Health literacy: A prescription to end confusion.* Washington, DC: National Academies Press.

John, M. T. (1988). *Geragogy: A theory for teaching the elderly.* New York: Haworth Press.

Kaiser Family Foundation. (2005). *E-health and the elderly: How seniors use the Internet for health information. Key findings from a national survey of older Americans.* Menlo Park, CA: Author.

Knowles, M. S. (1984). *Andragogy in action.* San Francisco: Jossey-Bass.

Leiner, M., Handal, G., & Williams, D. (2004). Patient communication: A multidisciplinary approach using animated cartoons. *Health Education Research, 19*(5), 591–595.

Monsivais, D., & Reynolds, A. (2003). Developing and evaluating patient education materials. *Journal of Continuing Education in Nursing, 34*(4), 172–176.

Moorhead, S., Johnson, H., & Maas, M. (2004). *Nursing outcomes classification (NOC)* (3rd ed.). St. Louis, MO: Mosby.

Munoz, C., & Luckmann, J. (2005). *Transcultural communication in nursing* (2nd ed.). Clifton Park, NY: Delmar Learning.

NANDA International. (2005). *NANDA nursing diagnoses: Definitions and classification 2005–2006.* Philadelphia: Author.

NANDA International. (2007). *NANDA nursing diagnoses: Definitions and classification 2007–2008.* Philadelphia: Author.

Pew Internet & American Life Project. (2005a). *Health information online.* Retrieved June 9, 2006, from http://www.pewinternet.org/PPF/ r/165/report_display.asp

Pew Internet & American Life Project. (2005b). *Digital divisions.* Retrieved June 9, 2006, from http://www.pewinternet.org/PPF/r/165/ report_display.asp

Pew Internet & American Life Project. (2006). *Demographics of Internet users.* Retrieved June 9, 2006, from http://www.pewinternet. org/trends.asp

Purnell, L. D., & Paulanka, B. J. (2005). *Guide to culturally competent health care.* Philadelphia: F. A. Davis.

Rankin, S. H., Stallings, K. D., & London, F. (2005). *Patient education in health and illness* (5th ed.). Philadelphia: Lippincott Williams & Wilkins.

Redman, B. K. (2004). *Advances in patient education.* New York: Springer.

Saarmann, L., Daugherty, J., & Riegel, B. (2000). Patient teaching to promote behavioral change. *Nursing Outlook, 48,* 281–287.

Schultz, M. (2002). Low literacy skills needn't hinder care. *RN, 65*(4), 45–48.

Smith, L. S. (2003). Help! My patient's illiterate. *Nursing, 33*(11), 32hn6–32hn8.

Stanley, M., Blair, K. A., & Beare, P. G. (2005). *Gerontological nursing: Promoting successful aging with older adults* (3rd ed.). Philadelphia: F. A. Davis.

Steward, D., & Steward, M. (1973). The observation of Anglo-Mexican and Chinese-American mothers teaching their young sons. *Child Development, 44,* 329–337.

Wilkinson, J. M. (2000). *Nursing diagnosis handbook with NIC interventions and NOC outcomes* (7th ed.). Upper Saddle River, NJ: Prentice Hall Health.

SELECTED BIBLIOGRAPHY

Using technology to transform patient education. (2004). *RN, 67*(2), 26nm1–26nm4.

Bandura, A. (1971). Analysis of modeling processes. In A. Bandura (Ed.), *Psychological modeling.* Chicago: Aldine.

London, F. (2004). How to prepare families for discharge in the limited time available. *Pediatric Nursing, 30*(3), 212–227.

Lorig, K. R. (2003). Taking patient ed to the next level. *RN, 66*(12), 35–38.

Mauk, K. L. (2006). Reaching and teaching older adults. *Nursing, 36*(2), 17.

McCray, A. T. (2005). Promoting health literacy. *Journal of the American Medical Informatics Association, 12*(2), 152–163.

Pavlov, I. P. (1927). *Conditioned reflexes* (G. V. Anrep, trans.). London: Oxford University Press.

Piaget, J. (1966). *Origins of intelligence in children.* New York: Norton.

Rogers, C. R. (1961). *On becoming a person.* Boston: Houghton-Mifflin.

Rogers, C. R. (1969). *Freedom to learn.* Columbus, OH: Chas. E. Merrill.

Skinner, B. F. (1953). *Science and human behavior.* New York: Macmillan.

Thomas, C., & Wolfe, H. (2005). Bulletin boards: Not just for kids anymore. *Nursing, 35*(7), 68.

Leading, Managing, and Delegating

LEARNING OUTCOMES

After completing this chapter, you will be able to:

1. Compare and contrast leadership and management.

2. Differentiate formal from informal leaders.

3. Compare and contrast different leadership styles.

4. Identify characteristics of an effective leader.

5. Compare and contrast the levels of management.

6. Describe the four functions of management.

7. Discuss the roles and functions of nurse managers.

8. Identify the skills and competencies needed by a nurse manager.

9. Describe the characteristics of tasks appropriate to delegate to unlicensed and licensed assistive personnel.

10. List the five rights of delegation.

11. Describe the role of the leader/manager in planning for and implementing change.

Although aspects of the individual nurse's role vary according to practice location and type, leadership, management, delegation, and change are consistent components of the role. Nurses function within health care systems, working with multiple clients and other health care providers. As a part of multidisciplinary teams, the nurse is often in a leadership position and frequently delegates aspects of care to others. There are opportunities in nursing to become leaders at various levels and also many situations in which the nurse functions as a manager and as a change agent.

THE NURSE AS LEADER AND MANAGER

The professional nurse frequently assumes the roles of leader and manager. These two roles are linked; that is, managers must have leadership abilities, and leaders often manage, but the two roles differ.

A **leader** influences others to work together to accomplish a specific goal. Leaders are often visionary; they are informed, articulate, confident, and self-aware. Leaders also usually have outstanding interpersonal skills and are excellent listeners and communicators. They have initiative and the ability and confidence to innovate change, motivate, facilitate, and mentor others. Within their organizations, nurse leaders participate in and guide teams that assess the effectiveness of care, implement evidence-based practice, and construct process improvement

strategies. They may be employed in a variety of positions—from shift team leader to institutional president. Leaders may also hold volunteer positions such as chairperson of a professional organization or a community board of directors.

A **manager** is an employee of an organization who is given authority, power, and responsibility for planning, organizing, coordinating, and directing the work of others, and for establishing and evaluating standards. Managers understand organizational structure and culture. They control human, financial, and material resources. Managers set goals, make decisions, and solve problems. They initiate and implement change.

The purposes of nursing leadership include (a) improving the health status of individuals or families, (b) increasing the effectiveness and level of satisfaction among professional colleagues, and (c) improving the attitudes of citizens and legislators toward the nursing profession and their expectations of it.

As managers, nurses are responsible for managing client care. Some nurses assume a position within the organization as nurse manager, supervisor, or executive. As a manager, the nurse is responsible for (a) efficiently accomplishing the goals of the organization, (b) efficiently using the organization's resources, (c) ensuring effective client care, and (d) ensuring compliance with institutional, professional, regulatory, and governmental standards. Managers are also responsible for development of licensed and unlicensed personnel within their work group. Table 28–1 further

TABLE 28–1 Comparison of Leader and Manager Roles

LEADERS	MANAGERS
May or may not be officially appointed to the position	Are appointed officially to the position
Have power and authority to enforce decisions only as long as followers are willing to be led	Have power and authority to enforce decisions
Influence others toward goal setting, either formally or informally	Carry out predetermined policies, rules, and regulations
Are interested in risk taking and exploring new ideas	Maintain an orderly, controlled, rational, and equitable structure
Relate to people personally in an intuitive and empathetic manner	Relate to people according to their roles
Feel rewarded by personal achievements	Feel rewarded when fulfilling organizational mission or goals
May or may not be successful as managers	Are managers as long as the appointment holds
Manage relationships	Manage resources
Focus on people	Focus on systems

compares the leader and manager roles. Figure 28-1 ■ illustrates some of the leading and managing roles.

LEADERSHIP

Leadership may be formal or informal. The **formal leader,** or appointed leader, is selected by an organization and given official

A

B

C

Figure 28-1 ■ Nurses as leaders and managers: *A,* The nurse manager discusses work assignments during change-of-shift report. *B,* The nurse delegates basic client care activities to the nursing assistant. *C,* The nurse consults the social worker during discharge planning.

(Patrick Watson)

authority to make decisions and act. An **informal leader** is not officially appointed to direct the activities of others, but because of seniority, age, or special abilities, is recognized by the group as its leader and plays an important role in influencing colleagues, co-workers, or other group members to achieve the group's goals.

Leadership Theory

Early leadership theories focused on what leaders are (trait theories), what leaders do (behavioral theories), and how leaders adapt their leadership style according to the situation (contingency theories). Theories about **leadership style** describe traits, behaviors, motivations, and choices used by individuals to effectively influence others.

Classic Leadership Theories

The trait theorists found that leaders often possess specific traits and abilities including good judgment, decisiveness, knowledge, adaptability, integrity, tact, self-confidence, and cooperativeness. The behaviorists believed that through education, training, and life experiences, leaders develop a particular leadership style. These styles have been characterized as autocratic, democratic, laissez-faire, and bureaucratic.

An **autocratic (authoritarian) leader** makes decisions for the group. The leader believes individuals are externally motivated (their driving force is extrinsic, they desire rewards from others) and are incapable of independent decision making. Likened to a dictator, the autocratic leader determines policies, giving orders and directions to the group. Under this leadership style, the group may feel secure because procedures are well defined and activities are predictable. Productivity may also be high. However, the group's needs for creativity, autonomy, and self-motivation are not met, and the degree of openness and trust between the leader and the group members is minimal or absent. Members are often dissatisfied with this leadership style; however, at times an autocratic style is the most effective. When urgent decisions are necessary (e.g., a cardiac arrest, a unit fire, or a terrorist attack), one person must assume the responsibility for making decisions without being challenged by other team members. When group members are unable or do not wish to participate in making a decision, the authoritarian style solves the problem and enables the individual or group to move on. This style can also be effective when a project must be completed quickly and efficiently.

A **democratic (participative, consultative) leader** encourages group discussion and decision making. This type of leader acts as a catalyst or facilitator, actively guiding the group toward achieving the group goals. Group productivity and satisfaction are high as group members contribute to the work effort. The democratic leader assumes individuals are internally motivated (their driving force is intrinsic, they desire self-satisfaction), are capable of making decisions, and value independence. Providing constructive feedback, offering information, making suggestions, and asking questions become the focus of the participative leader. This leadership style demands that the leader have faith in the group members to accomplish the goals. Although democratic leadership has been shown to be less efficient and more cumbersome than authoritarian leadership, it allows more self-motivation and more creativity among group members. It also calls for a great deal of cooperation and coordination among group members. This leadership style can be extremely effective in the health care setting.

The **laissez-faire (nondirective, permissive) leader** recognizes the group's need for autonomy and self-regulation. The leader assumes a "hands-off" approach. The leader presupposes the group is internally motivated. However, group members may act independently and at cross purposes because of a lack of cooperation and coordination. A laissez-faire style is most effective for groups whose members have both personal and professional maturity, so that once the group has made a decision, the members become committed to it and have the required expertise to implement it. Individual group members then perform tasks in their area of expertise while the leader acts as resource person. Table 28–2 compares the authoritarian, democratic, and laissez-faire leadership styles.

The **bureaucratic leader** does not trust self or others to make decisions and instead relies on the organization's rules, policies, and procedures to direct the group's work efforts. Group members are usually dissatisfied with the leader's inflexibility and impersonal relations with them.

According to contingency theorists, effective leaders adapt their leadership style to the situation. A popular contingency theory describes the situational leader. The **situational leader** (a) flexes task and relationship behaviors, (b) considers the staff members' abilities, (c) knows the nature of the task to be done, and (d) is sensitive to the context or environment in which the task takes place. The task-orientation focuses the leader on activities that encourage group productivity to get the work done. The relationship-orientation style is concerned with interpersonal relationships and focuses on activities that meet group members' needs.

Situational leaders adapt their leadership style to the readiness and willingness of the individual or group to perform the assigned task. When employees are insecure or unable or unwilling to perform the task, the leader uses a highly directive style, providing specific instructions and close supervision. If the group is motivated and willing but unable to perform the task, the leader again uses a highly directive style, but in this case, explains decisions and provides the opportunity for clarification. When the group is able but unwilling or lacking in confidence, the leader shares ideas and facilitates decision making. For a group that is willing, able, and confident to perform the task, the leader delegates, turning responsibility for decision making and implementation over to the group.

Contemporary Leadership Theories

Contemporary theorists have described charismatic leaders, transactional leaders, transformational leaders, and shared leadership.

A **charismatic leader** is rare and is characterized by an emotional relationship between the leader and the group members. The charming personality of the leader evokes strong feelings of commitment to both the leader and the leader's cause and beliefs. The followers of a charismatic leader often overcome extreme hardship to achieve the group's goals because of faith in the leader.

The **transactional leader** has a relationship with followers based on an exchange for some resource valued by the follower. These incentives are used to promote loyalty and performance. For example, in order to ensure adequate staffing on the night shift, the nurse manager entices a staff nurse to work the night shift in exchange for a weekend shift off. The transactional leader represents the traditional manager, focused on the day-to-day tasks of achieving organizational goals, and understanding and meeting the needs of the group.

In contrast, a **transformational leader** fosters creativity, risk taking, commitment, and collaboration by empowering the group to share in the organization's vision. The leader inspires others with a clear, attractive, and attainable goal and enlists them to participate in attaining the goal. Through shared values, honesty, trust, and continual learning the leader empowers the group. Independence, individual growth, and change are facilitated.

Shared leadership recognizes that a professional workforce is made up of many leaders. No one person is considered to have knowledge or ability beyond that of other members of the work group. Appropriate leadership is thought to emerge in relation to the challenges that confront the work group. Examples of shared leadership in nursing are self-directed work teams, coleadership, and shared governance. **Shared governance** is a method that aims to distribute decision making among a group of people.

Effective Leadership

Much has been written about effective leadership and style; some descriptive statements about effective leaders are listed in Box 28–1. Leadership is a learned process. To be an effective leader requires an understanding of factors such as needs, goals, and rewards that motivate people; knowledge of leadership skills and of the group's activities; and possession of the interpersonal skills to influence others. Principles of effective leadership include vision, influence, and acting as a role model.

TABLE 28–2	Comparison of Authoritarian, Democratic, and Laissez-Faire Leadership Styles		
	AUTHORITARIAN (AUTOCRATIC)	**DEMOCRATIC (PARTICIPATIVE)**	**LAISSEZ-FAIRE (PERMISSIVE)**
Degree of control	Makes decisions alone	Collaborative	No control
Leader activity level	High	High	Minimal
Assumption of responsibility	Primarily the leader	Shared	Relinquished
Output of the group	High quantity, good quality	Creative, high quality	Variable, may be of poor quality
Efficiency	Very efficient	Less efficient than authoritarian	Inefficient

MediaLink

Nurse as Manager and Delegator Case Study

BOX 28–1 **Characteristics of Effective Leaders**

Effective leaders

- Use a leadership style that is natural to them.
- Use a leadership style appropriate to the task and the members.
- Assess the effects of their behavior on others and the effects of others' behavior on themselves.
- Are sensitive to forces acting for and against change.
- Express an optimistic view about human nature.
- Are energetic.
- Are open and encourage openness, so that real issues are confronted.
- Facilitate personal relationships.
- Plan and organize activities of the group.
- Are consistent in behavior toward group members.
- Delegate tasks and responsibilities to develop members' abilities, not merely to get tasks performed.
- Involve members in all decisions.
- Value and use group members' contributions.
- Encourage creativity.
- Encourage feedback about their leadership style.
- Assess for and promote use of current technology.

Vision is a mental image of a possible and desirable future state. Leaders transform visions into realistic goals and communicate their visions to others who accept them as their own.

Influence is an informal strategy used to gain the cooperation of others without exercising formal authority. Influence is exercised through persuasion and excellent communication skills; it is based on a trusting relationship with the followers.

An effective leader needs to show sensitivity to being a positive **role model,** demonstrating caring toward co-workers and clients. As is appropriate for any health and caring profession, leadership can also be humanistic, that is, acting in a way that stresses individuals' dignity and worth. Being a good leader takes thought, care, insight, commitment, and energy. In this way, the leader sets the example for others to follow.

CLINICAL ALERT

Nurses generally move from first- to middle- to upper-level management positions through promotion. In addition, nursing administration graduate academic programs are available at some nursing schools. ■

MANAGEMENT

The manager's job is to accomplish the work of the organization. To this end, managers perform roles and functions that vary with the type of organization and the level of management.

Levels of Management

Traditional management is divided into three levels of responsibility. **First-level managers** are responsible for managing the work of nonmanagerial personnel and the day-to-day activities of a specific work group or groups. Their primary responsibil-

ity is to motivate staff to achieve the organization's goals. This level of manager communicates staff issues to upper administration and reports administrative messages back to staff. Titles may include primary care nurse, team leader, nurse case manager, or charge nurse.

Middle-level managers supervise a number of first-level managers and are responsible for the activities in the departments they supervise. Middle-level managers serve as liaisons between first-level managers and upper-level managers. They may be called supervisors, nurse managers, or head nurses.

Upper-level (top-level) managers are organizational executives who are primarily responsible for establishing goals and developing strategic plans. Nurse executives are registered nurses who are responsible for the management of nursing within the organization and the practice of nursing. Some nurse executives are also responsible for auxiliary units such as the pharmacy, laboratory, and dietary departments. Nurses in these positions may be called vice president for client care services, vice president for nursing, director of nursing, or chief nurse.

Management Functions

Four management functions are planning, organizing, directing, and coordinating. These four functions help to achieve the broad goal of quality client care.

Planning

Planning is an ongoing process that involves (a) assessing a situation, (b) establishing goals and objectives based on assessment of a situation or future trends, and (c) developing a plan of action that identifies priorities, delineates who is responsible, determines deadlines, and describes how the intended outcome is to be achieved and evaluated. In short, it involves deciding what, when, where, and how to do it, by whom, and with what resources. Distribution of money, personnel, equipment, and physical space are included in resource allocation. An upper-level manager spends considerable time planning the department's goals and services, determining numbers and types of nurses and other personnel needed to provide these services. On the other hand, a first-level manager such as a staff nurse spends less time planning but manages individual clients by use of the nursing process.

An example of the planning function is **risk management,** having in place a system to reduce danger to clients and staff. The steps of risk management include anticipating and seeking sources of risk; analyzing, classifying, and prioritizing risks; developing a plan to avoid and manage risk; gathering data that indicate success at avoiding or minimizing risk; and evaluating and modifying risk reduction programs. Central to the process of risk management is communication among all involved persons.

Organizing

Organizing is also an ongoing process. After identifying the work and evaluating human and material resources, the manager arranges the work into smaller units. Organizing involves determining responsibilities, communicating expectations, and establishing the chain of command for authority and communication. Although upper-level managers delegate much of the work and responsibility and accountability for the work to others, they need to ensure that department objectives, priorities, job descriptions, lines of communication, nursing standards, procedures, and policies clearly describe the expectations.

Directing

Directing is the process of getting the organization's work accomplished. Directing involves assigning and communicating expectations about the task to be completed, providing instruction and guidance, and ongoing decision making. Upper-level managers devote less time to directing than to planning, organizing, and controlling. Directing at this level of management generally involves supervision of the next level of managers such as those in middle management. Unit managers (charge nurses) and staff nurses devote more time to directing. For example, charge nurses direct shift work by assigning clients and scheduling meal and break times. Staff nurses direct the care of clients by ordering nursing care, communicating care in written care plans and shift reports, and supervising care that is given by others.

Coordinating

Coordinating is the process of ensuring that plans are carried out and evaluating outcomes. The manager measures results or actions against standards or desired outcomes and then reinforces effective actions or changes ineffective ones. For example, an upper-level manager evaluates the effectiveness of recruitment, staff turnover, and budget performance. The charge nurse appraises staff performance. The staff nurse determines whether nursing interventions have helped the client achieve desired outcomes.

Principles of Management

A manager has authority, accountability, and responsibility. **Authority** is defined as the legitimate right to direct the work of others. It is an integral component of managing. Authority is conveyed through leadership actions; it is determined largely by the situation, and it is always associated with responsibility and accountability. The manager must accept the authority granted.

Accountability is the ability and willingness to assume responsibility for one's actions and to accept the consequences of one's behavior. Accountability can be viewed as hierarchic, starting at the individual level, then the institutional or professional level, and finally the societal level. At the individual or client level, accountability is reflected in the nurse's ethical integrity. At the institutional level, it is reflected in the statement of philosophy and objectives of the nursing department and nursing audits. At the professional level, it is reflected in standards of practice developed by national or provincial nursing associations. At the societal level, it is reflected in legislated nurse practice acts.

Responsibility is an obligation to complete a task. Managers are responsible for utilization of resources, communication to subordinates, and implementation of organizational goals and objectives.

Skills and Competencies of Nurse Managers

To be effective managers, nurses need to think critically, communicate well, manage resources effectively and efficiently, enhance employee performance, build and manage teams, manage conflict, manage time, and initiate and manage change. Change is discussed on page 520.

Critical Thinking

Critical thinking is a creative cognitive process that includes problem solving and decision making. The nurse manager reasons with logic, exploring assumptions, alternatives, and the consequences of actions. See Chapter 10 ∞ for further discussion of critical thinking.

Communicating

Managers report spending much of their day communicating. Good communication is essential and often determines the manager's success as a leader. Managers use both verbal and written communication. Effective managers communicate assertively, expressing their ideas clearly, accurately, and honestly.

Managers use **networking,** a process whereby professional links are established through which people can share ideas, knowledge, and information, offer support and direction to each other, and facilitate accomplishment of professional goals.

Managing Resources

One of the greatest responsibilities of managers is their accountability for human, fiscal, and material resources. Budgeting and determining variances between the actual and budgeted expenses are crucial skills for any manager.

Enhancing Employee Performance

Several ways of enhancing employee performance are available to managers. Managers are responsible for ensuring that employees develop through appropriate learning opportunities, whether through in-service education, facilitating attendance at professional workshops and conventions, or encouraging achievement of advanced education such as higher degrees or certifications. The nurse manager who empowers the staff by providing information, support, resources, and opportunities to participate will find that employees have greater commitment to the institution, are more effective in their role, have increased self-esteem, and are better able to meet their goals.

In addition, the manager may provide day-to-day coaching or serve as a mentor or preceptor. **Mentors** "give their time, energy, and material support to teach, guide, assist, counsel, and inspire a younger nurse. It is a nurturing relationship . . . " (Tomey, 2004, p. 365). Having a mentor is recognized as important for career development.

In the clinical area, the term **preceptor** is used to describe relationships in which the experienced nurse assists the "new" nurse in improving clinical nursing skill and judgment. The preceptor also instills understanding of the routines, policies, and procedures of the institution and the unit.

MediaLink Motivating and Developing Staff Video

REAL WORLD PRACTICE

Whether you are in charge of a client assignment or nursing unit, delegating tasks to one person or fifty, or managing time and tasks for a shift, a project, or a multimillion dollar budget, the principles for achieving success remain the same. Respect each individual and the gifts that they bring to the experience. Being fair, valuing all members of the team, expressing gratitude for their contributions, being open to ideas, and the ability not only to admit your mistakes but learn from them are all qualities for success.

You must be willing to embrace change, encourage growth, celebrate success, and support one another through difficult times. Each interaction is unique and you get back what you put into each one throughout the course of your career.

—Catherine Tieva RN, OCN
Oncology Core Charge Nurse, St Cloud Hospital, St Cloud, MN

Building and Managing Teams

In addition to personnel development, the manager is responsible for building and managing the work team. Familiarity with group processes facilitates the manager's ability to lead the group and enhances development of the group into a work team. Groups develop in stages, during which roles and relationships are established. The purposes of the team as a whole and the role of each member must be clear. Each member must feel that the manager and the other members recognize his or her contributions. In health care, the team may consist of any health care providers: nurses, therapists, unlicensed personnel, clergy, and so on. All members of the team need to use effective communication skills.

Evaluating the group's work is another responsibility of the manager. Effectiveness, efficiency, and productivity are three outcome measures that are frequently used. In health care, **effectiveness** is a measure of the quality or quantity of services provided. **Efficiency** is a measure of the resources used in the provision of nursing services. In nursing, **productivity** is a performance measure of both the effectiveness and efficiency of nursing care. Productivity is frequently measured by the amount of nursing resources used per client or in terms of required versus actual hours of care provided.

Managing Conflict

Nurse managers are frequently in a position to manage conflict among people, groups, or teams. The conflict may arise from differing values, philosophies, or personalities. In health care, it can also arise due to competition for resources.

There are many methods the nurse can use to manage conflict and each has its advantages and disadvantages. Among the most common are compromise, negotiation, and collaboration. The new nurse manager may require training to become proficient in the use of these methods. Basic principles for all types of conflict management include demonstrating respect for all parties, avoiding blame, allowing full discussion, using ground rules during meetings to promote fairness, encouraging active listening, identifying the themes in the discussion, and exploring alternative solutions (Carroll, 2006).

Managing Time

The effective nurse manager uses time effectively and assists others to do the same. Many factors inhibit good use of time such as preference for doing things the nurse likes to do before things the nurse prefers not to have to do, emergencies or crises that divert one's attention, and unrealistic demands from others. Strategies that the manager, and all nurses, can use in order to use time well involve setting goals and priorities, delegating appropriately, examining how time is used, minimizing paperwork (automating whenever possible), and using regular schedules that avoid interruptions and set time limits on activities (Sullivan & Decker, 2005).

THE NURSE AS DELEGATOR

Delegation is the transference of responsibility and authority for an activity to a competent individual. The delegate assumes responsibility for the actual performance of the task or procedure.

RESEARCH NOTE   Does One's Generation Influence How Nurses Prefer to Be Managed?

In this study, 62 nurses, technicians, and secretaries from hospital units completed a survey to assess characteristics of the respondents' generation, significance of tasks, and their communication style. About half the respondents belonged to the Baby Boomers (born 1943–1960) and the other half belonged to Generation X or Generation Y (born 1961–1980). Respondents varied in their views regarding their preferred method of recognition. For example, older respondents preferred personal recognition while younger ones preferred public affirmation. Communication styles were similar between the groups. Not surprisingly, older respondents viewed technology as more complicated than younger ones. Baby Boomers reported good commitment to remaining in a particular job for a long time, while Generation Xers felt loyalty to their manager was of greater impor-

tance than length of employment. Based on the findings, the authors suggest areas in which nurse managers should consider approaching the generations differently.

IMPLICATIONS

All nurses interact with persons of the same and different generations, and information such as this can help us work together effectively. Understanding the viewpoint of others is a common and important role of the nurse in any position—leader, manager, or neither. In your work setting, it will be necessary to consider how the workforce is distributed among different generations with their unique perspectives.

Note: From "Managing the Multigenerational Nursing Team," by J. Hu, C. Herrick, and K. Allard Hodgin, 2004, *Health Care Manager, 23,* pp. 334–340.

MediaLink

Building and Managing Teams Video

MediaLink

Handling Conflict Video

BOX 28–2 Examples of Tasks that May and May Not Be Delegated to Unlicensed Assistive Personnel

Tasks that **May** Be Delegated to Unlicensed Assistive Personnel

- Taking of vital signs
- Measuring and recording intake and output
- Client transfers and ambulation
- Postmortem care
- Bathing
- Feeding
- Gastrostomy feedings in established systems
- Attending to safety
- Weighing
- Performing simple dressing changes
- Suctioning of chronic tracheostomies
- Performing basic life support (CPR)

Tasks that **May Not** Be Delegated to Unlicensed Assistive Personnel

- Assessment
- Interpretation of data
- Making a nursing diagnosis
- Creation of a nursing care plan
- Evaluation of care effectiveness
- Care of invasive lines
- Administering parenteral medications
- Insertion of nasogastric tubes
- Client education
- Performing triage
- Giving telephone advice

Managing Stress and Time Video

MediaLink

The delegator retains accountability for the outcome. Delegation is a tool that allows the delegator to devote more time to tasks that cannot be delegated. It also enhances the skills and abilities of the delegate, which builds self-esteem, promotes morale, and enhances teamwork and attainment of the organization's goals. In nursing, delegation refers to indirect care—the intended outcome is achieved through the work of someone supervised by the nurse—and involves defining the task, determining who can perform the task, describing the expectation, seeking agreement, monitoring performance, and providing feedback to the delegate regarding performance.

Registered nurses increasingly delegate components of nursing care to other health care workers, especially unlicensed assistive personnel (UAP). An RN who delegates a task to another health care worker is accountable for selecting an appropriately skilled caregiver and for continued evaluation of the client's care. These "nurse extenders" may be identified by a variety of titles including certified nursing aides/assistants, home health aides, patient care technicians, orderlies, or surgical technicians. They have had diverse degrees of training and experience. They are employees and do not include family members or friends who provide some client care.

Each state nurse practice act specifies which actions constitute the legal practice of nursing, which actions are the purview only of nurses, and which may be delegated to others. The National Council of State Boards of Nursing (NCSBN) published five "rights" of delegation: The nurse delegates the *right task*, under the *right circumstances*, to the *right person*, with the *right direction and communication*, and the *right supervision and evaluation* (1995).

It is not possible to generate an exhaustive list of exactly which actions may or may not be delegated to unlicensed personnel. Examples of tasks that may and may not be delegated are given in Box 28–2. A statement regarding delegation is included with the steps for each procedure in this book.

The unlicensed person may not delegate tasks to another person. Principles guiding the nurse's decision to delegate ensure the safety and quality of outcomes. These principles are listed in Box 28–3. Even if the task is one that may legally be delegated, the individual nurse must still determine if the task can be delegated to a particular UAP for a specific client. The NCSBN has created a grid to assist in this decision (see Figure 28-2 ■). Once the decision has been made to delegate, the nurse must communicate clearly to the UAP and verify that the UAP understands:

- The specific tasks to be done for each client.
- When each task is to be done.

BOX 28–3 Principles Used by the Nurse to Determine Delegation to Unlicensed Assistive Personnel

1. The nurse must assess the individual client prior to delegating tasks.
2. The client must be medically stable or in a chronic condition and not fragile.
3. The task must be considered routine for this client.
4. The task must not require a substantial amount of scientific knowledge or technical skill.
5. The task must be considered safe for this client.
6. The task must have a predictable outcome.
7. Learn the agency's procedures and policies about delegation.
8. Know the scope of practice and the customary knowledge, skills, and job description for each health care discipline represented on your team.
9. Be aware of individual variations in work abilities. Along with different categories of caregivers are individual variations. Each individual has different experiences and may not be capable of performing every task cited in the job description.
10. When unsure about an assistant's abilities to perform a task, observe while the person performs it, or demonstrate it to the person and get a return demonstration before allowing the person to perform it independently.
11. Clarify reporting expectations to ensure the task is accomplished.
12. Create an atmosphere that fosters communication, teaching, and learning. For example, encourage staff to ask questions, listen carefully to their concerns, and make use of every opportunity to teach.

Elements for Review		client A	client B	client C	client D
Activity/task	**Describe activity/task:**				
Level of Client Stability	**Score the client's level of stability:** 0. Client condition is chronic/stable/predictable 1. Client condition has minimal potential for change 2. Client condition has moderate potential for change 3. Client condition is unstable/acute/strong potential for change				
Level of UAP Competence	**Score the UAP competence in completing delegated nursing care activities in the defined client population:** 0. UAP - expert in activities to be delegated, in defined population 1. UAP - experienced in activities to be delegated, in defined population 2. UAP - experienced in activities but not in defined population 3. UAP - novice in performing activities and in defined population				
Level of Licensed Nurse Competence	**Score the licensed nurse's competence in relation to both knowledge of providing nursing care to a defined population and competence in implementation of the delegation process:** 0. Expert in the knowledge of nursing needs/activities of defined client population *and* expert in the delegation process 1. Either expert in knowledge of needs/activities of defined client population and competent in delegation *or* experienced in the needs/activities of defined client population and expert in the delegation process 2. Experienced in the knowledge of needs/activities of defined client population *and* competent in the delegation process 3. Either experienced in the knowledge of needs/activities of defined client population *or* competent in the delegation process 4. Novice in knowledge of defined population *and* novice in delegation				
Potential for Harm	**Score the potential level of risk the nursing care activity has for the client** *(risk is probability of suffering harm)*: 0. None 1. Low 2. Medium 3. High				
Frequency	**Score based on how often the UAP has performed the specific nursing care activity:** 0. Performed at least daily 1. Performed at least weekly 2. Performed at least monthly 3. Performed less than monthly 4. Never performed				
Level of Decision-making	**Score the decision-making needed, related to the specific nursing care activity, client (both cognitive and physical status) and client situation:** 0. Does not require decision making 1. Minimal level of decision making 2. Moderate level of decision making 3. High level of decision making				
Ability for Self Care	**Score the client's level of assistance needed for self-care activities:** 0. No assistance 1. Limited assistance 2. Extensive assistance 3. Total care or constant attendance				
	TOTAL SCORE				

Figure 28-2 ■ Delegation decision-making grid.

(*Note:* From *Delegation Decision-Making Grid,* by National Council of State Boards of Nursing, 1997, Chicago: Author. Reprinted with permission.)

- The expected outcomes for each task, including parameters outside of which the unlicensed person must immediately report to the nurse (and any action that must urgently be taken).
- Who is available to serve as a resource if needed.
- When and in what format (written or verbal) a report on the tasks is expected.

A specific task that can be delegated to one UAP may not be appropriate for a different UAP, depending on each UAP's experience and individual skill sets. Also, a task that is appropriate for the UAP to perform with one client may not be appropriate with a different client or the same client under altered circumstances. For example, the taking of routine vital signs may be delegated to the UAP for a client in stable condition but would not be delegated for the same client who has become unstable.

CLINICAL ALERT

Each nurse or other licensed or unlicensed health care provider is responsible for his or her own actions. Anyone who feels unqualified to perform a delegated task must decline to perform it. ■

The registered nurse delegates to licensed vocational/practical nurses (LVN/LPNs) and other RNs in additional to UAPs. The nurse must know the state-specific scope of practice for other licensed personnel in order to delegate effectively. LVN/LPNs require less direct supervision than UAPs. In some regions and some agencies, LVN/LPNs may perform tasks generally considered the role of the registered nurse if they have received special training (e.g., administration of intravenous fluids).

It is important to note that the nurse is not held legally responsible for the acts of the unlicensed person, but is accountable for the quality of the act of delegation and has ultimate responsibility to ensure that proper care is provided. Delegation can be an extremely useful strategy in providing thorough and effective nursing care. Skill in delegation, however, must be learned and developed over time. The nurse should not hesitate to consult with others regarding the appropriateness of delegation.

CHANGE

Change is the process of making something different from what it was. Change can involve gaining new knowledge or adapting what is currently known in the light of new information. It can also involve obtaining new skills. Change is an integral aspect of nursing, and nurses are often **change agents,** that is, individuals who initiate, motivate, and implement change. Change agents

- Have excellent communication and interpersonal skills with individuals, groups, administration, and all levels of the organization involved in change.
- Have knowledge of available resources and how to use them: people, time, money, facilities, and information.

- Are skilled in problem solving.
- Are skilled in teaching.
- Are respected by those involved in the change.
- Have the ability to encourage and nurture those going through change.
- Are self-confident, are able to take risks, and inspire trust in themselves and others.
- Are able to make decisions.
- Have a broad base of knowledge.
- Have a good sense of timing.

CLINICAL ALERT

Change that is viewed as a threat by one nurse may be viewed as an opportunity by another nurse. ■

Types of Change

Planned change is an intended, purposeful attempt by an individual, group, organization, or larger social system to influence its own current status. Problem-solving skills, decision-making skills, and interpersonal skills are important factors in planned change.

Change may be considered covert or overt. A covert change is hidden or occurs without the individual's awareness. An example is the gradual, subtle increase in the severity of an illness. Overt change is change of which a person is aware. An example might be that a piece of equipment will no longer be available since the agency has changed vendors. People who experience overt change may also experience anxiety. Overt change often necessitates behavioral changes that are in conflict with the person's needs or goals.

Unplanned change is an alteration imposed by external events or persons. It occurs when unexpected events force a reaction. It is usually haphazard, and the results can be unpredictable. Drift is a type of unplanned change in which change occurs without effort on anyone's part. Situational, or natural, change also may be considered unplanned and occurs without any control by the person or group impacted. An example is the change that occurs because of a war or a natural disaster. Not all situational changes are negative. For example, as agencies open or close units, the nurse may have the opportunity to change to a new workplace.

Models of Change

In his classic work, Lewin (1951) describes that change involves three stages: unfreezing, moving, and refreezing. During the unfreezing stage, the need for change is recognized, driving and restraining forces are identified, alternative solutions are generated, and participants are motivated to change. In the second stage, moving, participants agree the status quo is undesirable and the actual change is planned in detail and implemented. In the final stage, refreezing, the change is integrated and stabilized.

BOX 28–4 Common Driving and Restraining Forces

DRIVING FORCES

- Perception that the change is challenging
- Economic gain
- Perception that the change will improve the situation
- Visualization of the future impact of change
- Potential for self-growth, recognition, achievement, and improved relationships

RESTRAINING FORCES

- Fear that something of personal value will be lost (e.g., threat to job security or self-esteem)
- Misunderstanding of the change and its implications
- Low tolerance for change related to intellectual or emotional insecurity
- Perception that the change will not achieve goals; failure to see the big picture
- Lack of time or energy
- Perceived loss of freedom to engage in particular behaviors

BOX 28–5 Guidelines for Dealing with Resistance to Change

1. Communicate with those who oppose the change. Get to the root of their reasons for opposition.
2. Clarify information and provide accurate information.
3. Be open to revisions but clear about what must remain.
4. Present the negative consequences of resistance (threats to organizational survival, compromised client care, and so on).
5. Emphasize the positive consequences of the change and how the individual or group will benefit. However, do not spend too much energy on rational analysis of why the change is good and why the arguments against it do not hold up. People's resistance frequently flows from feelings that are not rational.
6. Keep resisters involved in face-to-face contact with supporters. Encourage proponents to empathize with opponents, recognize valid objections, and relieve unnecessary fears.
7. Maintain a climate of trust, support, and confidence.
8. Follow the "politics of change." (a) Analyze the organizational chart; know the formal lines of authority. Identify informal lines as well. (b) Identify key persons who will be affected by the change. Pay attention to those immediately above and below the point of change. (c) Find out as much as possible about these key people. What interests them, gets them excited, turns them off? What is on their personal and organizational agendas? Who typically aligns with whom on important decisions? (d) Begin to build a coalition of support before you start the change process. Identify the key people who will most likely support your idea and those who are most likely to be persuaded easily. Talk informally with them to flush out possible objections to your idea and potential opponents. What will the costs and benefits be to them— especially in political terms? Can your idea be modified in ways that retain your objectives but appeal to more key people?

Note: From *Effective Leadership and Management in Nursing*, 6th ed., by E. J. Sullivan and P. J. Decker, 2005, Upper Saddle River, NJ: Prentice Hall. Adapted with permission.

An important aspect of planning change is establishing the likelihood of the acceptance of the change and then determining the criteria by which that acceptance can be identified. Accepting change often takes time, particularly when it does not fit into a person's attitudinal framework. The course of acceptance is easier for people if they are involved in the process. If possible, change should be instituted on a small or pilot scale before full implementation. To facilitate acceptance of the change, the change agent needs to identify common driving and restraining forces (see Box 28–4). Guidelines for dealing with resistance to change are found in Box 28–5.

All nurses are affected by change; nobody can avoid it. Nurses knowledgeable about the historical and current trends in nursing and present political, social, technological, and economic issues make rational plans to deal with opportunities to initiate and guide needed change and to respond to change that affects them in the workplace, government, organizations, and the community.

CRITICAL THINKING CHECKPOINT

You have just interviewed for two nursing positions and are trying to decide which job to pursue. During your first interview for a team member position, the nurse manager, Mr. Caruso, was cheerful, spoke highly of his current staff and complimented them for their ability to set goals and participate in decision making, listened to your ideas, and explored ways in which you could contribute to this team's effectiveness. The second nurse manager, Mrs. Turner, was also cheerful and talkative. She provided you with a job description as a primary nurse caregiver, explained her expectations of you as a new employee, and spoke of new programs she was attempting to implement. Both nurse managers talked about changes taking place in their facilities and the need for employees to remain flexible.

1. Based on the brief data provided, speculate about the leadership style of each of these nurse managers.
2. Think about managers (or leaders) you have known and admired. What characteristics did they have that you would like to integrate into your own management style should you become a nurse manager?
3. Both nurse managers spoke of changes that were taking place in their facility. As a nurse, how can you assist your peers who are unhappy and seem to resist change even when it is positive?
4. How might the delegation of tasks to other nurses or UAPs be different in the two settings?

See Critical Thinking Possibilities in Appendix A.

CHAPTER 28 **REVIEW**

CHAPTER HIGHLIGHTS

- Delegation is a tool that a nurse can use to improve productivity. The nurse transfers responsibility and authority to another but retains accountability for the task.
- The professional nurse frequently assumes the roles of leader and manager. Leaders, as employees or volunteers, influence others to accomplish a specific goal, whereas managers have responsibility and accountability for accomplishing the tasks of an organization.
- Managers plan, organize, direct, and coordinate in order to accomplish the work of the organization.
- Several leadership styles have been described, including autocratic, democratic, laissez-faire, and bureaucratic. These styles are often blended to fit the situation. Nurses need to know which style is most consistent with their behavior and learn to incorporate aspects of other styles into their practice.

- Nurse managers work in the organizational framework of the employing agency. Principles of management include authority, accountability, and responsibility.
- Four major management functions are planning, organizing, directing, and coordinating.
- Effective managers need to be skilled at critical thinking, communication, resource management, enhancing employee performance, and managing teams, conflict, time, and change.
- Nurses function as change agents to initiate, motivate, and implement the change process.

TEST YOUR KNOWLEDGE

1. The nurse leader informs the staff of a local emergency and instructs them to stay at the hospital to prepare for major casualties. The staff display high levels of anxiety and disorganization. The most appropriate leadership style at this time is which of the following?
    1. Authoritarian
    2. Democratic
    3. Laissez-faire
    4. Bureaucratic

2. Which of the following approaches best illustrates transformational leadership?
    1. The leader stimulates group interest in establishing unit goals that contribute to the agency mission.
    2. The leader forms subgroups or task forces that make decisions about unit problems.
    3. The leader provides funding for continuing education conferences to staff who have not used any sick leave.
    4. The leader adjusts his/her strategies to fit the current situation.

3. Which of the following examples is reflective of a nurse manager with accountability but not authority?
    1. To reduce costs, administrators instruct the manager to inform the staff to reduce overtime.
    2. The manager evaluates the unit staff but cannot promote or terminate staff.

3. The manager is to recommend a new staffing procedure to the institution's nurse manager group.
    4. The manager prepares a monthly budget variance report that includes plans to correct overspending.

4. An unlicensed assistive person (UAP) has previously performed client transfers safely (bed to chair) on many occasions. It would be inappropriate to delegate this unsupervised task to the UAP under which of the following conditions?
    1. The unit had a new wheelchair.
    2. This was an elderly client.
    3. It was the client's first time out of bed after surgery.
    4. The UAP has just returned from an extended leave of absence.

5. The nurse manager plans to implement a new method for scheduling staff vacations. Senior staff members oppose the change while newer staff members are more accepting. Which of the following would be the most effective strategy for resolving this difference?
    1. Provide extensive and detailed rationale for the proposed change, then implement.
    2. Explain that the change will occur as designed, regardless of the staff's preference.
    3. Withdraw the proposal to prevent a decrease in staff morale.
    4. Encourage interaction between the opposing sides to attempt resolution.

See Answers to Test Your Knowledge in Appendix A.

EXPLORE MEDIALINK www.prenhall.com/berman

DVD-ROM
- Audio Glossary
- NCLEX Review
- End of Unit Concept Map Activity
- Videos
    - Introduction to Nursing Management
    - Leading and Managing
    - Motivating and Developing Staff
    - Building and Managing Teams
    - Handling Conflict
    - Managing Stress and Time
    - Delegating Successfully
    - Initiating and Managing Change

COMPANION WEBSITE
- Additional NCLEX Review
- Case Study: Nurse as Manager and Delegator
- Application Activity: Nursing World
- Links to Resources

READINGS AND REFERENCES

SUGGESTED READINGS

Case, B. (2004). Delegation skills. *Advance for Nurses* (Northern California and Reno, NV edition), *6*(16), 20–25. Retrieved July 3, 2006, from https://nursing.advanceweb.com/common/EditorialSearch/AViewer.aspx?AN=NW_04jul19_n1p23.html&AD=07-19-2004 *This article outlines the key aspects of delegation used by nurses including the need for knowledge of state law, professional organization standards, and agency policy. The NCSBN five rights of delegation are described as are the roles of UAPs and LVN/LPNs.*

RELATED RESEARCH

Gullo, S. R., & Gerstle, D. S. (2004). Transformational leadership and hospital restructuring: A descriptive study. *Policy Politics and Nursing Practice, 5,* 259–266.

Mrayyan, M. T. (2004). Nurses' autonomy: Influence of nurse managers' actions. *Journal of Advanced Nursing, 45,* 326–336.

REFERENCES

Carroll, P. (2006). *Nursing leadership and management: A practical guide.* Clifton Park, NY: Thomson Delmar Learning.

Hu, J., Herrick, C., & Allard Hodgin, K. (2004). Managing the multigenerational nursing team. *Health Care Manager, 23,* 334–340.

Lewin, K. (1951). *Field theory in social science.* New York: Harper & Row.

National Council of State Boards of Nursing. (1995). *Delegation: Concepts and decision-making process.* Chicago: Author.

National Council of State Boards of Nursing. (1997). *Delegation decision-making grid.* Chicago: Author. Retrieved May 12, 2006, from http://www.ncsbn.org/regulation/uap_delegation_documents.asp

Sullivan, E. J., & Decker, P. J. (2005). *Effective leadership and management in nursing* (6th ed.). Upper Saddle River, NJ: Prentice Hall.

Tomey, A. M. (2004). *Guide to nursing management and leadership* (7th ed.). St. Louis, MO: Mosby.

SELECTED BIBLIOGRAPHY

Bower, F. (2000). *Nurses taking the lead: Personal qualities of effective leadership.* St. Louis, MO: Mosby.

Carroll, P. L. (2006). *Nursing leadership and management: A practical guide.* Clifton Park, NY: Thomson Delmar Learning.

Hansten, R. I., & Jackson, M. (2004). *Clinical delegation skills: A handbook for professional practice* (3rd ed.). Philadelphia: Jones & Bartlett.

Kelly-Heidenthal, P., & Marthaler, M. T. (2004). *Nursing delegation and priority setting.* Clifton Park, NY: Thomson Delmar.

Marquis, B. L., & Huston, C. J. (2005). *Leading roles and management functions in nursing* (5th ed.). Philadelphia: Lippincott Williams & Wilkins.

Tappen, R. M., Weiss, S. A., & Whitehead, D. K. (2004). *Essentials of nursing leadership and management* (3rd ed.). Philadelphia: F. A. Davis.

Yoder-Wise, P. S. (2003). *Leading and managing in nursing* (3rd ed.). St. Louis, MO: Mosby.

UNIT 7

Assessing Health

Assessment is an interactive process of information gathering and analysis that nurses carry out to identify client strengths and actual and potential health problems and to evaluate effectiveness of care. A comprehensive assessment includes data about a client's psychosocial, spiritual, cultural, environmental, and developmental status as well as physiologic health. Nurses also regularly perform focused assessments as indicated by client needs.

CHAPTER
29

Vital Signs

LEARNING OUTCOMES

After completing this chapter, you will be able to:

1. Describe factors that affect the vital signs and accurate measurement of them.

2. Identify the variations in normal body temperature, pulse, respirations, and blood pressure that occur from infancy to old age.

3. Compare methods of measuring body temperature.

4. Describe appropriate nursing care for alterations in body temperature.

5. Identify nine sites used to assess the pulse and state the reasons for their use.

6. List the characteristics that should be included when assessing pulses.

7. Explain how to measure the apical pulse and the apical-radial pulse.

8. Describe the mechanics of breathing and the mechanisms that control respirations.

9. Identify the components of a respiratory assessment.

10. Differentiate systolic from diastolic blood pressure.

11. Describe five phases of Korotkoff's sounds.

12. Describe methods and sites used to measure blood pressure.

13. Discuss measurement of blood oxygenation using pulse oximetry.

14. Identify when it is appropriate to delegate measurement of vital signs to unlicensed assistive personnel.

KEY TERMS

The **vital signs** are body temperature, pulse, respirations, and blood pressure. Recently, many agencies such as the Veterans Administration have designated pain as a fifth vital sign, to be assessed at the same time as each of the other four. Pain assessment is covered in Chapter 46. ∞ Pulse oximetry is also commonly measured at the same time as the traditional vital signs. These signs, which should be looked at in total, are checked to monitor the functions of the body. The signs reflect changes in function that otherwise might not be observed. Monitoring a client's vital signs should not be an automatic or routine procedure; it should be a thoughtful, scientific assessment. Vital signs, which should be evaluated with reference to the client's present and prior health status, are compared to the client's usual (if known) and accepted normal standards.

When and how often to assess a specific client's vital signs are chiefly nursing judgments, depending on the client's health status. Some agencies have policies about taking clients' vital signs, and physicians may specifically order a vital sign (e.g., "Blood pressure q2h"). Ordered assessments, however, should be considered the minimum; a nurse should measure vital signs more often if the client's health status requires it. Examples of times to assess vital signs are listed in Box 29–1.

Often, someone other than the nurse measures the client's vital signs. The nurse must recall, however, that prior to delegating this task to unlicensed assistive personnel (UAP), the nurse must have assessed the individual client and determined that the client is medically stable or in a chronic condition and not frag-

BOX 29–1   Times to Assess Vital Signs

- On admission to a health care agency to obtain baseline data
- When a client has a change in health status or reports symptoms such as chest pain or feeling hot or faint
- Before and after surgery or an invasive procedure
- Before and/or after the administration of a medication that could affect the respiratory or cardiovascular systems, for example, before giving a digitalis preparation
- Before and after any nursing intervention that could affect the vital signs (e.g., ambulating a client who has been on bed rest)

ile and that the vital sign measurement is considered routine for this client. Under those circumstances, the UAP may measure, record, and report vital signs but interpretation of the measurements rests with the nurse.

BODY TEMPERATURE

Body temperature reflects the balance between the heat produced and the heat lost from the body, and is measured in heat units called degrees. There are two kinds of body temperature: core temperature and surface temperature. **Core temperature** is the temperature of the deep tissues of the body, such as the abdominal cavity and pelvic cavity. It remains relatively constant. The normal core body temperature is a range of temperatures (Figure 29-1 ■). The **surface temperature** is the temperature of

Oral °F °C **Rectal**

Hard exercise

Hard work, emotion
A few normal adults
Many active children

Emotion, moderate exercise
A few normal adults
Many active children

Usual range
of normal

Usual range of normal

Early morning
Cold weather

Early morning
Cold weather

Figure 29-1 ■ Estimated ranges of body temperatures in normal persons.

(*Note:* From *Fever and the Regulation of Body Temperature,* by E. F. DuBois, 1948, Springfield, IL: Charles C. Thomas. Reprinted with permission.)

the skin, the subcutaneous tissue, and fat. It, by contrast, rises and falls in response to the environment.

The body continually produces heat as a by-product of metabolism. When the amount of heat produced by the body equals the amount of heat lost, the person is in **heat balance** (Figure 29-2 ■).

A number of factors affect the body's heat production. The most important are these five:

1. *Basal metabolic rate (BMR).* The **basal metabolic rate (BMR)** is the rate of energy utilization in the body required to maintain essential activities such as breathing. Metabolic rates decrease with age. In general, the younger the person, the higher the BMR.

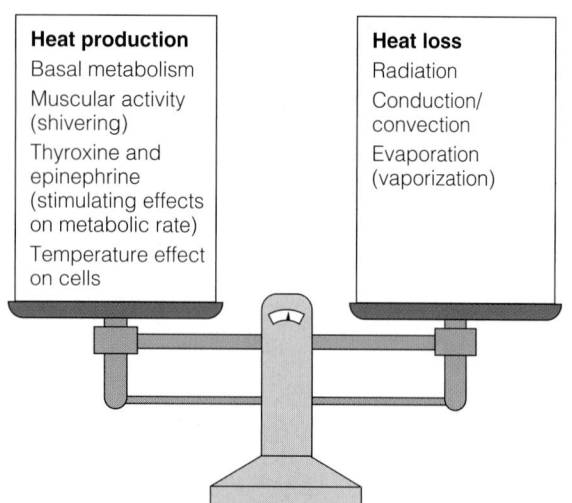

Heat production	Heat loss
Basal metabolism	Radiation
Muscular activity (shivering)	Conduction/ convection
Thyroxine and epinephrine (stimulating effects on metabolic rate)	Evaporation (vaporization)
Temperature effect on cells	

Figure 29-2 ■ As long as heat production and heat loss are properly balanced, body temperature remains constant. Factors contributing to heat production (and temperature rise) are shown on the left side of the scale; those contributing to heat loss (and temperature fall) are shown on the right side of the scale.

(*Note:* From *Human Anatomy and Physiology,* 7th ed. (p. 985), by E. N. Marieb and K. Hoehn, 2007, San Francisco: Pearson Benjamin Cummings. Adapted with permission.)

2. *Muscle activity.* Muscle activity, including shivering, increases the metabolic rate.
3. *Thyroxine output.* Increased thyroxine output increases the rate of cellular metabolism throughout the body. This effect is called **chemical thermogenesis,** the stimulation of heat production in the body through increased cellular metabolism.
4. *Epinephrine, norepinephrine, and sympathetic stimulation/ stress response.* These hormones immediately increase the rate of cellular metabolism in many body tissues. Epinephrine and norepinephrine directly affect liver and muscle cells, thereby increasing cellular metabolism.
5. *Fever.* Fever increases the cellular metabolic rate and thus increases the body's temperature further.

Heat is lost from the body through radiation, conduction, convection, and vaporization. **Radiation** is the transfer of heat from the surface of one object to the surface of another without contact between the two objects, mostly in the form of infrared rays. **Conduction** is the transfer of heat from one molecule to a molecule of lower temperature. Conductive transfer cannot take place without contact between the molecules and normally accounts for minimal heat loss except, for example, when a body is immersed in cold water. The amount of heat transferred depends on the temperature difference and the amount and duration of the contact.

Convection is the dispersion of heat by air currents. The body usually has a small amount of warm air adjacent to it. This warm air rises and is replaced by cooler air, and so people always lose a small amount of heat through convection.

Vaporization is continuous evaporation of moisture from the respiratory tract and from the mucosa of the mouth and from the skin. This continuous and unnoticed water loss is called **insensible water loss,** and the accompanying heat loss is called **insensible heat loss.** Insensible heat loss accounts for about 10% of basal heat loss. When the body temperature increases, vaporization accounts for greater heat loss.

Regulation of Body Temperature

The system that regulates body temperature has three main parts: sensors in the shell and in the core, an integrator in the hypothalamus, and an effector system that adjusts the production and loss of heat. Most sensors or sensory receptors are in the skin. The skin has more receptors for cold than warmth. Therefore, skin sensors detect cold more efficiently than warmth.

When the skin becomes chilled over the entire body, three physiologic processes to increase the body temperature take place:

1. Shivering increases heat production.
2. Sweating is inhibited to decrease heat loss.
3. Vasoconstriction decreases heat loss.

The hypothalamic integrator, the center that controls the core temperature, is located in the preoptic area of the hypothalamus. When the sensors in the hypothalamus detect heat, they send out signals intended to reduce the temperature, that is, to decrease heat production and increase heat loss. In contrast, when the cold sensors are stimulated, signals are sent out to increase heat production and decrease heat loss.

The signals from the cold-sensitive receptors of the hypothalamus initiate effectors, such as vasoconstriction, shivering, and the release of epinephrine, which increases cellular metabolism and hence heat production. When the warmth-sensitive receptors in the hypothalamus are stimulated, the effector system sends out signals that initiate sweating and peripheral vasodilatation. Also, when this system is stimulated, the person consciously makes appropriate adjustments, such as putting on additional clothing in response to cold or turning on a fan in response to heat.

Factors Affecting Body Temperature

Nurses should be aware of the factors that can affect a client's body temperature so that they can recognize normal temperature variations and understand the significance of body temperature measurements that deviate from normal. Among the factors that affect body temperature are the following:

1. *Age.* The infant is greatly influenced by the temperature of the environment and must be protected from extreme changes. Children's temperatures continue to be more variable than those of adults until puberty. Many older people, particularly those over 75 years, are at risk of hypothermia (temperatures below 36°C, or 96.8°F) for a variety of reasons, such as inadequate diet, loss of subcutaneous fat, lack of activity, and reduced thermoregulatory efficiency. Elders are also particularly sensitive to extremes in the environmental temperature due to decreased thermoregulatory controls.
2. *Diurnal variations (circadian rhythms).* Body temperatures normally change throughout the day, varying as much as 1.0°C (1.8°F) between the early morning and the late afternoon. The point of highest body temperature is usually reached between 1600 and 1800 hours (4:00 PM and 6:00 PM) (Mackowiak, Wasserman, & Levine, 1992), and the lowest point is reached during sleep between 0400 and 0600 hours (4:00 AM and 6:00 AM). (See Figure 29-3 ■).
3. *Exercise.* Hard work or strenuous exercise can increase body temperature to as high as 38.3°C to 40°C (101°F to 104°F) measured rectally.
4. *Hormones.* Women usually experience more hormone fluctuations than men. In women, progesterone secretion at the time of ovulation raises body temperature by about 0.3°C to 0.6°C (0.5°F to 1.0°F) above basal temperature.
5. *Stress.* Stimulation of the sympathetic nervous system can increase the production of epinephrine and norepinephrine, thereby increasing metabolic activity and heat production. Nurses may anticipate that a highly stressed or anxious client could have an elevated body temperature for that reason.
6. *Environment.* Extremes in environmental temperatures can affect a person's temperature regulatory systems. If the temperature is assessed in a very warm room and the body temperature cannot be modified by convection, conduction, or radiation, the temperature will be elevated. Similarly, if the client has been outside in cold weather without suitable clothing, or if there is a medical condition preventing the client from controlling the temperature in the environment (e.g. the client has altered mental status or cannot dress self), the body temperature may be low.

Figure 29-3 ■ Range of oral temperatures during 24 hours for a healthy young adult.

Alterations in Body Temperature

There are two primary alterations in body temperature: pyrexia and hypothermia.

Pyrexia

A body temperature above the usual range is called **pyrexia, hyperthermia,** or (in lay terms) **fever.** A very high fever, such as 41°C (105.8°F), is called **hyperpyrexia** (Figure 29-4 ■). The client who has a fever is referred to as **febrile;** the one who does not is **afebrile.**

Four common types of fevers are intermittent, remittent, relapsing, and constant. During an **intermittent fever,** the body temperature alternates at regular intervals between periods of fever and periods of normal or subnormal temperatures. An example is with the disease malaria. During a **remittent fever** such as with a cold or influenza, a wide range of temperature fluctuations (more

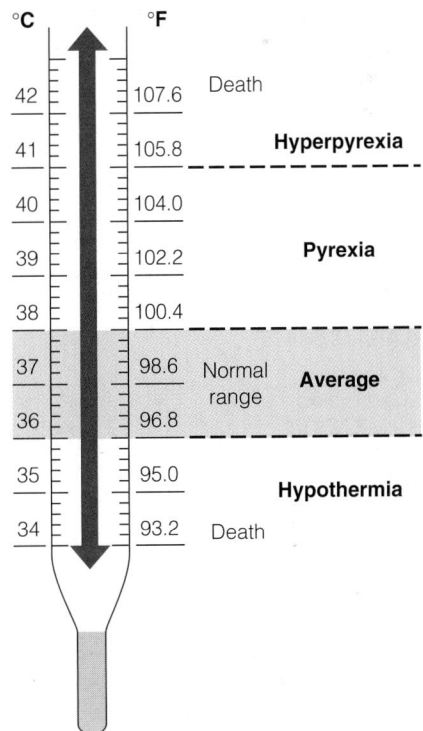

Figure 29-4 ■ Terms used to describe alterations in body temperature (oral measurements) and ranges in Celsius (centigrade) and Fahrenheit scales.

than 2°C [3.6°F]) occurs over the 24-hour period, all of which are above normal. In a **relapsing fever,** short febrile periods of a few days are interspersed with periods of 1 or 2 days of normal temperature. During a **constant fever,** the body temperature fluctuates minimally but always remains above normal. This can occur with typhoid fever. A temperature that rises to fever level rapidly following a normal temperature and then returns to normal within a few hours is called a **fever spike.** Bacterial blood infections often cause fever spikes.

In some conditions, an elevated temperature is not a true fever. Two examples are heat exhaustion and heat stroke. **Heat exhaustion** is a result of excessive heat and dehydration. Signs of heat exhaustion include paleness, dizziness, nausea, vomiting, fainting, and a moderately increased temperature (101°F–102°F). Persons experiencing **heat stroke** generally have been exercising in hot weather, have warm, flushed skin, and often do not sweat. They usually have a temperature of 106°F or higher, and may be delirious, unconscious, or having seizures.

The clinical signs of fever vary with the onset, course, and abatement stages of the fever (see Clinical Manifestations). These signs occur as a result of changes in the set point of the temperature control mechanism regulated by the hypothalamus. Under normal conditions, whenever the core temperature rises, the rate of heat loss is increased, resulting in a fall in temperature toward the set-point level. Conversely, when the core temperature falls, the rate of heat production is increased, resulting in a rise in temperature toward the set point.

In a fever, however, the set point of the hypothalamic thermostat changes suddenly from the normal level to a higher than normal value (e.g., 39.5°C [103.1°F]) as a result of the effects of tissue destruction, pyrogenic substances, or dehydration on the hypothalamus. Although the set point changes rapidly, the core body temperature (i.e., the blood temperature) reaches this new set point only after several hours. During this interval, the usual heat production responses that cause elevation of the body temperature occur: chills, feeling of coldness, cold skin due to vasoconstriction, and shivering. This is referred to as the chill phase.

When the core temperature reaches the new set point, the person feels neither cold nor hot and no longer experiences chills (the plateau phase). Depending on the degree of temperature elevation, other signs may occur during the course of the fever. Very high temperatures, such as 41°C to 42°C (106°F to 108°F), damage the parenchyma of cells throughout the body, particularly in the brain where destruction of neuronal cells is irreversible. Damage to the liver, kidneys, and other body organs can also be great enough to disrupt functioning and eventually cause death.

When the cause of the high temperature is suddenly removed, the set point of the hypothalamic thermostat is suddenly reduced to a lower value, perhaps even back to the original normal level. In this instance, the hypothalamus now attempts to lower the temperature, and the usual heat loss responses causing a reduction of the body temperature occur: excessive sweating and a hot, flushed skin due to sudden vasodilatation. This is referred to as the flush phase. Nursing interventions for a client who has a fever are designed to support the body's normal physiologic processes, provide comfort, and prevent complications. During the course of fever, the nurse needs to monitor the client's vital signs closely.

Nursing measures during the chill phase are designed to help the client decrease heat loss. At this time, the body's physiologic processes are attempting to raise the core temperature to the new set-point temperature. During the flush or crisis phase, the body processes are attempting to lower the core temperature to the reduced or normal set-point temperature. At this time, the nurse takes measures to increase heat loss and decrease heat production. Nursing interventions for a client with fever are shown in Box 29–2.

Hypothermia

Hypothermia is a core body temperature below the lower limit of normal. The three physiologic mechanisms of hypothermia are (a) excessive heat loss, (b) inadequate heat production to counteract heat loss, and (c) impaired hypothalamic thermoregulation. The clinical signs of hypothermia are listed in the Clinical Manifestations box.

CLINICAL MANIFESTATIONS FEVER

ONSET (COLD OR CHILL PHASE)
- Increased heart rate
- Increased respiratory rate and depth
- Shivering
- Pallid, cold skin
- Complaints of feeling cold
- Cyanotic nail beds
- "Gooseflesh" appearance of the skin
- Cessation of sweating

COURSE (PLATEAU PHASE)
- Absence of chills
- Skin that feels warm
- Photosensitivity
- Glassy-eyed appearance
- Increased pulse and respiratory rates
- Increased thirst
- Mild to severe dehydration
- Drowsiness, restlessness, delirium, or convulsions
- Herpetic lesions of the mouth
- Loss of appetite (if the fever is prolonged)
- Malaise, weakness, and aching muscles

DEFERVESCENCE (FEVER ABATEMENT/FLUSH PHASE)
- Skin that appears flushed and feels warm
- Sweating
- Decreased shivering
- Possible dehydration

CLINICAL MANIFESTATIONS HYPOTHERMIA

- Decreased body temperature, pulse, and respirations
- Severe shivering (initially)
- Feelings of cold and chills
- Pale, cool, waxy skin
- Frostbite (nose, fingers, toes)
- Hypotension
- Decreased urinary output
- Lack of muscle coordination
- Disorientation
- Drowsiness progressing to coma

BOX 29–2 Nursing Interventions for Clients with Fever

- Monitor vital signs.
- Assess skin color and temperature.
- Monitor white blood cell count, hematocrit value, and other pertinent laboratory reports for indications of infection or dehydration.
- Remove excess blankets when the client feels warm, but provide extra warmth when the client feels chilled.
- Provide adequate nutrition and fluids (e.g., 2,500–3,000 mL per day) to meet the increased metabolic demands and prevent dehydration.
- Measure intake and output.
- Reduce physical activity to limit heat production, especially during the flush stage.
- Administer antipyretics (drugs that reduce the level of fever) as ordered.
- Provide oral hygiene to keep the mucous membranes moist.
- Provide a tepid sponge bath to increase heat loss through conduction.
- Provide dry clothing and bed linens.

BOX 29–3 Nursing Interventions for Clients with Hypothermia

- Provide a warm environment.
- Provide dry clothing.
- Apply warm blankets.
- Keep limbs close to body.
- Cover the client's scalp with a cap or turban.
- Supply warm oral or intravenous fluids.
- Apply warming pads.

Hypothermia may be induced or accidental. Induced hypothermia is the deliberate lowering of the body temperature to decrease the need for oxygen by the body tissues such as during certain surgeries. Accidental hypothermia can occur as a result of (a) exposure to a cold environment, (b) immersion in cold water, and (c) lack of adequate clothing, shelter, or heat. In elders the problem can be compounded by a decreased metabolic rate and the use of sedatives. If skin and underlying tissues are damaged by freezing cold, this results in frostbite. Frostbite most commonly occurs in hands, feet, nose, and ears.

Managing hypothermia involves removing the client from the cold and rewarming the client's body. For the client with mild hypothermia, the body is rewarmed by applying blankets; for the client with severe hypothermia, a hyperthermia blanket (an electronically controlled blanket that provides a specified temperature) is applied, and warm intravenous fluids are given. Wet clothing, which increases heat loss because of the high conductivity of water, should be replaced with dry clothing. See Box 29–3 for nursing interventions for clients who have hypothermia.

See Identifying Nursing Diagnoses, Outcomes, and Interventions for examples of applying the nursing process to clients with temperature alterations.

Assessing Body Temperature

The most common sites for measuring body temperature are oral, rectal, axillary, tympanic membrane, and skin/temporal artery. Each of the sites has advantages and disadvantages (see Table 29–1).

IDENTIFYING NURSING DIAGNOSES, OUTCOMES, AND INTERVENTIONS
Imbalanced Body Temperature

NURSING DIAGNOSIS/ DEFINITION	SAMPLE DESIRED OUTCOMES* DEFINITION	INDICATORS†	SELECTED INTERVENTIONS* DEFINITION	SAMPLE ACTIVITIES (ALSO SEE BOXES 29–2 & 29–3)
Risk for Imbalanced Body Temperature/At risk for failure to maintain body temperature within normal range	Hydration [0602]/ *Adequate water in the intracellular and extracellular compartments of the body*	■ Moist mucous membranes ■ Urine output	Temperature Regulation [3900]/*Attaining and/or maintaining body temperature within a normal range*	Monitor temperature every 2 hours, as appropriate Promote adequate fluid and nutritional intake
Hyperthermia/Body temperature elevated above normal range	Thermoregulation [0800]/*Balance among heat production, heat gain, and heat loss*	■ Skin temperature in expected range ■ Body temperature in expected range ■ Sweating when hot	Fever Treatment [3740]/*Management of a patient with hyperpyrexia caused by nonenvironmental factors*	Monitor intake and output Apply ice bag covered with a towel to groin Cover the patient with only a sheet

*The NOC # for desired outcomes and the NIC # for nursing interventions are listed in brackets following the appropriate outcome or intervention. Outcomes, indicators, interventions, and activities seletected are only a sample of those suggested by NOC and NIC and should be further individualized for each client.

†The measurement scale for these indicators ranges from Extremely compromised to Not compromised. See Appendix B. ∞

TABLE 29–1	**Advantages and Disadvantages of Sites for Body Temperature Measurement**	
SITE	**ADVANTAGES**	**DISADVANTAGES**
Oral	Accessible and convenient	Thermometers can break if bitten. Inaccurate if client has just ingested hot or cold food or fluid or smoked. Could injure the mouth following oral surgery.
Rectal	Reliable measurement	Inconvenient and more unpleasant for clients; difficult for client who cannot turn to the side. Could injure the rectum following rectal surgery. Presence of stool may interfere with thermometer placement. If the stool is soft, the thermometer may be embedded in stool rather than against the wall of the rectum.
Axillary	Safe and noninvasive	The thermometer must be left in place a long time to obtain an accurate measurement.
Tympanic membrane	Readily accessible; reflects the core temperature. Very fast.	Can be uncomfortable and involves risk of injuring the membrane if the probe is inserted too far. Repeated measurements may vary. Right and left measurements can differ. Presence of cerumen can affect the reading.
Temporal artery	Safe and noninvasive; very fast.	Requires electronic equipment that may be expensive or unavailable; variation in technique needed if the client has perspiration on the forehead.

The body temperature may be measured *orally*. If a client has been taking cold or hot food or fluids or smoking, the nurse should wait 30 minutes before taking the temperature orally to ensure that the temperature of the mouth is not affected by the temperature of the food, fluid, or warm smoke.

Rectal temperature readings are considered to be very accurate. In some agencies, taking temperatures rectally is contraindicated for clients with myocardial infarction. It is believed that inserting a rectal thermometer can produce vagal stimulation, which in turn can cause abnormal heart rhythms. However, not all authorities share this belief. Rectal temperatures are contraindicated for clients who are undergoing rectal surgery, have diarrhea or diseases of the rectum, are immunosuppressed, have a clotting disorder, or have significant hemorrhoids.

The *axilla* is the preferred site for measuring temperature in newborns because it is accessible and safe. However, some research indicates that the axillary method is inaccurate when assessing a fever (Bindler & Ball, 2003). Nurses should check agency protocol when taking the temperature of newborns, infants, toddlers, and children. Adult clients for whom the axillary method of temperature assessment is appropriate include those for whom other temperature sites are contraindicated.

The *tympanic membrane*, or nearby tissue in the ear canal, is a frequent site for estimating core body temperature. Like the sublingual oral site, the tympanic membrane has an abundant arterial blood supply, primarily from branches of the external carotid artery. Because temperature sensors applied directly to the tympanic membrane can be uncomfortable and involve risk of membrane injury or perforation, noninvasive infrared thermometers are used. Electronic tympanic thermometers are found extensively in both inpatient and ambulatory care settings.

The temperature may also be measured on the forehead using a chemical thermometer or a temporal artery thermometer. Forehead temperature measurements are most useful for infants and children where a more invasive measurement is not necessary.

Types of Thermometers

Traditionally, body temperatures were measured using mercury-in-glass thermometers. Glass thermometers can be hazardous due to exposure to mercury, which is toxic to humans, and broken glass should the thermometer crack or break. In 1998, the U.S. Environmental Protection Agency and the American Hospital Association agreed to the goal of eliminating mercury from health care environments. Hospitals no longer use mercury-in-glass thermometers, and several cities have banned the sale and manufacture of them. In some cases, plastics have replaced glass and safer chemicals have replaced mercury in modern versions of the thermometer. However, the nurse may still encounter this type of thermometer.

Although the amount of mercury in a thermometer (or in a fluorescent light bulb) is minimal, should it break, cleanup involves several "dos and don'ts." Unsealed mercury slowly vaporizes into the air and these mercury vapors are toxic. Keep children and pets away from the area. Wearing rubber gloves, wipe mercury beads off clothing, skin, or disposable items with a paper towel placed immediately into a plastic bag. Discard the item. If the spill is on a porous material that cannot be discarded (e.g., carpet), a contractor trained in mercury disposal may be needed. If the mercury is on a hard surface, use folded stiff cardboard to slowly gather the beads and pour them into a wide-mouthed container. Use a flashlight to search for the beads since the light will reflect off the mercury. Dispose of all items used in the cleanup in a plastic bag that is sealed with tape. Shower or wash well. Keep the area well ventilated for several days. Do not use any type of vacuum cleaner or broom since these will disperse the mercury and be contaminated. Do not pour the mercury down a toilet or drain and do not wash or reuse contaminated materials.

Electronic thermometers can provide a reading in only 2 to 60 seconds, depending on the model. The equipment consists of a battery-operated portable electronic unit, a probe that the nurse attaches to the unit, and a probe cover, which is usually disposable (Figure 29-5 ■). Some models have a different circuit and probe for oral and rectal measurement.

Two specific types of oral thermometers that can be glass or electronic are basal and hypothermia. A basal thermometer is calibrated with 0.1°F intervals and is for fertility purposes, indicating the temperature rise that is associated with ovulation. Hypothermia thermometers have a greater low range than everyday thermometers, usually measuring temperatures from 81°F to 108°F.

Chemical disposable thermometers are also used to measure body temperatures. Chemical thermometers using liquid crystal dots or bars or heat-sensitive tape or patches applied to the forehead change color to indicate temperature. Some of these are single use and others may be reused several times. One type that has small chemical dots at one end is shown in Figure 29-6 ■. To read the temperature, the nurse notes the highest reading among the dots that have changed color.

Temperature-sensitive tape may also be used to obtain a general indication of body surface temperature. It does not indicate the core temperature. The tape contains liquid crystals that

Figure 29-5 ■ An electronic thermometer. Note the probe and probe cover.

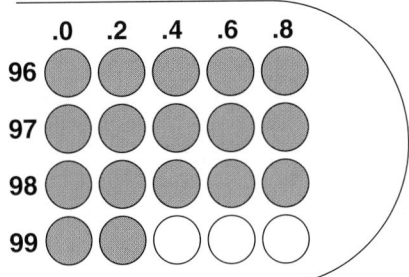

Figure 29-6 ■ A chemical thermometer showing a reading of 99.2°F.

Figure 29-7 ■ A temperature-sensitive skin tape.

Figure 29-8 ■ An infrared (tympanic) thermometer used to measure the tympanic membrane temperature.

change color according to temperature. When applied to the skin, usually of the forehead or abdomen, the temperature digits on the tape respond by changing color (Figure 29-7 ■). The skin area should be dry. After the length of time specified by the manufacturer (e.g., 15 seconds), a color appears on the tape. This method is particularly useful at home and for infants whose temperatures are to be monitored.

Infrared thermometers sense body heat in the form of infrared energy given off by a heat source, which in the ear canal, is primarily the tympanic membrane (Figure 29-8 ■). The infrared thermometer makes no contact with the tympanic membrane.

Temporal artery thermometers determine temperature using a scanning infrared thermometer that compares arterial temperature in the temporal artery of the forehead to the temperature in the room and calculates the heat balance to approximate the core temperature of the blood in the pulmonary artery (Roy, Powell, & Gerson, 2003). The probe is placed in the middle of the forehead and then drawn laterally to the hairline. If the client has perspiration on the forehead, the probe is also touched behind the earlobe so the thermometer can compensate for evaporative cooling (Figure 29-9 ■).

Temperature Scales

The body temperature is measured in degrees on two scales: Celsius (centigrade) and Fahrenheit. Sometimes a nurse needs

Figure 29-9 ■ A temporal artery thermometer.

to convert a Celsius reading to Fahrenheit, or vice versa. Although the conversion can be accomplished using several different formulas, the most common is described here. To convert from Fahrenheit to Celsius, deduct 32 from the Fahrenheit reading and then multiply by the fraction 5/9; that is:

$$C = (\text{Fahrenheit temperature} - 32) \times 5/9$$

For example, when the Fahrenheit reading is 100:

$$C = (100 - 32) \times 5/9 = (68) \times 5/9 = 37.8$$

To convert from Celsius to Fahrenheit, multiply the Celsius reading by the fraction 9/5 and then add 32; that is:

$$F = (\text{Celsius temperature} \times 9/5) + 32$$

For example, when the Celsius reading is 40:

$$F = (40 \times 9/5) + 32 = (72 + 32) = 104$$

Skill 29-1 explains how to measure body temperature.

SKILL 29-1

ASSESSING BODY TEMPERATURE

PURPOSES
- To establish baseline data for subsequent evaluation
- To identify whether the core temperature is within normal range
- To determine changes in the core temperature in response to specific therapies (e.g., antipyretic medication, immunosuppressive therapy, invasive procedure)
- To monitor clients at risk for imbalanced body temperature (e.g., clients at risk for infection or diagnosis of infection; those who have been exposed to temperature extremes)

ASSESSMENT
Assess

- Clinical signs of fever
- Clinical signs of hypothermia
- Site most appropriate for measurement
- Factors that may alter core body temperature

PLANNING

Delegation
Routine measurement of the client's temperature can be delegated to unlicensed assistive personnel (UAP)—or to family members/caregivers in nonhospital settings. The nurse must explain the appropriate type of thermometer and site to be used and ensure that the person knows when to report an abnormal temperature and how to record the finding. The interpretation of an abnormal temperature and determination of appropriate responses are done by the nurse.

Equipment
- Thermometer
- Thermometer sheath or cover
- Water-soluble lubricant for a rectal temperature
- Disposable gloves
- Towel for axillary temperature
- Tissues/wipes

IMPLEMENTATION
Preparation
Check that all equipment is functioning normally.

Performance
1. Prior to performing the procedure, introduce self and verify the client's identity using agency protocol. Explain to the client what you are going to do, why it is necessary, and how he or she can cooperate. Discuss how the results will be used in planning further care or treatments.
2. Perform hand hygiene and observe appropriate infection control procedures. Don gloves if performing a rectal temperature.
3. Provide for client privacy.
4. Place the client in the appropriate position (e.g., lateral or Sims' position for inserting a rectal thermometer).
5. Place the thermometer (see Box 29–4 on page 536).
   - Apply a protective sheath or probe cover if appropriate.
   - Lubricate a rectal thermometer.
6. Wait the appropriate amount of time. Electronic and tympanic thermometers will indicate that the reading is complete through a light or tone. Check package instructions for length of time to wait prior to reading chemical dot or tape thermometers.

CLINICAL ALERT

Be sure to record the temperature from an electronic thermometer before replacing the probe into the charging unit. With many models, replacing the probe erases the temperature from the display. ■

7. Remove the thermometer and discard the cover or wipe with a tissue if necessary.

8. Read the temperature and record it on your worksheet. If the temperature is obviously too high, too low, or inconsistent with the client's condition, recheck it with a thermometer known to be functioning properly.
9. Wash the thermometer if necessary and return it to the storage location.
10. Document the temperature in the client record. ❶ A rectal temperature may be recorded with an "R" next to the value or with the mark on a graphic sheet circled. An axillary temperature may be recorded with "AX" or marked on a graphic sheet with an X.

EVALUATION

■ Compare the temperature measurement to baseline data, normal range for age of client, and client's previous temperatures. Analyze considering time of day and any additional influencing factors and other vital signs.

■ Conduct appropriate follow-up such as notifying the primary care provider, giving a medication, or altering the client's environment. This includes teaching the client how to lower an elevated temperature through actions such as increasing fluid intake, coughing and deep breathing, or removing heavy coverings.

Date	6/24/07					
Temperature	23:00 – 07:00		07:00 – 15:00		15:00 – 23:00	
	24	4	8	12	16	20

❶ Vital signs graphic record.

BOX 29–4 Thermometer Placement

Oral Place the bulb on either side of the frenulum. ❶

❶ Oral thermometer placement.
(Patrick Watson)

Rectal Apply clean gloves.
Instruct the client to take a slow deep breath during insertion. ❷
Never force the thermometer if resistance is felt.
Insert 3.5 cm (11/2 in.) in adults.

❷ Inserting a rectal thermometer.
(Patrick Watson)

Axillary Pat the axilla dry if very moist.
The bulb is placed in the center of the axilla. ❸

❸ Placing the thermometer in the center of the axilla.
(Patrick Watson)

Tympanic Pull the pinna slightly upward and backward. ❹
Point the probe slightly anteriorly, toward the eardrum.
Insert the probe slowly using a circular motion until snug.

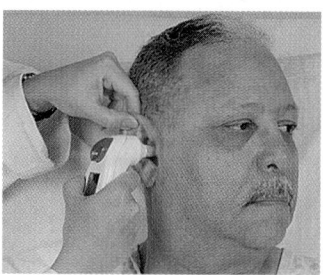

❹ Inserting the tympanic thermometer.

Temporal artery Brush hair aside if covering the TA area. With the probe flush on the center of the forehead, depress the red button; keep depressed. Slowly slide the probe midline across the forehead to the hair line, not down the side of the face. ❺ Lift the probe from the forehead and touch on the neck just behind the earlobe. ❻ Release the button.

❺ ❻ Positioning a temporal artery thermometer.

LIFESPAN CONSIDERATIONS Temperature

INFANTS

- The body temperature of newborns is extremely labile, and newborns must be kept warm and dry to prevent hypothermia.
- Using the axillary site, you need to hold the infant's arm against the chest (see Figure 29-10 ■).
- The axillary route may not be as accurate as other routes for detecting fevers in children (Bindler & Ball, 2003).
- The tympanic route is fast and convenient. Place the infant supine and stabilize the head. Pull the pinna straight back and slightly downward. Direct the probe tip anteriorly and insert far enough to seal the canal. The tip will not touch the tympanic membrane.
- Avoid the tympanic route in a child with active ear infections or tympanic membrane drainage tubes.

- The tympanic membrane route may be more accurate in determining temperature in febrile infants (Liu, Chang, & Chang, 2004; Nimah, Bshesh, Callahan, & Jacobs, 2006).
- When using a temporal artery thermometer, touching only the forehead or behind the ear is needed.
- The rectal route is least desirable in infants.

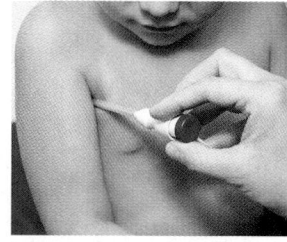

Figure 29-10 ■ Axillary thermometer placement.
(Patrick Watson)

LIFESPAN CONSIDERATIONS *continued*

CHILDREN

- Tympanic or temporal artery sites are preferred.
- For the tympanic route, have the child held on an adult's lap with the child's head held gently against the adult for support. Pull the pinna straight back and upward for children over age 3 (see Figure 29-11 ■).
- Avoid the tympanic route in a child with active ear infections or tympanic membrane drainage tubes.
- The oral route may be used for children over age 3, but nonbreakable, electronic thermometers are recommended.

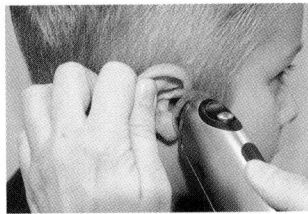

Figure 29-11 ■ Pull the pinna of the ear back and up for placement of a tympanic thermometer in a child over 3 years of age, back and down for children under age 3.
(Patrick Watson)

- For a rectal temperature, place the child prone across your lap or in a side-lying position with the knees flexed. Insert the thermometer 1 inch into the rectum.

ELDERS

- Elders' temperatures tend to be lower than those of middle-aged adults.
- Elders' temperatures are strongly influenced by both environmental and internal temperature changes. Their thermoregulation control processes are not as efficient as when they are younger, and they are at higher risk for both hypothermia and hyperthermia.
- Elders can develop significant buildup of ear cerumen that may interfere with tympanic thermometer readings.
- Elders are more likely to have hemorrhoids. Inspect the anus before taking a rectal temperature.
- Elders' temperatures may not be a valid indication of the seriousness of the pathology of a disease. They may have pneumonia or a urinary tract infection and have only a slight temperature elevation. Other symptoms, such as confusion and restlessness, may be displayed and need follow-up to determine if there is an underlying process.

HOME CARE CONSIDERATIONS Temperature

- Teach the client accurate use and reading of the type of thermometer to be used. Examine the thermometer used by the client in the home for safety and proper functioning. Facilitate the replacement of mercury thermometers with nonmercury ones. See page 532 for instructions regarding management of a broken mercury thermometer.
- Observe the client/caregiver taking and reading a temperature. Reinforce the importance of reporting the site and type of thermometer used and the value of using one consistently.
- Discuss means of keeping the thermometer clean, such as warm water and soap, and avoiding cross-contamination.

- Ensure that the client has water-soluble lubricant if using a rectal thermometer.
- Instruct the client or family member to notify the health care provider if the temperature is 37.7°C (100°F) or higher.
- When making a home visit, take a thermometer with you in case the clients do not have a functional thermometer of their own.
- Check that the client knows how to record the temperature. Provide a recording chart/table if indicated.
- Discuss environmental control modifications that should be taken during illness or extreme climate conditions (e.g., heating, air conditioning, appropriate clothing and bedding).

PULSE

The **pulse** is a wave of blood created by contraction of the left ventricle of the heart. Generally the pulse wave represents the stroke volume output or the amount of blood that enters the arteries with each ventricular contraction. **Compliance** of the arteries is their ability to contract and expand. When a person's arteries lose their distensibility, as can happen in old age, greater pressure is required to pump the blood into the arteries.

Cardiac output is the volume of blood pumped into the arteries by the heart and equals the result of the stroke volume (SV) times the heart rate (HR) per minute. For example, 65 mL × 70 beats per minute = 4.55 L per minute. When an adult is resting, the heart pumps about 5 liters of blood each minute.

In a healthy person, the pulse reflects the heartbeat; that is, the pulse rate is the same as the rate of the ventricular contractions of the heart. However, in some types of cardiovascular disease, the heartbeat and pulse rates can differ. For example, a client's heart may produce very weak or small pulse waves that are not detectable in a peripheral pulse far from the heart. In these instances, the nurse should assess the heartbeat and the peripheral pulse. A **peripheral pulse** is a pulse located away from the heart, for example, in the foot or wrist. The **apical pulse,** in contrast, is a central pulse; that is, it is located at the apex of the heart. It is also referred to as the **point of maximal impulse (PMI).**

Factors Affecting the Pulse

The rate of the pulse is expressed in beats per minute (BPM). A pulse rate varies according to a number of factors. The nurse should consider each of the following factors when assessing a client's pulse:

- *Age.* As age increases, the pulse rate gradually decreases overall. See Table 29–2 for specific variations in pulse rates from birth to adulthood.
- *Gender.* After puberty, the average male's pulse rate is slightly lower than the female's.
- *Exercise.* The pulse rate normally increases with activity. The rate of increase in the professional athlete is often less than in the average person because of greater cardiac size, strength, and efficiency.

TABLE 29-2 Variations in Pulse and Respirations by Age

AGE	PULSE AVERAGE (AND RANGES)	RESPIRATIONS AVERAGE (AND RANGES)
Newborn	130 (80–180)	35 (30–80)
1 year	120 (80–140)	30 (20–40)
5–8 years	100 (75–120)	20 (15–25)
10 years	70 (50–90)	19 (15–25)
Teen	75 (50–90)	18 (15–20)
Adult	80 (60–100)	16 (12–20)
Older adult	70 (60–100)	16 (15–20)

- *Fever.* The pulse rate increases (a) in response to the lowered blood pressure that results from peripheral vasodilatation associated with elevated body temperature and (b) because of the increased metabolic rate.
- *Medications.* Some medications decrease the pulse rate, and others increase it. For example, cardiotonics (e.g., digitalis preparations) decrease the heart rate, whereas epinephrine increases it.
- *Hypovolemia.* Loss of blood from the vascular system normally increases pulse rate. In adults the loss of circulating volume results in an adjustment of the heart rate to increase blood pressure as the body compensates for the lost blood volume. Adults can usually lose up to 10% of their normal circulating volume without adverse effects.
- *Stress.* In response to stress, sympathetic nervous stimulation increases the overall activity of the heart. Stress increases the rate as well as the force of the heartbeat. Fear and anxiety as well as the perception of severe pain stimulate the sympathetic system.
- *Position changes.* When a person is sitting or standing, blood usually pools in dependent vessels of the venous system. Pooling results in a transient decrease in the venous blood return to the heart and a subsequent reduction in blood pressure and increase in heart rate.
- *Pathology.* Certain diseases such as some heart conditions or those that impair oxygenation can alter the resting pulse rate.

Pulse Sites

A pulse may be measured in nine sites (see Figure 29-12 ■).

1. Temporal, where the temporal artery passes over the temporal bone of the head. The site is superior (above) and lateral to (away from the midline of) the eye.
2. Carotid, at the side of the neck where the carotid artery runs between the trachea and the sternocleidomastoid muscle.

CLINICAL ALERT

Never press both carotids at the same time because this can cause a reflex drop in blood pressure or pulse rate. ■

3. Apical, at the apex of the heart. In an adult this is located on the left side of the chest, about 8 cm (3 in.) to the left of the sternum (breastbone) and at the fourth, fifth, or sixth in-

Figure 29-12 ■ Nine sites for assessing pulse.

tercostal space (area between the ribs). In elders, the apex may be further left if there are conditions that have led to an enlarged heart. Before 4 years of age the apex is left of the midclavicular line (MCL); between 4 and 6 years, it is at the MCL (see Figure 29-13 ■). For a child 7 to 9 years of age, the apical pulse is located at the fourth or fifth intercostal space.

4. Brachial, at the inner aspect of the biceps muscle of the arm or medially in the antecubital space.
5. Radial, where the radial artery runs along the radial bone, on the thumb side of the inner aspect of the wrist.
6. Femoral, where the femoral artery passes alongside the inguinal ligament.
7. Popliteal, where the popliteal artery passes behind the knee.
8. Posterior tibial, on the medial surface of the ankle where the posterior tibial artery passes behind the medial malleolus.
9. Pedal (dorsalis pedis), where the dorsalis pedis artery passes over the bones of the foot, on an imaginary line drawn from the middle of the ankle to the space between the big and second toes. The radial site is most commonly used in adults. It is easily found in most people and readily accessible. Some reasons for use of each site are given in Table 29–3.

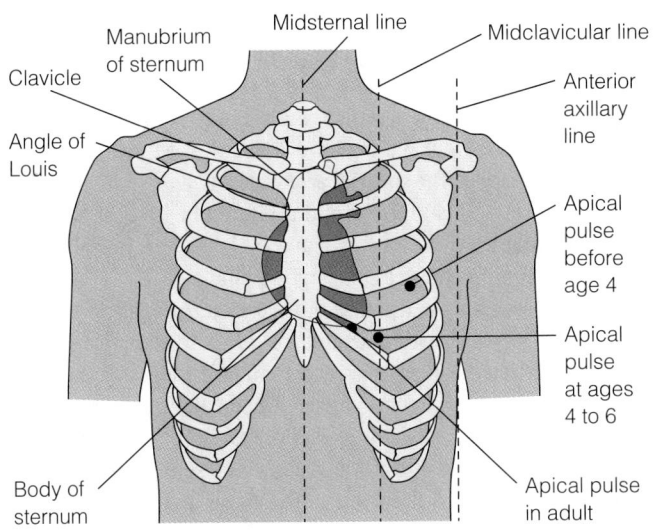

Figure 29–13 ■ Location of the apical pulse for a child under 4 years, a child 4 to 6 years, and an adult.

TABLE 29–3	**Reasons for Using Specific Pulse Site**
PULSE SITE	**REASONS FOR USE**
Radial	Readily accessible
Temporal	Used when radial pulse is not accessible
Carotid	Used during cardiac arrest/shock in adults Used to determine circulation to the brain
Apical	Routinely used for infants and children up to 3 years of age Used to determine discrepancies with radial pulse Used in conjunction with some medications
Brachial	Used to measure blood pressure Used during cardiac arrest for infants
Femoral	Used in cases of cardiac arrest/shock Used to determine circulation to a leg
Popliteal	Used to determine circulation to the lower leg
Posterior tibial	Used to determine circulation to the foot
Dorsal pedal	Used to determine circulation to the foot

Figure 29-14 ■ A Doppler ultrasound stethoscope (DUS).

See Identifying Nursing Diagnoses, Outcomes, and Interventions for examples of applying the nursing process to clients with pulse alterations.

Assessing the Pulse

A pulse is commonly assessed by palpation (feeling) or auscultation (hearing). The middle three fingertips are used for palpating all pulse sites except the apex of the heart. A stethoscope is used for assessing apical pulses. A Doppler ultrasound stethoscope (DUS; see Figure 29-14 ■) is used for pulses that are difficult to assess. The DUS headset has earpieces similar to standard stethoscope earpieces, but it has a long cord attached to a volume-controlled audio unit and an ultrasound transducer. The DUS detects movement of red blood cells through a blood vessel. In contrast to the conventional stethoscope, it excludes environmental sounds.

A pulse is normally palpated by applying moderate pressure with the three middle fingers of the hand. The pads on the most distal aspects of the finger are the most sensitive areas for detecting a pulse. With excessive pressure one can obliterate a pulse, whereas with too little pressure one may not be able to detect it. Before the nurse assesses the resting pulse, the client should assume a comfortable position. The nurse should also be aware of the following:

■ Any medication that could affect the heart rate.
■ Whether the client has been physically active. If so, wait 10 to 15 minutes until the client has rested and the pulse has slowed to its usual rate.

IDENTIFYING NURSING DIAGNOSES, OUTCOMES, AND INTERVENTIONS
Ineffective Peripheral Tissue Perfusion

NURSING DIAGNOSIS/ DEFINITION	SAMPLE DESIRED OUTCOMES* DEFINITION	INDICATORS†	SELECTED INTERVENTIONS* DEFINITION	SAMPLE ACTIVITIES
Ineffective Peripheral Tissue Perfusion/Decrease in oxygen resulting in the failure to nourish the tissues at the capillary level	Tissue Perfusion: Peripheral [0407]/ *Adequacy of blood flow through the small vessels of the extremities to maintain tissue function*	■ Distal peripheral pulses strong ■ Distal peripheral pulses symmetrical	Vital Signs Monitoring [6680]/*Collection and analysis of cardiovascular, respiratory, and body temperature data to determine and prevent complications*	Monitor presence and quality of pulses Take apical and radial pulses simultaneously and note the difference Monitor cardiac rhythm and rate

*The NOC # for desired outcomes and the NIC # for nursing interventions are listed in brackets following the appropriate outcome or intervention. Outcomes, indicators, interventions, and activities selected are only a sample of those suggested by NOC and NIC and should be further individualized for each client.

† The measurement scale for these indicators ranges from Extremely compromised to Not compromised. See Appendix B. ∞

- Any baseline data about the normal heart rate for the client. For example, a physically fit athlete may have a heart rate below 60 BPM.
- Whether the client should assume a particular position (e.g., sitting). In some clients, the rate changes with the position because of changes in blood flow volume and autonomic nervous system activity.

When assessing the pulse, the nurse collects the following data: the rate, rhythm, volume, arterial wall elasticity, and presence or absence of bilateral equality. An excessively fast heart rate (e.g., over 100 BPM in an adult) is referred to as **tachycardia.** A heart rate in an adult of less than 60 BPM is called **bradycardia.** If a client has either tachycardia or bradycardia, the apical pulse should be assessed.

The **pulse rhythm** is the pattern of the beats and the intervals between the beats. Equal time elapses between beats of a normal pulse. A pulse with an irregular rhythm is referred to as a **dysrhythmia** or **arrhythmia.** It may consist of random, irregular beats or a predictable pattern of irregular beats (documented as "regularly irregular"). When a dysrhythmia is detected, the apical pulse should be assessed. An electrocardiogram (ECG or EKG) is necessary to define the dysrhythmia further.

Pulse volume, also called the pulse strength or amplitude, refers to the force of blood with each beat. Usually, the pulse volume is the same with each beat. It can range from absent to bounding. A normal pulse can be felt with moderate pressure of the fingers and can be obliterated with greater pressure. A forceful or full blood volume that is obliterated only with difficulty is called a full or bounding pulse. A pulse that is readily obliterated with pressure from the fingers is referred to as weak, feeble, or thready.

The **elasticity of the arterial wall** reflects its expansibility or its deformities. A healthy, normal artery feels straight, smooth, soft, and pliable. Elders often have inelastic arteries that feel twisted (tortuous) and irregular upon palpation.

When assessing a peripheral pulse to determine the adequacy of blood flow to a particular area of the body (perfusion), the nurse should also assess the corresponding pulse on the other side of the body. The second assessment gives the nurse data with which to compare the pulses. For example, when assessing the blood flow to the right foot, the nurse assesses the right dorsalis pedis pulse and then the left dorsalis pedis pulse. If the client's right and left pulses are the same, the client's dorsalis pedis pulses are bilaterally equal. The pulse rate does not need to be counted when assessing for perfusion and equality.

When a peripheral pulse is located, it indicates that pulses more proximal to that location will also be present. For example, if the dorsalis pedis, the most distal pulse of the lower extremity, cannot be felt, the nurse next palpates for the posterior tibial pulse. If it is not felt, the popliteal pulse must be assessed. If the popliteal pulse is found, it is not necessary to assess the femoral pulse since it must also be present in order for the more distal pulse to exist.

Skill 29-2 provides guidelines for assessing a peripheral pulse.

SKILL 29-2 ASSESSING A PERIPHERAL PULSE

PURPOSES
- To establish baseline data for subsequent evaluation
- To identify whether the pulse rate is within normal range
- To determine whether the pulse rhythm is regular and the pulse volume is appropriate
- To determine the equality of corresponding peripheral pulses on each side of the body
- To monitor and assess changes in the client's health status
- To monitor clients at risk for pulse alterations (e.g., those with a history of heart disease or experiencing cardiac arrhythmias, hemorrhage, acute pain, infusion of large volumes of fluids, fever)
- To evaluate blood perfusion to the extremities

ASSESSMENT
Assess
- Clinical signs of cardiovascular alterations such as dyspnea (difficult respirations), fatigue, pallor, cyanosis (bluish discoloration of skin and mucous membranes), palpitations, syncope (fainting), or impaired peripheral tissue perfusion (as evidenced by skin discoloration and cool temperature)
- Factors that may alter pulse rate (e.g., emotional status and activity level)
- Which site is most appropriate for assessment based on the purpose

PLANNING

Delegation
Measurement of the client's radial or brachial pulse can be delegated to UAP—or family members/caregivers in nonhospital settings. Reports of abnormal pulse rates or rhythms require reassessment by the nurse, who also determines appropriate action if the abnormality is confirmed. UAPs are generally not delegated these techniques due to the skill required in locating and interpreting peripheral pulses other than the radial or brachial artery and in using Doppler ultrasound devices

Equipment
- Watch with a second hand or indicator
- If using a DUS: transducer probe, stethoscope headset, transmission gel, and tissues/wipes

ASSESSING A PERIPHERAL PULSE *continued*

IMPLEMENTATION

Preparation

If using a DUS, check that the equipment is functioning normally.

Performance

1. Prior to performing the procedure, introduce self and verify the client's identity using agency protocol. Explain to the client what you are going to do, why it is necessary, and how he or she can cooperate. Discuss how the results will be used in planning further care or treatments.
2. Perform hand hygiene and observe appropriate infection control procedures.
3. Provide for client privacy.
4. Select the pulse point. Normally, the radial pulse is taken, unless it cannot be exposed or circulation to another body area is to be assessed.
5. Assist the client to a comfortable resting position. When the radial pulse is assessed, with the palm facing downward, the client's arm can rest alongside the body or the forearm can rest at a 90-degree angle across the chest. For the client who can sit, the forearm can rest across the thigh, with the palm of the hand facing downward or inward.

6. Palpate and count the pulse. Place two or three middle fingertips lightly and squarely over the pulse point. **❶ Rationale:** *Using the thumb is contraindicated because the nurse's thumb has a pulse that could be mistaken for the client's pulse.*
   - Count for 15 seconds and multiply by 4. Record the pulse in beats per minute on your worksheet. If taking a client's pulse for the first time, when obtaining baseline data, or if the pulse is irregular, count for a full minute. If an irregular pulse is found, also take the apical pulse.
7. Assess the pulse rhythm and volume.
   - Assess the pulse rhythm by noting the pattern of the intervals between the beats. A normal pulse has equal time periods between beats. If this is an initial assessment, assess for 1 minute.
   - Assess the pulse volume. A normal pulse can be felt with moderate pressure, and the pressure is equal with each beat. A forceful pulse volume is full; an easily obliterated pulse is weak. Record the rhythm and volume on your worksheet.
8. Document the pulse rate, rhythm, and volume and your actions in the client record (see Figure ❶ in Skill 29-1). Also record pertinent related data such as variation in pulse rate compared to normal for the client and abnormal skin color and skin temperature in the nurse's notes.

❶ **A** Radial

❶ **B** Brachial

❶ **C** Carotid

❶ Assessing the pulses

❶ **D** Femoral

continued on page 542

ASSESSING A PERIPHERAL PULSE *continued*

❶ E Popliteal

❶ F Posterior tibial

Rationale: *Too much pressure can stop the blood flow and obliterate the signal.*

■ Adjust the volume if necessary. Distinguish artery sounds from vein sound. The artery sound (signal) is distinctively pulsating and has a pumping quality. The venous sound is intermittent and varies with respirations. Both artery and vein sounds are heard simultaneously through the DUS because major arteries and veins are situated close together throughout the body. If arterial sounds cannot be easily heard, reposition the probe.

■ After assessing the pulse, remove all gel from the probe to prevent damage to the surface. Clean the transducer with water-based solution. **Rationale:** *Alcohol or other disinfectants may damage the face of the transducer.* Remove all gel from the client.

❶ G Pedal (dorsalis pedis)

Variation: Using a DUS

■ If used, plug the stethoscope headset into one of the two output jacks located next to the volume control. DUS units may have two jacks so that a second person can listen to the signals.

■ Apply transmission gel either to the probe at the narrow end of the plastic case housing the transducer, or to the client's skin. **Rationale:** *Ultrasound beams do not travel well through air. The gel makes an airtight seal, which then promotes optimal ultrasound wave transmission.*

■ Press the "on" button.

■ Hold the probe against the skin over the pulse site. Use a light pressure, and keep the probe in contact with the skin. ❷

❷ Using a (Doppler) ultrasound stethoscope to assess the posterior tibial pulse.

EVALUATION

■ Compare the pulse rate to baseline data or normal range for age of client.

■ Relate pulse rate and volume to other vital signs; pulse rhythm and volume to baseline data and health status.

■ If assessing peripheral pulses, evaluate equality, rate, and volume in corresponding extremities.

■ Conduct appropriate follow-up such as notifying the primary care provider or giving medication.

Apical Pulse Assessment

Assessment of the apical pulse is indicated for clients whose peripheral pulse is irregular or unavailable as well as for clients with known cardiovascular, pulmonary, and renal diseases. It is commonly assessed prior to administering medications that affect heart rate. The apical site is also used to assess the pulse for newborns, infants, and children up to 2 to 3 years old. Skill 29-3 presents guidelines for assessing the apical pulse.

ASSESSING AN APICAL PULSE

PURPOSES
- To obtain the heart rate of newborns, infants, and children 2 to 3 years old or of an adult with an irregular peripheral pulse
- To establish baseline data for subsequent evaluation
- To determine whether the cardiac rate is within normal range and the rhythm is regular
- To monitor clients with cardiac, pulmonary, or renal disease and those receiving medications to improve heart action

ASSESSMENT
Assess
- Clinical signs of cardiovascular alterations (e.g., dyspnea, fatigue/weakness, pallor, cyanosis, syncope)
- Factors that may alter pulse rate (e.g., emotional status, activity level, and medications that affect heart rate such as digoxin, beta blockers, or calcium channel blockers)

PLANNING

> **Delegation**
> Due to the degree of skill and knowledge required, UAP are generally not responsible for assessing apical pulses.

Equipment
- Watch with a second hand or indicator
- Stethoscope
- Antiseptic wipes
- If using a DUS: the transducer probe, the stethoscope headset, transmission gel, and tissues/wipes

IMPLEMENTATION
Preparation
If using a DUS, check that the equipment is functioning normally.

Performance
1. Prior to performing the procedure, introduce self and verify the client's identity using agency protocol. Explain to the client what you are going to do, why it is necessary, and how he or she can cooperate. Discuss how the results will be used in planning further care or treatments.
2. Perform hand hygiene and observe appropriate infection control procedures.
3. Provide for client privacy.
4. Position the client appropriately in a comfortable supine position or in a sitting position. Expose the area of the chest over the apex of the heart.
5. Locate the apical impulse. This is the point over the apex of the heart where the apical pulse can be most clearly heard.
   - Palpate the angle of Louis (the angle between the manubrium, the top of the sternum, and the body of the sternum). It is palpated just below the suprasternal notch and is felt as a prominence (see Figure 29-13).
   - Slide your index finger just to the left of the sternum, and palpate the second intercostal space. ❶
   - Place your middle or next finger in the third intercostal space, and continue palpating downward until you locate the fifth intercostal space. ❷
   - Move your index finger laterally along the fifth intercostal space toward the MCL. ❸ Normally, the apical impulse is palpable at or just medial to the MCL (see Figure 29-18 ■).
6. Auscultate and count heartbeats.
   - Use antiseptic wipes to clean the earpieces and diaphragm of the stethoscope if their cleanliness is in doubt. **Rationale:** *The diaphragm needs to be cleaned and disinfected if soiled with body substances.*

❶ Second intercostal space.
(Patrick Watson)

❷ Third intercostal space.
(Patrick Watson)

continued on page 544

ASSESSING AN APICAL PULSE *continued*

❸ Fifth intercostal space, MCL.
(Patrick Watson)

❹ A stethoscope with both a bell-shaped and flat-disc amplifier.

❹ B Close-up of a flat-disc amplifier (left) and a bell amplifier (right).

- Warm the diaphragm (flat-disc) of the stethoscope by holding it in the palm of the hand for a moment. **Rationale:** *The metal of the diaphragm is usually cold and can startle the client when placed immediately on the chest.*
- Insert the earpieces of the stethoscope into your ears in the direction of the ear canals, or slightly forward, *to facilitate hearing.*
- Tap your finger lightly on the diaphragm *to be sure it is the active side of the head.* If necessary, rotate the head to select the diaphragm side. ❹
- Place the diaphragm of the stethoscope over the apical impulse and listen for the normal S_1 and S_2 heart sounds, which are heard as "lub-dub". ❺ **Rationale:** *The heartbeat is normally loudest over the apex of the heart.* Each lub-dub is counted as one heartbeat. **Rationale:** *The two heart sounds are produced by closure of the heart valves. The S_1 heart sound (lub) occurs when the atrioventricular valves close after the ventricles have been sufficiently filled. The S_2 heart sound (dub) occurs when the semilunar valves close after the ventricles empty.*
- If you have difficulty hearing the apical pulse, ask the supine client to roll onto his or her left side or the sitting client to lean slightly forward. **Rationale:** *This positioning moves the apex of the heart closer to the chest wall.*
- If the rhythm is regular, count the heartbeats for 30 seconds and multiply by 2. If the rhythm is irregular or for giving certain medications such as digoxin, count the beats for 60 seconds. **Rationale:** *A 60-second count provides a more accurate assessment of an irregular pulse than a 30-second count.*

7. Assess the rhythm and the strength of the heartbeat.
   - Assess the rhythm of the heartbeat by noting the pattern of intervals between the beats. A normal pulse has equal time periods between beats.
   - Assess the strength (volume) of the heartbeat. Normally, the heartbeats are equal in strength and can be described as strong or weak.

❺ Taking an apical pulse using the flat disc of the stethoscope. Note how the amplifier is held against the chest.

8. Document the pulse site, rate, rhythm, and volume and nursing actions in the client record. Also record pertinent related data such as variation in pulse rate compared to normal for the client and abnormal skin color and skin temperature.

ASSESSING AN APICAL PULSE *continued*

EVALUATION

■ Relate the pulse rate to other vital signs. Relate the pulse rhythm to baseline data and health status.

■ Report to the primary care provider any abnormal findings such as irregular rhythm, and reduced ability to hear the heartbeat, pallor, cyanosis, dyspnea, tachycardia, or bradycardia.

■ Conduct appropriate follow-up such as administering medication ordered based on apical heart rate.

Apical-Radial Pulse Assessment

An **apical-radial pulse** may need to be assessed for clients with certain cardiovascular disorders. Normally, the apical and radial rates are identical. An apical pulse rate greater than a radial pulse rate can indicate that the thrust of the blood from the heart is too weak for the wave to be felt at the peripheral pulse site, or it can indicate that vascular disease is preventing impulses from being transmitted. Any discrepancy between the two pulse rates is called a **pulse deficit** and needs to be reported promptly. In no instance is the radial pulse greater than the apical pulse.

An apical-radial pulse can be taken by two nurses or one nurse, although the two-nurse technique may be more accurate. Skill 29-4 outlines the steps for assessing an apical-radial pulse.

ASSESSING AN APICAL-RADIAL PULSE

PURPOSE

■ To determine adequacy of peripheral circulation or presence of pulse deficit

ASSESSMENT

Assess

■ Clinical signs of hypovolemic shock (hypotension, pallor, cyanosis, and cold, clammy skin)

PLANNING

Delegation

UAP are generally not responsible for assessing apical-radial pulses using the one-nurse technique. UAP may perform the radial pulse count for the two-nurse technique.

Equipment

■ Watch with a second hand or indicator
■ Stethoscope
■ Antiseptic wipes

IMPLEMENTATION

Preparation

If using the two-nurse technique, ensure that the other nurse is available at this time.

Performance

1. Prior to performing the procedure, introduce self and verify the client's identity using agency protocol. Explain to the client what you are going to do, why it is necessary, and how he or she can cooperate. Discuss how the results will be used in planning further care or treatments.

2. Perform hand hygiene and observe appropriate infection control procedures.

3. Provide for client privacy.

4. Position the client appropriately. Assist the client to a comfortable supine or sitting position. Expose the area of the chest over the apex of the heart. If previous measurements were taken, determine what position the client assumed, and use the same position. **Rationale:** *This ensures an accurate comparative measurement.*

5. Locate the apical and radial pulse sites. In the two-nurse technique, one nurse locates the apical impulse by palpation or with the stethoscope while the other nurse palpates the radial pulse site (see Skills 29-2 and 29-3).

6. Count the apical and radial pulse rates.

Two-Nurse Technique

● Place the watch where both nurses can see it. The nurse who is taking the radial pulse may hold the watch.

● Decide on a time to begin counting. A time when the second hand is on 12, 3, 6, or 9 or an even number on digital clocks is usually selected. The nurse taking the radial pulse says "Start." **Rationale:** *This ensures that simultaneous counts are taken.*

● Each nurse counts the pulse rate for 60 seconds. Both nurses end the count when the nurse taking the radial pulse says "Stop." **Rationale:** *A full 60-second count is necessary for accurate assessment of any discrepancies between the two pulse sites.*

● The nurse who assesses the apical rate also assesses the apical pulse rhythm and volume (i.e., whether the heartbeat is strong or weak). If the pulse is irregular, note whether the irregular beats come at random or at predictable times.

● The nurse assessing the radial pulse rate also assesses the radial pulse rhythm and volume.

One-Nurse Technique

● Assess the apical pulse for 60 seconds.
● Assess the radial pulse for 60 seconds.

continued on page 546

ASSESSING AN APICAL-RADIAL PULSE *continued*

7. Document the apical and radial (AR) pulse rates, rhythm, volume, and any pulse deficit in the client record. Also record related data such as variation in pulse rate compared to normal

for the client and other pertinent observations, such as pallor, cyanosis, or dyspnea.

EVALUATION

- Relate pulse rate and rhythm to other vital signs, to baseline data, and to general health status.
- Report to the primary care provider any changes from previous measurements or any discrepancy between the two pulses.

- Conduct appropriate follow-up such as administering medication or other actions to be taken for a discrepancy in the AR pulse rates.

LIFESPAN CONSIDERATIONS Pulse

INFANTS

- Use the apical pulse for the heart rate of newborns, infants, and children 2 to 3 years old to establish baseline data for subsequent evaluation, to determine whether the cardiac rate is within normal range, and to determine if the rhythm is regular.
- Place a baby in a supine position, and offer a pacifier if the baby is crying or restless. Crying and physical activity will increase the pulse rate. For this reason, take the apical pulse rate of infants and small children before assessing body temperatures.
- Locate the apical pulse in the fourth intercostal space, lateral to the midclavicular line during infancy.
- Brachial, popliteal, and femoral pulses may be palpated. Due to a normally low blood pressure and rapid heart rate, infants' other distal pulses may be hard to feel.
- Newborn infants may have heart murmurs that are not pathological, but reflect functional incomplete closure of fetal heart structures (ductus arteriosus or foramen ovale).

CHILDREN

- To take a peripheral pulse, position the child comfortably in the adult's arms, or have the adult remain close by. This may decrease anxiety and yield more accurate results.
- To assess the apical pulse, assist a young child to a comfortable supine or sitting position.

- Demonstrate the procedure to the child using a stuffed animal or doll, and allow the child to handle the stethoscope before beginning the procedure. This will decrease anxiety and promote cooperation.
- The apex of the heart is normally located in the fourth intercostal space in young children; fifth intercostal space in children 7 years of age and over.
- Locate the apical impulse along the fourth intercostal space, between the MCL and the anterior axillary line (see Figure 29-13).
- Count the pulse prior to other uncomfortable procedures so that the rate is not artificially elevated by the discomfort.

ELDERS

- If the client has severe hand or arm tremors, the radial pulse may be difficult to count.
- Cardiac changes in elders, such as decrease in cardiac output, sclerotic changes to heart valves, and dysrhythmias often indicate that obtaining an apical pulse will be more accurate.
- Elders often have decreased peripheral circulation, so pedal pulses should also be checked for regularity, volume, and symmetry.
- The pulse returns to baseline after exercise more slowly than with other age groups.

HOME CARE CONSIDERATIONS Pulse

- Assist in obtaining and using an electronic pulse device if indicated.
- Teach the client to monitor the pulse prior to taking medications that affect the heart rate. Tell the client to report any notable

changes in heart rate or rhythm (regularity) to the health care provider.

RESPIRATIONS

Respiration is the act of breathing. **Inhalation** or **inspiration** refers to the intake of air into the lungs. **Exhalation** or **expiration** refers to breathing out or the movement of gases from the lungs to the atmosphere. **Ventilation** is also used to refer to the movement of air in and out of the lungs.

There are basically two types of breathing: **costal (thoracic) breathing** and **diaphragmatic (abdominal) breathing.** Costal breathing involves the external intercostal muscles and other accessory muscles, such as the sternocleidomastoid muscles. It

can be observed by the movement of the chest upward and outward. By contrast, diaphragmatic breathing involves the contraction and relaxation of the diaphragm, and it is observed by the movement of the abdomen, which occurs as a result of the diaphragm's contraction and downward movement.

Mechanics and Regulation of Breathing

During inhalation, the following processes normally occur (Figure 29-15 ■): The diaphragm contracts (flattens), the ribs

DRUG CAPSULE *Cardiac Glycoside or Digitalis Glycoside* **digoxin (Lanoxin)**

CLIENT WITH CARDIAC MEDICATIONS THAT AFFECT HEART RATE

Cardiac glycosides increase cardiac contractility, which increases cardiac output. As a result, perfusion to the kidneys is increased, which increases the production of urine. Cardiac glycosides also decrease heart rate by prolonging cardiac conduction, especially at the AV node. Digoxin is commonly used for the clinical management of heart failure, atrial fibrillation, atrial flutter, and paroxysmal atrial tachycardia.

NURSING RESPONSIBILITIES

- Take the apical pulse for one minute before administering the dose. If the apical pulse is < 60 or another specific parameter set by the health care provider, retake the pulse in one hour. If pulse remains < 60, call the prescriber.
- Monitor electrolyte levels: low potassium and low magnesium and high levels of calcium place the client at risk for digitalis toxicity. Check the client's most recent electrolyte lab work before administering the dose.
- Avoid giving with meals as this will delay absorption.
- Monitor for therapeutic drug levels: 0.5–2 ng/mL. Digoxin has a narrow therapeutic index, which means that there is not much difference between a therapeutic effect and a toxic effect.
- Assess for signs of digoxin toxicity: anorexia, nausea, vomiting, diarrhea, blurred or "yellow" vision, unusual tiredness and weakness.

CLIENT AND FAMILY TEACHING

- Explain the reason for taking digoxin and the importance of medical checkups that may include lab work to evaluate the effects and dosage of the drug.
- Teach the client and/or family how to check the radial or carotid pulse for a full minute. Inform them to take the pulse at the same time each day and to write it on the calendar. Provide pulse parameters and tell them when it is appropriate to call the health care provider.
- Caution the client not to stop taking the digoxin without approval of the health care provider.
- Caution the client to avoid over-the-counter drugs, except on the advice of the health care provider, as many can interact with digoxin.
- Explain the signs and symptoms of digoxin toxicity and the importance of calling the health care provider.

Note: Prior to administering any medication, review all aspects with a current drug handbook or other reliable source.

REAL WORLD PRACTICE

I received report on a client transfer who was being rushed to my unit from a general medical floor. The client was a 42-year-old male admitted for gastrointestinal bleeding and currently in tachycardia at a rate of 200 beats per minute. He received a fluid challenge prior to transfer with no change on the cardiac monitor. A stat CBC was pending. When the client arrived on my unit the resident physician immediately ordered adenosine for his rapid heart rate. While another nurse was preparing to administer the medication, I assessed the client. He was alert and oriented. Blood pressure and oxygen saturation were stable. He denied chest pain, palpitations, or shortness of breath. His skin was pink, warm, and moist. I could feel him trembling. As I auscultated his breath sounds, I could hear his heart beating. It wasn't the fast beat we saw racing across the monitor. His apical pulse was only 92. The perfect textbook tachycardia we saw on the cardiac monitor was simply artifact from the fine tremors the client was having secondary to alcohol withdrawal. He was an alcoholic and hadn't consumed any alcohol in over three days. In this great era of advancements in medical technology, always remember a thorough client history and physical assessment are still our most useful tools.

—Kelly S. Flavin, RN, PCCN,
OSF Saint Francis Medical Center, Peoria, IL

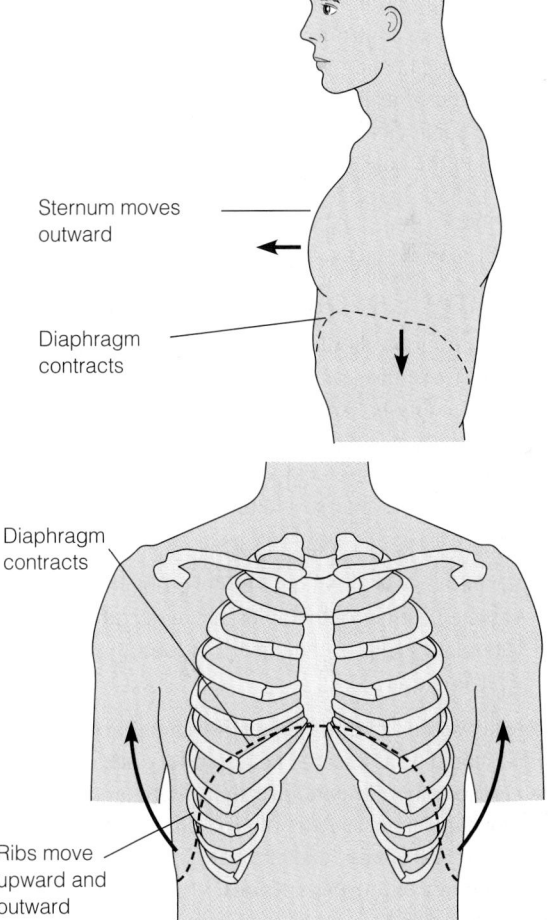

Sternum moves outward

Diaphragm contracts

Diaphragm contracts

Ribs move upward and outward

Figure 29-15 ■ Respiratory inhalation. *Top*: lateral view; *Bottom*: anterior view.

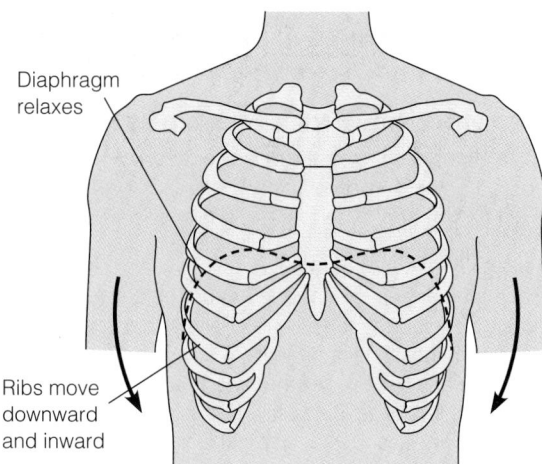

Figure 29-16 ■ Respiratory exhalation. *Left*: lateral view; *Right*: anterior view.

move upward and outward, and the sternum moves outward, thus enlarging the thorax and permitting the lungs to expand. During exhalation (Figure 29-16 ■), the diaphragm relaxes, the ribs move downward and inward, and the sternum moves inward, thus decreasing the size of the thorax as the lungs are compressed. Normally breathing is carried out automatically and effortlessly. A normal adult inspiration lasts 1 to 1.5 seconds, and an expiration lasts 2 to 3 seconds.

Respiration is controlled by (a) respiratory centers in the medulla oblongata and the pons of the brain and (b) chemoreceptors located centrally in the medulla and peripherally in the carotid and aortic bodies. These centers and receptors respond to changes in the concentrations of oxygen (O_2), carbon dioxide (CO_2), and hydrogen (H^+) in the arterial blood. See Chapter 50 ∞ for details.

Assessing Respirations

Resting respirations should be assessed when the client is relaxed because exercise affects respirations, increasing their rate and depth. Anxiety is likely to affect respiratory rate and depth as well. Respirations may also need to be assessed after exercise to identify the client's tolerance to activity. Before assessing a client's respirations, a nurse should be aware of the following:

■ The client's normal breathing pattern
■ The influence of the client's health problems on respirations
■ Any medications or therapies that might affect respirations
■ The relationship of the client's respirations to cardiovascular function

The rate, depth, rhythm, and quality and effectiveness of respirations should be assessed. The respiratory rate is normally described in breaths per minute. Breathing that is normal in rate and depth is called eupnea. Abnormally slow respirations are referred to as **bradypnea,** and abnormally fast respirations are called **tachypnea** or **polypnea. Apnea** is the absence of breathing. For the respiratory rates for different age groups, see Table 29–2 on page 538.

Factors Affecting Respirations

Several factors influence respiratory rate. Those that increase the rate include exercise (increases metabolism), stress (readies the body for "fight or flight"), increased environmental temperature, and lowered oxygen concentration at increased altitudes. Factors that may decrease the respiratory rate include decreased environmental temperature, certain medications (e.g., narcotics), and increased intracranial pressure.

CLINICAL ALERT

An adult sleeping client's respirations can fall to fewer than 10 shallow breaths per minute. Use other vital signs to validate the client's condition. ■

The depth of a person's respirations can be established by watching the movement of the chest. Respiratory depth is generally described as normal, deep, or shallow. Deep respirations are those in which a large volume of air is inhaled and exhaled, inflating most of the lungs. Shallow respirations involve the exchange of a small volume of air and often the minimal use of lung tissue. During a normal inspiration and expiration, an adult takes in about 500 mL of air. This volume is called the **tidal volume.** For further information about pulmonary volumes and pulmonary capacities, see Chapter 50. ∞

Body position also affects the amount of air that can be inhaled. People in a supine position experience two physiologic processes that suppress respiration: an increase in the volume of blood inside the thoracic cavity and compression of the chest. Consequently, clients lying on their back have poorer lung aeration, which predisposes them to the stasis of fluids and subsequent infection. Certain medications also affect the respiratory depth. For example, narcotics such as morphine and large doses of barbiturates such as secobarbital sodium depress the respiratory centers in the brain, thereby depressing the respiratory rate and depth. **Hyperventilation** refers to very deep, rapid respirations; **hypoventilation** refers to very shallow respirations.

BOX 29–5   Altered Breathing Patterns and Sounds

BREATHING PATTERNS

Rate
- *Tachypnea*—quick, shallow breaths
- *Bradypnea*—abnormally slow breathing
- *Apnea*—cessation of breathing

Volume
- *Hyperventilation*—overexpansion of the lungs characterized by rapid and deep breaths
- *Hypoventilation*—underexpansion of the lungs, characterized by shallow respirations

Rhythm
- *Cheyne-Stokes breathing*—rhythmic waxing and waning of respirations, from very deep to very shallow breathing and temporary apnea

Ease or Effort
- *Dyspnea*—difficult and labored breathing during which the individual has a persistent, unsatisfied need for air and feels distressed
- *Orthopnea*—ability to breathe only in upright sitting or standing positions

BREATH SOUNDS

Audible without Amplification
- *Stridor*—a shrill, harsh sound heard during inspiration with laryngeal obstruction
- *Stertor*—snoring or sonorous respiration, usually due to a partial obstruction of the upper airway
- *Wheeze*—continuous, high-pitched musical squeak or whistling sound occurring on expiration and sometimes on inspiration when air moves through a narrowed or partially obstructed airway
- *Bubbling*—gurgling sounds heard as air passes through moist secretions in the respiratory tract

Chest Movements
- *Intercostal retraction*—indrawing between the ribs
- *Substernal retraction*—indrawing beneath the breastbone
- *Suprasternal retraction*—indrawing above the clavicles

Secretions and Coughing
- *Hemoptysis*—the presence of blood in the sputum
- *Productive cough*—a cough accompanied by expectorated secretions
- *Nonproductive cough*—a dry, harsh cough without secretions

---

Respiratory rhythm refers to the regularity of the expirations and the inspirations. Normally, respirations are evenly spaced. Respiratory rhythm can be described as regular or irregular. An infant's respiratory rhythm may be less regular than an adult's. See Chapter 50 ∞ for details about abnormal respiratory rhythms.

Respiratory quality or **character** refers to those aspects of breathing that are different from normal, effortless breathing. Two of these aspects are the amount of effort a client must exert to breathe and the sound of breathing. Usually, breathing does not require noticeable effort. Sometimes, however, clients can breathe only with substantial effort—this is referred to as labored breathing.

The sound of breathing is also significant. Normal breathing is silent, but a number of abnormal sounds such as a wheeze are obvious to the nurse's ear. Many sounds occur as a result of the presence of fluid in the lungs and are most clearly heard with a stethoscope. See Chapter 30 ∞ for methods used to assess lung sounds. For details about altered breathing patterns and terms used to describe various patterns and sounds, see Box 29–5.

The effectiveness of respirations is measured in part by the uptake of oxygen from the air into the blood and the release of carbon dioxide from the blood into expired air. The amount of hemoglobin in arterial blood that is saturated with oxygen can be measured indirectly through pulse oximetry. A pulse oximeter provides a digital readout of both the client's pulse rate and the oxygen saturation (see Skill 29-7). See the Identifying Nursing Diagnoses, Outcomes, and Interventions for an example of applying the nursing process to a client with a breathing disorder.

Skill 29-5 outlines the steps for assessing respirations.

IDENTIFYING NURSING DIAGNOSES, OUTCOMES, AND INTERVENTIONS

Ineffective Breathing Pattern

NURSING DIAGNOSIS/ DEFINITION	SAMPLE DESIRED OUTCOMES*/ DEFINITION	INDICATORS†	SELECTED INTERVENTIONS*/ DEFINITION	SAMPLE ACTIVITIES
Ineffective Breathing Pattern/Inspiration and/or expiration that does not provide adequate ventilation	Respiratory Status: Ventilation [0403]/*Movement of air in and out of the lungs*	▪ Respiratory rate IER (in expected range) ▪ Ease of breathing	Respiratory Monitoring [3350]/*Collection and analysis of respiratory data to ensure airway patency and adequate gas exchange*	▪ Monitor for noisy respirations such as snoring ▪ Monitor rate, rhythm, depth, and effort of respirations

*The NOC # for desired outcomes and the NIC # for nursing interventions are listed in brackets following the appropriate outcome or intevention. Outcomes, indicators, interventions, and activities selected are only a sample of those suggested by NOC and NIC and should be further individualized for each client.

†The measurement scale ranges from Extremely compromised to Not compromised. See Appendix B. ∞

SKILL 29-5

ASSESSING RESPIRATIONS

PURPOSES

- To acquire baseline data against which future measurements can be compared
- To monitor abnormal respirations and respiratory patterns and identify changes
- To monitor respirations before or following the administration of a general anesthetic or any medication that influences respirations
- To monitor clients at risk for respiratory alterations (e.g., those with fever, pain, acute anxiety, chronic obstructive pulmonary disease, asthma, respiratory infection, pulmonary edema or emboli, chest trauma or constriction, brain stem injury)

ASSESSMENT

Assess

- Skin and mucous membrane color (e.g., cyanosis or pallor)
- Position assumed for breathing (e.g., use of orthopneic position)
- Signs of cerebral anoxia (e.g., irritability, restlessness, drowsiness, or loss of consciousness)
- Chest movements (e.g., retractions between the ribs or above or below the sternum)
- Activity tolerance
- Chest pain
- Dyspnea
- Medications affecting respiratory rate

PLANNING

Delegation

Counting and observing respirations may be delegated to UAP. The follow-up assessment, interpretation of abnormal respirations, and determination of appropriate responses are done by the nurse.

Equipment

- Watch with a second hand or indicator

IMPLEMENTATION

PREPARATION

For a routine assessment of respirations, determine the client's activity schedule and choose a suitable time to monitor the respirations. A client who has been exercising will need to rest for a few minutes to permit the accelerated respiratory rate to return to normal.

Performance

1. Prior to performing the procedure, introduce self and verify the client's identity using agency protocol. Explain to the client what you are going to do, why it is necessary, and how he or she can cooperate. Discuss how the results will be used in planning further care or treatments.
2. Perform hand hygiene and observe appropriate infection control procedures.
3. Provide for client privacy.
4. Observe or palpate and count the respiratory rate.
   - The client's awareness that the nurse is counting the respiratory rate could cause the client to purposefully alter the respiratory pattern. If you anticipate this, place a hand against the client's chest to feel the chest movements with breathing, or place the client's arm across the chest and observe the chest movements while supposedly taking the radial pulse.

   - Count the respiratory rate for 30 seconds if the respirations are regular. Count for 60 seconds if they are irregular. An inhalation and an exhalation count as one respiration.
5. Observe the depth, rhythm, and character of respirations.
   - Observe the respirations for depth by watching the movement of the chest. **Rationale:** *During deep respirations, a large volume of air is exchanged; during shallow respirations, a small volume is exchanged.*
   - Observe the respirations for regular or irregular rhythm. **Rationale:** *Normally, respirations are evenly spaced.*
   - Observe the character of respirations—the sound they produce and the effort they require. **Rationale:** *Normally, respirations are silent and effortless.*
6. Document the respiratory rate, depth, rhythm, and character on the appropriate record (see page 535).

SAMPLE DOCUMENTATION

5/17/07 1320 Respirations irregular, varying from 18–34/min. in past hour. Shallower resp. during tachypnea. Slight wheezing noted. Resp. therapist called to provide treatment. D. Katano, RN

EVALUATION

- Relate respiratory rate to other vital signs, in particular pulse rate; relate respiratory rhythm and depth to baseline data and health status.
- Report to the primary care provider a respiratory rate significantly above or below the normal range and any notable change in respirations from previous assessments; irregular respiratory rhythm; inadequate respiratory depth; abnormal character of breathing—orthopnea, wheezing, stridor, or bubbling; and any complaints of dyspnea.
- Conduct appropriate follow-up such as administering oxygen or other appropriate medications or treatments, positioning the client to ease breathing, and requesting involvement of other members of the health care team such as the respiratory therapist.

LIFESPAN CONSIDERATIONS   Respirations

INFANTS

- An infant or child who is crying will have an abnormal respiratory rate and rhythm and needs to be quieted before respirations can be accurately assessed.
- Infants and young children use their diaphragms for inhalation and exhalation. If necessary, place your hand gently on the infant's abdomen to feel the rapid rise and fall during respirations.
- Most newborns are complete nose breathers, and nasal obstruction can be life-threatening.
- Some newborns display "periodic breathing" in which they pause for a few seconds between respirations. This condition can be normal, but parents should be alert to prolonged or frequent pauses (apnea) that require medical attention.
- Compared to adults, infants have fewer alveoli and their airways

have a smaller diameter. As a result, infants' respiratory rate and effort of breathing will increase with respiratory infections.

CHILDREN

- Because young children are diaphragmatic breathers, observe the rise and fall of the abdomen. If necessary, place your hand gently on the abdomen to feel the rapid rise and fall during respirations.
- Count respirations prior to other uncomfortable procedures so that the respiratory rate is not artificially elevated by the discomfort.

ELDERS

- Ask the client to remain quiet, or count respirations after taking the pulse.
- Elders experience anatomic and physiologic changes that cause the respiratory system to be less efficient. Any changes in rate or type of breathing should be reported immediately.

HOME CARE CONSIDERATIONS   Respirations

- Monitor respiratory rate following the administration of respiratory depressants such as morphine.
- Assess the home setting for factors that could interfere with breathing such as exhaust, gas, or paint fumes or persons who smoke.

- If the client has just come in from another room, allow the client to rest a minute or two before counting respirations.
- Have an adult hold a child gently to reduce movement while counting respirations.

BLOOD PRESSURE

Arterial blood pressure is a measure of the pressure exerted by the blood as it flows through the arteries. Because the blood moves in waves, there are two blood pressure measures. The **systolic pressure** is the pressure of the blood as a result of contraction of the ventricles, that is, the pressure of the height of the blood wave. The **diastolic pressure** is the pressure when the ventricles are at rest. Diastolic pressure, then, is the lower pressure, present at all times within the arteries. The difference between the diastolic and the systolic pressures is called the **pulse pressure.** A normal pulse pressure is about 40 mm Hg but can be as high as 100 mm Hg during exercise. A consistently elevated pulse pressure occurs in arteriosclerosis. A low pulse pressure (e.g., less than 25 mm Hg) occurs in conditions such as severe heart failure.

Blood pressure is measured in millimeters of mercury (mm Hg) and recorded as a fraction: systolic pressure over the diastolic pressure. A typical blood pressure for a healthy adult is 120/80 mm Hg (pulse pressure of 40). A number of conditions are reflected by changes in blood pressure. Because blood pressure can vary considerably among individuals, it is important for the nurse to know a specific client's baseline blood pressure. For example, if a client's usual blood pressure is 180/100 mm Hg, and it is assessed following surgery to be 120/80 mm Hg, this significant drop in pressure may indicate complications and must be reported to the primary care provider.

Determinants of Blood Pressure

Arterial blood pressure is the result of several factors: the pumping action of the heart, the peripheral vascular resistance (the re-

sistance supplied by the blood vessels through which the blood flows), and the blood volume and viscosity.

Pumping Action of the Heart

When the pumping action of the heart is weak, less blood is pumped into arteries (lower cardiac output), and the blood pressure decreases. When the heart's pumping action is strong and the volume of blood pumped into the circulation increases (higher cardiac output), the blood pressure increases.

Peripheral Vascular Resistance

Peripheral resistance can increase blood pressure. The diastolic pressure especially is affected. Some factors that create resistance in the arterial system are the capacity of the arterioles and capillaries, the compliance of the arteries, and the viscosity of the blood.

The internal diameter or capacity of the arterioles and the capillaries determines in great part the peripheral resistance to the blood in the body. The smaller the space within a vessel, the greater the resistance. Normally, the arterioles are in a state of partial constriction. Increased vasoconstriction, such as occurs with smoking, raises the blood pressure, whereas decreased vasoconstriction lowers the blood pressure.

If the elastic and muscular tissues of the arteries are replaced with fibrous tissue, the arteries lose much of their ability to constrict and dilate. This condition, most common in middle-aged and elderly adults, is known as **arteriosclerosis.**

Blood Volume

When the blood volume decreases (for example, as a result of a hemorrhage or dehydration), the blood pressure decreases because of decreased fluid in the arteries. Conversely, when the volume increases (for example, as a result of a rapid intravenous infusion), the blood pressure increases because of the greater fluid volume within the circulatory system.

Blood Viscosity

Blood pressure is higher when the blood is highly **viscous** (thick), that is, when the proportion of red blood cells to the blood plasma is high. This proportion is referred to as the **hematocrit.** The viscosity increases markedly when the hematocrit is more than 60% to 65%.

Factors Affecting Blood Pressure

Among the factors influencing blood pressure are age, exercise, stress, race, obesity, sex, medications, diurnal variations, and disease processes.

- *Age.* Newborns have a mean systolic pressure of about 75 mm Hg. The pressure rises with age, reaching a peak at the onset of puberty, and then tends to decline somewhat. In elders, elasticity of the arteries is decreased—the arteries are more rigid and less yielding to the pressure of the blood. This produces an elevated systolic pressure. Because the walls no longer retract as flexibly with decreased pressure, the diastolic pressure may also be high.
- *Exercise.* Physical activity increases the cardiac output and hence the blood pressure; thus 20 to 30 minutes of rest following exercise is indicated before the resting blood pressure can be reliably assessed.
- *Stress.* Stimulation of the sympathetic nervous system increases cardiac output and vasoconstriction of the arterioles, thus increasing the blood pressure reading; however, severe pain can decrease blood pressure greatly by inhibiting the vasomotor center and producing vasodilatation.
- *Race.* African American males over 35 years have higher blood pressures than European American males of the same age.
- *Gender.* After puberty, females usually have lower blood pressures than males of the same age; this difference is thought to be due to hormonal variations. After menopause, women generally have higher blood pressures than before.
- *Medications.* Many medications, including caffeine, may increase or decrease the blood pressure.
- *Obesity.* Both childhood and adult obesity predispose to hypertension.
- *Diurnal variations.* Pressure is usually lowest early in the morning, when the metabolic rate is lowest, then rises throughout the day and peaks in the late afternoon or early evening.
- *Disease process.* Any condition affecting the cardiac output, blood volume, blood viscosity, and/or compliance of the arteries has a direct effect on the blood pressure.

Hypertension

A blood pressure that is persistently above normal is called **hypertension.** A single elevated blood pressure reading indicates the need for reassessment. Hypertension cannot be diag-

TABLE 29–4 Classification of Blood Pressure

CATEGORY	SYSTOLIC BP MM HG		DIASTOLIC BP MM HG
Normal	<120	and	<80
Prehypertension	120–139	or	80–89
Hypertension, stage 1	140–159	or	90–99
Hypertension, stage 2	>160	or	>100

Note: From the "Seventh Report of the Joint National Committee for the Detection, Evaluation, and Treatment of High Blood Pressure," by National Institutes of Health, National Heart, Lung, and Blood Institute, 2004.

nosed unless an elevated blood pressure is found when measured twice at different times. It is usually asymptomatic and is often a contributing factor to myocardial infarctions (heart attacks). An elevated blood pressure of unknown cause is called *primary hypertension.* An elevated blood pressure of known cause is called *secondary hypertension.* Hypertension is a widespread health problem. Individuals with diastolic blood pressures of 80 to 89 mm Hg or systolic blood pressures of 120 to 139 mm Hg should be considered prehypertensive and, without intervention, may develop cardiac disease. Hypertension is when either the diastolic blood pressure is 90 mm Hg or higher or when the systolic blood pressure is higher than 140 mm Hg (see Table 29–4). The stage of hypertension is determined by the higher of the two values. For example, if either the systolic or diastolic values fall in the stage 2 range, stage 2 hypertension is assigned. Factors associated with hypertension include thickening of the arterial walls, which reduces the size of the arterial lumen, and inelasticity of the arteries as well as such lifestyle factors as cigarette smoking, obesity, heavy alcohol consumption, lack of physical exercise, high blood cholesterol levels, and continued exposure to stress. Follow-up care should include lifestyle changes conducive to lowering the blood pressure as well as monitoring the pressure itself.

Hypotension

Hypotension is a blood pressure that is below normal, that is, a systolic reading consistently between 85 and 110 mm Hg in an adult whose normal pressure is higher than this. **Orthostatic hypotension** is a blood pressure that falls when the client sits or stands. It is usually the result of peripheral vasodilatation in which blood leaves the central body organs, especially the brain, and moves to the periphery, often causing the person to feel faint. Hypotension can also be caused by analgesics such as meperidine hydrochloride (Demerol), bleeding, severe burns, and dehydration. It is important to monitor hypotensive clients carefully to prevent falls. When assessing for orthostatic hypotension:

- Place the client in a supine position for 10 minutes.
- Record the client's pulse and blood pressure.
- Assist the client to slowly sit or stand. Support the client in case of faintness.
- Immediately recheck the pulse and blood pressure in the same sites as previously.

- Repeat the pulse and blood pressure after 3 minutes.
- Record the results. A rise in pulse of 15 to 30 beats per minute or a drop in blood pressure of 20 mm Hg systolic or 10 mm Hg diastolic indicates orthostatic hypotension (Irvin & White, 2004).

Assessing Blood Pressure

Blood pressure is measured with a blood pressure cuff, a sphygmomanometer, and a stethoscope. The blood pressure cuff consists of a rubber bag that can be inflated with air called the bladder (Figure 29-17 ■). It is covered with cloth and has two tubes attached to it. One tube connects to a rubber bulb that inflates the bladder. A small valve on the side of this bulb traps and releases the air in the bladder.

The other tube is attached to a sphygmomanometer. The sphygmomanometer indicates the pressure of the air within the bladder. There are two types of sphygmomanometers: aneroid and digital. The aneroid sphygmomanometer is a calibrated dial with a needle that points to the calibrations (Figure 29-18 ■).

Many agencies use digital (electronic) sphygmomanometers (Figure 29-19 ■), which eliminate the need to listen for the sounds of the client's systolic and diastolic blood pressures through a stethoscope. Electronic blood pressure devices should be calibrated periodically to check accuracy. All health care facilities should have manual blood pressure equipment available as backup.

Doppler ultrasound stethoscopes are also used to assess blood pressure (see Figure 29-14 earlier in the chapter). These are of particular value when blood pressure sounds are difficult to hear, such as in infants, obese clients, and clients in shock. Systolic pressure may be the only blood pressure obtainable with some ultrasound models.

Figure 29-18 ■ An aneroid sphygmomanometer and cuff.

Figure 29-19 ■ Blood pressure monitors register systolic and diastolic blood pressures and often other vital signs.

(Patrick Watson)

Blood pressure cuffs come in various sizes because the bladder must be the correct width and length for the client's arm (Figure 29-20 ■). If the bladder is too narrow, the blood pressure reading will be erroneously elevated; if it is too wide, the reading will be erroneously low. The width should be 40% of the circumference, or 20% wider than the diameter of the midpoint, of the limb on which it is used. The arm circumference, not the age of the client, should always be used to determine bladder size. The nurse can determine whether the width of a blood pressure cuff is appropriate: Lay the cuff lengthwise at the midpoint of the upper arm, and hold the outermost side of the bladder edge laterally on the arm. With the other hand, wrap the width of the cuff around the arm, and ensure that the width is 40% of the arm circumference (Figure 29-21 ■).

The length of the bladder also affects the accuracy of measurement. The bladder should be sufficiently long to cover at least two-thirds of the limb's circumference.

Blood pressure cuffs are made of nondistensible material so that an even pressure is exerted around the limb. Most cuffs are held in place by hooks, snaps, or Velcro. Others have a cloth bandage that is long enough to encircle the limb several times;

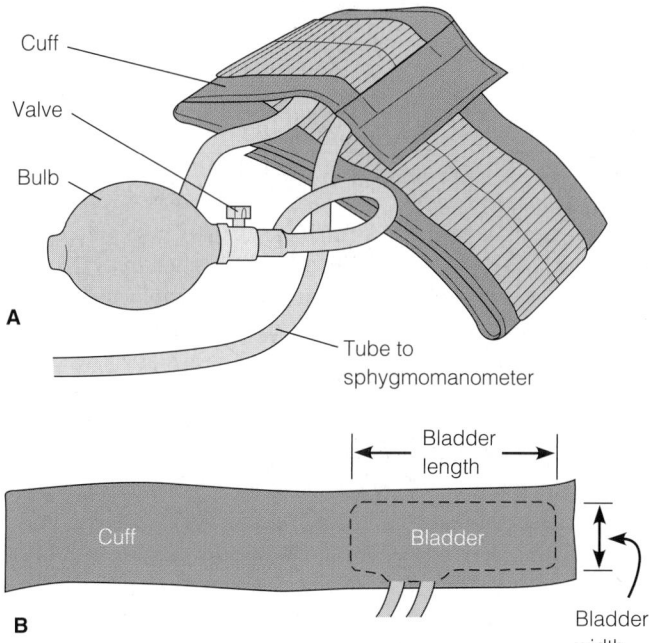

Figure 29-17 ■ *A*, A blood pressure cuff and bulb; *B*, the bladder inside the cuff.

Figure 29-20 ■ Three standard cuff sizes: a small cuff for an infant, small child, or frail adult; a normal adult-size cuff; and a large cuff for measuring the blood pressure on the leg or on the arm of an obese adult.

this type is closed by tucking the end of the bandage into one of the bandage folds.

Blood Pressure Sites

The blood pressure is usually assessed in the client's upper arm using the brachial artery and a standard stethoscope. Assessing the blood pressure on a client's thigh is indicated in these situations:

■ The blood pressure cannot be measured on either arm (e.g., because of burns or other trauma).

■ The blood pressure in one thigh is to be compared with the blood pressure in the other thigh.

Blood pressure is not measured on a particular client's limb in the following situations:

■ The shoulder, arm, or hand (or the hip, knee, or ankle) is injured or diseased.

■ A cast or bulky bandage is on any part of the limb.

■ The client has had surgical removal of axilla (or hip) lymph nodes on that side, such as for cancer.

■ The client has an intravenous infusion in that limb.

■ The client has an arteriovenous fistula (e.g., for renal dialysis) in that limb.

Methods

Blood pressure can be assessed directly or indirectly. Direct (invasive monitoring) measurement involves the insertion of a catheter into the brachial, radial, or femoral artery. Arterial pressure is represented as wavelike forms displayed on a monitor. With correct placement, this pressure reading is highly accurate.

Two noninvasive indirect methods of measuring blood pressure are the auscultatory and palpatory methods. The auscultatory method is most commonly used in hospitals, clinics, and homes. Required equipment is a sphygmomanometer, a cuff, and a stethoscope. When carried out correctly, the auscultatory method is relatively accurate.

When taking a blood pressure using a stethoscope, the nurse identifies phases in the series of sounds called **Korotkoff's**

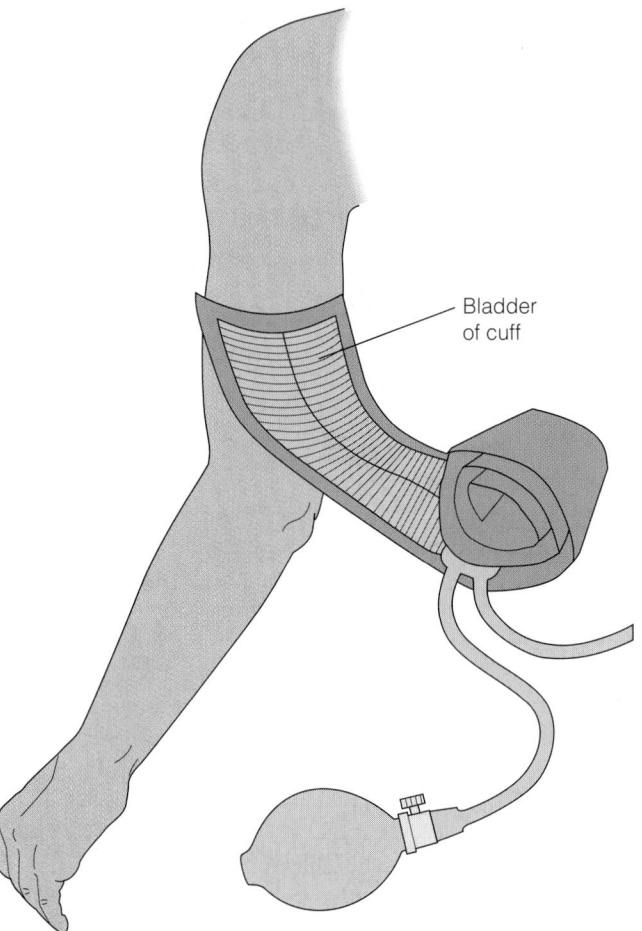

Figure 29-21 ■ Determining that the bladder of a blood pressure cuff is 40% of the arm circumference or 20% wider than the diameter of the midpoint of the limb.

sounds (Figure 29-22 ■). First the nurse pumps the cuff up to about 30 mm Hg above the point where the pulse is no longer felt; that is the point when the blood flow in the artery is stopped. Then the pressure is released slowly (2 to 3 mm Hg per second) while the nurse observes the readings on the manometer and relates them to the sounds heard through the stethoscope. Five phases occur but may not always be audible (see Box 29–6).

The palpatory method is sometimes used when Korotkoff's sounds cannot be heard and electronic equipment to amplify the sounds is not available, or to prevent misdirection from the presence of an auscultatory gap. An **auscultatory gap,** which occurs particularly in hypertensive clients, is the temporary disappearance of sounds normally heard over the brachial artery when the cuff pressure is high followed by the reappearance of the sounds at a lower level. This temporary disappearance of sounds occurs in the latter part of phase 1 and phase 2 and may cover a range of 40 mm Hg. If a palpated estimation of the systolic pressure is not made prior to auscultation, the nurse may begin listening in the middle of this range and underestimate the systolic pressure. In the palpatory method of blood pressure determination, instead of listening for the blood flow sounds, the nurse uses light to moderate pressure to palpate the pulsations of the artery as the pressure in the cuff is released. The pressure is read from the sphygmomanometer when the first pulsation is felt.

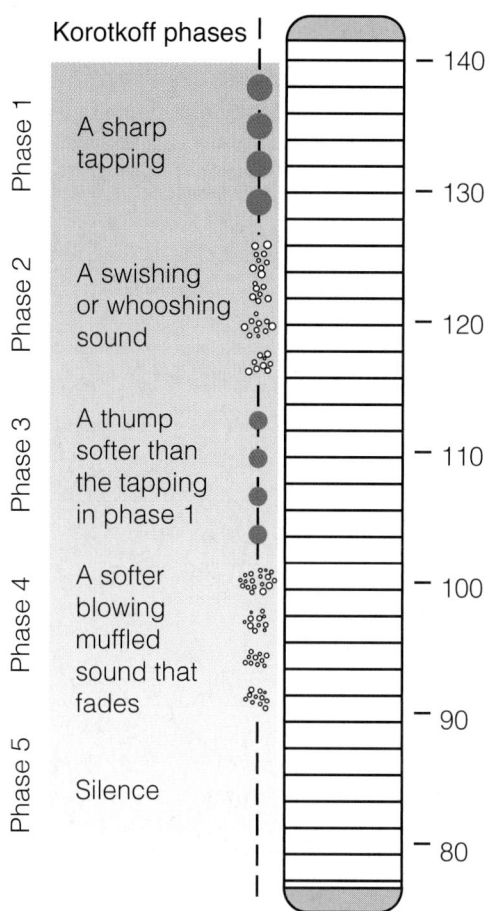

Korotkoff phases

Phase 1 — A sharp tapping — 140, 130

Phase 2 — A swishing or whooshing sound — 120

Phase 3 — A thump softer than the tapping in phase 1 — 110

Phase 4 — A softer blowing muffled sound that fades — 100, 90

Phase 5 — Silence — 80

Figure 29-22 ■ Korotkoff's sounds can be differentiated into five phases. In the illustration the blood pressure is 138/90 or 138/102/90.

BOX 29–6 Korotkoff's Sounds

■ *Phase 1* The pressure level at which the first faint, clear tapping or thumping sounds are heard. These sounds gradually become more intense. To ensure that they are not extraneous sounds, the nurse should identify at least two consecutive tapping sounds. The first tapping sound heard during deflation of the cuff is the systolic blood pressure.

■ *Phase 2* The period during deflation when the sounds have a muffled, whooshing, or swishing quality.

■ *Phase 3* The period during which the blood flows freely through an increasingly open artery and the sounds become crisper and more intense and again assume a thumping quality but softer than in phase 1.

■ *Phase 4* The time when the sounds become muffled and have a soft, blowing quality.

■ *Phase 5* The pressure level when the last sound is heard. This is followed by a period of silence. The pressure at which the last sound is heard is the diastolic blood pressure in adults.*

*In agencies where the fourth phase is considered the diastolic pressure, three measures are recommended (systolic pressure, diastolic pressure, and phase 5). These may be referred to as systolic, first diastolic, and second diastolic pressures. The phase 5 (second diastolic pressure) reading may be zero; that is, the muffled sounds are heard even when there is no air pressure in the blood pressure cuff. In some instances, muffled sounds are never heard, in which case a dash is inserted where the reading would normally be recorded (e.g.,/–/110).

Common Errors in Assessing Blood Pressure

The importance of the accuracy of blood pressure assessments cannot be overemphasized. Many judgments about a client's health are made on the basis of blood pressure. It is an important indicator of the client's condition and is used extensively as a basis for nursing interventions. Two possible reasons for blood pressure errors are haste on the part of the nurse and subconscious bias. For example, a nurse may be influenced by the client's previous blood pressure measurements or diagnosis and "hear" a value consonant with the practitioner's expectations. Some reasons for erroneous blood pressure readings are given in Table 29–5.

Skill 29-6 provides guidelines for assessing blood pressure.

TABLE 29–5 Selected Sources of Error in Blood Pressure Assessment

ERROR	EFFECT
Bladder cuff too narrow	Erroneously high
Bladder cuff too wide	Erroneously low
Arm unsupported	Erroneously high
Insufficient rest before the assessment	Erroneously high
Repeating assessment too quickly	Erroneously high systolic or low diastolic readings
Cuff wrapped too loosely or unevenly	Erroneously high
Deflating cuff too quickly	Erroneously low systolic and high diastolic readings
Deflating cuff too slowly	Erroneously high diastolic reading
Failure to use the same arm consistently	Inconsistent measurements
Arm above level of the heart	Erroneously low
Assessing immediately after a meal or while client smokes or has pain	Erroneously high
Failure to identify auscultatory gap	Erroneously low systolic pressure and erroneously low diastolic pressure

SKILL 29-6

ASSESSING BLOOD PRESSURE

PURPOSES
- To obtain a baseline measure of arterial blood pressure for subsequent evaluation
- To determine the client's hemodynamic status (e.g., cardiac output: stroke volume of the heart and blood vessel resistance)
- To identify and monitor changes in blood pressure resulting from a disease process or medical therapy (e.g., presence or history of cardiovascular disease, renal disease, circulatory shock, or acute pain; rapid infusion of fluids or blood products)

ASSESSMENT
Assess
- Signs and symptoms of hypertension (e.g., headache, ringing in the ears, flushing of face, nosebleeds, fatigue)
- Signs and symptoms of hypotension (e.g., tachycardia, dizziness, mental confusion, restlessness, cool and clammy skin, pale or cyanotic skin)
- Factors affecting blood pressure (e.g., activity, emotional stress, pain, and time the client last smoked or ingested caffeine)
- Some blood pressure cuffs contain latex. Assess the client for latex allergy and obtain a latex-free cuff if indicated.

PLANNING

Delegation
Blood pressure measurement may be delegated to UAP. The interpretation of abnormal blood pressure readings and determination of appropriate responses are done by the nurse.

Equipment
- Stethoscope or DUS
- Blood pressure cuff of the appropriate size
- Sphygmomanometer

IMPLEMENTATION
Preparation
1. Ensure that the equipment is intact and functioning properly. Check for leaks in the tubing of the sphygmomanometer.
2. Make sure that the client has not smoked or ingested caffeine within 30 minutes prior to measurement. **Rationale:** *Smoking constricts blood vessels, and caffeine increases the pulse rate. Both of these cause a temporary increase in blood pressure.*

Performance
1. Prior to performing the procedure, introduce self and verify the client's identity using agency protocol. Explain to the client what you are going to do, why it is necessary, and how he or she can cooperate. Discuss how the results will be used in planning further care or treatments.
2. Perform hand hygiene and observe appropriate infection control procedures.
3. Provide for client privacy.
4. Position the client appropriately.
   - The adult client should be sitting unless otherwise specified. Both feet should be flat on the floor. **Rationale:** *Legs crossed at the knee result in elevated systolic and diastolic blood pressures* (Pinar, Sabuncu, & Oksay, 2004).
   - The elbow should be slightly flexed with the palm of the hand facing up and the forearm supported at heart level. Readings in any other position should be specified. The blood pressure is normally similar in sitting, standing, and lying positions, but it can vary significantly by position in certain persons. **Rationale:** *The blood pressure increases when the arm is below heart level and decreases when the arm is above heart level.*
   - Expose the upper arm.
5. Wrap the deflated cuff evenly around the upper arm. Locate the brachial artery (see page 538). Apply the center of the bladder directly over the artery. **Rationale:** *The bladder inside the cuff must be directly over the artery to be compressed if the reading is to be accurate.*
   - For an adult, place the lower border of the cuff approximately 2.5 cm (1 in.) above the antecubital space.
6. If this is the client's initial examination, perform a preliminary palpatory determination of systolic pressure. **Rationale:** *The initial estimate tells the nurse the maximal pressure to which the manometer needs to be elevated in subsequent determinations. It also prevents underestimation of the systolic pressure or overestimation of the diastolic pressure should an auscultatory gap occur.*
   - Palpate the brachial artery with the fingertips.
   - Close the valve on the bulb.
   - Pump up the cuff until you no longer feel the brachial pulse. At that pressure the blood cannot flow through the artery. Note the pressure on the sphygmomanometer at which pulse is no longer felt. **Rationale:** *This gives an estimate of the systolic pressure.*
   - Release the pressure completely in the cuff, and wait 1 to 2 minutes before making further measurements. **Rationale:** *A waiting period gives the blood trapped in the veins time to be released. Otherwise, false high systolic readings will occur.*
7. Position the stethoscope appropriately.
   - Cleanse the earpieces with antiseptic wipe.
   - Insert the ear attachments of the stethoscope in your ears so that they tilt slightly forward. **Rationale:** *Sounds are heard more clearly when the ear attachments follow the direction of the ear canal.*
   - Ensure that the stethoscope hangs freely from the ears to the diaphragm. **Rationale:** *If the stethoscope tubing rubs against an object, the noise can block the sounds of the blood within the artery.*
   - Place the bell side of the amplifier of the stethoscope over the brachial pulse site. **Rationale:** *Because the blood pressure is a low-frequency sound, it is best heard with the bell-shaped diaphragm.*
   - Place the stethoscope directly on the skin, not on clothing over the site. **Rationale:** *This is to avoid noise made from rubbing the amplifier against cloth.*
   - Hold the diaphragm with the thumb and index finger.
8. Auscultate the client's blood pressure.

ASSESSING BLOOD PRESSURE *continued*

- Pump up the cuff until the sphygmomanometer reads 30 mm Hg above the point where the brachial pulse disappeared.
- Release the valve on the cuff carefully so that the pressure decreases at the rate of 2 to 3 mm Hg per second. **Rationale:** *If the rate is faster or slower, an error in measurement may occur.*
- As the pressure falls, identify the manometer reading at Korotkoff phases I, IV, and V. **Rationale:** *There is no clinical significance to phases II and III* (Pickering et al., 2005).
- Deflate the cuff rapidly and completely.
- Wait 1 to 2 minutes before making further determinations. **Rationale:** *This permits blood trapped in the veins to be released.*
- Repeat the above steps to confirm the accuracy of the reading—especially if it falls outside the normal range (although this may not be routine procedure for hospitalized or well clients). If there is > 5 mm Hg difference between the two readings, additional measurements may be taken and the results averaged (Pickering et al., 2005).

9. If this is the client's initial examination, repeat the procedure on the client's other arm. There should be a difference of no more than 10 mm Hg between the arms. The arm found to have the higher pressure should be used for subsequent examinations.

Variation: Obtaining a Blood Pressure by the Palpation Method

If it is not possible to use a stethoscope to obtain the blood pressure or if the Korotkoff sounds cannot be heard, palpate the radial or brachial pulse site as the cuff pressure is released. The manometer reading at the point where the pulse reappears represents a value between auscultated systolic and diastolic values.

Variation: Taking a Thigh Blood Pressure

- Help the client to assume a prone position. If the client cannot assume this position, measure the blood pressure while the client is in a supine position with the knee slightly flexed. Slight flexing of the knee will facilitate placing the stethoscope on the popliteal space. ❶
- Expose the thigh, taking care not to expose the client unduly.
- Locate the popliteal artery (Figure 29-12).
- Wrap the cuff evenly around the midthigh with the compression bladder over the posterior aspect of the thigh and the bottom edge above the knee. **Rationale:** *The bladder must be directly over the posterior popliteal artery if the reading is to be accurate.*
- If this is the client's initial examination, perform a preliminary palpatory determination of systolic pressure by palpating the popliteal artery.
- In adults, the systolic pressure in the popliteal artery is usually 20 to 30 mm Hg higher than that in the brachial artery because of use of a larger bladder; the diastolic pressure is usually the same.

❶ Measuring blood pressure in the client's thigh—location of the popliteal artery and application of the cuff.

Variation: Using an Electronic Indirect Blood Pressure Monitoring Device (Figure 29-19)

- Place the blood pressure cuff on the extremity according to the manufacturer's guidelines.
- Turn on the blood pressure switch.
- If appropriate, set the device for the desired number of minutes between blood pressure determinations.
- When the device has determined the blood pressure reading, note the digital results.

CLINICAL ALERT

Electronic/automatic blood pressure cuffs can be left in place for many hours. Remove the cuff and check skin condition periodically. ■

10. Remove the cuff.
11. Wipe the cuff with an approved disinfectant. **Rationale:** *Cuffs can become significantly contaminated.* Many institutions use disposable blood pressure cuffs. The client uses it for the length of stay and then it is discarded. This decreases the risk of spreading infection by sharing cuffs.
12. Document and report pertinent assessment data according to agency policy. Record two pressures in the form "130/80" where "130" is the systolic (phase 1) and "80" is the diastolic (phase 5) pressure. Record three pressures in the form "130/90/0," where "130" is the systolic, "90" is the first diastolic (phase 4), and sounds are audible even after the cuff is completely deflated (Pickering et al., 2005). Use the abbreviations RA or RL for right arm or right leg and LA or LL for left arm or left leg. Record a difference of greater than 10 mm Hg between the two arms or legs.

EVALUATION

- Relate blood pressure to other vital signs, to baseline data, and to health status.
- Report any significant change in the client's blood pressure. Also report these findings:
  - Systolic blood pressure (of an adult) above 120 mm Hg
  - Diastolic blood pressure (of an adult) above 80 mm Hg
  - Systolic blood pressure (of an adult) below 100 mm Hg
- Conduct appropriate follow-up such as administration of medication. If the blood pressure is significantly higher or lower than usual, implement appropriate safety precautions.

LIFESPAN CONSIDERATIONS Blood Pressure

INFANTS

- Use a pediatric stethoscope with a small diaphragm.
- The lower edge of the blood pressure cuff can be closer to the antecubital space of an infant.
- Use the palpation method if auscultation with a stethoscope or DUS is unsuccessful.
- Arm and thigh pressures are equivalent in children under 1 year of age.
- One quick way to determine the normal systolic blood pressure of a child is to use the following formula:

    Normal systolic BP = 80 + (2 × child's age in years)

CHILDREN

- Blood pressure should be measured in all children over 3 years of age and in children under 3 years of age with certain medical conditions (e.g., congenital heart disease, renal malformation, medications that affect blood pressure).
- Explain each step of the process and what it will feel like. Demonstrate on a doll.
- Use the palpation technique for children under 3 years old.
- Cuff bladder width should be 40% and length should be 80% to 100% of the arm circumference (Figure 29-23 ■).
- Take the blood pressure prior to other uncomfortable procedures so that the blood pressure is not artificially elevated by the discomfort.
- In children, the diastolic pressure is considered to be the onset of phase 4, where the sounds become muffled.
- In children, the thigh pressure is about 10 mm Hg higher than the arm.

Figure 29-23 ■ Pediatric blood pressure cuffs (with manometers).

ELDERS

- Skin may be very fragile. Do not allow cuff pressure to remain high any longer than necessary.
- Determine if the client is taking antihypertensives and, if so, when the last dose was taken.
- Medications that cause vasodilation (antihypertensive medications) along with the loss of baroreceptor efficiency in the elderly place them at increased risk for having orthostatic hypotension. Measuring blood pressure while the client is in the lying, sitting, and standing positions, and noting any changes can determine this.
- If the client has arm contractures, assess the blood pressure by palpation, with the arm in a relaxed position. If this is not possible, take a thigh blood pressure.

HOME CARE CONSIDERATIONS Blood Pressure

- If the client takes blood pressure readings at home, use the same equipment or calibrate it against a system known to be accurate.
- Observe the client or family member taking the blood pressure and provide feedback if further instruction is needed.
- Home blood pressure measurement done by the client or family can detect elevated pressures not identified when the client is seen in a medical office (Bobrie et al., 2004).
- If the client is in a chair or low bed, position yourself so that you maintain the client's arm at heart level and you can read the sphygmomanometer at eye level.

OXYGEN SATURATION

A **pulse oximeter** is a noninvasive device that estimates a client's arterial blood oxygen saturation (SaO_2) by means of a sensor attached to the client's finger (Figure 29-24 ■), toe, nose, earlobe, or forehead (or around the hand or foot of a neonate). The pulse oximeter can detect hypoxemia before clinical signs and symptoms, such as dusky skin color and dusky nailbeds color develop.

The pulse oximeter's sensor has two parts: (a) two light-emitting diodes (LEDs)—one red, the other infrared—that transmit light through nails, tissue, venous blood, and arterial blood; and (b) a photodetector placed directly opposite the LEDs (e.g., the other side of the finger, toe, or nose). The photodetector measures the amount of red and infrared light absorbed by oxygenated and deoxygenated hemoglobin in peripheral arterial blood and reports it as SpO_2. Normal SaO_2 is 95% to 100%, and an SaO_2 below 70% is life threatening. The values for SaO_2 and SpO_2 are the same.

Pulse oximeters with various types of sensors are available from several manufacturers. The oximeter unit consists of an inlet connection for the sensor cable, and a faceplate that indicates (a) the oxygen saturation measurement (expressed as a percentage) and (b) the pulse rate. Cordless units are also available (Figure 29-25 ■). A preset alarm system signals high and low SpO_2 measurements and a high and low pulse rate. The high and low SpO_2 levels are generally preset at 100% and 85%, respectively, for adults. The high and low pulse rate alarms are usually preset at 140 and 50 BPM for adults. These alarm limits can, however, be changed according to the manufacturer's directions.

Factors Affecting Oxygen Saturation Readings

- *Hemoglobin.* If the hemoglobin is fully saturated with oxygen, the SaO_2 will appear normal even if the total

Figure 29-24 ■ Fingertip oximeter sensor (adult).

hemoglobin level is low. Thus, the client could be severely anemic and have inadequate oxygen to supply the tissues but the pulse oximeter would return a normal value.

■ *Circulation.* The oximeter will not return an accurate reading if the area under the sensor has impaired circulation.

■ *Activity.* Shivering or excessive movement of the sensor site may interfere with accurate readings.

■ *Carbon monoxide poisoning.* Pulse oximeters cannot discriminate between hemoglobin saturated with carbon

Figure 29-25 ■ Fingertip oximeter sensor (cordless).
(Courtesy of Nonin Medical, Inc.)

monoxide versus oxygen. In this case, other measures of oxygenation are needed.

Skill 29-7 outlines the steps in measuring oxygen saturation.

MEASURING OXYGEN SATURATION

SKILL 29-7

PURPOSES
■ To estimate the arterial blood oxygen saturation (SaO_2)

■ To detect the presence of hypoxemia before visible signs develop

ASSESSMENT
Assess
■ The best location for a pulse oximeter sensor based on the client's age and physical condition (Unless contraindicated, the finger is usually selected for adults.)

■ The client's overall condition including risk factors for development of hypoxemia (e.g., respiratory or cardiac disease) and hemoglobin level
■ Vital signs, skin color and temperature, nail bed color, and tissue perfusion of extremities as baseline data
■ Adhesive allergy

PLANNING
Many hospitals and clinics have pulse oximeters readily available for use with other vital signs equipment (or even as an integrated part of the electronic blood pressure device). Other facilities may have a limited supply of oximeters, and the nurse may need to request it from the central supply department.

Delegation
Application of the pulse oximeter sensor and recording of the SpO_2 value may be delegated to UAP. The interpretation of the oxygen saturation value and determination of appropriate responses are done by the nurse.

Equipment
■ Nail polish remover as needed
■ Alcohol wipe
■ Sheet or towel
■ Pulse oximeter

IMPLEMENTATION
Preparation
Check that the oximeter equipment is functioning normally.

Performance
1. Prior to performing the procedure, introduce self and verify the client's identity using agency protocol. Explain to the client what

continued on page 560

SKILL 29-7

MEASURING OXYGEN SATURATION *continued*

you are going to do, why it is necessary, and how he or she can cooperate. Discuss how the results will be used in planning further care or treatments.

2. Perform hand hygiene and observe appropriate infection control procedures.

3. Provide for client privacy.

4. Choose a sensor appropriate for the client's weight, size, and desired location. Because weight limits of sensors overlap, a pediatric sensor could be used for a small adult.
   - If the client is allergic to adhesive, use a clip or sensor without adhesive. If using an extremity, assess the proximal pulse and capillary refill at the point closest to the site.
   - If the client has low tissue perfusion due to peripheral vascular disease or therapy using vasoconstrictive medications, use a nasal sensor or a reflectance sensor on the forehead. Avoid using lower extremities that have a compromised circulation and extremities that are used for infusions or other invasive monitoring.

5. Prepare the site.
   - Clean the site with an alcohol wipe before applying the sensor.
   - It may be necessary to remove a female client's dark nail polish. **Rationale:** *It can interfere with accurate measurements.*
   - Alternatively, position the sensor on the side of the finger rather than perpendicular to the nail bed (Chan, Chan, & Chan, 2003).

6. Apply the sensor, and connect it to the pulse oximeter.
   - Make sure the LED and photodetector are accurately aligned, that is, opposite each other on either side of the finger, toe, nose, or earlobe. Many sensors have markings to facilitate correct alignment of the LEDs and photodetector.
   - Attach the sensor cable to the connection outlet on the oximeter. Turn on the machine according to the manufacturer's directions. Appropriate connection will be confirmed by an

audible beep indicating each arterial pulsation. Some devices have a wheel that can be turned clockwise to increase the pulse volume and counterclockwise to decrease it.
   - Ensure that the bar of light or waveform on the face of the oximeter fluctuates with each pulsation.

7. Set and turn on the alarm when using continuous monitoring.
   - Check the preset alarm limits for high and low oxygen saturation and high and low pulse rates. Change these alarm limits according to the manufacturer's directions as indicated. Ensure that the audio and visual alarms are on before you leave the client. A tone will be heard and a number will blink on the faceplate.

8. Ensure client safety.
   - Inspect and/or move or change the location of an adhesive toe or finger sensor every 4 hours and a spring-tension sensor every 2 hours.
   - Inspect the sensor site tissues for irritation from adhesive sensors.

9. Ensure the accuracy of measurement.
   - Minimize motion artifacts by using an adhesive sensor, or immobilize the client's monitoring site. **Rationale:** *Movement of the client's finger or toe may be misinterpreted by the oximeter as arterial pulsations.*
   - If indicated, cover the sensor with a sheet or towel to block large amounts of light from external sources (e.g., sunlight, procedure lamps, or bilirubin lights in the nursery). **Rationale:** *Bright room light may be sensed by the photodetector and alter the SpO$_2$ value* (Popovich, Richiuso, & Danek, 2004).
   - Compare the pulse rate indicated by the oximeter to the radial pulse periodically. **Rationale:** *A large discrepancy between the two values may indicate oximeter malfunction.*

10. Document the oxygen saturation on the appropriate record at designated intervals.

EVALUATION

■ Compare the oxygen saturation to the client's previous oxygen saturation level. Relate to pulse rate and other vital signs.

■ Conduct appropriate follow-up such as notifying the primary care provider, adjusting oxygen therapy, or providing breathing treatments.

MediaLink Client with Pneumonia Care Plan Activity

LIFESPAN CONSIDERATIONS Pulse Oximetry

INFANTS

■ If an appropriate-sized finger or toe sensor (Figure 29-26 ■) is not available, consider using an earlobe or forehead sensor.

■ The high and low SpO$_2$ levels are generally preset at 95% and 80% for neonates.

■ The high and low pulse rate alarms are usually preset at 200 and 100 for neonates.

■ The oximeter may need to be taped, wrapped with an elastic bandage, or covered by a stocking to keep it in place.

CHILDREN

■ Instruct the child that the sensor does not hurt. Disconnect the probe whenever possible to allow for movement.

ELDERS

■ Use of vasoconstrictive medications, poor circulation, or thickened nails may make finger or toe sensors inaccurate.

Figure 29-26 ■ Fingertip oximeter sensor (child).
(Courtesy of Nonin Medical, Inc.)

HOME CARE CONSIDERATIONS **Pulse Oximetry**

■ Pulse oximetry is a quick, inexpensive, noninvasive method of assessing oxygenation. Like an automatic blood pressure cuff, it also provides a pulse rate reading. Use in the ambulatory or home setting whenever indicated.

■ If the client requires frequent or continuous home monitoring, teach the client and family how to apply and maintain the equipment. Remind them to rotate the site periodically and assess for skin trauma.

RESEARCH NOTE **What Do Health Care Providers Know About Pulse Oximetry?**

This study assessed knowledge of pulse oximetry and interpretation of the data given. Sixty-eight nurses, respiratory therapists, and resident physicians at a large general pediatric unit of a children's hospital were surveyed. The majority (84%) felt they received adequate training in the use of the device; 84% correctly identified what a pulse oximeter measured; 40% correctly identified how a pulse oximeter worked; but only 15% had a correct understanding of the physiology of oxygen saturation of hemoglobin. Clinicians identified a wide range of normal arterial oxygen saturation values and made numerous errors in evaluating saturation readings in hypothetical clinical situations.

IMPLICATIONS

Although this study was conducted in a pediatric setting, it is likely that similar findings would result from a study of health care providers of adults. It is worrisome that so few providers understood the underlying processes involved in what the device measures. Even 16% of the providers not feeling adequately trained in use of the monitor or correct in regard to what the device measures is also of concern. The results indicate a strong need for enhanced orientation and training. In addition, the study was self-report only. It would also be beneficial to observe health care providers' use of the device to ensure that they are applying and reading it accurately.

Note: From "Pediatric Health Care Providers' Knowledge of Pulse Oximetry" by D. M. Popovich, N. Richiuso, & G. Danek, 2004, *Pediatric Nursing, 30*(1), pp. 14–20.

CRITICAL THINKING CHECKPOINT

1. When you approach your elderly client to take her blood pressure, she tells you she doesn't want you to take it. What questions will you ask the client at this time?
2. After much exploration, the client agrees to let you take the blood pressure. After pumping up the cuff, you are unable to hear any sounds during release of the valve. What would you say to her?
3. Once you are able to measure the blood pressure, your reading is 180/110. Before taking any action on this blood pressure, what do you need to know?
4. The pulse oximeter on the client's finger reads 85%. Her skin is warm and has normal color, she is awake and oriented, temperature is 37.1°C (98.8°F), and apical pulse is 78. What would be your next actions and why?

See Critical Thinking Possibilities in Appendix A. ∞

CHAPTER 29 **REVIEW**

CHAPTER HIGHLIGHTS

■ Vital signs reflect changes in body function that otherwise might not be observed.
■ Body temperature is the balance between heat produced by the body and heat lost from the body.
■ Factors affecting body temperature include age, diurnal variations, exercise, hormones, stress, and environmental temperatures.
■ Four common types of fever are intermittent, remittent, relapsing, and constant.
■ During a fever, the set point of the hypothalamic thermostat changes suddenly from the normal level to a higher than normal level, but several hours elapse before the core temperature reaches the new set point.
■ Hypothermia involves three mechanisms: excessive heat loss, inadequate heat production by body cells, and increasing impairment of hypothalamic thermoregulation.
■ The nurse selects the most appropriate site to measure temperature according to the client's age and condition.

■ Pulse rate and volume reflect the stroke volume output, the compliance of the client's arteries, and the adequacy of blood flow.
■ Normally a peripheral pulse reflects the client's heartbeat, but it may differ from the heartbeat in clients with certain cardiovascular diseases; in these instances, the nurse takes an apical pulse and compares it to the peripheral pulse.
■ Many factors may affect a person's pulse rate: age, gender, exercise, presence of fever, certain medications, hypovolemia, stress (in some situations), position changes, and pathology.
■ Although the radial pulse is the site most commonly used, eight other sites may be used in certain situations.
■ The difference between the apical and radial pulses is called pulse deficit.

- Respirations are normally quiet, effortless, and automatic and are assessed by observing respiratory rate, depth, rhythm, quality, and effectiveness.
- Blood pressure reflects cardiac output, peripheral vascular resistance, blood volume, and blood viscosity.
- Among the factors influencing blood pressure are age, exercise, stress, race, gender, medications, obesity, diurnal variations, and disease processes.

- Orthostatic hypotension occurs when the blood pressure falls as the client assumes an upright position.
- A blood pressure cuff too large or too small will give false readings.
- During blood pressure measurement, the artery must be held at heart level.
- A pulse oximeter measures the percent of hemoglobin saturated with oxygen. A normal result is 95% to 100%.
- Pulse oximeter sensors may be placed on the finger, hand, foot, or nose.

TEST YOUR KNOWLEDGE

1. The client's temperature at 8:00 AM using an oral electronic thermometer is 36.1°C (97.2°F). If the respiration, pulse, and blood pressure are within normal range, what would the nurse do *next*?
   1. Wait 15 minutes and retake it.
   2. Check what the client's temperature was the last time.
   3. Retake it using a different thermometer.
   4. Chart the temperature; it is normal.

2. Which of the following clients meets the criteria for selection of the apical site for assessment of the pulse rather than a radial pulse?
   1. A client is in shock
   2. The pulse changes with body position changes
   3. A client with an arrhythmia
   4. It is less than 24 hours since a client's surgical operation

3. When the nurse enters the room to measure vital signs in preparing the client for a diagnostic test, the client is on the phone. What technique should the nurse use to determine the respiratory rate?
   1. Count the respirations during conversational pauses.
   2. Ask the client to end the phone call now and resume it at a later time.
   3. Wait at the client's bedside until the phone call is completed and then count respirations.
   4. Since there is no evidence of distress or urgency, defer the measurement.

4. For a client with a previous blood pressure of 138/74 and pulse of 64, approximately how long should the nurse take to release the blood pressure cuff in order to obtain an accurate reading?
   1. 10–20 seconds
   2. 30–45 seconds
   3. 1–1.5 minutes
   4. 3–3.5 minutes

5. It would be appropriate to delegate the taking of vital signs of which of the following clients to a UAP?
   1. A client being prepared for elective facial surgery with a history of stable hypertension
   2. A client receiving a blood transfusion with a history of transfusion reactions
   3. A client recently started on a new antiarrhythmic agent
   4. A client who is admitted frequently with asthma attacks

6. An 85-year-old client has had a stroke resulting in right-sided facial drooping, difficulty swallowing, and is unable to move self or maintain position unaided. The nurse determines that which of the following sites is appropriate for taking the temperature (select all that apply)?
   1. Oral
   2. Rectal

3. Axillary
4. Tympanic
5. Temporal artery

7. A nursing diagnosis of *Ineffective Peripheral Tissue Perfusion* would be validated by which one of the following:
   1. Bounding radial pulse
   2. Irregular apical pulse
   3. Carotid pulse stronger on the left side than the right
   4. Absent posterior tibial and pedal pulses

8. The nurse reports that the client has dyspnea when ambulating. The nurse is most likely to have assessed which of the following?
   1. Shallow respirations
   2. Wheezing
   3. Shortness of breath
   4. Coughing up blood

9. When auscultating the blood pressure, the nurse hears the following:
   From 200 mm Hg to 180 mm Hg: silence; then:
   a thumping sound continuing down to 150 mm Hg:
   muffled sounds continuing down to 130 mm Hg;
   soft thumping sounds continuing down to 105 mm Hg;
   muffled sounds continuing down to 95 mm Hg;
   then silence

The nurse records the blood pressure as _____.

10. In Figure 29-27 ■, which number indicates the client's oxygen saturation as measured by pulse oximetry? _____

Figure 29-27 ■ Vital signs monitor.

(Patrick Watson)

See Answers to Test Your Knowledge in Appendix A. ∞

EXPLORE MEDIALINK www.prenhall.com/berman

DVD-ROM
- Audio Glossary
- NCLEX Review
- Skills Checklists
- Animation: Digoxin

COMPANION WEBSITE
- Additional NCLEX Review
- Case Study: Assessing Vital Signs
- Care Plan Activity: Client with Pneumonia
- Application Activity: Joanna Briggs Institute
- Links to Resources

READINGS AND REFERENCES

SUGGESTED READINGS

U.S. Preventive Services Task Force. (2004). Screening for high blood pressure: Recommendations and rationale. *American Journal of Nursing, 104*(11), 82–85, 87.
This is the official statement updating the 1996 recommendations from the Guide to Clinical Preventive Services. *It recommends screening for high blood pressure in all individuals over age 18 but is neutral on screening those younger than 18. The report contains data supporting or refuting recommendations in the areas of epidemiology, accuracy and reliability of screening tests, effectiveness of early treatment, and potential harms of screening and treatment.*

Woodrow, P. (2004). Assessing blood pressure in older people. *Nursing Older People, 16*(1), 29–31.
This is a clear, concise review of the physiological issues of blood pressure monitoring in elders. The author reviews factors affecting blood pressure; the accuracy of devices; impact of aging and age-related factors on systolic, diastolic, mean, and pulse pressure; and orthostatic blood pressures.

RELATED RESEARCH

Smith, L. S. (2004). Temperature measurement in critical care adults: A comparison of thermometry and measurement routes. *Biological Research for Nursing, 6*(2), 117–125.

Sund Levander, M., Grodzinsky, E., Loyd, D., & Wahren, L. K. (2004). Errors in body temperature assessment related to individual variation, measuring technique and equipment. *International Journal of Nursing Practice, 10*, 216–223.

REFERENCES

Bindler, R. C., & Ball, J. W. (2003). *Clinical skills manual for pediatric nursing: Caring for children* (3rd ed.). Upper Saddle River, NJ: Prentice Hall Health.

Bobrie, G., Chatellier, G., Genes, N., Clerson, P., Vaur, L., Vaisse, B., et al. (2004). Cardiovascular prognosis of "masked hypertension" detected by blood pressure self-measurement in elderly treated hypertensive patients. *Journal of the American Medical Association, 291*, 1342–1349.

Chan, M. M., Chan, M. D., & Chan, E. D. (2003). What is the effect of nail polish on pulse oximetry? *Chest, 123*, 2163–2164.

DuBois, E. F. (1948). *Fever and the regulation of body temperature.* Springfield, IL: Charles C. Thomas.

Irvin, D. J., & White, M. (2004). The importance of accurately assessing orthostatic hypotension. *Geriatric Nursing, 25*, 99–101.

Liu, C. C., Chang, R. E., & Chang, W. C. (2004). Limitations of forehead infrared body temperature detection for fever screening for severe acute respiratory syndrome. *Infection Control Hospital Epidemiology, 25*, 1109–1111.

Mackowiak, P. A., Wasserman, S. S., & Levine, M. M. (1992). A critical appraisal of 98.6 degrees F, the upper limit of the normal body temperature, and other legacies of Carl Reinhold August Wunderlich. *Journal of the American Medical Association, 268*, 1578–1580.

Marieb, E. N. & Hoehn, K. (2007). *Human anatomy and physiology* (7th ed.). San Francisco: Benjamin Cummings.

National Institutes of Health, National Heart, Lung, and Blood Institute. (2004). *The seventh report of the Joint National Committee on Prevention, Detection, Evaluation, and Treatment of High Blood Pressure* (NIH Publication No. 04–5230). Retrieved May 19, 2006, from http://www.nhlbi.nih.gov/guidelines/hypertension/jnc7full.htm

Nimah, M. M., Bshesh, K., Callahan, J., & Jacobs, B. R. (2006). Infrared tympanic thermometry in comparison with other temperature measurement techniques in febrile children. *Pediatric Critical Care Medicine, 7*, 48–55.

Pickering, T. G., Hall, J. E., Appel, L. J., Falkner, B. E., Graves, J., Hill, M. N., et al. (2005). Recommendations for blood pressure measurement in humans and experimental animals: Part 1: Blood pressure measurement in humans: A statement for professionals from the Subcommittee of Professional and Public Education of the American Heart Association Council on High Blood Pressure Research. *Circulation, 111*, 697–716.

Pinar, R., Sabuncu, N., & Oksay, A. (2004). Effects of crossed leg on blood pressure. *Blood Pressure, 13*, 252–254.

Popovich, D. M., Richiuso, N., & Danek, G. (2004). Pediatric health care providers' knowledge of pulse oximetry. *Pediatric Nursing, 30*(1), 14–20.

Roy, S., Powell, K., & Gerson, L. W. (2003). Temporal artery temperature measurements in healthy infants, children, and adolescents. *Clinical Pediatrics, 42*, 433–437.

SELECTED BIBLIOGRAPHY

Artinian, N. T. (2004). Innovations in blood pressure monitoring, new, automated devices provide in home or around the clock readings. *American Journal of Nursing, 104*(8), 52–60.

Davidhizar, R., & Shearer, R. (2004). Assisting patients to maintain a healthy blood pressure. *Journal of Practical Nursing, 54*(3), 5–8.

Kempainen, R. R., & Brunette, D. D. (2004). The evaluation and management of accidental hypothermia. *Respiratory Care, 49*, 192–205.

Rushing, J. (2004). Clinical do's & don'ts. Taking blood pressure accurately. *Nursing, 34*(11), 26.

Rushing, J. (2005). Clinical do's & don'ts. Assessing for orthostatic hypotension. *Nursing, 35*(1), 30.

Sclater, A., & Kannayiram. A. (2004). Orthostatic hypotension: A primary care primer for assessment and treatment. *Geriatrics, 59*(8), 22–27.

Smith, L. S. (2004). Temperature monitoring in newborns, a comparison of thermometry and measurement sites. *Journal of Neonatal Nursing, 10*, 157–165.

Viverais-Dresler, G., & Bakker, D. A. (2004). Blood pressure monitoring: Older adults' perceptions. *Journal of Gerontological Nursing, 30*, 44–52.

Woods, A. (2004). Loosening the grip of hypertension. *Nursing, 34*(12), 36–43.

CHAPTER 30

Health Assessment

LEARNING OUTCOMES

After completing this chapter, you will be able to:

1. Identify the purposes of the physical examination.

2. Explain the four methods used in physical examination.

3. Explain the significance of selected physical findings.

4. Identify expected outcomes of health assessment.

5. Identify the steps in selected examination procedures.

6. Describe suggested sequencing to conduct a physical health examination in an orderly fashion.

7. Discuss variations in examination techniques appropriate for clients of different ages.

adventitious breath sounds, *613*
alopecia, *581*
angle of Louis, *611*
antihelix, *594*
aphasia, *642*
astigmatism, *586*
auricle, *594*
auscultation, *571*
blanch test, *583*
bruit, *620*
caries, *601*
cataracts, *586*
cerumen, *595*
clubbing, *582*
cochlea, *595*
conduction hearing loss, *595*
conjunctivitis, *586*
crepitations, *613*
cyanosis, *576*
dacryocystitis, *586*
diastole, *619*
dullness, *571*
duration, *571*
edema, *576*
erythema, *576*
eustachian tube, *595*
exophthalmos, *584*
external auditory meatus, *594*
extinction, *643*
flatness, *571*
gingivitis, *601*
glaucoma, *586*
glossitis, *601*

goniometer, *641*
helix, *594*
hernia, *657*
hordeolum (sty), *586*
hyperopia, *586*
hyperresonance, *571*
incus, *595*
inspection, *568*
intensity, *571*
intention tremor, *639*
jaundice, *576*
lift, *619*
lobule, *594*
malleus, *595*
manubrium, *611*
mastoid, *594*
miosis, *587*
mixed hearing loss, *595*
mydriasis, *587*
myopia, *586*
normocephalic, *584*
nystagmus, *592*
one-point discrimination, *643*
ossicles, *595*
otoscope, *594*
pallor, *576*
palpation, *568*
parotitis, *601*
periodontal disease, *601*
percussion, *570*
perfusion, *624*
pinna, *594*
pitch, *571*

plaque, *601*
pleximeter, *570*
plexor, *570*
precordium, *619*
presbyopia, *586*
proprioceptors, *643*
pyorrhea, *601*
quality, *571*
reflex, *643*
resonance, *571*
resting tremor, *639*
S$_1$, *619*
S$_2$, *619*
semicircular canals, *595*
sensorineural hearing loss, *595*
sordes, *601*
stapes, *595*
stereognosis, *643*
sternum, *611*
systole, *619*
tartar, *601*
thrill, *620*
tragus, *594*
tremor, *639*
triangular fossa, *594*
two-point discrimination, *643*
tympanic membrane, *594*
tympany, *571*
vestibule, *595*
visual acuity, *586*
visual fields, *586*
vitiligo, *576*

Assessing a client's health status is a major component of nursing care and has two aspects: (1) the nursing health history discussed in Chapter 11 ∞ and (2) the physical examination discussed in this chapter. A physical examination can be any of three types: (a) a complete assessment (e.g., when a client is admitted to a health care agency); (b) examination of a body system (e.g., the cardiovascular system); or (c) examination of a body area (e.g., the lungs, when difficulty with breathing is observed). *Note:* Some nurses consider *assessment* to be the broad term used in applying the nursing process to health data and *examination* to be the physical process used to gather the data. In this text, the terms *assessment* and *examination* are sometimes used interchangeably—both referring to a critical investigation and evaluation of client status.

PHYSICAL HEALTH ASSESSMENT

A complete health assessment may be conducted starting at the head and proceeding in a systematic manner downward (head-to-toe assessment). However, the procedure can vary according to the age of the individual, the severity of the illness, the preferences of the nurse, the location of the examination, and the agency's priorities and procedures. The order of head-to-toe assessment is given in Box 30–1. Regardless of the procedure used, the client's energy and time need to be considered. The health assessment is therefore conducted in a systematic and efficient manner that results in the fewest position changes for the client.

Frequently, nurses assess a specific body area instead of the entire body. These specific assessments are made in relation to client complaints, the nurse's own observation of problems, the client's presenting problem, nursing interventions provided, and medical therapies. Examples of these situations and assessments are provided in Table 30–1.

These are some of the purposes of the physical examination:

- To obtain baseline data about the client's functional abilities
- To supplement, confirm, or refute data obtained in the nursing history
- To obtain data that will help establish nursing diagnoses and plans of care

BOX 30–1 Head-to-Toe Framework

- General survey
- Vital signs
- Head
  - Hair, scalp, cranium, face
  - Eyes and vision
  - Ears and hearing
  - Nose and sinuses
  - Mouth and oropharynx
  - Cranial nerves
- Neck
  - Muscles
  - Lymph nodes
  - Trachea
  - Thyroid gland
  - Carotid arteries
  - Neck veins
- Upper extremities
  - Skin and nails
  - Muscle strength and tone
  - Joint range of motion
  - Brachial and radial pulses
  - Biceps tendon reflexes
  - Tendon reflexes
  - Sensation

- Chest and back
  - Skin
  - Chest shape and size
  - Lungs
  - Heart
  - Spinal column
  - Breasts and axillae
- Abdomen
  - Skin
  - Abdominal sounds
  - Specific organs (e.g., liver, bladder)
  - Femoral pulses
- Genitals
  - Testicles
  - Vagina
  - Urethra
- Anus and rectum
- Lower extremities
  - Skin and toenails
  - Gait and balance
  - Joint range of motion
  - Popliteal, posterior tibial, and pedal pulses
  - Tendon and plantar reflexes

TABLE 30–1 Nursing Assessments Addressing Selected Client Situations

SITUATION	PHYSICAL ASSESSMENT
Client complains of abdominal pain.	Inspect, auscultate, and palpate the abdomen; assess vital signs.
Client is admitted with a head injury.	Assess level of consciousness using Glasgow Coma Scale (see Table 30–10 later in this chapter); assess pupils for reaction to light and accommodation; assess vital signs.
The nurse prepares to administer a cardiotonic drug to a client.	Assess apical pulse and compare with baseline data.
The client has just had a cast applied to the lower leg.	Assess peripheral perfusion of toes, capillary blanch test, pedal pulse if able, and vital signs.
The client's fluid intake is minimal.	Assess tissue turgor, fluid intake and output, and vital signs.

- To evaluate the physiologic outcomes of health care and thus the progress of a client's health problem
- To make clinical judgments about a client's health status
- To identify areas for health promotion and disease prevention

Nurses use national guidelines and evidence-based practice to focus health assessment on specific conditions. For example, when screening for cancer, nurses should keep in mind the American Cancer Society's guidelines for early detection (see Box 30–2).

Preparing the Client

Most people need an explanation of the physical examination. Often clients are anxious about what the nurse will find. They can be reassured during the examination by explanations at each step. The nurse should explain when and where the examination will take place, why it is important, and what will happen. Instruct the client that all information gathered and documented during the assessment is kept confidential in accordance with the Health Insurance Portability and Accountability Act (HIPAA). This means that only those health care providers who have a legitimate need to know the client's information will have access to it.

Health examinations are usually painless; however, it is important to determine in advance any positions that are contraindicated for a particular client. The nurse assists the client as needed to undress and put on a gown. Clients should empty their bladders before the examination. Doing so helps them feel more relaxed and facilitates palpation of the abdomen and pubic area. If a urinalysis is required, the urine should be collected in a container for that purpose.

When assessing adults it is important to recognize that people of the same age differ markedly. Box 30–3 provides special considerations for assessing adults, especially elders.

BOX 30-2   Cancer Screening Guidelines for Asymptomatic People

COLORECTAL CANCER (MALES AND FEMALES)
- Fecal occult blood test or fecal immunochemical test annually beginning at age 50
- Flexible sigmoidoscopy every 5 years beginning at age 50
- Colonoscopy every 10 years
- Double contrast barium enema every 5 years

BREAST CANCER (FEMALES)
- Monthly breast self-examination beginning at age 20
- Clinical breast examination every 3 years from age 20 to 40, and then annually beginning at age 40
- Mammogram annually at age 40 and over

CERVICAL AND UTERINE CANCER (FEMALES)
- Papanicolaou (Pap) smear 3 years after beginning vaginal intercourse or by age 21; annually or every 2 years using liquid-based Pap (After age 30, if a woman has had three or more consecutive satisfactory annual examinations, the Pap test may be performed less frequently at the discretion of her primary care provider.)

- Pap smears may be stopped at age 70 if no abnormal results in the past 10 years.
- Pap smears may be stopped following total hysterectomy.

PROSTATE CANCER (MALES)
- Prostate-specific antigen (PSA) and digital rectal examination annually beginning at age 50 for men who have at least a 10-year life expectancy and for younger men who are at high risk

HEALTH COUNSELING AND CANCER CHECKUP (MALES AND FEMALES)
- Examination for cancers of the thyroid, testicles, ovaries, lymph nodes, oral region, and skin every 3 years over age 20 and annually over age 40

Note: From "American Cancer Society Recommendations for the Early Detection of Cancer, 2006" by R. A. Smith, V. Cokkinides, & H. J. Eyre, 2006, *CA: A Cancer Journal for Clinicians, 56,* pp. 11–25.

BOX 30-3   Health Assessment of the Adult

- Be aware of normal physiologic changes that occur with age.
- Be aware of stiffness of muscles and joints from aging changes or history of orthopedic surgery. The client may need modification of the usual positioning necessary for examination and assessment.
- Expose only areas of the body to be examined in order to avoid chilling.
- Permit ample time for the client to answer your questions and assume the required positions.
- Be aware of cultural differences. The client may want a family member present during disrobing.
- Arrange for an interpreter if the client's language differs from that of the nurse.
- Ask clients how they wish to be addressed, such as Mrs. or Miss.
- Adapt assessment techniques to any sensory impairment; for example, make sure eyeglasses or hearing aids are nearby.
- If clients are elderly and/or frail it is wise to plan several assessment times in order to not overtire them.

The sequence of the assessment differs with children and adults. With children, always proceed from the least invasive or uncomfortable to the more invasive. Examination of the head and neck, heart and lungs, and range of motion can be done early in the process, while the ears, mouth, abdomen, and genitals should be left for the end of the exam.

Preparing the Environment

It is important to prepare the environment before starting the assessment. The time for the physical assessment should be convenient to both the client and the nurse. The environment needs to be well lighted and the equipment should be organized for efficient use. A client who is physically relaxed will usually experience little discomfort. The room should be warm enough to be comfortable for the client.

Providing privacy is important. Most people are embarrassed if their bodies are exposed or if others can overhear or view them during the assessment. Culture, age, and gender of both the client and the nurse influence how comfortable the client will be and what special arrangements might be needed. For example, if the client and nurse are of different genders, the nurse should ask if it is acceptable to perform the physical examination or if a nurse of the same gender is preferred. Family and friends should not be present unless the client asks for someone.

Positioning

Several positions are frequently required during the physical assessment. It is important to consider the client's ability to assume a position. The client's physical condition, energy level, and age should also be taken into consideration. Some positions are embarrassing and uncomfortable and therefore should not be maintained for long. The assessment is organized so that several body areas can be assessed in one position, thus minimizing the number of position changes needed (see Table 30–2).

Draping

Drapes should be arranged so that the area to be assessed is exposed and other body areas are covered. Exposure of the body is frequently embarrassing to clients. Drapes provide not only a degree of privacy but also warmth. Drapes are made of paper, cloth, or bed linen.

Instrumentation

All equipment required for the health assessment should be clean, in good working order, and readily accessible. Equipment is frequently set up on trays, ready for use.

Various instruments are shown in Table 30–3.

TABLE 30–2 Client Positions and Body Areas Assessed

POSITION	DESCRIPTION	AREAS ASSESSED	CAUTIONS
Dorsal recumbent	Back-lying position with knees flexed and hips externally rotated; small pillow under the head; soles of feet on the surface	Female genitals, rectum, and female reproductive tract	May be contraindicated for clients who have cardiopulmonary problems.
Supine (horizontal recumbent)	Back-lying position with legs extended; with or without pillow under the head	Head, neck, axillae, anterior thorax, lungs, breasts, heart, vital signs, abdomen, extremities, peripheral pulses	Tolerated poorly by clients with cardiovascular and respiratory problems.
Sitting	A seated position, back unsupported and legs hanging freely	Head, neck, posterior and anterior thorax, lungs, breasts, axillae, heart, vital signs, upper and lower extremities, reflexes	Elders and weak clients may require support.
Lithotomy	Back-lying position with feet supported in stirrups; the hips should be in line with the edge of the table	Female genitals, rectum, and female reproductive tract	May be uncomfortable and tiring for elders and often embarrassing.
Sims	Side-lying position with lowermost arm behind the body, uppermost leg flexed at hip and knee, upper arm flexed at shoulder and elbow	Rectum, vagina	Difficult for elders and people with limited joint movement.
Prone	Lies on abdomen with head turned to the side, with or without a small pillow	Posterior thorax, hip joint movement	Often not tolerated by elders and people with cardiovascular and respiratory problems.

Methods of Examining

Four primary techniques are used in the physical examination: inspection, palpation, percussion, and auscultation. These techniques are discussed throughout this chapter as they apply to each body system.

Inspection

Inspection is the visual examination, that is, assessing by using the sense of sight. It should be deliberate, purposeful, and systematic. The nurse inspects with the naked eye and with a lighted instrument such as an otoscope (used to view the ear). In addition to visual observations, olfactory (smell) and auditory (hearing) cues are noted. Nurses frequently use visual inspection to assess moisture, color, and texture of body surfaces, as well as shape, position, size, color, and symmetry of the body. Lighting must be sufficient for the nurse to see clearly; either natural or artificial light can be used. When using the auditory senses it is important to have a quiet environment for accurate hearing. Observation can be combined with the other assessment techniques.

Palpation

Palpation is the examination of the body using the sense of touch. The pads of the fingers are used because their concentration of nerve endings makes them highly sensitive to tactile discrimination. Palpation is used to determine (a) texture (e.g., of the hair); (b) temperature (e.g., of a skin area); (c) vibration (e.g., of a joint); (d) position, size, consistency, and mobility of organs or masses; (e) distention (e.g., of the urinary bladder); (f) pulsation; and (g) the presence of pain upon pressure.

There are two types of palpation: light and deep. *Light (superficial) palpation* should always precede *deep palpa-*

TABLE 30–3 Equipment and Supplies Used for a Health Examination

SUPPLIES		PURPOSE
Flashlight or penlight		To assist viewing of the pharynx and cervix or to determine the reactions of the pupils of the eye
Nasal speculum		To permit visualization of the lower and middle turbinates; usually, a penlight is used for illumination
Ophthalmoscope		A lighted instrument to visualize the interior of the eye
Otoscope		A lighted instrument to visualize the eardrum and external auditory canal (a nasal speculum may be attached to the otoscope to inspect the nasal cavities)
Percussion (reflex) hammer		An instrument with a rubber head to test reflexes
Tuning fork		A two-pronged metal instrument used to test hearing acuity and vibratory sense
Vaginal speculum		To assess the cervix and the vagina
Cotton applicators		To obtain specimens
Gloves		To protect the nurse
Lubricant		To ease insertion of instruments (e.g., vaginal speculum)
Tongue blades (depressors)		To depress the tongue during assessment of the mouth and pharynx

tion because heavy pressure on the fingertips can dull the sense of touch. For light palpation, the nurse extends the dominant hand's fingers parallel to the skin surface and presses gently while moving the hand in a circle (see Figure 30-1 ■ on page 570). With light palpation, the skin is slightly depressed. If it is necessary to determine the details of a mass, the nurse presses lightly several times rather than holding the pressure. See Box 30–4 on page 570 for the characteristics of masses.

Deep palpation is done with two hands (bimanually) or one hand. In deep bimanual palpation, the nurse extends the dominant hand as for light palpation, then places the finger pads of the nondominant hand on the dorsal surface of the distal interphalangeal joint of the middle three fingers of the dominant hand (Figure 30-2 ■). The top hand applies pressure while the lower hand remains relaxed to perceive the tactile sensations. For deep palpation using one hand, the finger pads of the dominant hand press over the area to be palpated. Often the other

Figure 30-1 ■ The position of the hand for light palpation.

BOX 30–4 Characteristics of Masses

Location—Site on the body, dorsal/ventral surface
Size—Length and width in centimeters
Shape—Oval, round, elongated, irregular
Consistency—Soft, firm, hard
Surface—Smooth, nodular
Mobility—Fixed, mobile
Pulsatility—Present or absent
Tenderness—Degree of tenderness to palpation

---

hand is used to support a mass or organ from below (Figure 30-3 ■). *Deep palpation is usually not done during a routine examination and requires significant practitioner skill. It is performed with extreme caution because pressure can damage internal organs. It is usually not indicated in clients who have acute abdominal pain or pain that is not yet diagnosed.*

To test skin temperature, it is best to use the dorsum or back of the hand and fingers, where the examiner's skin is thinnest. To test for vibration, the nurse should use the palmar surface of the hand. General guidelines for palpation include the following:

Figure 30-2 ■ The position of the hands for deep bimanual palpation.

Figure 30-3 ■ Deep palpation using the lower hand to support the body while the upper hand palpates the organ.

- The nurse's hands should be clean and warm, and the fingernails short.
- Areas of tenderness should be palpated last.
- Deep palpation should be done after superficial palpation.

The effectiveness of palpation depends largely on the client's relaxation. Nurses can assist a client to relax by (a) gowning and/or draping the client appropriately, (b) positioning the client comfortably, and (c) ensuring that their own hands are warm before beginning. During palpation, the nurse should be sensitive to the client's verbal and facial expressions indicating discomfort.

Percussion

Percussion is the act of striking the body surface to elicit sounds that can be heard or vibrations that can be felt. There are two types of percussion: direct and indirect. In *direct percussion,* the nurse strikes the area to be percussed directly with the pads of two, three, or four fingers or with the pad of the middle finger. The strikes are rapid, and the movement is from the wrist (see Figure 30-4 ■). This technique is not generally used to percuss the thorax but is useful in percussing an adult's sinuses.

Indirect percussion is the striking of an object (e.g., a finger) held against the body area to be examined. In this technique, the middle finger of the nondominant hand, referred to as the **pleximeter,** is placed firmly on the client's skin. Only the distal phalanx and joint of this finger should be in contact with the skin. Using the tip of the flexed middle finger of the other hand, called the **plexor,** the nurse strikes the pleximeter, usually at the distal interphalangeal joint (see Figure 30-5 ■). Some nurses may find a point between the distal and proximal joints to be a more comfortable pleximeter point. The motion comes from the wrist; the forearm remains stationary. The angle between the plexor and the pleximeter should be 90 degrees, and the blows must be firm, rapid, and short to obtain a clear sound.

Percussion is used to determine the size and shape of internal organs by establishing their borders. It indicates whether tissue is fluid filled, air filled, or solid. Percussion elicits five types of sound: flatness, dullness, resonance, hyperresonance, and

Figure 30-4 ■ **Direct percussion.** Using one hand to strike the surface of the body.

Figure 30-5 ■ **Indirect percussion.** Using the finger of one hand to tap the finger of the other hand.

tympany. **Flatness** is an extremely dull sound produced by very dense tissue, such as muscle or bone. **Dullness** is a thudlike sound produced by dense tissue such as the liver, spleen, or heart. **Resonance** is a hollow sound such as that produced by lungs filled with air. **Hyperresonance** is not produced in the normal body. It is described as booming and can be heard over an emphysematous lung. **Tympany** is a musical or drumlike sound produced from an air-filled stomach. On a continuum, flatness

reflects the most dense tissue (the least amount of air) and tympany the least dense tissue (the greatest amount of air). A percussion sound is described according to its intensity, pitch, duration, and quality (see Table 30–4).

Auscultation

Auscultation is the process of listening to sounds produced within the body. Auscultation may be direct or indirect. *Direct auscultation* is the use of the unaided ear, for example, to listen to a respiratory wheeze or the grating of a moving joint. *Indirect auscultation* is the use of a stethoscope, which transmits the sounds to the nurse's ears. A stethoscope is used primarily to listen to sounds from within the body, such as bowel sounds or valve sounds of the heart and blood pressure.

The stethoscope tubing should be 30 to 35 cm (12 to 14 in.) long, with an internal diameter of about 0.3 cm (1/8 in.). It should have both a flat disc diaphragm and a bell-shaped amplifier (see Figure ❹ in Skill 29-3 on page 544). The diaphragm best transmits high-pitched sounds (e.g., bronchial sounds), and the bell best transmits low-pitched sounds such as some heart sounds. The earpieces of the stethoscope should fit comfortably into the nurse's ears, facing forward. The amplifier of the stethoscope is placed firmly but lightly against the client's skin. If the client has excessive hair, it may be necessary to dampen the hairs with a moist cloth so that they will lie flat against the skin and not interfere with clear sound transmission.

Auscultated sounds are described according to their pitch, intensity, duration, and quality. The **pitch** is the frequency of the vibrations (the number of vibrations per second). Low-pitched sounds, such as some heart sounds, have fewer vibrations per second than high-pitched sounds, such as bronchial sounds. The **intensity** (amplitude) refers to the loudness or softness of a sound. Some body sounds are loud, for example, bronchial sounds heard from the trachea; others are soft, for example, normal breath sounds heard in the lungs. The **duration** of a sound is its length (long or short). The **quality** of sound is a subjective description of a sound, for example, whistling, gurgling, or snapping.

GENERAL SURVEY

Health assessment begins with a general survey that involves observation of the client's general appearance and mental status, and measurement of vital signs, height, and weight. Many components of the general survey are assessed while taking the client's health history, such as the client's body build, posture, hygiene, and mental status.

TABLE 30–4	**Percussion Sounds and Tones**				
SOUND	**INTENSITY**	**PITCH**	**DURATION**	**QUALITY**	**EXAMPLE OF LOCATION**
Flatness	Soft	High	Short	Extremely dull	Muscle, bone
Dullness	Medium	Medium	Moderate	Thudlike	Liver, heart
Resonance	Loud	Low	Long	Hollow	Normal lung
Hyperresonance	Very loud	Very low	Very long	Booming	Emphysematous lung
Tympany	Loud	High (distinguished mainly by musical timbre)	Moderate	Musical	Stomach filled with gas (air)

Appearance and Mental Status

The general appearance and behavior of an individual must be assessed in relationship to culture, educational level, socioeconomic status, and current circumstances. For example, an individual who has recently experienced a personal loss may appropriately appear depressed (sad expression, slumped posture). The client's age, sex, and race are also useful factors in interpreting findings that suggest increased risk for known conditions. Skill 30-1 describes how to assess general appearance and mental status.

SKILL 30-1

ASSESSING APPEARANCE AND MENTAL STATUS

PLANNING

Delegation

Due to the substantial knowledge and skill required, assessment of general appearance and mental status is not delegated to unlicensed assistive personnel (UAP). However, many aspects are observed during usual care and may be recorded by persons other than the nurse. Abnormal findings must be validated and interpreted by the nurse.

Equipment

None

IMPLEMENTATION

Performance

1. Prior to performing the procedure, introduce self and verify the client's identity using agency protocol. Explain to the client what you are going to do, why it is necessary, and how he or she can cooperate. Discuss how the results will be used in planning further care or treatments.

2. Perform hand hygiene and observe appropriate infection control procedures.

3. Provide for client privacy.

ASSESSMENT	NORMAL FINDINGS	DEVIATIONS FROM NORMAL
4. Observe body build, height, and weight in relation to the client's age, lifestyle, and health.	Proportionate, varies with lifestyle	Excessively thin or obese
5. Observe client's posture and gait, standing, sitting, and walking.	Relaxed, erect posture; coordinated movement	Tense, slouched, bent posture; uncoordinated movement; tremors
6. Observe client's overall hygiene and grooming. Relate these to the person's activities prior to the assessment.	Clean, neat	Dirty, unkempt
7. Note body and breath odor in relation to activity level.	No body odor or minor body odor relative to work or exercise; no breath odor	Foul body odor; ammonia odor; acetone breath odor; foul breath
8. Observe for signs of distress in posture or facial expression.	No distress noted	Bending over because of abdominal pain, wincing, frowning, or labored breathing
9. Note obvious signs of health or illness (e.g., in skin color or breathing).	Healthy appearance	Pallor; weakness; lesions
10. Assess the client's attitude.	Cooperative, able to follow instructions	Negative, hostile, withdrawn
11. Note the client's affect/mood; assess the appropriateness of the client's responses.	Appropriate to situation	Inappropriate to situation
12. Listen for quantity of speech (amount and pace), quality (loudness, clarity, inflection), and organization (coherence of thought, overgeneralization, vagueness).	Understandable, moderate pace; clear tone and inflection; exhibits thought association	Rapid or slow pace; overly loud or soft; uses generalizations; lacks association
13. Listen for relevance and organization of thoughts.	Logical sequence; makes sense; has sense of reality	Illogical sequence; flight of ideas; confusion; vague

14. Document findings in the client record using handwritten or electronic forms and checklists supplemented by narrative notes when appropriate. ❶

EVALUATION

- Perform a detailed follow-up examination of other individual systems based on findings that deviated from expected or normal for the client. Relate findings to previous assessment data if available.

- Report significant deviations from normal to the primary care provider.

SKILL 30-1

ASSESSING APPEARANCE AND MENTAL STATUS *continued*

ADMISSION DATA

Date 4-16-07 Time 3:15 p.m. Primary Language English
Arrived Via: ☐ Wheelchair ☐ Stretcher ☑ Ambulatory
From: ☐ Admitting ☐ ER ☑ Home ☐ Nursing Home ☐ Other
Admitting M.D. R. Katz Time Notified 5 p.m.

ORIENTATION TO UNIT

	YES	NO		YES	NO
Arm Band Correct	☑	☐	Visiting Hours	☑	☐
Allergy Band	☑	☐	Smoking Policy	☑	☐
Telephone	☑	☐	TV, Lights, Bed Controls,		
Electrical Policy	☑	☐	Call Lights, Side Rails	☑	☐
Educational Mat'l	☑	☐	Nurses Station	☑	☐
(TV Brochure)	☑	☐			

Family M.D. R. Katz
Weight 125 lb. Height 5 ft. 2 in. BP:R — L 122/80
Temp. 103F Pulse 92, weak Resp 28, shallow
Source Providing Information ☑ Patient ☐ Other
Unable to Obtain History ☐
Reason for Admission (Onset, Duration, Pt.'s Perception) "Chest cold" X 2 weeks S.O.B on exertion. "Lung pain, fever," "Dr. says I have pneumonia."

ALLERGIES & REACTIONS

Drugs Penicillin
Food/Other
Signs & Symptoms rash, nausea
Blood Reaction ☐ Yes ☑ No Dyes/Shellfish ☐ Yes ☑ No

MEDICATIONS

Current Meds	Dose/Freq.	Last Dose
Synthroid	0.1 mg. daily	4-16, 8 a.m.

Disposition of Meds: ☒ Home ☐ Pharmacy ☐ Safe *At Bedside

MEDICAL HISTORY

☑ No Major Problems   ☐ Gastro
☐ Cardiac   ☐ Arthritis
☐ Hyper/Hypotension   ☐ Stroke
☐ Diabetes   ☐ Seizures
☐ Cancer   ☐ Glaucoma
☐ Respiratory   ☑ Other Childbirth-1998

Surgery/Procedures	Date
Appendectomy	1989
Partial thyroidectomy	1996

SPECIAL ASSISTIVE DEVICES

☐ Wheelchair ☐ Contacts ☐ Venous ☐ Dentures
☐ Braces ☐ Hearing Aid Access ☐ Partial
☐ Cane/Crutches ☐ Prosthesis Device ☐ Upper
☐ Walker ☐ Glasses ☐ Epidural Catheter ☐ Lower
☐ Other None

VALUABLES

Patient informed Hospital not responsible for personal belongings.
Valuables Disposition: ☐ Patient ☐ Safe ☐ Given to
Patient/SO Signature None

PSYCHOSOCIAL HISTORY

Recent Stress None
Coping Mechanism Not assessed because of fatigue
Support System Husband, coworkers, friends
Calm: ☑ Yes ☐ No
Anxious: ☐ Yes ☐ No Facial muscles tense; trembling
Religion Catholic, Would want Last Rites
Tobacco Use: ☐ Yes ☑ No
Alcohol Use: ☐ Yes ☑ No
Drug Use: ☐ Yes ☑ No

NEUROLOGICAL

Oriented: ☑ Person ☑ Place ☑ Time ☐ Confused ☐ Sedated
☐ Alert ☐ Restless ☑ Lethargic ☐ Comatose
Pupils: ☑ Equal ☐ Unequal ☑ Reactive ☐ Sluggish
☐ Other 3mm.
Extremity Strength: ☑ Equal ☐ Unequal
Speech: ☑ Clear ☐ Slurred ☐ Other

MUSCULO-SKELETAL

Normal ROM of Extremities ☑ Yes ☐ No
☑ Weakness ☐ Paralysis ☐ Contractures ☐ Joint Swelling ☑ Pain
☐ Other ↓ related to fatigue when coughing

RESPIRATORY

Pattern: ☐ Even ☐ Uneven ☑ Shallow ☑ Dyspnea
☑ Other diminished breath sounds
Breathing Sounds: ☐ Clear ☑ Other inspiratory crackles
Secretions: ☐ None ☑ Other pink, thick sputum
Cough: ☐ None ☑ Productive ☐ Nonproductive

CARDIOVASCULAR

Pulses: Apical Rate 92-W ☑ Reg. ☐ Irregular ☐ Pacemaker
S = Strong W = Weak A = Absent D = Doppler
Radial R 92 L ___ Pedal R ___ L ___
Edema: ☑ Absent ☐ Present Site
Perfusion: ☐ Warm ☐ Dry ☑ Diaphoretic ☐ Cool (Hot)

GASTROINTESTINAL

Oral Mucosa ☐ Normal ☑ Other pale and dry
Bowel Sounds: ☑ Normal ☐ Other Abd. soft
Wt. Change: ☐ ☑ N/V Stool Frequency/Character 1/day; soft
Last B/M 4-15-07 ☐ Ostomy (type)
Equip.

GENITOURINARY

Urine: Last Voided This morning
☐ Normal ☐ Anuria ☐ Hematuria ☐ Dysuria ☐ Incontinent
☒ Other ↓ amount & frequency since ill
☐ Catheter (type) Other
LMP 4-1-07 ☐ Vaginal/Penile Discharge
Other

SELF CARE

Need Assist with: ☐ Ambulating ☐ Elimination
☐ Meals ☒ Hygiene ☐ Dressing
While fatigued

Amanda Aquilini [F. age 28]
#4637651 DOB 11-02-79

✖ **NORTH BROWARD HOSPITAL DISTRICT**
NURSING ADMINISTRATION ASSESSMENT

❶ Nursing assessment form.

continued on page 574

SKILL 30-1

ASSESSING APPEARANCE AND MENTAL STATUS *continued*

NUTRITION

General Appearance: ☑ Well Nourished ☐ Emaciated
☐ Other _____

Appetite: ☐ Good ☐ Fair ☑ Poor -x2 days
Diet _Liquid_ Meal Pattern _3/day_
☐ Feeds Self ☐ Assist ☐ Total Feed

SKIN ASSESSMENT

Color: ☐ Normal ☐ Flushed ☑ Pale ☐ Dusky ☐ Cyanotic
☐ Jaundiced ☑ Other _Cheeks flushed, hot_
General Description _Surgical scars:_
RLQ abdomen; anterior neck
_____
_____
_____

Note Cultures Obtained _____
_____
_____

PRESSURE SORE ™AT RISK∫ SCREENING CRITERIA

OVERALL SKIN CONDITION
Grade
0	Turgor (elasticity adequate, skin warm and moist)
✓ 1	Poor turgor, skin cold & dry
2	Areas mottled, red or denuded
3	Existing skin ulcer/lesions

BOWEL AND BLADDER CONTROL
Grade
✓ 0	Always able to ask for bedpan
1	Incontinence of urine
2	Incontinence of feces
3	Totally incontinent Confined to bed

REHABILITATIVE STATE
Grade
0	Fully ambulatory
✓ 1	Ambulated with assistance
2	Chair to bed ambulation only
3	Confined to bed
4	Immobile in bed

NUTRITIONAL STATE
Grade
0	Eats all
✓ 1	Eats very little
2	Refuses food often
3	Tube feeding
4	Intravenous feeding

MENTAL STATE
Grade
✓ 0	Alert and clear
1	Confused
2	Disoriented/senile
3	Stuporous
4	Unconcious

CHRONIC DISEASE STATUS (i.e. COPD, ASCVD, Peripheral Vascular Disease, Diabetes, or Renal Disease, Cancer, Motor or Sensory Deficits, Elderly, Other)
Grade
✓ 0	Absent
1	One Present
2	Two Present
3	Three or more Present

TOTAL _____ Refer to Skin Care Protocol

FALLS SCREENING

If one or more of the following are checked institute fall precautions/plan of care
☐ History of Falls ☐ Unsteady Gait ☐ Confusion/Disorientation ☐ Dizziness

If two or more of the following are checked institute fall precautions/plan of care
☐ Age over 80 ☐ Utilizes cane, walker, w/c ☐ Sleeplessness
☐ Impaired vision ☐ Urgency/frequency in elimination
☐ Multiple Diagnoses ☐ Impaired hearing
☐ Inability to understand or follow directions ☐ Medication/Sedative /Diuretic etc.

NURSE SIGNATURE/TITLE	DATE	TIME
Mary Medina, RN	4-16-07	3:30pm
NURSE SIGNATURE/TITLE	DATE	TIME

EDUCATION/DISCHARGE PLANNING

1. What do you know about your present illness? _"Dr. says I have pneumonia." "I will have an I.V."_
2. What information do you want or need about your illness? _____
3. Would you like family/SO involved in your care? _Husband, Michael_
4. How long do you expect to be in the hospital? _"1-2 days"_
5. What concerns do you have about leaving the hospital? ____

CHECK APPROPRIATE BOX

Will patient need post discharge assistance with ADLs/physical functioning? ☐ Yes ☑ No ☐ Unknown

Does patient have family capable of and willing to provide assistance post discharge?
☑ Yes ☐ No ☐ Unknown ☐ No family

Is assistance needed beyond that which family can provide?
☐ Yes ☑ No ☐ Unknown

Previous admission in the last six months?
☐ Yes ☑ No ☐ Unknown

Patient lives with _Husband and 1 child_
Planned discharge to _Home_
Comments: _Fatigue and anxiety may have interfered with learning. Re-teach anything covered at admission, later._

Social Services Notified ☐ Yes ☑ No

NARRATIVE NOTES

S--c/o sharp chest pain when coughing and dyspnea on exertion. States unable to carry out regular daily exercise for past week. Coughing relieved "if I sit up and sit still." Nausea associated with coughing. Having occasional "chills." Occasionally becomes frightened, stating, "I can't breathe." Well groomed but "too tired to put on make-up." Assesses own supports as "good" (eg, relationship c̄ husband). Is "worried" about daughter. States husband will be out of town until tomorrow. Left 8-year-old daughter with neighbor. Concerned too about her work (is attorney). "I'll never get caught up." Had water at noon—no food today.

O--Chest expansion < 3cm, no nasal flaring or use of accessory muscles. Breath sounds and insp. crackles in ® upper and lower chest. Capillary refill 5 seconds.

✱✱ **NORTH BROWARD HOSPITAL DISTRICT**
NURSING ADMINISTRATION ASSESSMENT

❶ Nursing Assesment Form (continued)

Vital Signs

Vital signs are measured (a) to establish baseline data against which to compare future measurements and (b) to detect actual and potential health problems. See Chapter 29 ∞ for measurements of temperature, pulse, respirations, blood pressure, and oxygen saturation. See Chapter 46 ∞ for pain assessment.

Height and Weight

In adults, the ratio of weight to height provides a general measure of health. By asking clients about their height and weight before actually measuring them, the nurse obtains some idea of the person's self-image. Excessive discrepancies between the client's responses and the measurements may provide clues to actual or potential problems in self-concept. Be aware of any significant unintentional weight gain or loss.

The nurse measures height with a measuring stick attached to weight scales or to a wall. The client should remove the shoes and stand erect, with heels together, and the heels, buttocks, and back of the head against the measuring stick; eyes should be looking straight ahead. The nurse raises the L-shaped sliding arm on the weight scale until it rests on top of the client's head, or places a small flat object such as a ruler or book on the client's head. The edge of the flat object should abut the measuring guide.

Weight is usually measured when a client is admitted to a health agency and often regularly, for example, each morning before breakfast. Scales measure in pounds (lb) or kilograms

Figure 30-7 ■ Bed scale.

(kg), and the nurse may need to convert between the two systems. One kilogram is equal to 2.2 pounds. When accuracy is essential, the nurse should use the same scale each time (because every scale weighs slightly differently), take the measurements at the same time each day, and make sure the client has on a similar kind of clothing and no footwear. The client stands on a platform, and the weight is read from a digital display panel or a balancing arm. Clients who cannot stand are weighed on chair (Figure 30-6 ■) or bed scales. The bed scales (Figure 30-7 ■) have canvas straps or a stretcher-like apparatus. A machine lifts the client above the bed, and the weight is reflected either on a digital display panel or on a balance arm like that of a standing scale. Some agencies may have beds with built-in scales.

> **CLINICAL ALERT**
>
> Review the agency charting form before beginning your assessment to ensure that you have all of the equipment you need and know how to perform the assessment in a systematic approach. ■

THE INTEGUMENT

The integument includes the skin, hair, and nails. The examination begins with a generalized inspection using a good source of lighting, preferably indirect natural daylight.

Skin

Assessment of the skin involves inspection and palpation. The entire skin surface may be assessed at one time or as each aspect of the body is assessed. In some instances, the nurse may also use the olfactory sense to detect unusual skin odors; these are usually

Figure 30-6 ■ Chair scale.

LIFESPAN CONSIDERATIONS   General Survey

INFANTS

- Observation of children's behavior can provide important data for the general survey, including physical development, neuromuscular function, and social and interactional skills.
- It may be helpful to have parents hold older infants and very young children for part of the assessment.
- Measure height of children under age 2 in the supine position with knees fully extended.
- Weigh without clothing.
- Include measurement of head circumference until age 2. Standardized growth charts include head circumference up to age 3.

CHILDREN

- Anxiety in preschool-age children can be decreased by letting them handle and become familiar with examination equipment.

- School-age children may be very modest and shy about exposing parts of the body.
- Adolescents should be examined without parents present.
- Weigh children without shoes and with as little clothing as possible.

ELDERS

- Allow extra time for clients to answer questions.
- Adapt questioning techniques as appropriate for clients with hearing or visual limitations.
- Elders with osteoporosis can lose several inches in height. Be sure to document height and ask if they are aware of becoming shorter in height.
- When asking about weight loss, be specific about amount and time frame, e.g., "Have you lost more than five pounds in the last two months?"

HOME CARE CONSIDERATIONS   General Survey

- Assess the client in private whenever possible. If a family member is needed to assist with recall of events or translation, obtain the client's permission to have the family member present.

- Use your own equipment when possible in measuring vital signs. Bring a tape measure for measuring height. Recognize that the client's home scale for measuring weight may not be accurate.

---

most evident in the skinfolds or in the axillae. Pungent body odor is frequently related to poor hygiene, hyperhidrosis (excessive perspiration), or bromhidrosis (foul-smelling perspiration).

Pallor is the result of inadequate circulating blood or hemoglobin and subsequent reduction in tissue oxygenation. In clients with dark skin, it is usually characterized by the absence of underlying red tones in the skin and may be most readily seen in the buccal mucosa. In brown-skinned clients, pallor may appear as a yellowish brown tinge; in black-skinned clients, the skin may appear ashen gray. Pallor in all people is usually most evident in areas with the least pigmentation such as the conjunctiva, oral mucous membranes, nail beds, palms of the hand, and soles of the feet.

Cyanosis (a bluish tinge) is most evident in the nail beds, lips, and buccal mucosa. In dark-skinned clients, close inspection of the palpebral conjunctiva (the lining of the eyelids) and palms and soles may also show evidence of cyanosis. **Jaundice** (a yellowish tinge) may first be evident in the sclera of the eyes and then in the mucous membranes and the skin. Nurses should take care not to confuse jaundice with the normal yellow pigmentation in the sclera of a dark-skinned client. If jaundice is suspected, the posterior part of the hard palate should also be inspected for a yellowish color tone. **Erythema** is a redness associated with a variety of rashes.

Dark-skinned clients have areas of lighter pigmentation, such as the palms, lips, and nail beds. Localized areas of hyperpigmentation (increased pigmentation) and hypopigmentation (decreased pigmentation) may also occur as a result of changes in the distribution of melanin (the dark pigment) or in the function of the melanocytes in the epidermis. An example of hyperpigmentation in a defined area is a birthmark; an example of hypopigmentation is vitiligo. **Vitiligo,** seen as patches of hypopigmented skin, is caused by the destruction of melanocytes in the area. Albinism is the complete or partial lack of melanin in the skin, hair, and eyes. Other localized color changes may indicate a problem such as edema or a localized infection. **Edema** is the presence of excess interstitial fluid. An area of edema appears swollen, shiny, and taut and tends to blanch the skin color or, if accompanied by inflammation, may redden the skin. Generalized edema is most often an indication of impaired venous circulation and in some cases reflects cardiac dysfunction or venous abnormalities.

A skin lesion is an alteration in a client's normal skin appearance. Primary skin lesions are those that appear initially in response to some change in the external or internal environment of the skin (see Figure 30-8 ■, *A–H*). Secondary skin lesions are those that do not appear initially but result from modifications such as chronicity, trauma, or infection of the primary lesion. For example, a vesicle or blister (primary lesion) may rupture and cause an erosion (secondary lesion). Table 30–5 illustrates secondary lesions. Nurses are responsible for describing skin lesions accurately in terms of location (e.g., face), distribution (i.e., body regions involved), and configuration (the arrangement or position of several lesions) as well as color, shape, size, firmness, texture, and characteristics of individual lesions.

CLINICAL ALERT

If possible and the client agrees, take a digital or instant photograph of significant skin lesions for the client record. Include a measuring guide (ruler or tape) in the picture to demonstrate lesion size. ■

Skill 30-2 describes how to assess the skin.

Macule, Patch Flat, unelevated change in color. Macules are 1 mm to 1 cm in size and circumscribed. Examples: freckles, measles, petechiae, flat moles. Patches are larger than 1 cm and may have an irregular shape. Examples: port wine birthmark, vitiligo (white patches), rubella. ❶

❶ **Multiple café-au-lait macules**

Nodule, Tumor Elevated, solid, hard mass that extends deeper into the dermis than a papule. Nodules have a circumscribed border and are 0.5 to 2 cm. Examples: squamous cell carcinoma, fibroma. Tumors are larger than 2 cm and may have an irregular border. Examples: malignant melanoma, hemangioma. ❹

❹ **Peripheral neurofibromas**

❼ **Digital mucous cyst**

Papule Circumscribed, solid elevation of skin. Papules are less than 1 cm. Examples: warts, acne, pimples, elevated moles. ❷

❷ **Papular drug eruption** (Courtesy Scott D. Bennion, MD.)

Pustule Vesicle or bulla filled with pus. Examples: acne vulgaris, impetigo. ❺

❺ **Chronic pustular psoriasis**

Cyst A 1-cm or larger, elevated, encapsulated, fluid-filled or semisolid mass arising from the subcutaneous tissue or dermis. Examples: sebaceous and epidermoid cysts, chalazion of the eyelid. ❼

Plaque Plaques are larger than 1 cm. Examples: psoriasis, rubeola. ❸

❸ **Psoriasis vulgaris**

Vesicle, Bulla A circumscribed, round or oval, thin translucent mass filled with serous fluid or blood. Vesicles are less than 0.5 cm. Examples: herpes simplex, early chicken pox, small burn blister. Bullae are larger than 0.5 cm. Examples: large blister, second-degree burn, herpes simplex. ❻

❻ **Bullous pemphigoid**

Wheal A reddened, localized collection of edema fluid; irregular in shape. Size varies. Examples: hives, mosquito bites. ❽

❽ **Allergic wheals, urticaria**

Figure 30-8 ■ Primary skin lesions.

(*Note:* (❶–❼) from *Dermatology Secrets in Color,* 2nd ed., by J. E. Fitzpatrick and J. L. Aeling, 2001, Philadelphia: Hanley & Belfus, Inc.; (❽) Reprinted with permission from the American Academy of Dermatology. All rights reserved.)

TABLE 30–5 Secondary Skin Lesions

Atrophy

A translucent, dry, paperlike, sometimes wrinkled skin surface resulting from thinning or wasting of the skin due to loss of collagen and elastin.
Examples Striae, aged skin.

Erosion

Wearing away of the superficial epidermis causing a moist, shallow depression. Because erosions do not extend into the dermis, they heal without scarring.
Examples Scratch marks, ruptured vesicles.

Lichenification

Rough, thickened, hardened area of epidermis resulting from chronic irritation such as scratching or rubbing.
Example Chronic dermatitis.

Scales

Shedding flakes of greasy, keratinized skin tissue. Color may be white, gray, or silver. Texture may vary from fine to thick.
Examples Dry skin, dandruff, psoriasis, and eczema.

Crust

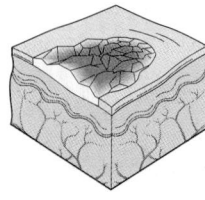

Dry blood, serum, or pus left on the skin surface when vesicles or pustules burst. Can be red-brown, orange, or yellow. Large crusts that adhere to the skin surface are called scabs.
Examples Eczema, impetigo, herpes, or scabs following abrasion.

Ulcer

Deep, irregularly shaped area of skin loss extending into the dermis or subcutaneous tissue. May bleed. May leave scar.
Examples Decubitus ulcers (pressure sores), stasis ulcers, chancres.

Fissure

Linear crack with sharp edges, extending into the dermis.
Examples Cracks at the corners of the mouth or in the hands, athlete's foot.

Scar

Flat, irregular area of connective tissue left after a lesion or wound has healed. New scars may be red or purple; older scars may be silvery or white.
Examples Healed surgical wound or injury, healed acne.

Keloid

Elevated, irregular, darkened area of excess scar tissue caused by excessive collagen formation during healing. Extends beyond the site of the original injury. Higher incidence in people of African descent.
Examples Keloid from ear piercing or surgery.

Excoriation

Linear erosion.
Examples Scratches, some chemical burns

ASSESSING THE SKIN

PLANNING
- Review characteristics of primary and secondary skin lesions if necessary (see Figure 30-8 and Table 30–5).
- Ensure that adequate lighting is available.

Delegation
Due to the substantial knowledge and skill required, assessment of the skin is not delegated to UAP. However, the skin is observed during usual care and these persons should record their findings. Abnormal findings must be validated and interpreted by the nurse.

Equipment
- Millimeter ruler
- Clean gloves
- Magnifying glass

ASSESSING THE SKIN *continued*

IMPLEMENTATION
Performance

1. Prior to performing the procedure, introduce self and verify the client's identity using agency protocol. Explain to the client what you are going to do, why it is necessary, and how he or she can cooperate. Discuss how the results will be used in planning further care or treatments.

2. Perform hand hygiene and observe appropriate infection control procedures.

3. Provide for client privacy.

4. Inquire if the client has any history of the following: pain or itching; presence and spread of lesions, bruises, abrasions, pigmented spots; previous experience with skin problems; associated clinical signs; family history; presence of problems in other family members; related systemic conditions; use of medications, lotions, home remedies; excessively dry or moist feel to the skin; tendency to bruise easily; association of the problem to season of year, stress, occupation, medications, recent travel, housing, and so on; recent contact with allergens, e.g., metal paint.

ASSESSMENT	NORMAL FINDINGS	DEVIATIONS FROM NORMAL
5. Inspect skin color (best assessed under natural light and on areas not exposed to the sun).	Varies from light to deep brown; from ruddy pink to light pink; from yellow overtones to olive	Pallor, cyanosis, jaundice, erythema
6. Inspect uniformity of skin color.	Generally uniform except in areas exposed to the sun; areas of lighter pigmentation (palms, lips, nail beds) in dark-skinned people	Areas of either hyperpigmentation or hypopigmentation
7. Assess edema, if present (i.e., location, color, temperature, shape, and the degree to which the skin remains indented or pitted when pressed by a finger). Measuring the circumference of the extremity with a millimeter tape may be useful for future comparison.	No edema	See the scale for describing edema. ❶
8. Inspect, palpate, and describe skin lesions. Apply gloves if lesions are open or draining. Palpate lesions to determine shape and texture. Describe lesions according to location, distribution, color, configuration, size, shape, type, or structure (see Box 30–5 on page 581).	Freckles, some birthmarks, some flat and raised nevi; no abrasions or other lesions	Various interruptions in skin integrity; irregular, multicolored, or raised nevi
9. Observe and palpate skin moisture.	Moisture in skin folds and the axillae (varies with environmental temperature and humidity, body temperature, and activity)	Excessive moisture (e.g., in hyperthermia); excessive dryness (e.g., in dehydration)
10. Palpate skin temperature. Compare the two feet and the two hands, using the backs of your fingers.	Uniform; within normal range	Generalized hyperthermia (e.g., in fever); generalized hypothermia (e.g., in shock); localized hyperthermia (e.g., in infection); localized hypothermia (e.g., in arteriosclerosis)

❶ Scale for grading edema.

continued on page 580

SKILL 30-2

ASSESSING THE SKIN *continued*

ASSESSMENT	NORMAL FINDINGS	DEVIATIONS FROM NORMAL
11. Note skin turgor (fullness or elasticity) by lifting and pinching the skin on an extremity.	When pinched, skin springs back to previous state; may be slower in elders	Skins stays pinched or tented or moves back slowly (e.g., in dehydration)

12. Document findings in the client record using forms or checklists supplemented by narrative notes when appropriate. Draw location of skin lesions on body surface diagrams. ❷

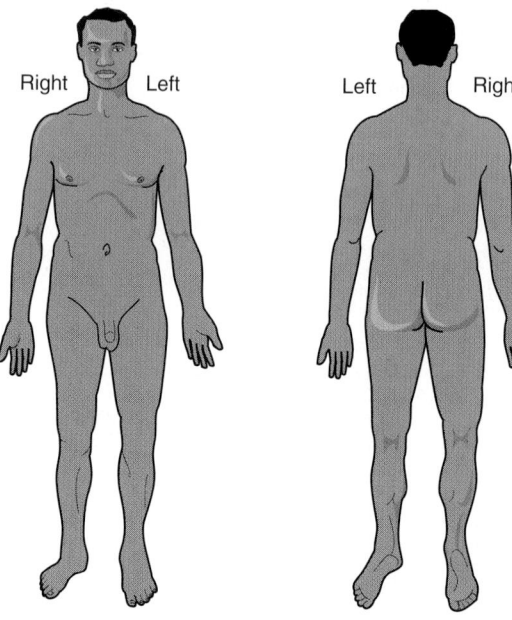

Right   Left   Left   Right

❷ Diagram for charting skin lesions.

EVALUATION
- Compare findings to previous skin assessment data if available to determine if lesions or abnormalities are changing.
- Report significant deviations from normal to the primary care provider.

LIFESPAN CONSIDERATIONS Assessing the Skin

INFANTS
- Physiologic jaundice may appear in newborns 2 to 3 days after birth and usually lasts about 1 week. Pathologic jaundice, or that which indicates a disease, appears within 24 hours of birth and may last more than 8 days.
- Newborns may have milia (whiteheads), small white nodules over the nose and face, and vernix caseosa (white cheesy, greasy material on the skin).
- Premature infants may have lanugo, a fine downy hair covering their shoulders and back.
- In dark-skinned infants, areas of hyperpigmentation may be found on the back, especially in the sacral area.
- Diaper dermatitis may be seen in infants.
- If a rash is present, inquire in detail about immunization history.
- Assess skin turgor by pinching the skin on the abdomen.

CHILDREN
- Children normally have minor skin lesions (e.g., bruising or abrasions) on arms and legs due to their high activity level. Lesions on other parts of the body may be signs of disease or abuse, and a thorough history should be taken.
- Secondary skin lesions may occur frequently as children scratch or expose a primary lesion to microbes.

- With puberty, oil glands become more productive, and children may develop acne. Most persons 12 to 24 years have some acne.
- In dark-skinned children, areas of hyperpigmentation may be found on the back, especially in the sacral area.
- If a rash is present, inquire in detail about immunization history.

ELDERS
- Changes in white skin occur at an earlier age than in black skin.
- The skin loses its elasticity and wrinkles. Wrinkles first appear on the skin of the face and neck, which are abundant in collagen and elastic fibers.
- The skin appears thin and translucent because of loss of dermis and subcutaneous fat.
- The skin is dry and flaky because sebaceous and sweat glands are less active. Dry skin is more prominent over the extremities.
- The skin takes longer to return to its natural shape after being tented between the thumb and finger.
- Due to the normal loss of peripheral skin turgor in elders, assess for hydration by checking skin turgor over the sternum or clavicle.
- Flat tan to brown-colored macules, referred to as *senile lentigines* or *melanotic freckles,* are normally apparent on the back of the hand and other skin areas that are exposed to the sun. These macules may be as large as 1 to 2 cm.

LIFESPAN CONSIDERATIONS Assessing the Skin—*continued*

- Warty lesions (*seborrheic keratosis*) with irregularly shaped borders and a scaly surface often occur on the face, shoulders, and trunk. These benign lesions begin as yellowish to tan and progress to a dark brown or black.
- *Vitiligo* tends to increase with age and is thought to result from an autoimmune response.
- Cutaneous tags (*acrochordons*) are most commonly seen in the neck and axillary regions. These skin lesions vary in size and are soft, often flesh colored, and pedicled.

- Visible, bright red, fine dilated blood vessels (*telangiectasias*) commonly occur as a result of the thinning of the dermis and the loss of support for the blood vessel walls.
- Pink to slightly red lesions with indistinct borders (*actinic keratoses*) may appear at about age 50, often on the face, ears, backs of the hands, and arms. They may become malignant if untreated.

HOME CARE CONSIDERATIONS Assessing the Skin

- When making a home visit, take a penlight or examination lamp with you in case the home has inadequate lighting.
- If skin lesions are suggestive of physical abuse, follow state regulations for follow-up and reporting. Signs of abuse may include a pattern of bruises, unusual location of burns, or lesions that are not easily explainable. If lesions are present in adults or verbal-age children, conduct the interview and assessment in private.

- Document lesions by taking a photo (if client consents). Another method that can be used is to lay clean double-thick clear plastic (such as a grocery bag) over the lesion or wound and trace the shape with a permanent marker. Cut away and dispose of the bottom layer that came in contact with the client and place the top layer in the client record. Use this method only if contact with the plastic does not contaminate the wound.

BOX 30–5 Describing Skin Lesions

- *Type or structure.*   Skin lesions are classified as *primary* (those that appear initially in response to some change in the external or internal environment of the skin) and *secondary* (those that do not appear initially but result from modifications such as chronicity, trauma, or infection of the primary lesion). For example, a vesicle (primary lesion) may rupture and cause an erosion (secondary lesion).
- *Size, shape, and texture.*   Note size in millimeters and whether the lesion is circumscribed or irregular; round or oval shaped; flat, elevated, or depressed; solid, soft, or hard; rough or thickened; fluid filled or has flakes.
- *Color.*   There may be no discoloration, one discrete color (e.g., red, brown, or black), several colors, as with *ecchymosis* (a bruise), in which an initial dark red or blue color fades to a yellow color. When

color changes are limited to the edges of a lesion, they are described as *circumscribed;* when spread over a large area, they are described as *diffuse.*
- *Distribution.*   Distribution is described according to the location of the lesions on the body and symmetry or asymmetry of findings in comparable body areas.
- *Configuration.*   Configuration refers to the arrangement of lesions in relation to each other. Configurations of lesions may be annular (arranged in a circle), may be clustered together or grouped, may be linear (arranged in a line), may be arc or bow shaped, may be merged together or indiscrete, may follow the course of cutaneous nerves, or may be meshed in the form of a network.

Hair

Assessing a client's hair includes inspecting the hair, considering developmental changes and ethnic differences, and determining the individual's hair care practices and factors influencing them. Much of the information about hair can be obtained by questioning the client.

Normal hair is resilient and evenly distributed. In people with severe protein deficiency (kwashiorkor), the hair color is faded and appears reddish or bleached, and the texture is coarse and dry. Some therapies cause **alopecia** (hair loss), and some disease conditions and medications affect the coarseness of hair. For example, hypothyroidism can cause very thin and brittle hair.

Skill 30-3 describes how to assess the hair.

ASSESSING THE HAIR

PLANNING

Delegation
Assessment of the hair is not delegated to UAP. However, many aspects are observed during usual care and may be recorded by persons other than the nurse. Abnormal findings must be validated and interpreted by the nurse.

Equipment
- Clean gloves

SKILL 30-3

continued on page 582

ASSESSING THE HAIR *continued*

IMPLEMENTATION
Performance

1. Prior to performing the procedure, introduce self and verify the client's identity using agency protocol. Explain to the client what you are going to do, why it is necessary, and how he or she can cooperate. Discuss how the results will be used in planning further care or treatments.

2. Perform hand hygiene, apply gloves, and observe other appropriate infection control procedures.
3. Provide for client privacy.
4. Inquire if the client has any history of the following: recent use of hair dyes, rinses, or curling or straightening preparations; recent chemotherapy (if alopecia is present); presence of disease, such as hypothyroidism, which can be associated with dry, brittle hair.

ASSESSMENT	NORMAL FINDINGS	DEVIATIONS FROM NORMAL
5. Inspect the evenness of growth over the scalp.	Evenly distributed hair	Patches of hair loss (i.e., alopecia)
6. Inspect hair thickness or thinness.	Thick hair	Very thin hair (e.g., in hypothyroidism)
7. Inspect hair texture and oiliness.	Silky, resilient hair	Brittle hair (e.g., hypothyroidism); excessively oily or dry hair
8. Note presence of infections or infestations by parting the hair in several areas, checking behind the ears and along the hairline at the neck.	No infection or infestation	Flaking, sores, lice, nits (louse eggs), and ringworm
9. Inspect amount of body hair.	Variable	Hirsutism (abnormal hairiness) in women; naturally absent or sparse leg hair (poor circulation)

10. Document findings in the client record using forms or checklists supplemented by narrative notes when appropriate.

EVALUATION
■ Report significant deviations from normal to the primary care provider.

LIFESPAN CONSIDERATIONS Assessing the Hair

INFANTS

■ It is normal for infants to have either very little or a great deal of body and scalp hair.

CHILDREN

■ As puberty approaches, axillary and pubic hair will appear (see Box 30–9 later in this chapter).

ELDERS

■ There may be loss of scalp, pubic, and axillary hair.
■ Hairs of the eyebrows, ears, and nostrils become bristle-like and coarse.

HOME CARE CONSIDERATIONS Assessing the Hair

■ When making a home visit, ask to see the products the client usually uses on the hair. Assist the client to determine if the products are appropriate for the client's type of hair and scalp, e.g., for dry or oily hair. Provide education regarding hygiene of the hair and scalp.

■ When making a home visit, examine the equipment that the client uses on the hair. Provide client teaching regarding appropriate combs and brushes and regarding safety in using electric hair styling appliances such as hair dryers.

Nails

Nails are inspected for nail plate shape, angle between the nail and the nail bed (fingernails), nail texture, nail bed color, and the intactness of the tissues around the nails. The parts of the nail are shown in Figure 30-9 ■.

The nail plate is normally colorless and has a convex curve. The angle between the fingernail and the nail bed is normally 160 degrees (Figure 30-10 ■, *A*). One nail abnormality is the spoon shape, in which the nail curves upward from the nail bed (Figure 30-10 ■, *B*). This condition, called koilonychia, may be seen in clients with iron deficiency anemia. **Clubbing** is a condition in which the angle between the nail and the nail bed is 180 degrees or greater (Figure 30-10 ■, *C* and ■ *D*). Clubbing may be caused by a long-term lack of oxygen.

Nail texture is normally smooth. Excessively thick nails can appear in elders, in the presence of poor circulation, or in relation to a chronic fungal infection. Excessively thin nails or the

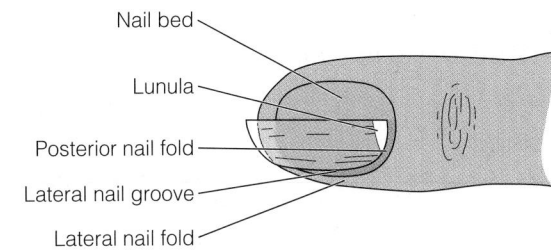

Figure 30-9 ■ The parts of a nail.

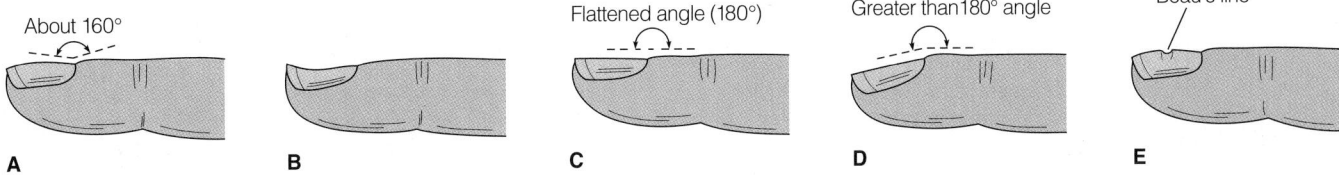

Figure 30-10 ■ *A,* A normal nail, showing the convex shape and the nail plate angle of about 160 degrees; *B,* a spoon-shaped nail, which may be seen in clients with iron deficiency anemia; *C,* early clubbing; *D,* late clubbing (may be caused by long-term oxygen lack); *E,* Beau's line on nail (may result from severe injury or illness).

presence of grooves or furrows can reflect prolonged iron deficiency anemia. Beau's lines are horizontal depressions in the nail that can result from injury or severe illness (Figure 30-10 ■, *E*). The nail bed is highly vascular, a characteristic that accounts for its color. A bluish or purplish tint to the nail bed may reflect cyanosis, and pallor may reflect poor arterial circulation. Should the client report a history of nail fungus (onychomycosis), a referral to a podiatrist or dermatologist for treatment of nail fungus may be appropriate. Symptoms of nail fungus include brittleness, discoloration, thickening, distortion of nail shape, crumbling of the nail, and loosening (detaching) of the nail.

The tissue surrounding the nails is normally intact epidermis. Paronychia is an inflammation of the tissues surrounding a nail (often referred to as an "ingrown nail"). The tissues appear inflamed and swollen, and tenderness is usually present. A **blanch test** can be carried out to test the capillary refill, that is, peripheral circulation. Normal nail bed capillaries blanch when pressed but quickly turn pink or their usual color when pressure is released. A slow rate of capillary refill may indicate circulatory problems.

Skill 30-4 describes how to assess the nails.

ASSESSING THE NAILS

PLANNING

Delegation
Assessment of the nails is not delegated to UAP. However, many aspects are observed during usual care and may be recorded by persons other than the nurse. Abnormal findings must be validated and interpreted by the nurse.

Equipment
None

IMPLEMENTATION
Performance
1. Prior to performing the procedure, introduce self and verify the client's identity using agency protocol. Explain to the client what you are going to do, why it is necessary, and how he or she can cooperate. Discuss how the results will be used in planning further care or treatments. In most situations, clients with artificial nails or polish on fingernails or toenails are not required to remove these for assessment. If the assessment cannot be conducted due to the presence of polish or artificial nails, document this in the record.
2. Observe appropriate infection control procedures.
3. Provide for client privacy.
4. Inquire if the client has any history of the following: presence of diabetes mellitus, peripheral circulatory disease, previous injury, or severe illness.

ASSESSMENT	NORMAL FINDINGS	DEVIATIONS FROM NORMAL
5. Inspect fingernail plate shape to determine its curvature and angle.	Convex curvature; angle of nail plate about 160° (Figure 30-10, *A*)	Spoon nail (Figure 30-10, *B*); clubbing (180° or greater) (Figure 30-10, *C* and *D*)
6. Inspect fingernail and toenail texture.	Smooth texture	Excessive thickness or thinness or presence of grooves or furrows; Beau's lines (Figure 30-10, *E*); discolored or detached nail—often due to fungus

continued on page 584

SKILL 30-4

SKILL 30-4

ASSESSING THE NAILS *continued*

ASSESSMENT	NORMAL FINDINGS	DEVIATIONS FROM NORMAL
7. Inspect fingernail and toenail bed color.	Highly vascular and pink in light-skinned clients; dark-skinned clients may have brown or black pigmentation in longitudinal streaks	Bluish or purplish tint (may reflect cyanosis); pallor (may reflect poor arterial circulation)
8. Inspect tissues surrounding nails.	Intact epidermis	Hangnails; paronychia (inflammation)
9. Perform blanch test of capillary refill. Press two or more nails between your thumb and index finger; look for blanching and return of pink color to nail bed.	Prompt return of pink or usual color (generally less than 4 seconds)	Delayed return of pink or usual color (may indicate circulatory impairment)

10. Document findings in the client record using forms or checklists supplemented by narrative notes when appropriate.

EVALUATION
- Perform a detailed follow-up examination of other individual systems based on findings that deviated from expected or normal for the client. Relate findings to previous assessment data if available.
- Report significant deviations from normal to the primary care provider.

LIFESPAN CONSIDERATIONS Assessing the Nails

INFANTS
- Newborns nails grow very quickly, are extremely thin, and tear easily.

CHILDREN
- Bent, bruised, or ingrown toenails may indicate shoes that are too tight.
- Nail biting should be discussed with a family member.

ELDERS
- The nails grow more slowly and thicken.
- Longitudinal bands commonly develop, and the nails tend to split.
- Bands across the nails may indicate protein deficiency; white spots, zinc deficiency; and spoon-shaped nails, iron deficiency.
- Toenail fungus is more common and difficult to eliminate (although not dangerous to health).

HOME CARE CONSIDERATIONS Assessing the Nails

- If indicated, teach the client or family member about proper nail care including how to trim and shape the nails to avoid paronychia.
- Refer the client to a podiatrist or manicurist if the client requires assistance with nail care.

THE HEAD

During assessment of the head, the nurse inspects and palpates simultaneously and also auscultates. The nurse examines the skull, face, eyes, ears, nose, sinuses, mouth, and pharynx.

Skull and Face

There is a large range of normal shapes of skulls. A normal head size is referred to as **normocephalic.** Names of areas of the head are derived from names of the underlying bones: frontal, parietal, occipital, mastoid process, mandible, maxilla, and zygomatic (Figure 30-11 ■).

Many disorders cause a change in facial shape or condition. Kidney or cardiac disease can cause edema of the eyelids. Hyperthyroidism can cause **exophthalmos,** a protrusion of the eyeballs with elevation of the upper eyelids, resulting in a startled or staring expression. Hypothyroidism, or myxedema, can cause a dry, puffy face with dry skin and coarse features and thinning of scalp hair and eyebrows. Increased adrenal hormone production or administration can cause a round face with reddened cheeks, referred

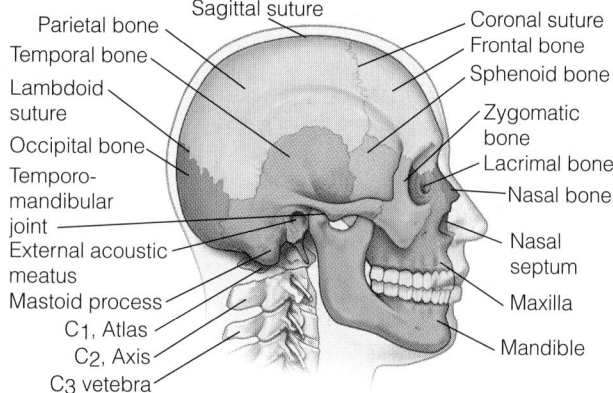

Figure 30-11 ■ Bones of the head.

to as *moon face,* and excessive hair growth on the upper lips, chin, and sideburn areas. Prolonged illness, starvation, and dehydration can result in sunken eyes, cheeks, and temples. Skill 30-5 describes how to assess the skull and face.

ASSESSING THE SKULL AND FACE

PLANNING

Delegation

Assessment of the skull and face is not delegated to UAP. However, many aspects are observed during usual care and may be recorded by persons other than the nurse. Abnormal findings must be validated and interpreted by the nurse.

Equipment

None

IMPLEMENTATION

Performance

1. Prior to performing the procedure, introduce self and verify the client's identity using agency protocol. Explain to the client what you are going to do, why it is necessary, and how he or she can cooperate. Discuss how the results will be used in planning further care or treatments.

2. Perform hand hygiene and observe appropriate infection control procedures.

3. Provide for client privacy.

4. Inquire if the client has any history of the following: past problems with lumps or bumps, itching, scaling, or dandruff; history of loss of consciousness, dizziness, seizures, headache, facial pain, or injury; when and how any lumps occurred; length of time any other problem existed; any known cause of problem; associated symptoms, treatment, and recurrences.

ASSESSMENT	NORMAL FINDINGS	DEVIATIONS FROM NORMAL
5. Inspect the skull for size, shape, and symmetry.	Rounded (normocephalic and symmetric, with frontal, parietal, and occipital prominences); smooth skull contour	Lack of symmetry; increased skull size with more prominent nose and forehead; longer mandible (may indicate excessive growth hormone or increased bone thickness)
6. Palpate the skull for nodules or masses and depressions. Use a gentle rotating motion with the fingertips. Begin at the front and palpate down the midline, then palpate each side of the head.	Smooth, uniform consistency; absence of nodules or masses	Sebaceous cysts; local deformities from trauma; masses, nodules
7. Inspect the facial features (e.g., symmetry of structures and of the distribution of hair).	Symmetric or slightly asymmetric facial features; palpebral fissures equal in size; symmetric nasolabial folds	Increased facial hair; thinning of eyebrows; asymmetric features; exophthalmos; myxedema facies; moon face
8. Inspect the eyes for edema and hollowness.		Periorbital edema; sunken eyes
9. Note symmetry of facial movements. Ask the client to elevate the eyebrows, frown, or lower the eyebrows, close the eyes tightly, puff the cheeks, and smile and show the teeth. See Skill 30-17, Assessing the Neurologic System, on page 644.	Symmetric facial movements	Asymmetric facial movements (e.g., eye on affected side cannot close completely); drooping of lower eyelid and mouth; involuntary facial movements (i.e., tics or tremors)

10. Document findings in the client record using forms or checklists supplemented by narrative notes when appropriate.

EVALUATION

- Perform a detailed follow-up examination of other systems based on findings that deviated from expected or normal for the client. Relate findings to previous assessment data if available.

- Report significant deviations from normal to the primary care provider.

LIFESPAN CONSIDERATIONS   Assessing the Skull and Face

INFANTS

- Newborns delivered vaginally can have elongated, molded heads, which take on more rounded shapes after a week or two. Infants born by cesarean section tend to have smooth, rounded heads.

- The posterior fontanel (soft spot) is about 1 cm in size and usually closes by 8 weeks. The anterior fontanel is larger, about 2 to 3 cm in size. It closes by 18 months.

- Newborns can lift their heads slightly and turn them from side to side. Voluntary head control is well established by 4 to 6 months.

Eyes and Vision

To maintain optimum vision, people need to have their eyes examined regularly throughout life. It is recommended that people under age 40 have their eyes tested every 3 to 5 years, or more frequently if there is a family history of diabetes, hypertension, blood dyscrasia, or eye disease (e.g., glaucoma). After age 40, an eye examination is recommended every 2 years to rule out the possibility of glaucoma.

An eye assessment should be carried out as part of the client's initial physical examination; periodic reassessments need to be made for clients in long-term care. Examination of the eyes includes assessment of the external structures, **visual acuity** (the degree of detail the eye can discern in an image), ocular movement, and **visual fields** (the area an individual can see when looking straight ahead). Most eye assessment procedures involve inspection. Consideration is also given to developmental changes and to individual hygienic practices, if the client wears contact lenses or has an artificial eye. For the anatomical structures of the eye, see Figure 30-12 ■ and 30-13 ■.

Many people wear eyeglasses or contact lenses to correct common refractive errors of the lens of the eye. These errors include **myopia** (nearsightedness), **hyperopia** (farsightedness), and **presbyopia** (loss of elasticity of the lens and thus loss of ability to see close objects). Presbyopia begins at about 45 years of age. People notice that they have difficulty reading newsprint. When both far and near vision require correction, two lenses (bifocals) are required. **Astigmatism,** an uneven curvature of the cornea that prevents horizontal and vertical rays from focusing on the retina, is a common problem that may occur in conjunction with myopia and hyperopia. Astigmatism may be corrected with glasses or surgery.

Three types of eye charts are available to test visual acuity (see Figure 30-14 ■). People with denominators of 40 or more on the Snellen chart with or without corrective lenses need to be referred to an ophthalmologist.

Common inflammatory visual problems that nurses may encounter in clients include conjunctivitis, dacryocystitis, hordeolum, iritis, and contusions or hematomas of the eyelids and surrounding structures. **Conjunctivitis** (inflammation of the bulbar and palpebral conjunctiva) may result from foreign bodies, chemicals, allergenic agents, bacteria, or viruses. Redness, itching, tearing, and discharge occur. During sleep, the eyelids may become encrusted and matted together. **Dacryocystitis** (inflammation of the lacrimal sac) is manifested by tearing and a discharge from the nasolacrimal duct. **Hordeolum (sty)** is a redness, swelling, and tenderness of the hair follicle and glands that empty at the edge of the eyelids. *Iritis* (inflammation of the iris) may be caused by local or systemic infections and results in pain, tearing, and photophobia (sensitivity to light). Contusions or hematomas are "black eyes" resulting from injury.

Cataracts tend to occur in persons over 65 years old. This opacity of the lens or its capsule, which blocks light rays, is frequently removed and replaced by a lens implant. Cataracts may also occur in infants due to a malformation of the lens if the mother contracted rubella in the first trimester of pregnancy. **Glaucoma** (a disturbance in the circulation of aqueous fluid, which causes an increase in intraocular pressure) is the most frequent cause of blindness in people over 40. It can be controlled if diagnosed early. Danger signs of glaucoma include blurred or foggy vision, loss of peripheral vision, difficulty focusing on close objects, difficulty adjusting to dark rooms, and seeing rainbow-colored rings around lights.

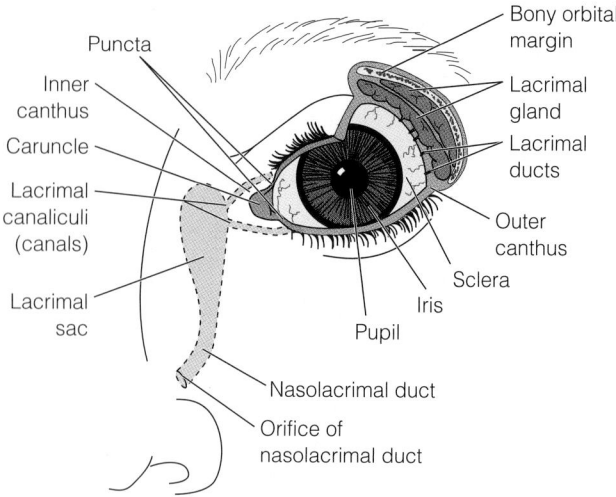

Figure 30-12 ■ The external structures and lacrimal apparatus of the left eye.

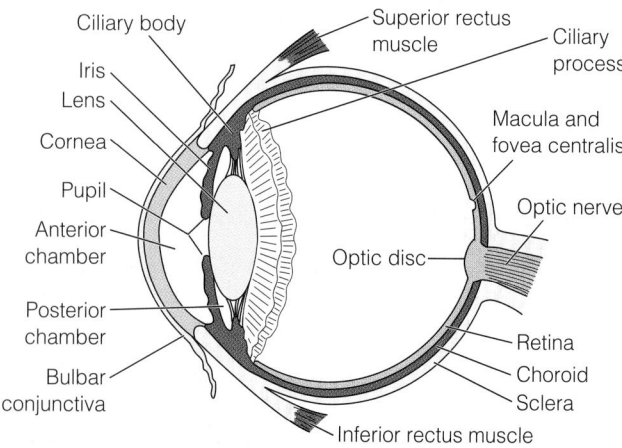

Figure 30-13 ■ Anatomic structures of the right eye, lateral view.

Figure 30-14 ■ Three types of eye charts: the preschool children's chart (*left*), the Snellen standard chart (*center*), and the Snellen E chart for clients unable to read (*right*).

Eyelids that lie at or below the pupil margin are referred to as ptosis and are usually associated with aging, edema from drug allergy or systemic disease (e.g., kidney disease), congenital lid muscle dysfunction, neuromuscular disease (e.g., myasthenia gravis), and third cranial nerve impairment. Eversion, an outturning of the eyelid, is called ectropion; inversion, an inturning of the lid, is called entropion. These abnormalities are often associated with scarring injuries or the aging process.

Pupils are normally black, are equal in size (about 3 to 7 mm in diameter), and have round, smooth borders. Cloudy pupils

are often indicative of cataracts. **Mydriasis** (enlarged pupils) may indicate injury or glaucoma, or result from certain drugs (e.g., atropine). **Miosis** (constricted pupils) may indicate an inflammation of the iris or result from such drugs as morphine or pilocarpine. It is also an age-related change in older adults. Anisocoria (unequal pupils) may result from a central nervous system disorder; however, slight variations may be normal. The iris is normally flat and round. A bulging toward the cornea can indicate increased intraocular pressure.

Skill 30-6 describes how to assess a client's eye structures and visual acuity.

ASSESSING THE EYE STRUCTURES AND VISUAL ACUITY

PLANNING

Place the client in an appropriate room for assessing the eyes and vision. The nurse must be able to control natural and overhead lighting during some portions of the examination.

Delegation

Due to the substantial knowledge and skill required, assessment of the eyes and vision is not delegated to UAP. However, many aspects are observed during usual care and may be recorded by persons other than the nurse. Abnormal findings must be validated and interpreted by the nurse.

Equipment

- Cotton tip applicator
- Gauze square
- Clean gloves
- Millimeter ruler
- Penlight
- Snellen's or E chart
- Opaque card

SKILL 30-6

continued on page 588

SKILL 30-6

ASSESSING THE EYE STRUCTURES AND VISUAL ACUITY *continued*

IMPLEMENTATION

Performance

1. Prior to performing the procedure, introduce self and verify the client's identity using agency protocol. Explain to the client what you are going to do, why it is necessary, and how he or she can cooperate. Discuss how the results will be used in planning further care or treatments.

2. Perform hand hygiene, apply gloves, and observe appropriate infection control procedures.

3. Provide for client privacy.

4. Inquire if the client has any history of the following: family history of diabetes, hypertension, blood dyscrasia, or eye disease, injury, or surgery; client's last visit to an ophthalmologist; current use of eye medications; use of contact lenses or eyeglasses; hygienic practices for corrective lenses; current symptoms of eye problems (e.g., changes in visual acuity, blurring of vision, tearing, spots, photophobia, itching, or pain).

ASSESSMENT	NORMAL FINDINGS	DEVIATIONS FROM NORMAL
External Eye Structures		
5. Inspect the eyebrows for hair distribution and alignment and skin quality and movement (ask client to raise and lower the eyebrows).	Hair evenly distributed; skin intact Eyebrows symmetrically aligned; equal movement	Loss of hair; scaling and flakiness of skin Unequal alignment and movement of eyebrows
6. Inspect the eyelashes for evenness of distribution and direction of curl.	Equally distributed; curled slightly outward	Turned inward
7. Inspect the eyelids for surface characteristics (e.g., skin quality and texture), position in relation to the cornea, ability to blink, and frequency of blinking. For proper visual examination of the upper eyelids, elevate the eyebrows with your thumb and index fingers, and have the client close the eyes. ❶ Inspect the lower eyelids while the client's eyes are closed.	Skin intact; no discharge; no discoloration Lids close symmetrically Approximately 15 to 20 involuntary blinks per minute; bilateral blinking When lids open, no visible sclera above corneas, and upper and lower borders of cornea are slightly covered	Redness, swelling, flaking, crusting, plaques, discharge, nodules, lesions Lids close asymmetrically, incompletely, or painfully Rapid, monocular, absent, or infrequent blinking Ptosis, ectropion, or entropion; rim of sclera visible between lid and iris

❶ Inspecting the upper eyelids.

ASSESSMENT	NORMAL FINDINGS	DEVIATIONS FROM NORMAL
8. Inspect the bulbar conjunctiva (that lying over the sclera) for color, texture, and the presence of lesions. Retract the eyelids with your thumb and index finger, exerting pressure over the upper and lower bony orbits, and ask the client to look up, down, and from side to side.	Transparent; capillaries sometimes evident; sclera appears white (darker or yellowish and with small brown macules in dark-skinned clients)	Jaundiced sclera (e.g., in liver disease); excessively pale sclera (e.g., in anemia); reddened sclera; lesions or nodules (may indicate damage by mechanical, chemical, allergenic, or bacterial agents)
9. Inspect the palpebral conjunctiva (that lining the eyelids) by everting the lids. Evert both lower lids, and ask the client to look up. Then gently retract the lower lids with the index fingers.	Shiny, smooth, and pink or red	Extremely pale (possible anemia); extremely red (inflammation); nodules or other lesions
10. Evert the upper lids if a problem is suspected. • Ask the client to look down while keeping the eyes slightly open.		

ASSESSING THE EYE STRUCTURES AND VISUAL ACUITY *continued*

ASSESSMENT	NORMAL FINDINGS	DEVIATIONS FROM NORMAL

ASSESSMENT

    Rationale: *Closing the eyelids contracts the orbicular muscle, which prevents lid eversion.*

- Gently grasp the client's eyelashes with the thumb and index finger. Pull the lashes gently downward. **Rationale:** *Upward or outward pulling on the eyelashes causes muscle contraction.*
- Place a cotton-tipped applicator stick about 1 cm above the lid margin, and push it gently downward while holding the eyelashes. ❷ **Rationale:** *These actions evert the lid, that is, flip the lower part of the lid over on top of itself.*
- Hold the margin of the everted lid or the eyelashes against the ridge of the upper bony orbit with the applicator stick or the thumb. ❸
- Inspect the conjunctiva for color, texture, lesions, and foreign bodies.
- To return the lid to its normal position, gently pull the lashes forward, and ask the client to look up and blink.

11. Inspect and palpate the lacrimal gland.
    - Using the tip of your index finger, palpate the lacrimal gland. ❹
    - Observe for edema between the lower lid and the nose.

12. Inspect and palpate the lacrimal sac and nasolacrimal duct.
    - Observe for evidence of increased tearing.
    - Using the tip of your index finger, palpate inside the lower orbital rim near the inner canthus. ❺

13. Inspect the cornea for clarity and texture. Ask the client to look straight ahead. Hold a penlight at an oblique angle to the eye, and move the light slowly across the corneal surface.

14. Perform the corneal sensitivity (reflex) test to determine the function of the fifth (trigeminal) cranial nerve. Ask the client to keep both eyes open and look straight ahead. Extend your hand behind the client's field of vision, then bring the gauze toward the outer canthus. Lightly touch the cornea with a corner of the gauze. ❻

NORMAL FINDINGS

❷ Everting the upper eyelid.

❹ Palpating the lacrimal gland.

No edema or tenderness over lacrimal gland

No edema or tearing

Transparent, shiny, and smooth; details of the iris are visible

In older people, a thin, grayish white ring around the margin, called arcus senilis, may be evident

Client blinks when the cornea is touched, indicating that the trigeminal nerve is intact

DEVIATIONS FROM NORMAL

❸ Holding the margin of the everted upper eyelid.

❺ Palpating the lacrimal sac and the nasolacrimal duct.

Swelling or tenderness over lacrimal gland

Evidence of increased tearing; regurgitation of fluid on palpation of lacrimal sac

Opaque; surface not smooth (may be the result of trauma or abrasion)

Arcus senilis in clients under age 40

One or both eyelids fail to respond

❻ Testing the corneal reflex.
(Patrick Watson, Pearson Education/PH)

continued on page 590

ASSESSING THE EYE STRUCTURES AND VISUAL ACUITY *continued*

ASSESSMENT	NORMAL FINDINGS	DEVIATIONS FROM NORMAL
15. Inspect the anterior chamber for transparency and depth. Use the same oblique lighting as used to test the cornea.	Transparent No shadows of light on iris Depth of about 3 mm	Cloudy Crescent-shaped shadows on far side of iris Shallow chamber (possible glaucoma)
16. Inspect the pupils for color, shape, and symmetry of size. Pupil charts are available in some agencies. See ❼ for variations in pupil diameters.	Black in color; equal in size; normally 3 to 7 mm in diameter; round, smooth border, iris flat and round	Cloudiness, mydriasis, miosis, anisocoria; bulging of iris toward cornea

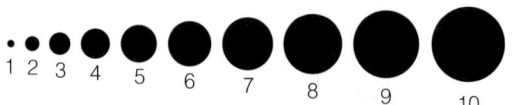

❼ Variations in pupil diameters in millimeters.

ASSESSMENT	NORMAL FINDINGS	DEVIATIONS FROM NORMAL
17. Assess each pupil's direct and consensual reaction to light to determine the function of the third (oculomotor) and fourth (trochlear) cranial nerves. • Partially darken the room. • Ask the client to look straight ahead. • Using a penlight and approaching from the side, shine a light on the pupil. • Observe the response of the illuminated pupil. It should constrict (direct response). • Shine the light on the pupil again, and observe the response of the other pupil. It should also constrict (consensual response).	Illuminated pupil constricts (direct response) Nonilluminated pupil constricts (consensual response)	Neither pupil constricts Unequal responses Absent responses
18. Assess each pupil's reaction to accommodation. • Hold an object (a penlight or pencil) about 10 cm (4 in.) from the bridge of the client's nose. • Ask the client to look first at the top of the object and then at a distant object (e.g., the far wall) behind the penlight. Alternate the gaze from the near to the far object. • Observe the pupil response. The pupils should constrict when looking at the near object and dilate when looking at the far object. • Next, move the penlight or pencil toward the client's nose. The pupils should converge. To record normal assessment of the pupils, use the abbreviation PERRLA (pupils equally round and react to light and accommodation).	Pupils constrict when looking at near object; pupils dilate when looking at far object; pupils converge when near object is moved toward nose	One or both pupils fail to constrict, dilate, or converge

ASSESSING THE EYE STRUCTURES AND VISUAL ACUITY *continued*

ASSESSMENT	NORMAL FINDINGS	DEVIATIONS FROM NORMAL

Visual Fields

19. Assess peripheral visual fields to determine function of the retina and neuronal visual pathways to the brain and second (optic) cranial nerve.

   - Have the client sit directly facing you at a distance of 60 to 90 cm (2 to 3 ft).
   - Ask the client to cover the right eye with a card and look directly at your nose.
   - Cover or close your eye directly opposite the client's covered eye (i.e., your left eye), and look directly at the client's nose.
   - Hold an object (e.g., a penlight or pencil) in your fingers, extend your arm, and move the object into the visual field from various points in the periphery. ❽ The object should be at an equal distance from the client and yourself. Ask the client to tell you when the moving object is first spotted.

     a. To test the temporal field of the left eye, extend and move your right arm in from the client's right periphery. Temporally, peripheral objects can be seen at right angles (90 degrees) to the central point of vision.

     b. To test the upward field of the left eye, extend and move the right arm down from the upward periphery. The upward field of vision is normally 50 degrees because the orbital ridge is in the way.

     c. To test the downward field of the left eye, extend and move the right arm up from the lower periphery. The downward field of vision is normally 70 degrees because the cheekbone is in the way.

     d. To test the nasal field of the left eye, extend and move your left arm in from the periphery. The nasal field of vision is normally 50 degrees away from the central point of vision because the nose is in the way.

   - Repeat the above steps for the right eye, reversing the process.

When looking straight ahead, client can see objects in the periphery

Visual field smaller than normal (possible glaucoma); one-half vision in one or both eyes (possible nerve damage)

❽ Assessing the client's left peripheral visual field.

(Patrick Watson, Pearson Education/PH)

continued on page 592

SKILL 30-6

ASSESSING THE EYE STRUCTURES AND VISUAL ACUITY *continued*

ASSESSMENT	NORMAL FINDINGS	DEVIATIONS FROM NORMAL
Extraocular Muscle Tests		
20. Assess six ocular movements to determine eye alignment and coordination. These can be performed on clients over 6 months of age.	Both eyes coordinated, move in unison, with parallel alignment	Eye movements not coordinated or parallel; one or both eyes fail to follow a penlight in specific directions, e.g., strabismus (cross-eye)
• Stand directly in front of the client and hold the penlight at a comfortable distance, such as 30 cm (1 ft) in front of the client's eyes.		**Nystagmus** (rapid involuntary rhythmic eye movement) other than at end point may indicate neurologic impairment
• Ask the client to hold the head in a fixed position facing you and to follow the movements of the penlight with the eyes only.		
• Move the penlight in a slow, orderly manner through the six cardinal fields of gaze, that is, from the center of the eye along the lines of the arrows in ❾ and back to the center.		
• Stop the movement of the penlight periodically so that nystagmus can be detected.		
21. Assess for location of light reflex by shining penlight on pupil in corneal surface (Hirschberg test).	Light falls symmetrically on both pupils (e.g., at "6 o'clock" on both pupils)	Light falls off center on one eye (indicates misalignment)
22. Have client fixate on a near or far object. Cover one eye and observe for movement in the uncovered eye (cover test).	Uncovered eye does not move	If misalignment is present, when dominant eye is covered, the uncovered eye will move to focus on object
Visual Acuity		
23. Assess near vision by providing adequate lighting and asking the client to read from a magazine or newspaper held at a distance of 36 cm (14 in.). If the client normally wears corrective lenses, the glasses or lenses should be worn during the test.	Able to read newsprint	Difficulty reading newsprint unless due to aging process

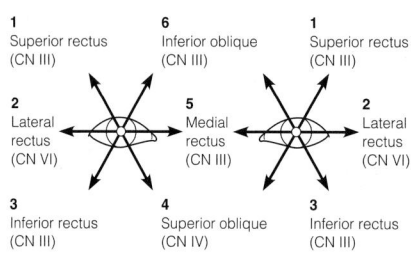

❾ The six muscles that govern eye movement.

1 Superior rectus (CN III)
6 Inferior oblique (CN III)
1 Superior rectus (CN III)
2 Lateral rectus (CN VI)
5 Medial rectus (CN III)
2 Lateral rectus (CN VI)
3 Inferior rectus (CN III)
4 Superior oblique (CN IV)
3 Inferior rectus (CN III)

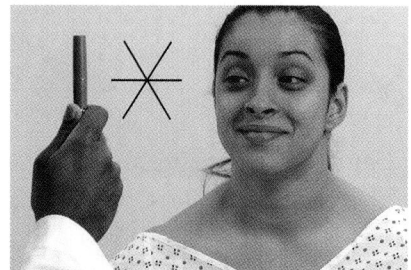

CLINICAL ALERT

A Rosenbaum eye chart may be used to test near vision. It consists of paragraphs of text or characters in different sizes on a 3½ × 6½ inch card. Be sure the client has a literacy level appropriate for the text used. ■

24. Assess distance vision by asking the client to wear corrective lenses, unless they are used for reading only, i.e., for distances of only 36 cm (12 to 14 in.).	20/20 vision on Snellen-type chart	Denominator of 40 or more on Snellen-type chart with corrective lenses
• Ask the client to stand or sit 6 m (20 ft) from a Snellen or character chart ❿, cover the eye not being tested, and identify the letters or characters on the chart.		

❿ Testing distance vision.

ASSESSING THE EYE STRUCTURES AND VISUAL ACUITY *continued*

ASSESSMENT	NORMAL FINDINGS	DEVIATIONS FROM NORMAL
• Take three readings: right eye, left eye, both eyes. • Record the readings of each eye and both eyes (i.e., the smallest line from which the person is able to read one-half or more of the letters).		

At the end of each line of the chart are standardized numbers (fractions). The top line is 20/200. The numerator (top number) is always 20, the distance the person stands from the chart. The denominator (bottom number) is the distance from which the normal eye can read the chart. Therefore, a person who has 20/40 vision can see at 20 feet from the chart what a normal-sighted person can see at 40 feet from the chart. Visual acuity is recorded as "$\overline{s}$–c" (without correction), or "$\overline{c}$–c" (with correction). You can also indicate how many letters were misread in the line, e.g., "visual acuity 20/40 − 2 $\overline{c}$–c" indicates that two letters were misread in the 20/40 line by a client wearing corrective lenses.

25. If the client is unable to see even the top line (20/200) of the Snellen-type chart, perform functional vision tests (see Box 30–6).

26. Document findings in the client record using forms or checklists supplemented by narrative notes when appropriate.

Deviation (item 25): Functional vision only (e.g., light perception, hand movements, counting fingers at 1 ft)

EVALUATION
- Perform a detailed follow-up examination of other systems based on findings that deviated from expected or normal for the client. Relate findings to previous assessment data if available.
- Report significant deviations from normal to the primary care provider. Persons with denominators of 40 or more on the Snellen or character chart, with or without corrective lenses, may need to be referred to an optometrist or ophthalmologist.

LIFESPAN CONSIDERATIONS Assessing the Eyes and Vision

INFANTS
- Infants 4 weeks of age should gaze at and follow objects.
- Ability to focus with both eyes should be present by 6 months of age.
- Infants do not have tears until about 3 months of age.
- A cover test and the corneal light reflex (Hirschberg) test should be conducted on infants to detect misalignment early and prevent amblyopia.
- Visual acuity is about 20/300 at 4 months and progressively improves.

CHILDREN
- Epicanthal folds, common in persons of Asian cultures, may cover the medial canthus and cause eyes to appear misaligned. Epicanthal folds may also be seen in young children of any race before the bridge of the nose begins to elevate.
- Preschool children's acuity can be checked with picture cards or the E chart. Acuity should approach 20/20 by 6 years of age.
- A cover test and the corneal light reflex (Hirschberg) test should be conducted on young children to detect misalignment early and prevent amblyopia.

continued on page 594

LIFESPAN CONSIDERATIONS   Assessing the Eyes and Vision—continued

- Always perform the acuity test with glasses on if a child has a prescription to wear lenses.
- Children should be tested for color vision deficit. From 8% to 10% of Caucasian males and from 0.5% to 1% of Caucasian females have this deficit; it is much less common in non-Caucasian children. The Ishihara or Hardy-Rand-Rittler test can be used.

ELDERS

Visual Acuity

- Visual acuity decreases as the lens of the eye ages and becomes more opaque and loses elasticity.
- The ability of the iris to accommodate to darkness and dim light diminishes.
- Peripheral vision diminishes.
- The adaptation to light (glare) and dark decreases.
- Accommodation to far objects often improves, but accommodation to near objects decreases.
- Color vision declines; older people are less able to perceive purple colors and to discriminate pastel colors.
- Many elders wear corrective lenses; they are most likely to have hyperopia. Visual changes are due to loss of elasticity (presbyopia) and transparency of the lens.

External Eye Structures

- The skin around the orbit of the eye may darken.
- The eyeball may appear sunken because of the decrease in orbital fat.
- Skin folds of the upper lids may seem more prominent, and the lower lids may sag.
- The eyes may appear dry and lusterless because of the decrease in tear production from the lacrimal glands.
- A thin, grayish white arc or ring (*arcus senilis*) appears around part or all of the cornea. It results from an accumulation of a lipid substance on the cornea. The cornea tends to cloud with age.
- The iris may appear pale with brown discolorations as a result of pigment degeneration.
- The conjunctiva of the eye may appear paler than that of younger adults and may take on a slightly yellow appearance because of the deposition of fat.
- Pupil reaction to light and accommodation is normally symmetrically equal but may be less brisk.
- The pupils can appear smaller in size, unequal, and irregular in shape because of sclerotic changes in the iris.

HOME CARE CONSIDERATIONS   Assessing the Eyes and Vision

- When making a home visit, take your equipment and charts with you. Also include a tape measure to lay out the 20 feet for distance vision testing.
- Use the assessment as an opportunity to reinforce proper eye care and need for regular vision testing.

BOX 30–6   Performing Functional Vision Tests

LIGHT PERCEPTION

Shine a penlight into the client's eye from a lateral position, and then turn the light off. Ask the client to tell you when the light is on or off. If the client knows when the light is on or off, the client has light perception, and the vision is recorded as "LP."

HAND MOVEMENTS (H/M)

Hold your hand 30 cm (1 ft) from the client's face and move it slowly back and forth, stopping it periodically. Ask the client to tell you when your hand stops moving. If the client knows when your hand stops moving, record the vision as "H/M 1 ft."

COUNTING FINGERS (C/F)

Hold up some of your fingers 30 cm (1 ft) from the client's face, and ask the client to count your fingers. If the client can do so, note on the vision record "C/F 1 ft."

Middle Ear Dynamics Animation

MediaLink

Ears and Hearing

Assessment of the ear includes direct inspection and palpation of the external ear, inspection of the remaining parts of the ear by an **otoscope** (instrument for examining the interior of the ear, especially the eardrum, consisting essentially of a magnifying lens and a light), and determination of auditory acuity. The ear is usually assessed during an initial physical examination; periodic reassessments may be necessary for long-term clients or those with hearing problems. In some practice settings, only advanced practice nurses perform otoscopic examinations.

The ear is divided into three parts: external ear, middle ear, and inner ear. Most of the structures mentioned next are illustrated in Figure 30-15 ■. The external ear includes the **auricle** or **pinna,** the external auditory canal, and the **tympanic membrane,** or eardrum. Landmarks of the auricle include the **lobule** (earlobe), **helix** (the posterior curve of the auricle's upper aspect), **antihelix** (the anterior curve of the auricle's upper aspect), **tragus** (the cartilaginous protrusion at the entrance to the ear canal), **triangular fossa** (a depression of the antihelix), and **external auditory meatus** (the entrance to the ear canal). Although not part of the ear, the **mastoid,** a bony prominence behind the ear, is another important landmark. The external ear canal is curved, is about 2.5 cm (1 in.) long in the adult, and ends at the tympanic membrane. It is covered with skin that has many

Figure 30-15 ■ Anatomic structures of the external, middle, and inner ear.

fine hairs, glands, and nerve endings. The glands secrete **cerumen** (earwax), which lubricates and protects the canal.

The curvature of the external ear canal differs with age. In the infant and toddler, the canal has an upward curvature. By age 3, the ear canal assumes the more downward curvature of adulthood.

The middle ear is an air-filled cavity that starts at the tympanic membrane and contains three **ossicles** (bones of sound transmission): the **malleus** (hammer), the **incus** (anvil), and the **stapes** (stirrups). The **eustachian tube,** another part of the middle ear, connects the middle ear to the nasopharynx. The tube stabilizes the air pressure between the external atmosphere and the middle ear, thus preventing rupture of the tympanic membrane and discomfort produced by marked pressure differences.

The inner ear contains the **cochlea,** a seashell-shaped structure essential for sound transmission and hearing, and the **vestibule** and **semicircular canals,** which contain the organs of equilibrium.

Sound transmission and hearing are complex processes. In brief, sound can be transmitted by air conduction or bone conduction. Air-conducted transmission occurs by this process:

1. A sound stimulus enters the external canal and reaches the tympanic membrane.
2. The sound waves vibrate the tympanic membrane and reach the ossicles.
3. The sound waves travel from the ossicles to the opening in the inner ear (oval window).
4. The cochlea receives the sound vibrations.
5. The stimulus travels to the auditory nerve (the eighth cranial nerve) and the cerebral cortex.

Bone-conducted sound transmission occurs when skull bones transport the sound directly to the auditory nerve.

Audiometric evaluations, which measure hearing at various decibels, are recommended for children and elders. A common hearing deficit with age is loss of ability to hear high-frequency sounds, such as *f, s, sh,* and *ph.* This neurosensory hearing deficit does not respond well to use of a hearing aid.

Conduction hearing loss is the result of interrupted transmission of sound waves through the outer and middle ear structures. Possible causes are a tear in the tympanic membrane or an obstruction, due to swelling or other causes, in the auditory canal. **Sensorineural hearing loss** is the result of damage to the inner ear, the auditory nerve, or the hearing center in the brain. **Mixed hearing loss** is a combination of conduction and sensorineural loss. Skill 30-7 describes how to assess the ears and hearing.

ASSESSING THE EARS AND HEARING

PLANNING
It is important to conduct the ear and hearing examination in an area that is quiet. In addition, the location should allow the client to be positioned sitting or standing at the same level as the nurse.

Delegation
Assessment of the ears and hearing is not delegated to UAP. However, many aspects are observed during usual care and may be recorded by persons other than the nurse. Abnormal findings must be validated and interpreted by the nurse.

Equipment
■ Otoscope with several sizes of ear specula

IMPLEMENTATION
Performance
1. Prior to performing the procedure, introduce self and verify the client's identity using agency protocol. Explain to the client what you are going to do, why it is necessary, and how he or she can cooperate. Discuss how the results will be used in planning further care or treatments.
2. Perform hand hygiene and observe appropriate infection control procedures.
3. Provide for client privacy.
4. Inquire if the client has any history of the following: family history of hearing problems or loss; presence of ear problems or pain; medication history, especially if there are complaints of ringing in ears; hearing difficulty: its onset, factors contributing to it, and how it interferes with activities of daily living; use of a corrective hearing device: when and from whom it was obtained.
5. Position the client comfortably, seated if possible.

continued on page 596

SKILL 30-7

ASSESSING THE EARS AND HEARING *continued*

ASSESSMENT	NORMAL FINDINGS	DEVIATIONS FROM NORMAL

Auricles

6. Inspect the auricles for color, symmetry of size, and position. To inspect position, note the level at which the superior aspect of the auricle attaches to the head in relation to the eye.

Color same as facial skin

Symmetrical

Auricle aligned with outer canthus of eye, about 10° from vertical. ❶

Bluish color of earlobes (e.g., cyanosis); pallor (e.g., frostbite); excessive redness (inflammation or fever)

Asymmetry

Low-set ears (associated with a congenital abnormality, such as Down syndrome)

Normal alignment   Low-set ears and deviation in alignment

❶ Alignment of ears.

7. Palpate the auricles for texture, elasticity, and areas of tenderness.
   - Gently pull the auricle upward, downward, and backward.
   - Fold the pinna forward (it should recoil).
   - Push in on the tragus.
   - Apply pressure to the mastoid process.

Mobile, firm, and not tender; pinna recoils after it is folded

Lesions (e.g., cysts); flaky, scaly skin (e.g., seborrhea); tenderness when moved or pressed (may indicate inflammation or infection of external ear)

External Ear Canal
and Tympanic Membrane

8. Using an otoscope, inspect the external ear canal for cerumen, skin lesions, pus, and blood.
   - Attach a speculum to the otoscope. Use the largest diameter that will fit the ear canal without causing discomfort. **Rationale:** *This achieves maximum vision of the entire ear canal and tympanic membrane.*
   - Tip the client's head away from you, and straighten the ear canal. For an adult, straighten the ear canal by pulling the pinna up and back. ❷ **Rationale:** *Straightening the ear canal facilitates vision of the ear canal and the tympanic membrane.*
   - Hold the otoscope either (a) right side up, with your fingers between the otoscope handle and the client's head or (b) upside down, with your fingers and the ulnar sur-

Distal third contains hair follicles and glands

Dry cerumen, grayish-tan color; or sticky, wet cerumen in various shades of brown

Redness and discharge

Scaling

Excessive cerumen obstructing canal

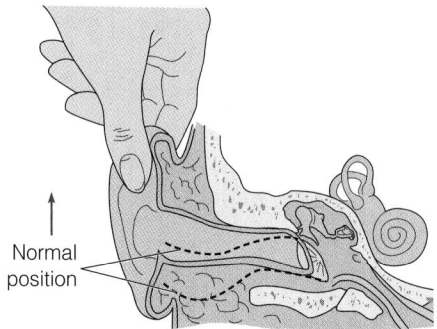

Normal position

❷ Straightening the ear canal of an adult by pulling the pinna up and back.

ASSESSING THE EARS AND HEARING *continued*

ASSESSMENT	NORMAL FINDINGS	DEVIATIONS FROM NORMAL

face of your hand against the client's head. ❸
Rationale: *This stabilizes the head and protects the eardrum and canal from injury if a quick head movement occurs.*

- Gently insert the tip of the otoscope into the ear canal, avoiding pressure by the speculum against either side of the ear canal.
Rationale: *The inner two-thirds of the ear canal is bony; if the speculum is pressed against either side, the client will experience discomfort.*

❸ Inserting an otoscope.
(Both photos: Patrick Watson, Pearson Education/PH)

9. Inspect the tympanic membrane for color and gloss.

Pearly gray color, semitransparent ❹

Pink to red, some opacity
Yellow-amber
White
Blue or deep red
Dull surface

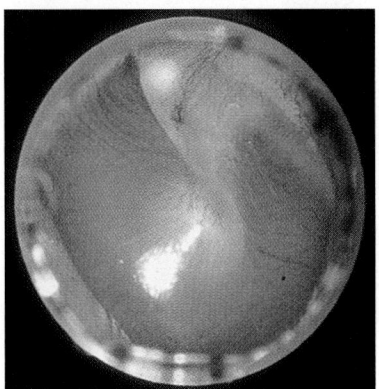

❹ Normal tympanic membrane.

Gross Hearing Acuity Tests

10. Assess client's response to normal voice tones. If client has difficulty hearing the normal voice, proceed with the following tests.

Normal voice tones audible

Normal voice tones not audible (e.g., requests nurse to repeat words or statements, leans toward the speaker, turns the head, cups the ears, or speaks in loud tone of voice)

10A. Perform the watch tick test. The ticking of a watch has a higher pitch than the human voice.
- Have the client occlude one ear. Out of the client's sight, place a ticking watch 2 to 3 cm (1 to 2 in.) from the unoccluded ear.
- Ask what the client can hear. Repeat with the other ear.

Able to hear ticking in both ears

Unable to hear ticking in one or both ears

10B. *Tuning Fork Tests*
Perform Weber's test to assess bone conduction by examining the lateralization (sideward transmission) of sounds.
- Hold the tuning fork at its base. Activate it by tapping the fork gently against the back of your hand near the knuckles or by stroking the fork between your thumb and index fingers. It should be made to ring softly.

Sound is heard in both ears or is localized at the center of the head (Weber negative)

Sound is heard better in impaired ear, indicating a bone-conductive hearing loss; or sound is heard better in ear without a problem, indicating a sensorineural disturbance (Weber positive)

continued on page 598

SKILL 30-7

ASSESSING THE EARS AND HEARING *continued*

ASSESSMENT	NORMAL FINDINGS	DEVIATIONS FROM NORMAL
• Place the base of the vibrating fork on top of the client's head ❺ and ask where the client hears the noise. Conduct the Rinne test to compare air conduction to bone conduction. • Ask the client to block the hearing in one ear intermittently by moving a fingertip in and out of the ear canal. • Hold the handle of the activated tuning fork on the mastoid process of one ear ❻ until the client states that the vibration can no longer be heard. • Immediately hold the still vibrating fork prongs in front of the client's ear canal. ❼ Push aside the client's hair if necessary. Ask whether the client now hears the sound. Sound conducted by air is heard more readily than sound conducted by bone. The tuning fork vibrations conducted by air are normally heard longer. 11. Document findings in the client record using forms or checklists supplemented by narrative notes when appropriate.	Air-conducted (AC) hearing is greater than bone-conducted (BC) hearing, i.e., AC > BC (positive Rinne) ❺ Rinne test tuning fork placement. Placing the base of a tuning fork on the client's skull (Weber's test). (❺, ❻, ❼ Patrick Watson, Pearson Education/PH)	Bone conduction time is equal to or longer than the air conduction time, i.e., BC > AC or BC = AC (negative Rinne; indicates a conductive hearing loss) ❻ Base of the tuning fork on the mastoid process. ❼ Tuning fork prongs placed in front of the client's ear.

EVALUATION
▪ Perform a detailed follow-up examination of the neurologic system based on findings that deviated from expected or normal for the client. Relate findings to previous assessment data if available.
▪ Report significant deviations from normal to the primary care provider.

LIFESPAN CONSIDERATIONS Assessing the Ears and Hearing

INFANTS
To assess gross hearing, ring a bell from behind the infant or have the parent call the child's name to check for a response. Newborns will quiet to the sound and may open their eyes wider. By 3 to 4 months of age, the child will turn head and eyes toward the sound.

▪ All newborns should be assessed for hearing using auditory brain response testing prior to discharge from the hospital.

CHILDREN
▪ To inspect the external canal and tympanic membrane in children less than 3 years old, pull the pinna down and back. Insert the speculum only 1/4 to 1/2 inch.
▪ Hearing loss is becoming more common in adolescents and young adults, probably as a result of exposure to loud music and prolonged use of headsets at loud volumes.

ELDERS
▪ The skin of the ear may appear dry and be less resilient because of the loss of connective tissue.
▪ Increased coarse and wire-like hair growth occurs along the helix, antihelix, and tragus.
▪ The pinna increases in both width and length, and the earlobe elongates.
▪ Earwax is drier.
▪ The tympanic membrane is more translucent and less flexible. The intensity of the light reflex may diminish slightly.
▪ Sensorineural hearing loss occurs.
▪ Generalized hearing loss (presbycusis) occurs in all frequencies, although the first symptom is the loss of high-frequency sounds: the *f, s, sh,* and *ph* sounds. To such persons, conversation can be distorted and result in what appears to be inappropriate or confused behavior.

> **HOME CARE CONSIDERATIONS Assessing the Ears and Hearing**
>
> - Ensure that the examination is conducted in a quiet place. In particular, elders will have difficulty accurately reporting results of hearing tests if there is excessive outside noise.
> - If necessary, ask the adult present with an infant or child to assist in holding the child still during the examination.

Nose and Sinuses

A nurse can inspect the nasal passages very simply with a flashlight. However, a nasal *speculum* and a penlight or an otoscope with a nasal attachment facilitates examination of the nasal cavity.

Assessment of the nose includes inspection and palpation of the external nose (the upper third of the nose is bone; the remainder is cartilage); patency of the nasal cavities; and inspection of the nasal cavities.

If the client reports difficulty or abnormality in smell, the nurse may test the client's olfactory sense by asking the client to identify common odors such as coffee or mint. This is done by asking the client to close the eyes and placing vials containing the scent under the client's nose.

The nurse also inspects and palpates the facial sinuses (Figure 30-16 ■). Skill 30–8 describes how to assess the nose and sinuses.

Lateral view

Frontal view

Figure 30-16 ■ The facial sinuses.

ASSESSING THE NOSE AND SINUSES

PLANNING

Delegation
Assessment of the nose and sinuses is not delegated to UAP. However, many aspects are observed during usual care and may be recorded by persons other than the nurse. Abnormal findings must be validated and interpreted by the nurse.

Equipment
- Nasal speculum
- Flashlight/penlight

IMPLEMENTATION
Performance

1. Prior to performing the procedure, introduce self and verify the client's identity using agency protocol. Explain to the client what you are going to do, why it is necessary, and how he or she can cooperate. Discuss how the results will be used in planning further care or treatments.

2. Perform hand hygiene and observe appropriate infection control procedures.
3. Provide for client privacy.
4. Inquire if the client has any history of the following: allergies, difficulty breathing through the nose, sinus infections, injuries to nose or face, nosebleeds; medications taken; changes in sense of smell.
5. Position the client comfortably, seated if possible.

SKILL 30-8

continued on page 600

SKILL 30-8

ASSESSING THE NOSE AND SINUSES *continued*

ASSESSMENT	NORMAL FINDINGS	DEVIATIONS FROM NORMAL
Nose		
6. Inspect the external nose for any deviations in shape, size, or color and flaring or discharge from the nares.	Symmetric and straight No discharge or flaring Uniform color	Asymmetric Discharge from nares Localized areas of redness or presence of skin lesions
7. Lightly palpate the external nose to determine any areas of tenderness, masses, and displacements of bone and cartilage.	Not tender; no lesions	Tenderness on palpation; presence of lesions
8. Determine patency of both nasal cavities. Ask the client to close the mouth, exert pressure on one naris, and breathe through the opposite naris. Repeat the procedure to assess patency of the opposite naris.	Air moves freely as the client breathes through the nares	Air movement is restricted in one or both nares
9. Inspect the nasal cavities using a flashlight or a nasal speculum. • Hold the speculum in your right hand to inspect the client's left nostril and your left hand to inspect the client's right nostril. • Tip the client's head back. • Facing the client, insert the tip of the closed speculum (blades together) about 1 cm or up to the point at which the blade widens. Care must be taken to avoid pressure on the sensitive nasal septum. ❶ • Stabilize the speculum with your index finger against the side of the nose. Use the other hand to position the head and then to hold the light. • Open the speculum as much as possible and inspect the floor of the nose (vestibule), the anterior portion of the septum, the middle meatus, and the middle turbinates. The posterior turbinate is rarely visualized because of its position. ❷ • Inspect the lining of the nares and the integrity and the position of the nasal septum.		

❶ Using a nasal speculum to inspect the nasal passages.

❷ The inferior and middle turbinates of the nasal passage.

ASSESSMENT	NORMAL FINDINGS	DEVIATIONS FROM NORMAL
10. Observe for the presence of redness, swelling, growths, and discharge.	Mucosa pink Clear, watery discharge No lesions	Mucosa red, edematous Abnormal discharge (e.g., pus) Presence of lesions (e.g., polyps)
11. Inspect the nasal septum between the nasal chambers.	Nasal septum intact and in midline	Septum deviated to the right or to the left
Facial Sinuses		
12. Palpate the maxillary and frontal sinuses for tenderness.	Not tender	Tenderness in one or more sinuses
13. Document findings in the client record using forms or checklists supplemented by narrative notes when appropriate.		

ASSESSING THE NOSE AND SINUSES *continued*

EVALUATION

- Perform a detailed follow-up examination of other systems based on findings that deviated from expected or normal for the client. Relate findings to previous assessment data if available.

- Report significant deviations from normal to the primary care provider.

LIFESPAN CONSIDERATIONS **Assessing the Nose and Sinuses**

INFANTS

- A speculum is usually not necessary to examine the septum, turbinates, and vestibule. Instead, push the tip of the nose upward with the thumb and shine a light into the nares.
- Ethmoid and maxillary sinuses are present at birth; frontal sinuses begin to develop by 1 to 2 years of age; and sphenoid sinuses develop later in childhood. Infants and young children have fewer sinus problems than older children and adolescents.

CHILDREN

- A speculum is usually not necessary to examine the septum, turbinates, and vestibule. It might cause the child to be apprehensive. Instead, push the tip of the nose upward with the thumb and shine a light into the nares.

- Ethmoid sinuses develop by age 6. Sinus problems in children under this age are rare.
- Cough and runny nose are the most common signs of sinusitis in preadolescent children.
- Adolescents may have headaches, facial tenderness, and swelling, similar to the signs seen in adults.

ELDERS

- The sense of smell markedly diminishes because of a decrease in the number of olfactory nerve fibers and atrophy of the remaining fibers. Elders are less able to identify and discriminate odors.
- Nosebleeds may result from hypertensive disease or other arterial vessel changes.

Mouth and Oropharynx

The mouth and oropharynx are composed of a number of structures: lips, inner and buccal mucosa, the tongue and floor of the mouth, teeth and gums, hard and soft palate, uvula, salivary glands, tonsillar pillars, and tonsils. Anatomic structures of the mouth are shown in Figure 30-17 ■.

By age 25, most people have all their permanent teeth. For information about structures of the teeth, see Chapter 33 ∞ .

Normally, three pairs of salivary glands empty into the oral cavity: the parotid, submandibular, and sublingual glands. The *parotid gland* is the largest and empties through the Stensen's duct opposite the second molar. The *submandibular gland* empties through Wharton's duct, which is situated on either side of the frenulum on the floor of the mouth. The *sublingual salivary gland* lies in the floor of the mouth and has numerous openings.

Dental **caries** (cavities) and **periodontal disease (pyorrhea)** are the two problems that most frequently affect the teeth. Both problems are commonly associated with plaque and tartar deposits. **Plaque** is an invisible soft film that adheres to the enamel surface of teeth; it consists of bacteria, molecules of saliva, and remnants of epithelial cells and leukocytes. When plaque is unchecked, tartar (dental calculus) forms. **Tartar** is a visible, hard deposit of plaque and dead bacteria that forms at the gum lines. Tartar buildup can alter the fibers that attach the teeth to the gum and eventually disrupt bone tissue. Periodontal disease is characterized by **gingivitis** (red, swollen gingiva, i.e., gum), bleeding, receding gum lines, and the formation of

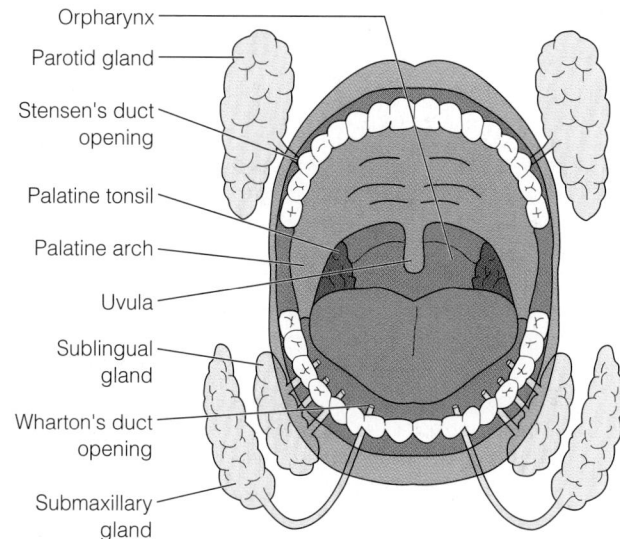

Figure 30-17 ■ Anatomic structures of the mouth.

pockets between the teeth and gums. In advanced periodontal disease, the teeth are loose and pus is evident when the gums are pressed.

Other problems nurses may see are **glossitis** (inflammation of the tongue), stomatitis (inflammation of the oral mucosa), and **parotitis** (inflammation of the parotid salivary gland). The accumulation of foul matter (food, microorganisms, and epithelial elements) on the teeth and gums is referred to as **sordes.**

Skill 30-9 describes assessment of the mouth and oropharynx.

ASSESSING THE MOUTH AND OROPHARYNX

PLANNING

If possible, arrange for the client to sit with the head against a firm surface such as a headrest or examination table. This makes it easier for the client to hold the head still during the examination.

Delegation

Assessment of the mouth and oropharynx is not delegated to UAP. However, many aspects are observed during usual care and may be recorded by persons other than the nurse. Abnormal findings must be validated and interpreted by the nurse.

Equipment

- Clean gloves
- Tongue depressor
- 2×2 gauze pads
- Penlight

IMPLEMENTATION

Performance

1. Prior to performing the procedure, introduce self and verify the client's identity using agency protocol. Explain to the client what you are going to do, why it is necessary, and how he or she can cooperate. Discuss how the results will be used in planning further care or treatments.

2. Perform hand hygiene and observe appropriate infection control procedures.
3. Provide for client privacy.
4. Inquire if the client has any history of the following: routine pattern of dental care, last visit to dentist; length of time ulcers or other lesions have been present; denture discomfort; medications client is receiving.
5. Position the client comfortably, seated if possible.

ASSESSMENT	NORMAL FINDINGS	DEVIATIONS FROM NORMAL
Lips and Buccal Mucosa		
6. Inspect the outer lips for symmetry of contour, color, and texture. Ask the client to purse the lips as if to whistle.	Uniform pink color (darker, e.g., bluish hue, in Mediterranean groups and dark-skinned clients) Soft, moist, smooth texture Symmetry of contour Ability to purse lips	Pallor; cyanosis Blisters; generalized or localized swelling; fissures, crusts, or scales (may result from excessive moisture, nutritional deficiency, or fluid deficit) Inability to purse lips (may indicate facial nerve damage)
7. Inspect and palpate the inner lips and buccal mucosa for color, moisture, texture, and the presence of lesions. • Apply clean gloves. • Ask the client to relax the mouth, and, for better visualization, pull the lip outward and away from the teeth. • Grasp the lip on each side between the thumb and index finger. ❶ • Palpate any lesions for size, tenderness, and consistency. • Inspect the front teeth and gums.	Uniform pink color (freckled brown pigmentation in dark-skinned clients) Moist, smooth, soft, glistening, and elastic texture (drier oral mucosa in elderly due to decreased salivation)	Pallor; leukoplakia (white patches), red, bleeding Excessive dryness Mucosal cysts; irritations from dentures; abrasions, ulcerations; nodules

❶ Inspecting the mucosa of the lower lip.

Teeth and Gums		
8. Inspect the teeth and gums while examining the inner lips and buccal mucosa. • Ask the client to open the mouth. Using a tongue depressor, retract the cheek. ❷ View the surface buccal mucosa from top to bottom and back to front. A flashlight or penlight will help illuminate the surface. Repeat the procedure for the other side.	32 adult teeth Smooth, white, shiny tooth enamel Pink gums (bluish or brown patches in dark-skinned clients) Moist, firm texture to gums No retraction of gums (pulling away from the teeth)	Missing teeth; ill-fitting dentures Brown or black discoloration of the enamel (may indicate staining or the presence of caries) Excessively red gums Spongy texture; bleeding; tenderness (may indicate periodontal disease) Receding, atrophied gums; swelling that partially covers the teeth

SKILL 30-9

ASSESSING THE MOUTH AND OROPHARYNX *continued*

ASSESSMENT	NORMAL FINDINGS	DEVIATIONS FROM NORMAL
• Ask the client to open the mouth again. Using a penlight to assist visualization, move a finger along the inside cheek. Another finger may be moved outside the cheek. • Examine the back teeth. For proper vision of the molars, use the index fingers of both hands to retract the cheek. ❸ Ask the client to relax the lips and first close, then open, the jaw. **Rationale:** *Closing the jaw assists in observation of tooth alignment and loss of teeth; opening the jaw assists in observation of dental fillings and caries.* Observe the number of teeth, tooth color, the state of fillings, dental caries, and tartar along the base of the teeth. Note the presence and fit of partial or complete dentures. • Inspect the gums around the molars. Observe for bleeding, color, retraction (pulling away from the teeth), edema, and lesions. • Assess the texture of the gums by gently pressing the gum tissue with a tongue depressor.	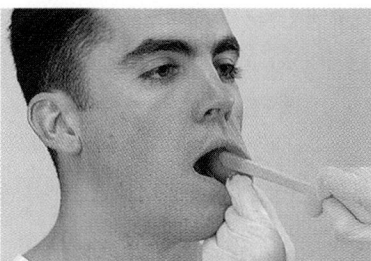 ❷ Inspecting the buccal mucosa using a tongue depressor. ❸ Inspecting the back teeth.	
9. Inspect the dentures. Ask the client to remove complete or partial dentures. Inspect their condition, noting in particular broken or worn areas.	Smooth, intact dentures	Ill-fitting dentures; irritated and excoriated area under dentures

Tongue/Floor of the Mouth

ASSESSMENT	NORMAL FINDINGS	DEVIATIONS FROM NORMAL
10. Inspect the surface of the tongue for position, color, and texture. Ask the client to protrude the tongue.	Central position Pink color (some brown pigmentation on tongue borders in dark-skinned clients); moist; slightly rough; thin whitish coating Smooth, lateral margins; no lesions Raised papillae (taste buds)	Deviated from center (may indicate damage to hypoglossal [twelfth cranial] nerve); excessive trembling Smooth red tongue (may indicate iron, vitamin B_{12}, or vitamin B_3 deficiency) Dry, furry tongue (associated with fluid deficit), white coating (may be oral yeast infection) Nodes, ulcerations, discolorations (white or red areas); areas of tenderness
11. Inspect tongue movement. Ask the client to roll the tongue upward and move it from side to side.	Moves freely; no tenderness	Restricted mobility
12. Inspect the base of the tongue, the mouth floor, and the frenulum. Ask the client to place the tip of the tongue against the roof of the mouth.	Smooth tongue base with prominent veins	Swelling, ulceration

continued on page 604

ASSESSING THE MOUTH AND OROPHARYNX *continued*

ASSESSMENT	NORMAL FINDINGS	DEVIATIONS FROM NORMAL
13. Palpate the tongue and floor of the mouth for any nodules, lumps, or excoriated areas. To palpate the tongue, use a piece of gauze to grasp its tip (stabilize it), and with the index finger of your other hand, palpate the back of the tongue, its borders, and its base. ❹ To assess function of the glossopharyngeal and hypoglossal nerves, see the neurologic assessment, later in this chapter.	Smooth with no palpable nodules	Swelling, nodules

❹ Palpating the tongue.

ASSESSMENT	NORMAL FINDINGS	DEVIATIONS FROM NORMAL
Salivary Glands		
14. Inspect salivary duct openings for any swelling or redness. See Figure 30-17.	Same as color of buccal mucosa and floor of mouth	Inflammation (redness and swelling)
Palates and Uvula		
15. Inspect the hard and soft palate for color, shape, texture, and the presence of bony prominences. Ask the client to open the mouth wide and tilt the head backward. Then, depress tongue with a tongue depressor as necessary, and use a penlight for appropriate visualization.	Light pink, smooth, soft palate Lighter pink hard palate, more irregular texture	Discoloration (e.g., jaundice or pallor) Palates the same color Irritations Exostoses (bony growths) growing from the hard palate
16. Inspect the uvula for position and mobility while examining the palates. To observe the uvula, ask the client to say "ah" so that the soft palate rises.	Positioned in midline of soft palate	Deviation to one side from tumor or trauma; immobility (may indicate damage to trigeminal [fifth cranial] nerve or vagus [tenth cranial] nerve)
Oropharynx and Tonsils		
17. Inspect the oropharynx for color and texture. Inspect one side at a time to avoid eliciting the gag reflex. To expose one side of the oropharynx, press a tongue depressor against the tongue on the same side about halfway back while the client tilts the head back and opens the mouth wide. Use a penlight for illumination, if needed.	Pink and smooth posterior wall	Reddened or edematous; presence of lesions, plaques, or drainage
18. Inspect the tonsils (behind the fauces) for color, discharge, and size.	Pink and smooth No discharge Of normal size or not visible ■ *Grade 1 (normal):* The tonsils are behind the tonsillar pillars (the soft structures supporting the soft palate).	Inflamed Presence of discharge Swollen ■ *Grade 2:* The tonsils are between the pillars and the uvula. ■ *Grade 3:* The tonsils touch the uvula. ■ *Grade 4:* One or both tonsils extend to the midline of the oropharynx.
19. Elicit the gag reflex by pressing the posterior tongue with a tongue depressor.	Present	Absent—may indicate problems with glossopharyngeal (ninth cranial) or vagus (tenth cranial) nerves

20. Document findings in the client record using forms or checklists supplemented by narrative notes when appropriate.

ASSESSING THE MOUTH AND OROPHARYNX *continued*

EVALUATION

▪ Perform a detailed follow-up examination of neurological and other systems based on findings that deviated from expected or normal for the client. Relate findings to previous assessment data if available.

▪ Report significant deviations from normal to the primary care provider.

LIFESPAN CONSIDERATIONS **Assessing the Mouth and Oropharynx**

INFANTS

▪ Inspect the palate and uvula for a cleft. A bifid (forked) uvula may indicate an unsuspected cleft palate (i.e., a cleft in the cartilage that is covered by skin).
▪ Newborns may have a pearly white nodule on their gums, which resolves without treatment.
▪ The first teeth erupt at about 6 to 7 months of age. Assess for dental hygiene; parents should cleanse the infant's teeth daily with a soft cloth or soft toothbrush.
▪ Fluoride supplements should be given by 6 months if the child's drinking water contains less than 0.3 parts per million (ppm) fluoride.
▪ Children should see a dentist by 1 year of age.

CHILDREN

▪ Tooth development should be appropriate for age.
▪ White spots on the teeth may indicate excessive fluoride ingestion.
▪ Drooling is common up to 2 years of age.
▪ The tonsils are normally larger in children than in adults and commonly extend beyond the palatine arch until the age of 11 or 12 years.

ELDERS

▪ The oral mucosa may be drier than that of younger persons because of decreased salivary gland activity. Decreased salivation oc-curs in elderly people taking prescribed medications such as antidepressants, antihistamines, decongestants, diuretics, antihypertensives, tranquilizers, antispasmodics, and antineoplastics. Extreme dryness is associated with dehydration.
▪ Some receding of the gums occurs, giving an appearance of increased toothiness.
▪ Taste sensations diminish. Sweet and salty tastes are lost first. Elderly persons may add more salt and sugar to food than they did when they were younger. Diminished taste sensation is due to atrophy of the taste buds and a decreased sense of smell. It indicates diminished function of the fifth and seventh cranial nerves.
▪ Tiny purple or bluish black swollen areas (varicosities) under the tongue, known as *caviar spots,* are not uncommon.
▪ The teeth may show signs of staining, erosion, chipping, and abrasions due to loss of dentin.
▪ Tooth loss occurs as a result of dental disease but is preventable with good dental hygiene.
▪ The gag reflex may be slightly sluggish.
▪ Elders who are homebound or are in long-term care facilities often have teeth or dentures in need of repair, due to the difficulty of obtaining dental care in these situations. Do a thorough assessment of missing teeth and those in need of repair, whether they are natural teeth or dentures.

HOME CARE CONSIDERATIONS **Assessing the Mouth and Oropharynx**

▪ Although clients may be sensitive to discussion of their personal hygiene practices, use the assessment as an opportunity to provide teaching regarding appropriate oral and dental care for the entire family. Refer clients to a dentist if indicated.

THE NECK

Examination of the neck includes the muscles, lymph nodes, trachea, thyroid gland, carotid arteries, and jugular veins. Areas of the neck are defined by the sternocleidomastoid muscles, which divide each side of the neck into two triangles: the anterior and posterior (Figure 30-18 ▪). The trachea, thyroid gland, anterior cervical nodes, and carotid artery lie within the anterior triangle (Figure 30-19 ▪); the carotid artery runs parallel and anterior to the sternocleidomastoid muscle. The posterior lymph nodes lie within the posterior triangle (Figure 30-20 ▪).

Each sternocleidomastoid muscle extends from the upper sternum and the medial third of the clavicle to the mastoid process of the temporal bone behind the ear. These muscles turn and laterally flex the head. Each trapezius muscle extends from the occipital bone of the skull to the lateral third of the

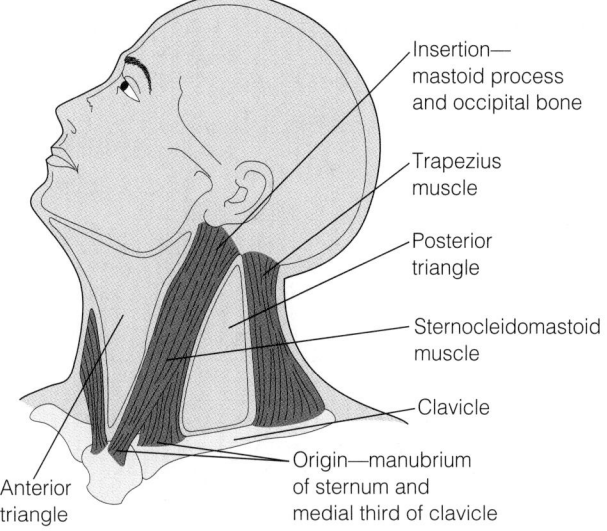

Figure 30-18 ▪ Major muscles of the neck.

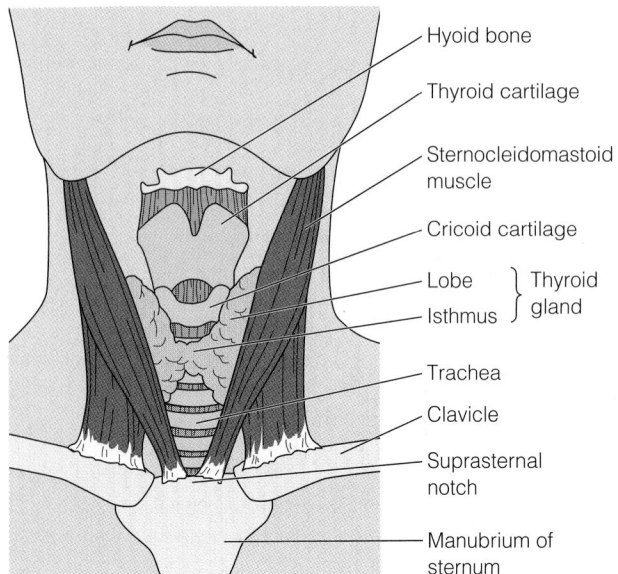

Figure 30-19 ■ Structures of the neck.

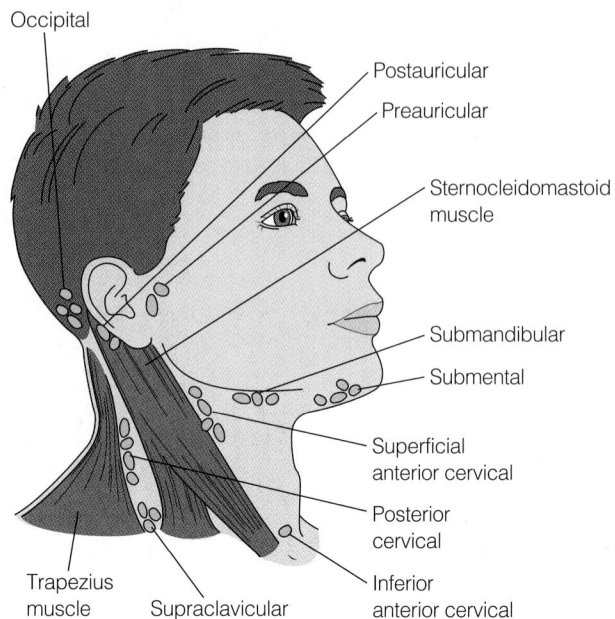

Figure 30-20 ■ Lymph nodes of the neck.

clavicle. These muscles draw the head to the side and back, elevate the chin, and elevate the shoulders to shrug them.

Lymph nodes in the neck that collect lymph from the head and neck structures are grouped serially and referred to as *chains*. See Figure 30-20 and Table 30–6. The deep cervical chain is not shown in Figure 30-20 because it lies beneath the sternocleidomastoid muscle.

Skill 30-10 describes how to assess the neck.

TABLE 30–6 Lymph Nodes of the Head and Neck

NODE CENTER	LOCATION	AREA DRAINED
Head		
Occipital	At the posterior base of the skull	The occipital region of the scalp and the deep structures of the back of the neck
Postauricular (mastoid)	Behind the auricle of the ear or in front of the mastoid process	The parietal region of the head and part of the ear
Preauricular	In front of the tragus of the ear	The forehead and upper face
Floor of Mouth		
Submandibular (submaxillary)	Along the medial border of the mandible, halfway between the angle of the jaw and the chin	The chin, upper lip, cheek, nose, teeth, eyelids, part of the tongue and of the floor of the mouth
Submental	Behind the tip of the mandible in the midline, under the chin	The anterior third of the tongue, gums, and floor of the mouth
Neck		
Superficial anterior cervical (tonsillar)	Along the mandible, anterior to the sternocleidomastoid muscle	The skin and neck
Posterior cervical	Along the anterior aspect of the trapezius muscle	The posterior and lateral regions of the neck, occiput, and mastoid
Deep cervical	Under the sternocleidomastoid muscle	The larynx, thyroid gland, trachea, and upper part of the esophagus
Supraclavicular	Above the clavicle, in the angle between the clavicle and the sternocleidomastoid muscle	The lateral regions of the neck and lungs

ASSESSING THE NECK

PLANNING

Delegation
Assessment of the neck is not delegated to UAP. However, many aspects are observed during usual care and may be recorded by persons other than the nurse. Abnormal findings must be validated and interpreted by the nurse.

Equipment
None

IMPLEMENTATION
Performance
1. Prior to performing the procedure, introduce self and verify the client's identity using agency protocol. Explain to the client what you are going to do, why it is necessary, and how he or she can cooperate. Discuss how the results will be used in planning further care or treatments.

2. Perform hand hygiene and observe appropriate infection control procedures.
3. Provide for client privacy.
4. Inquire if the client has any history of the following: problems with neck lumps; neck pain or stiffness; when and how any lumps occurred; previous diagnoses of thyroid problems; and other treatments provided (e.g., surgery, radiation).

ASSESSMENT	NORMAL FINDINGS	DEVIATIONS FROM NORMAL
Neck Muscles		
5. Inspect the neck muscles (sternocleidomastoid and trapezius) for abnormal swellings or masses. Ask the client to hold the head erect.	Muscles equal in size; head centered	Unilateral neck swelling; head tilted to one side (indicates presence of masses, injury, muscle weakness, shortening of sternocleidomastoid muscle, scars)
6. Observe head movement. Ask client to:	Coordinated, smooth movements with no discomfort	Muscle tremor, spasm, or stiffness
• Move the chin to the chest. **Rationale:** *This determines function of the sternocleidomastoid muscle.*	Head flexes 45°	Limited range of motion; painful movements; involuntary movements (e.g., up-and-down nodding movements associated with Parkinson's disease)
• Move the head back so that the chin points upward. **Rationale:** *This determines function of the trapezius muscle.*	Head hyperextends 60°	Head hyperextends less than 60°
• Move the head so that the ear is moved toward the shoulder on each side. **Rationale:** *This determines function of the sternocleidomastoid muscle.*	Head laterally flexes 40°	Head laterally flexes less than 40°
• Turn the head to the right and to the left. **Rationale:** *This determines function of the sternocleidomastoid muscle.*	Head laterally rotates 70°	Head laterally rotates less than 70°
7. Assess muscle strength.		
• Ask the client to turn the head to one side against the resistance of your hand. Repeat with the other side. **Rationale:** *This determines the strength of the sternocleidomastoid muscle.*	Equal strength	Unequal strength
• Ask the client to shrug the shoulders against the resistance of your hands. **Rationale:** *This determines the strength of the trapezius muscles.*	Equal strength	Unequal strength
Lymph Nodes		
8. Palpate the entire neck for enlarged lymph nodes.	Not palpable	Enlarged, palpable, possibly tender (associated with infection and tumors)

continued on page 608

ASSESSING THE NECK *continued*

ASSESSMENT	NORMAL FINDINGS	DEVIATIONS FROM NORMAL

- Face the client, and bend the client's head forward slightly or toward the side being examined. **Rationale:** *This relaxes the soft tissue and muscles.*
- Palpate the nodes using the pads of the fingers. Move the fingertips in a gentle rotating motion.
- When examining the submental and submandibular nodes, place the fingertips under the mandible on the side nearest the palpating hand, and pull the skin and subcutaneous tissue laterally over the mandibular surface so that the tissue rolls over the nodes.
- When palpating the supraclavicular nodes, have the client bend the head forward to relax the tissues of the anterior neck and to relax the shoulders so that the clavicles drop. Use your hand nearest the side to be examined when facing the client (i.e., your left hand for the client's right nodes). Use your free hand to flex the client's head forward if necessary. Hook your index and third fingers over the clavicle lateral to the sternocleidomastoid muscle. ❶
- When palpating the anterior cervical nodes and posterior cervical nodes, move your fingertips slowly in a forward circular motion against the sternocleidomastoid and trapezius muscles, respectively.
- To palpate the deep cervical nodes, bend or hook your fingers around the sternocleidomastoid muscle.

❶ Palpating the supraclavicular lymph nodes.

Trachea

9. Palpate the trachea for lateral deviation. Place your fingertip or thumb on the trachea in the suprasternal notch (see Figure 30-19, earlier), and then move your finger laterally to the left and the right in spaces bordered by the clavicle, the anterior aspect of the sternocleidomastoid muscle, and the trachea.

Central placement in midline of neck; spaces are equal on both sides

Deviation to one side, indicating possible neck tumor; thyroid enlargement; enlarged lymph nodes

Thyroid Gland

10. Inspect the thyroid gland.
- Stand in front of the client.
- Observe the lower half of the neck overlying the thyroid gland for symmetry and visible masses.

Not visible on inspection

Visible diffuseness or local enlargement

SKILL 30-10

ASSESSING THE NECK *continued*

ASSESSMENT

- Ask the client to extend the head and swallow. If necessary, offer a glass of water to make it easier for the client to swallow. **Rationale:** *This action determines how the thyroid and cricoid cartilages move and whether swallowing causes a bulging of the gland.*

11. Palpate the thyroid gland for smoothness. Note any areas of enlargement, masses, or nodules.

    Stand in front of or behind the client, and ask the client to lower the chin slightly. **Rationale:** *Lowering the chin relaxes the neck muscles, facilitating palpation.*

Posterior Approach

- Place your hands around the client's neck, with your fingertips on the lower half of the neck over the trachea. ❷
- Ask the client to swallow (taking a sip of water, if necessary), and feel for any enlargement of the thyroid isthmus as it rises. The isthmus lies across the trachea, below the cricoid cartilage. See Figure 30-19, earlier.
- To examine the right thyroid lobe, have the client lower the chin slightly and turn the head slightly to the right (the side being examined). With your left fingers, displace the trachea slightly to the right. With your right fingers, palpate the right thyroid lobe. Have the client swallow while you are palpating.
- Repeat the last step, in reverse, to examine the left thyroid lobe.

Anterior Approach

- Place the tips of your index and middle fingers over the trachea, and palpate the thyroid isthmus as the client swallows.
- To examine the right thyroid lobe, have the client lower the chin slightly and turn the head slightly to the right. With your right fingers, displace the trachea slightly to the client's right (your left). With your left fingers, palpate the right thyroid lobe. ❸
- To examine the left thyroid lobe, repeat the above step in reverse.

NORMAL FINDINGS

Gland ascends during swallowing but is not visible

Lobes may not be palpated

If palpated, lobes are small, smooth, centrally located, painless, and rise freely with swallowing

DEVIATIONS FROM NORMAL

Gland is not fully movable with swallowing

Solitary nodules

❷ Placement of the fingertips over the trachea to begin palpation of the thyroid gland (posterior approach).

❸ Palpating the thyroid (anterior approach).

continued on page 610

ASSESSING THE NECK *continued*

ASSESSMENT	NORMAL FINDINGS	DEVIATIONS FROM NORMAL
12. If enlargement of the gland is suspected, auscultate over the thyroid area for a bruit (a soft rushing sound created by turbulent blood flow). Use the bell of the stethoscope. **Rationale:** *The bell transmits this low-frequency sound better than the diaphragm does.*	Absence of bruit	Presence of bruit
13. Document findings in the client record using forms or checklists supplemented by narrative notes when appropriate.		

EVALUATION

■ Perform a detailed follow-up examination of other systems based on findings that deviated from expected or normal for the client. Relate findings to previous assessment data if available.

■ Report significant deviations from normal to the primary care provider.

LIFESPAN CONSIDERATIONS Assessing the Neck

INFANTS AND CHILDREN

■ Examine the neck while the infant or child is lying supine. Lift the head and turn it from side to side to determine neck mobility.

■ An infant's neck is normally short, lengthening by about age 3 years. This makes palpation of the trachea difficult.

THE THORAX AND LUNGS

Assessing the thorax and lungs is frequently critical to assessing the client's oxygenation status. Changes in the respiratory system can come about slowly or quickly. In clients with chronic obstructive pulmonary disease (COPD), such as chronic bronchitis, emphysema, and asthma, changes are frequently gradual. The onset of conditions such as pneumonia or pulmonary embolus is generally more acute or sudden.

Chest Landmarks

Before beginning the assessment, the nurse must be familiar with a series of imaginary lines on the chest wall and be able to locate the position of each rib and some spinous processes. These landmarks help the nurse to identify the position of underlying organs (e.g., lobes of the lung) and to record abnormal assessment findings. Figure 30-21 ■ shows the anterior, lateral, and posterior series of lines. The midsternal line is a vertical line running through the center of the sternum. The midclavicular lines (right and left) are vertical lines from the midpoints of the clavicles. The anterior axillary lines (right and left) are vertical lines from the anterior axillary folds (Figure 30-21, *A*). Figure 30-21, *B*, shows the three imaginary lines of the lateral chest. The posterior axillary line is a vertical line from the posterior axillary fold. The midaxillary line is a vertical line from the apex of the axilla. Figure 30-21, *C*, shows the posterior chest landmarks. The vertebral line

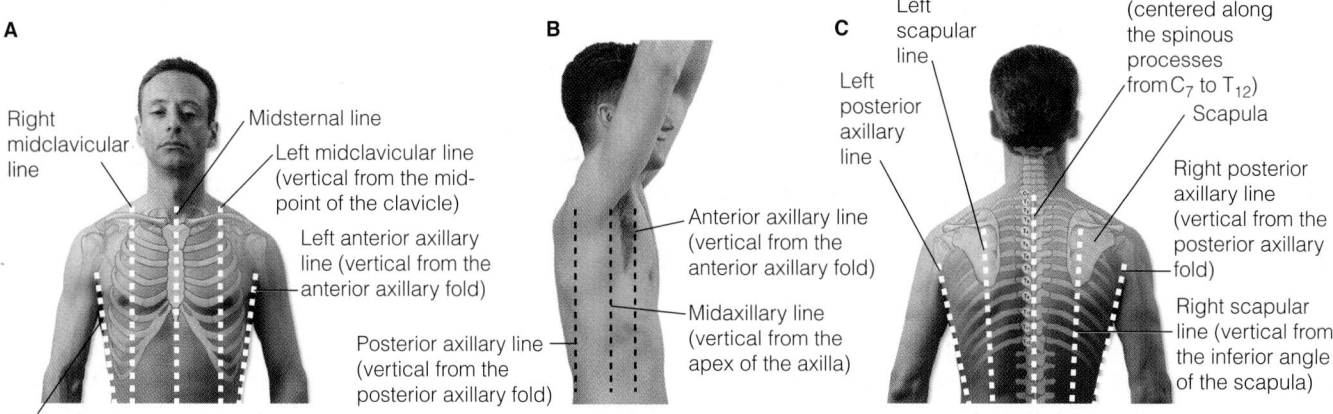

Figure 30-21 ■ Chest wall landmarks: *A*, anterior chest; *B*, lateral chest; *C*, posterior chest.

A

Horizontal
fissure
Right oblique
fissure
5th rib
midaxillary
line
6th rib

Left
midclavicular
line
6th rib
Left
oblique
fissure

B

Left upper lobe
Left oblique fissure
6th rib
midaxillary
line
Left
lower
lobe

Right upper lobe
Spinous process
of T$_3$
Right oblique
fissure
Right
lower
lobe

C

Spinous
process of T$_3$
Fifth rib at
midaxillary line
Right oblique
fissure

Fourth rib at
sternal border
Horizontal
fissure
Sixth rib at
midclavicular line

Left oblique
fissure

Apex
Spinous process
of T$_3$

Base

RUL
RML
RLL

LUL
LLL

Figure 30-22 ■ Chest landmarks: *A,* anterior chest landmarks and underlying lungs; *B,* posterior chest landmarks and underlying lungs; *C,* lateral chest landmarks and underlying lungs.

is a vertical line along the spinous processes. The scapular lines (right and left) are vertical lines from the inferior angles of the scapulae.

Locating the position of each rib and certain spinous processes is essential for identifying underlying lobes of the lung. Figure 30-22 ■, *A,* shows an anterior view of the chest and underlying lungs; Figure 30-22, *B,* a posterior view; and Figure 30-22, *C,* right and left lateral views. Each lung is first divided into the upper and lower lobes by an oblique fissure that runs from the level of the spinous process of the third thoracic vertebra (T-3) to the level of the sixth rib at the midclavicular line. The right upper lobe is abbreviated RUL; the right lower lobe, RLL. Similarly, the left upper lobe is abbreviated LUL; the left lower lobe, LLL. The right lung is further divided by a minor fissure into the right upper lobe and right middle lobe (RML). This fissure runs anteriorly from the right midaxillary line at the level of the fifth rib to the level of the fourth rib.

These specific landmarks, that is, T-3 and the fourth, fifth, and sixth ribs, are located as follows. The starting point for locating the ribs anteriorly is the **angle of Louis,** the junction between the body of the **sternum** (breastbone) and the **manubrium** (the handlelike superior part of the sternum that joins with the clavicles). The superior border of the second rib attaches to the sternum at this manubriosternal junction (Figure 30-23 ■). The nurse can identify the manubrium by first palpating the clavicle and following its course to its attachment at the manubrium. The nurse then palpates and counts distal ribs and intercostal spaces (ICSs) from the second rib. It is important to note that an ICS is numbered according to the number of the rib immediately *above* the space. When palpating for rib identification, the nurse should palpate along the midclavicular line rather than the sternal border because the rib cartilages are very close at the sternum. Only the first seven ribs attach directly to the sternum.

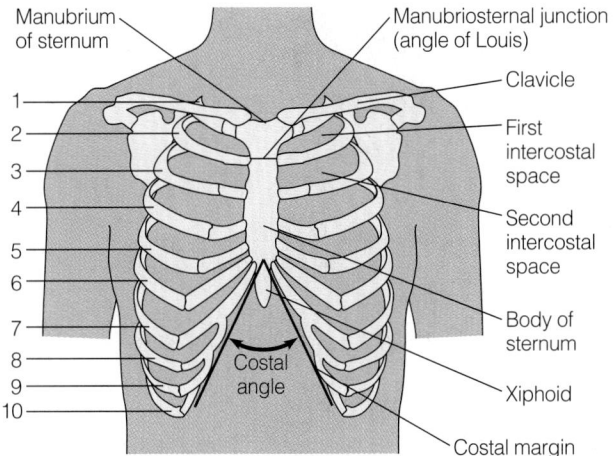

Manubrium
of sternum

Manubriosternal junction
(angle of Louis)
Clavicle
First
intercostal
space
Second
intercostal
space
Body of
sternum
Xiphoid
Costal margin

1
2
3
4
5
6
7
8
9
10

Costal
angle

Figure 30-23 ■ Location of the anterior ribs, the angle of Louis, and the sternum.

The counting of ribs is more difficult on the posterior than on the anterior thorax. For identifying underlying lung lobes, the pertinent landmark is T-3. The starting point for locating T-3 is the spinous process of the seventh cervical vertebra (C-7) (Figure 30-24 ■). When the client flexes the neck anteriorly, a prominent process can be observed and palpated. This is the spinous process of the seventh cervical vertebra. If two spinous processes are observed, the superior one is C-7, and the inferior one is the spinous process of the first thoracic vertebra (T-1). The nurse then palpates and counts the spinous processes from C-7 to T-3. Each spinous process up to T-4 is adjacent to the corresponding rib number; for example, T-3 is adjacent to the third rib. After T-4, however, the spinous processes project obliquely, causing the spinous process of the vertebra to lie, not over its correspondingly numbered rib, but over the rib below. Thus, the spinous process of T-5 lies over the body of T-6 and is adjacent to the sixth rib.

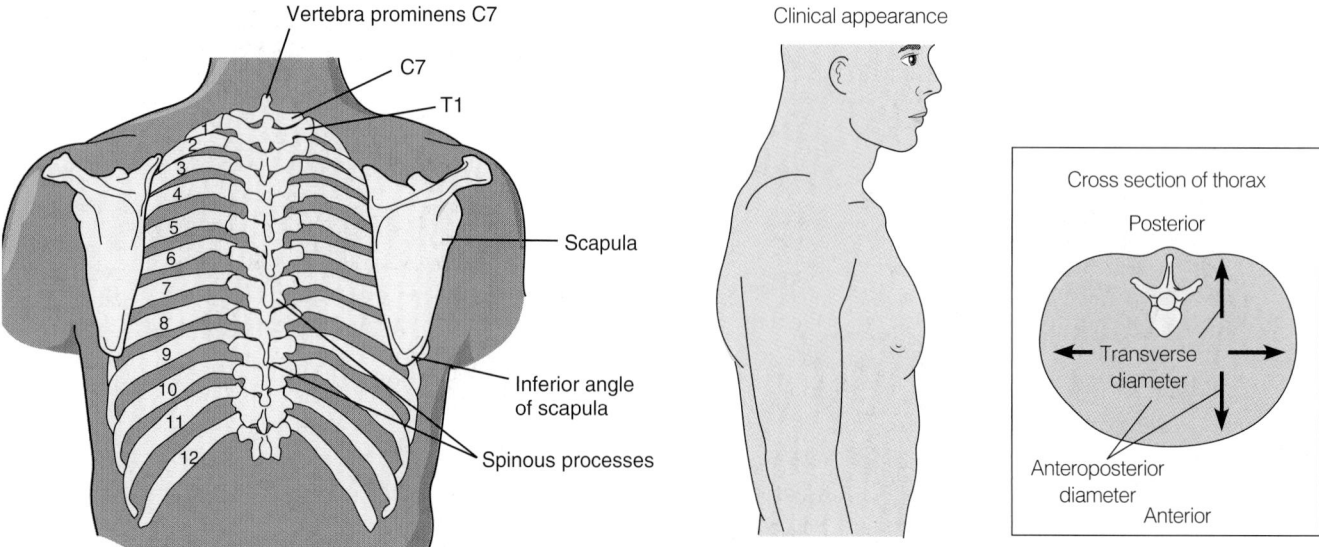

Vertebra prominens C7

C7

T1

2
3
4
5
6
7
8
9
10
11
12

Scapula

Inferior angle
of scapula

Spinous processes

Figure 30-24 ■ Location of the posterior ribs in relation to the spinous processes.

Clinical appearance

Cross section of thorax

Posterior

Transverse
diameter

Anteroposterior
diameter

Anterior

Figure 30-25 ■ Configurations of the thorax showing anteroposterior diameter and transverse diameter.

A

Posterior

Pigeon

Anterior

B

Posterior

Funnel

Anterior

C

Posterior

Barrel

Anterior

D

E

Figure 30-26 ■ Chest deformities: *A,* pigeon chest; *B,* funnel chest; *C,* barrel chest; *D,* kyphosis; *E,* scoliosis.

Chest Shape and Size

In adults, the thorax is oval. Its anteroposterior diameter is half its transverse diameter (Figure 30-25 ■). The overall shape of the thorax is elliptical; that is, its diameter is smaller at the top than at the base. In older adults, kyphosis and osteoporosis alter the size of the chest cavity as the ribs move downward and forward.

There are several deformities of the chest (Figure 30-26 ■). Pigeon chest (*pectus carinatum*), a permanent deformity, may be caused by rickets. A narrow transverse diameter, an increased anteroposterior diameter, and a protruding sternum characterize pigeon chest. A funnel chest (*pectus excavatum*), a congenital defect, is the opposite of pigeon chest in that the sternum is depressed, narrowing the anteroposterior diameter. Because the sternum points posteriorly in clients with a funnel chest, abnormal pressure on the heart may result in altered function. A barrel chest, in which the ratio of the anteroposterior to transverse diameter is 1 to 1, is seen in clients with thoracic kyphosis (excessive convex curvature of the thoracic spine) and emphysema (chronic pul-

monary condition in which the air sacs, or alveoli, are dilated and distended). Scoliosis is a lateral deviation of the spine.

Breath Sounds

Abnormal breath sounds, called **adventitious breath sounds,** occur when air passes through narrowed airways or airways filled with fluid or mucus, or when pleural linings are inflamed. Table 30–7 describes normal breath sounds. Adventitious sounds are often superimposed over normal sounds. The four types of adventitious sounds—crackles (referred to as rales or **crepitations**), gurgles, pleural friction rubs, and wheezes—are described in Table 30–8. Absence of breath sounds over some lung areas is also a significant finding that is associated with collapsed and surgically removed lobes or severe pneumonia.

Assessment of the lungs and thorax includes all methods of examination: inspection, palpation, percussion, and auscultation. Skill 30-11 describes how to assess the thorax and lungs.

TABLE 30–7 Normal Breath Sounds

TYPE	DESCRIPTION	LOCATION	CHARACTERISTICS
Vesicular	Soft-intensity, low-pitched, "gentle sighing" sounds created by air moving through smaller airways (bronchioles and alveoli)	Over peripheral lung; best heard at base of lungs	Best heard on inspiration, which is about 2.5 times longer than the expiratory phase (5:2 ratio)
Broncho-vesicular	Moderate-intensity and moderate-pitched "blowing" sounds created by air moving through larger airway (bronchi)	Between the scapulae and lateral to the sternum at the first and second intercostal spaces	Equal inspiratory and expiratory phases (1:1 ratio)
Bronchial (tubular)	High-pitched, loud, "harsh" sounds created by air moving through the trachea	Anteriorly over the trachea; not normally heard over lung tissue	Louder than vesicular sounds; have a short inspiratory phase and long expiratory phase (1:2 ratio)

TABLE 30–8 Adventitious Breath Sounds

NAME	DESCRIPTION	CAUSE	LOCATION
Crackles (rales)	Fine, short, interrupted crackling sounds; alveolar rales are high pitched. Sound can be simulated by rolling a lock of hair near the ear. Best heard on inspiration but can be heard on both inspiration and expiration. May not be cleared by coughing.	Air passing through fluid or mucus in any air passage	Most commonly heard in the bases of the lower lung lobes
Gurgles (rhonchi)	Continuous, low-pitched, coarse, gurgling, harsh, louder sounds with a moaning or snoring quality. Best heard on expiration but can be heard on both inspiration and expiration. May be altered by coughing.	Air passing through narrowed air passages as a result of secretions, swelling, tumors	Loud sounds can be heard over most lung areas but predominate over the trachea and bronchi
Friction rub	Superficial grating or creaking sounds heard during inspiration and expiration. Not relieved by coughing.	Rubbing together of inflamed pleural surfaces	Heard most often in areas of greatest thoracic expansion (e.g., lower anterior and lateral chest)
Wheeze	Continuous, high-pitched, squeaky musical sounds. Best heard on expiration. Not usually altered by coughing.	Air passing through a constricted bronchus as a result of secretions, swelling, tumors	Heard over all lung fields

SKILL 30-11

ASSESSING THE THORAX AND LUNGS

PLANNING

For efficiency, the nurse usually examines the posterior chest first, then the anterior chest. For posterior and lateral chest examinations, the client is uncovered to the waist and in a sitting position. A sitting or lying position may be used for anterior chest examination. The sitting position is preferred because it maximizes chest expansion. Good lighting is essential, especially for chest inspection.

Delegation

Assessment of the thorax and lungs is not delegated to UAP. However, many aspects of breathing are observed during usual care and may be recorded by persons other than the nurse. Abnormal findings must be validated and interpreted by the nurse.

Equipment

- Stethoscope
- Skin marker/pencil
- Centimeter ruler

IMPLEMENTATION

Performance

1. Prior to performing the procedure, introduce self and verify the client's identity using agency protocol. Explain to the client what you are going to do, why it is necessary, and how he or she can cooperate. Discuss how the results will be used in planning further care or treatments.
2. Perform hand hygiene and observe appropriate infection control procedures.
3. Provide for client privacy. In women, drape the anterior chest when it is not being examined.
4. Inquire if the client has any history of the following: family history of illness, including cancer, allergies, tuberculosis; lifestyle habits such as smoking and occupational hazards (e.g., inhaling fumes); medications being taken; current problems (e.g., swellings, coughs, wheezing, pain).

ASSESSMENT	NORMAL FINDINGS	DEVIATIONS FROM NORMAL
Posterior Thorax		
5. Inspect the shape and symmetry of the thorax from posterior and lateral views. Compare the anteroposterior diameter to the transverse diameter.	Anteroposterior to transverse diameter in ratio of 1:2 Chest symmetric	Barrel chest; increased anteroposterior to transverse diameter Chest asymmetric
6. Inspect the spinal alignment for deformities. Have the client stand. From a lateral position, observe the three normal curvatures: cervical, thoracic, and lumbar.	Spine vertically aligned	Exaggerated spinal curvatures (kyphosis, lordosis)
• To assess for lateral deviation of spine (scoliosis), observe the standing client from the rear. Have the client bend forward at the waist and observe from behind.	Spinal column is straight, right and left shoulders and hips are at same height.	Spinal column deviates to one side, often accentuated when bending over. Shoulders or hips not even.
7. Palpate the posterior thorax.		
• For clients who have no respiratory complaints, rapidly assess the temperature and integrity of all chest skin.	Skin intact; uniform temperature	Skin lesions; areas of hyperthermia
• For clients who do have respiratory complaints, palpate all chest areas for bulges, tenderness, or abnormal movements. Avoid deep palpation for painful areas, especially if a fractured rib is suspected. In such a case, deep palpation could lead to displacement of the bone fragment against the lungs.	Chest wall intact; no tenderness; no masses	Lumps, bulges; depressions; areas of tenderness; movable structures (e.g., rib)

ASSESSING THE THORAX AND LUNGS *continued*

ASSESSMENT	**NORMAL FINDINGS**	**DEVIATIONS FROM NORMAL**

8. Palpate the posterior chest for respiratory excursion (thoracic expansion). Place the palms of both your hands over the lower thorax with your thumbs adjacent to the spine and your fingers stretched laterally. ❶ Ask the client to take a deep breath while you observe the movement of your hands and any lag in movement.

Full and symmetric chest expansion (i.e., when the client takes a deep breath, your thumbs should move apart an equal distance and at the same time; normally the thumbs separate 3 to 5 cm [1 1/2 to 2 in.] during deep inspiration)

❶ Position of the nurse's hands when assessing respiratory excursion on the posterior thorax.

Asymmetric and/or decreased chest expansion

9. Palpate the chest for vocal (tactile) fremitus, the faintly perceptible vibration felt through the chest wall when the client speaks.

- Place the palmar surfaces of your fingertips or the ulnar aspect of your hand or closed fist on the posterior chest, starting near the apex of the lungs (see ❷, position A).
- Ask the client to repeat such words as "blue moon" or "one, two, three."
- Repeat the two steps, moving your hands sequentially to the base of the lungs, through positions B–E in. ❷
- Compare the fremitus on both lungs and between the apex and the base of each lung, using either one hand and moving it from one side of the client to the corresponding area on the other side *or* using two hands that are placed simultaneously on the corresponding areas of each side of the chest.

Bilateral symmetry of vocal fremitus

Fremitus is heard most clearly at the apex of the lungs

Low-pitched voices of males are more readily palpated than higher pitched voices of females

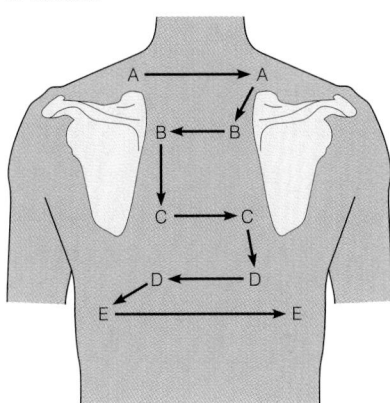

❷ Areas and sequence for palpating tactile fremitus on the posterior chest.

Decreased or absent fremitus (associated with pneumothorax)

Increased fremitus (associated with consolidated lung tissue, as in pneumonia)

10. Percuss the thorax.
Percussion of the thorax is performed to determine whether underlying lung tissue is filled with air, liquid, or solid material and to determine the positions and boundaries of certain organs. Because percussion penetrates

Percussion notes resonate, except over scapula

Lowest point of resonance is at the diaphragm (i.e., at the level of the eighth to tenth rib posteriorly)

Note: Percussion on a rib normally elicits dullness.

Asymmetry in percussion

Areas of dullness or flatness over lung tissue (associated with consolidation of lung tissue or a mass)

continued on page 616

ASSESSING THE THORAX AND LUNGS *continued*

ASSESSMENT	NORMAL FINDINGS	DEVIATIONS FROM NORMAL

to a depth of 5 to 7 cm (2 to 3 in.), it detects superficial rather than deep lesions. Percussion sounds and tones are described in Table 30–4, earlier. ❸

- Ask the client to bend the head and fold the arms forward across the chest. **Rationale:** *This separates the scapula and exposes more lung tissue to percussion.*

- Percuss in the intercostal spaces at about 5 cm (2 in.) intervals in a systematic sequence. ❹

- Compare one side of the lung with the other.

- Percuss the lateral thorax every few inches, starting at the axilla and working down to the eighth rib.

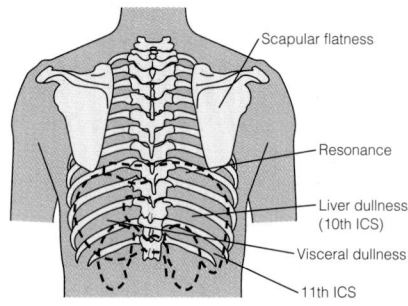

❸ Normal percussion sounds on the posterior chest.

Scapular flatness
Resonance
Liver dullness (10th ICS)
Visceral dullness
11th ICS

❹ Sequence for posterior chest percussion.

11. Percuss for diaphragmatic excursion (movement of the diaphragm during maximal inspiration and expiration).

- Ask the client to take a deep breath and hold it while you percuss downward along the scapular line until dullness is produced at the level of the diaphragm. Mark this point with a marking pencil, and repeat the procedure on the other side of the chest.

- Ask the client to take a few normal breaths and then expel the last breath completely and hold it while you percuss upward from the marked point to assess and mark the diaphragmatic excursion during deep expiration on each side.

- Measure the distance between the two marks.

Excursion is 3 to 5 cm (1 1/2 to 2 in.) bilaterally in women and 5 to 6 cm (2 to 3 in.) in men

Diaphragm is usually slightly higher on the right side

Restricted excursion (associated with lung disorder)

12. Auscultate the chest using the flat-disc diaphragm of the stethoscope (*best for transmitting the high-pitched breath sounds*).

- Use the systematic zigzag procedure used in percussion

- Ask the client to take slow, deep breaths through the mouth. Listen at each point to the breath sounds during a complete inspiration and expiration.

- Compare findings at each point with the corresponding point on the opposite side of the chest.

Vesicular and bronchovesicular breath sounds (see Table 30–7)

Adventitious breath sounds (e.g., crackles, gurgles, wheeze, friction rub; see Table 30–8)

Absence of breath sounds

ASSESSING THE THORAX AND LUNGS *continued*

ASSESSMENT	NORMAL FINDINGS	DEVIATIONS FROM NORMAL
Anterior Thorax		
13. Inspect breathing patterns (e.g., respiratory rate and rhythm).	Quiet, rhythmic, and effortless respirations (see Chapter 29, page 549)	See Chapter 29, Box 29–5, on page 549 for abnormal breathing patterns and sounds
14. Inspect the costal angle (angle formed by the intersection of the costal margins) and the angle at which the ribs enter the spine.	Costal angle is less than 90°, and the ribs insert into the spine at approximately a 45° angle (see Figure 30-23, earlier)	Costal angle is widened (associated with chronic obstructive pulmonary disease)
15. Palpate the anterior chest (see posterior chest palpation).		
16. Palpate the anterior chest for respiratory excursion.	Full symmetric excursion; thumbs normally separate 3 to 5 cm (11/2 to 2 in.)	Asymmetric and/or decreased respiratory excursion

- Place the palms of both your hands on the lower thorax, with your fingers laterally along the lower rib cage and your thumbs along the costal margins. ❺
- Ask the client to take a deep breath while you observe the movement of your hands.

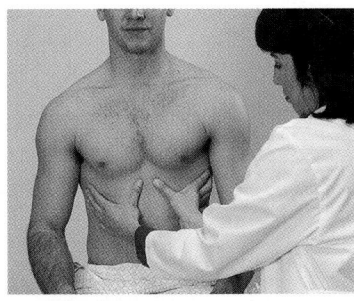

❺ Position of nurse's hands when assessing respiratory excursion on the anterior thorax.

17. Palpate tactile fremitus in the same manner as for the posterior chest and using the sequence shown in. ❻ If the breasts are large and cannot be retracted adequately for palpation, this part of the examination is usually omitted.	Same as posterior vocal fremitus; fremitus is normally decreased over heart and breast tissue	Same as posterior fremitus

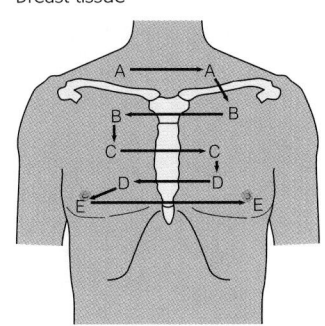

❻ Areas and sequence for palpating tactile fremitus on the anterior chest.

18. Percuss the anterior chest systematically.	Percussion notes resonate down to the sixth rib at the level of the diaphragm but are flat over areas of heavy muscle and bone, dull on areas over the heart and the liver, and tympanic over the underlying stomach ❽.	Asymmetry in percussion notes
		Areas of dullness or flatness over lung tissue

- Begin above the clavicles in the supraclavicular space, and proceed downward to the diaphragm. ❼
- Compare one side of the lung to the other.
- Displace female breasts for proper examination.

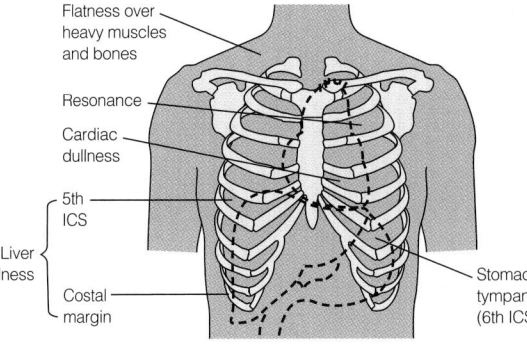

Flatness over heavy muscles and bones
Resonance
Cardiac dullness
5th ICS
Liver dullness
Costal margin
Stomach tympany (6th ICS)

❼ Sequence for anterior chest percussion.

❽ Normal percussion sounds on the anterior chest.

continued on page 618

ASSESSING THE THORAX AND LUNGS *continued*

ASSESSMENT	NORMAL FINDINGS	DEVIATIONS FROM NORMAL
19. Auscultate the trachea.	Bronchial and tubular breath sounds (see Table 30–7 on page 613)	Adventitious breath sounds (see Table 30–8 on page 613)
20. Auscultate the anterior chest. Use the sequence used in percussion ❼, beginning over the bronchi between the sternum and the clavicles.	Bronchovesicular and vesicular breath sounds (see Table 30–7)	Adventitious breath sounds (see Table 30–8)
21. Document findings in the client record using forms or checklists supplemented by narrative notes when appropriate.		

SAMPLE DOCUMENTATION

5/28/07 0830 Lungs clear to auscultation except for fine crackles both lower lobes, lessened p̄ coughing. Rarely moves in bed. Assisted to a chair and reviewed deep breathing exercises. Effective return demonstration. ————— N. Schmidt, RN

EVALUATION

▨ Relate findings to previous assessment data if available. Report significant deviations from normal to the primary care provider.

LIFESPAN CONSIDERATIONS Assessing the Thorax and Lungs

INFANTS

▨ The thorax is rounded; that is, the diameter from the front to the back (anteroposterior) is equal to the transverse diameter. See Figure 30-27. ■ It is also cylindrical, having a nearly equal diameter at the top and the base. This makes it harder for infants to expand their thoracic space.

▨ To assess tactile fremitus, place the hand over the crying infant's chest.

▨ Infants tend to breathe using their diaphragm; assess rate and rhythm by watching the abdomen, rather than the thorax, rise and fall.

▨ The right bronchial branch is short and angles down as it leaves the trachea, making it easy for small objects to be inhaled. Sudden onset of cough or other signs of respiratory distress may indicate the infant has inhaled a foreign object.

CHILDREN

▨ By about 6 years of age, the anteroposterior diameter has decreased in proportion to the transverse diameter, with a 1:2 ratio present.

▨ Children tend to breathe more abdominally than thoracically up to age 6.

▨ During the rapid growth spurts of adolescence, spinal curvature and rotation (scoliosis) may appear. Children should be assessed for scoliosis by age 12 and annually until their growth slows. Curvature greater than 10% should be referred for further medical evaluation.

ELDERS

▨ The thoracic curvature may be accentuated (kyphosis) because of osteoporosis and changes in cartilage, resulting in collapse of the vertebrae. This can also compromise and decrease normal respiratory effort.

▨ Kyphosis and osteoporosis alter the size of the chest cavity as the ribs move downward and forward.

▨ The anteroposterior diameter of the chest widens, giving the person a barrel-chested appearance. This is due to loss of skeletal muscle strength in the thorax and diaphragm and constant lung inflation from excessive expiratory pressure on the alveoli.

▨ Breathing rate and rhythm are unchanged at rest; the rate normally increases with exercise but may take longer to return to the preexercise rate.

▨ Inspiratory muscles become less powerful, and the inspiration reserve volume decreases. A decrease in depth of respiration is therefore apparent.

▨ Expiration may require the use of accessory muscles. The expiratory reserve volume significantly increases because of the increased amount of air remaining in the lungs at the end of a normal breath.

▨ Deflation of the lung is incomplete.

▨ Small airways lose their cartilaginous support and elastic recoil; as a result, they tend to close, particularly in basal or dependent portions of the lung.

▨ Elastic tissue of the alveoli loses its stretchability and changes to fibrous tissue. Exertional capacity decreases.

▨ Cilia in the airways decrease in number and are less effective in removing mucus; elderly clients are therefore at greater risk for pulmonary infections.

Clinical appearance

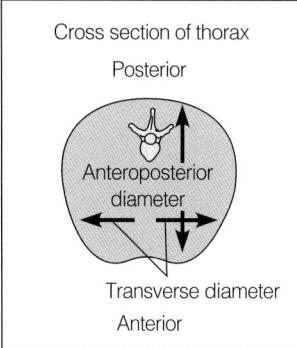

Cross section of thorax

Posterior

Anteroposterior diameter

Transverse diameter

Anterior

Figure 30-27 ■ Configurations of the child's thorax showing anteroposterior diameter and transverse diameter.

THE CARDIOVASCULAR AND PERIPHERAL VASCULAR SYSTEMS

Heart

Nurses assess the heart through inspection, palpation, and auscultation, in that sequence. Auscultation is more meaningful when other data are obtained first. The heart is usually assessed during an initial physical assessment; periodic reassessments may be necessary for long-term or at-risk clients or those with cardiac problems. Heart examinations are usually performed while the client is in a semireclined position.

In the average adult, most of the heart lies behind and to the left of the sternum. A small portion (the right atrium) extends to the right of the sternum. The upper portion of the heart (both atria), referred to as its *base,* lies toward the back. The lower portion (the ventricles), referred to as its *apex,* points anteriorly. The apex of the left ventricle actually touches the chest wall at or medial to the left midclavicular line (MCL) and at or near the fifth left intercostal space (LICS), which is slightly below the left nipple (see ❸ on page 544 ∞). This point is the point of maximal impulse (PMI).

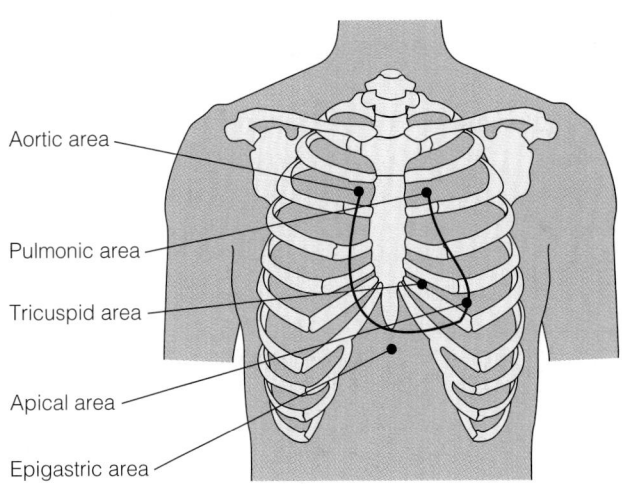

Figure 30-28 ■ Anatomic sites of the precordium.

CLINICAL ALERT

Remember that the base of the lungs is the lower (inferior) portion, and the base of the heart is the upper (superior) portion. ■

The **precordium,** the area of the chest overlying the heart, is inspected and palpated for the presence of abnormal pulsations or lifts or heaves. The terms **lift** and heave, often used interchangeably, refer to a rising along the sternal border with each heartbeat. A lift occurs when cardiac action is very forceful. It should be confirmed by palpation with the palm of the hand. Enlargement or overactivity of the left ventricle produces a heave lateral to the apex, whereas enlargement of the right ventricle produces a heave at or near the sternum.

Heart sounds can be heard by auscultation. The normal first two heart sounds are produced by closure of the valves of the heart. The first heart sound, **S₁,** occurs when the atrioventricular (A-V) valves close. These valves close when the ventricles have been sufficiently filled. Although the A-V valves do not close simultaneously, the closure occurs closely enough to be heard as one sound. S_1 is a dull, low-pitched sound described as "lub." After the ventricles empty the blood into the aorta and pulmonary arteries, the semilunar valves close, producing the second heart sound, **S₂,** described as "dub." S_2 has a higher pitch than S_1 and is shorter in duration. These two sounds, S_1 and S_2 ("lub-dub"), occur within 1 second or less, depending on the heart rate.

The two heart sounds are audible anywhere on the precordial area, but they are best heard over the aortic, pulmonic, tricuspid, and apical areas (see Figure 30-28 ■). Each area is associated with the closure of heart valves: the aortic area with the aortic valve (inside the aorta as it arises from the left ventricle); the

pulmonic area with the pulmonic valve (inside the pulmonary artery as it arises from the right ventricle); the tricuspid area with the tricuspid valve (between the right atrium and ventricle); and the apical area with the mitral valve (between the left atrium and ventricle).

Associated with these sounds are systole and diastole. **Systole** is the period in which the ventricles contract. It begins with S_1 and ends at S_2. Systole is normally shorter than diastole. **Diastole** is the period in which the ventricles relax. It starts with S_2 and ends at the subsequent S_1. Normally no sounds are audible during these periods (see Figure 30-29 ■). The experienced nurse, however, may perceive extra heart sounds (S_3 and S_4) during diastole. Both sounds are low in pitch and heard best at the apex, with the bell of the stethoscope, and with the client lying on the left side. S_3 occurs early in diastole right after S_2 and sounds like "lub-dub-*ee*" (S_1, S_2, S_3) or "Kentuc-*ky.*" It often disappears when the client sits up. S_3 is normal in children and young adults. In older adults, it may indicate heart failure. S_4 occurs near the very end of diastole just before S_1 and creates the sound of "*dee*-lub-dub" (S_4, S_1, S_2) or "*Ten*-nessee." S_4 is rarely heard in healthy young adults. S_4 may be heard in many elderly clients and can be a sign of hypertension.

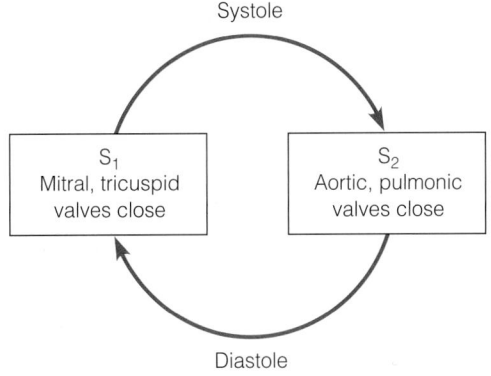

Figure 30-29 ■ Relationship of heart sounds to systole and diastole.

TABLE 30–9 Normal Heart Sounds

SOUND OR PHASE	DESCRIPTION	AREA			
		AORTIC	PULMONIC	TRICUSPID	APICAL
S_1	Dull, low pitched, and longer than S_2; sounds like "lub"	Less intensity than S_2	Less intensity than S_2	Louder than or equal to S_2	Louder than or equal to S_2
Systole	Normally silent interval between S_1 and S_2				
S_2	Higher pitch than S_1; sounds like "dub"	Louder than S_1	Louder than S_1; abnormal if louder than the aortic S_2 in adults over 40 years of age	Less intensity than or equal to S_1	Less intensity than or equal to S_1
Diastole	Normally silent interval between S_2 and next S_1				

Normal heart sounds are summarized in Table 30–9. The nurse may also hear abnormal heart sounds, such as clicks, rubs, and murmurs. These are caused by valve disorders or impaired blood flow within the heart and require advanced training to diagnose.

Central Vessels

The carotid arteries supply oxygenated blood to the head and neck (see Figure 30-30 ■). Because they are the only source of blood to the brain, prolonged occlusion of these arteries can result in serious brain damage. The carotid pulses correlate with central aortic pressure, thus reflecting cardiac function better than the peripheral pulses. When cardiac output is diminished, the peripheral pulses may be difficult or impossible to feel, but the carotid pulse should be felt easily.

The carotid is also auscultated for a bruit. A **bruit** (a blowing or swishing sound) is created by turbulence of blood flow due either to a narrowed arterial lumen (a common development in older people) or to a condition, such as anemia or hyperthyroidism, which elevates cardiac output. If a bruit is found, the carotid artery is then palpated for a thrill. A **thrill,** which frequently accompanies a bruit, is a vibrating sensation like the purring of a cat or water running through a hose. It, too, indicates turbulent blood flow due to arterial obstruction.

The jugular veins drain blood from the head and neck directly into the superior vena cava and right side of the heart. The external jugular veins are superficial and may be visible above the clavicle. The internal jugular veins lie deeper along the carotid artery and may transmit pulsations onto the skin of the neck. Normally, external neck veins are distended and visible

Figure 30-30 ■ Arteries and veins of the right side of the neck.

Sternocleidomastoid muscle
Internal jugular vein
Internal carotid artery
External carotid artery
Carotid sinus
External jugular vein
Common carotid artery
Aortic arch
Superior vena cava

when a person lies down; they are flat and not as visible when a person stands up, because gravity encourages venous drainage. By inspecting the jugular veins for pulsations and distention, the nurse can assess the adequacy of function of the right side of the heart and venous pressure. Bilateral jugular vein distention (JVD) may indicate right-sided heart failure.

Skill 30-12 describes how to assess the heart and central vessels.

ASSESSING THE HEART AND CENTRAL VESSELS

PLANNING

Heart examinations are usually performed while the client is in a semi-reclined position. The practitioner stands at the client's right side, where palpation of the cardiac area is facilitated and optimal inspection allowed.

Delegation
Assessment of the heart and central vessels is not delegated to UAP. However, many aspects of cardiac function are observed during usual care and may be recorded by persons other than the nurse. Abnormal findings must be validated and interpreted by the nurse.

Equipment
- Stethoscope
- Centimeter ruler

IMPLEMENTATION

Performance

1. Prior to performing the procedure, introduce self and verify the client's identity using agency protocol. Explain to the client what you are going to do, why it is necessary, and how he or she can cooperate. Discuss how the results will be used in planning further care or treatments.
2. Perform hand hygiene and observe appropriate infection control procedures.
3. Provide for client privacy.
4. Inquire if the client has any history of the following: family history of incidence and age of heart disease, high cholesterol levels, high blood pressure, stroke, obesity, congenital heart disease, arterial disease, hypertension, and rheumatic fever; client's past history of rheumatic fever, heart murmur, heart attack, varicosities, or heart failure; present symptoms indicative of heart disease, e.g., fatigue, dyspnea, orthopnea, edema, cough, chest pain, palpitations, syncope, hypertension, wheezing, hemoptysis; presence of diseases that affect heart, e.g., obesity, diabetes, lung disease, endocrine disorders; lifestyle habits that are risk factors for cardiac disease, e.g., smoking, alcohol intake, eating and exercise patterns, areas and degree of stress perceived.

ASSESSMENT	NORMAL FINDINGS	DEVIATIONS FROM NORMAL
5. Simultaneously inspect and palpate the precordium for the presence of abnormal pulsations, lifts, or heaves. Locate the valve areas of the heart:		
• Locate the angle of Louis. It is felt as a prominence on the sternum.		
• Move your fingertips down each side of the angle until you can feel the second intercostal spaces. The client's right second intercostal space is the aortic area, and the left second intercostal space is the pulmonic area.		
• From the pulmonic area, move your fingertips down three left intercostal spaces along the side of the sternum. The left fifth intercostal space close to the sternum is the tricuspid or right ventricular area.		
• From the tricuspid area, move your fingertips laterally 5 to 7 cm (2 to 3 in.) to the left middavicular line (LMCL). This is the apical or mitral area, or point of maximal impulse (PMI). If you have difficulty locating the PMI, have the client roll onto the left side to move the apex closer to the chest wall.		
• Inspect and palpate the aortic and pulmonic areas, observing them at an angle and to the side, to note the presence or absence of	No pulsations	Pulsations

continued on page 622

ASSESSING THE HEART AND CENTRAL VESSELS *continued*

ASSESSMENT	NORMAL FINDINGS	DEVIATIONS FROM NORMAL
pulsations. Observing these areas at an angle increases the likelihood of seeing pulsations.		
• Inspect and palpate the tricuspid area for pulsations and heaves or lifts.	No pulsations No lift or heave	Pulsations Diffuse lift or heave, indicating enlarged or overactive right ventricle
• Inspect and palpate the apical area for pulsation, noting its specific location (it may be displaced laterally or lower) and diameter. If displaced laterally, record the distance between the apex and the MCL in centimeters.	Pulsations visible in 50% of adults and palpable in most PMI in fifth LICS at or medial to MCL Diameter of 1 to 2 cm (1/3 to 1/2 in.) No lift or heave	PMI displaced laterally or lower (indicates enlarged heart) Diameter over 2 cm (indicates enlarged heart or aneurysm) Diffuse lift or heave lateral to apex (indicates enlargement or overactivity of left ventricle)
• Inspect and palpate the epigastric area at the base of the sternum for abdominal aortic pulsations.	Aortic pulsations	Bounding abdominal pulsations (e.g., aortic aneurysm)
6. Auscultate the heart in all four anatomic sites: aortic, pulmonic, tricuspid, and apical (mitral). Auscultation need not be limited to these areas; however, the nurse may need to move the stethoscope to find the most audible sounds for each client.	S_1: Usually heard at all sites Usually louder at apical area S_2: Usually heard at all sites Usually louder at base of heart Systole: silent interval; slightly shorter duration than diastole at normal heart rate (60 to 90 beats/min) Diastole: silent interval; slightly longer duration than systole at normal heart rates S_3 in children and young adults S_4 in many older adults	Increased or decreased intensity Varying intensity with different beats Increased intensity at aortic area Increased intensity at pulmonic area Sharp-sounding ejection clicks S_3 in older adults S_4 may be a sign of hypertension
• Eliminate all sources of room noise. **Rationale:** *Heart sounds are of low intensity, and other noise hinders the nurse's ability to hear them.*		
• Keep the client in a supine position with head elevated 30° to 45°.		
• Use both the diaphragm and the bell to listen to all areas.		
• In every area of auscultation, distinguish both S_1 and S_2 sounds.		
• When auscultating, concentrate on one particular sound at a time in each area: the first heart sound, followed by systole, then the second heart sound, then diastole. Systole and diastole are normally silent intervals.		
• Later, reexamine the heart while the client is in the upright sitting position. **Rationale:** *Certain sounds are more audible in certain positions.*		

Carotid Arteries

ASSESSMENT	NORMAL FINDINGS	DEVIATIONS FROM NORMAL
7. Palpate the carotid artery, using extreme caution.	Symmetric pulse volumes Full pulsations, thrusting quality	Asymmetric volumes (possible stenosis or thrombosis)
• Palpate only one carotid artery at a time. **Rationale:** *This ensures adequate blood flow through the other artery to the brain.*	Quality remains same when client breathes, turns head, and changes from sitting to supine position	Decreased pulsations (may indicate impaired left cardiac output) Increased pulsations
• Avoid exerting too much pressure and massaging the area. **Rationale:** *Pres-*	Elastic arterial wall	Thickening, hard, rigid, beaded, inelastic walls (indicate arteriosclerosis)

ASSESSING THE HEART AND CENTRAL VESSELS *continued*

ASSESSMENT	NORMAL FINDINGS	DEVIATIONS FROM NORMAL
sure can occlude the artery, and carotid sinus massage can precipitate bradycardia. The carotid sinus is a small dilation at the beginning of the internal carotid artery just above the bifurcation of the common carotid artery, in the upper third of the neck.		
• Ask the client to turn the head slightly toward the side being examined. This makes the carotid artery more accessible.		
8. Auscultate the carotid artery.	No sound heard on auscultation	Presence of bruit in one or both arteries (suggests occlusive artery disease)
• Turn the client's head slightly away from the side being examined. **Rationale:** *This facilitates the placement of the stethoscope.*		
• Auscultate the carotid artery on one side and then the other.		
• Listen for the presence of a bruit. If you hear a bruit, gently palpate the artery to determine the presence of a thrill.		

Jugular Veins

ASSESSMENT	NORMAL FINDINGS	DEVIATIONS FROM NORMAL
9. Inspect the jugular veins for distention while the client is placed in a semi-Fowler's position (30° to 45° angle), with the head supported on a small pillow.	Veins not visible (indicating right side of heart is functioning normally)	Veins visibly distended (indicating advanced cardiopulmonary disease)
10. If jugular distention is present, assess the jugular venous pressure (JVP).		Bilateral measurements above 3 to 4 cm are considered elevated (may indicate right-sided heart failure)
• Locate the highest visible point of distention of the internal jugular vein. Although either the internal or the external jugular vein can be used, the internal jugular vein is more reliable. **Rationale:** *The external jugular vein is more easily affected by obstruction or kinking at the base of the neck.*		Unilateral distention (may be caused by local obstruction)
• Measure the vertical height of this point in centimeters from the sternal angle, the point at which the clavicles meet. ❶		
• Repeat the preceding steps on the other side.		
11. Document findings in the client record using forms or checklists supplemented by narrative notes when appropriate.		

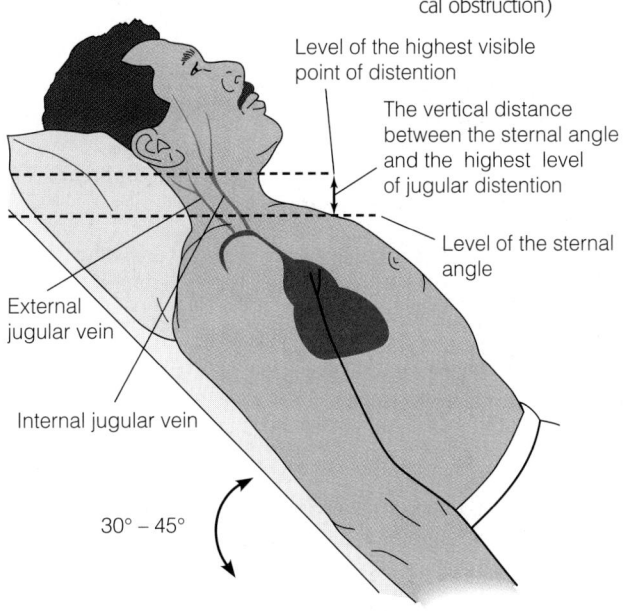

❶ Assessing the highest point of distention of the jugular vein.

continued on page 624

ASSESSING THE HEART AND CENTRAL VESSELS *continued*

EVALUATION

■ Perform a detailed follow-up examination based on findings that deviated from expected or normal for the client. Relate findings to previous assessment data if available.

■ Report significant deviations from normal to the primary care provider.

LIFESPAN CONSIDERATIONS **Assessing the Heart and Central Vessels**

INFANTS

■ Physiologic splitting of the second heart sound (S_2) may be heard when the child takes a deep breath and the aortic valve closes a split second before the pulmonic valve. If splitting of S_2 is heard during normal respirations, it is abnormal and may indicate an atrial-septal defect, pulmonary stenosis, or another heart problem.

■ Infants may normally have sinus arrhythmia that is related to respiration. The heart rate slows during expiration and increases when the child breathes in.

■ Murmurs may be heard in newborns as the structures of fetal circulation, especially the ductus arteriosus, close.

CHILDREN

■ Heart sounds may be louder because of the thinner chest wall.

■ A third heart sound (S_3), caused as the ventricles fill, is best heard at the apex and is present in about one-third of all children.

■ The PMI is higher and more medial in children under 8 years old.

ELDERS

■ If no disease is present, heart size remains the same size throughout life.

■ Cardiac output and strength of contraction decrease, thus lessening the older person's activity tolerance.

■ The heart rate returns to its resting rate more slowly after exertion than it did when the individual was younger.

■ S_4 heart sound is considered normal in older adults.

■ Extra systoles commonly occur. Ten or more systoles per minute are considered abnormal.

■ Sudden emotional and physical stresses may result in cardiac arrhythmias and heart failure.

Peripheral Vascular System

Assessing the peripheral vascular system includes measuring the blood pressure, palpating peripheral pulses, and inspecting the skin and tissues to determine **perfusion** (blood supply to an area) to the extremities. Certain aspects of peripheral vascular assessment are often incorporated into other parts of the assessment procedure. For example, blood pressure is usually measured at the beginning of the physical examination (see the section on assessing blood pressure in Chapter 29 ∞). Pulse sites and pulse assessments are described in Chapter 29 ∞ .

Skill 30-13 describes how to assess the peripheral vascular system.

ASSESSING THE PERIPHERAL VASCULAR SYSTEM

PLANNING

Delegation
Due to the substantial knowledge and skill required, assessment of the peripheral vascular system is not delegated to UAP. However, many aspects of the vascular system are observed during usual care and may be recorded by persons other than the nurse. Abnormal findings must be validated and interpreted by the nurse.

Equipment
None

IMPLEMENTATION
Performance

1. Prior to performing the procedure, introduce self and verify the client's identity using agency protocol. Explain to the client what you are going to do, why it is necessary, and how he or she can cooperate. Discuss how the results will be used in planning further care or treatments.

2. Perform hand hygiene and observe appropriate infection control procedures.

3. Provide for client privacy.

4. Inquire if the client has any history of the following: past history of heart disorders, varicosities, arterial disease, and hypertension; lifestyle habits such as exercise patterns, activity patterns and tolerance, smoking, and use of alcohol.

ASSESSING THE PERIPHERAL VASCULAR SYSTEM *continued*

ASSESSMENT	NORMAL FINDINGS	DEVIATIONS FROM NORMAL
Peripheral Pulses		
5. Palpate the peripheral pulses on both sides of the client's body individually, simultaneously (except the carotid pulse), and systematically to determine the symmetry of pulse volume. If you have difficulty palpating some of the peripheral pulses, use a Doppler ultrasound probe.	Symmetric pulse volumes Full pulsations	Asymmetric volumes (indicate impaired circulation) Absence of pulsation (indicates arterial spasm or occlusion) Decreased, weak, thready pulsations (indicate impaired cardiac output) Increased pulse volume (may indicate hypertension, high cardiac output, or circulatory overload)
Peripheral Veins		
6. Inspect the peripheral veins in the arms and legs for the presence and/or appearance of superficial veins when limbs are dependent and when limbs are elevated.	In dependent position, presence of distention and nodular bulges at calves When limbs elevated, veins collapse (veins may appear tortuous or distended in older people)	Distended veins in the thigh and/or lower leg or on posterolateral part of calf from knee to ankle
7. Assess the peripheral leg veins for signs of phlebitis. • Inspect the calves for redness and swelling over vein sites. • Palpate the calves for firmness or tension of the muscles, the presence of edema over the dorsum of the foot, and areas of localized warmth. **Rationale:** *Palpation augments inspection findings, particularly in greater pigmented people in whom redness may not be visible.* • Push the calves from side to side to test for tenderness. • Firmly dorsiflex the client's foot while supporting the entire leg in extension (Homans' test), or have the person stand or walk.	Limbs not tender Symmetric in size	Tenderness on palpation Pain in calf muscles with forceful dorsiflexion of the foot (positive Homans' test) Warmth and redness over vein Swelling of one calf or leg
Peripheral Perfusion		
8. Inspect the skin of the hands and feet for color, temperature, edema, and skin changes.	Skin color pink Skin temperature not excessively warm or cold No edema Skin texture resilient and moist	Cyanotic (venous insufficiency) Pallor that increases with limb elevation Dependent rubor, a dusky red color when limb is lowered (arterial insufficiency) Brown pigmentation around ankles (arterial or chronic venous insufficiency) Skin cool (arterial insufficiency) Marked edema (venous insufficiency) Mild edema (arterial insufficiency) Skin thin and shiny or thick, waxy, shiny, and fragile, with reduced hair and ulceration (venous or arterial insufficiency)
9. Assess the adequacy of arterial flow if arterial insufficiency is suspected.		

continued on page 626

ASSESSING THE PERIPHERAL VASCULAR SYSTEM *continued*

ASSESSMENT	NORMAL FINDINGS	DEVIATIONS FROM NORMAL
Buerger's Test (Arterial Adequacy Test) • Assist the client to a supine position. Ask the client to raise one leg or one arm about 30 cm (1 ft) above heart level, move the foot or hand briskly up and down for about 1 minute, and then sit up and dangle the leg or arm. • Observe the time elapsed until return of original color and vein filling.	Buerger's test: Original color returns in 10 seconds; veins in feet or hands fill in about 15 seconds	Delayed color return or mottled appearance; delayed venous filling; marked redness of arms or legs (indicates arterial insufficiency)
Capillary Refill Test • Squeeze the client's fingernail and toenail between your fingers sufficiently to cause blanching (about 5 seconds). • Release the pressure, and observe how quickly normal color returns. Color normally returns immediately (less than 2 seconds).	Capillary refill test: Immediate return of color	Delayed return of color (arterial insufficiency)
Other Assessments • Inspect the fingernails for changes indicative of circulatory impairment. See the section on assessment of nails, earlier in this chapter. • See also peripheral pulse assessment, earlier. 10. Document findings in the client record using forms or checklists supplemented by narrative notes when appropriate.		

SAMPLE DOCUMENTATION

5/28/07 0830 Legs mottled red bilaterally toes to mid-calf. States "actually looks a bit better." Capillary refill 4-5 seconds in toes on both feet. Pedal pulses present but weak. Homans' test negative. c/o pain in calves after walking 100 feet.

—N. Schmidt, RN

EVALUATION

■ Perform a detailed follow-up examination of the heart or central vessels, integument, or other systems based on findings that deviated from expected or normal for the client. Relate findings to previous assessment data if available.

■ Report significant deviations from normal to the primary care provider.

LIFESPAN CONSIDERATIONS   **Assessing the Peripheral Vascular System**

INFANTS

■ Screen for coarctation of the aorta by palpating the peripheral pulses and comparing the strength of the femoral pulses with the radial pulses and apical pulse. If coarctation is present, femoral pulses will be diminished and radial pulses will be stronger.

CHILDREN

■ Changes in the peripheral vasculature, such as bruising, petechiae, and purpura, can indicate serious systemic diseases in children (e.g., leukemia, meningococcemia).

ELDERS

■ The overall effectiveness of blood vessels decreases as smooth muscle cells are replaced by connective tissue. The lower extremities are more likely to show signs of arterial and venous impairment because of the more distal and dependent position.

■ Peripheral vascular assessment should always include upper and lower extremities' temperature, color, pulses, edema, skin integrity, and sensation. Any differences in symmetry of these findings should be noted.

■ Proximal arteries become thinner and dilate.

LIFESPAN CONSIDERATIONS **Assessing the Peripheral Vascular System—*continued***

- Peripheral arteries become thicker and dilate less effectively because of arteriosclerotic changes in the vessel walls.
- Blood vessels lengthen and become more tortuous and prominent. Varicosities occur more frequently.
- In some instances, arteries may be palpated more easily because of the loss of supportive surrounding tissues. Often, however, the most distal pulses of the lower extremities are more difficult to palpate because of decreased arterial perfusion.

- Systolic and diastolic blood pressures increase, but the increase in the systolic pressure is greater. As a result, the pulse pressure widens. Any client with a blood pressure reading above 140/90 should be referred for follow-up assessments.
- Peripheral edema is frequently observed and is most commonly the result of chronic venous insufficiency or low protein levels in the blood (hypoproteinemia).

HOME CARE CONSIDERATIONS **Assessing the Peripheral Vascular System**

- Use the assessment as an opportunity to provide teaching regarding appropriate care of the extremities in those at high risk for or with actual vascular impairment. Educate clients and families regarding skin and nail care, exercise, and positioning to promote circulation.

THE BREASTS AND AXILLAE

The breasts of men and women need to be inspected and palpated. Men have some glandular tissue beneath each nipple, a potential site for malignancy, whereas mature women have glandular tissue throughout the breast. In females, the largest portion of glandular breast tissue is located in the upper outer quadrant of each breast. A projection of breast tissue from this quadrant extends into the axilla, called the *axillary tail of Spence* (see Figure 30-31 ■). The majority of breast tumors are located in this upper outer breast quadrant including the tail of Spence. During assessment, the nurse can localize specific findings by using this division of the breast into quadrants and the axillary tail. Skill 30-14 describes how to assess the breasts and axillae.

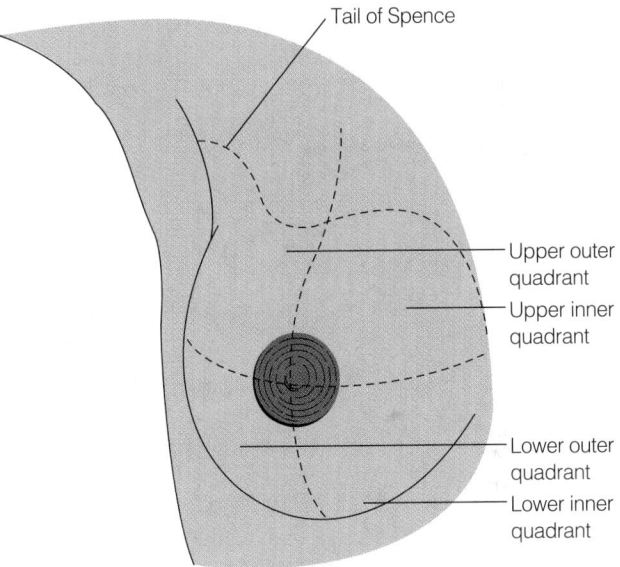

Figure 30-31 ■ Four breast quadrants and the axillary tail of Spence.

ASSESSING THE BREASTS AND AXILLAE

SKILL 30-14

PLANNING

Delegation
Assessment of the breasts and axillae is not delegated to UAP. However, persons other than the nurse may record aspects observed during usual care. Abnormal findings must be validated and interpreted by the nurse.

Equipment
- Centimeter ruler

IMPLEMENTATION
Performance
1. Prior to performing the procedure, introduce self and verify the client's identity using agency protocol. Explain to the client what you are going to do, why it is necessary, and how he or she can cooperate. Inquire whether the client has ever had a clinical breast exam previously. Discuss how the results will be used in planning further care or treatments.

2. Perform hand hygiene and observe appropriate infection control procedures.
3. Provide for client privacy.
4. Inquire if the client has a history of breast masses and what was done about them; pain or tenderness in the breasts and relation to the woman's menstrual cycle; discharge from the nipple; medication history (some medications, e.g., oral contraceptives, steroids, digitalis, and diuretics, may cause nipple discharge;

continued on page 628

ASSESSING THE BREASTS AND AXILLAE *continued*

estrogen replacement therapy may be associated with the development of cysts or cancer); risk factors that may be associated with development of breast cancer (e.g., mother, sister, aunt with breast cancer; alcohol consumption, high-fat diet, obesity, use of oral contraceptives, menarche before age 12, menopause after age 55, age 30 or more at first pregnancy). Inquire if the client performs breast self-examination; technique used and when performed in relation to the menstrual cycle.

ASSESSMENT	NORMAL FINDINGS	DEVIATIONS FROM NORMAL
5. Inspect the breasts for size, symmetry, and contour or shape while the client is in a sitting position.	*Females:* Rounded shape; slightly unequal in size; generally symmetric *Males:* Breasts even with the chest wall; if obese, may be similar in shape to female breasts	Recent change in breast size; swellings; marked asymmetry
6. Inspect the skin of the breast for localized discolorations or hyperpigmentation, retraction or dimpling, localized hypervascular areas, swelling or edema. ❶	Skin uniform in color (same in appearance as skin of abdomen or back) Skin smooth and intact Diffuse symmetric horizontal or vertical vascular pattern in light-skinned people Striae (stretch marks); moles and nevi	Localized discolorations or hyperpigmentation Retraction or dimpling (result of scar tissue or an invasive tumor) Unilateral, localized hypervascular areas (associated with increased blood flow) Swelling or edema appearing as pig skin or orange peel due to exaggeration of the pores

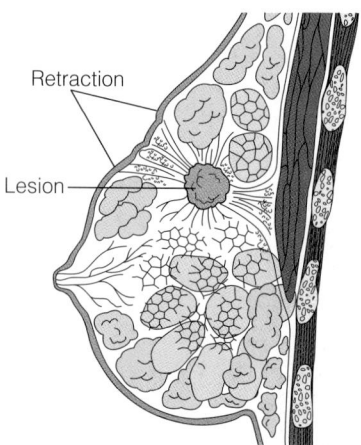

Retraction

Lesion

❶ A lesion causing retraction of the skin.

7. Emphasize any retraction by having the client
   - Raise the arms above the head.
   - Push the hands together, with elbows flexed. ❷
   - Press the hands down on the hips. ❸

❷ Pushing the hands together to accentuate retraction of the breast tissue.

(Patrick Watson, Pearson Education/PH)

❸ Pressing the hands down on the hips to accentuate retraction of the breast tissue.

(Patrick Watson, Pearson Education/PH)

ASSESSMENT	NORMAL FINDINGS	DEVIATIONS FROM NORMAL
8. Inspect the areola area for size, shape, symmetry, color, surface characteristics, and any masses or lesions.	Round or oval and bilaterally the same Color varies widely, from light pink to dark brown Irregular placement of sebaceous glands on the surface of the areola (Montgomery's tubercles)	Any asymmetry, mass, or lesion
9. Inspect the nipples for size, shape, position, color, discharge, and lesions.	Round, everted, and equal in size; similar in color; soft and smooth; both nipples point in same direction (out in young women and men, downward in older women) No discharge, except from pregnant or breast-feeding females Inversion of one or both nipples that is present from puberty	Asymmetrical size and color Presence of discharge, crusts, or cracks Recent inversion of one or both nipples

ASSESSING THE BREASTS AND AXILLAE *continued*

ASSESSMENT	NORMAL FINDINGS	DEVIATIONS FROM NORMAL

ASSESSMENT

10. Palpate the axillary, subclavicular, and supraclavicular lymph nodes ❹ while the client sits with the arms abducted and supported on the nurse's forearm. For palpation of clavicular lymph nodes, see page 607. Use the flat surfaces of all fingertips to palpate the four areas of the axilla:

- the edge of the greater pectoral muscle (musculus pectoralis major) along the anterior axillary line
- the thoracic wall in the midaxillary area
- the upper part of the humerus, and
- the anterior edge of the latissimus dorsi muscle along the posterior axillary line.

11. Palpate the breast for masses, tenderness, and any discharge from the nipples. Palpation of the breast is generally performed while the client is supine. **Rationale:** *In the supine position, the breasts flatten evenly against the chest wall, facilitating palpation.* For clients who have a past history of breast masses, who are at high risk for breast cancer, or who have pendulous breasts, examination in both a supine and a sitting position is recommended.

- If the client reports a breast lump, start with the "normal" breast to obtain baseline data that will serve as a comparison to the reportedly involved breast.

- To enhance flattening of the breast, instruct the client to abduct the arm and place her hand behind her head. Then place a small pillow or rolled towel under the client's shoulder.

- For palpation, use the palmar surface of the middle three fingertips (held together) and make a gentle rotary motion on the breast.

- Choose one of three patterns for palpation:

  a. Hands-of-the-clock or spokes-on-a-wheel ❹

NORMAL FINDINGS

No tenderness, masses, or nodules

❹ Location and palpation of the lymph nodes that drain the lateral breast. *A,* Lymph nodes; *B,* Palpating the axilla.

(*B,* Patrick Watson, Pearson Education/PH)

No tenderness, masses, nodules, or nipple discharge

❹ Hands-of-the-clock or spokes-on-a-wheel pattern of breast palpation.

DEVIATIONS FROM NORMAL

Tenderness, masses, or nodules

No tenderness, masses, nodules, or nipple discharge

Tenderness, masses, nodules, or nipple discharge

- If you detect a mass, record the following data:
  a. **Location:** the exact location relative to the quadrants and axillary tail, or the clock ❹ and the distance from the nipple in centimeters.
  b. **Size:** the length, width, and thickness of the mass in centimeters. If you are able to determine the discrete edges, record this fact.
  c. **Shape:** whether the mass is round, oval, lobulated, indistinct, or irregular.
  d. **Consistency:** whether the mass is hard or soft.
  e. **Mobility:** whether the mass is movable or fixed.
  f. **Skin over the lump:** whether it is reddened, dimpled, or retracted.
  g. **Nipple:** whether it is displaced or retracted.
  h. **Tenderness:** whether palpation is painful.

continued on page 630

SKILL 30-14

ASSESSING THE BREASTS AND AXILLAE *continued*

ASSESSMENT	**NORMAL FINDINGS**	**DEVIATIONS FROM NORMAL**

ASSESSMENT

   b. Concentric circles ❺

   c. Vertical strips pattern ❻

● Start at one point for palpation, and move systematically to the end point to ensure that all breast surfaces are assessed.

● Pay particular attention to the upper outer quadrant area and the tail of Spence.

NORMAL FINDINGS

❺ Concentric circles pattern for breast palpation.

No tenderness, masses, nodules, or nipple discharge

DEVIATIONS FROM NORMAL

Start here

❻ Vertical strips pattern of breast palpation.

Tenderness, masses, nodules, or nipple discharge

12. Palpate the areola and the nipples for masses. Compress each nipple to determine the presence of any discharge. If discharge is present, milk the breast along its radius to identify the discharge-producing lobe. Assess any discharge for amount, color, consistency, and odor. Note also any tenderness on palpation.

13. Teach the client the technique of breast self-examination (see Chapter 40 ∞).

14. Document findings in the client record using forms or checklists supplemented by narrative notes when appropriate.

EVALUATION

■ Perform a detailed follow-up examination based on findings that deviated from expected or normal for the client. Relate findings to previous assessment data if available.

■ Report significant deviations from normal to the primary care provider.

LIFESPAN CONSIDERATIONS **Assessing the Breasts and Axillae**

INFANTS

■ Newborns, both boys and girls, up to 2 weeks of age may have breast enlargement and white discharge from the nipples (witch's milk).

■ Supernumerary ("extra") nipples infrequently are present as small dimples along the mammary chain; these may be associated with renal anomalies.

CHILDREN

■ Female breast development begins between 9 and 13 years of age and occurs in five stages (Tanner stages). One breast may develop more rapidly than the other, but at the end of development, they are more or less the same size.

   Stage 1 Prepubertal with no noticeable change

   Stage 2 Breast bud with elevation of nipple and enlargement of the areola

   Stage 3 Enlargement of the breast and areola with no separation of contour

   Stage 4 Projection of the areola and nipple

   Stage 5 Recession of the areola by about age 14 or 15, leaving only the nipple projecting

■ Boys may develop breast buds and have slight enlargement of the areola in early adolescence. Further enlargement of breast tissue (gynecomastia) can occur. This growth is transient, usually lasting about 2 years, resolving completely by late puberty.

■ Axillary hair usually appears in Tanner stages 3 or 4 and is related to adrenal rather than gonadal changes.

PREGNANT FEMALES

■ Breast, areola, and nipple size increase.

■ The areolae and nipples darken; nipples may become more erect; areolae contain small, scattered, elevated Montgomery's glands.

■ Superficial veins become more prominent, and jagged linear stretch marks may develop.

■ A thick yellow fluid (colostrum) may be expressed from the nipples after the first trimester.

LIFESPAN CONSIDERATIONS   **Assessing the Breasts and Axillae–continued**

ELDERS

■ In the postmenopausal female, breasts change in shape and often appear pendulous or flaccid; they lack the firmness they had in younger years.

■ The presence of breast lesions may be detected more readily because of the decrease in connective tissue.

■ General breast size remains the same. Although glandular tissue atrophies, the amount of fat in breasts (predominantly in the lower quadrants) increases in most women.

THE ABDOMEN

The nurse locates and describes abdominal findings using two common methods of subdividing the abdomen: quadrants and regions. To divide the abdomen into quadrants, the nurse imagines two lines: a vertical line from the xiphoid process to the pubic symphysis, and a horizontal line across the umbilicus (see Figure 30-32 ■). These quadrants are labeled right upper quadrant (*1*), left upper quadrant (*2*), right lower quadrant (*3*), and left lower quadrant (*4*). Using the second method, division into nine regions, the nurse imagines two vertical lines that extend superiorly from the midpoints of the inguinal ligaments, and two horizontal lines, one at the level of the edge of the lower ribs and the other at the level of the iliac crests (see Figure 30-33 ■). Specific organs or parts of organs lie in each abdominal region (see Boxes 30–7 and 30–8).

In addition, practitioners often use certain landmarks to locate abdominal signs and symptoms. These are the xiphoid process of the sternum, the costal margins, the anterosuperior iliac spine, the inguinal ligaments (Poupart's ligaments), and the superior margin of the pubic symphysis (see Figure 30-34 ■).

Assessment of the abdomen involves all four methods of examination (inspection, auscultation, palpation, and percussion). When assessing the abdomen, the nurse performs inspection first, followed by auscultation, percussion, and/or palpation. Auscultation is done before palpation and percussion because palpation and percussion cause movement or stimulation of the bowel, which can increase bowel motility and thus heighten bowel sounds, creating false results. Skill 30-15 describes how to assess the abdomen.

Figure 30-32 ■ The four abdominal quadrants and the underlying organs: *RUQ,* right upper quadrant; *LUQ,* left upper quadrant; *RLQ,* right lower quadrant; *LLQ,* left lower quadrant.

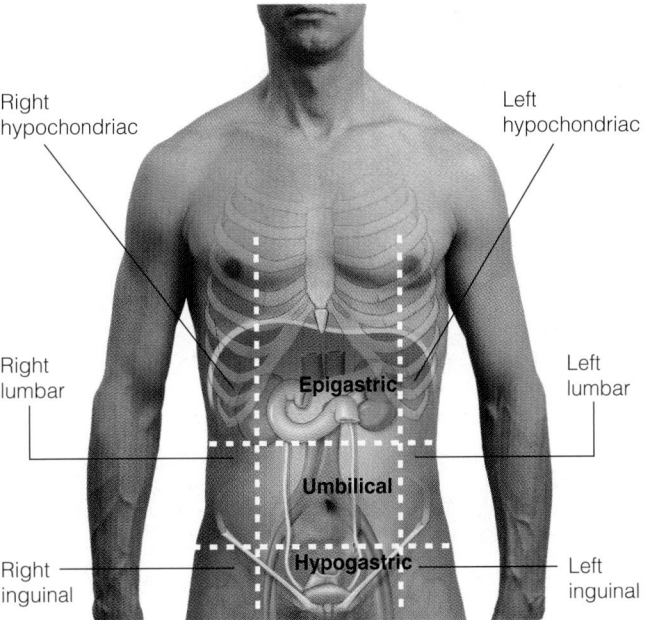

Figure 30-33 ■ The nine abdominal regions: epigastric; left and right hypochondriac; umbilical; left and right lumbar; suprapubic and hypogastric; left and right inguinal or iliac.

BOX 30–7 Organs in the Four Abdominal Quadrants

RIGHT UPPER QUADRANT

Liver
Gallbladder
Duodenum
Head of pancreas
Right adrenal gland
Upper lobe of right kidney
Hepatic flexure of colon
Section of ascending colon
Section of transverse colon

LEFT UPPER QUADRANT

Left lobe of liver
Stomach
Spleen
Upper lobe of left kidney
Pancreas
Left adrenal gland
Splenic flexure of colon
Section of transverse colon
Section of descending colon

RIGHT LOWER QUADRANT

Lower lobe of right kidney
Cecum
Appendix
Section of ascending colon
Right ovary
Right fallopian tube
Right ureter
Right spermatic cord
Part of uterus

LEFT LOWER QUADRANT

Lower lobe of left kidney
Sigmoid colon
Section of descending colon
Left ovary
Left fallopian tube
Left ureter
Left spermatic cord
Part of uterus

BOX 30–8 Organs in the Nine Abdominal Regions

RIGHT HYPOCHONDRIAC

Right lobe of liver
Gallbladder
Part of duodenum
Hepatic flexure of colon
Upper half of right kidney
Suprarenal gland

RIGHT LUMBAR

Ascending colon
Lower half of right kidney
Part of duodenum and
jejunum

RIGHT INGUINAL

Cecum
Appendix
Lower end of ileum
Right ureter
Right spermatic cord
Right ovary

EPIGASTRIC

Aorta
Pyloric end of stomach
Part of duodenum
Pancreas
Part of liver

UMBILICAL

Omentum
Mesentery
Lower part of duodenum
Part of jejunum and ileum

HYPOGASTRIC (PUBIC)

Ileum
Bladder
Uterus

LEFT HYPOCHONDRIAC

Stomach
Spleen
Tail of pancreas
Splenic flexure of colon
Upper half of left kidney
Suprarenal gland

LEFT LUMBAR

Descending colon
Lower half of left kidney
Part of jejunum and ileum

LEFT INGUINAL

Sigmoid colon
Left ureter
Left spermatic cord
Left ovary

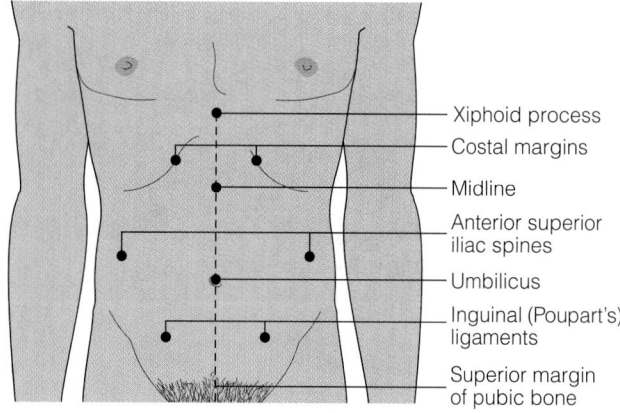

Xiphoid process
Costal margins
Midline
Anterior superior iliac spines
Umbilicus
Inguinal (Poupart's) ligaments
Superior margin of pubic bone

Figure 30-34 ■ Landmarks commonly used to identify abdominal areas.

SKILL 30-15

ASSESSING THE ABDOMEN

PLANNING

- Ask the client to urinate since an empty bladder makes the assessment more comfortable.
- Ensure that the room is warm since the client will be exposed.

Delegation

Assessment of the abdomen is not delegated to UAP. However, signs and symptoms of problems may be observed during usual care and should be recorded by those persons. Abnormal findings must be validated and interpreted by the nurse.

Equipment

- Examining light
- Tape measure (metal or unstretchable cloth)
- Water-soluble skin-marking pencil
- Stethoscope

IMPLEMENTATION

Performance

1. Prior to performing the procedure, introduce self and verify the client's identity using agency protocol. Explain to the client what you are going to do, why it is necessary, and how he or she can cooperate. Discuss how the results will be used in planning further care or treatments.
2. Perform hand hygiene and observe appropriate infection control procedures.
3. Provide for client privacy.

ASSESSING THE ABDOMEN *continued*

4. Inquire if the client has any history of the following: incidence of abdominal pain; its location, onset, sequence, and chronology; its quality (description); its frequency; associated symptoms (e.g., nausea, vomiting, diarrhea); bowel habits; incidence of constipation or diarrhea (have client describe what client means by these terms); change in appetite, food intolerances, and foods ingested in last 24 hours; specific signs and symptoms (e.g., heartburn, flatulence and/or belching, difficulty swallowing, hematemesis [vomiting blood], blood or mucus in stools, and aggravating and alleviating factors); previous problems and treatment (e.g., stomach ulcer, gallbladder surgery, history of jaundice).

5. Assist the client to a supine position, with the arms placed comfortably at the sides. Place small pillows beneath the knees and the head to reduce tension in the abdominal muscles. Expose the client's abdomen only from the chest line to the pubic area to avoid chilling and shivering, which can tense the abdominal muscles.

ASSESSMENT	NORMAL FINDINGS	DEVIATIONS FROM NORMAL
Inspection of the Abdomen		
6. Inspect the abdomen for skin integrity (refer to the discussion of skin assessment, earlier in this chapter).	Unblemished skin Uniform color Silver-white striae (stretch marks) or surgical scars	Presence of rash or other lesions Tense, glistening skin (may indicate ascites, edema) Purple striae (associated with Cushing's disease or rapid weight gain and loss)
7. Inspect the abdomen for contour and symmetry:		
• Observe the abdominal contour (profile line from the rib margin to the pubic bone) while standing at the client's side when the client is supine.	Flat, rounded (convex), or scaphoid (concave)	Distended
• Ask the client to take a deep breath and to hold it. **Rationale:** *This makes an enlarged liver or spleen more obvious.*	No evidence of enlargement of liver or spleen	Evidence of enlargement of liver or spleen
• Assess the symmetry of contour while standing at the foot of the bed.	Symmetric contour	Asymmetric contour, e.g., localized protrusions around umbilicus, inguinal ligaments, or scars (possible hernia or tumor)
• If distention is present, measure the abdominal girth by placing a tape around the abdomen at the level of the umbilicus. ❶		

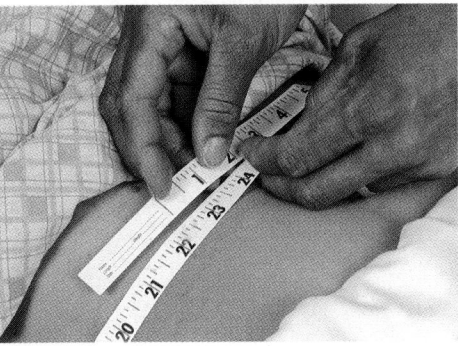

❶ Measuring abdominal girth.
(Al Dodge, Pearson Education/PH)

ASSESSMENT	NORMAL FINDINGS	DEVIATIONS FROM NORMAL
8. Observe abdominal movements associated with respiration, peristalsis, or aortic pulsations.	Symmetric movements caused by respiration Visible peristalsis in very lean people Aortic pulsations in thin persons at epigastric area	Limited movement due to pain or disease process Visible peristalsis in nonlean clients (possible bowel obstruction) Marked aortic pulsations

continued on page 634

ASSESSING THE ABDOMEN *continued*

ASSESSMENT	NORMAL FINDINGS	DEVIATIONS FROM NORMAL
9. Observe the vascular pattern.	No visible vascular pattern	Visible venous pattern (dilated veins) is associated with liver disease, ascites, and venocaval obstruction

Auscultation of the Abdomen

10. Auscultate the abdomen for bowel sounds, vascular sounds, and peritoneal friction rubs.

Warm the hands and the stethoscope diaphragms. **Rationale:** *Cold hands and a cold stethoscope may cause the client to contract the abdominal muscles, and these contractions may be heard during auscultation.*

For Bowel Sounds

- Use the flat-disc diaphragm. **Rationale:** *Intestinal sounds are relatively high pitched and best accentuated by the diaphragm.* Light pressure with the stethoscope is adequate.
- Ask when the client last ate. **Rationale:** *Shortly after or long after eating, bowel sounds may normally increase. They are loudest when a meal is long overdue.* Four to 7 hours after a meal, bowel sounds may be heard continuously over the ileocecal valve area while the digestive contents from the small intestine empty through the valve into the large intestine.
- Place diaphragm of the stethoscope in each of the four quadrants of the abdomen over all of the auscultatory sites shown in. ❷
- Listen for active bowel sounds—irregular gurgling noises occurring about every 5 to 20 seconds. The duration of a single sound may range from less than a second to more than several seconds.

For Vascular Sounds

- Use the bell of the stethoscope over the aorta, renal arteries, iliac arteries, and femoral arteries. ❸
- Listen for bruits .

Peritoneal Friction Rubs

- Peritoneal friction rubs are rough, grating sounds like two pieces of leather rubbing together. Friction rubs may be caused by inflammation, infection, or abnormal growths.

Audible bowel sounds

Absence of arterial bruits

Absence of friction rub

Hypoactive, i.e., extremely soft and infrequent (e.g., one per minute). Hypoactive sounds indicate decreased motility and are usually associated with manipulation of the bowel during surgery, inflammation, paralytic ileus, or late bowel obstruction.

Hyperactive/increased, i.e., high-pitched, loud, rushing sounds that occur frequently (e.g., every 3 seconds) also known as borborygmi.

Hyperactive sounds indicate increased intestinal motility and are usually associated with diarrhea, an early bowel obstruction, or the use of laxatives.

True absence of sounds (none heard in 3 to 5 minutes) indicates a cessation of intestinal motility.

❷ Auscultating the abdomen for bowel sounds.

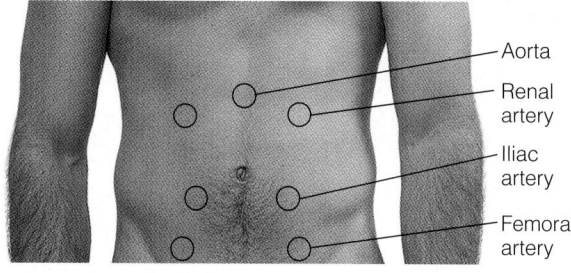

❸ Sites for auscultating the abdomen.

Loud bruit over aortic area (possible aneurysm)

Bruit over renal or iliac arteries

ASSESSING THE ABDOMEN *continued*

ASSESSMENT	NORMAL FINDINGS	DEVIATIONS FROM NORMAL
• To auscultate the splenic site, place the stethoscope over the left lower rib cage in the anterior axillary line, and ask the client to take a deep breath. A deep breath may accentuate the sound of a friction rub area. • To auscultate the liver site, place the stethoscope over the lower right rib cage.		

Percussion of the Abdomen

11. Percuss several areas in each of the four quadrants to determine presence of tympany (gas in stomach and intestines) and dullness (decrease, absence, or flatness of resonance over solid masses or fluid). Use a systematic pattern: Begin in the lower right quadrant, proceed to the upper right quadrant, the upper left quadrant, and the lower left quadrant. ❹

Tympany over the stomach and gas-filled bowels; dullness, especially over the liver and spleen, or a full bladder

Large dull areas (associated with presence of fluid or a tumor)

❹ Systematic percussion sites for all four quadrants.

Percussion of the Liver

12. Percuss the liver to determine its size. Begin in the right midclavicular line below the level of the umbilicus and proceed as follows:

• Percuss upward over tympanic areas until a dull percussion sound indicates the lower liver border. Mark the site with a skin-marking pencil. ❺

• Then percuss downward at the right midclavicular line, beginning from an area of lung resonance and progressing downward until a dull percussion sound indicates the upper liver border (usually at the fifth to seventh interspace). Mark this site.

• Measure the distance between the two marks (upper and lower liver border) in centimeters to establish the liver span or size.

• Repeat steps 1 to 3 at the midsternal line.

6 to 12 cm (2 1/2 to 3 1/2 in.) in the midclavicular line; 4 to 8 cm (1 1/2 to 3 in.) at the midsternal line

Enlarged size (associated with liver disease)

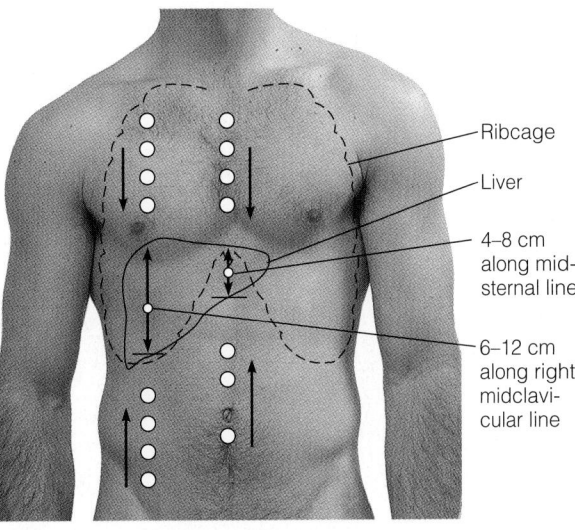

Ribcage
Liver
4–8 cm along midsternal line
6–12 cm along right midclavicular line

❺ Percussion pattern to determine liver size.

continued on page 636

ASSESSING THE ABDOMEN *continued*

ASSESSMENT	NORMAL FINDINGS	DEVIATIONS FROM NORMAL
Palpation of the Abdomen		

13. Perform light palpation first to detect areas of tenderness and/or muscle guarding. Systematically explore all four quadrants. Ensure that the client's position is appropriate for relaxation of the abdominal muscles, and warm the hands. **Rationale:** *Cold hands can elicit muscle tension and thus impede palpatory evaluation.*

	NORMAL FINDINGS	DEVIATIONS FROM NORMAL
	No tenderness; relaxed abdomen with smooth, consistent tension	Tenderness and hypersensitivity
		Superficial masses
		Localized areas of increased tension

Light Palpation

- Hold the palm of your hand slightly above the client's abdomen, with your fingers parallel to the abdomen.

- Depress the abdominal wall lightly, about 1 cm or to the depth of the subcutaneous tissue, with the pads of your fingers. ❻

- Move the finger pads in a slight circular motion.

- Note areas of tenderness or superficial pain, masses, and muscle guarding. To determine areas of tenderness, ask the client to tell you about them and watch for changes in the client's facial expressions.

- If the client is excessively ticklish, begin by pressing your hand on top of the client's hand while pressing lightly. Then slide your hand off the client's and onto the abdomen to continue the examination.

❻ Light palpation of the abdomen.

14. Perform deep palpation over all four quadrants.

- Palpate sensitive areas last.

- Press the distal half of the palmar surface of the fingers of one hand into the abdominal wall.

  or

  Use the bimanual method of palpation discussed earlier in this chapter, page 569.

- Depress the abdominal wall about 4 to 5 cm (1 1/2 to 2 in.). ❼

- Note masses and the structure of underlying contents. If a mass is present, determine its size, location, mobility, contour, consistency, and tenderness. Normal abdominal structures that may be mistaken for masses include the lateral borders of the rectus abdominis muscles,

	NORMAL FINDINGS	DEVIATIONS FROM NORMAL
	Tenderness may be present near xiphoid process, over cecum, and over sigmoid colon	Generalized or localized areas of tenderness
		Mobile or fixed masses

❼ Deep palpation of the abdomen.

ASSESSING THE ABDOMEN *continued*

ASSESSMENT	NORMAL FINDINGS	DEVIATIONS FROM NORMAL
the feces-filled colon, the aorta, and the uterus.		

- Check for rebound tenderness in areas where the client complains of pain. With one hand, press slowly and deeply over the area indicated and then lift the hand quickly. If the client does not complain of pain during the deep pressure but indicates pain at the release of the pressure, rebound tenderness is present. This can indicate peritoneal inflammation and should be reported to the primary care provider immediately.

Palpation of the Liver

15. Palpate the liver to detect enlargement and tenderness.

   Two bimanual approaches are used in palpation of the liver. In using the first method, place one hand along the anterior rib cage and the other hand on the posterior rib cage.

- Stand on the client's right side.

- Place your left hand on the posterior thorax at about the 11th or 12th rib. This hand is used to push upward and provide support of underlying structures for the subsequent anterior palpation.

- Place your right hand along the rib cage at about a 45° angle to the right of the rectus abdominis muscle or parallel to the rectus muscle with the fingers pointing toward the rib cage. ❽

- While the client exhales, exert a gradual and gentle downward and forward pressure beneath the costal margin until you reach a depth of 4 to 5 cm (1 1/2 to 2 in.). During expiration, the abdominal wall relaxes, facilitating deep palpation.

- Maintain your hand position, and ask the client to inhale deeply. This makes the liver border descend and moves the liver into a palpable position.

- While the client inhales, feel the liver border move against your hand. It should feel firm and have a regular contour. If you do not palpate the liver initially, ask the client

Normal Findings:

May not be palpable

Border feels smooth

Deviations from Normal:

Enlarged (abnormal finding, even if liver is smooth and not tender)

Smooth but tender; nodular or hard

❽ Palpating the liver.

continued on page 638

SKILL 30-15

ASSESSING THE ABDOMEN *continued*

ASSESSMENT	NORMAL FINDINGS	DEVIATIONS FROM NORMAL
to take two or three more deep breaths while you maintain or apply slightly more palpation pressure. Livers are harder to palpate in obese, tense, or very physically fit people.		

- If the liver is enlarged (i.e., palpable below the costal margin), measure the number of centimeters it extends below the costal region.

A second method is the bimanual palpation method discussed on page 569, in which one hand is superimposed on the other (Figure 30-2, earlier). The techniques and principles used for palpating the liver with one hand apply to the two-hand method as well.

❾ Palpating the bladder.

Palpation of the Bladder

16. Palpate the area above the pubic symphysis if the client's history indicates possible urinary retention. ❾

17. Document findings in the client record using forms or checklists supplemented by narrative notes when appropriate.

NORMAL FINDINGS (Bladder)

Not palpable

DEVIATIONS FROM NORMAL (Bladder)

Distended and palpable as smooth, round, tense mass (indicates urinary retention)

SAMPLE DOCUMENTATION

5/28/07 0945 c/o "gassy" pain LRQ. No BM x 48 hrs. Ate 75% regular diet yesterday. Abd flat. Active bowels sounds all 4 quadrants. Tympany above umbilicus, dull below. Liver 7 cm @ MCL. No masses palpated. 30 mL MOM given.———N. Schmidt, RN

EVALUATION

- Perform a detailed follow-up examination of other systems based on findings that deviated from expected or normal for the client. Relate findings to previous assessment data if available.

- Report significant deviations from normal to the primary care provider.

LIFESPAN CONSIDERATIONS   Assessing the Abdomen

INFANTS

- Internal organs of newborns and infants are proportionately larger than those of older children and adults, so their abdomens are rounded and tend to protrude.
- The infant's liver may be palpable 1 to 2 cm below the right costal margin.
- Umbilical hernias may be present at birth.

CHILDREN

- Toddlers have a characteristic "pot belly" appearance, which can persist until age 3 to 4 years.
- Late preschool and school-age children are leaner and have a flat abdomen.
- Peristaltic waves may be more visible than in adults.
- Children may not be able to pinpoint areas of tenderness; by observing facial expressions the examiner can determine areas of maximum tenderness.

- The liver is relatively larger than in adults. It can be palpated 1 to 2 cm below the right costal margin.
- If the child is ticklish, guarding, or fearful, use a task that requires concentration (such as squeezing the hands together) to distract the child, or have the child place his or her hands on yours as you palpate the abdomen, "helping" you to do the exam.

ELDERS

- The rounded abdomens of elders are due to an increase in adipose tissue and a decrease in muscle tone.
- The abdominal wall is slacker and thinner, making palpation easier and more accurate than in younger clients. Muscle wasting and loss of fibroconnective tissue occur.
- The pain threshold in elders is often higher; major abdominal problems such as appendicitis or other acute emergencies may therefore go undetected.

LIFESPAN CONSIDERATIONS **Assessing the Abdomen**–*continued*

- Gastrointestinal pain needs to be differentiated from cardiac pain. Gastrointestinal pain may be located in the chest or abdomen, whereas cardiac pain is usually located in the chest. Factors aggravating gastrointestinal pain are usually related to either ingestion or lack of food intake; gastrointestinal pain is usually relieved by antacids, food, or assuming an upright position. Common factors that can aggravate cardiac pain are activity or anxiety; rest or nitroglycerin relieves cardiac pain.
- Stool passes through the intestines at a slower rate in elders, and the perception of stimuli that produce the urge to defecate often diminishes.
- Fecal incontinence may occur in confused or neurologically impaired older adults.

- Many elders erroneously believe that the absence of a daily bowel movement signifies constipation. When assessing for constipation, the nurse must consider the client's diet, activity, medications, and characteristics and ease of passage of feces as well as the frequency of bowel movements.
- The incidence of colon cancer is higher among elders than younger adults. Symptoms include a change in bowel function, rectal bleeding, and weight loss. Changes in bowel function, however, are associated with many factors, such as diet, exercise, and medications.
- Decreased absorption of oral medications often occurs with aging.
- In the liver, impaired metabolism of some drugs may occur with aging.

HOME CARE CONSIDERATIONS **Assessing the Abdomen**

- Be sure you have the required equipment on a home visit, including a tape measure and skin-marking pen.
- Use pillows to position the client.

- Undressing the client to perform a complete abdominal examination may not be necessary. Focus the assessment on areas indicated by the history and present complaint.

THE MUSCULOSKELETAL SYSTEM

The musculoskeletal system encompasses the muscles, bones, and joints. The completeness of an assessment of this system depends largely on the needs and problems of the individual client. The nurse usually assesses the musculoskeletal system for muscle strength, tone, size, and symmetry of muscle development, and for tremors. A **tremor** is an involuntary trembling of a limb or body part. Tremors may involve large groups of muscle fibers or small bundles of muscle fibers. An **intention tremor** becomes more apparent when an individual attempts a voluntary movement, such as holding a cup of coffee. A **resting tremor** is more apparent when the client is at rest and diminishes with activity.

Bones are assessed for normal form. Joints are assessed for tenderness, swelling, thickening, crepitation (the sound of bone grating on bone), presence of nodules, and range of motion. Body posture is assessed for normal standing and sitting positions. For information about body posture, see Chapter 44.

Skill 30-16 describes how to assess the musculoskeletal system.

ASSESSING THE MUSCULOSKELETAL SYSTEM

SKILL 30-16

PLANNING

Delegation
Assessment of the musculoskeletal system is not delegated to UAP. However, many aspects of its functioning are observed during usual care and may be recorded by persons other than the nurse. Abnormal findings must be validated and interpreted by the nurse.

Equipment
- Goniometer

IMPLEMENTATION
Performance
1. Prior to performing the procedure, introduce self and verify the client's identity using agency protocol. Explain to the client what you are going to do, why it is necessary, and how he or she can cooperate. Discuss how the results will be used in planning further care or treatments.
2. Perform hand hygiene and observe appropriate infection control procedures.
3. Provide for client privacy.
4. Inquire if the client has any history of the following: presence of muscle pain: onset, location, character, associated phenomena (e.g., redness and swelling of joints), and aggravating and alleviating factors; limitations to movement or inability to perform activities of daily living; previous sports injuries; loss of function without pain.

continued on page 640

ASSESSING THE MUSCULOSKELETAL SYSTEM *continued*

ASSESSMENT	NORMAL FINDINGS	DEVIATIONS FROM NORMAL
Muscles		
5. Inspect the muscles for size. Compare the muscles on one side of the body (e.g., of the arm, thigh, and calf) to the same muscle on the other side. For any discrepancies, measure the muscles with a tape.	Equal size on both sides of body	Atrophy (a decrease in size) or hypertrophy (an increase in size), asymmetry
6. Inspect the muscles and tendons for contractures (shortening).	No contractures	Malposition of body part, e.g., foot drop (foot flexed downward)
7. Inspect the muscles for tremors, for example by having the client hold the arms out in front of the body.	No tremors	Presence of tremor
8. Palpate muscles at rest to determine muscle tonicity (the normal condition of tension, or tone, of a muscle at rest).	Normally firm	Atonic (lacking tone)
9. Palpate muscles while the client is active and passive for flaccidity, spasticity, and smoothness of movement.	Smooth coordinated movements	Flaccidity (weakness or laxness) or spasticity (sudden involuntary muscle contraction)
10. Test muscle strength. Compare the right side with the left side. *Sternocleidomastoid:* Client turns the head to one side against the resistance of your hand. Repeat with the other side. *Trapezius:* Client shrugs the shoulders against the resistance of your hands. *Deltoid:* Client holds arm up and resists while you try to push it down. *Biceps:* Client fully extends each arm and tries to flex it while you attempt to hold arm in extension. *Triceps:* Client flexes each arm and then tries to extend it against your attempt to keep arm in flexion. *Wrist and finger muscles:* Client spreads the fingers and resists as you attempt to push the fingers together. *Grip strength:* Client grasps your index and middle fingers while you try to pull the fingers out. *Hip muscles:* Client is supine, both legs extended; client raises one leg at a time while you attempt to hold it down. *Hip abduction:* Client is supine, both legs extended. Place your hands on the lateral surface of each knee; client spreads the legs apart against your resistance. *Hip adduction:* Client is in same position as for hip abduction. Place your hands between the knees; client brings the legs together against your resistance.	Equal strength on each body side	25% or less of normal strength **Grading Muscle Strength** 0: 0% of normal strength; complete paralysis 1: 10% of normal strength; no movement, contraction of muscle is palpable or visible 2: 25% of normal strength; full muscle movement against gravity, with support 3: 50% of normal strength; normal movement against gravity 4: 75% of normal strength; normal full movement against gravity and against minimal resistance 5: 100% of normal strength; normal full movement against gravity and against full resistance

ASSESSING THE MUSCULOSKELETAL SYSTEM *continued*

ASSESSMENT	NORMAL FINDINGS	DEVIATIONS FROM NORMAL
Hamstrings: Client is supine, both knees bent. Client resists while you attempt to straighten the legs.		
Quadriceps: Client is supine, knee partially extended; client resists while you attempt to flex the knee.		
Muscles of the ankles and feet: Client resists while you attempt to dorsiflex the foot and again resists while you attempt to flex the foot.		

Bones

11. Inspect the skeleton for structure.	No deformities	Bones misaligned
12. Palpate the bones to locate any areas of edema or tenderness.	No tenderness or swelling	Presence of tenderness or swelling (may indicate fracture, neoplasms, or osteoporosis)

Joints

13. Inspect the joint for swelling. Palpate each joint for tenderness, smoothness of movement, swelling, crepitation, and presence of nodules.	No swelling No tenderness, swelling, crepitation, or nodules Joints move smoothly	One or more swollen joints Presence of tenderness, swelling, crepitation, or nodules
14. Assess joint range of motion. See Chapter 44 for the types of joint movements. ∞	Varies to some degree in accordance with person's genetic makeup and degree of physical activity	Limited range of motion in one or more joints
• Ask the client to move selected body parts. The amount of joint movement can be measured by a **goniometer,** a device that measures the angle of the joint in degrees. ❶		

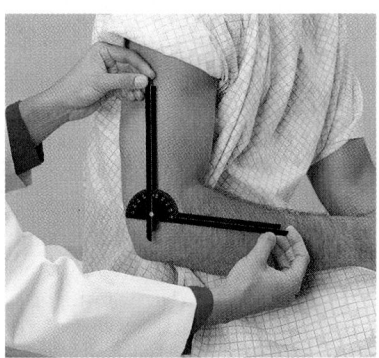

❶ A goniometer is used to measure joint range of motion.

15. Document findings in the client record using forms or checklists supplemented by narrative notes when appropriate.

EVALUATION

- Perform a detailed follow-up examination of other systems based on findings that deviated from expected or normal for the client. Relate findings to previous assessment data if available.

- Report significant deviations from normal to the primary care provider.

LIFESPAN CONSIDERATIONS Assessing the Musculoskeletal System

INFANTS

- Palpate the clavicles of newborns. A mass and crepitus may indicate a fracture experienced during vaginal delivery. The newborn may also have limited movement of the arm and shoulder on the affected side.

- When the arms and legs of newborns are pulled to extension and released, newborns naturally return to the flexed fetal position.
- Check muscle strength by holding the infant lightly under the arms with feet placed lightly on a table. Infants should not fall through the hands and should be able to bear body weight on their legs if normal muscle strength is present.

continued on page 642

LIFESPAN CONSIDERATIONS   Assessing the Musculoskeletal System—*continued*

- Check infants for developmental dysplasia of the hip (congenital dislocation) by examining for asymmetric gluteal folds, asymmetric abduction of the legs (Ortolani and Barlow tests), or apparent shortening of the femur.
- Infants should be able to sit without support by 8 months of age, crawl by 7 to 10 months, and walk by 12 to 15 months.
- Observe for symmetry of muscle mass, strength, and function.

CHILDREN

- Pronation and "toeing in" of the feet is common in children between 12 and 30 months of age.
- Genu varum (bowleg) is normal in children for about 1 year after beginning to walk.
- Genu valgus (knock-knee) is normal in preschool and early school-age children.
- Lordosis (swayback) is common in children before age 5.
- Observe the child in normal activities to determine motor function.
- During the rapid growth spurts of adolescence, spinal curvature and rotation (scoliosis) may appear. Children should be assessed for scoliosis by age 12 and annually until their growth slows. Curvature greater than 10% should be referred for further medical evaluation.

- Muscle mass increases in adolescence, especially as children engage in strenuous physical activity, and requires increased nutritional intake.
- Children are at risk for injury related to physical activity and should be assessed for nutritional status, physical conditioning, and safety precautions in order to prevent injury.
- Adolescent girls who participate in strenuous athletic activities are at risk for delayed menses, osteoporosis, and eating disorders; assessment should include a history of these factors.

ELDERS

- Muscle mass decreases progressively with age, but there are wide variations among different individuals.
- The decrease in speed, strength, resistance to fatigue, reaction time, and coordination in the older person is due to a decrease in nerve conduction and muscle tone.
- The bones become more fragile and osteoporosis leads to a loss of total bone mass. As a result, elders are predisposed to fractures and compressed vertebrae.
- In most elders, osteoarthritic changes in the joints can be observed.
- Note any surgical scars from joint replacement surgeries.

HOME CARE CONSIDERATIONS   Assessing the Musculoskeletal System

- When making a home visit, observe the client in natural movement around the living area. To assess children, have them remove their clothes down to the underwear.

- A complete examination of joints, bone, and muscles may not be necessary. Focus the assessment on areas indicated by the history and present complaint.

THE NEUROLOGIC SYSTEM

A thorough neurologic examination may take 1 to 3 hours; however, routine screening tests are usually done first. If the results of these tests raise questions, more extensive evaluations are made. Three major considerations determine the extent of a neurologic exam: (a) the client's chief complaints, (b) the client's physical condition (i.e., level of consciousness and ability to ambulate) because many parts of the examination require movement and coordination of the extremities, and (c) the client's willingness to participate and cooperate.

Examination of the neurologic system includes assessment of (a) mental status including level of consciousness, (b) the cranial nerves, (c) reflexes, (d) motor function, and (e) sensory function. Parts of the neurologic assessment are performed throughout the health examination. For example, the nurse performs a large part of the mental status assessment during the taking of the history and when observing the client's general appearance. Also, the nurse assesses the function of cranial nerves. Cranial nerves II, III, IV, V, and VI (ophthalmic branch) are assessed with the eyes and vision, and cranial nerve VIII (cochlear branch) is assessed with the ears and hearing.

Mental Status

Assessment of mental status reveals the client's general cerebral function. These functions include intellectual (cognitive) as well as emotional (affective) functions.

If problems with use of language, memory, concentration, or thought processes are noted during the nursing history, a more extensive examination is required during neurologic assessment. Major areas of mental status assessment include language, orientation, memory, and attention span and calculation.

Language

Any defects in or loss of the power to express oneself by speech, writing, or signs, or to comprehend spoken or written language due to disease or injury of the cerebral cortex, is called **aphasia.** Aphasias can be categorized as sensory or receptive aphasia, and motor or expressive aphasia.

Sensory or receptive aphasia is the loss of the ability to comprehend written or spoken words. Two types of sensory aphasia are auditory (or acoustic) aphasia and visual aphasia. Clients with auditory aphasia have lost the ability to understand the symbolic content associated with sounds. Clients with visual aphasia have lost the ability to understand printed or written figures.

Motor or expressive aphasia involves loss of the power to express oneself by writing, making signs, or speaking. Clients may find that even though they can recall words, they have lost the ability to combine speech sounds into words.

Orientation

This aspect of the assessment determines the client's ability to recognize other persons (*person*), awareness of when and where they presently are (*time* and *place*), and who they, themselves, are (*self*).

Memory

The nurse assesses the client's recall of information presented seconds previously (immediate recall), events or information from earlier in the day or examination (recent memory), and knowledge recalled from months or years ago (remote or long-term memory).

Attention Span and Calculation

This component determines the client's ability to focus on a mental task that is expected to be able to be performed by persons of normal intelligence.

Level of Consciousness

Level of consciousness (LOC) can lie anywhere along a continuum from a state of alertness to coma. A fully alert client responds to questions spontaneously; a comatose client may not respond to verbal stimuli. The Glasgow Coma Scale was originally developed to predict recovery from a head injury; however, it is used by many professionals to assess LOC. It tests in three major areas: eye response, motor response, and verbal response. An assessment totaling 15 points indicates the client is alert and completely oriented. A comatose client scores 7 or less.

Cranial Nerves

The nurse needs to be aware of specific nerve functions and assessment methods for each cranial nerve to detect abnormalities. In some cases, each nerve is assessed; in other cases only selected nerve functions are evaluated.

Reflexes

A **reflex** is an automatic response of the body to a stimulus. It is not voluntarily learned or conscious. The deep tendon reflex (DTR) is activated when a tendon is stimulated (tapped) and its associated muscle contracts. The quality of a reflex response varies among individuals and by age. As a person ages, reflex responses may become less intense.

Reflexes are tested using a percussion hammer. The response is described on a scale of 0 to 14. Experience is necessary to determine appropriate scoring for an individual. Several reflexes are normally tested during the physical examination: (a) the biceps reflex, (b) the triceps reflex, (c) the brachioradialis reflex, (d) the patellar reflex, (e) the Achilles reflex, and (f) the plantar (Babinski) reflex.

Motor Function

Neurologic assessment of the motor system evaluates proprioception and cerebellar function. Structures involved in proprioception are the proprioceptors, the posterior columns of the spinal cord, the cerebellum, and the vestibular apparatus (which is innervated by cranial nerve VIII) in the labyrinth of the internal ear.

Proprioceptors are sensory nerve terminals, occurring chiefly in the muscles, tendons, joints, and the internal ear, that give information about movements and the position of the body. Stimuli from the proprioceptors travel through the posterior columns of the spinal cord. Deficits of function of the posterior columns of the spinal cord result in impairment of muscle and position sense. Clients with such an impairment often must watch their own arm and leg movements to ascertain the position of the limbs.

The cerebellum (a) helps to control posture, (b) acts with the cerebral cortex to make body movements smooth and coordinated, and (c) controls skeletal muscles to maintain equilibrium.

Sensory Function

Sensory functions include touch, pain, temperature, position, and tactile discrimination. The first three are routinely tested. Generally, the face, arms, legs, hands, and feet are tested for touch and pain, although all parts of the body can be tested. If the client complains of numbness, peculiar sensations, or paralysis, the practitioner should check sensation more carefully over flexor and extensor surfaces of limbs, mapping out clearly any abnormality of touch or pain by examining responses in the area about every 2 cm (1 in.). This is a lengthy procedure and may be performed by a specialist. Abnormal responses to touch stimuli include loss of sensation (anesthesia); more than normal sensation (hyperesthesia); less than normal sensation (hypoesthesia); or an abnormal sensation such as burning, pain, or an electric shock (paresthesia).

A variety of common health conditions, including diabetes and arteriosclerotic heart disease, result in loss of the protective sensation in the lower extremities. This loss can lead to severe tissue damage. In efforts to identify clients at increased risk for damage to the feet, the Bureau of Primary Health Care of the U.S. government has established the Lower Extremity Amputation Prevention (LEAP) program. The most important aspect of LEAP is assessment of sensation using a special monofilament that delivers 10 grams of force. Health care providers should perform an initial foot screen on all clients with diabetes and at least annually thereafter. Clients who are at risk should have their feet and shoes evaluated at least four times a year to help prevent foot problems from occurring.

A detailed neurologic examination includes position sense, temperature sense, and tactile discrimination. Three types of tactile discrimination are generally tested: **one-** and **two-point discrimination,** the ability to sense whether one or two areas of the skin are being stimulated by pressure; **stereognosis,** the act of recognizing objects by touching and manipulating them; and **extinction,** the failure to perceive touch on one side of the body when two symmetric areas of the body are touched simultaneously.

Skill 30-17 describes how to assess the neurologic system.

ASSESSING THE NEUROLOGIC SYSTEM

PLANNING

If possible, determine whether a screening or full neurologic examination is indicated. This will impact preparation of the client, equipment, and timing.

Delegation

Due to the substantial knowledge and skill required, assessment of the neurologic system is not delegated to UAP. However, many aspects of neurologic behavior are observed during usual care and may be recorded by persons other than the nurse. Abnormal findings must be validated and interpreted by the nurse.

Equipment (Depending on Components of Examination)

- Sugar, salt, lemon juice, quinine flavors
- Percussion hammer
- Tongue depressors (one broken diagonally for testing pain sensation)
- Wisps of cotton to assess light-touch sensation
- Test tubes of hot and cold water for skin temperature assessment (optional)
- Pins or needles for tactile discrimination

IMPLEMENTATION

Performance

1. Prior to performing the procedure, introduce self and verify the client's identity using agency protocol. Explain to the client what you are going to do, why it is necessary, and how he or she can cooperate. Discuss how the results will be used in planning further care or treatments.
2. Perform hand hygiene and observe appropriate infection control procedures.
3. Provide for client privacy.
4. Inquire if the client has any history of the following: presence of pain in the head, back, or extremities, as well as onset and aggravating and alleviating factors; disorientation to time, place, or person; speech disorder; history of loss of consciousness, fainting, convulsions, trauma, tingling or numbness, tremors or tics, limping, paralysis, uncontrolled muscle movements, loss of memory, mood swings, or problems with smell, vision, taste, touch, or hearing.

CLINICAL ALERT

All questions and tests used in a neurologic examination must be age, language, education level, and culturally appropriate. Individualize questions and tests before using them. ■

Language

5. If the client displays difficulty speaking,
   - Point to common objects, and ask the client to name them.
   - Ask the client to read some words and to match the printed and written words with pictures.
   - Ask the client to respond to simple verbal and written commands, e.g., "point to your toes" or "raise your left arm."

Orientation

6. Determine the client's orientation to *person, time,* and *place* by tactful questioning. Ask the client the city and state of residence, time of day, date, day of the week, duration of illness, and names of family members. To evaluate the response, you must know the correct answer. More direct questioning may be necessary for some people, e.g., "Where are you now?" "What day is it today?" Most people readily accept these questions if initially the nurse asks, "Do you get confused at times?" If the client cannot answer these questions accurately, also include assessment of the *self* by asking the client to state his or her full name.

Memory

7. Listen for lapses in memory. Ask the client about difficulty with memory. If problems are apparent, three categories of memory are tested: immediate recall, recent memory, and remote memory.

   To assess immediate recall:
   - Ask the client to repeat a series of three digits, e.g., 7–4–3, spoken slowly.
   - Gradually increase the number of digits, e.g., 7–4–3–5, 7–4–3–5–6, and 7–4–3–5–6–7–2, until the client fails to repeat the series correctly.
   - Start again with a series of three digits, but this time ask the client to repeat them backward. The average person can repeat a series of five to eight digits in sequence and four to six digits in reverse order.

   To assess recent memory:
   - Ask the client to recall the recent events of the day, such as how the client got to the clinic. This information must be validated, however.
   - Ask the client to recall information given early in the interview, e.g., the name of a doctor.
   - Provide the client with three facts to recall, e.g., a color, an object, and an address; or a three-digit number, and ask the client to repeat all three. Later in the interview, ask the client to recall all three items.

   To assess remote memory, ask the client to describe a previous illness or surgery, e.g., 5 years ago, or a birthday or anniversary.

Attention Span and Calculation

8. Test the ability to concentrate or maintain *attention span* by asking the client to recite the alphabet or to count backward from 100. Test the ability to calculate by asking the client to subtract 7 or 3 progressively from 100, i.e., 100, 93, 86, 79, or 100, 97, 94, 91 (referred to as *serial sevens* or *serial threes*). Normally, an adult can complete the serial sevens test in about 90 seconds with three or fewer errors. Because educational level, language, or cultural differences affect calculating ability, this test may be inappropriate for some people.

Level of Consciousness

9. Apply the Glasgow Coma Scale: eye response, motor response, and verbal response. An assessment totaling 15 points indicates the client is alert and completely oriented. A comatose client scores 7 or less (see Table 30–10 on page 652).

ASSESSING THE NEUROLOGIC SYSTEM *continued*
Cranial Nerves

10. For the specific functions and assessment methods of each cranial nerve, see Table 30–11 on page 653. Test each nerve not already evaluated in another component of the health assessment.

CLINICAL ALERT

The names and order of the cranial nerves can be recalled by a mnemonic device: "On old Olympus's treeless top, a Finn and German viewed a hop." The first letter of each word in the sentence is the same as the first letter of the name of the cranial nerve, in order. ■

Reflexes

11. Test reflexes using a percussion hammer, comparing one side of the body with the other to evaluate the symmetry of response.

0	No reflex response
+1	Minimal activity (hypoactive)
+2	Normal response
+3	More active than normal
+4	Maximal activity (hyperactive)

Biceps Reflex The biceps reflex tests the spinal cord level C-5, C-6.
- Partially flex the client's arm at the elbow, and rest the forearm over the thighs, placing the palm of the hand down.
- Place the thumb of your nondominant hand horizontally over the biceps tendon.
- Deliver a blow (slight downward thrust) with the percussion hammer to your thumb. ❶
- Observe the normal slight flexion of the elbow, and feel the bicep's contraction through your thumb.

Triceps Reflex The triceps reflex tests the spinal cord level C-7, C-8.
- Flex the client's arm at the elbow, and support it in the palm of your nondominant hand. ❷
- Palpate the triceps tendon about 2 to 5 cm (1 to 2 in.) above the elbow.

- Deliver a blow with the percussion hammer directly to the tendon.
- Observe the normal slight extension of the elbow.

Brachioradialis Reflex The brachioradialis reflex tests the spinal cord level C-5, C-6.
- Rest the client's forearm in a relaxed position externally rotated on a firm surface.
- Deliver a blow with the percussion hammer directly on the radius 2 to 5 cm (1 to 2 in.) above the wrist or the styloid process, the bony prominence on the thumb side of the wrist. ❸
- Observe the normal flexion and supination of the forearm. The fingers of the hand may also extend slightly.

Patellar Reflex The patellar reflex tests the spinal cord level L-2, L-3, L-4.
- Ask the client to sit on the edge of the examining table so that the legs hang freely.
- Locate the patellar tendon directly below the patella (kneecap).
- Deliver a blow with the percussion hammer directly to the tendon. ❹
- Observe the normal extension or kicking out of the leg as the quadriceps muscle contracts.
- If no response occurs and you suspect the client is not relaxed, ask the client to interlock the fingers and pull.
  Rationale: *This action often enhances relaxation so that a more accurate response is obtained.*

Achilles Reflex The Achilles reflex tests the spinal cord level S-1, S-2.
- With the client in the same position as for the patellar reflex, slightly dorsiflex the client's ankle by supporting the ball of the foot lightly in the hand.
- Deliver a blow with the percussion hammer directly to the Achilles tendon just above the heel. ❺
- Observe and feel the normal plantar flexion (downward jerk) of the foot.

Plantar (Babinski) Reflex The plantar, or Babinski, reflex is superficial. It may be absent in adults without pathology or overridden by voluntary control.

❶ the biceps reflex

❷ the triceps reflex

❸ the brachioradialis reflex

❹ the patellar reflex

❺ the Achilles reflex

❻ the plantar (Babinski) reflex

continued on page 646

ASSESSING THE NEUROLOGIC SYSTEM *continued*

- Use a moderately sharp object, such as the handle of the percussion hammer, a key, or an applicator stick.
- Stroke the lateral border of the sole of the client's foot, starting at the heel, continuing to the ball of the foot, and then proceeding across the ball of the foot toward the big toe. ❻

- Observe the response. Normally, all five toes bend downward; this reaction is negative Babinski. In an abnormal (positive) Babinski response the toes spread outward and the big toe moves upward.

Motor Function

ASSESSMENT	NORMAL FINDINGS	DEVIATIONS FROM NORMAL
12. *Gross Motor and Balance Tests* Generally, the Romberg test and one other gross motor function and balance tests are used.		
Walking Gait Ask the client to walk across the room and back, and assess the client's gait.	Has upright posture and steady gait with opposing arm swing; walks unaided, maintaining balance	Has poor posture and unsteady, irregular, staggering gait with wide stance; bends legs only from hips; has rigid or no arm movements
Romberg Test Ask the client to stand with feet together and arms resting at the sides, first with eyes open, then closed. Stand close during this test *to prevent the client from falling.*	*Negative Romberg:* may sway slightly but is able to maintain upright posture and foot stance	*Positive Romberg:* cannot maintain foot stance; moves the feet apart to maintain stance. If client cannot maintain balance with the eyes shut, client may have sensory ataxia (lack of coordination of the voluntary muscles). If balance cannot be maintained whether the eyes are open or shut, client may have cerebellar ataxia.
Standing on One Foot with Eyes Closed Ask the client to close the eyes and stand on one foot. Repeat on the other foot. Stand close to the client during this test.	Maintains stance for at least 5 seconds	Cannot maintain stance for 5 seconds
Heel-Toe Walking Ask the client to walk a straight line, placing the heel of one foot directly in front of the toes of the other foot. ❼	Maintains heel-toe walking along a straight line	Assumes a wider foot gait to stay upright

❼ Heel-toe walking test.

(Al Dodge, Pearson Education/PH)

ASSESSING THE NEUROLOGIC SYSTEM *continued*

ASSESSMENT	NORMAL FINDINGS	DEVIATIONS FROM NORMAL
Toe or Heel Walking Ask the client to walk several steps on the toes and then on the heels.	Able to walk several steps on toes or heels	Cannot maintain balance on toes and heels

13. *Fine Motor Tests for the Upper Extremities*

ASSESSMENT	NORMAL FINDINGS	DEVIATIONS FROM NORMAL
Finger-To-Nose Test Ask the client to abduct and extend the arms at shoulder height and then rapidly touch the nose alternately with one index finger and then the other. The client repeats the test with the eyes closed if the test is performed easily. **8**	Repeatedly and rhythmically touches the nose	Misses the nose or gives slow response

8 Finger-to-nose test.

ASSESSMENT	NORMAL FINDINGS	DEVIATIONS FROM NORMAL
Alternating Supination and Pronation of Hands on Knees Ask the client to pat both knees with the palms of both hands and then with the backs of the hands alternately at an ever-increasing rate. **9**	Can alternately supinate and pronate hands at rapid pace	Performs with slow, clumsy movements and irregular timing; has difficulty alternating from supination to pronation

9 Alternating supination and pronation of hands on knees test.

(Al Dodge, Pearson Education/PH)

continued on page 648

ASSESSING THE NEUROLOGIC SYSTEM *continued*

ASSESSMENT	NORMAL FINDINGS	DEVIATIONS FROM NORMAL

Finger to Nose and to the Nurse's Finger

Ask the client to touch the nose and then your index finger, held at a distance of about 45 cm (18 in.), at a rapid and increasing rate. ❿

Performs with coordination and rapidity

Misses the finger and moves slowly

❿ Finger-to-nose and to the nurse's finger test.

Fingers To Fingers

Ask the client to spread the arms broadly at shoulder height and then bring the fingers together at the midline, first with the eyes open and then closed, first slowly and then rapidly. ⓫

Performs with accuracy and rapidity

Moves slowly and is unable to touch fingers consistently

⓫ Fingers-to-fingers test.

Fingers to Thumb (Same Hand)

Ask the client to touch each finger of one hand to the thumb of the same hand as rapidly as possible. ⓬

14. *Fine Motor Tests for the Lower Extremities*

   Ask the client to lie supine and to perform these tests.

Rapidly touches each finger to thumb with each hand

Cannot coordinate this fine discrete movement with either one or both hands

⓬ Fingers-to-thumb (same hand) test.

Heel Down Opposite Shin

Ask the client to place the heel of one foot just below the opposite knee and run the heel down the shin to the foot. Repeat with the other foot. The client may also use a sitting position for this test. ⓭

Demonstrates bilateral equal coordination

Has tremors or is awkward; heel moves off shin

⓭ Heel down opposite shin test.

ASSESSING THE NEUROLOGIC SYSTEM *continued*

ASSESSMENT	NORMAL FINDINGS	DEVIATIONS FROM NORMAL
Toe or Ball of Foot to the Nurse's Finger Ask the client to touch your finger with the large toe of each foot. ⑭	Moves smoothly, with coordination	Misses your finger; cannot coordinate movement

⑭ Toe or ball of foot to the nurse's finger test.

15. *Light-Touch Sensation* Compare the light-touch sensation of symmetric areas of the body. **Rationale:** *Sensitivity to touch varies among different skin areas.*	Light tickling or touch sensation	Anesthesia, hyperesthesia, hypoesthesia, or paresthesia

- Ask the client to close the eyes and to respond by saying "yes" or "now" whenever the client feels the cotton wisp touching the skin.
- With a wisp of cotton, lightly touch one specific spot and then the same spot on the other side of the body. ⑮
- Test areas on the forehead, cheek, hand, lower arm, abdomen, foot, and lower leg. Check a distal area of the limb first (i.e., the hand before the arm and the foot before the leg). **Rationale:** *The sensory nerve may be assumed to be intact if sensation is felt at its most distal part.*
- Ask the client to point to the spot where the touch was felt. **Rationale:** *This demonstrates whether the client is able to determine tactile location (point localization), i.e., can accurately perceive where the client was touched.*
- If areas of sensory dysfunction are found, determine the boundaries of sensation by testing responses about every 2.5 cm (1 in.) in the area. Make a sketch of the sensory loss area for recording purposes.

⑮ Assessing light-touch sensation.

16. *Pain Sensation* Assess pain sensation as follows:	Able to discriminate "sharp" and "dull" sensations	Areas of reduced, heightened, or absent sensation (map them out for recording purposes)

- Ask the client to close the eyes and to say "sharp," "dull," or "don't know" when the sharp or dull end of the broken tongue depressor is felt.

continued on page 650

SKILL 30-17

ASSESSING THE NEUROLOGICAL SYSTEM *continued*

ASSESSMENT	NORMAL FINDINGS	DEVIATIONS FROM NORMAL

- Alternately, use the sharp and dull end to lightly prick designated anatomic areas at random, e.g., hand, forearm, foot, lower leg, abdomen. ⓰ The face is not tested in this manner.
- Allow at least 2 seconds between each test to prevent summation effects of stimuli, i.e., several successive stimuli perceived as one stimulus.

⓰ Assessing pain sensation using a broken tongue depressor.

17. *Temperature Sensation*
Temperature sensation is not routinely tested if pain sensation is found to be within normal limits. If pain sensation is not normal or is absent, testing sensitivity to temperature may prove more reliable.
- Touch skin areas with test tubes filled with hot or cold water.
- Have the client respond by saying "hot," "cold," or "don't know."

Able to discriminate between "hot" and "cold" sensations

Areas of dulled or lost sensation (when sensations of pain are dulled, temperature sense is usually also impaired because distribution of these nerves over the body is similar)

18. *Position or Kinesthetic Sensation*
Commonly, the middle fingers and the large toes are tested for the kinesthetic sensation (sense of position).
- To test the fingers, support the client's arm and hand with one hand. To test the toes, place the client's heels on the examining table.
- Ask the client to close the eyes.
- Grasp a middle finger or a big toe firmly between your thumb and index finger, and exert the same pressure on both sides of the finger or toe while moving it. ⓱
- Move the finger or toe until it is up, down, or straight out, and ask the client to identify the position.
- Use a series of brisk up-and-down movements before bringing the finger or toe suddenly to rest in one of the three positions.

Can readily determine the position of fingers and toes

Unable to determine the position of one or more fingers or toes

⓱ Position or kinesthetic sensation.
(Patrick Watson, Pearson Education/PH)

19. *Tactile Discrimination*
For all tests, the client's eyes need to be closed.

ASSESSING THE NEUROLOGIC SYSTEM *continued*

ASSESSMENT	NORMAL FINDINGS	DEVIATIONS FROM NORMAL
One- and Two-Point Discrimination Alternately stimulate the skin with two pins simultaneously and then with one pin. Ask whether the client feels one or two pinpricks.	Perception varies widely in adults over different parts of the body. Normally, a person can distinguish between a one- and two-point stimulus within the following minimum distances: Fingertips, 2.8 mm Palms of hands, 8–12 mm Chest, forearm, 40 mm Back, 50–70 mm Upper arm, thigh, 75 mm Toes, 3–8 mm	Unable to sense whether one or two areas of the skin are being stimulated by pressure
Stereognosis (Ability to Recognize Objects by Touching Them) Place familiar objects, such as a key, paper clip, or coin, in the client's hand, and ask the client to identify them.	Recognizes common objects	Unable to recognize common objects
If the client has a motor impairment of the hand and is unable to manipulate an object, write a number or letter on the client's palm, using a blunt instrument, and ask the client to identify it (graphesthesia).	Able to identify numbers or letters written on palm	Unable to identify numbers or letters written on palm
Extinction Phenomenon Simultaneously stimulate two symmetric areas of the body, such as the thighs, the cheeks, or the hands.	Both points of stimulus are felt	Failure to perceive touch on one side of the body when two symmetric areas of the body are touched simultaneously (frequently noted in clients with lesions of the sensory cortex)

20. Document findings in the client record using forms or checklists supplemented by narrative notes when appropriate. Describe any abnormal findings in objective terms, e.g., "When asked to count backwards by threes, client made seven errors and completed the task in 4 minutes."

EVALUATION

- Perform a detailed follow-up examination of other systems based on findings that deviated from expected or normal for the client. Relate findings to previous assessment data if available.

- Report significant deviations from normal to the primary care provider.

LIFESPAN CONSIDERATIONS Assessing the Neurologic System

INFANTS

- Reflexes commonly tested in newborns include:
  - *Rooting:* Stroke the side of the face near mouth; infant opens mouth and turns to the side that is stroked.
  - *Sucking:* Place nipple or finger 3 to 4 cm into mouth; infant sucks vigorously.
  - *Tonic neck:* Place infant supine, turn head to one side; arm on side to which head is turned extends; on opposite side, arm curls up (fencer's pose).
  - *Palmar grasp:* Place finger in infant's palm and press; infant curls fingers around.
  - *Stepping:* Hold infant as if weight bearing on surface; infant steps along, one foot at a time.

  - *Moro:* Present loud noise or unexpected movement; infant spreads arms and legs, extends fingers, then flexes and brings hands together; may cry.
- Most of these reflexes disappear between 4 and 6 months of age.

CHILDREN

- Present the procedures as games whenever possible.
- Positive Babinski reflex is abnormal after the child ambulates or at age 2.
- For children under age 5, the Denver Developmental Screening Test II provides a comprehensive neurologic evaluation—particularly for motor function.
- Note the child's ability to understand and follow directions.

continued on page 652

LIFESPAN CONSIDERATIONS   Assessing the Neurologic System—*continued*

- Assess immediate recall or recent memory by using names of cartoon characters. Normal recall in children is one less than age in years.
- Assess for signs of hyperactivity or abnormally short attention span.
- Children should be able to walk backward by age 2, balance on one foot for 5 seconds by age 4, heel-toe walk by age 5, and heel-toe walk backward by age 6.
- The Romberg test is appropriate over age 3.

ELDERS

- A full neurologic assessment can be lengthy. Conduct in several sessions if indicated, and cease the tests if the client is noticeably fatigued.
- A decline in mental status is not a normal result of aging. Changes are more the result of physical or psychologic disorders (e.g., fever, fluid and electrolyte imbalances, medications). Acute, abrupt-onset mental status changes are usually caused by delirium. These changes are often reversible with treatment. Chronic subtle insidious mental health changes are usually caused by dementia and are usually irreversible.
- Intelligence and learning ability are unaltered with age. Many factors, however, inhibit learning (e.g., anxiety, illness, pain, cultural barrier).
- Short-term memory is often less efficient. Long-term memory is usually unaltered.
- Because old age is often associated with loss of support persons, depression is a common disorder. Mood changes, weight loss,

anorexia, constipation, and early morning awakening may manifest it.
- The stress of being in unfamiliar situations can cause confusion in elders.
- As a person ages, reflex responses may become less intense.
- Because elders tire more easily than younger clients, a total neurologic assessment is often done at a different time than the other parts of the physical assessment.
- Although there is a progressive decrease in the number of functioning neurons in the central nervous system and in the sense organs, elders usually function well because of the abundant reserves in the number of brain cells.
- Impulse transmission and reaction to stimuli are slower.
- Many elders have some impairment of hearing, vision, smell, temperature and pain sensation, memory, and mental endurance.
- Coordination changes, including a reduced speed of fine finger movements. Standing balance remains intact, and Romberg's test remains negative.
- Reflex responses may slightly increase or decrease. Many show loss of Achilles reflex, and the plantar reflex may be difficult to elicit.
- When testing sensory function, the nurse needs to give elders time to respond. Normally, elders have unaltered perception of light touch and superficial pain, decreased perception of deep pain, and decreased perception of temperature stimuli. Many also reveal a decrease or absence of position sense in the large toes.

TABLE 30–10 Levels of Consciousness: Glasgow Coma Scale		
FACULTY MEASURED	**RESPONSE**	**SCORE**
Eye opening	Spontaneous	4
	To verbal command	3
	To pain	2
	No response	1
Motor response	To verbal command	6
	To localized pain	5
	Flexes and withdraws	4
	Flexes abnormally	3
	Extends abnormally	2
	No response	1
Verbal response	Oriented, converses	5
	Disoriented, converses	4
	Uses inappropriate words	3
	Makes incomprehensible sounds	2
	No response	1

TABLE 30–11 **Cranial Nerve Functions and Assessment Methods**

CRANIAL NERVE	NAME	TYPE	FUNCTION	ASSESSMENT METHOD
I	Olfactory	Sensory	Smell	Ask client to close eyes and identify different mild aromas, such as coffee, vanilla, peanut butter, orange/lemon, chocolate.
II	Optic	Sensory	Vision and visual fields	Ask client to read Snellen-type chart; check visual fields by confrontation; and conduct an ophthalmoscopic examination (see Skill 30-6).
III	Oculomotor	Motor	Extraocular eye movement (EOM); movement of sphincter of pupil; movement of ciliary muscles of lens	Assess six ocular movements and pupil reaction (see Skill 30-6).
IV	Trochlear	Motor	EOM; specifically, moves eyeball downward and laterally	Assess six ocular movements (see Skill 30-6).
V	Trigeminal Ophthalmic branch	Sensory	Sensation of cornea, skin of face, and nasal mucosa	While client looks upward, lightly touch the lateral sclera of the eye with sterile gauze to elicit blink reflex. To test light sensation, have client close eyes, wipe a wisp of cotton over client's forehead and paranasal sinuses. To test deep sensation, use alternating blunt and sharp ends of a safety pin over same areas.
	Maxillary branch	Sensory	Sensation of skin of face and anterior oral cavity (tongue and teeth)	Assess skin sensation as for ophthalmic branch above.
	Mandibular branch	Motor and sensory	Muscles of mastication; sensation of skin of face	Ask client to clench teeth.
VI	Abducens	Motor	EOM; moves eyeball laterally	Assess directions of gaze.
VII	Facial	Motor and sensory	Facial expression; taste (anterior two-thirds of tongue)	Ask client to smile, raise the eyebrows, frown, puff out cheeks, close eyes tightly. Ask client to identify various tastes placed on tip and sides of tongue: sugar (sweet), salt, lemon juice (sour), and quinine (bitter); identify areas of taste.
VIII	Auditory Vestibular branch	Sensory	Equilibrium	Romberg test (see page 646).
	Cochlear branch	Sensory	Hearing	Assess client's ability to hear spoken word and vibrations of tuning fork.
IX	Glossopharyngeal	Motor and sensory	Swallowing ability, tongue movement, taste (posterior tongue)	Apply tastes on posterior tongue for identification. Ask client to move tongue from side to side and up and down.
X	Vagus	Motor and sensory	Sensation of pharynx and larynx; swallowing; vocal cord movement	Assessed with cranial nerve IX; assess client's speech for hoarseness.
XI	Accessory	Motor	Head movement; shrugging of shoulders	Ask client to shrug shoulders against resistance from your hands and turn head to side against resistance from your hand (repeat for other side).
XII	Hypoglossal	Motor	Protrusion of tongue; moves tongue up and down and side to side	Ask client to protrude tongue at midline, then move it side to side.

THE FEMALE GENITALS AND INGUINAL AREA

The examination of the genitals and reproductive tract of women includes assessment of the inguinal lymph nodes and inspection and palpation of the external genitals. Completeness of the assessment of the genitals and reproductive tract depends on the needs and problems of the individual client. In most practice settings, generalist nurses perform only inspection of the external genitals and palpation of the inguinal lymph nodes.

For sexually active adolescent and adult women, a Papanicolaou test (Pap test) is used to detect cancer of the cervix. If there is an increased or abnormal vaginal discharge, specimens should be taken to check for sexually transmitted disease.

Examination of the genitals usually creates uncertainty and apprehension in women, and the lithotomy position required can cause embarrassment. The nurse must explain each part of the examination in advance and perform the examination in an objective, supportive, and efficient manner. Not all agencies permit male practitioners to examine the female genitals. Some agencies may require the presence of another woman during the examination so that there is no question of unprofessional behavior. Most female clients accept examination by a male, especially if he is emotionally comfortable about performing it and does so in a matter-of-fact and competent manner. If the male nurse does not feel comfortable about this part of the examination or if the client is reluctant to be examined by a man, the nurse should refer this part of the examination to a female practitioner.

Skill 30-18 describes how to assess the female genitals and inguinal area.

SKILL 30-18

ASSESSING THE FEMALE GENITALS AND INGUINAL AREA

PLANNING

Delegation

Due to the substantial knowledge and skill required, assessment of the female genitals and inguinal lymph nodes is not delegated to UAP. However, persons other than the nurse may record any aspect that is observed during usual care. Abnormal findings must be validated and interpreted by the nurse.

Equipment
- Clean gloves
- Drape
- Supplemental lighting, if needed

IMPLEMENTATION

Performance

1. Prior to performing the procedure, introduce self and verify the client's identity using agency protocol. Explain to the client what you are going to do, why it is necessary, and how she can cooperate. Discuss how the results will be used in planning further care or treatments.
2. Perform hand hygiene, apply gloves, and observe appropriate infection control procedures.
3. Provide for client privacy. Request the presence of another woman if desired, required by agency policy, or requested by the client.

4. Inquire regarding the following: age of onset of menstruation, last menstrual period (LMP), regularity of cycle, duration, amount of daily flow, and whether menstruation is painful; incidence of pain during intercourse; vaginal discharge; number of pregnancies, number of live births, labor or delivery complications; urgency and frequency of urination at night; blood in urine, painful urination, incontinence; history of sexually transmitted disease, past and present.
5. Cover the pelvic area with a sheet or drape at all times when not actually being examined. Position the client supine with feet elevated on the stirrups of an examination table. Alternatively, assist the client into the dorsal recumbent position with knees flexed and thighs externally rotated.

ASSESSMENT	NORMAL FINDINGS	DEVIATIONS FROM NORMAL
6. Inspect the distribution, amount, and characteristics of pubic hair.	There are wide variations; generally kinky in the menstruating adult, thinner and straighter after menopause	Scant pubic hair (may indicate hormonal problem)
	Distributed in the shape of an inverse triangle	Hair growth should not extend over the abdomen
7. Inspect the skin of the pubic area for parasites, inflammation, swelling, and lesions. To assess pubic skin adequately, separate the labia majora and labia minora.	Pubic skin intact, no lesions	Lice, lesions, scars, fissures, swelling, erythema, excoriations, varicosities, or leukoplakia
	Skin of vulva area slightly darker than the rest of the body	
	Labia round, full, and relatively symmetric in adult females	
8. Inspect the clitoris, urethral orifice, and vaginal orifice when separating the labia minora.	Clitoris does not exceed 1 cm in width and 2 cm in length	Presence of lesions
	Urethral orifice appears as a small slit and is the same color as surrounding tissues	Presence of inflammation, swelling, or discharge
	No inflammation, swelling, or discharge	

ASSESSING THE FEMALE GENITALS AND INGUINAL AREA *continued*

ASSESSMENT	NORMAL FINDINGS	DEVIATIONS FROM NORMAL
9. Palpate the inguinal lymph nodes ❶. Use the pads of the fingers in a rotary motion, noting any enlargement or tenderness.	No enlargement or tenderness	Enlargement and tenderness

Superior or horizontal group

Inferior or vertical group

❶ Lymph nodes of the groin area.

10. Document findings in the client record using forms or checklists supplemented by narrative notes when appropriate.

EVALUATION

- Perform a detailed follow-up examination based on findings that deviated from expected or normal for the client. Relate findings to previous assessment data if available.
- Significant deviations from normal indicate the need for an internal vaginal examination.

LIFESPAN CONSIDERATIONS   Assessing the Female Genitals and Inguinal Lymph Nodes

INFANTS

- Infants can be held in a supine position on the parent's lap with the knees supported in a flexed position and separated.
- In newborns, because of maternal estrogen, the labia and clitoris may be edematous and enlarged, and there may be a small amount of white or bloody vaginal discharge.
- Assess the mons and inguinal area for swelling or tenderness that may indicate presence of an inguinal hernia.

CHILDREN

- Ensure that you have the parent or guardian's approval to perform the examination and then tell the child what you are going to do. Preschool children are taught not to allow others to touch their "private parts."
- Assessment of adolescent girls is limited to inspection of the external genitals, unless the girl is sexually active. The exam should be conducted with the parent out of the room.
- Girls should be assessed for Tanner staging of pubertal development (see Box 30–9).
- Girls should have a Papanicolaou (Pap) test done if sexually active, or by age 18 years.
- Sexually active girls with abnormal vaginal discharge should be tested for sexually transmitted disease.

- The clitoris is a common site for syphilitic chancres in younger females.

ELDERS

- Labia are atrophied and flatter in older females.
- The clitoris is a potential site for cancerous lesions in older females.
- The vulva atrophies as a result of a reduction in vascularity, elasticity, adipose tissue, and estrogen levels. Because the vulva is more fragile, it is more easily irritated.
- The vaginal environment becomes drier and more alkaline, resulting in an alteration of the type of flora present and a predisposition to vaginitis. Dyspareunia (difficult or painful intercourse) is also a common occurrence.
- The cervix and uterus decrease in size.
- The fallopian tubes and ovaries atrophy.
- Ovulation and estrogen production cease.
- Vaginal bleeding unrelated to estrogen therapy is abnormal in older women.
- Prolapse of the uterus can occur in older females, especially those who have had multiple pregnancies.
- Older females may be arthritic and find the examination position uncomfortable.

MediaLink · Physical Exam Study Guides Application

In many agencies only nurse practitioners examine the internal genitals. However, generalist nurses often assist with this examination and need to be familiar with the procedure. Examination of the internal genitals involves (a) palpating Skene's and Bartholin's glands, (b) assessing the pelvic mus-culature, (c) inserting a vaginal speculum to inspect the cervix and vagina, and (d) obtaining a Papanicolaou smear.

The speculum examination of the vagina involves the insertion of a plastic or metal speculum that consists of two blades and an adjustable thumb screw (Figure 30-35 ■). Various sizes

Figure 30-35 ■ A vaginal speculum.
(Patrick Watson)

are available (small, medium, and large); the appropriate size needs to be selected for each client. The speculum may be lubricated with water-soluble lubricant if specimens are not being collected. Most examiners lubricate the speculum with warm water. After visualizing the cervix, the examiner takes smear specimens from one or more of the sites.

The nurse's responsibilities when assisting with an examination of the internal female genitals include the following:

1. *Assembling equipment.* These include drapes, gloves, vaginal speculum, warm water or lubricant, and supplies for cytology and culture studies.
2. *Preparing the client.* Advise the client not to douche prior to the procedure. Explain the procedure. It should take only 5 minutes and is normally not painful. Assist the client to a lithotomy position as needed, and drape her appropriately.
3. *Supporting the client during the procedure.* This involves explaining the procedure as needed, and encouraging the

client to take deep breaths that will help the pelvic muscles relax.

4. *Monitoring and assisting the client after the procedure.* Assist the client from the lithotomy position and with perineal care as needed.
5. *Documenting the procedure.* Include the date and time it was performed, the name of the examiner, and any nursing assessments and interventions.

THE MALE GENITALS AND INGUINAL AREA

In adult men, a complete examination includes assessment of the external genitals, the presence of any hernias, and the prostate gland. Nurses in some practice settings performing routine assessment of clients may assess only the external genitals. The male reproductive and urinary systems (see Figure 30-37 ■) share the urethra, which is the passageway for both urine and semen. Therefore, in physical assessment of the male these two systems are frequently assessed together.

Examination of the male genitals by a female practitioner is becoming increasingly common, although not all agencies permit a female practitioner to examine the male genitals. Some agencies may require the presence of another person during the examination so that there is no question of unprofessional behavior. Most male clients accept examination by a female, especially if she is emotionally comfortable about performing it and does so in a matter-of-fact and competent manner. If the female nurse does not feel comfortable about this part of the examination or if the client is reluctant to be examined by a woman, the nurse should refer this part of the examination to a male practitioner.

Development of secondary sex characteristics is assessed in relationship to the client's age. See Table 30–12 for the five Tanner stages of the development of pubic hair, the penis, and the testes and scrotum during puberty.

BOX 30—9 Five Stages of Pubic Hair Development in Females

Stage 1   Preadolescence. No pubic hair except for fine body hair.

Stage 2   Usually occurs at ages 11 and 12. Sparse, long, slightly pigmented curly hair develops along the labia.

Stage 3   Usually occurs at ages 12 and 13. Hair becomes darker in color and curlier and develops over the pubic symphysis.

Stage 4   Usually occurs between ages 13 and 14. Hair assumes the texture and curl of the adult but is not as thick and does not appear on the thighs.

Stage 5   Sexual maturity. Hair assumes adult appearance and appears on the inner aspect of the upper thighs (see Figure 30-36 ■).

1   2

3   4   5

Figure 30-36 ■ Stages of female pubic hair development.

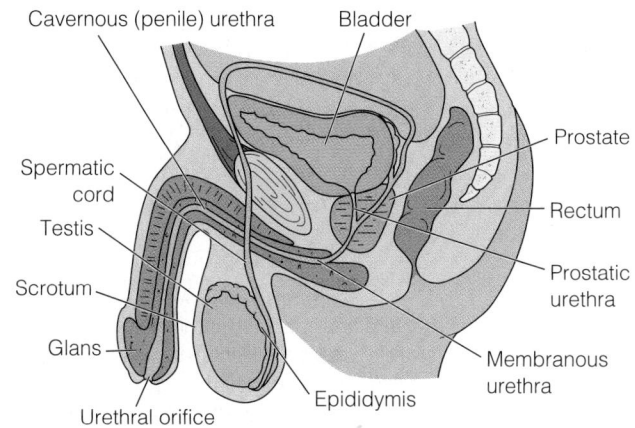

Cavernous (penile) urethra Bladder

Spermatic cord

Testis

Scrotum

Glans

Urethral orifice Epididymis

Prostate

Rectum

Prostatic urethra

Membranous urethra

Figure 30-37 ■ The male urogenital tract.

All male clients should be screened for the presence of inguinal or femoral hernias. A **hernia** is a protrusion of the intestine through the inguinal wall or canal. Cancer of the prostate gland is the most common cancer in adult men and occurs primarily in men over age 50. Examination of the prostate gland is performed with the examination of the rectum and anus (see Skill 30-20).

Testicular cancer is much rarer than prostate cancer and occurs primarily in young men ages 15 to 35. Testicular cancer is most commonly found on the anterior and lateral surfaces of the testes. Testicular self-examination should be conducted monthly (see Chapter 40 ∞).

The techniques of inspection and palpation are used to examine the male genitals. Skill 30-19 describes how the nurse can conduct an assessment of the male genitals and inguinal area.

TABLE 30–12	**Tanner Stages of Male Pubic Hair and External Genital Development (12 to 16 Years)**		
STAGE	PUBIC HAIR	PENIS	TESTES/SCROTUM
1	None, except for body hair like that on the abdomen	Size is relative to body size, as in childhood	Size is relative to body size, as in childhood
2	Scant, long, slightly pigmented at base of penis	Slight enlargement occurs	Becomes reddened in color and enlarged
3	Darker, begins to curl and becomes more coarse; extends over pubic symphysis	Elongation occurs	Continuing enlargement
4	Continues to darken and thicken; extends on the sides, above and below	Increase in both breadth and length; glans develops	Continuing enlargement; color darkens
5	Adult distribution that extends to inner thighs, umbilicus, and anus	Adult appearance	Adult appearance

ASSESSING THE MALE GENITALS AND INGUINAL AREA

PLANNING

Delegation
Due to the substantial knowledge and skill required, assessment of the male genitals and inguinal area is not delegated to UAP. However, persons other than the nurse may record any aspect that is observed during usual care. Abnormal findings must be validated and interpreted by the nurse.

Equipment
- Clean gloves

IMPLEMENTATION

Performance

1. Prior to performing the procedure, introduce self and verify the client's identity using agency protocol. Explain to the client what you are going to do, why it is necessary, and how he can co-operate. Discuss how the results will be used in planning further care or treatments.
2. Perform hand hygiene, apply gloves, and observe appropriate infection control procedures.
3. Provide for client privacy. Request the presence of another person if desired, required by agency policy, or requested by the client.
4. Inquire if the client has any history of the following: usual voiding patterns and changes, bladder control, urinary incontinence, frequency, urgency, abdominal pain; symptoms of sexually transmitted disease; swellings that could indicate presence of hernia; family history of nephritis, malignancy of the prostate, or malignancy of the kidney.
5. Cover the pelvic area with a sheet or drape at all times when not actually being examined.

ASSESSMENT	NORMAL FINDINGS	DEVIATIONS FROM NORMAL
Pubic Hair		
6. Inspect the distribution, amount, and characteristics of pubic hair.	Triangular distribution, often spreading up the abdomen	Scant amount or absence of hair
Penis		
7. Inspect the penile shaft and glans penis for lesions, nodules, swellings, and inflammation.	Penile skin intact	Presence of lesions, nodules, swellings, or inflammation
	Appears slightly wrinkled and varies in color as widely as other body skin	
	Foreskin easily retractable from the glans penis	
	Small amount of thick white smegma between the glans and foreskin	
8. Inspect the urethral meatus for swelling, inflammation, and discharge.	Pink and slitlike appearance	Inflammation; discharge
● Compress or ask the client to compress the glans slightly to open the urethral meatus to inspect it for discharge.	Positioned at the tip of the penis	Variation in meatal locations (e.g., hypospadias, on the underside of the penile shaft, and epispadias, on the upper side of the penile shaft)
9. Palpate the penis for tenderness, thickening, and nodules. Use your thumb and first two fingers.	Smooth and semifirm	Presence of tenderness, thickening, or nodules
	Is slightly movable over the underlying structures	Immobility
Scrotum		
10. Inspect the scrotum for appearance, general size, and symmetry.	Scrotal skin is darker in color than that of the rest of the body and is loose	Discolorations; any tightening of skin (may indicate edema or mass)
● To facilitate inspection of the scrotum during a physical examination, ask the client to hold the penis out of the way.	Size varies with temperature changes (the dartos muscles contract when the area is cold and relax when the area is warm)	Marked asymmetry in size
● Inspect all skin surfaces by spreading the rugated surface skin and lifting the scrotum as needed to observe posterior surfaces.	Scrotum appears asymmetric (left testis is usually lower than right testis)	

ASSESSING THE MALE GENITALS AND INGUINAL AREA *continued*

ASSESSMENT	NORMAL FINDINGS	DEVIATIONS FROM NORMAL
11. Palpate the scrotum to assess status of underlying testes, epididymis, and spermatic cord. Palpate both testes simultaneously for comparative purposes.	Testicles are rubbery, smooth, and free of nodules and masses	Testicles are enlarged, with uneven surface (possible tumor)
• Using your first two fingers and thumb, palpate each testis for size, consistency, shape, smoothness, and presence of masses. During assessment of male adolescents, establish the descent of the testicles into the scrotum; note undescended testes.	Testis is about 2 × 4 cm (0.7 × 1.5 in.)	Epididymis is nonresilient and painful
• Palpate the epididymis between your thumb and index finger. It is located at the top of the testis and extends behind it.	Epididymis is resilient, normally tender, and softer than the spermatic cord	
• Palpate the spermatic cord between thumb and index finger. It is usually found at the top lateral portion of the scrotum and feels firm.	Spermatic cord is firm	
• If swelling, irregularities, or nodules are detected during the scrotal examination, attempt to transilluminate the lesion. This is done by darkening the room and shining a flashlight behind the scrotum through the mass. **Rationale:** *Serous fluid causes the light to show with a red glow; tissue or blood does not transilluminate.*		
• Describe all scrotal masses in terms of their size, shape, placement, consistency, tenderness, and presence of transillumination.		
Inguinal Area		
12. Inspect both inguinal areas for bulges while the client is standing, if possible.	No swelling or bulges	Swelling or bulge (possible inguinal or femoral hernia)
• First, have the client remain at rest.		
• Next, have the client hold his breath and strain or bear down as though having a bowel movement. Bearing down may make the hernia more visible.		

13. Document findings in the client record using forms or checklists supplemented by narrative notes when appropriate.

EVALUATION

■ Perform a detailed follow-up examination based on findings that deviated from expected or normal for the client. Relate findings to previous assessment data if available.

■ Report significant deviations from normal to the primary care provider.

LIFESPAN CONSIDERATIONS ⟩ Assessing the Male Genitals and Inguinal Area

INFANTS
- The foreskin of the uncircumcised infant is normally tight at birth and should not be retracted. It will gradually loosen as the baby grows and is usually fully retractable by 2 to 3 years of age. Assess for cleanliness, redness, or irritation.
- Assess for placement of the urethral meatus.
- Palpate the scrotum to determine if the testes are descended; in the newborn and infant, the testes may retract into the inguinal canal, especially with stimulation of the cremasteric reflex.
- Assess the inguinal area for swelling or tenderness that may indicate presence of an inguinal hernia.

CHILDREN
- Ensure that you have the parent or guardian's approval to perform the examination and then tell the child what you are going to do. Preschool children are taught to not allow others to touch their "private parts."

- In young boys, the cremasteric reflex can cause the testes to ascend into the inguinal canal. If possible have the boy sit cross-legged, which stretches the muscle and decreases the reflex.
- Table 30–12 on page 657 shows the five Tanner stages of development of pubic hair, penis, and testes/scrotum.

ELDERS
- The penis decreases in size with age; the size and firmness of the testes decrease.
- Testosterone is produced in smaller amounts.
- More time and direct physical stimulation are required for an older man to achieve an erection, but he can maintain the erection for a longer period before ejaculation than he could at a younger age.
- Seminal fluid is reduced in amount and viscosity.
- Urinary frequency, nocturia, dribbling, and problems with beginning and ending the stream are usually the result of prostatic enlargement.

THE RECTUM AND ANUS

Rectal examination, an essential part of every comprehensive physical examination, involves inspection and palpation (digital examination). The extent of the assessment of the rectum and anus depends on the rectal problems stated by the client in the nursing history. In many practice settings, the nurse performs only inspection of the anus.

Skill 30-20 describes how to assess the rectum and anus.

ASSESSING THE RECTUM AND ANUS

PLANNING

Delegation
Assessment of the rectum and anus is not delegated to UAP. However, many aspects are observed during usual care and may be recorded by persons other than the nurse. Abnormal findings must be validated and interpreted by the nurse.

Equipment
- Clean gloves
- Water-soluble lubricant

IMPLEMENTATION
Performance
1. Prior to performing the procedure, introduce self and verify the client's identity using agency protocol. Explain to the client what you are going to do, why it is necessary, and how he or she can cooperate. Discuss how the results will be used in planning further care or treatments. Because digital examination can cause apprehension and embarrassment in the client, it is important that the nurse help the client relax by encouraging the client to take slow, deep breaths (tension can cause spasms of the anal sphincters, making the examination uncomfortable) and inform the client about potential sensations such as feelings of defecation or passing gas.
2. Perform hand hygiene, apply gloves, and observe appropriate infection control procedures for all rectal examinations.
3. Provide for client privacy. Drape the client appropriately to prevent undue exposure of body parts.

4. Inquire if the client has any history of the following: bright blood in stools, tarry black stools, diarrhea, constipation, abdominal pain, excessive gas, hemorrhoids, or rectal pain; family history of colorectal cancer; when last stool specimen for occult blood was performed and the results; and for males, if not obtained during the genitourinary examination, signs or symptoms of prostate enlargement (e.g., slow urinary stream, hesitance, frequency, dribbling, and nocturia).
5. Position the client. In adults, a left lateral or Sims' position with the upper leg acutely flexed is required for the examination. For females, a dorsal recumbent position with hips externally rotated and knees flexed or a lithotomy position may be used. ❶ For males, a standing position while the client bends over the examining table may also be used. This position is commonly used to examine the prostate gland.

ASSESSING THE RECTUM AND ANUS *continued*

Position	Description
Sims'	Side-lying position with lowermost arm behind the body, uppermost leg flexed at hip and knee, upper arm flexed at shoulder and elbow.
Lithotomy	Back-lying position with feet supported in stirrups; the hips should be in line with the edge of the table.
Dorsal recumbent	Back-lying position with knees flexed and hips externally rotated; small pillow under the head; soles of feet on the surface.

❶ Left Sims' lithotomy, and dorsal recumbent positions.

ASSESSMENT

6. Inspect the anus and surrounding tissue for color, integrity, and skin lesions. Then, ask the client to bear down as though defecating. Bearing down creates slight pressure on the skin that may accentuate rectal fissures, rectal prolapse, polyps, or internal hemorrhoids. Describe the location of all abnormal findings in terms of a clock, with the 12 o'clock position toward the pubic symphysis.

7. Palpate the rectum for anal sphincter tonicity, nodules, masses, and tenderness.
   - Lubricate your gloved index finger, and instruct the client to bear downward as though having a bowel movement. **Rationale:** *This relaxes the anal sphincter.*
   - Slowly insert your finger into the anus and into the rectum in the direction of the umbilicus. The anal canal (distance from the anal opening to the anorectal junction) is short (less than 3 cm [about 1 in.]). The posterior wall of the rectum follows the curve of the coccyx and sacrum. The nurse's finger is usually able to palpate a distance of 6 to 10 cm (2 to 4 in.).
   - Never force digital insertion. If lesions are painful or bleeding occurs, discontinue the examination.

NORMAL FINDINGS

Intact perianal skin; usually slightly more pigmented than the skin of the buttocks Anal skin is normally more pigmented, coarser, and moister than perianal skin and is usually hairless

Anal sphincter has good tone

DEVIATIONS FROM NORMAL

Presence of fissures (cracks), ulcers, excoriations, inflammations, abscesses, protruding hemorrhoids (dilated veins seen as reddened protrusions of the skin), lumps or tumors, fistula openings, or rectal prolapse (varying degrees of protrusion of the rectal mucous membrane through the anus)

Hypertonicity of the anal sphincter (may occur in the presence of an anal fissure or other lesion that causes contraction)

Hypotonicity of anal sphincter (may occur after rectal surgery or result from a neurologic deficiency)

MediaLink Client Care After Motor Vehicle Crash Care Plan

continued on page 662

SKILL 30-20

ASSESSING THE RECTUM AND ANUS *continued*

- Ask the client to tighten the anal sphincter around your finger, and note the tone of the anal sphincter.
- Rotate the pad of the index finger along the anal and the rectal walls, feeling for nodules, masses, and tenderness.

Rectal wall is smooth and not tender | Rectal wall is tender and nodular

- Note the location of any abnormalities of the rectum (e.g., "anterior wall, 2 cm proximal to the internal anal sphincter").

8. On withdrawing the finger from the rectum and anus, observe it for feces. If ordered, perform a test for occult blood on the stool (see Chapter 34 ∞ , page 809).

Brown color | Presence of mucus, blood, or black tarry stool

9. Document findings in the client record using forms or checklists supplemented by narrative notes when appropriate.

EVALUATION

- Perform a detailed follow-up examination based on findings that deviated from expected or normal for the client. Relate findings to previous assessment data if available.

- Report significant deviations from normal to the primary care provider.

LIFESPAN CONSIDERATIONS Assessing the Rectum and Anus

INFANTS

- Lightly touching the anus should result in a brief anal contraction ("wink" reflex).
- If the infant has normal bowel function, a rectal examination is not routinely performed.

CHILDREN

- Erythema and scratch marks around the anus may indicate a pinworm parasite. Children with this condition may be disturbed by itching during sleep.
- A rectal examination is not routinely performed on children.

ELDERS

- Chronic constipation and straining at stool cause an increase in the frequency of hemorrhoids and rectal prolapse.

CRITICAL THINKING CHECKPOINT

A 75-year-old woman is admitted to your unit for evaluation after being found in her apartment unconscious on the floor. She is now awake but moving slowly. Her vital signs are within normal limits.

1. In the hospital, it is unrealistic to expect to be able to spend an uninterrupted 30 to 60 minutes with a single client performing an admission assessment. Which three systems would have top priority for her initial assessment and why?
2. While gathering relevant history data, what should you do if the client answers with simple one-word answers or gestures?

3. Because the client may be in significant discomfort from her fall, it is not easy for her to move about for the examination. How might you organize your assessment to minimize her need to change positions frequently?
4. If the client is unable to provide a detailed recent history, what other sources of these data could you consider?

See Critical Thinking Possibilities in Appendix A.

CHAPTER 30 **REVIEW**

CHAPTER HIGHLIGHTS

- The health examination is conducted to assess the function and integrity of the client's body parts.
- The health examination may entail a complete head-to-toe assessment or individual assessment of a body system or body part.
- The health assessment is conducted in a systematic manner that requires the fewest position changes for the client.
- Aspects of the physical assessment procedures should be incorporated in the assessment, intervention, and evaluation phases of the nursing process.
- Data obtained in the physical health examination supplement, confirm, or refute data obtained during the nursing history.
- Nursing history data help the nurse focus on specific aspects of the physical health examination.
- Data obtained in the physical health examination help the nurse establish nursing diagnoses, plan the client's care, and evaluate the outcomes of nursing care.

- Initial assessment findings provide baseline data about the client's functional abilities against which subsequent assessment findings are compared.
- Skills in inspection, palpation, percussion, and auscultation are required for the physical health examination; these skills are used in that order throughout the examination except during abdominal assessment, when auscultation follows inspection and precedes percussion and palpation.
- Knowledge of the normal structure and function of body parts and systems is an essential requisite to conducting physical assessment.

TEST YOUR KNOWLEDGE

1. Which of the following indicates a normal finding on auscultation of the lungs?
    1. Tympany over the right upper lobe
    2. Resonance over the left upper lobe
    3. Hyperresonance over the left lower lobe
    4. Dullness above the left 10th intercostal space

2. The nurse positions the client sitting upright during palpation of which of the following areas?
    1. Abdomen
    2. Genitals
    3. Breast
    4. Head and neck

3. After auscultating the abdomen, the nurse should report which of the following to the primary care provider?
    1. Bruit over the aorta
    2. Absence of bowel sounds for 60 seconds
    3. Continuous bowel sounds over the ileocecal valve
    4. A completely irregular pattern of bowel sounds

4. If unable to locate the client's popliteal pulse during a routine examination, the nurse should perform which of the following next?
    1. Check for a pedal pulse.
    2. Check for a femoral pulse.
    3. Take the client's blood pressure on that thigh.
    4. Ask another nurse to try to locate the pulse.

5. Which of the following is an expected finding during assessment of the older adult?
    1. Facial hair becomes finer and softer
    2. Decreased peripheral, color, and night vision
    3. Increased sensitivity to odors
    4. Respiratory rate and rhythm are irregular at rest

6. List five aspects of the skin that the nurse assesses during a routine examination.
    1.
    2.
    3.
    4.
    5.

7. If the client reports loss of short-term memory, the nurse would assess this using which one of the following?
    1. Have the client repeat a series of three numbers, increasing to eight if possible.
    2. Have the client describe his or her childhood illnesses.
    3. Ask the client to describe how he or she arrived at this location.
    4. Ask the client to count backwards from 100 subtracting seven each time.

8. Refer back to Figure 30-14. If the client can accurately read only lines 1, 2, 3, and 4, an appropriate nursing diagnosis would be
   1. *Deficient Knowledge.*
   2. *Impaired Memory.*
   3. *Ineffective Tissue Perfusion.*
   4. *Risk for Injury.*

9. In order to palpate lymph nodes, the nurse uses which of the following techniques?
   1. Use the flat of all four fingers in a vertical and then side-to-side motion.
   2. Use the back of the hand and feel for temperature variation between the right and left sides.
   3. Use the pads of two fingers in a circular motion.
   4. Compress the nodes between the index fingers of both hands.

10. For a client whose assessment of the musculoskeletal system is normal, the nurse checks which of the following on the medical record? (Check all that apply.)
   1. _____ Atrophied
   2. _____ Contractured
   3. _____ Crepitation
   4. _____ Equal
   5. _____ Firm
   6. _____ Flaccid
   7. _____ Hypertrophied
   8. _____ Spastic
   9. _____ Symmetrical
   10. _____ Tremor

See Answers to Test Your Knowledge in Appendix A.

EXPLORE MEDIALINK www.prenhall.com/berman

DVD-ROM
- Audio Glossary
- NCLEX Review
- End of Unit Concept Map Activity
- Animations:
    Middle Ear Dynamics
    Otoscope Examination
    Ear Abnormalities
    Mouth and Throat
    Lung Sounds
    Heart Sounds

COMPANION WEBSITE
- Additional NCLEX Review
- Case Study: Performing Physical Assessments
- Care Plan Activity: Client Care After Motor Vehicle Crash
- Application Activity: Physical Exam Study Guide
- Links to Resources

READINGS AND REFERENCES

SUGGESTED READINGS
Dulak, S. B. (2004). A practical guide to a thorough history. *RN, 67*(1), 14–21. *Obtaining a thorough history during an initial meeting with a client is vital since this information is used to guide future medical and nursing care decisions. This review of the essentials will help you get the most out of your next nursing history.*

RELATED RESEARCH
Davidson, L. J., Bennett, S. E., Hamera, E. K., & Raines, B. K. (2004). What constitutes advanced assessment? *Journal of Nursing Education, 43*, 421–425.

REFERENCES
Smith, R. A., Cokkinides, V., & Eyre, H. J. (2006). American Cancer Society recommendations for the early detection of cancer, 2006. *CA: A Cancer Journal for Clinicians, 56,* 11–25.

SELECTED BIBLIOGRAPHY
Carter, K. F., Dufour, L. T., & Ballard, C. N. (2003). Wound & skin care. Identifying primary skin lesions. *Nursing, 33*(12), 68–69.
Carter, K. F., Dufour, L. T., & Ballard, C. N. (2004). Wound & skin care. Identifying secondary skin lesions. *Nursing, 34*(1), 68.
D'Amico, D., & Barbarito, C. (2007). *Health and physical assessment in nursing.* Upper Saddle River, NJ: Pearson Education.

Mehta, M. (2003). Assessing the abdomen. *Nursing, 33*(5), 54–55.
Mehta, M. (2003). Assessing respiratory status. *Nursing, 33*(2), 54–56.
Rushing, J. (2005). Clinical do's & don'ts. Assessing for ascites. *Nursing, 35*(2), 68.
Peacock, S. (2004). Systematic health assessment: A case study. *Practice Nursing, 15*(6), 270, 271–274.
Pullen, R. L. (2004). Clinical do's & don'ts. Neurologic assessment for pronator drift. *Nursing, 34*(3), 22.
Pullen, R. L. (2005). Clinical do's & don'ts. Testing the corneal reflex. *Nursing, 35*(11), 68.

UNIT
8

Integral Components of Client Care

Of all the components that are integral to caring for clients, safety is paramount. Concern for safety permeates every element of nursing practice. Nursing activities that promote safety include assessing risk, preventing infection, providing a safe environment, and preventing injury in hospital, outpatient, home, or community-based settings.

CHAPTER 31

Asepsis

LEARNING OUTCOMES

After completing this chapter, you will be able to:

1. Explain the concepts of medical and surgical asepsis.

2. Identify signs of localized and systemic infections.

3. Identify risks for nosocomial infections.

4. Identify factors influencing a microorganism's capability to produce an infectious process.

5. Identify anatomic and physiologic barriers that defend the body against microorganisms.

6. Differentiate active from passive immunity.

7. Identify relevant nursing diagnoses and contributing factors for clients at risk for infection and who have an infection.

8. Identify interventions to reduce risks for infections.

9. Identify measures that break each link in the chain of infection.

10. Compare and contrast category-specific, disease-specific, universal, body substance, standard, and transmission-based isolation precaution systems.

11. Correctly implement aseptic practices, including hand washing; donning and removing a facemask, gown, and disposable gloves; managing equipment used for isolation clients; and maintaining a sterile field.

12. Describe the steps to take in the event of a bloodborne pathogen exposure.

Nurses are directly involved in providing a biologically safe environment. Microorganisms exist everywhere: in water, in soil, and on body surfaces such as the skin, intestinal tract, and other areas open to the outside (e.g., mouth, upper respiratory tract, vagina, and lower urinary tract). Most microorganisms are harmless, and some are even beneficial in that they perform essential functions in the body. Some microorganisms found in the intestines (e.g., enterobacteria) produce substances called *bacteriocins*, which are lethal to related strains of bacteria. Others produce substances that repress the growth of other microorganisms. Some microorganisms are normal **resident flora** (the collective vegetation in a given area) in one part of the body, yet produce infection in another. For example, *Escherichia coli* is a normal inhabitant of the large intestine but a common cause of infection of the urinary tract. Table 31–1 provides a list of common resident microorganisms.

An **infection** is an invasion of body tissue by microorganisms and their growth there. Such a microorganism is called an *infectious agent*. If the microorganism produces no clinical evidence of disease, the infection is called *asymptomatic* or *subclinical*. Some subclinical infections can cause considerable damage, for example, cytomegalovirus (CMV) infection in a pregnant woman can lead to significant disease in the unborn child. A detectable alteration in normal tissue function, however, is called **disease.**

Microorganisms vary in their **virulence** (i.e., their ability to produce disease). Microorganisms also vary in the severity of

TABLE 31–1 Examples of Common Resident Microorganisms

BODY AREA	MICROORGANISMS
Skin	*Staphylococcus epidermidis* *Propionibacterium acnes* *Staphylococcus aureus* *Corynebacterium xerosis* *Pityrosporum oxale* (yeast)
Nasal passages	*Staphylococcus aureus* *Staphylococcus epidermidis*
Oropharynx	*Streptococcus pneumoniae*
Mouth	*Streptococcus mutans* *Lactobacillus* *Bacteroides* *Actinomyces*
Intestine	*Bacteroides* *Fusobacterium* *Eubacterium* *Lactobacillus* *Streptococcus* Enterobacteriaceae *Shigella* *Escherichia coli*
Urethral orifice	*Staphylococcus epidermidis*
Urethra (lower)	*Proteus*
Vagina	*Lactobacillus* *Bacteroides* *Clostridium* *Candida albicans*

the diseases they produce and their degree of communicability. For example, the common cold virus is more readily transmitted than the bacillus that causes leprosy (*Mycobacterium leprae*). If the infectious agent can be transmitted to an individual by direct or indirect contact or as an airborne infection, the resulting condition is called a **communicable disease.**

Pathogenicity is the ability to produce disease; thus a pathogen is a microorganism that causes disease. Many microorganisms that are normally harmless can cause disease under certain circumstances. A "true" pathogen causes disease or infection in a healthy individual. An **opportunistic pathogen** causes disease only in a susceptible individual.

Infectious diseases are a major cause of death worldwide. The control of the spread of microorganisms and the protection of people from communicable diseases and infections are carried out on the international, national, state, community, and individual level. The World Health Organization is the major regulatory agency at the international level. In the United States, the Centers for Disease Control and Prevention (CDC) is the principal public health agency at the national level concerned with disease prevention and control. At the state level, health departments track epidemics and illnesses as reports are made throughout that area.

Asepsis is the freedom from disease-causing microorganisms. To decrease the possibility of transferring microorganisms from one place to another, aseptic technique is used. There are two basic types of asepsis: medical and surgical. **Medical asepsis** includes all practices intended to confine a specific microorganism to a specific area, limiting the number, growth, and transmission of microorganisms. In medical asepsis, objects are referred to as **clean,** which means the absence of almost all microorganisms, or **dirty** (soiled, contaminated), which means likely to have microorganisms, some of which may be capable of causing infection.

Surgical asepsis, or **sterile technique,** refers to those practices that keep an area or object free of all microorganisms; it includes practices that destroy all microorganisms and spores (microscopic dormant structures formed by some pathogens that are very hardy and often survive common cleaning techniques). Surgical asepsis is used for all procedures involving the sterile areas of the body. **Sepsis** is the state of infection and can take many forms, including septic shock.

TYPES OF MICROORGANISMS CAUSING INFECTIONS

Four major categories of microorganisms cause infection in humans: bacteria, viruses, fungi, and parasites. **Bacteria** are by far the most common infection-causing microorganisms. Several hundred species can cause disease in humans and can live and be transported through air, water, food, soil, body tissues and fluids, and inanimate objects. Most of the microorganisms in Table 31–1 are bacteria. **Viruses** consist primarily of nucleic acid and therefore must enter living cells in order to reproduce. Common virus families include the rhinovirus (causes the common cold), hepatitis, herpes, and human immunodeficiency

virus. **Fungi** include yeasts and molds. *Candida albicans* is a yeast considered to be normal flora in the human vagina. **Parasites** live on other living organisms. They include protozoa such as the one that causes malaria, helminths (worms), and arthropods (mites, fleas, ticks).

TYPES OF INFECTIONS

Colonization is the process by which strains of microorganisms become resident flora. In this state, the microorganisms may grow and multiply but do not cause disease. Infection occurs when newly introduced or resident microorganisms succeed in invading a part of the body where the host's defense mechanisms are ineffective and the pathogen causes tissue damage. The infection becomes a disease when the signs and symptoms of the infection are unique and can be differentiated from other conditions.

Infections can be local or systemic. A **local infection** is limited to the specific part of the body where the microorganisms remain. If the microorganisms spread and damage different parts of the body, it is a **systemic infection.** When a culture of the person's blood reveals microorganisms, the condition is called **bacteremia.** When bacteremia results in systemic infection, it is referred to as **septicemia.** Unfortunately, these infections have become more common over time.

There are also **acute** or **chronic infections.** Acute infections generally appear suddenly or last a short time. A chronic infection may occur slowly, over a very long period, and may last months or years.

NOSOCOMIAL INFECTIONS

Nosocomial infections are classified as infections that are associated with the delivery of health care services in a health care facility. Nosocomial infections can either develop during a client's stay in a facility or manifest after discharge. Nosocomial microorganisms may also be acquired by health personnel working in the facility and can cause significant illness and time lost from work.

Nosocomial infections have received increasing attention in recent years and are believed to involve about 2 million clients per year. The Joint Commission on Accreditation of Healthcare Organizations included reducing the risk of health care associated infections as one of the 2006 National Patient Safety Goals. The most common settings where nosocomial infections develop are hospital surgical or medical intensive care units. Reports from the National Nosocomial Infection Surveillance (NNIS) System have revealed that the urinary tract, the respiratory tract, bloodstream, and wounds are the most common nosocomial infection sites (see the NNIS website). The microorganisms that cause nosocomial infections can originate from the clients themselves (an **endogenous** source) or from the hospital environment and hospital personnel (**exogenous** sources). Most nosocomial infections appear to have endogenous sources. *Escherichia coli, Staphylococcus aureus,* and enterococci are the most common infecting microorganisms.

A number of factors contribute to nosocomial infections. **Iatrogenic infections** are the direct result of diagnostic or therapeutic procedures. One example of an iatrogenic infection is bacteremia that results from an intravascular line. Not all nosocomial infections are iatrogenic, nor are all nosocomial infections preventable.

Another factor contributing to the development of nosocomial infections is the compromised host, that is, a client whose normal defenses have been lowered by surgery or illness.

The hands of personnel are a common vehicle for the spread of microorganisms. Insufficient hand cleansing is thus an important factor contributing to the spread of nosocomial microorganisms.

CLINICAL ALERT

A person does not need to have an identified infection in order to pass potentially infective microorganisms to another person. Even normal microorganisms for one person can infect another person. ■

The cost of nosocomial infections to the client, the facility, and funding sources (e.g., insurance companies and federal, state, or local governments) is great. Nosocomial infections extend hospitalization time, increase clients' time away from work, cause disability and discomfort, and even result in loss of life (see Table 31–2).

CHAIN OF INFECTION

Six links make up the chain of infection (Figure 31-1 ■): the etiologic agent, or microorganism; the place where the organism naturally resides (reservoir); a portal of exit from the reservoir; a method (mode) of transmission; a portal of entry into a host; and the susceptibility of the host.

Etiologic Agent

The extent to which any microorganism is capable of producing an infectious process depends on the number of microorganisms present, the virulence and potency of the microorganisms (pathogenicity), the ability of the microorganisms to enter the body, the susceptibility of the host, and the ability of the microorganisms to live in the host's body.

Some microorganisms, such as the smallpox virus, have the ability to infect almost all susceptible people after exposure. By contrast, microorganisms such as the tuberculosis bacillus infect a relatively small number of the population who are susceptible and exposed, usually people who are poorly nourished, who are living in crowded conditions, or whose immune systems are less competent (such as elders or those with HIV or cancer).

Reservoir

There are many **reservoirs,** or sources of microorganisms. Common sources are other humans, the client's own microorganisms, plants, animals, or the general environment. People are the

TABLE 31–2 **Nosocomial Infections**	
MOST COMMON MICROORGANISMS	**CAUSES**
Urinary Tract	
Escherichia coli	Improper catheterization technique
Enterococcus species	Contamination of closed drainage system
Pseudomonas aeruginosa	Inadequate hand cleansing
Surgical Sites	
Staphylococcus aureus (including methicillin-resistant strains—MRSA)	Inadequate hand cleansing
Enterococcus species (including vancomycin-resistant strains—VRE)	Improper dressing change technique
Pseudomonas aeruginosa	
Bloodstream	
Coagulase-negative staphylococci	Inadequate hand cleansing
Staphylococcus aureus	Improper intravenous fluid, tubing, and site care technique
Enterococcus species	
Pneumonia	
Staphylococcus aureus	Inadequate hand cleansing
Pseudomonas aeruginosa	Improper suctioning technique
Enterobacter species	

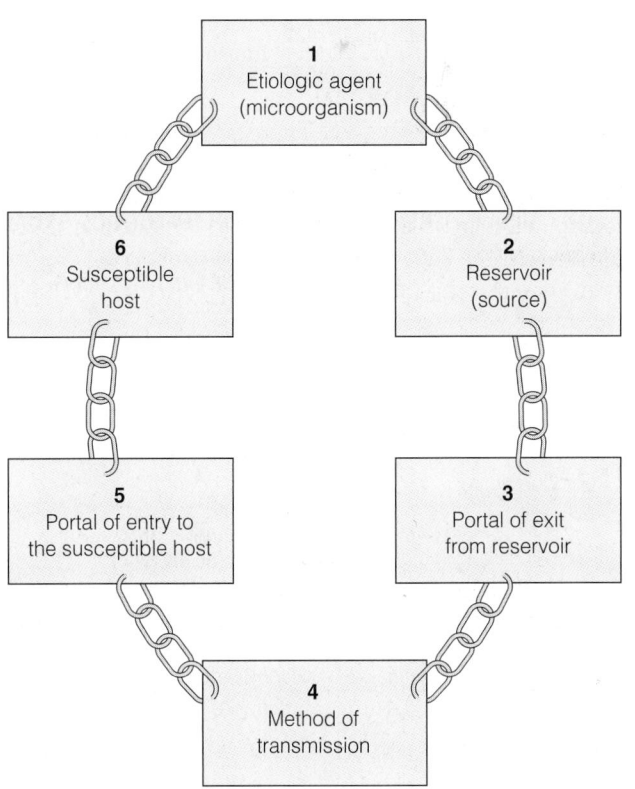

Figure 31-1 ■ The chain of infection.

most common source of infection for others and for themselves. For example, the person with an influenza virus frequently spreads it to others. A **carrier** is a person or animal reservoir of a specific infectious agent that usually does not manifest any clinical signs of disease. The *Anopheles* mosquito reservoir carries the malaria parasite but is unaffected by it. The carrier state may also exist in individuals with a clinically recognizable disease such as the dog with rabies. Under either circumstance, the carrier state may be of short duration (temporary or transient carrier) or long duration (chronic carrier). Food, water, and feces also can be reservoirs.

Portal of Exit from Reservoir

Before an infection can establish itself in a host, the microorganisms must leave the reservoir. Common human reservoirs and their associated portals of exit are summarized in Table 31–3.

Method of Transmission

After a microorganism leaves its source or reservoir, it requires a means of transmission to reach another person or host through a receptive portal of entry. There are three mechanisms:

1. *Direct transmission.* Direct transmission involves immediate and direct transfer of microorganisms from person to person through touching, biting, kissing, or sexual intercourse. Droplet spread is also a form of direct transmission but can occur only if the source and the host are within 3 feet of each other. Sneezing, coughing, spitting, singing, or talking can project droplet spray into the conjunctiva or onto the mucous membranes of the eye, nose, or mouth of another person.
2. *Indirect transmission.* Indirect transmission may be either vehicle-borne or vector-borne.
   a. **Vehicle-borne transmission.** A *vehicle* is any substance that serves as an intermediate means to transport and introduce an infectious agent into a susceptible host through a suitable portal of entry. Fomites (inanimate materials or objects), such as handkerchiefs, toys, soiled clothes, cooking or eating utensils, and surgical instruments or dressings, can act as vehicles. Water, food, blood, serum, and plasma are other vehicles. For example, food or water may become contaminated by a food handler who carries the hepatitis A virus. The food is then ingested by a susceptible host.
   b. **Vector-borne transmission.** A *vector* is an animal or flying or crawling insect that serves as an intermediate means of transporting the infectious agent. Transmission may occur by injecting salivary fluid during biting or by depositing feces or other materials on the skin through the bite wound or a traumatized skin area.
3. *Airborne transmission.* Airborne transmission may involve droplets or dust. **Droplet nuclei,** the residue of evaporated droplets emitted by an infected host such as someone with tuberculosis, can remain in the air for long periods. Dust particles containing the infectious agent (e.g., *Clostridium difficile,* commonly referred to as *C. difficile,* spores from the soil) can also become airborne. The material is transmitted by air currents to a suitable portal of entry, usually the respiratory tract, of another person.

Portal of Entry to the Susceptible Host

Before a person can become infected, microorganisms must enter the body. The skin is a barrier to infectious agents; however, any break in the skin can readily serve as a portal of entry. Often, microorganisms enter the body of the host by the same route they used to leave the source.

TABLE 31–3 Human Body Area Reservoirs, Common Infectious Microorganisms, and Portals of Exit

BODY AREA RESERVOIR	COMMON INFECTIOUS ORGANISMS	PORTALS OF EXIT
Respiratory tract	Parainfluenza virus *Mycobacterium tuberculosis* *Staphylococcus aureus*	Nose or mouth through sneezing, coughing, breathing, or talking
Gastrointestinal tract	Hepatitis A virus *Salmonella* species *Clostridium difficile*	Mouth: saliva, vomitus; anus: feces; ostomies Anus: feces, colostomies
Urinary tract	*Escherichia coli* enterococci *Pseudomonas aeruginosa*	Urethral meatus and urinary diversion
Reproductive tract	*Neisseria gonorrhoeae* *Treponema pallidum* Herpes simplex virus type 2 Hepatitis B virus (HBV)	Vagina: vaginal discharge; urinary meatus: semen, urine
Blood	Hepatitis B virus Human immunodeficiency virus (HIV) *Staphylococcus aureus* *Staphylococcus epidermidis*	Open wound, needle puncture site, any disruption of intact skin or mucous membrane surfaces
Tissue	*Staphylococcus aureus* *Escherichia coli* *Proteus* species *Streptococcus* beta-hemolytic A or B	Drainage from cut or wound

Susceptible Host

A susceptible host is any person who is at risk for infection. A **compromised host** is a person at increased risk, an individual who for one or more reasons is more likely than others to acquire an infection. Impairment of the body's natural defenses and a number of other factors can affect susceptibility to infection. Examples include age (the very young or the very old); clients receiving immune suppression treatment for cancer, for chronic illness, or following a successful organ transplant; and those with immune deficiency conditions.

BODY DEFENSES AGAINST INFECTION

Individuals normally have defenses that protect the body from infection. These defenses can be categorized as nonspecific and specific. **Nonspecific defenses** protect the person against all microorganisms, regardless of prior exposure. **Specific (immune) defenses,** by contrast, are directed against identifiable bacteria, viruses, fungi, or other infectious agents.

Nonspecific Defenses

Nonspecific body defenses include anatomic and physiologic barriers, and the inflammatory response.

Anatomic and Physiologic Barriers

Intact skin and mucous membranes are the body's first line of defense against microorganisms. Unless the skin and mucosa become cracked and broken, they are an effective barrier against bacteria. Fungi can live on the skin, but they cannot penetrate it. The dryness of the skin also is a deterrent to bacteria. Bacteria are most plentiful in moist areas of the body, such as the perineum and axillae. Resident bacteria of the skin also prevent other bacteria from multiplying. They use up the available nourishment, and the end products of their metabolism inhibit other bacterial growth. Normal secretions make the skin slightly acidic; acidity also inhibits bacterial growth.

The nasal passages have a defensive function. As entering air follows the tortuous route of the passage, it comes in contact with moist mucous membranes and cilia. These trap microorganisms, dust, and foreign materials. The lungs have alveolar macrophages (large phagocytes). Phagocytes are cells that ingest microorganisms, other cells, and foreign particles.

Each body orifice also has protective mechanisms. The oral cavity regularly sheds mucosal epithelium to rid the mouth of colonizers. The flow of saliva and its partially buffering action help prevent infections. Saliva contains microbial inhibitors, such as lactoferrin, lysozyme, and secretory IgA.

The eye is protected from infection by tears, which continually wash microorganisms away and contain inhibiting lysozyme. The gastrointestinal tract also has defenses against infection. The high acidity of the stomach normally prevents microbial growth. The resident flora of the large intestine help prevent the establishment of disease-producing microorganisms. Peristalsis also tends to move microbes out of the body.

The vagina also has natural defenses against infection. When a girl reaches puberty, lactobacilli ferment sugars in the vaginal secretions, creating a vaginal pH of 3.5 to 4.5. This low pH inhibits the growth of many disease-producing microorganisms. The entrance to the urethra normally harbors many microorganisms. These include *Staphylococcus epidermidis coagulase* (from the skin) and *Escherichia coli* (from feces). It is believed that the urine flow has a flushing and bacteriostatic action that keeps the bacteria from ascending the urethra. An intact mucosal surface also acts as a barrier.

Inflammatory Response

Inflammation is a local and nonspecific defensive response of the tissues to an injurious or infectious agent. It is an adaptive mechanism that destroys or dilutes the injurious agent, prevents further spread of the injury, and promotes the repair of damaged tissue. It is characterized by five signs: (a) pain, (b) swelling, (c) redness, (d) heat, and (e) impaired function of the part, if the injury is severe. Commonly, words with the suffix *-itis* describe an inflammatory process. For example, *appendicitis* means inflammation of the appendix; *gastritis* means inflammation of the stomach.

> ### CLINICAL ALERT
>
> An easy way to remember the signs of inflammation are the rhyming Latin words: *rubor* (redness), *tumor* (swelling), *color/calor* (heat), and *dolor* (pain). ■

Injurious agents can be categorized as physical agents, chemical agents, and microorganisms. *Physical agents* include mechanical objects causing trauma to tissues, excessive heat or cold, and radiation. *Chemical agents* include external irritants (e.g., strong acids, alkalis, poisons, and irritating gases) and internal irritants (substances manufactured within the body such as excessive hydrochloric acid in the stomach). *Microorganisms* include the broad groups of bacteria, viruses, fungi, and parasites.

A series of dynamic events is commonly referred to as the three stages of the inflammatory response:

First stage: Vascular and cellular responses
Second stage: Exudate production
Third stage: Reparative phase

VASCULAR AND CELLULAR RESPONSES. At the start of the first stage of inflammation, blood vessels at the site of injury constrict. This is rapidly followed by dilation of small blood vessels (occurring as a result of histamine released by the injured tissues). Thus, more blood flows to the injured area. This marked increase in blood supply is referred to as **hyperemia** and is responsible for the characteristic signs of redness and heat.

Vascular permeability increases at the site with dilation of the vessels in response to cell death, the release of chemical mediators (e.g., bradykinin, serotonin, and prostaglandin), and the release of histamine. Fluid, proteins, and **leukocytes** (white blood cells) leak into the interstitial spaces, and the signs of inflammation swelling (edema) and pain appear. Pain is caused by the pressure of accumulating fluid on nerve endings and the irritating chemical mediators. Fluid pouring into areas such as the pleural or pericardial cavity can seriously affect organ function. In other areas, such as joints, mobility is impaired.

Blood flow slows in the dilated vessels, allowing more leukocytes to arrive at the injured tissues. When the blood flow slows, leukocytes aggregate or line up along this inner surface of the blood vessels. This process is known as margination. Leukocytes then move through the blood vessel wall into the affected tissue spaces, a process called emigration.

In response to the exit of leukocytes from the blood, the bone marrow produces large numbers of leukocytes and releases them into the bloodstream. This is called **leukocytosis.** A normal leukocyte count of 4,500 to 11,000 per cubic millimeter of blood can rise to 20,000 or more when inflammation occurs.

EXUDATE PRODUCTION. In the second stage of inflammation, the inflammatory **exudate** is produced, consisting of fluid that escaped from the blood vessels, dead phagocytic cells, and dead tissue cells and products that they release. The plasma protein fibrinogen (which is converted to fibrin when it is released into the tissues), thromboplastin (released by injured tissue cells), and platelets together form an interlacing network to wall off the area, and prevent spread of the injurious agent. During this stage, the injurious agent is overcome, and the exudate is cleared away by lymphatic drainage.

The nature and amount of exudate vary according to the tissue involved and the intensity and duration of the inflammation. The major types of exudate are serous, purulent, and hemorrhagic (sanguineous). Descriptions of these exudates are provided in Chapter 36. ∞

REPARATIVE PHASE. The third stage of the inflammatory response involves the repair of injured tissues by regeneration or replacement with fibrous tissue (scar) formation. **Regeneration** is the replacement of destroyed tissue cells by cells that are identical or similar in structure and function. Damaged cells are replaced one by one but also cells are organized so that the architectural pattern and function of the tissue are restored. The ability to regenerate cells varies considerably from one type of tissue to another. For example, epithelial tissues of the skin and of the digestive and respiratory tracts have a good regenerative capacity, if their underlying support structures are intact. The same holds true for osseous, lymphoid, and bone marrow tissues. Tissues that have little regenerative capacity include nervous, muscular, and elastic tissues.

When regeneration is not possible, repair occurs by fibrous (scar) tissue formation. The inflammatory exudate with its interlacing network of fibrin provides the framework for this tissue to develop. Damaged tissues are replaced with the connective tissue elements of collagen, blood capillaries, lymphatics, and other tissue-bound substances. In the early stages of this process, the tissue is called **granulation tissue.** It is a fragile, gelatinous tissue, appearing pink or red because of the many newly formed capillaries. Later in the process, the tissue shrinks (the capillaries are constricted, even obliterated) and the collagen fibers contract, so that a firmer fibrous tissue remains. This is called cicatrix, or scar.

Specific Defenses

Specific defenses of the body involve the immune system. An **antigen** is a substance that induces a state of sensitivity or immune responsiveness (**immunity**). If the proteins originate in a person's own body, the antigen is called an **autoantigen.**

The immune response has two components: antibody-mediated defenses and cell-mediated defenses. These two systems provide distinct but overlapping protection.

Antibody-Mediated Defenses

Another name for the *antibody-mediated defenses* is **humoral** (or **circulating**) **immunity** because these defenses reside ultimately in the B lymphocytes and are mediated by antibodies produced by B cells. **Antibodies,** also called **immunoglobulins,** are part of the body's plasma proteins. The antibody-mediated responses defend primarily against the extracellular phases of bacterial and viral infections.

There are two major types of immunity: active and passive (see Table 31–4). In **active immunity,** the host produces antibodies in response to natural antigens (e.g., infectious microorganisms) or artificial antigens (e.g., vaccines). B cells are activated when they recognize the antigen. They then differentiate into plasma cells, which secrete the antibodies and serum proteins that bind specifically to the foreign substance and initiate a variety of elimination responses. The B cell may produce antibody molecules of five classes of immunoglobulins designated by letters and usually written as IgM, IgG, IgA, IgD, and IgE. The

TABLE 31–4	**Types of Immunity**		
TYPE	**ANTIGEN OR ANTIBODY SOURCE**		**DURATION**
1. Active	Antibodies are produced by the body in response to an antigen.		Long
a. Natural	Antibodies are formed in the presence of active infection in the body.		Lifelong
b. Artificial	Antigens (vaccines or toxoids) are administered to stimulate antibody production.		Many years; the immunity must be reinforced by booster
2. Passive	Antibodies are produced by another source, animal or human.		Short
a. Natural	Antibodies are transferred naturally from an immune mother to her baby through the placenta or in colostrum.		6 months to 1 year
b. Artificial	Immune serum (antibody) from an animal or another human is injected.		2 to 3 weeks

presence of IgM in a laboratory analysis shows current infection. Before the antibody response can become effective, the phagocytic cells of the blood bind and ingest foreign substances. The rate of binding and phagocytosis increases if IgG antibodies (which indicate past infection and subsequent immunity) are present. With **passive** (or **acquired**) **immunity,** the host receives natural (e.g., from a nursing mother) or artificial (e.g., from an injection of immune serum) antibodies produced by another source.

Cell-Mediated Defenses

The **cell-mediated defenses,** or **cellular immunity,** occur through the T-cell system. On exposure to an antigen, the lymphoid tissues release large numbers of activated T cells into the lymph system. These T cells pass into the general circulation. There are three main groups of T cells: (a) helper T cells, which help in the functions of the immune system; (b) cytotoxic T cells, which attack and kill microorganisms and sometimes the body's own cells; and (c) suppressor T cells, which can suppress the functions of the helper T cells and the cytotoxic T cells. When cell-mediated immunity is lost, as occurs with human immunodeficiency virus (HIV) infection, an individual is "defenseless" against most viral, bacterial, and fungal infections.

FACTORS INCREASING SUSCEPTIBILITY TO INFECTION

Whether a microorganism causes an infection depends on a number of factors already mentioned. One of the most important factors is host susceptibility, which is affected by age, heredity, level of stress, nutritional status, current medical therapy, and preexisting disease processes.

Age influences the risk of infection. Newborns and older adults have reduced defenses against infection. Infections are a major cause of death of newborns, who have immature immune systems and are protected only for the first 2 or 3 months by immunoglobulins passively received from the mother. Between 1 and 3 months of age, infants begin to synthesize their own immunoglobulins. Immunizations against diphtheria, tetanus, and pertussis are usually started at 2 months, when the infant's immune system can respond (see Table 31–5, page 676).

With advancing age, the immune responses again become weak. Although there is still much to learn about aging, it is known that immunity to infection decreases with advancing age. Because of the prevalence of influenza and its potential for causing death, the CDC recommends annual immunization against influenza for older adults and for persons with chronic cardiac, respiratory, metabolic, and renal disease. Pneumococcal vaccine is recommended for elders last vaccinated more than 5 years previously (see Table 31–6, page 677).

Heredity influences the development of infection in that some people have a genetic susceptibility to certain infections. For example, some may be deficient in serum immunoglobulins, which play a significant role in the internal defense mechanism of the body.

The nature, number, and duration of physical and emotional stressors can influence susceptibility to infection. Stressors elevate blood cortisone. Prolonged elevation of blood cortisone decreases anti-inflammatory responses, depletes energy stores, leads to a state of exhaustion, and decreases resistance to infection. For example, a person recovering from a major operation or injury is more likely to develop an infection than a healthy person.

Resistance to infection depends on adequate nutritional status. Because antibodies are proteins, the ability to synthesize antibodies may be impaired by inadequate nutrition, especially when protein reserves are depleted (e.g., as a result of injury, surgery, or debilitating diseases such as cancer).

Some medical therapies predispose a person to infection. For example, radiation treatments for cancer destroy not only cancerous cells but also some normal cells, thereby rendering them more vulnerable to infection. Some diagnostic procedures may also predispose the client to an infection, especially when the skin is broken or sterile body cavities are penetrated during the procedure.

Certain medications also increase susceptibility to infection. Antineoplastic (anticancer) medications may depress bone marrow function, resulting in inadequate production of white blood cells necessary to combat infections. Anti-inflammatory medications, such as adrenal corticosteroids, inhibit the inflammatory response, an essential defense against infection. Even some antibiotics used to treat infections can have adverse effects. Antibiotics may kill resident flora, allowing the proliferation of strains that would not grow and multiply in the body under normal conditions. An important example of this is *C. difficile*-associated disease, an infection of the colon almost always caused initially by treatment with an antibiotic for another infection (Sunenshine & McDonald, 2006).

Certain antibiotics can also induce resistance in some strains of organisms. This resistance has become so widespread that the CDC has created a 12-step Campaign to Prevent Antimicrobial Resistance in Healthcare Settings consisting of four strategies: preventing infection, diagnosing and treating infection effectively, using antimicrobials wisely, and preventing transmission.

Any disease that lessens the body's defenses against infection places the client at risk. Examples are chronic pulmonary disease, which impairs ciliary action and weakens the mucous barrier; peripheral vascular disease, which restricts blood flow; burns, which impair skin integrity; chronic or debilitating diseases, which deplete protein reserves; and such immune system diseases as leukemia and aplastic anemia, which alter the production of white blood cells. Diabetes mellitus is a major underlying disease predisposing clients to infection because compromised peripheral vascular status and increased serum glucose levels increase susceptibility.

CLINICAL ALERT

Some common medications such as aspirin and ibuprofen are analgesic (pain relieving), antipyretic (fever reducing), and anti-inflammatory. Acetaminophen, however, is analgesic and antipyretic, but not anti-inflammatory. ■

TABLE 31–5 Recommended Childhood and Adolescent Immunization Schedule—United States, 2006

Vaccine ▼ / Age ▶	Birth	1 month	2 months	4 months	6 months	12 months	15 months	18 months	24 months	4–6 years	11–12 years	13–14 years	15 years	16–18 years
Hepatitis B[1]	HepB	HepB		HepB[1]		HepB					HepB Series			
Diphtheria, Tetanus, Pertussis[2]			DTaP	DTaP	DTaP		DTaP			DTaP	Tdap		Tdap	
Haemophilus influenzae type b[3]			Hib	Hib	Hib[3]	Hib								
Inactivated Poliovirus			IPV	IPV		IPV				IPV				
Measles, Mumps Rubella[4]						MMR				MMR		MMR		
Varicella[5]						Varicella					Varicella			
Meningococcal[6]									Vaccines within broken line are for selected populations	MPSV4	MCV4		MCV4 / MCV4	
Pneumococcal[7]			PCV	PCV	PCV	PCV				PCV	PPV			
Influenza[8]					Influenza (Yearly)						Influenza (Yearly)			
Hepatitis A[9]									HepA Series					

Legend: Range of recommended ages | Catch-up immunization | 11–12 year old assessment

This schedule indicates the recommended ages for routine administration of currently licensed childhood vaccines, as of December 1, 2005, for children through age 18 years. Any dose not administered at the recommended age should be administered at any subsequent visit when indicated and feasible. ▓ Indicates age groups that warrant special effort to administer those vaccines not previously administered. Additional vaccines may be licensed and recommended during the year. Licensed combination vaccines may be used whenever any components of the combination are indicated and other components of the vaccine are not contraindicated and if approved by the Food and Drug Administration for that dose of the series. Providers should consult the respective ACIP statement for detailed recommendations. Clinically significant adverse events that follow immunization should be reported to the Vaccine Adverse Event Reporting System (VAERS). Guidance about how to obtain and complete a VAERS form is available at www.vaers.hhs.gov or by telephone, 800-822-7967.

1. **Hepatitis B vaccine (HepB). AT BIRTH: All newborns** should receive monovalent HepB soon after birth and before hospital discharge. **Infants born to mothers who are HBsAg-positive** should receive HepB and 0.5 mL of hepatitis B immune globulin (HBIG) within 12 hours of birth. **Infants born to mothers whose HBsAg status is unknown** should receive HepB within 12 hours of birth. The mother should have blood drawn as soon as possible to determine her HBsAg status; if HBsAg-positive, the infant should receive HBIG as soon as possible (no later than age 1 week). **For infants born to HBsAg-negative mothers,** the birth dose can be delayed in rare circumstances but only if a physician's order to withhold the vaccine and a copy of the mother's original HBsAg-negative laboratory report are documented in the infant's medical record. **FOLLOWING THE BIRTHDOSE:** The HepB series should be completed with either monovalent HepB or a combination vaccine containing HepB. The second dose should be administered at age 1–2 months. The final dose should be administered at age ≥24 weeks. It is permissible to administer 4 doses of HepB (e.g., when combination vaccines are given after the birth dose); however, if monovalent HepB is used, a dose at age 4 months is not needed. **Infants born to HBsAg-positive mothers** should be tested for HBsAg and antibody to HBsAg after completion of the HepB series, at age 9–18 months (generally at the next well-child visit after completion of the vaccine series).

2. **Diphtheria and tetanus toxoids and acellular pertussis vaccine (DTaP).** The fourth dose of DTaP may be administered as early as age 12 months, provided 6 months have elapsed since the third dose and the child is unlikely to return at age 15–18 months. The final dose in the series should be given at age ≥4 years.
Tetanus and diphtheria toxoids and acellular pertussis vaccine (Tdap – adolescent preparation) is recommended at age 11–12 years for those who have completed the recommended childhood DTP/DTaP vaccination series and have not received a Td booster dose. Adolescents 13–18 years who missed the 11–12-year Td/Tdap booster dose should also receive a single dose of Tdap if they have completed the recommended childhood DTP/DTaP vaccination series. Subsequent **tetanus and diphtheria toxoids (Td)** are recommended every 10 years.

3. **Haemophilus influenzae type b conjugate vaccine (Hib).** Three Hib conjugate vaccines are licensed for infant use. If PRP-OMP (PedvaxHIB® or ComVax® [Merck]) is administered at ages 2 and 4 months, a dose at age 6 months is not required. DTaP/Hib combination products should not be used for primary immunization in infants at ages 2, 4 or 6 months but can be used as boosters after any Hib vaccine. The final dose in the series should be administered at age ≥12 months.

4. **Measles, mumps, and rubella vaccine (MMR).** The second dose of MMR is recommended routinely at age 4–6 years but may be administered during any visit, provided at least 4 weeks have elapsed since the first dose and both doses are administered beginning at or after age 12 months. Those who have not previously received the second dose should complete the schedule by age 11–12 years.

5. **Varicella vaccine.** Varicella vaccine is recommended at any visit at or after age 12 months for susceptible children (i.e., those who lack a reliable history of chickenpox). Susceptible persons aged ≥13 years should receive 2 doses administered at least 4 weeks apart.

6. **Meningococcal vaccine (MCV4).** Meningococcal conjugate vaccine (MCV4) should be given to all children at the 11–12 year old visit as well as to unvaccinated adolescents at high school entry (15 years of age). Other adolescents who wish to decrease their risk for meningococcal disease may also be vaccinated. All college freshmen living in dormitories should also be vaccinated, preferably with MCV4, although **meningococcal polysaccharide vaccine (MPSV4)** is an acceptable alternative. Vaccination against invasive meningococcal disease is recommended for children and adolescents aged ≥2 years with terminal complement deficiencies or anatomic or functional asplenia and certain other high risk groups (see *MMWR* 2005;54 [RR-7]:1-21); use MPSV4 for children aged 2–10 years and MCV4 for older children, although MPSV4 is an acceptable alternative.

7. **Pneumococcal vaccine.** The heptavalent **pneumococcal conjugate vaccine (PCV)** is recommended for all children aged 2–23 months and for certain children aged 24–59 months. The final dose in the series should be given at age ≥12 months. **Pneumococcal polysaccharide vaccine (PPV)** is recommended in addition to PCV for certain high-risk groups. See *MMWR* 2000; 49(RR-9):1-35.

8. **Influenza vaccine.** Influenza vaccine is recommended annually for children aged ≥6 months with certain risk factors (including, but not limited to, asthma, cardiac disease, sickle cell disease, human immunodeficiency virus [HIV], diabetes, and conditions that can compromise respiratory function or handling of respiratory secretions or that can increase the risk for aspiration), healthcare workers, and other persons (including household members) in close contact with persons in groups at high risk (see *MMWR* 2005;54[RR-8]:1-55). In addition, healthy children aged 6–23 months and close contacts of healthy children aged 0–5 months are recommended to receive influenza vaccine because children in this age group are at substantially increased risk for influenza-related hospitalizations. For healthy persons aged 5–49 years, the intranasally administered, live, attenuated influenza vaccine (LAIV) is an acceptable alternative to the intramuscular trivalent inactivated influenza vaccine (TIV). See *MMWR* 2005;54(RR-8):1-55. Children receiving TIV should be administered a dosage appropriate for their age (0.25 mL if aged 6–35 months or 0.5 mL if aged ≥3 years). Children aged ≤8 years who are receiving influenza vaccine for the first time should receive 2 doses (separated by at least 4 weeks for TIV and at least 6 weeks for LAIV).

9. **Hepatitis A vaccine (HepA).** HepA is recommended for all children at 1 year of age (i.e.,12–23 months). The 2 doses in the series should be administered at least 6 months apart. States, counties, and communities with existing HepA vaccination programs for children 2–18 years of age are encouraged to maintain these programs. In these areas, new efforts focused on routine vaccination of 1-year-old children should enhance, not replace, ongoing programs directed at a broader population of children. HepA is also recommended for certain high risk groups (see *MMWR* 1999; 48[RR-12]1-37).

TABLE 31–6 Recommended Adult Immunization Schedule—United States, 2006

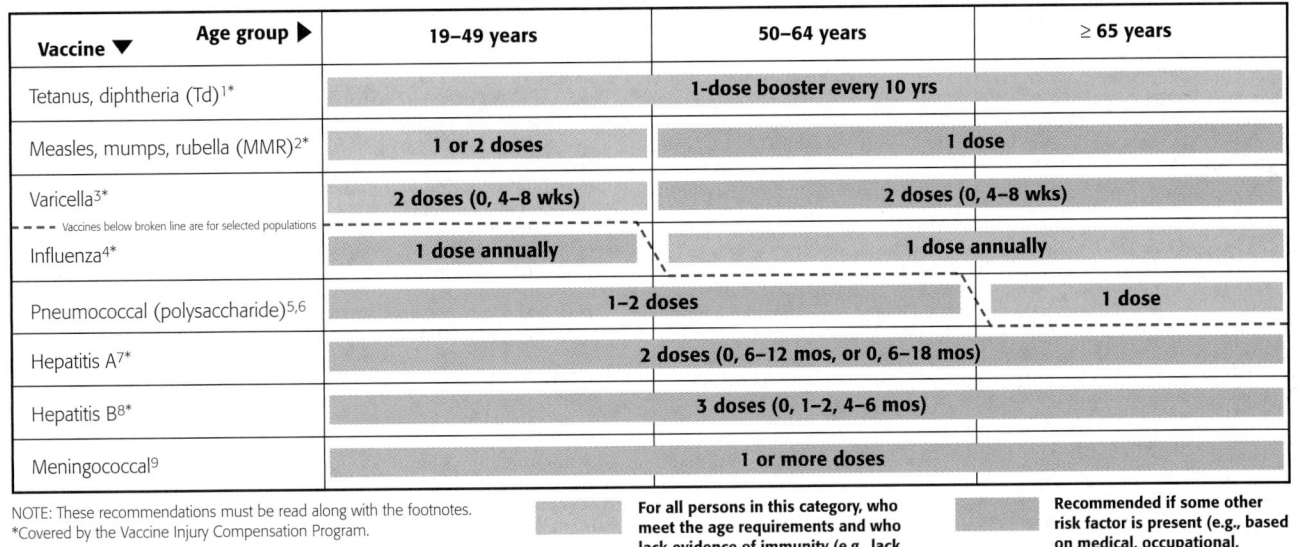

Vaccine ▼ / Age group ▶	19–49 years	50–64 years	≥ 65 years
Tetanus, diphtheria (Td)[1*]	1-dose booster every 10 yrs		
Measles, mumps, rubella (MMR)[2*]	1 or 2 doses	1 dose	
Varicella[3*]	2 doses (0, 4–8 wks)	2 doses (0, 4–8 wks)	
Influenza[4*]	1 dose annually	1 dose annually	
Pneumococcal (polysaccharide)[5,6]	1–2 doses		1 dose
Hepatitis A[7*]	2 doses (0, 6–12 mos, or 0, 6–18 mos)		
Hepatitis B[8*]	3 doses (0, 1–2, 4–6 mos)		
Meningococcal[9]	1 or more doses		

Vaccines below broken line are for selected populations

NOTE: These recommendations must be read along with the footnotes.
*Covered by the Vaccine Injury Compensation Program.

For all persons in this category, who meet the age requirements and who lack evidence of immunity (e.g., lack documentation of vaccination or have no evidence of prior infection)

Recommended if some other risk factor is present (e.g., based on medical, occupational, lifestyle, or other indications)

This schedule indicates the recommended age groups and medical indications for routine administration of currently licensed vaccines for persons aged ≥19 years. Licensed combination vaccines may be used whenever any components of the combination are indicated and when the vaccine's other components are not contraindicated. For detailed recommendations, consult the manufacturers' package inserts and the complete statements from the ACIP (www.cdc.gov/nip/publications/acip-list.htm).

Report all clinically significant postvaccination reactions to the Vaccine Adverse Event Reporting System (VAERS). Reporting forms and instructions on filing a VAERS report are available by telephone, 800-822-7967, or from the VAERS website at www.vaers.hhs.gov.

Information on how to file a Vaccine Injury Compensation Program claim is available at www.hrsa.gov/osp/vcip or by telephone, 800-338-2382. To file a claim for vaccine injury, contact the U.S. Court of Federal Claims, 717 Madison Place, N.W., Washington D.C. 20005, telephone 202-357-6400.

Additional information about the vaccines listed above and contraindications for vaccination is also available at www.cdc.gov/nip or from the CDC-INFO Contact Center at 800-CDC-INFO (232-4636) in English and Spanish, 24 hours a day, 7 days a week.

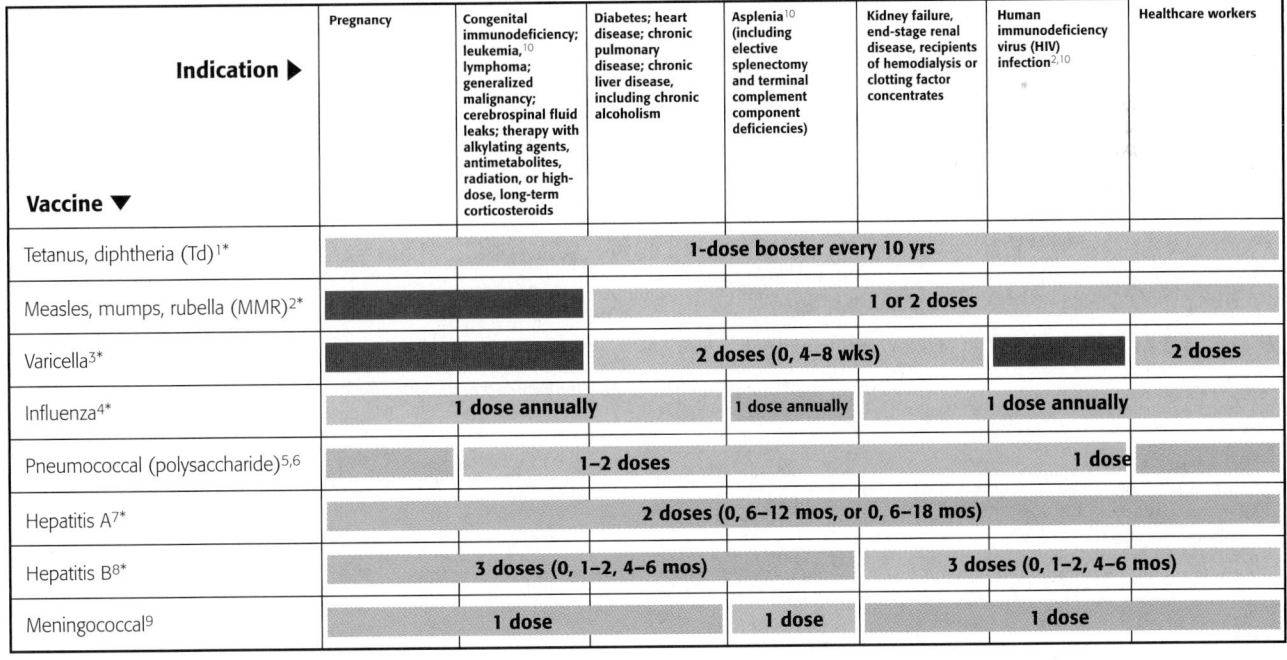

Vaccine ▼ / Indication ▶	Pregnancy	Congenital immunodeficiency; leukemia,[10] lymphoma; generalized malignancy; cerebrospinal fluid leaks; therapy with alkylating agents, antimetabolites, radiation, or high-dose, long-term corticosteroids	Diabetes; heart disease; chronic pulmonary disease; chronic liver disease, including chronic alcoholism	Asplenia[10] (including elective splenectomy and terminal complement component deficiencies)	Kidney failure, end-stage renal disease, recipients of hemodialysis or clotting factor concentrates	Human immunodeficiency virus (HIV) infection[2,10]	Healthcare workers
Tetanus, diphtheria (Td)[1*]	1-dose booster every 10 yrs						
Measles, mumps, rubella (MMR)[2*]	Contraindicated	1 or 2 doses					
Varicella[3*]	Contraindicated	2 doses (0, 4–8 wks)				Contraindicated	2 doses
Influenza[4*]	1 dose annually		1 dose annually		1 dose annually		
Pneumococcal (polysaccharide)[5,6]		1–2 doses				1 dose	
Hepatitis A[7*]	2 doses (0, 6–12 mos, or 0, 6–18 mos)						
Hepatitis B[8*]	3 doses (0, 1–2, 4–6 mos)			3 doses (0, 1–2, 4–6 mos)			
Meningococcal[9]	1 dose		1 dose		1 dose		

NOTE: These recommendations must be read along with the footnotes.
*Covered by the Vaccine Injury Compensation Program.

For all persons in this category, who meet the age requirements and who lack evidence of immunity (e.g., lack documentation of vaccination or have no evidence of prior infection)

Recommended if some other risk factor is present (e.g., based on medical, occupational, lifestyle, or other indications)

Contraindicated

Approved by the Advisory Committee on Immunization Practices (ACIP)
the American College of Obstetricians and Gynecologists (ACOG), and the American Academy of Family Physicians (AAFP)

(continued)

TABLE 31–6 Recommended Adult Immunization Schedule—United States, 2006—continued

Footnotes
Recommended Adult Immunization Schedule, UNITED STATES, OCTOBER 2005–SEPTEMBER 2006

1. **Tetanus and Diphtheria (Td) vaccination.** Adults with uncertain histories of a complete primary vaccination series with diphtheria and tetanus toxoid-containing vaccines should receive a primary series using combined Td toxoid. A primary series for adults is 3 doses; administer the first 2 doses at least 4 weeks apart and the third dose 6–12 months after the second. Administer 1 dose if the person received the primary series and if the last vaccination was received ≥10 years previously. Consult ACIP statement for recommendations for administering Td as prophylaxis in wound management (www.cdc.gov/mmwr/preview/mmwrhtml/00041645.htm). The American College of Physicians Task Force on Adult Immunization supports a second option for Td use in adults: a single Td booster at age 50 years for persons who have completed the full pediatric series, including the teenage/young adult booster. A newly licensed tetanus-diphtheria-acellular pertussis vaccine is available for adults. ACIP recommendations for its use will be published.

2. **Measles, Mumps, Rubella (MMR) vaccination.** *Measles component:* adults born before 1957 can be considered immune to measles. Adults born during or after 1957 should receive ≥1 dose of MMR unless they have a medical contraindication, documentation of ≥1 dose, history of measles based on healthcare provider diagnosis, or laboratory evidence of immunity. A second dose of MMR is recommended for adults who 1) were recently exposed to measles or in an outbreak setting, 2) were previously vaccinated with killed measles vaccine, 3) were vaccinated with an unknown type of measles vaccine during 1963–1967, 4) are students in postsecondary educational institutions, 5) work in a healthcare facility, or 6) plan to travel internationally. Withhold MMR or other measles-containing vaccines from HIV-infected persons with severe immunosuppression. *Mumps component:* 1 dose of MMR vaccine should be adequate for protection for those born during or after 1957 who lack a history of mumps based on healthcare provider diagnosis or who lack laboratory evidence of immunity. *Rubella component:* administer 1 dose of MMR vaccine to women whose rubella vaccination history is unreliable or who lack laboratory evidence of immunity. For women of childbearing age, regardless of birth year, routinely determine rubella immunity and counsel women regarding congenital rubella syndrome. Do not vaccinate women who are pregnant or might become pregnant within 4 weeks of receiving the vaccine. Women who do not have evidence of immunity should receive MMR vaccine upon completion or termination of pregnancy and before discharge from the healthcare facility.

3. **Varicella vaccination.** Varicella vaccination is recommended for all adults without evidence of immunity to varicella. Special consideration should be given to those who 1) have close contact with persons at high risk for severe disease (healthcare workers and family contacts of immunocompromised persons) or 2) are at high risk for exposure or transmission (e.g., teachers of young children; child care employees; residents and staff members of institutional settings, including correctional institutions; college students; military personnel; adolescents and adults living in households with children; nonpregnant women of childbearing age; and international travelers). Evidence of immunity to varicella in adults includes any of the following: 1) documented age-appropriate varicella vaccination (i.e., receipt of 1 dose before age 13 years or receipt of 2 doses [administered at least 4 weeks apart] after age 13 years); 2) born in the United States before 1966; 3) history of varicella disease based on healthcare provider diagnosis or self- or parental report of typical varicella disease for non-U.S.-born persons born before 1966 and all persons born during 1966–1997 (for a patient reporting a history of an atypical, mild case, healthcare providers should seek either an epidemiologic link with a typical varicella case or evidence of laboratory confirmation, if it was performed at the time of acute disease); 4) history of herpes zoster based on healthcare provider diagnosis; or 5) laboratory evidence of immunity. Do not vaccinate women who are pregnant or might become pregnant within 4 weeks of receiving the vaccine. Assess pregnant women for evidence of varicella immunity. Women who do not have evidence of immunity should receive dose 1 of varicella vaccine upon completion or termination of pregnancy and before discharge from the healthcare facility. Dose 2 should be given 4–8 weeks after dose 1.

4. **Influenza vaccination.** *Medical indications:* chronic disorders of the cardiovascular or pulmonary systems, including asthma; chronic metabolic diseases, including diabetes mellitus, renal dysfunction, hemoglobinopathies, or immunosuppression (including immunosuppression caused by medications or by HIV); any condition (e.g., cognitive dysfunction, spinal cord injury, seizure disorder or other neuromuscular disorder) that compromises respiratory function or the handling of respiratory secretions or that can increase the risk of aspiration; and pregnancy during the influenza season. No data exist on the risk for severe or complicated influenza disease among persons with asplenia; however, influenza is a risk factor for secondary bacterial infections that can cause severe disease among persons with asplenia. *Occupational indications:* healthcare workers and employees of long-term care and assisted living facilities. *Other indications:* residents of nursing homes and other long-term care and assisted living facilities; persons likely to transmit influenza to persons

at high risk (i.e., in-home household contacts and caregivers of children birth through 23 months of age, or persons of all ages with high-risk conditions); and anyone who wishes to be vaccinated.

For healthy nonpregnant persons aged 5–49 years without high-risk conditions who are not contacts of severely immunocompromised persons in special care units, intranasally administered influenza vaccine (FluMist®) may be administered in lieu of inactivated vaccine.

5. **Pneumococcal polysaccharide vaccination.** *Medical indications:* chronic disorders of the pulmonary system (excluding asthma); cardiovascular diseases; diabetes mellitus; chronic liver diseases, including liver disease as a result of alcohol abuse (e.g., cirrhosis); chronic renal failure or neuphrotic syndrome; functional or anatomic asplenia (e.g., sickle cell disease or splenectomy [if elective splenectomy is planned, vaccinate at least 2 weeks before surgery]); immunosuppressive conditions (e.g., congenital immunodeficiency, HIV infection [vaccinate as close to diagnosis as possible when CD4 cell counts are highest], leukemia, lymphoma, multiple myeloma, Hodgkin disease, generalized malignancy, organ or bone marrow transplantation); chemotherapy with alkylating agents, antimetabolites, or high-dose, long-term corticosteroids; and cochlear implants. *Other indications:* Alaska Natives and certain American Indian populations; residents of nursing homes and other long-term care facilities.

6. **Revaccination with pneumococcal polysaccharide vaccine.** One-time revaccination after 5 years for persons with chronic renal failure or nephrotic syndrome; functional or anatomic asplenia (e.g., sickle cell disease or splenectomy); immunosuppressive conditions (e.g., congenital immunodeficiency, HIV infection, leukemia, lymphoma, multiple myeloma, Hodgkin disease, generalized malignancy, organ or bone marrow transplanation); or chemotherapy with alkylating agents, antimetabolites, or high-dose, long-term corticosteroids. For persons aged ≥65 years, one-time revaccination if they were vaccinated ≥5 years previously and were aged, <65 years at the time of primary vaccination.

7. **Hepatitis A vaccination.** *Medical indications:* persons with clotting factor disorders or chronic liver disease. *Behavioral indications:* men who have sex with men or users of illegal drugs. *Occupational indications:* persons working with hepatitis A virus (HAV)-infected primates or with HAV in a research laboratory setting. *Other indications:* persons traveling to or working in countries that have high or intermediate endemicity of hepatitis A (for list of countries, visit ww.cdc.gov/travel/diseases.htm#hepa) as well as any person wishing to obtain immunity. Current vaccines should be given in a 2-dose series at either 0 and 6–18 months, if the combined hepatitis A and hepatitis B vaccine is used, administer 3 doses at 0, 1, and 6 months.

8. **Hepatitis B vaccination.** *Medical indications:* hemodialysis patients (use special formulation [40 μg/mL] or two 20-μg/mL doses) or patients who receive clotting factor concentrates. *Occupational indications:* healthcare workers and public-safety workers who have exposure to blood in the workplace; and persons in training in schools of medicine, dentistry, nursing, laboratory technology, and other allied health professions. *Behavioral indications:* injection-drug users; persons with more than one sex partner in the previous 6 months; persons with a recently acquired sexually transmitted diseases (STD); and men who have sex with men. *Other indications:* household contacts and sex partners of persons with chronic hepatitis B virus (HBV) infection; clients and staff of institutions for the developmentally disabled; all clients of STD clinics; inmates of correctional facilities; or international travelers who will be in countries with high or intermediate prevalence of chronic HBV infection for >6 months (for list of countries, visit www.cdc.gov/travel/diseases.htm#hepa).

9. **Meningococcal vaccination.** *Medical indications:* adults with anatomic or functional asplenia, or terminal complement component deficiencies. *Other indications:* first-year college students living in dormitories; microbiologists who are routinely exposed to isolates of *Neisseria meningitidis;* military recruits; and persons who travel to or reside in countries in which meningococcal disease is hyperendemic or epidemic (e.g., the "meningitis belt" of sub-Saharan Africa during the dry season [Dec–June]), particularly if contact with the local populations will be prolonged. Vaccination is required by the government of Saudi Arabia for all travelers to Mecca during the annual Hajj. Meningococcal conjugate vaccine is preferred for adults meeting any of the above indications who are aged ≤55 years, although meningococcal polysaccharide vaccine (MPSV4) is an acceptable alternative. Revaccination after 5 years may be indicated for adults previously vaccinated with MPSV4 who remain at high risk for infection (e.g., persons residing in areas in which disease is epidemic).

10. **Selected conditions for which *Haemophilus influenzae* type b (Hib) vaccine may be used.** *Haemophilus influenzae* type b conjugate vaccines are licensed for children aged 6 weeks–71 months. No efficacy data are available on which to base a recommendation concerning use of Hib vaccine for older children and adults with the chronic conditions associated with an increased risk for Hib disease. However, studies suggest good immunogenicity in patients who have sickle cell disease, leukemia, or HIV infection, or have had splenectomies; administering vaccine to these patients is not contraindicated.

LIFESPAN CONSIDERATIONS Infections

CHILDREN

Infections are an expected part of childhood, with most children experiencing some kind of infection from time to time. The majority of these infections are caused by viruses, and for the most part are transient, relatively benign, and able to be overcome by the body's natural defenses and supportive care. In some cases, severe, even life-threatening infections occur. Considerations related to children include the following:

- Newborns may not be able to respond to infections due to an underdeveloped immune system. As a result, in the first few months of life, infections may not be associated with typical signs and symptoms (e.g., an infant with an infection may not have a fever).
- Newborns are born with some naturally acquired immunity transferred from the mother across the placenta.
- Breast-fed infants enjoy higher levels of immunity against infections than formula-fed infants.
- Fevers less than 39°C (102.2°F) in children should not be treated, except for comfort of the child.
- Children between 6 months and 5 years are at higher risk for fever-induced (febrile) seizures. Febrile seizures are not associated with neurological seizure disorders (e.g., epilepsy).
- Children who are immune-compromised (e.g., leukemia, HIV) or have a chronic health condition (e.g., cystic fibrosis, sickle cell disease, congenital heart disease) need extra precautions to prevent exposure to infectious agents.
- Hand hygiene, comprehensive immunizations, good nutrition, adequate hydration, and appropriate rest are essential to preventing and/or treating infections in children.
- Hand washing and good hygiene in day care and schools are important to prevent the spread of infections.
- Adolescents are at high risk for sexually transmitted diseases and should be well educated about how to prevent infections.

ELDERS

Normal aging may predispose elders to increased risk of infection and delayed healing. Anatomical and physiological agents that are protective when a person is younger often change in structure and function with increasing age and then provide a decrease in their protective ability. Changes take place in the skin, respiratory tract, gastrointestinal system, kidneys, and immune system. If unchallenged, these systems work well to maintain homeostasis for the individual, but if compromised by stress, illness, infections, treatments, or surgeries, they find it difficult to keep up and therefore are not able to provide adequate protection. Special considerations for elders include the following:

- Nutrition is often poor in older adults. Certain components, especially adequate protein, are necessary to build up and maintain the immune system.
- Diabetes mellitus, which occurs more frequently in elders, increases the risk of infection and delayed healing by causing an alteration in nutrition and impaired peripheral circulation, which decrease the oxygen transport to the tissues.
- The immune system reacts slowly to the introduction of antigens, allowing the antigen to reproduce itself several times before it is recognized by the immune system. T-cell effectiveness is often decreased due to immaturity.
- The normal inflammatory response is delayed. This often causes atypical responses to infections with unusual presentations. Instead of displaying redness, swelling, and fever usually associated with infections, atypical symptoms such as confusion and disorientation, agitation, incontinence, falls, lethargy, and general fatigue are often seen first.

Recognizing these changes in elders is important in early detection and treatment of related potential for infections and delayed healing. Nursing interventions to promote prevention include the following:

- Provide and teach ways to improve nutritional status.
- Use strict aseptic technique to decrease chance of infections (especially nosocomial infections in health care facilities).
- Encourage elders to have regular immunizations for flu and pneumonia.
- Be alert to subtle atypical signs of infection and act quickly to diagnose and treat.

NURSING MANAGEMENT

Assessing

During the assessing phase of the nursing process, the nurse obtains the client's history, conducts the physical assessment, and gathers laboratory data.

Nursing History

During the nursing history, the nurse assesses (a) the degree to which a client is at risk of developing an infection and (b) any client complaints suggesting the presence of an infection. To identify clients at risk, the nurse reviews the client's chart and structures the nursing interview to collect data regarding the factors influencing the development of infection, especially existing disease process, history of recurrent infections, current medications and therapeutic measures, current emotional stressors, nutritional status, and history of immunizations (see the Assessment Interview).

Physical Assessment

Signs and symptoms of an infection vary according to the body area involved. For example, sneezing, watery or mucoid discharge from the nose, and nasal stuffiness commonly occur with an infection of the nose and sinuses; urinary frequency and possible cloudy or discolored urine often occur with a urinary infection. Commonly the skin and mucous membranes are involved in a local infectious process, resulting in the following:

- Localized swelling
- Localized redness
- Pain or tenderness with palpation or movement
- Palpable heat at the infected area
- Loss of function of the body part affected, depending on the site and extent of involvement

ASSESSMENT INTERVIEW
Client at Risk for Infections

- When were you last immunized for diphtheria, tetanus, poliomyelitis, rubella, measles, influenza, hepatitis, and pneumococcal pneumonia?
- When did you last have a tuberculin skin test?
- What infections have you had in the past, and how were these treated?
- Have any of these infections recurred?
- Are you taking any antibiotics, anti-inflammatory medications such as aspirin or ibuprofen, or medications for cancer?
- Have you had any recent diagnostic procedure or therapy that penetrated through your skin or a body cavity?
- What past surgeries have you had?
- How would you describe your eating habits? Do you eat a variety of different types of foods?
- Do you take vitamins?
- On a scale of 1 to 10, how would you rate the stress you have experienced in the last 6 months?
- Have you experienced any loss of energy, loss of appetite, nausea, headache, or other signs associated with specific body systems (e.g., difficulty urinating, urinary frequency, or a sore throat)?

Note: As with all history taking, the nurse must individualize the specific terms used, examples given to the client, and teaching techniques used to validate agreement on the meaning of words according to the client's culture, language spoken, and education or intellectual abilities.

In addition, open wounds may exude drainage of various colors. Signs of systemic infection include the following:

- Fever
- Increased pulse and respiratory rate if the fever is high
- Malaise and loss of energy
- Anorexia and, in some situations, nausea and vomiting
- Enlargement and tenderness of lymph nodes that drain the area of infection

Laboratory Data

Laboratory data that indicate the presence of an infection include the following:

- Elevated leukocyte (white blood cell or WBC) count (4,500 to 11,000/mL is normal).
- Increases in specific types of leukocytes as revealed in the differential WBC count. Specific types of white blood cells are increased or decreased in certain infections. See Chapter 34 ∞ for normal values for the adult.
- Elevated *erythrocyte sedimentation rate (ESR)*. Red blood cells normally settle slowly, but the rate increases in the presence of an inflammatory process.
- Urine, blood, sputum, or other drainage **cultures** (laboratory cultivations of microorganisms in a special growth medium) that indicate the presence of pathogenic microorganisms.

Diagnosing

The NANDA nursing diagnostic label for problems associated with the transmission of microorganisms is *Risk for Infection:* the state in which an individual is at increased risk for being invaded by pathogenic microorganisms.

When using this label, the nurse should identify risk factors:

1. *Inadequate primary defenses* such as broken skin, traumatized tissue, decreased ciliary action, stasis of body fluids, change in pH of secretions, or altered peristalsis
2. *Inadequate secondary defenses* such as leukopenia, immunosuppression, decreased hemoglobin, or suppressed inflammatory response

Clients who have or are at risk for an existing infection are prime candidates for other physical and psychologic problems. Examples of nursing diagnoses or collaborative problems that may arise from the actual presence of an infection include the following:

- *Potential Complication of Infection: Fever*
- *Imbalanced Nutrition: Less Than Body Requirements* if the client is too ill to eat adequately
- *Acute Pain* if the client is experiencing tissue damage and discomfort
- *Impaired Social Interaction or Social Isolation* if the client is required to be separated from others during a contagious episode
- *Anxiety* if the client is apprehensive regarding changes in life activities resulting from the infection or its treatment such as absence from work or inability to perform usual functions

Examples of nursing diagnoses and related outcomes and interventions are shown in Identifying Nursing Diagnoses, Outcomes, and Interventions.

Planning

The major goals for clients susceptible to infection are to

- Maintain or restore defenses.
- Avoid the spread of infectious organisms.
- Reduce or alleviate problems associated with the infection.

Desired outcomes depend on the individual client's condition. Examples of desired outcomes, established in the planning phase, are provided in Identifying Nursing Diagnoses, Outcomes, and Interventions. Nursing strategies to meet the three broad goals generally include using meticulous medical and surgical aseptic techniques to prevent the spread of potentially infectious microorganisms, implementing measures to support the defenses of a susceptible host, and teaching clients about protective measures to prevent infections and the spread of infectious agents when an infection is present.

Planning for Home Care

Clients being discharged following hospital care for an infection often require continued care to completely eliminate the infection or to adapt to a chronic state. In addition, such clients may be at increased risk for reinfection or development of an opportunistic infection following therapy for existing pathogens.

In preparation for discharge, the nurse needs to know the client's and family's risks, needs, strengths, and resources. The Home Care Assessment box describes the specific assessment data required before establishing a discharge plan. Using the data gathered about the home situation, the nurse tailors the teaching plan for the client and family (see Client Teaching: Infection Control on page 682).

IDENTIFYING NURSING DIAGNOSES, OUTCOMES, AND INTERVENTIONS

Client at Risk for Infection

NURSING DIAGNOSIS/ DEFINITION	SAMPLE DESIRED OUTCOMES*/ DEFINITION	INDICATORS†	SELECTED INTERVENTIONS*/ DEFINITION	SAMPLE ACTIVITIES
Risk for Infection/At increased risk for being invaded by pathogenic organisms	Knowledge: Infection Control [1807]/*Extent of understanding conveyed about prevention and control of infection*	▪ Description of factors contributing to transmission ▪ Description of practices that reduce transmission ▪ Description of activities to increase resistance to infection	Infection Control [6540]/*Minimizing the acquisition and transmission of infectious agents*	▪ Description of signs and symptoms ▪ Description of treatment for diagnosed infection ▪ Instruct patient on proper hand cleansing techniques ▪ Institute standard precautions ▪ Promote appropriate nutritional intake ▪ Administer antibiotic therapy as indicated

*The NOC # for desired outcomes and the NIC # for nursing interventions are listed in brackets following the appropriate outcome or intervention. Outcomes, indicators, interventions, and activities are only a sample of those suggested by NOC and NIC and should be further individualized for each client.

†The measurement scale for these indicators ranges from None to Extensive. See Appendix B. ∞

HOME CARE ASSESSMENT
Infection

CLIENT AND ENVIRONMENT

▪ *Self-care abilities for wound care:* Understanding of rationale for wound care as well as wound care technique; ability to gather and use supplies for clean or aseptic technique to change dressings or care for wounds
▪ *Self-care abilities for hygiene and toileting:* Understanding of rationale for hygiene in the home setting; ability to contain potentially infectious material, such as that from coughing or sneezing, and body fluids (urine, stool, drainage); ability to cleanse hands and implement any required isolation practices
▪ *Self-care abilities for medication administration:* Understanding of medication therapy, expected outcomes, and potential side effects; physical dexterity to take pills, administer intravenous antibiotics, and store medications safely
▪ *Facilities:* Presence of running water, trash containers and disposal, bathroom to facilitate wound care and contain potentially infectious materials

FAMILY

▪ *Caregiver availability, skills, and responses:* Understanding of rationale for wound care as well as wound care technique; persons able to assist with wound care, medication administration, and shopping if client has restricted activity; people able to comprehend infection control activities without excessive personal anxiety
▪ *Other susceptible cohabitants:* Presence and immunization status of children, elders, or others who may be at risk of infection from the client

COMMUNITY

▪ *Resources:* Availability of and familiarity with possible sources of assistance for finances, supplies, and home health aid (such as public health department and visiting nurses)

Implementing

Whenever possible, the nurse implements strategies to prevent infection. If infection cannot be prevented, the nurse's goal is to prevent the spread of the infection within and between persons, and to treat the existing infection. In the sections that follow, specific nursing activities are described that interfere in the chain of infection to prevent and control transmission of infectious organisms, and that promote care of the infected client. These activities are summarized in Table 31–7.

Preventing Nosocomial Infections

Meticulous use of medical and surgical asepsis is necessary to prevent transport of potentially infectious microorganisms. As discussed previously in this chapter, nosocomial infections are those acquired in relation to health care services. Many nosocomial infections can be prevented using proper hand hygiene techniques, environmental controls, sterile technique when warranted, and identification and management of clients at risk for infections. Many research studies investigate the effectiveness of aseptic technique. Not all, however, show what would have been thought to be intuitive results. For example, no controlled studies have shown that removing nail polish or rings influences the rate of infection following surgical hand scrubbing and gloving (Arrowsmith, Maunder, Sargent, & Taylor, 2005). A number of studies have shown a link between artificial fingernails and infection transmission, especially fungal. In any case, the nurse uses critical thinking and agency policy in implementing infection control procedures.

Hand Hygiene

Hand hygiene is important in every setting, including hospitals. It is considered one of the most effective infection control measures. Any client may harbor microorganisms that are currently harmless to the client yet potentially harmful to another

CLIENT TEACHING Infection Control

ENVIRONMENTAL MANAGEMENT

- Discuss injury-proofing the home to prevent the possibility of further tissue injury (e.g., use of padding, handrails, removal of hazards).
- Explore ways to control the environmental temperature and airflow (especially if client has an airborne pathogen).
- Determine the advisability of visitors and family members in proximity to the client.
- Describe ways to manipulate the bed, the room, and other household facilities to prevent additional injury or to contain possible cross-contamination.
- Instruct to clean obviously soiled linen separately from other laundry. Rinse in cold water, wash in hot water if possible, and add a cup of bleach or phenol-based disinfectant such as Lysol concentrate to the wash.

INFECTION CONTROL

- Based on assessment of client and family knowledge, teach proper hand hygiene (e.g., before handling foods, before eating, after toileting, before and after any required home care treatment, and after touching any body substances such as wound drainage) and related hygienic measures to all family members.
- Promote nail care: keep fingernails short, clean, and well manicured to eliminate rough edges or hangnails, which can harbor microorganisms.
- Instruct not to share personal care items such as toothbrushes, washcloths, and towels. Describe the rationale of how infections can be transmitted from shared personal items.
- Discuss antimicrobial soaps and effective disinfectants.
- Ensure access to and proper use of gloves and other barriers as indicated by the type of infection or risk.
- Discuss the relationship between hygiene, rest, activity, and nutrition in the chain of infection.
- Instruct about proper administration of medication.
- Instruct about cleaning reusable equipment and supplies. Use soap and water, and disinfect with a chlorine bleach solution.

INFECTION PROTECTION

- Teach the client and family members the signs and symptoms of infection, and when to contact a health care provider. Determine by verbal questions the level of understanding on the topic after each teaching session.
- Teach the client and family members how to avoid infections.
- Suggest techniques for safe food preservation and preparation (e.g., wash raw fruits and vegetables before eating them, refrigerate all opened and unpackaged foods).
- Remind to avoid coughing, sneezing, or breathing directly on others. Cover the mouth and nose to prevent the transmission of airborne microorganisms.
- Inform of the importance of maintaining sufficient fluid intake to promote urine production and output. This helps flush the bladder and urethra of microorganisms.
- Emphasize the need for proper immunizations of all family members.

WOUND CARE

- Teach the client and family the signs of wound healing and of wound infection and why monitoring of the wound is important.
- Delineate the factors that promote wound healing.
- Explain the proper technique for changing the dressing and disposing of the soiled one. Reinforce the need to place contaminated dressings and other disposable items containing body fluids in moisture-proof plastic bags.
- Advise to put used needles in a puncture-resistant container with a screw-top lid. Label so as not to discard in the garbage.
- Have client or family repeat instructions and demonstrate skills.

REFERRALS

- Provide appropriate information regarding how to access community resources, home care agencies, sources of supplies, and community or public health departments for immunizations.

person or to the same client if they find a portal of entry. It is important that both the nurses' and the clients' hands be cleansed at the following times to prevent the spread of microorganisms: before eating, after using the bedpan or toilet, and after the hands have come in contact with any body substances, such as sputum or drainage from a wound. In addition, health care workers should cleanse their hands before and after giving care of any kind.

For routine client care, the World Health Organization (2005) recommends hand washing under a stream of water for at least 20 seconds using plain granule soap, soap-filled sheets, or liquid soap when hands are visibly soiled, after using the restroom, after removing gloves, before handling invasive devices (such as intravenous tubing), and after contact with medical equipment or furniture.

However, soap and water are inadequate to sufficiently remove pathogens. The CDC recommends use of alcohol-based antiseptic hand rubs (rinses, gels, or foams) for use before and after direct client contact. Recently, placement of alcohol-based

antiseptic hand rub dispensers has been approved for agency corridors (Centers for Medicare and Medicaid Services, 2005). Previous concerns that this represented a fire hazard have been addressed in the regulations. Proper application of alcohol-based products includes the following steps.

- Apply a palmful of the product to a cupped hand. An adequate amount to completely cover both hands, palms and backs, is essential.
- Rub palms against palms.
- Interlace fingers palm to palm.
- Rub palms to back of hands.
- Rub each finger individually on all sides with the other hand.
- Continue until product is dry—about 20 to 30 seconds.

Antimicrobial soaps are usually provided in high-risk areas, such as the newborn nursery, and are frequently supplied in dispensers at the sink. Studies have shown that the convenience of antimicrobial foams and gels, which do not require soap and water, may increase health care workers' adherence to hand cleansing.

TABLE 31–7 Nursing Interventions that Break the Chain of Infection

LINK	INTERVENTIONS	RATIONALES
Etiologic agent (microorganism)	Ensure that articles are correctly cleaned and disinfected or sterilized before use.	Correct cleaning, disinfecting, and sterilizing reduce or eliminate microorganisms.
	Educate clients and support persons about appropriate methods to clean, disinfect, and sterilize articles.	Knowledge of ways to reduce or eliminate microorganisms reduces the numbers of microorganisms present and the likelihood of transmission.
Reservoir (source)	Change dressings and bandages when they are soiled or wet.	Moist dressings are ideal environments for microorganisms to grow and multiply.
	Assist clients to carry out appropriate skin and oral hygiene.	Hygienic measures reduce the numbers of resident and transient microorganisms and the likelihood of infection.
	Dispose of damp, soiled linens appropriately.	Damp, soiled linens harbor more microorganisms than dry linens.
	Dispose of feces and urine in appropriate receptacles.	Urine and feces in particular contain many microorganisms.
	Ensure that all fluid containers, such as bedside water jugs and suction and drainage bottles, are covered or capped.	Prolonged exposure increases the risk of contamination and promotes microbial growth.
	Empty suction and drainage bottles at the end of each shift or before they become full, or according to agency policy.	Drainage harbors microorganisms that, if left for long periods, proliferate and can be transmitted to others.
Portal of exit from the reservoir	Avoid talking, coughing, or sneezing over open wounds or sterile fields, and cover the mouth and nose when coughing and sneezing.	These measures limit the number of microorganisms that escape from the respiratory tract.
Method of transmission	Cleanse hands between client contacts, after touching body substances, and before performing invasive procedures or touching open wounds.	Hand cleansing is an important means of controlling and preventing the transmission of microorganisms.
	Instruct clients and support persons to cleanse hands before handling food or eating, after eliminating, and after touching infectious material.	Hand cleansing helps prevent transfer of microorganisms from one person to another.
	Wear gloves when handling secretions and excretions.	Gloves and gowns prevent soiling of the hands and clothing.
	Wear gowns if there is danger of soiling clothing with body substances.	
	Place discarded soiled materials in moisture-proof refuse bags.	Moisture-proof bags prevent the spread of microorganisms to others.
	Hold used bedpans steadily to prevent spillage, and dispose of urine and feces in appropriate receptacles.	Feces in particular contain many microorganisms.
	Initiate and implement aseptic precautions for all clients.	All clients may harbor potentially infectious microorganisms that can be transmitted to others.
	Wear masks and eye protection when in close contact with clients who have infections transmitted by droplets from the respiratory tract.	Masks and eyewear reduce the spread of droplet-transmitted microorganisms.
	Wear masks and eye protection when sprays of body fluid are possible (e.g., during irrigation procedures).	Masks and eye protection provide protection from microorganisms in clients' body substances.
Portal of entry to the susceptible host	Use sterile technique for invasive procedures (e.g., injections, catheterizations).	Invasive procedures penetrate the body's natural protective barriers to microorganisms.
	Use sterile technique when exposing open wounds or handling dressings.	Open wounds are vulnerable to microbial infection.
	Place used disposable needles and syringes in puncture-resistant containers for disposal.	Injuries from needles contaminated by blood or body fluids from an infected client or carrier are a primary cause of HBV and HIV transmission to health care workers.
	Provide all clients with their own personal care items.	People have less resistance to another person's microorganisms than to their own.
Susceptible host	Maintain the integrity of the client's skin and mucous membranes.	Intact skin and mucous membranes protect against invasion by microorganisms.
	Ensure that the client receives a balanced diet.	A balanced diet supplies proteins and vitamins necessary to build or maintain body tissues.
	Educate the public about the importance of immunizations.	Immunizations protect people against virulent infectious diseases.

The CDC recommends antimicrobial hand cleansing agents in the following situations:

- When there are known multiple resistant bacteria
- Before invasive procedures
- In special care units, such as nurseries and ICUs
- Before caring for severely immunocompromised clients

It is important to recognize that performing hand hygiene with either soap or alcohol-based cleansers can damage the skin through the drying effect of the detergents or chemicals. If the nurse develops dermatitis, the client may be at higher risk because hand washing does not decrease bacterial counts on skin with dermatitis. The nurse is also at higher risk because the normal skin barrier has been broken. Although lotions, moisturizers, and emollients have been tried, no research has yet confirmed their effectiveness in decreasing the problem.

Skill 31-1 describes proper hand hygiene techniques using soap and water.

HAND WASHING

PURPOSES
- To reduce the number of microorganisms on the hands
- To reduce the risk of transmission of microorganisms to clients
- To reduce the risk of cross-contamination among clients
- To reduce the risk of transmission of infectious organisms to oneself

ASSESSMENT
Determine the client's

- Presence of factors increasing susceptibility to infection and possibility of undiagnosed infection (e.g., HIV).
- Use of immunosuppressive medications.
- Recent diagnostic procedures or treatments that penetrated the skin or a body cavity.
- Current nutritional status.
- Signs and symptoms indicating the presence of an infection:
- Localized signs, such as swelling, redness, pain or tenderness with palpation or movement, palpable heat at site, loss of function of affected body part, presence of exudate
- Systemic indications, such as fever, increased pulse and respiratory rates, lack of energy, anorexia, enlarged lymph nodes

PLANNING
Determine the location of running water and soap or soap substitutes.

Delegation
The technique of hand washing is identical for all health care providers, including unlicensed assistive personnel (UAP). Health care team members are accountable for the implementation of appropriate hand washing procedures by themselves and others.

Equipment
- Soap
- Warm running water
- Disposable or sanitized towels

IMPLEMENTATION
Preparation
Assess the hands.

- Nails should be kept short. **Rationale:** *Short, natural nails are less likely to harbor microorganisms, scratch a client, or puncture gloves.* Most agencies do not permit health care workers in direct contact with clients to have any form of artificial nails.
- Remove all jewelry. **Rationale:** *Microorganisms can lodge in the settings of jewelry and under rings. Removal facilitates proper cleaning of the hands and arms.*
- Check hands for breaks in the skin, such as hangnails or cuts. **Rationale:** *A nurse who has open sores may require a work assignment with decreased risk for transmission of infectious organisms due to the chance of acquiring or passing on an infection.*

Performance
1. If you are washing your hands where the client can observe you, introduce yourself and explain to the client what you are going to do and why it is necessary.
2. Turn on the water and adjust the flow.
   - There are five common types of faucet controls:
     a. Hand-operated handles.
     b. Knee levers. Move these with the knee to regulate flow and temperature. ❶

❶ A knee-lever faucet control.

HAND WASHING *continued*

    c. Foot pedals. Press these with the foot to regulate flow and temperature. ❷

    d. Elbow controls. Move these with the elbows instead of the hands.

    e. Infrared control. Motion in front of the sensor causes water to start and stop flowing automatically.

- Adjust the flow so that the water is warm. **Rationale:** *Warm water removes less of the protective oil of the skin than hot water.*

3. Wet the hands thoroughly by holding them under the running water and apply soap to the hands.

- Hold the hands lower than the elbows so that the water flows from the arms to the fingertips. **Rationale:** *The water should flow from the least contaminated to the most contaminated area; the hands are generally considered more contaminated than the lower arms.* Note that this is a different technique than is used when performing surgical hand washing. Nurses will learn to perform that level of hand washing if they are working in the operating room.
- If the soap is liquid, apply 2 to 4 mL (1 tsp). If it is bar soap, granules, or sheets, rub them firmly between the hands.

4. Thoroughly wash and rinse the hands.

- Use firm, rubbing, and circular movements to wash the palm, back, and wrist of each hand. Be sure to include the heel of the hand. Interlace the fingers and thumbs, and move the hands back and forth. ❸

    Continue this motion for at least 15 seconds (Boyce & Pittet, 2002; Houghton, 2006). **Rationale:** *The circular action creates friction that helps remove microorganisms mechanically. Interlacing the fingers and thumbs cleans the interdigital spaces.*

- Rub the fingertips against the palm of the opposite hand. **Rationale:** *The nails and fingertips are commonly missed during hand washing.*
- Rinse the hands.

5. Thoroughly pat dry the hands and arms.

- Dry hands and arms thoroughly with a paper towel without scrubbing. **Rationale:** *Moist skin becomes chapped readily as does dry skin that is rubbed vigorously; chapping produces lesions.*
- Discard the paper towel in the appropriate container.

6. Turn off the water.

- Use a new paper towel to grasp a hand-operated control. ❹ **Rationale:** *This prevents the nurse from picking up microorganisms from the faucet handles.*

❷ A foot-pedal faucet control.

❸ Interlacing the fingers during hand washing.

❹ Using a paper towel to grasp the handle of a hand-operated faucet.

continued on page 686

HAND WASHING *continued*

VARIATION: HAND WASHING BEFORE STERILE TECHNIQUES

■ Apply the soap and wash as described in step 4, but hold the hands higher than the elbows during this hand wash. Wet the hands and forearms under the running water, letting it run from the fingertips to the elbows so that the hands become cleaner than the elbows. ❺ **Rationale:** *In this way, the water runs from the area that now has the fewest microorganisms to areas with a relatively greater number.*

■ After washing and rinsing, use a towel to dry one hand thoroughly in a rotating motion from the fingers to the elbow. Use a new towel to dry the other hand and arm. **Rationale:** *A clean towel prevents the transfer of microorganisms from one elbow (least clean area) to the other hand (cleanest area).*

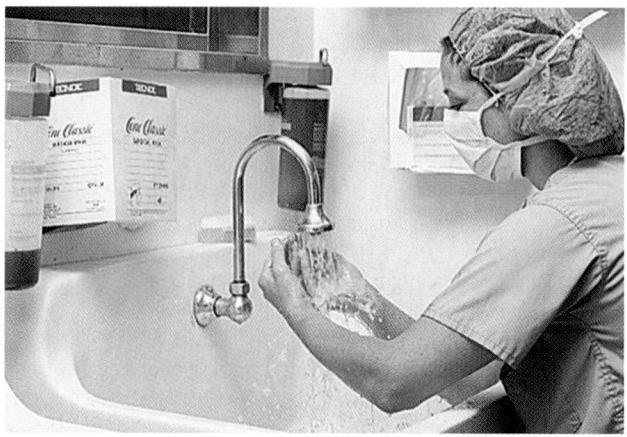

❺ The hands are held higher than the elbows during a hand wash before sterile technique.

EVALUATION

There is no traditional evaluation of the effectiveness of the individual nurse's hand washing. Institutional quality control departments monitor the occurrence of client infections and investigate those situations in which health care providers are implicated in the transmission of infectious organisms. Research has repeatedly shown the positive impact of careful hand cleansing on client health associated with prevention of infection (see Readings and References at the end of this chapter).

RESEARCH NOTE
Does Frequency of Hand Washing Vary According to Risk of Infection Transmission?

In this Canadian study, all visits by nurses in an acute care hospital to selected client rooms were recorded for 3 days and 2 nights to assess compliance with hand washing. The highest level of infection transmission risk was contact with body fluids in 11% of visits and skin in 40% of visits. The overall rate of hand washing was 46%; however, the rate for visits involving contact with body fluids was 81% and skin 61%. Nurses returned immediately to the same client 45% of the time. The rate of hand washing was higher for the last of a series of visits to a patient's room. The researchers concluded that nurses adjusted their hand washing rates in accordance with the risk level of each visit.

IMPLICATIONS

Many studies have examined compliance with hand washing policies among health care workers. In almost every case, the rates were far below what is recommended. This study suggests that raw data of compliance are less useful than examining the use and pattern of hand washing in those instances in which the care provider recognizes highest risk of infection transmission. Education programs about hand hygiene may be more effective if patterns of care and levels of risk are incorporated into recommendations.

Note: From "Patterns of Handwashing Behavior and Visits to Patients on a General Medical Ward of Healthcare Workers," by J. Raboud, R. Saskin, K. Wong, C. Moore, G. Parucha, J. Bennett, et al., 2004, *Infection Control and Hospital Epidemiology, 25*, pp. 198–202.

Supporting Defenses of a Susceptible Host

People are constantly in contact with microorganisms in the environment. Normally a person's natural defenses ward off the development of an infection. *Susceptibility* is the degree to which an individual can be affected, that is, the likelihood of an organism causing an infection in that person. The following measures can reduce a person's susceptibility:

■ *Hygiene.* Intact skin and mucous membranes are one barrier against microorganisms entering the body. In addition, good oral care, including flossing the teeth, reduces the likelihood of an oral infection. Regular and thorough bathing and shampooing remove microorganisms and dirt that can result in an infection.

■ *Nutrition.* A balanced diet enhances the health of all body tissues, helps keep the skin intact, and promotes the skin's ability to repel microorganisms. Adequate nutrition enables tissues to maintain and rebuild themselves and helps keep the immune system functioning well.

■ *Fluid.* Fluid intake permits fluid output that flushes out the bladder and urethra, removing microorganisms that could cause an infection.

■ *Sleep.* Adequate sleep is essential to health and to renewing energy. See Chapter 45. ∞

■ *Stress.* Excessive stress predisposes people to infections. Nurses can assist clients to learn stress-reducing techniques. See Chapter 42. ∞

DRUG CAPSULE **Macrolide Antibiotic** *azithromycin* (Zithromax)

Macrolide antibiotics prevent bacteria from growing by interfering with their ability to make proteins. Due to the differences in the way proteins are made in bacteria and humans, the macrolide antibiotics do not interfere with humans' ability to make proteins. They are effective against a wide variety of bacteria organisms, such as *Haemophilus influenzae, Streptococcus pneumoniae, Mycoplasma pneumoniae, Staphylococcus aureus, Mycobacterium avium*, and many others. Azithromycin is unusual in that it stays in the body for quite a while, allowing for once a day dosing and for shorter treatment courses for most infections. It may be prescribed for infections from susceptible microorganisms such as those that occur in the lungs (bronchitis), ears, skin, and throat.

NURSING RESPONSIBILITIES

- Assess the client for any drug allergies—especially to other antibiotics and particularly those from the erythromycin family. Do not administer azithromycin to clients with stated allergies unless the primary care provider has given approval.
- Assess for signs of possible allergic reaction: rash, hives, itching, swelling of the face or mouth, and difficulty breathing or swallowing. If any are detected, contact the primary care provider immediately—this is an emergency.
- Azithromycin may be given with meals or on an empty stomach.
- It is available in capsules or oral liquid suspension.
- Drug interactions can occur with anticoagulants, digoxin, and several other medications. Always check the list of client medications for possible interactions.
- Adverse effects are generally limited to gastrointestinal upset.

CLIENT AND FAMILY TEACHING

- Assess and document client's level of understanding related to medication therapy. Develop a teaching plan to augment any lack of knowledge on the part of the client or family caregiver.
- Teach the client to take azithromycin with a full glass of water, with or without food, but at least 2 hours after antacids.
- Teach the client to complete the entire course of therapy—not to stop taking the medication even if the client feels better before then.
- Instruct to store the medication away from heat and moisture—not in the bathroom.
- Be sure the client understands not to keep leftover medication or share it with other persons.

Note: Prior to administering any medication, review all aspects with a current drug handbook or other reliable source.

- *Immunizations.* The use of immunizations has dramatically decreased the incidence of infectious diseases. It is recommended that immunizations begin shortly after birth and be completed in early childhood except for boosters. (See Table 31–5 earlier in this chapter.) Immunizations may be given by injection, inhalation, oral solutions, or nasal sprays. They are frequently given in combination to minimize multiple injections. Because there are frequent changes to immunization schedules, it is advisable to update immunization schedules yearly.

There are immunization programs for high-risk groups such as health care personnel, older adults who are chronically ill, and people traveling to foreign countries. For example, hepatitis B vaccine is recommended for all health care workers.

Disinfecting and Sterilizing

The first links in the chain of infection, the etiologic agent and the reservoir, are interrupted by the use of **antiseptics** (agents that inhibit the growth of some microorganisms) and **disinfectants** (agents that destroy pathogens other than spores), and by sterilization.

Disinfecting

A disinfectant is a chemical preparation, such as phenol or iodine compounds, used on inanimate objects. Disinfectants are frequently caustic and toxic to tissues. An antiseptic is a chemical preparation used on skin or tissue. Disinfectants and antiseptics often have similar chemical components, but the disinfectant is a more concentrated solution.

Both antiseptics and disinfectants are said to have bactericidal or bacteriostatic properties. A *bactericidal* preparation destroys bacteria, whereas a *bacteriostatic* preparation prevents the growth and reproduction of some bacteria. An agent known to be effective against it should be selected. Spore-forming bacteria such as *C. difficile*, which is a frequent cause of nosocomial diarrhea, and *Bacillus anthracis* (anthrax) may be inhibited by only a few of the agents normally effective against other forms of bacteria. Table 31–8 lists commonly used antiseptics and disinfectants.

TABLE 31–8 Commonly Used Antiseptics and Disinfectants, Effectiveness, and Use

AGENT	BACTERIA	TUBERCULOSIS	SPORES	FUNGI	VIRUSES	USE ON
Isopropyl and ethyl alcohol	X	X		X	X	Hands, vial stoppers
Chlorine (bleach)	X	X	X	X	X	Blood spills
Hydrogen peroxide	X	X	X	X	X	Surfaces
Iodophors	X	X	X	X	X	Equipment; intact skin and tissues if diluted
Phenol	X	X		X	X	Surfaces
Chlorhexidine gluconate (Hibiclens)	X				X	Hands
Triclosan (Bacti-Stat)	X					Hands, intact skin

When disinfecting articles, nurses need to follow agency protocol and consider the following:

1. The type and number of infectious organisms. Some microorganisms are readily destroyed, whereas others require longer contact with the disinfectant.
2. The recommended concentration of the disinfectant and the duration of contact.
3. The presence of soap. Some disinfectants are ineffective in the presence of soap or detergent.
4. The presence of organic materials. The presence of saliva, blood, pus, or excretions can readily inactivate many disinfectants.
5. The surface areas to be treated. The disinfecting agent must come into contact with all surfaces and areas.

Sterilizing

Sterilization is a process that destroys all microorganisms, including spores and viruses. Four commonly used methods of sterilization are moist heat, gas, boiling water, and radiation.

MOIST HEAT. To sterilize with moist heat (such as with an autoclave), steam under pressure is used because it attains temperatures higher than the boiling point.

GAS. Ethylene oxide gas destroys microorganisms by interfering with their metabolic processes. It is also effective against spores. Its advantages are good penetration and effectiveness for heat-sensitive items. Its major disadvantage is its toxicity to humans.

BOILING WATER. This is the most practical and inexpensive method for sterilizing in the home. The main disadvantage is that spores and some viruses are not killed by this method. Boiling a minimum of 15 minutes is advised for disinfection of articles in the home.

RADIATION. Both ionizing (such as alpha, beta, and x-rays) and nonionizing (ultraviolet light) radiation are used for disinfection and sterilization. The main drawback to ultraviolet light is that the rays do not penetrate deeply. Ionizing radiation is used effectively in industry to sterilize foods, drugs, and other items that are sensitive to heat. Its main advantage is that it is effective for items difficult to sterilize; its chief disadvantage is that the equipment is very expensive.

ISOLATION PRECAUTIONS

Isolation refers to measures designed to prevent the spread of infections or potentially infectious microorganisms to health personnel, clients, and visitors. Several sets of guidelines have been used in hospitals and other health care settings.

Category-specific isolation precautions use seven categories: strict isolation, contact isolation, respiratory isolation, tuberculosis isolation, enteric precautions, drainage/secretions precautions, and blood/body fluid precautions.

Disease-specific isolation precautions provide precautions for specific diseases. These precautions delineate use of private rooms with special ventilation, having the client share a room with other clients infected with the same organism, and gowning to prevent gross soilage of clothes for specific infectious diseases (Garner & Simmons, 1983).

Figure 31-2 ■ Biohazard alert.

Universal precautions (UP) are techniques to be used with all clients to decrease the risk of transmitting unidentified pathogens (CDC, 1987; U.S. Department of Health and Human Services [USDHHS], 1988). Universal precautions obstruct the spread of **bloodborne pathogens,** those microorganisms carried in blood and body fluids that are capable of infecting other persons with serious and difficult to treat viral infections, namely, hepatitis B virus, hepatitis C virus, and HIV. The CDC did not recommend that universal precautions replace disease-specific or category-specific precautions, but that they be used in conjunction with them.

The **body substance isolation (BSI)** system employs generic infection control precautions for all clients except those with the few diseases transmitted through the air. The BSI system (Jackson, 1993) is based on three premises:

1. All people have an increased risk for infection from microorganisms placed on their mucous membranes and nonintact skin.
2. All people are likely to have potentially infectious microorganisms in all of their moist body sites and substances.
3. An unknown portion of clients and health care workers will always be colonized or infected with potentially infectious microorganisms in their blood and other moist body sites and substances.

The term *body substance* includes blood, some body fluids, urine, feces, wound drainage, oral secretions, and any other body product or tissue.

In addition to other actions and precautions discussed in this chapter, significant emphasis is placed on avoiding injury due to sharp instruments (see Chapter 35 ∞), measures to be taken in case of exposure to bloodborne pathogens, and communication about biohazards to employees. Federal regulations require that in most cases warning labels be affixed to containers of regulated waste and to refrigerators and freezers containing blood or other potentially infectious materials. The labels required are fluorescent orange or orange-red and feature the biohazard legend shown in Figure 31-2 ■.

CDC (HICPAC) Isolation Precautions (1996)

The Hospital Infection Control Practices Advisory Committee (HICPAC) of the CDC presented new guidelines for isolation precautions in hospitals in 1996 (Garner & HICPAC, 1996). These guidelines designate two tiers of precautions:

Standard Precautions
Transmission-Based Precautions

Standard Precautions

These precautions are used in the care of all hospitalized persons regardless of their diagnosis or possible infection status. They apply to blood, all body fluids, secretions, and excretions except sweat (whether or not blood is present or visible), nonintact skin, and mucous membranes. Thus they combine the major features of UP and BSI. Recommended practices for standard precautions are shown in Box 31–1.

Transmission-Based Precautions

These precautions are used in addition to standard precautions for clients with known or suspected infections that are spread in one of three ways: by airborne or droplet transmission, or by contact. The three types of transmission-based precautions may be used alone or in combination but always in addition to standard precautions. They encompass all of the conditions or diseases previously listed in the category-specific or

---

BOX 31–1 Recommended Isolation Precautions in Hospitals

STANDARD PRECAUTIONS

- Designed for all clients in hospital.
- These precautions apply to (a) blood; (b) all body fluids, excretions, and secretions except sweat; (c) nonintact (broken) skin; and (d) mucous membranes.
- Designed to reduce risk of transmission of microorganisms from recognized and unrecognized sources.

1. Perform proper hand hygiene after contact with blood, body fluids, secretions, excretions, and contaminated objects whether or not gloves are worn.
   a. Perform proper hand hygiene immediately after removing gloves.
   b. Use a nonantimicrobial product for routine hand cleansing.
   c. Use an antimicrobial agent or an antiseptic agent for the control of specific outbreaks of infection.
2. Wear clean gloves when touching blood, body fluids, secretions, excretions, and contaminated items (i.e., soiled gowns).
   a. Clean gloves can be unsterile unless their use is intended to prevent the entrance of microorganisms into the body. See the discussion of sterile gloves in this chapter.
   b. Remove gloves before touching noncontaminated items and surfaces.
   c. Perform proper hand hygiene immediately after removing gloves.
3. Wear a mask, eye protection, or a face shield if splashes or sprays of blood, body fluids, secretions, or excretions can be expected.
4. Wear a clean, nonsterile gown if client care is likely to result in splashes or sprays of blood, body fluids, secretions, or excretions. The gown is intended to protect clothing.
   a. Remove a soiled gown carefully to avoid the transfer of microorganisms to others (i.e., clients or other health care workers).
   b. Cleanse hands after removing gown.
5. Handle client care equipment that is soiled with blood, body fluids, secretions, or excretions carefully to prevent the transfer of microorganisms to others and to the environment.
   a. Make sure reusable equipment is cleaned and reprocessed correctly.
   b. Dispose of single-use equipment correctly.
6. Handle, transport, and process linen that is soiled with blood, body fluids, secretions, or excretions in a manner to prevent contamination of clothing and the transfer of microorganisms to others and to the environment.
7. Prevent injuries from used scalpels, needles, or other equipment, and place in puncture-resistant containers.

TRANSMISSION-BASED PRECAUTIONS

Airborne Precautions

Use standard precautions as well as the following:

1. Place client in a private room that has negative air pressure, 6 to 12 air changes per hour, and either discharge of air to the outside or a filtration system for the room air.

2. If a private room is not available, place client with another client who is infected with the same microorganism.
3. Wear a respiratory device (N95 respirator) when entering the room of a client who is known or suspected of having primary tuberculosis.
4. Susceptible people should not enter the room of a client who has rubeola (measles) or varicella (chickenpox). If they must enter, they should wear a respirator.
5. Limit movement of client outside the room to essential purposes. Place a surgical mask on the client during transport.

Droplet Precautions

Use standard precautions as well as the following:

1. Place client in private room.
2. If a private room is not available, place client with another client who is infected with the same microorganism.
3. Wear a mask if working within 3 feet of the client.
4. Limit movement of client outside the room to essential purposes. Place a surgical mask on the client during transport.

Contact Precautions

Use standard precautions as well as the following:

1. Place client in private room.
2. If a private room is not available, place client with another client who is infected with the same microorganism.
3. Wear gloves as described in standard precautions.
   a. Change gloves after contact with infectious material.
   b. Remove gloves before leaving client's room.
   c. Cleanse hands immediately after removing gloves. Use an antimicrobial agent. Note: If the client is infected with *C. difficile*, do not use an alcohol-based hand rub as it may not be effective on these spores. Use soap and water.
   d. After hand cleansing, do not touch possibly contaminated surfaces or items in the room.
4. Wear a gown (see standard precautions) when entering a room if there is a possibility of contact with infected surfaces or items, or if the client is incontinent, or has diarrhea, a colostomy, or wound drainage not contained by a dressing.
   a. Remove gown in the client's room.
   b. Make sure uniform does not contact possible contaminated surfaces.
5. Limit movement of client outside the room.
6. Dedicate the use of noncritical client care equipment to a single client or to clients with the same infecting microorganisms.

Note: Adapted from "Guidelines for Isolation Precautions in Hospitals," by J. S. Garner and the Hospital Infection Control Practices Advisory Committee (HICPAC), 1996, *Infection Control Hospital Epidemiology, 17,* pp. 53–80, and 1996, *American Journal of Infection Control, 24,* pp. 24–52.

disease-specific classifications developed by the CDC in 1983. Recommended practices for Transmission-Based Precautions are shown in Box 31–1.

Airborne precautions are used for clients known to have or suspected of having serious illnesses transmitted by airborne droplet nuclei smaller than 5 microns. Examples of such illnesses include measles (rubeola), varicella (including disseminated zoster), and tuberculosis. The CDC has prepared special guidelines for preventing the transmission of tuberculosis. The most current information may be found on the CDC Division of Tuberculosis Elimination website.

Droplet precautions are used for clients known or suspected to have serious illnesses transmitted by particle droplets larger than 5 microns. Examples of such illnesses are diphtheria (pharyngeal); mycoplasma pneumonia; pertussis; mumps; rubella; streptococcal pharyngitis, pneumonia, or scarlet fever in infants and young children; and pneumonic plague.

Contact precautions are used for clients known or suspected to have serious illnesses easily transmitted by direct client contact or by contact with items in the client's environment. According to the CDC (Garner & HICPAC, 1996), such illnesses include gastrointestinal, respiratory, skin, or wound infections or colonization with multidrug-resistant bacteria; specific enteric infections such as *C. difficile*, and enterohemorrhagic *Escherichia coli 0157:H7, Shigella,* and hepatitis A, for diapered or incontinent clients; respiratory syncytial virus, parainfluenza virus, or enteroviral infections in infants and young children; and highly contagious skin infections such as herpes simplex virus, impetigo, pediculosis, and scabies.

In addition to the preceding conditions, special contact precautions are used for vancomycin-resistant enterococci (VRE) infections. The CDC recommends use of an antimicrobial soap for hand washing and no sharing of equipment among clients with and without VRE. The client should have a private room (or a room with other clients who have VRE), and such isolation should continue until at least three cultures taken 1 week apart are negative (HICPAC, 1995).

Some diseases require a combination of transmission-based precautions. For clients infected with the coronavirus that causes severe acute respiratory syndrome (SARS-CoV), standard (including eye protection), contact, and airborne precautions are indicated (CDC, 2005).

Compromised Clients

Compromised clients (those highly susceptible to infection) are often infected by their own microorganisms, by microorganisms on the inadequately cleansed hands of health care personnel, and by nonsterile items (food, water, air, and client-care equipment). Clients who are severely compromised include those who

- Have diseases, such as leukemia, that depress the client's resistance to infectious organisms.
- Have extensive skin impairments, such as severe dermatitis or major burns, which cannot be effectively covered with dressings.

The 1997 CDC guidelines for severely compromised (immunocompromised) clients include the use of standard precautions as described earlier.

ISOLATION PRACTICES

Initiation of practices to prevent the transmission of microorganisms is generally a nursing responsibility and is based on a comprehensive assessment of the client. This assessment takes into account the status of the client's normal defense mechanisms, the client's ability to implement necessary precautions, and the source and mode of transmission of the infectious agent. The nurse then decides whether to wear gloves, gowns, masks, and protective eyewear. In all client situations, *nurses must cleanse their hands before and after giving care.*

In addition to the precautions cited within this chapter, the nurse implements aseptic precautions when performing many specific therapies discussed throughout this book. The following are some examples:

- Use strict aseptic technique when performing any invasive procedure (e.g., inserting an intravenous needle or catheter) and when changing surgical dressings.
- Change intravenous tubing and solution containers according to hospital policy (e.g., every 48 to 72 hours).
- Check all sterile supplies for expiration date and intact packaging.
- Prevent urinary infections by maintaining a closed urinary drainage system with a downhill flow of urine. Keep the drainage bag and spout off the floor.
- Implement measures to prevent impaired skin integrity and to prevent accumulation of secretions in the lungs (for example, encourage the client to move, cough, and breathe deeply at least every 2 hours).

Personal Protective Equipment

All health care providers must apply clean or sterile gloves, gowns, masks, and protective eyewear according to the risk of exposure to potentially infective materials.

Gloves

Gloves are worn for three reasons: First, they protect the hands when the nurse is likely to handle any body substances, for example, blood, urine, feces, sputum, and nonintact skin. Second, gloves reduce the likelihood of nurses transmitting their own endogenous microorganisms to individuals receiving care. Nurses who have open sores or cuts on the hands must wear gloves for protection. Third, gloves reduce the chance that the nurse's hands will transmit microorganisms from one client or a fomite to another client. In all situations, gloves are changed between client contacts. The hands are cleansed each time gloves are removed for two primary reasons: (a) the gloves may have imperfections or be damaged during wearing so that they could allow microorganism entry and (b) the hands may become contaminated during glove removal.

Some of the gloves used in infection control may be made of latex rubber, as are various other items used in health care (catheters, blood pressure cuffs, rubber sheets, intravenous tubing, stockings and binders, adhesive bandages, and dental dams). Because of the frequent use of gloves, clients with chronic illnesses and health care workers have increasingly reported allergic reactions to latex. Latex gloves lubricated by powder or cornstarch are particularly allergenic because the latex allergen adheres to the powder, which is aerosolized during glove use and inhaled by the user. Latex gloves that are labeled "hypoallergenic" still contain measurable latex and should not be used by or on persons with known latex sensitivity. Recent studies show some level of latex allergy in 8% to 12% of health care personnel (Occupational Safety and Health Administration, 2005). The people at greatest risk for developing latex al-

lergies are those with other allergic conditions and those who have had frequent or long-term exposure to latex.

Latex allergies can be either local or systemic and may take the form of dermatitis, urticaria (hives), asthma, or anaphylaxis. Clients and health care workers should be assessed for possible allergies through a thorough history taking. Ask clients if they have had any adverse reactions to items such as balloons, condoms, or dishwashing or utility gloves. Strategies to avoid sensitization or exposure to latex include use of nonlatex products, nonlatex barriers between latex products and the skin, and gloves that are unpowdered or washed before use. People with significant allergies should have no contact with latex products. Most hospitals have eliminated latex products wherever possible and have established a "latex-free environment" goal.

Skill 31-2 describes application and removal of gloves.

DONNING AND REMOVING PERSONAL PROTECTIVE EQUIPMENT (GLOVES, GOWN, MASK, EYEWEAR)

PURPOSES
- To protect health care workers and clients from transmission of potentially infective materials

ASSESSMENT
Consider which activities will be required while the nurse is in the client's room at this time. **Rationale:** *This will determine which equipment is required.*

PLANNING
- Application and removal of personal protective equipment (PPE) can be time consuming. Prioritize care and arrange for personnel to care for your other clients if indicated.

- Determine which supplies are present within the client's room and which must be brought to the room.
- Consider if special handling is indicated for removal of any specimens or other materials from the room.

Delegation
Use of PPE is identical for all health care providers. Clients whose care requires use of PPE may be delegated to UAP. Health care team members are accountable for proper implementation of these procedures by themselves and others.

Equipment
As indicated according to which activities will be performed. Ensure that extra supplies are easily available.

- Gown
- Mask
- Eyewear
- Clean gloves

IMPLEMENTATION
Preparation
Remove or secure all loose items such as name tags or jewelry.

Performance
1. Prior to performing the procedure, introduce self and verify the client's identity using agency protocol. Explain to the client what you are going to do, why it is necessary, and how he or she can cooperate.
2. Perform proper hand hygiene.
3. Don a clean gown.
   - Pick up a clean gown, and allow it to unfold in front of you without allowing it to touch any area soiled with body substances.
   - Slide the arms and the hands through the sleeves.
   - Fasten the ties at the neck to keep the gown in place.
   - Overlap the gown at the back as much as possible, and fasten the waist ties or belt. ❶ **Rationale:** *Overlapping securely covers the uniform at the back. Waist ties keep the gown from falling away from the body which can cause inadvertent soiling of the uniform.*

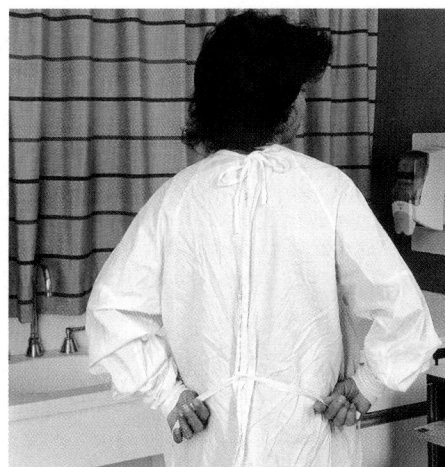

❶ Overlapping the gown at the back to cover the nurse's uniform.

(Al Dodge, Pearson Education/PH College)

continued on page 692

DONNING AND REMOVING PERSONAL PROTECTIVE EQUIPMENT (GLOVES, GOWN, MASK, EYEWEAR) *continued*

4. Don the face mask.
   - Locate the top edge of the mask. The mask usually has a narrow metal strip along the edge.
   - Hold the mask by the top two strings or loops.
   - Place the upper edge of the mask over the bridge of the nose, and tie the upper ties at the back of the head or secure the loops around the ears. If glasses are worn, fit the upper edge of the mask under the glasses. **Rationale:** *With the edge of the mask under the glasses, clouding of the glasses is less likely to occur.*
   - Secure the lower edge of the mask under the chin, and tie the lower ties at the nape of the neck. ❷ **Rationale:** *To be effective, a mask must cover both the nose and the mouth, because air moves in and out of both.*
   - If the mask has a metal strip, adjust this firmly over the bridge of the nose. **Rationale:** *A secure fit prevents both the escape and the inhalation of microorganisms around the edges of the mask and the fogging of eyeglasses.*
   - Wear the mask only once, and do not wear any mask longer than the manufacturer recommends or once it becomes wet. **Rationale:** *A mask should be used only once because it becomes ineffective when moist.*
   - Do not leave a used face mask hanging around the neck.
5. Don protective eyewear if it is not combined with the face mask.
6. Don clean disposable gloves.
   - No special technique is required.
   - If wearing a gown, pull the gloves up to cover the cuffs of the gown. If not wearing a gown, pull the gloves up to cover the wrists.
7. To remove soiled PPE, remove the gloves first since they are the most soiled.
   - If wearing a gown that is tied at the waist in front, undo the ties before removing gloves.
   - Remove the first glove by grasping it on its palmar surface, taking care to touch only glove to glove. ❸ **Rationale:** *This keeps the soiled parts of the used gloves from touching the skin of the wrist or hand.*
   - Pull the first glove completely off by inverting or rolling the glove inside out.
   - Continue to hold the inverted removed glove by the fingers of the remaining gloved hand. Place the first two fingers of the bare hand inside the cuff of the second glove. ❹ **Rationale:** *Touching the outside of the second soiled glove with the bare hand is avoided.*
   - Pull the second glove off to the fingers by turning it inside out. This pulls the first glove inside the second glove. **Rationale:** *The soiled part of the glove is folded to the inside to reduce the chance of transferring any microorganisms by direct contact.*

❷ A facemask and eye protection covering the nose, mouth, and eyes.

❸ Plucking the palmar surface below the cuff of a contaminated glove.

(Al Dodge, Pearson Education/PH College)

❹ Inserting fingers to remove the second contaminated glove.

(Al Dodge, Pearson Education/PH College)

DONNING AND REMOVING PERSONAL PROTECTIVE EQUIPMENT (GLOVES, GOWN, MASK, EYEWEAR) *continued*

- Using the bare hand, continue to remove the gloves, which are now inside out, and dispose of them in the refuse container. ⑤
8. Perform proper hand hygiene.
9. Remove protective eyewear and dispose of properly or place in the appropriate receptacle for cleaning.
10. Remove the gown when preparing to leave the room. Unless a gown is grossly soiled with body substances, no special precautions are needed to remove it. If a gown is grossly soiled:
    - Avoid touching soiled parts on the outside of the gown, if possible. **Rationale:** *The top part of the gown may be soiled, for example, if you have been holding an infant with a respiratory infection.*
    - Grasp the gown along the inside of the neck and pull down over the shoulders.
    - Roll up the gown with the soiled part inside, and discard it in the appropriate container.
11. Remove the mask.
    - Remove the mask at the doorway to the client's room. If using a respirator mask, remove it after leaving the room and closing the door.
    - If using a mask with strings, first untie the *lower* strings of the mask. **Rationale:** *This prevents the top part of the mask from falling onto the chest.*

⑤ Holding contaminated gloves, which are inside out.
(Al Dodge, Pearson Education/PH College)

- Untie the top strings and, while holding the ties securely, remove the mask from the face. If side loops are present, lift the side loops up and away from the ears and face. Do not touch the front of the mask. **Rationale:** *The front of the mask through which the nurse has been breathing is contaminated.*
- Discard a disposable mask in the waste container.
- Perform proper hand hygiene again.

EVALUATION

Conduct any follow-up indicated during your care of the client. If there has been any failure of the equipment and exposure to potentially infective materials is suspected, follow the procedure in the Practice Guidelines: Steps to Follow after Exposure to Bloodborne Pathogens later in this chapter.

Ensure that an adequate supply of equipment is available for the next health care provider.

HOME CARE CONSIDERATIONS Sterile Field

- Clean and wipe dry a flat surface for the sterile field.
- Keep pets and noninvolved small children out of the area when setting up for and performing sterile procedures.
- Dispose of all soiled materials in a waterproof bag. Check with the agency as to how to dispose of medical refuse.
- Remove all instruments from the home or other setting where others might accidentally find them. *New or used instruments can be sharp or capable of causing injury. Used instruments may transmit infection.* Check with the agency for instructions on cleansing of reusable supplies and disposal of single-use instruments.
- If appropriate, teach the client and family members the principles and rationale underlying the use of a sterile field.

Gowns

Clean or disposable impervious (water-resistant) gowns or plastic aprons are worn during procedures when the nurse's uniform is likely to become soiled. Sterile gowns may be indicated when the nurse changes the dressings of a client with extensive wounds (e.g., burns). *Single-use gown technique* (using a gown only once before it is discarded or laundered) is the usual practice in hospitals. After the gown is worn, the nurse discards it (if it is paper) or places it in a laundry hamper. See Skill 31-2. Before leaving the client's room, the nurse cleanses his or her hands.

CLINICAL ALERT

Wearing a client hospital gown over your uniform does not serve any infection control purpose. ■

Face Masks

Masks are worn to reduce the risk for transmission of organisms by the droplet contact and airborne routes, and by splatters of body substances. The CDC recommends that masks be worn:

1. By those close to the client if the infection (e.g., measles, mumps, or acute respiratory diseases in children) is

transmitted by large-particle aerosols (droplets). Large-particle aerosols are transmitted by close contact and generally travel short distances (about 1 m, or 3 ft).

2. By all persons entering the room if the infection (e.g., pulmonary tuberculosis and SARS-CoV) is transmitted by small-particle aerosols (droplet nuclei). Small-particle aerosols remain suspended in the air and thus travel greater distances by air. Special masks that provide a tighter face seal and better filtration may be used for these infections.

Various types of masks differ in their filtration effectiveness and fit. Single-use disposable surgical masks are effective for use while the nurse provides care to most clients but should be changed if they become wet or soiled. These masks are discarded in the waste container after use. Disposable particulate respirators of different types may be effective for droplet transmission, splatters, and airborne microorganisms. Some respirators now available are effective in preventing inhalation of tuberculin organisms. The National Institute for Occupational Safety and Health (NIOSH) tests and certifies such respirators. Currently, the category "N" respirator at 95% efficiency (referred to as an N95 respirator) meets tuberculosis and SARS control criteria.

During certain techniques requiring surgical asepsis (sterile technique), masks are worn (a) to prevent droplet contact transmission of exhaled microorganisms to the sterile field or to a client's open wound and (b) to protect the nurse from splashes of body substances from the client.

Guidelines for donning and removing face masks are shown in Skill 31-2.

Eyewear

Protective eyewear (goggles, glasses, or face shields) and masks are indicated in situations where body substances may splatter the face (see Skill 31-2). If the nurse wears prescription eyeglasses, goggles must still be worn over the glasses because the protection must extend around the sides of the glasses.

Disposal of Soiled Equipment and Supplies

Many pieces of equipment are supplied for single use only and are disposed of after use. Some items, however, are reusable. Agencies have specific policies and procedures for handling soiled equipment (e.g., disposal, cleaning, disinfecting, and sterilizing); the nurse needs to become familiar with these practices in the employing agency. Appropriate handling of soiled equipment and supplies is essential for these reasons:

- To prevent inadvertent exposure of health care workers to articles contaminated with body substances
- To prevent contamination of the environment

Bagging

Articles contaminated, or likely to have been contaminated, with infective material such as pus, blood, body fluids, feces, or respiratory secretions need to be enclosed in a sturdy bag impervious to microorganisms before they are removed from the room of any client. Some agencies use labels or bags of a particular color that designates them as infective wastes.

CDC guidelines recommend the following methods:

- A single bag, if it is sturdy and impervious to microorganisms, and if the contaminated articles can be placed in the bag without soiling or contaminating its outside
- Double-bagging if the above conditions are not met

Follow agency protocol, or use the following CDC guidelines to handle and bag soiled items:

- Place garbage and soiled *disposable* equipment, including dressings and tissues, in the plastic bag that lines the waste container. Some agencies separate dry and wet waste material and incinerate dry items, such as paper towels and disposable items. No special precautions are required for disposable equipment that is not contaminated.
- Place *nondisposable* or *reusable* equipment that is visibly soiled in a labeled bag before removing it from the client's room or cubicle, and send it to a central processing area for decontamination. Some agencies may require that glass bottles or jars and metal items be placed in separate bags from rubber and plastic items. Glass and metal can be sterilized in an autoclave, but rubber and plastic are damaged by this process and must be cleaned by other methods, such as gas sterilization.
- Disassemble special procedure trays into component parts. Some components are disposable; others need to be sent to the laundry or central services for cleaning and decontaminating.
- Bag soiled clothing before sending it home or to the agency laundry.

Linens

Handle soiled linen as little as possible and with the least agitation possible before placing it in the laundry hamper. This prevents gross microbial contamination of the air and persons handling the linen. Close the bag before sending it to the laundry in accordance with agency practice.

Laboratory Specimens

Laboratory specimens, if placed in a leakproof container with a secure lid with a biohazard label, need no special precautions. Use care when collecting specimens to avoid contaminating the outside of the container. Containers that are visibly contaminated on the outside should be placed inside a sealable plastic bag before sending them to the laboratory. This prevents personnel from having hand contact with potentially infective material.

Dishes

Dishes require no special precautions. Soiling of dishes can largely be prevented by encouraging clients to cleanse their hands before eating. Some agencies use paper dishes for convenience, which are disposed of in the refuse container.

Blood Pressure Equipment

Blood pressure equipment needs no special precautions unless it becomes contaminated with infective material. If it does become contaminated, follow agency policy to decontaminate it. Cleaning procedures vary according to whether it is a wall or portable unit. In some agencies, a disposable cuff is used for clients placed on contact precautions.

Thermometers

Nondisposable used thermometers are generally disinfected after use. Check agency practice.

Disposable Needles, Syringes, and Sharps

Place needles, syringes, and "sharps" (e.g., lancets, scalpels, and broken glass) into a puncture-resistant container. To avoid puncture wounds, use approved safety or needleless systems and do not detach needles from the syringe or recap the needle before disposal. See Chapter 35 for how to prevent needlestick injuries. ∞

CLINICAL ALERT

Federal rules protecting the privacy of personal health information may extend to the client labels placed on disposable supplies such as intravenous fluid containers. Agencies may require that these be returned to the pharmacy so that personal information may be removed before disposal. Check agency policy. ■

Transporting Clients with Infections

Transporting clients with infections outside their own rooms is avoided unless absolutely necessary. If a client must be moved, the nurse implements appropriate precautions and measures to prevent soilage of the environment. For example, the nurse ensures that any draining wound is securely covered or places a surgical mask on the client who has an airborne infection. In addition, the nurse notifies personnel at the receiving area of any infection risk so that they can maintain necessary precautions. Follow agency protocol.

Psychosocial Needs of Isolation Clients

Clients requiring isolation precautions can develop several problems as a result of the separation from others and of the special precautions taken in their care. Two of the most common are sensory deprivation and decreased self-esteem related to feelings of inferiority. *Sensory deprivation* occurs when the environment lacks normal stimuli for the client, for example, communication with others. Nurses should therefore be alert to common clinical signs of sensory deprivation: boredom, inactivity, slowness of thought, daydreaming, increased sleeping, thought disorganization, anxiety, hallucinations, and panic.

Chapter 39 ∞ provides information on the development of self-esteem and self-esteem disturbances. A client's *feeling of inferiority* can be due to the perception of the infection itself or to the required precautions. In North America, many people place a high value on cleanliness, and the idea of being "soiled," "contaminated," or "dirty" can give clients the feeling that they are at fault and substandard. Although this is obviously not true, the infected persons may feel "not as good" as others and blame themselves. An appropriate nursing diagnosis may be *Risk for Situational Low Self-Esteem.*

Nurses need to provide care that prevents these two problems or that deals with them positively. Nursing interventions include the following:

1. Assess the individual's need for stimulation.
2. Initiate measures to help meet the need, including regular communication with the client and diversionary activities, such as toys for a child, and books, television, or radio for an adult; provide a variety of foods to stimulate the client's sense of taste; stimulate the client's visual sense by providing a view or an activity to watch.
3. Explain the infection and the associated procedures to help clients and their support people understand and accept the situation.
4. Demonstrate warm, accepting behavior. Avoid conveying to the client any sense of annoyance about the precautions or any feelings of revulsion about the infection.
5. Do not use stricter precautions than are indicated by the diagnosis or the client's condition.

STERILE TECHNIQUE

An object is sterile only when it is free of all microorganisms. It is well known that sterile technique is practiced in operating rooms and special diagnostic areas. Less known perhaps is that sterile technique is also employed for many procedures in general care areas (such as administering injections, changing wound dressings, performing urinary catheterizations, and administering intravenous therapy). In these situations, all of the principles of surgical asepsis are applied as in the operating or delivery room; however, not all of the sterile techniques that follow are always required. For example, before an operating room procedure, the "scrub" nurse generally puts on a mask and cap, performs a surgical hand scrub, and then dons a sterile gown and gloves. In a general care area, the nurse may only perform hand cleansing and don sterile gloves. The basic principles of surgical asepsis, and practices that relate to each principle, appear in Table 31–9.

Sterile Field

A **sterile field** is a microorganism-free area. Nurses often establish a sterile field by using the innermost side of a sterile wrapper or by using a sterile drape. When the field is established, sterile supplies and sterile solutions can be placed on it. Sterile forceps are used in many instances to handle and transfer sterile supplies.

So that sterility can be maintained, supplies may be wrapped in a variety of materials. Commercially prepared items are frequently wrapped in plastic, paper, or glass. In the past, it was not unusual for sterile liquids (e.g., sterile water for irrigations) to be supplied in large containers and used many times. This practice is considered undesirable today because once a container has been opened, there can be no assurance that it will remain sterile. Liquids are preferably packaged in amounts adequate for one use only. Any leftover liquid is discarded.

Skill 31-3 describes how to establish and maintain a sterile field.

TABLE 31–9 Principles and Practices of Surgical Asepsis

PRINCIPLES	PRACTICES
All objects used in a sterile field must be sterile.	All articles are sterilized appropriately by dry or moist heat, chemicals, or radiation before use. Always check a package containing a sterile object for intactness, dryness, and expiration date. Sterile articles can be stored for only a prescribed time; after that, they are considered unsterile. Any package that appears already open, torn, punctured, or wet is considered unsterile. Storage areas should be clean, dry, off the floor, and away from sinks. Always check chemical indicators of sterilization before using a package. The indicator is often a tape used to fasten the package or contained inside the package. The indicator changes color during sterilization, indicating that the contents have undergone a sterilization procedure. If the color change is not evident, the package is considered unsterile. Commercially prepared sterile packages may not have indicators but are marked with the word *sterile*.
Sterile objects become unsterile when touched by unsterile objects.	Handle sterile objects that will touch open wounds or enter body cavities only with sterile forceps or sterile gloved hands. Discard or resterilize objects that come into contact with unsterile objects. Whenever the sterility of an object is questionable, assume the article is unsterile.
Sterile items that are out of vision or below the waist or table level are considered unsterile.	Once left unattended, a sterile field is considered unsterile. Sterile objects are always kept in view. Nurses do not turn their backs on a sterile field. Only the front part of a sterile gown, from shoulder to waist (or table height, whichever is higher), and the cuff of the sleeves to 2 inches above the elbows are considered sterile. Always keep sterile gloved hands in sight and above waist/table level; touch only objects that are sterile. Sterile draped tables in the operating room or elsewhere are considered sterile only at surface level.
Sterile objects can become unsterile by prolonged exposure to airborne microorganisms.	Keep doors closed and traffic to a minimum in areas where a sterile procedure is being performed, because moving air can carry dust and microorganisms. Keep areas in which sterile procedures are carried out as clean as possible by frequent damp cleaning with detergent germicides to minimize contaminants in the area. Keep hair clean and short or enclose it in a net to prevent hair from falling on sterile objects. Microorganisms on the hair can make a sterile field unsterile. Wear surgical caps in operating rooms, delivery rooms, and burn units. Refrain from sneezing or coughing over a sterile field. This can make it unsterile because droplets containing microorganisms from the respiratory tract can travel 1 m (3 ft). Some agencies recommend that masks covering the mouth and the nose should be worn by anyone working over a sterile field or an open wound. Nurses with mild upper respiratory tract infections refrain from carrying out sterile procedures or wear masks. When working over a sterile field, keep talking to a minimum. Avert the head from the field if talking is necessary. To prevent microorganisms from falling over a sterile field, refrain from reaching over a sterile field unless sterile gloves are worn and refrain from moving unsterile objects over a sterile field.
Fluids flow in the direction of gravity.	Unless gloves are worn, always hold wet forceps with the tips below the handles. When the tips are held higher than the handles, fluid can flow onto the handle and become contaminated by the hands. When the forceps are again pointed downward, the contaminated fluid flows back down and contaminates the tips. During a surgical hand wash, hold the hands higher than the elbows to prevent contaminants from the forearms from reaching the hands.
Moisture that passes through a sterile object draws microorganisms from unsterile surfaces above or below to the sterile surface by capillary action. The edges of a sterile field are considered unsterile.	Sterile moisture-proof barriers are used beneath sterile objects. Liquids (sterile saline or antiseptics) are frequently poured into containers on a sterile field. If they are spilled onto the sterile field, the barrier keeps the liquid from seeping beneath it. Keep the sterile covers on sterile equipment dry. Damp surfaces can attract microorganisms in the air. Replace sterile drapes that do not have a sterile barrier underneath when they become moist. A 2.5-cm (1-in.) margin at each edge of an opened drape is considered unsterile because the edges are in contact with unsterile surfaces. Place all sterile objects more than 2.5 cm (1 in.) inside the edges of a sterile field. Any article that falls outside the edges of a sterile field is considered unsterile.
The skin cannot be sterilized and is unsterile.	Use sterile gloves or sterile forceps to handle sterile items. Prior to a surgical aseptic procedure, cleanse the hands to reduce the number of microorganisms on them.
Conscientiousness, alertness, and honesty are essential qualities in maintaining surgical asepsis.	When a sterile object becomes unsterile, it does not necessarily change in appearance. The person who sees a sterile object become contaminated must correct or report the situation. Do not set up a sterile field ahead of time for future use.

ESTABLISHING AND MAINTAINING A STERILE FIELD

PURPOSES
▨ To ensure that sterile items remain sterile

ASSESSMENT

Review the client's record or discuss with the client or other health care team member exactly what procedure will be performed that requires a sterile field. Determine the client's presence or risk for infection and ability to cooperate with the procedure.

PLANNING

Determine, if possible, what supplies and techniques have been used in the past to perform the procedures for this client. Also, attempt to determine if the procedure will be performed again in the future, so appropriate client teaching can be done and adequate supplies will be available.

Schedule the procedure at a time consistent with the order, the need for the procedure, and the client's other activities.

Delegation
Sterile procedures are not delegated to UAP in most states.

Equipment
▨ Package containing a sterile drape
▨ Sterile equipment as needed (e.g., wrapped sterile gauze, wrapped sterile bowl, antiseptic solution, sterile forceps)

IMPLEMENTATION

Preparation

▨ Ensure that the package is clean and dry; if moisture is noted on the inside of a plastic-wrapped package or the outside of a cloth-wrapped package, it is considered contaminated and must be discarded.
▨ Check the sterilization expiration dates on the package, and look for any indications that it has been previously opened. Spots or stains on cloth or paper-wrapped objects may indicate contamination, and the objects should not be used.
▨ Follow agency practice for disposal of possibly contaminated packages.

Performance

1. Prior to performing the procedure, introduce self and verify the client's identity using agency protocol. Explain to the client what you are going to do, why it is necessary, and how he or she can cooperate. Discuss how the results will be used in planning further care or treatments.
2. Observe other appropriate infection control procedures (see Skills 31-1 and 31-2).
3. Provide for client privacy.
4. Open the package. If the package is inside a plastic cover, remove the cover.

   To Open a Wrapped Package on a Surface
   • Place the package in the work area so that the top flap of the wrapper opens away from you.
   • Reaching around the package (not over it), pinch the first flap on the outside of the wrapper between the thumb and index finger. ❶ **Rationale:** *Touching only the outside of the wrapper maintains the sterility of the inside of the wrapper.* Pull the flap open, laying it flat on the far surface.
   • Repeat for the side flaps, opening the top one first. Use the right hand for the right flap, and the left hand for the left flap. ❷ **Rationale:** *By using both hands, you avoid reaching over the sterile contents.*

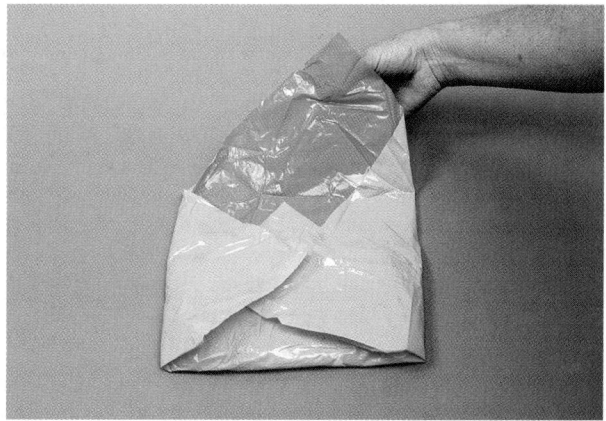

❶ Opening the first flap of a sterile wrapped package.
(Al Dodge, Pearson Education/PH College)

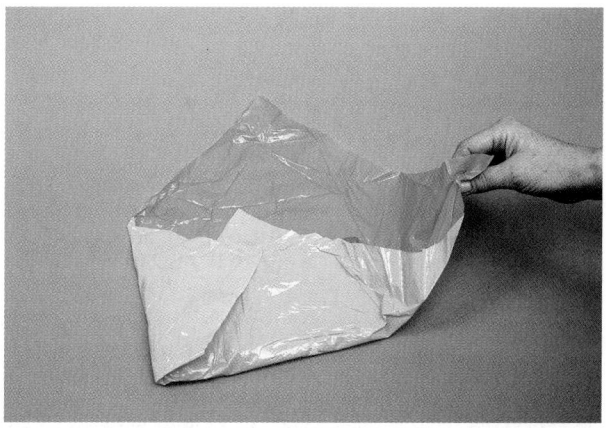

❷ Opening the second flap to the side.
(Al Dodge, Pearson Education/PH College)

continued on page 698

SKILL 31-3

ESTABLISHING AND MAINTAINING A STERILE FIELD *continued*

❸ Pulling the last flap toward oneself by grasping the corner.
(Al Dodge, Pearson Education/PH College)

❹ Opening a wrapped package while holding it.
(Al Dodge, Pearson Education/PH College)

- Pull the fourth flap toward you by grasping the corner that is turned down. ❸ Make sure that the flap does not touch any object. **Rationale:** *If the inner surface touches any unsterile article, it is contaminated.*

Variation: Opening a Wrapped Package While Holding It
- Hold the package in one hand with the top flap opening away from you.
- Using the other hand, open the package as described above, pulling the corners of the flaps well back. ❹ Tuck each of the corners into the hand holding the package so that they do not flutter and contaminate sterile objects. **Rationale:** *The hands are considered contaminated, and at no time should they touch the contents of the package.*

Variation: Opening Commercially Prepared Packages
- If the flap of the package has an unsealed corner, hold the container in one hand, and pull back on the flap with the other hand. ❺
- If the package has a partially sealed edge, grasp both sides of the edge, one with each hand, and pull apart gently. ❻

5. Establish a sterile field by using a drape.
   - Open the package containing the drape as described above.
   - With one hand, pluck the corner of the drape that is folded back on the top touching only one side of the drape.

❺ Opening a sterile package that has an unsealed corner.

- Lift the drape out of the cover, and allow it to open freely without touching any articles. ❼ **Rationale:** *If the drape touches the outside of the package or any unsterile surface, it is considered contaminated.*
- With the other hand, carefully pick up another corner of the drape, holding it well away from you, and again, touching only the same side of the drape as the first hand.

❻ Opening a sterile package that has a partially sealed edge.

❼ Allowing a drape to open freely without touching any objects.
(Patrick Watson)

ESTABLISHING AND MAINTAINING A STERILE FIELD *continued*

- Lay the drape on a clean and dry surface, placing the bottom (i.e., the freely hanging side) farthest from you. ❽ **Rationale:** *By placing the lowermost side farthest away, you avoid leaning over the sterile field and contaminating it.*
6. Add necessary sterile supplies, being careful not to touch the drape with the hands.

To Add Wrapped Supplies to a Sterile Field
- Open each wrapped package as described in the preceding steps.
- With the free hand, grasp the corners of the wrapper, and hold them against the wrist of the other hand. ❾ **Rationale:** *The sterile wrapper now covers the unsterile hand.*
- Place the sterile bowl, drape, or other supply on the sterile field by approaching from an angle rather than holding the arm over the field.
- Discard the wrapper.

Variation: Adding Commercially Packaged Supplies to a Sterile Field
- Open each package as previously described.
- Hold the package 15 cm (6 in.) above the field, and allow the contents to drop on the field. ❿ Keep in mind that 2.5 cm (1 in.) around the edge of the field is considered contaminated. **Rationale:** *At a height of 15 cm (6 in.), the outside of the package is not likely to touch and contaminate the sterile field.*

Adding Solution to a Sterile Bowl
7. Liquids (e.g., normal saline) may need to be poured into containers within a sterile field. Unwrapped bottles that contain sterile solution are considered sterile on the inside and contaminated on the outside because the bottle may have been handled. Bottles used in an operating room may be sterilized on the outside as well as the inside, however, and these are handled with sterile gloves.
- Before pouring any liquid, read the label three times to make sure you have the correct solution and concentration (strength). Wipe the outside of the bottle with a damp towel to remove any large particles that could fall into the bowl or field.
- Obtain the exact amount of solution, if possible. **Rationale:** *Once a sterile bottle has been opened, its sterility cannot be ensured for future use.* Follow agency policy for reuse of opened sterile solution bottles.

- Remove the lid or cap from the bottle and invert the lid before placing it on a surface that is not sterile. **Rationale:** *Inverting the lid maintains the sterility of the inside surface because it is not allowed to touch an unsterile surface.*
- Hold the bottle at a slight angle so that the label is uppermost. ⓫ **Rationale:** *Any solution that flows down the outside of the bottle during pouring will not damage or obliterate the label.*

❾ Adding wrapped sterile supplies to a sterile field.

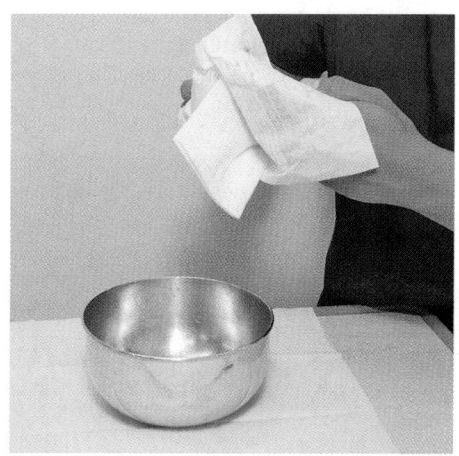

❿ Adding commercially packaged gauze to a sterile field.
(Patrick Watson)

❽ Placing a drape on a surface.
(Patrick Watson)

⓫ Adding a liquid to a sterile bowl.
(Patrick Watson)

continued on page 700

SKILL 31-3

ESTABLISHING AND MAINTAINING A STERILE FIELD *continued*

- Hold the bottle of fluid at a height of 10 to 15 cm (4 to 6 in.) over the bowl and to the side of the sterile field so that as little of the bottle as possible is over the field. **Rationale:** *At this height, there is less likelihood of contaminating the sterile field by touching the field or by reaching an arm over it.*
- Pour the solution gently to avoid splashing the liquid. **Rationale:** *If a barrier drape (one that has a water-resistant layer) is not used and the drape is on an unsterile surface, moisture will contaminate the field by wicking microorganisms through the drape.*
- Tilt the neck of the bottle back to vertical quickly when done pouring so that none of the liquid flows down the outside of the bottle. **Rationale:** *Such drips would contaminate the sterile field if the outside of the bottle is not sterile.*
- If the bottle will be used again, replace the lid securely and write on the label the date and time of opening. **Rationale:** *Replacing the lid immediately maintains the sterility of the inner aspect of the lid and the solution.*
- Depending on agency policy, a sterile container of solution that is opened may be used only once and is then discarded (such as in the operating room). In other settings, policy may permit recapped bottles to be reused within 24 hours.

8. Use sterile forceps to handle sterile supplies. Forceps are usually used to move a sterile article from one place to another, for example, transferring sterile gauze from its package to a sterile dressing tray. Forceps may be disposable or resterilized after use. Commonly used forceps include hemostats ❶❷ and tissue forceps. ❶❸
   - If forceps tips are wet, keep the tips lower than the wrist at all times, unless you are wearing sterile gloves. ❶❹ **Rationale:** *Gravity prevents liquids on the tips of the forceps from flowing to the unsterile handles and later back to the tips.*
   - Hold sterile forceps above waist or table level, whichever is higher. **Rationale:** *Items held below waist or table level are considered contaminated.*

- Hold sterile forceps within sight. **Rationale:** *While out of sight, forceps may, unknown to the user, become unsterile. Any forceps that go out of sight should be considered unsterile.*
- When using forceps to lift sterile supplies, be sure that the forceps do not touch the edges or outside of the wrapper. **Rationale:** *The edges and outside of the sterile field are considered unsterile.*
- When placing forceps whose handles were in contact with the bare hand, position the handles outside the sterile area. **Rationale:** *The handles of these forceps harbor microorganisms from the bare hand.*
- Deposit a sterile item on a sterile field without permitting moist forceps to touch the sterile field when the surface under the absorbent sterile field is unsterile and a barrier drape is not used.

9. Document that sterile technique was used in the performance of the procedure.

❶❸ Tissue forceps: *A,* plain; *B,* toothed.

(Alexandra Truitt &
Terry Marshall)

❶❹ Holding forceps with an ungloved hand, keeping the tips lower than the wrist.

(Al Dodge, Pearson Education/PH College)

❶❷ Hemostats: *A,* straight; *B,* curved.

(Alexandra Truitt & Terry Marshall)

EVALUATION

Conduct any follow-up indicated during your care of the client. Ensure that adequate numbers and types of sterile supplies are available for the next health care provider.

Sterile Gloves

Sterile gloves may be donned by the open method or the closed method. The open method is most frequently used outside the operating room because the closed method requires that the nurse wear a sterile gown. Gloves are worn during many procedures to maintain the sterility of equipment and to protect a client's wound.

Sterile gloves are packaged with a cuff of about 5 cm (2 in.) and with the palms facing upward when the package is opened. The package usually indicates the size of the glove (e.g., size 6 or 7½).

Latex and latex-free (e.g., nitrile and vinyl) sterile gloves are available to protect the nurse from contact with blood and body fluids. Latex and nitrile are more flexible than vinyl, mold to the wearer's hands, allow freedom of movement, and have the added feature of resealing tiny punctures automatically. Therefore, wear latex or nitrile gloves when performing tasks (a) that demand flexibility, (b) that place stress on the material (e.g., turning stopcocks, handling sharp instruments or tape), and (c) that involve a high risk of exposure to pathogens. Vinyl gloves should be chosen for tasks unlikely to stress the glove material, requiring minimal precision, and with minimal risk of exposure to pathogens.

Skill 31-4 describes how to don and remove sterile gloves by the open method.

SKILL 31-4

DONNING AND REMOVING STERILE GLOVES (OPEN METHOD)

PURPOSES
- To enable the nurse to handle or touch sterile objects freely without contaminating them
- To prevent transmission of potentially infective organisms from the nurse's hands to clients at high risk for infection

ASSESSMENT
Review the client's record and orders to determine exactly what procedure will be performed that requires sterile gloves. Check the client record and ask about latex allergies. Use nonlatex gloves whenever possible.

PLANNING
Think through the procedure, planning which steps need to be completed before the gloves can be applied. Determine what additional supplies are needed to perform the procedure for this client. Always have an extra pair of sterile gloves available.

Delegation
Sterile procedures are not delegated to UAP in most states.

Equipment
- Packages of sterile gloves

IMPLEMENTATION
Preparation
Ensure the sterility of the package of gloves.

Performance
1. Prior to performing the procedure, introduce self and verify the client's identity using agency protocol. Explain to the client what you are going to do, why it is necessary, and how he or she can cooperate. Discuss how the results will be used in planning further care or treatments.
2. Observe other appropriate infection control procedures (see Skills 31-1, 31-2, and 31-3).
3. Provide for client privacy.
4. Open the package of sterile gloves.
   - Place the package of gloves on a clean, dry surface. **Rationale:** *Any moisture on the surface could contaminate the gloves.*
   - Some gloves are packed in an inner as well as an outer package. Open the outer package without contaminating the gloves or the inner package. See Skill 31-3.
   - Remove the inner package from the outer package.
   - Open the inner package as in step 4 of Skill 31-3 or according to the manufacturer's directions. Some manufacturers provide a numbered sequence for opening the flaps and folded tabs to grasp for opening the flaps. If no tabs are provided, pluck the flap so that the fingers do not touch the inner surfaces. **Rationale:** *The inner surfaces, which are next to the sterile gloves, will remain sterile.*
5. Put the first glove on the dominant hand.
   - If the gloves are packaged so that they lie side by side, grasp the glove for the dominant hand by its folded cuff edge (on the palmar side) with the thumb and first finger of the nondominant hand. Touch only the inside of the cuff. **❶ Rationale:** *The hands are not sterile. By touching only the inside of the glove, the nurse avoids contaminating the outside.*

❶ Picking up the first sterile glove.
(Al Dodge, Pearson Education/PH)

continued on page 702

DONNING AND REMOVING STERILE GLOVES (OPEN METHOD) *continued*

or

- If the gloves are packaged one on top of the other, grasp the cuff of the top glove as above, using the opposite hand.
- Insert the dominant hand into the glove and pull the glove on. Keep the thumb of the inserted hand against the palm of the hand during insertion. ❷ **Rationale:** *If the thumb is kept against the palm, it is less likely to contaminate the outside of the glove.*
- Leave the cuff in place once the unsterile hand releases the glove. **Rationale:** *Attempting to further unfold the cuff is likely to contaminate the glove.*

6. Put the second glove on the nondominant hand.
    - Pick up the other glove with the sterile gloved hand, inserting the gloved fingers under the cuff and holding the gloved thumb close to the gloved palm. ❸ **Rationale:** *This helps prevent accidental contamination of the glove by the bare hand.*
    - Pull on the second glove carefully. Hold the thumb of the gloved first hand as far as possible from the palm. ❹ **Rationale:** *In this position, the thumb is less likely to touch the arm and become contaminated.*
    - Adjust each glove so that it fits smoothly, and carefully pull the cuffs up by sliding the fingers under the cuffs.

7. Remove and dispose of used gloves.

- There is no technique for removing sterile gloves that is different from removing unsterile gloves. If they are soiled with secretions, remove them by turning them inside out. See removal of disposable gloves in Skill 31-2 on page 692.

8. Document that sterile technique was used in the performance of the procedure.

❸ Picking up the second sterile glove.
(Al Dodge, Pearson Education/PH College)

❷ Putting on the first sterile glove.
(Al Dodge, Pearson Education/PH College)

❹ Putting on the second sterile glove.
(Al Dodge, Pearson Education/PH College)

EVALUATION
Conduct any follow-up indicated during your care of the client. Ensure that adequate numbers and types of sterile supplies are available for the next health care provider.

Sterile Gowns

Sterile gowning and closed gloving are chiefly carried out in operating or delivery rooms, where surgical asepsis is necessary. The closed method of gloving can be used only when a sterile gown is worn because the gloves are handled through the sleeves of the gown. Before these procedures, the nurse dons a hair cover and a mask, and performs a surgical hand wash.

Skill 31-5 describes the steps in donning a sterile gown and sterile gloves by the closed method.

DONNING A STERILE GOWN AND GLOVES (CLOSED METHOD)

PURPOSES
- To enable the nurse to work close to a sterile field and handle sterile objects freely
- To protect clients from becoming contaminated with microorganisms on the nurse's hands, arms, and clothing

ASSESSMENT
Review the client's record and orders to determine exactly what procedure will be performed that requires sterile gloves. Check the client record and ask about latex allergies. Use nonlatex gloves whenever possible.

PLANNING
Think through the procedure, planning which steps need to be completed before the gloves and gown can be applied. Determine what additional supplies are needed to perform the procedure for this client. Always have an extra pair of sterile gloves available.

Equipment
- Sterile pack containing a sterile gown
- Sterile gloves

Delegation
Sterile procedures are not delegated to UAP in most states.

IMPLEMENTATION

Preparation
Ensure the sterility of the package of gloves.

Performance
1. Prior to performing the procedure, introduce self and verify the client's identity using agency protocol. Explain to the client what you are going to do, why it is necessary, and how he or she can cooperate. Discuss how the results will be used in planning further care or treatments.
2. Observe other appropriate infection control procedures (see Skills 31-1, 31-2, and 31-3).
3. Provide for client privacy.

Donning a Sterile Gown
4. Open the package of sterile gloves.
   - Remove the outer wrap from the sterile gloves and leave the gloves in their inner sterile wrap on the sterile field. **Rationale:** *If the inner wrapper is not touched, it will remain sterile. See Skill 31-3, step 4.*
5. Unwrap the sterile gown pack.
6. Perform proper hand hygiene.
     See "Variation" at the end of Skill 31-1 and review agency practice.
7. Put on the sterile gown.
   - Grasp the sterile gown at the crease near the neck, hold it away from you, and permit it to unfold freely without touching anything, including the uniform. **Rationale:** *The gown will be unsterile if its outer surface touches any unsterile objects.*
   - Put the hands inside the shoulders of the gown without touching the outside of the gown. ❶
   - If donning sterile gloves by using the closed method (see below), work the hands down the sleeves only to the beginning of the cuffs.
       or
   - If donning sterile gloves by using the open method, work the hands down the sleeves and through the cuffs.
   - Have a co-worker grasp the neck ties without touching the outside of the gown and pull the gown upward to cover the neckline of your uniform in front and back. The co-worker ties the neck ties. Gowning continues at step 11.

Donning Sterile Gloves (Closed Method)
8. Open the sterile glove wrapper while the hands are still covered by the sleeves. ❷

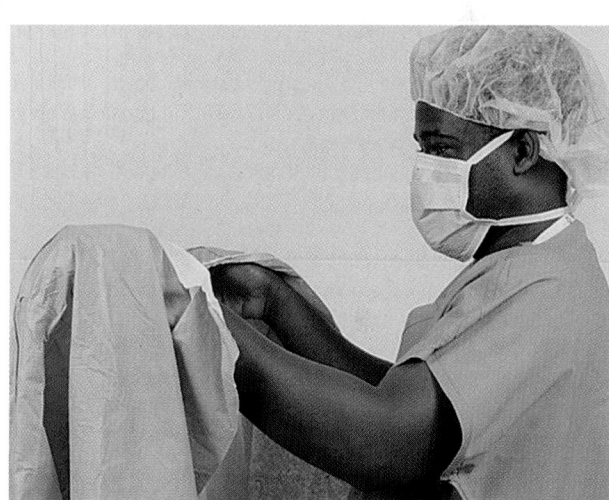

❶ Putting on a sterile gown.

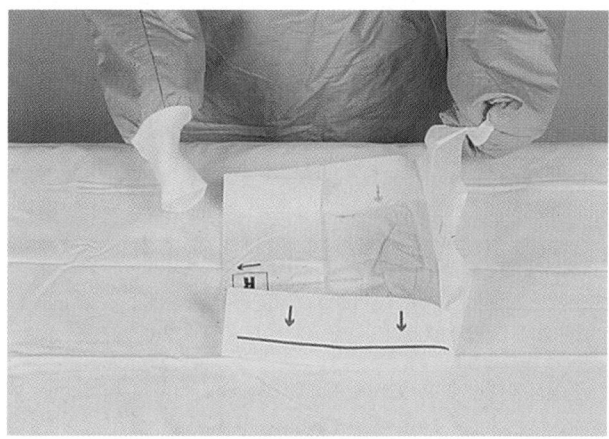

❷ Opening the sterile glove wrapper.

continued on page 704

DONNING A STERILE GOWN AND GLOVES (CLOSED METHOD) *continued*

9. Put the glove on the nondominant hand. Figures ❸ through ❺ show a right-handed person.
   - With the dominant hand, pick up the opposite glove with the thumb and index finger, handling it through the sleeve.
   - Position the dominant hand palm upward inside the sleeve. Lay the glove on the opposite gown cuff, thumb side down, with the glove opening pointed toward the fingers. ❸
   - Use the nondominant hand to grasp the cuff of the glove through the gown cuff, and firmly anchor it.
   - With the dominant hand working through its sleeve, grasp the upper side of the glove's cuff, and stretch it over the cuff of the gown.
   - Pull the sleeve up to draw the cuff over the wrist as you extend the fingers of the nondominant hand into the glove's fingers. ❹
10. Put the glove on the dominant hand.
    - Place the fingers of the gloved hand under the cuff of the remaining glove.
    - Place the glove over the cuff of the second sleeve.
    - Extend the fingers into the glove as you pull the glove up over the cuff. ❺

Completion of Gowning

11. Complete gowning as follows.
    - Have a co-worker hold the waist tie of your gown, using sterile gloves or a sterile forceps or drape. **Rationale:** *This approach keeps the ties sterile.*
    - Make a three-quarter turn, then take the tie and secure it in front of the gown.
      or
    - Have a co-worker take the two ties at each side of the gown and tie them at the back of the gown, making sure that your uniform is completely covered.
    - When worn, sterile gowns should be considered sterile in front from the waist to the shoulder. Once the nurse approaches a table, the gown is considered contaminated from the waist or table down, whichever is higher. The sleeves should be considered sterile from the cuff to 2 inches above the elbow, since the arms of a scrubbed person must move across a sterile field. Moisture collection and friction areas such as the neckline, shoulders, underarms, back, and sleeve cuffs should be considered unsterile.
12. Remove and dispose of used gown and gloves.
    - If soiled, remove the attire by turning it inside out. See removal of disposable gowns and gloves in Skill 31-2 for the sequence of when to remove the gown.
13. If appropriate, document that sterile technique was used in the performance of the procedure.

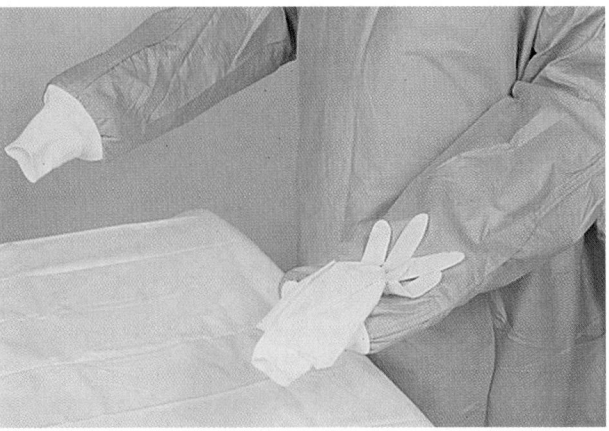

❸ Positioning the first sterile glove for the nondominant hand.

❹ Pulling on the first sterile glove.

❺ Extending the fingers into the second glove of the dominant hand.

EVALUATION

Conduct any follow-up indicated during your care of the client. Ensure that adequate numbers and types of sterile supplies are available for the next health care provider.

INFECTION CONTROL FOR HEALTH CARE WORKERS

NIOSH is part of the CDC and is a research agency of the U.S. Department of Health and Human Services. NIOSH investigates potentially hazardous working conditions and publishes recommendations for preventing workplace illnesses and injuries. For example, NIOSH published a study on preventing needlestick injuries in health care settings in 1999 that found that the majority of needlestick injuries were preventable. This, in part, led to the Needlestick Safety and Prevention Act that went into effect in April 2001.

The Occupational Safety and Health Administration (OSHA), an agency of the U.S. Department of Labor, publishes and enforces regulations to protect health care workers from occupational injuries, including exposure to bloodborne pathogens in the workplace. **Occupational exposure** is defined as skin, eye, mucous membrane, or parenteral contact with blood or other potentially infectious materials that may result from the performance of an employee's duties.

There are three major modes of transmission of infectious materials in the clinical setting:

■ Puncture wounds from contaminated needles or other sharps
■ Skin contact, which allows infectious fluids to enter through wounds and broken or damaged skin
■ Mucous membrane contact, which allows infectious fluids to enter through mucous membranes of the eyes, mouth, or nose

Using proper precautions with general medical asepsis, appropriately using PPE (gloves, masks, gowns, goggles, special resuscitative equipment), and avoiding carelessness in the clinical area will place the caregiver at significantly less risk for injury. The chance of a health care worker becoming infected following exposure to pathogens varies widely—estimates range from 30% for hepatitis B (nonimmune workers), to 1.8% for hepatitis C, to 0.3% for HIV (CDC, 2003). Measures to be taken in case of possible exposure to these viruses are delineated by the CDC and outlined in the accompanying Practice Guidelines feature. Hepatitis C, a worldwide epidemic greater than HIV, has become a significant concern to all health care workers since there is currently no vaccine against the virus or postexposure prophylaxis. Prevention remains the primary goal.

OSHA requires that health care employers make the hepatitis B vaccine and vaccination series available to all employees. Other vaccinations may also be made available (e.g., nurses working in an obstetric area should be vaccinated against rubella to protect pregnant clients and their fetuses).

CLINICAL ALERT

The nurse should consider in advance whether he or she would want prophylaxis for HIV exposure since this is optimally begun within 1 hour of exposure. ■

PRACTICE GUIDELINES Steps to Follow after Exposure to Bloodborne Pathogens

■ Report the incident immediately to appropriate personnel within the agency.
■ Complete an injury report.
■ Seek appropriate evaluation and follow-up. This includes:
  • Identification and documentation of the source individual when feasible and legal.
  • Testing of the source for hepatitis B, hepatitis C, and HIV when feasible and consent is given.
  • Making results of the test available to the source individual's health care provider.
  • Testing of blood of exposed nurse (with consent) for hepatitis B, hepatitis C, and HIV antibodies.
  • Postexposure prophylaxis if medically indicated.
  • Medical and psychologic counseling regarding personal risk of infection or risk of infecting others.
■ For a puncture/laceration:
  • Encourage bleeding.
  • Wash/clean the area with soap and water.
  • Initiate first-aid and seek treatment if indicated.
  • For a mucous membrane exposure (eyes, nose, mouth), saline or water flush for 5 to 10 minutes.

POSTEXPOSURE PROTOCOL (PEP)

HIV
■ Treatment should be started as soon as possible, preferably within hours after exposure. Treatment may be less effective

when started more than 24 hours after exposure. Starting treatment after a longer period (e.g., 1 week) should be considered for high-risk exposures previously untreated.
■ For "high-risk" exposure (high blood volume *and* source with a high HIV titer): three-drug treatment is recommended.
■ For "increased risk" exposure (high blood volume *or* source with a high HIV titer): three-drug treatment is recommended.
■ For "low-risk" exposure (neither high blood volume nor source with a high HIV titer): two-drug treatment is considered.
■ Drug prophylaxis continues for 4 weeks.
■ Drug regimens vary and new drugs and regimens are continuously being developed.
■ HIV antibody tests should be done shortly after exposure (baseline), and 6 weeks, 3 months, and 6 months afterward.

Hepatitis B
■ Anti-HBs testing 1 to 2 months after last vaccine dose.
■ HBIG and/or hepatitis B vaccine within 1 to 7 days following exposure for nonimmune workers.

Hepatitis C
■ Anti-HCV and ALT at baseline and 4 to 6 months after exposure.

ROLE OF THE INFECTION CONTROL NURSE

All health care organizations must have interdisciplinary infection control committees. Representatives from the clinical laboratory, housekeeping, maintenance, dietary, and client care areas are included. An important member of this committee is the infection control nurse. This nurse is specially trained to be knowledgeable about the latest research and practices in preventing, detecting, and treating infections. All infections are reported to the nurse in a manner that allows for recording and analyzing statistics that can assist in improving infection control practices. In addition, the infection control nurse may be involved in employee education and implementation of the bloodborne pathogen exposure control plan mandated by OSHA.

EVALUATING

Using data collected during care—vital signs, lung sounds, skin status, characteristics of urine or other drainage, laboratory blood values, and so on—the nurse judges whether client outcomes have been achieved. Examples of client outcomes and indicators are shown in Identifying Nursing Diagnoses, Outcomes, and Interventions on page 681.

If outcomes are not achieved, the nurse may need to consider questions such as the following:

- Were appropriate measures implemented to prevent skin breakdown and lung infection?
- Was strict aseptic technique implemented for invasive procedures?
- Are prescribed medications affecting the immune system?
- Is client placement appropriate to reduce the risk of transmission of microorganisms?
- Did the client and family misunderstand or fail to comply with necessary instructions?

CRITICAL THINKING CHECKPOINT

Mrs. Cortez is a 76-year-old woman who is independent, lives alone, and prefers not to rely on others unless absolutely necessary. She was active and healthy until about 6 months ago, at which time she developed a persistent upper respiratory infection. Because she was unable to obtain or prepare foods, she lost weight and became very weak. She finally sought medical attention, but she has not yet fully recovered. Her primary care provider has admitted Mrs. Cortez to the acute care facility for shortness of breath, productive cough, dehydration, and nutritional deficiency.

1. Mrs. Cortez's primary care provider suspects that Mrs. Cortez has pneumonia. What data support Mrs. Cortez's increased risk for such an infection?
2. What other information or assessment data would be helpful to you when planning care for Mrs. Cortez?
3. You recognize that standard precautions are instituted for all hospitalized clients. Explain why the use of such precautions may not prevent the spread of Mrs. Cortez's respiratory infection to other susceptible clients.
4. What can you do to prevent the spread of Mrs. Cortez's infection to other hospitalized clients and at the same time prevent Mrs. Cortez from getting infections from other clients?
5. You see the nursing assistant leaving Mrs. Cortez's room. The assistant stops to wash her hands. She turns on the water handles and soaps and rubs her hands together under running water for about 5 seconds. She then turns off the faucets with her bare hands and proceeds with drying her hands. Should you intervene and, if so, what should you do?

See Critical Thinking Possibilities in Appendix A.

CHAPTER 31 REVIEW

CHAPTER HIGHLIGHTS

- Microorganisms are everywhere. Most are harmless and some are beneficial; however, many can cause infection in susceptible persons.
- Effective control of infectious disease is an international, national, community, and individual responsibility.
- Asepsis is the freedom from infection or infectious material.
- Medical aseptic practices limit the number, growth, and transmission of microorganisms.
- Surgical aseptic practices keep an area or objects free of all microorganisms.
- The incidence of nosocomial infections is significant. Major sites for these infections are the respiratory and urinary tracts, the bloodstream, and wounds.
- Factors that contribute to nosocomial infection risks are invasive procedures, medical therapies, the existence of a large number of susceptible persons, inappropriate use of antibiotics, and insufficient hand cleansing after client contact and after contact with body substances.
- An infection can develop if the links in the chain of infection—infectious agent, reservoir, portal of exit, mode of transmission, portal of entry, and susceptible host—are not interrupted.
- Intact skin and mucous membranes are the body's first line of defense against microorganisms.
- Some normal body flora release bacteriocins and antibiotic-like substances that inhibit microbial growth and destroy foreign bacteria.
- Some body secretions (e.g., saliva and tears) contain enzymes that act as antibacterial agents.
- The inflammatory response limits physical, chemical, and microbial injury and promotes repair of injured tissue.

- Immunity is the specific resistance of the body to infectious agents.
- Acquired immunity is active or passive and in either case may be naturally or artificially induced.
- Especially at risk of acquiring an infection are the very young or old; those with poor nutritional status, a deficiency of serum immunoglobulins, multiple stressors, insufficient immunizations, or an existing disease process; and those receiving certain medical therapies.
- Preventing infections in healthy or ill persons and preventing the transmission of microorganisms from infected clients to others are major nursing functions.

- The nurse must be knowledgeable about sources and modes of transmission of microorganisms.
- Microorganisms are invisible, and nurses have an ethical obligation to ensure that appropriate aseptic measures are taken to protect clients, support people, and health personnel, including themselves.
- All health care providers must apply clean or sterile gloves, gowns, masks, and protective eyewear according to the risk of exposure to potentially infective materials.
- Should a health care worker be exposed to substances with high risk of transmitting bloodborne pathogens, postexposure practices and consideration of prophylactic treatment must be followed immediately.

TEST YOUR KNOWLEDGE

1. The client is a chronic carrier of infection. To prevent the spread of the infection to other clients or health care providers, the nurse emphasizes interventions that do which of the following?
   1. Eliminate the reservoir.
   2. Block the portal of exit from the reservoir.
   3. Block the portal of entry into the host.
   4. Decrease the susceptibility of the host.

2. The most effective nursing action for controlling the spread of infection includes which of the following?
   1. Thorough hand cleansing
   2. Wearing gloves and masks when providing direct client care
   3. Implementing appropriate isolation precautions
   4. Administering broad-spectrum prophylactic antibiotics

3. In caring for a client on contact precautions for a draining infected foot ulcer, the nurse should perform which of the following?
   1. Wear a mask during dressing changes
   2. Provide disposable meal trays and silverware
   3. Follow standard precautions in all interactions with the client
   4. Use surgical aseptic technique for all direct contact with the client

4. When caring for a single client during one shift, it is appropriate for the nurse to reuse which of the following personal protective equipment?
   1. Goggles
   2. Gown
   3. Surgical mask
   4. Clean gloves

5. While donning sterile gloves (open method), the cuff of the first glove rolls under itself about 1/4 inch. The best action for the nurse is to
   1. Remove the glove and start over with a new pair.
   2. Wait until the second glove is in place and then unroll the cuff with the other sterile hand.
   3. Ask a colleague to assist by unrolling the cuff.
   4. Leave the cuff rolled under.

6. After evaluating the client's chart, the nurse concludes that a 65-year-old client's immunizations are current. What evidence supports this conclusion?
   1. Last tetanus booster was at age 50
   2. Receives a flu shot every year
   3. Has not received the hepatitis B vaccine
   4. Has not received the hepatitis A vaccine

7. A client with poor nutrition enters the hospital for treatment of a puncture wound. An appropriate nursing diagnosis would be

   _____.

8. After teaching a client and family strategies to prevent infection prevention, which statement by the client would indicate effective learning has occurred?
   1. "We will use antimicrobial soap and hot water to wash our hands at least three times per day."
   2. "We must wash or peel all raw fruits and vegetables before eating."
   3. "A wound or sore is not infected unless we see it draining pus."
   4. "We should not share toothbrushes but it is OK to share towels and washcloths."

9. Which of the numbered areas is considered sterile on a person in the operating room? You may assume that all articles were sterile when applied. _____

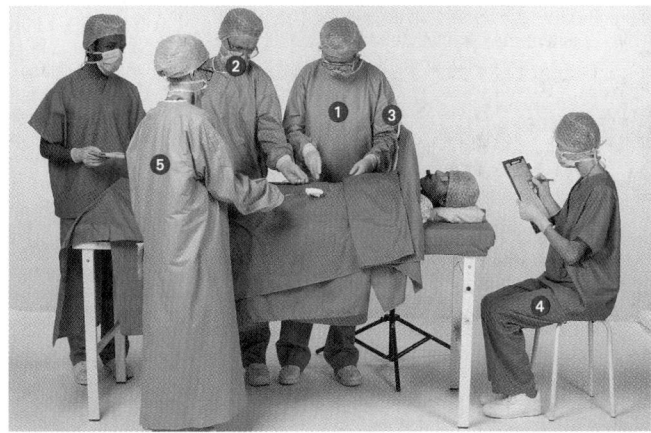

(Dorling Kindersley Media Library)

10. The nurse determines that a field remains sterile if which of the following conditions exist?
   1. Tips of wet forceps are held upward when held in ungloved hands.
   2. The field was set up 1 hour before the procedure.
   3. Sterile items are 2 inches from the edge of the field.
   4. The nurse reaches over the field rather than around the edges.

See Answers to Test Your Knowledge in Appendix A.

EXPLORE MEDIALINK www.prenhall.com/berman

DVD-ROM
- Audio Glossary
- NCLEX Review
- Skills Checklists
- Video: Gloving Techniques

COMPANION WEBSITE
- Additional NCLEX Review
- Case Study: Client with Mycoplasma Pneumonia
- Care Plan Activity: Client on Radiation Therapy and Medication
- Application Activity: Infection Control Today
- Links to Resources

READINGS AND REFERENCES

SUGGESTED READINGS

Doody, L. (2004). Action stat. Bloodborne pathogen exposure. *Nursing, 34*(9), 88. *This brief article clearly describes immediate actions to take if experiencing a potential bloodborne pathogen exposure from a needlestick.*

Jarvis, W. R. (2004). The state of the science of health care epidemiology, infection control, and patient safety, 2004. *American Journal of Infection Control, 32*, 496–503. *As indicated in the title, this article reviews infection control publications from May 2003 to May 2004 and summarizes the guidelines for prevention and control of diseases such as SARS-CoV and West Nile virus.*

Scott, A. (2003). Hand hygiene. *Advance for Providers of Post-Acute Care, 6*(4), 67–68. *This article provides clear and succinct discussion of when to use nonmicrobial soaps, alcohol-based hand rubs, and antibacterial agents.*

RELATED RESEARCH

Korniewicz, D., Garzon, L., & Feinleib, M. (2004). Failure rates in non latex and latex surgical gloves. *American Journal of Infection Control, 32*, 268–273.

REFERENCES

Arrowsmith, V. A., Maunder, J. A., Sargent, R. J., & Taylor, R. (2005). Removal of nail polish and finger rings to prevent surgical infection. *The Cochrane Library* (Oxford) (ID #CD003325).

Boyce, J. M., & Pittet, D. (2002). Guideline for hand hygiene in health-care settings: Recommendations of the Healthcare Infection Control Practices Advisory Committee and the HICPAC/SHEA/APIC/IDSA Hand Hygiene Task Force. *Morbidity and Mortality Weekly Report, 51*(RR-16), 1–44.

Centers for Disease Control. (1987). Recommendations for prevention of HIV transmission in health-care settings. *Morbidity and Mortality Weekly Report (suppl.), 36*(2s), 1S–18S.

Centers for Disease Control. (1997). 1997 USPHS/IDSA guidelines for the prevention of opportunistic infections in persons infected with human immunodeficiency virus. *Morbidity and Mortality Weekly Report, 46*(RR-12), 1–46.

Centers for Disease Control and Prevention. (2003). *Exposure to blood: What healthcare personnel need to know.* Atlanta, GA: Author.

Centers for Disease Control and Prevention. (2005). *Public health guidance for community-level preparedness and response to severe acute respiratory syndrome (SARS) version 2: Supplement I: Infection control in healthcare, home, and community settings.* Retrieved June 3, 2006, from http://www.cdc.gov/ncidod/sars/guidance/I/healthcare.htm

Centers for Disease Control and Prevention. (2006a). *Recommended childhood and adolescent immunization schedule, United States, 2005.* Retrieved June 1, 2006, from http://www.cdc.gov/nip/recs/child-schedule.htm#printable

Centers for Disease Control and Prevention. (2006b). *Recommended adult immunization schedule, United States, 2006.* Retrieved June 1, 2006, from http://www.cdc.gov/nip/recs/adult-schedule.htm#print

Centers for Medicare and Medicaid Services. (2005). Alcohol based hand rub solutions TIA 00-1 (101). *Federal Register, 70*(57), 15229–15239.

Garner, J. S., & Hospital Infection Control Practices Advisory Committee. (1996). Guidelines for isolation precautions in hospitals. *Infection Control Hospital Epidemiology, 17*, 53–80, and *American Journal of Infection Control, 24*, 24–52.

Garner, J. S., & Simmons, B. P. (1983). *CDC guideline for isolation precautions in hospitals* (HHS Publication No. CDC 83-8314). Atlanta, GA: U.S. Department of Health and Human Services, Public Health Service, Centers for Disease Control.

Hospital Infection Control Practices Advisory Committee. (1995). Recommendations for preventing the spread of vancomycin resistance. *American Journal of Infection Control, 23*, 87–94; *Infection Control and Hospital Epidemiology, 16*, 105–113; and *Morbidity and Mortality Weekly Report, 44* (RR-12), 1–13.

Houghton, D. (2006). HAI prevention: The power is in your hands. *Nursing Management, 37*(Suppl.), 1–7.

Jackson, M. M. (1993). Infection precautions: What works and what does not. *CRNA: The Clinical Forum for Nurse Anesthetists, 4*(2), 77–82.

Joint Commission on Accreditation of Healthcare Organizations. (2006). *National patient safety goals.* Oakbrook Terrace, IL: Author. Retrieved June 3, 2006, from http://www.jointcommission.org/Standards/NationalPatientSafetyGoals/

National Institute for Occupational Safety and Health. (1999). *Preventing needlestick injuries in health care settings.* (DHHS Publication No. 2000-108) Cincinnati, OH: U.S. Department of Health and Human Services, Public Health Service, Centers for Disease Control and Prevention, National Institute for Occupational Safety and Health.

Occupational Safety & Health Administration. (2005). *Latex allergy.* Retrieved June 3, 2006, from http://www.osha.gov/SLTC/latexallergy/

Raboud, J., Saskin, R., Wong, K., Moore, C., Parucha, G., Bennett, J., et al. (2004). Patterns of handwashing behavior and visits to patients on a general medical ward of healthcare workers. *Infection Control and Hospital Epidemiology, 25*, 198–202.

Sunenshine, R. H., & McDonald, L. C. (2006). *Clostridium difficile*-associated disease: New challenges from an established pathogen. *Cleveland Clinical Journal of Medicine, 73*, 187–197.

U.S. Department of Health and Human Services, Public Health Service. (1988). Update: Universal precautions for prevention of transmission of human immunodeficiency virus, hepatitis B virus, and other bloodborne pathogens in health care settings. *Morbidity and Mortality Weekly Report, 37*(24), 377–388.

World Health Organization. (2005). *WHO guidelines on hand hygiene in health care.* Geneva, Switzerland: Author.

SELECTED BIBLIOGRAPHY

Barbacane, J. L. (2004). Back to the basics: Handwashing. *Geriatric Nursing, 25*(2), 90–92.

Carr, M. P. (2004). Waterless hand washing: A new era in hand hygiene. *Journal of Practical Hygiene, 13*(2), 33–36.

Centers for Disease Control and Prevention. (2001). Updated U.S. Public Health Service guidelines for the management of occupational exposures to HBV, HCV, and HIV and recommendations for postexposure prophylaxis. *Morbidity and Mortality Weekly Report 50*(RR-11), 1–67.

Centers for Disease Control and Prevention. (2004). *Sequence for donning and removing personal protective equipment.* Retrieved July 16, 2006, from www.cdc.gov/ncidod/dhqp/ppe.html

Garcia-Martin, M., Lardelli-Claret, P., Jimenez-Moleon, J. J., Bueno-Cavanillas, A., de Dios Luna del Castillo, J., & Galvez-Vargas, R. (2001). Proportion of hospital deaths potentially attributable to nosocomial infection. *Infection Control and Hospital Epidemiology, 22*, 708–714.

Goldrick, B. A. (2003). Adult respiratory infections. *American Journal of Nursing, 103*(10), 65–66.

Goldrick, B. A. (2004). 21st century emerging and reemerging infections. *American Journal of Nursing, 104*(1), 67–70.

Goldrick, B. A. (2004). MRSA, VRE, and VRSA: How do we control them in nursing homes? *American Journal of Nursing, 104*(8), 50–51.

Jarvis, J. R. (2001). Infection control and changing health-care delivery systems. *Emerging Infectious Diseases, 7*, 170–173.

National Center for HIV, STD, and TB Prevention, Division of Tuberculosis Elimination. (2004). *Self-study modules on tuberculosis.* Retrieved July 16, 2006, from http://www.phppo.cdc.gov/phtn/tbmodules/Default.htm

Peate, I. (2004). Infection control. Occupational exposure of staff to HIV and prophylaxis therapy. *British Journal of Nursing, 13,* 1146–1150.

Sehulster, L. M., Chinn, R. Y. W., Arduino, M. J., Carpenter, J., Donlan, R., Ashford, D., et al. (2004). *Guidelines for environmental infection control in health-care facilities. Recommendations from CDC and the Healthcare Infection Control Practices Advisory Committee (HICPAC).* Chicago: American Society for Healthcare Engineering/American Hospital Association.

Srinivasan, A., McDonald, L. C., Jernigan, D., Helfand, R., Ginsheimer, K., Jernigan, J., et al. (2004). Foundations of the severe acute respiratory syndrome preparedness and response plan for healthcare facilities. *Infection Control and Hospital Epidemiology, 25,* 1020–1025.

Stirling, B., Littlejohn, P., & Willbond, M. L. (2004). Nurses and the control of infectious disease: Understanding epidemiology and disease transmission is vital to nursing care. *Canadian Nurse, 100(9),* 16–20.

CHAPTER 32

Safety

A fundamental concern of nurses, which extends from the bedside to the home to the community, is prevention of accidents and injury, as well as assisting the injured. Motor vehicle accidents, falls, drowning, fire and burns, poisoning, inhalation and ingestion of foreign objects, and firearm use are major causes of accidental injury and death.

Nurses need to be aware of what constitutes a safe environment for a particular person or for a group of people in home and community settings. Accidents are often caused by human conduct and can be prevented.

FACTORS AFFECTING SAFETY

The ability of people to protect themselves from injury is affected by such factors as age and development, lifestyle, mobility and health status, sensory-perceptual alterations, cognitive awareness, psychosocial state, ability to communicate, safety awareness, and environmental factors. Nurses need to assess each of these factors when they plan care or teach clients to protect themselves.

Age and Development

Through knowledge and accurate assessment of the environment, people learn to protect themselves from many injuries.

Children walking to school learn to stop before crossing the street and wait for oncoming traffic. They also learn not to touch a hot stove. For the very young, learning about the environment is essential. Only through knowledge and experience do children learn what is potentially harmful.

Elders can have difficulty with movement and diminished sensory acuity that contributes to the likelihood of injury. Specific age-related potential hazards and preventive measures are discussed later in this chapter. Box 32–1 summarizes selected hazards for each age group.

Lifestyle

Lifestyle factors that place people at risk include unsafe work environments; residence in neighborhoods with high crime rates; access to guns and ammunition; insufficient income to buy safety equipment or make necessary repairs; and access to illicit drugs, which may also be contaminated by harmful additives. Risk-taking behavior is a factor in some accidents.

Mobility and Health Status

People who have impaired mobility due to paralysis, muscle weakness, and poor balance or coordination are obviously prone to injury. Clients with spinal cord injury and paralysis of both legs may be unable to move even when they perceive discomfort.

LIFESPAN CONSIDERATIONS
Preventing Falls

ELDERS

- Assess for potential personal causes of falls: hypotension, unsteady gait, altered mental responsiveness (such as from medications), poor vision, foot pathology, cognitive changes, and fear.
- In the home or community setting, assess for potential environmental causes of falls:
  - *Lighting:* inadequate amount, inaccessible or inconvenient switches
  - *Floors:* presence of electrical cords, loose rugs, clutter, slippery surfaces
  - *Stairs:* absent or unsteady railings, uneven step height or surfaces
  - *Furniture:* unsteady base, lack of armrests, cabinets too high or too low
  - *Bathroom:* inappropriate toilet height, slippery floors or tub, absence of grab bars
- In the home, consider alternatives to hospital or regular bed if client is extremely prone to fall out of bed:
  - Place the mattress directly onto the floor.
  - Use a water mattress.
  - Place padding on floor next to bed or between client and side rails.

BOX 32–1 Selected Safety Hazards Throughout the Life Span*

- *Developing fetus:* Exposure to maternal smoking, alcohol consumption, addictive drugs, x-rays (first trimester), certain pesticides
- *Newborns and infants:* Falling, suffocation in crib, choking from aspirated milk or ingested objects, burns from hot water or other spilled hot liquids, automobile accidents, crib or playpen injuries, electric shock, poisoning
- *Toddlers:* Physical trauma from falling, banging into objects, or getting cut by sharp objects; automobile accidents; burns; poisoning; drowning; and electric shock
- *Preschoolers:* Injury from traffic, playground equipment, and other objects; choking, suffocation, and obstruction of airway or ear canal by foreign objects; poisoning; drowning; fire and burns; harm from other people or animals
- *Adolescents:* Vehicular (automobile, bicycle) accidents, recreational accidents, firearms, substance abuse
- *Older adults:* Falling, burns, and pedestrian and automobile accidents

*Preventive measures are discussed later in this chapter.

Hemiplegic clients or clients with leg casts often have poor balance and fall easily. Clients weakened by illness or surgery are not always fully aware of their condition.

Sensory-Perceptual Alterations

Accurate sensory perception of environmental stimuli is vital to safety. People with impaired touch perception, hearing, taste, smell, and vision are highly susceptible to injury. A person who does not see well may trip over a toy or not see an electric cord. Deaf people do not hear a siren in traffic, and people with impaired olfactory sense may not smell burning food or the sulfur aroma of escaping gas.

Cognitive Awareness

Awareness is the ability to perceive environmental stimuli and body reactions and to respond appropriately through thought and action. Clients with impaired awareness include people lacking sleep; unconscious or semiconscious persons; disoriented people who may not understand where they are or what to do to help themselves; people who perceive stimuli that do not exist; and people whose judgment is altered by disease or medications, such as narcotics, tranquilizers, hypnotics, and sedatives. Mildly confused clients may momentarily forget where they are, wander from their rooms, misplace personal belongings, and so forth.

Emotional State

Extreme emotional states can alter the ability to perceive environmental hazards. Stressful situations can reduce a person's level of concentration, cause errors of judgment, and decrease awareness of external stimuli. People with depression may think and react to environmental stimuli more slowly than usual.

Ability to Communicate

Individuals with diminished ability to receive and convey information are at risk for injury. They include aphasic clients, people with language barriers, and those unable to read. For example, the person unable to interpret the sign "No smoking—oxygen in use" could cause a fire.

Safety Awareness

Information is crucial to safety. Clients in unfamiliar environments frequently need specific safety information. Lack of knowledge about unfamiliar equipment, such as oxygen tanks, intravenous tubing, and hot packs, is a potential hazard. Healthy clients need information about water safety, car safety, fire prevention, ways to prevent the ingestion of harmful substances, and many preventive measures related to specific age-related hazards.

Environmental Factors

Depending on the client situation, the nurse may need to assess the environment of the home, workplace, or community. Client safety is affected by the health care setting. Bioterrorism has recently become a national safety concern.

Home

A safe home requires well-maintained flooring and carpets, a nonskid bathtub or shower surface, functioning smoke alarms that are strategically placed, and knowledge of fire escape routes. Outdoor areas, such as swimming pools, need to be safely secured and maintained. Adequate lighting, both inside and out, will minimize the potential for accidents.

Workplace

In the workplace, machinery, industrial belts and pulleys, and chemicals may create danger. Worker fatigue, noise and air pollution, or working at great heights or in subterranean areas may also create occupational hazards. The work environment of the nurse may also be unsafe. Health care workers need to maintain an awareness of the potential risks of their work environment.

Community

Adequate street lighting, safe water and sewage treatment, and regulation of sanitation in food buying and handling all contribute to a healthy, hazard-free community. A safe and secure community strives to be free of excess noise, crime, traffic congestion, dilapidated housing, or unprotected creeks and landfills.

Health Care Setting

The 2000 Institute of Medicine (IOM) report *To Err Is Human: Building a Safer Health System* estimated that 44,000 to 98,000 people die in the United States each year due to medical errors in hospitals. This means that more people die in a given year as a result of medical errors than from motor vehicle accidents, breast cancer, or AIDS (Kohn, Corrigan, & Donaldson, 2000, p. 1). Client safety problems can include a variety of errors such as medication errors, wrong-site surgery, restraint-related injuries or death, falls, burns, pressure ulcers, and mistaken identity (p. 35). The IOM report defines *safety* as "freedom from accidental injury" (p. 58) and *error* as the "failure of a planned action to be completed as intended or the use of a wrong plan to achieve an aim" (p. 54).

The IOM reviewed many studies that investigated adverse events. An adverse event includes an injury caused by medical management rather than the underlying disease or condition of the client. It noted that over 50% of the adverse events were preventable. The committee who put together the report emphasized that while some of the errors were due to incompetent or impaired providers, the majority of the errors could have been avoided had better systems of care been in place (p. 30). Leonard, Frankel, Simmonds, and Vega (2004) echoed this belief by stating that an ever-increasing body of evidence indicates that at least 80% of medical error is system derived—meaning that system flaws set good people up to fail (p. 5). These same authors state that when people perform complex tasks, errors will occur.

The hospital environment is quite complex. Leonard et al. (2004) identified the following factors that increase the risk of human error:

- *Limited short-term memory.* Nurses have rapidly changing information coming at them continuously in busy hospital environments. Systems that rely on human memory are prone to failure.

- *Being late or in a hurry.* People start cutting corners when they are late or in a hurry. This may get the work done quicker; however, it also contributes to the possibility of missing an important detail or piece of information that could cause client harm.
- *Limited ability to multitask.* People perform better at a single task. For example, consider the number of accidents caused when someone uses a cell phone while driving.
- *Interruptions.* Many interruptions occur in complex environments such as a hospital (e.g., alarms, call lights, telephone calls). It is more difficult to get back on task or to remember what you were thinking with frequent interruptions.
- *Stress.* Stress causes anxiety, and anxiety affects performance. Also, stress affects a person's thinking by filtering information (e.g., only hearing the information you want to hear or missing all of the information), which subsequently affects problem-solving ability.
- *Fatigue and other physiological factors.* Studies show that fatigue affects a person's ability to process complex information.
- *Environmental factors.* Heat, noise, distractions, visual stimuli, and lighting can affect performance and lead to mistakes. Workplace design is a part of keeping clients and staff safe (p. 18–22).

Another IOM report, *Keeping Patients Safe—Transforming the Work Environment of Nurses* (2004), established a link between nurses' work environment and client safety. The report found that the usual work environment of nurses is characterized by many serious threats to client safety (p. 3). Examples in this report include:

- Inconsistent staffing levels.
- Long work hours.
- Some nursing work processes. For example, medication administration and hand washing are two common nursing activities well documented as involving threats to client safety (p. 239).
- Inefficient nurse work processes. Multiple demands for documentation and paperwork consume very large amounts of nurses' time. This takes time away from providing therapeutic nursing care.
- Physical design of the workplace. Examples identified as potential sources of errors include poor layout of client care units, poor design of communication technologies where nurses spend much time hunting down other nurses and primary care providers, and the increasing practice of transferring clients to other units.

Bioterrorism

In the past, being prepared for a disaster pertained to natural events such as hurricanes and earthquakes. However, the United States has significantly increased its preparedness for terrorism attacks since the events of September 11, 2001, and subsequent episodes where letters containing anthrax spores were sent through the U.S. postal system.

Terrorism can include chemical, biological, or nuclear weapons. **Bioterrorism** is an intentional attack using weapons

of viruses, bacteria, and other germs (Weber, 2004, p. 417). It is thought that biological threats such as bioterrorism are of greatest concern because of the potential far-reaching effects such as easy transmission, high mortality rate, and public panic. Nurses are important members of the community's disaster-preparedness team. As a result, nurses must be prepared and able to respond appropriately to all types of disasters.

 NURSING MANAGEMENT

Assessing

Assessing clients at risk for accidents and injury involves (a) noting pertinent indicators in the nursing history and physical examination, (b) using specifically developed risk assessment tools, and (c) evaluating the client's home environment.

Nursing History and Physical Examination

The nursing history and physical examination can reveal considerable data about the client's safety practices and risks for injury. Data include age and developmental level; general health status; mobility status; presence or absence of physiologic or perceptual deficits such as olfactory, visual, tactile, taste, or other sensory impairments; altered thought processes or other impaired cognitive or emotional capabilities; substance abuse; any indications of abuse or neglect; and an accident and injury history. A safety history also needs to include the client's awareness of hazards, knowledge of safety precautions both at home and at work, and any perceived threats to safety (Figure 32-1■).

RISK ASSESSMENT TOOLS. Risk assessment tools are available to determine clients at risk both for specific kinds of injury, such as falls, or for the general safety of the home and health care setting. In general, these tools direct the nurse to appraise the factors affecting safety as previously discussed. The tools summarize specific data contained in the client's nursing history and physical examination. Client risk factors and environmental hazards for falls are discussed later in this chapter (see "Falls").

HOME HAZARD APPRAISAL. Hazards in the home are major causes of falls, fire, poisoning, suffocation, and other accidents, such as those caused by improper use of household equipment, tools, and cooking utensils. See Chapter 8 ∞ for a summary of specific data necessary for a home hazard appraisal.

National Patient Safety Goals

As a result of IOM's report *To Err Is Human*, the health care industry and national organizations (e.g., National Patient Safety Foundation) increased their awareness of the need to improve client safety. For example, the Joint Commission on Accreditation of Healthcare Organizations (JCAHO) requires its accredited agencies to meet specific National Patient Safety Goals (NPSGs). See Box 32–2 for JCAHO's 2006 National Patient Safety Goals. It is important to remember that the focus of the NPSGs is on system-wide solutions. This is an important change from the traditional method of finding out who made the error (e.g., creating an environment of fear and scapegoating) to analyzing the system to find out why the error was made (e.g., creating an environment of learning and improvement).

Figure 32-1 ■ Nurses need to teach clients about safety and how to prevent accidents such as using smoke detectors, safety covers for electrical outlets, childproof locks on drawers and cabinets, Mr. Yuk stickers on toxic substances, infant car seats, and by placing poison control information near or on the telephone.

(Top: Courtesy of Tony Freeman/PhotoEdit; Jerry Marshall; Michael Newman/PhotoEdit; Bottom: Grantpix/Photo Researchers Inc.; Geri Engberg; Children's Hospital Pittsburgh.)

Bioterrorism Attacks

Nurses are considered frontline health care providers. As a result, they need education and training to be able to assess and detect potential bioterrorism attacks. The Centers for Disease Control and Prevention (CDC, 2001) defined three categories of biological pathogens that can be used for bioterrorism. The agents of highest concern are anthrax, botulism, plague, viral hemorrhagic fevers, smallpox, and tularemia. See Table 32–1 for additional information on these agents.

Health care workers need to sustain a heightened awareness and alertness of circumstances or patterns that may indicate potential bioterrorism. The CDC (2001) and Massey (2004) have provided the following examples of when it is important to become suspicious:

- Is there an unusual geographic clustering of illness (e.g., persons who attended the same public event)?
- Is the emergency department receiving an increase of clients with similar symptoms?
- Is the ICU caring for an unusual number of elderly clients with pneumonia?
- Is there an unusual age distribution for common diseases (e.g., an increase in chickenpox-like symptoms among adults)?

The health problems that nurses and other health care workers are seeing and caring for in one facility may only be one part of the big picture. Calling the local public health department and reporting observations and suspicions may reveal a larger pattern. Early detection and management is needed to help stop a bioterrorism attack.

BOX 32–2 JCAHO 2006 National Patient Safety Goals

Improve the accuracy of patient identification.

- Use at least two patient identifiers (neither to be the patient's room number) whenever administering medications or blood products, taking blood samples and other specimens for clinical testing, or providing any other treatments or procedures.
- Prior to the start of any invasive procedure, conduct a final verification process to confirm the correct patient, procedure, site, and availability of appropriate documents. This verification process uses active—not passive—communication techniques.

Improve the effectiveness of communication among caregivers.

- For verbal or telephone orders or for telephonic reporting of critical test results, verify the complete order or test result by having the person receiving the order or test result "read-back" the complete order or test result.
- Standardize a list of abbreviations, acronyms, and symbols that are not to be used throughout the organization.
- Measure, assess, and, if appropriate, take action to improve the timeliness of reporting, and the timeliness of receipt by the responsible licensed caregiver of critical test results and values.
- All values defined as critical by the laboratory are reported to a responsible licensed caregiver within time frames established by the laboratory (defined in cooperation with nursing and medical staff). When the patient's responsible licensed caregiver is not available within the time frames, there is a mechanism to report the critical information to an alternative responsible caregiver.
- Implement a standardized approach to "hand off" communications, including an opportunity to ask and respond to questions.

Improve the safety of using medications.

- Standardize and limit the number of drug concentrations available in the organization.
- Identify and, at a minimum, annually review a list of look-alike/sound-alike drugs used in the organization, and take action to prevent errors involving the interchange of these drugs.
- Label all medications, medication containers (e.g., syringes, medicine cups, basins), or other solutions on and off the sterile field in perioperative and other procedural settings.

Reduce the risk of health care–associated infections.

- Comply with current Centers for Disease Control and Prevention (CDC) hand hygiene guidelines.
- Manage as sentinel events all identified cases of unanticipated death or major permanent loss of function associated with a health care–associated infection.

Accurately and completely reconcile medications across the continuum of care.

- Implement a process for obtaining and documenting a complete list of the patient's current medications upon the patient's admission to the organization and with the involvement of the patient. This process includes a comparison of the medications the organization provides to those on the list.
- A complete list of the patient's medications is communicated to the next provider of service when it refers or transfers a patient to another setting, service, practitioner, or level of care within or outside the organization.

Reduce the risk of patient harm resulting from falls.

- Implement a fall reduction program and evaluate the effectiveness of the program.

Reduce the risk of influenza and pneumococcal disease in institutionalized older adults.

- Develop and implement a protocol for administration and documentation of the flu vaccine.
- Develop and implement a protocol for administration and documentation of the pneumococcus vaccine.
- Develop and implement a protocol to identify new cases of influenza and to manage an outbreak.

Reduce the risk of surgical fires.

- Educate staff, including operating licensed independent practitioners and anesthesia providers, on how to control heat sources and manage fuels, and establish guidelines to minimize oxygen concentration under drapes.

Implement applicable National Patient Safety Goals and associated requirements by components and practitioner sites.

- Inform and encourage components and practitioner sites to implement the applicable National Patient Safety Goals and associated requirements.

Encourage the active involvement of patients and their families in the patient's care as a patient safety strategy.

- Define and communicate the means for patients to report concerns about safety and encourage them to do so.

Prevent health care–associated pressure ulcers (decubitus ulcers).

- Assess and periodically reassess each patient's risk for developing a pressure ulcer (decubitus ulcer) and take action to address any identified risks.

Note: © Joint Commission Resources: *Facts about 2006 National Patient Safety Goals* Oakbrook Terrace, IL: Joint Commission on Accreditation of Healthcare Organizations, 2006. Reprinted with permission.

Diagnosing

NANDA offers a broad diagnostic label related to safety issues:

- *Risk for Injury:* A state in which the individual is at risk for injury as a result of environmental conditions interacting with the individual's adaptive and defense resources.

This broad label consists of seven subcategories that may be preferred when the nurse wants to describe injury more specifically or isolate suitable interventions (Wilkinson, 2005):

- *Risk for Poisoning:* Accentuated risk of accidental exposure to, or ingestion of, drugs or dangerous products in doses sufficient to cause poisoning

- *Risk for Suffocation:* Accentuated risk of accidental suffocation (inadequate air available for inhalation)
- *Risk for Trauma:* Accentuated risk of accidental tissue injury (e.g., wound, burn, or fracture)
- *Latex Allergy Response:* A hypersensitive reaction to natural latex rubber products
- *Risk for Latex Allergy Response:* Risk of hypersensitivity to natural latex rubber products
- *Contamination:* Exposure to environmental contaminants in doses sufficient to cause adverse health effects.
- *Risk for Contamination:* Accentuated risk of exposure to environmental contaminants in doses sufficient to cause adverse health effects.

TABLE 32–1	**Biological Pathogens of Highest Concern for Bioterrorism Attacks**	
Anthrax	Cause	Spore-forming bacterium—*Bacillus anthracis*
	Transmission	■ Not known to spread from one person to another ■ Cutaneous/skin: direct skin contact with spores (most common) ■ Respiratory: inhalation of aerosolized spores (rare) ■ GI: consumption of undercooked or raw meat products or dairy products from infected animals (rare)
	Symptoms of cutaneous anthrax	■ Localized itching followed by a lesion that turns vesicular and subsequent development of black eschar (scab) within 7 to 10 days of initial lesion ■ Fever, flulike symptoms, nonproductive cough, sore throat
Botulism	Cause	By a toxin made by a bacterium called *Clostridium botulinum*
	Transmission	■ Not spread from one person to another ■ Foodborne—person ingests preformed toxin ■ Infant—occurs in small number of infants who harbor *C. botulinum* in their intestinal tract ■ Wound—occurs when wounds are infected with *C. botulinum*
	Symptoms of foodborne botulism	Between 12 and 36 hours after eating toxin-containing food: double and blurred vision, slurred speech, difficulty swallowing, muscle weakness that always descends through the body
Plague	Cause	A bacterium found in rodents and their fleas—*Yersinia pestis*
	Transmission	■ Bubonic plague is transmitted through the bite of an infected flea or exposure to infected material through a break in the skin. Bubonic plague is not transmitted person to person. ■ Pneumonic plague would be caused by an aerosol attack (bioweapon). Pneumonic plague can be transmitted person to person.
	Symptoms of pneumonic plague	Fever, weakness, rapidly developing pneumonia with dyspnea, chest pain, cough, and sometimes bloody or watery sputum
Viral Hemorrhagic Fevers (VHF)	Cause	■ Virus. Ebola and yellow fever are two examples. ■ Viruses of most VHFs reside in an animal reservoir host or arthropod host (e.g., rodents are hosts and ticks and mosquitoes can be vectors). However, the hosts of some VHF, (e.g., Ebola and Marburg) are unknown.
	Transmission	Humans are not natural reservoirs for VHFs. People are infected when they come in contact with infected hosts. However, with some VHFs, after the accidental transmission from the host, humans can transmit the virus to one another.
	Symptoms	After an incubation period of 5 to 10 days: abrupt onset of fever, myalgia, headache, nausea and vomiting, abdominal pain, diarrhea, chest pain. A rash on the trunk develops approximately 5 days after onset. Bleeding (e.g., petechiae, bruises, and hemorrhages) occur as disease progresses.
Smallpox	Cause	Variola virus
	Transmission	Droplet nuclei expelled from the mouth of an infected person or by aerosol. Contaminated clothing or bed linen could also spread the disease. Humans are the only natural host of variola.
	Symptoms	■ Incubation period can range from 7 to 17 days where the person has no symptoms and is not contagious. ■ Initial symptoms include high fever, head and body aches, and possibly vomiting. These symptoms last 2 to 4 days and the person may be contagious. ■ A rash then appears—first on the tongue and in the mouth. These red spots develop into sores that break open and spread large amounts of the virus into the mouth and throat. The person is highly contagious at this point. ■ The rash then spreads to the entire body. By the third day of the rash, the rash becomes raised bumps which fill with thick, opaque fluid and have a depression in the center. The bumps become pustules which begin to form a crust and then scab. ■ The scabs fall off leaving pitted scars. The person is contagious until all the scabs have fallen off.
Tularemia	Cause	The bacterium *Francisella tularensis* found in animals (especially rodents, rabbits, and hares)
	Transmission	Not known to be spread from person to person It is spread in different ways: ■ Being bitten by an infected tick, deer-fly, or other insect ■ Handling infected animal carcasses ■ Eating or drinking contaminated food or water ■ Breathing in/inhaling the *F. tularensis*
	Symptoms	■ Sudden fever, chills, headache, diarrhea, muscle aches, joint pain, dry cough, and progressive weakness. ■ If *F. tularensis* was used as a bioweapon and made airborne for exposure by inhalation, the infected people would experience severe respiratory illness, including life-threatening pneumonia and systemic infection.

IDENTIFYING NURSING DIAGNOSES, OUTCOMES, AND INTERVENTIONS
Clients at Risk for Safety

DATA CLUSTER   Mrs. H. has adopted a toddler. Home assessment reveals many cleaning supplies at floor level, and paint peeling off the walls.

NURSING DIAGNOSIS/ DEFINITION	SAMPLE DESIRED OUTCOMES*/ *DEFINITION*	INDICATORS	SELECTED INTERVENTIONS*/ *DEFINITION*	SAMPLE NIC ACTIVITIES
Risk for Poisoning related to dangerous products within reach of a child/ *Accentuated risk of accidental exposure to, or ingestion of, drugs or dangerous products in doses sufficient to cause poisoning*	Safe Home Physical Environment [1910]/ *Physical arrangements to minimize environmental factors that might cause physical harm or injury in the home*	Totally adequate • Placement of appropriate hazard warning labels • Storage of hazardous materials to prevent injury • Correction of lead hazard risks • Provision of safe play area	Environmental Management: Safety [6486]/*Monitoring and manipulation of the physical environment to promote safety*	• Identify safety hazards • Remove hazards from the environment, when possible • Initiate and/or conduct screening programs for environmental hazards (e.g., lead) • Educate about environmental hazards • Provide emergency phone numbers (e.g., poison control center)

DATA CLUSTER   Mr. P. suffered a stroke resulting in left-sided weakness. As a result, his gait is unsteady. The nurse noticed that his home has several throw rugs and much furniture impeding his mobility. The bathroom does not have grab bars by the toilet or shower.

NURSING DIAGNOSIS/ DEFINITION	SAMPLE DESIRED OUTCOMES*/ *DEFINITION*	INDICATORS	SELECTED INTERVENTIONS*/ *DEFINITION*	SAMPLE NIC ACTIVITIES
Risk for Injury related to impaired mobility and potential home hazards/*At risk of injury as a result of environmental conditions interacting with the individual's adaptive and defense resources*	Safe Home Environment [1910]/*Physical arrangements to minimize environmental factors that might cause physical harm or injury in the home*	Totally adequate • Placement of handrails in bathroom • Arrangement of furniture to reduce risks	Environmental Management: Safety [6486]/*Monitoring and manipulation of the physical environment to promote safety*	• Identify safety needs of client • Identify safety hazards • Modify the environment to minimize hazards and risks • Provide adaptive devices (e.g., handrails) to increase safety of the environment • Monitor the environment for changes in safety status • Educate about environmental hazards

*The NOC # for desired outcomes and the NIC # for nursing interventions are listed in brackets following the appropriate outcome or intervention. Outcomes, indicators, interventions, and activities selected are only a sample of those suggested by NOC and NIC and should be further individualized for each client.

■ *Risk for Aspiration:* At risk for the entry of gastrointestinal secretions, oropharyngeal secretions, solids, or fluids into tracheobronchial passages
■ *Risk for Disuse Syndrome:* At risk for deterioration of body systems as the result of prescribed or unavoidable musculoskeletal inactivity

Another diagnosis the nurse may choose to use is

■ *Deficient Knowledge (Accident Prevention):* Inability to state or explain information or demonstrate a required skill related to safety of self and others

See Identifying Nursing Diagnoses, Outcomes, and Interventions for examples of applying the nursing process for clients at risk for injury.

Planning

When planning care to prevent accidents and injury, the nurse considers all factors affecting the client's safety, specifies desired outcomes, and selects nursing activities to meet these outcomes. The major goal for clients with safety risks is to prevent accidents and injury. To meet this goal, clients often need to change their health behavior and may need to modify the environment.

Desired outcomes associated with preventing injury depend on the individual client. Examples of desired outcomes, although established in the planning phase, are provided in the "Evaluating" section on page 736.

Nursing interventions to meet desired outcomes are largely directed toward helping the client and family to accomplish the following:

■ Identify environmental hazards in the home and community.

- Demonstrate safety practices appropriate to the home health care agency, community, and workplace.
- Experience a decrease in the frequency or severity of injury.
- Demonstrate safe child-rearing practices or lifestyle practices.

Implementing

Hazards to safety occur at all ages and vary according to the age and development level of the individual.

Promoting Safety across the Life Span

Measures to ensure the safety of people of all ages focus on (a) observation or prediction of potentially harmful situations so that harm can be avoided and (b) client education that empowers clients to protect themselves and their families from injury. Safety measures covering the life span from infancy to elders are listed in the accompanying Client Teaching.

CLIENT TEACHING **Safety Measures throughout the Life Span**

NEWBORNS AND INFANTS

- Use a federally approved car seat at all times (including coming home from hospital). It should be in the back seat, facing backward.
- Never leave the infant unattended on a raised surface.
- Check the temperature of the infant's bath water and formula prior to using.
- Hold the infant upright during feeding. Do not prop the bottle. Cut food in small pieces, and do not feed the infant peanuts or popcorn.
- Investigate the infant's crib for compliance with federal safety regulations: slats no more than 2 3/8 inches apart, lead-free paint, height of crib sides, tight fit of mattress to crib.
- Use a playpen with sides made of small-size netting. Never leave playpen sides down.
- Provide large soft toys with no small detachable or sharp-edged parts.
- Use guard gates on stairs and screens on windows. Supervise the infant in swings and highchairs.
- Cover electric outlets. Coil cords out of reach.
- Place plants, household cleaners, and wastebaskets out of reach. Lock away potential poisons, such as medicines, paint, and gasoline.

TODDLERS

- Continue to use federally approved car seats at all times. Place children in back seat when traveling in a car.
- Teach children not to put objects in the mouth, including pills (unless given by parent).
- Keep objects with sharp edges (such as furniture and knives) out of children's reach.
- Place hot pots on back burners with handles turned inward.
- Keep cleaning solutions, insecticides, and medicines in locked cupboards.
- Keep windows and balconies screened.
- Supervise toddlers in the tub.
- Fence in pools, and supervise toddlers at all times when in or near pools. Do not overfill bathtub. Do not let toddlers play near ditches or wells.
- Teach children not to run or ride a tricycle into the street.
- Obtain a low bed when the child begins to climb.
- Cover outlets with safety covers or plugs.

PRESCHOOLERS

- Do not allow children to run with candy or other objects in the mouth.
- Teach children not to put small objects in the mouth, nose, and ears.
- Remove doors from unused equipment such as refrigerators.

- Always supervise preschoolers crossing streets and begin safety teaching about obeying traffic signals and looking both ways.
- Check Halloween treats before allowing children to eat them. Discard loose or open candy.
- Teach children to play in "safe" areas, not on streets and railroad tracks.
- Teach preschoolers the dangers of playing with matches and playing near charcoal, fire, and heating appliances.
- Teach children to avoid strangers and keep parents informed of their whereabouts.
- Teach preschoolers not to walk in front of swings and not to push others off playground equipment.

SCHOOL-AGE CHILDREN

- Teach children safety rules for recreational and sports activities: never swim alone, always wear a life jacket when in a boat, and wear a protective helmet and knee and elbow pads when needed.
- Supervise contact sports and activities in which children aim at a target.
- Teach children to obey all traffic and safety rules for bicycling, skateboarding, and roller skating.
- Teach children to use light or reflective clothing when walking or cycling at night.
- Teach children safe ways to use the stove, garden tools, and other equipment.
- Supervise children when they use saws, electric appliances, tools, and other potentially dangerous equipment.
- Teach children not to play with fireworks, gunpowder, or firearms. Keep firearms unloaded, locked up, and out of reach.
- Teach children to avoid excavations, quarries, vacant buildings, and playing around heavy machinery.
- Teach children the health hazards of smoking. If you smoke, stop.
- Teach children the effects of drugs and alcohol on judgment and coordination.

ADOLESCENTS

- Have adolescents complete a drivers' education course, and take practice drives with them in various kinds of weather.
- Set firm limits on automobile use, namely, never to drive after drinking or using drugs, and never to ride with a driver who has done so. Encourage adolescents to call home for a ride if they have been drinking, assuring them they can do so without a reprimand.
- Restrict number of passengers in car during the first year of driving.
- Teach adolescents to wear a safety helmet when riding motorcycles, scooters, and other sports vehicles. Teach safety rules for water sports.
- Encourage adolescents to use proper equipment when participating in sports. Schedule a physical examination before participation, and be certain there is medical supervision for all athletic activities.

CLIENT TEACHING   Safety Measures throughout the Life Span—*continued*

- Encourage adolescents to swim, jog, and go boating in groups so they can obtain help in case of an accident.
- Teach safety measures for use of power tools.
- Teach rules for hunting and the proper care and use of firearms.
- Inform the adolescent of the dangers of drugs, alcohol, and unprotected sex. Include teaching about date rape prevention and defense.
- Teach dangers of sunbathing and tanning beds, as well as use of sun block and protective clothing when doing outdoor activities.
- Be alert to changes in the adolescent's mood and behavior. Listen to and maintain open communication with the adolescent. Open communication is a powerful preventive measure.
- Set a good example of behavior that the adolescent can follow.

YOUNG ADULTS

- Reinforce motor vehicle safety: Drive defensively, use "designated drivers" if alcohol is consumed, routinely check brakes and tires, and use seat and shoulder belts or car seats for all passengers.
- Remind the young adult to repair potential fire hazards, such as electric wiring.
- Reinforce water safety: Know the depth of a pool or lake before diving; supervise backyard pools and other water activities.
- Discuss evaluating the potential for workplace injuries or death when making decisions about a career or occupation. Encourage the young adult to participate actively in programs that reduce occupational hazards.
- Discuss avoiding excessive sun radiation by limiting exposure, using sun-blocking agents, and wearing protective clothing. Explain the skin changes that may indicate a cancerous condition.
- Encourage young adults who are unable to cope with the pressures, responsibilities, and expectations of adulthood to seek counseling.

MIDDLE-AGED ADULTS

- Reinforce motor vehicle safety: Use seat belts and drive within the speed limit, especially at night. Test visual acuity periodically.
- Make certain stairways are well lighted and uncluttered.
- Equip bathrooms with hand grasps and nonskid bath mats.
- Test smoke detectors and fire alarms regularly.
- Keep all machines and tools in good working condition at work and at home. Follow safety precautions when using machinery.

- Reinforce safety measures taught earlier in life, such as the hazards of excessive sun exposure.

ELDERS

- Encourage the client to have regular vision and hearing tests.
- Assist the client to have a home hazard appraisal.
- Encourage the client to keep as active as possible.

PREVENTIVE MEASURES

- Ensure eyeglasses are functional.
- Ensure appropriate lighting.
- Mark doorways and edges of steps as needed.
- Keep environment tidy and uncluttered.
- Set safe limits to activities.
- Remove unsafe objects.
- Wear shoes or well-fitted slippers with nonskid soles.
- Use ambulatory devices as necessary (cane, crutches, walker, braces, wheelchair).
- Provide assistance with ambulation as needed.
- Monitor gait and balance.
- Adapt living arrangements to one floor if necessary.
- Encourage exercise and activity as tolerated to maintain muscle strength, joint flexibility, and balance.
- Ensure uncluttered environment with securely fastened rugs.
- Encourage client to request assistance.
- Keep bed in the low position.
- Install grab bars in bathroom.
- Provide raised toilet seat.
- Instruct client to rise slowly from a lying to sitting to standing position, and to stand in place for several seconds before walking.
- Provide a bedside commode as needed.
- Assist with voiding on a frequent and scheduled basis.
- Encourage client to summon help.
- Monitor activity tolerance.
- Attach side rails to the bed.
- Keep rails in place when the bed is in the lowest position.
- Monitor orientation and alertness status.
- Encourage annual or more frequent review of all medications prescribed.

NEWBORNS AND INFANTS. Accidents are a leading cause of death during infancy, especially during the first year of life. Infants are completely dependent on others for care; they are oblivious to such dangers as falling or ingesting harmful substances. Parents need to learn the amount of observation necessary to maintain infant safety. They also need help to identify and remove common hazards in and around the home, and first-aid information that includes cardiopulmonary resuscitation and interventions for airway obstruction. Common accidents during infancy include burns, suffocation or choking, automobile accidents, falls, and poisoning. Education and support of parents can make them more knowledgeable and better prepared to protect their children from accidents and injuries.

TODDLERS. Toddlers are curious and like to feel and taste everything. They are fascinated by potential dangers, such as pools and busy streets, so they need constant supervision and

protection (Figure 32-2 ■). Parents prevent many accidents by "toddler-proofing" the home or other setting where the child will be. This practice extends to the use of federally approved car restraints and removing or securing all items that can pose a safety hazard to the child in any setting. It may be necessary to inspect for and remove sources of lead from the environment. Lead poisoning (plumbism) is a risk for children exposed to lead paint chips, fumes from leaded gasoline, or any "leaded" substances. The ingestion of lead-based paint chips is the most common cause of lead poisoning in children.

CLINICAL ALERT

The remodeling and renovation of older homes (e.g., those built before 1978) accounts for most of the lead poisoning seen today. Nurses need to educate families living in older homes about their children's risk for lead poisoning and provide lead poisoning prevention advice. ■

Figure 32-2 ■ Promoting safety (e.g., by placing hot pots on back burners with handles turned inward) is required to keep children from injury.

PRESCHOOLERS. Children of preschool age are active and often very clumsy, making them susceptible to injury. Control of the environment must continue, keeping hazards such as matches, medicines, and other potential poisons out of reach. Safety education for the child must begin now. Education of the preschooler involves learning how to cross streets, what traffic signals mean, and how to ride bicycles and other wheeled toys safely. Children must be cautioned to avoid hazards, such as busy streets, swimming pools, and other potentially dangerous areas. Parents must maintain careful surveillance; the developmental level of the preschooler does not allow for self-reliance in matters of safety. Parents must also keep in mind that their child's cognitive and motor skills increase quickly; hence, safety measures must keep up with the acquisition of new skills.

SCHOOL-AGE CHILDREN. By the time children attend school, they are learning to think before they act. They often prefer adult equipment to toys. They want to play with other children in such activities as bicycling, hiking, swimming, and boating. Although sensitive to peer pressure, the school-age child will respond to rules. Children of this age engage in fantasy and magical thinking. They often imitate actions of parents and superheroes with whom they identify.

Injuries are the leading cause of death in school-age children. The most frequent causes of fatalities, in descending order, are motor vehicle crashes, drownings, fires, and firearms. School-age children are also involved in many minor injuries, frequently resulting from outdoor activities and recreational equipment such as swings, bicycles, skateboards, and swimming pools.

ADOLESCENTS. Obtaining a driver's license is an important event in the life of an adolescent in United States, but the privilege is not always wisely handled. Teenagers may use driving as an outlet for stress, as a way to assert independence, or as a way to impress peers. When setting limits on automobile use, parents need to assess the teenager's level of responsibility, common sense, and ability to resist peer pressure. The age of the teenager alone does not determine readiness to handle this responsibility.

Adolescents are at risk for sports injuries because their coordination skills are not fully developed. However, sports activities are important to the adolescent's self-esteem and overall development. In addition to providing beneficial exercise, sports activities enhance social and personal development. They help the adolescent experience competition, teamwork, and conflict resolution.

Suicide and homicide are two leading causes of death among teenagers. Adolescent males commit suicide at a higher rate than adolescent females, and African Americans commit homicide at a higher rate than European Americans. Suicides by firearms, drugs, and automobile exhaust gases are the most common. Factors influencing the high suicide and homicide rates include economic deprivation, family breakup, and the availability of firearms, which are the most frequently used weapons. Cutting or stabbing tools are the next most frequently used weapons.

YOUNG ADULTS. Motor vehicle crashes are by far the leading cause of mortality for this group; other causes of death for young adults include drowning, fires, burns, and firearms.

One safety hazard for many young adults is exposure to natural radiation from sunbathing or outdoor activities. Exposure to the sun is directly related to skin cancer. Suicide is another leading cause of death in young adults. Many suicides may actually be mistaken for unintentional death (automobile crashes, alcohol intoxication, and drug overdose). In general, suicide results from the young adult's inability to cope with the pressures, responsibilities, and expectations of adulthood.

The nurse's role in the prevention of suicide includes identifying behaviors that may indicate potential problems: depression; a variety of physical complaints including weight loss, sleep disturbances, and digestive disorders; and decreased interest in social and work roles along with an increase in isolation. A young adult identified as at risk for suicide should be referred to a mental health professional or a crisis center. Nurses can also reduce the incidence of suicide by participating in educational programs that provide information about the early signs of suicide.

MIDDLE-AGED ADULTS. Changing physiologic factors, as well as concern over personal and work-related responsibilities, may contribute to the injury rate of middle-aged persons. Motor vehicle crashes are the most common cause of accidental death in this age group. Decreased reaction times and visual acuity may make the middle-aged adult prone to accidents. Other unintentional causes of death for middle-aged adults include falls, fires, burns, poisonings, and drownings. Occupational injuries continue to be a significant safety hazard during the middle years.

ELDERS. Injury prevention is a major concern for elders. Because vision is limited, reflexes are slowed, and bones are brittle, climbing stairs, driving a car, and even walking require caution. Driving, particularly night driving, requires caution because accommodation of the eye to light is impaired and peripheral vision is diminished. Elders need to learn to turn their head before changing lanes and should not rely on side vision, for example, when crossing a street or changing lanes. Driving in fog or other hazardous conditions should be avoided.

Fires are a hazard for the elderly person with a failing memory. The older person may forget that the iron or stove has been left on or may not extinguish a cigarette completely. Because of reduced sensitivity to pain and heat, care must be taken to prevent burns when the person bathes or uses heating devices.

Elders at risk for wandering due to organic brain syndromes need to wear identification devices. They can also be registered with the local Alzheimer's Association's Wanderer's Alert Program.

Because elders who take analgesics or sedatives may become lethargic or confused, they should be monitored regularly and closely. Other measures to induce sleep should be used whenever possible. Nurses can help elderly clients make the home environment safe. Specific hazards should be identified and corrected; for example, handrails can be installed on staircases. The nurse teaches the importance of taking only prescribed medications and contacting a health professional at the first indication of medication intolerance.

CLINICAL ALERT

Elders have trouble seeing the edges of stairs. Painting white stripes on the edges of the steps will help increase contrast and may prevent falls. ∎

The incidence of suicide in elders is increasing and often goes unnoticed when the causes are due to hidden self-destructive behaviors, such as starvation, overdosing with medications, and noncompliance with medical care, treatments, and medications. In older individuals, the suicide attempt is usually more serious, because it is truly intended to end the life, not just

to get attention as is often seen in other age groups. Also, the method of suicide is generally more violent in the elderly, such as a gunshot wound to the head, or hanging.

Ebersole, Hess, Touhy, and Jett (2005) have listed important facts regarding suicide of the older adult: (a) White men are the most likely to commit suicide; (b) uncontrollable pain, loss of a loved one, and major life changes can be contributing factors; (c) major depression and social isolation increase the risk of suicide and; (d) elderly people rarely threaten to commit suicide; they just do it.

Nurses need to be aware of the symptoms and risk factors of suicide. They should direct the client to the appropriate professional or agency for treatment and counseling.

SAFETY PROBLEMS ACROSS THE LIFE SPAN. Domestic violence is increasing at an alarming rate and involving individuals of all ages. It includes child abuse, intimate partner abuse, and elder abuse and affects the health and safety of families and the community. Statistics are inaccurate due to the underreporting of incidents. Nurses should be involved in working with all phases of domestic violence: prevention, screening, referrals for treatment, and follow-up care. This usually necessitates collaborative planning with primary care providers, law enforcement agencies, social services, and other community agencies.

Nurses also have the opportunity to become advocates for community support programs for domestic violence and can become involved in educating other professionals regarding prevention, screening, and treatment.

Domestic violence takes on extra importance because it is known that people who were abused as children often display abusive behavior as an adult. This points to the need for prevention and early intervention to prevent the cycle from continuing. Nurses can be of assistance in restoring dignity, health, and safety to vulnerable individuals.

Promoting Safety in the Health Care Setting

As stated previously, the IOM report *To Err Is Human* provided proof that errors in the health care industry are at an unacceptably high level (p. 69). Recent health care literature (Leonard et al, 2004; Page, 2004; Kohn et al., 2000) suggests that new systems to improve client safety are needed. Examples include

- Establishing a National Center for Patient Safety to provide leadership for safety improvements and expand the knowledge base for improving safety and preventing errors in health care (Kohn et al., 2000).
- Establishing a reporting system. This information would be used to design systems that are safer for clients. Literature discussions (Berntsen, 2004; Kohn et al., 2000) suggest both a mandatory reporting system for errors causing serious injury or death and a voluntary reporting system for errors that result in no harm, sometimes called "near misses" or "close calls."
- Promoting effective teamwork and communication. Health care practitioners are part of a team and client safety may be at risk if critical, relevant information is not communicated

appropriately. Successful nurse–primary care provider communication is critical. See Chapter 26. ∞

- Creating a culture of trust. There is a need to change the culture in health care from placing blame to examining how to improve. Trust needs to be developed and sustained for people to feel open to discuss and share experiences about their safety near misses and/or errors.
- Involving health care workers in the design of work processes and work spaces to promote efficiency and safety.

Preventing Specific Hazards

Implementing measures to prevent specific hazards or injuries such as burns, fires, falls, poisoning, suffocation, electrocution, and so on are critical aspects of nursing care. Teaching clients about safety is another important aspect. Nurses usually have opportunities to teach while providing care.

SCALDS AND BURNS. A **scald** is a burn from a hot liquid or vapor, such as steam. A **burn** results from excessive exposure to thermal, chemical, electric, or radioactive agents.

Common home hazards causing scalds include the following:

- Pot handles that protrude over the edge of a stove
- Electric appliances used to heat liquids or oils, especially those with dangling cords that are within reach of crawling infants and young children
- Excessively hot bath water

In health care agencies, the risk of scalds and burns is greater for clients whose skin sensitivity to temperature is impaired. Scalds can occur from overly hot bath water, and burns can occur from therapeutic applications of heat (see Chapter 36 ∞). It is important for the nurse to assess how well clients can protect themselves and what special precautions, if any, need to be taken.

FIRES. Fires continue to be a constant risk in both health care settings and homes. Agency fires usually result from malfunctioning electric equipment or combustion of anesthetic gas. Home fires most frequently result from careless disposal of burning cigarettes or matches, from grease, or from faulty electric wiring.

Agency Fires. In health care agencies, fire is particularly hazardous when people are incapacitated and unable to leave the building without assistance. This incapacity makes it extremely important for nurses to be aware of the fire safety regulations and fire prevention practices of the agency in which they work. When a fire occurs the nurse follows four sequential priorities:

1. Protect and evacuate clients who are in immediate danger.
2. Report the fire.
3. Contain the fire.
4. Extinguish the fire.

Extinguishing the fire requires knowledge of three categories of fire, classified according to the type of material that is burning:

Class A: Paper, wood, upholstery, rags, ordinary rubbish
Class B: Flammable liquids and gases
Class C: Electrical

The right type of extinguisher must be used to fight the fire. Extinguishers have picture symbols showing the type of fire for which they are to be used. Directions for use are also attached.

Home Fires. Nursing interventions for home fires focus on teaching fire safety. Preventive measures include the following:

- Keep emergency numbers near the telephone, or stored for speed dialing.
- Be sure the smoke alarms are operable and appropriately located.
- Teach clients to change the batteries in their smoke alarms annually on a special day such as a birthday or January 1.
- Have a family "fire drill" plan. Every member needs to know the plan for the nearest exit from different locations of the home.
- Keep fire extinguishers available and in working order.
- Close windows and doors if possible; cover the mouth and nose with a damp cloth when exiting through a smoke-filled area; and avoid heavy smoke by assuming a bent position with the head as close to the floor as possible.

FALLS. People of any age can fall, but infants and elders are particularly prone to falling and causing serious injury. Falls are the leading cause of injuries among older adults. They are also a major cause of hospital and nursing home admissions. Most falls occur in the home and are a major threat to the independence of older adults. Fear of falling is common in elders, even in those who have not experienced a fall. This fear is of particular concern for those who live alone and who anticipate being helpless and unable to summon help after a fall. For these individuals the nurse should encourage daily or more frequent contact with a friend or family member, installation of a personal emergency response system, and measures to maintain a physical environment that prevents falls. Risk factors and associated preventive measures are shown in Table 32–2.

CLINICAL ALERT

Falls can break bones and self-confidence, leading to fear of falling causing a decreased activity level and decreased muscle strength. All increase the risk of falling. ■

Weak leg muscles, weak knees, poor balance, and loss of flexibility contribute to falls in the elderly. The nurse can use an assessment tool, called the "Get Up and Go" test, in a hospital, subacute, or home setting. Kimbell (2001) describes the following steps of the test:

1. Observe the client's posture while he sits in a straight-backed chair.
2. Ask the client to stand. Observe if the client stands using only his leg muscles or if he needs to push himself up with his hands.
3. Once the client is comfortable standing, ask him to close his eyes. Does he sway?
4. Ask him to open his eyes, walk 10 feet, turn around, and return to the chair. Observe his gait, balance, speed, and stability. How smoothly does he turn?

TABLE 32–2 Risk Factors and Preventive Measures for Falls

RISK FACTOR	PREVENTIVE MEASURES
Poor vision	Ensure eyeglasses are functional. Ensure appropriate lighting. Mark doorways and edges of steps as needed. Keep the environment tidy.
Cognitive dysfunction (confusion, disorientation, impaired memory, or judgment)	Set safe limits to activities. Remove unsafe objects.
Impaired gait or balance and difficulty walking because of lower extremity dysfunction (e.g., arthritis)	Wear shoes or well-fitted slippers with nonskid soles. Use ambulatory devices as necessary (cane, crutches, walker, braces, wheelchair). Provide assistance with ambulation as needed. Monitor gait and balance. Adapt living arrangements to one floor if necessary. Encourage exercise and activity as tolerated to maintain muscle strength, joint flexibility, and balance. Ensure uncluttered environment with securely fastened rugs.
Difficulty getting in and out of chair or in and out of bed	Encourage client to request assistance. Keep the bed in the low position. Install grab bars in bathroom. Provide raised toilet seat.
Orthostatic hypotension	Instruct client to rise slowly from a lying to sitting to standing position, and to stand in place for several seconds before walking.
Urinary frequency or receiving diuretics	Provide a bedside commode. Assist with voiding on a frequent and scheduled basis.
Weakness from disease process or therapy	Encourage client to summon help. Monitor activity tolerance.
Current medication regimen that includes sedatives, hypnotics, tranquilizers, narcotic analgesics, diuretics	Attach side rails to the bed if appropriate. Keep the rails in place when the bed is in the lowest position. Monitor orientation and alertness status. Discuss how alcohol contributes to fall-related injuries. Encourage client not to mix alcohol and medications and to avoid alcohol when necessary. Encourage annual or more frequent review of all medications prescribed.

5. When he gets to the chair, ask him to turn and sit down. Observe how smoothly the client performs this motion.

This quick assessment along with an assessment of the client's environment can help the nurse recommend safety measures to the client and family.

Prevention of falls in health care agencies is an ongoing concern. Health care environments are designed with many safety features to reduce the risk of falls, such as railings along corridors; call bells at each bedside; safety bars in toilet areas; locks on beds, wheelchairs, and stretchers; side rails on beds; night-lights; and so on. In addition, nurses can implement measures to decrease the incidence of falls (see the Practice Guidelines box).

CLINICAL ALERT

When a client falls, the nurse's first duty is to the client. First, assess for injuries. Then, notify the primary care provider. ■

Although it may seem that raising the side rails on a bed is an effective method of preventing falls, rails should not be raised

PRACTICE GUIDELINES Preventing Falls in Health Care Agencies

■ On admission, orient clients to their surroundings and explain the call system.

■ Carefully assess the client's ability to ambulate and transfer. Provide walking aids and assistance as required.

■ Closely supervise the clients at risk for falls, especially at night.

■ Encourage the client to use the call bell to request assistance. Ensure that the bell is within easy reach.

■ Place beside tables and overbed tables near the bed or chair so that clients do not overreach and consequently lose their balance.

■ Always keep hospital beds in the low position and wheels locked when not providing care so that clients can move in or out of bed easily.

■ Encourage clients to use grab bars mounted in toilet and bathing areas and railings along corridors.

■ Make sure nonskid bath mats are available in tubs and showers.

■ Encourage the client to wear nonskid footwear.

■ Keep the environment tidy; especially keep light cords from underfoot and furniture out of the way.

■ Use individualized interventions (e.g., alarm sensitive to client position) rather than side rails for confused clients.

routinely for this purpose. Research has shown that persons with memory impairment, altered mobility, nocturia, and other sleep disorders are prone to becoming entrapped in side rails and may, in fact, be more likely to fall trying to get out of bed by going around or over the raised rails (Marcy-Edwards, 2005).

Electronic devices are available to detect that clients are attempting to move or get out of bed. A bed or chair **safety monitoring device** has a position-sensitive switch that triggers an audio alarm when the client attempts to get out of the bed or chair. Skill 32-1 describes how to use these devices.

USING A BED OR CHAIR EXIT SAFETY MONITORING DEVICE

PURPOSES
- To alert the nurse that the client is attempting to get out of bed
- To help decrease the risk of client falls

ASSESSMENT

Assess
- Mobility status
- Judgment about ability to get out of bed safely
- Proximity of client's room to nurses' station
- Position of side rails
- Functioning status of call light

PLANNING

Determine the appropriate location for the device. If the device will be applied to a thigh, ensure that the location has intact skin.

Delegation
Risk factors for falls may be observed and recorded by persons other than the nurse. The nurse is responsible for assessing the client and confirming that there is a risk of the client falling when getting out of a chair or bed unassisted. The nurse develops a plan of care that includes a variety of interventions that will protect the client. If indicated, use of a safety monitoring device may be delegated to unlicensed assistive personnel (UAP) who have been trained in their application and monitoring.

Equipment
- Alarm and control device
- Sensor
- Connection to nurse call system

IMPLEMENTATION

Performance
1. Prior to performing the procedure, introduce self and verify the client's identity using agency protocol. Explain to client and family the purpose and procedure of using a safety monitoring device. Explain that the device does not limit mobility in any manner; rather, it alerts the staff when the client is about to get out of bed. Explain that the nurse must be called when the client needs to get out of bed.
2. Perform hand hygiene and observe appropriate infection control procedures.
3. Provide for client privacy.
4. Test the battery device and alarm sound. **Rationale:** *Testing ensures that the device is functioning properly prior to use.*

❶ Placing the leg band alarm.
(Courtesy of Alert Care, Mill Valley, CA.)

5. Apply the sensor pad or leg band.
   - Place the leg band according to the manufacturer's recommendation. ❶ Place the client's leg in a straight horizontal position. **Rationale:** *The alarm device is position sensitive; that is, when it approaches a near-vertical position (such as in walking, crawling, or kneeling as the client attempts to get out of bed), the audio alarm will be triggered.*
   - For the bed or chair device, the sensor is usually placed under the buttocks area. ❷
   - For a bed or chair device, set the time delay for determining the client's movement patterns from 1 to 12 seconds.
   - Connect the sensor pad to the control unit and the nurse call system.
6. Instruct the client to call the nurse when the client wants or needs to get up, and assist as required.
   - When assisting the client up, deactivate the alarm.
   - Assist the client back to bed, and reattach the alarm device.
7. Ensure client safety with additional safety precautions.
   - Place call light within client reach, lift side rails per agency policy, and lower the bed to its lowest position. **Rationale:** *The alarm device is not a substitute for other precautionary measures.*
   - Place ambulation monitoring stickers on the client's door, chart, and Kardex.
8. Document the type of alarm used, where it was placed, and its effectiveness in the client record using forms or checklists supplemented by narrative notes when appropriate. Record all additional safety precautions and interventions discussed and employed.

SKILL 32-1

USING A BED OR CHAIR EXIT SAFETY MONITORING DEVICE *continued*

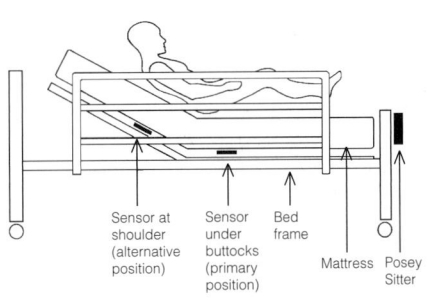

Sensor at shoulder (alternative position) Sensor under buttocks (primary position) Bed frame Mattress Posey Sitter

❷ Placement of a bed exit monitoring device.
(Courtesy of J.T. Posey, Co.)

SAMPLE DOCUMENTATION

7/2/07 Found out of bed again despite frequent reminders given to use call light for assistance. Explained about using a leg band alarm to ensure own safety from possible fall. Verbalized agreement. Alarm device applied. Reminded again of importance to call the nurse for assistance. ———— T. Kyle, RN

EVALUATION

- If the alarm is too sensitive to client movement that is not an attempt to move from bed or chair, reassess and modify alarm controls accordingly.

- Conduct appropriate follow-up relating to effectiveness of safety precautions.
- Report any difficulties using the device or any falls to the primary care practitioner.

HOME CARE CONSIDERATIONS   **Using a Bed or Chair Exit Safety Monitoring Device**

If the device is used in the home, instruct caregivers to do the following:
- Test the monitoring device every 12 to 24 hours to ensure that it is working.
- Check the volume of the alarm to ascertain they can hear it.

Use of the device does not take the place of proper supervision of clients at risk for falling. Assessment of the reasons for falling, especially among elders, can lead to effective prevention.

SEIZURES A **seizure** is a sudden onset of excessive electrical discharges in one or more areas of the brain. Seizures can develop at any time during a person's life and can occur at any time (Gambrell & Flynn, 2004). Clients may be prone to seizures due to permanent or temporary medical conditions such as drug reactions, epilepsy, or extreme fever. However, about 50% of seizures have no known cause (Cross, 2004).

Seizures are classified into two categories: partial and generalized. Partial seizures (also called focal) involve electrical discharges from one area of the brain. In contrast, generalized seizures affect the whole brain. Each of these seizure categories includes different types of seizure, depending on the characteristics of the seizure activity (e.g., loss of consciousness versus no impairment to consciousness). Thus, it is important for nurses to thoroughly describe their observations before, during, and after a client's seizure episode. Clients are at risk for injury if they experience seizures that involve the entire body such as *grand mal* (tonic-clonic) seizures or any seizure that includes loss of consciousness. **Seizure precautions** are safety measures taken by the nurse to protect clients from injury should they have a seizure. Skill 32-2 describes how to implement seizure precautions.

IMPLEMENTING SEIZURE PRECAUTIONS

SKILL 32-2

PURPOSE
- Protect the client from injury

ASSESSMENT
Assess history of seizures during the admission assessment. If the client has experienced a seizure previously, ask for detailed information, including characteristics of an aura or warning symptoms that indicate the seizure is beginning, duration and frequency of the seizures, consequences of the seizures (e.g., incontinence or difficulty breathing), and actions that should be taken to prevent or reduce seizure activity.

continued on page 726

SKILL 32-2

IMPLEMENTING SEIZURE PRECAUTIONS *continued*

PLANNING

Review emergency procedures as a respiratory arrest or other injury can result from a seizure.

> **Delegation**
> UAP should be familiar with establishing and implementing seizure precautions and methods of obtaining assistance during a client's seizure. Care of the client during a seizure, however, is the responsibility of the nurse due to the importance of careful assessment of respiratory status and potential need for intervention.

Equipment
- Blankets or other linens to pad side rails
- Oral suction equipment
- Oxygen equipment

IMPLEMENTATION

Performance

1. Prior to performing the procedure, introduce self and verify the client's identity using agency protocol.
   Explain to the client what you are going to do, why it is necessary, and how he or she can cooperate.
2. Perform hand hygiene and observe appropriate infection control procedures. If the client is actively seizing, apply clean gloves in preparation for performing respiratory care measures.
3. Provide for client privacy.
4. Pad the bed of any client who might have a seizure. Secure blankets or other linens around the head, foot, and side rails of the bed. ❶
5. Put oral suction equipment in place and test to ensure that it is functional. **Rationale:** *Suctioning may be needed to prevent aspiration of oral secretions.*
6. If a seizure occurs:
   - Remain with the client and call for assistance. Do not restrain the client.
   - If the client is not in bed, assist client to the floor and protect the head in your lap or on a pillow. Loosen any clothing around the neck and chest.
   - Turn the client to a lateral position if possible. **Rationale:** *Turning to the side allows secretions to drain out of the mouth, decreasing the risk of aspiration, and helps keep the tongue from occluding the airway.*
   - Move items in the environment to ensure the client does not experience an injury.
   - Do not insert anything into the client's mouth.
   - Time the seizure duration.
   - Observe the progression of the seizure, noting the sequence and type of limb involvement. Observe skin color. When the seizure allows, check pulse and respirations.
   - Apply oxygen.
   - Use equipment to suction the oral airway if the client vomits or has excessive oral secretions.
   - Administer anticonvulsant medications, as ordered.
   - When the seizure has subsided, assist client to a comfortable position. Reorient. Explain what happened. Reassure the

❶ Padding a bed for seizure precautions.

client. Provide hygiene as necessary. Allow the client to verbalize feelings about the seizure.
7. Document the event in the client record using forms or checklists supplemented by narrative notes when appropriate.

SAMPLE DOCUMENTATION

7/8/07 1815 Upon entering room, observed generalized muscle spasms/contractions of arms and legs lasting 25 seconds. Seizure padding previously placed on bed. Incontinent of urine. Cyanotic. Placed on left side. Suctioned. Airway clear. Respirations slightly irregular at 14/min. Oxygen applied at 4L/min via mask. Oxygen sat 90% on O2. Not currently responding to verbal stimuli. Dr. Smith notified. Diazepam 10 mg given IV per order. VS taken every 15 min. See neuro flow sheet. ———————————————— *B. Gill, RN*

EVALUATION

- Perform a detailed follow-up examination of the client. Administer medications if indicated and ordered.
- Report significant deviations from normal to the primary care practitioner.

LIFESPAN CONSIDERATIONS   Implementing Seizure Precautions

INFANTS

- About 24% of children experience seizures, most during infancy (Ball & Bindler, 2003).

CHILDREN

- Febrile seizures occur more commonly than in adults and are usually preventable through antipyretics and tepid baths.

- Determine oxygenation. Apply oxygen if pulse oximetry reading is less than 95% (see Chapter 50). ∞
- Children who have frequent seizures may need to wear helmets for protection.
- Children on anticonvulsant medications should wear a medical identification tag (bracelet or necklace).

HOME CARE CONSIDERATIONS   Implementing Seizure Precautions

- If clients have frequent or recurrent seizures or take anticonvulsant medications, they should wear a medical identification tag (bracelet or necklace) and carry a card delineating any medications they take.
- When making home visits, inspect anticonvulsant medications and confirm that clients are taking them correctly. Blood level measurements may be required periodically.
- Assist clients in determining which persons in the community should/must be informed of their seizure disorder (e.g., employ-

ers, health care providers such as dentists, motor vehicle department if driving, companions).
- Discuss safety precautions for inside and out of the home. If seizures are not well controlled, activities that may require restriction or direct supervision by others include tub bathing, swimming, cooking, using electric equipment or machinery, and driving.
- Discuss with the client and family factors that may precipitate a seizure.

POISONING. Inadequate supervision and improper storage of many household toxic substances are the major reasons for poisoning in children. Implementing poison prevention for children is focused on teaching parents to "childproof" the environment, including disposing of unused medications properly by flushing them down a drain. Adolescent and adult poisonings are usually caused by insect or snake bites and drugs used for recreation or in suicide attempts. Implementing poison prevention in these age groups focuses on providing information and counseling. Poisoning in elders usually results from accidental ingestion of a toxic substance (e.g., due to failing eyesight) or an overdose of a prescribed medication (e.g., due to impaired memory). Implementing poison prevention with elders focuses on safeguarding the environment and monitoring the underlying problems.

In elders who have dementia, poisoning is often a safety problem. As cognitive abilities deteriorate, the same precautions need to be taken as with children. Elders who have dementia have the need to feel everything and will put anything in their mouths, including plants, flowers, candles, small objects, and medications. These and other potentially dangerous items need to be locked up or kept out of reach. A telephone number for the nearest poison control center should be readily available. These precautions are important whether the individual with dementia is being cared for at home or in an institution.

In response to the ever-increasing number of poison hazards, many countries have established poison control centers that provide accurate, up-to-date information about potential hazards and recommend treatment as needed. For certain poisons, specific antidotes or treatments are available; for many, there is no specific therapy.

Nurses intervene in community settings by educating the public about what to do in the event of poisoning: Identify the specific poison by searching for an opened container, empty bottle, or other evidence. Contact the poison control center, indicate the exact quantity of poison the person ingested, and state the person's age and apparent symptoms. Keep the person as quiet as possible and lying on the side or sitting with head placed between the legs to prevent aspiration of vomitus. The Client Teaching feature provides additional guidelines for teaching clients to prevent poisoning.

CARBON MONOXIDE POISONING. **Carbon monoxide** (CO) is an odorless, colorless, tasteless gas that is very toxic. Exposure to CO can cause symptoms including headaches, dizziness, weakness, nausea, vomiting, or loss of muscle control. Prolonged exposure to CO can lead to unconsciousness, brain damage, or death. Learning the steps to prevent CO exposure is particularly important because all gasoline-powered vehicles, lawn mowers, kerosene stoves, barbecues, and burning wood emit CO. Incomplete or faulty combustion of any fuel, including natural gas used in furnaces, also produces CO. Carbon monoxide detectors are available for the home.

SUFFOCATION OR CHOKING. Suffocation, or **asphyxiation,** is lack of oxygen due to interrupted breathing. Suffocation occurs when the air source is cut off for any reason. One common reason for choking is that food or a foreign object has become lodged in the throat. The universal sign of distress is the victim's grasping the anterior neck and being unable to speak or cough. The emergency response is the **Heimlich maneuver.** or abdominal thrust, which can dislodge the foreign object and reestablish an airway. See Figure 32-3 ∎.

CLIENT TEACHING   Preventing Poisoning

- Lock potentially toxic agents, including drugs and cleaning agents, in a cupboard, or attach special plastic hooks to the insides of cabinet doors to keep them securely closed. Unlatching these hooks requires firmer thumb pressure than small children can usually exert. Don't let children watch you open the latches. Kids learn fast!
- Avoid storing toxic liquids or solids in food containers, such as soft drink bottles, peanut butter jars, or milk cartons.
- Do not remove container labels or reuse empty containers to store different substances. Laws mandate that the labels of all poisons specify antidotes.
- Do not rely on cooking to destroy toxic chemicals in plants. Never use anything prepared from nature as a medicine or "tea."
- Teach children never to eat any part of an unknown plant or mushroom and not to put leaves, stems, bark, seeds, nuts, or berries from any plant into their mouths.

- Place poison warning stickers designed for children on containers of bleach, lye, kerosene, solvent, and other toxic substances.
- Do not refer to medicine as candy or pretend false enjoyment when taking medications in front of children; allow them to see the necessity of the medicine without glamorizing it.
- Read and follow label directions on all products before using them.
- Keep syrup of ipecac on hand at all times. Syrup of ipecac is a nonprescription emetic available in single-dose 15-mL vials in all drugstores. Use it only after advice from the local poison control center or the family primary care provider.
- Do not keep poisonous plants in the home, and avoid planting poisonous plants in the yard. The cooperative extension agency in your county can provide a list of poisonous plants.
- Display the phone number of the poison control center near or on all telephones in the home so that it is available to baby-sitters, family, and friends.

Figure 32-3 ■ Performing the Heimlich maneuver.

Other causes of suffocation are drowning, gas or smoke inhalation, accidental coverage of the nose and mouth by a piece of plastic, accidental strangulation by the shoulder harness of a seat belt, and being trapped in a confined space (e.g., a discarded refrigerator). If a person does not receive immediate relief from suffocation, the interrupted breathing leads to respiratory and cardiac arrest and death. Any obstruction to the air passages must be immediately removed and life support measures instituted when an arrest occurs.

EXCESSIVE NOISE. Excessive noise is a health hazard that can cause hearing loss, depending on (a) the overall level of noise, (b) the frequency range of the noise, and (c) the duration of exposure and individual susceptibility. Sound levels above 120 decibels (units of loudness) are painful and may cause hearing damage even if a person is exposed for only a short period. Exposure to 85 to 95 decibels for several hours a day can lead to progressive or permanent hearing loss. Noise levels below 85 decibels usually do not affect hearing.

Tolerance of noise is largely individual. The rural dweller may find the city noisy, whereas the city dweller may be oblivious to urban sounds.

When ill or injured, people are frequently sensitive to noises that normally would not disturb them. Loud voices, the clatter of dishes, and even a nearby television can disturb clients, some of whom react angrily. Physiologic effects of noise include (a) increased heart and respiratory rates, (b) increased muscular activity, (c) nausea, and (d) hearing loss, if the noise is sufficiently loud.

Noise can be minimized in several ways. Acoustic tile on ceilings, walls, and floors as well as drapes and carpeting absorb sound. Background music can mask noise and have a calming effect on some people. It is important for nurses to minimize noise in the hospital setting and to encourage clients to protect their hearing as much as possible.

ELECTRICAL HAZARDS. All electric equipment must be properly grounded. The electric plug of grounded equipment has three prongs. The two short prongs transmit the power to the equipment. The third, longer prong is the grounding device, which carries short circuits or stray electric current to the ground (Figure 32-4 ■). Grounding prongs offer a path of least resistance to stray electric currents.

Faulty equipment such as equipment with a frayed cord presents a danger of electric shock or may start a fire. For example, an electric spark near certain anesthetic gases or a high concentration of oxygen can cause a serious fire. Actions to reduce electrical hazards are described in Client Teaching.

When major electrical injury (macroshock) does occur, the victim may sustain both superficial and deep burns, muscle contractions, and cardiac and respiratory arrest, necessitating car-

Figure 32-4 ■ Three-pronged grounded plug.

CLIENT TEACHING **Reducing Electrical Hazards**

- Check cords for fraying or other signs of damage before using an appliance. Do not use if damage is apparent.
- Avoid overloading outlets and fuse boxes with too many appliances.
- Use only grounded outlets and plugs.
- Always pull a plug from the wall outlet by firmly grasping the plug and pulling it straight out. Pulling a plug by its cord can damage the cord and plug unit.
- Never use electric appliances near sinks, bathtubs, showers, or other wet areas, because water readily conducts electricity.
- Keep electric cords and appliances out of the reach of young children.

- Place protective covers over wall outlets to protect young children.
- Have all noninsulated wiring in the home altered to meet safety standards.
- Carefully read instructions before operating electric equipment. Clients who do not understand how to operate the equipment should seek advice.
- Always disconnect appliances before cleaning or repairing them.
- Unplug any appliance that has given a tingling sensation or shock and have an electrician evaluate it for stray current.
- Keep electric cords coiled or taped to the ground away from areas of traffic to prevent others from damaging the cords or tripping over them.

---

diopulmonary resuscitation and life support. **Electric shock** occurs when a current travels through the body to the ground rather than through electric wiring, or from static electricity that builds up on the body. Using machines in good repair, wearing shoes with rubber soles, standing on a nonconductive floor, and using nonconductive gloves can prevent macroshock. However, even with such precautions the rescuer must know that the victim is not to be touched until the electricity is shut off or the victim has been removed from contact with the electric current; otherwise the rescuer may also receive electrical injury.

FIREARMS. Parents who bring a handgun into the home must accept full responsibility for teaching safety rules to any children who have knowledge of the presence of firearms. The following basic firearm safety rules must be implemented for any gun:

- Store all guns in sturdy locked cabinets without glass and make sure the keys are inaccessible to children.
- Store the bullets in a different location from the guns.
- Tell children never to touch a gun or stay in a friend's house where a gun is accessible.
- Teach children never to point the barrel of a gun at anyone.
- Ensure the firearm is unloaded and the action is open when handing it to someone else.
- Don't handle firearms while affected by alcohol or drugs of any kind, including pharmaceuticals.
- When cleaning or dry firing a firearm, remove all ammunition to another room, and double-check the firearm when you enter the room you will be using to clean the firearm.
- Have firearms that are regularly used inspected by a qualified gunsmith at least every 2 years.

RADIATION. Radiation injury can occur from overexposure to radioactive materials used in diagnostic and therapeutic procedures. Clients being examined using radiography or fluoroscopy generally receive minimal exposure and few precautions are necessary. Nurses need to protect themselves, however, from radiation when some clients are receiving radiation therapy. Exposure to radiation can be minimized by (a) limiting the time near the source, (b) providing as much distance as possible from the source, and (c) using shielding devices such as lead aprons when near the source. Nurses need

to become familiar with agency protocols related to radiation therapy.

BIOTERRORISM ATTACK. No one knows when a bioterrorism attack will occur. Thus, it is important that health care personnel and facilities plan and prepare for the unknown. JCAHO requires its accredited health care organizations to meet established disaster preparedness standards. In 2001, these standards were expanded to introduce the concepts of emergency management and community involvement in the preparedness process. Health care organizations are now expected to address four specific phases of disaster planning—mitigation, preparedness, response, and recovery—as well as to participate annually in at least one community-wide practice drill (JCAHO, 2005a, p. 4). A major part of being prepared is knowledge. See Box 32–3 for a list of content that nurses should know about terrorism. These elements are imperative for an appropriate response to a potential bioterrorism attack.

BOX 32–3 Key Knowledge Content about Bioterrorism

- Detection and reporting of an unusual outbreak or syndrome (e.g., CDC's categorization of biological agents and the process for reporting to public health authorities)
- Treatment of casualties (e.g., basic prophylactic guidelines, nursing care needs for each biological agent)
- Implementation of control measures (e.g., using standard precautions for every patient, isolation procedures, cleaning, disinfection and sterilization of equipment, linen, and the environment)
- Resource acquisition and preparedness planning (e.g., how to obtain resources such as medical equipment, medications, personnel during a crisis)
- Management of public reactions to bioterrorism (e.g., clear communication to victims, mental health professional support, treatment of anxiety in people not exposed but concerned)

Note: From "Integrating Bioterrorism Education into Nursing School Curricula," by C. Steed, L. Howe, R. Pruitt, and W. Sherrill, 2004, *Journal of Nursing Education.* Copyright © 2004 SLACK, Inc. Reprinted with permission.

MediaLink   Disaster Nursing and the Red Cross

Procedure- and Equipment-Related Accidents

Risk assessment in the health care setting must include risks related to procedures and equipment. Whether giving a medication or assisting a client out of bed, nurses need to follow safeguards to prevent errors or accidents. Most health care agencies establish protocols that are designed to prevent accidents. When in doubt about a course of action, the nurse should consult the appropriate written guidelines before proceeding.

When an accident or error does occur, most agencies require that the incident be reported. The nurse completes the report immediately after taking whatever action is required to safeguard the client and notifying the charge nurse. For additional information about incident reports, see Chapter 4. ∞

Restraining Clients

Restraints are protective devices used to limit the physical activity of the client or a part of the body. They can be classified as physical or chemical. **Physical restraints** are any manual method or physical or mechanical device, material, or equipment attached to the client's body; they cannot be removed easily and they restrict the client's movement. **Chemical restraints** are medications such as neuroleptics, anxiolytics, sedatives, and psychotropic agents used to control socially disruptive behavior. The purpose of restraints is to prevent the client from injuring self or others.

Restraints, however, can injure. In 1998, JCAHO sent out a sentinel event alert warning of the need to prevent restraint deaths. This alert resulted after a tracking study of sentinel events, which are unexpected occurrences that resulted in death or serious injury. The results indicated that 20 clients who were being physically restrained had died, with the majority of deaths caused by asphyxiation and strangulation. In addition to the physical safety concerns, many consider restraints to be de-

meaning and psychologically harmful. Some believe they limit a client's autonomy. The current focus in health care is to explore ways to prevent, reduce, and hopefully eliminate the use of restraints while protecting a client's safety, rights, and dignity.

LEGAL IMPLICATIONS OF RESTRAINTS. Increasingly, determining the need for safety measures is viewed as an independent nursing function. However, because restraints restrict the individual's freedom, their use has legal implications. Nurses need to know their agency's policies and state laws about restraining clients. The U.S. Centers for Medicare and Medicaid Services published revised standards for use of restraints in the United States in 2001. These standards apply to all health care organizations and specify two standards for applying restraints: the behavior management standard when the client is a danger to self or others, and the acute medical and surgical care standard when temporary immobilization of a client is required to perform a procedure. In the case of the behavior management standard, the nurse may apply restraints but the primary care provider or other licensed independent practitioner must see the client within 1 hour for evaluation. A written restraint order for an adult, following evaluation, is valid for only 4 hours. If the client must be restrained and secluded, there must be continual visual and audio monitoring of the client's status. The medical surgical care standard permits up to 12 hours for obtaining the primary care provider written order for the restraints. All orders must be renewed daily. See Figure 32-5 ■ for an example of a restraint monitoring and intervention flow sheet.

Standards require that a primary care provider's order for restraints state the reason and time period. The use of a prn order for restraints is prohibited. In all cases, restraints should be used *only* after every other possible means of ensuring safety have been unsuccessful and documented. See alternatives to the use

---

RESEARCH NOTE   **Does the Use of Restraints Vary between Hospitals in the United States and Other Countries?**

This observational research study used a descriptive, correlational design to compare the relationship between clients' characteristics, environment, and actual use of restraints in critical care units in Norway and the United States. Fifty ICU clients in each country were observed for 10 weeks. During this time the researchers collected data on the level of activity and use of physical restraints. Other collected data included a description of the ICU environment, the nurse-to-client ratio, and nursing workload.

The results indicated that the use of restraints was associated with client activity. Restraints were used 40% of the time in U.S. subjects and not at all in the Norwegian sample. The Norwegian subjects were more sedated. The client characteristics between the two countries did not significantly differ. The activity level, however, differed significantly. The clients in the United States were more active, and the most common restraint used was soft wrist restraints. The activity that led to restraints being applied was interference with an invasive device. Seven incidents of unplanned removal of an invasive device occurred in the United States sample—all in restrained clients. The activity level was less in the Norwegian sample as morphine sulfate was administered at a substantially higher dose.

The nursing workload per client and nurse-to-client ratio differed significantly between the two samples. The nursing workload was higher in the Norwegian sample, and the Norwegian nurse-to-client ratio remained higher than the ratio in the U.S. critical care units.

In the discussion of the study, the researchers pointed out that there was a cultural norm in Norway for nurses to remain within a distance that allows direct visual observation of clients, respiratory therapists are not used at all, and unlicensed personnel are used infrequently.

IMPLICATIONS

Additional research and larger scale studies are needed to determine the effectiveness of restraint-free care. Comparing health care practices in different cultural settings helps nurses become more aware of their own environment.

Note: American Journal of Critical Care by B. Martin and L. Mathisen. Copyright 2005 by American Association of Critical-Care Nurses. Reproduced with permission of American Association of Critical Care Nurses in the format Textbook via Copyright Clearance Center.

Medical Center

ACUTE MEDICAL/SURGICAL CARE
RESTRAINT FLOW SHEET

Restraint Initiated: Date: _____   Time: _____

Order Expires: Date: _____   Time: _____
New verbal order required every 24 hours.

Assessment should be based on individual needs. Patients must be assessed at least every 2 hours.

	0700	0800	0900	1000	1100	1200	1300	1400	1500	1600	1700	1800	1900	2000	2100	2200	2300	2400	0100	0200	0300	0400	0500	0600
Restraints Removed																								
Skin & Circulation Assessed																								
Toileting Offered																								
Food/Fluids Offered																								
Range of Motion & Patient Repositioned																								
Patient Response — R=Restless C=Calm S=Sleeping U=Unaware																								
Effect of Restraint — A=Adequate I=Inadequate (explain)																								
Continued Need — Y=Yes N=No																								
Restraint Reapplied																								
Initials																								

Explain: _____

_____

INIT	SIGNATURE	TITLE

©HRC 2003
HSPI F9440

Figure 32-5 ■ Restraint monitoring and intervention flow sheet.

(Courtesy of Health South Medical Center, Birmingham, Alabama.)

BOX 32–4 **Alternatives to Restraints**

- Assign nurses in pairs to act as "buddies" so that one nurse can observe the client when the other leaves the unit.
- Place unstable clients in an area that is constantly or closely supervised.
- Prepare clients before a move to limit relocation shock and resultant confusion.
- Stay with a client using a bedside commode or bathroom if the client is confused or sedated or has a gait disturbance or a high risk score for falling.
- Monitor all the client's medications and, if possible, attempt to lower or eliminate dosages of sedatives or psychotropics.
- Position beds at their lowest level to facilitate getting in and out of bed.
- Replace full-length side rails with half- or three-quarter-length rails to prevent confused clients from climbing over rails or falling from the end of the bed.
- Use rocking chairs to help confused clients expend some of their energy so that they will be less inclined to wander.
- Wedge pillows or pads against the sides of wheelchairs to keep clients well positioned.
- Place a removable lap tray on a wheelchair to provide support and help keep the client in place.
- To quiet agitated clients, try a warm beverage, soft lights, a back rub, or a walk.
- Use "environmental restraints," such as pieces of furniture or large plants as barriers, to keep clients from wandering beyond appropriate areas.
- Place a picture or other personal item on the door to clients' rooms to help them identify their room.
- Try to determine the causes of the client's sundowner syndrome (nocturnal wandering and disorientation as darkness falls, associated with dementia). Possible causes include poor hearing, poor eyesight, or pain.
- Establish ongoing assessment to monitor changes in physical and cognitive functional abilities and risk factors.

of restraints in Box 32–4. Restrained clients often become more restless and anxious as a result of the loss of self-control. Nurses must document that the need for the restraint was made clear both to the client and family.

Clients have the right to be free from restraints that are not medically necessary. As a result, there must be justification that the use of restraints will protect the client and that less restrictive measures were attempted and found not effective. Restraints *cannot* be used for staff convenience or client punishment. Given that the above conditions are met and restraints are needed, it is important for the nurse to be able to correctly apply restraints without endangering client safety.

SELECTING A RESTRAINT. Before selecting a restraint, nurses need to understand its purpose clearly and measure it against the following five criteria:

1. It restricts the client's movement as little as possible. If a client needs to have one arm restrained, do not restrain the entire body.
2. It does not interfere with the client's treatment or health problem. If a client has poor blood circulation to the hands, apply a restraint that will not aggravate that circulatory problem.
3. It is readily changeable. Restraints need to be changed frequently, especially if they become soiled. Keeping other guidelines in mind, choose a restraint that can be changed with minimal disturbance to the client.
4. It is safe for the particular client. Choose a restraint with which the client cannot self-inflict injury. For example, a physically restrained person could be injured trying to climb out of bed if one wrist is tied to the bed frame. A jacket restraint would restrain the person more safely.
5. It is the least obvious to others. Both clients and visitors are often embarrassed by a restraint, even though they understand why it is being used. The less obvious the restraint, the more comfortable people feel.

KINDS OF RESTRAINTS. There are several kinds of restraints. Among the most common for adults are jacket restraints, belt restraints, mitt or hand restraints, and limb restraints. Geri chairs, wheelchairs with lap trays, and bed rails can also be considered restraints. Restraints for infants and children include mummy restraints, elbow restraints, and crib nets (see Lifespan Considerations later in the chapter). When using restraints, the nurse may find the Practice Guidelines box helpful.

When evaluating if a device is a restraint or not, determine the intended use (e.g., physical restriction), its involuntary application, and/or the client need for the restraint (JCAHO, 2005b). For example, if all of the bed's side rails are up and restrict the client's freedom to leave the bed, and the client did not voluntarily request all rails to be up, they are a restraint. If, however, one side rail is up to assist the client to get in and out of the bed, it is not a restraint. Also, if the client can release or remove a device, it would not be considered a restraint.

There are several types of vest restraints, but all are essentially sleeveless jackets or vests with straps (tails) that can be tied to the bed frame under the mattress. These body restraints are used to ensure the safety of confused or sedated clients in beds or wheelchairs. The U.S. Food and Drug Administration (FDA) advises that manufacturers place "front" and "back" labels on vest restraints.

Belt or safety strap body restraints (Figure 32-6 ■) are used to ensure the safety of all clients who are being moved on stretchers or in wheelchairs. Some wheelchairs have a soft, padded safety bar that attaches to side brackets that are installed under the arm rests. To prevent the person from slumping forward, the nurse then attaches a shoulder "Y" strap to the bar and over the client's shoulders to the rear handles. Other safety belt models have a three-loop design. One loop surrounds the person's waist and attaches to the rear handles. If such restraints are unavailable, the nurse can place a folded towel or small sheet around the client's waist and fasten it at the back of the wheel-

PRACTICE GUIDELINES Applying Restraints

- Obtain consent from the client or guardian.
- Ensure that a primary care provider's order has been provided or, in an emergency, obtain one within 24 hours after applying the restraint.
- Assure the client and the client's support people that the restraint is temporary and protective. A restraint must never be applied as punishment for any behavior or merely for the nurse's convenience.
- Apply the restraint in such a way that the client can move as freely as possible without defeating the purpose of the restraint.
- Ensure that limb restraints are applied securely but not so tightly that they impede blood circulation to any body area or extremity.
- Pad bony prominences (e.g., wrists and ankles) before applying a restraint over them. The movement of a restraint without padding over such prominences can quickly abrade the skin.
- Always tie a limb restraint with a knot (e.g., a clove hitch) that will not tighten when pulled.
- Tie the ends of a body restraint to the part of the bed that moves to elevate the head. Never tie the ends to a side rail or to the fixed frame of the bed if the bed position is to be changed.
- Assess the restraint per agency protocol time frame. Some facilities have specific forms to be used to record ongoing assess-
ment. This may be a visual check to ensure client safety and no signs of injury.
- Assess skin integrity per agency protocol (e.g., every 2 hours), and provide range-of-motion (ROM) exercises (see Chapter 44 ∞) and skin care when restraints are removed (see Chapter 36 ∞).
- Assess and assist with basic needs: nutrition, hydration, hygiene, elimination.
- Reassess the continued need for the restraint. Include an assessment of the underlying cause of the behavior necessitating use of the restraints.
- When a restraint is temporarily removed, do not leave the client unattended.
- Immediately report to the nurse in charge and record on the client's chart any persistent reddened or broken skin areas under the restraint.
- At the first indication of cyanosis or pallor, coldness of a skin area, or a client's complaint of a tingling sensation, pain, or numbness, loosen the restraint and exercise the limb.
- Apply a restraint so that it can be released quickly in case of an emergency and with the body part in a normal anatomic position.
- Provide emotional support verbally and through touch.

chair. Belt restraints may also be used for certain clients confined to bed or to chairs.

A mitt or hand restraint (Figure 32-7 ■) is used to prevent confused clients from using their hands or fingers to scratch and injure themselves. For example, a confused client may need to be prevented from pulling at intravenous tubing or a head bandage following brain surgery. Hand or mitt restraints allow the client to be ambulatory and/or to move the arm freely rather than be confined to a bed or a chair. Mittens need to be removed on a regular basis to permit the client to wash and exercise the

hands. The nurse also needs to take off the mitten to check the circulation to the hand.

Limb restraints (Figure 32-8 ■), which are generally made of cloth, may be used to immobilize a limb, primarily for therapeutic reasons (e.g., to maintain an intravenous infusion). See Skill 32-3 for applying restraints.

Figure 32-7 ■ A mitt restraint.

Figure 32-6 ■ A belt restraint.

Figure 32-8 ■ A limb restraint.

APPLYING RESTRAINTS

PURPOSES
- To promote safety and prevent injury
- To allow a medical or surgical treatment to proceed without client interference (e.g., to prevent movements that would disrupt therapy to a limb connected to tubes or appliance)

ASSESSMENT
Assess

- The behavior indicating the possible need for a restraint
- Underlying cause for assessed behavior

- What other protective measures may be implemented before applying a restraint
- Status of skin to which restraint is to be applied
- Circulatory status distal to restraints and of extremities
- Effectiveness of other available safety precautions

PLANNING
Review institutional policy for restraints and seek consultation as appropriate before independently deciding to apply a restraint. All other possible interventions that are less restrictive *must* have been tried. The primary care practitioner must be notified prior to using a restraint, unless there is a danger to self or others. In that case the primary care practitioner must be notified within the prescribed time frame per the agency protocol.

Delegation
The nurse must make the determination that restraints are appropriate in specific situations, select the proper type of restraints, evaluate the effectiveness of the restraints, and assess for potential complications from their use. Application of ordered restraints and their temporary removal for skin assessment and care may be delegated to UAP who have been trained in their use.

Equipment
- Appropriate type and size of restraint

IMPLEMENTATION
Performance

1. Prior to performing the procedure, introduce self and verify the client's identity using agency protocol. Explain to the client and family what you are going to do, why it is necessary, and how they can cooperate. Discuss how the results will be used in planning further care or treatments. Allow time for the client to express feelings about being restrained. Provide needed emotional reassurance that the restraints will be used only when absolutely necessary and that there will be close contact with the client in case assistance is required.
2. Perform hand hygiene and observe appropriate infection control procedures.
3. Provide for client privacy if indicated.
4. Apply the selected restraint.

   Belt Restraint (Safety Belt)
   - Determine that the safety belt is in good order. If a Velcro safety belt is to be used, make sure that both pieces of Velcro are intact.
   - If the belt has a long portion and a shorter portion, place the long portion of the belt behind (under) the bedridden client and secure it to the movable part of the bed frame. **Rationale:** *The long attached portion will then move up when the head of the bed is elevated and will not tighten around the client.* Place the shorter portion of the belt around the client's waist, over the gown. There should be a finger's width between the belt and the client.
      or
   - Attach the belt around the client's waist, and fasten it at the back of the chair.
      or
   - If the belt is attached to a stretcher, secure the belt firmly over the client's hips or abdomen. **Rationale:** *Belt restraints*

must be applied to all clients on stretchers even when the side rails are up.

Jacket Restraint
- Place vest on client, with opening at the front or the back, depending on the type.
- Pull the tie on the end of the vest flap across the chest, and place it through the slit in the opposite side of the chest.
- Repeat for the other tie.

Use a half-bow knot to secure each tie around the movable bed frame or behind the chair to a chair leg ❶ ❷).

A

B

C Pull here to untie

❶ To make a half-bow knot (quick-release knot), first place the restraint tie under the side frame of the bed (or around a chair leg). *A,* Bring the free end up, around, under, and over the attached end of the tie and pull it tight. *B,* Again take the free end over and under the attached end of the tie, but this time make a half-bow loop. *C,* Tighten the free end of the tie and the bow until the knot is secure. To untie the knot, pull the end of the tie and then loosen the first cross over the tie.

SKILL 32-3

APPLYING RESTRAINTS *continued*

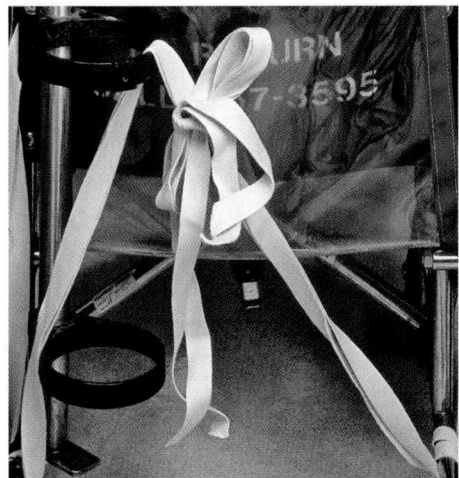

❷ Quick-release knot.
(Al Dodge, Pearson Education/PH College)

Rationale *A half-bow knot does not tighten or slip when the attached end is pulled but unties easily when the loose end is pulled.*

or

- Fasten the ties together behind the chair using a slip or quick-release knot.
- Ensure that the client is positioned appropriately to enable maximum chest expansion for breathing.

Mitt Restraint

- Apply the commercial thumbless mitt (Figure 32-7 ■) to the hand to be restrained. Make sure the fingers can be slightly flexed and are not caught under the hand.
- Follow the manufacturer's directions for securing the mitt.
- If a mitt is to be worn for several days, remove it at regular intervals per agency protocol. Wash and exercise the client's hand, then reapply the mitt. Check agency practices about recommended intervals for removal.
- Assess the client's circulation to the hands shortly after the mitt is applied and at regular intervals. **Rationale:** *Client complaints of numbness, discomfort, or inability to move the fingers could indicate impaired circulation to the hand.*

Wrist or Ankle Restraint

- Pad bony prominences on the wrist or ankle if needed to prevent skin breakdown.
- Apply the padded portion of the restraint around the ankle or wrist.
- Pull the tie of the restraint through the slit in the wrist portion or through the buckle. ❸
- Using a half-bow knot (quick-release knot), attach the other end of the restraint to the movable portion of the bed frame.

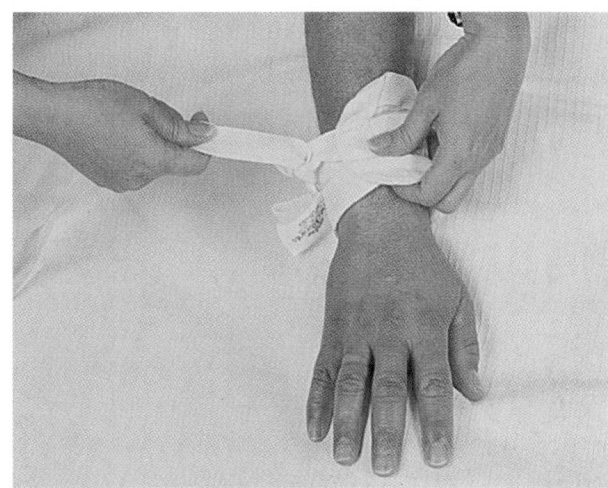

❸ Ensure that a finger can be inserted between the restraint and the wrist or ankle.

Rationale: *If the ties are attached to the movable portion, the wrist or ankle will not be pulled when the bed position is changed.*

5. Adjust the plan of care as required, for example, to include releasing the restraint, providing skin care, range-of-motion exercises, and attending to the client's physical needs by providing fluids, nutrition, and toileting.
6. Record on the client's chart the behavior(s) indicating the need for the restraint, all other interventions implemented in an attempt to avoid the use of restraints and their outcomes, and the time the primary care providers was notified of the need for restraint. Also record:
   - The type of restraint applied, the time it was applied, and the goal for its application.
   - The client's response to the restraint.
   - The times that the restraints were removed and skin care given.
   - Any other assessments and interventions.
   - Explanations given to the client and significant others.

SAMPLE DOCUMENTATION

7/10/2007 2000 Confused. Disoriented to time and place. Reoriented frequently. Pulling at central IV line, NG tube and chest tube. Medicated for pain relief. Lights dimmed. Continues to pull at IV and tubes. Dr. Jones called. Received an order to apply mitt restraints. Family called and explained the situation. Stated someone will come in and sit with the client. Mitt restraints applied till family member arrives. ——— *C. Murphy, RN*

EVALUATION

- Perform a detailed follow-up of the need for the restraints and the client's response. Relate these findings to previous data if available.
- Evaluate circulatory status of restrained limbs.

- Evaluate skin status beneath restraints.
- Remove the restraints as soon as they are no longer needed and document.
- Report significant deviations from normal to the physician.

LIFESPAN CONSIDERATIONS **Restraints**

INFANTS

Elbow restraints (Figure 32-9 ■) are used to prevent infants or small children from flexing their elbows to touch or reach their face or head, especially after surgery. Ready-made elbow restraints are available commercially.

A mummy restraint (Figure 32-10 ■) is a special folding of a blanket or sheet around the infant to prevent movement during a procedure such as gastric washing, eye irrigation, or collection of a blood specimen.

- Obtain a blanket or sheet large enough so that the distance between opposite corners is about twice the length of the infant's body. Lay the blanket or sheet on a flat, dry surface.
- Fold down one corner, and place the baby on it in the supine position.
- Fold the right side of the blanket over the infant's body, leaving the left arm free (Figure 32-10 *A* ■,). The right arm is in a natural position at the side.

- Fold the excess blanket at the bottom up under the infant (Figure 32-10 , *B,* 2 ■).
- With the left arm in a natural position at the baby's side, fold the left side of the blanket over the infant, including the arm, and tuck the blanket under the body (Figure 32-10, *B,* 3 ■).
- Remain with the infant who is in a mummy restraint until the specific procedure is completed.

CHILDREN

A crib net is simply a device placed over the top of a crib to prevent active young children from climbing out of the crib. At the same time, it allows them freedom to move about in the crib. The crib net or dome is not attached to the movable parts of the crib so that the caregiver can have access to the child without removing the dome or net.

- Place the net over the sides and ends of the crib.
- Secure the ties to the springs or frame of the crib. The crib sides can then be freely lowered without removing the net.
- Test with your hand that the net will stretch if the child stands against it in the crib.

Figure 32-9 ■ Infant with elbow restraints.
(Roy Ramsey, Pearson Education/PH College)

A   **B**

Figure 32-10 ■ Making a mummy restraint.

HOME CARE CONSIDERATIONS **Applying Restraints**

Restraints may be necessary for clients in wheelchairs or in the home. Safety guidelines apply in all cases. Assess the knowledge and skill of all caregivers in the use of restraints and educate as indicated.

- Use means other than restraints as much as possible, and stay with the client.
- Pad bony prominences, such as wrists and ankles, if needed before applying a restraint over them.

- Tie restraints with knots that will not tighten when pulled and to parts of the wheelchair that do not move and release quickly in case of emergency.
- Assess restrained limbs for signs of impaired blood circulation.
- Always stay with a client whose restraint is temporarily removed.

Evaluating

To prevent client injury, the nurse's role is largely educative and desired outcomes reflect the client's acquisition of knowledge of hazards, behaviors that incorporate safety practices, and skills to perform in the event of certain emergencies. The nurse needs to individualize these for clients. Examples of desired outcomes include the client being able to do the following:

- Describe methods to prevent specific hazards (e.g., falls, suffocation, choking, fires, drowning, electric shock).
- Report use of home safety measures (e.g., fire safety measures, smoke detector maintenance, fall prevention strategies, burn prevention measures, poison prevention measures, safe storage of hazardous materials, firearm safety precautions, electrocution prevention, water safety precautions, bicycle safety, motor vehicle safety).

- Alter home physical environment to reduce the risk of injury.
- Describe emergency procedures for poisoning and fire.
- Describe age-specific risks, work safety risks, or community safety risks.

- Demonstrate correct use of child safety seats.
- Demonstrate correct administration of cardiopulmonary resuscitation.

LIFESPAN CONSIDERATIONS Safety

ELDERS

Some of the changes due to aging that place the elder at higher risk for safety concerns are

- Decrease in hearing and sight.
- Decrease in response of reflexes.
- Fragility of bones and decrease in flexibility of joints and muscles.
- Decrease in temperature regulation, increasing the risk of hypothermia and hyperthermia.

- Decrease in kidney function, which increases risk of toxicity from medications.

A home environment that was safe when they were younger may need modifications for elders to decrease the risk of injury. A plan and telephone numbers of those to call should be available for emergency situations.

CRITICAL THINKING CHECKPOINT

Mr. Moore is a 72-year-old widower who is recovering from a fall in which he fractured his hip and underwent surgical repair 1 week ago. He will be staying with his son for 2 weeks after he is discharged from the hospital, but he is eager to return to his own home. Once he is home, his son will visit nightly after work, he will receive Meals on Wheels once a day, and a home health care attendant will visit weekly to assist him with hygienic care until he is more independent. Mr. Moore's wife died 3 years ago, but he has remained independent and continued his social functions. He lives in a small single-level house with his dog and cat, and he enjoys gardening. Prior to fracturing his hip he walked his dog daily. You will be his home health care nurse.

1. While hospitalized, Mr. Moore experienced some mild confusion during the night, but his nurses decided not to restrain him. What are the best reasons for avoiding the use of restraints for clients such as Mr. Moore?
2. What are some of the more obvious factors that may affect Mr. Moore's safety as he returns home?
3. What do you need to assess in regard to Mr. Moore's safety and what suggestions can you make for enhancing his safety?
4. What strengths do you note about Mr. Moore that may protect him from injury when he returns home?

See Critical Thinking Possibilities in Appendix A. ∞

CHAPTER 32 **REVIEW**

CHAPTER HIGHLIGHTS

- Injuries are a major cause of death among individuals of all ages in the United States.
- Nurses need awareness of what constitutes a safe environment for specific individuals and for groups of people in the home, community, and workplace.
- Hazards to safety occur at all ages and vary according to the age and development of the individual.
- Nursing assessment of safety includes assessing factors that can affect safety, for example, age, lifestyle, mobility, sensory alterations, level of awareness, emotional state, and environmental factors.
- Nurses assess clients at risk for injury through methods such as nursing history and physical examination, risk assessment tools, and home hazard appraisal.
- Recent studies and reports (e.g., *To Err Is Human*) indicate that the incidence of medical errors in hospitals is too high and half are preventable. At least 80% of the medical errors are system related. As a result, National Patient Safety Goals (NPSGs) were initiated and are required to be implemented by JCAHO-accredited agencies. The focus of the NPSGs is on system-wide solutions.
- Nurses need to sustain a heightened awareness and alertness of circumstances or patterns that may indicate potential bioterrorism.

Early detection and management is needed to help stop a bioterrorism attack.

- Major nursing diagnoses for clients at risk for accidental injury can be categorized as *Risk for Injury,* with seven subcategories: *Risk for Poisoning, Risk for Suffocation, Risk for Trauma, Latex Allergy Response, Risk for Latex Allergy Response, Contamination, Risk for Contamination, Risk for Aspiration,* and *Risk for Disuse Syndrome.*
- When planning to meet safety needs of clients, nurses need to consider physical factors in the environment and the psychologic and physiologic state of the individual. Clients often need to change their health behavior and may need to modify the environment.
- Measures to ensure the safety of people of all ages focus on (a) observation or prediction of situations that are potentially harmful and (b) client education that empowers clients to safeguard themselves and their families from injury. Education is a major health protection strategy in preventing accidents.
- Nurses must be familiar with the fire procedures in the health care agency where they practice. In the event of a fire, the nurse must

(a) protect clients from injury, (b) report, (c) contain, and (d) put out the fire.

■ Falls are a common cause of injury among older adults.

■ Prevention of falls in health care agencies is a continuous concern.

■ Side rails do not protect hospitalized clients from falls. It is more likely the client will fall trying to get around or over the side rail.

■ Seizure precautions are safety measures taken by the nurse to protect clients from injury should they have a seizure.

■ Major reasons for poisoning in children are inadequate supervision and improper storage of household toxic substances.

■ Suffocation can occur when foreign objects are swallowed or inhaled, cutting off the person's oxygen supply.

■ Prolonged exposure to excessive noise can produce hearing loss.

■ Faulty electric equipment and improper grounding pose health hazards in the hospital and the home. Accidents can be prevented by using grounded outlets and plugs, putting protective covers over outlets, keeping appliances in good repair, and making sure that electric wiring and circuits meet safety standards.

■ Firearms pose a risk to individuals of all ages. Adults must take full responsibility for following safety procedures when keeping firearms in the home, including storage of ammunition in a separate location.

■ In hospitals, radioactive substances are used for both diagnostic and treatment purposes; agency policy should be followed to safeguard clients and staff from unsafe exposure.

■ Various alternatives to restraints must be considered before a restraint is applied.

■ Because restraints restrict a client's basic freedom to move, careful assessment and accurate, complete documentation are important when restraints are used.

TEST YOUR KNOWLEDGE

1. Place the following nursing priorities in correct sequence if a fire occurs in a health setting.
   1. Report the fire.
   2. Extinguish the fire.
   3. Protect the clients.
   4. Contain the fire.

2. What is the leading cause of accidents in young and middle-aged adults?
   1. Automobile crashes
   2. Drowning and firearms
   3. Falls
   4. Suicide and homicide

3. Because a hospitalized elderly female client, who ambulates with a walker, is receiving diuretics which results in frequent trips to the bathroom at night, the nurse should perform which of the following?
   1. Leave the bathroom light on.
   2. Withhold the client's diuretic medication.
   3. Provide a bedside commode.
   4. Keep the side rails up.

4. Which NANDA nursing diagnosis is most applicable for toddlers?
   1. *Risk for Suffocation*
   2. *Risk for Injury*
   3. *Risk for Poisoning*
   4. *Risk for Disuse Syndrome*

5. A 75-year-old client, hospitalized with a cerebral vascular accident (stroke), becomes disoriented at times and tries to get out of bed, but is unable to ambulate without help. What is the most appropriate safety measure?
   1. Restrain the client in bed.
   2. Ask a family member to stay with the client.
   3. Check the client every 15 minutes.
   4. Use a bed exit safety monitoring device.

6. A client is being admitted to the hospital because of a seizure that occurred at his home. The client has no previous history of seizures. In planning the client's nursing care, which of the following measures is most essential at this time of admission? Select all that apply.
   1. Place a padded tongue depressor at the head of the bed.
   2. Pad the bed with blankets.
   3. Inform the client about the importance of wearing a medical identification tag.
   4. Teach the client about epilepsy.
   5. Test oral suction equipment.

7. Which of the following nursing interventions is the highest in priority for a client at risk for falls in a hospital setting?
   1. Keep all of the side rails up.
   2. Review prescribed medications.
   3. Complete the "get up and go" test.
   4. Place the bed in the lowest position.

8. Medication errors can place the client at significant risk. Which of the following practices will help decrease the possibility of errors? Select all that apply.
   1. Hire only competent nurses.
   2. Improve the nurse's ability to multitask.
   3. Establish a reporting system for "near misses."
   4. Communicate effectively.
   5. Create a culture of trust.

9. When planning to teach health care topics to a group of male adolescents, the nurse should consider which of the following topics a priority?
   1. Sports contribute to an adolescent's self-esteem.
   2. Sunbathing and tanning beds can be dangerous.
   3. Guns are the most frequently used weapon for adolescent suicide.
   4. A driver's education course is mandatory for safety.

10. The nurse, at change-of-shift report, learns that one of the clients in his care has bilateral soft wrist restraints. The client is confused, is trying to get out of bed, and had pulled out the IV line which was subsequently reinserted. Which of the following actions by the nurse is appropriate? Select all that apply.
    1. Document the behavior(s) that require continued use of the restraints.
    2. Ensure that the restraints are tied to the side rails.
    3. Provide range-of-motion exercises when the restraints are removed.
    4. Orient the client.
    5. Assess the tightness of the restraints.

See Answers to Test Your Knowledge in Appendix A. ∞

EXPLORE MEDIALINK www.prenhall.com/berman

DVD-ROM
- Audio Glossary
- NCLEX Review
- Skills Checklists
- Animation: Lead Poisoning

COMPANION WEBSITE
- Additional NCLEX Review
- Case Study: Ensuring Client Safety
- Care Plan Activity: Safety at Home
- Application Activities:
  - Disaster Nursing and the Red Cross
  - Safety in Nursing Issues
- Links to Resources

READINGS AND REFERENCES

SUGGESTED READINGS

Cross, C. (2004). Seizures. Regaining control. *RN, 67*(12), 44–50.
The author provides a comprehensive summary of the different types of seizures, how to protect the client during a seizure, diagnostic tests, drug therapy, and important teaching points.

Joint Commission International Center for Patient Safety.
This website, http://www.jcipatientsafety.org, provides a wide array of practical solutions that can be used to improve the safety and quality of patient care in health care environments.

Marcy-Edwards, D. (2005). Bed rails. Is there an up side? *Canadian Nurse, 101*(1), 30–34.
This is a fascinating historical perspective of bed rail use in Canada, Great Britain, and the United States. The author also discusses how bed rail use is influenced not only by the nurse's knowledge base but also by the moral and ethical belief systems of the nurse.

McCarter-Bayer, A., Bayer, F., & Hall, K. (2005). Preventing falls in acute care: An innovative approach. *Journal of Gerontological Nursing, 31*(3), 25–33.
This article describes a fall prevention program instituted in an acute care setting in southern Arizona that produced encouraging results.

Tsilimingras, D., Rosen, A. K., & Berlowitz, D. R. (2003). Patient safety in geriatrics: A call for action. *Journals of Gerontology, 58A*(9), 813–819.
The authors point out that the IOM reports To Err Is Human and Crossing the Quality Chasm did not address the safety implications of elderly clients. This article describes aging and medical errors and recommendations for improving the safety of geriatric care.

Walker-Cillo, G. (2006). Bioterrorism! We put our plan to the test. *RN, 69*(4), 36–41.
The author and her colleagues participated in the largest terrorism response drill the United States has ever conducted. What they learned from the 2-day experience is helpful information.

RELATED RESEARCH

Hart-Hughes, S., Quigley, P., Bulat, T., Palacios, P., & Scott, S. (2004). An interdisciplinary approach to reducing fall risks and falls. *Journal of Rehabilitation, 70*(4), 46–51.

Johnson, K., & Hudson, M. A. (2004). Keeping patients safe: An analysis of organizational culture and caregiver training. *Journal of Healthcare Management, 49*(3), 171–179.

Li, F., Harmer, P., Fisher, J., McAuley, E., Chaumeton, N., Eckstrom, E., & Wilson, N. L. (2005). Tai chi and fall reductions in older adults: A randomized controlled trial. *Journals of Gerontology, 60A*(2), 187–194.

Morgan, R. O., Virnig, B. A., Duque, M., Abdel-Moty, E., & DeVito, C. A. (2004). Low-intensity exercise and reduction of the risk for falls among at-risk elders. *Journals of Gerontology, 59A*(10), 1062–1067.

Wang, W., & Moyle, W. (2005). Physical restraint use on people with dementia: A review of the literature. *Australian Journal of Advanced Nursing, 22*(4), 46–52.

REFERENCES

Ball, J., & Bindler, R. (2003). *Pediatric nursing: Caring for children* (3rd ed.). Upper Saddle River, NJ: Prentice Hall Health.

Berntsen, K. J. (2004). Valuable lessons in patient safety. Reporting near misses in healthcare. *Journal of Nursing Care Quality, 19*(3), 177–179.

Cross, C. (2004). Seizures. Regaining control. *RN, 67*(12), 44–50.

Ebersole, P., Hess, P., Touhy, T., & Jett, K. (2005). *Gerontological nursing & healthy aging* (2nd ed.). St. Louis, MO: Mosby.

Gambrell, M., & Flynn, N. (2004). Seizures 101: Brush up on the essentials about seizures, so you can remain calm and provide effective care. *Nursing, 34*(8), 36–41.

Institute of Medicine, (2000). *To err is human. Building a safer health system.* Washington, DC: National Academy of Sciences.

Institute of Medicine. (2004). *Keeping patients safe. Transforming the work environment of nurses.* Washington, DC: National Academies Press.

Joint Commission on Accreditation of Healthcare Organizations. (2006). *Facts about 2006 National Patient Safety Goals.* Retrieved June 19, 2006, from http://www.jointcommission.org/PatientSafety/NationalPatientSafetyGoals/06_npsg_facts.htm

Joint Commission on Accreditation of Healthcare Organizations (JCAHO). (2005a). *Setting the standard.* Oakbrook Terrace, IL: Author.

Joint Commission on Accreditation of Healthcare Organizations (JCAHO). (2005b). *Restraint and seclusion.* Retrieved June 11, 2006, from http://www.jointcommission.org/AccreditationPrograms/BehavioralHealthCare/Standards/FAQs/Provision+of+Care+Treatment+and+Services/Restraint+and+Seclusion/Restraint_Seclusion.htm

Kimbell, S. (2001). Before the fall. Keeping your patient on his feet. *Nursing, 3*(8), 44–45.

Kohn, L. T., Corrigan, J. M., & Donaldson, M. S. (Eds.). (2000). *To err is human. Building a safer health system.* Washington, DC: National Academy Press.

Leonard, M., Frankel, A., Simmonds, T., & Vega, K. B. (2004). *Achieving safe and reliable healthcare.* Chicago: Health Administration Press.

Marcy-Edwards, D. (2005). Bed rails: Is there an up side? *Canadian Nurse, 101*(1), 30–34.

Martin, B., & Mathisen, L. (2005). Use of physical restraints in adult critical care: A bicultural study. *American Journal of Critical Care, 14*(2), 133–142.

Massey, M. (2004, October 11). Battling bioterrorism. *Advance for Nurses–Northern California and Reno, NV,* 30–31.

Moorhead, S., Johnson, M., & Mao, S. M. (2004). *Nursing outcomes classification* (3rd ed.). St Louis: Mosby.

Dochterman, J. M., & Bulechek, G. M. (Eds.). (2004). *Nursing interventions classification (NIC)* (4th ed.). St. Louis, MO: Mosby.

NANDA International. (2007). *NANDA nursing diagnoses: Definitions and classification 2007–2008.* Philadelphia: Author.

Page, A. (Ed.). (2004). *Keeping patients safe. Transforming the work environment of nurses.* Washington, DC: National Academies Press.

Steed, C. J., Howe, L. A., Pruitt, R. H., & Sherrill, W. W. (2004). Integrating bioterrorism education into nursing school curricula. *Journal of Nursing Education, 43*(8), 362–367.

Weber, C. J. (2004). Update on bioterrorism preparedness. *Urologic Nursing, 24*(5), 417–419.

Wilkinson, J. M. (2005). *Nursing diagnosis handbook with NIC interventions and NOC outcomes* (8th ed.). Upper Saddle River, NJ: Prentice Hall Health.

SELECTED BIBLIOGRAPHY

American Geriatrics Society. (2006). *Falls in older adults. Management in primary practice.* Retrieved June 18, 2006, from http://www.americangeriatrics.org/education/falls.shtml

Beyea, S. C. (2004). A critical partnership–Safety for nurses and patients. *AORN Journal, 79*(6), 1299–1302.

Beyea, S. C. (2005). Patient advocacy–Nurses keeping patients safe. *AORN Journal, 81*(5), 1046–1047.

Centers for Disease Control and Prevention. (2001). Recognition of illness associated with the intentional release of a biologic agent. *Morbidity and Mortality Weekly Report, 50*(41), 893–897.

Centers for Disease Control and Prevention. (2001). *Facts about botulism.* Retrieved June 18, 2006, from http://www.bt.cdc.gov/agent/botulism/factsheet.asp

Centers for Disease Control and Prevention. (2002). *Fact sheet: Anthrax information for health care providers.* Retrieved June 18, 2006, from http://www.bt.cdc.gov/agent/anthrax/anthrax-hcp-factsheet.asp

Centers for Disease Control and Prevention. (2003). *Key facts about tularemia.* Retrieved June 18, 2006, from http://www.bt.cdc.gov/agent/tularemia/facts.asp

Centers for Disease Control and Prevention. (2003). *Frequently asked questions (FAQ) about tularemia.* Retrieved June 18, 2006, from http://www.bt.cdc.gov/agent/tularemia/faq.asp

Centers for Disease Control and Prevention. (2004). *Viral hemorrhagic fevers.* Retrieved June 19, 2006, from http://www.cdc.gov/ncidod/dvrd/spb/mnpages/dispages/Fact_Sheets/Viral_Hemorrhagic_Fevers_Fact_Sheet.pdf

Centers for Disease Control and Prevention. (2004). *Frequently asked questions about smallpox.* Retrieved June 19, 2006, from http://www.bt.cdc.gov/agent/smallpox/disease/faq.asp

Centers for Disease Control and Prevention. (2004). *Smallpox disease overview.* Retrieved June 18, 2006, from http://www.bt.cdc.gov/agent/smallpox/overview/disease-facts.asp

Centers for Disease Control and Prevention. (2005). *Frequently asked questions (FAQ) about plague.* Retrieved June 19, 2006, from http://www.bt.cdc.gov/agent/plague/faq.asp

Centers for Disease Control and Prevention. (2005). *Questions and answers about anthrax.* Retrieved June 18, 2006, from http://www.bt.cdc.gov/agent/anthrax/faq/index.asp

Jasniewski, J. (2006). Take steps to protect your patient from falls. *Nursing, 36*(4), 24–25.

Joint Commission on Accreditation of Healthcare Organizations. (2006). *2007 critical access hospital and hospital national patient safety goals.* Retrieved June 19, 2006, from http://www.jointcommission.org/PatientSafety/NationalPatientSafetyGoals/07_hap_cah_npsgs.htm

Joint Commission on Accreditation of Healthcare Organizations. (2006). *2007 Long term care national patient safety goals.* Retrieved June 19, 2006, from http://www.jointcommission.org/PatientSafety/NationalPatientSafetyGoals/07_ltc_npsgs.htm

Joint Commission on Accreditation of Healthcare Organizations (JCAHO). (2003). *Health care at the crossroads. Strategies for creating and sustaining community-wide emergency preparedness systems.* Oakbrook Terrace, IL: Author.

Karber, S., & Fasano, N. (2003). What you need to know about the smallpox vaccine. *Nursing, 33*(6), 36–42.

Kleen, K. (2004). Restraint regulation: The tie that binds. *Nursing Management, 35*(11), 36–38.

Lyons, S. S. (2005). Evidence-based protocol: Fall prevention for older adults. *Journal of Gerontological Nursing, 31*(11), 9–14.

Manno, M., Hogan, P., Heberlein, V., Nyakiti, J., & Mee, C. L. (2006). Patient-safety survey report. *Nursing, 36*(3), 54–63.

Marthaler, M. T. (2004). Seizures revisited. *Nursing Management, 35*(4), 71–74.

McBeth, S. (2004). Get a firmer grasp on restraints. *Nursing Management, 35*(10), 20–22.

Morath, J., & Leary, M. (2004). Creating safe spaces in organizations to talk about safety. *Nursing Economics, 22*(6), 344–354.

Murphy, J. K. (2004). After 9/11: Priority focus areas for bioterrorism preparedness in hospitals. *Journal of Healthcare Management, 49*(4), 227–235.

Napierkowski, D. (2002). Using restraints with restraint. *Nursing, 32*(11), 58–62.

National Safety Council. (2004). How to prevent poisonings in your home. Retrieved June 18, 2006, from http://www.nsc.org/library/facts/poisong.htm

National Safety Council. (2004). *Carbon monoxide.* Retrieved June 18, 2006, from http://www.nsc.org/library/facts/carbmono.htm

National Safety Council. (2004). *Lead poisoning.* Retrieved June 22, 2005, from http://www.nsc.org/library/facts/lead.htm

Pena, C. G. (2003). Seizure. A calm response and careful observation are crucial. *American Journal of Nursing, 103*(11), 73–81.

Rowell, P. (2003, September 30). The professional nursing association's role in patient safety. *Online Journal of Issues in Nursing, 8*(3), manuscript 3. Retrieved June 18, 2006, from http://nursingworld.org/ojin/topic22/tpc22_3.htm

Todd, J. F. (2004). Burning beds. *Nursing, 34*(9), 23.

Hygiene

LEARNING OUTCOMES

After completing this chapter, you will be able to:

1. Describe hygienic care that nurses provide to clients.

2. Identify factors influencing personal hygiene.

3. Identify normal and abnormal assessment findings while providing hygiene care.

4. Apply the nursing process to common problems related to hygienic care of the skin, feet, nails, mouth, hair, eyes, ears, and nose.

5. Identify the purposes of bathing.

6. Describe various types of baths.

7. Explain specific ways in which nurses help hospitalized clients with hygiene.

8. Describe steps for identified hygienic-care procedures.

9. Identify steps in removing contact lenses and inserting and removing artificial eyes.

10. Describe steps for removing, cleaning, and inserting hearing aids.

11. Identify safety and comfort measures underlying bed-making procedures.

Hygiene is the science of health and its maintenance. Personal **hygiene** is the self-care by which people attend to such functions as bathing, toileting, general body hygiene, and grooming. Hygiene is a highly personal matter determined by individual values and practices. It involves care of the skin, hair, nails, teeth, oral and nasal cavities, eyes, ears, and perineal-genital areas.

It is important for nurses to know exactly how much assistance a client needs for hygienic care. Clients may require help after urinating or defecating, after vomiting, and whenever they become soiled, for example, from wound drainage or from profuse perspiration. Table 33–1 lists factors that influence hygiene practices.

HYGIENIC CARE

Nurses commonly use the following terms to describe types of hygienic care. *Early morning care* is provided to clients as they awaken in the morning. This care consists of providing a urinal or bedpan to the client confined to bed, washing the face and hands, and giving oral care. *Morning care* is often provided after clients have breakfast, although it may be provided before breakfast. It usually includes providing for elimination needs, a bath or shower, perineal care, back massages, and oral, nail, and hair care. Making the client's bed is part of morning care. *Hour of sleep (HS)* or *PM care* is provided to clients before they re-

tire for the night. It usually involves providing for elimination needs, washing face and hands, giving oral care, and giving a back massage. *As-needed (prn) care* is provided as required by the client. For example, a client who is diaphoretic (sweating profusely) may need more frequent bathing and a change of clothes and linen.

SKIN

The skin is the largest organ of the body. It serves five major functions:

1. It protects underlying tissues from injury by preventing the passage of microorganisms. The skin and mucous membranes are considered the body's first line of defense.
2. It regulates the body temperature. Cooling of the body occurs through the heat loss processes of evaporation of perspiration, and by radiation and conduction of heat from the body when the blood vessels of the skin are vasodilated. Body heat is conserved through lack of perspiration and vasoconstriction of the blood vessels. See Chapter 30. ∞
3. It secretes **sebum,** an oily substance that (a) softens and lubricates the hair and skin, (b) prevents the hair from becoming brittle, and (c) decreases water loss from the skin

TABLE 33–1 Factors Influencing Individual Hygienic Practices

FACTOR	VARIABLES
Culture	North American culture places a high value on cleanliness. Many North Americans bathe or shower once or twice a day, whereas people from some other cultures bathe once a week. Some cultures consider privacy essential for bathing, whereas others practice communal bathing. Body odor is offensive in some cultures and accepted as normal in others.
Religion	Ceremonial washings are practiced by some religions.
Environment	Finances may affect the availability of facilities for bathing. For example, homeless people may not have warm water available; soap, shampoo, shaving lotion, and deodorants may be too expensive for people who have limited resources.
Developmental level	Children learn hygiene in the home. Practices vary according to the individual's age; for example, preschoolers can carry out most tasks independently with encouragement.
Health and energy	Ill people may not have the motivation or energy to attend to hygiene. Some clients who have neuromuscular impairments may be unable to perform hygienic care.
Personal preferences	Some people prefer a shower to a tub bath. People have different preferences regarding the time of bathing (e.g., morning versus evening).

when the external humidity is low. Because fat is a poor conductor of heat, sebum (d) lessens the amount of heat lost from the skin. Sebum also (e) has a **bactericidal** (bacteria-killing) action.

4. It transmits sensations through nerve receptors, which are sensitive to pain, temperature, touch, and pressure.
5. It produces and absorbs vitamin D in conjunction with ultraviolet rays from the sun, which activate a vitamin D precursor present in the skin.

The normal skin of a healthy person has transient and resident microorganisms that are not usually harmful. See Chapter 36. ∞

Sudoriferous (sweat) glands are on all body surfaces except the lips and parts of the genitals. The body has from 2 to 5 million, which are all present at birth. They are most numerous on the palms of the hands and the soles of the feet. Sweat glands are classified as apocrine and eccrine. The **apocrine glands,** located largely in the axillae and anogenital areas, begin to function at puberty under the influence of androgens. Although they produce sweat almost constantly, apocrine glands are of little use in thermoregulation. The secretion of these glands is odorless, but when decomposed or acted on by bacteria on the skin, it takes on a musky, unpleasant odor. The **eccrine glands** are important physiologically. They are more numerous than the apocrine glands and are found chiefly on the palms of the hands, the soles of the feet, and the forehead. The sweat they produce cools the body through evaporation. Sweat is made up of water, sodium, potassium, chloride, glucose, urea, and lactate.

NURSING MANAGEMENT

Assessing

Assessment of the client's skin and hygienic practices includes (a) a nursing health history to determine the client's skin care practices, self-care abilities, and past or current skin problems; (b) physical assessment of the skin; and (c) identification of clients at risk for developing skin impairments.

Nursing History

Data about the client's skin care practices enable the nurse to incorporate the client's needs and preferences as much as possible in the plan of care. According to Andrews and Boyle (2003, p. 55), people in most cultures in the United States try to disguise natural body odors by bathing frequently and using deodorant, cologne, or perfumes. Immigrants from other countries where water is scarce may bathe less often than people from countries where water is more accessible.

Assessment of the client's self-care abilities determines the amount of nursing assistance and the type of bath (e.g., bed, tub, or shower) best suited for the client. Important considerations include the client's balance (for tub and shower), ability to sit unsupported (in the tub or bed), activity tolerance, coordination, adequate muscle strength, appropriate joint range of motion, vision, and the client's preferences. Cognition and motivation are

---

CULTURALLY COMPETENT CARE
Biocultural Variations in Body Secretions

- Most Asians and Native North Americans have a mild to absent body odor, whereas Whites and African Americans tend to have strong body odor.
- Eskimos have made an environmental adaptation where they sweat less than Whites on their trunks and extremities but more on their faces. This adaptation allows for temperature regulation without the need to change clothes because of perspiration.
- The amount of chloride excreted by sweat glands varies widely. African Americans have lower salt concentrations in their sweat than Whites.

Note: From M. M. Andrews and J. S. Boyle, *Transcultural Concepts in Nursing Care,* 4th ed. Lippincott, Williams & Wilkins, 2003. Reprinted with permission.

---

also essential. Clients whose cognitive function is impaired or whose illness alters energy levels and motivation will usually need more assistance. It is important for the nurse to determine the client's functional level and to maintain and promote as much client independence as possible. This also enables the nurse to identify the client's potential for growth and rehabilitation. There are several models of functional levels of self-care. One example is shown in Table 33–2.

The presence of past or current skin problems alerts the nurse to specific nursing interventions or referrals the client may require. Many skin care conditions have implications for hygienic care. The client may provide descriptions of these problems during the nursing health history, or the nurse may observe some during the physical examination that follows. Common skin problems and implications for nursing interventions are shown in Table 33–3. Questions to elicit data about the client's skin care practices, self-care abilities, and skin problems are shown in the accompanying Assessment Interview.

Physical Assessment

Physical assessment of the skin, which involves inspection and palpation, is described in Chapter 30. ∞ When assisting with bathing and other hygienic care, the nurse often has the opportunity to collect data about skin color, uniformity of color, texture, turgor, temperature, intactness, and lesions.

Diagnosing

Self-Care Deficit diagnoses are used for clients who have problems performing hygiene care. Three of NANDA's four self-care deficit diagnoses, specified as *Self-Care Deficit: Bathing/Hygiene, Self-Care Deficit: Dressing/Grooming,* and *Self-Care Deficit: Toileting* are discussed in this chapter. The fourth diagnosis, *Self-Care Deficit: Feeding,* is discussed in Chapter 47. ∞

Difficulties encountered by the client in performing bathing activities include the inability to wash the body or body parts, to obtain or get to a water source, and to regulate water temperature

TABLE 33-2	**Definitions and Descriptors for Functional Level**				
	(0) **COMPLETELY INDEPENDENT**	**(+ 1)** **REQUIRES USE OF EQUIPMENT OR DEVICE**	**SEMIDEPENDENT (+ 2)** **REQUIRES HELP FROM ANOTHER PERSON FOR ASSISTANCE, SUPERVISION, OR TEACHING**	**MODERATELY DEPENDENT (+ 3)** **REQUIRES HELP FROM ANOTHER PERSON AND EQUIPMENT OR DEVICE**	**TOTALLY DEPENDENT (+ 4)** **DEPENDENT, DOES NOT PARTICIPATE IN ACTIVITY**
Bathing			Nurse provides all equipment; positions client in bed/bathroom. Client completes bath, except for back and feet.	Nurse supplies all equipment; positions client; washes back, legs, perineum, and all other parts, as needed. Client can assist.	Client needs complete bath; cannot assist at all.
Oral hygiene			Nurse provides equipment; client does task.	Nurse prepares brush, rinses mouth, positions client.	Nurse completes entire procedure.
Dressing/ grooming			Nurse gathers items for client; may button, zip, or tie clothing. Client dresses self.	Nurse combs client's hair, assists with dressing, buttons and zips clothing, ties shoes.	Client needs to be dressed and cannot assist the nurse; nurse combs client's hair.
Toileting			Client can walk to bathroom/commode with assistance; nurse helps with clothing.	Nurse provides bedpan, positions client on or off bedpan, places client on commode.	Client is incontinent; nurse places client on bedpan or commode.

Note: From *Nursing Diagnosis Handbook with NIC Interventions and NOC Outcomes,* 8th ed. (pp. 424, 428, 435), by J. M. Wilkinson, 2005. Upper Saddle River, NJ: Prentice Hall Health. Adapted with permission.

TABLE 33-3	**Common Skin Problems**
PROBLEM AND APPEARANCE	**NURSING IMPLICATIONS**
Abrasion Superficial layers of the skin are scraped or rubbed away. Area is reddened and may have localized bleeding or serous weeping.	1. Prone to infection; therefore, wound should be kept clean and dry. 2. Do not wear rings or jewelry when providing care to avoid causing abrasions to clients. 3. Lift, do not pull, a client across a bed. 4. Use two or more people for assistance.
Excessive Dryness Skin can appear flaky and rough.	1. Prone to infection if the skin cracks; therefore, provide alcohol-free lotions to moisturize the skin and prevent cracking. 2. Bathe client less frequently; use no soap, or use nonirritating soap and limit its use. Rinse skin thoroughly because soap can be irritating and drying. 3. Encourage increased fluid intake if health permits to prevent dehydration.
Ammonia Dermatitis (Diaper Rash) Caused by skin bacteria reacting with urea in the urine. The skin becomes reddened and is sore.	1. Keep skin dry and clean by applying protective ointments containing zinc oxide to areas at risk (e.g., buttocks and perineum). 2. Boil an infant's diapers or wash them with an antibacterial detergent to prevent infection. Rinse diapers well because detergent is irritating to an infant's skin.
Acne Inflammatory condition with papules and pustules.	1. Keep the skin clean to prevent secondary infection. 2. Treatment varies widely.
Erythema Redness associated with a variety of conditions, such as rashes, exposure to sun, elevated body temperature.	1. Wash area carefully to remove excess microorganisms. 2. Apply antiseptic spray or lotion to prevent itching, promote healing, and prevent skin breakdown.
Hirsutism Excessive hair on a person's body and face, particularly in women.	1. Remove unwanted hair by using depilatories, shaving, electrolysis, or tweezing. 2. Enhance client's self-concept.

ASSESSMENT INTERVIEW **Skin Hygiene**

SKIN CARE PRACTICES

- What are your usual showering or bathing times?
- What hygienic products do you routinely use (e.g., bath oils, powder, facial cleansing creams, body lotions or creams, deodorants, antiperspirants)?
- What facial cosmetic products do you use?
- How and when do you clean makeup applicators and puffs? (Applicators should be kept clean, and products used around the eyes in particular should be discarded after 4 months to prevent bacterial and fungal infections.)
- What hygienic or cosmetic products do you not use because of the skin problems they create (e.g., skin dryness or allergic reactions)?

SELF-CARE ABILITIES

- Do you have any problems managing your hygienic practices (e.g., baths and facial care)? If so, what are these?
- How can the nurses best help you?

SKIN PROBLEMS

- Do you have any tendency toward skin dryness, itchiness, rashes, bruising, excessive perspiration, or lack of perspiration? Have you had skin or scalp lesions in the past?
- Do you have any allergic tendencies? If so, what?

Positive responses to any of these require further exploration in terms of duration (When did it start?); frequency (How often have you had this?); description of lesion or rash; any associated signs, such as fever or nausea; aggravating factors (e.g., season of the year, stress, occupation, medication, recent travel, housing, personal contact); alleviating factors (e.g., medications, lotions, home remedies); and any family history of the problem.

---

or flow. Difficulties in dressing and grooming include inability to obtain, put on, take off, fasten, or replace articles of clothing; and to maintain appearance at a satisfactory level. Toileting problems may involve difficulties getting to the toilet or commode or sitting on and rising from it. In addition, the client may experience problems manipulating clothing for toileting, carrying out proper toilet hygiene, or flushing the toilet or emptying the commode. The reasons (etiologies or related factors) for these problems are varied (see Box 33–1).

Clinical examples of assessment data clusters, related nursing diagnoses, outcomes, and interventions are shown in the accompanying Identifying Nursing Diagnoses, Outcomes, and Interventions.

Examples of associated diagnoses include the following:

- *Deficient Knowledge* related to
  a. Lack of experience with skin condition (acne) and need to prevent secondary infection
  b. New therapeutic regimen to manage skin problems
  c. Lack of experience in providing hygiene care to dependent person
  d. Unfamiliarity with devices available to facilitate sitting on or rising from toilet

---

BOX 33–1 **Etiologies of Self-Care Deficits**

- Decreased or lack of motivation
- Weakness or tiredness
- Pain or discomfort
- Perceptual or cognitive impairment
- Inability to perceive body part or spatial relationship
- Neuromuscular or musculoskeletal impairment
- Medically imposed restriction
- Therapeutic procedure restraining mobility (e.g., intravenous infusion, cast)
- Severe anxiety
- Environmental barriers

- *Situational Low Self-Esteem* related to
  a. Visible skin problem (e.g., acne or alopecia)
  b. Body odor

The diagnoses *Risk for Impaired Skin Integrity* and *Impaired Skin Integrity* are discussed in Chapter 36. ∞

Planning

In planning care, the nurse and, if appropriate, the client and/or family set outcomes for each nursing diagnosis. The nurse then performs nursing interventions and activities to achieve the client outcomes.

The specific, detailed nursing activities taken by the nurse may include assisting dependent clients with bathing, skin care, and perineal care; providing back massages to promote circulation; instructing clients/families about appropriate hygienic practices and alternative methods for dressing; and demonstrating use of assistive equipment and adaptive activities. Although the nursing interventions discussed in this chapter focus on hygienic measures, the etiology of the nursing diagnoses established may point to other interventions that promote circulation, promote self-esteem, restore nutritional status, correct fluid deficits or excesses, or prevent problems associated with immobility. Nursing strategies to deal with these etiologies are provided in other chapters.

Planning to assist a client with personal hygiene includes consideration of the client's personal preferences, health, and limitations; the best time to give the care; and the equipment, facilities, and personnel available. A client's personal preferences—about when and how to bathe, for example—should be followed as long as they are compatible with the client's health and the equipment available. Another consideration for the nurse is to assess the client's comfort level with the gender of the caregiver. Hygienic care, particularly bathing, can be embarrassing and stressful to modest individuals. Women in some cultures (e.g., Hindu, Iranian, Korean, Arab, and Navajo Indian) are generally modest. Nurses must respect a person's modesty,

IDENTIFYING NURSING DIAGNOSES, OUTCOMES, AND INTERVENTIONS
Clients With Skin Problems

DATA CLUSTER   Stan Bailey, 75 years old, suffered a "stroke" 2 weeks ago resulting in paralysis of his left side. He states, "I don't want a bath. I can wash myself. I just want to be left alone." He is withdrawn and uncommunicative.

NURSING DIAGNOSIS/ DEFINITION	SAMPLE DESIRED OUTCOME*/ DEFINITION	INDICATORS	SELECTED INTERVENTIONS*/ DEFINITION	SAMPLE NIC ACTIVITIES
Self-Care Deficit: Bathing/Hygiene related to paralyzed left upper and lower limbs and lack of motivation/*Impaired ability to perform or complete bathing/hygiene activities for oneself*	Self-Care: Bathing [0301]/*Ability to cleanse own body independently with or without assistive device*	Mildly compromised: ■ Gets in and out of bathroom ■ Regulates water temperature ■ Bathes in shower ■ Washes body ■ Dries body	Self-Care Assistance: Bathing/Hygiene [1801]/*Assisting client to perform personal hygiene*	■ Place towels, soap, deodorant, shaving equipment, and other needed accessories at bedside/bathroom ■ Facilitate client's bathing self, as appropriate ■ Provide assistance until client is fully able to assume self-care ■ Assist client to identify the impact of peer group on feelings of self-worth

DATA CLUSTER   Mark Drake, 15 years old, has facial pustules and papules. Facial skin is inflamed. He states, "I hate going to school or anywhere looking like this. I don't think any girl wants to go out with me. Can you do something to get rid of this?"

Situational Low Self-Esteem related to acne/*Development of a negative perception of self-worth in response to a current situation (Specify)*	Self-Esteem [1205]/ *Personal judgment of self-worth*	Often positive ■ Verbalizations of self acceptance ■ Maintenance of grooming/hygiene ■ Description of success in social groups	Self-Esteem Enhancement [5400]/*Assisting a client to increase his/her personal judgment of self-worth*	■ Encourage client to identify strengths ■ Convey confidence in client's ability to handle situation ■ Assist client to reexamine negative perceptions of self-worth

*The NOC # for desired outcomes and the NIC# for nursing interventions are listed in brackets following the appropriate outcome or intervention. Outcomes, indicators, interventions, and activities selected are only a sample of those suggested by NOC and NIC and should be further individualized for each client.

whether male or female, and provide adequate privacy and sensitivity. If possible, try to provide a caregiver of the same gender (Purnell & Paulanka, 2005). Nurses need to provide whatever assistance the client requires, either directly or by delegating this task to other nursing personnel.

Planning for Home Care

To provide for continuity of care, it is important that the nurse assess the client's and family's abilities for care and the need for referrals and home health services (see Home Care Assessment on page 747.) In addition, the nurse needs to determine the client's learning needs.

Implementing

The nurse applies the general guidelines for skin care while providing one of the various types of baths available to clients. Skill 33-1 describes how to bathe an adult or pediatric client.

General Guidelines for Skin Care

1. *An intact, healthy skin is the body's first line of defense.* Nurses need to ensure that all skin care measures prevent

injury and irritation. Scratching the skin with jewelry or long, sharp fingernails must be avoided. Harsh rubbing or use of rough towels and washcloths can cause tissue damage, particularly when the skin is irritated or when circulation or sensation is diminished. Bottom bedsheets are kept taut and free from wrinkles to reduce friction and abrasion to the skin. Top bed linens are arranged to prevent undue pressure on the toes. When necessary, bed cradles on footboards are used to keep bedclothes off the feet.

2. *The degree to which the skin protects the underlying tissues from injury depends on the general health of the cells, the amount of subcutaneous tissue, and the dryness of the skin.* Skin that is poorly nourished and dry is less easily protected and more vulnerable to injury. When the skin is dry, lotions or creams with lanolin can be applied, and bathing is limited to once or twice a week because frequent bathing removes the natural oils of the skin and causes dryness.

3. *Moisture in contact with the skin for more than a short time can result in increased bacterial growth and irritation.* After a bath, the client's skin is dried carefully. Particular

HOME CARE ASSESSMENT Hygiene

CLIENT AND ENVIRONMENT

- *Self-care abilities for hygiene:* Assess the client's ability to bathe, to regulate water faucets, to dress and undress, to groom, and to use the toilet.
- *Self-care aids required:* Determine if there is a need for a tub/shower seat (see Figure 33-1 ■) a hand shower, a nonskid surface or mat in the tub or shower, hand bars on the sides of the tub (see Figure 33-2 ■), or a raised toilet seat.
- *Facilities:* Check for the presence of laundry facilities and running water.
- *Mechanical barriers:* Note furniture obstructing access to the bathroom and toilet, or a doorway too narrow for a wheelchair.

FAMILY

- *Caregiver availability, skills, and responses:* Determine whether individuals are available and able to assist with bathing, dressing, toileting, nail care, hair shampoo, or shopping for hygienic or grooming aids.

- *Education needs:* Assess whether the caregiver needs instruction in how to assist the client in and out of the tub, on and off the toilet, and so on.
- *Family roles changes and coping:* Assess effects of client's illness on financial status, parenting, spousal roles, sexuality, and social roles.

COMMUNITY

- Explore resources that will provide assistance with bathing, laundry, and foot care (e.g., home health aid, podiatrist).
- Consult a social worker as needed to coordinate placement of a client unable to remain in the home or to identify community resources that will help the client stay in the home.
- Consider a consult with (a) a physical therapist to assess, develop, and improve the client's motor function; (b) a home health nurse to provide follow-up for care, teaching, and support; and (c) an occupational therapist to assess and develop abilities to perform activities of daily living.

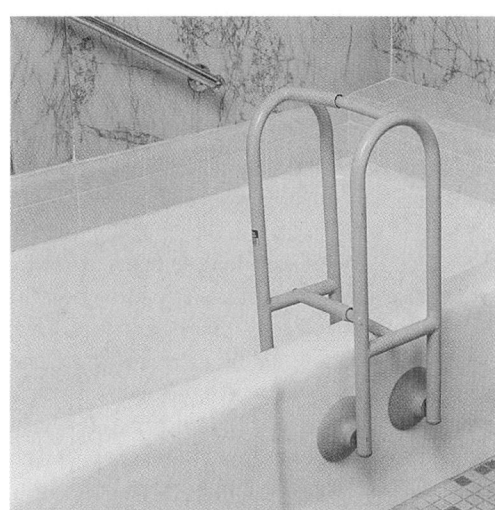

Figure 33-1 ■ Tub/shower seat in the home.

Figure 33-2 ■ Hand bars on the sides of the bathtub.

attention is paid to areas such as the axillae, the groin, beneath the breasts, and between the toes, where the potential for irritation is greatest. A nonirritating dusting powder tends to reduce moisture and can be applied to these areas after they are dried. Clients who are incontinent of urine or feces or who perspire excessively are provided with immediate skin care to prevent skin irritation.

4. *Body odors are caused by resident skin bacteria acting on body secretions.* Cleanliness is the best deodorant. Commercial deodorants and antiperspirants can be applied only after the skin is cleaned. Deodorants diminish odors, whereas antiperspirants reduce the amount of perspiration. Neither is applied immediately after shaving, because of the possibility of skin irritation, nor are they used on skin that is already irritated.

5. *Skin sensitivity to irritation and injury varies among individuals and in accordance with their health.* Generally speaking, skin sensitivity is greater in infants, very young children, and older people. A person's nutritional status also affects sensitivity. Emaciated and obese persons tend to experience more skin irritation and injury. The same tendency is seen in individuals with poor dietary habits and insufficient fluid intake. Even in healthy persons, skin sensitivity is highly variable. Some people's skin is sensitive to chemicals in skin care agents and cosmetics. Hypoallergenic cosmetics and soaps or soap substitutes are now available for these people. The nurse needs to ascertain whether the client has any sensitivities and what agents are appropriate to use.

6. *Agents used for skin care have selective actions and purposes.* Commonly used agents are described in Table 33–4.

TABLE 33–4	**Agents Commonly Used on the Skin**
Soap	Lowers surface tension and thus helps in cleaning. Some soaps contain antibacterial agents, which can change the natural flora of the skin.
Detergent	Used instead of soap for cleaning. Some people who are allergic to soaps may not be allergic to detergents, and vice versa. Do not use on elderly clients.
Bath oil	Used in bathwater; provides an oily film on the skin that softens and prevents chapping. Oils can make the tub surface slippery, and clients should be instructed about safety measures (e.g., using nonskid tub surface or mat).
Skin cream, lotion	Provides a film on the skin that prevents evaporation and therefore chapping.
Powder	Can be used to absorb water and prevent friction. For example, powder under the breasts can prevent skin irritation. Some powders are antibacterial.
Deodorant	Masks or diminishes body odors.
Antiperspirant	Reduces the amount of perspiration.

Bathing

Bathing removes accumulated oil, perspiration, dead skin cells, and some bacteria. The nurse can appreciate the quantity of oil and dead skin cells produced when observing a person after the removal of a cast that has been on for 6 weeks. The skin is crusty, flaky, and dry underneath the cast. Applications of oil over several days are usually necessary to remove the debris.

Excessive bathing, however, can interfere with the intended lubricating effect of the sebum, causing dryness of the skin. This is an important consideration, especially for elders, who produce less sebum.

In addition to cleaning the skin, bathing also stimulates circulation. A warm or hot bath dilates superficial arterioles, bringing more blood and nourishment to the skin. Vigorous rubbing has the same effect. Rubbing with long smooth strokes from the distal to proximal parts of extremities (from the point farthest from the body to the point closest) is particularly effective in facilitating venous blood flow unless there is some underlying condition (e.g., blood clot) that would preclude this.

Bathing also produces a sense of well-being. It is refreshing and relaxing and frequently improves morale, appearance, and self-respect. Some people take a morning shower for its refreshing, stimulating effect. Others prefer an evening bath because it is relaxing. These effects are more evident when a person is ill.

REAL WORLD PRACTICE

Many clients, especially those from ethnic cultures, have the support of their family, including extended family members, throughout their hospital stay. Most family members want to assist the client, but do not know how to do so. The nurse can facilitate the client's recovery by teaching family members how to provide certain basic care functions. Appropriate tasks to delegate to family members, after their expression of wanting to assist, and proper instruction, can include mouth care, range of motion, skin care, and assisting the client with meals. For the client who will be hospitalized for an extended period, the family can be asked to bring in music that the client likes, pictures of family members, a favorite pillow from home, or even a stuffed animal.

—Marie Lasater, MSN, RN, CCRN,
Barnes-Jewish Hospital, St. Louis, MO

For example, it is not uncommon for clients who have had a restless or sleepless night to feel relaxed, comfortable, and sleepy after a morning bath.

Bathing offers an excellent opportunity for the nurse to assess all clients. The nurse can observe the condition of the client's skin and physical conditions such as sacral edema or rashes. While assisting a client with a bath, the nurse can also assess the client's psychosocial needs, such as orientation to time and ability to cope with the illness. Learning needs, such as a diabetic client's need to learn foot care, can also be assessed.

CATEGORIES. Two categories of baths are given to clients: cleaning and therapeutic. **Cleaning baths** are given chiefly for hygiene purposes and include these types:

- *Complete bed bath.* The nurse washes the entire body of a dependent client in bed.
- *Self-help bed bath.* Clients confined to bed are able to bathe themselves with help from the nurse for washing the back and perhaps the feet.
- *Partial bath (abbreviated bath).* Only the parts of the client's body that might cause discomfort or odor, if neglected, are washed: the face, hands, axillae, perineal area, and back. Omitted are the arms, chest, abdomen, legs, and feet. The nurse provides this care for dependent clients and assists self-sufficient clients confined to bed by washing their backs. Some ambulatory clients prefer to take a partial bath at the sink. The nurse can assist them by washing their backs.
- *Bag bath.* This bath is a commercially prepared product that contains 10 to 12 presoaked disposable washcloths that contain no-rinse cleanser solution. The package is warmed in a microwave. The warming time is about 1 minute, but the nurse needs to determine how long it takes to attain a desirable temperature. Each area of the body is cleaned with a different cloth and then air dried. Because the body is not rubbed dry, the emollient in the solution remains on the skin.
- *Tub bath.* Tub baths are often preferred to bed baths because it is easier to wash and rinse in a tub. Tubs are also used for therapeutic baths. The amount of assistance the nurse offers depends on the abilities of the client. There are specially designed tubs for dependent clients. These tubs greatly reduce the work of the nurse in lifting clients in and out of the tub and offer greater benefits than a sponge bath in bed.

Sponge baths are suggested for the newborn because daily tub baths are not considered necessary. After the bath, the infant should be immediately dried and wrapped to prevent heat loss. Parents need to be advised that the infant's ability to regulate body temperature has not yet fully developed. Infants perspire minimally, and shivering starts at a lower temperature than it does in adults; therefore, infants lose more heat before shivering begins. In addition, because the infant's body surface area is very large in relation to body mass, the body loses heat readily.

■ *Shower.* Many ambulatory clients are able to use shower facilities and require only minimal assistance from the nurse. Clients in long-term care settings are often given showers with the aid of a shower chair. The wheels on the shower chair allow clients to be transported from their room to the shower. The shower chair also has a commode seat to facilitate cleansing of the client's perineal area during the shower process (see Figure 33–3 ■).

The water for a bath should feel comfortably warm to the client. People vary in their sensitivity to heat; generally, the temperature should be 43°C to 46°C (110°F to 115°F). Most clients will verify a suitable temperature. Clients with decreased circulation or cognitive problems will not be able to verify the temperature. Therefore, the nurse must check the water temperature to avoid burning the client with water that is too hot. The water for a bed bath should be changed when it becomes dirty or cold.

Therapeutic baths are given for physical effects, such as to soothe irritated skin or to treat an area (e.g., the perineum). Medications may be placed in the water. A therapeutic bath is generally taken in a tub one-third or one-half full. The client remains in the bath for a designated time, often 20 to 30 minutes. If the client's back, chest, and arms are to be treated, these areas need to be immersed in the solution. The bath temperature is generally included in the order; 37.7°C to 46°C (100°F to 115°F) may be ordered for adults, and 40.5°C (105°F) is usually ordered for infants. Skill 33-1 provides guidelines for bathing clients.

Figure 33–3 ■ A shower chair.

BATHING AN ADULT OR PEDIATRIC CLIENT

PURPOSES
- To remove transient microorganisms, body secretions and excretions, and dead skin cells
- To stimulate circulation to the skin
- To promote a sense of well-being
- To produce relaxation and comfort
- To prevent and eliminate unpleasant body odors

ASSESSMENT
Assess

- Condition of the skin (color, texture and turgor, presence of pigmented spots, temperature, lesions, excoriations, abrasions, and bruises)
- Physical or emotional factors (e.g., fatigue, sensitivity to cold, need for control, anxiety or fear)
- Presence of pain and need for adjunctive measures (e.g., an analgesic) before the bath
- Range of motion of the joints
- Any other aspect of health that may affect the client's bathing process (e.g., mobility, strength, cognition)
- Need for use of clean gloves during the bath

PLANNING

Delegation

The nurse often delegates the skill of bathing to UAP. However, the nurse remains responsible *for assessment and client care.* The nurse needs to do the following:

- Inform the UAP of the type of bath appropriate for the client and precautions, if any, specific to the needs of the client.
- Remind the UAP to notify the nurse of any concerns or changes (e.g., redness, skin breakdown, rash) so the nurse can assess, intervene if needed, and document.
- Instruct the UAP to encourage the client to perform as much self-care as appropriate in order to promote independence and self-esteem.
- Obtain a complete report about the bathing experience from the UAP.

SKILL 33-1

continued on page 750

SKILL 33-1

BATHING AN ADULT OR PEDIATRIC CLIENT *continued*

Equipment

- Basin or sink with warm water (between 43°C and 46°C or 110°F and 115°F)
- Soap and soap dish
- Linens: bath blanket, two bath towels, washcloth, clean gown or pajamas or clothes as needed, additional bed linen and towels, if required
- Gloves, if appropriate (e.g., presence of body fluids or open lesions)
- Personal hygiene articles (e.g., deodorant, powder, lotions)
- Shaving equipment
- Table for bathing equipment
- Laundry hamper

IMPLEMENTATION

Preparation

Before bathing a client, determine (a) the purpose and type of bath the client needs; (b) self-care ability of the client; (c) any movement or positioning precautions specific to the client; (d) other care the client may be receiving, such as physical therapy or x-rays, in order to coordinate all aspects of health care and prevent unnecessary fatigue; (e) the client's comfort level with being bathed by someone else; and (f) necessary bath equipment and linens.

Caution is needed when bathing clients who are receiving intravenous therapy. Easy-to-remove gowns that have Velcro or snap fasteners along the sleeves may be used. If a special gown is not available, the nurse needs to pay special attention when changing the client's gown after the bath (or whenever the gown becomes soiled).

Performance

1. Prior to performing the procedure, introduce self and verify the client's identity using agency protocol. Explain to the client what you are going to do, why it is necessary, and how he or she can cooperate. Discuss with the client the plan for bathing and explain any unfamiliar procedures to the client.

2. Perform hand hygiene and observe other appropriate infection control procedures.

3. Provide for client privacy by drawing the curtains around the bed or closing the door to the room. Some agencies provide signs indicating the need for privacy. **Rationale:** *Hygiene is a personal matter.*

4. Prepare the client and the environment.
   - Invite a family member or significant other to participate if desired.
   - Close windows and doors to ensure the room is a comfortable temperature. **Rationale:** *Air currents increase loss of heat from the body by convection.*
   - Offer the client a bedpan or urinal or ask whether the client wishes to use the toilet or commode. **Rationale:** *Warm water and activity can stimulate the need to void. The client will be more comfortable after voiding, and voiding before cleaning the perineum is advisable.*
   - Encourage the client to perform as much personal self-care as possible. **Rationale:** *This promotes independence, exercise, and self-esteem.*
   - During the bath, assess each area of the skin carefully.

FOR A BED BATH

5. Prepare the bed and position the client appropriately.
   - Position the bed at a comfortable working height. Lower the side rail on the side close to you. Keep the other side rail *up.* Assist the client to move near you. **Rationale:** *This avoids undue reaching and straining and promotes good body mechanics.*

❶ Remove top sheet from under the bath blanket.
(Al Dodge, Pearson Education/PH College)

   - Place a bath blanket over the top sheet. Remove the top sheet from under the bath blanket by starting at the client's shoulders and moving linen down toward the client's feet. **❶** Ask the client to grasp and hold the top of the bath blanket while pulling linen to the foot of the bed. **Rationale:** *The bath blanket provides comfort, warmth, and privacy. Note:* If the bed linen is to be reused, place it over the bedside chair. If it is to be changed, place it in the linen hamper, not on the floor.
   - Remove client's gown while keeping the client covered with the bath blanket. Place gown in linen hamper.

6. Make a bath mitt with the washcloth. **Rationale:** *A bath mitt retains water and heat better than a cloth loosely held and prevents ends of washcloth from dragging across the skin.* See **❷** for the triangular method and **❸** for the rectangular method.

7. Wash the face. **Rationale:** *Begin the bath at the cleanest area and work downward toward the feet.*
   - Place towel under client's head.
   - Wash the client's eyes with water only and dry them well. Use a separate corner of the washcloth for each eye. **Rationale:** *Using separate corners prevents transmitting microorganisms from one eye to the other.* Wipe from the inner to the outer canthus. **❹ Rationale:** *This prevents secretions from entering the nasolacrimal ducts.*
   - Ask whether the client wants soap used on the face. **Rationale:** *Soap has a drying effect, and the face, which is exposed to the air more than other body parts, tends to be drier.*
   - Wash, rinse, and dry the client's face, ears, and neck.
   - Remove the towel from under the client's head.

8. Wash the arms and hands. (Omit the arms for a partial bath.)
   - Place a towel lengthwise under the arm away from you. **Rationale:** *It protects the bed from becoming wet.*

BATHING AN ADULT OR PEDIATRIC CLIENT *continued*

A   B   C   D

❷ Making a bath mitt, triangular method. *A,* Lay your hand on the washcloth; *B,* fold the top corner over your hand; *C,* fold the side corners over your hand; *D,* tuck the second corner under the cloth on the palm side to secure the mitt.

(Al Dodge, Pearson Education/PH College)

  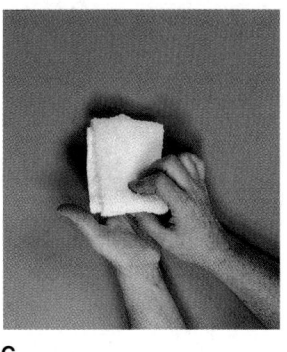

A   B   C

❸ Making a bath mitt, rectangular method. *A,* Lay your hand on the washcloth and fold one side over your hand; *B,* fold the second side over your hand; *C,* fold the top of the cloth down and tuck it under the folded side against your palm to secure the mitt.

(Al Dodge, Pearson Education/PH College)

 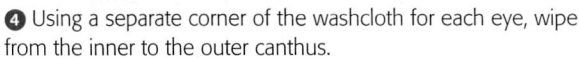

❹ Using a separate corner of the washcloth for each eye, wipe from the inner to the outer canthus.

(Al Dodge, Pearson Education/PH College)

❺ Washing the far arm using long, firm strokes from wrist to shoulder area.

(Al Dodge, Pearson Education/PH College)

- Wash, rinse, and dry the arm by elevating the client's arm and supporting the client's wrist and elbow. ❺ Use long, firm strokes from wrist to shoulder, including the axillary area. **Rationale:** *Firm strokes from distal to proximal areas promote circulation by increasing venous blood return.*
- Apply deodorant or powder if desired.

- (Optional) Place a towel on the bed and put a washbasin on it. Place the client's hands in the basin. **Rationale:** *Many clients enjoy immersing their hands in the basin and washing themselves. Soaking loosens dirt under the nails.* Assist the client as needed to wash, rinse, and dry the hands, paying particular attention to the spaces between the fingers.

continued on page 752

BATHING AN ADULT OR PEDIATRIC CLIENT *continued*

- Repeat for hand and arm nearest you. Exercise caution if an intravenous infusion is present, and check its flow after moving the arm.

9. Wash the chest and abdomen. (Omit the chest and abdomen for a partial bath. However, the areas under a woman's breast may require bathing if this area is irritated or if the client has significant perspiration under the breast.)
   - Place the bath towel lengthwise over the chest. Fold the bath blanket down to the client's pubic area. **Rationale:** *This keeps the client warm while preventing unnecessary exposure of the chest.*
   - Lift the bath towel off the chest, and bathe the chest and abdomen with your mitted hand using long, firm strokes. ❻ Give special attention to the skin under the breasts and any other skin folds particularly if the client is overweight. Rinse and dry well.
   - Replace the bath blanket when the areas have been dried.

10. Wash the legs and feet. (Omit legs and feet for a partial bath.)
    - Expose the leg farthest from you by folding the bath blanket toward the other leg being careful to keep the perineum covered. **Rationale:** *Covering the perineum promotes privacy and maintains the client's dignity.*
    - Lift leg and place the bath towel lengthwise under the leg. Wash, rinse, and dry the leg using long, smooth, firm strokes from the ankle to the knee to the thigh. ❼ **Rationale:** *Washing from the distal to proximal areas promotes circulation by stimulating venous blood flow.*
    - Reverse the coverings and repeat for the other leg.
    - Wash the feet by placing them in the basin of water. ❽
    - Dry each foot. Pay particular attention to the spaces between the toes. If preferred, wash one foot after that leg before washing the other leg.
    - Obtain fresh, warm bathwater now or when necessary. **Rationale:** *Water may become dirty or cold.* Because surface skin cells are removed with washing, the bathwater from dark-skinned clients may be dark, however, this does not mean the client is dirty. Lower the bed when refilling basin. **Rationale:** *This ensures the safety of the client.*

11. Wash the back and then the perineum.
    - Assist the client into a prone or side-lying position facing away from you. Place the bath towel lengthwise alongside the back and buttocks while keeping the client covered with the bath blanket as much as possible. **Rationale:** *This provides warmth and prevents undue exposure.*
    - Wash and dry the client's back, moving from the shoulders to the buttocks, and upper thighs, paying attention to the gluteal folds. ❾
    - Perform a back massage now or after completion of bath. (See Skill 43-1. ∞)
    - Assist the client to the supine position and determine whether the client can wash the perineal area independently. If the client cannot do so, drape the client as shown in Skill 45-2 and wash the area. ∞

12. Assist the client with grooming aids such as powder, lotion, or deodorant.
    - Use powder sparingly. Release as little as possible into the atmosphere. **Rationale:** *This will avoid irritation of the respiratory tract by powder inhalation. Excessive powder can cause caking, which leads to skin irritation.*

❻ Washing the chest and abdomen.
(Patrick Watson)

❼ Washing far leg.
(Al Dodge, Pearson Education/PH College)

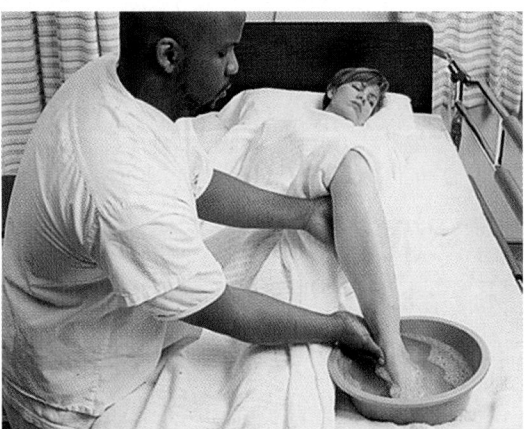

❽ Soaking a foot in a basin.

❾ Washing the back.
(Al Dodge, Pearson Education/PH College)

BATHING AN ADULT OR PEDIATRIC CLIENT *continued*

- Help the client put on a clean gown or pajamas.
- Assist the client to care for hair, mouth, and nails. Some people prefer or need mouth care prior to their bath.

FOR A TUB BATH OR SHOWER

13. Prepare the client and the tub.
    - Fill the tub about one-third to one-half full of water at 43° to 46°C (110°F to 115°F). **Rationale:** *Sufficient water is needed to cover the perineal area.*
    - Cover all intravenous catheters or wound dressings with plastic coverings, and instruct the client to prevent wetting these areas if possible.
    - Put a rubber bath mat or towel on the floor of the tub if safety strips are not on the tub floor. **Rationale:** *These prevent slippage of the client during the bath or shower.*

14. Assist the client into the shower or tub.
    - Assist the client taking a standing shower with the initial adjustment of the water temperature and water flow pressure, as needed. Some clients need a chair to sit on in the shower because of weakness. Hot water can cause elderly people to feel faint.
    - If the client requires considerable assistance with a tub bath, a hydraulic bathtub chair may be required (see "Variation").
    - Explain how the client can signal for help, leave the client for 2 to 5 minutes, and place an "occupied" sign on the door. For safety reasons, do not leave a client with decreased cognition or clients who may be at risk (e.g., history of seizures, syncope).

15. Assist the client with washing and getting out of the tub.
    - Wash the client's back, lower legs, and feet, if necessary.
    - Assist the client out of the tub. If the client is unsteady, place a bath towel over the client's shoulders and drain the tub of water before the client attempts to get out of it. **Rationale:** *Draining the water first lessens the likelihood of a fall. The towel prevents chilling.*

16. Dry the client, and assist with follow-up care.
    - Follow step 12.
    - Assist the client back to his or her bed.
    - Clean the tub or shower in accordance with agency practice, discard the used linen in the laundry hamper, and place the "unoccupied" sign on the door.

17. Document
    - Type of bath given (i.e., complete, partial, or self-help). This is usually recorded on a flow sheet.
    - Skin assessment, such as excoriation, erythema, exudates, rashes, drainage, or skin breakdown.

- Nursing interventions related to skin integrity.
- Ability of the client to assist or cooperate with bathing.
- Client response to bathing.
- Educational needs regarding hygiene.
- Information or teaching shared with the client or the family.

VARIATION: BATHING USING A HYDRAULIC BATHTUB CHAIR

A hydraulic lift, often used in long-term care or rehabilitation settings, can facilitate the transfer of a client who is unable to ambulate to a tub. The lift also helps eliminate strain on the nurse's back.

- Bring the client to the tub room in a wheelchair or shower chair.
- Fill the tub and check the water temperature with a bath thermometer *to avoid thermal injury to the client.*
- Lower the hydraulic chair lift to its lowest point, outside the tub.
- Transfer the client to the chair lift and secure the seat belt. ⑩
- Raise the chair lift above the tub.
- Support the client's legs as the chair is moved over the tub *to avoid injury to the legs.*
- Position the client's legs down into the water and slowly lower the chair lift into the tub.
- Assist in bathing the client, if appropriate.
- Reverse the procedure when taking the client out of the tub.
- Dry the client and transport him or her to the room.

⑩ Secure the seat belt before moving the client in a hydraulic bathtub chair.

EVALUATION

- Note the client's tolerance of the procedure (e.g., respiratory rate and effort, pulse rate, behaviors of acceptance or resistance, statements regarding comfort).
- Conduct appropriate follow-up, such as
  - Condition and integrity of skin (dryness, turgor, redness, lesions, and so on).

  - Client strength.
  - Percentage of bath done without assistance.
- Relate to prior assessment data, if available.

LIFESPAN CONSIDERATIONS Bathing

INFANTS

■ Sponge baths are suggested for the newborn because daily tub baths are not considered necessary. After the bath, the infant should be immediately dried and wrapped. Parents need to be advised that the infant's ability to regulate body temperature has not yet fully developed and newborns' bodies lose heat readily.

CHILDREN

■ Encourage a child's participation appropriate for developmental level.
■ Closely supervise children in the bathtub. Do not leave them unattended.

ADOLESCENTS

■ Assist adolescents as needed to choose deodorants and antiperspirants. Secretions from newly active sweat glands react with bacteria on the skin, causing a pungent odor.

ELDERS

■ Changes of aging can decrease the protective function of the skin in elders. These changes include fragile skin, less oil and moisture, and a decrease in elasticity.
■ To minimize skin dryness in elders, avoid excessive use of soap. The ideal time to moisturize the skin is immediately after bathing.
■ Avoid powder because it causes moisture loss and is a hazardous inhalant. Cornstarch should also be avoided because in the presence of moisture it breaks down into glucose and can facilitate the growth of organisms.
■ Protect elders and children from injury related to hot water burns.

HOME CARE CONSIDERATIONS Hygiene

Suggest that the client or family do the following:

■ Consider purchasing a bath seat that fits in the tub or shower.
■ Install a hand shower for use with a bath seat and shampooing.
■ Use a nonskid surface on the tub or shower.

■ Install hand bars on both sides of the tub or shower to facilitate transfers in and out of the tub or shower.
■ Carefully monitor the temperature of the bathwater.
■ Apply lotion and oil *after* a bath, not during, because these solutions can make a tub surface slippery.

LONG-TERM CARE SETTING. From a historical perspective, the bath has always been a part of nursing care and considered a component of the "art" of nursing. In today's nursing world, however, the bath is seen as a necessary, routine task and is often delegated to nonprofessionals.

In spite of the previously listed beneficial values associated with bathing, the choice of bathing procedure often depends on the amount of time available to the nurse or unlicensed assistive personnel (UAP) and the client's self-care ability. Nursing authors (Barrick & Rader, 2000; Dunn, Thiru-Chelvam, & Beck, 2002; Rasin & Barrick, 2004; Rader et al., 2006) have challenged nurses to switch from a task-centered approach to a person-centered approach to bathing, especially for the older person in a long-term care setting. The bath routine (e.g., day, time, and number/week) for clients in health care settings is often determined by agency policy, which often results in the bath becoming routine and depersonalized versus therapeutic, satisfying, and person focused.

Rader et al. (2006) encourage nurses in the long-term care setting to view the bath from the individual's perspective. Rader, who was showered during a preliminary study, realized that behaviors previously labeled "aggressive" or "resistive" were actually defensive actions from feeling threatened and anxious during a cold and distressing shower experience (p. 44). A nurse who provides person-centered care asks such questions as: What is the client's usual method of maintaining cleanli-

ness? Are there any past negative experiences related to bathing? Are factors such as pain or fatigue increasing the client's difficulty with the demands and stimuli associated with bathing or showering? A client's resistance to the bathing experience can be a cue to the nurse to consider other methods of maintaining cleanliness. For example, if the shower causes distress, is there another form of bathing (such as the bag bath) that may be more therapeutic and comforting?

An individualized approach focusing on therapeutic and comforting outcomes of bathing is especially important for clients with dementia. Alzheimer's disease is the most common cause of dementia among people age 65 and older. Given the current population trends, it is estimated that 14 million Americans will have Alzheimer's disease by 2050 (Alzheimer's Disease Education & Referral Center, n.d.). This statistic has implications for nursing care. For example, Rasin and Barrick (2004) reported that in an observational study of people with dementia, more than 90% became agitated as soon as they were told it was time to bathe (p. 30). See Box 33–2 for possible strategies that can reduce the stress of the bathing experience for both the person with dementia and the caregiver.

Providing personal hygiene to clients with dementia is often an ongoing challenge. Being sensitive to the rhythm of their behavior and looking for cues can often offset problems related to this. Clients with dementia, whether they are at home or in a health care facility, often have certain times of

MediaLink Client with Chickenpox Application

the day when they are more agitated—these are times to avoid doing things that will increase their fear and agitation. It is sometimes helpful to wait (e.g., half an hour or so) and then

---

BOX 33–2 General Guidelines for Bathing Persons with Dementia

■ Focus on the person rather than the task.
  ● Cover! Keep the person covered as much as possible to keep him or her warm.
  ● Time the bath to fit the person's history, preferences, and mood.
  ● Move slowly and let the person know when you are going to move him or her.
  ● Evaluate to determine if the person needs pain control before the bath.
  ● Use a gentle touch. Use soft cloths. Pat dry rather than rubbing.
■ Be flexible. Adapt your approach to meet the needs of the person.
  ● Consider adapting your methods (e.g., distracting the person with singing while bathing), the environment (e.g., correct size of shower chair, reducing noise, playing music), and the procedure (e.g., consistently assigning same caregiver, inviting family to help).
  ● Encourage flexibility in scheduling of bath based on person's preference.
■ Use persuasion, not coercion.
  ● Give choices and respond to individual requests.
  ● Help the person feel in control.
  ● Use a supportive, calm approach and praise the person often.
■ Be prepared.
  ● Gather everything that you will need for the bath (e.g., towels, washcloths, clothes) before approaching the person.
■ Stop when a person becomes distressed. It is *not* normal to have cries, screams, or protests from the person.
  ● Stop what you are doing and assess for causes of the distress.
  ● Adjust your approach.
  ● Shorten or stop the bath.
  ● Try to end on a positive note.
  ● Reapproach later to wash critical areas if necessary.
■ Ask for help.
  ● Talk with others, including the family, about different ways to help make the bath more comfortable for the person.

Note: Adapted From *Bathing Without a Battle: Personal Care of Individuals with Dementia,* by A. L. Barrick, J. Rader, B. Hoeffer, & P. D. Sloane, 2002. Copyright © 2002 Springer Publishing Company, Inc., New York, New York, 10036. Used by permission.

---

try giving the bath because they may forget that they were protesting and be willing to participate.

In addition, collaboration between the nurse and UAP is a critical element to implementing the individualized person-focused approach for cognitively impaired clients who exhibit aggressive behavior during bathing. The nurse, after observing a difficult bathing situation, should discuss with the UAP possible alternative strategies or methods they might implement for the client. More than one intervention may be required (e.g., reassurance, simple explanations, moving slowly). It is important for the nurse to subsequently evaluate the person's response to the new intervention(s).

PERINEAL-GENITAL CARE. Perineal-genital care is also referred to as *perineal care* or *pericare.* Perineal care as part of the bed bath is embarrassing for many clients. Nurses also may find it embarrassing initially, particularly with clients of the opposite sex. Most clients who require a bed bath from the nurse are able to clean their own genital areas with minimal assistance. The nurse may need to hand a moistened washcloth and soap to the client, rinse the washcloth, and provide a towel.

Because some clients are unfamiliar with terminology for the genitals and perineum, it may be difficult for nurses to explain what is expected. Most clients, however, understand what is meant if the nurse simply says, "I'll give you a washcloth to finish your bath." Some older clients may be familiar with the term *private parts.* Whatever expression the nurse uses, it needs to be one that the client understands and one that is comfortable for the nurse to use.

The nurse needs to provide perineal care efficiently and matter-of-factly. Nurses should wear gloves while providing this care for the comfort of the client and to protect themselves from infection. Skill 33-2 explains how to provide perineal-genital care.

CLINICAL ALERT

Always wash or wipe from "clean to dirty." For a female, cleanse the perineal area from front to back. For a male, cleanse the urinary meatus by moving in a circular motion from center of urethral opening around the glans. ■

PROVIDING PERINEAL-GENITAL CARE

PURPOSES
■ To remove normal perineal secretions and odors
■ To promote client comfort

ASSESSMENT
Assess for the presence of

■ Irritation, excoriation, inflammation, swelling
■ Excessive discharge
■ Odor; pain or discomfort
■ Urinary or fecal incontinence
■ Recent rectal or perineal surgery
■ Indwelling catheter

Determine
■ Perineal-genital hygiene practices
■ Self-care abilities

SKILL 33-2

continued on page 756

SKILL 33-2

PROVIDING PERINEAL-GENITAL CARE *continued*

PLANNING

> **Delegation**
> Perineal-genital care can be delegated to UAP. If the client has recently had perineal, rectal, or genital surgery, the nurse needs to assess if it is appropriate for the UAP to perform perineal-genital care.

Equipment
Perineal-genital care provided in conjunction with the bed bath:

- Bath towel
- Bath blanket
- Clean gloves

- Bath basin with water at 43°C to 46°C (110°F to 115°F)
- Soap
- Washcloth

  Special perineal-genital care:

- Bath towel
- Bath blanket
- Clean gloves
- Cotton balls or swabs
- Solution bottle, pitcher, or container filled with warm water or a prescribed solution
- Bedpan to receive rinse water
- Moisture-resistant bag or receptacle for used cotton swabs
- Perineal pad

IMPLEMENTATION
Preparation

- Determine whether the client is experiencing any discomfort in the perineal-genital area.
- Obtain and prepare the necessary equipment and supplies.

Performance

1. Prior to performing the procedure, introduce self and verify the client's identity using agency protocol. Explain to the client what you are going to do, why it is necessary, and how he or she can cooperate, being particularly sensitive to any embarrassment felt by the client.
2. Perform hand hygiene and observe other appropriate infection control procedures (e.g., clean gloves).
3. Provide for client privacy by drawing the curtains around the bed or closing the door to the room. Some agencies provide signs indicating the need for privacy. **Rationale:** *Hygiene is a personal matter.*
4. Prepare the client:
   - Fold the top bed linen to the foot of the bed and fold the gown up to expose the genital area.
   - Place a bath towel under the client's hips. **Rationale:** *The bath towel prevents the bed from becoming soiled.*
5. Position and drape the client and clean the upper inner thighs.

   For Females
   - Position the female in a back-lying position with the knees flexed and spread well apart.
   - Cover her body and legs with the bath blanket positioned so a corner is at her head, the opposite corner at her feet, and the other two on the sides. Drape the legs by tucking the bottom corners of the bath blanket under the inner sides of the legs. ❶ **Rationale:** *Minimum exposure lessens embarrassment and helps to provide warmth.* Bring the middle portion of the base of the blanket up over the pubic area.
   - Put on gloves, wash and dry the upper inner thighs.

   For Males
   - Position the male client in a supine position with knees slightly flexed and hips slightly externally rotated.
   - Put on gloves; wash and dry the upper inner thighs.
6. Inspect the perineal area.
   - Note particular areas of inflammation, excoriation, or swelling, especially between the labia in females and the scrotal folds in males.
   - Also note excessive discharge or secretions from the orifices and the presence of odors.
7. Wash and dry the perineal-genital area.

   For Females
   - Clean the labia majora. Then spread the labia to wash the folds between the labia majora and the labia minora. ❷ **Rationale:** *Secretions that tend to collect around the labia minora facilitate bacterial growth.*
   - Use separate quarters of the washcloth for each stroke, and wipe from the pubis to the rectum. For menstruating women and clients with indwelling catheters, use clean wipes. Take a clean wipe for each stroke. **Rationale:** *Using separate quarters of the washcloth or new wipes prevents the transmission of microorganisms from one area to the other. Wipe from the area of least contamination (the pubis) to that of greatest (the rectum).*

❶ Draping the client for perineal-genital care.

Mons pubis
Labia majora
Labia minora
Orifice of urethra
Orifice of vagina
Perineum
Anus

❷ Female genitals.

PROVIDING PERINEAL-GENITAL CARE *continued*

- Rinse the area well. You may place the client on a bedpan and use a periwash or solution bottle to pour warm water over the area. Dry the perineum thoroughly, paying particular attention to the folds between the labia. **Rationale:** *Moisture supports the growth of many microorganisms.*

For Males

- Wash and dry the penis, using firm strokes.
- If the client is uncircumcised, retract the prepuce (foreskin) to expose the glans penis (the tip of the penis) for cleaning. Replace the foreskin after cleaning the glans penis. ❸ **Rationale:** *Retracting the foreskin is necessary to remove the smegma (thick, cheesy secretion) that collects under the foreskin and facilitates bacterial growth. Replacing the foreskin prevents constriction of the penis, which may cause edema.*
- Wash and dry the scrotum. The posterior folds of the scrotum may need to be cleaned when the buttocks are cleaned (see step 9). **Rationale:** *The scrotum tends to be more soiled than the penis because of its proximity to the rectum; thus it is usually cleaned after the penis.*

8. Inspect perineal orifices for intactness.

- Inspect particularly around the urethra in clients with indwelling catheters. **Rationale:** *A catheter may cause excoriation around the urethra.*

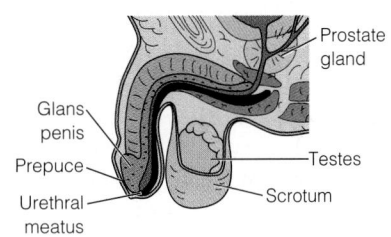

❸ Male genitals.

9. Clean between the buttocks.

- Assist the client to turn onto the side facing away from you.
- Pay particular attention to the anal area and posterior folds of the scrotum in males. Clean the anus with toilet tissue before washing it, if necessary.
- Dry the area well.
- For postdelivery or menstruating females, apply a perineal pad as needed from front to back. **Rationale:** *This prevents contamination of the vagina and urethra from the anal area.*

10. Document any unusual findings such as redness, excoriation, skin breakdown, discharge or drainage, and any localized areas of tenderness.

EVALUATION

- Relate current assessments to previous assessments.
- Conduct appropriate follow-up such as prescribed ointment for excoriation.
- Report any deviation from normal to the primary care provider.

CLIENT TEACHING. Clients often need information about dry skin, skin rashes, and acne.

Evaluating

Using data collected during care, the nurse judges whether desired outcomes have been achieved. If the outcomes are not achieved, the nurse explores reasons why. For example:

- Did the nurse overestimate the client's functional abilities (physical, mental, emotional) for self-care?
- Were provided instructions not clear?
- Were appropriate assistive devices or supplies not available to the client?
- Did the client's condition change?
- Were required analgesics provided before hygienic care?

CLIENT TEACHING **Skin Problems and Care**

DRY SKIN

- Use cleansing creams to clean the skin rather than soap or detergent, which cause drying and, in some cases, allergic reactions.
- Use bath oils, but take precautions to prevent falls caused by slippery tub surfaces.
- Thoroughly rinse soap or detergent, if used, from the skin.
- Bathe less frequently when environmental temperature and humidity are low.
- Increase fluid intake.
- Humidify the air with a humidifier or by keeping a tub or sink full of water.
- Use moisturizing or emollient creams that contain lanolin, petroleum jelly, or cocoa butter to retain skin moisture.

SKIN RASHES

- Keep the area clean by washing it with a mild soap. Rinse the skin well, and pat it dry.

- To relieve itching, try a tepid bath or soak. Some over-the-counter preparations, such as Caladryl lotion, may help but should be used with full knowledge of the product.
- Avoid scratching the rash to prevent inflammation, infection, and further skin lesions.
- Choose clothing carefully. Too much can cause perspiration and aggravate a rash.

ACNE

- Wash the face frequently with soap or detergent and hot water to remove oil and dirt.
- Avoid using oily creams, which aggravate the condition.
- Avoid using cosmetics that block the ducts of the sebaceous glands and the hair follicles.
- Never squeeze or pick at the lesions. This increases the potential for infection and scarring.

■ What currently prescribed medications and therapies could affect the client's abilities or tissue integrity?

■ Is the client's fluid and food intake adequate or appropriate to maintain skin and mucous membrane moisture and integrity?

FEET

The feet are essential for ambulation and merit attention even when people are confined to bed. Each foot contains 26 bones, 107 ligaments, and 19 muscles. These structures function together for both standing and walking.

Developmental Variations

At birth, a baby's foot is relatively unformed. The arches are supported by fatty pads and do not take their full shape until 5 to 6 years of age. During childhood, the bones and small muscles of the feet are easily damaged by tight, binding stockings and ill-fitting shoes. For normal development, it is important that the arches be supported and that the bony structure and the feet grow with no external restrictions. Feet are not fully grown until about age 20. The average person takes 10,000 steps per day. Each step places 2 to 3 times the force of the body weight on the feet. This repetitive use leads to normal changes associated with aging. These include wider and longer feet, mild settling of the arches, and loss of natural padding on the bottom of the heels. The cartilage around the joints also deteriorates, producing loss of normal range of motion of the foot and ankle (Pattillo, 2004, p. 27). All elderly persons should know about foot care. However, some elderly individuals require special attention for their feet. For example, reduced blood supply and accompanying arteriosclerosis can make a foot prone to ulcers and infection following trauma.

CLINICAL ALERT

Clients with diabetes are at high risk for lower extremity amputations (LEA). Routine foot assessment and client education in proper foot care can significantly reduce the risk for LEA. ■

 NURSING MANAGEMENT

Assessing

Assessment of the client's feet includes a nursing health history, physical assessment of the feet, and identifying clients at risk for foot problems.

Nursing Health History

The nurse determines the client's history of (a) normal nail and foot care practices, (b) type of footwear worn, (c) self-care abilities, (d) presence of risk factors for foot problems, (e) any foot discomfort, and (f) any perceived problems with foot mobility. To obtain such data, the nurse asks the client the questions provided in the accompanying Assessment Interview.

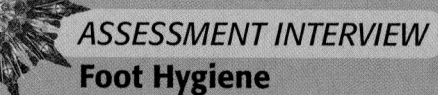

ASSESSMENT INTERVIEW
Foot Hygiene

FOOT CARE PRACTICES

■ How often do you wash your feet and cut your toenails?

■ What hygiene products do you usually use on your feet (e.g., soap, foot powder or deodorant, lotion, or cream)?

■ What type of shoes and socks do you wear?

■ How often do you change your socks or put on clean socks?

■ Do you ever go barefoot? If so, when, where, and how often?

SELF-CARE ABILITIES

■ Do you have any problems managing your foot care? If so, what are these?

■ How can the nurses best help you?

FOOT PROBLEMS AND RISK FACTORS

■ Do you have any problems with foot odor?

■ Do you have any foot discomfort? If so, where? When does this occur? What do you do to relieve the discomfort? Does this discomfort affect how you walk?

■ Have you noticed any problems with foot mobility (e.g., joint stiffness)?

■ Do you have diabetes, any circulatory problems with feet (e.g., swelling, changes in skin color, arthritis), or any instances of prolonged exposure to chemicals or water?

Physical Assessment

Each foot and toe is inspected for shape, size, and presence of lesions and is palpated to assess areas of tenderness, edema, and circulatory status. Normally, the toes are straight and flat. Table 33–5 lists physical assessment methods for the feet. Common foot problems include calluses, corns, unpleasant odors, plantar warts, fissures between the toes, and fungal infections such as athlete's foot.

A **callus** is a thickened portion of epidermis, a mass of keratotic material. Most calluses are painless and flat and are found on the bottom or side of the foot over a bony prominence. Calluses are usually caused by pressure from shoes. They can be softened by soaking the foot in warm water with Epsom salts, and abraded with pumice stones or similar abrasives. Creams with lanolin help to keep the skin soft and prevent the formation of calluses.

A **corn** is a keratosis caused by friction and pressure from a shoe. It commonly occurs on the fourth or fifth toe, usually on a bony prominence such as a joint. Corns are usually conical (circular and raised). The base is the surface of the corn. The apex is in deeper tissues, sometimes even attached to bone. Corns are generally removed surgically. They are prevented from re-forming by relieving the pressure on the area (i.e., wearing comfortable shoes) and massaging the tissue to promote circulation. The use of oval corn pads should be avoided because they increase pressure and decrease circulation.

Unpleasant odors occur as a result of perspiration and its interaction with microorganisms. Regular and frequent washing of the feet and wearing clean hosiery help to minimize odor. Foot powders and deodorants also help to prevent this problem.

Plantar warts appear on the sole of the foot. These warts are caused by the virus papovavirus hominis. They are moderately

TABLE 33–5 Assessment of the Feet

METHOD	NORMAL FINDINGS	DEVIATIONS FROM NORMAL
Inspect all skin surfaces, particularly between the toes, for cleanliness, odor, dryness, inflammation, swelling, abrasions, or other lesions.	Intact skin Absence of swelling or inflammation	Excessive dryness Areas of inflammation or swelling (e.g., corns, calluses) Fissures Scaling and cracking of skin (e.g., athlete's foot) Plantar warts
Palpate anterior and posterior surfaces of ankles and feet for edema.	No swelling	Swelling or pitting edema
Palpate the dorsalis pedis pulse on the dorsal surface of the foot.	Strong, regular pulses in both feet	Weak or absent pulses
Compare skin temperature of both feet.	Warm skin temperature	Cool skin temperature in one or both feet

contagious. The warts are frequently painful and often make walking difficult. The primary care provider may curettage the warts, freeze them with solid carbon dioxide several times, or apply salicylic acid.

Fissures, or deep grooves, frequently occur between the toes as a result of dryness and cracking of the skin. The treatment of choice is good foot hygiene and application of an antiseptic to prevent infection. Often a small piece of gauze is inserted between the toes in applying the antiseptic and left in place to assist healing by allowing air to reach the area.

CLINICAL ALERT

Clients with diabetes often have extremely dry skin. Tell them to use a nonperfumed lotion and to avoid putting lotion between the toes. Advise to not soak their feet in water because it is drying to the skin. ■

Athlete's foot, or **tinea pedis** (ringworm of the foot), is caused by a fungus. The symptoms are scaling and cracking of the skin, particularly between the toes. Sometimes small blisters form, containing a thin fluid. In severe cases, the lesions may also appear on other parts of the body, particularly the hands. Treatments usually involve the application of commercial antifungal ointments or powders. Prevention is important. Common preventive measures are keeping the feet well ventilated, drying the feet well after bathing, wearing clean socks or stockings, and not going barefoot in public showers.

An **ingrown toenail,** the growing inward of the nail into the soft tissues around it, most often results from improper nail trimming. Pressure applied to the area causes localized pain. Treatment involves frequent, hot antiseptic soaks and surgical removal of the portion of nail embedded in the skin. Preventing recurrence involves appropriate instruction and adherence to proper nail-trimming techniques.

Identifying Clients at Risk

Because of reduced peripheral circulation to the feet, clients with diabetes or peripheral vascular disease are particularly prone to infection if skin breakage occurs. Many foot problems can be prevented by teaching the client simple foot care guidelines (see Client Teaching).

CLIENT TEACHING Foot Care

■ Wash the feet daily, and dry them well, especially between the toes.

■ When washing, inspect the skin of the feet for breaks or red or swollen areas. Use a mirror if needed to visualize all areas.

■ To prevent burns, check the water temperature before immersing the feet.

■ Cover the feet, except between the toes, with creams or lotions to moisten the skin. Lotion will also soften calluses. A lotion that reduces dryness effectively is a mixture of lanolin and mineral oil.

■ To prevent or control an unpleasant odor due to excessive foot perspiration, wash the feet frequently and change socks and shoes at least daily. Special deodorant sprays or absorbent foot powders are also helpful.

■ File the toenails rather than cutting them to avoid skin injury. File the nails straight across the ends of the toes. If the nails are too thick or misshapen to file, consult a podiatrist.

■ Wear clean stockings or socks daily. Avoid socks with holes or darns that can cause pressure areas.

■ Wear comfortable, well-fitting shoes that neither restrict the foot nor rub on any area; rubbing can cause corns and calluses. Check worn shoes for rough spots in the lining. Break in new shoes gradually by increasing the wearing time 30 to 60 minutes each day.

■ Avoid walking barefoot, because injury and infection may result. Wear slippers in public showers and in change areas to avoid contracting athlete's foot or other infections.

■ Several times each day exercise the feet to promote circulation. Point the feet upward, point them downward, and move them in circles.

■ Avoid wearing constricting garments such as knee-high elastic stockings and avoid sitting with the legs crossed at the knees, which may decrease circulation.

■ When the feet are cold, use extra blankets and wear warm socks rather than using heating pads or hot water bottles, which may cause burns. Test bathwater before stepping into it.

■ Wash any cut on the foot thoroughly, apply a mild antiseptic, and notify the primary care provider.

■ Avoid self-treatment for corns or calluses. Pumice stones and some callus and corn applications are injurious to the skin. Do not cut calluses or corns. Consult a podiatrist or primary care provider first.

■ Notify the primary care provider if you notice abnormal sores or drainage, pain, or changes in temperature, color, and sensation of the foot.

Diagnosing

A number of nursing diagnoses may apply to clients with foot or foot care problems. The most common diagnostic labels, along with possible related or contributing factors, are as follows:

- *Self-Care Deficit: Hygiene* (foot care) related to
  a. Visual impairment
  b. Impaired hand coordination
  c. Other related or contributing factors (see Box 33–1).

- *Risk for Impaired Skin Integrity* related to
  a. Altered tissue perfusion: peripheral (associated with edema, inadequate arterial circulation)
  b. Poorly fitting shoes
- *Risk for Infection* related to
  a. Impaired skin integrity (ingrown toenail, corn, trauma)
  b. Deficient nail or foot care
- *Deficient Knowledge* (diabetic foot care) related to
  a. Lack of teaching/learning activities about diabetic foot care

---

IDENTIFYING NURSING DIAGNOSES, OUTCOMES, AND INTERVENTIONS
Clients With Foot Problems

DATA CLUSTER Sally Brown, an 83-year-old widow, lives alone. Has home-maker services twice a week and Meals on Wheels service daily. Manages to shower once a week with daughter's help. Has pronounced hand tremors and obvious cataracts. States, "I can't see well enough to cut my nails and even if I could see, my hands shake so badly."

NURSING DIAGNOSIS/ DEFINITION	SAMPLE DESIRED OUTCOME*/ DEFINITION	INDICATORS	SELECTED INTERVENTIONS*/ DEFINITION	SAMPLE NIC ACTIVITIES
Self-Care Deficit: Hygiene (Foot Care) related to impaired hand coordination and visual impairment/ *Impaired ability to perform or complete bathing/hygiene activities for oneself*	Self-Care: Hygiene [0305]/*Ability to maintain own personal cleanliness and kempt appearance independently with or without assistive device*	Severely compromised: ■ Cares for nails	Foot Care [1660]/*Cleansing and inspecting the feet for the purposes of relaxation, cleanliness, and healthy skin*	■ Inspect skin for irritation, cracking, lesions, corns, calluses, or edema ■ Instruct family on the importance of foot care ■ Cut normal-thickness toenails when soft, using a toenail clipper and using the curve of the toe as a guide ■ Refer to podiatrist for trimming of thickened nails, as appropriate

DATA CLUSTER Kyle Stevens, 14 years old, lives with his mother and eight sisters and brothers in a three-room walk-up. Bathroom down the hall is shared with other tenants in the building. Shoes are ragged and fit poorly. States, "I can't get new ones."

Risk for Impaired Skin Integrity related to poorly fitting shoes and limited access to bathing facilities/*At risk for skin being adversely altered*	Tissue Integrity: Skin & Mucous Membranes [1101]/*Structural intactness and normal physiologic function of skin and mucous membranes*	Not compromised ■ Skin intactness	Skin Surveillance [3590]/*Collection and analysis of client data to maintain skin and mucous membrane integrity*	■ Monitor skin for areas of redness and breakdown ■ Monitor skin for excessive dryness and moisture ■ Institute measures to prevent deterioration of skin ■ Instruct client and family about signs of skin breakdown

DATA CLUSTER Jim Wakefield, 64 years old, was recently diagnosed with diabetes mellitus. States he has heard of "diabetes" and is worried because a friend of his father's had diabetes and, after cutting his foot, had his leg amputated.

Deficient Knowledge (Diabetic Foot Care) related to misinterpretation of information/*Absence or deficiency of cognitive information related to a specific topic*	Knowledge: Diabetes Management [1820]/*Extent of understanding conveyed about diabetes mellitus and the precaution of complication*	Substantial knowledge ■ Description of preventive foot care practices	Teaching: Disease Process [5602]/*Assisting the client to understand information related to a specific disease process*	■ Appraise the client's current level of knowledge related to diabetes ■ Provide information to the client about diabetes, as appropriate ■ Discuss lifestyle changes that may be required to prevent future complications or control the disease process ■ Describe rationale behind foot care management ■ Instruct the client on which signs and symptoms to report to health care provider, as appropriate

*The NOC # for desired outcomes and the NIC# for nursing interventions are listed in brackets following the appropriate outcome or intervention. Outcomes, indicators, interventions, and activities selected are only a sample of those suggested by NOC and NIC and should be further individualized for each client.

b. Newly established medical diagnosis (diabetes) and necessary foot hygiene practices.

Examples of assessment data clusters, related nursing diagnoses, outcomes, and interventions are shown in Identifying Nursing Diagnoses, Outcomes, and Interventions.

Planning

Planning involves (a) identifying nursing interventions that will help the client maintain or restore healthy foot care practices and (b) establishing desired outcomes for each client. Interventions may include teaching the client about correct nail and foot care, proper footwear, wearing the correct size, and ways to prevent potential foot problems (e.g., infection, injury, and decreased circulation). For clients with self-care difficulties, the nurse plans a schedule for soaking the client's feet and assisting with regular cleaning and trimming of nails (if not contraindicated). Foot and nail care is often provided during the client's bath but may be provided at any time in the day to accommodate the client's preference or schedule. The frequency of foot care is determined by the nurse and client and is based on objective assessment data and the client's specific problems. For some clients, the feet need to be bathed daily; for those whose feet perspire excessively, bathing more than once a day may be necessary.

Implementing

Skill 33-3 describes how to provide foot care. See also the discussion of nails. During these procedures, the nurse has the opportunity to teach the client appropriate methods for foot care, that is, methods designed to prevent tissue injury and infection (see earlier Client Teaching feature).

SKILL 33-3

PROVIDING FOOT CARE

PURPOSES
- To maintain the skin integrity of the feet
- To prevent foot infections
- To prevent foot odors
- To assess or monitor foot problems

ASSESSMENT
Determine
- History of any problems with foot discomfort, foot odor, foot mobility, circulatory problems (e.g., swelling, changes in skin color and/or temperature, and pain), structural problems (e.g., bunion, hammer toe, or overlapping digits)
- Usual foot care practices (e.g., frequency of washing feet and cutting nails, foot hygiene products used, how often socks are changed, whether the client ever goes barefoot, whether the client sees a podiatrist)

Assess
- Skin surfaces for cleanliness, odor, dryness, and intactness
- Each foot and toe for shape, size, presence of lesions (e.g., corn, callus, wart, or rash), and areas of tenderness, ankle edema
- Skin temperatures of both feet to assess circulatory status
- Pedal pulses: dorsalis pedis and posterior tibialis
- Self-care abilities (e.g., any problems managing foot care)

PLANNING

Delegation
Foot care for the *nondiabetic* client can be delegated to UAP. Remind the UAP to notify the nurse of anything that looks out of the ordinary. Review with the UAP the agency policy about cutting or trimming nails.

Equipment
- Washbasin containing warm water
- Pillow
- Moisture-resistant disposable pad
- Towels
- Soap
- Washcloth
- Toenail cleaning and trimming equipment, if agency policy permits
- Lotion or foot powder

IMPLEMENTATION
Performance
1. Prior to performing the procedure, introduce self and verify the client's identity using agency protocol. Explain to the client what you are going to do, why it is necessary, and how he or she can cooperate.
2. Perform hand hygiene and observe other appropriate infection control procedures.
3. Provide for client privacy by drawing the curtains around the bed or closing the door to the room. Some agencies provide signs indicating the need for privacy. **Rationale:** *Hygiene is a personal matter.*
4. Prepare the equipment and the client.

- Fill the washbasin with warm water at about 40°C to 43°C (105°F to 110°F). **Rationale:** *Warm water promotes circulation, comforts, and refreshes.*
- Assist the ambulatory client to a sitting position in a chair, or the bed client to a supine or semi-Fowler's position.
- Place a pillow under the bed client's knees. **Rationale:** *This provides support and prevents muscle fatigue.*
- Place the washbasin on the moisture-resistant pad at the foot of the bed for a bed client or on the floor in front of the chair for an ambulatory client.
- For a bed client, pad the rim of the washbasin with a towel. **Rationale:** *The towel prevents undue pressure on the skin.*
5. Wash the foot and soak it.

continued on page 762

PROVIDING FOOT CARE *continued*

- Place one of the client's feet in the basin and wash it with soap, paying particular attention to the interdigital areas. Prolonged soaking is generally not recommended for diabetic clients or individuals with peripheral vascular disease. **Rationale:** *Prolonged soaking may remove natural skin oils, thus drying the skin and making it more susceptible to cracking and injury.*
- Rinse the foot well to remove soap. **Rationale:** *Soap irritates the skin if not completely removed.*
- Rub callused areas of the foot with the washcloth. **Rationale:** *This helps remove dead skin layers.*
- If the nails are brittle or thick and require trimming, replace the water and allow the foot to soak for 10 to 20 minutes. **Rationale:** *Soaking softens the nails and loosens debris under them.*
- Clean the nails as required with an orange stick. **Rationale:** *This removes excess debris that harbors microorganisms.*
- Remove the foot from the basin and place it on the towel.

6. Dry the foot thoroughly and apply lotion or foot powder.
   - Blot the foot gently with the towel to dry it thoroughly, particularly between the toes. **Rationale:** *Harsh rubbing can damage the skin. Thorough drying reduces the risk of infection.*

- Apply lotion or lanolin cream to the foot but not between the toes. **Rationale:** *This lubricates dry skin and keeps the area between the toes dry.*

   or
- Apply a foot powder containing a nonirritating deodorant if the feet tend to perspire excessively. **Rationale:** *Foot powders have greater absorbent properties than regular bath powders; some also contain menthol, which makes the feet feel cool.*

7. If agency policy permits, trim the nails of the first foot while the second foot is soaking.
   - See the discussion on nails for the appropriate method to trim nails. Note that in many agencies, toenail trimming requires a primary care provider's order or is contraindicated for clients with diabetes mellitus, toe infections, and peripheral vascular disease, unless performed by a podiatrist, general practice physician, or advanced practice provider such as a nurse practitioner.

8. Document any foot problems observed.
   - Foot care is not generally recorded unless problems are noted.
   - Record any signs of inflammation, infection, breaks in the skin, corns, troublesome calluses, bunions, and pressure areas. This is of particular importance for clients with peripheral vascular disease and diabetes.

EVALUATION
- Inspect nails and skin after the soak.
- Compare to prior assessment data.
- Report any abnormalities to the primary care provider.

Evaluating

Examples of desired outcomes for foot hygiene include the client being able to

- Participate in self-care (foot hygiene) to optimal level of capacity (specify).
- Describe hygienic and other interventions (e.g., proper footwear) to maintain skin integrity, prevent infection, and maintain peripheral tissue perfusion.
- Demonstrate optimal foot hygiene, as evidenced by
   a. Intact, pink, smooth, soft, hydrated, and warm skin.
   b. Intact cuticles and skin surrounding nails.
   c. Correct foot care and nail care practices.

NAILS

Nails are normally present at birth. They continue to grow throughout life and change very little until people are elderly. At that time, the nails tend to be tougher, more brittle, and in some cases thicker. The nails of an older person normally grow less quickly than those of a younger person and may be ridged and grooved.

 NURSING MANAGEMENT

Assessing

During the nursing health history, the nurse explores the client's usual nail care practices, self-care abilities, and any problems associated with them (see accompanying Assessment Interview). Physical assessment involves inspection of the nails (e.g., nail shape and texture, nail bed color, and tissues surrounding the nails). See Chapter 28. ∞

Diagnosing

Nursing diagnoses related to nail care and nail problems include *Self-Care Deficit* and *Risk for Infection*. Examples of these nursing diagnoses and contributing factors follow:

- *Self-Care Deficit: Grooming* related to
   a. Impaired vision
- *Risk for Infection* around the nail bed related to
   a. Impaired skin integrity of cuticles
   b. Altered peripheral circulation

- What are your usual nail care practices?
- Do you have any problems managing your nail care? If so, what are these?
- Have you had any problems associated with your nails (e.g., inflammation of the tissue surrounding the nail, injury, prolonged exposure to water or chemicals, circulatory problems)?

- Describe preventive interventions for the specific nail problem.
- Demonstrate nail care as instructed.

In addition, the client should have pink nail beds and quick return of nail bed color after the blanch test.

Planning

The nurse identifies measures that will assist the client to develop or maintain healthy nail care practices. A schedule of nail care needs to be established.

Implementing

To provide nail care, the nurse needs a nail cutter or sharp scissors, a nail file, an orange stick to push back the cuticle, hand lotion or mineral oil to lubricate any dry tissue around the nails, and a basin of water to soak the nails if they are particularly thick or hard. Check the agency's policy regarding nail care. Often, podiatrists must be consulted for clients with diabetes.

One hand or foot is soaked, if needed, and dried; then the nail is cut or filed straight across beyond the end of the finger or toe (see Figure 33-4 ■). Avoid trimming or digging into nails at the lateral corners. This predisposes the client to ingrown toenails. Clients who have diabetes or circulatory problems should have their nails filed rather than cut; inadvertent injury to tissues can occur if scissors are used. After the initial cut or filing, the nail is filed to round the corners, and the nurse cleans under the nail. The nurse then gently pushes back the cuticle, taking care not to injure it. The next finger or toe is cared for in the same manner. Any abnormalities, such as an infected cuticle or inflammation of the tissue around the nail, are recorded and reported.

Evaluating

Examples of desired outcomes for nail hygiene include the client being able to

- Demonstrate healthy nail care practices, as shown by
  a. Clean, short nails with smooth edges.
  b. Intact cuticles and hydrated surrounding skin.
- Describe factors contributing to the nail problem.

MOUTH

Each tooth has three parts: the crown, the root, and the pulp cavity (Figure 33-5 ■). The crown is the exposed part of the tooth, which is outside the gum. It is covered with a hard substance called enamel. The ivory-colored internal part of the crown below the enamel is the dentin. The root of a tooth is embedded in the jaw and covered by a bony tissue called cementum. The pulp cavity in the center of the tooth contains the blood vessels and nerves.

Developmental Variations

Teeth usually appear 5 to 8 months after birth. Baby-bottle syndrome may result in decay of all of the upper teeth and the lower posterior teeth (Pillitteri, 2003, p. 824). This syndrome occurs when an infant is put to bed with a bottle of sugar water, formula, milk, or fruit juice. The carbohydrates in the solutions cause demineralization of the tooth enamel, which leads to tooth decay.

By the time children are 2 years old, they usually have all 20 of their temporary teeth (Figure 33-6 ■). At about age 6 or 7, children start losing their deciduous teeth, and these are gradually replaced by the 33 permanent teeth (Figure 33-7 ■). By age 25, most people have all of their permanent teeth.

The incidence of periodontal disease increases during pregnancy because the rise in female hormones affects gingival tissue and increases its reaction to bacterial plaque. Many pregnant women experience more bleeding from the gingival sulcus during brushing and increased redness and swelling of the **gingiva** (the gum).

Teeth turn yellowish in color as a part of the aging process. Teeth are normally off-white. With age, the enamel thins and the yellow-gray color of the inner portion of the teeth begins to

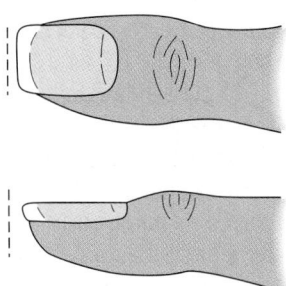

Figure 33-4 ■ Fingernails are trimmed straight across.

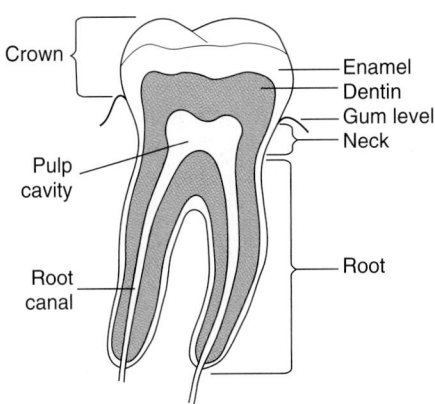

Figure 33-5 ■ The anatomic parts of a tooth.

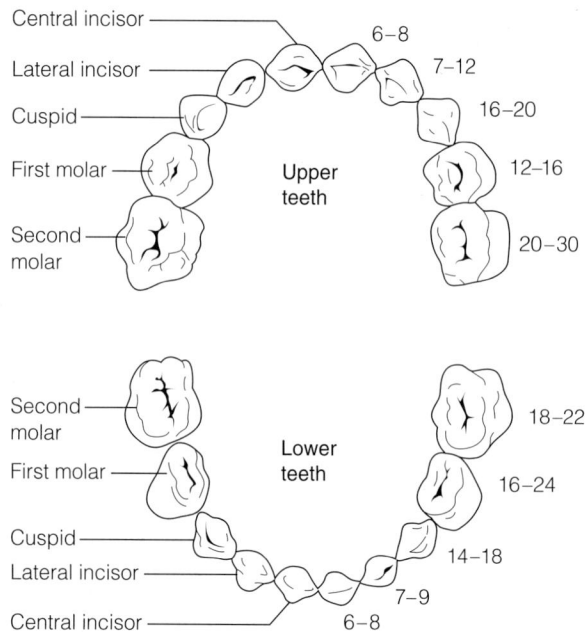

Figure 33-6 ■ Temporary teeth and their times of eruption (stated in months).

show. In addition, coffee drinking and cigarette smoking can stain the teeth. Commercial teeth whitening products and whitening treatments offered at dental offices are available to consumers who desire whiter teeth for cosmetic reasons.

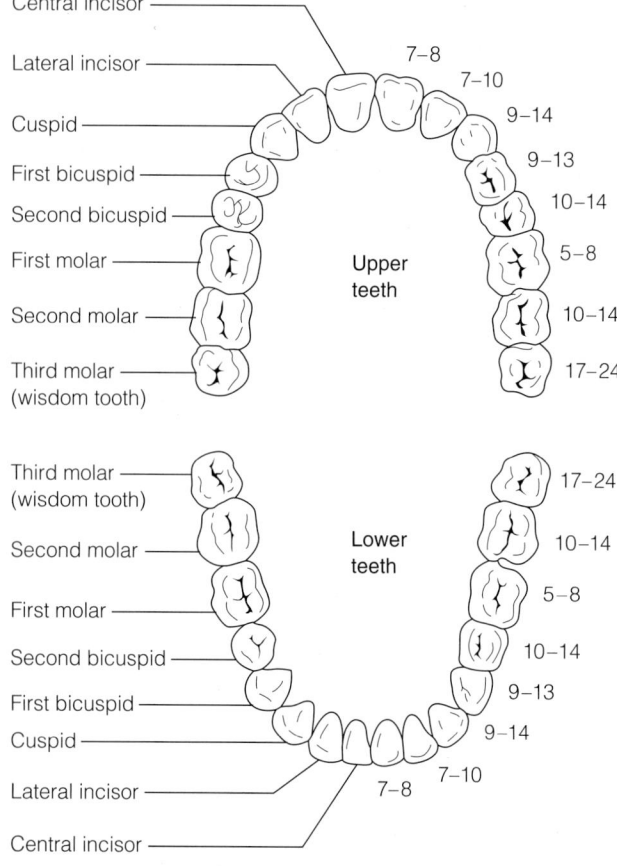

Figure 33-7 ■ Permanent teeth and their times of eruption (stated in years).

CULTURALLY COMPETENT CARE
Biocultural Variation in Teeth

■ It is rare for a White baby to be born with teeth; however, the incidence exists among Alaskan Tlingit Indian and Canadian Eskimo infants.

■ The size of teeth varies with the teeth of Whites being the smallest, followed by Blacks and then Asians and Native North Americans.

■ Whites have more tooth decay than Blacks. Complete tooth loss occurs more often in Whites than in African Americans even though African Americans have a higher incidence of periodontal disease. The difference in tooth decay may be explained by the fact that African Americans have harder and denser tooth enamel.

Note: From M. M. Andrews and S. J. Boyle, *Transcultural Concepts in Nursing Care,* 4th ed. (p. 62), Lippincott, Williams & Wilkins, 2003. Reprinted with permission.

Lack of fluoridated water and preventive dentistry during their developmental years caused tooth and gum problems in older adults (Edelman & Mandle, 2006, p. 582). As a result, some elders may have few permanent teeth left, and some have dentures. Loss of teeth occurs mainly because of **periodontal disease** (gum disease) rather than **dental caries** (cavities); however, caries are also common in middle-aged adults.

Some receding of the gums and a brownish pigmentation of the gums occur with age. Because saliva production decreases with age, dryness of the oral mucosa is a common finding in older people.

NURSING MANAGEMENT

Assessing

Assessment of the client's mouth and hygiene practices includes (a) a nursing health history, (b) physical assessment of the mouth, and (c) identification of clients at risk for developing oral problems.

Nursing History

During the nursing health history, the nurse obtains data about the client's oral hygiene practices, including dental visits, self-care abilities, and past or current mouth problems. Data about the client's oral hygiene help the nurse determine learning needs and incorporate the client's needs and preferences in the plan of care. Assessment of the client's self-care abilities determines the amount and type of nursing assistance to provide. Clients whose hand coordination is impaired, whose cognitive function is impaired, whose illness alters energy levels and motivation, or whose therapy imposes restrictions on activities will need assistance from the nurse. Information about past or current problems alerts the nurse to specific interventions required or referrals that may be necessary. Questions to elicit this information are shown in the accompanying Assessment Interview.

ASSESSMENT INTERVIEW
Oral Hygiene

ORAL HYGIENE PRACTICES

- What are your usual mouth care and/or denture care practices?
- What oral hygiene products do you routinely use (e.g., mouthwash, type of toothpaste, dental floss, denture cleaner)?
- When was your last dental examination, and how often do you see your dentist?

SELF-CARE ABILITIES

- Do you have any problems managing your mouth care?

PAST OR CURRENT MOUTH PROBLEMS

- Have you had or do you have any problems such as bleeding, swollen or reddened gums, ulcerations, lumps, or tooth pain?

Physical Assessment

For information about mouth assessment, see Chapter 30. ∞ Dental caries (cavities) and periodontal disease are the two problems that most frequently affect the teeth. Both problems are commonly associated with plaque and tartar deposits. **Plaque** is an *invisible* soft film that adheres to the enamel surface of teeth; it consists of bacteria, molecules of saliva, and remnants of epithelial cells and leukocytes. When plaque is unchecked, tartar (dental calculus) is formed. **Tartar** is a visible, hard deposit of plaque and dead bacteria that forms at the gum lines. Tartar buildup can alter the fibers that attach teeth to the gum and eventually disrupt bone tissue. Periodontal disease is characterized by **gingivitis** (red, swollen gingiva), bleeding, receding gum lines, and the formation of pockets between the teeth and gums. In advanced periodontal disease (**pyorrhea**), the teeth are loose and pus is evident when the gums are pressed. Table 33–6 lists additional problems of the mouth.

Identifying Clients at Risk

Certain clients are prone to oral problems because of lack of knowledge or the inability to maintain oral hygiene. Among these are seriously ill, confused, comatose, depressed, and dehydrated clients. In addition, people with nasogastric tubes or receiving oxygen are likely to develop dry oral mucous membranes, especially if they breathe through their mouths. Clients who have had oral or jaw surgery must have meticulous oral hygiene care to prevent the development of infections.

CLINICAL ALERT

Clients in long-term care settings are at high risk for oral health problems. The nurse must assess the client's oral health and teach the UAP about the importance of and methods to promote oral hygiene. ■

Healthy-appearing individuals, too, may be at risk. High-risk variables such as inadequate nutrition, lack of money and/or insurance for dental care, excessive intake of refined sugars, and family history of periodontal disease also need to be identified. Some older people may also be at risk, for example, those who choose salty and enamel-eroding sugary foods because of a decline in their number of taste buds. The decreased saliva production in older adults, which produces a dry mouth and thinning of the oral mucosa, is another factor.

A dry mouth can be aggravated by poor fluid intake, heavy smoking, alcohol use, high salt intake, anxiety, and many medications. Medications that can cause dryness of the mouth include diuretics; laxatives, if used excessively; and tranquilizers, such as chlorpromazine (Thorazine) and diazepam (Valium). Some chemotherapeutic agents used to treat cancer also cause oral dryness and lesions. A common side effect of the anticonvulsant drug phenytoin (Dilantin) is gingival hyperplasia. Optimal oral hygiene (e.g., brushing with a soft toothbrush and flossing) is needed.

TABLE 33–6 Common Problems of the Mouth

PROBLEM	DESCRIPTION	NURSING IMPLICATIONS
Halitosis	Bad Breath	Teach or provide regular oral hygiene.
Glossitis	Inflammation of the tongue	As above.
Gingivitis	Inflammation of the gums	As above.
Periodontal disease	Gums appear spongy and bleeding	As above.
Reddened or excoriated mucosa		Check for ill-fitting dentures.
Excessive dryness of the buccal mucosa		Increase fluid intake as health permits.
Cheilosis	Cracking of lips	Lubricate lips, use antimicrobial ointment to prevent infection.
Dental caries	Teeth have darkened areas, may be painful	Advise client to see a dentist.
Sordes	Accumulation of foul matter (food, microorganisms, and epithelial elements) on the teeth and on the lips	Teach or provide regular cleaning.
Stomatitis	Inflammation of the oral mucosa	Teach or provide regular cleaning.
Parotitis	Inflammation of the parotid salivary glands	Teach or provide regular oral hygiene.

Clients who are receiving or have received radiation treatments to the head and neck may have permanent damage to salivary glands. This results in a very dry mouth and can often be treated by providing a thick liquid called *artificial saliva*. Some clients prefer to just sip on liquids to moisten their mouth. Radiation can also cause damage to teeth and jaw structure, with actual damage occurring years after the radiation.

Diagnosing

Three nursing diagnoses related to problems with oral hygiene and the oral cavity are *Self-Care Deficit, Impaired Oral Mucous Membrane,* and *Deficient Knowledge.* Note that the North American Nursing Diagnosis Association (NANDA, 2007) includes oral hygiene in the diagnostic label *Self-Care Deficit: Bathing/Hygiene.* In this book the diagnosis *Self-Care Deficit: Oral Hygiene* will be used for clients unable to perform oral care independently. This includes the inability to brush or floss teeth or clean dentures.

The nursing diagnosis *Impaired Oral Mucous Membrane* refers to the state in which an individual experiences disruptions in the tissue layers of the oral cavity. Manifestations include a coated tongue; dry mouth; halitosis; gingivitis; oral pain, discomfort, erythema, oral lesions, or ulcers; and dry mouth. These may be the result of ineffective oral hygiene, physical injury or drying effect (e.g., mouth breathing, oxygen therapy, dehydration), mechanical trauma (e.g., oral surgery, braces or ill-fitting dentures), chemical trauma (e.g., side effects of medications), or radiation therapy. The diagnosis *Deficient Knowledge* is discussed in Chapter 27. ∞

Clinical examples of assessment data clusters, related nursing diagnoses, outcomes, and interventions are shown in the Identifying Nursing Diagnoses, Outcomes, and Interventions box.

Planning

In planning care, the nurse and, if appropriate, the client and/or family set outcomes for each nursing diagnosis. The nurse then performs nursing interventions and activities to achieve the client outcomes.

During the planning phase, the nurse also identifies interventions that will help the client achieve these goals. Spe-

IDENTIFYING NURSING DIAGNOSES, OUTCOMES, AND INTERVENTIONS
Clients With Oral Cavity Problems

DATA CLUSTER Mary Brown, 77 years old, suffered a cerebrovascular accident. Is unconscious and breathing through the mouth via O₂ face mask. 2,500 mL intravenous fluid ordered daily.

NURSING DIAGNOSIS/ DEFINITION	SAMPLE DESIRED OUTCOME*/ DEFINITION	INDICATORS	SELECTED INTERVENTIONS*/ DEFINITION	SAMPLE NIC ACTIVITIES
Self-Care Deficit: Oral Hygiene related to cognitive inability (unconsciousness)/*Impaired ability to perform or complete bathing/hygiene activities for oneself*	Self-Care: Oral Hygiene [0308]/*Ability to care for own mouth and teeth independently with or without assistive device*	Severely compromised: ■ Cleans mouth, gums, and tongue	Oral Health Maintenance [1710]/ *Maintenance and promotion of oral hygiene and dental health for the client at risk for developing oral or dental lesions*	■ Establish a mouth care routine ■ Apply lubricant to moisten lips and oral mucosa, as needed ■ Monitor for signs and symptoms of glossitis and stomatitis

DATA CLUSTER Joe Kwan, 46 years old, was admitted with a fractured femur. Teeth stained from heavy smoking. One large cavity evident in 2nd lower left molar, tartar buildup along gum margins, and pronounced halitosis. Gums are reddened in some areas and bleed when flossed. States, "I can't remember when I last saw a dentist."

Impaired Oral Mucous Membrane related to ineffective oral hygiene/*Disruption of the lips and soft tissue of the oral cavity*	Oral Hygiene [1100]/*Condition of the mouth, teeth, gums, and tongue*	Not compromised: ■ Cleanliness of teeth ■ Cleanliness of gums ■ No: Halitosis ■ Bleeding	Oral Health Restoration [1730]/*Promotion of healing for a client who has an oral mucosa or dental lesion*	■ Use a soft toothbrush for removal of dental debris ■ Use toothettes or disposable foam swabs to stimulate gums and clean oral cavity ■ Encourage flossing between teeth twice daily with unwaxed dental floss, if platelet levels are above 50,000/mm³ ■ Discourage smoking ■ Reinforce oral hygiene regimen as part of discharge teaching

*The NOC # for desired outcomes and the NIC # for nursing interventions are listed in brackets following the appropriate outcome or intervention. Outcomes, indicators, interventions, and activities selected are only a sample of those suggested by NOC and NIC and should be further individualized for each client.

cific, detailed nursing activities taken by the nurse may include the following:

- Monitor every shift for dryness of the oral mucosa.
- Monitor for signs and symptoms of glossitis (inflammation of the tongue) and stomatitis (inflammation of the mouth).
- Assist dependent clients with oral care.
- Provide special oral hygiene for clients who are debilitated, are unconscious, or have lesions of the mucous membranes or other oral tissues.
- Teach clients about good oral hygiene practices and other measures to prevent tooth decay.
- Reinforce the oral hygiene regimen as part of discharge teaching.

Implementing

Good oral hygiene includes daily stimulation of the gums, mechanical brushing and flossing of the teeth, and flushing of the mouth. The nurse is often in a position to help people maintain oral hygiene by helping or teaching them to clean the teeth and oral cavity, by inspecting whether clients (especially children) have done so, or by actually providing mouth care to clients who are ill or incapacitated. The nurse can also be instrumental in identifying problems that require the intervention of a dentist or oral surgeon and arranging a referral.

Promoting Oral Health Through the Life Span

A major role of the nurse in promoting oral health is to teach clients about specific oral hygienic measures.

INFANTS AND TODDLERS. Most dentists recommend that dental hygiene should begin when the first tooth erupts and be practiced after each feeding. Cleaning can be accomplished by using a wet washcloth or small gauze moistened with water.

Dental caries occur frequently during the toddler period, often as a result of the excessive intake of sweets or a prolonged use of the bottle during naps and at bedtime. The nurse should give parents the following instructions to promote and maintain dental health:

- Beginning at about 18 months of age, brush the child's teeth with a soft toothbrush. Use only a toothbrush moistened with water at first and introduce toothpaste later. Use one that contains fluoride.
- Give a fluoride supplement daily or as recommended by the primary care provider or dentist, unless the drinking water is fluoridated.
- Schedule an initial dental visit for the child at about 2 or 3 years of age, as soon as all 20 primary teeth have erupted.
- Some dentists recommend an inspection type of visit when the child is about 18 months old to provide an early pleasant introduction to the dental examination.
- Seek professional dental attention for any problems such as discoloring of the teeth, chipping, or signs of infection such as redness and swelling.

PRESCHOOLERS AND SCHOOL-AGE CHILDREN. Because deciduous teeth guide the entrance of permanent teeth, dental care is essential to keep these teeth in good repair. Abnormally placed or lost deciduous teeth can cause misalignment of permanent teeth. Fluoride remains important at this stage to prevent dental caries. Preschoolers need to be taught to brush their teeth after eating and to limit their intake of refined sugars. Parental supervision may be needed to ensure the completion of these self-care activities. Regular dental checkups are required during these years when permanent teeth appear.

ADOLESCENTS AND ADULTS. Proper diet and tooth and mouth care should be evaluated and reinforced to adolescents

---

RESEARCH NOTE **What Factors Affect Access for Dental Care Among Medicaid-Enrolled Children?**

Poor oral health is the most unmet health need, and tooth decay is the most common chronic childhood disease in the United States. The researchers wanted to examine factors that affected caregivers of diverse racial/ethnic backgrounds who did not seek preventive dental care for their Medicaid-enrolled children. The study was limited to one county in Kentucky. The researchers conducted eight focus groups with 76 caregivers of Medicaid-enrolled children in the specified county. Forty-six of the caregivers were African American and 30 were White.

Belief in the importance of oral health for overall health emerged as a major theme. Caregivers who used Medicaid dental care for their children emphasized prevention of dental problems while nonutilizing caregivers perceived both dental and general health care in emergency terms rather than preventive. They often relied on home remedies and believed that dental care was more important for older children. Nonutilizing White caregivers believed that tooth loss was expected with aging.

Another major factor that emerged between the caregivers that used the Medicaid oral health services and those who did not was the belief about responsibility for children's professional preventive dental care. Those who used the services believed that it was part of being a "good parent." Those caregivers who did not use the oral health services did not view preventive dental health with a child's overall health. They set poor examples and reported that they lacked knowledge about child dental care and oral health.

The study also confirmed previously identified structural barriers that included difficulty in locating Medicaid providers, scheduling convenient appointments, transportation, and discrimination.

IMPLICATIONS

The researchers suggest that interventions to improve use of professional dental care among Medicaid-enrolled children should include educating the caregivers about the importance of oral health and that preventive dental care is part of a caregiver's responsibility for their child's overall health.

Note: From "Barriers to Care-Seeking for Children's Oral Health Among Low-Income Caregivers" by S. E. Kelly, C. J. Binkley, W. P. Neace, and B. S. Gale, 2005, *American Journal of Public Health, 95*(8), pp. 1345–1351.

CLIENT TEACHING
Measures to Prevent Tooth Decay

- Brush the teeth thoroughly after meals and at bedtime. Assist children or inspect their mouths to be sure the teeth are clean. If the teeth cannot be brushed after meals, vigorous rinsing of the mouth with water is recommended.
- Floss the teeth daily.
- Ensure an adequate intake of nutrients, particularly calcium, phosphorus, vitamins A, C, and D, and fluoride.
- Avoid sweet foods and drinks between meals. Take them in moderation at meals.
- Eat coarse, fibrous foods (cleansing foods), such as fresh fruits and raw vegetables.
- Have topical fluoride applications as prescribed by the dentist.
- Have a checkup by a dentist every 6 months.

---

and adults. Specific measures to prevent tooth decay and periodontal disease are listed in Client Teaching.

OLDER ADULTS. Over 50% of older adults have their own teeth (Gooch, Eke, & Malvitz, 2004). As a result, older adults are at risk for dental cavities and periodontal disease. Older adults who have self-care deficits are at an increased risk because they cannot maintain their oral hygiene practices and/or may not be able to visit the dentist on a routine basis. Furthermore, those who suffer the worst oral health and hygiene include older adults residing in nursing homes (Coleman, 2002, 2004). Coleman (2004) reported that poor oral hygiene among the frail and dependent nursing home residents can place them at risk for serious illness such as pneumonia (p. 3). Nurses have an important role in promoting optimal geriatric oral health care.

Brushing and Flossing the Teeth

Thorough brushing of the teeth is important in preventing tooth decay. The mechanical action of brushing removes food particles that can harbor and incubate bacteria. It also stimulates circulation in the gums, thus maintaining their healthy firmness. One of the techniques recommended for brushing teeth is called the sulcular technique, which removes plaque and cleans under the gingival margins. Many toothpastes are marketed. Fluoride toothpaste is often recommended because of its antibacterial protection.

Caring for Artificial Dentures

Some people have artificial teeth in the form of a plate—a complete set of teeth for one jaw. A person may have a lower plate or an upper plate or both. When only a few artificial teeth are needed, the individual may have a bridge rather than a plate. A bridge may be fixed or removable. Artificial teeth are fitted to the individual and usually will not fit another person. People who wear dentures or other types of oral prostheses should be encouraged to use them. Ill-fitting dentures or other oral prostheses can cause discomfort and chewing difficulties. They may also contribute to oral problems as well as poor nutrition and enjoyment

of food. Those who do not wear their prostheses are prone to shrinkage of the gums, which results in further tooth loss.

Like natural teeth, artificial dentures collect microorganisms and food. They need to be cleaned regularly, at least once a day. They can be removed from the mouth, scrubbed with a toothbrush, rinsed, and reinserted. Some people use a dentifrice for cleaning teeth, and others use commercial cleaning compounds for plates.

Assisting Clients with Oral Care

When providing mouth care for partially or totally dependent clients, the nurse should wear gloves to guard against infections. Other required equipment includes a curved basin that fits snugly under the client's chin (e.g., a kidney basin) to receive the rinse water, and a towel to protect the client and the bedclothes. See Skill 33-4.

Foam swabs are often used in health care agencies to clean the mouths of dependent clients (Figure 33-8 ■). These swabs are convenient and effective in removing excess debris from the teeth and mouth but should be used infrequently and for short periods (i.e., less than 3 days) because they do not remove plaque that is at the base of the teeth.

Most people prefer privacy when they take their artificial teeth out to clean them. Many do not like to be seen without their teeth; one of the first requests of many postoperative clients is "May I have my teeth in, please?" The "Variation" section in Skill 33-4 describes how to clean artificial dentures.

Clients with Special Oral Hygiene Needs

For the client who is debilitated or unconscious or who has excessive dryness, sores, or irritations of the mouth, it may be necessary to clean the oral mucosa and tongue in addition to the teeth. Agency practices differ in regard to special mouth care and the frequency with which it is provided. Depending on the health of the client's mouth, special care may be needed every 2 to 8 hours.

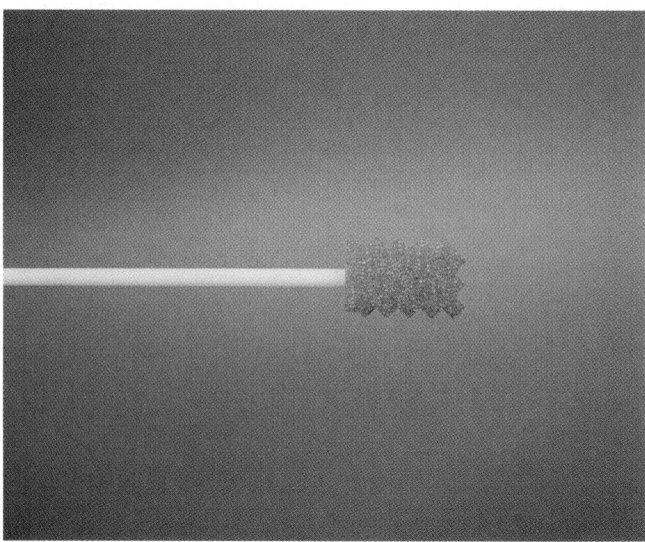

Figure 33-8 ■ Example of a foam swab used to clean the mouth of a dependent client.

BRUSHING AND FLOSSING THE TEETH

PURPOSES
- To remove food particles from around and between the teeth
- To remove dental plaque
- To promote the client's feelings of well-being
- To prevent sores and infection of the oral tissues

ASSESSMENT
- Determine the extent of the client's self-care abilities.
- Assess the client's usual mouth care practices.
- Inspect lips, gums, oral mucosa, and tongue for deviations from normal.
- Identify presence of oral problems such as tooth caries, halitosis, gingivitis, and loose or broken teeth.
- Check if the client has bridgework or wears dentures. If the client has dentures, ask if any tenderness or soreness is present and, if so, the location of the area(s) for ongoing assessment.

PLANNING

Delegation
Oral care, brushing and flossing of teeth, and denture care can be delegated to the UAP. After performing the above assessment, the nurse should instruct the UAP as to the type of oral care and amount of assistance needed by the client. Remind the UAP to report changes in the client's oral mucosa.

Equipment
Brushing and Flossing
- Towel
- Disposable gloves
- Curved basin (emesis basin)
- Toothbrush (soft bristle)
- Cup of tepid water
- Dentifrice (toothpaste)
- Mouthwash
- Dental floss, at least two pieces 20 cm (8 in.) in length
- Floss holder (optional)

For Cleaning Artificial Dentures
- Disposable gloves
- Tissue or piece of gauze
- Denture container
- Clean washcloth
- Toothbrush or stiff-bristled brush
- Dentifrice or denture cleaner
- Tepid water
- Container of mouthwash
- Curved basin (emesis basin)
- Towel

IMPLEMENTATION

Preparation
Assemble all the necessary equipment.

Performance
1. Prior to performing the procedure, introduce self and verify the client's identity using agency protocol. Explain to the client what you are going to do, why it is necessary, and how he or she can cooperate.
2. Perform hand hygiene and observe other appropriate infection control procedures (e.g., disposable gloves). **Rationale:** *Wearing gloves while providing mouth care prevents the nurse from acquiring infections. Gloves also prevent transmission of microorganisms to the client.*
3. Provide for client privacy by drawing the curtains around the bed or closing the door to the room. Some agencies provide signs indicating the need for privacy. **Rationale:** *Hygiene is a personal matter.*
4. Prepare the client.
   - Assist the client to a sitting position in bed, if health permits. If not, assist the client to a side-lying position with the head turned *so liquid may be prevented from draining down the client's throat.*
5. Prepare the equipment.
   - Place the towel under the client's chin.
   - Put on disposable gloves.
   - Moisten the bristles of the toothbrush with tepid water and apply the dentifrice to the toothbrush.
   - Use a soft toothbrush (a small one for a child) and the client's choice of dentifrice.
   - For the client who must remain in bed, place or hold the curved basin under the client's chin, fitting the small curve around the chin or neck.
   - Inspect the mouth and teeth.
6. Brush the teeth.
   - Hand the toothbrush to the client, or brush the client's teeth as follows:
     a. Hold the brush against the teeth with the bristles at a 45-degree angle. The tips of the outer bristles should rest against and penetrate under the gingival sulcus. ❶ The

❶ The sulcular technique: Place the bristles at a 45-degree angle with the tips of the outer bristles under the gingival margins.
(Al Dodge, Pearson Education/PH College)

continued on page 770

bicarbonate toothpaste will help dissolve mucus and reduce the saliva's acidity, which helps decrease bacteria (Nainar & Mohummed, 2004). If the client cannot tolerate the use of a toothbrush, the nurse can use an oral swab or a gauze soaked with saline to swab the teeth and tongue. A foam swab (Figure 33-28) can be used to provide oral hygiene to dependent clients. The swab, however, is not effective for plaque removal (Munro, Grap, & Kleinpell, 2004). Lemon-glycerin swabs are not recommended as they irritate and dry the oral mucosa and can decalcify teeth. Mouthwashes containing alcohol can irritate the oral mucosa as well as cause dryness. Hydrogen peroxide is approved as a mouth rinse by the Food and Drug Administration (Anonymous, 2003, p. 12). It provides a cleaning action as well as an antimicrobial effect. Diluting the hydrogen peroxide with saline or a non-alcohol–based mouthwash will help decrease a possible burning sensation experienced by the client. Mineral oil is contraindicated as a moisturizer for the lips or inside the mouth because aspiration of it can initiate an infection (lipid pneumonia). A water-soluble moisturizer, absorbed by the skin and tissue, provides important hydration. Saliva substitutes can also help moisturize the oral cavity.

Skill 33-5 focuses on oral care for the unconscious person but may be adapted for conscious persons who are seriously ill or have mouth problems.

SKILL 33-5

PROVIDING SPECIAL ORAL CARE FOR THE UNCONSCIOUS CLIENT

PURPOSES
- To maintain the intactness and health of the lips, tongue, and mucous membranes of the mouth
- To prevent oral infections
- To clean and moisten the membranes of the mouth and lips

ASSESSMENT
- Inspect lips, gums, oral mucosa, and tongue for deviations from normal.
- Identify presence of oral problems such as tooth caries, halitosis, gingivitis, and loose or broken teeth.
- Assess for gag reflex, when appropriate.

PLANNING

Delegation

Special oral care may be delegated to UAP; however, the nurse needs to assess for the gag reflex. Dependent on this assessment, the nurse needs to inform the UAP of the correct positioning of the client and how to use the oral suction catheter, if needed. Remind the UAP to report changes in the client's oral mucosa.

Equipment
- Towel
- Curved basin (emesis basin)
- Disposable clean gloves
- Bite-block to hold the mouth open and teeth apart (optional)
- Toothbrush
- Cup of tepid water
- Dentifrice or denture cleaner
- Tissue or piece of gauze to remove dentures (optional)
- Denture container as needed
- Mouthwash
- Rubber-tipped bulb syringe
- Suction catheter with suction apparatus when aspiration is a concern
- Foam swabs and cleaning solution for cleaning the mucous membranes
- Water-soluble lip moisturizer

Performance

1. Prior to performing the procedure, introduce self and verify the client's identity using agency protocol. Explain to the client and the family what you are going to do and why it is necessary.
2. Perform hand hygiene and observe other appropriate infection control procedures (e.g., disposable gloves).
3. Provide for client privacy by drawing the curtains around the bed or closing the door to the room. Some agencies provide signs indicating the need for privacy. **Rationale:** *Hygiene is a personal matter.*
4. Prepare the client.
   - Position the unconscious client in a side-lying position, with the head of the bed lowered. **Rationale:** *In this position, the saliva automatically runs out by gravity rather than being aspirated into the lungs.* This position is chosen for the unconscious client receiving mouth care. If the client's head cannot be lowered, turn it to one side. **Rationale:** *The fluid will readily run out of the mouth or pool in the side of the mouth, where it can be suctioned.*
   - Place the towel under the client's chin.
   - Place the curved basin against the client's chin and lower cheek to receive the fluid from the mouth. ❶
   - Put on gloves.
5. Clean the teeth and rinse the mouth.
   - If the person has natural teeth, brush the teeth as described in Skill 33-4. Brush gently and carefully to avoid injuring the gums. If the client has artificial teeth, clean them as described in the "Variation" component of Skill 33-4.
   - Rinse the client's mouth by drawing about 10 mL of water or alcohol-free mouthwash into the syringe and injecting it gently into each side of the mouth. **Rationale:** *If the solution is injected with force, some of it may flow down the client's throat and be aspirated into the lungs.*
   - Watch carefully to make sure that all the rinsing solution has run out of the mouth into the basin. If not, suction the fluid from the mouth. **Rationale:** *Fluid remaining in the mouth may be aspirated into the lungs.*
   - Repeat rinsing until the mouth is free of dentifrice, if used.
6. Inspect and clean the oral tissues.
   - If the tissues appear dry or unclean, clean them with the foam swabs or gauze and cleaning solution following agency policy.

SKILL 33-5

PROVIDING SPECIAL ORAL CARE FOR THE UNCONSCIOUS CLIENT *continued*

1 Position of client and placement of curved basin when providing special mouth care.

- Picking up a moistened foam swab, wipe the mucous membrane of one cheek. Discard the swab in a waste container; use a fresh one to clean the next area. **Rationale:** *Using separate applicators for each area of the mouth prevents the transfer of microorganisms from one area to another.*
- Clean all mouth tissues in an orderly progression, using separate applicators: the cheeks, roof of the mouth, base of the mouth, and tongue.
- Observe the tissues closely for inflammation and dryness.
- Rinse the client's mouth as described in step 5.
- Remove and discard gloves.
7. Ensure client comfort.
   - Remove the basin, and dry around the client's mouth with the towel. Replace artificial dentures, if indicated.
   - Lubricate the client's lips with water-soluble moisturizer. **Rationale:** *Lubrication prevents cracking and subsequent infection.*
8. Document assessment of the teeth, tongue, gums, and oral mucosa. Include any problems such as sores or inflammation and swelling of the gums.

EVALUATION

- Consider the client's medical diagnosis and treatment (e.g., chemotherapy, oxygen) and the necessary nursing interventions related to oral hygiene.
- Conduct an ongoing assessment, if appropriate, of the oral mucosa, gums, tongue, and lips.
- Report deviations from normal to the primary care provider.
- Conduct appropriate follow-up such as a referral to a dentist for dental caries.

LIFESPAN CONSIDERATIONS **Oral Hygiene**

INFANTS

- Most dentists recommend that dental hygiene should begin when the first tooth erupts and be practiced after each feeding. Cleaning can be accomplished by using a wet washcloth or small gauze moistened with water.

CHILDREN

- Beginning at about 18 months of age, brush the child's teeth with a soft toothbrush. Use only a toothbrush moistened with water. Introduce toothpaste later and use one that contains fluoride.
- Frequent snacking of products containing sugar increases the child's risk for developing cavities.

ELDERS

- Oral care is often difficult for certain elders to perform due to problems with dexterity or cognitive problems with dementia.
- Most long-term health care facilities have dentists that come on a regular basis to see clients with special needs.
- Dryness of the oral mucosa is a common finding in elders. Because this can lead to tooth decay, advise clients to discuss it with their dentist or primary care provider.
- Decay of the tooth root is common among elders. When the gums recede, the tooth root is more vulnerable to decay.
- Promoting good oral hygiene can have a positive effect on the elders' ability to eat.

HOME CARE CONSIDERATIONS **Oral Hygiene**

- Assess the oral hygiene practices and attitude toward oral hygiene of family members and the client.
- Remind adults to replace their toothbrush every 3 to 4 months and a child's toothbrush more frequently.
- The client with a nasogastric tube or who is receiving oxygen is likely to develop dry oral mucous membranes, especially if the client breathes through the mouth. More frequent oral hygiene will be needed.

Evaluating

Using data collected during care—status of oral mucosa, lips, tongue, teeth, and so on—the nurse judges whether desired outcomes have been achieved.

If outcomes are not achieved, the nurse and client need to explore the reasons before modifying the care plan. Examples of questions to consider are as follows:

- Did the nurse overestimate the client's functional abilities?
- Is the client's hand coordination or cognitive function impaired?
- Did the client's condition change?
- Has there been a change in the client's energy level and/or motivation?

HAIR

The appearance of the hair often reflects a person's feelings of self-concept and sociocultural well-being. Becoming familiar with hair care needs and practices that may be different from our own is an important aspect of providing competent nursing care to all clients. People who feel ill may not groom their hair as before. A dirty scalp and hair are itchy and uncomfortable, and can have an odor. The hair may also reflect state of health (e.g., excessive coarseness and dryness may be associated with endocrine disorders such as hypothyroidism).

Each person has particular ways of caring for hair. Many dark-skinned people need to oil their hair daily because it tends to be dry. Oil prevents the hair from breaking and the scalp from drying. A wide-toothed comb is usually used because finer combs pull and break the hair. Some people brush their hair vigorously before retiring; others comb their hair frequently.

Developmental Variations

Newborns may have **lanugo** (the fine hair on the body of the fetus, also referred to as *down* or *woolly hair*) over their shoulders, back, and sacrum. This generally disappears, and the hair distribution on the eyebrows, head, and eyelashes of young children subsequently becomes noticeable. Some newborns have hair on their scalps; others are free of hair at birth but grow hair over the scalp during the first year of life.

Pubic hair usually appears in early puberty, followed in about 6 months by the growth of axillary hair. Boys develop facial hair in later puberty.

In adolescence, the sebaceous glands increase in activity as a result of increased hormone levels. As a result, hair follicle openings enlarge to accommodate the increased amount of sebum, which can make the adolescent's hair more oily.

In older adults, the hair is generally thinner, grows more slowly, and loses its color as a result of aging tissues and diminishing circulation. Men often lose their scalp hair and may become completely bald. This phenomenon may occur even when a man is relatively young. The older person's hair also tends to be drier than normal. With age, axillary and pubic hair becomes finer and scanter, in contrast to the eyebrows, which become bristly and coarse. Many women develop hair on their faces, which may be a concern to them.

 NURSING MANAGEMENT

Assessing

Assessment of the client's hair, hair care practices, and potential problems includes a nursing health history and physical assessment.

Nursing History

During the nursing history the nurse elicits data about usual hair care, self-care abilities, history of hair or scalp problems, and conditions known to affect the hair. Chemotherapeutic agents and radiation of the head may cause **alopecia** (hair loss). Hy-

---

pothyroidism may cause the hair to be thin, dry, and/or brittle. Use of some hair dyes and curling or straightening preparations can cause the hair to become dry and brittle. Questions to elicit these data are shown in the accompanying Assessment Interview.

Physical Assessment

Physical assessment of the hair is discussed in Chapter 30. ∞ Problems include dandruff, hair loss, ticks, pediculosis, scabies, and hirsutism.

DANDRUFF. Often accompanied by itching, **dandruff** appears as a diffuse scaling of the scalp. In severe cases it involves the auditory canals and the eyebrows. Dandruff can usually be treated effectively with a commercial shampoo. In severe or persistent cases, the client may need the advice of a primary care provider.

HAIR LOSS. Hair loss and growth are continual processes. Some permanent thinning of hair normally occurs with aging. Baldness, common in men, is thought to be a hereditary problem for which there is no known remedy other than the wearing of a hairpiece or a costly surgical hair transplant, in which hair is taken from the back or the sides of the scalp and surgically moved to the hairless area. Although some medications are being developed, their long-term outcomes are unknown.

TICKS. Small gray-brown parasites that bite into tissue and suck blood, **ticks** transmit several diseases to people, in particular Rocky Mountain spotted fever, Lyme disease, and tularemia. To remove a tick, use a blunt tweezers or gloved fingers and grasp the tick as close to the skin as possible. Gently pull the tick away using perpendicular traction to remove the tick. Be careful to not twist or squeeze the tick's body. If the head breaks off and remains in the skin, use tweezers to remove in a manner similar to that used for removing a splinter. Wash the area with antibacterial soap. Save the tick in a bottle of rubbing alcohol in case the primary care provider wants to identify the type of tick. The following practices to remove a tick are ineffective or dangerous: applying heat with a match and applying substances such as petroleum jelly or gasoline (Gammons & Salam, 2002).

PEDICULOSIS (LICE). Lice are parasitic insects that infest mammals. Infestation with lice is called **pediculosis.** Hundreds of varieties of lice infest humans. Three common kinds are *Pediculus capitis* (the head louse), *Pediculus corporis* (the body louse), and *Pediculus pubis* (the crab louse).

Pediculus capitis is found on the scalp and tends to stay hidden in the hairs; similarly, *Pediculus pubis* stays in pubic hair. *Pediculus corporis* tends to cling to clothing, so that when a client undresses, the lice may not be evident on the body; these lice suck blood from the person and lay their eggs on the clothing. The nurse can suspect their presence in the clothing if (a) the person habitually scratches, (b) there are scratches on the skin, and (c) there are hemorrhagic spots on the skin where the lice have sucked blood.

Head and pubic lice lay their eggs on the hairs; the eggs look like oval particles, similar to dandruff, clinging to the hair. Bites and pustular eruptions may also be noticed at the hair lines and behind the ears.

Lice are very small, grayish white, and difficult to see. The crab louse in the pubic area has red legs. Lice may be contracted from infested clothes and direct contact with an infested person.

The treatment often includes topical pediculicides such as pyrethrins (e.g., RID, Pyrinate), permethrin (e.g., Nix), and lindane (e.g., Kwell). The current recommended treatment of choice for head lice is Nix because it is the least toxic (Frankowski & Weiner, 2002; Goldsmith, 2003). Natural products offered by health food stores are also available (e.g., Lice B Gone, Lice Away Enzyme Shampoo). Moses (2003) advocates using these natural vegetable extracts first because they are nontoxic, safe for children and pregnant or nursing women, inexpensive, and effective (p. 11). Clients, however, need to be reminded that natural products are not required to meet the Food and Drug Administration standards. Some home remedies suggest applying an oily substance such as olive oil or petroleum jelly to smother the lice. This practice, according to the Centers for Disease Control and Prevention, can be dangerous or cause infections (Goldsmith, 2003, p. 23).

Removal of nits (eggs) after applying the treatment is not necessary to prevent spread but most people remove them for aesthetic reasons (Frankowski & Weiner, 2002). Fine-toothed "nit" combs are available. Transmission is from head-to-head contact, and it is suggested that the hair care items and bedding of the person who has the lice infestation be washed with hot water.

SCABIES. **Scabies** is a contagious skin infestation by the itch mite. The characteristic lesion is the burrow produced by the female mite as it penetrates into the upper layers of the skin. Burrows are short, wavy, brown or black, threadlike lesions most commonly observed between the fingers, in the creases of the wrists and elbows, beneath breast tissue, and in the groin area (Stewart, 2000). The mites cause intense itching that is more pronounced at night because the increased warmth of the skin has a stimulating effect on the parasites. Secondary lesions caused by scratching include vesicles, papules, pustules, excoriations, and crusts. Treatment involves thorough cleansing of the body with soap and water to remove scales and debris from crusts, and then an application of a scabicide lotion. All bed linens and clothing should be washed in very hot or boiling water.

HIRSUTISM. The growth of excessive body hair is called **hirsutism.** The acceptance of body hair in the axillae and on the legs is largely dictated by culture. In North America, the well-groomed woman, as depicted in magazines, has no hair on her legs or under her axillae. In many European cultures, it is not customary for well-groomed women to remove this hair.

Excessive facial hair on a woman is thought unattractive in most Western and Asian cultures. For example, some Japanese brides follow the custom of shaving their faces the day before the wedding.

The cause of excessive body hair is not always known. Older women may have some on their faces, and women in menopause may also experience the growth of facial hair. Excessive body hair may be due to the action of the endocrine system. Heredity is also thought to influence the pattern of hair distribution.

Diagnosing

Nursing diagnoses related to hair hygiene and hair and scalp problems include *Self-Care Deficit: Grooming, Impaired Skin Integrity, Risk for Infection,* and *Disturbed Body Image.* Examples of these nursing diagnoses with contributing factors follow:

- *Self-Care Deficit: Grooming* related to
  a. Activity intolerance
  b. Imposed immobility (bed rest)
  c. Pain in upper extremities
  d. Altered level of consciousness
  e. Lack of motivation associated with depression
- *Impaired Skin Integrity* related to
  a. Scalp laceration
  b. Insect bite
- *Risk for Infection* related to
  a. Scalp laceration
  b. Insect bite
- *Disturbed Body Image* related to alopecia

Planning

In planning care, the nurse and, if appropriate, the client and/or family set outcomes for each nursing diagnosis. The nurse then performs nursing interventions and activities to achieve the client outcomes. Identifying Nursing Diagnoses, Outcomes, and Interventions provides suggested outcomes and interventions for hair grooming.

The specific, detailed nursing activities taken by the nurse to assist the client should take into account the client's personal preferences, health, and energy resources as well as the time, equipment, and personnel available. Often, clients like to receive hair care after a bath, before receiving visitors, and before retiring. Nursing interventions may include instructing the client/family in alternative methods for hair care including facilitating the assistance of a barber or beautician, as necessary. At some agencies, shampoos can be given to clients only after a primary care provider's order.

Implementing

Hair needs to be brushed or combed daily and washed, as needed, to keep it clean. Nurses may need to provide hair care for clients who cannot meet their own self-care needs.

IDENTIFYING NURSING DIAGNOSES, OUTCOMES, AND INTERVENTIONS

Hair Grooming

NURSING DIAGNOSIS/ DEFINITION	SAMPLE DESIRED OUTCOME*/ DEFINITION	INDICATORS†	SELECTED INTERVENTIONS*/ DEFINITION	SAMPLE NIC ACTIVITIES
Self-Care Deficit: Dressing/Grooming/Impaired ability to perform or complete dressing and grooming activities for self	Self-Care: Hygiene [0305]/*Ability to maintain own personal cleanliness and kempt appearance independently with or without assistive device*	Not compromised: • Shampoos hair • Combs or brushes hair • Maintains neat appearance	Hair Care [1670]/*Promotion of neat, clean, attractive hair*	• Wash hair, as needed and desired • Dry hair with hair dryer • Brush/comb hair daily or more frequently, as needed • Monitor scalp daily • Braid or otherwise arrange hair as client wishes • Use hair care products of client's preference, as available

*The NOC # for desired outcomes and the NIC # for nursing interventions are listed in brackets following the appropriate outcome or intervention. Outcomes, indicators, interventions, and activities selected are only a sample of those suggested by NOC and NIC and should be further individualized for each client.

† The measurement scale ranges from Dependent, does not participate to Completely independent. See *Appendix B.* ∞

Brushing and Combing Hair

To be healthy, hair needs to be brushed daily. Brushing has three major functions: It stimulates the circulation of blood in the scalp, it distributes the oil along the hair shaft, and it helps to arrange the hair.

Long hair may present a problem for clients confined to bed because it may become matted. It should be combed and brushed at least once a day to prevent this. A brush with stiff bristles provides the best stimulation to blood circulation in the scalp. The bristles should not be so sharp that they injure the client's scalp, however. A comb with dull, even teeth is advisable. A comb with sharp teeth might injure the scalp; combs that are too fine can pull and break the hair. Some clients are pleased to have their hair tied neatly in the back or braided until other assistance is available or until they feel better and can look after it themselves. Braiding also prevents tangling and matting for clients confined to bed.

CLINICAL ALERT

Excessively matted or tangled hair may be infested with lice. ■

Dark-skinned people often have thicker, drier, curlier hair than light-skinned people. Very curly hair may stand out from the scalp. Although the shafts of curly or kinky hair look strong and wiry, they have less strength than straight hair shafts and can break easily. Many African American people have hair that is naturally curly, and it can easily become matted and tangled in a short period of time (Jackson, 1998). African Americans generally wash their hair less often than other ethnic groups because the hair is drier. Shampooing often could damage their hair.

Some African Americans have their hair straightened. Even if straightened, the hair tends to tangle and mat easily, especially at the back and the sides if the client is confined to bed. Other African Americans style their hair in small braids (see Figure 33-9 ■). These braids do not have to be unbraided for shampooing and washing. If, however, unbraiding becomes necessary,

Figure 33-9 ■ An African American's hair styled with braids.

the nurse should obtain the client's permission to do so. Some African American clients may use oil by applying it between the braids and massaging it into the scalp. The oil prevents the hair strands from breaking and the scalp from becoming too dry. Not all African American individuals have curly or kinky hair. Some have naturally straight hair. Keeping the scalp and hair clean and oiled remains important and necessary. Skill 33-6 describes how to provide hair care for clients.

Shampooing the Hair

Hair should be washed as often as needed to keep it clean. There are several ways to shampoo clients' hair, depending on their health, strength, and age. The client who is well enough to take a shower can shampoo while in the shower. The client who is unable to shower may be given a shampoo while sitting on a chair in front of a sink. The back-lying client who can move to a stretcher can be given a shampoo on a stretcher wheeled to a sink. The client who must remain in bed can be

PROVIDING HAIR CARE FOR CLIENTS

PURPOSES
- To stimulate the blood circulation to the scalp
- To distribute hair oils and provide a healthy sheen
- To increase the client's comfort
- To assess or monitor hair or scalp problems (e.g., matted hair or dandruff)

ASSESSMENT
Determine
- History of the following conditions or therapies: recent chemotherapy, hypothyroidism, radiation of the head, unexplained hair loss, and growth of excessive body hair
- Usual hair care practices and routinely used hair care products (e.g., hair spray, shampoo, conditioners, hair oil preparation, hair dye, curling or straightening preparations).
- Whether wetting the hair will make it difficult to comb. Kinky hair is easier to comb when wet and is very difficult to comb when it dries (Jackson, 1998, p. 102).

Assess
- Condition of the hair and scalp. Is the hair straight, curly, kinky? Is the hair matted or tangled? Is the scalp dry?
- Evenness of hair growth over the scalp, in particular, any patchy loss of hair; hair texture, oiliness, thickness, or thinness; presence of lesions, infections, or infestations on the scalp; presence of hirsutism.
- Self-care abilities (e.g., any problems managing hair care).

PLANNING

Delegation
Brushing and combing hair, shampooing hair, and shaving facial hair can be delegated to UAP unless the client has a condition in which the procedure would be contraindicated (e.g., cervical spinal injury or trauma). The nurse needs to assess the UAP's knowledge and experience of hair care for clients of other cultures, if appropriate.

Equipment
- Clean brush and comb
- A wide-toothed comb is usually used for many black-skinned people because finer combs pull the hair into knots and may also break the hair
- Towel
- Hair oil preparation, if appropriate

IMPLEMENTATION
Performance
1. Prior to performing the procedure, introduce self and verify the client's identity using agency protocol. Explain to the client what you are going to do, why it is necessary, and how he or she can cooperate.
2. Perform hand hygiene and observe other appropriate infection control procedures.
3. Provide for client privacy by drawing the curtains around the bed or closing the door to the room. Some agencies provide signs indicating the need for privacy. **Rationale:** *Hygiene is a personal matter.*
4. Position and prepare the client appropriately.
   - Assist the client who can sit to move to a chair. **Rationale:** *Hair is more easily brushed and combed when the client is in a sitting position.* If health permits, assist a client confined to a bed to a sitting position by raising the head of the bed. Otherwise, assist the client to alternate side-lying positions, and do one side of the head at a time.
   - If the client remains in bed, place a clean towel over the pillow and the client's shoulders. Place it over the sitting client's shoulders. **Rationale:** *The towel collects any removed hair, dirt, and scaly material.*
   - Remove any pins or ribbons in the hair.
5. Remove any mats or tangles gradually.
   - Mats can usually be pulled apart with fingers or worked out with repeated brushings.
   - If the hair is very tangled, rub alcohol or an oil, such as mineral oil, on the strands to help loosen the tangles.
   - Comb out tangles in a small section of hair toward the ends. Stablilize the hair with one hand and comb toward the ends of the hair with the other hand. **Rationale:** *This avoids scalp trauma.*
6. Brush and comb the hair.
   - For short hair, brush and comb one side at a time. Divide long hair into two sections by parting it down the middle from the front to the back. If the hair is very thick, divide each section into front and back subsections or into several layers.
7. Arrange the hair as neatly and attractively as possible, according to the individual's desires.
   - Braiding long hair helps prevent tangles.
8. Document assessments and special nursing interventions. Daily combing and brushing of the hair are not normally recorded.

VARIATION: HAIR CARE FOR AFRICAN AMERICAN CLIENTS
- Position and prepare the client.
- Separate the hair into four sections, proceeding from one section to the next.
- Untangle the hair first, if appropriate.
  - Use fingers to reduce hair breakage and discomfort. Move fingers in a circular motion starting at the roots and gently moving up to the tip of the hair.
- Comb the hair.
  - Dampen the hair with water or a leave-in conditioner. **Rationale:** *This will help loosen any tangles.*
- Apply hair oil preparation as the client indicates.
  - Using a large and open-toothed comb, grasp a small section of hair and, holding the hair at the tip, start untangling at the tip and work down toward the scalp (Jackson, 1998, p. 102).
- Ask the client if he or she would like the hair braided. **Rationale:** *Braiding will decrease tangling; however, the choice is the client's.*

EVALUATION
- Conduct ongoing assessments for problems such as dandruff, alopecia, pediculosis, scalp lesions, or excessive dryness or matting.
- Evaluate effectiveness of medication (e.g., for treating pediculosis), if appropriate.

given a shampoo with water brought to the bedside. A commercial product, similar to the bag bath, called a "head bath" is another approach. It consists of a specially designed cap (looks like a shower cap) placed over the hair. The cap contains shampoo and conditioner, and gently massaging the cap cleans the hair and scalp. In some agencies, volunteer beauticians with portable shampoo chairs may be available to assist with hair care.

Shampoo basins to catch the water and direct it to the washbasin or other receptacle are usually made of plastic or metal. A pail or large washbasin can be used as a receptacle for the shampoo water. If possible, the receptacle should be large enough to hold all shampoo water so that it does not have to be emptied during the shampoo.

Water used for the shampoo should be 40.5°C (105°F) for an adult or child to be comfortable and not injure the scalp. Usually the client will supply a liquid or cream shampoo. If the shampoo is being given to destroy lice, a medicated shampoo should be used. Dry shampoos are also available. They will remove some of the dirt, odor, and oil. Their main disadvantage is that they dry the hair and scalp.

How often a person needs a shampoo is highly individual, depending largely on the person's activities and the amount of sebum secreted by the scalp. Oily hair tends to look stringy and dirty, and it feels unclean to the person. Skill 33-7 explains how to provide a shampoo for a client confined to bed.

SKILL 33-7

SHAMPOOING THE HAIR OF A CLIENT CONFINED TO BED

PURPOSES
- To stimulate the blood circulation to the scalp through massage
- To clean the hair and increase the client's sense of well-being

ASSESSMENT
- Determine routinely used shampoo products
- Assess:
- Any scalp problems
- Activity tolerance of the client

PLANNING

Delegation (see Skill 33-6)

Equipment
- Comb and brush
- Plastic sheet or pad
- Two bath towels
- Shampoo basin
- Washcloth or pad
- Bath blanket
- Receptacle for the shampoo water
- Pitcher of water
- Bath thermometer
- Liquid or cream shampoo
- Hair dryer

IMPLEMENTATION

Preparation
- Determine whether a primary care provider's order is needed before a shampoo can be given. **Rationale:** *Some agencies require an order.*
- Determine the type of shampoo to be used (e.g., medicated shampoo).
- Determine the best time of day for the shampoo. Discuss this with the client. A person who must remain in bed may find the shampoo tiring. Choose a time when the client is rested and can rest after the procedure.

Performance
1. Prior to performing the procedure, introduce self and verify the client's identity using agency protocol. Explain to the client what you are going to do, why it is necessary if appropriate, and how he or she can cooperate.
2. Perform hand hygiene and observe other appropriate infection control procedures as needed.
3. Provide for client privacy by drawing the curtains around the bed or closing the door to the room. Some agencies provide signs indicating the need for privacy. **Rationale:** *Hygiene is a personal matter.*
4. Position and prepare the client appropriately.
   - Assist the client to the side of the bed from which you will work.
   - Remove pins and ribbons from the hair, and brush and comb it to remove any tangles.

5. Arrange the equipment.
   - Put the plastic sheet or pad on the bed under the head. **Rationale:** *The plastic keeps the bedding dry.*
   - Remove the pillow from under the client's head, and place it under the shoulders unless there is some underlying condition (e.g., neck surgery, arthritis of the neck). **Rationale:** *This hyperextends the neck.*
   - Tuck a bath towel around the client's shoulders. **Rationale:** *This keeps the shoulders dry.*
   - Place the shampoo basin under the head ❶, putting a folded washcloth or pad where the client's neck rests on the edge of the basin. If the client is on a stretcher, the neck can rest on the edge of the sink with the washcloth as padding. **Rationale:** *Padding supports the muscles of the neck and prevents undue strain and discomfort.*
   - Fanfold the top bedding down to the waist, and cover the upper part of the client with the bath blanket. **Rationale:** *The folded bedding will stay dry, and the bath blanket, which can be discarded after the shampoo, will keep the client warm.*
   - Place the receiving receptacle on a table or chair at the bedside. Put the spout of the shampoo basin over the receptacle.
6. Protect the client's eyes.
   - Place a damp washcloth over the client's eyes. **Rationale:** *The washcloth protects the eyes from soapy water. A damp washcloth will not slip.*

SHAMPOOING THE HAIR OF A CLIENT CONFINED TO BED *continued*

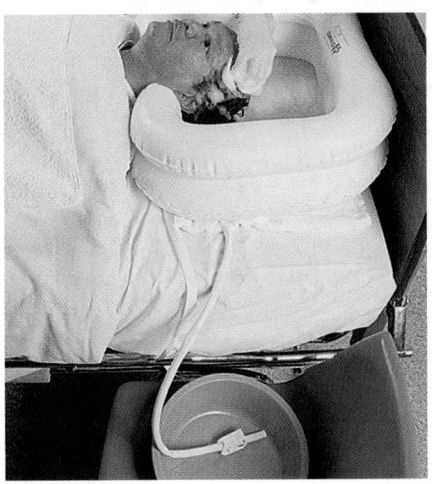

❶ Shampooing the hair of a client confined to bed. Note the shampoo basin and the receptacle below.

7. Shampoo the hair.
   - Wet the hair thoroughly with the water.
   - Apply shampoo to the scalp. Make a good lather with the shampoo while massaging the scalp with the pads of your fingertips. Massage all areas of the scalp systematically, for example, starting at the front and working toward the back of the head. **Rationale:** *Massaging stimulates the blood circulation in the scalp. The pads of the fingers are used so that the fingernails will not scratch the scalp.*
   - Rinse the hair briefly, and apply shampoo again.
   - Make a good lather and massage the scalp as before.
   - Rinse the hair thoroughly this time to remove all shampoo. **Rationale:** *Shampoo remaining in the hair may dry and irritate the hair and scalp.*
   - Squeeze as much water as possible out of the hair with your hands.
8. Dry the hair thoroughly.
   - Rub the client's hair with a heavy towel.
   - Dry the hair with the dryer. Set the temperature at "warm."
   - Continually move the dryer to prevent burning the client's scalp.
9. Ensure client comfort.
   - Assist the person confined to bed to a comfortable position.
   - Arrange the hair using a clean brush and comb.
10. Document the shampoo and any assessments.

EVALUATION

■ Conduct ongoing assessments such as any scalp problems or intolerance to the procedure. Report any problems noted to the nurse in charge.

LIFESPAN CONSIDERATIONS   Hair Care

INFANTS

■ Shampoo an infant's hair daily to prevent seborrhea.

CHILDREN

■ Monitor school-age children for nits (pediculosis).

ELDERS

■ Ensure adequate warmth for elders when shampooing their hair, because they are susceptible to chilling.

Beard and Mustache Care

Beards and mustaches also require daily care. The most important aspect of the care is to keep them clean. Food particles tend to collect in beards and mustaches, and they need washing and combing periodically. Clients may also wish a beard or mustache trim to maintain a well-groomed appearance.

CLINICAL ALERT

A beard or mustache should not be shaved off without the client's consent. ■

Male clients often shave or are shaved after a bath. Frequently clients supply their own electric or safety razors. See Box 33–3 for the steps involved in shaving facial hair with a safety razor. If a client is taking an anticoagulant (e.g., Warfarin [Coumadin], heparin), an electric shaver should be used.

Evaluating

Using data collected during care, the nurse judges whether desired outcomes have been achieved. Examples of client outcomes that are measurable or observable include the client being able to

■ Perform hair grooming with assistance (specify).
■ Exhibit clean, well-groomed, resilient hair with a healthy sheen.
■ Reduce or get rid of scalp lesions or infestations.
■ Describe factors, interventions, and preventive measures for a specific hair problem (e.g., dandruff).

BOX 33–3 Using a Safety Razor to Shave Facial Hair

- Wear gloves in case facial nicks occur and you come in contact with blood.
- Apply shaving cream or soap and water to soften the bristles and make the skin more pliable.
- Hold the skin taut, particularly around creases, to prevent cutting the skin.
- Hold the razor so that the blade is at a 45-degree angle to the skin, and shave in short, firm strokes in the direction of hair growth (Figure 33-10 ■).
- After shaving the entire area, wipe the client's face with a wet washcloth to remove any remaining shaving cream and hair.
- Dry the face well, then apply aftershave lotion or powder as the client prefers.
- To prevent irritating the skin, pat on the lotion with the fingers and avoid rubbing the face.

Figure 33-10 ■ Shaving in the direction of hair growth.

EYES

Normally eyes require no special hygiene, because lacrimal fluid continually washes the eyes, and the eyelids and lashes prevent the entrance of foreign particles. Special interventions are needed, however, for unconscious clients and for clients recovering from eye surgery or having eye injuries, irritations, or infections. In unconscious clients, the blink reflex may be absent, and excessive drainage may accumulate along eyelid margins. In clients with eye trauma or eye infections, excessive discharge or drainage is common. Excessive secretions on the lashes need to be removed before they dry on the lashes as crusts. Clients who wear eyeglasses, contact lenses, or an artificial eye also may require instruction from and care by the nurse.

 NURSING MANAGEMENT

Assessing

Assessment of the client's eyes includes a nursing health history and physical assessment.

Nursing Health History

During the nursing history, the nurse obtains data about the client's eyeglasses or contact lenses, recent examination by an ophthalmologist, and any history of eye problems and related treatments. Questions to elicit these data are shown in the accompanying Assessment Interview.

Physical Assessment

In physical assessment, all external eye structures are inspected for signs of inflammation, excessive drainage, encrustations, or other obvious abnormalities. Inspection of the external eye structures is discussed in Chapter 30. ∞

Diagnosing

Nursing diagnoses related to eye problems may include *Self-Care Deficit, Risk for Infection,* and *Risk for Injury.* Examples of these diagnoses and possible contributing factors follow:

- *Self-Care Deficit* (contact lens insertion, removal, and cleaning) related to
  a. Deficient knowledge
  b. Impaired vision associated with cataracts
- *Risk for Infection* related to
  a. Improper contact lens hygiene
  b. Accumulation of secretions on eyelids

ASSESSMENT INTERVIEW
Eyes

FOR CLIENTS WHO WEAR EYEGLASSES
- When do you use your glasses?
- What is your vision like with and without the glasses?

FOR CLIENTS WHO WEAR CONTACT LENSES
- How often do you wear lenses? Daily? On special occasions?
- How long do you wear your lenses in a given day, including sleep time?
- Do you have any problems with the lenses (e.g., cleaning, insertion, removal, damage)?
- Do you carry an emergency identification label to alert others to remove the lenses and ensure appropriate care in an emergency? (If not, advise the client to acquire one.)
- What are your insertion and removal procedures?
- What are your cleaning and storage procedures?
- Have you had any problems with either or both eyes or eyelids, such as excessive tearing, burning, redness, sensitivity to light, swelling, or feelings of dryness? Describe them.
- Are you using any eyedrops or ointments? (These medications can combine chemically with soft lenses and cause lens damage and eye irritation.)

FOR ALL CLIENTS
- When did you last have your eyesight tested?
- Are you currently taking any eye medication? If so, provide name, dosage, and frequency.
- Do you have any of the following eye problems: difficulty reading or seeing objects, blurring of vision, tearing, spots or floaters, photophobia (sensitivity to light), burning, itching, pain, double vision, flashing lights, or halos around lights?

■ *Risk for Injury* related to
   a. Prolonged wearing of contact lenses
   b. Absence of blink reflex associated with unconsciousness

Planning

In planning care, the nurse identifies nursing activities that will assist the client to maintain the integrity of the eye structures or a prosthesis and to prevent eye injury and infection.

Implementing

Nursing activities may include teaching clients about how to insert, clean, and remove contact lenses or a prosthesis and ways to protect the eyes from injury and strain.

Eye Care

Dried secretions that have accumulated on the lashes need to be softened and wiped away. Soften dried secretions by placing a sterile cotton ball moistened with sterile water or normal saline over the lid margins. Wipe the loosened secretions from the inner canthus of the eye to the outer canthus to prevent the particles and fluid from draining into the lacrimal sac and nasolacrimal duct.

If the client is unconscious and lacks a blink reflex or cannot close the eyelids completely, drying and irritation of the cornea must be prevented. Lubricating eye drops may be ordered. Box 33–4 gives suggestions for providing eye care for the comatose client.

Eyeglass Care

It is essential that the nurse exercise caution when cleaning eyeglasses to prevent breaking or scratching the lenses. Glass lenses can be cleaned with warm water and dried with a soft tissue that will not scratch the lenses. Plastic lenses are easily scratched and may require special cleaning solutions and drying tissues. When not being worn, all glasses should be placed in an appropriately labeled case and stored in the client's bedside table drawer.

Contact Lens Care

Contact lenses, thin curved discs of hard or soft plastic, fit on the cornea of the eye directly over the pupil. They float on the

---

BOX 33–4   Eye Care for the Comatose Client

When a comatose client's corneal reflex is impaired, eye care is essential to keep moist the areas of the cornea that are exposed to air.
■ Administer moist compresses to cover the eyes every 2 to 4 hours.
■ Clean the eyes with saline solution and cotton balls. Wipe from the inner to outer canthus. This prevents debris from being washed into the nasolacrimal duct.
■ Use a new cotton ball for each wipe. This prevents extending infection in one eye to the other eye.
■ Instill ophthalmic ointment or artificial tears into the lower lids as ordered. This keeps the eyes moist.
■ If the client's corneal reflex is absent, keep the eyes moist with artificial tears and protect the eye with a protective shield. These should be ordered by a primary care provide.
■ Monitor the eyes for redness, exudate, or ulceration.

---

tear layer of the eye. For some people, contact lenses offer several advantages over eyeglasses: (a) They cannot be seen and thus have cosmetic value; (b) they are highly effective in correcting some astigmatisms; (c) they are safer than glasses for some physical activities; (d) they do not fog, as eyeglasses do; and (e) they provide better vision in many cases.

Contact lenses may be either hard or soft or a compromise between the two types—gas-permeable lenses. *Hard contact lenses* are made of a rigid, unwettable, airtight plastic that does not absorb water or saline solutions. They usually cannot be worn for more than 12 to 14 hours and are rarely recommended for first-time wearers.

Soft contact lenses cover the entire cornea. Being more pliable and soft, they mold to the eye for a firmer fit. The duration of extended wear varies by brand from 1 to 30 days or more. Eye specialists recommend that long-wear brands be removed and cleaned at least once a week. These lenses require scrupulous care and handling.

Gas-permeable lenses are rigid enough to provide clear vision but are more flexible than the traditional hard lens. They permit oxygen to reach the cornea, thus providing greater comfort, and will not cause serious damage to the eye if left in place for several days.

Most clients normally care for their own contact lenses. In general, each lens manufacturer provides detailed cleaning instructions. Depending on the type of lens and cleaning method used, warm tap water, normal saline, or special rinsing or soaking solutions may be used.

All users should have a special container for their lenses. Some contain a solution so that the lenses are stored wet; in others, the lenses are dry. Each lens container has a slot or cup with a label indicating whether it is for the right or left lens. It is essential that the correct lens be stored in the appropriate slot so that it will be placed in the correct eye.

REMOVING CONTACT LENSES. Hard contact lenses must be positioned directly over the cornea for proper removal. If the lens is displaced, the nurse asks the client to look straight ahead, and gently exerts pressure on the upper and lower lids to move the lens back onto the cornea. Figure 33-11 ■ shows the steps needed to remove a hard lens. To avoid lens mixups, the nurse places the first lens in its designated cup in the storage base before removing the second lens (Figure 33-12 ■).

Removal of soft lenses differs in two ways. First, have the client look forward. Retract the lower lid with one hand. Using the pad of the index finger of the other hand, move the lens down to the inferior part of the sclera. This reduces the risk of damage to the cornea. Second, remove the lens by gently pinching the lens between the pads of the thumb and index finger. Pinching causes the lens to double up, so that air enters underneath the lens, overcoming the suction and allowing removal. Use the pads of the fingers to prevent scratching the eye or the lens with the fingernails. Figure 33-13 ■ shows a client removing her own contact lens using the method described. Please note that a nurse would need to wear gloves.

INSERTING CONTACT LENSES. Seriously ill clients whose contact lenses have been removed will not need them reinserted until they become more active in their care and require the lenses

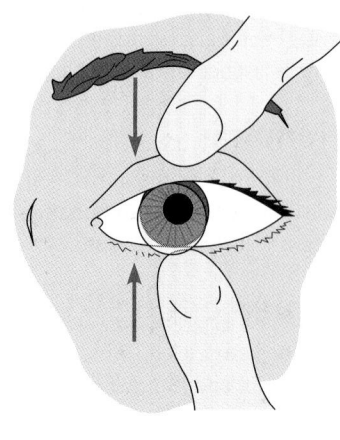

A

B

C

Figure 33-11 ■ Removing hard contact lenses.

Figure 33-12 ■ Storing lenses. Place the first lens in its designated cup in the storage case before removing the second lens. This avoids mixing up two potentially different lenses.

(David Parker/Science Photo Library/Photo Researchers, Inc.)

Figure 33-13 ■ Removing a soft lens by pinching it between the pads of the thumb and index finger.

(Lester Lefkowitz/Corbis.)

to see properly. Contact lenses need to be lubricated in a sterile, nonirritating wetting solution (usually a saline solution) before they are inserted. The wetting solution helps the lens glide over the cornea, thus reducing the risk of injury. Most clients, when well, will reinsert the lenses independently.

Artificial Eyes

Artificial eyes are usually made of glass or plastic. Some are permanently implanted; others are removed regularly for cleaning. Most clients who wear a removable artificial eye follow their own care regimen. Even for an unconscious client, daily removal and cleaning are not necessary.

To remove an artificial eye, the nurse puts on clean gloves and retracts the client's lower eyelid down over the infraorbital bone while exerting slight pressure below the eyelid to overcome the suction (Figure 33-14 ■). An alternative method is to compress a small rubber bulb and apply the tip directly to the eye. As the nurse gradually releases the finger pressure on the bulb, the suction of the bulb counteracts the suction holding the eye in the socket and draws the eye out of the socket.

The eye is cleaned with warm normal saline and placed in a container filled with water or saline solution. The socket and tissues around the eye are usually cleaned with cotton wipes and

Figure 33-14 ■ Removing an artificial eye by retracting the lower eyelid and exerting slight pressure below the eyelid.

Figure 33-15 ■ Holding an artificial eye between the thumb and index finger for insertion.

normal saline. To reinsert the eye, the nurse uses the thumb and index finger of one hand to retract the eyelids, exerting pressure on the supraorbital and infraorbital bones. Holding the eye between the thumb and index finger of the other hand, the nurse slips the eye gently into the socket (Figure 33-15 ■).

General Eye Care

Many clients may need to learn specific information about care of the eyes. Some examples follow:

■ Avoid home remedies for eye problems. Eye irritations or injuries at any age should be treated medically and immediately.
■ If dirt or dust gets into the eyes, clean them copiously with clean, tepid water as an emergency treatment.
■ Take measures to guard against eyestrain and to protect vision, such as maintaining adequate lighting for reading and obtaining shatterproof lenses for glasses.
■ Schedule regular eye examinations, particularly after age 40, to detect problems such as cataracts and glaucoma.

Evaluating

Using data collected during care, the nurse judges whether desired outcomes have been achieved. Examples of desired outcomes to evaluate the effectiveness of nursing interventions follow:

■ Conjunctiva and sclera free of inflammation
■ Eyelids free of secretions
■ No tearing
■ No eye discomfort
■ Demonstrates appropriate methods of caring for contact lenses
■ Describes interventions to prevent eye injury and infection

EARS

Normal ears require minimal hygiene. Clients who have excessive **cerumen** (earwax) and dependent clients who have hearing aids may require assistance from the nurse. Hearing aids are usually removed before surgery.

CLINICAL ALERT

Cerumen impaction is a common cause of hearing loss in elders. Nearly 35% of elders in the community have cerumen impaction in one or both ears, and the incidence is higher in institutionalized older adults (Stone, 1999). ■

Cleaning the Ears

The auricles of the ear are cleaned during the bed bath. The nurse or client must remove excessive cerumen that is visible or that causes discomfort or hearing difficulty. Visible cerumen may be loosened and removed by retracting the auricle up and back. If this measure is ineffective, irrigation is necessary. Clients need to be advised never to use bobby pins, toothpicks, or cotton-tipped applicators to remove cerumen. Bobby pins and toothpicks can injure the ear canal and rupture the tympanic membrane; cotton-tipped applicators can cause wax to become impacted within the canal.

Care of Hearing Aids

A hearing aid is a battery-powered, sound-amplifying device used by persons with hearing impairments. It consists of a microphone that picks up sound and converts it to electric energy, an amplifier that magnifies the electric energy electronically, a receiver that converts the amplified energy back to sound energy, and an earmold that directs the sound into the ear. There are several types of hearing aids:

■ *Behind-the-ear (BTE, or postaural) aid.* This is the most widely used type because it fits snugly behind the ear. The hearing aid case, which holds the microphone, amplifier, and receiver, is attached to the earmold by a plastic tube (Figure 33-16 ■).
■ *In-the-ear aid (ITE, or intra-aural).* This one-piece aid has all its components housed in the earmold (Figure 33-17 ■).

A

B

Figure 33-16 ■ *A*, A behind-the-ear hearing aid. *B*, A behind-the-ear hearing aid attached to glasses.

(Jane Schemilt/Science Photo Library, Photo Researchers, Inc.)

A **B** **C**

Figure 33-17 ■ *A,* An in-the-ear hearing aid. *B,* Small hearing aid in ear canal. *C,* Large hearing aid in ear canal.

Source: Jane Schemilt; Science Photo Library/Photo Researcher's, Inc.

■ *In-the-canal (ITC) aid.* This is the most compact and least visible aid, fitting completely inside the ear canal. In addition to having cosmetic appeal, the ITC does not interfere with telephone use or the wearing of eyeglasses. However, it is not suitable for clients with progressive hearing loss; it requires adequate ear canal diameter and length for a good fit; and it tends to plug with cerumen more than other aids.

■ *Eyeglasses aid.* This is similar to the behind-the-ear aid, but the components are housed in the temple of the eyeglasses. A hearing aid can be in one or both temples of the glasses.

■ *Body hearing aid.* This pocket-sized aid, used for more severe hearing losses, clips onto an undergarment, shirt pocket, or harness carrier supplied by the manufacturer. The case, containing the microphone and amplifier, is connected by a cord to the receiver, which snaps into the earpiece.

For correct functioning, hearing aids require appropriate handling during insertion and removal, regular cleaning of the earmold, and replacement of dead batteries. With proper care, hearing aids generally last 5 to 10 years. Earmolds generally need readjustment every 2 to 3 years. Skill 33-8 describes how to remove, clean, and insert a hearing aid.

SKILL 33-8

REMOVING, CLEANING, AND INSERTING A HEARING AID

PURPOSE
■ To maintain proper hearing aid function

ASSESSMENT
Determine if the client has experienced any problems with the hearing aid and hearing aid practices. Assess for the presence of inflammation, excessive wax, drainage, or discomfort in the external ear.

PLANNING

Delegation

A nurse can delegate the task of caring for a hearing aid to the UAP. It is important, however, for the nurse to first determine that the UAP knows the correct way to care for a hearing aid. Inform the UAP to report the presence of ear inflammation, discomfort, excess wax, or drainage to the RN.

Equipment
■ Client's hearing aid
■ Soap, water, and towels or a damp cloth
■ Pipe cleaner or toothpick (optional)
■ New battery (if needed)

IMPLEMENTATION
Performance
1. Prior to performing the procedure, introduce self and verify the client's identity using agency protocol. Explain to the client what you are going to do, why it is necessary, and how he or she can cooperate.
2. Perform hand hygiene and observe other appropriate infection control procedures.
3. Provide for client privacy by drawing the curtains around the bed or closing the door to the room. Some agencies provide signs indicating the need for privacy. **Rationale:** *Hygiene is a personal matter.*
4. Remove the hearing aid.
   ● Turn the hearing aid off and lower the volume. The on/off switch may be labeled "O" (off), "M" (microphone), "T" (tele-

phone), or "TM" (telephone/microphone). **Rationale:** *The batteries continue to run if the hearing aid is not turned off.*
   ● Remove the earmold by rotating it slightly forward and pulling it outward.
   ● If the hearing aid is not to be used for several days, remove the battery. **Rationale:** *Removal prevents corrosion of the hearing aid from battery leakage.*
   ● Store the hearing aid in a safe place and label with client's name. Avoid exposure to heat and moisture. **Rationale:** *Proper storage prevents loss or damage.*
5. Clean the earmold.
   ● Detach the earmold if possible. Disconnect the earmold from the receiver of a body hearing aid or from the hearing aid case of behind-the-ear and eyeglass hearing aids where the tubing meets the hook of the case. Do not remove the

REMOVING, CLEANING, AND INSERTING A HEARING AID *continued*

earmold if it is glued or secured by a small metal ring. **Rationale:** *Removal facilitates cleaning and prevents inadvertent damage to the other parts.*

- If the earmold is detachable, soak it in a mild soapy solution. Rinse and dry it well. Do not use isopropyl alcohol. **Rationale:** *Alcohol can damage the hearing aid.*
- If the earmold is not detachable or is for an in-the-ear aid, wipe the earmold with a damp cloth.
- Check that the earmold opening is patent. Blow any excess moisture through the opening or remove debris (e.g., earwax) with a pipe cleaner or toothpick.
- Reattach the earmold if it was detached from the rest of the hearing aid.

6. Insert the hearing aid.
   - Determine from the client if the earmold is for the left or the right ear.
   - Check that the battery is inserted in the hearing aid. Turn off the hearing aid, and make sure the volume is turned all the way down. **Rationale:** *A volume that is too loud is distressing.*
   - Inspect the earmold to identify the ear canal portion. Some earmolds are fitted for only the ear canal and concha; others are fitted for all the contours of the ear. The canal portion, common to all, can be used as a guide for correct insertion.
   - Line up the parts of the earmold with the corresponding parts of the client's ear.
   - Rotate the earmold slightly forward, and insert the ear canal portion.
   - Gently press the earmold into the ear while rotating it backward.

- Check that the earmold fits snugly by asking the client if it feels secure and comfortable.
- Adjust the other components of a behind-the-ear or body hearing aid.
- Turn the hearing aid on, and adjust the volume according to the client's needs.

7. Correct problems associated with improper functioning.
   - If the sound is weak or there is no sound:
     a. Ensure that the volume is turned high enough.
     b. Ensure that the earmold opening is not clogged.
     c. Check the battery by turning the hearing aid on, turning up the volume, cupping your hand over the earmold, and listening. A constant whistling sound indicates the battery is functioning. If necessary, replace the battery. Be sure that the negative (−) and positive (+) signs on the battery match those where indicated on the hearing aid.
     d. Ensure that the ear canal is not blocked with wax, which can obstruct sound waves.
   - If the client reports a whistling sound or squeal after insertion:
     a. Turn the volume down.
     b. Ensure that the earmold is properly attached to the receiver.
     c. Reinsert the earmold.

8. Document pertinent data.
   - The removal and the insertion of a hearing aid are not normally recorded.
   - Report and record any problems the client has with the hearing aid.

EVALUATION

- Speak to the client in a normal conversational tone and observe client behaviors.
- Compare the client's hearing ability to previous assessments.
- Report to the primary care provider any deviations from normal for the client.

HOME CARE CONSIDERATIONS **Hearing Aids**

- People who need a hearing aid may not wear one because they view the hearing aid as a stigma of old age.
- It is important for the client who just purchased a hearing aid to know that it often takes weeks or even months to adjust to the hearing aid. At first, the sounds will seem shrill as they start hearing high-frequency sounds that had been forgotten. Remind them that it is a hearing aid, not a hearing cure. Encourage them to not give up.

- The client needs to adjust to the hearing aid gradually by increasing the amount of time each day until the aid can be worn for a full day (Anderson, 1998).
- Encourage clients to purchase their hearing aids from a company that has a minimum warranty of a 30-day return policy.
- Emphasize the importance of maintaining the hearing aid, that is, having it cleaned and checked regularly.

NOSE

Nurses usually need not provide special care for the nose, because clients can ordinarily clear nasal secretions by blowing gently into a soft tissue. When the external nares are encrusted with dried secretions, they should be cleaned with a cotton-tipped applicator or moistened with saline or water. The applicator should not be inserted beyond the length of the cotton tip; inserting it further may cause injury to the mucosa.

SUPPORTING A HYGIENIC ENVIRONMENT

Because people are usually confined to bed when ill, often for long periods, the bed becomes an important element in the client's life. A place that is clean, safe, and comfortable contributes to the client's ability to rest and sleep and to a sense of well-being. Basic furniture in a health care facility includes the bed, bedside table, overbed table, one or more chairs, and a storage space for clothing. Most bed units also have a call light, light fixtures, electric outlets, and hygienic equipment in the bedside table. Three types of equipment often installed in an acute care facility are a suction outlet for several kinds of suction, an oxygen outlet for most oxygen equipment, and a sphygmomanometer to measure the client's blood pressure. Some long-term care agencies also permit clients to have personal furniture, such as a television, a chair, and lamps, at the bedside. In the home a client often has personal and medical equipment.

Environment

When providing a comfortable environment it is important to consider the client's age, severity of illness, and level of activity.

Room Temperature

The very young, the very old, and the acutely ill frequently need a room temperature higher than normal. A room temperature between 20°C and 23°C (68°F and 74°F) is comfortable for most clients.

Ventilation

Good ventilation is important to remove unpleasant odors and stale air. Odors caused by urine, draining wounds, or vomitus, for example, can be offensive to people. Room deodorizers can help eliminate odors. However, good hygienic practices are the best way to prevent offensive body and breath odors. Hospitals are required to monitor smoking. Hospitals often have a smoking area for clients and prohibit smoking in client rooms.

Noise

Ill persons are sensitive to noise such as clanging of metal equipment, loud talking, and laughter. Nurses should try to control noise in health care settings.

Hospital Beds

The frame of a hospital bed is divided into three sections. This permits the head and the foot to be elevated separately. Most hospital beds have electric motors to operate the movable joints. The motor is activated by pressing a button or moving a small lever, located either at the side of the bed or on a small panel separate from the bed but attached to it by a cable, which the client can readily use. Common bed positions are shown in Table 33–7.

Hospital beds are usually 66 cm (26 in.) high and 0.9 m (3 ft) wide, narrower than the usual bed, so that the nurse can reach the client from either side of the bed without undue stretching.

TABLE 33–7 Commonly Used Bed Positions

Flat Foot of bed / Head of bed	Mattress is completely horizontal.	Client sleeping in a variety of bed positions, such as back-lying, side-lying, and prone (face down) To maintain spinal alignment for clients with spinal injuries To assist clients to move and turn in bed Bed-making by nurse
Fowler's position 	Semisitting position in which head of bed is raised to angle of at least 45°. Knees may be flexed or horizontal.	Convenient for eating, reading, visiting, watching TV Relief from lying positions To promote lung expansion for client with respiratory problem To assist a client to a sitting position on the edge of the bed
Semi-Fowler's position 	Head of bed is raised only to 30° angle.	Relief from lying position To promote lung expansion
Trendelenburg's position 	Head of bed is lowered and the foot raised in a straight incline.	To promote venous circulation in certain clients To provide postural drainage of basal lung lobes
Reverse Trendelenburg's position 	Head of bed raised and the foot lowered. Straight tilt in direction opposite to Trendelenburg's position.	To promote stomach emptying and prevent esophageal reflux in client with hiatal hernia

The length is usually 1.9 m (6.5 ft). Some beds can be extended in length to accommodate very tall clients. Long-term care facilities for ambulatory clients usually have low beds to facilitate movement in and out of bed. Most hospital beds have "high" and "low" positions that can be adjusted either mechanically or electrically by a button or lever. The high position permits the nurse to reach the client without undue stretching or stooping. The low position allows the client to step easily to the floor.

Mattresses

Mattresses are usually covered with a water-repellent material that resists soiling and can be cleaned easily. Most mattresses have handles on the sides called lugs by which the mattress can be moved.

Many special mattresses are also used in hospitals to relieve pressure on the body's bony prominences, such as the heels. They are particularly helpful for clients confined to bed for a long time. For additional information about mattresses, see Chapter 36. ∞

Side Rails

Side rails, or safety sides, are used on both hospital beds and stretchers. They are of various shapes and sizes and are usually made of metal. A bed can have two full-length side rails or four half- or quarter-length side rails (also called split rails). Devices to raise and lower side rails differ. Often one or two knobs are pulled to release the side and permit it to be moved. When side rails are being used, it is important that the nurse never leave the bedside while the rail is lowered. Some side rails have two positions: up and down. Others have three: high, intermediate, and low.

For decades, the use of side rails has been routine practice with the rationale that the side rails serve as a safe and effective means of preventing clients from falling out of bed. Research, however, has not validated this assumption. In fact, several studies have shown that raised side rails do not deter older clients from getting out of bed unassisted and have led to more serious falls, injuries, and even death (Capezuti, 2004; Talerico & Capezuti, 2001). The Health Care Financing Administration now mandates that nurses in both acute care and long-term care decrease the routine use of side rails. Alternatives to side rails do exist and can include low-height bed, mats placed at the side of the beds, motion sensors, and bed alarms (see Chapter 32). ∞

CLINICAL ALERT

Side rail entrapment, injuries, and deaths do occur. When side rails are used, the nurse must assess the client's physical and mental status and closely monitor high-risk (frail, elderly, or confused) clients. ■

Footboard or Footboot

These are used to support the immobilized client's foot in a normal right angle to the legs to prevent plantar flexion contractures (see Chapter 44). ∞

Bed Cradles

A bed cradle is a device designed to keep the top bedclothes off the feet, legs, and even abdomen of a client. The bedclothes are arranged over the device and may be pinned in place. There are several types of bed cradles. One of the most common is a curved metal rod that fits over the bed. Part of the cradle fits under the mattress, and small metal brackets press down on each side of the mattress to keep the cradle in place. The frame of some cradles extends over half of the width of the bed, above one leg.

Intravenous Rods

Intravenous rods (poles, stands, standards), usually made of metal, support intravenous (IV) infusion containers while fluid is being administered to a client. These rods were traditionally freestanding on the floor beside the bed. Now, intravenous rods are often attached to the hospital beds. Some hospital units have overhead hanging rods on a track for IVs.

MAKING BEDS

Nurses need to be able to prepare hospital beds in different ways for specific purposes. In most instances, beds are made after the client receives certain care and when beds are unoccupied. At times, however, nurses need to make an occupied bed or prepare a bed for a client who is having surgery (an anesthetic, postoperative, or surgical bed). Regardless of what type of bed equipment is available, whether the bed is occupied or unoccupied, or the purpose for which the bed is being prepared, certain practice guidelines pertain to all bed-making.

Unoccupied Bed

An unoccupied bed can be either closed or open. Generally the top covers of an open bed are folded back (thus the term *open bed*) to make it easier for a client to get in. Open and closed beds are made the same way, except that the top sheet, blanket, and bedspread of a *closed bed* are drawn up to the top of the bed and under the pillows.

PRACTICE GUIDELINES   Bed-Making

- Wash hands thoroughly after handling a client's bed linen. Linens and equipment that have been soiled with secretions and excretions harbor microorganisms that can be transmitted to others directly or by the nurse's hands or uniform.
- Hold soiled linen away from uniform.
- Linen for one client is never (even momentarily) placed on another client's bed.
- Place soiled linen directly in a portable linen hamper or tucked into a pillow case at the end of the bed before it is gathered up for disposal.
- Do not shake soiled linen in the air because shaking can disseminate secretions and excretions and the microorganisms they contain.
- When stripping and making a bed, conserve time and energy by stripping and making up one side as much as possible before working on the other side.
- To avoid unnecessary trips to the linen supply area, gather all linen before starting to strip a bed.

A

B

C

D

E

Figure 33-18 ■ Mitering the corner of a bed.

Beds are often changed after bed baths. The linen can be collected before the bath. The linen is not usually changed unless it is soiled. Check the policy at each clinical agency. Unfitted sheets, blankets, and bedspreads are mitered at the corners of the bed. The purpose of mitering is to secure the bedclothes while the bed is occupied. Figure 33-18 ■ shows how to miter the corner of a bed. Skill 33-9 explains how to change an unoccupied bed.

SKILL 33-9

CHANGING AN UNOCCUPIED BED

PURPOSES
- To promote the client's comfort
- To provide a clean neat environment for the client
- To provide a smooth, wrinkle-free bed foundation, thus minimizing sources of skin irritation

ASSESSMENT
- Assess the client's health status to determine that the person can safely get out of bed. In some hospitals it is necessary to have a written order if the client has been in bed continuously.
- Assess the client's pulse and respirations if indicated.
- Note all the tubes and equipment connected to the client. **Rationale:** *This may influence the need for additional linens or waterproof pads.*

PLANNING

Delegation
Bed-making is usually delegated to UAP. If appropriate, inform the UAP of the proper disposal method of linens that contain drainage. Ask the UAP to inform you immediately if any tubes or dressings become dislodged or removed. Stress the importance of the call light being readily available while the client is out of bed.

Equipment
- Two flat sheets or one fitted and one flat sheet
- Cloth drawsheet (optional)
- One blanket
- One bedspread
- Waterproof pads (optional)
- Pillowcase(s) for the head pillow(s)
- Plastic laundry bag or portable linen hamper, if available

IMPLEMENTATION
Preparation
Determine what linens the client may already have in the room *to avoid stockpiling of unnecessary extra linens.*

Performance
1. Prior to performing the procedure, introduce self and verify the client's identity using agency protocol. Explain to the client what you are going to do, why it is necessary, and how he or she can cooperate.
2. Perform hand hygiene and observe other appropriate infection control procedures.
3. Provide for client privacy.
4. Place the fresh linen on the client's chair or overbed table; do not use another client's bed. **Rationale:** *This prevents cross-*

CHANGING AN UNOCCUPIED BED *continued*

❶ Fold reusable linens into fourths when removing them from the bed.

(Al Dodge, Pearson Education/PH College)

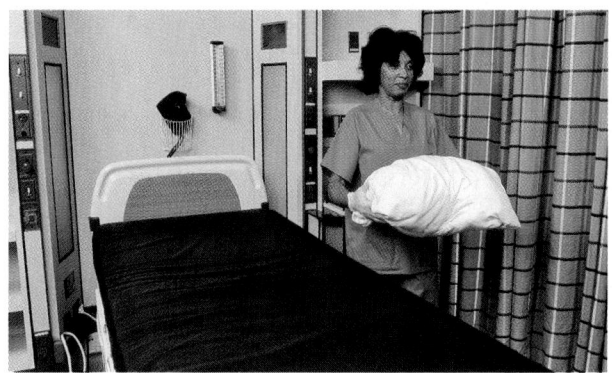

❷ Roll soiled linen inside the bottom sheet and hold away from the body.

(Al Dodge, Pearson Education/PH College)

contamination *(the movement of microorganisms from one client to another) via soiled linen.*

5. Assess and assist the client out of bed.
   - Make sure that this is an appropriate and convenient time for the client to be out of bed.
   - Assist the client to a comfortable chair.
6. Raise the bed to a comfortable working height.
7. Strip the bed.
   - Check bed linens for any items belonging to the client, and detach the call bell or any drainage tubes from the bed linen.
   - Loosen all bedding systematically, starting at the head of the bed on the far side and moving around the bed up to the head of the bed on the near side. **Rationale:** *Moving around the bed systematically prevents stretching and reaching and possible muscle strain.*
   - Remove the pillowcases, if soiled, and place the pillows on the bedside chair near the foot of the bed.
   - Fold reusable linens, such as the bedspread and top sheet on the bed, into fourths. First, fold the linen in half by bringing the top edge even with the bottom edge, and then grasp it at the center of the middle fold and bottom edges. ❶ **Rationale:** *Folding linens saves time and energy when reapplying the linens on the bed and keeps them clean.*
   - Remove the waterproof pad and discard it if soiled.
   - Roll all soiled linen inside the bottom sheet, hold it away from your uniform, and place it directly in the linen hamper, not on the floor. ❷ **Rationale:** *These actions are essential to prevent the transmission of microorganisms to the nurse and others.*
   - Grasp the mattress securely, using the lugs if present, and move the mattress up to the head of the bed.
8. Apply the bottom sheet and drawsheet.
   - Place the folded bottom sheet with its center fold on the center of the bed. Make sure the sheet is hem side down for a smooth foundation. Spread the sheet out over the mattress, and allow a sufficient amount of sheet at the top to tuck under the mattress. ❸ **Rationale:** *The top of the sheet needs to be well tucked under to remain securely in place, especially when the head of the bed is elevated.* Place the sheet along the edge of the mattress at the foot of the bed and do not tuck it in (unless it is a contour or fitted sheet).
   - Miter the sheet at the top corner on the near side (Figure 33–18, earlier) and tuck the sheet under the mattress, working from the head of the bed to the foot.

❸ Placing bottom sheet on bed.

(Patrick Watson)

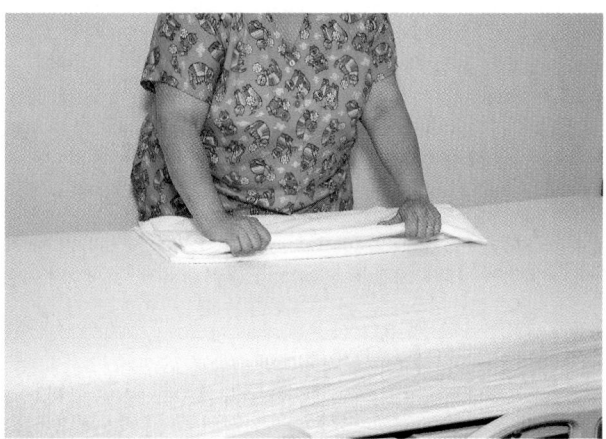

❹ Placing a clean drawsheet on the bed.

(Patrick Watson)

- If a waterproof drawsheet is used, place it over the bottom sheet so that the centerfold is at the centerline of the bed and the top and bottom edges extend from the middle of the client's back to the area of the midthigh or knee. Fanfold the uppermost half of the folded drawsheet at the center or far edge of the bed and tuck in the near edge. ❹

continued on page 790

CHANGING AN UNOCCUPIED BED *continued*

- Lay the cloth drawsheet over the waterproof sheet in the same manner.
- *Optional:* Before moving to the other side of the bed, place the top linens on the bed hemside up, unfold them, tuck them in, and miter the bottom corners. **Rationale:** *Completing one entire side of the bed at a time saves time and energy.*

9. Move to the other side and secure the bottom linens.
   - Tuck in the bottom sheet under the head of the mattress, pull the sheet firmly, and miter the corner of the sheet.
   - Pull the remainder of the sheet firmly so that there are no wrinkles. **Rationale:** *Wrinkles can cause discomfort for the client and breakdown of skin. Tuck the sheet in at the side.*
   - Complete this same process for the drawsheet(s).

10. Apply or complete the top sheet, blanket, and spread.
    - Place the top sheet, hemside up, on the bed so that its centerfold is at the center of the bed and the top edge is even with the top edge of the mattress.
    - Unfold the sheet over the bed.
    - *Optional:* Make a vertical or a horizontal toe pleat in the sheet to provide additional room for the client's feet.
      a. *Vertical toe pleat:* Make a fold in the sheet 5 to 10 cm (2 to 4 in.) perpendicular to the foot of the bed. ❺
      b. *Horizontal toe pleat:* Make a fold in the sheet 5 to 10 cm (2 to 4 in.) across the bed near the foot. ❻
      Loosening the top covers around the feet after the client is in bed is another way to provide additional space.
    - Follow the same procedure for the blanket and the spread, but place the top edges about 15 cm (6 in.) from the head of the bed to allow a cuff of sheet to be folded over them.
    - Tuck in the sheet, blanket, and spread at the foot of the bed, and miter the corner, using all three layers of linen. Leave the sides of the top sheet, blanket, and spread hanging freely unless toe pleats were provided.
    - Fold the top of the top sheet down over the spread, providing a cuff. ❼ **Rationale:** *The cuff of sheet makes it easier for the client to pull the covers up.*
    - Move to the other side of the bed and secure the top bedding in the same manner.

11. Put clean pillowcases on the pillows as required.
    - Grasp the closed end of the pillowcase at the center with one hand.
    - Gather up the sides of the pillowcase and place them over the hand grasping the case. Then grasp the center of one short side of the pillow through the pillowcase. ❽
    - With the free hand, pull the pillowcase over the pillow.
    - Adjust the pillowcase so that the pillow fits into the corners of the case and the seams are straight. **Rationale:** *A smoothly fitting pillowcase is more comfortable than a wrinkled one.*
    - Place the pillows appropriately at the head of the bed.

12. Provide for client comfort and safety.
    - Attach the signal cord so that the client can conveniently reach it. Some cords have clamps that attach to the sheet or pillowcase. Others are attached by a safety pin.
    - If the bed is currently being used by a client, either fold back the top covers at one side or fanfold them down to the cen-

❺ A vertical toe pleat.

❻ A horizontal toe pleat.

❼ Making a cuff of the top linens.

(Patrick Watson)

CHANGING AN UNOCCUPIED BED *continued*

❽ Method for putting a clean pillowcase on a pillow.

❾ Fold up the two outer corners of the top linens, forming a triangle.

ter of the bed. **Rationale:** *This makes it easier for the client to get into the bed.*
- Place the bedside table and the overbed table so that they are available to the client.
- Leave the bed in the high position if the client is returning by stretcher, or place in the low position if the client is returning to bed after being up.
13. Document and report pertinent data.
    - Bed-making is not normally recorded.
    - Record any nursing assessments, such as the client's physical status and pulse and respiratory rates before and after being out of bed, as indicated.

VARIATION: SURGICAL BED
While the client is in the operating room, the client's bed is prepared for the postoperative phase. In some agencies, the client is brought back to the unit on a stretcher and transferred to the bed in the room. In other agencies, the client's bed is brought to the surgery suite and the client is transferred there. In the latter situation, the bed needs to be made with clean linens as soon as the client goes to surgery so that it can be taken to the operating room when needed.
- Strip the bed.
- Place and leave the pillows on the bedside chair. **Rationale:** *Pillows are left on a chair to facilitate transferring the client into the bed.*
- Apply the bottom linens as for an unoccupied bed. Place a bath blanket on the foundation of the bed if this is agency practice. **Rationale:** *A flannel bath blanket provides additional warmth.*
- Place the top covers (sheet, blanket, and bedspread) on the bed as you would for an unoccupied bed. Do not tuck them in, miter the corners, or make a toe pleat.

❿ Surgical bed. The linens are horizontally fanfolded to the other side of the bed to facilitate transfer of the client into the bed.

- Make a cuff at the top of the bed as you would for an unoccupied bed. Fold the top linens up from the bottom.
- On the side of the bed where the client will be transferred, fold up the two outer corners of the top linens so they meet in the middle of the bed forming a triangle. ❾
- Pick up the apex of the triangle and fanfold the top linens lengthwise to the other side of the bed *to facilitate the client's transfer into the bed.* ❿
- Leave the bed in high position with the side rails down. **Rationale:** *The high position facilitates the transfer of the client.*
- Lock the wheels of the bed if the bed is not to be moved. **Rationale:** *Locking the wheels keeps the bed from rolling when the client is transferred from the stretcher to the bed.*

EVALUATION
- Make sure the call light is accessible to the client.
- Relate client parameters of activity (e.g., pulse and respirations) to previous assessment data, particularly if the client has been

on bed rest for an extended period of time or if it is the first time that the client is getting out of bed after surgery.

Changing an Occupied Bed

Some clients may be too weak to get out of bed. Either the nature of their illness may contraindicate their sitting out of bed, or they may be restricted in bed by the presence of traction or other therapies. When changing an occupied bed, the nurse works quickly and disturbs the client as little as possible to conserve the client's energy, using the following guidelines:

■ Maintain the client in good body alignment. Never move or position a client in a manner that is contraindi-

cated by the client's health. Obtain help if necessary to ensure safety.
■ Move the client gently and smoothly. Rough handling can cause the client discomfort and abrade the skin.
■ Explain what you plan to do throughout the procedure before you do it. Use terms that the client can understand.
■ Use the bed-making time, like the bed bath time, to assess and meet the client's needs.

See Skill 33-10 for instructions on changing an occupied bed.

CHANGING AN OCCUPIED BED

PURPOSES
■ To conserve the client's energy
■ To promote client comfort
■ To provide a clean, neat environment for the client
■ To provide a smooth, wrinkle-free bed foundation, thus minimizing sources of skin irritation

ASSESSMENT
■ Note specific orders or precautions for moving and positioning the client.
■ Determine presence of incontinence or excessive drainage from other sources indicating the need for protective waterproof pads.
■ Assess skin condition and need for special mattress (e.g., egg crate), footboard, or heel protectors.

PLANNING

Delegation
Bed-making is usually delegated to UAP. Inform the UAP to what extent the client can assist or if another person will be needed to assist the UAP. Instruct the UAP about the handling of any dressings and/or tubes of the client and also the need for special equipment (e.g., footboard, heel protectors), if appropriate.

Equipment
■ Two flat sheets or one fitted and one flat sheet
■ Cloth drawsheet (optional)
■ One blanket
■ One bedspread
■ Waterproof drawsheet or waterproof pads (optional)
■ Pillowcase(s) for the head pillow(s)
■ Plastic laundry bag or portable linen hamper, if available

IMPLEMENTATION
Performance
1. Explain to the client what you are going to do, why it is necessary, and how he or she can cooperate.
2. Perform hand hygiene and observe other appropriate infection control procedures. Put on disposable gloves if linen is soiled with body fluids.
3. Provide for client privacy.
4. Remove the top bedding.
   ● Remove any equipment attached to the bed linen, such as a signal light.
   ● Loosen all the top linen at the foot of the bed, and remove the spread and the blanket.
   ● Leave the top sheet over the client (the top sheet can remain over the client if it is being changed and if it will provide sufficient warmth), or replace it with a bath blanket as follows:
      Spread the bath blanket over the top sheet.
   a. Ask the client to hold the top edge of the blanket.
   b. Reaching under the blanket from the side, grasp the top edge of the sheet and draw it down to the foot of the bed, leaving the blanket in place. ❶
   c. Remove the sheet from the bed and place it in the soiled linen hamper.
5. Change the bottom sheet and drawsheet.
   ● Assist the client to turn on the side facing away from the side where the clean linen is.

● Raise the side rail nearest the client. **Rationale:** *This protects the client from falling.* If there is no side rail, have another nurse support the client at the edge of the bed.
● Loosen the foundation of the linen on the side of the bed near the linen supply.
● Fanfold the drawsheet and the bottom sheet at the center of the bed ❷, as close to and under the client as possible. **Rationale:** *Doing this leaves the near half of the bed free to be changed.*
● Place the new bottom sheet on the bed, and vertically fanfold the half to be used on the far side of the bed as close to the client as possible. ❸ Tuck the sheet under the near

❶ Removing top linens under a bath blanket.

(Al Dodge, Pearson Education/PH College)

CHANGING AN OCCUPIED BED *continued*

❷ Moving soiled linen as close to the client as possible.

(Al Dodge, Pearson Education/PH College)

❸ Placing a new bottom sheet on half of the bed.

(Al Dodge, Pearson Education/PH College)

half of the bed and miter the corner if a contour sheet is not being used.

- Place the clean drawsheet on the bed with the center fold at the center of the bed. Fanfold the uppermost half vertically at the center of the bed and tuck the near side edge under the side of the mattress. ❹
- Assist the client to roll over toward you onto the clean side of the bed. The client rolls over the fanfolded linen at the center of the bed.
- Move the pillows to the clean side for the client's use. Raise the side rail before leaving the side of the bed.
- Move to the other side of the bed and lower the side rail.
- Remove the used linen and place it in the portable hamper.
- Unfold the fanfolded bottom sheet from the center of the bed.
- Facing the side of the bed, use both hands to pull the bottom sheet so that it is smooth and tuck the excess under the side of the mattress.
- Unfold the drawsheet fanfolded at the center of the bed and pull it tightly with both hands. Pull the sheet in three sections: (a) Face the side of the bed to pull the middle section, (b) face the far top corner to pull the bottom section, and (c) face the far bottom corner to pull the top section.
- Tuck the excess drawsheet under the side of the mattress.

6. Reposition the client in the center of the bed.
   - Reposition the pillows at the center of the bed.
   - Assist the client to the center of the bed. Determine what position the client requires or prefers and assist the client to that position.

7. Apply or complete the top bedding.
   - Spread the top sheet over the client and either ask the client to hold the top edge of the sheet or tuck it under the shoulders. The sheet should remain over the client when the bath blanket or used sheet is removed. ❺
   - Complete the top of the bed.

8. Ensure continued safety of the client.
   - Raise the side rails. Place the bed in the low position before leaving the bedside.

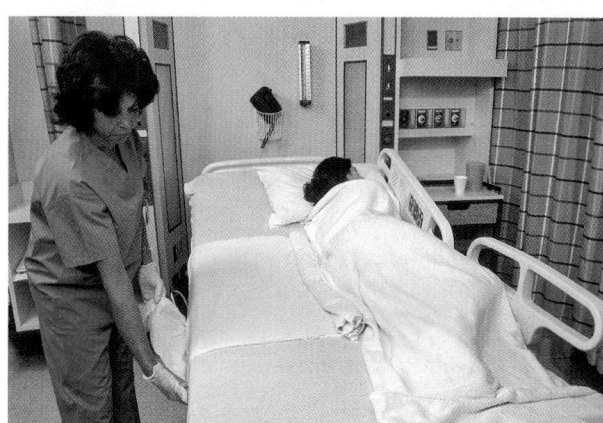

❹ Placing a clean drawsheet on the bed.

(Al Dodge, Pearson Education/PH College)

❺ Client holds top edge of sheet while nurse removes bath blanket.

- Attach the signal cord to the bed linen within the client's reach.
- Put items used by the client within easy reach.

9. Bed-making is not normally recorded.

EVALUATION

■ Conduct appropriate follow-up, such as determining client's comfort and safety, patency of all drainage tubes, and client's access to call light to summon help when needed.

CRITICAL THINKING CHECKPOINT

It is the fourth day following a female client's abdominal surgery. She is progressing well, is ambulating several times each day, has been providing for her own hygienic needs, and is planning on going home tomorrow. During your early morning assessment you note that the client's hair is oily and matted and she has an unpleasant body odor. Her dentures in a container at the bedside are in need of cleaning. You check her abdominal incision and verify that there is no drainage, redness, or signs of infection. You inquire about her ability to take care of her own bath and personal needs, and offer to assist her with her bath. She replies that she had a bath yesterday, doesn't feel that she needs another one today, and requests to omit her personal care for the day.

1. You are considering *Self-Care Deficit: Bathing/Hygiene* as an appropriate nursing diagnosis for the client. You review the defining characteristics and related factors and discover what?
2. What else should you ask the client?
3. Why is it important that you obtain the assessments you have already completed along with the above questions you asked?
4. What approaches might you use if you feel that the client does need her hair shampooed and needs to have her personal care attended to?
5. What advantages does performing baths and personal hygiene for clients offer to the nurse?

See Critical Thinking Possibilities in Appendix A.

CHAPTER 33 **REVIEW**

CHAPTER HIGHLIGHTS

- Clients' hygienic practices are influenced by numerous factors, including culture, religion, environment, developmental level, health and energy, and personal preferences.
- The major functions of the skin are to protect underlying tissues, to help regulate body temperature, to secrete sebum, to transmit sensations through nerve receptors for sensory perception, and to produce and absorb vitamin D in conjunction with ultraviolet rays from the sun.
- When planning hygiene care, the nurse must take the client's preferences into consideration.
- Nurses provide perineal-genital care for clients who are unable to do so for themselves.
- Nurses can often teach clients how to prevent foot problems.
- Oral hygiene should include daily dental flossing and mechanical brushing of the teeth.

- Regular dental checkups and fluoride supplements are recommended to maintain healthy teeth.
- Nurses provide special oral care to clients who are unconscious or debilitated.
- Hair care includes daily combing and brushing and regular shampooing.
- African American clients' hair may require special care.
- Nurses may need to assist dependent clients with their artificial eyes, eyeglasses, and contact lenses.
- Clients with a hearing aid may require nursing assistance with the device.
- Changing bed linens is a part of maintaining hygiene.
- It is important to keep beds clean and comfortable for clients.

TEST YOUR KNOWLEDGE

1. A client can bathe independently except for the back and feet, walk to and from the bathroom and dress if the clothing is provided. What is the most appropriate functional level for this client?
1. Totally dependent (+4)
2. Moderately dependent (+3)
3. Semidependent (+2)
4. Independent (0)

2. The client is unresponsive and requires total care. Prior to providing oral care, the nurse should assess for which of the following?
1. Presence of pain
2. Condition of the skin
3. Gag reflex
4. Range of motion

3. A client with diabetes has very dry skin on her feet and lower extremities. To maintain intact skin the nurse teaches which of the following?
1. Soak her feet frequently.

2. Use a nonperfumed lotion.
3. Apply foot powder.
4. Avoid knee-high elastic stockings.

4. The client wears an in-the-ear hearing aid and because of arthritis needs someone to insert the hearing aid. The nurse teaches the unlicensed assistive personnel (UAP) to do which of the following actions before inserting the client's hearing aid?
1. Turn the hearing aid off.
2. Soak the hearing aid in soapy solution to clean it.
3. Turn the volume all the way up.
4. Remove the batteries.

5. The client is in surgery and will be returning to his bed via a stretcher. The nurse plans ahead by making which type of bed and placing the bed in which position?
1. An open bed in low position
2. An occupied bed in low position
3. A closed bed in high position
4. A surgical bed in high position

6. Which of the following strategies are most appropriate for client with dementia? Select all that apply.
1. Cover the client as much as possible.
2. Sing or talk to the client.
3. Complete the bath as quickly as possible.
4. Be organized.
5. Expect the client to protest—finish quickly.

7. The nurse observed the UAP performing perineal care for a client. Which of the following actions indicates that further teaching is required?
1. Used a clean portion of the washcloth for each stroke.
2. Wiped from the pubis to the rectum.
3. Used clean gloves.
4. Did not retract the foreskin.

8. Which of the following statements will be important to include during a presentation on oral health at an intergenerational community center? Select all that apply.
1. Using a bottle during naps and at bedtime can cause dental caries in a toddler.
2. Schedule a visit to the dentist when your child is ready to go to school.

3. It is important for parents to supervise a child's brushing of their teeth.
4. Most elders have dentures and don't need to worry about oral care.
5. Elders are at risk for periodontal disease.

9. The nurse is discussing foot care with a client who was recently diagnosed with diabetes. Which of the following statements indicates a need for further teaching?
1. "I am going to use a mirror to check my feet."
2. "I enjoy walking barefoot around the house."
3. "I will file my nails."
4. "I will increase the time that I wear new shoes each day."

10. The client experiencing labored, shortness of breath has a respiratory rate of 28. The bed is currently in the flat position. The best nursing intervention includes putting the bed in which of the following positions?
1. Fowler's
2. Semi-Fowler's
3. Trendelenburg
4. Reverse Trendelenburg

See Answers to Test your knowledge in Appendix A.

EXPLORE MEDIALINK www.prenhall.com/berman

DVD-ROM
- Audio Glossary
- NCLEX Review
- Skills Checklists

COMPANION WEBSITE
- Additional NCLEX Review
- Case Study: Providing Basic Hygiene Care
- Care Plan Activity: Client on Radiation Therapy
- Application Activities:
  Client with Chickenpox
  Caring for Dentures
- Links to Resources

READINGS AND REFERENCES

SUGGESTED READINGS
Bailey, R., Gueldner, S., Ledikwe, J., & Smiciklas-Wright, H. (2005). The oral health of older adults. *Journal of Gerontological Nursing, 31*(7), 11–17.
The authors bring attention to the silent epidemic of poor oral health in the older population and that oral care is not viewed as a priority by many health care givers. A model for solving the problem with a multidisciplinary approach is offered to the reader.
Barrick, A. L., Rader, J., Hoeffer, B., & Sloane, P. D. (2002). *Bathing without a battle: Personal care of individuals with dementia.* New York: Springer.
The purpose of this informative book is to change current bathing practices that create distress and discomfort for people with dementia. The book is divided into three parts. Part I explores a general overview of bathing. Part II looks at special concerns that occur during bathing (e.g., pain, skin care, transfer techniques, level of assistance needed, and the environment). Part III explores ways to support the caregivers. Throughout the book are "Caregiver Wisdom" boxes, written by certified nurses assistants (CNAs), which describe caring, helpful hints based on their experiences. A must-read book for anyone who cares for clients with dementia.

Rader, J., Barrick, A. L., Hoeffer, B., Sloane, P. D., McKenzie, D., Talerico, K. A., & Glover, J. U. (2006). The bathing of older adults with dementia. Easing the unnecessarily unpleasant aspects of assisted bathing. *American Journal of Nursing, 106*(4), 40–48.
The authors propose eliminating forced bathing. As they say: Bathing people routinely against their wishes—"for their own good"—should become part of nursing history. Instead of a task that must be done, bathing should be viewed as a human interaction. Inexpensive, practical, and evidence-based alternatives are discussed.
Rados, C. (2005). Sound advice about age-related hearing loss. *FDA Consumer, 39*(3), 29–27.
This article reviews age-related hearing loss, how to lessen the severity of age-related hearing loss, and different types of hearing devices.

RELATED RESEARCH
El-Solh, A. A., Pietrantoni, C., Bhat, A., Okada, M., Zambon, J., Aquilina, A., & Berbary, E. (2004). Colonization of dental plaques. A reservoir of respiratory pathogens for hospital-acquired pneumonia in institutionalized elders. *Chest, 126*(5), 1575–1582.
Jones, K., & Tomar, S. L. (2005). Estimated impact of competing policy recommendations for age of first dental visit. *Pediatrics, 115*(4), 906–914.

McNamara, M. E., Burnham, D. C., Smith, C., & Carroll, D. L. (2003). The effects of back massage before diagnostic cardiac catheterization. *Alternative Therapies in Health and Medicine, 9*(1), 50–57.
Somboontanont, W., Sloane, P. D., Floyd, F. J., Holditch-Davis, D., Hogue, C. C., & Mitchell, M. (2004). Assaultive behavior in Alzheimer's disease: Identifying immediate antecedents during bathing. *Journal of Gerontological Nursing, 30*(9), 22–29.
Stiefel, K. A., Damron, S., Sowers, N. J., & Velez, L. (2000). Improving oral hygiene for the seriously ill patient: Implementing research-based practice. *Medsurg Nursing, 9*(1), 40–46.

REFERENCES
Alzheimer's Disease Education & Referral Center. (n.d.). *2001-2002 Alzheimer's disease progress report.* Retrieved June 13, 2006, from http://www.nia.nih.gov/NR/rdonlyres?7049AF18-6827-4DCE-95FA-B853D171C974/0/2002_ALZ_PR.pdf
American Dental Association. (n.d.). *Cleaning your teeth and gums (oral hygiene).* Retrieved June 13, 2006, from http://www.ada.org/public/topics/cleaning_faq.asp
American Dental Association. (n.d.). *Oral changes with age.* Retrieved June 13, 2006, from http://www.ada.org/public/topics/oral_changes_faq.asp

Anderson, E. G. (1998). Deafness is a scourge and you can say that again. *Geriatrics, 53*(8), 65–69.

Andrews, M. M., & Boyle, J. S. (2003). *Transcultural concepts in nursing care* (4th ed.). Philadelphia: Lippincott Williams & Wilkins.

Anonymous. (2003). Oral care update. *Nursing Management, 34*(5), S1–S16.

Barrick, A. L., & Rader, J. (2000). Bathing without a battle [Electronic Version]. *Alzheimer's Care Quarterly, 1*(4), 35–49.

Barrick, A. L., Rader, J., Hoeffer, B., & Sloane, P. (Eds.). (2002). *Bathing without a battle: Personal care of individuals with dementia.* New York: Springer.

Capezuti, E. (2004). Guidelines address side rail entrapment. *American Journal of Nursing, 104*(5), 74.

Coleman, P. R. (2002). Improving oral health care for the frail elderly: A review of widespread problems and best practices. *Geriatric Nursing, 23,* 189–199.

Coleman, P. R. (2004). Promoting oral health in elder care: Challenges and opportunities. *Journal of Gerontological Nursing, 30*(4), 3.

Dochterman, J. M. & Bulechek, G. M. (2004). *Nursing interventions classification (NIC)* (4th ed.). St. Louis, MO: Mosby.

Dunn, J. C., Thiru-Chelvam, B., & Beck, C. H. M. (2002). Bathing: Pleasure or pain? *Journal of Gerontological Nursing, 28*(11), 6–13.

Edelman, C. L., & Mandle, C. L. (2006). *Health promotion throughout the life span* (6th ed.). St. Louis, MO: Mosby Elsevier.

Frankowski, B. L., & Weiner, L. B. (2002). Head lice. *Pediatrics, 110*(3), 638–643.

Gammons, M., & Salam, G. (2002). Tick removal. *American Family Physician, 66*(4), 643–645.

Goldsmith, J. (2003). Nit-picking. *American Journal of Nursing, 103*(9), 22–23.

Gooch, B. F., Eke, P. I., & Malvitz, D. M. (2004). Public health and aging: Retention of natural teeth among older adults—United States, 2002. *Journal of the American Medical Association, 291*(3), 292.

Jackson, F. (1998). The ABC's of black hair and skin care. *ABNF Journal, 9*(5), 100–104.

Kelly, S. E., Binkley, C. J., Neace, W. P., & Gale, B. S. (2005). Barriers to care-seeking for children's oral health among low-income caregivers.

American Journal of Public Health, 95(8), 1345–1351.

Moorhead, S., Johnson, M., & Maas, M. (2004). *Nursing outcomes classification (NOC)* (2nd ed.). St. Louis, MO: Mosby.

Moses, M. (2003). A simple matter of grooming. Stop using toxic pesticides to treat head lice. *American Journal of Nursing, 103*(9), 11.

Munro, C. L., Grap, M. J., & Kleinpell, R. (2004). Oral health and care in the intensive care unit: State of the science. *American Journal of Critical Care, 13*(1), 25–34.

Nainar, S. M., & Mohummed, S. (2004). Role of infant feeding practices on the dental health of children. *Clinical Pediatrics, 43*(2), 129–133.

NANDA International (2007). *NANDA nursing diagnoses: Definitions & Classification 2007–2008.* Philadelphia. Author.

Pattillo, M. M. (2004). Therapeutic and healing foot care: A healthy feet clinic for older adults. *Journal of Gerontological Nursing, 30*(12), 25–32.

Pillitteri, A. (2003). *Maternal and child health nursing: Care of the childbearing and childrearing family* (2nd ed.). Philadelphia: Lippincott, Williams & Wilkins.

Purnell, L. D., & Paulanka, B. J. (2005). *Guide to culturally competent health care.* Philadelphia: F. A. Davis.

Rader, J., Barrick, A. L., Hoeffer, B., Sloane, P. D., McKenzie, D., Talerico, K. A., & Glover, J. U. (2006). The bathing of older adults with dementia. Easing the unnecessarily unpleasant aspects of assisted bathing. *American Journal of Nursing, 106*(4), 40–48.

Rasin, J., & Barrick, A. L. (2004). Bathing patients with dementia: Concentrating on the patient's needs rather than merely the task. *American Journal of Nursing, 104*(3), 30–33.

Stewart, K. B. (2000). Stopping the itch of scabies and lice. *Nursing, 30*(7), 30–31.

Stone, C. M. (1999). Preventing cerumen impaction in nursing facility residents. *Journal of Gerontological Nursing, 25*(5), 43–45.

Talerico, K. A., & Capezuti, E. (2001). Myths and facts about side rails. *American Journal of Nursing, 101*(7), 43–48.

Walton, J. C., Miller, J., & Tordecilla, L. (2001). Elder oral assessment and care. *Medsurg Nursing, 10*(1), 37–44.

Wilkinson, J. M. (2005). *Nursing diagnosis handbook with NIC interventions and NOC outcomes* (8th ed.). Upper Saddle River, NJ: Prentice Hall Health.

SELECTED BIBLIOGRAPHY

Chalmer, J., Johnson, V., Hsiao-Chen, J., & Titler, M. G. (2004). Evidence-based protocol: Oral hygiene care for functionally dependent and cognitively impaired older adults. *Journal of Gerontological Nursing, 30*(11), 5–12.

Dougherty, J., & Long, C. O. (2003). Techniques for bathing without a battle. *Home Healthcare Nurse, 21*(1), 38–39.

Ficorelli, C. T., & Edelman, M. (2005). Foot care for patients with diabetes. *Nursing, 35*(10), 43.

Forrester, D. A., Nash-Luchenback, D., & Tistler, M. (2004). Help your patient manage dry mouth. *Nursing, 34*(4), 32hn10.

Hilgers, J. (2003). Comforting a confused patient. *Nursing, 33*(1), 48–50.

Hoffman, S. B., Powell-Cope, G., MacClellan, L., & Bero, K. (2003). BedSAFE: A bed safety project for frail older adults. *Journal of Gerontological Nursing, 29*(11), 34–42.

Lamster, I. B. (2004). Oral health care services for older adults: A looming crisis. *American Journal of Public Health, 94*(5), 699–703.

Lucas, L. J., & Mathews-Flint, L. J. (2003). Heed the word about hearing impairment. *Nursing, 33*(10), 32hn1–32hn2.

Parker, L. (2004). Infection control: Maintaining the personal hygiene of patients and staff. *British Journal of Nursing, 13*(8), 474–478.

Perlmutter, J. S., & Camberg, L. (2004). Better bathing for residents with Alzheimer's. *Nursing Homes, 53*(4), 40–43.

Sieggreen, M. Y. (2005). Stepping up care for diabetic foot ulcers. *Nursing, 35*(10), 36–41.

Yetzer, E. A. (2004). Incorporating foot care education into diabetic foot screening. *Rehabilitation Nursing, 29*(3), 80–84.

Zulkowski, K., & Albrecht, D. (2003). How dental status affects healing in older adults. *Nursing, 33*(10), 22.

Diagnostic Testing

LEARNING OUTCOMES

After completing this chapter, you will be able to:

1. Describe the nurse's role for each of the phases involved in diagnostic testing.

2. List common blood tests.

3. Accurately measure blood glucose from a capillary blood specimen using a blood glucose meter.

4. Discuss the nursing responsibilities for specimen collection.

5. Explain the rationale for the collection of each type of specimen.

6. Collect and test stool specimens.

7. Compare and contrast the different types of urine specimens.

8. Collect sputum and throat specimens.

9. Describe visualization procedures that may be used for the client with gastrointestinal, urinary, and cardiopulmonary alterations.

10. Compare and contrast CT, MRI, and nuclear imaging studies.

11. Describe the nurse's role in caring for clients undergoing aspiration/biopsy procedures.

KEY TERMS

abdominal paracentesis, *821*
angiography, *818*
anoscopy, *817*
arterial blood gases, *802*
ascites, *821*
aspiration, *819*
biopsy, *819*
blood chemistry, *802*
blood urea nitrogen (BUN), *802*
cannula, *821*
clean-catch urine specimen, *810*
clean voided urine specimen, *810*
colonoscopy, *817*
complete blood count (CBC), *799*
computed tomography (CT), *818*
creatinine, *802*
cystoscope, *817*
cystoscopy, *817*
echocardiogram, *818*
electrocardiogram (ECG), *817*
electrocardiography, *817*
expectorate, *816*

guaiac test, *808*
hematocrit, *799*
hemoglobin, *799*
hemoglobin A_{1c} (HbA$_1$), *802*
hemoptysis, *816*
intravenous pyelography (IVP), *817*
kidneys/ureters/bladder (KUB), *817*
leukocyte, *801*
lumbar puncture, *819*
lung scan, *818*
magnetic resonance imaging (MRI), *818*
manometer, *820*
midstream urine specimen, *810*
occult blood, *808*
peak level, *802*
phlebotomist, *799*
polycythemia, *801*
positron emission tomography (PET), *819*

proctoscopy, *817*
proctosigmoidoscopy, *817*
radiopharmaceutical, *819*
reagent, *809*
red blood cell (RBC) count, *801*
red blood cell (RBC) indices, *801*
retrograde pyelography, *817*
saliva, *815*
serum osmolality, *802*
specific gravity, *815*
sputum, *815*
steatorrhea, *808*
stress electrocardiography, *818*
thoracentesis, *821*
trocar, *821*
trough level, *802*
ultrasonography, *817*
urine osmolality, *815*
venipuncture, *799*
white blood cell (WBC), *801*

Diagnostic and laboratory tests (commonly called lab tests) are tools that provide information about the client. Tests may be used as basic screening as part of a wellness check. Frequently tests are used to help confirm a diagnosis, monitor an illness, and provide valuable information about the client's response to treatment. Nurses require knowledge of the most common lab and diagnostic tests because one primary role of the nurse is to teach the client and family or significant other how to prepare for the test and the care that may be required following the test. Nurses must also know the implications of the test results in order to provide the most appropriate nursing care for the client.

DIAGNOSTIC TESTING PHASES

Diagnostic testing occurs in many environments. The traditional sites include hospitals, clinics, and the primary care provider's office. Many test sites, however, are moving to the community. Examples include the home, workplace, shopping malls, and mobile units. The more complex diagnostic tests are performed at diagnostic centers specifically built for those tests.

Diagnostic testing involves three phases: pretest, intratest, and post-test.

Pretest

The major focus of the pretest phase is client preparation. A thorough assessment and data collection (e.g., biologic, psychologic, sociologic, cultural, and spiritual) assist the nurse in determining communication and teaching strategies. Prior to radiologic studies it is important to ask female clients if pregnancy is possible. Special precautions may be necessary or the test may need to be postponed.

The nurse also needs to know what equipment and supplies are needed for the specific test. Common questions include the following: What type of sample will be needed and how will it be collected? Does the client need to stop oral intake for a certain number of hours prior to the test? Does the test include administration of dye (contrast media) and, if so, is it injected or swallowed? Are fluids restricted or forced? Are medications given or withheld? How long is the test? Is a consent form required? Answers to these type of questions can help avoid costly mistakes and reduce inconvenience to all involved. Most facilities have information about the tests available to the health care team. The laboratory at the facility can also act as a resource for information.

CULTURALLY COMPETENT CARE
Drawing Blood Samples

In Asian traditional medicine, blood is not drawn for medical purposes (Salimbene, 2000, p. 23). An Asian client practicing traditional medicine views blood as a source of life and believes that the body cannot replace lost blood (Spector, 2004). As a result, Asian clients may be upset by venipuncture or the drawing of blood for testing, especially if there are numerous tests. They may view this as upsetting the body's normal balance and weakening the body. Also, blood represents a person's essence and they may fear that their essence is being given away. Therefore, Asian clients may also need to be informed that their blood will not be given to anyone else.

Note: From What Language Does Your Patient Hurt In? A Practical Guide to Culturally Competent Patient Care *by S. Salimbene, 2000, EMCParadigm; and* Cultural Diversity in Health & Illness *by R. E. Spector, 2004, Prentice Hall. Adapted with permission.*

CLIENT TEACHING **Preparing for Diagnostic Testing**

- Instruct the client and family about requirements or restrictions (e.g., when and what to eat or drink, how long to fast).
- Provide information about what the client may feel (e.g., a temporary flushing and feeling of warmth when the dye is injected).
- Ask the client if a description or pictures of the involved equipment would help prepare him or her for the test.
- Encourage questions and dialogue about fears and apprehensions. Find out what the client may have heard about the test from others.

- Inform the client of the time period before the results will be available.
- Document teaching. Include the client's response. Record names of audiovisual and reading materials, if used.

Note: From *A Manual of Laboratory & Diagnostic Tests,* 7th ed., by F. Fischbach, 2004, Philadelphia: Lippincott Williams & Wilkins. Reprinted with permission.

Intratest

This phase focuses on specimen collection and performing or assisting with certain diagnostic testing. The nurse uses standard precautions and sterile technique as appropriate. During the procedure the nurse provides emotional and physical support while monitoring the client as needed (e.g., vital signs, pulse oximetry, ECG). The nurse ensures correct labeling, storage, and transportation of the specimen to avoid invalid test results.

Post-Test

The focus of this phase is on nursing care of the client and follow-up activities and observations. As appropriate, the nurse compares the previous and current test results and modifies nursing interventions as needed. The nurse also reports the results to appropriate health team members.

Nursing Diagnoses

Nursing diagnoses are based on client data and need. Examples can include

- *Anxiety* or *Fear* related to possible diagnosis of acute or chronic illness pending conclusion of diagnostic testing.
- *Impaired Physical Mobility* related to prescribed bed rest and restricted movement of involved extremity after testing.
- *Deficient Knowledge* (state diagnostic test) related to misperceptions received from others regarding process for test.

BLOOD TESTS

Blood tests are one of the most commonly used diagnostic tests and can provide valuable information about the hematologic system and many other body systems. A **venipuncture** (puncture of a vein for collection of a blood specimen) can be performed by various members of the health care team. Usually a **phlebotomist,** a person from a laboratory who performs venipuncture, collects the blood specimen for the tests ordered by the primary care provider. In some institutions, nurses may draw blood samples. The nurse needs to know the guidelines for drawing blood samples for the facility and also the state's nurse practice act.

Complete Blood Count

Specimens of venous blood are taken for a **complete blood count (CBC),** which includes hemoglobin and hematocrit measurements, erythrocyte (RBC) count, leukocyte (WBC) count, red blood cell (RBC) indices, and a differential white cell count. The CBC is a basic screening test and one of the most frequently ordered blood tests (see Table 34–1).

Hemoglobin is the main intracellular protein of erythrocytes. It carries oxygen to and removes carbon dioxide from red blood cells (Van Leeuwen et al, 2006, p. 732). The hemoglobin test is a measure of the total amount of hemoglobin in the blood. The **hematocrit** measures the percentage of red blood cells in the total blood volume. Normal values for both hemoglobin and hematocrit vary, with males having higher levels than females.

TABLE 34–1 **Complete Blood Count with Clinical Implications**			
COMPONENT	**NORMAL FINDINGS (ADULT)**	**POSSIBLE CAUSES OF ABNORMAL FINDINGS**	
		INCREASED	**DECREASED**
Red blood cell count (RBC) The number of RBCs per cubic millimeter (mm³).	M: 4.5–5.3 million/mm³ F: 4.1–5.1 million/mm³	Primary polycythemia (e.g., polycythemia vera) Secondary polycythemia or erythrocytosis—usually caused by oxygen need (e.g., chronic lung disease, congenital heart defects)	Abnormal loss of erythrocytes Abnormal destruction of erythrocytes Lack of needed elements or hormones for erythrocyte production Bone marrow suppression
Hemoglobin (Hgb) Composed of a pigment (heme), which contains iron, and a protein (globin).	M: 13.8–18 g/dL F: 12–16 g/dL	Polycythemia	Blood loss Hemolytic anemia Bone marrow suppression Sickle cell anemia

(continued on page 800)

TABLE 34–1   **Complete Blood Count with Clinical Implications—*continued***

COMPONENT	NORMAL FINDINGS (ADULT)	POSSIBLE CAUSES OF ABNORMAL FINDINGS	
		INCREASED	**DECREASED**
Hematocrit (Hct) The hematocrit or packed cell volume (Hct, PCV, or crit) is a fast way to determine the percentage of RBCs in the plasma. The Hct is reported as a percentage because it is the proportion of RBCs to the plasma.	M: 37–49% F: 36–46%	Polycythemia Dehydration Burns	Blood loss Overhydration Dietary deficiency Anemia
Red blood cell indices (RBC indices) *Mean corpuscular volume (MCV)* The mean or average size of the individual RBC.	M: 78–100 μm^3 F: 78–102 μm^3	Liver disease Alcoholism Pernicious anemia	Iron deficiency anemia Lead poisoning
Mean corpuscular hemoglobin (MCH) Amount of Hgb present in one cell.	25–35 pg	Rarely seen	Iron deficiency anemia
Mean corpuscular hemoglobin concentration (MCHC) The proportion of each cell occupied by Hgb.	31–37%	Rarely seen	Iron deficiency anemia
White blood cell count (WBC) Count of the total number of WBCs in a cubic millimeter of blood.	4,500–11,000/mm^3	Leukocytosis Infection	Leukopenia Autoimmune disease
Differential count: The proportion of each of the five types of WBCs in a sample of 100 WBCs.			
Neutrophils	55–70%	Stress Acute infection	Viral diseases Some drugs (e.g., chemotherapy, antibiotics such as nafcillin, penicillin, and cephalosporins) Radiation therapy
Lymphocytes	20–40%	Viral infection Mononucleosis Tuberculosis Chronic bacterial infections Lymphocytic leukemia	Adrenal corticosteroids and other immunosuppressive drugs Autoimmune diseases (e.g., lupus erythematosus) Severe malnutrition
Monocytes	2–8%	Chronic inflammatory disorders Tuberculosis Protozoan infections (e.g., malaria, Rocky Mountain spotted fever) Chronic ulcerative colitis	Drug therapy: Prednisone
Eosinophils	1–4%	Allergic reactions (e.g., asthma, hay fever, or hypersensitivity to a drug) Parasitic infestations (e.g., round worms)	Corticosteroid therapy
Basophils	0–2%	Leukemia	Acute allergic reaction Corticosteroids Acute infections
Platelet count Platelets are fragments of cytoplasm that function in blood coagulation.	150,000–350,000/mm^3	Malignant tumors Polycythemia vera	Idiopathic (unknown cause) Thrombocytopenic purpura Viral infections AIDS Systemic lupus erythematosus Chemotherapy drugs Some types of anemias

Note: From *Laboratory Tests and Diagnostic Procedures with Nursing Diagnoses,* 6th ed., by J. V. Corbett, 2004, Upper Saddle River, NJ: Pearson Prentice Hall. Reproduced with permission of Pearson Education, Inc., Upper Saddle River, New Jersey.

Hemoglobin and hematocrit increase with dehydration as the blood becomes more concentrated, and decrease with hypervolemia and resulting hemodilution. Hemoglobin and hematocrit are often ordered together and commonly referred to as "H & H" when ordering lab tests. Both the hemoglobin and hematocrit are related to the **red blood cell (RBC) count,** which is the number of RBCs per cubic millimeter of whole blood. It also varies by gender and age. Low RBC counts are indicative of anemia. Clients with chronic hypoxia may develop higher than normal counts, a condition known as **polycythemia. Red blood cell (RBC) indices** may be performed as part of the CBC to evaluate the size, weight, and hemoglobin concentration of RBCs.

The **leukocyte** or **white blood cell (WBC)** count determines the number of circulating WBCs per cubic millimeter of whole

> ### *CULTURALLY COMPETENT CARE*
> **Biocultural Considerations**
>
> There are some cultural variations in hemoglobin (Hgb) and hematocrit (Hct) values. For example, the normal hemoglobin level for African American people is 1 g lower than for other groups.

blood. High WBC counts are often seen in the presence of a bacterial infection; by contrast, WBC counts may be low if a viral infection is present. In the WBC differential, leukocytes are identified by type, and the percentage of each type is determined. This information is useful in diagnosing certain disorders that have characteristic patterns of distribution (see Figure 34-1 ■).

Figure 34-1 ■ Composition of blood.

Serum Electrolytes

Serum electrolytes are often routinely ordered for any client admitted to a hospital as a screening test for electrolyte and acid–base imbalances. Serum electrolytes also are routinely assessed for clients at risk in the community, for example, clients who are being treated with a diuretic for hypertension or heart failure. The most commonly ordered serum tests are for sodium, potassium, chloride, and bicarbonate ions. Serum electrolytes may be ordered as a Chem 7 or BMP (basic metabolic panel). The lab terminology varies depending on the lab. Normal values of commonly measured electrolytes are shown in Box 34–1.

Blood levels of two metabolically produced substances, urea and creatinine, are routinely used to evaluate renal function. The kidneys, through filtration and tubular secretion, normally eliminate both. Urea, the end product of protein metabolism, is measured as **blood urea nitrogen (BUN). Creatinine** is produced in relatively constant quantities by the muscles and is excreted by the kidneys. Thus, the amount of creatinine in the blood relates to renal excretory function.

Serum Osmolality

Serum osmolality is a measure of the solute concentration of the blood. The particles included are sodium ions, glucose, and urea (BUN). Serum osmolality can be estimated by doubling the serum sodium, because sodium and its associated chloride ions are the major determinants of serum osmolality. Serum osmolality values are used primarily to evaluate fluid balance. Normal values are 280 to 300 mOsm/kg. An increase in serum osmolality indicates a fluid volume deficit; a decrease reflects a fluid volume excess.

Drug Monitoring

Therapeutic drug monitoring is often conducted when a client is taking a medication with a narrow therapeutic range (e.g, digoxin, theophylline, aminoglycosides). This monitoring includes drawing blood samples for peak and trough levels to determine if the blood serum levels of a specific drug are at a therapeutic level and not a subtherapeutic or toxic level. The **peak level** indicates the highest concentration of the drug in the

blood serum, and the **trough level** represents the lowest concentration. Ideally, a client's peak and trough levels fall within the therapeutic range.

Arterial Blood Gases

Measurement of **arterial blood gases** is another important diagnostic procedure (see Chapter 50 ∞). Specialty nurses, medical technicians, and respiratory therapists normally take specimens of arterial blood from the radial, brachial, or femoral arteries. Because of the relatively great pressure of the blood in these arteries, it is important to prevent hemorrhaging by applying pressure to the puncture side for about 5 to 10 minutes after removing the needle.

Blood Chemistry

A number of other tests may be performed on blood serum (the liquid portion of the blood). These are often referred to as a **blood chemistry.** In addition to serum electrolytes, common chemistry examinations include determining certain enzymes that may be present (including lactic dehydrogenase [LDH], creatine kinase [CK], aspartate aminotransferase [AST], and alanine aminotransferase [ALT]), serum glucose, hormones such as thyroid hormone, and other substances such as cholesterol and triglycerides. These tests provide valuable diagnostic cues. For example, cardiac markers (e.g., CPK-MB, myoglobin, Troponin T, and Troponin I) are released into the blood during a myocardial infarction (MI, or heart attack). Elevated levels of these markers in the venous blood can help differentiate between an MI and chest pain from a different cause such as angina or pleuritic pain.

A common lab test is the glycosylated hemoglobin or **hemoglobin A$_{1C}$ (HbA$_{1C}$),** which is a measurement of blood glucose that is bound to hemoglobin. Hemoglobin A$_{1C}$ is a reflection of how well blood glucose levels have been controlled during the prior 3 to 4 months. The normal range is 4.0% to 5.5%. An elevated HbA$_{1C}$ reflects hyperglycemia in diabetics.

The first specific blood test to detect and guide treatment for heart failure is the BNP (B-type natriuretic peptide) test. B-type natriuretic peptide is secreted primarily by the left ventricle in response to increased ventricular volume and pressure. BNP levels increase as the heart failure becomes more severe.

See Table 34–2 for normal values of common blood chemistry tests.

Metabolic Screening

Newborns are routinely screened for congenital metabolic conditions. Tests for phenylketonuria (PKU) and congenital hypothyroidism are required in all states in the United States. Other conditions that are frequently screened include sickle cell disease and galactosemia. Screening involves collecting peripheral venous blood (via a heel-stick) on a prepared blotting paper and sending the specimen to the state laboratory for analysis. Discovered abnormalities allow the provider and parents to plan early care (e.g., special diets for children with PKU) that can prevent long-term complications.

BOX 34–1 **Normal Electrolyte Values for Adults ***	
VENOUS BLOOD	
Sodium	135–145 mEq/L
Potassium	3.5–5.0 mEq/L
Chloride	95–105 mEq/L
Calcium (total) (ionized)	4.5–5.5 mEq/L or 8.5–10.5 mg/dL 56% of total calcium (2.5 mEq/L or 4.0–5.0 mg/dL)
Magnesium	1.5–2.5 mEq/L or 1.6–2.5 mg/dL
Phosphate	1.8–2.6 mEq/L (phosphorus)
Serum osmolality	280–300 mOsm/kg water

* Normal laboratory values vary from agency to agency.

TABLE 34–2 Common Blood Chemistry Tests with Clinical Implications

TEST	NORMAL FINDINGS (ADULT)	SIGNIFICANCE	POSSIBLE CAUSES OF INCREASED	POSSIBLE CAUSES OF DECREASED
Liver Function Tests:				
ALT, (alanine amino transferase) formerly known as serum pyretic transaminase (SGPT)	Men: 10–55 U/L Women: 7–30 U/L	Marker of hepatic injury; more specific of liver damage than AST.	Hepatitis; infectious mononucleosis; acute pancreatitis; acute myocardial infarction; heart failure.	Not clinically significant.
AST, (Aspartate amino transferase) formerly known as serum gluctamic-oxaloacetic transaminase (SGOT)	Men: 10–40 U/L Women: 9–25 U/L	Found in heart, liver, and skeletal muscle. Can also be used to indicate liver injury.	Liver diseases (e.g., hepatitis, alcoholism, drug toxicity); acute myocardial infarction, anemias, skeletal muscle diseases.	Chronic renal dialysis, vitamin B_6 deficiency.
Albumin	Adults: 3.5–4.8 g/dL or 35–48 g/L Panic value: <1.5 g/dL	Is a protein produced by the liver.	No pathology causes the liver to produce more albumin. An increased level reflects dehydration.	Chronic liver dysfunction; AIDS, severe burns, malnutrition, renal disease; acute and chronic infections.
Alkaline phosphatase	Adults: 25–100 U/L	Found in the tissues of the liver, bone, intestine, kidney, and placenta. Used as an index of liver and bone disease when correlated with other clinical findings.	Liver disease; bone disease; hyperparathyroidism; myocardial infarction; chronic renal failure; heart failure.	Malnutrition; pernicious anemia and severe anemias; hypothyroidism; magnesium and zinc deficiency (nutritional).
Ammonia	Adults: 35–65 µg/dL	The liver converts ammonia, a by-product of protein metabolism, into urea which is excreted by the kidneys.	Liver disease, cirrhosis; Reye's syndrome; GI hemorrhage.	Renal failure.
Bilirubin	Adults: Total: 0.3–1.0 mg/dL Direct: 0.0–0.2 mg/dL Indirect: 0.1–1/0 mg/dL Panic value: >12 mg/dL	Results from the breakdown of hemoglobin in the red blood cells; removed from the body by the liver, which excretes it into the bile.	Total: Hepatitis; obstruction of the common bile or hepatic ducts; pernicious anemia; sickle cell anemia. Direct: Cancer of the head of the pancreas; choledocholithiasis. Indirect: Hemolytic anemias; drug toxicity; transfusion reaction.	Not clinically significant.
GGT (Gamma-glutamyl transferase)	Men: 1–94 U/L Women: 1–70 U/L	Found primarily in the liver, kidney, prostate, and spleen. Is more specific for the hepatobiliary system.	Liver disease; alcohol abuse.	Not clinically significant.
Prothrombin	11–13 seconds Critical value: > 20 seconds for non-anticoagulated persons	A protein produced by the liver for clotting of blood.	Liver disease, damage; vitamin K deficiency; obstruction of common bile duct; deficiency of factors II, V, VII, or X.	Thrombophlebitis; malignant tumor.
Cardiac Markers:				
CK (creatine kinase)	Total: Men: 38–174 U/L Women: 26–140 U/L Isoenzymes: MM (CK_3): 96%–100% MB (CK_2): 0% –6% BB (CK_1): 0%	An enzyme found in the heart and skeletal muscles. Has three isoenzymes: BB or CK_1, MB or CK_2, and MM or CK_3.	Total: Acute myocardial infarction (MI); myocarditis; after open heart surgery; acute cerebrovascular disease, muscular dystrophy; chronic alcoholism CK Isoenzymes: MB (CK_2): Myocardial infarct; myocardial ischemia, angina pectoris.	Not clinically significant.

(continued on page 804)

TABLE 34–2 **Common Blood Chemistry Tests with Clinical Implications**—*continued*

TEST	NORMAL FINDINGS (ADULT)	SIGNIFICANCE	POSSIBLE CAUSES OF INCREASED	POSSIBLE CAUSES OF DECREASED
Cardiac Markers: (continued)				
Myoglobin	5–70 ng/mL	After an MI, serum levels of myoglobin rise in 2–4 hours, making it an early marker for muscle damage in MI.	Myocardial infarction, angina, other muscle injury (e.g., trauma), renal failure, rhabdomyolysis.	Rheumatoid arthritis; myasthenia gravis.
Troponin I Troponin T	Troponin I: <0.35 ng/mL Critical value: >1.5 ng/mL Troponin T: <0.2 ng/mL	Cardiac troponin is highly concentrated in the heart muscle. This test is used in the early diagnosis of MI. After an MI, troponin I begins to increase in 4–6 hours and remains elevated for 5–7 days. Troponin T begins to increase in 3–4 hours and remains elevated for 10–14 days.	Troponin I: Small infarct; myocardial injury. Troponin T: Acute MI, unstable angina, myocarditis.	Not clinically significant.
BNP (brain natriuretic peptide)	<100 pg/mL or <100 ng/L	A hormone produced by the ventricles of the heart and is a marker of ventricular systolic and diastolic dysfunction. This test is useful in diagnosing and guiding treatment of heart failure.	Heart failure; symptomatic cardiac volume overload; paroxysmal atrial tachycardia.	Not clinically significant.
Lipoprotein Profile:				
Cholesterol	Adults: Desirable: < 200 mg/dL	This test is an important screening test for heart disease.	Type II familial hypercholesterolemia; biliary cirrhosis; chronic renal failure; poorly controlled diabetes mellitus; alcoholism; diet high in cholesterol and fats.	Severe hepatocellular disease; hyperthyroidism; malnutrition, chronic anemias, severe burns.
HDL-C (high-density lipoprotein cholesterol)	Men: 35–65 mg/dL Women: 35–80 mg/dL	A class of lipoproteins produced by the liver and intestines. The "good" cholesterol.	HDL excess; chronic liver disease; long-term aerobic or vigorous exercise.	Familial hypo-lipoproteinemia; hypertriglyceridemia (familial), poorly controlled diabetes mellitus, chronic renal failure.
LDL (low-density lipoprotein)	Adults: Desirable: <130 mg/dL	Up to 70% of the total serum cholesterol is present in the LDL. The "bad" cholesterol.	Familial type 2 hyperlipidemia; Secondary causes can include: diet high in cholesterol and saturated fat, nephritic syndrome, multiple myeloma, diabetes mellitus, chronic renal failure.	Hypolipoproteinemia; hyperthyroidism, chronic anemias, severe hepatocellular disease.
Triglycerides	Desirable: <150 mg/dL	This test evaluates suspected atherosclerosis and measures the body's ability to metabolize fat.	Hyperlipoproteinemia; liver disease; renal disease; hypothyroidism; pancreatitis; myocardial infarction.	Malnutrition; hyperthyroidism, brain infarction, chronic obstructive lung disease.

Capillary Blood Glucose

A capillary blood specimen is often taken to measure blood glucose when frequent tests are required or when a venipuncture cannot be performed. This technique is less painful than a venipuncture and easily performed. Hence, clients can perform this technique on themselves.

The development of home glucose test kits and reagent strips has simplified the testing of blood glucose and greatly facilitated the management of home care by clients with diabetes. A number of manufacturers have developed blood glucose meters or monitors (Figure 34-2 ■).

Advances in technology have resulted in clients having greater choices for a glucose meter that meets their needs. For example, a person with a vision impairment could choose a voice-activated glucose meter. If a client has a physical impairment, an available meter can rest on the arm and perform the lancing and testing automatically (Mensing, 2004, p. 43). For high-tech clients, there are software programs that analyze their trends in glucose control.

Glucose meters can vary in the following ways: amount of blood needed, testing speed, size, ability to store results, cost of the meter, and test strips (U.S. Food and Drug Administration, n.d.). Choosing the right glucose meter that matches the client's needs will help the client to be comfortable and confident in using the meter and thus promote control of his or her diabetes. Once the client chooses a blood glucose meter, it is imperative that the nurse or client review the manufacturer's operating

Figure 34-2 ■ Blood glucose monitor, test strips, and lancet injector.

guidelines. Being familiar with the proper use of the equipment helps ensure accurate readings.

Capillary blood specimens are commonly obtained from the lateral aspect or side of the finger in adults. This site avoids the nerve endings and calloused areas at the fingertip. The earlobe may be used if the client is in shock or the fingers are edematous. Some newer monitors allow for obtaining specimens from less sensitive areas on the arms, legs, or abdomen.

Skill 34-1 describes how to obtain a capillary blood specimen and measure blood glucose using a portable meter.

REAL WORLD REFLECTION

THE STORY

During one clinical day, I was provided with an opportunity to assess data on an hourly basis, and I became GREAT at performing blood glucose checks. The client was a 36-year-old woman who had been diagnosed 10 years earlier with diabetes. Following surgery her blood glucose levels became very erratic, and she was placed on a sliding insulin scale requiring hourly glucose checks. The amount of insulin she was to receive was based on her glucose levels, so I knew I had to be accurate.

STUDENT REFLECTION

When I started the shift, I just wanted to "do it right." I was concerned about all the mechanics of which finger to choose, getting enough blood on the strip, not forgetting the reading, etc. . . . But after so many sticks, I started to notice small things. I saw all of the little stick marks on her finger tips. I was more considerate about which finger I chose and asked her if her fingers felt sore. I realized that even the small procedures I do for clients can be uncom-

fortable and painful. In the future, as I hurry from client room to client room or try to get things done before the end of my shift, I need to take time to focus on the client and his or her feelings.

FACULTY REFLECTION

Lisa learned several valuable lessons that day. She became an expert in the skill of blood glucose monitoring and insulin injections. Lisa knew she needed to be proficient and accurate in order to provide the correct insulin dosage, and she wanted to "do it right." But as she grew more comfortable in her psychomotor skills, Lisa began to see beyond her own world and the business of the shift. She began to notice both the physical and emotional world of her client. As Lisa reflects on this client and the care she delivered in those 8 hours, she takes another step toward becoming a competent and caring practitioner.

—Student: Lisa Lindley
—Faculty Member: Deb Filer, PhD, RN
College of St. Catherine, St Paul, MN

SKILL 34-1

OBTAINING A CAPILLARY BLOOD SPECIMEN TO MEASURE BLOOD GLUCOSE

PURPOSES
- To determine or monitor blood glucose levels of clients at risk for hyperglycemia or hypoglycemia
- To promote blood glucose regulation by the client
- To evaluate the effectiveness of insulin administration

ASSESSMENT
- Before obtaining a capillary blood specimen, determine
- The frequency and type of testing.
- The client's understanding of the procedure.
- The client's response to previous testing.
- Assess the client's skin at the puncture site to determine if it is intact and the circulation is not compromised. Check color, warmth, and capillary refill.
- Review the client's record for medications that may prolong bleeding such as anticoagulants.
- Assess the client's self-care abilities that may affect accuracy of test results, such as visual impairment and finger dexterity.

PLANNING

Delegation
Check the applicable nurse practice act and the facility policy and procedure manual to determine who can perform this skill. It is usually considered an invasive technique and one that requires problem solving and application of knowledge. It is the responsibility of the nurse to know the results of the test.

Equipment
- Blood glucose meter (glucometer)
- Blood glucose reagent strip compatible with the meter
- 2 × 2 gauze
- Warm cloth or other warming device (optional)
- Antiseptic swab
- Disposable gloves
- Sterile lancet
- Lancet injector

IMPLEMENTATION

Preparation
Review the type of meter and the manufacturer's instructions. Assemble the equipment at the bedside.

Performance
1. Prior to performing the procedure, introduce self and verify the client's identity using agency protocol. Explain to the client what you are going to do, why it is necessary, and how he or she can cooperate. Discuss how the results will be used in planning further care or treatments.
2. Perform hand hygiene and observe other appropriate infection control procedures (e.g., gloves).
3. Provide for client privacy.
4. Prepare the equipment.
   - Calibrate the meter and run a control sample according to the manufacturer's instructions.
5. Select and prepare the vascular puncture site.
   - Choose a vascular puncture site (e.g., the side of an adult's finger). Avoid sites beside bone. Wrap the finger first in a warm cloth, *or* hold a finger in a dependent position. If the earlobe is used, rub it gently with a small piece of gauze. **Rationale:** *These actions increase the blood flow to the area, ensure an adequate specimen, and reduce the need for a repeat puncture.*
   - Clean the site with the antiseptic swab or soap and water and allow it to dry completely. **Rationale:** *Alcohol can affect accuracy and the site burns when punctured when wet with alcohol.*
6. Obtain the blood specimen.
   - Put on gloves.
   - Place the injector, if used, against the site, and release the needle, thus permitting it to pierce the skin. Make sure the lancet is perpendicular to the site. **Rationale:** *The lancet is designed to pierce the skin at a specific depth when it is in a perpendicular position relative to the skin.* ❶

❶ Place the injector against the site.

     or
- Prick the site with a lancet or needle, using a darting motion.
- Gently squeeze (but do not touch) the puncture site until a large drop of blood forms. The size of the drop of blood can vary depending on the meter. Some meters require as little as 0.3 mL (Passanza, 2001) or not much larger than the period at the end of this sentence (Mensing, 2004).
- Hold the reagent strip under the puncture site until adequate blood covers the indicator square. The pad will absorb the blood and a chemical reaction will occur. Do not smear the blood. **Rationale:** *This will cause an inaccurate reading.* ❷ Some meters wick the blood by just touching the puncture site with the strip.
- Ask the client to apply pressure to the skin puncture site with a 2 × 2 or 4 × 4 gauze. **Rationale:** *Pressure will assist hemostasis.*
7. Expose the blood to the test strip for the period and the manner specified by the manufacturer. As soon as the blood is placed on the test strip:

OBTAINING A CAPILLARY BLOOD SPECIMEN TO MEASURE BLOOD GLUCOSE *continued*

❷ Gently squeeze a drop of blood onto the reagent strip.

- Follow the manufacturer's recommendations on the glucose meter and monitor for the amount of time indicated by the manufacturer. **Rationale:** *The blood must remain in contact with the test pad for a prescribed time to obtain accurate results.*
Some glucometers have the test strip placed in the machine before the specimen is obtained.
8. Measure the blood glucose.
- Place the strip into the meter according to the manufacturer's instructions. Some devices require that the strip be wiped or blotted after a designated period of time before being inserted in the meter. Other strips do not require blotting or wiping. Refer to the specific manufacturer's recommendations for the specific procedure.

❸ The glucose meter will display the glucose reading.

- After the designated time, most glucose meters will display the glucose reading automatically. Correct timing ensures accurate results. ❸
- Turn off the meter and discard the test strip and 2 x 2 gauze in a biohazard container. Discard the lancet into a sharps container.
9. Document the method of testing and results on the client's record. If appropriate, record the client's understanding and ability to demonstrate the technique. The client's record may also include a flow sheet on which capillary blood glucose results and the amount, type, route, and time of insulin administration are recorded.
10. Check for orders for sliding scale insulin based on capillary blood glucose results. Administer insulin as prescribed.

EVALUATION

- Compare glucose meter reading with normal blood glucose level, status of puncture site, and motivation of the client to perform the test independently.
- Relate blood glucose reading to previous readings and the client's current health status.

- Report abnormal results to the primary care provider.
- Conduct appropriate follow-up such as asking the client to explain the meaning of the results and/or demonstrating the procedure at the next scheduled test.

LIFESPAN CONSIDERATIONS **Capillary Blood Glucose**

INFANTS

- The outer aspect of the heel is the most common site for neonates and infants. Placing a warm cloth on the infant's heel often increases the blood flow to the area.

CHILDREN

- Use the side of a fingertip for a young client older than age 2, unless contraindicated.
- Allow the child to choose the puncture site, when possible.
- Praise the young client for cooperating and assure the child that the procedure is not a punishment.

ELDERS

- Elders may have arthritic joint changes, poor vision, or hand tremors and may need assistance using the glucose meter or obtaining a meter that accommodates their limitations.
- Elders may have difficulty obtaining diabetic supplies due to financial concerns or homebound status.
- Elders often have poor circulation. Warming the hands by wrapping with a warm washcloth for 3 to 5 minutes or placing the hand dependent for a few moments may help in obtaining a blood sample.

HOME CARE CONSIDERATIONS **Capillary Blood Glucose**

- Assess the client or caregiver's ability and willingness to perform blood glucose monitoring at home.
- Teach the proper use of the lancet and glucose monitor, and provide written guidelines. Allow time for a return demonstration. The client may need several visits to completely learn the procedure.
- Ensure the client's ability to obtain supplies and purchase reagent strips. The strips are relatively expensive and may not be covered by the client's insurance.

- Stress the importance of record keeping. Instruct the client on when to do glucose monitoring, how to record the blood glucose levels, and when to notify the primary care provider.
- Diabetic children who need to perform finger-sticks should be taught about safe practices for cleaning blood from surfaces (household bleach is best) and about safe storage of equipment to prevent young children from having access to it. Identify a place in the school where the child can store glucose-monitoring equipment and perform the procedure in private.

SPECIMEN COLLECTION

The nurse contributes to the assessment of a client's health status by collecting specimens of body fluids. All hospitalized clients have at least one laboratory specimen collected during their stay at the health care facility. Laboratory examination of specimens such as urine, blood, stool, sputum, and wound drainage provides important adjunct information for diagnosing health care problems and also provides a measure of the responses to therapy.

Nurses often assume the responsibility for specimen collection. Depending on the type of specimen and skill required, the nurse may be able to delegate this task to unlicensed assistive personnel (UAP) under the supervision of the professional nurse.

Nursing responsibilities associated with specimen collection include the following:

- Explain the purpose of the specimen collection and the procedure for obtaining the specimen. Clients may experience anxiety about the procedure, especially if it is perceived as being intrusive or if they fear an unknown test result. A clear explanation will facilitate the client's cooperation in the collection of the specimen. With proper instruction, many clients are able to collect their own specimen, which promotes independence and reduces or avoids embarrassment.
- Provide client comfort, privacy, and safety. Clients may experience embarrassment or discomfort when providing a specimen. The nurse should provide the client with as much privacy as possible and handle the specimen discreetly. The nurse needs to be nonjudgmental and sensitive to possible sociocultural beliefs that may affect the client's willingness to participate in the specimen collection.
- Use the correct procedure for obtaining a specimen or ensure that the client or staff follows the correct procedure. Aseptic technique is used in specimen collection to prevent contamination that can cause inaccurate test results. A nursing procedure or laboratory manual is often available if the nurse is unfamiliar with the procedure. If there is any question about the procedure, the nurse calls the laboratory for directions before collecting the specimen.
- Note relevant information on the laboratory requisition slip, for example, medications the client is taking that may affect the results.

- Transport the specimen to the laboratory promptly. Fresh specimens provide more accurate results.
- Report abnormal laboratory findings to the health care provider in a timely manner consistent with the severity of the abnormal results.

Stool Specimens

Analysis of stool specimens can provide information about a client's health condition. Some of the reasons for testing feces include the following:

- To determine the presence of **occult** (hidden) **blood.** Bleeding can occur as a result of ulcers, inflammatory disease, or tumors. The test for occult blood, often referred to as the **guaiac test,** can be readily performed by the nurse in the clinical area or by the client at home. Guaiac paper used in the test is sensitive to fecal blood content.
- To analyze for dietary products and digestive secretions. For example, an excessive amount of fat in the stool (**steatorrhea**) can indicate faulty absorption of fat from the small intestine. A decreased amount of bile can indicate obstruction of bile flow from the liver and gallbladder into the intestine. For these kinds of tests, the nurse needs to collect and send the total quantity of stool expelled at one time instead of a small sample.
- To detect the presence of ova and parasites. When collecting specimens for parasites, it is important that the sample be transported immediately to the lab while it is still warm. Usually three stool specimens, over a period of days, are evaluated to confirm the presence of and to identify the organism so that appropriate treatment can be ordered.
- To detect the presence of bacteria or viruses. Only a small amount of feces is required because the specimen will be cultured. Collection containers or tubes must be sterile and aseptic technique used during collection. Stools need to be sent immediately to the laboratory. The nurse needs to note on the lab requisition if the client is receiving any antibiotics.

Collecting Stool Specimens

The nurse is responsible for collecting stool specimens ordered for laboratory analysis. Before obtaining a specimen, the nurse needs to determine the reason for collecting the stool specimen and the correct method of obtaining and handling (i.e., how much stool to obtain, whether a preservative needs to be added to the stool, and whether it needs to be sent immediately to the laboratory). It may be necessary to confirm this information by checking with the agency laboratory. In many situations only a single specimen is required; in others, timed specimens are necessary, and every stool passed is collected within a designated time period.

UAP may obtain and collect stool specimen(s). The nurse, however, needs to consider the collection process before delegating this task. For example, a random stool specimen collected in a specimen container may be delegated, but a stool culture requiring a sterile swab in a test tube should be done by the nurse. An incorrect collection technique can cause inaccurate test results.

The task of obtaining and testing a stool specimen for occult blood may be performed by UAP. It is important that the nurse instruct the UAP to tell the nurse if blood is detected and/or whether the test is positive. In addition, the stool specimen should be saved to allow the nurse to repeat the test.

Nurses need to give clients the following instructions:

- Defecate in a clean bedpan or bedside commode.
- If possible, do not contaminate the specimen with urine or menstrual discharge. Void before the specimen collection.
- Do not place toilet tissue in the bedpan after defecation. Contents of the paper can affect the laboratory analysis.
- Notify the nurse as soon as possible after defecation, particularly for specimens that need to be sent to the laboratory immediately.

When obtaining stool samples—that is, when handling the client's bedpan, when transferring the stool sample to a specimen container, and when disposing of the bedpan contents—the nurse follows medical aseptic technique meticulously. Wear disposable gloves to prevent hand contamination and take care not to contaminate the outside of the specimen container. Use one or two clean tongue blades to transfer the specimen to the container and then wrap them in a paper towel before disposing of them in the waste container. This practice reduces the chance of contact with other articles and the spread of microorganisms. The amount of stool to be sent depends on the purpose for which the specimen is collected. Usually about 2.5 cm (1 in.) of formed stool or 15 to 30 mL of liquid stool is adequate. For some timed specimens, however, the entire stool passed may need to be sent. Visible pus, mucus, or blood should be included in sample specimens. For a stool culture, the nurse dips a sterile swab into the specimen, preferably where purulent fecal matter is present and, using sterile technique, places the swab in a sterile test tube.

Ensure that the specimen label and the laboratory requisition have the correct information on them and are securely attached to the specimen container. Inappropriate identification of the specimen risks errors of diagnosis or therapy for the client.

Because fresh specimens provide the most accurate results, the nurse sends the specimen to the laboratory immediately. If this is not possible, the nurse follows the directions on the specimen container. In some instances refrigeration is indicated, because bacteriologic changes take place in stool specimens left at room temperature. To prevent contamination, never place a stool specimen in a refrigerator that contains food or medication.

Document all relevant information. Record the collection of the specimen on the client's chart and on the nursing care plan. Include in the recording the date and time of the collection and all nursing assessments (e.g., color, odor, consistency, and amount of feces); presence of abnormal constituents, such as blood or mucus; results of test for occult blood if obtained; discomfort during or after defecation; status of perianal skin; and any bleeding from the anus after defecation.

Testing Feces for Occult Blood

A commonly used test product to measure occult blood is the Hemoccult test, which uses a chemical **reagent** (substance used in a chemical reaction to detect a specific substance). This reagent detects the presence of the enzyme peroxidase in the hemoglobin molecule. To perform the test, the nurse or client uses a tongue blade to place a small amount of stool on a slide or card and then closes the card. The card is turned over and a few drops of a reagent are placed onto the smear on the back of the card. The nurse then observes for a color change (Figure 34-3 ■). A

A

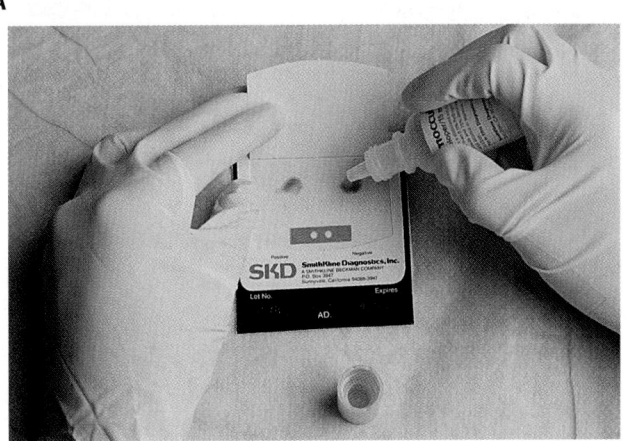

B

Figure 34-3 ■ *A,* Opening the front cover of a Hemoccult slide and applying a thin smear of feces on the slide. *B,* Opening the flap on the back of the slide and applying two drops of developing fluid over each smear.

Photographer: Elena Dorfman

blue color indicates a guaiac positive result, that is, the presence of occult blood. No color change or any color other than blue is a negative finding, indicating the absence of blood in the stool.

Certain foods, medications, and vitamin C can produce inaccurate test results. False-positive results can occur if the client has recently ingested (a) red meat (beef, lamb, liver, and processed meats); (b) raw vegetables or fruits, particularly radishes, turnips, horseradish, and melons; or (c) certain medications that irritate the gastric mucosa and cause bleeding, such as aspirin or other nonsteroidal anti-inflammatory drugs, steroids, iron preparations, and anticoagulants. False-negative results can occur if the client has taken more than 250 mg per day of vitamin C from all sources (dietary and supplemental) up to 3 days before the test—even if bleeding is present. Guidelines for instructing clients to assess their stool for occult blood are listed in Client Teaching.

CLIENT TEACHING
Assessing Stool for Occult Blood

- Avoid restricted foods, medications, and vitamin C for the period recommended by the manufacturer and during the test. Usually specified foods and vitamin C are restricted for 3 days before the test and specified medications for 7 days before the test.
- Use a ballpoint pen to label the specimens with your name, address, age, and date of specimen. Usually three specimens are collected from consecutive and different bowel movements. Each specimen must be dated accurately.
- Avoid collecting specimens during your menstrual period and for 3 days afterward, and while you have bleeding hemorrhoids or blood in your urine.
- Remove toilet bowl cleaners from the toilet bowl. Flush the toilet twice before proceeding with the test.
- Avoid contaminating the specimen with urine or toilet tissue. Empty your bladder before the test. To facilitate specimen collection, transfer the stool to a clean, dry container. Wear disposable gloves.
- Use the tongue blade provided to transfer the specimen to the test folder or tape. Only a small amount of stool is required. Take the sample from the center of a formed stool to ensure a uniform sample.
- Wrap the tongue blade in a paper towel and dispose of it in the waste receptacle. Do not flush the stick.
- Follow the manufacturer's directions explicitly for the test product being used. Test products vary. For example, for the Hemoccult test, a thin layer of feces is smeared over the boxes inside the envelope, and a drop of developing solution is applied on the opposite side of the specimen paper. For the Hematest, a thin layer of feces is smeared onto guaiac filter paper, a tablet is placed in the middle of the specimen, and two or three drops of water are added to the tablet. If there is space for two specimens in the test folder, take the sample from two different areas of the stool specimen.
- Consult your health care provider if there is any problem understanding the instructions.
- Return completed specimens to your primary care provider or laboratory as instructed.

LIFESPAN CONSIDERATIONS
Stool Specimen

INFANTS

- To collect a stool specimen for an infant, the stool is scraped from the diaper, being careful not to contaminate the stool with urine.

CHILDREN

- A child who is toilet trained should be able to provide a fecal specimen, but may prefer being assisted by a parent.
- When explaining the procedure to the child, use words appropriate for the child's age rather than medical terms. Ask the parent what words the family normally uses to describe a bowel movement.
- A specimen for pinworms is collected by the parent early in the morning, after sleep and before the child has a bowel movement. Scotch tape is attached to a tongue blade and the sticky side is laid flat against the perineum and anus to pick up any eggs or small worms. The tongue blade is then examined under a microscope.

ELDERS

- Elders may need assistance if serial stool specimens are required.

HOME CARE CONSIDERATIONS
Stool Specimen

- Ask the client or caregiver to call when the stool specimen is obtained. If a laboratory test is needed, the home health nurse can pick up the specimen or a family member may take it to the laboratory.
- Place the stool specimen inside a plastic biohazard bag. Carry the bag in a sealed container marked "biohazard" and take it to the laboratory promptly. Do not expose the specimen to extreme temperatures in the car.

Urine Specimens

The nurse is responsible for collecting urine specimens for a number of tests: **clean voided** specimens for routine urinalysis, **clean-catch** or **midstream urine specimens** for urine culture, and timed urine specimens for a variety of tests that depend on the client's specific health problem. Urine specimen collection may require collection via straight catheter insertion. If this is necessary, refer to Chapter 48, Skill 48-2. ∞

Clean Voided Urine Specimen

A clean voided specimen is usually adequate for routine examination. Many clients are able to collect a clean voided specimen and provide the specimen independently with minimal instructions. Male clients generally are able to void directly into the specimen container, and female clients usually sit or squat over the toilet, holding the container between their legs during voiding. Routine urine examination is usually done on the first voided specimen in the morning because it tends to have a higher, more uniform concentration and a more acidic pH than specimens later in the day.

At least 10 mL of urine is generally sufficient for a routine urinalysis. Clients who are seriously ill, physically incapacitated, or disoriented may need to use a bedpan or urinal in bed; others may require supervision or assistance in the bathroom. Whatever the situation, clear and specific directions are required:

- The specimen must be free of fecal contamination, so urine must be kept separate from feces.
- Female clients should discard the toilet tissue in the toilet or in a waste bag rather than in the bedpan because tissue in the specimen makes laboratory analysis more difficult.
- Put the lid tightly on the container to prevent spillage of the urine and contamination of other objects.
- If the outside of the container has been contaminated by urine, clean it with a disinfectant.

The nurse must (a) make sure that the specimen label and the laboratory requisition carry the correct information and (b) attach them securely to the specimen. Inappropriate identification of the specimen can lead to errors of diagnosis or therapy for the client.

UAP may be assigned to collect a routine urine specimen. Provide the UAP with clear directions on how to instruct the client to collect his or her own urine specimen or how to correctly collect the specimen for the client who may need to use a bedpan or urinal.

CLINICAL ALERT

Kidney function directly relates to cardiac output. Therefore, any health problem that changes cardiac output may affect urine output. ■

Figure 34-4 ■ Disposable clean-catch specimen equipment.
Photographer: Jenny Thomas

Clean-Catch or Midstream Urine Specimen

Clean-catch or midstream voided specimens are collected when a urine culture is ordered to identify microorganisms causing urinary tract infection. Although some contamination by skin bacteria may occur with a clean-catch specimen, the risk of introducing microorganisms into the urinary tract through catheterization is more significant. Care is taken to ensure that the specimen is as free as possible from contamination by microorganisms around the urinary meatus. Clean-catch specimens are collected into a sterile specimen container with a lid. Disposable clean-catch kits are available (Figure 34-4 ■). Skill 34-2 explains how to collect a clean-catch urine specimen for culture.

Timed Urine Specimen

Some urine examinations require collection of all urine produced and voided over a specific period of time, ranging from 1 to 2 hours to 24 hours. Timed specimens generally either are refrigerated or contain a preservative to prevent bacterial growth or decomposition of urine components. Each voiding of urine is collected in a small, clean container and then emptied immediately into the large refrigerated bottle or carton.

COLLECTING A URINE SPECIMEN FOR CULTURE AND SENSITIVITY BY CLEAN CATCH

SKILL 34-2

PURPOSE
- To determine the presence of microorganisms, the type of organism(s), and the antibiotics to which the organisms are sensitive

ASSESSMENT
- Determine the ability of the client to provide the specimen.
- Assess the color, odor, and consistency of the urine and the presence of clinical signs of urinary tract infection (e.g., frequency, urgency, dysuria, hematuria, flank pain, cloudy urine with foul odor).

PLANNING

Delegation

UAP may perform the collection of a clean-catch or midstream urine specimen. It is important, however, that the nurse inform the unlicensed person about how to instruct the client in the correct process for obtaining the specimen. Proper cleansing of the urethra should be emphasized to avoid contaminating the urine specimen.

Equipment

Equipment used varies from agency to agency. Some agencies use commercially prepared disposable clean-catch kits. Others are

agency-prepared sterile trays. Both prepared trays and kits generally contain the following items:

- Clean gloves
- Antiseptic towelettes
- Sterile specimen container
- Specimen identification label

In addition the nurse needs to obtain the following:

- Completed laboratory requisition form
- Urine receptacle, if the client is not ambulatory
- Basin of warm water, soap, washcloth, and towel for the nonambulatory client

continued on page 812

- Record collection of the specimen, time started and completed, and any pertinent observations of the urine on appropriate records.

CLINICAL ALERT

If the client or staff forgets and discards the client's urine during a timed collection, the procedure must be restarted from the beginning. ■

Indwelling Catheter Specimen

Sterile urine specimens can be obtained from closed drainage systems by inserting a sterile needle attached to a syringe through a drainage port in the tubing. Aspiration of urine from catheters can be done only with self-sealing rubber catheters—not plastic, silicone, or Silastic catheters. When self-sealing rubber catheters are used, the needle is inserted just above the location where the catheter is attached to the drainage tubing. The area from which to obtain urine may be marked by a patch on the catheter (see Figure 34-5 ■). Newer closed drainage urinary systems now have needleless ports which avoids having to use a needle to obtain a sample. This protects the nurse from a needle-stick injury and maintains the integrity and sterility of the catheter system by eliminating the need to puncture the tubing (Davis, 2004). The needleless port accepts a Luer-Lok syringe (Figure 34-6 ■). Position the syringe perpendicular to the center of the port and insert, twist, and lock into the port. When the specimen is obtained and the syringe removed, the port seals itself.

To collect a specimen from a Foley (retention) catheter or a drainage tube, follow these steps:

- Put on disposable gloves.
- If there is no urine in the catheter, clamp the drainage tubing at least 3 inches below the sampling port for about 30 minutes. This allows fresh urine to collect in the catheter.
- Wipe the area where the needle or Luer-Lok syringe will be inserted with a disinfectant swab. The site should be distal to the tube leading to the balloon to avoid puncturing this tube. Disinfecting the needle insertion site re-

Figure 34-6 ■ A needleless port that allows for needle-free aspiration of urine.

moves any microorganisms on the surface of the catheter, thereby avoiding contamination of the needle and the entrance of microorganisms into the catheter.

- Insert the needle at a 30- to 45-degree angle (Figure 34-6). This angle of entrance facilitates self-sealing of the rubber. Insert the Luer-Lck syringe at a 90-degree angle for the needleless port.
- Unclamp the catheter.
- Withdraw the required amount of urine, for example, 3 mL for a urine culture or 30 mL for a routine urinalysis.
- Transfer the urine to the specimen container. If a sterile culture tube is used, make sure the needle or syringe (depending on the system) does not touch the outside of the container.
- Discard the syringe and needle or syringe (depending on the system) in an appropriate sharps container.
- Cap the container.
- Remove gloves and discard appropriately.
- Label the container, and send the urine to the laboratory immediately for analysis or refrigeration.
- Record collection of the specimen and any pertinent observations of the urine on the appropriate records.

Urine Testing

Several simple urine tests are often done by nurses on the nursing units. These include tests for specific gravity, pH, and the presence of abnormal constituents such as glucose, ketones, protein, and occult blood.

Nurses in a health care facility or clients in the home setting can use commercially prepared kits to test abnormal constituents in the urine. These kits contain the required equipment and an appropriate reagent which may be in the form of a tablet, fluid, or paper test strip or dipstick. When the urine contacts the reagent a chemical reaction occurs, causing a color change that is then compared with a chart to interpret the significance of the color (Figure 34-7 ■). Specific directions for the amount of urine needed, the time required for the chemical reaction, and the meaning of the colors produced vary among manufacturers.

Figure 34-5 ■ Obtaining a urine specimen from a retention catheter. *A,* From a specific area near the end of the catheter; *B,* from an access port in the tubing.

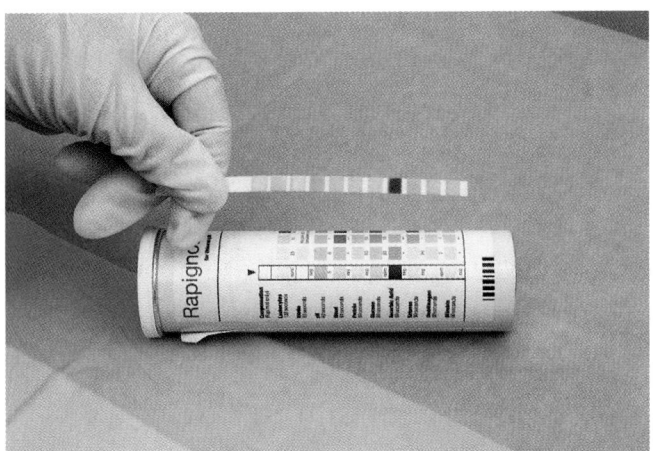

Figure 34-7 ■ After dipping the reagent strip (dipstick) into fresh urine, wait the stated time period and compare the results to the color chart.

Thus it is essential that nurses and clients read and follow directions supplied by each manufacturer. In addition, testing materials need to be checked to ascertain that they are not outdated.

Urine testing may be performed by UAP. It is important that the UAP understands the specific specimen collection procedure and reports the results of the test to the nurse. Inform the UAP to save the urine sample to allow the nurse to repeat the test if necessary.

SPECIFIC GRAVITY. **Specific gravity** is an indicator of urine concentration, or the amount of solutes (metabolic wastes and electrolytes) present in the urine. The specific gravity of distilled water is 1.00; the specific gravity of urine normally ranges from 1.010 to 1.025. As urine becomes more concentrated, its specific gravity increases. Excess fluid intake or diseases affecting the ability of the kidneys to concentrate urine can result in low specific gravity readings. A high specific gravity may indicate fluid deficit or dehydration, or excess solutes such as glucose in the urine. Specific gravity can be measured with the use of a multiple-test dipstick that has a separate reagent area for specific gravity.

URINARY pH. Urinary pH is measured to determine the relative acidity or alkalinity of urine and assess the client's acid–base status. Quantitative measurements of urine pH can be performed in the laboratory, but dipsticks or litmus paper often are used on nursing units or in clinics to obtain less precise pH measurements. Urine normally is slightly acidic, with an average pH of 6 (7 is neutral, less than 7 is acidic, greater than 7 is alkaline). Because the kidneys play a critical role in regulating acid–base balance, assessment of urine pH can be useful in determining whether the kidneys are responding appropriately to acid–base imbalances. In metabolic acidosis, urine pH should decrease as the kidneys excrete hydrogen ions; in metabolic alkalosis, the pH should increase (see Chapter 52 ∞).

GLUCOSE. Urine is tested for glucose to screen clients for diabetes mellitus and to assess clients during pregnancy for abnormal glucose tolerance. Normally, the amount of glucose in the urine is negligible, although individuals who have ingested large amounts of sugar may show small amounts of glucose in their urine.

Testing urine for glucose is not a measure of current blood glucose level and is considered an inadequate measurement. The American Diabetes Association (2000, p. 66) states that testing urine for glucose is *only* for people who *cannot or will not* test their blood glucose levels. It is important for clients to understand that urine testing is considered an inadequate measurement of blood glucose.

KETONES. Ketone bodies, a product of the breakdown of fatty acids, normally are not present in the urine. They may, however, be found in the urine of clients with poorly controlled diabetes. Urine testing for ketone level is advised for type 1 diabetics who are at home and not feeling well, who are running a fever, or who have blood glucose consistently over 240 mg/dL (American Diabetes Association, 2000). Urine ketone testing with reagent tablets or a dipstick is also used to evaluate ketoacidosis in clients who are alcoholic, fasting, starving, or consuming high-protein diets.

PROTEIN. Protein molecules normally are too large to escape from glomerular capillaries into the filtrate. If the glomerular membrane has been damaged, however (e.g., because of an inflammatory process such as glomerulonephritis), it can become "leaky," allowing proteins to escape. Urine testing for the presence of protein generally is done with a reagent strip (commonly referred to as a *dipstick*).

OCCULT BLOOD. Normal urine is free from blood. When blood is present, it may be clearly visible or not visible (occult). Commercial reagent strips are used to test for occult blood in the urine.

CLINICAL ALERT

Blood in urine is always an indicator of damage to the kidney or urinary tract (Fischbach, 2004, p. 189). ■

OSMOLALITY. **Urine osmolality** is a measure of the solute concentration of urine that is a more exact measurement of urine concentration than specific gravity. It is also used to monitor fluid and electrolyte balance. The particles included are nitrogenous wastes, such as creatinine, urea, and uric acid. Normal values are 500 to 800 mOsm/kg. An increased urine osmolality indicates a fluid volume deficit; a decreased urine osmolality reflects a fluid volume excess. This test is sent to the laboratory rather than being tested at the bedside like the previous tests.

Sputum Specimens

Sputum is the mucous secretion from the lungs, bronchi, and trachea. It is important to differentiate it from **saliva,** the clear liquid secreted by the salivary glands in the mouth, sometimes referred to as "spit." Healthy individuals do not produce sputum. Clients need to cough to bring sputum up from the lungs, bronchi, and trachea into the mouth in order to expectorate it into a collecting container.

A UAP can obtain a sputum specimen that is expectorated by a client. It is important to instruct the UAP on when to collect the specimen, how to position the client, and how to correctly collect the specimen. Obtaining a sputum specimen by use of pharyngeal suctioning, however, should be performed by the nurse because it is an invasive, sterile process and requires knowledge application and problem solving. A "sputum trap" is used when the specimen is obtained by suctioning. (See Chapter 50, Skill 50-2.) ∞

Sputum specimens are usually collected for one or more of the following reasons:

- For culture and sensitivity to identify a specific microorganism and its drug sensitivities.
- For cytology to identify the origin, structure, function, and pathology of cells. Specimens for cytology often require serial collection of three early-morning specimens and are tested to identify cancer in the lung and its specific cell type.
- For acid-fast bacillus (AFB), which also requires serial collection, often for 3 consecutive days, to identify the presence of tuberculosis (TB). Some agencies use a special glass container when the presence of AFB is suspected.
- To assess the effectiveness of therapy.

Sputum specimens are often collected in the morning. Upon awakening, the client can cough up the secretions that have accumulated during the night. Sometimes specimens are collected during postural drainage, when the client can usually produce sputum. When a client cannot cough, the nurse must sometimes use pharyngeal suctioning to obtain a specimen.

To collect a sputum specimen, the nurse follows these steps:

- Offer mouth care so that the specimen will not be contaminated with microorganisms from the mouth.
- Ask the client to breathe deeply and then cough up 1 to 2 tablespoons, or 15 to 30 mL (4 to 8 fluid drams), of sputum.
- Wear gloves and personal protective equipment to avoid direct contact with the sputum. Follow special precautions if tuberculosis is suspected, obtaining the specimen in a room equipped with a special airflow system or ultraviolet light, or outdoors. If these options are not available, wear a mask capable of filtering droplet nuclei.
- Ask the client to **expectorate** (spit out) the sputum into the specimen container. Make sure the sputum does not contact the outside of the container (Figure 34-8 ■). If the outside of the container does become contaminated, wash it with a disinfectant.
- Following sputum collection, offer mouthwash to remove any unpleasant taste.
- Label and transport the specimen to the laboratory. Ensure that the specimen label and the laboratory requisition contain the correct information. Arrange for the specimen to be sent to the laboratory immediately or refrigerated. Bacterial cultures must be started immediately before any contaminating organisms can grow, multiply, and produce false results.
- Document the collection of the sputum specimen on the client's chart. Include the amount, color, consistency (thick, tenacious, watery), presence of **hemoptysis** (blood in the sputum), odor of the sputum, any measures needed to obtain the specimen (e.g., postural drainage), and any discomfort experienced by the client.

Figure 34-8 ■ Sputum specimen container.
Photographer: Elena Dorfman

Throat Culture

A throat culture sample is collected from the mucosa of the oropharynx and tonsillar regions using a culture swab. The sample is then cultured and examined for the presence of disease-producing microorganisms. Obtaining a throat culture is an invasive procedure that requires the application of scientific knowledge and potential problem solving to ensure client safety. Thus, it is best for the nurse to perform this procedure.

To obtain a throat culture specimen, the nurse puts on clean gloves, then inserts the swab into the oropharynx and runs the swab along the tonsils and areas on the pharynx that are reddened or contain exudate. The gag reflex, active in some clients, may be decreased by having the client sit upright if health permits, open the mouth, extend the tongue, and say "ah," and by taking the specimen quickly. The sitting position and extension of the tongue help expose the pharynx; saying "ah" relaxes the throat muscles and helps minimize contraction of the constrictor muscle of the pharynx (the gag reflex). If the posterior pharynx cannot be seen, use a light and depress the tongue with a tongue blade (see Figure 34-9 ■).

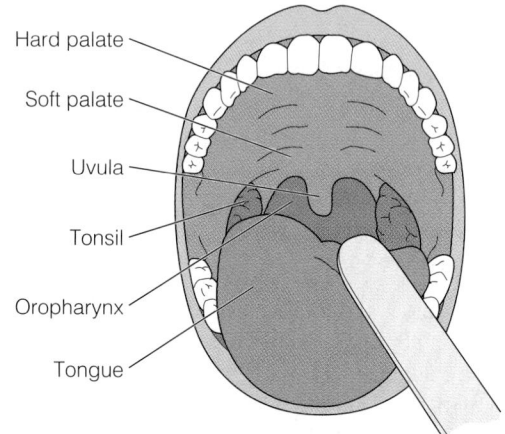

Hard palate
Soft palate
Uvula
Tonsil
Oropharynx
Tongue

Figure 34-9 ■ Depressing the tongue to view the pharynx.

Figure 34-10 ■ Enhanced color x-ray of the colon during a barium enema exam.

(CNRI/Science Photo Library; Photo Researchers, Inc.)

VISUALIZATION PROCEDURES

Visualization procedures include *indirect visualization* (noninvasive) and *direct visualization* (invasive) techniques for visualizing body organ and system functions.

Clients with Gastrointestinal Alterations

Direct visualization techniques include **anoscopy,** the viewing of the anal canal; **proctoscopy,** the viewing of the rectum; **proctosigmoidoscopy,** the viewing of the rectum and sigmoid colon; and **colonoscopy,** the viewing of the large intestine. Indirect visualization of the gastrointestinal tract is achieved by roentgenography. X-rays of the gastrointestinal tract can detect strictures, obstructions, tumors, ulcers, inflammatory disease, or other structural changes such as hiatal hernias. Visualization of the tract is enhanced by the introduction of a radiopaque substance such as barium. For examination of the upper gastrointestinal tract or small bowel, the client drinks the barium sulfate. This examination is often referred to as a *barium swallow.* For examination of the lower gastrointestinal tract, the client is given an enema containing the barium. This examination is commonly referred to as a *barium enema.* These x-rays usually include fluoroscopic examination; that is, projection of the x-ray films onto a screen, which permits continuous observation of the flow of barium (Figure 34-10 ■). Nurses are responsible for preparing clients before these studies and for follow-up care.

Clients with Urinary Alterations

Visualization procedures also may be used to evaluate urinary function. An x-ray of the **kidneys/ureters/bladder** is commonly referred to as a **KUB. Intravenous pyelography (IVP)** and **retrograde pyelography** also are radiographic studies used to evaluate the urinary tract. In an intravenous pyelogram, contrast medium is injected intravenously; during retrograde pyelography, the contrast medium is instilled directly into the kidney pelvis via the urethra, bladder, and ureters. Following injection or instillation of the contrast medium, x-rays are taken to evaluate urinary tract structures. Renal **ultrasonography** is a noninvasive test that uses reflected sound waves to visualize the kidneys. During a **cystoscopy,** the bladder, ureteral orifices, and urethra can be directly visualized using a **cystoscope,** a lighted instrument inserted through the urethra. Nurses are responsible for preparing clients before these studies and for follow-up care.

Clients with Cardiopulmonary Alterations

A number of visualization procedures can be done to examine the cardiovascular system and respiratory tract.

Electrocardiography provides a graphic recording of the heart's electrical activity. Electrodes placed on the skin transmit the electrical impulses to an oscilloscope or graphic recorder. With the wave forms recorded, the **electrocardiogram (ECG)** can then be examined to detect dysrhythmias and alterations in conduction indicative of myocardial damage, enlargement of the heart, or drug effects.

Stress electrocardiography uses ECGs to assess the client's response to an increased cardiac workload during exercise. As the body's demand for oxygen increases with exercising, the cardiac workload increases, as does the oxygen demand of the heart muscle itself. Clients with coronary artery disease may develop chest pain and characteristic ECG changes during exercise.

Angiography is an invasive procedure requiring informed consent of the client. A radiopaque dye is injected into the vessels to be examined. Using fluoroscopy and x-rays, the flow through the vessels is assessed and areas of narrowing or blockage can be observed. Coronary angiography is performed to evaluate the extent of coronary artery disease; pulmonary angiography may be performed to assess the pulmonary vascular system, particularly if pulmonary emboli are suspected. Other vessels that may be studied include the carotid and cerebral arteries, the renal arteries, and the vessels of the lower extremities.

An **echocardiogram** is a noninvasive test that uses ultrasound to visualize structures of the heart and evaluate left ventricular function. Images are produced as ultrasound waves reflect back to a transducer after striking cardiac structures. The nurse should tell the client that this test causes no discomfort, although the conductive gel used may be cold.

X-ray examination of the chest is done both to diagnose disease and to assess the progress of a disease. For an x-ray examination, the nurse needs to inform the client that jewelry and clothing from the waist up must be removed.

A **lung scan,** also known as a V/Q (ventilation/perfusion) scan, records the emissions from radioisotopes that indicate how well gas and blood are traveling through the lungs. The *perfusion scan* (Q scan—P usually stands for "pulmonary," so apparently the next letter in the alphabet was used for "perfusion") is used to assess blood flow through the pulmonary vascular system. For this, the radioisotope is injected intravenously and measured as it circulates through the lung. The *ventilation scan* (V scan) detects ventilation abnormalities, particularly in clients with emphysema. For this scan, the client inhales a radioactive gas through a mask and then exhales it into room air. The client needs to be informed that no radiation precautions are necessary because the amount of radioactivity is very small. The scan may take 20 to 40 minutes.

Laryngoscopy and bronchoscopy are sterile procedures that are conducted with a laryngoscope and bronchoscope, respectively. Tissue samples may also be taken for biopsy. A local anesthetic is usually given before the examination. A local anesthetic is sprayed on the client's pharynx to prevent gagging; alternatively, the client gargles with an anesthetic to anesthetize the throat. The bronchoscope is then inserted to visualize the larynx or bronchi (Figure 34-11 ■). Informed consent is required for these procedures.

Computed Tomography

Computed tomography (CT), also called *CT scanning, computerized tomography,* or *computerized axial tomography (CAT),*

Figure 34-11 ■ Bronchoscopy.

(From Fremgen, Bonnie F., Frucht, Suzanne S., *Medical Terminology: A Living Language,* 3rd ed. © 2005. Electronically reproduced by permission of Pearson Education, Inc., Upper Saddle River, New Jersey.)

is a painless, noninvasive x-ray procedure that has the unique capability of distinguishing minor differences in the density of tissues. The CT produces a three-dimensional image of the organ or structure, making it more sensitive than the x-ray machine.

Magnetic Resonance Imaging

Magnetic resonance imaging (MRI) is a noninvasive diagnostic scanning technique in which the client is placed in a magnetic field. Clients with implanted metal devices (e.g., pacemaker, metal hip prosthesis) cannot undergo an MRI because of the strong magnetic field. There is no exposure to radiation. If a contrast media is injected during the procedure, it is not an iodine contrast. Another advantage to the MRI is that it provides a better contrast between normal and abnormal tissue than the CT scan. It is, however, more costly.

Reports have shown that body art may cause problems to the client during an MRI (Armstrong & Elkins, 2005). Tattoo pigments may contain metal substances which create an electric current that can cause redness and swelling similar to a first-degree burn at the site of the tattoo. Permanent cosmetics (e.g., tattooed eyeliner, eyebrows, lip liner) may cause similar problems. The Society of Permanent Cosmetic Professionals (SPCP) (2005) states that the concentration of zinc oxide is low and the chances of diagnostic imaging problems are remote. Potential problems, however, can be avoided by wearing goggles to cover permanent cosmetics around the eyes. Metal body-piercing jewelry should be removed before an MRI. If the client is worried about the piercing tract closing, a sterile plastic IV catheter can be used to replace the jewelry and the pierced area can be covered by a sterile dressing during the MRI.

Many transdermal patches contain a foil backing which creates an electric current that can lead to intense heat and a burn (Karch, 2004). Again, it is important to ask clients if they are using a transdermal patch before undergoing an MRI. Because the patch may lose its adhesiveness, advise the client to apply a new patch after the MRI.

CLINICAL ALERT

Advise clients to inform the MRI operator if they have a tattoo or permanent makeup and to let the operator know of any unusual sensations felt at the site of the tattoo during the MRI. ■

The MRI is commonly used for visualization of the brain, spine, limbs and joints, heart, blood vessels, abdomen, and pelvis. The procedure involves the client lying on a platform that moves into either a narrow, closed, high-magnet scanner, or into an open, low-magnet scanner. The client must lie very still. A two-way communication system is used to monitor the client's response and to help relieve feelings of claustrophobia. Earplugs are offered to the client to reduce the discomfort from the loud noises that occur during the test. The procedure lasts between 60 and 90 minutes (Figure 34-12 ■).

Nuclear Imaging Studies

Fischbach (2004, p. 655) states that nuclear scans study the "physiology or function" of an organ system in contrast to other studies (e.g., CT, MRI, x-ray) which visualize "anatomic" structures. A **radiopharmaceutical,** a pharmaceutical (targeted to a specific organ) labeled with a radioisotope, is administered through various routes for the test. Clients retain the radioisotope for a relatively short time with the most common radio-

Figure 34-13 ■ PET scan comparing the metabolic activity levels of a normal brain and the brain of an individual with Alzheimer's disease. Red and yellow colors indicate high activity levels; blue colors represent low activity levels.

(Monte S. Buchsbaum, M. D.)

pharmaceutical having a half-life of 6 hours. A gamma camera is placed over the part of the body under study. The camera, which is networked with a computer, converts the emission of the radioisotope and forms a detailed image. An equal distribution of color is normal; however, darker spots ("hot" spots) indicate hyperfunction and lighter areas ("cold" spots) indicate hypofunction (Fischbach, 2004). **Positron emission tomography (PET)** is a noninvasive radiologic study that involves the injection or inhalation of a radioisotope. Images are created as the radioisotope is distributed in the body. This allows study of various aspects of organ function and may include evaluation of blood flow and tumor growth, for example (Figure 34-13 ■).

ASPIRATION/BIOPSY

Aspiration is the withdrawal of fluid that has abnormally collected (e.g., pleural cavity, abdominal cavity) or to obtain a specimen (e.g., cerebral spinal fluid). A **biopsy** is the removal and examination of tissue. Usually the biopsy is performed to determine a diagnosis or to detect malignancy. Both aspiration and biopsy are invasive procedures and require strict sterile technique.

CLINICAL ALERT

Determine if the facility requires a signed informed-consent form for the aspiration/biopsy procedure. ■

Lumbar Puncture

In a **lumbar puncture** (LP, or spinal tap), cerebrospinal fluid (CSF) is withdrawn through a needle (Figure 34-14 ■) inserted into the subarachnoid space of the spinal canal between the third

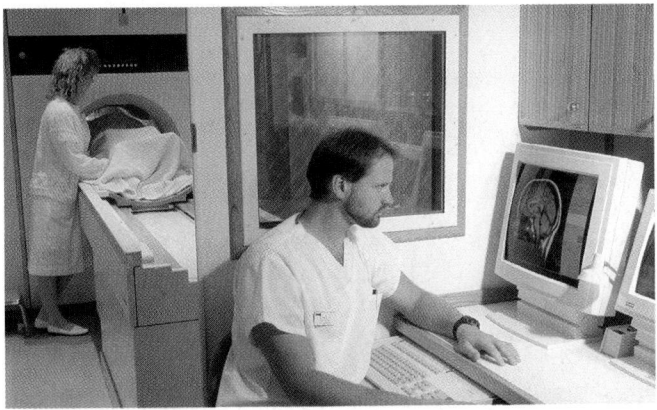

Figure 34-12 ■ MRI lab.

(Will and Deni McIntyre/Photo Researchers, Inc.)

MediaLink

PET and SPECT Scans Animation

Figure 34-14 ■ A spinal needle with the stylet protruding from the hub.

and fourth lumbar vertebrae or between the fourth and fifth lumbar vertebrae. At this level the needle avoids damaging the spinal cord and major nerve roots (Figure 34-15 ■). The client is positioned laterally with the head bent toward the chest, the knees flexed onto the abdomen, and the back at the edge of the

bed or examining table (Figure 34-16 ■). In this position the back is arched, increasing the spaces between the vertebrae so that the spinal needle can be inserted readily. During a lumbar puncture, the primary care provider frequently takes CSF pressure readings using a **manometer,** a glass or plastic tube calibrated in millimeters (Figure 34-17 ■).

LIFESPAN CONSIDERATIONS
Lumbar Puncture

CHILDREN

- Briefly demonstrate the procedure on a doll or stuffed animal. Allow time to answer questions.
- One member of the health care team should stay in close physical contact with the child, maintain eye contact, and talk to and reassure the child during the procedure.

ELDERS

- Some clients need help maintaining the flexed position due to arthritis, weakness, or tremors.
- Provide an extra blanket to keep the client warm during the procedure. Elders have a decreased metabolism and less subcutaneous fat.
- If the client has a hearing loss, speak slowly, distinctly, and loud enough, especially when unable to make eye contact.

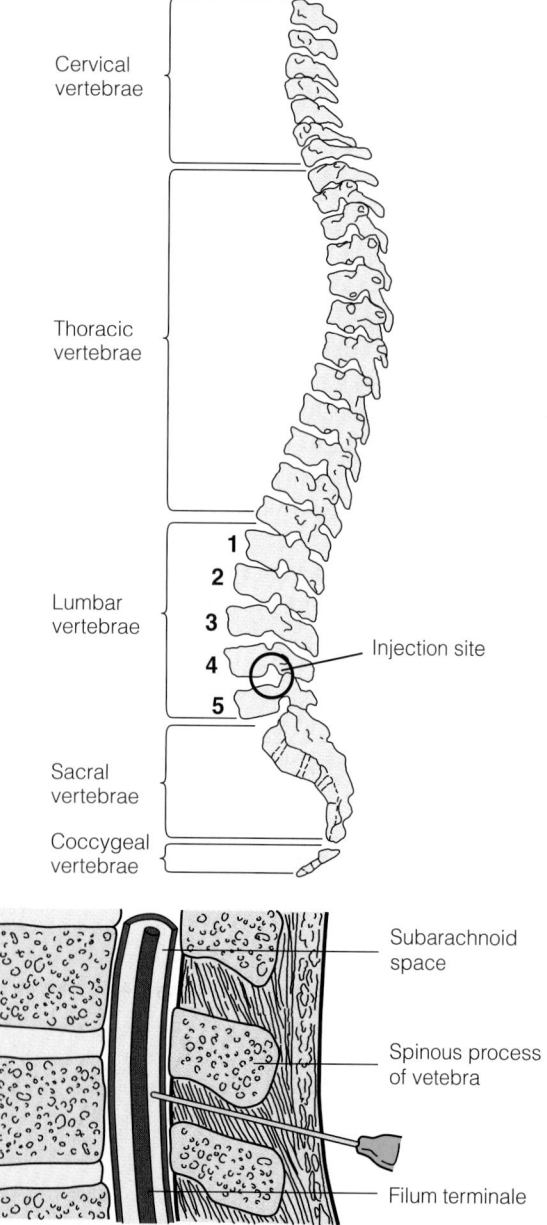

Figure 34-15 ■ A diagram of the vertebral column, indicating a site for insertion of the lumbar puncture needle into the subarachnoid space of the spinal canal.

Figure 34-16 ■ Supporting the client for a lumbar puncture.

Figure 34-17 ■ A preassembled lumbar puncture set. Note the manometer at the top of the set.

Abdominal Paracentesis

Normally the body creates just enough peritoneal fluid for lubrication. The fluid is continuously formed and absorbed into the lymphatic system. However, in some disease processes, a large amount of fluid accumulates in the abdominal cavity; this condition is called **ascites.** Normal ascitic fluid is serous, clear, and light yellow in color. An **abdominal paracentesis** is carried out to obtain a fluid specimen for laboratory study and to relieve pressure on the abdominal organs due to the presence of excess fluid.

A primary care provider performs the procedure with the assistance of a nurse. Strict sterile technique is followed. A common site for abdominal paracentesis is midway between the umbilicus and the symphysis pubis on the midline (Figure 34-18 ■). The primary care provider makes a small incision with a scalpel, inserts the **trocar** (a sharp, pointed instrument) and **cannula** (tube), and then withdraws the trocar, which is inside the cannula (Figure 34-19 ■). Tubing is attached to the cannula and the fluid flows through the tubing into a receptacle. If the purpose of the paracentesis is to obtain a specimen, the primary care provider may use a long aspirating needle attached to a syringe rather than making an incision and using a trocar and cannula. Normally about 1,500 mL is the maximum amount of fluid drained at one time to avoid hypovolemic shock. The fluid is drained very slowly for the same reason. Some fluid is placed in the specimen container before the cannula is withdrawn. The small incision may or may not be sutured; in either case, it is covered with a small sterile bandage.

Figure 34-18 ■ A common site for an abdominal paracentesis.

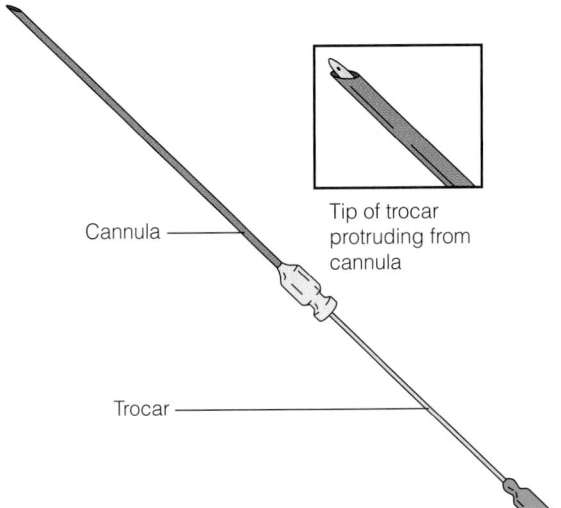

Figure 34-19 ■ A trocar and cannula may be used for an abdominal paracentesis.

Thoracentesis

Normally, only sufficient fluid to lubricate the pleura is present in the pleural cavity. However, excessive fluid can accumulate as a result of injury, infection, or other pathology. In such a case or in the case of pneumothorax, a primary care provider may perform a **thoracentesis** to remove the excess fluid or air to ease breathing. Thoracentesis is also performed to introduce chemotherapeutic drugs intrapleurally.

The nurse assists the client to assume a position that allows easy access to the intercostal spaces. This is usually a sitting position with the arms above the head, which spreads the ribs and enlarges the intercostal space. Two positions commonly used are one in which the arm is elevated and stretched forward (Figure 34-20 ■, A) and one in which the client leans forward over a pillow (Figure 34-20 ■, B). To make sure that the needle is inserted below the fluid level when fluid is to be removed (or above any fluid if air is to be removed), the primary care provider will palpate and percuss the chest and select the exact site for insertion of the needle. A site on the lower posterior chest is often used to remove fluid, and a site on the upper anterior chest is used to remove air (Figure 34-21 ■). A chest x-ray prior to the procedure will help pinpoint the best insertion site.

The primary care provider and the assisting nurse follow strict sterile technique. The primary care provider attaches a syringe and/or stopcock to the aspirating needle. The stopcock must be in the closed position so that no air will enter the pleural space. The primary care provider inserts the needle through the intercostal space to the pleural cavity. In some instances, the primary care provider threads a small plastic tube through the needle and then withdraws the needle. (The tubing is less likely to puncture the pleura.)

If a syringe is used to collect the fluid, the plunger is pulled out to withdraw the pleural fluid as the stopcock is opened. If a large container is used to receive the fluid, the tubing is attached from the stopcock to the adapter on the receiving bottle. When the adapter and stopcock are opened, gravity allows fluid to

A   **B**

Figure 34-20 ■ Two positions commonly used for a thoracentesis. *A,* Sitting on one side with arm held to the front and up; *B,* sitting and leaning forward over a pillow.

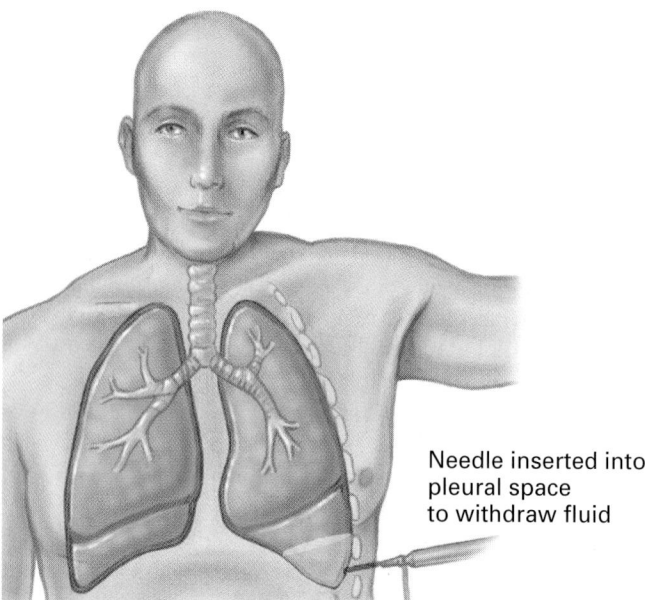

Needle inserted into
pleural space
to withdraw fluid

Figure 34-21 ■ Needle is inserted into the pleural space on the lower posterior chest to withdraw fluid.

(From Fremgen, Bonnie F., Frucht, Suzanne S., *Medical Terminology: A Living Language*, 3rd ed. © 2005. Electronically reproduced by permission of Pearson Education, Inc., Upper Saddle River, New Jersey.)

drain from the pleural cavity into the container, which should be kept below the level of the client's lungs. After the fluid has been withdrawn, the primary care provider removes the needle or plastic tubing.

LIFESPAN CONSIDERATIONS
Thoracentesis

ELDERS

■ Some elders will need help maintaining the proper position due to arthritis, tremors, or weakness.

■ Provide support with pillows during the procedure.

■ Absence of body fat in elders can help the primary care provider locate the intercostal spaces.

■ Provide an extra blanket to keep your client warm during the procedure. Elders have a decreased metabolism and less sub-cutaneous fat.

Bone Marrow Biopsy

Another type of diagnostic study is the *biopsy*. A biopsy is a procedure whereby tissue is obtained for examination. Biopsies are performed on many different types of tissues, for example, bone marrow, liver, breast, lymph nodes, and lung.

A bone marrow biopsy is the removal of a specimen of bone marrow for laboratory study. The biopsy is used to detect specific diseases of the blood, such as pernicious anemia and leukemia. The bones of the body commonly used for a bone marrow biopsy are the sternum, iliac crests, anterior or posterior iliac spines, and proximal tibia in children. The *posterior superior iliac crest* is the preferred site with the client placed prone or on the side (Figure 34-22 ■).

After injecting a local anesthetic, a small incision may be made with a scalpel to avoid tearing the skin or pushing skin into the bone marrow with a needle. The primary care provider then introduces a bone marrow needle with stylet into the red marrow of the spongy bone (Figure 34-23 ■).

Once the needle is in the marrow space, the stylet is removed and a 10-mL syringe is attached to the needle. The plunger is withdrawn until 1 to 2 mL of marrow has been obtained. The primary care provider replaces the stylet in the needle, withdraws the needle, and places the specimen in test tubes and/or on glass slides.

LIFESPAN CONSIDERATIONS
Bone Marrow Biopsy

CHILDREN

■ Young clients need emotional support due to the pain and pressure associated with this procedure.

■ Young clients may require gentle restraint to prevent movement during the procedure.

ELDERS

■ Elders with osteoporosis will experience less needle pressure.

■ Ask the client to empty the bladder for comfort before the procedure.

■ Provide pillows and blankets to help elders remain comfortable during the procedure.

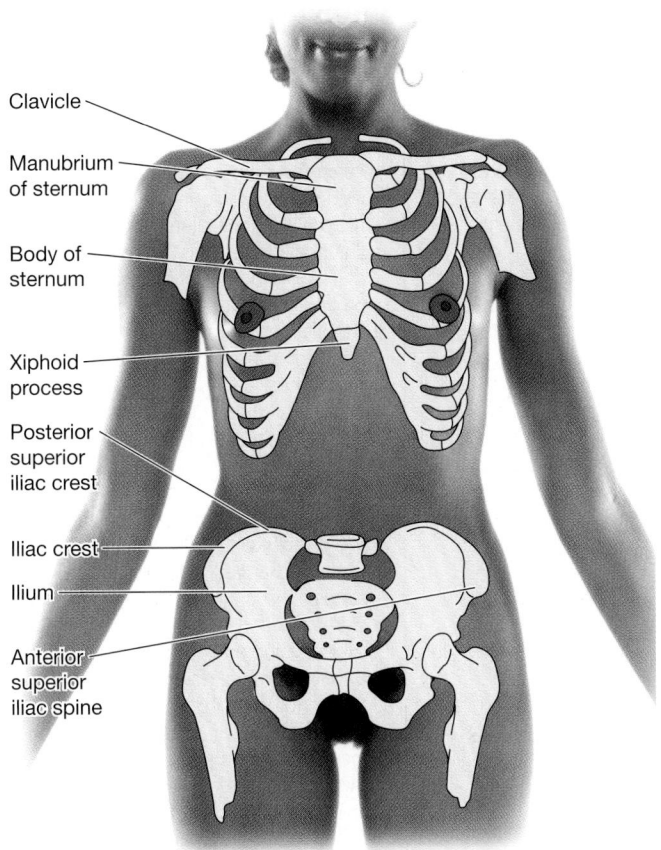

Clavicle

Manubrium of sternum

Body of sternum

Xiphoid process

Posterior superior iliac crest

Iliac crest

Ilium

Anterior superior iliac spine

Figure 34-22 ■ The sternum and the iliac crests are common sites for a bone marrow biopsy.

Periosteum

Compact Bone

Spongy Bone

Figure 34-23 ■ A cross section of a bone.

Liver Biopsy

A liver biopsy is a short procedure, generally performed at the client's bedside, in which a sample of liver tissue is aspirated. A primary care provider inserts a needle in the intercostal space between

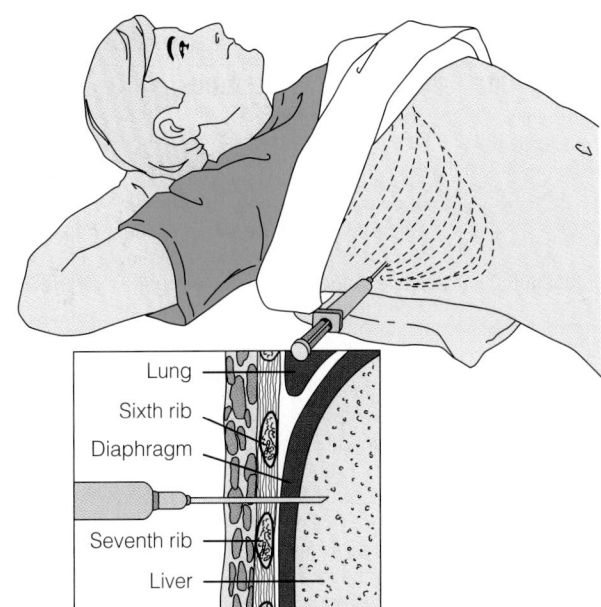

Lung

Sixth rib

Diaphragm

Seventh rib

Liver

Figure 34-24 ■ A common site for a liver biopsy.

two of the right lower ribs and into the liver (Figure 34-24 ■) or through the abdomen below the right rib cage (subcostally).

The client exhales and stops breathing while the primary care provider inserts the biopsy needle, injects a small amount of sterile normal saline to clear the needle of blood or particles of tissue picked up during insertion, and aspirates liver tissue by drawing back on the plunger of the syringe. After the needle is withdrawn, the nurse applies pressure to the site to prevent bleeding, often by positioning the client on the biopsy site (Figure 34-25 ■).

Because many clients with liver disease have blood clotting defects and are prone to bleeding, prothrombin time and platelet count are normally taken well in advance of the test. If the test results are abnormal, the biopsy may be contraindicated.

Table 34–3 describes how the nurse assists with the above aspiration/biopsy procedures.

Figure 34-25 ■ The position to provide pressure on a liver biopsy site.

TABLE 34–3   Assisting with Aspiration and Biopsy

PROCEDURE	BEFORE THE PROCEDURE	DURING THE PROCEDURE	AFTER THE PROCEDURE
Lumbar puncture	Prepare the client: ■ Explain the procedure to the client and support persons. The primary care provider will be taking a small sample of spinal fluid from the lower spine. A local anesthetic will be given to minimize discomfort. Explain when and where the procedure will occur (e.g., the bedside or in a treatment room) and who will be present (e.g., the primary care provider and the nurse). Explain that it will be necessary to lie in a certain position without moving for about 15 minutes. A slight pinprick will be felt when the local anesthetic is injected and a sensation of pressure as the spinal needle is inserted. ■ Have the client empty the bladder and bowels prior to the procedure to prevent unnecessary discomfort. ■ Position and drape the client. ■ Open the lumbar puncture set.	Support and monitor the client throughout: ■ Stand in front of the client and support the back of the neck and knees if the client needs help remaining still. ■ Reassure the client throughout the procedure by explaining what is happening. Encourage normal breathing and relaxation. ■ Observe the client's color, respirations, and pulse during the procedure. Ask the client to report headache or persistent pain at the insertion site. Handle specimen tubes appropriately: ■ Wear gloves when handling test tubes. ■ Label the specimen tubes in sequence. ■ Send the CSF specimens to the lab immediately. Place a small sterile dressing over the puncture site.	Ensure the client's comfort and safety: ■ Assist the client to a dorsal recumbent position with only one head pillow. The client remains in this position for 1 to 12 hours, depending on the primary care provider orders. ■ Determine whether analgesics are ordered and can be given for headaches. ■ Offer oral fluids frequently, unless contraindicated, to help restore the volume of CSF. Monitor the client: ■ Observe for swelling or bleeding at the puncture site. ■ Monitor changes in neurologic status. ■ Determine whether the client is experiencing any numbness, tingling, or pain radiating down the legs. Document the procedure on the client's chart: ■ Include date and time performed; the primary care provider's name; the color, character, and amount of CSF; and the number of specimens obtained. Also document CSF pressure and the nurse's assessments and interventions.
Abdominal paracentesis	Prepare the client: ■ Explain the procedure: obtaining the specimen usually takes about 15 minutes. Emphasize the importance of remaining still during the procedure. Tell the client when and where the procedure will occur and who will be present. ■ Have the client void just before the paracentesis to reduce the possibility of puncturing the urinary bladder. ■ Help the client assume a sitting position in bed, in a chair, or on the edge of the bed supported by pillows. ■ Maintain the client's privacy and provide blankets for warmth.	Assist and monitor the client: ■ Support the client verbally and describe the steps of the procedure as needed. ■ Observe the client closely for signs of distress (e.g., abnormal pulse rate, skin color, and blood pressure). ■ Observe for signs of hypovolemic shock induced by the loss of fluid: pallor, dyspnea, diaphoresis, drop in BP, and restlessness or increased anxiety. ■ Place a small sterile dressing over the site of the incision after the cannula or aspirating needle is withdrawn.	Monitor the client closely: ■ Observe for hypovolemic shock. ■ Observe for scrotal edema with male clients. ■ Monitor VS, urine output, and drainage from the puncture site every 15 minutes for at least 2 hours and every hour for 4 hours or as the client's condition indicates. ■ Measure the abdominal girth at the level of the umbilicus. Document all relevant information: ■ Include date and time performed; the primary care provider's name; abdominal girth before and after; the color, clarity, and amount of drained fluid; and the nurse's assessments and interventions. Transport the correctly labeled specimens to the laboratory.
Thoracentesis	Prepare the client: ■ Explain the procedure to the client. Normally, the client may experience some discomfort and a feeling of pressure when the needle is inserted. The procedure may bring considerable relief if breathing has been difficult. The procedure takes only a few minutes, depending primarily on the time it takes for the fluid to drain from the pleural cavity.	Support and monitor the client throughout: ■ Support the client verbally and describe the steps of the procedure as needed. ■ Observe the client for signs of distress, such as dyspnea, pallor, and coughing. Collect drainage and laboratory specimens. Place a small sterile dressing over the site of the puncture.	Monitor the client: ■ Assess pulse rate and respiratory rate and skin color. ■ Don't remove more than 1,000 mL of fluid from the pleural cavity within the first 30 minutes. ■ Observe changes in the client's cough, sputum, respiratory depth, and breath sounds, and note complaints of chest pain.

TABLE 34–3 **Assisting with Aspiration and Biopsy—***continued*

PROCEDURE	BEFORE THE PROCEDURE	DURING THE PROCEDURE	AFTER THE PROCEDURE
Thoracentesis—(continued)	To avoid puncturing the lungs, it is important for the client not to cough while the needle is inserted. Explain when and where the procedure will occur and who will be present. ■ Help position the client and cover the client as needed with a bath blanket.		Position the client appropriately: ■ Some agency protocols recommend that the client lie on the unaffected side with the head of the bed elevated 30 degrees for at least 30 minutes because this position facilitates expansion of the affected lung and eases respirations. Document all relevant information: ■ Include date and time performed; the primary care provider's name; the amount, color, and clarity of fluid drained; and nursing assessments and interventions provided. Transport the specimens to the laboratory.
Bone marrow biopsy	Prepare the client: ■ Explain the procedure. The client may experience pain when the marrow is aspirated and hear a crunching sound as the needle is pushed through the cortex of the bone. The procedure usually takes 15 to 30 minutes. Explain when and where the procedure will occur, who will be present, and which site will be used. ■ Help the client assume a supine position (with one pillow if desired) for a biopsy of the sternum (sternal puncture) or a prone position for a biopsy of either iliac crest. Fold the bedclothes back or drape the client to expose the area. ■ Administer a sedative as ordered.	Monitor and support the client throughout: ■ Describe the steps of the procedure as needed and provide verbal support. ■ Observe the client for pallor, diaphoresis, and faintness due to bleeding or pain. Place a small dressing over the site of the puncture after the needle is withdrawn: ■ Some agency protocols recommend direct pressure over the site for 5 to 10 minutes to prevent bleeding. Assist with preparing specimens as needed.	Monitor the client: ■ Assess for discomfort and bleeding from the site. The client may experience some tenderness in the area. Bleeding and hematoma formation need to be assessed for several days. Report bleeding or pain to the nurse in charge. ■ Provide an analgesic as needed and ordered. Document all relevant information: ■ Include date and time of the procedure, the primary care provider's name; and any nursing assessments and interventions. Document any specimens obtained. Transport the specimens to the laboratory.
Liver biopsy	Prepare the client: ■ Give preprocedural medications as ordered. Vitamin K may be given for several days before the biopsy to reduce the risk of hemorrhage. ■ Explain the procedure and tell the client that the primary care provider will take a small sample of liver tissue by putting a needle into the client's side or abdomen. Explain that a sedative and local anesthetic will be given, so the client will feel no pain. Explain when and where the procedure will occur, who will be present, the time required, and what to expect as the procedure is being performed (e.g., the client may experience mild discomfort when the local anesthetic is injected and slight pressure when the biopsy needle is inserted). ■ Ensure that the client fasts for at least 2 hours before the procedure. ■ Administer the appropriate sedative about 30 minutes beforehand or at the specified time. ■ Help the client assume a supine position with the upper right quadrant of the abdomen exposed. Cover the client with the bedclothes so that only the abdominal area is exposed.	Monitor and support the client throughout: ■ Support the client in a supine position. ■ Instruct the client to take a few deep inhalations and exhalations and to hold the breath after the final exhalation for up to 10 seconds as the needle is inserted, the biopsy obtained, and the needle withdrawn. Holding the breath after exhalation immobilizes the chest wall and liver and keeps the diaphragm in its highest position, avoiding injury to the lung and laceration of the liver. ■ Instruct the client to resume breathing when the needle is withdrawn. ■ Apply pressure to the site of the puncture to help stop any bleeding. Apply a small dressing to the site of the puncture.	Position the client appropriately: ■ Assist the client to a right side-lying position with a small pillow or folded towel under the biopsy site. Instruct the client to remain in this position for several hours. Monitor the client: ■ Assess the client's VS every 15 minutes for the first hour following the test or until the signs are stable. Then monitor vital signs every hour for 24 hours or as needed. ■ Determine whether the client is experiencing abdominal pain. Severe abdominal pain may indicate bile peritonitis. ■ Check the biopsy site for localized bleeding. Pressure dressings may be required if bleeding does occur. Document all relevant information: ■ Include date and time performed; the primary care provider's name; and all nursing assessments and interventions. Transport the specimens to the laboratory.

LIFESPAN CONSIDERATIONS   Liver Biopsy

ELDERS

■ Observe for skin irritation from tape applied to the sterile dressing. Elders often have fragile skin.

■ Ask the client to empty the bladder before the procedure. Elders may need to void more often and in smaller amounts.

LIFESPAN CONSIDERATIONS   General Considerations

CHILDREN

■ Children may be frightened of even noninvasive procedures to collect specimens if they are not sure what is going to happen. Cooperation can be maximized by:

  • Demonstrating on dolls or teddy bears.
  • Allowing the child to examine and explore the collection materials being used.
  • Explaining in age-appropriate language what will be done.
  • Having parents actively involved in gently holding and comforting the child during and after the procedure.
  • Being well prepared to conduct the procedure.
  • Performing the procedure quickly, competently, and as gently as possible.

ELDERS

■ In elders, homeostatic mechanisms are not as efficient as in the younger person. When undergoing diagnostic tests that challenge these functions, care must be taken to accurately monitor functions and note any changes. Examples:

  • Dehydration and electrolyte imbalance can occur from laxative preps given before bowel diagnostic tests, such as a colonoscopy.
  • Fluid restrictions and NPO status for a length of time can lead to hypovolemia and electrolyte imbalances.
  • Many dye contrasts used for x-rays and scans can cause renal damage (especially in clients with diabetes).
  • Sedation used for certain procedures may require a longer recovery time for older clients.
  • Having several tests at a time or for several days compounds these potential problems and increases fatigue.

Interventions should focus on ensuring that the client is hydrated during and after these diagnostic tests, monitoring intake and output and vital signs frequently and accurately, and noting any mental status changes that might suggest electrolyte imbalance. Identification of clients at risk (persons with diabetes, kidney disease, or on certain medications) will help initiate measures to prevent injuries or complications from diagnostic tests.

CRITICAL THINKING CHECKPOINT

Ms. Angyal, 68, is admitted with fever, nausea, vomiting, and abdominal pain. She informs you that she is a "borderline diabetic" and "only has to watch what she eats." She tells you that she has not eaten for 3 days and has had difficulty "keeping liquids down." While doing the nursing history, she describes her urine as dark and foul smelling. Upon further questions, she states she does have some burning upon urination. She describes her abdominal pain as constant, generalized, and rates it as a 5 or 6 on a scale of 0 to 10. The primary care provider called in the following orders:

    CBC and electrolytes STAT
    Capillary blood glucose STAT and q 4 hr
    VS and TPR q 4 hr
    Urine specimen for C & S
    CXR
    Flat plate abdominal x-ray

1. When measuring Ms. Angyal's capillary blood glucose, you do not obtain enough blood to cover the indicator square on the

reagent strip. What could be possible reasons and what should you do?

The lab work returns with the following results:
WBC = $17 \times 10^3/mL^3$ with neutrophils = 80%; Hct = 43.2.

1. Based on the above lab work, what are your nursing interventions?
2. The primary care provider orders IV fluids and an antibiotic with the first dose to be given STAT. You have not obtained the urine specimen yet. Which has priority (e.g., starting the IV, administrating the antibiotic, or obtaining the urine specimen) and why?
3. Three days later, Ms. Angyal has the following lab results: Hct = 39.2 and WBC = $10.8 \times 10^3/mL^3$. What do those results indicate to you?
4. The abdominal x-ray shows a possible mass. An MRI of the abdomen is ordered. Ms. Angyal is quite anxious because she has heard from her friend that the procedure is claustrophobic for people. How will you respond?

See Critical Thinking Possibilities in Appendix A.

CHAPTER 34 **REVIEW**

CHAPTER HIGHLIGHTS

- Diagnostic testing involves three phases. Client preparation is the focus during the pretest phase. During the intratest phase, the nurse performs or assists with the diagnostic test and collects the specimen. Providing nursing care of the client and follow-up activities and observations are the role of the nurse during the post-test phase.
- Blood tests are one of the most commonly used diagnostic tests. Routinely ordered blood tests can include complete blood count (CBC) and serum electrolytes.
- A capillary blood glucose is a frequent test performed by nurses and clients. This test is used to monitor glucose levels of clients at risk for hyper- and hypoglycemia. It also evaluates the effectiveness of insulin administration.
- Nursing responsibilities associated with specimen collection include (a) providing client comfort, privacy, and safety; (b) explaining the purpose of and procedure for the specimen collection; (c) using correct procedure for obtaining the specimen; (d) noting relevant information on the laboratory requisition slip; (e) transporting the specimen promptly; and (f) reporting abnormal findings.
- Clients may need assistance to obtain stool specimens for laboratory analysis. In many agencies, nurses test the stool for occult blood.
- Nurses collect urine specimens for a number of tests. A clean voided specimen is used for routine examination. A clean-catch or

midstream voided specimen is collected when a urine culture is ordered to identify microorganisms. Timed urine specimens are collected for a variety of tests, depending on the client's health problem. Nurses can complete some simple urine tests (e.g., specific gravity, pH, ketones, protein) at the bedside.
- Sputum and throat culture specimens help determine the presence of disease-producing organisms.
- Visualization procedures include indirect visualization (noninvasive) and direct visualization (invasive) techniques for visualizing body organs and system functions. Examples of invasive procedures include colonoscopy, barium enema, intravenous pyelography, and angiography. Noninvasive procedures include lung scan, echocardiogram, electrocardiography, x-ray, CT, and MRI.
- Examples of aspiration/biopsy tests include lumbar puncture, abdominal paracentesis, thoracentesis, bone marrow biopsy, and liver biopsy. These tests are invasive procedures and require strict sterile technique. After the procedure, the nurse assesses the client for possible complications and provides appropriate nursing interventions as needed.

TEST YOUR KNOWLEDGE

1. The nurse would call the primary care provider immediately for which of the following lab results?
   1. Hgb = 16 g/dL for male client
   2. Hct = 22% for female client
   3. WBC = $9 \times 10^3/mL^3$
   4. platelets = $300 \times 10^3/mL^3$

2. Mr. Jones, 78, needs to complete a 24-hour urine specimen. In planning his care, which of the following measures is most important?
   1. At the beginning of the test, instruct him to empty his bladder and save this voiding to start the collection.
   2. Use a sterile receptacle to collect the urine.
   3. Place a sign stating "Save All Urine" in the bathroom.
   4. Keep the urine specimen in the refrigerator.

3. The client has a urinary health problem. Which of the following procedures is performed using indirect visualization?
   1. IVP
   2. KUB
   3. Retrograde pyelography
   4. Cystoscopy

4. Which procedure provides information regarding the physiology of an organ?
   1. x-ray
   2. Computerized Tomography (CT)
   3. Magnetic Resonance Imagery (MRI)
   4. Nuclear scan

5. When assisting with a bone marrow biopsy, the nurse should take which of the following actions?
   1. Assist the client to a right side-lying position after the procedure.
   2. Observe for signs of dyspnea, pallor, and coughing.

   3. Assess for bleeding and hematoma formation for several days after the procedure.
   4. Stand in front of the client and support the back of the neck and knees.

6. During an assessment, the nurse learns that the client has a history of liver disease. Which of the following diagnostic tests might be indicated for this client? Select all that apply.
   1. Alanine aminotransferase (ALT)
   2. Myoglobin
   3. Cholesterol
   4. Ammonia
   5. BNP

7. The nurse practitioner requests a laboratory blood test to determine how well a client has controlled her diabetes over the past three months. Which blood test will provide this information?
   1. Fasting blood glucose
   2. Capillary blood specimen
   3. Glycosylated hemoglobin
   4. Glucose tolerance test

8. The client is supposed to have a fecal occult blood test done on a stool sample. The nurse is going to use the Hemoccult test. Which of the following indicates that the nurse is using the correct procedure? Select all that apply.
   1. Mixes the reagent with the stool sample before applying to the card
   2. Collects a sample from two different areas of the stool specimen
   3. Assesses for a blue color change
   4. Asks a colleague to verify the pink color results
   5. Asks the client if he has taken vitamin C in the past few days

9. A primary care provider is going to perform a thoracentesis. The nurse's role will include which of the following?
1. Place the client supine in the trendelenburg position.
2. Position the client in a seated position with elbows on the overbed table.
3. Instruct the UAP to measure vital signs.
4. Administer narcotic analgesic.

10. The nurse needs to collect a sputum specimen to identify the presence of TB. Which of the following is indicated for this type of specimen? Select all that apply.
1. Collect the specimen in the evening.
2. Send the specimen immediately to the lab.
3. Ask the client to spit into the sputum container.
4. Offer mouthcare before and after collection of the sputum specimen.
5. Collect a specimen for 3 consecutive days.

See Answers to Test Your Knowledge in Appendix A.

EXPLORE MEDIALINK www.prenhall.com/berman

DVD-ROM
- Audio Glossary
- NCLEX Review
- Skills Checklists
- Animation: PET and SPECT Scans

COMPANION WEBSITE
- Additional NCLEX Review
- Case Study: Checking Lab Results
- Care Plan Activity: Client Waiting for Diagnosis
- Application Activity: Diagnostic Tests
- Links to Resources

READINGS AND REFERENCES

SUGGESTED READINGS
Dale, L. (2006). Make a point about alternate site blood glucose sampling. *Nursing, 36*(2), 52–53.
The author shows the technique for blood sampling from one of the alternate sites—the palm of the hand. Pictures show the process and the narrative provides important teaching points.
Fox, V. J. (2005). Deciphering diagnostics: Get the inside story with spiral CT. *Nursing Made Incredibly Easy, 3*(3), 60–62.
The author outlines how a spiral CT works, what it can detect, and why it is helpful for critically ill clients. The before and after client care tips are helpful.
Moshang, J. (2005). Making a point about insulin pens. *Nursing, 35*(2), 46–47.
This article has many photos that detail how to use an insulin pen. It should be helpful for teaching nurses as well as clients.
Simerville, J. A., Maxted, W. C., & Pahira, J. J. (2005). Urinalysis: A comprehensive review. *American Family Physician, 71*(6), 1153–1162.
This comprehensive article is clearly written and informative about how to interpret urinalysis results correctly.

RELATED RESEARCH
Mulhall, B. P., Veerappan, G. R., & Jackson, J. L. (2005). Meta-analysis: Computed tomographic colonography. *Annals of Internal Medicine, 142*(8), 635–650.
Sharma, V., Dowd, D., Swanson, D. S., Slaughter, A. J., & Simon, S. D. (2003). Influence of the news media on diagnostic testing in the emergency department. *Archives of Pediatrics & Adolescent Medicine, 157*, 257–260.

REFERENCES
American Diabetes Association. (2000, January). Resource guide 2000: Urine testing. *Diabetes Forecast Supplement,* 66–67.
Armstrong, M. L. & Elkins, L. (2005). Body art and MRI. *American Journal of Nursing, 105*(3), 65–66.
Ball, J. W., & Bindler, R. C. (2006). *Child health nursing.* Upper Saddle River, NJ: Prentice Hall Health.
Bindler, R. C., Ball, J. W., London, M. L., & Ladewig, P. W. (2007). *Clinical skills manual for maternal & child nursing care.* (2nd ed.). Upper Saddle River, NJ: Pearson Prentice Hall.
Corbett, J. V. (2004). *Laboratory tests and diagnostic procedures with nursing diagnoses* (6th ed.). Upper Saddle River, N.J.: Pearson Prentice Hall.
Davis, K. (2004). Need urine from a catheter system? Forget the needle! *Nursing, 34*(12), 64.
Fischbach, F. T. (2004). *A manual of laboratory & diagnostic tests* (7th ed.). Philadelphia: Lippincott.
Karch, A. M. (2004). Don't get burnt by the MRI. *American Journal of Nursing, 104*(8), 31.
Kim, J. (2005). What does a B-type natriuretic peptide test show? *Nursing, 35*(1), 26.
Mensing, C. (2004). Helping patients choose the right blood glucose meter. *Nurse Practitioner, 29*(5), 43–45.
NANDA International. (2007). *Nursing diagnosis: Definitions and classification 2007–2008.* Philadelphia: Author.
Passanza, C. (2001). Diabetes update: Monitor options *RN, 64*(6), 36–42.
Penharlow, C., & Spader, C. (2005). Liver function tests: Pieces of a complex diagnostic puzzle. *NurseWeek-MountainWest, 6*(3), 13–15.

Salimbene, S. (2000). *What language does your patient hurt in? A practical guide to culturally competent patient care.* Rockford, IL: EMC Paradigm.
Society of Permanent Cosmetic Professionals. (2005). *MRI facts.* Retrieved June 15, 2006, from http://www.spcp.org/MRIinfo.htm
Spector, R. E. (2004). *Cultural diversity in health and illness* (6th ed.). Upper Saddle River, NJ: Pearson Prentice Hall.
U.S. Food and Drug Administration. (n.d.). *Glucose meters & diabetes management.* Retrieved June 15, 2006, from http://www.fda.gov/diabetes/glucose.html
Van Leeuwen, A. M., Kranpitz, T. R., & Smith, L. (2006). *Laboratory and diagnostic tests with nursing implications* (2nd ed.). Philadelphia: F. A. Davis.

SELECTED BIBLIOGRAPHY
Ahmed, D. S. (2000). Hidden factors in occult blood testing. *American Journal of Nursing, 100*(12), 25.
Anonymous. (2004). Blood glucose monitors and data management systems. *Diabetes Forecast, 57*(1), RG39–RG58.
Anonymous. (2004). Deciphering diagnostics: Every picture tells a story. *Nursing Made Incredibly Easy, 2*(6), 56–57.
DiNella, J. V. (2005). The ins and outs of pulmonary function testing. *Nursing, 35*(12), 70–71.
Fain, J. A. (2004). Blood glucose meters: Different strokes for different folks. *Nursing, 34*(11), 48–51.
George, E. L., & Panos, A. (2005). Does a high WBC count signal infection? *Nursing, 35*(1), 20–21.
Li, C. Z. (2004). Viewing the small intestine via capsule endoscopy. *Nursing, 34*(4), 70–71.

Medications

LEARNING OUTCOMES

After completing this chapter, you will be able to:

1. Define selected terms related to the administration of medications.

2. Describe legal aspects of administering medications.

3. Identify physiologic factors and individual variables affecting medication action.

4. Describe various routes of medication administration.

5. Identify essential parts of a medication order.

6. List examples of various types of medication orders.

7. State systems of measurement that are used in the administration of medications.

8. List six essential steps to follow when administering medication.

9. State the "rights" to accurate medication administration.

10. Describe physiologic changes in older adults that alter medication administration and effectiveness.

11. Outline steps required to administer oral medications safely.

12. Outline steps required for nasogastric and gastrostomy tube medication administration.

13. Identify equipment required for parenteral medications.

14. Describe how to prepare selected drugs from ampules and vials.

15. Identify sites used for intradermal, subcutaneous, and intramuscular injections.

16. Describe essential steps for safely administering parenteral medications by intradermal, subcutaneous, intramuscular, and intravenous routes.

17. Describe essential steps in safely administering topical medications: dermatologic, ophthalmic, otic, nasal, vaginal, respiratory inhalation, and rectal preparations.

A **medication** is a substance administered for the diagnosis, cure, treatment, or relief of a symptom or for prevention of disease. In the health care context, the words *medication* and *drug* are generally used interchangeably. The term **drug** also has the connotation of an illicitly obtained substance such as heroin, cocaine, or amphetamines. Medications have been known and used since antiquity. Crude drugs, such as opium, castor oil, and vinegar, were used in ancient times. Over the centuries the number of drugs available has increased greatly, and knowledge about these drugs has become correspondingly more accurate and detailed.

In the United States and Canada, medications are usually dispensed on the order of physicians and dentists. In some U.S. states, specially qualified nurse practitioners or other advanced practice nurses and physician's assistants may prescribe drugs. The written direction for the preparation and administration of a drug is called a **prescription.** One drug can have as many as four kinds of names: its generic name, official name, chemical name, and trademark or brand name. The **generic name** is given before a drug becomes officially an approved medication. The generic name is generally used throughout the drug's use. The **official name** is the name under which it is listed in one of the official publications (e.g., the *United States Pharmacopeia*). The **chemical name** is the name by which a chemist knows it; this name describes the constituents of the drug precisely. A drug's **trade name** is the name given by the drug manufacturer. The name is usually selected to be short and easy to remember. The trade name is sometimes called the **brand name.** Because one drug may be manufactured by several companies, it can have several trade names; for example, the drug hydrochlorothiazide (official name) is known by the trade names Esidrix and HydroDIURIL. Medications are often available in a variety of forms (see Table 35–1).

Pharmacology is the study of the effect of drugs on living organisms. **Pharmacy** is the art of preparing, compounding, and dispensing drugs. The word also refers to the place where drugs

TABLE 35-1	**Types of Drug Preparation**
TYPE	**DESCRIPTION**
Aerosol spray or foam	A liquid, powder, or foam deposited in a thin layer on the skin by air pressure
Aqueous solution	One or more drugs dissolved in water
Aqueous suspension	One or more drugs finely divided in a liquid such as water
Caplet	A solid form, shaped like a capsule, coated and easily swallowed
Capsule	A gelatinous container to hold a drug in powder, liquid, or oil form
Cream	A nongreasy, semisolid preparation used on the skin
Elixir	A sweetened and aromatic solution of alcohol used as a vehicle for medicinal agents
Extract	A concentrated form of a drug made from vegetables or animals
Gel or jelly	A clear or translucent semisolid that liquefies when applied to the skin
Liniment	A medication mixed with alcohol, oil, or soapy emollient and applied to the skin
Lotion	A medication in a liquid suspension applied to the skin
Lozenge (troche)	A flat, round, or oval preparation that dissolves and releases a drug when held in the mouth
Ointment (salve, unction)	A semisolid preparation of one or more drugs used for application to the skin and mucous membrane
Paste	A preparation like an ointment, but thicker and stiff, that penetrates the skin less than an ointment
Pill	One or more drugs mixed with a cohesive material, in oval, round, or flattened shapes
Powder	A finely ground drug or drugs; some are used internally, others externally
Suppository	One or several drugs mixed with a firm base such as gelatin and shaped for insertion into the body (e.g., the rectum); the base dissolves gradually at body temperature, releasing the drug
Syrup	An aqueous solution of sugar often used to disguise unpleasant-tasting drugs
Tablet	A powdered drug compressed into a hard small disc; some are readily broken along a scored line; others are enteric coated to prevent them from dissolving in the stomach
Tincture	An alcoholic or water-and-alcohol solution prepared from drugs derived from plants
Transdermal patch	A semipermeable membrane shaped in the form of a disc or patch that contains a drug to be absorbed through the skin over a long period of time

are prepared and dispensed. Drugs are prepared by a **pharmacist,** a person licensed to prepare and dispense drugs and to make up prescriptions. A clinical pharmacist is a specialist who often guides the physician in prescribing drugs. A pharmacy technician is a member of the health team who in some states administers drugs to clients.

DRUG STANDARDS

Drugs may have natural (e.g., plant, mineral, and animal) sources, or they may be synthesized in the laboratory. For example, digitalis and opium are plant derived, iron and sodium chloride are minerals, insulin and vaccines have animal or human sources, and the sulfonamides and propoxyphene hydrochloride (the analgesic Darvon) are the products of laboratory synthesis. Early drugs were derived from the three natural sources only. More and more drugs, however, are being produced synthetically.

Drugs vary in strength and activity. Drugs derived from plants, for example, vary in strength according to the age of the plant, the variety, the place in which it is grown, and the method by which it is preserved. Drugs must be pure and of uniform strength if drug dosages are to be predictable in their effect. Drug standards have therefore been developed to ensure uniform quality. In the United States, official drugs are those so designated by the federal Food, Drug, and Cosmetic Act. These drugs are officially listed in the *United States Pharmacopeia (USP)* and described according to their source, physical and chemical properties, tests for purity and identity, method of storage, assay, category, and normal dosages. In Canada, the *British Pharmacopoeia* is used for the same purpose, although some drugs used in Canada conform to the *USP* because they are obtained from the United States. There is a trend for people to purchase "natural" vitamins and supplements from health food stores or over the counter at pharmacies. An example of this is a thyroid supplement. The natural form varies in strength and is difficult to regulate, while the synthetic thyroid is much more predictable in strength and management of symptoms for clients who need to take a thyroid supplement.

A **pharmacopoeia** (also spelled *pharmacopeia*) is a book containing a list of products used in medicine, with descriptions of the product, chemical tests for determining identity and purity, and formulas and prescriptions. The United States' *National Formulary* lists drugs and their therapeutic value and can include drugs that may still be used but not listed in the *USP.* The *Canadian Formulary* lists drugs used extensively in Canada but not necessarily listed in the *British Pharmacopoeia.*

Pharmacopoeias and formularies are invaluable reference sources for nurses and nursing students. Nurses not only administer thousands of medications but also are responsible for assessing their effectiveness and recognizing unfavorable reactions to drugs. Medication or drug handbooks and agency formularies are valuable resources for nurses. Because it is impossible to commit to memory all pertinent information about a very large number of drugs, nurses must have a reliable reference readily available.

LEGAL ASPECTS OF DRUG ADMINISTRATION

The administration of drugs in both the United States and Canada is controlled by law. Table 35–2 provides a summary of U.S. drug legislation. Table 35–3 summarizes Canadian drug legislation.

Nurses need to (a) know how nursing practice acts in their areas define and limit their functions and (b) be able to recognize the limits of their own knowledge and skill. To function beyond the limits of nursing practice acts or one's ability is to endanger clients' lives and leave oneself open to malpractice suits. Under the law, nurses are responsible for their own actions regardless of whether there is a written order. If a physician writes an incorrect order (e.g., Demerol 500 mg instead of Demerol 50 mg), *a nurse who administers the written incorrect dosage is responsible for the error as well as the physician.* Therefore, nurses should question any order that appears unreasonable and refuse to give the medication until the order is clarified.

Another aspect of nursing practice governed by law is the use of controlled substances. In hospitals, controlled substances are kept in a locked drawer, cupboard, medication cart, or computer-controlled dispensing system. Agencies may have special inventory forms for recording the use of controlled substances. The information required usually includes the name of the client, the date and time of administration, the name of the drug, the dosage, and the signature of the person who prepared and gave the drug. The name of the physician who ordered the drug may also be part of the record. Some agencies may require a verifying signature of another registered nurse for administration of a controlled substance. Most health care agencies maintain a list of high-alert medications, including controlled substances, which require the verification of two registered nurses. Before removing a controlled substance, the nurse verifies the number actually available with the number indicated on the narcotic or controlled substance inventory record (Figure 35-1 ■). If the number is not the same, the nurse must investigate and correct the discrepancy before proceeding.

Figure 35-1 ■ Some narcotics are kept in specially designed packages or plastic containers that are sectioned and numbered.

TABLE 35–2 United States Drug Legislation

LEGISLATION	CONTENT
Food, Drug, and Cosmetic Act (1938)	Implemented by Food and Drug Administration (FDA); requires that labels be accurate and that all drugs be tested for harmful effects.
Durkham-Humphrey Amendment (1952)	Clearly differentiates drugs that can be sold only with a prescription, those that can be sold without a prescription, and those that should not be refilled without a new prescription.
Kefauver-Harris Amendment (1962)	Requires proof of safety and efficacy of a drug for approval.
Comprehensive Drug Abuse Prevention and Control Act (1970) (Controlled Substances Act)	Categorizes controlled substances and limits how often a prescription can be filled; established government-funded programs to prevent and treat drug dependence.

TABLE 35–3 Canadian Drug Legislation

LEGISLATION	CONTENT
Proprietary or Patent Medicine Act (1908)	Protects the public against unsafe and ineffective over-the-counter drugs.
Canada Food and Drugs Act (1953)	Prohibits advertising any food, drug, cosmetic, or device as a cure for certain specified diseases. Sets standards for manufacture, distribution, and sale of all drugs, with the exception of narcotics.
Canadian Narcotic Control Act (1961)	Allows only authorized people to possess narcotics. Specifies records about narcotics that must be kept.

Included on the record are the controlled substances wasted during preparation. When a portion or all of a controlled substance dose is discarded, the nurse must ask a second nurse to witness the discarding. Both nurses must sign the control inventory form.

In most agencies, counts of controlled substances are taken at the end of each shift. The count total should tally with the total at the end of the last shift minus the number used. If the totals do not tally and the discrepancy cannot be resolved, it must be reported immediately to the nurse manager, nursing supervisor, and pharmacy according to agency policy. In facilities that use a computerized dispensing system, manual counts are not required, because the dispensing system runs a continuous count; however, discrepancies must be accounted for.

EFFECTS OF DRUGS

The **therapeutic effect** of a drug, also referred to as the **desired effect,** is the primary effect intended, that is, the reason the drug is prescribed. For example, the therapeutic effect of morphine sulfate is analgesia, and the therapeutic effect of diazepam is relief of anxiety. See Table 35–4 for kinds of therapeutic actions.

A **side effect,** or secondary effect, of a drug is one that is unintended. Side effects are usually predictable and may be either harmless or potentially harmful. For example, digitalis increases the strength of myocardial contractions (desired effect), but it can have the side effect of inducing nausea and vomiting. Some side effects are tolerated for the drug's therapeutic effect; more severe side effects, also called **adverse effects** or reac-

tions, may justify the discontinuation of a drug. The nurse should monitor for dose-related side or adverse effects and report these to the health care provider who may discontinue the medication or change the dosage.

Drug toxicity (deleterious effects of a drug on an organism or tissue) results from overdosage, ingestion of a drug intended for external use, and buildup of the drug in the blood because of impaired metabolism or excretion (cumulative effect). Some toxic effects are apparent immediately; some are not apparent for weeks or months. Fortunately, most drug toxicity is avoidable if careful attention is paid to dosage and monitoring for toxicity. An example of a toxic effect is respiratory depression due to the cumulative effect of morphine sulfate in the body.

A **drug allergy** is an immunologic reaction to a drug. When a client is first exposed to a foreign substance (antigen), the body may react by producing antibodies. A client can react to a drug as to an antigen and thus develop symptoms of an allergic reaction.

Allergic reactions can be either mild or severe. A mild reaction has a variety of symptoms, from skin rashes to diarrhea (see Table 35–5). An allergic reaction can occur anytime from a few minutes to 2 weeks after the administration of the drug. A severe allergic reaction usually occurs immediately after the administration of the drug and is called an **anaphylactic reaction.** This response can be fatal if the symptoms are not noticed immediately and treatment is not obtained promptly. The earliest symptoms are a subjective feeling of swelling in the mouth and tongue, acute shortness of breath, acute hypotension, and tachycardia.

Drug tolerance exists in a person who has unusually low physiologic response to a drug and who requires increases in the

TABLE 35–4 Therapeutic Actions of Drugs

DRUG TYPE	DESCRIPTION	EXAMPLES
Palliative	Relieves the symptoms of a disease but does not affect the disease itself.	Morphine sulfate, aspirin for pain
Curative	Cures a disease or condition.	Penicillin for infection
Supportive	Supports body function until other treatments or the body's response can take over.	Norepinephrine bitartrate for low blood pressure; aspirin for high body temperature
Substitutive	Replaces body fluids or substances.	Thyroxine for hypothyroidism, insulin for diabetes mellitus
Chemotherapeutic	Destroys malignant cells.	Busulfan for leukemia
Restorative	Returns the body to health.	Vitamin, mineral supplements

TABLE 35–5 Common Mild Allergic Responses

SYMPTOM	DESCRIPTION/RATIONALE
Skin rash	Either an intraepidermal vesicle rash or a rash typified by an urticarial wheal or macular eruption; rash is usually generalized over the body
Pruritus	Itching of the skin with or without a rash
Angioedema	Edema due to increased permeability of the blood capillaries
Rhinitis	Excessive watery discharge from the nose
Lacrimal tearing	Excessive tearing
Nausea, vomiting	Stimulation of these centers in the brain
Wheezing and dyspnea	Shortness of breath and wheezing on inhalation and exhalation due to accumulated fluids and swelling of the respiratory tissues
Diarrhea	Irritation of the mucosa of the large intestine

dosage to maintain a given therapeutic effect. Drugs that commonly produce tolerance are opiates, barbiturates, ethyl alcohol, and tobacco. A **cumulative effect** is the increasing response to repeated doses of a drug that occurs when the rate of administration exceeds the rate of metabolism or excretion. As a result, the amount of the drug builds up in the client's body unless the dosage is adjusted. Toxic symptoms may occur. An **idiosyncratic effect** is one that is unexpected and may be individual to a client. Underresponse and overresponse to a drug may be idiosyncratic. Also, the drug may have a completely different effect from the normal one or cause unpredictable and unexplainable symptoms in a particular client.

A **drug interaction** occurs when the administration of one drug before, at the same time as, or after another drug alters the effect of one or both drugs. Drug interactions may be beneficial or harmful. The effect of one or both drugs may be either increased (**potentiating effect**) or decreased (**inhibiting effect**). Potentiating effects may be additive or synergistic. When two of the same types of drug increase the action of each other it is known as additive. **Synergistic** is when two different drugs increase the action of one or another drug. For example, probenecid, which blocks the excretion of penicillin, can be given with penicillin to increase blood levels of the penicillin for longer periods (synergistic effect). Two analgesics, such as aspirin and codeine, are often given together because together they provide greater pain relief (additive effect). In this example of aspirin and codeine, using a combination of drugs often decreases the total dose of narcotics needed. In addition, certain foods may interact adversely with a medication (see Table 47–1 in Chapter 47). ∞

Iatrogenic disease (disease caused unintentionally by medical therapy) can be due to drug therapy. Hepatic toxicity resulting in biliary obstruction, renal damage, and malformations of the fetus as a result of specific drugs taken during pregnancy are examples.

DRUG MISUSE

Drug misuse is the improper use of common medications in ways that lead to acute and chronic toxicity. Both over-the-counter drugs and prescription drugs may be misused. Laxatives, antacids, vitamins, headache remedies, and cough and cold medications are often self-prescribed and overused. Most people suffer no harmful effects from these drugs, but some people do. A persistent cough may go undiagnosed until the underlying problem becomes serious and advanced.

Drug abuse is inappropriate intake of a substance, either continually or periodically. By definition, drug use is abusive when society considers it abusive. For example, the intake of alcohol at work may be considered alcohol abuse, but intake at a social gathering may not. Drug abuse has two main facets, drug dependence and habituation. **Drug dependence** is a person's reliance on or need to take a drug or substance. The two types of dependence, physiologic and psychologic, may occur separately or together. **Physiologic dependence** is due to biochemical changes in body tissues, especially the nervous system. These tissues come to require the substance for normal functioning. A dependent person who stops using the drug experiences withdrawal symptoms. **Psychologic dependence** is emotional reliance on a drug to maintain a sense of well-being, accompanied by feelings of need or cravings for that drug. There are varying degrees of psychologic dependence, ranging from mild desire to craving and compulsive use of the drug.

Drug habituation denotes a mild form of psychologic dependence. The individual develops the habit of taking the substance and feels better after taking it. The habituated individual tends to continue the habit even though it may be injurious to health.

Illicit drugs, also called *street drugs,* are those sold illegally. Illicit drugs are of two types: (a) drugs unavailable for purchase under any circumstances, such as heroin (in the United States), and (b) drugs normally available with a prescription that are being obtained through illegal channels. Illicit drugs often are taken because of their mood-altering effect; that is, they make the person feel happy or relaxed.

ACTIONS OF DRUGS ON THE BODY

The action of a drug in the body can be described in terms of its half-life, the time interval required for the body's elimination processes to reduce the concentration of the drug in the body by one-half. For example, if a drug's half-life is 8 hours, then the amount of drug in the body is as follows:

Initially: 100%
After 8 hours: 50%
After 16 hours: 25%
After 24 hours: 12.5%
After 32 hours: 6.25%

Because the purpose of most drug therapy is to maintain a constant drug level in the body, repeated doses are required to maintain that level. When an orally administered drug is absorbed from the gastrointestinal tract into the blood plasma, its concentration in the plasma increases until the elimination rate equals the rate of absorption. This point is known as the *peak plasma level* (Figure 35-2 ■). When a drug is given intra-

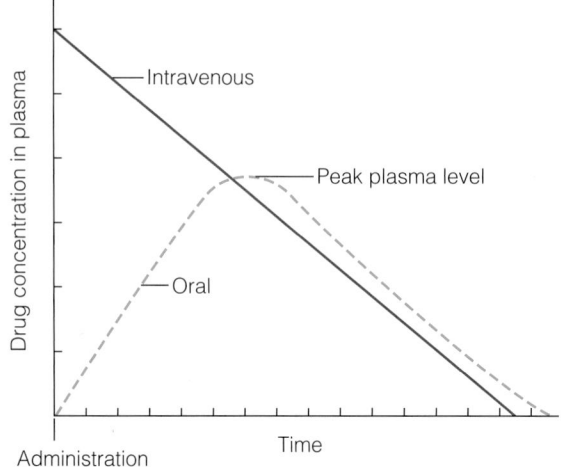

Figure 35-2 ■ A graphic plot of drug concentration in the blood plasma following a single dose.

venously (IV), its level is high immediately after administration and decreases through time. Another dose is given in order to maintain therapeutic levels. If the client does not receive another dose of the drug (either orally or IV), the concentration steadily decreases. Key terms related to drug actions are as follows:

- **Onset of action:** The time after administration when the body initially responds to the drug
- **Peak plasma level:** The highest plasma level achieved by a single dose when the elimination rate of a drug equals the absorption rate
- **Drug half-life (elimination half-life):** The time required for the elimination process to reduce the concentration of the drug to one-half what it was at initial administration
- **Plateau:** A maintained concentration of a drug in the plasma during a series of scheduled doses

Pharmacodynamics

Pharmacodynamics is the process by which a drug changes the body (e.g., alters cell physiology). Such changes require that the drug interact with specific molecules and chemicals normally found in the body (Adams, Josephson, & Holland, 2005). A **receptor,** usually a protein, is located on the surface of a cell membrane or within the cell. A cell membrane contains receptors for physiologic or endogenous substances such as hormones and neurotransmitters (Abrams, 2004, p. 16).

Most drugs exert their effects by chemically binding with receptors at the cellular level. When a drug binds to its receptor, the pharmacologic effects are either agonism or antagonism. A drug that produces the same type of response as the physiologic or endogenous substance is called an **agonist.** For example, epinephrine-like drugs act on the heart to increase the heart rate. Conversely, a drug that inhibits cell function by occupying receptor sites is called an **antagonist.** The antagonist prevents natural body substances or other drugs from activating the functions of the cell by occupying the receptor sites. For example, naloxone (Narcan) is an opioid antagonist used as an antidote for respiratory depression caused by an opioid drug (e.g., morphine). This drug competes with opioids for opioid receptor sites in the brain and thereby prevents opioids binding with receptors or displaces opioids already occupying receptor sites (Abrams, 2004, p. 87).

Pharmacokinetics

Pharmacokinetics is the study of the absorption, distribution, biotransformation, and excretion of drugs.

Absorption

Absorption is the process by which a drug passes into the bloodstream. Unless the drug is administered directly into the bloodstream, absorption is the first step in the movement of the drug through the body. For absorption to occur, the correct form of the drug must be given by the route intended.

The rate of absorption of a drug in the stomach is variable. Food, for example, can delay the dissolution and absorption of some drugs as well as their passage into the small intestine, where most drug absorption occurs. Food can also combine with molecules of certain drugs, thereby changing their molecular structure and subsequently inhibiting or preventing their absorption. Another factor that affects the absorption of some drugs is the acid medium in the stomach. Acidity can vary according to the time of day, foods ingested, use of antacid medications, and the age of the client. Some drugs do not dissolve or have limited ability to dissolve in the gastrointestinal fluids, decreasing their absorption into the bloodstream. Some drugs are absorbed by tissues before they reach the stomach. For example, nitroglycerin is administered under the tongue, where it is absorbed into the blood vessels that carry it directly to the heart, the intended site of action. If swallowed, this drug will be absorbed into the bloodstream and carried to the liver, where it will be destroyed. This is known as the first-pass effect, in which oral drugs first pass through the liver and are partially metabolized prior to reaching the target organ. This requires higher oral doses in order to achieve the appropriate effect.

A drug administered directly into the bloodstream, that is, intravenously, is immediately in the vascular system without having to be absorbed. This, then, is the route of choice for rapid action. The intramuscular route is the next most rapid route due to the highly vascular nature of muscle tissue. Because subcutaneous tissue has a poorer blood supply than muscle tissue, absorption from subcutaneous tissue is slower. The rate of absorption of a drug can be accelerated by the application of heat, which increases blood flow to the area; conversely, absorption can be slowed by the application of cold. In addition, the injection of a vasoconstrictor drug such as epinephrine into the tissue can slow absorption of other drugs. Some drugs intended to be absorbed slowly are suspended in a low-solubility medium, such as oil. The absorption of drugs from the rectum into the bloodstream tends to be unpredictable. Therefore, this route is normally used when other routes are unavailable or when the intended action is localized to the rectum or sigmoid colon.

Distribution

Distribution is the transportation of a drug from its site of absorption to its site of action. When a drug enters the bloodstream, it is carried to the most vascular organs—that is, liver, kidneys, and brain. Body areas with lower blood supply—that is, skin and muscles—receive the drug later. The chemical and physical properties of a drug largely determine the area of the body to which the drug will be attracted. For example, fat-soluble drugs will accumulate in fatty tissue, whereas other drugs may bind with plasma proteins.

Biotransformation

Biotransformation, also called **detoxification** or **metabolism,** is a process by which a drug is converted to a less active form. Most biotransformation takes place in the liver, where many drug-metabolizing enzymes in the cells detoxify the drugs. The products of this process are called **metabolites.** There are two types of metabolites: active and inactive. An *active metabolite* has a pharmacologic action itself, whereas an *inactive metabolite* does not.

Biotransformation may be altered if a person is very young, is older, or has an unhealthy liver. Nurses must be alert to the

ANATOMY & PHYSIOLOGY REVIEW   Pharmacokinetics of an Oral Medication

GI System: Stomach, Small Intestine

The oral medication reaches the systemic circulation through the GI system. As a result, numerous factors can affect the absorption of the pill.

QUESTIONS

1. Which would be absorbed the fastest: pill, capsule, or liquid?
2. A client is experiencing diarrhea. How could this affect absorption of an oral drug?
3. How does the presence of food in the stomach affect the rate of absorption?

Cardiovascular System

Once the pill is absorbed into the bloodstream, it is carried or delivered to the sites of pharmacologic action where the drug produces its effects.

QUESTION

1. How is distribution of the oral medication affected if a client has less than normal cardiac output (e.g., low BP, prolonged capillary refill)?

Liver

Most biotransformation takes place in the liver. Any decrease in the ability of the liver to metabolize medication could lead to an accumulation of the active drug in the bloodstream. This could put the client at risk for toxic effects and adverse reactions.

QUESTIONS

1. What are risk factors that can affect liver function?
2. A client is suspected of having decreased liver function. What information would be essential for the nurse to know about the oral medication that is to be given?

Kidneys

Drug excretion occurs mainly through the kidneys into the urine. If there is any impairment in kidney function, medications may not be excreted at the anticipated speed. Subsequent medication administration may lead to accumulation and potential toxicity.

QUESTIONS

1. Why would the very young and very old clients need to be closely monitored by the nurse for signs and symptoms of drug toxicity?
2. How can the nurse assess kidney function?

---

accumulation of the active drug in these clients and to subsequent toxicity.

Excretion

Excretion is the process by which metabolites and drugs are eliminated from the body. Most metabolites are eliminated by the kidneys in the urine; however, some are excreted in the feces, the breath, perspiration, saliva, and breast milk. Certain drugs, such as general anesthetic agents, are excreted in an unchanged form via the respiratory tract. The efficiency with which the kidneys excrete drugs and metabolites diminishes with age. Older people may require smaller doses of a drug because the drug and its metabolites may accumulate in the body.

FACTORS AFFECTING MEDICATION ACTION

A number of factors other than the drug itself can affect its action. A person may not respond in the same manner to successive doses of a drug. In addition, the identical drug and dosage may affect different clients differently.

Developmental Factors

During pregnancy women must be very careful about taking medications. Drugs taken during pregnancy pose a risk throughout the pregnancy, but pose the highest risk during the first trimester, due to the formation of vital organs and functions of the fetus during this time. Most drugs are contraindicated because of the possible adverse effects on the fetus.

Infants usually require small dosages because of their body size and the immaturity of their organs, especially the liver and kidneys. Differences in gastric acidity and liver enzymes required for drug metabolism may require different medication choices and dosages than adults. In adolescence or adulthood, allergic reactions may occur to drugs formerly tolerated.

Older adults have different responses to medications due to physiologic changes that accompany aging. These changes include decreased liver and kidney function, which can result in the accumulation of the drug in the body. In addition, the older person may be on multiple drugs and incompatibilities may occur.

Older adults often experience decreased gastric motility and decreased gastric acid production and blood flow, which can impair drug absorption. Increased adipose tissue and decreased total body fluid proportionate to the body mass can increase the possibility of drug toxicity. Older adults may also experience a decreased number of protein-binding sites and changes in the blood–brain barrier. The latter permits fat-soluble drugs to move readily to the brain, often resulting in dizziness and confusion. This is particularly evident with beta blockers.

Gender

Differences in the way men and women respond to drugs are chiefly related to the distribution of body fat and fluid and hormonal differences. Because most drug research is done on men, more research on women is required to reflect the effects of hormonal changes on drug actions in women.

Cultural, Ethnic, and Genetic Factors

A client's response to a drug is influenced by genetic variations such as gender, size, and body composition. This variation in response is called **pharmacogenetics.**

According to Lea (2005), drug metabolism and variations in enzymes are genetically determined and, as a result, may affect a drug response. For example, the genes that control liver metabolism vary. Some clients may have slow liver metabolism and not achieve an adequate response to a medication, whereas others are rapid metabolizers and may require lower doses of a medication to avoid adverse reactions. A new genetic blood test, approved in 2004, analyzes genes in a client's blood for variations that could cause the variations in metabolism of certain drugs. This information can help health care providers to individualize medication treatment and avoid adverse reactions.

A new field of study, **ethnopharmacology,** is the study of the effect of ethnicity on responses to prescribed medication (Munoz & Hilgenberg, 2005). Research has shown that certain medications may work well at usual therapeutic dosages for certain ethnic groups but be toxic for others. Ethnopharmacology also incorporates pharmacogenetics which is the study of the genetic ability to produce enzymes that affect drug metabolism. Pharmacogenetics can also vary by race or ethnic group.

Cultural factors and practices (e.g., values and beliefs) can also affect a drug's action. For example, an herbal remedy (e.g.,

the Chinese herb ginseng) may speed up or slow down the metabolism of prescribed medications. The Culturally Competent Care feature provides guidelines for nurses who care for clients from other cultures.

Diet

Nutrients can affect the action of a medication. For example, vitamin K found in green leafy vegetables can counteract the effect of an anticoagulant such as warfarin (Coumadin) (see Table 47–1 in Chapter 47). ∞

CULTURALLY COMPETENT CARE
Ethnopharmacology

Knowing that ethnicity can affect drug response helps the nurse provide culturally competent care. In the past, clinical drug research was conducted on Caucasian males even when the health disorder being studied was prevalent in other ethnic groups. Ethnopharmacologic research has focused on two major classifications: psychotropic and antihypertensive medications.

PSYCHOTROPIC MEDICATIONS

Research has found that African American clients experienced faster therapeutic responses, to tricyclic antidepressants, higher serum concentrations, and more adverse reactions than Caucasian clients.

African American clients may require lower doses of lithium than white clients.

ANTIHYPERTENSIVE MEDICATIONS

Studies have shown that certain angiotensin-converting enzyme (ACE) inhibitors (i.e., captopril and enalapril) and the angiotensin II receptor antagonist (i.e., losartan) were found to be less effective in African Americans than in Whites.

Thiazide diuretics appear to be more effective antihypertensives in African Americans than in Whites.

Beta blockers can vary among ethnic groups. African Americans may require higher dosages than Whites, and Asians usually require lower doses than Whites.

IMPLICATIONS FOR NURSING INTERVENTIONS

Remember that there may be differences in medication responses among different ethnic groups and differences *within* ethnic groups.

Ask about health beliefs, values, and customs/practices.

Conduct a cultural assessment with each client.

Learn about drugs that are likely to elicit varied responses in people from different ethnic groups, as well as the potential for adverse effects.

Ask the client direct, specific questions to reveal the presence or absence of potential adverse effects of medications.

Monitor the client and document findings carefully as it may be possible to maintain therapeutic benefit at a lower dosage of a given drug.

Keep cultural context in mind when planning education for clients and families.

Note: From "Ethnopharmacology" by C. Munoz and C. Hilgenberg, 2005, *American Journal of Nursing, 105*(8), pp. 40–48. Adapted with permission.

RESEARCH NOTE   Is There an Intervention to Improve Medication Adherence in Minority Women?

The purpose of this 12-month study was to determine the effectiveness of several strategies to promote medication adherence in older women from a variety of minority groups. The total sample of 109 women older than 65 years from Caucasian, African American, and Hispanic origins received standardized teaching about osteoporosis and their medication (estrogen and calcium) and provided opportunities for questions and clarification.

The Caucasian women used pillboxes marked with the days of the week and times of the day for 12 months. The African American and Hispanic women used the pillboxes for 6 months and then switched to using electronic monitoring medication bottles that recorded each bottle opening and closing as the administration of a dose for the remaining 6 months. A nurse contacted each participant on a monthly basis.

Results: Caucasian women were found to be the most adherent to their medication regimen. Hispanic women demonstrated significantly higher levels of adherence using the electronic bottles, while the African American women had higher levels of adherence using both the pillboxes and electronic monitoring devices.

IMPLICATIONS

Older clients, especially those from minority groups, may benefit from innovative medication adherence programs.

Note: From "Multicultural Medication Adherence: A Comparative Study," by B. Robbins, K. J. Rausch, R. I. Garcia, & K. W. Prestwood, 2004, *Journal of Gerontological Nursing, 30*(7), 25–32. Copyright © 2004 SLACK, Inc. Reprinted with permission.

Environment

The client's environment can affect the action of drugs, particularly those used to alter behavior and mood. Therefore, nurses assessing the effects of a drug need to consider the drug in the context of the client's personality and milieu.

Environmental temperature may also affect drug activity. When environmental temperature is high the peripheral blood vessels dilate, thus intensifying the action of vasodilators. In contrast, a cold environment and the consequent vasoconstriction inhibit the action of vasodilators but enhance the action of vasoconstrictors. A client who takes a sedative or analgesic in a busy, noisy environment may not benefit as fully as if the environment were quiet and peaceful.

Psychologic Factors

A client's expectations about what a drug can do can affect the response to the medication. For example, a client who believes that codeine is ineffective as an analgesic may experience no relief from pain after it is given.

Illness and Disease

Illness and disease can also affect the action of drugs. For example, aspirin can reduce the body temperature of a feverish client but has no effect on the body temperature of a client without fever. Drug action is altered in clients with circulatory, liver, or kidney dysfunction.

Time of Administration

The time of administration of oral medications affects the relative speed with which they act. Orally administered medications are absorbed more quickly if the stomach is empty. Thus, oral medications taken 2 hours before meals act faster than those taken after meals. However, some medications, for example iron preparations, irritate the gastrointestinal tract and are given after a meal, when they will be better tolerated.

ROUTES OF ADMINISTRATION

Pharmaceutical preparations are generally designed for one or two specific routes of administration (see Table 35–6). The route of administration should be indicated when the drug is ordered. When administering a drug, the nurse should ensure that the pharmaceutical preparation is appropriate for the route specified.

Oral

Oral administration is the most common, least expensive, and most convenient route for most clients. In oral administration, the drug is swallowed. Because the skin is not broken as it is for an injection, oral administration is also a safe method.

The major disadvantages are possibly unpleasant taste of the drugs, irritation of the gastric mucosa, irregular absorption from the gastrointestinal tract, slow absorption, and, in some cases, harm to the client's teeth. For example, the liquid preparation of ferrous sulfate (iron) can stain the teeth.

Sublingual

In **sublingual** administration a drug is placed under the tongue, where it dissolves (Figure 35-3 ■). In a relatively short time, the drug is largely absorbed into the blood vessels on the underside of the tongue. The medication should not be swallowed. Nitroglycerin is one example of a drug commonly given in this manner.

Tablet

Figure 35-3 ■ Sublingual administration of a tablet.

TABLE 35–6   Routes of Administration

ROUTE	ADVANTAGES	DISADVANTAGES
Oral	Most convenient Usually least expensive Safe, does not break skin barrier Administration usually does not cause stress Some new oral medications are designed to rapidly dissolve on the tongue, allowing for faster absorption and action	Inappropriate for clients with nausea or vomiting Drug may have unpleasant taste or odor Inappropriate when gastrointestinal tract has reduced motility Inappropriate if client cannot swallow or is unconscious Cannot be used before certain diagnostic tests or surgical procedures Drug may discolor teeth, harm tooth enamel Drug may irritate gastric mucosa Drug can be aspirated by seriously ill clients
Sublingual	Same as for oral, *plus:* Drug can be administered for local effect More potent than oral route because drug directly enters the blood and bypasses the liver	If swallowed, drug may be inactivated by gastric juice Drug must remain under tongue until dissolved and absorbed. May cause stinging or irritation of the mucous membranes Drug is rapidly absorbed into the bloodstream
Buccal	Same as for sublingual	Same as for sublingual
Rectal	Can be used when drug has objectionable taste or odor Drug released at slow, steady rate Provides a local therapeutic effect	Dose absorbed is unpredictable May be perceived as unpleasant by the client Limited use
Vaginal	Provides a local effect	May be messy and may soil clothes
Topical	Few side effects	Drug can enter body through abrasions and cause systemic effects Leaves residue on the skin that may soil clothes
Transdermal	Prolonged systemic effect Few side effects Avoids gastrointestinal absorption problems	
Subcutaneous	Onset of drug action faster than oral	Must involve sterile technique because breaks skin barrier More expensive than oral Can administer only small volume Slower than intramuscular administration Some drugs can irritate tissues and cause pain Can produce anxiety Breaks skin barrier
Intramuscular	Can administer larger volume than subcutaneous Drug is rapidly absorbed	Can produce anxiety
Intradermal	Absorption is slow (this is an advantage in testing for allergies)	Amount of drug administered must be small Breaks skin barrier
Intravenous	Rapid effect	Limited to highly soluble drugs Drug distribution inhibited by poor circulation
Inhalation	Introduces drug throughout respiratory tract Rapid localized relief Drug can be administered to unconscious client	Drug intended for localized effect can have systemic effect Of use only for the respiratory system

Buccal

Buccal means "pertaining to the cheek." In buccal administration, a medication (e.g., a tablet) is held in the mouth against the mucous membranes of the cheek until the drug dissolves (Figure 35-4 ■). The drug may act locally on the mucous membranes of the mouth or systemically when it is swallowed in the saliva.

Parenteral

The **parenteral** route is defined as other than through the alimentary or respiratory tract; that is, by needle. The following are some of the more common routes for parenteral administration:

- **Subcutaneous (hypodermic)**—into the subcutaneous tissue, just below the skin
- **Intramuscular**—into a muscle
- **Intradermal**—under the epidermis (into the dermis)
- **Intravenous**—into a vein

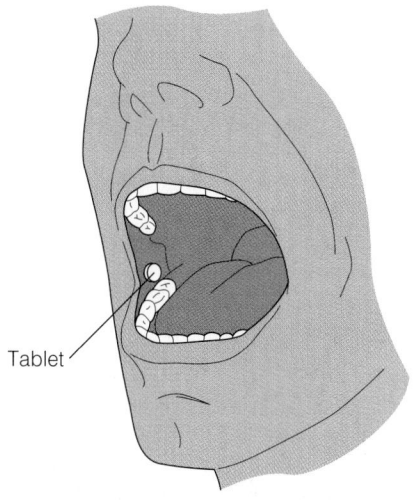

Tablet

Figure 35-4 ■ Buccal administration of a tablet.

Some of the less commonly used routes for parenteral administration are intra-arterial (into an artery), intracardiac (into the heart muscle), intraosseous (into a bone), **intrathecal** or **intraspinal** (into the spinal canal), intrapleural (into the pleural space), **epidural** (into the epidural space), and intra-articular (into a joint). Sterile equipment and sterile drug solution are essential for all parenteral therapy. The main advantage is fast absorption.

Topical

Topical applications are those applied to a circumscribed surface area of the body. They affect only the area to which they are applied. Topical applications include the following:

- Dermatologic preparations—applied to the skin
- Instillations and irrigations—applied into body cavities or orifices, such as the urinary bladder, eyes, ears, nose, rectum, or vagina
- Inhalations—administered into the respiratory tract by a nebulizer or positive pressure breathing apparatus. Air, oxygen, and vapor are generally used to carry the drug into the lungs.

MEDICATION ORDERS

A physician usually determines the client's medication needs and orders medications, although in some settings nurse practitioners and physician's assistants now order some drugs. Each health agency will have its own policies. Usually the order is written, although telephone and verbal orders are acceptable in a number of agencies. Nursing students need to know the agency policies about medication orders. In some hospitals, for example, only licensed nurses are permitted to accept telephone and verbal orders.

Policies about primary care providers' orders vary considerably from agency to agency. For example, a client's orders may be automatically canceled after surgery or an examination involving an anesthetic agent. The primary care provider must then write new orders. Most agencies also have lists of abbreviations officially accepted for use in the agency. Recently, in order to prevent medication errors, the Joint Commission on Accreditation of Healthcare Organizations (JCAHO) mandated that agencies must standardize abbreviations, acronyms, and symbols used throughout the organization and *must* list abbreviations that are never to be used (Karch, 2004; JCAHO, n.d.). See Table 35–7 for the list of unacceptable abbreviations.

TABLE 35–7 Unacceptable Abbreviations—"Do Not Use" List

ABBREVIATION	POTENTIAL PROBLEM	USE INSTEAD
U (unit)	Mistaken for "0" (zero), the number "4" (four), or "cc"	Write "unit"
IU (international unit)	Mistaken for IV (intravenous) or the number 10 (ten)	Write "International Unit"
Q.D., QD, q.d., qd (daily)	Mistaken for each other	Write "daily"
Q.O.D., QOD, q.o.d., qod (every other day)	Period after the Q mistaken for "I" and the "O" mistaken for "I"	Write "every other day"
Trailing zero (X.0 mg)	Decimal point is missed	Write X mg
Lack of leading zero (.X mg)		Write 0.X mg
MS	Can mean morphine sulfate or magnesium sulfate	Write "morphine sulfate"
MSO₄ and MgSO₄		Write "magnesium sulfate"

For Possible Future Inclusion in the Official "Do Not Use" List		
>(greater than)	Misinterpreted as the number "7" (seven) or the letter "L"	Write "greater than"
<(less than)	Confused for one another	Write "less than"
Abbreviations for drug names	Misinterpreted due to similar abbreviations for multiple drugs	Write drug names in full
Apothecary units	Unfamiliar to many practitioners Confused with metric units	Use metric units
@	Mistaken for the number "2" (two)	Write "at"
cc	Mistaken for U (units) when poorly written	Write "ml" or "milliliters"
μg	Mistaken for mg (milligrams) resulting in one thousand-fold overdose	Write "mcg" or "micrograms"

Others to Consider		
TIW (three times a week)	Has been misinterpreted as "two times a week" or "three times a day" resulting in misdosing	Write "three times weekly"
AS (left ear) AD (right ear) AU (both ears)	Mistaken for OS (left eye), OD (either "overdose" or "optic density"), and OU ("each eye" or "both eyes")	Write "left ear," "right ear," or "both ears," as appropriate
HS	Has been used to indicate "half strength" and "bedtime" or "hour of sleep"	Write out "half strength" or "at bedtime", as appropriate
SC and SQ (subcutaneous)	Have been read as "SL" (sublingual) and as "5 every hour"	Write "subq" or "subcutaneous"
D/C	Can mean either "discharge" or "discontinue"	Write "discharge" or "discontinue" as appropriate

Types of Medication Orders

Four common medication orders are the stat order, the single order, the standing order, and the prn order.

1. A **stat order** indicates that the medication is to be given immediately and only once (e.g., Demerol 100 mg IM stat).
2. The **single order** or *one-time order* is for medication to be given once at a specified time (e.g., Seconal 100 mg hs before surgery).
3. The **standing order** may or may not have a termination date. A standing order may be carried out indefinitely (e.g., multiple vitamins daily) until an order is written to cancel it, or it may be carried out for a specified number of days (e.g., Demerol 100 mg IM q4h × 5 days). In some agencies, standing orders are automatically canceled after a specified number of days and must be reordered.
4. A **prn order,** or *as-needed order,* permits the nurse to give a medication when, in the nurse's judgment, the client requires it (e.g., Amphojel 15 mL prn). The nurse must use good judgment about when the medication is needed and when it can be safely administered.

Essential Parts of a Drug Order

The drug order has seven essential parts, as listed in Box 35–1. In addition, unless it is a standing order it should state the number of doses or the number of days the drug is to be administered.

The *client's full name,* that is, the first and last names and middle initials or names, should always be used to avoid confusion between two clients who have the same last name. In some agencies, the client's identification number and physician's name are put on the order as further identification. Some hospitals imprint the client's name, identification number, and room number on all forms; some agencies use stickers with similar information.

In addition to the *day,* the *month,* and the *year* the order was written, some agencies also require that the time of day be written. Writing the *time of day* on the order can eliminate errors when the nursing shifts change and makes clear when certain orders automatically terminate. For example, in some settings narcotics can be ordered only for 48 hours after surgery. Therefore, a drug that is ordered at 1600 hours November 1, 2008, is automatically canceled at 1600 hours November 3, 2008. Many health agencies use the 24-hour clock, which eliminates confusion between morning and afternoon times. Time with the 24-hour clock starts at midnight, which is 0000 hours (see Chapter 15). ∞

The *name of the drug to be administered* must be clearly written. In some settings only generic names are permitted;

however, trade names are widely used in hospitals and health agencies.

The *dosage of the drug* includes the amount, the times or *frequency of administration,* and in many instances the strength; for example, tetracycline 250 mg (amount) four times a day (frequency); potassium chloride 10% (strength) 5 mL (amount) three times a day with meals (time and frequency). Dosages can be written in apothecary or metric systems. The metric system, however, is strongly suggested for safety reasons because many practitioners are unfamiliar with apothecary units.

Also included in the order is the *route of administration* of the drug. This part of the order, like other parts, is frequently abbreviated. It is not unusual for a drug to have several possible routes of administration; therefore, it is important that the route be included in the order.

The *signature* of the ordering primary care provider or nurse makes the drug order a legal request. *An unsigned order has no validity,* and the ordering physician or nurse practitioner needs to be notified if the order is unsigned.

When a primary care provider writes a prescription for a client, the prescription also includes information for the pharmacist. Therefore, a prescription's content differs from that of a medication order in a hospital. Compare the parts of a prescription listed in Box 35–2 with those shown in Figure 35–5 ■.

Communicating a Medication Order

A drug order is written on the client's chart by a primary care provider or by a nurse receiving a telephone or verbal order from a primary care provider. Most acute care agencies have a specified time frame (e.g., 24 or 48 hours) in which the primary care provider issuing the telephone or verbal order must cosign the order written by the nurse. The medication order is then copied by a nurse or clerk to a Kardex or medication administration record (MAR). Increasingly, nurses receive computer printouts of a client's medications instead of a copy of the primary care provider's order. This method avoids errors and saves nursing time.

CLINICAL ALERT

If your assigned client receives new medication orders, double-check the transcribed information with the primary care provider's order. This ensures client safety. ■

BOX 35–2 Parts of a Prescription

- Descriptive information about the client: name, address, and sometimes age
- Date on which the prescription was written
- The Rx symbol, meaning "take thou"
- Medication name, dosage, and strength
- Route of administration
- Dispensing instructions for the pharmacist, for example, "Dispense 30 capsules"
- Directions for administration to be given to the client, for example, "one tablet with meals"
- Refill and/or special labeling, for example, "Refill × 1"
- Prescriber's signature

BOX 35–1 Essential Parts of a Drug Order

- Full name of the client
- Date and time the order is written
- Name of the drug to be administered
- Dosage of the drug
- Frequency of administration
- Route of administration
- Signature of the person writing the order

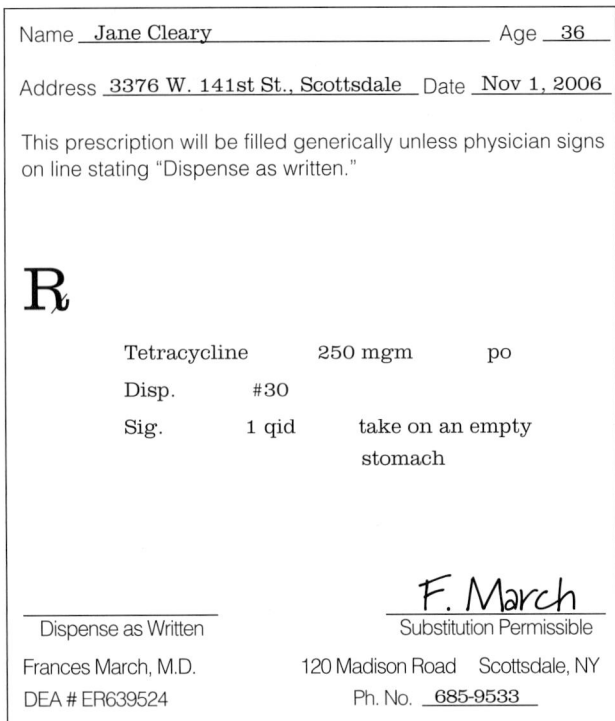

```
Name  Jane Cleary                                    Age   36

Address  3376 W. 141st St., Scottsdale  Date  Nov 1, 2006

This prescription will be filled generically unless physician signs
on line stating "Dispense as written."


R

        Tetracycline        250 mgm         po

        Disp.       #30

        Sig.        1 qid        take on an empty
                                 stomach




                                        F. March
  _____              _____
    Dispense as Written               Substitution Permissible

  Frances March, M.D.          120 Madison Road   Scottsdale, NY
  DEA # ER639524                    Ph. No.  685-9533
```

Figure 35-5 ■ A prescription filled out by a primary care provider.

Medication administration records (MARs) vary in form, but all include the client's name, room, and bed number; drug name and dose; and times and method of administration (Figure 35-6 ■). In some agencies, the date the order was prescribed and the date the order expires are also included.

The nurse should always question the primary care provider about any order that is ambiguous, unusual (e.g., an abnormally high dosage of a medication), or contraindicated by the client's condition. When the nurse judges a primary care provider-ordered medication inappropriate, the following actions are required:

- Contact the primary care provider and discuss the rationale for believing the medication or dosage to be inappropriate.
- Document in notes the following: when the primary care provider was notified, what was conveyed to the primary care provider, and how the primary care provider responded.
- If the primary care provider cannot be reached, document all attempts to contact the primary care provider and the reason for withholding the medication.
- If someone else gives the medication, document data about the client's condition before and after the medication.
- If an incident report (see Chapter 4 ∞) is indicated, clearly document factual information.

SYSTEMS OF MEASUREMENT

Three systems of measurement are used in North America: the metric system, the apothecaries' system, and the household system, which is similar to the apothecaries' system.

Metric System

The metric system, devised by the French in the latter part of the 18th century, is the system prescribed by law in most European countries and in Canada. The metric system is logically organized into units of 10; it is a decimal system. Basic units can be multiplied or divided by 10 to form secondary units. Multiples are calculated by moving the decimal point to the right, and division is accomplished by moving the decimal point to the left.

Basic units of measurement are the *meter,* the *liter,* and the *gram.* Prefixes derived from Latin designate subdivisions of the basic unit: *deci* (1/10 or 0.1), *centi* (1/100 or 0.01), and *milli* (1/1,000 or 0.001). Multiples of the basic unit are designated by prefixes derived from Greek: *deka* (10), *hecto* (100), and *kilo* (1,000). Only the measurements of volume (the liter) and of weight (the gram) are discussed in this chapter. These are the measures used in medication administration (see Figure 35-7 ■). The *kilogram* (kg) is the only multiple of the gram used, and the *milligram* (mg) and *microgram* (mcg) are subdivisions. Fractional parts of the liter are usually expressed in *milliliters* (mL), for example, 600 mL; multiples of the liter are usually expressed as *liters* or milliliters, for example, 2.5 liters or 2,500 mL. In nursing practice it is important to understand the difference between weight and volume. A drug dosage may be ordered by weight (i.e, grams, mg, mcg) and administered by volume (mL). For example, a health care provider prescribes 20 mg (weight) of codeine elixir. The codeine elixir bottle is labeled 10 mg per 5 mL The nurse administers 10 mL (volume) of codeine elixir.

Apothecaries' System

The apothecaries' system, older than the metric system, was brought to the United States from England during the colonial period. The basic unit of weight in the apothecaries' system is the *grain* (gr), likened to a grain of wheat, and the basic unit of volume is the *minim,* a volume of water equal in weight to a grain of wheat. The word *minim* means "the least." In ascending order, the other units of weight are the *scruple,* the *dram,* the *ounce,* and the *pound.* Today, the scruple is seldom used. The units of volume are, in ascending order, the fluid dram, the fluid ounce, the pint, the quart, and the gallon.

Quantities in the apothecaries' system are often expressed by lowercase Roman numerals, particularly when the unit of measure is abbreviated. The Roman numeral follows rather than precedes the unit of measure. For example, two grains are written as gr ii. Quantities less than 1 are expressed as a fraction, for example, gr 1/6. As stated earlier, apothecary units are unfamiliar to many practitioners and they may be confused with metric units. It is advisable to *not* use apothecary units. Use metric units instead to avoid medication errors.

Household System

Household measures may be used when more accurate systems of measure are not required. Included in household measures are drops, teaspoons, tablespoons, cups, and glasses. Although pints and quarts are often found in the home, they are defined as apothecaries' measures.

MEDICATION ADMINISTRATION RECORD				PAGE 1 OF 1

MEDICATION ADMINISTRATION RECORD

PRN#:
MRN#:   AGE:
ADM: 08-04-07   SEX:
DOB: HT:
DR.   HT:

VERIFIED BY: _____ DATE: _____

DIAGNOSIS: ALOC
            PNEUMONIA
ALLERGIES: NO KNOWN DRUG ALLERGIES

GENERATED: 08-07-07   07:32
FOR PERIOD: 08-07-07   08:00
THROUGH: 08-08-07   07:59

START	STOP	MEDICATION/I.V./IVPB/IRRIGATION	0800-1559	1600-2359	0000-0759
08-06	09-05	FERROUS SULFATE 300MG=5ML TWICE A DAY PO (FESO4) (973539)	09	17	
08-06	09-05	DOCUSATE SODIUM 100MG=1UDCUP TWICE A DAY PO (COLACE) 100MG/30ML UD (973532) HOLD FOR LOOSE STOOL	09	17	
08-05	09-04	ASCORBIC ACID 500MG=1TAB TWICE A DAY PO (VITAMIN C) 500MG TAB (972096)	09	17	
08-05	09-04	LEVOTHYROXINE 0.05MG=1TAB DAILY PO (SYNTHROID) 0.05MG TAB (972095)	09		
08-05	09-04	ASPIRIN 325MG=1 TAB DAILY PO (ASPIRIN) 325MG TAB (972094) *W/FOOD TO AVOID GI UPSET	09		
08-04	08-14	CEFUROXIME ADDV. 1.500GM=1VIAL EVERY 8 HOURS IV (KEFUROX) 1.5GM ADDV (971776) *ATTACH TO D5W 50ML ADDV BAG *ACTIVATE BEFORE INFUSION* * INFUSE OVER 30 MINS*	14	22	06
		——— PRN ORDERS ———			
08-04	09-03	ACETAMINOPHEN 650MG=1SUPP EVERY 4 HOURS AS NEEDED PR (TYLENOL) 650MG SUPP (971779)			

INITIALS	SIGNATURE	SHIFT	INITIALS	SIGNATURE	SHIFT	INITIALS	SIGNATURE	SHIFT

SITE CODES:
A. Right Upper Outer Quadrant Gluteus   C. Right Outer Aspect Arm   E. Right Ventrogluteal   G. Abdomen   I. Left Thigh
B. Left Upper Outer Quadrant Gluteus   D. Left Outer Aspect Arm   F. Left Ventrogluteal   H. Right Thigh

Figure 35-6 ■ Sample medication administration record (MAR).

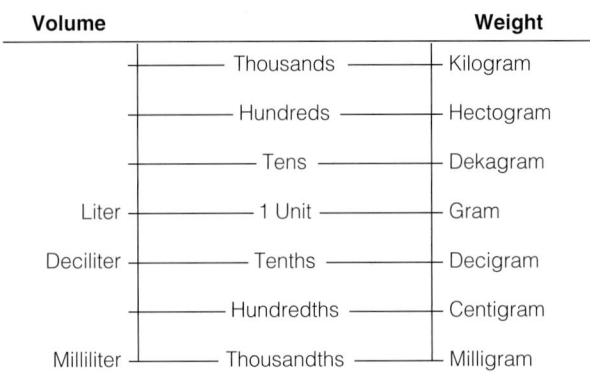

Figure 35-7 ■ Basic metric measurements of volume and weight.

Converting Units of Weight and Measure

Sometimes drugs are dispensed from the pharmacy in grams when the order specifies milligrams, or they are dispensed in milligrams though ordered in grains. For example, a physician orders morphine gr 1/4. The medication is available labeled only in milligrams. The nurse knows that 1 mg = 1/60 gr or 60 mg = 1 grain. To convert the ordered dose to milligrams, the nurse calculates as follows:

$$\text{If } 60 \text{ mg} = 1 \text{ gr}$$
$$\text{Then } x \text{ mg} = 1/4 \text{ gr } (0.25 \text{ gr})$$
$$x = \frac{(60 \times 0.25)}{1}$$
$$x = 15 \text{ mg}$$

Converting Weights within the Metric System

It is relatively simple to arrive at equivalent units of weight within the metric system because the system is based on units of 10. Only three metric units of weight are used for drug dosages, the gram (g), milligram (mg), and microgram (mcg): 1,000 mg or 1,000,000 mcg equals 1 gram (g). Equivalents are computed by dividing or multiplying; for example, to change milligrams to grams, the nurse divides the number of milligrams by 1,000. The simplest way to divide by 1,000 is to move the decimal point three places to the left:

$$500 \text{ mg} = ? \text{ g}$$

Move the decimal point three places to the *left:*

$$\text{Answer} = 0.5 \text{ g}$$

Conversely, to convert grams to milligrams, multiply the number of grams by 1,000, or move the decimal point three places to the right:

$$0.006 \text{ g} = ? \text{ mg}$$

Move the decimal point three places to the *right:*

$$\text{Answer} = 6 \text{ mg}$$

Converting Weights and Measures between Systems

When preparing client medications, a nurse may need to convert weights or volumes from one system to another. As an example, the pharmacy may dispense milligrams or grams of chloral hydrate, yet the nurse must administer an order that reads "chloral hydrate gr viiss." To prepare the correct dose, the nurse must convert from the apothecaries' to the metric system. To give clients a useful, realistic measure for home use, the nurse may have to convert from the apothecaries' or metric system to the household system. All conversions are approximate, that is, not totally precise.

Converting Units of Volume

Commonly used approximate equivalents are shown in Table 35–8. By learning these equivalents, the nurse can make many conversions readily. For example, 15 minims = approximately 15 drops (gtt); therefore, 1 minim is approximately 1 drop. Similarly, 1 quart approximates 1,000 mL, and 1 gallon approximates 4,000 mL.

The following are some situations in which nurses need to apply knowledge of volume conversion:

- Fluid drams and ounces are commonly used in prescribing liquid medications, such as cough syrups, laxatives, antacids, and antibiotics for children. The fluid ounce is frequently converted to milliliters when measuring a client's fluid intake or output.
- Liters and milliliters are the volumes commonly used in preparing solutions for enemas, irrigating solutions for bladder irrigations, and solutions for cleaning open wounds. In some situations, the nurse needs to convert the volumes of such solutions.

Converting Units of Weight

The units of weight most commonly used in nursing practice are the gram, milligram, and kilogram and the grain and the pound. Household units of weight are generally not applicable.

MediaLink Calculating Dosages Application

TABLE 35–8		Approximate Volume Equivalents: Metric, Apothecaries', and Household Systems		
METRIC		**APOTHECARIES'**		**HOUSEHOLD**
1 mL	=	15 minims (min or m)	=	15 drops (gtt)
4–5 mL	=	1 fluid dram	=	1 teaspoon
15 mL	=	4 fluid drams	=	1 tablespoon (Tbsp)
30 mL	=	1 fluid ounce	=	same
500 mL	=	1 pint (pt)	=	same
1,000 mL	=	1 quart (qt)	=	same
4,000 mL	=	1 gallon (gal)	=	same

TABLE 35–9 Approximate Weight Equivalents: Metric and Apothecaries' Systems

METRIC		APOTHECARIES'
1 mg	=	1/60 grain
60 mg	=	1 grain
1 g	=	15 grains
4 g	=	1 dram
30 g	=	1 ounce
500 g	=	1.1 pound (lb)
1,000 g (1 kg)	=	2.2 lb

Table 35–9 shows metric and apothecaries' approximate equivalents. Learning these equivalents helps the nurse make weight conversions readily, as for example in the following situations:

- Converting milligrams to grains and vice versa, for example, when preparing medications
- Converting pounds to kilograms and vice versa, for example, a person's weight

When converting units of weight from the metric system to the apothecaries' system, the nurse should keep in mind that a milligram is smaller than a grain (1 mg = 1/60 grain and 1 grain = 60 mg). The result of converting a smaller unit (milligram) to a larger unit (grain) is a smaller number. Thus, the nurse must divide (by 60 if converting from milligrams to grains). Conversely, when converting from a larger unit to a smaller unit, the nurse multiplies (by 60 if converting from grains to milligrams), and the product is a larger number. In other words:

$$\text{Small units (mg) to large units (grains)} = \text{a smaller number}$$
$$\text{Large units (grains) to small units (mg)} = \text{a larger number}$$
$$\frac{3,000 \text{ mg}}{60} = 50 \text{ grains}$$
$$50 \text{ grains} \times 60 = 3,000 \text{ mg}$$

When converting pounds to kilograms, the nurse applies the same rule. The pound is a smaller unit than the kilogram, and the nurse converts by dividing or multiplying by 2.2:

$$2.2 \text{ lb} = 1 \text{ kg}$$
$$110 \text{ lb} = x \text{ kg}$$
$$x = \frac{110 \times 1}{2.2}$$
$$= 50 \text{ kg}$$

or

$$50 \text{ kg} = x \text{ lb}$$
$$1 \text{ kg} = 2.2 \text{ lb}$$
$$x = \frac{2.2 \times 50}{1}$$
$$= 110 \text{ lb}$$

The conversion of milligrams to grams was previously discussed. The decimal point is moved three spaces to the left:

$$3,000 \text{ mg} = 3 \text{ g}$$

Calculating Dosages

Several formulas can be used to calculate drug dosages. One formula uses ratios:

$$\frac{\text{Dose on hand}}{\text{Quantity on hand}} = \frac{\text{desired dose}}{\text{quantity desired } (x)}$$

For example, erythromycin 500 mg is ordered. It is supplied in a liquid form containing 250 mg in 5 mL. To calculate the dosage, the nurse uses the formula

$$\frac{\text{Dose on hand (250 mg)}}{\text{Quantity on hand (5 mL)}} = \frac{\text{desired dose (500 mg)}}{\text{quantity desired } (x)}$$

Then the nurse cross multiplies:

$$250\,x = 5 \text{ mL} \times 500 \text{ mg}$$
$$x = \frac{5 \text{ mL} \times 500 \text{ mg}}{250 \text{ mg}}$$
$$x = 10 \text{ mL}$$

Therefore, the dose ordered is 10 mL. The nurse can also use this formula to calculate dosages:

$$\text{Amount to administer } (x) =$$
$$\frac{\text{desired dose}}{\text{dose on hand}} \times \text{quantity on hand}$$

For example, heparin is often distributed in vials in prepared dilutions of 10,000 units per milliliter. If the order calls for 5,000 units, the nurse can use the preceding formula to calculate

$$x = \frac{5,000}{10,000} \times 1$$
$$x = 1/2 \text{ mL}$$

Therefore, the nurse injects 0.5 mL for a 5,000-unit dose.

Dosages for Children

Although dosage is stated in the medication order, nurses must understand something about the safe dosage for children and verify dosages as within a safe range. Unlike adult dosages, children's dosages are not always standard. Body size significantly affects dosage; therefore, dosages are calculated. Dosages based on weight use kilograms of body weight and per kilogram medication recommendations to arrive at appropriate and safe doses. Recommendations for surface area dosing are also standardized.

Body Surface Area

Body surface area is determined by using a nomogram and the child's height and weight. This is considered to be the most accurate method of calculating a child's dose. Standard nomograms give a child's body surface area according to weight and height (Figure 35-8 ■). The formula is the ratio of the child's body surface area to the surface area of an average adult (1.7 square meters, or 1.7 m^2), multiplied by the normal adult dose of the drug:

$$\text{Child's dose} = \frac{\text{surface area of child (m}^2)}{1.7 \text{ m}^2} \times \text{normal adult dose}$$

Figure 35-8 ■ Nomogram with estimated body surface area. A straight line is drawn between the child's height (on the left) and the child's weight (on the right). The point at which the line intersects the surface area column is the estimated body surface area.

For example, a child who weighs 10 kg and is 50 cm tall has a body surface area of 0.4 m^2. Therefore, the child's dose of tetracycline corresponding to an adult dose of 250 mg would be as follows:

$$\text{Child's dose} = \frac{0.4 \text{ m}^2}{1.7 \text{ m}^2} \times 250 \text{ mg}$$

$$= 0.23 \times 250 = 58.82 \text{ mg}$$

ADMINISTERING MEDICATIONS SAFELY

The nurse should always assess a client's health status and obtain a medication history prior to giving any medication. The extent of the assessment depends on the client's illness or current condition, the intended drug, and the route of administration. For example, if a client has dyspnea, the nurse assesses respirations carefully before administering any medication that might affect breathing. It is important to determine whether the route of administration is suitable. For example, a client who is nauseated may not be able to keep down a drug taken orally. In general, the nurse assesses the client *prior* to administering any medication to obtain baseline data by which to evaluate the effectiveness of the medication.

The medication history includes information about the drugs the client is taking currently or has taken recently. This includes prescription drugs; over-the-counter drugs such as antacids, alcohol, and tobacco; and nonsanctioned drugs such as marijuana. Sometimes an incompatibility with one or more of these drugs affects the choice of a new medication.

Elders often take vitamins, herbs, and food supplements, and/or use folk remedies that they do not list in their medication history. Because many of these have unknown or unpredictable actions and side effects, they need to be noted, with attention paid to possible incompatibilities with other prescribed medications.

An important part of the history is clients' knowledge of their drug allergies. Some clients can tell a nurse, "I am allergic to penicillin, adhesive tape, and curry." The nurse should clarify with the client any side effects, adverse reactions, or allergic responses due to medications. Other clients may not be sure about allergic reactions. An illness occurring after a drug was taken may not be identified as an allergy, but the client may associate

PRACTICE GUIDELINES
Administering Medications

- Nurses who administer medications are responsible for their own actions. Question any order that is illegible or that you consider incorrect. Call the person who prescribed the medication for clarification.
- Be knowledgeable about the medications you administer. You need to know why the client is receiving the medication. Look up the necessary information if you are not familiar with the medication.
- Federal laws govern the use of narcotics and barbiturates. Keep these medications in a locked place.
- Use only medications that are in a clearly labeled container.
- Do not use liquid medications that are cloudy or have changed color.
- Calculate drug doses accurately. If you are uncertain, ask another nurse to double-check your calculations.
- Administer only medications personally prepared.
- Before administering a medication, identify the client correctly using the appropriate means of identification, such as checking the identification bracelet.
- Do not leave medications at the bedside, with certain exceptions (e.g., nitroglycerin, cough syrup). Check agency policy.
- If a client vomits after taking an oral medication, report this to the nurse in charge, or the primary care provider, or both.
- Take special precautions when administering certain medications; for example, have another nurse check the dosages of anticoagulants, insulin, and certain IV preparations.
- Most hospital policies require new orders from the primary care provider a for a client's postsurgery care.
- When a medication is omitted for any reason, record the fact together with the reason.
- When a medication error is made, report it immediately to the nurse in charge, the primary care provider, or both.

the drug with an illness or unusual reaction. The client's primary care provider can often give information about allergies. During the history, the nurse tries to elicit information about drug dependencies. How often drugs are taken and the client's perceived need for them are measures of dependence.

Also included in the history are the client's normal eating habits. Sometimes the medication schedule needs to be coordinated with mealtimes or the ingestion of foods. Where a medication must be taken with food on a specified schedule, clients can often adjust their mealtime or have a snack (e.g., with a bedtime medication). In addition, certain foods are incompatible with certain medications; for example, milk is incompatible with tetracycline.

It is also important for the nurse to identify any problems the client may have in self-administering a medication. A client with poor eyesight, for example, may require special labels for the medication container; elderly clients with unsteady hands may not be able to hold a syringe or to inject themselves or another person. Obtaining information as to how and where clients store their medications is also important. If clients have difficulty opening certain containers, they may change containers, but leave old labels on, which increases the risk of medication errors.

The nurse needs to consider socioeconomic factors for all clients, but especially for elders. Two common problems are lack of transportation to obtain medications and inadequate finances to purchase medications. When aware of these problems, the nurse can refer proper resources for the client.

Medication Reconciliation

Another safety issue that affects the nurse is to ensure that clients receive the appropriate medications and dosages on admission, during transfer, and at discharge. According to the Institute for Healthcare Improvement (IHI), poorly communicated medical information at admission and other health care transition points is responsible for as many as 50% of all medication errors in hospitals (Manno & Hayes, 2006, p. 63). Furthermore, one out of five drugs administered in hospitals and skilled nursing facilities is in error and nearly 34% of preventable adverse drug events (ADEs) can be traced back to the administration process (Ketchum, Grass, & Padwojski, 2005, p. 78).

As a result, the IHI campaigned for medication reconciliation, and JCAHO incorporated medication reconciliation into their National Patient Safety Goals. The IHI defines **medication reconciliation** as "the process of creating the most accurate list possible of all medications a patient is taking—including drug name, dosage, frequency, and route—and comparing that list against the physician's admission, transfer, and/or discharge orders, with the goal of providing correct medications to the patient at all transition points within the hospital" (IHI, n.d.).

As of January 2006, all JCAHO-accredited facilities must have protocols and processes in place for medication reconciliation, particularly in three transition areas: on admission; during transfer between units, in shift reports, and in new MARs; and at discharge. The nurse needs to make a complete list of the client's medications (including prescriptions, vitamins, supplements, and over-the-counter) on admission. This current list needs to be compared to any new medications ordered by the physician on admission and during the client's hospital stay. Medications that are to be administered around the time of shift report need to be discussed at the report. For example, insulin is a common medication scheduled between night and day shifts. It is important that the oncoming nurse know if the medication was given or not. If a client is transferred to another setting, within or outside of the facility, a complete list of the client's medications must be communicated to the next provider of care. This list is also provided to clients on discharge from the facility. In addition, the client should receive, at discharge, written and oral information on each medication to be taken at home. It is important for the nurse to emphasize to the client the importance of keeping the list of their medications and taking it with them to their follow-up visits and to future hospitalizations, if any. Maintaining their list of current medications helps improve communication and avoid potential errors in medication administration.

Medication Dispensing Systems

Medical facilities vary in their medication dispensing systems. The systems can include the following:

- *Medication cart.* The medication cart is on wheels allowing the nurse to move the cart to outside the client's room. The cart contains small numbered drawers that correlate to the room numbers on the nursing unit. The small drawer is labeled with the name of the client currently in that room and holds the client's medications for the shift or 24 hours (Figure 35-9 ■). The medication is usually in

Figure 35-9 ■ Medication cart.

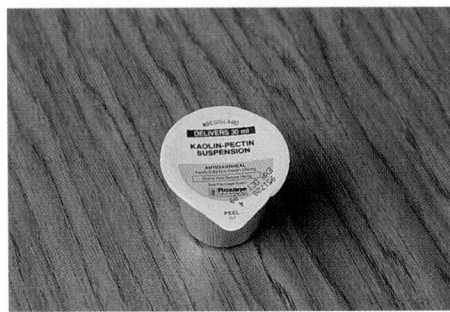

Figure 35-10 ■ Unit-dose packages: *A,* tablets; *B,* liquid medications.

Photographer: Elena Dorfman

unit-dose packaging; that is, the individual drug package states the drug name, dose, and expiration date (Figure 35-10 ■). A larger locked drawer in the cart contains the controlled substances rather than keeping them in the client's individual drawer. The cart may also include a supply drawer that contains client-labeled bulk containers, such as Metamucil, that are too large for the small individual drawer. The MAR is usually located in a binder or a computer located on top of the medication cart. The nurse either carries a key for the medication cart or enters a special code to open the cart, because it must be kept locked when not in use (Figure 35-11 ■).

■ *Medication cabinet.* Some facilities have a locked cabinet in the client's room. This cabinet holds the client's unit-dose medications and MAR. Controlled substances are not kept in this cabinet but at another location on the nursing unit. The nurse uses either a key or a special code for opening the client's medication cabinet, because it must be locked when not in use.

■ *Medication room.* Depending on the facility, a medication room may be used for a variety of purposes. For example, the medication carts, when not in use, may be placed in this room. The medication room may also be the central location for stock medications, controlled medications, and/or drugs used for emergencies. The medication room may have a refrigerator for intravenous and other medications needing a cold environment. The room may also contain other medication administration supplies (syringes, needles, etc.). Nurses access the medication room by either a key or a special code as the room is often kept locked. Check agency policy.

■ *Automated dispensing cabinet (ADC).* This computerized access system (Figure 35-12 ■) automates the distribution, management, and control of medications. Similar to automated teller machines, the nurse uses a password to access the system, selects the client's name from an on-screen list, and selects the medication(s) (Figure 35-13 ■).

Process of Administering Medications

When administering any drug, regardless of the route of administration, the nurse must do the following:

1. *Identify the client.* Errors can and do occur, usually because one client gets a drug intended for another. One of the Joint Commission's National Patient Safety Goals is to improve the accuracy of client identification. This goal

Figure 35-11 ■ The medication cart is kept locked when not in use. The nurse is using a key to access client medications.

Figure 35-12 ■ Computerized medication access system.

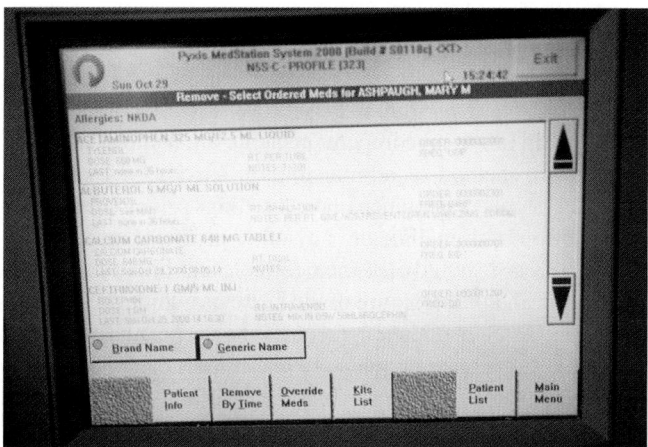

Figure 35-13 ■ Client profile in a computerized medication access system.

A

B

C

Figure 35-14 ■ *A,* A sample bar code. *B,* The nurse scans the bar code on the medication package and *C,* the bar code on the client's wristband before administering the medication.

(Shirlee Synder)

requires a nurse to use at least two client identifiers whenever administering medications. Neither identifier can be the client's room number. Acceptable identifiers may be the person's name, assigned identification number, telephone number, photograph, or other person-specific identifier (JCAHO, 2006). In hospitals, most clients wear some sort of identification, such as a wristband with name and hospital identification number. Before giving the client any drug, always check the client's identification band. Some hospitals use bar-code technology for medication administration. A nurse preparing to administer a medication using bar-code technology scans or enters the nurse's own ID, the client's wristband, and each package of medication to be administered (Grissinger, & Globus, 2004, p. 39). Bar coding often includes two or more person-specific identifiers, which meets the identifier requirement (Figure 35-14 ■).

CLINICAL ALERT

Do not ask "Are you John Jones?" because the client may answer "yes" to the wrong name. ■

2. *Inform the client.* If the client is unfamiliar with the medication, the nurse should explain the intended action as well as any side effects or adverse effects that might occur. Listen to the client. It is easy to get so focused on the task of timely medication administration that the nurse may miss relevant information provided by the client. For example, if the client says that he doesn't take a pill for high blood pressure, this should be an "alert" for the nurse to stop and check if this is the correct medication for that client.

3. *Administer the drug.* Read the MAR carefully and perform three checks with the labeled medications (see Box 35–3). Then administer the medication in the prescribed dosage, by the route ordered, at the correct time. There are aspects of medication administration that are important for the nurse to check each time a medication is administered. These are referred to as the "rights." Traditionally, there

were five rights to medication administration. More rights have been added over the last few years with the latest being the ten rights (Przybycien, 2005). See Box 35–4.

4. *Provide adjunctive interventions as indicated.* Clients may need help when receiving medications. They may require

---

BOX 35–3 *Check Three Times for Safe Medication Administration*

FIRST CHECK
- Read the medication administration record (MAR) and remove the medication(s) from the client's drawer. Verify that the client's name and room number match the MAR.
- Compare the label of the medication against the MAR.
- If the dosage does not match the MAR, determine if you need to do a math calculation.
- Check the expiration date of the medication.

SECOND CHECK
- While preparing the medication (e.g., pouring, drawing up, or placing unopened package in a medication cup), look at the medication label and check against the MAR.

THIRD CHECK
- Recheck the label on the container (e.g., vial, bottle, or unused unit-dose medications) before returning to its storage place.

or
- Check the label on the medication against the MAR before opening the package at the bedside.

Note: Reprinted from "*Safe Meds: An Interactive Guide to Safe Medication Practices*," by P. Przybycien. Copyright © 2005, with permission of Elsevier.

---

physical assistance, for instance, in assuming positions for intramuscular injections, or they may need guidance about measures to enhance drug effectiveness and prevent complications, such as drinking fluids. Some clients convey fear about their medications. The nurse can allay fears by listening carefully to clients' concerns and giving correct information.

5. *Record the drug administered.* The facts recorded in the chart, in ink or by computer printout, are name of the drug, dosage, method of administration, specific relevant data such as pulse rate (taken in most settings prior to the administration of digitalis), and any other pertinent information. The record should also include the exact time of administration and the signature of the nurse providing the medication. Many medication records are designed so that the nurse signs once on the page and initials each medication administered. Often, medications that are given regularly are recorded on a special flow record. PRN (as needed) or stat (at once) medications are recorded separately.

6. *Evaluate the client's response to the drug.* The kinds of behavior that reflect the action or lack of action of a drug and its untoward effects (both minor and major) are as variable as the purposes of the drugs themselves. The anxious client may show the desired effects of a tranquilizer by behavior that reflects a lowered stress level (e.g., slower speech or fewer random movements). The effectiveness of a sedative can often be measured by how well a client slept, and the effectiveness of an antispasmodic by how much pain the client feels. In all nursing activities, nurses need to be aware of the medications that a client is taking and record their effectiveness as assessed by the client and the nurse on the client's chart. The nurse may also report the client's response directly to the nurse manager and primary care provider.

BOX 35–4 **Ten "Rights" of Medication Administration**

RIGHT MEDICATION
- The medication given was the medication ordered.

RIGHT DOSE
- The dose ordered is appropriate for the client.
- Give special attention if the calculation indicates multiple pills/tablets or a large quantity of a liquid medication. This can be a "cue" that the math calculation may be incorrect.
- Double-check calculations that appear questionable.
- Know the usual dosage range of the medication.
- Question a dose outside of the usual dosage range.

RIGHT TIME
- Give the medication at the right frequency and at the time ordered according to agency policy.
- Medications given within 30 minutes before or after the scheduled time are considered to meet the right time standard.

RIGHT ROUTE
- Give the medication by the ordered route.
- Make certain that the route is safe and appropriate for the client.

RIGHT CLIENT
- Medication is given to the intended client.
- Check the client's identification band with each administration of a medication.
- Know the agency's name alert procedure when clients with the same or similar last names are on the nursing unit.

RIGHT CLIENT EDUCATION
- Explain information about the medication to the client (e.g., why receiving, what to expect, any precautions).

RIGHT DOCUMENTATION
- Document medication administration after giving it, not before.
- If time of administration differs from prescribed time, note the time on the MAR and explain reason and follow-through activities (e.g., pharmacy states medication will be available in 2 hours) in nursing notes.
- If a medication is not given, follow the agency's policy for documenting the reason why.

RIGHT TO REFUSE
- Adult clients have the right to refuse any medication.
- The nurse's role is to ensure that the client is fully informed of the potential consequences of refusal and to communicate the client's refusal to the health care provider.

RIGHT ASSESSMENT
- Some medications require specific assessments prior to administration (e.g., apical pulse, blood pressure, lab results).
- Medication orders may include specific parameters for administration (e.g., do not give if pulse less than 60 or systolic blood pressure less than 100).

RIGHT EVALUATION
- Conduct appropriate follow-up (e.g., was the desired effect achieved or not? Did the client experience any side effects or adverse reactions?).

Developmental Considerations

It is important for the nurse to be aware of how growth and development affects administration of medications for all age groups, particularly the very young and the very old.

Infants and Children

Knowledge of growth and development is essential for the nurse administering medications to children. Oral medications for children are usually prepared in sweetened liquid form to make them more palatable. The parents may provide suggestions about what method is best for their child. Do not use necessary foods such as milk or orange juice to mask the taste of medications, because the child may develop unpleasant associations and refuse that food in the future.

Children tend to fear any procedure in which a needle is used because they anticipate pain or because the procedure is unfamiliar and threatening. The nurse needs to acknowledge that the child will feel some pain; denying this fact only deepens the child's distrust. After the injection, the nurse (or the parent) can cuddle and speak softly to the infant and give the child a toy to dispel the child's association of the nurse only with pain.

Elders

Elders can have special problems, most of which are related to physiologic changes, to past experiences, and to established attitudes toward medications. See Box 35–5 for a list of the physiologic changes in elders that may affect the administration and effectiveness of medications.

Many of these changes enhance the possibility of cumulative effects and toxicity. For example, impaired circulation delays the action of medications given intramuscularly or subcutaneously. Digitalis, which is frequently taken by elders, can accumulate to toxic levels and be lethal. It is not uncommon for elders to take several different medications daily. The possibility of error increases with the number of medications taken, whether self-administered at home or administered in a hospital. The greater number of medications also compounds the problem of drug interactions. A general rule to follow is that elders should take as few medications as possible.

Elders usually require smaller dosages of drugs, especially sedatives and other central nervous system depressants. Reactions of elders to medications, particularly sedatives, are unpredictable and often bizarre. It is not uncommon to see irritability, confusion, disorientation, restlessness, and incontinence as a result of sedatives. Nurses therefore need to observe clients carefully for untoward reactions. Prescribers often follow the unwritten rule to "start low and go slow" when prescribing medications for elders. The initial prescribed dosage will often be low and then gradually increased with careful monitoring of actions and side effects of the drug.

Attitudes of elders toward medical care and medications vary. Elders tend to believe in the wisdom of the health care provider more readily than younger people. Some older people are bewildered by the prescription of several medications and may passively accept their medications from nurses but not swallow them, spitting out tablets or capsules after the nurse leaves the room. For this reason, the nurse is advised to stay with clients until they have swallowed the medications. Others may be suspicious of medications and actively refuse them.

Elders are mature adults capable of reasoning. Therefore, the nurse needs to explain the reasons for and the effects of medications. This education can prevent clients from continuing to take a medication long after there is a need for it or discontinuing a drug too quickly. For example, clients should know that diuretics will cause them to urinate more frequently and may reduce ankle edema. All clients need instructions about medications. These instructions should include when to take the drugs, what effects to expect, and when to consult a primary care provider.

Because some clients are required to take several medications daily and because visual acuity and memory may be impaired, the nurse needs to develop simple, realistic plans for clients to follow at home. For example, remembering to take drugs can be difficult for most people, including elders. Scheduling medications at mealtime or at bedtime helps clients to remember to take their medications. Some clients may take their medications and then an hour later not remember whether they took them. One solution to forgetfulness is to use a special container or glass strictly for medications. An empty glass or container indicates that the person took the pills. Special containers with individual slots and markings for each day can reduce confusion. Loss of visual acuity presents problems that can be overcome by writing out the plan in block letters large enough to be read. In some situations, enlisting the help of a spouse, son, or daughter can be helpful.

Elders often have a decrease in dexterity due to arthritis or stiffness of their hands and fingers due to aging. This causes difficulty in opening medication containers or in self-administration of other medications such as eyedrops, eardrops, insulin injections, and inhalers. Nurses can help clients make the necessary changes or enlist the assistance of another person to help them administer their medications.

BOX 35–5 Physiologic Changes Associated with Aging That Influence Medication Administration and Effectiveness

- Altered memory
- Decreased visual acuity
- Decrease in renal function, resulting in slower elimination of drugs and higher drug concentrations in the bloodstream for longer periods
- Less complete and slower absorption from the gastrointestinal tract
- Increased proportion of fat to lean body mass, which facilitates retention of fat-soluble drugs and increases potential for toxicity
- Decreased liver function, which hinders biotransformation of drugs
- Decreased organ sensitivity, which means that the response to the same drug concentration in the vicinity of the target organ is less in older people than in the young
- Altered quality of organ responsiveness, resulting in adverse effects becoming pronounced before therapeutic effects are achieved
- Decrease in manual dexterity due to arthritis and/or decrease in flexibility

---

RESEARCH NOTE **Can Changing the Health Care Workplace to Avoid Interruptions Prevent Medication Errors?**

Nursing units are complex units in which nurses are often hurried, distracted, and interrupted during medication administration. This process improvement project implemented a program to decrease distractions on the nursing unit through "Do not Disturb" reminder signs at medication carts and medication dispensing machines. They also designed a medication administration protocol checklist that was given to the nurses and also placed on medication carts. Nurses were asked to avoid conversation and prevent distractions during medication administration.

Researchers conducted medication administration observations during 7 AM to 7 PM shifts during the week. The observations revealed decreased episodes of distraction, more focus on the administration process, and decreased reported medication errors. The researchers found that interruptions by other nurses and personnel, conversation, and loud noises caused the highest number of distractions when nurses administered medications.

IMPLICATIONS

"Do Not Disturb" signs and protocol checklists represent easy and inexpensive strategies to reduce distractions and keep nurses focused during the process of medication administration with the outcome of enhancing client safety.

Note: From: "Innovative Approaches to Reducing Nurses': Distractions during Medication Administration," by T. M. Pape et al., 2005, *Journal of Continuing Education in Nursing, 36*(3), 108–116. Copyright © 2005 SLACK, Inc. Reprinted with permission.

ORAL MEDICATIONS

The oral route is the most common route by which medications are given. As long as a client can swallow and retain the drug in the stomach, this is the route of choice (see Skill 35-1). Oral medications are contraindicated when a client is vomiting, has gastric or intestinal suction, or is unconscious and unable to swallow. Such clients in a hospital are usually on orders for "nothing by mouth" (Latin is *nil per os:* **NPO**).

SKILL 35-1

ADMINISTERING ORAL MEDICATIONS

PURPOSE
- To provide a medication that has systemic effects or local effects on the gastrointestinal tract or both (see specific drug action).

ASSESSMENT
Assess
- Allergies to medication(s)
- Clients' ability to swallow the medication
- Presence of vomiting or diarrhea that would interfere with the ability to absorb the medication
- Specific drug action, side effects, interactions, and adverse reactions
- Client's knowledge of and learning needs about the medication

Perform appropriate assessments (e.g., vital signs, laboratory results) specific to the medication.

Determine if the assessment data influence administration of the medication (i.e., is it appropriate to administer the medication or does the medication need to be held and the prescriber notified?).

PLANNING

Delegation
In acute care settings, administration of oral/enteral medications is performed by the nurse and is not delegated to unlicensed assistive personnel (UAP). The nurse can inform the UAP of the intended therapeutic effects and/or specific side effects of the medication and request the UAP to report specific client observations to the nurse for follow-up. In some long-term care settings, trained UAP may administer certain medications to stable clients. It is important, however, for the nurse to remember that the medication knowledge of the UAP is limited and *assessment and evaluation of the effectiveness of the medication remains the responsibility of the nurse.*

Equipment
- Dispensing system
- Disposable medication cups: small paper or plastic cups for tablets and capsules, waxed or plastic calibrated medication cups for liquids
- MAR or computer printout
- Pill crusher/cutter
- Straws to administer medications that may discolor the teeth or to facilitate the ingestion of liquid medication for certain clients
- Drinking glass and water or juice
- Applesauce or pudding to use for crushed medications for clients who may choke on liquids

IMPLEMENTATION
Preparation
1. Know the reason why the client is receiving the medication, the drug classification, contraindications, usual dosage range, side effects, and nursing considerations for administering and evaluating the intended outcomes for the medication.

ADMINISTERING ORAL MEDICATIONS *continued*

2. Check the medication administration record (MAR).
   - Check the MAR for the drug name, dosage, frequency, route of administration, and expiration date for administering the medication, if appropriate. **Rationale:** *Certain medications (e.g., narcotics, antibiotics) have a specified time frame at which they expire and need to be reordered by the primary care provider.*
   - If the MAR is unclear or pertinent information is missing, compare the MAR with the most recent prescriber's written order.
   - Report any discrepancies to the charge nurse or the prescriber, as agency policy dictates.
3. Verify the client's ability to take medication orally.
   - Determine whether the client can swallow, is NPO, is nauseated or vomiting, has gastric suction, or has diminished or absent bowel sounds.
4. Organize the supplies.
   - Assemble the MAR(s) for each client together so that medications can be prepared for one client at a time. **Rationale:** *Organization of supplies saves time and reduces the chance of error.*

Performance

1. Perform hand hygiene and observe other appropriate infection control procedures.
2. Unlock the dispensing system.
3. Obtain appropriate medication.
   - Read the MAR and take the appropriate medication from the shelf, drawer, or refrigerator. The medication may be dispensed in a bottle, box, or unit-dose package.
   - Compare the label of the medication container or unit-dose package against the order on the MAR or computer printout. **Rationale:** *This is a safety check to ensure that the right medication is given.* If these are not identical, recheck the prescriber's written order in the client's chart. If there is still a discrepancy, check with the nurse in charge or the pharmacist. ❶
   - Check the expiration date of the medication. Return expired medications to the pharmacy. **Rationale:** *Outdated medications are not safe to administer.*

- Use only medications that have clear, legible labels *to ensure accuracy.*
4. Prepare the medication.
   - Calculate the medication dosage accurately.
   - Prepare the correct amount of medication for the required dose, without contaminating the medication. **Rationale:** *Aseptic technique maintains drug cleanliness.*
   - While preparing the medication, recheck each prepared drug and container with the MAR again. **Rationale:** *This second safety check reduces the chance of error.*

Tablets or Capsules

- Place packaged unit-dose capsules or tablets directly into the medicine cup. Do not remove the medication from the package until at the bedside. **Rationale:** *The wrapper keeps the medication clean. Not removing the medication facilitates identification of the medication in the event the client refuses the drug or assessment data indicate to hold the medication. Unopened unit-dose packages can usually be returned to the medication cart.*
- If using a stock container, pour the required number into the bottle cap, and then transfer the medication to the disposable cup without touching the tablets.
- Keep narcotics and medications that require specific assessments, such as pulse measurements, respiratory rate or depth, or blood pressure, separate from the others. **Rationale:** *This reminds the nurse to complete the needed assessment(s) in order to decide whether to give the medication or to withhold the medication if indicated.*
- Break only scored tablets if necessary to obtain the correct dosage. Use a cutting or splitting device if needed. Check the agency policy as to whether unused portions of a medication can be discarded and, if so, how they are to be discarded. ❷
- If the client has difficulty swallowing, crush the tablets to a fine powder with a pill crusher or between two medication cups. Then, mix the powder with a small amount of soft food (e.g., custard, applesauce). Some medications should not be crushed (e.g., time-released and enteric coated). An

❶ Compare the medication label to the MAR.

❷ A cutting device can be used to divide tablets.

Photographer: Elena Dorfman

continued on page 854

ADMINISTERING ORAL MEDICATIONS *continued*

example of tablets that should not be crushed is oxycodone (OxyContin), a long-acting narcotic that normally lasts 12 hours after administration. If the tablet is crushed, the client gets a surge of action in the first 2 hours, then may start having severe pain again in 4 to 6 hours, as the effects wear off too soon. The crushing of these tablets causes an uneven effect, and the long action of the medication is lost.

CLINICAL ALERT

Check with the pharmacy before crushing tablets. Sustained-action, enteric-coated, buccal, or sublingual tablets should not be crushed. ∎

Liquid Medication

- Thoroughly mix the medication before pouring. Discard any medication that has changed color or turned cloudy.
- Remove the cap and place it upside down on the counter-top *to avoid contaminating the inside of the cap.*
- Hold the bottle so the label is next to your palm and pour the medication away from the label. **Rationale:** *This prevents the label from becoming soiled and illegible as a result of spilled liquids.* ❸
- Place the medication cup on a flat surface at eye level and fill it to the desired level, using the *bottom* of the **meniscus** (crescent-shaped upper surface of a column of liquid) to align with the container scale. ❹ **Rationale:** *This method ensures accuracy of measurement.*
- Before capping the bottle, wipe the lip with a paper towel. **Rationale:** *This prevents the cap from sticking.*
- When giving small amounts of liquids (e.g., < 5 mL), prepare the medication in a sterile syringe without the needle or in a specially designed oral syringe. Label the syringe with the name of the medication and the route (PO). **Rationale:** *Any oral solution removed from the original container and placed into a syringe should be labeled to avoid medications being given by the wrong route (e.g., IV). This practice facilitates client safety and avoids tragic errors.*
- Keep unit-dose liquids in their package and open them at the bedside.

❸ Pouring a liquid medication from a bottle.
(Patrick Watson)

Oral Narcotics

- If an agency uses a manual recording system for controlled substances, check the narcotic record for the previous drug count and compare it with the supply available. Some medications, including narcotics, are kept in plastic containers that are sectioned and numbered.
- Remove the next available tablet and drop it in the medicine cup.
- After removing a tablet, record the necessary information on the appropriate narcotic control record and sign it.
- *Note:* Computer-controlled dispensing systems allow access only to the selected drug and automatically record its use.

All Medications

- Place the prepared medication and MAR together on the medication cart.
- Recheck the label on the container before returning the bottle, box, or envelope to its storage place. **Rationale:** *This third check further reduces the risk of error.*
- Avoid leaving prepared medications unattended. **Rationale:** *This precaution prevents potential mishandling errors.*
- Lock the medication cart before entering the client's room. **Rationale:** *This is a safety measure because medication carts are not to be left open when unattended.*
- Check the room number against the MAR if agency policy does not allow the MAR to be removed from the medication cart. **Rationale:** *This is another safety measure to ensure that the nurse is entering the correct client room.*

5. Provide for client privacy.
6. Prepare the client.
   - Check the client's identification band. **Rationale:** *This ensures that the right client receives the medication.*
   - Assist the client to a sitting position or, if not possible, to a side-lying position. **Rationale:** *These positions facilitate swallowing and prevent aspiration.*
   - If not previously assessed, take the required assessment measures, such as pulse and respiratory rates or blood pressure. Take the apical pulse rate before administering digitalis preparations. Take blood pressure before giving antihypertensive drugs. Take the respiratory rate prior to administering narcotics. **Rationale:** *Narcotics depress the respiratory center.* If any of the findings are above or below the predetermined parameters, consult the primary care provider before administering the medication.

Base of meniscus

❹ The *bottom* of the meniscus is the measuring guide.

ADMINISTERING ORAL MEDICATIONS *continued*

7. Explain the purpose of the medication and how it will help, using language that the client can understand. Include relevant information about effects; for example, tell the client receiving a diuretic to expect an increase in urine output. **Rationale:** *Information can facilitate acceptance of and compliance with the therapy.*

8. Administer the medication at the correct time.
   - Take the medication to the client within the period of 30 minutes before or after the scheduled time.
   - Give the client sufficient water or preferred juice to swallow the medication. Before using juice, check for any food and medication incompatibilities. **Rationale:** *Fluids ease swallowing and facilitate absorption from the gastrointestinal tract.* Liquid medications other than antacids or cough preparations may be diluted with 15 mL (1/2 oz) of water to facilitate absorption.
   - If the client is unable to hold the pill cup, use the pill cup to introduce the medication into the client's mouth, and give only one tablet or capsule at a time. **Rationale:** *Putting the cup to the client's mouth maintains the cleanliness of the nurse's hands. Giving one medication at a time eases swallowing.*
   - If an older child or adult has difficulty swallowing, ask the client to place the medication on the back of the tongue before taking the water. **Rationale:** *Stimulation of the back of the tongue produces the swallowing reflex.*
   - If the medication has an objectionable taste, ask the client to suck a few ice chips beforehand, or give the medication with juice, applesauce, or bread if there are no contraindications. **Rationale:** *The cold of the ice chips will desensitize the taste buds, and juices or bread can mask the taste of the medication.*
   - If the client says that the medication you are about to give is different from what the client has been receiving, do not give the medication without first checking the original order. **Rationale:** *Most clients are familiar with the appearance of medications taken previously. Unfamiliar medications may signal a possible error.*
   - Stay with the client until all medications have been swallowed. **Rationale:** *The nurse must see the client swallow the medication before the drug administration can be recorded.* The nurse may need to check the client's mouth to ensure that the medication was swallowed and not hidden inside the cheek. A primary care provider's order or agency policy is required for medications left at the bedside.

9. Document each medication given.
   - Record the medication given, dosage, time, any complaints or assessments of the client, and your signature.
   - If medication was refused or omitted, record this fact on the appropriate record; document the reason, when possible, and the nurse's actions according to agency policy.

10. Dispose of all supplies appropriately.
    - Replenish stock (e.g., medication cups) and return the cart to the appropriate place.
    - Discard used disposable supplies.

11. Evaluate the effects of the medication.
    - Return to the client when the medication is expected to take effect (usually 30 minutes) to evaluate the effects of the medication on the client.

EVALUATION
- Conduct appropriate follow-up.
- Observe for desired effect (e.g., relief of pain or decrease in body temperature).
- Note any adverse effects or side effects (e.g., nausea, vomiting, skin rash, change in vital signs).
- Relate to previous findings, if available.
- Report significant deviations from normal to the primary care provider.

LIFESPAN CONSIDERATIONS Administering Oral Medications

- Knowledge of growth and development is essential for the nurse administering medications to infants and children.
- Nurses must know the range of safe medication dosages for infants and children.

INFANTS
- Oral medications can be effectively administered in several ways:
  - A syringe or dropper
  - A medication nipple which allows the infant to suck the medication
  - Mixed in small amounts of food
  - A spoon or medication cup, for older children
- Never mix medications into foods that are essential, since the infant may associate the food with an unpleasant taste and refuse that food in the future. Never mix medications with formula.
- Place a small amount of liquid medication along the inside of the baby's cheek and wait for the infant to swallow before giving more to prevent aspiration or spitting out.
- When using a spoon, retrieve and refeed medication that is thrust outward by the infant's tongue.

CHILDREN
- Whenever possible, give children a choice between the use of a spoon, dropper, or syringe.
- Dilute the oral medication, if indicated, with a small amount of water. Many oral medications are readily swallowed if they are diluted with a small amount of water. If large quantities of water are used, the child may refuse to drink the entire amount and receive only a portion of the medication.
- Oral medications for children are usually prepared in sweetened liquid form to make them more palatable. Crush medications that are not supplied in liquid form and mix them with substances available on most pediatric units, such as honey, flavored syrup, jam, or a fruit puree.
- Necessary foods such as milk or orange juice should not be used to mask the taste of medications because the child may develop unpleasant associations and refuse that food in the future.

continued on page 856

LIFESPAN CONSIDERATIONS Administering Oral Medications—*continued*

- Disguise disagreeable-tasting medications with sweet-tasting substances mentioned previously. However, present any altered medication to the child honestly and not as a food or treat.
- Place the young child or toddler on your lap or a parent's lap in a sitting position.
- Administer the medication slowly with a measuring spoon, plastic syringe, or medicine cup.
- To prevent nausea, pour a carbonated beverage over finely crushed ice and give it before or immediately after the medication is administered.
- Follow medication with a drink of water, juice, a soft drink, or a Popsicle or frozen juice bar. This removes any unpleasant aftertaste.
- For children who take sweetened medications on a long-term basis, follow the medication administration with oral hygiene. These children are at high risk for dental caries.

ELDERS

- The physiologic changes associated with aging influence medication administration and effectiveness. Examples include altered memory, less acute vision, decrease in renal function, less complete and slower absorption from the gastrointestinal tract, and decreased liver function. Many of these changes enhance the possibility of cumulative effects and toxicity.
- Elders usually require smaller dosages of drugs, especially sedatives and other central nervous system depressants.
- Elders are mature adults capable of reasoning. The nurse, therefore, needs to explain the reasons for and the effects of the client's medications.
- Socioeconomic factors such as lack of transportation and decreased finances may influence obtaining medications when needed.
- An increase in marketing and availability of vitamins, herbs, and supplements alerts the nurse to include this information in a medication history.

HOME CARE CONSIDERATIONS Administering Medications

The nurse should instruct the client to:

- Learn the names of the medications as well as their actions and possible adverse effects. Carry a complete list of all prescriptions, OTC medications, and home remedies at all times.
- Keep all medications out of reach of children and pets.
- If using a syringe to administer the medication to an infant or child, remove and dispose of the plastic cap that fits on the end of the syringe. Infants and small children have been known to choke on these caps.
- Take the medications only as prescribed. Know which medications need to be taken on an empty stomach and which can be taken with food/meals. Immediately consult the nurse, pharmacist, or primary care provider about any problems with the medication.
- Always check the medication label to make sure the correct medication is being taken.
- Request labels printed with larger type on medication containers if there is difficulty reading the label.

- Check the expiration date and discard outdated medications by flushing them down the toilet. Do not throw the medication(s) into the trash.
- Ask the pharmacist to substitute childproof caps with ones that are more easily opened, as necessary.
- If a dose or more is missed, do not take two or more doses; ask the pharmacist or primary care provider for directions.
- Do not crush or cut a tablet or capsule without first checking with the primary care provider or pharmacist. Doing so may affect the medication's absorption.
- Never stop taking the medication without first discussing it with the primary care provider.
- Always check with the pharmacist before taking any nonprescription medications. Some OTC medications can interact with the prescribed medication.

Additionally, the nurse can set up a medication plan to assist clients and family members to remember a schedule. Weekly pill containers (available at pharmacies) or a written plan may be helpful.

NASOGASTRIC AND GASTROSTOMY MEDICATIONS

For clients who cannot take anything by mouth (NPO) and have a **nasogastric tube** or a **gastrostomy tube** in place, an alternative route for administering medications is through the nasogastric or gastrostomy tube. A nasogastric (NG) tube is inserted by way of the nasopharynx and is placed into the client's stomach for the purpose of feeding the client or to remove gastric secretions. A gastrostomy tube is surgically placed directly into the client's stomach and provides another route for administering medications and nutrition (see Chapter 47 ∞). Guidelines for administering medications by nasogastric tubes and gastrostomy tubes are shown in the Practice Guidelines box.

PARENTERAL MEDICATIONS

Parenteral administration of medications is a common nursing procedure. Nurses give parenteral medications intradermally (ID), subcutaneously, intramuscularly (IM), or intravenously (IV). Because these medications are absorbed more quickly than oral medications and are irretrievable once injected, the nurse must prepare and administer them carefully and accurately. Administering parenteral drugs requires the same nursing

PRACTICE GUIDELINES   Administering Medications by Nasogastric or Gastrostomy Tube

■ Always check with the pharmacist to see if the client's medications come in a liquid form because these are less likely to cause tube obstruction.

■ If medications do not come in liquid form, check to see if they may be crushed. (Note that enteric-coated, sustained action, buccal, and sublingual medications should never be crushed.)

■ Crush a tablet into a fine powder and dissolve in at least 30 mL of warm water. Cold liquids may cause client discomfort. Use only water for mixing and flushing. Some medications are mixed with other fluids, such as normal saline, in order to maximize dissolution. Nurses are encouraged to consult with a pharmacist.

■ Read medication labels carefully before opening a capsule. Open capsules and mix the contents with water only with the pharmacist's advice.

■ Do not administer whole or undissolved medications because they will clog the tube.

■ Assess tube placement (see Chapter 47 ∞ for methods to verify tube placement).

■ Before giving the medication, aspirate all the stomach contents and measure the residual volume. Check agency policy if residual volume is greater than 100 mL.

■ When administering the medication(s):
  • Remove the plunger from the syringe and connect the syringe to a pinched or kinked tube. *Pinching or kinking the tube prevents excess air from entering the stomach and causing distention.*
  • Put 15 to 30 mL (5 to 10 mL for children) of water into the syringe barrel to flush the tube before administering the first medication. Raise or lower the barrel of the syringe to adjust the flow as needed. Pinch or clamp the tubing before all the water is instilled to avoid excess air entering the stomach.
  • Pour liquid or dissolved medication into the syringe barrel and allow to flow by gravity into the enteral tube.
  • If you are giving several medications, administer each one separately and flush with at least 15 to 30 mL (5 mL for children) of tap water between each medication.
  • When you have finished administering all medications, flush with another 15 to 30 mL (5 to 10 mL for children) of warm water to clear the tube.

■ If the tube is connected to suction, disconnect the suction and keep the tube clamped for 20 to 30 minutes after giving the medication to enhance absorption.

---

knowledge as for oral and topical drugs; however, because injections are invasive procedures, aseptic technique must be used to minimize the risk of infection.

Equipment

To administer parenteral medications, nurses use syringes and needles to withdraw medication from ampules and vials.

Syringes

Syringes have three parts: the tip, which connects with the needle; the barrel, or outside part, on which the scales are printed; and the plunger, which fits inside the barrel (Figure 35-15 ■). When handling a syringe, the nurse may touch the outside of the barrel and the handle of the plunger; however, the nurse must *avoid letting any unsterile object touch the tip or inside of the barrel, the shaft of the plunger, or the shaft or tip of the needle.*

There are several kinds of syringes, differing in size, shape, and material. The three most commonly used types are the standard hypodermic syringe, the insulin syringe, and the tuberculin syringe (Figure 35-16 ■). A **hypodermic syringe** comes in 2-, 2.5-, 3-, and 5-mL sizes. The syringe may have two scales marked on it: the minim and the milliliter. The milliliter scale is the one normally used; the minim scale is used for very small dosages.

An **insulin syringe** is similar to a hypodermic syringe, but the scale is specially designed for insulin: a 100-unit calibrated scale intended for use with U-100 insulin. This is the only syringe that should be used to administer insulin. Several low-dose insulin

Tip
Barrel
Plunger

Figure 35-15 ■ The three parts of a syringe.

A
B
C

Figure 35-16 ■ Three kinds of syringes: *A,* hypodermic syringe marked in tenths (0.1) of milliliters and in minims; *B,* insulin syringe marked in 100 units; *C,* tuberculin syringe marked in tenths and hundredths (0.01) of cubic millimeters and in minims.

Figure 35-17 ■ Different insulin syringes based on the amount of insulin required.
(Patrick Watson)

Figure 35-19 ■ A 50-mL non-Luer-Lok syringe which can be used for irrigation of tubes or wounds.
(Patrick Watson)

syringes are also available. These syringes frequently have a nonremovable needle. All insulin syringes are calibrated on the 100-unit scale in North America. The correct choice of syringe is based on the amount of insulin required (Figure 35-17 ■).

The **tuberculin syringe** was originally designed to administer tuberculin solution. It is a narrow syringe, calibrated in tenths and hundredths of a milliliter (up to 1 mL) on one scale and in sixteenths of a minim (up to 1 minim) on the other scale. This type of syringe can also be useful in administering other drugs, particularly when small or precise measurement is indicated (e.g., pediatric dosages).

Syringes are made in other sizes as well (e.g., 10, 20, and 50 mL). These are not generally used to administer drugs di-

rectly but can be useful for adding medications to intravenous solutions or for irrigating wounds. The tip of a syringe varies and is classified as either a Luer-Lok or non-Luer-Lok. A Luer-Lok syringe has a tip that requires the needle to be twisted onto it to avoid accidental removal of the needle (see Figure 35-18 ■). The non-Luer-Lok syringe has a smooth graduated tip, and needles are slipped onto it. The larger 50-mL non-Luer-Lok syringe is often used for irrigation purposes (e.g., wounds, tubes). See Figure 35-19 ■.

Most syringes used today are made of plastic, are individually packaged for sterility in a paper wrapper or a rigid plastic container (Figure 35-20 ■), and are disposable. The syringe and needle may be packaged together or separately. Needleless sys-

A

B

Figure 35-18 ■ Tips of syringes: *A,* Luer-Lok syringe (note threaded tip); *B,* non-Luer-Lok syringe (note the smooth graduated tip).

Figure 35-20 ■ Disposable plastic syringes and needles: *Top,* with syringe and needle exposed; *Middle,* with plastic cap over the needle; *Bottom,* with plastic case over the needle and syringe.
Photographer: Elena Dorfman

tems are also available in which the needle is replaced by a plastic cannula.

Injectable medications are frequently supplied in disposable **prefilled unit-dose systems.** These are available as (a) prefilled syringes ready for use or (b) prefilled sterile cartridges and needles that require the attachment of a reusable holder (injection system) before use (Figure 35-21 ■). Examples of the latter system are the Tubex and Carpuject injection systems. The manufacturers provide specific directions for use. Because most

A

B

C

Figure 35-21 ■ *A,* Syringe and prefilled sterile cartridge with needle; *B,* assembling the device; *C,* the cartridge slides into the syringe barrel, turns, and locks at the needle end. The plunger then screws into the cartridge end.

Photographer: Elena Dorfman

prefilled cartridges are overfilled, excess medication must be ejected before the injection to ensure the right dosage. Because the needle is fused to the syringe, the nurse cannot change the gauge or length of the needle. The nurse, however, can transfer the medication into a regular syringe if the assessment of the client necessitates a different needle gauge or length.

Needles

Needles are made of stainless steel, and most are disposable. Reusable needles (e.g., for special procedures) need to be sharpened periodically before resterilization because the points become dull with use and are occasionally damaged or acquire burrs on the tips. A dull or damaged needle should *never* be used.

A needle has three discernible parts: the **hub,** which fits onto the syringe; the **cannula,** or **shaft,** which is attached to the hub; and the **bevel,** which is the slanted part at the tip of the needle (Figure 35-22 ■). A disposable needle has a plastic hub. Needles used for injections have three variable characteristics:

1. *Slant or length of the bevel.* The bevel of the needle may be short or long. Longer bevels provide the sharpest needles and cause less discomfort. They are commonly used for subcutaneous and intramuscular injections. Short bevels are used for intradermal and intravenous injections because a long bevel can become occluded if it rests against the side of a blood vessel.
2. *Length of the shaft.* The shaft length of commonly used needles varies from 1/2 to 2 inches. The appropriate needle length is chosen according to the client's muscle development, the client's weight, and the type of injection.
3. **Gauge** *(or diameter) of the shaft.* The gauge varies from #18 to #28. The larger the gauge number, the smaller the diameter of the shaft. Smaller gauges produce less tissue trauma, but larger gauges are necessary for viscous medications, such as penicillin.

For an adult requiring a subcutaneous injection, it is appropriate to use a needle of #24 to #26 gauge and 3/8 to 5/8 inch long. Obese clients may require a 1-inch needle. For intramuscular injections, a longer needle (e.g., 1 to 1 1/2 inches) with a larger gauge (e.g., #20 to #22 gauge) is used. Slender adults and children usually require a shorter needle. The nurse must assess the client to determine the appropriate needle length.

Preventing Needlestick Injuries

One of the most potentially hazardous procedures that health care personnel face is using and disposing of needles and sharps. Needlestick injuries present a major risk for infection with hepatitis B virus, human immunodeficiency virus (HIV), and many other pathogens. Standards have been set by OSHA

Figure 35-22 ■ The parts of a needle.

BOX 35-6   *Avoiding Puncture Injuries*

■ Use appropriate puncture-proof disposal containers to dispose of uncapped needles and sharps. These are provided in all client areas (Figure 35-23 ■). Never throw sharps in wastebaskets. Sharps include any items that can cut or puncture skin such as:

 Needles
 Surgical blades

 Lancets
 Razors
 Broken glass
 Broken capillary pipettes
 Exposed dental wires
 Reusable items (e.g., large-bore needles, hooks, rasps, drill points)
 ANY SHARP INSTRUMENT!

■ Never bend or break needles before disposal.
■ Never recap *used* needles (i.e., has been inserted into a client) except under specified circumstances (e.g., when transporting a syringe to the laboratory for an arterial blood gas or blood culture).
■ When recapping a needle (i.e., drawing up a medication into a syringe *prior* to administration):
  ● Use a safety mechanical device that firmly grips the needle cap and holds it in place until it is ready to recap.
  ● Use a one-handed "scoop" method. This is performed by (a) placing the needle cap and syringe with needle horizontally on a flat surface, (b) inserting the needle into the cap, using one hand (Figure 35-24 ■), and then (c) using your other hand to pick up the cap and tighten it to the needle hub. Be careful not to contaminate the needle. If the needle becomes contaminated, replace the needle with a new one.

Figure 35-23 ■ A disposal container for contaminated needles and other sharps.

Photographer: Elena Dorfman

Figure 35-24 ■ Recapping a used needle using the one-handed scoop method.

Photographer: Elena Dorfman

---

to prevent such injuries. Some of these are summarized in Box 35–6. If an accidental needlestick injury occurs, the nurse needs to follow specific steps outlined by the agency.

Safety syringes have been designed in recent years to protect health care workers. Safety devices are categorized as either *passive* or *active*. The nurse does not need to activate the passive safety device. For example, for some syringes, after injection, the needle retracts immediately into the barrel (Figure 35-25 ■). In contrast, the active safety device requires the nurse to manually activate the safety feature. For example, the nurse

Before injection.

After injection, pull sheath over needle.

Figure 35-26 ■ Active safety device. The nurse manually pulls the sheath or guard over the needle after injection.

activates a mechanism to retract the needle into the syringe barrel, or the nurse, after injection, manually pulls a plastic sheath or guard over the needle (Figure 35-26 ■).

Preparing Injectable Medications

Injectable medications can be prepared by withdrawing the medication from an ampule or vial into a sterile syringe, using prefilled syringes, or using needleless injection systems. Figure 35-27 ■ shows an example of a needleless system used to access medication from a vial.

Before injection.

After injection.

Figure 35-25 ■ Passive safety device. The needle retracts immediately into the barrel after injection.

Figure 35-27 ■ A needleless system can extract medication from a vial.

A

B

Figure 35-28 ■ *A*, Ampules; *B*, vials.

Ampules and Vials

Ampules and vials (Figure 35-28 ■) are frequently used to package sterile parenteral medications. An **ampule** is a glass container usually designed to hold a single dose of a drug. It is made of clear glass and has a distinctive shape with a constricted neck. Ampules vary in size from 1 to 10 mL or more. Most ampule necks have colored marks around them, indicating where they are prescored for easy opening.

To access the medication in an ampule, the ampule must be broken at its constricted neck. Traditionally, files have been used to score the ampule. Today plastic ampule openers are available that prevent injury from broken glass. The device consists of a plastic cap that fits over the top of an ampule. The head of the ampule, when broken, remains inside the cap and is placed into a sharps container (Figure 35-29 ■). If an ampule opener is not available, the neck should be filed with a small file, then broken off at that point. Once the ampule is broken, the fluid is aspirated into a syringe using a filter needle. This prevents aspiration of any glass particles.

A **vial** is a small glass bottle with a sealed rubber cap. Vials come in different sizes, from single to multidose vials. They usually have a metal or plastic cap that protects the rubber seal and must be removed to access the medication. To access the medication in a vial, the vial must be pierced with a needle. In addition, air must be injected into a vial before the medication can be withdrawn. Failure to inject air before withdrawing the medication leaves a vacuum within the vial that makes withdrawal difficult.

Several drugs (e.g., penicillin) are dispensed as powders in vials. A liquid (diluent) must be added to a powdered medication before it can be injected. The technique of adding a diluent

to a powdered drug to prepare it for administration is called **reconstitution.** Powdered drugs usually have printed instructions (enclosed with each packaged vial) that describe the amount and kind of solvent to be added. Commonly used diluents are sterile water or sterile normal saline. Some preparations are supplied in individual-dose vials; others come in multidose vials. The following are two examples of the preparation of powdered drugs:

1. *Single-dose vial:* Instructions for preparing a single-dose vial state that 1.5 mL of sterile water be added to the sterile dry powder, thus providing a single dose of 2 mL. The volume of the drug powder was 0.5 mL. Therefore, the 1.5 mL of water plus the 0.5 mL of powder results in 2 mL of solution. In other instances, the addition of a solution does not increase the volume. Therefore, it is important to follow the manufacturer's directions.

Figure 35-29 ■ *A,* Ampule opener. *B,* Plastic opener is placed over top of ampule. *C,* Top of ampule remains in opener after ampule is broken open.

(Patrick Watson)

2. *Multidose vial:*   A dose of 750 mg of a certain drug is ordered for a client. On hand is a 10-g multidose vial. The directions for preparation read: "Add 8.5 mL of sterile water, and each milliliter will contain 1.0 g or 1,000 mg." To determine the amount to inject, the nurse calculates as follows:

$$1 \text{ mL} = 1,000 \text{ mg}$$
$$x \text{ mL} = 750 \text{ mg}$$
$$(\text{cross multiply})$$
$$x = \frac{750 \times 1}{1,000}$$
$$x = 0.75$$

The nurse will give 0.75 mL of the medication.

Glass and rubber particulate have been found in medications withdrawn from ampules and vials using a regular needle. As a result, it is strongly recommended that the nurse use a filter needle when withdrawing medications from ampules and vials to prevent withdrawing glass and rubber particles. After drawing the medication into the syringe, the filter needle is replaced with the regular needle for injection. This prevents tracking of the medication through the client's tissues during the insertion of the needle, which minimizes discomfort. Research validates this practice, especially in clients receiving intramuscular injections on a repeated basis or with injections that use larger bore needles (Preston & Hegadoren, 2004).

Skills 35-2 and 35-3 describe how to prepare medications from ampules and vials. Additionally, it is important to remember that when powdered drugs have been reconstituted, the date and time should be written on the label of the vial. Many of these drugs have to be used within a certain time period following reconstitution, so nurses need to know the expiration time after it has been reconstituted.

Mixing Medications in One Syringe

Frequently, clients need more than one drug injected at the same time. To spare the client the experience of being injected twice, two drugs (if compatible) are often mixed in one syringe and given as one injection. It is common, for instance, to combine two types of insulin in this manner or to combine

---

SKILL 35-2

PREPARING MEDICATIONS FROM AMPULES

PLANNING

Delegation
Preparing medications from ampules and vials involves knowledge and use of sterile technique. Therefore, these techniques are not delegated to UAP.

Equipment
- MAR or computer printout
- Ampule of sterile medication
- File (if ampule is not scored) and small gauze square or plastic ampule opener

- Antiseptic swabs
- Syringe
- Needle for administering the medication
- Filter needle for withdrawing medication from the ampule

PREPARING MEDICATIONS FROM AMPULES *continued*

IMPLEMENTATION
Preparation
1. Check the medication administration record (MAR).
   - Check the label on the ampule carefully against the MAR to make sure that the correct medication is being prepared.
   - Follow the three checks for administering medications. Read the label on the medication (1) when it is taken from the medication cart, (2) before withdrawing the medication, and (3) after withdrawing the medication.
2. Organize the equipment.

Performance
1. Perform hand hygiene and observe other appropriate infection control procedures.
2. Prepare the medication ampule for drug withdrawal.
   - Flick the upper stem of the ampule several times with a fingernail. **Rationale:** *This will bring all medication down to the main portion of the ampule.*
   - Use an ampule opener or place a piece of sterile gauze or alcohol wipe between your thumb and the ampule neck or around the ampule neck, and break off the top by *bending it toward you to ensure the ampule is broken away from yourself and away from others.* **Rationale:** *The sterile gauze protects the fingers from the broken glass, and any glass fragments will spray away from the nurse.* ❶

or
   - Place the antiseptic wipe packet over the top of the ampule before breaking off the top. **Rationale:** *This method ensures that all glass fragments fall into the packet and reduces the risk of cuts.*
   - Dispose of the top of the ampule in the sharps container.
3. Withdraw the medication.
   - Place the ampule on a flat surface.
   - Attach the filter needle to the syringe. **Rationale:** *The filter needle prevents glass particles from being withdrawn with the medication.*
   - Remove the cap from the filter needle and insert the needle into the center of the ampule. Do not touch the rim of the ampule with the needle tip or shaft. **Rationale:** *This will keep the needle sterile.* Withdraw the amount of drug required for the dosage.
   - With a single-dose ampule, hold the ampule slightly on its side, if necessary, to obtain more than the ordered amount of medication. ❷
   - Dispose of the filter needle by placing in a sharps container.
   - If giving an injection replace the filter needle with a regular needle, tighten the cap at the hub of the needle, and push solution into the needle, to the prescribed amount.

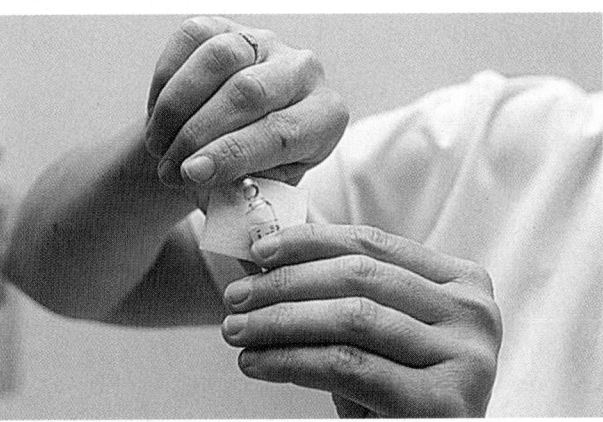

❶ Breaking the neck of an ampule.
Photographer: Jenny Thomas

❷ Withdrawing a medication from an ampule.
(Patrick Watson)

PREPARING MEDICATIONS FROM VIALS

PLANNING
Equipment
- MAR or computer printout
- Vial of sterile medication
- Antiseptic swabs
- Safety needle and syringe
- Filter needle (check agency policy)
- Sterile water or normal saline, if drug is in powdered form

IMPLEMENTATION
Preparation
- Follow the same preparation as described in Skill 35-2.

Performance
1. Perform hand hygiene and observe other appropriate infection control procedures.
2. Prepare the medication vial for drug withdrawal.
   - Mix the solution, if necessary, by rotating the vial between the palms of the hands, not by shaking. **Rationale:** *Some vials contain aqueous suspensions, which settle when they stand. In some instances, shaking is contraindicated because it may cause the mixture to foam.*

continued on page 864

PREPARING MEDICATIONS FROM VIALS *continued*

- Remove the protective cap, or clean the rubber cap of a previously opened vial with an antiseptic wipe by rubbing in a circular motion. **Rationale:** *The antiseptic cleans the cap and reduces the number of microorganisms.*

3. Withdraw the medication.
   - Attach a filter needle, as agency practice dictates, to draw up premixed liquid medications from multidose vials. **Rationale:** *Using the filter needle prevents any solid particles from being drawn up through the needle.*
   - Ensure that the needle is firmly attached to the syringe.
   - Remove the cap from the needle, then draw up into the syringe the amount of air equal to the volume of the medication to be withdrawn.
   - Carefully insert the needle into the upright vial through the center of the rubber cap, maintaining the sterility of the needle.
   - Inject the air into the vial, keeping the bevel of the needle above the surface of the medication. ❶ **Rationale:** *The air will allow the medication to be drawn out easily because negative pressure will not be created inside the vial. The bevel is kept above the medication to avoid creating bubbles in the medication.*
   - Withdraw the prescribed amount of medication using either of the following methods:
     a. Hold the vial down (i.e., with the base lower than the top), move the needle tip so that it is below the fluid level, and withdraw the medication. Avoid drawing up the last drops of the vial. **Rationale:** *Proponents of this method say that keeping the vial in the upright position while withdrawing the medication allows particulate matter to precipitate out of the solution. Leaving the last few drops reduces the chance of withdrawing foreign particles.* ❷

or

   b. Invert the vial, ensure the needle tip is *below* the fluid level; and gradually withdraw the medication. **Rationale:** *Keeping the tip of the needle below the fluid level prevents air from being drawn into the syringe.* ❸
   - Hold the syringe and vial at eye level to determine that the correct dosage of drug is drawn into the syringe. Eject air remaining at the top of the syringe into the vial.
   - When the correct volume of medication plus a little more (e.g., 0.25 mL) is obtained, withdraw the needle from the vial, and replace the cap over the needle using the scoop method, thus maintaining its sterility.
   - If necessary, tap the syringe barrel to dislodge any air bubbles present in the syringe. **Rationale:** *The tapping motion will cause the air bubbles to rise to the top of the syringe where they can be ejected out of the syringe.*
   - If giving an injection, replace the filter needle, if used, with a regular or safety needle of the correct gauge and length. Eject air from the new needle and verify correct medication volume before injecting the client.

VARIATION: PREPARING AND USING MULTIDOSE VIALS
- Read the manufacturer's directions.
- Withdraw an equivalent amount of air from the vial before adding the diluent, unless otherwise indicated by the directions.
- Add the amount of sterile water or saline indicated in the directions.

❶ Injecting air into a vial.
(Patrick Watson)

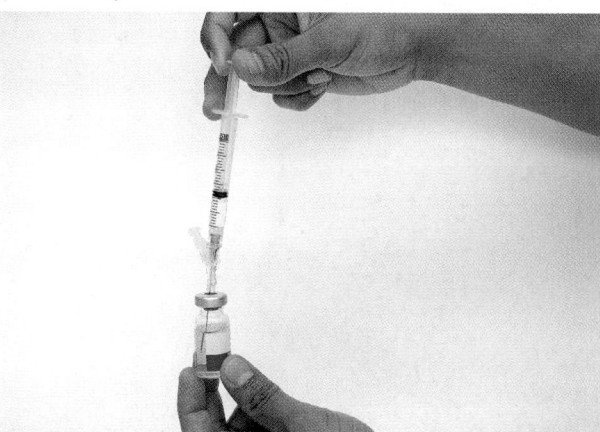

❷ Withdrawing a medication from a vial that is held with the base down.
(Patrick Watson)

❸ Withdrawing a medication from an inverted vial.
(Patrick Watson)

- If a multidose vial is reconstituted, label the vial with the date and time it was prepared, the amount of drug contained in each milliliter of solution, and your initials. **Rationale:** *Time is an important factor to consider in the expiration of these medications.*
- Once the medication is reconstituted, store it in a refrigerator or as recommended by the manufacturer.

injectable preoperative medications such as morphine or meperidine (Demerol) with atropine or scopolamine. Drugs can also be mixed in intravenous solutions. When uncertain about drug compatibilities, the nurse should consult a pharmacist or check a compatibility chart before mixing the drugs.

The nurse must also exercise caution when mixing short- and long-acting insulins, because they vary in content. Chemically, insulin is a protein that, when hydrolyzed in the body, yields a number of amino acids. Some insulin prepara-

tions contain an additional modifying protein, such as globulin or protamine, that slows absorption. This fact is particularly relevant to mixing two insulin preparations for injection because many insulin syringes have needles that cannot be changed. A vial of insulin that does not have the added protein (i.e., regular insulin) should *never* be contaminated with insulin that does have the added protein (i.e., Lente or NPH insulin). Skill 35-4 describes how to mix medications in one syringe.

MIXING MEDICATIONS USING ONE SYRINGE

PLANNING

Delegation
Mixing medications in one syringe involves knowledge and use of aseptic technique. Therefore, this procedure is not delegated to UAP.

Equipment
- MAR or computer printout
- Two vials of medication; one vial and one ampule; two ampules; or one vial or ampule and one cartridge
- Antiseptic swabs
- Sterile syringe and safety needle or insulin syringe and needle (If insulin is being given, use a small-gauge hypodermic needle, e.g., #26 gauge.)
- Additional sterile subcutaneous or intramuscular safety needle (optional)

IMPLEMENTATION

Preparation
1. Check the medication administration record (MAR).
   - Check the label on the medications carefully against the MAR to make sure that the correct medication is being prepared.
   - Follow the three checks for administering medications. Read the label on the medication (1) when it is taken from the medication cart, (2) before withdrawing the medication, and (3) after withdrawing the medication.
   - Before preparing and combining the medications, ensure that the total volume of the injection is appropriate for the injection site.
2. Organize the equipment.

Performance
1. Perform hand hygiene and observe other appropriate infection control procedures.
2. Prepare the medication ampule or vial for drug withdrawal.
   - See Skill 35-2, step 2, for an ampule.
   - Inspect the appearance of the medication for clarity. Some medications are always cloudy. **Rationale:** *Preparations that have changed in appearance should be discarded.*
   - If using insulin, thoroughly mix the solution in each vial prior to administration. Rotate the vials between the palms of the hands and invert the vials. **Rationale:** *Mixing ensures an adequate concentration and thus an accurate dose. Shaking insulin vials can make the medication frothy, making precise measurement difficult.*
   - Clean the tops of the vials with antiseptic swabs.
3. Withdraw the medications.

MIXING MEDICATIONS FROM TWO VIALS
- Take the syringe and draw up a volume of air equal to the volume of medications to be withdrawn from both vials A *and* B.
- Inject a volume of air equal to the volume of medication to be withdrawn into vial A. Make sure the needle does not touch the

solution. **Rationale:** *This prevents cross-contamination of the medications.*
- Withdraw the needle from vial A and inject the remaining air into vial B.
- Withdraw the required amount of medication from vial B. **Rationale:** *The same needle is used to inject air into and withdraw medication from the second vial. It must not be contaminated with the medication in vial A.*
- Using a newly attached sterile needle, withdraw the required amount of medication from vial A. Avoid pushing the plunger as that will introduce medication B into vial A. If using a syringe with a fused needle, withdraw the medication from vial A. The syringe now contains a mixture of medications from vials A and B. **Rationale:** *With this method, neither vial is contaminated by microorganisms or by medication from the other vial.* Be careful to withdraw only the ordered amount and to not create air bubbles. **Rationale:** *The syringe now contains two medications and an excess amount cannot be returned to the vial.*

See also the Variation later in this Skill.

MIXING MEDICATIONS FROM ONE VIAL AND ONE AMPULE
- First prepare and withdraw the medication from the vial. **Rationale:** *Ampules do not require the addition of air prior to withdrawal of the drug.*
- Then withdraw the required amount of medication from the ampule.

MIXING MEDICATIONS FROM ONE CARTRIDGE AND ONE VIAL OR AMPULE
- First ensure that the correct dose of the medication is in the cartridge. Discard any excess medication and air.
- Draw up the required medication from a vial or ampule into the cartridge. Note that when withdrawing medication from a vial, an equal amount of air must first be injected into the vial.
- If the total volume to be injected exceeds the capacity of the cartridge, use a syringe with sufficient capacity to withdraw the de-

continued on page 866

MIXING MEDICATIONS USING ONE SYRINGE *continued*

sired amount of medication from the vial or ampule, and transfer the required amount from the cartridge to the syringe.

VARIATION: MIXING INSULINS

The following is an example of mixing 10 units of regular insulin and 30 units of neutral protamine Hagedorn (NPH) insulin, which contains protamine.

- Inject 30 units of air into the NPH vial and withdraw the needle. (There should be no insulin in the needle.) The needle should not touch the insulin. ❶
- Inject 10 units of air into the regular insulin vial and immediately withdraw 10 units of regular insulin. ❷ and ❸ Always withdraw the regular insulin first *to minimize the possibility of the regular insulin becoming contaminated with the additional protein in the NPH.*
- Reinsert the needle into the NPH insulin vial and withdraw 30 units of NPH insulin. ❹ (The air was previously injected into the

vial.) Be careful to withdraw only the ordered amount and to not create air bubbles. If excess medication has been drawn up, discard the syringe and begin the procedure over again. **Rationale:** *The syringe now contains two medications, and an excess amount cannot be returned to the vial because the syringe contains regular insulin, which, if returned to the NPH vial, would dilute the NPH with regular insulin. The NPH vial would not provide accurate future dosages of NPH insulin.*

By using this method, you avoid adding NPH insulin to the regular insulin.

CLINICAL ALERT

One way to determine which insulin to *withdraw* first is to remember the saying "Clear before cloudy." (Regular insulin is clear and NPH is cloudy due to the proteins in the insulin.) ■

❶ ❷ ❸ ❹

(Patrick Watson)

Intradermal Injections

An **intradermal (ID) injection** is the administration of a drug into the dermal layer of the skin just beneath the epidermis. Usually only a small amount of liquid is used, for example, 0.1 mL. This method of administration is frequently used for allergy testing and tuberculosis (TB) screening. Common sites for intradermal injections are the inner lower arm, the upper chest, and the back beneath the scapulae (Figure 35-30 ■). The left arm is commonly used for TB screening and the right arm is used for all other tests. The steps for administering an intradermal are described in Skill 35-5.

Subcutaneous Injections

Among the many kinds of drugs administered subcutaneously (just beneath the skin) are vaccines, insulin, and heparin. Common sites for subcutaneous injections are the outer aspect of the upper arms and the anterior aspect of the thighs. These areas are

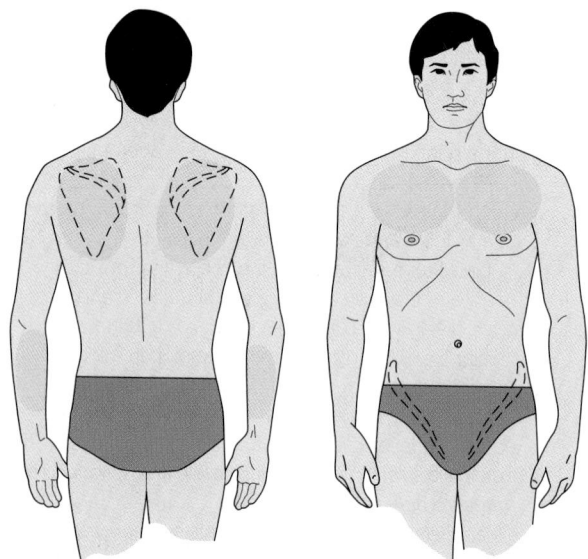

Figure 35-30 ■ Body sites commonly used for intradermal injections.

ADMINISTERING AN INTRADERMAL INJECTION FOR SKIN TESTS

PURPOSE
■ To provide a medication that the client requires for allergy testing and TB screening

ASSESSMENT
Assess
■ Appearance of injection site
■ Specific drug action and expected response
■ Client's knowledge of drug action and response

Check agency protocol about sites to use for skin tests.

PLANNING

Delegation
The administration of intradermal injections is an invasive technique that involves the application of nursing knowledge, problem solving, and sterile technique. This technique is not delegated to UAP. The nurse, however, can inform the UAP about symptoms of allergic reactions and the necessity to report those observations immediately to the nurse.

Equipment
■ Vial or ampule of the correct medication
■ Sterile 1-mL syringe calibrated into hundredths of a milliliter (i.e., tuberculin syringe) and a #25- to #27-gauge safety needle that is 1/4 to 5/8 inch long
■ Alcohol swabs
■ 2-in. × 2-in. sterile gauze square (optional)
■ Clean gloves (according to agency protocol)
■ Bandage (optional)
■ Epinephrine on hand in case of allergic anaphylactic reaction

IMPLEMENTATION
Preparation
1. Check the medication administration record (MAR).
   ● Check the label on the medication carefully against the MAR to make sure that the correct medication is being prepared.
   ● Follow the three checks for administering medications. Read the label on the medication (1) when it is taken from the medication cart, (2) before withdrawing the medication, and (3) after withdrawing the medication.
2. Organize the equipment.

Performance
1. Perform hand hygiene and observe other appropriate infection control procedures (e.g., clean gloves).
2. Prepare the medication from the vial or ampule for drug withdrawal.
   ● See Skills 35-2 and 35-3.
3. Prepare the client
   ● Prior to performing the procedure, introduce self and verify the client's identity using agency protocol. **Rationale:** *This ensures that the right client receives the medication.*
4. Explain to the client that the medication will produce a small wheal, sometimes called a *bleb*. A *wheal* is a small raised area, like a blister. The client will feel a slight prick as the needle enters the skin. Some medications are absorbed slowly through the capillaries into the general circulation, and the bleb gradually disappears. Other drugs remain in the area and interact with the body tissues to produce redness and induration (hardening), which will need to be interpreted at a particular time (e.g., in 24 or 48 hours). This reaction will also gradually disappear. **Rationale:** *Information can facilitate acceptance of and compliance with the therapy.*
5. Provide for client privacy.

6. Select and clean the site.
   ● Select a site (e.g., the forearm about a hand's width above the wrist and three or four fingerwidths below the antecubital space).
   ● Avoid using sites that are tender, inflamed, or swollen and those that have lesions.
   ● Put on gloves as indicated by agency policy.
   ● Cleanse the skin at the site using a firm circular motion starting at the center and widening the circle outward. Allow the area to dry thoroughly.
7. Prepare the syringe for the injection.
   ● Remove the needle cap while waiting for the antiseptic to dry.
   ● Expel any air bubbles from the syringe. Small bubbles that adhere to the plunger are of no consequence. **Rationale:** *A small amount of air will not harm the tissues.*
   ● Grasp the syringe in your dominant hand, close to the hub, holding it between thumb and forefinger. Hold the needle almost parallel to the skin surface, with the bevel of the needle up. **Rationale:** *The possibility of the medication entering the subcutaneous tissue increases when using an angle greater than 15 degrees. The bevel up position provides more comfort for the nurse and is faster to administer (Tarnow & King, 2004).*
8. Inject the fluid.
   ● With the nondominant hand, pull the skin at the site until it is taut. For example, if using the ventral forearm, grasp the client's dorsal forearm and gently pull it to tighten the ventral skin. **Rationale:** *Taut skin allows for easier entry of the needle and less discomfort for the client.*
   ● Insert the tip of the needle far enough to place the bevel through the epidermis into the dermis. The outline of the bevel should be visible under the skin surface.

continued on page 868

ADMINISTERING AN INTRADERMAL INJECTION FOR SKIN TESTS *continued*

1 A

1 B

Epidermis
Dermis
Subcutaneous
tissue

1 C

For an intradermal injection: *A,* the needle enters the skin at a 5- to 15-degree angle; *B, C,* the medication forms a bleb or wheal under the epidermis.

- Stabilize the syringe and needle. Inject the medication carefully and slowly so that it produces a small wheal on the skin. **Rationale:** *This verifies that the medication entered the dermis.* **1**
- Withdraw the needle quickly at the same angle at which it was inserted. Activate the needle safety device. Apply a bandage if indicated.
- Do not massage the area. **Rationale:** *Massage can disperse the medication into the tissue or out through the needle insertion site.*

- Dispose of the syringe and needle into the sharps container. **Rationale:** *Do not recap the needle in order to prevent needlestick injuries.*
- Remove gloves.
- Circle the injection site with ink to observe for redness or induration (hardening), per agency policy.
9. Document all relevant information.
- Record the testing material given, the time, dosage, route, site, and nursing assessments.

EVALUATION

- Evaluate the client's response to the testing substance. **Rationale:** *Some medications used in testing may cause allergic reactions.* Epinephrine may need to be used.

- Evaluate the condition of the site in 24 or 48 hours, depending on the test. Measure the area of redness and induration in millimeters at the largest diameter and document findings.

LIFESPAN CONSIDERATIONS **Administering an Intradermal Injection**

CHILDREN

- Children should be gently restrained during the procedure in order to prevent injury from a sudden movement.

- Make sure the child understands that the injection is not a punishment.
- Ask the child not to rub or scratch the injection site. *Rubbing the site can interfere with test results by irritating the underlying tissue.*

HOME CARE CONSIDERATIONS **Administering an Intradermal Injection**

- Assess the client's knowledge about the intradermal injection and the reason for follow-up with the health care professional. Set up an appointment for the visit.

- Instruct and explain why the injection site should not be washed, rubbed, or scratched.

---

convenient and normally have good blood circulation. Other areas that can be used are the abdomen, the scapular areas of the upper back, and the upper ventrogluteal and dorsogluteal areas (Figure 35-31 ■). Only small doses (0.5 to 1 mL) of medication are usually injected via the subcutaneous route. Check agency policy.

The type of syringe used for subcutaneous injections depends on the medication to be given. Generally a 2-mL syringe is used for most subcutaneous injections. However, if insulin is being administered, an insulin syringe is used; and if heparin is being administered, a tuberculin syringe or prefilled cartridge may be used.

RESEARCH NOTE   Should the Bevel Be Up or Down?

The tradition in nursing practice is to administer an intradermal injection with the bevel up. The authors point out that only one 1997 study investigated intradermal technique and it found the bevel-down technique to be superior to the bevel-up technique. However, the sample size of that study was small (e.g., three volunteers). Therefore, these researchers decided to replicate the study with tighter control and improved research methods.

This study used qualitative and quantitative methods to examine differences regarding correct placement of injectate, leaking or bleeding, time to administer injection, and comfort of persons administering and receiving an intradermal injection. Each of the 98 subjects administered and received two injections. The subjects evaluated their comfort in administering and in receiving a bevel-up injection and a bevel-down injection using a Likert scale.

The results indicated that there was no significant difference related to comfort for client preference for bevel up or bevel down.

There was, however, a statistically significant difference for the subjects in the nurse role citing that there was more comfort with the bevel being up. The subjects administered the bevel-up injections faster than the bevel-down injections. Client outcomes (e.g., wheal, leakage, and bleeding) with regard to bevel-up or bevel-down technique were equivalent. There was no statistical difference.

IMPLICATIONS

The researchers suggest that nurses continue to use bevel-up technique as the preferred way to administer intradermal injections because of the increased comfort for the person in the nurse role and because it was faster to administer. They also suggest that more research be done as there are only two studies and they differ in results.

Note: Reprinted from *Applied Nursing Research, 17*(4) K. Tarnow and N. King, "Intradermal Injections: Traditional Bevel Up Versus Bevel Down," pp. 275–282. Copyright 2004, with permission from Elsevier.

Needle sizes and lengths are selected based on the client's body mass, the intended angle of insertion, and the planned site. Generally a #25-gauge, 5/8-inch needle is used for adults of normal weight and the needle is inserted at a 45-degree angle; a 3/8-inch needle is used at a 90-degree angle. A child may need a 1/2-inch needle inserted at a 45-degree angle.

Figure 35-31 ■ Body sites commonly used for subcutaneous injections.

One method nurses use to determine length of needle is to pinch the tissue at the site and select a needle length that is half the width of the skinfold. To determine the angle of insertion, a general rule to follow relates to the amount of tissue that can be pinched or grasped at the site. A 45-degree angle is used when 1 inch of tissue can be grasped at the site; a 90-degree angle is used when 2 inches of tissue can be grasped.

When administering insulin to adults, the current standard needle gauge is #30 gauge. Short needles (5/16 inch) are available with 0.3-, 0.5-, 1.0-, and 2.0-mL capacities (American Diabetes Association, 2004). Most clients prefer the shorter and thinner needles because they are less painful. The risk of injecting into the muscle is lessened with the shorter needle.

Subcutaneous injection sites need to be rotated in an orderly fashion to minimize tissue damage, aid absorption, and avoid discomfort. This is especially important for clients who must receive repeated injections, such as diabetics. Because insulin is absorbed at different rates at different parts of the body, the diabetic client's blood glucose levels can vary when various sites are used. Insulin is absorbed most quickly when injected into the abdomen and then into the arms, and most slowly when injected into the thighs and buttocks. Current recommendations include rotating injections within one area to prevent lipoatrophy and lipohypertrophy (American Diabetes Association, 2004).

Nurses have traditionally been taught to aspirate by pulling back on the plunger after inserting the needle and before injecting the medication. The nurse could then determine whether the needle had entered a blood vessel. Absence of blood was believed to indicate that the needle was in subcutaneous tissue and not in the more vascular muscular tissue. According to the American Diabetes Association (2004), routine aspiration is no longer recommended with insulin administration. It is likely that students will observe that the practice of aspirating subcutaneous injections will vary among nurses.

The steps for administering a subcutaneous injection are described in Skill 35-6.

MediaLink Client on Insulin Care Plan Activity

SKILL 35-6

ADMINISTERING A SUBCUTANEOUS INJECTION

PURPOSES

- To provide a medication the client requires (see specific drug action)
- To allow slower absorption of a medication compared with either the intramuscular or intravenous route

ASSESSMENT

Assess

- Allergies to medication
- Specific drug action, side effects, and adverse reactions
- Client's knowledge and learning needs about the medication
- Status and appearance of subcutaneous site for lesions, erythema, swelling, ecchymosis, inflammation, and tissue damage from previous injections
- Ability of client to cooperate during the injection
- Previous injection sites used

PLANNING

Delegation

The administration of subcutaneous injections is an invasive technique that involves the application of nursing knowledge, problem solving, and sterile technique. Therefore, this skill is not delegated to UAP. The nurse, however, can inform the UAP of the intended therapeutic effects and/or specific side effects of the medication and direct the UAP to report specific client observations to the nurse for follow-up.

Equipment

- Client's MAR or computer printout
- Vial or ampule of the correct sterile medication
- Syringe and needle (e.g., 3-mL syringe, #25-gauge needle or smaller, 3/8 or 5/8 inch long)
- Antiseptic swabs
- Dry sterile gauze for opening an ampule (optional)
- Clean gloves

IMPLEMENTATION

Preparation

1. Check the medication administration record (MAR).
   - Check the label on the medication carefully against the MAR to make sure that the correct medication is being prepared.
   - Follow the three checks for administering medications. Read the label on the medication (1) when it is taken from the medication cart, (2) before withdrawing the medication, and (3) after withdrawing the medication.
2. Organize the equipment.

Performance

1. Perform hand hygiene and observe other appropriate infection control procedures (e.g., clean gloves).
2. Prepare the medication from the ampule or vial for drug withdrawal.
   - See Skill 35-2 (ampule) or 35-3 (vial).
3. Provide for client privacy.
4. Prepare the client.
   - Prior to performing the procedure, introduce self and verify the client's identity using agency protocol. **Rationale:** *This ensures that the right client receives the medication.*
   - Assist the client to a position in which the arm, leg, or abdomen can be relaxed, depending on the site to be used. **Rationale:** *A relaxed position of the site minimizes discomfort.*
   - Obtain assistance in holding an uncooperative client. **Rationale:** *This prevents injury due to sudden movement after needle insertion.*
5. Explain the purpose of the medication and how it will help, using language that the client can understand. Include relevant information about effects of the medication. **Rationale:** *Information can facilitate acceptance of and compliance with the therapy.*
6. Select and clean the site.
   - Select a site free of tenderness, hardness, swelling, scarring, itching, burning, or localized inflammation. Select a site that has not been used frequently. **Rationale:** *These conditions could hinder the absorption of the medication and may also*

increase the likelihood of injury and discomfort at the injection site.
   - Put on clean gloves.
   - As agency protocol indicates, clean the site with an antiseptic swab. Start at the center of the site and clean in a widening circle to about 5 cm (2 in.). Allow the area to dry thoroughly. **Rationale:** *The mechanical action of swabbing removes skin secretions, which contain microorganisms.*
   - Place and hold the swab between the third and fourth fingers of the nondominant hand, or position the swab on the client's skin above the intended site. **Rationale:** *Using this technique keeps the swab readily accessible when the needle is withdrawn.*
7. Prepare the syringe for injection.
   - Remove the needle cap while waiting for the antiseptic to dry. Pull the cap straight off to avoid contaminating the needle by the outside edge of the cap. **Rationale:** *The needle will become contaminated if it touches anything but the inside of the cap, which is sterile.*
   - Dispose of the needle cap.
8. Inject the medication.
   - Grasp the syringe in your dominant hand by holding it between your thumb and fingers. With palm facing to the side or upward for a 45-degree angle insertion, or with the palm downward for a 90-degree angle insertion, prepare to inject. ❶

❶ Inserting a needle into the subcutaneous tissue using 90- and 45-degree angles.

ADMINISTERING A SUBCUTANEOUS INJECTION *continued*

- Using the nondominant hand, pinch or spread the skin at the site, and insert the needle using the dominant hand and a firm steady push. Recommendations vary about whether to pinch or spread the skin and at what angle to administer subcutaneous injections. The most important consideration is the depth of the subcutaneous tissue in the area to be injected. If the client has more than ½ inch of adipose tissue in the injection site, it would be safe to administer the injection at a 90-degree angle with the skin spread. If the client is thin or lean and lacks adipose tissue, the subcutaneous injection should be given with the skin pinched and at a 45- to 60-degree angle. One way to check that the pinch of skin is subcutaneous tissue is to ask the client to flex and extend the elbow. If any muscle is being held in the pinch, you will feel it contract and relax. If so, release the pinch and try again. ❷
- When the needle is inserted, move your nondominant hand to the end of the plunger. Some nurses find it easier to move the nondominant hand to the barrel of the syringe and the dominant hand to the end of the plunger.
- Inject the medication by holding the syringe steady and depressing the plunger with a slow, even pressure. **Rationale:** *Holding the syringe steady and injecting the medication at an even pressure minimizes discomfort for the client.*
- It is recommended that with many subcutaneous injections, especially insulin, the needle "should be embedded within the skin for five seconds after complete depression of the plunger to ensure complete delivery of the dose" (American Diabetes Association, 2004, p. S108).

9. Remove the needle.
   - Remove the needle smoothly, pulling along the line of insertion while depressing the skin with your nondominant hand. **Rationale:** *Depressing the skin places countertraction on it and minimizes the client's discomfort when the needle is withdrawn.*
   - If bleeding occurs, apply pressure to the site with dry sterile gauze until it stops. *Bleeding rarely occurs after subcutaneous injection.*
10. Dispose of supplies appropriately.
    - Activate the needle safety device or discard the uncapped needle and attached syringe into designated receptacles. **Rationale:** *Proper disposal protects the nurse and others from injury and contamination. The Centers for Disease Control and Prevention (CDC) recommends not capping the needle before disposal to reduce the risk of needlestick injuries.*
    - Remove gloves and perform hand hygiene.
11. Document all relevant information.
    - Document the medication given, dosage, time, route, and any assessments.
    - Many agencies prefer that medication administration be recorded on the medication record. The nurse's notes are used when prn medications are given or when there is a special problem.
12. Assess the effectiveness of the medication at the time it is expected to act and document it.

VARIATION: ADMINISTERING A HEPARIN INJECTION

The subcutaneous administration of heparin and low molecular weight heparin (i.e., enoxaparin [Lovenox]) requires special precautions because of the drug's anticoagulant properties.

- Select a site on the abdomen at least 2 inches *away* from the umbilicus and above the level of the iliac crests. Some agencies support the practice of subcutaneous injection of heparin in the thighs or arms as alternate sites to the abdomen.
- Use a 3/8-inch, #25- or #26-gauge needle or smaller, and insert it at a 90-degree angle. If a client is very lean or wasted, use a needle longer than 3/8 inch and insert it at a 45-degree angle. The arms or thighs may be used as alternate sites.
- Do *not* aspirate when giving heparin by subcutaneous injection. **Rationale:** *Aspiration can possibly damage the surrounding tissue and cause bleeding as well as bruising.*
- Do not massage the site after the injection. **Rationale:** *Massaging could cause bleeding and ecchymoses (bruises) and hasten drug absorption.*
- Alternate the sites of subsequent injections.

❷ Administering a subcutaneous injection into pinched tissue.
Photographer: Elena Dorfman

EVALUATION

- Conduct appropriate follow-up such as desired effect (e.g., relief of pain, sedation, lowered blood sugar, a prothrombin time within preestablished limits), any adverse effects (e.g., nausea, vomiting, skin rash), and clinical signs of side effects.
- Relate to previous findings if available.
- Report deviations from normal to the primary care provider.

HOME CARE CONSIDERATIONS **Subcutaneous Injections**

- If the client has impaired vision, consider prefilling syringes and storing them in an appropriate environment (e.g., the refrigerator) or obtaining prefilled medication syringes from pharmaceutical companies.
- For frequent injections, develop a plan for site rotation with the client and explain the reason for injection site rotation.
- For cost-saving measures, teach able clients to safely reuse disposable syringes. Clients with diabetes can be taught to use the same syringe two to three times. They should be instructed to change syringes when the needle appears dull. Clients should be encouraged to maintain needle asepsis, practice safe recapping, and

assess for needle dullness with each injection (American Diabetes Association, 2004). However, clients with poor personal hygiene, acute concurrent illness, open wounds on the hands, or decreased resistance to infection should be discouraged from reusing syringes.
- Explore with the client and primary care provider the appropriateness of the new inhaled version of insulin in place of the injectable version.
- For insulin-dependent clients, ensure that at least one knowledgeable support person can correctly inject insulin in an emergency situation and recognize and treat hypoglycemia.

Intramuscular Injections

Injections into muscle tissue, or **intramuscular (IM) injections,** are absorbed more quickly than subcutaneous injections because of the greater blood supply to the body muscles. Muscles can also take a larger volume of fluid without discomfort than subcutaneous tissues can, although the amount varies among individuals, chiefly based on muscle size and condition and the site used. An adult with well-developed muscles can usually safely tolerate up to 3 mL of medication in the gluteus medius and gluteus maximus muscles (Figure 35-32 ■). A volume of 1 to 2 mL is usually recommended for adults with less developed muscles. In the deltoid muscle, volumes of 0.5 to 1 mL are recommended.

Usually a 3- to 5-mL syringe is needed. The size of syringe used depends on the amount of medication being administered. The standard prepackaged intramuscular needle is 1½ inches and #21 or #22 gauge. Several factors indicate the size and length of the needle to be used:

- The muscle
- The type of solution

- The amount of adipose tissue covering the muscle
- The age of the client

For example, a smaller needle such as a #23- to #25-gauge needle 1 inch long is commonly used for the deltoid muscle. More viscous solutions require a larger gauge (e.g., #20 gauge). Very obese clients may require a needle longer than 1½ inches (e.g., 2 inches), and emaciated clients may require a shorter needle (e.g., 1 inch).

A major consideration in the administration of intramuscular injections is the selection of a safe site located away from large blood vessels, nerves, and bone. Several body sites can be used for intramuscular injections. These sites are discussed in detail next. Contraindications for using a specific site include tissue injury and the presence of nodules, lumps, abscesses, tenderness, or other pathology.

Ventrogluteal Site

The ventrogluteal site is in the gluteus medius muscle, which lies over the gluteus minimus (Figure 35-32). The ventrogluteal site is the *preferred* site for intramuscular injections because the area:

- Contains no large nerves or blood vessels.
- Provides the greatest thickness of gluteal muscle consisting of both the gluteus medius and gluteus minimus.
- Is sealed off by bone.
- Contains consistently less fat than the buttock area, thus eliminating the need to determine the depth of subcutaneous fat.

This site is suitable for children over 1 year and adults (Nicoll & Hesby, 2002). The client position for the injection can be a back, prone, or side-lying position. The side-lying position, however, helps locate the ventrogluteal site more easily. Position the client on his or her side with the knee bent and raised slightly toward the chest. The trochanter will protrude, which facilitates locating the ventrogluteal site. To establish the exact site, the nurse places the heel of the hand on the client's greater trochanter, with the fingers pointing toward the client's head. The right hand is used for the left hip, and the left hand for the right hip. With the index finger on the client's anterior superior iliac spine, the nurse stretches the middle finger dorsally (toward the buttocks), palpating the crest of the ilium and then pressing below it. The triangle formed by the index finger, the

Iliac crest

Anterior superior iliac spine

Gluteus medius

Gluteus minimus (underlying medius)

Gluteus maximus

Greater trochanter of femur

Figure 35-32 ■ Lateral view of the right buttock showing the three gluteal muscles used for intramuscular injections.

(Custom Medical Stock Photo, Inc.)

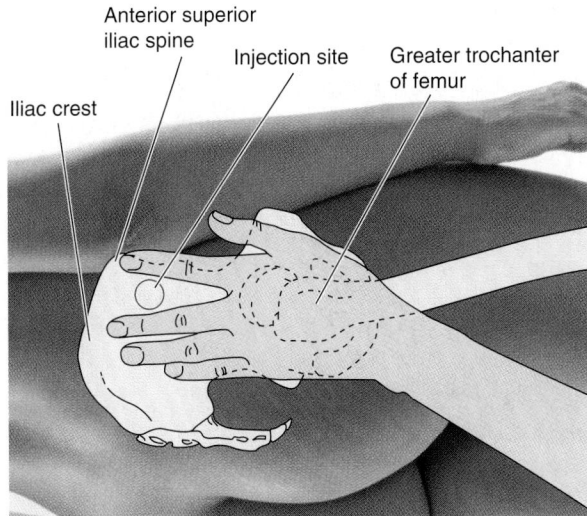

Figure 35-33 ■ Landmarks for the ventrogluteal site for an intramuscular injection.

Figure 35-34 ■ Administering an intramuscular injection into the ventrogluteal site.

Photographer: Jenny Thomas

third finger, and the crest of the ilium is the injection site (Figures 35-33 ■ and Figure 35-34 ■).

Vastus Lateralis Site

The vastus lateralis muscle is usually thick and well developed in both adults and children. It is recommended as the site of choice for intramuscular injections for infants 1 year and younger (Nicoll & Hesby, 2002). Because there are no major blood vessels or nerves in the area, it is desirable for infants whose gluteal muscles are poorly developed. It is situated on the anterior lateral aspect of the infant's thigh (Figure 35-35 ■). The middle third of the muscle is suggested as the site. In the adult, the landmark is established by dividing the area between the greater trochanter of the femur and the lateral femoral condyle into thirds and selecting the middle third (Figures 35-36 ■ and 35-37 ■). The client can assume a back-lying or a sitting position for an injection into this site.

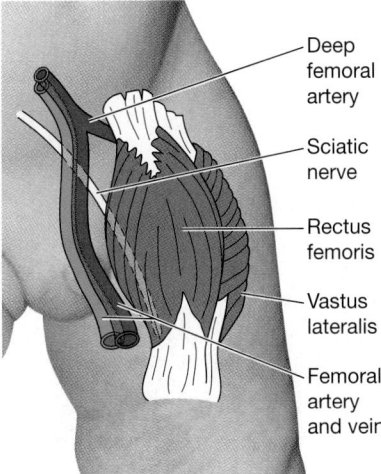

Figure 35-35 ■ The vastus lateralis muscle of an infant's upper thigh, used for intramuscular injections.

(Custom Medical Stock Photo, Inc.)

Dorsogluteal Site

The dorsogluteal site is composed of the thick gluteal muscles of the buttocks (Figure 35–32). The dorsogluteal site can be used for adults and for children with well-developed gluteal muscles. Because these muscles are developed by walking, this site should not be used for children under 3 years unless the child has been walking for at least 1 year. The nurse must choose

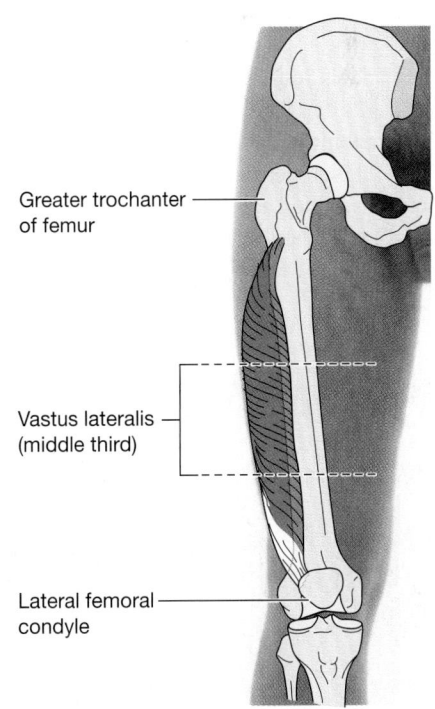

Figure 35-36 ■ Landmarks for the vastus lateralis site of an adult's right thigh, used for an intramuscular injection.

(Custom Medical Stock Photo, Inc.)

A

B

Figure 35-37 ■ *A,* Determining landmarks and *B,* administering an intramuscular injection into the vastus lateralis site.

the injection site carefully to avoid striking the sciatic nerve, major blood vessels, or bone.

The nurse palpates the posterior superior iliac spine, then draws an imaginary line to the greater trochanter of the femur. This line is lateral to and parallel to the sciatic nerve. The injection site is lateral and superior to this line (Figure 35-38 ■). Palpating the ilium and the trochanter is important; visual calculations alone can result in an injection that is placed too low and injures other structures.

The client needs to assume a prone position with the toes pointed inward or a side-lying position with the upper knee flexed and in front of the lower leg. These positions promote muscle relaxation and therefore minimize discomfort from the injection.

Deltoid Site

The deltoid muscle is found on the lateral aspect of the upper arm. It is not used often for intramuscular injections because it is a relatively small muscle and is very close to the radial nerve and radial artery. It is sometimes considered for use in adults because of rapid absorption from the deltoid area, but no more than 1 mL of solution can be administered. This site is recommended for the administration of hepatitis B vaccine in adults.

The upper landmark for the deltoid site is located by the nurse placing four fingers across the deltoid muscle with the first finger on the acromion process. The top of the axilla is the line that marks the lower border landmark (Figure 35-39 ■). A triangle within these boundaries indicates the deltoid muscle about 5 cm (2 in.) below the acromion process (Figures 35-40 ■ and 35-41 ■).

Nicoll and Hesby (2002) reported that researchers found that "applying pressure to the site for ten seconds prior to injection reduced injection pain" (p. 158). Further research is needed to determine additional techniques that will minimize the degree of pain at the time of injection.

Rectus Femoris Site

The rectus femoris muscle, which belongs to the quadriceps muscle group, is used only occasionally for intramuscular in-

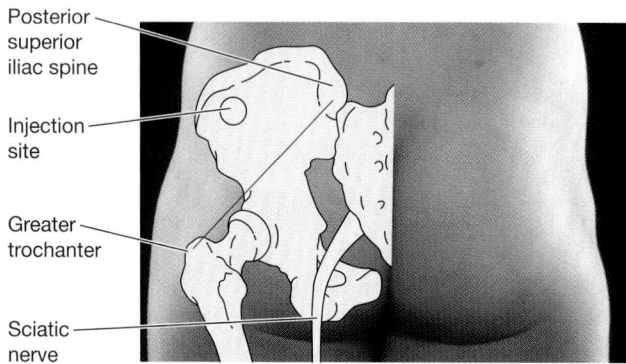

Figure 35-38 ■ Landmarks for the dorsogluteal site for an intramuscular injection.

(Custom Medical Stock Photo, Inc.)

Posterior superior iliac spine

Injection site

Greater trochanter

Sciatic nerve

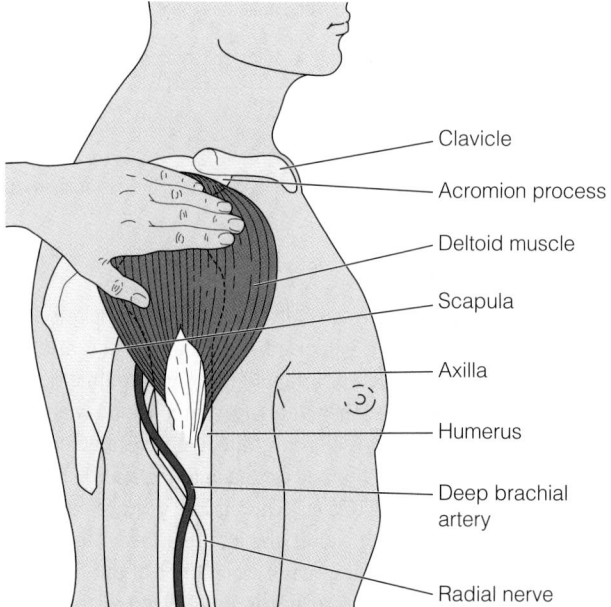

Clavicle

Acromion process

Deltoid muscle

Scapula

Axilla

Humerus

Deep brachial artery

Radial nerve

Figure 35-39 ■ A method of establishing the deltoid muscle site for an intramuscular injection.

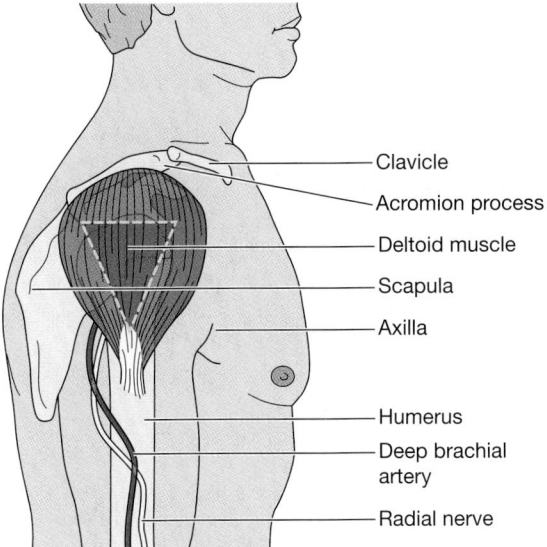

Figure 35-40 ■ Landmarks for the deltoid muscle of the upper arm, used for intramuscular injections.
(Custom Medical Stock Photo, Inc.)

Figure 35-42 ■ Landmarks for the rectus femoris muscle of the upper right thigh, used for intramuscular injections.

jections. It is situated on the anterior aspect of the thigh (Figure 35-42 ■). Its chief advantage is that clients who administer their own injections can reach this site easily. Its main disadvantage is that an injection here may cause considerable discomfort for some people.

IM Injection Technique

Skill 35-7 describes how to administer an intramuscular injection using the Z-track technique, which is recommended for all intramuscular injections (Nicoll & Hesby, 2002, p. 157). The Z-track method has been found to be less painful than the tradi-

tional injection technique and decreases leakage of irritating and discoloring medications into the subcutaneous tissue (Nicoll & Hesby, 2002; Pullen, 2005). Although the Z-track technique is not always used in practice, research evidence does support its effectiveness and recommends its routine use.

Intravenous Medications

Because intravenous (IV) medications enter the client's bloodstream directly by way of a vein, they are appropriate when a rapid effect is required. This route is also appropriate when medications are too irritating to tissues to be given by other routes. When an intravenous line is already established, this route is desirable because it avoids the discomfort of other parenteral routes. Following are methods to administer medications intravenously:

- Large-volume infusion of intravenous fluid
- Intermittent intravenous infusion (piggyback or tandem setups)
- Volume-controlled infusion (often used for children)
- Intravenous push or bolus
- Intermittent injection ports (device)

In all of these methods, the client has an existing intravenous line or an IV access site such as a saline or heparin lock. Most agencies have procedures and policies about who may administer an IV medication. Chapter 52 describes the technique for performing a venipuncture and establishing an IV line. ∞

With all IV medication administration, it is very important to observe clients closely for signs of adverse reactions. Because

Figure 35-41 ■ Administering an intramuscular injection into the deltoid site.

ADMINISTERING AN INTRAMUSCULAR INJECTION

PURPOSE
- To provide a medication the client requires (see specific drug action)

ASSESSMENT

Assess
- Client allergies to medication(s)
- Specific drug action, side effects, and adverse reactions
- Client's knowledge of and learning needs about the medication
- Tissue integrity of the selected site
- Client's age and weight to determine site and needle size
- Client's ability or willingness to cooperate

Determine whether the size of the muscle is appropriate to the amount of medication to be injected. An average adult's deltoid muscle can usually absorb 0.5 mL of medication, although some authorities believe 1 mL can be absorbed by a well-developed deltoid muscle. The gluteus medius muscle can often absorb 1 to 4 mL, although 4 mL may be very painful and may be contraindicated by agency protocol.

PLANNING

Delegation
The administration of IM injections is an invasive technique that involves the application of nursing knowledge, problem solving, and sterile technique. Delegation to UAP would be inappropriate. The nurse, however, can inform the UAP of the intended therapeutic effects and/or specific side effects of the medication and direct the UAP to report specific client observations to the nurse for follow-up.

Equipment
- MAR or computer printout
- Sterile medication (usually provided in an ampule or vial or prefilled syringe)
- Syringe and needle of a size appropriate for the amount and type of solution to be administered
- Antiseptic swabs
- Clean gloves

IMPLEMENTATION

Preparation
1. Check the medication administration record (MAR).
   - Check the label on the medication carefully against the MAR to make sure that the correct medication is being prepared.
   - Follow the three checks for administering the medication and dose. Read the label on the medication (1) when it is taken from the medication cart, (2) before withdrawing the medication, and (3) after withdrawing the medication.
   - Confirm that the dose is correct.
2. Organize the equipment.

PERFORMANCE
1. Perform hand hygiene and observe other appropriate infection control procedures (e.g., clean gloves).
2. Prepare the medication from the ampule or vial for drug withdrawal.
   - See Skill 35-2 (ampule) or 35-3 (vial).
   - Whenever feasible, change the needle on the syringe before the injection. **Rationale:** *Because the outside of a new needle is free of medication, it does not irritate subcutaneous tissues as it passes into the muscle.*
   - Invert the syringe needle uppermost and expel all excess air.
3. Provide for client privacy.
4. Prepare the client.
   - Prior to performing the procedure, introduce self and verify the client's identity using agency protocol. **Rationale:** *This ensures that the right client receives the medication.*
   - Assist the client to a supine, lateral, prone, or sitting position, depending on the chosen site. If the target muscle is the gluteus medius (ventrogluteal site), have the client in the supine position flex the knee(s); in the lateral position, flex the upper leg; and in the prone position, toe in. **Rationale:** *Appropriate positioning promotes relaxation of the target muscle.*
   - Obtain assistance in holding an uncooperative client. **Rationale:** *This prevents injury due to sudden movement after needle insertion.*

5. Explain the purpose of the medication and how it will help, using language that the client can understand. Include relevant information about effects of the medication. **Rationale:** *Information can facilitate acceptance of and compliance with the therapy.*
6. Select, locate, and clean the site.
   - Select a site free of skin lesions, tenderness, swelling, hardness, or localized inflammation and one that has not been used frequently.
   - If injections are to be frequent, alternate sites. Avoid using the same site twice in a row. **Rationale:** *This is to reduce the discomfort of intramuscular injections.* If necessary, discuss with the prescribing primary care provider an alternative method of providing the medication.
   - Locate the exact site for the injection. See the discussion of sites earlier in this chapter.
   - Put on clean gloves.
   - Clean the site with an antiseptic swab. Using a circular motion, start at the center and move outward about 5 cm (2 in.).
   - Transfer and hold the swab between the third and fourth fingers of your nondominant hand in readiness for needle withdrawal, or position the swab on the client's skin above the intended site. Allow skin to dry prior to injecting medication. **Rationale:** *This will help reduce the discomfort of the injection.*
7. Prepare the syringe for injection.
   - Remove the needle cover and discard without contaminating the needle.
   - If using a prefilled unit-dose medication, take caution to avoid dripping medication on the needle prior to injection. If this does occur, wipe the medication off the needle with a sterile gauze. Some sources recommend changing the needle if possible. **Rationale:** *Medication left on the needle can cause pain when it is tracked through the subcutaneous tissue (Nicoll & Hesby, 2002, p. 156).*
8. Inject the medication using a Z-track technique.
   - Use the ulnar side of the nondominant hand to pull the skin approximately 2.5 cm (1 inch) to the side. Under some cir-

❶ Inserting an intramuscular needle at a 90-degree angle using the Z-track method: *A,* skin pulled to the side; *B,* skin released. *Note:* When the skin returns to its normal position after the needle is withdrawn, a seal is formed over the intramuscular site. This prevents seepage of the medication into the subcutaneous tissues and subsequent discomfort.

Skin
Subcutaneous tissue
Muscle
Medication

A   B

cumstances, such as for an emaciated client or an infant, the muscle may be pinched. **Rationale:** *Pulling the skin and subcutaneous tissue or pinching the muscle makes it firmer and facilitates needle insertion.* ❶

- Holding the syringe between the thumb and forefinger (as if holding a pencil), pierce the skin quickly and smoothly at a 90-degree angle (Figure 35-34), and insert the needle into the muscle. **Rationale:** *Using a quick motion lessens the client's discomfort.*
- Hold the barrel of the syringe steady with your nondominant hand and aspirate by pulling back on the plunger with your dominant hand. Aspirate for 5 to 10 seconds. **Rationale:** *If the needle is in a small blood vessel, it takes time for the blood to appear.* If blood appears in the syringe, withdraw the needle, discard the syringe, and prepare a new injection. **Rationale:** *This step determines whether the needle has been inserted into a blood vessel.* Although some controversy exists with subcutaneous aspiration practices, aspiration continues to be recommended with IM injection to avoid medication injection into the bloodstream (Barr & Thomas, 2005).
- If blood does not appear, inject the medication steadily and slowly (approximately 10 seconds per milliliter) while holding the syringe steady. **Rationale:** *Injecting medica-*

tion slowly promotes comfort and allows time for tissue to expand and begin absorption of the medication (Nicoll & Hesby, 2002). Holding the syringe steady minimizes discomfort.
- After injection, wait 10 seconds *to permit the medication to disperse into the muscle tissue, thus decreasing the client's discomfort.*

9. Withdraw the needle.
   - Withdraw the needle smoothly at the same angle of insertion. **Rationale:** *This minimizes tissue injury.* Release the skin.
   - Apply gentle pressure at the site with a dry sponge. **Rationale:** *Use of an alcohol swab may cause pain or a burning sensation.*
   - If bleeding occurs, apply pressure with a dry sterile gauze until it stops.
10. Activate the needle safety device or discard the uncapped needle and attached syringe into the proper receptacle.
    - Remove gloves. Perform hand hygiene.
11. Document all relevant information.
    - Include the time of administration, drug name, dose, route, and the client's reactions.
12. Assess effectiveness of the medication at the time it is expected to act.

EVALUATION
- Conduct appropriate follow-up, such as
  - Desired effect (e.g., relief of pain or vomiting).
  - Any adverse reactions or side effects.

- Local skin or tissue reactions at injection site (e.g., redness, swelling, pain, or other evidence of tissue damage).
- Relate to previous findings, if available.
- Report significant deviation from normal to the primary care provider.

LIFESPAN CONSIDERATIONS   Intramuscular Injections

INFANTS

- The vastus lateralis site is recommended as the site of choice for intramuscular injections for infants. There are no major blood vessels or nerves in this area, and it is the infant's largest muscle mass. It is situated on the anterior lateral aspect of the thigh.
- Obtain assistance to immobilize an infant or young child. The parent may hold the child. This prevents accidental injury during the procedure.

CHILDREN

- Use needles that will place medication in the main muscle mass; infants and children usually require smaller, shorter needles (#22 to #25 gauge, 5/8 to 1 inch long) for intramuscular injections.

- The vastus lateralis is recommended as the site of choice for toddlers and children.
- For the older child and adolescent, the recommended sites are the same as for the adult: ventrogluteal or deltoid. Ask which arm they would like the injection in.

ELDERS

- Older clients may have a decreased muscle mass or muscle atrophy. A shorter needle may be needed. Assessment of appropriate injection site is critical. Absorption of medication may occur more quickly than expected.

the drug enters the bloodstream directly and acts immediately, there is no way it can be withdrawn or its action terminated. Therefore, the nurse must take special care to avoid any errors about the preparation of the drug and the calculation of the dosage. When the administered drug is particularly potent, an antidote to the drug should be available. In addition, assess the vital signs before, during, and after infusion of the drug.

Before adding any medications to an existing intravenous infusion, the nurse must check for the "rights" and check compatibility of the drug and the existing intravenous fluid. Be aware of any incompatibilities of the drug and the fluid that is infusing. For example, the drug phenytoin (Dilantin) is incompatible with glucose and will form a precipitate if injected through a port in an intravenous line with glucose/dextrose infusing.

Large-Volume Infusions

Mixing a medication into a large-volume IV container is the safest and easiest way to administer a drug intravenously. The drugs are diluted in volumes of 1,000 mL or 500 mL of compatible fluids. It may be necessary to consult a pharmacist to confirm compatibility. Fluids such as IV normal saline or Ringer's lactate are frequently used. Commonly added drugs are potassium chloride and vitamins. It may also be necessary to ensure the compatibility of some drugs with the plastic IV bag and tubing. A glass IV bottle and special tubing may be used in special situations. See Skill 35-8.

The main danger of infusing a large volume of fluid is circulatory overload (hypervolemia) (see Chapter 51 ∞).

SKILL 35-8

ADDING MEDICATIONS TO INTRAVENOUS FLUID CONTAINERS

PURPOSES
- To provide and maintain a constant level of a medication in the blood
- To administer well-diluted medications at a continuous and slow rate

ASSESSMENT
- Inspect and palpate the intravenous insertion site for signs of infection, infiltration, or a dislocated catheter.
- Inspect the surrounding skin for redness, pallor, or swelling.
- Palpate the surrounding tissues for coldness and the presence of edema, which could indicate leakage of the IV fluid into the tissues.
- Take vital signs for baseline data for medication that is particularly potent.
- Determine if the client has allergies to the medication(s).
- Check the compatibility of the medication(s) and IV fluid.

PLANNING

Delegation

Adding medications to IV fluid containers involves the application of nursing knowledge and critical thinking. The nurse does not delegate this procedure to UAP. However, the nurse can inform the UAP of the intended therapeutic effects and/or specific side effects of the medication(s) in the IV and direct the UAP to report specific client observations to the nurse for follow-up.

Equipment
- MAR or computer printout
- Correct sterile medication
- Diluent for medication in powdered form (see manufacturer's instructions)
- Correct solution container, if a new one is to be attached
- Antiseptic swabs
- Sterile syringe of appropriate size (e.g., 5 or 10 mL) and a 1- to 1 1/2-inch, #20- or #21-gauge sterile safety needle if not using a needleless system
- IV additive label

IMPLEMENTATION
Preparation
1. Check the medication administration record (MAR).
   - Check the label on the medication carefully against the MAR to make sure that the correct medication is being prepared.
   - Follow the three checks for administering medications. Read the label on the medication (1) when it is taken from the medication cart, (2) before withdrawing the medication, and (3) after withdrawing the medication.
   - Confirm that the dosage and route is correct.
   - Verify which infusion solution is to be used with the medication.
   - Consult a pharmacist, if required, to confirm compatibility of the drugs and solutions being mixed.
2. Organize the equipment.

Performance
1. Perform hand hygiene and observe other appropriate infection control procedures.

2. Prepare the medication ampule or vial for drug withdrawal.
   - See Skill 35-2 (ampule) or 35-3 (vial).
   - Check the agency's practice for using a filter needle to withdraw premixed liquid medications from multidose vials or ampules.
3. Add the medication.

   To New IV Container
   - Locate the injection port. Clean the port with the antiseptic or alcohol swab. **Rationale:** *This reduces the risk of introducing microorganisms into the container when the needle is inserted.*
   - Remove the needle cap from the syringe, insert the needle through the center of the injection port, and inject the medication into the bag. Activate the needle safety device. ❶
   - Mix the medication and solution by gently rotating the bag or bottle. **Rationale:** *This should disperse the medication throughout the solution.* ❷

ADDING MEDICATION TO INTRAVENOUS FLUID CONTAINERS *continued*

❶ Inserting a medication through the injection port of an infusing container.
Photographer: Elena Dorfman

❷ Rotating an intravenous bag to distribute a medication.
Photographer: Elena Dorfman

- Complete the IV additive label with name and dose of medication, date, time, and nurse's initials. Attach it upside down on the bag or bottle. **Rationale:** *This documents that medication has been added to the solution. When the label is attached upside down, it is easily read when the bag is hanging up.* ❸
- Clamp the IV tubing. Spike the bag or bottle with IV tubing and hang the IV. **Rationale:** *Clamping prevents rapid infusion of the solution.*
- Regulate infusion rate as ordered.

To an Existing Infusion
- Determine that the IV solution in the container is sufficient for adding the medication. **Rationale:** *Sufficient volume is necessary to dilute the medication adequately.*
- Confirm the desired dilution of the medication, that is, the amount of medication per milliliter of solution.
- Close the infusion clamp. **Rationale:** *This prevents the medication from infusing directly into the client as it is injected into the bag or bottle.*
- Wipe the medication port with the alcohol or disinfectant swab. **Rationale:** *This reduces the risk of introducing microorganisms into the container when the needle is inserted.*
- Remove the needle cover from the medication syringe.
- While supporting and stabilizing the bag with your thumb and forefinger, carefully insert the syringe needle through the port and inject the medication. **Rationale:** *The bag is supported during the injection of the medication to avoid punctures. If the bag is too high to reach easily, lower it from the IV pole.* Activate the needle safety device.
- Remove the bag from the pole and gently rotate the bag. **Rationale:** *This will mix the medication and solution.*

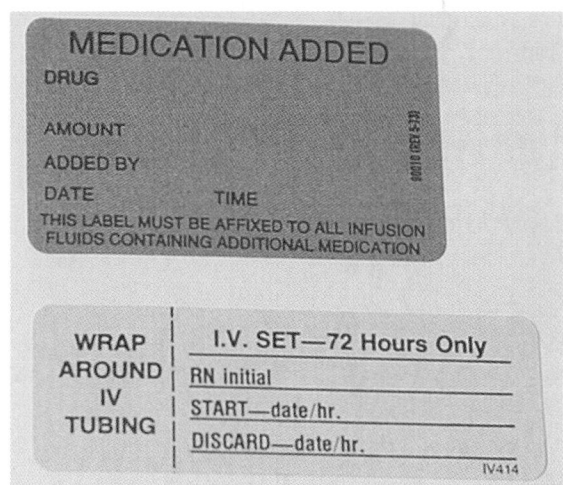

❸ *Top,* label indicating a medication added to an IV infusion; *Bottom,* label indicating time for IV tubing change.
Photographer: Elena Dorfman

- Rehang the container and regulate the flow rate. **Rationale:** *This establishes the correct flow rate.*
- Complete the medication label and apply to the IV container.
4. Dispose of the equipment and supplies according to agency practice. **Rationale:** *This prevents inadvertent injury to others and the spread of microorganisms.*
5. Document the medication(s) on the appropriate form in the client's record.

The nurse adds the medication to the infusing fluid container or before it is hung for infusion. In some hospitals, the pharmacist adds the medication to the IV container.

Intermittent Intravenous Infusions

An intermittent infusion is a method of administering a medication mixed in a small amount of IV solution, such as 50 or 100 mL (Figure 35-43 ■). The drug is administered at regular intervals, such as every 4 hours, with the drug being infused for a short period of time such as 30 to 60 minutes. Two commonly used additive or secondary IV setups are the **tandem** and the **piggyback.**

In a tandem setup, a second container is attached to the line of the first container at the lower, secondary port

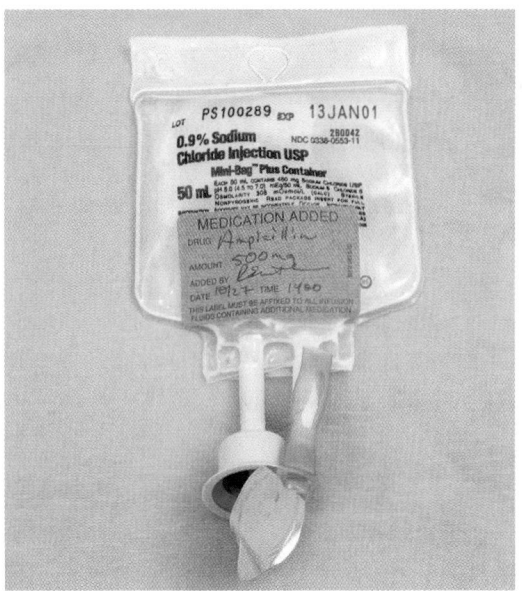

Figure 35-43 ■ Medication in a labeled infusion bag.

(Figure 35-44 ■, *A*). It permits medications to be administered intermittently or simultaneously with the primary solution.

In the piggyback alignment, a second set connects the second container to the tubing of the primary container at the upper port (Figure 35-44 ■, *B*). This setup is used solely for intermittent drug administration. Various manufacturers describe these sets differently, so the nurse must check the manufacturer's labeling and directions carefully. Traditionally the tubing of the secondary set has been attached to ports of the primary infusion by inserting a needle through the port and taping it in place. Needleless systems are now available. These needleless systems can use threaded-lock or lever-lock cannulae to connect the secondary set to the ports of the primary infusion (Figure 35-45 ■). This design prevents needlestick injuries and also prevents touch contamination at the IV connection site.

Another method of intermittently administering an IV medication is by a syringe pump or mini-infuser. The medication is mixed in a syringe that is connected to the primary IV line via a mini-infuser (see Figure 35-46 ■).

Figure 35-44 ■ Secondary intravenous lines: *A,* a tandem intravenous alignment; *B,* an intravenous piggyback (IVPB) alignment.

Figure 35-45 ■ Needleless cannulae used to connect the tubing of secondary sets to primary infusions: *A,* threaded-lock cannula; *B,* lever-lock cannula.

(photo a) Photograph reprinted courtesy of (BD) Becton, Dickinson and Company and courtesy of Baxter Healthcare Corporation. All rights reserved. (photo b) Photograph reprinted courtesy of (BD) Becton, Dickinson and Company and courtesy of Baxter Healthcare Corporation. All rights reserved

Figure 35-46 ■ Syringe pump or mini-infuser for administration of IV medications.

Volume-Control Infusions

Intermittent medications may also be administered by a **volume-control infusion set** such as Buretrol, Soluset, Volutrol, and Pediatrol (Figure 35-47 ■). They are small fluid containers (100 to 150 mL in size) attached below the primary infusion container so that the medication is administered through the client's IV line. Volume-control sets are frequently used to infuse solutions into children and older clients when the volume administered is critical and must be carefully monitored. Box 35–7 provides additional information.

Intravenous Push

Intravenous push (IVP) (bolus) is the intravenous administration of an undiluted drug directly into the systemic circulation. It is used when a medication cannot be diluted or in an emergency. An IV bolus can be introduced directly into a vein by venipuncture or into an existing IV line through an injection port or through an IV lock.

There are two major disadvantages to this method of drug administration: Any error in administration cannot be corrected after the drug has entered the client, and the drug may be irritating to the lining of the blood vessels. Before administering a bolus, the nurse should look up the maximum concentration recommended for the particular drug and the rate of administration. The administered medication takes effect immediately (see Skill 35-9).

Figure 35-47 ■ A volume-control infusion set.

BOX 35–7	**Adding a Medication to a Volume-Control Infusion Set**

- Withdraw the required dose of the medication into a syringe.
- Ensure that there is sufficient fluid in the volume-control fluid chamber to dilute the medication. Generally, at least 50 mL of fluid is used. Check the directions from the drug manufacturer or consult the pharmacist.
- Close the inflow to the fluid chamber by adjusting the upper roller or slide clamp above the fluid chamber; also ensure that the clamp on the air vent of the chamber is open.

- Clean the medication port on the volume-control fluid chamber with an antiseptic swab.
- Inject the medication into the port of the partially filled volume-control set.
- Gently rotate the fluid chamber until the fluid is well mixed.
- Open the line's upper clamp, and regulate the flow by adjusting the lower roller or slide clamp below the fluid chamber.
- Attach a medication label to the volume-control fluid chamber.
- Document relevant data, and monitor the client and the infusion.

Intermittent Infusion Devices

Intermittent infusion devices (Figure 35-48 ■) may be affixed to an intravenous catheter or needle to allow medications to be administered intravenously without requiring repeated needle-sticks or a continuous intravenous infusion.

Intermittent injection ports have either a resealable latex injection site for needle access or a port that allows a syringe or a needleless adapter to be connected for administering medications. Needleless systems are preferred, because they significantly reduce the risk of needlestick injuries among health care workers. Skill 52-5 in Chapter 52 ∞ describes how to convert an intravenous infusion to an intermittent injection port. With the needleless system, the injection adapter may be attached at the time of intravenous catheter placement, allowing a closed system to be maintained.

Intermittent injection ports may be flushed with sterile saline prior to and after medication. Most agencies use saline flushes with medication administration through peripheral IV lines. When administering a medication through a central venous access devices (CVAD), some agencies use the SASH (saline–adminster drug–saline–heparin) flushing procedure (Bunce, 2003). Flushing the port maintains patency of the intravenous catheter and port, and reduces the risks of mixing incompatible medications within the system (see Skill 35-9).

Clients who require long-term venous access for administering medications (e.g., people receiving chemotherapy for can-

Figure 35-48 ■ Intermittent infusion device with injection port.

cer treatment) may have a specialized catheter or port to allow central venous access. The catheter may be tunneled subcutaneously and accessed through an intermittent injection port attached to the distal end of the venous catheter. Other devices have an implantable port or vascular access port surgically inserted under the skin so that no portion of the device exits the body. To administer medications, the port is accessed using a specialized needle through the skin. See Chapter 52 ∞ for more information about central venous lines.

SKILL 35-9

ADMINISTERING INTRAVENOUS MEDICATIONS USING IV PUSH

PURPOSE
- To achieve immediate and maximum effects of a medication

ASSESSMENT
- Inspect and palpate the IV insertion site for signs of infection, infiltration, or a dislocated catheter.
- Inspect the surrounding skin for redness, pallor, or swelling.
- Palpate the surrounding tissues for coldness and the presence of edema, which could indicate leakage of the IV fluid into the tissues.

- Take vital signs for baseline data if the medication being administered is particularly potent.
- Determine if the client has allergies to the medication(s).
- Check the compatibility of the medication(s) and IV fluid.
- Determine specific drug action, side effects, normal dosage, recommended administration time, and peak action time.
- Check patency of IV.

ADMINISTERING INTRAVENOUS MEDICATIONS USING IV PUSH *continued*

PLANNING

Delegation

The administration of intravenous medication via IV push involves the application of nursing knowledge and critical thinking. This procedure is not delegated to UAP. The nurse, however, can inform the UAP of the intended therapeutic effects and/or specific side effects of the medication and direct the UAP to report specific client observations to the nurse for follow-up. *Note:* Administration of IV push medications varies by state nurse practice acts. For example, some states may allow the RN to delegate certain medications to be given by an LPN/LVN while other states may allow only the RN to administer IV push medications. The nurse needs to know his or her scope of practice according to the state's nurse practice act and agency policies.

Equipment
IV Push for an Existing Line

- Medication in a vial or ampule
- Sterile syringe (3 to 5 mL) (to prepare the medication)

- Sterile needles #21 to #25 gauge, 2.5 cm (1 in.) (needle not needed if using a needleless system)
- Antiseptic swabs
- Watch with a digital readout or second hand
- Clean gloves

IV Push for an IV Lock

- Medication in a vial or ampule
- Sterile syringe (3 to 5 mL) (to prepare the medication)
- Sterile syringe (3 mL) (for the saline or heparin flush)
- Vial of normal saline to flush the IV catheter or vial of heparin flush solution or both depending on agency practice. **Rationale:** *These maintain the patency of the IV lock. Saline is frequently used for peripheral locks.*
- Sterile needles (#21 gauge) (needle not needed if using a needleless system)
- Antiseptic swabs
- Watch with a digital readout or second hand
- Disposable gloves

IMPLEMENTATION
Preparation

1. Check the medication administration record (MAR).
   - Check the label on the medication carefully against the MAR to make sure that the correct medication is being prepared.
   - Follow the three checks for correct medication and dose. Read the label on the medication (1) when it is taken from the medication cart, (2) before withdrawing the medication, and (3) after withdrawing the medication.
   - Calculate medication dosage accurately.
   - Confirm that the route is correct.
2. Organize the equipment.

Performance

1. Perform hand hygiene and observe other appropriate infection control procedures.
2. Prepare the medication.

   Existing Line
   - Prepare the medication according to the manufacturer's direction. **Rationale:** *It is important to have the correct dose and the correct dilution.*

   IV Lock
   a. Flushing with saline
      - Prepare two syringes, each with 1 mL of sterile normal saline.
   b. Flushing with heparin (if indicated by agency policy) and saline
      - Prepare one syringe with 1 mL of heparin flush solution (if indicated by agency policy).
      - Prepare two syringes with 1 mL each of sterile, normal saline.
      - Draw up the medication into a syringe.

3. Put a small-gauge needle on the syringe if using a needle system.
4. Perform hand hygiene and put on clean gloves. **Rationale:** *This reduces the transmission of microorganisms and reduces the likelihood of the nurse's hands contacting the client's blood.*
5. Provide for client privacy.
6. Prepare the client.
   - Prior to performing the procedure, introduce self and verify the client's identity using agency protocol. **Rationale:** *This ensures that the right client receives the medication.*
   - If not previously assessed, take the appropriate assessment measures necessary for the medication. If any of the findings are above or below the predetermined parameters, consult the primary care provider before administering the medication.
7. Explain the purpose of the medication and how it will help, using language that the client can understand. Include relevant information about the effects of the medication.
8. Administer the medication by IV push. Bunce (2003) reported that the use of the "push-stop-push-stop" technique is helpful, especially for central venous catheters. **Rationale:** *This creates a turbulence in the flow through the catheter which reduces the residue buildup in the line and the potential for occlusion.*

   IV Lock with Needle
   - Clean the diaphragm with the antiseptic swab. **Rationale:** *This prevents microorganisms from entering the circulatory system during the needle insertion.*
   - Insert the needle of the syringe containing normal saline through the center of the diaphragm and aspirate for blood. **Rationale:** *The presence of blood confirms that the catheter*

continued on page 884

ADMINISTERING INTRAVENOUS MEDICATIONS USING IV PUSH *continued*

❶ Inserting a needle through the diaphragm of an IV lock.

❷ A blunt plastic cannula replaces the sharp steel needle.
(Photograph reprinted courtesy of (BD) Becton, Dickinson and Company.)

or needle is in the vein. In some situations, blood will not return even though the lock is patent. ❶

- Flush the lock by injecting 1 mL of saline slowly. **Rationale:** *This removes blood and heparin (if present) from the needle and the lock.*
- Remove the needle and syringe. Activate the needle safety device.
- Clean the lock's diaphragm with an antiseptic swab. **Rationale:** *This prevents the transfer of microorganisms.*
- Insert the needle of the syringe containing the prepared medication through the center of the diaphragm.
- Inject the medication slowly at the recommended rate of infusion. Use a watch or digital readout to time the injection. Observe the client closely for adverse reactions. Remove the needle and syringe when all medication is administered. **Rationale:** *Injecting the drug too rapidly can have a serious untoward reaction.*
- Activate the needle safety device.
- Clean the diaphragm of the lock.
- Attach the second saline syringe, and inject 1 mL of saline. **Rationale:** *The saline injection flushes the medication through the catheter and prepares the lock for heparin if this medication is used. Heparin is incompatible with many medications.*
- If heparin is to be used, insert the heparin syringe and inject the heparin slowly into the lock.

IV Lock with Needleless System
- Remove the protective cap from the needleless port.
- Insert syringe containing normal saline into the lock.
- Flush the lock with 1 mL of sterile saline. **Rationale:** *This clears the lock of blood.*
- Remove the syringe.
- Insert the syringe containing the medication into the valve. ❷
- Inject the medication following the precautions described previously.
- Withdraw the syringe.
- Repeat injection of 1 mL of saline.
- Place a new sterile cap over the lock.

Existing Line
- Identify the injection port closest to the client. Some ports have a circle indicating the site for the needle insertion. **Rationale:** *An injection port must be used because it is self-sealing. Any puncture to the plastic tubing will leak.*
- Clean the port with an antiseptic swab.
- Stop the IV flow by closing the clamp or pinching the tubing above the injection port.
- Connect the syringe to the IV system.
  a. Needle system
    - Hold the port steady.
    - Insert the needle of the syringe that contains the medication through the center of the port. **Rationale:** *This prevents damage to the IV line and to the diaphragm of the port.* ❸
  b. Needleless system
    - Remove the cap from the needleless injection port. Connect the tip of the syringe directly to the port. ❹
    - Inject the medication at the ordered rate. Use the watch or digital readout to time the medication administration. **Rationale:** *This ensures safe drug administration because a too rapid injection could be dangerous.*

❸ Injecting a medication by IV push to an existing IV using a needle system.

ADMINISTERING INTRAVENOUS MEDICATIONS USING IV PUSH *continued*

❹ Injecting a medication by IV push to an existing IV using a needleless system.

Photographer: Jenny Thomas

- Release the clamp or tubing.
- After injecting the medication, withdraw the needle and activate the needle safety device. For a needleless system, detach the syringe and attach a new sterile cap to the port.
9. Dispose of equipment according to agency practice. **Rationale:** *This reduces needlestick injuries and spread of microorganisms.*
10. Remove and dispose of gloves. Perform hand hygiene.
11. Observe the client closely for adverse reactions.
12. Determine agency practice about recommended times for changing the IV lock. Some agencies advocate a change every 48 to 72 hours for peripheral IV devices.
13. Document all relevant information.
    - Record the date, time, drug, dose, and route; client response; and assessments of infusion or heparin lock site if appropriate.

EVALUATION

- Conduct appropriate follow-up such as desired effect of medication, any adverse reactions or side effects, or change in vital signs.
- Reassess status of IV lock site and patency of IV infusion, if running.
- Relate to previous findings, if available.
- Report significant deviations from normal to the primary care provider.

HOME CARE CONSIDERATIONS   Administering IV Push Antibiotics

Shortened hospital stays and the need to cut costs have led to clients or their caregivers being taught to administer IV push antibiotics at home. The antibiotic is delivered IV push directly into a venous access device with pre- and post-administration flushing.

The nurse must

- Know which antibiotics are unsuitable for IV push administration.
- Know the adverse side effects:
  - Phlebitis (pain and tenderness over the vein, erythema, swelling, and warmth)
  - Speed shock (systemic reaction when a drug is given too rapidly)
  - Venous spasm (cramping and pain above infusion site)
  - Infiltration

- Assess caregiver or client's eyesight and manual dexterity. Both are needed for safe administration of the antibiotic.
- Provide thorough teaching about:
  - Venous access device
  - Administration rate (minutes/dose)
  - Schedule for medication administration
  - Flushing technique
  - Adverse reactions
  - Signs that indicate an emergency and the need to call 911
  - Proper storage of medication
- Inspect appearance of medication and check expiration date.

Topical Medications

A topical medication is applied locally to the skin or to mucous membranes in areas such as the eye, external ear canal, nose, vagina, and rectum. Most topical applications used therapeutically are not absorbed well, completely, or predictably when applied to intact skin because the skin's thick outer layer serves as a natural barrier to drug diffusion. This route of absorption through the skin, called **percutaneous,** can be increased if the skin is altered by a laceration, burn, or some other problem. However, if high concentrations or large amounts of a topical medication are applied to the skin, especially if it is done repeat-

edly, sufficient amounts of the drug can enter the bloodstream to cause systemic effects, usually undesirable ones.

A particular type of topical or dermatologic medication delivery system is the **transdermal patch.** This system administers sustained-action medications (e.g., nitroglycerin, estrogen, and nicotine) via multilayered films containing the drug and an adhesive layer. The rate of delivery of the drug is controlled and varies with each product (e.g., from 12 hours to 1 week). Generally, the patch is applied to a hairless, clean area of skin that is not subject to excessive movement or wrinkling (i.e., the trunk or lower abdomen). It may also be applied on the side, lower back, or buttocks. Patches should not be applied to areas with

A   **B**

Figure 35-49 ■ Transdermal patch administration: *A,* protective coating removed from patch; *B,* patch immediately applied to clean, dry, hairless skin and labeled with date, time, and initials.

Source: From *Pharmacology for Nurses* (p. 38), by Adams, Josephson, & Holland, 2005, Upper Saddle River, NJ: Pearson Education.

cuts, burns, or abrasions, or on distal parts of extremities (e.g., the forearms). If hair is likely to interfere with patch adhesion or removal, clipping (not shaving) may be necessary before application (Figure 35-49 ■).

CLINICAL ALERT

It is important to keep track of the transdermal patches. Some patches are clear and may be difficult to see and, as a result, be overlooked. If the client is obese, patches may be difficult to find in the skin folds. Duplication of patches may cause adverse reactions. Remove the old patch before applying a new one. ■

Reddening of the skin with or without mild local itching or burning, as well as allergic contact dermatitis, may occasionally occur. Upon removal of the patch, any slight reddening of the skin usually disappears within a few hours. All applications should be changed regularly to prevent local irritation, and each successive application should be placed on a different site. All clients need to be assessed for allergies to the drug and to materials in the patch before the patch is applied. If a client has a transdermal patch on and develops a fever, the medication may be absorbed and metabolize at a faster rate than normal. The client will need to be monitored for changes in effects of the medication.

When transdermal patches are removed, care needs to be taken as to how and where they are discarded. In the home environment, if they are simply discarded into a trash can, pets or children can be exposed to them, causing effects from any drug remaining on the patch. When removed, they should be folded with the medication side to the inside, put into a closed container, and kept out of reach of children and pets.

CLINICAL ALERT

The nurse should wear gloves when applying a transdermal patch to avoid getting any of the medication on his or her skin, which can result in the nurse receiving the effect of the medication. ■

Skin Applications

Topical skin or dermatologic preparations include ointments, pastes, creams, lotions, powders, sprays, and patches. See Table 35–1 earlier in this chapter. See Practice Guidelines for applying topical medications. Before applying a dermatologic preparation, thoroughly clean the area with soap and water and dry it with a patting motion. Skin encrustations harbor microorganisms and these as well as previously applied applications can prevent the medication from coming in contact with the area to be treated. Nurses should wear gloves when administering skin applications and always use surgical asepsis when an open wound is present.

Ophthalmic Medications

Medications may be administered to the eye using irrigations or instillations. An eye irrigation is administered to wash out the conjunctival sac to remove secretions or foreign bodies or to remove chemicals that may injure the eye. Medications for the eyes, called **ophthalmic** medications, are instilled in the form of liquids or ointments. Eyedrops are packaged in monodrip plastic containers that are used to administer the preparation. Ointments are usually supplied in small tubes. All containers must state that the medication is for ophthalmic use. Sterile preparations and sterile technique are indicated. Prescribed liquids are usually dilute, for example, less than 1% strength.

Skill 35-10 illustrates how to administer ophthalmic instillations.

MediaLink   Preparing Medications Case Study

PRACTICE GUIDELINES   Applying Skin Preparations

POWDER
Make sure the skin surface is dry. Spread apart any skin folds, and sprinkle the site until the area is covered with a fine *thin* layer. Cover the site with a dressing if ordered.

SUSPENSION-BASED LOTION
Shake the container before use to distribute suspended particles. Put a little lotion on a small gauze dressing or pad, and apply the lotion to the skin by stroking it evenly in the direction of the hair growth.

CREAMS, OINTMENTS, PASTES, AND OIL-BASED LOTIONS
Warm and soften the preparation in gloved hands to make it easier to apply and to prevent chilling (if a large area is to be treated). Smear it evenly over the skin using long strokes that follow the direction of the hair growth. Explain that the skin may feel somewhat greasy after application. Apply a sterile dressing if ordered by the primary care provider.

AEROSOL SPRAY
Shake the container well to mix the contents. Hold the spray container at the recommended distance from the area (usually about 15 to 30 cm [6 to 12 inches] but check the label). Cover the client's face with a towel if the upper chest or neck is to be sprayed. Spray the medication over the specified area.

TRANSDERMAL PATCHES
Select a clean, dry area that is free of hair and matches the manufacturer's recommendations. Remove the patch from its protective covering, holding it without touching the adhesive edges, and apply it by pressing firmly with the palm of the hand for about 10 seconds. Advise the client to avoid using a heating pad over the area to prevent an increase in circulation and the rate of absorption. Remove the patch at the appropriate time, folding the medicated side to the inside so it is covered.

ADMINISTERING OPHTHALMIC INSTILLATIONS

SKILL 35-10

PURPOSE
■ To provide an eye medication the client requires (e.g., an antibiotic) to treat an infection or for other reasons (see specific drug action)

ASSESSMENT
In addition to the assessment performed by the nurse related to the administration of any medication, prior to applying ophthalmic medications, assess:

■ Appearance of eye and surrounding structures for lesions, exudate, erythema, or swelling
■ The location and nature of any discharge, lacrimation, and swelling of the eyelids or of the lacrimal gland

■ Client complaints (e.g., itching, burning pain, blurred vision, and photophobia)
■ Client behavior (e.g., squinting, blinking excessively, frowning, or rubbing the eyes)

Determine if assessment data influence administration of the medication (i.e., is it appropriate to administer the medication or does the medication need to be held and the primary care provider notified?).

PLANNING

Delegation
Due to the need for assessment, interpretation of client status, and use of sterile technique, ophthalmic medication administration is not delegated to UAP.

Equipment
■ Clean gloves
■ Sterile absorbent sponges soaked in sterile normal saline

■ Medication
■ Sterile eye dressing (pad) as needed and paper tape to secure it
For irrigation, add:
■ Irrigating solution (e.g., normal saline) and irrigating syringe or tubing
■ Dry sterile absorbent sponges
■ Moisture-resistant towel
■ Basin (e.g., emesis basin)

IMPLEMENTATION
Preparation
1. Check the medication administration record (MAR).
   ● Check the MAR for the drug name, dose, and strength. Also confirm the prescribed frequency of the instillation and which eye is to be treated.
   ● If the MAR is unclear or pertinent information is missing, compare it with the most recent primary care provider's written order.
   ● Report any discrepancies to the charge nurse or physician, as agency policy dictates.

2. Know the reason why the client is receiving the medication, the drug classification, contraindications, usual dose range, side effects, and nursing considerations for administering and evaluating the intended outcomes of the medication.

Performance
1. Compare the label on the medication tube or bottle with the medication record and check the expiration date.
2. If necessary, calculate the medication dosage.
3. Introduce self and explain to the client what you are going to do, why it is necessary, and how he or she can cooperate. The administration of an ophthalmic medication is not usually

continued on page 888

SKILL 35-10

ADMINISTERING OPHTHALMIC INSTILLATIONS *continued*

painful. Ointments are often soothing to the eye, but some liquid preparations may sting initially. Discuss how the results will be used in planning further care or treatments.

4. Perform hand hygiene and observe appropriate infection control procedures.
5. Provide for client privacy.
6. Prepare the client.
   - Prior to performing the procedure, verify the client's identity using agency protocol. **Rationale:** *This ensures that the right client receives the medication.*
   - Assist the client to a comfortable position, either sitting or lying.
7. Clean the eyelid and the eyelashes.
   - Put on clean gloves.
   - Use sterile cotton balls moistened with sterile irrigating solution or sterile normal saline, and wipe from the inner canthus to the outer canthus. **Rationale:** *If not removed, material on the eyelid and lashes can be washed into the eye. Cleaning toward the outer canthus prevents contamination of the other eye and the lacrimal duct.*
8. Administer the eye medication.
   - Check the ophthalmic preparation for the name, strength, and number of drops if a liquid is used. **Rationale:** *Checking medication data is essential to prevent a medication error.* Draw the correct number of drops into the shaft of the dropper if a dropper is used. If ointment is used, discard the first bead. **Rationale:** *The first bead of ointment from a tube is considered to be contaminated.*
   - Instruct the client to look up to the ceiling. Give the client a dry sterile absorbent sponge. **Rationale:** *The person is less likely to blink if looking up. While the client looks up, the cornea is partially protected by the upper eyelid. A sponge is needed to press on the nasolacrimal duct after a liquid instillation to prevent systemic absorption or to wipe excess ointment from the eyelashes after an ointment is instilled.*
   - Expose the lower conjunctival sac by placing the thumb or fingers of your nondominant hand on the client's cheekbone just below the eye and gently drawing down the skin on the cheek. If the tissues are edematous, handle the tissues carefully to avoid damaging them. **Rationale:** *Placing the fingers on the cheekbone minimizes the possibility of touching the cornea, avoids putting any pressure on the eyeball, and prevents the person from blinking or squinting.*
   - Holding the medication in the dominant hand, place hand on client's forehead to stabilize hand. Approach the eye from the side and instill the correct number of drops onto the outer third of the lower conjunctival sac. Hold the dropper 1 to 2 cm (0.4 to 0.8 in.) above the sac. ❶ **Rationale:** *The client is less likely to blink if a side approach is used. When instilled into the conjunctival sac, drops will not harm the cornea as they might if dropped directly on it. The dropper must not touch the sac or the cornea.*
   or
   - Holding the tube above the lower conjunctival sac, squeeze 2 cm (0.8 in.) of ointment from the tube into the lower conjunctival sac from the inner canthus outward. ❷
   - Instruct the client to close the eyelids but not to squeeze them shut. **Rationale:** *Closing the eye spreads the medica-*

❶ Instilling an eyedrop into the lower conjunctival sac.

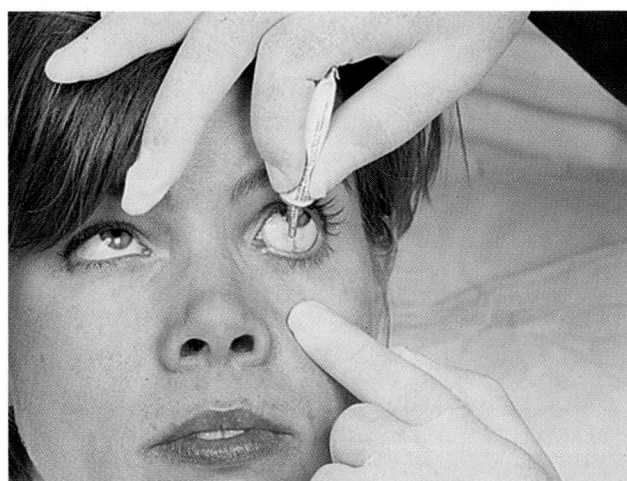

❷ Instilling an eye ointment into the lower conjunctival sac.
Photographer: Jenny Thomas

❸ Pressing on the nasolacrimal duct.
Photographer: Jenny Thomas

SKILL 35-10

ADMINISTERING OPHTHALMIC INSTILLATIONS *continued*

tion over the eyeball. *Squeezing can injure the eye and push out the medication.*
- For liquid medications, press firmly or have the client press firmly on the nasolacrimal duct for at least 30 seconds. **Rationale:** *Pressing on the nasolacrimal duct prevents the medication from running out of the eye and down the duct, preventing systemic absorption* ❸

Variation: Irrigation
- Place absorbent pads under the head, neck, and shoulders. Place an emesis basin next to the eye to catch drainage. Some eye medications cause systemic reactions such as confusion or a decrease in heart rate and blood pressure if the eyedrops go down the nasolacrimal duct and get into the systemic circulation.
- Expose the lower conjunctival sac. Or, to irrigate in stages, first hold the lower lid down, then hold the upper lid up. Exert pressure on the bony prominences of the cheekbone and beneath the eyebrow when holding the eyelids. **Rationale:** *Separating the lids prevents reflex blinking. Exerting pressure on the bony prominences minimizes the possibility of pressing the eyeball and causing discomfort.*

- Fill and hold the eye irrigator about 2.5 cm (1 in.) above the eye. **Rationale:** *At this height the pressure of the solution will not damage the eye tissue, and the irrigator will not touch the eye.*
- Irrigate the eye, directing the solution onto the lower conjunctival sac and from the inner canthus to the outer canthus. **Rationale:** *Directing the solution in this way prevents possible injury to the cornea and prevents fluid and contaminants from flowing down the nasolacrimal duct.*
- Irrigate until the solution leaving the eye is clear (no discharge is present) or until all the solution has been used.
- Instruct the client to close and move the eye periodically. **Rationale:** *Eye closure and movement help to move secretions from the upper to the lower conjunctival sac.*
9. Clean and dry the eyelids as needed. Wipe the eyelids gently from the inner to the outer canthus to collect excess medication.
10. Apply an eye pad if needed, and secure it with paper eye tape.
11. Assess the client's response immediately after the instillation or irrigation and again after the medication should have acted.
12. Document all relevant assessments and interventions. Include the name of the drug or irrigating solution, the strength, the number of drops if a liquid medication, the time, and the response of the client.

EVALUATION
- Perform follow-up based on findings of the effectiveness of the administration or outcomes that deviated from expected or normal for the client. Relate findings to previous data if available.
- Report significant deviations from normal to the primary care provider.

LIFESPAN CONSIDERATIONS Administering Ophthalmic Medications

INFANTS/CHILDREN
- Explain the technique to the parents of an infant or child.
- For a young child or infant, obtain assistance to immobilize the arms and head. The parent may hold the infant or young child. *This prevents accidental injury during medication administration.*
- For a young child, use a doll to demonstrate the procedure. *This facilitates cooperation and decreases anxiety.*
- Drops may be tolerated better by children than ointment since they are less likely to cause blurred vision.
- An intravenous (IV) bag and tubing may be used to deliver irrigating fluid to the eye (Figure 35-50 ■).

Figure 35-50 ■ Eye irrigation using IV tubing.

Otic Medications

Instillations or irrigations of the external auditory canal are referred to as **otic** and are generally carried out for cleaning purposes. Sometimes applications of heat and antiseptic solutions are prescribed. Irrigations performed in a hospital require aseptic technique so that microorganisms will not be introduced into the ear. Sterile technique is used if the eardrum is perforated. The position of the external auditory canal varies with age. In the child under 3 years of age, it is directed upward. In the adult, the external auditory canal is an S-shaped structure about 2.5 cm (1 inch) long.

Skill 35-11 explains how to administer otic instillations.

ADMINISTERING OTIC INSTILLATIONS

PURPOSE
- To soften earwax so that it can be readily removed at a later time
- To provide local therapy to reduce inflammation, destroy infective organisms in the external ear canal, or both
- To relieve pain

ASSESSMENT
In addition to the assessment performed by the nurse related to the administration of any medications, prior to applying otic medications, assess:

- Appearance of the pinna of the ear and meatus for signs of redness and abrasions
- Type and amount of any discharge

Determine if assessment data influence administration of the medication (i.e., is it appropriate to administer the medication or does the medication need to be held and the primary care provider notifed?)

PLANNING

> ### Delegation
> Due to the need for assessment, interpretation of client status, and use of sterile technique, otic medication administration is not delegated to UAP.

Equipment
- Clean gloves
- Cotton-tipped applicator
- Correct medication bottle with a dropper
- Flexible rubber tip (optional) for the end of the dropper, which prevents injury from sudden motion, for example, by a disoriented client
- Cotton fluff

For irrigation, add:

- Moisture-resistant towel
- Basin (e.g., emesis basin)
- Irrigating solution at the appropriate temperature, about 500 mL (16 oz) or as ordered
- Container for the irrigating solution
- Syringe (rubber bulb or Asepto syringe is frequently used)

IMPLEMENTATION
Preparation
1. Check the medication administration record (MAR).
   - Check the MAR for the drug name, strength, number of drops, and prescribed frequency.
   - If the MAR is unclear or pertinent information is missing, compare it with the most recent primary care provider's written order.
   - Report any discrepancies to the charge nurse or physician, as agency policy dictates.
2. Know the reason why the client is receiving the medication, the drug classification, contraindications, usual dose range, side effects, and nursing considerations for administering and evaluating the intended outcomes of the medication.

Performance
1. Compare the label on the medication container with the medication record and check the expiration date.
2. If necessary, calculate the medication dosage.
3. Explain to the client what you are going to do, why it is necessary, and how he or she can cooperate. The administration of an otic medication is not usually painful. Discuss how the results will be used in planning further care or treatments.
4. Perform hand hygiene and observe appropriate infection control procedures.
5. Provide for client privacy.
6. Prepare the client.
   - Prior to performing the procedure, introduce self and verify the client's identity using agency protocol. **Rationale:** *This ensures that the right client receives the medication.*
   - Assist the client to a comfortable position for eardrops, lying with the ear being treated uppermost.

7. Clean the pinna of the ear and the meatus of the ear canal.
   - Put on gloves if infection is suspected.
   - Use cotton-tipped applicators and solution to wipe the pinna and auditory meatus. **Rationale:** *This removes any discharge present before the instillation so that it won't be washed into the ear canal.*
8. Administer the ear medication.
   - Warm the medication container in your hand, or place it in warm water for a short time. **Rationale:** *This promotes client comfort.*
   - Partially fill the ear dropper with medication.
   - Straighten the auditory canal. Pull the pinna upward and backward for clients over 3 years of age. **Rationale:** *The auditory canal is straightened so that the solution can flow the entire length of the canal.* ❶
   - Instill the correct number of drops along the side of the ear canal. ❷

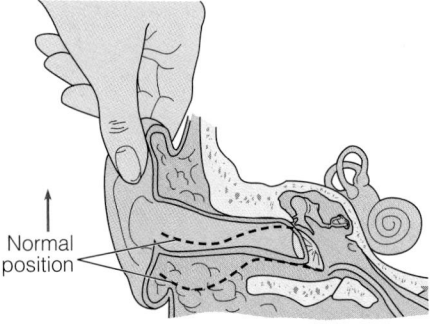

❶ Straightening the adult ear canal by pulling pinna upward and backward.

ADMINISTERING OTIC INSTILLATIONS *continued*

❷ Instilling eardrops.

Photographer: Jenny Thomas

❸ Ear irrigation.

(Patrick Watson)

- Press gently but firmly a few times on the tragus of the ear (the cartilaginous projection in front of the exterior meatus of the ear). **Rationale:** *Pressing on the tragus assists the flow of medication into the ear canal.*
- Ask the client to remain in the side-lying position for about 5 minutes. **Rationale:** *This prevents the drops from escaping and allows the medication to reach all sides of the canal cavity.*
- Insert a small piece of cotton fluff loosely at the meatus of the auditory canal for 15 to 20 minutes. Do not press it into the canal. **Rationale:** *The cotton helps retain the medication when the client is up. If pressed tightly into the canal, the cotton would interfere with the action of the drug and the outward movement of normal secretions.*

Variation: Ear Irrigation
- Explain that the client may experience a feeling of fullness, warmth, and, occasionally, discomfort when the fluid comes in contact with the tympanic membrane.
- Assist the client to a sitting or lying position with head tilted toward the affected ear. **Rationale:** *The solution can then flow from the ear canal to a basin.* ❸
- Place the moisture-resistant towel around the client's shoulder under the ear to be irrigated, and place the basin under the ear to be irrigated.
- Fill the syringe with solution.
     or

- Hang up the irrigating container, and run solution through the tubing and the nozzle. **Rationale:** *Solution is run through to remove air from the tubing and nozzle.*
- Straighten the ear canal.
- Insert the tip of the syringe into the auditory meatus, and direct the solution gently upward against the top of the canal. **Rationale:** *The solution will flow around the entire canal and out at the bottom. The solution is instilled gently because strong pressure from the fluid can cause discomfort and damage the tympanic membrane.*
- Continue instilling the fluid until all the solution is used or until the canal is cleaned, depending on the purpose of the irrigation. Take care not to block the outward flow of the solution with the syringe.
- Assist the client to a side-lying position on the affected side. **Rationale:** *Lying with the affected side down helps drain the excess fluid by gravity.*
- Place a cotton fluff in the auditory meatus to absorb the excess fluid.
9. Assess the client's response and the character and amount of discharge, appearance of the canal, discomfort, and so on, immediately after the instillation and again when the medication is expected to act. Inspect the cotton ball for any drainage.
10. Document all nursing assessments and interventions relative to the procedure. Include the name of the drug or irrigating solution, the strength, the number of drops if a liquid medication, the time, and the response of the client.

EVALUATION
- Perform follow-up based on findings of the effectiveness of the administration or outcomes that deviated from expected or normal for the client. Relate findings to previous data if available.
- Report significant deviations from normal to the primary care provider.

LIFESPAN CONSIDERATIONS **Administering Otic Medications**

INFANTS/CHILDREN

- Obtain assistance to immobilize an infant or young child. This prevents accidental injury due to sudden movement during the procedure.
- Because in infants and children under 3 years of age, the ear canal is directed upward, to administer medication, gently pull the pinna down and back (Figure 35-51 ■). For a child *older* than 3 years of age, pull the pinna upward and backward.

Figure 35-51 ■ Straightening the ear canal of a child by pulling the pinna down and back.

Nasal Medications

Nasal instillations (nose drops and sprays) usually are instilled for their astringent effect (to shrink swollen mucous membranes), to loosen secretions and facilitate drainage, or to treat infections of the nasal cavity or sinuses. Nasal decongestants are the most common nasal instillations. Many of these products are available without a prescription. Clients need to be taught to use these agents with caution. Chronic use of nasal decongestants may lead to a rebound effect, that is, an increase in nasal congestion. If excess decongestant solution is swallowed, serious systemic effects may also develop, especially in children. Saline drops are safer as a decongestant for children.

Usually clients self-administer sprays. In the supine position with the head tilted back, the client holds the tip of the container just inside the nares and inhales as the spray enters the nasal passages. For clients who use nasal sprays repeatedly, the nares need to be assessed for irritation. In children, nasal sprays are given with the head in an upright position to prevent excess spray from being swallowed.

Nasal drops may be used to treat sinus infections. Clients need to learn ways to position themselves to effectively treat the affected sinus:

- To treat the ethmoid and sphenoid sinuses, instruct the client to lie back with the head over the edge of the bed or a pillow under the shoulders so that the head is tipped backward (Figure 35-52 ■).
- To treat the maxillary and frontal sinuses, instruct the client to assume the same back-lying position, with the head turned toward the side to be treated (Figure 35-53 ■). The client should also be instructed to (a) breathe through the mouth to prevent aspiration of medication into the trachea and bronchi, (b) remain in a back-lying position for at least 1 minute so that the solution will come into contact with all of the nasal surface, and (c) avoid blowing the nose for several minutes.

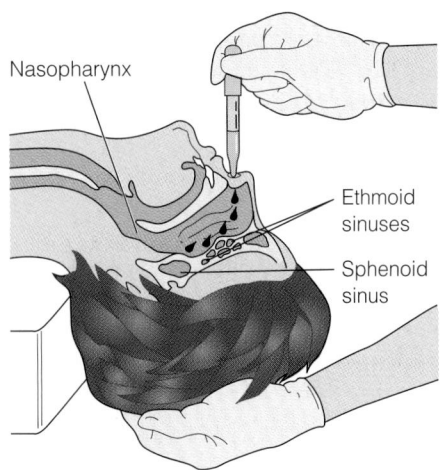

Nasopharynx

Ethmoid sinuses

Sphenoid sinus

Figure 35-52 ■ Position of the head to instill drops into the ethmoid and sphenoid sinuses.

Maxillary sinuses

Frontal sinuses

Figure 35-53 ■ Position of the head to instill drops into the maxillary and frontal sinuses.

Vaginal Medications

Vaginal medications, or instillations, are inserted as creams, jellies, foams, or suppositories to treat infection or to relieve vaginal discomfort (e.g., itching or pain). Medical aseptic technique is usually used. Vaginal creams, jellies, and foams are applied by using a tubular applicator with a plunger. Suppositories are inserted with the index finger of a gloved hand. Suppositories are designed to melt at body temperature, so they are generally stored in the refrigerator to keep them firm for insertion. See Skill 35-12 for administering vaginal instillations.

A vaginal irrigation (douche) is the washing of the vagina by a liquid at a low pressure. Vaginal irrigations are not necessary for ordinary female hygiene but are used to prevent infection by applying an antimicrobial solution that discourages the growth of microorganisms, to remove an offensive or irritating discharge, and to reduce inflammation or prevent hemorrhage by the application of heat or cold. In hospitals, sterile supplies and equipment are used; in a home, sterility is not usually necessary because people are accustomed to the microorganisms in their environments. Sterile technique, however, is indicated if there is an open wound.

ADMINISTERING VAGINAL INSTILLATIONS

SKILL 35-12

PURPOSE
- To treat or prevent infection
- To reduce inflammation
- To relieve vaginal discomfort

ASSESSMENT
In addition to the assessment performed by the nurse related to the administration of any medications, prior to applying vaginal medications, assess:

- The vaginal orifice for inflammation; amount, character, and odor of vaginal discharge
- For complaints of vaginal discomfort (e.g., burning or itching)

Determine if assessment data influence administration of the medication (i.e., is it appropriate to administer the medication or does the medication need to be held and the primary care provider notified?).

PLANNING

Delegation
Due to the need for assessments and interpretation of client status, vaginal medication administration is not delegated to UAP.

Equipment
- Drape
- Correct vaginal suppository or cream
- Applicator for vaginal cream

- Clean gloves
- Lubricant for a suppository
- Disposable towel
- Clean perineal pad

  For an irrigation, add:

- Moisture-proof pad
- Vaginal irrigation set (these are often disposable) containing a nozzle, tubing and a clamp, and a container for the solution
- Irrigating solution

IMPLEMENTATION
Preparation
1. Check the medication administration record (MAR).
   - Check the MAR for the drug name, strength, and prescribed frequency.
   - If the MAR is unclear or pertinent information is missing, compare it with the most recent primary care provider's written order.
   - Report any discrepancies to the charge nurse or primary care provider, as agency policy dictates.
2. Know the reason why the client is receiving the medication, the drug classification, contraindications, usual dose range, side effects, and nursing considerations for administering and evaluating the intended outcomes of the medication.

Performance
1. Compare the label on the medication container with the medication record and check the expiration date.
2. If necessary, calculate the medication dosage.
3. Explain to the client what you are going to do, why it is necessary, and how she can cooperate. Explain to the client that a

vaginal instillation is normally a painless procedure, and in fact may bring relief from itching and burning if an infection is present. Many people feel embarrassed about this procedure, and some may prefer to perform the procedure themselves if instruction is provided. Discuss how the results will be used in planning further care or treatments.
4. Perform hand hygiene and observe appropriate infection control procedures.
5. Provide for client privacy.
6. Prepare the client.
   - Prior to performing the procedure, introduce self and verify the client's identity using agency protocol. **Rationale:** *This ensures that the right client receives the medication.*
   - Ask the client to void. **Rationale:** *If the bladder is empty, the client will have less discomfort during the treatment, and the possibility of injuring the vaginal lining is decreased.*
   - Assist the client to a back-lying position with the knees flexed and the hips rotated laterally.
   - Drape the client appropriately so that only the perineal area is exposed.

continued on page 894

ADMINISTERING VAGINAL INSTILLATIONS *continued*

7. Prepare the equipment.
   - Unwrap the suppository, and put it on the opened wrapper.
     or
   - Fill the applicator with the prescribed cream, jelly, or foam. Directions are provided with the manufacturer's applicator.
8. Assess and clean the perineal area.
   - Put on gloves. **Rationale:** *Gloves prevent contamination of the nurse's hands from vaginal and perineal microorganisms.*
   - Inspect the vaginal orifice, note any odor of discharge from the vagina, and ask about any vaginal discomfort.
   - Provide perineal care to remove microorganisms. **Rationale:** *This decreases the chance of moving microorganisms into the vagina.*
9. Administer the vaginal suppository, cream, foam, jelly, or irrigation.

Suppository
- Lubricate the rounded (smooth) end of the suppository, which is inserted first. **Rationale:** *Lubrication facilitates insertion.*
- Lubricate your gloved index finger.
- Expose the vaginal orifice by separating the labia with your nondominant hand.
- Insert the suppository about 8 to 10 cm (3 to 4 in.) along the posterior wall of the vagina, or as far as it will go. **Rationale:** *The posterior wall of the vagina is about 2.5 cm (1 in.) longer than the anterior wall because the cervix protrudes into the uppermost portion of the anterior wall.* ❶
- Ask the client to remain lying in the supine position for 5 to 10 minutes following insertion. The hips may also be elevated on a pillow. **Rationale:** *This position allows the medication to flow into the posterior fornix after it has melted.*

Vaginal Cream, Jelly, or Foam
- Gently insert the applicator about 5 cm (2 in.).
- Slowly push the plunger until the applicator is empty. ❷
- Remove the applicator and place it on the towel. **Rationale:** *The applicator is put on the towel to prevent the spread of microorganisms.*
- Discard the applicator if disposable or clean it according to the manufacturer's directions.
- Ask the client to remain lying in the supine position for 5 to 10 minutes following the insertion.

Irrigation
- Place the client on a bedpan.
- Clamp the tubing. Hold the irrigating container about 30 cm (12 in.) above the vagina. **Rationale:** *At this height, the pressure of the solution should not be great enough to injure the vaginal lining.*
- Run fluid through the tubing and nozzle into the bedpan. **Rationale:** *Fluid is run through the tubing to remove air and to moisten the nozzle.*
- Insert the nozzle carefully into the vagina. Direct the nozzle toward the sacrum, following the direction of the vagina.

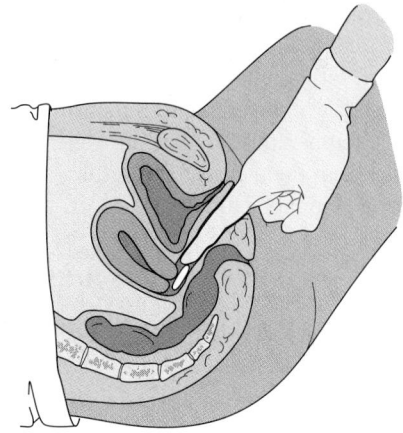

❶ Instilling a vaginal suppository.

❷ Using an applicator to instill a vaginal cream.

- Insert the nozzle about 7 to 10 cm (3 to 4 in.), start the flow, and rotate the nozzle several times. **Rationale:** *Rotating the nozzle irrigates all parts of the vagina.*
- Use all of the irrigating solution, permitting it to flow out freely into the bedpan.
- Remove the nozzle from the vagina.
- Assist the client to a sitting position on the bedpan. **Rationale:** *Sitting on the bedpan will help drain the remaining fluid by gravity.*
10. Ensure client comfort.
    - Dry the perineum with tissues as required.
    - Apply a clean perineal pad if there is excessive drainage.
11. Document all nursing assessments and interventions relative to the Skill. Include the name of the drug or irrigating solution, the strength, the time, and the response of the client.

EVALUATION
- Perform follow-up based on findings of the effectiveness of the administration or outcomes that deviated from expected or normal for the client. Relate findings to previous data if available.

- Report significant deviations from normal to the primary care provider.

Rectal Medications

Insertion of medications into the rectum in the form of suppositories is a frequent practice. Rectal administration is a convenient and safe method of giving certain medications. Advantages include the following:

- It avoids irritation of the upper gastrointestinal tract in clients who encounter this problem (e.g., in clients who are nauseated or vomiting).
- It is advantageous when the medication has an objectionable taste or odor.
- The drug is released at a slow but steady rate.
- Rectal suppositories are thought to provide higher bloodstream levels (titers) of medication because the venous blood from the lower rectum is not transported through the liver.

To insert a rectal suppository:

- Assist the client to a left lateral or left Sims' position, with the upper leg flexed.
- Fold back the top bedclothes to expose the buttocks.
- Put a glove on the hand used to insert the suppository.
- Unwrap the suppository and lubricate the smooth rounded end, or see the manufacturer's instructions. The rounded end is usually inserted first and lubricant reduces irritation of the mucosa.
- Lubricate the gloved index finger.
- Encourage the client to relax by breathing through the mouth. This usually relaxes the external anal sphincter.
- Insert the suppository gently into the anal canal, rounded end first (or according manufacturer's instructions), along the rectal wall using the gloved index finger. For an adult, insert the suppository beyond the internal sphincter (i.e., 10 cm [4 in.]) (see Figure 35-54 ■).
- Avoid embedding the suppository in feces in order for the suppository to be absorbed effectively.
- Press the client's buttocks together for a few minutes.
- Ask the client to remain in the left lateral or supine position for at least 5 minutes to help retain the suppository. The suppository should be retained for varying lengths of time according the manufacturer's instructions.

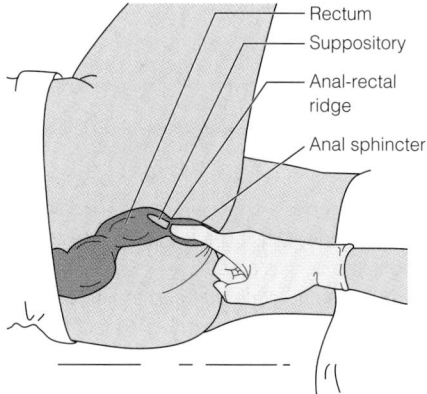

Figure 35-54 ■ Inserting a rectal suppository beyond the internal sphincter and along the rectal wall.

LIFESPAN CONSIDERATIONS
Administering Rectal Medications

INFANTS/CHILDREN

- Obtain assistance to immobilize an infant or young child. This prevents accidental injury due to sudden movement during the procedure.
- For a child under 3 years, the nurse should use the gloved fifth finger for insertion. After this age, the index finger can usually be used.
- For a child or infant, insert a suppository 5 cm (2 in.) or less.

RESPIRATORY INHALATION

Nebulizers deliver most medications administered through the inhaled route. A nebulizer is used to deliver a fine spray (fog or mist) of medication or moisture to a client. There are two kinds of nebulization: *atomization* and *aerosolization*. In atomization, a device called an *atomizer* produces rather large droplets for inhalation. In aerosolization, the droplets are suspended in a gas, such as oxygen. The smaller the droplets, the further they can be inhaled into the respiratory tract. When a medication is intended for the nasal mucosa, it is inhaled through the nose; when it is intended for the trachea, bronchi, and/or lungs, it is inhaled through the mouth.

A large-volume nebulizer can provide a heated or cool mist. It is used for long-term therapy, such as that following a tracheostomy. The ultrasonic nebulizer (Figure 35-55 ■) provides

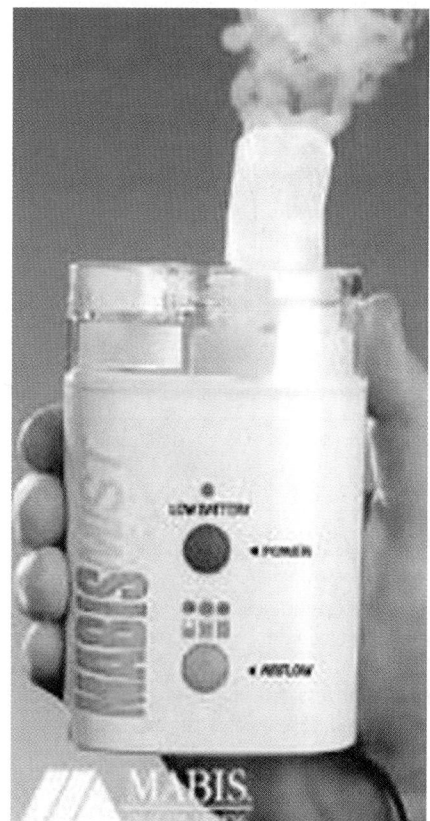

Figure 35-55 ■ Ultrasonic nebulizer.

(Courtesy of Mabis Healthcare, Inc.)

Figure 35-56 ■ Metered-dose inhaler.

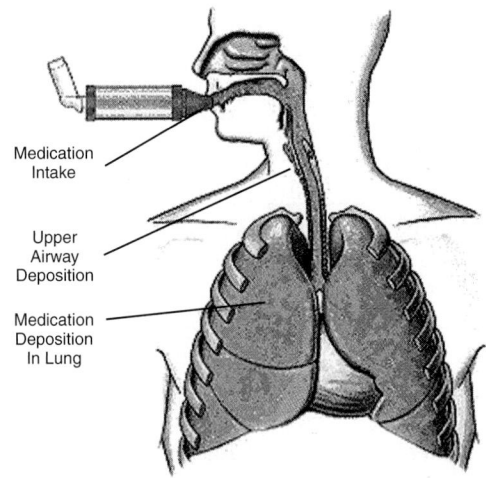

Figure 35-57 ■ Delivery of medication to the lungs using a metered-dose inhaler extender.
(Courtesy of Trudell Medical International.)

100% humidity and can provide particles small enough to be inhaled deeply into the respiratory tract.

The **metered-dose inhaler (MDI),** a handheld nebulizer (Figure 35-56 ■), is a pressurized container of medication that can be used by the client to release the medication through a nosepiece or mouthpiece. The force with which the air moves through the nebulizer causes the large particles of medicated solution to break up into finer particles, forming a mist or fine spray. According to Bower (2005), metered-dose inhalers can deliver accurate doses, provide for target action at the needed sites, and sustain less systemic effects than medication delivered by other routes.

To ensure correct delivery of the prescribed medication by MDIs, nurses need to instruct clients to use aerosol inhalers correctly. The client compresses the medication canister by hand to release medication through a mouthpiece. An extender or spacer may be attached to the mouthpiece to facilitate medication absorption for better results (Figure 35-57 ■). Spacers are holding chambers into which the medication is fired and from which the client inhales, so that the dose is not lost by exhalation. The Client Teaching feature provides instructions for clients about using an MDI. Newer breath-activated MDIs are being produced in which inhalation triggers the release of a premeasured dose of medication.

CLINICAL ALERT

It is important for the nurse to assess if the client is using the MDI correctly. A client's ability to use an MDI correctly can decrease over time. ■

LIFESPAN CONSIDERATIONS   **Administering Metered-Dose Inhalers and Nebulizers**

CHILDREN

■ Spacers hold a medication in suspension and provide the child an opportunity to take several deep breaths in order to inhale all the medication.

■ A mask is used for nebulizer treatments, allowing the child to breathe naturally. Some infants and children may be frightened or uncomfortable with the mask and become resistant. Use a doll or stuffed animal to demonstrate its use, and allow them to play with the equipment before putting it in place. Having the child sit in the parent's lap during the procedure can help the child relax and be more cooperative.

HOME CARE CONSIDERATIONS   **Metered-Dose Inhalers**

■ Disinfect the metered-dose inhaler mouthpieces weekly by soaking for 20 minutes in one pint of water with 2 ounces of vinegar added.

■ Teach clients how to determine the amount of medication remaining in a metered-dose inhaler canister:
  • Calculate the number of days' doses in a canister. Divide the number of doses (puffs) in the canister (on the label) by the number of puffs taken per day (Bower, 2005). The previous method of floating the canister in water is not considered accurate because some of the propellant may remain (even after the medication is gone), which leads the client to incorrectly believe he or she is receiving medication.

■ Review instructions and periodically assess the client's techniques for using an inhaler spacer or chamber correctly. Research shows that these devices assist in delivering the medication deeply into the lungs rather than only to the oropharynx.

CLIENT TEACHING   Using a Metered-Dose Inhaler

- Ensure that the canister is firmly and fully inserted into the inhaler.
- Remove the mouthpiece cap. Holding the inhaler upright, shake the inhaler vigorously for 3 to 5 seconds to mix the medication evenly.
- Exhale comfortably (as in a normal full breath).
- Hold the canister upside down.
  - a. Hold the MDI 2 to 4 cm (1 to 2 in.) from the open mouth (Figure 35-58 ■).

    or
  - b. Put the mouthpiece far enough into the mouth with its opening toward the throat such that the lips can tightly close around the mouthpiece. An MDI with a spacer or extender is always placed in the mouth (Figure 35-59 ■). This method should not be used for steroid medications via an MDI because it is not considered as efficient in delivery of the medication (Bower, 2005).

ADMINISTERING THE MEDICATION

- Press down *once* on the MDI canister (which releases the dose) and inhale slowly (for 3 to 5 seconds) and deeply through the mouth.
- Hold your breath for 10 seconds or as long as possible. *This allows the aerosol to reach deeper airways.*
- Remove the inhaler from or away from the mouth.
- Exhale slowly through *pursed* lips. *Controlled exhalation keeps the small airways open during exhalation.*

- Repeat the inhalation if ordered. Wait 20 to 30 seconds between inhalations of bronchodilator medications *so the first inhalation has a chance to work and the subsequent dose reaches deeper into the lungs.*
- Following use of the inhaler, rinse mouth with tap water to remove any remaining medication and reduce irritation and risk of infection.
- Clean the MDI mouthpiece after each use. Use mild soap and water, rinse it, and let it air dry before replacing it on the device.
- Store the canister at room temperature. Avoid extremes of temperature.
- Report adverse reactions such as restlessness, palpitations, nervousness, or rash to the physician.
- Many MDIs contain steroids for an anti-inflammatory effect. Prolonged use increases the risk of fungal infections in the mouth, indicating a need for attentive mouth care.

If two inhalers are to be used, the bronchodilator medication (which opens the airways) should be given prior to other medications. Bower (2005) recommends the use of the mnemonic *B before C* to remember bronchodilator before corticosteroid.

Inhaled steroids may not be correctly used by clients because they do not associate these medications with immediate symptom relief. The bronchodilators act to open the airways in the short term. However, it is the inhaled steroids that act as "chemical Band-Aids" to keep airway inflammation under control.

Figure 35-58 ■ Inhaler positioned away from the open mouth.

Photographer: Jenny Thomas

Figure 35-59 ■ An extender spacer attached to a mouthpiece placed in the mouth.

Photographer: Jenny Thomas

IRRIGATIONS

An **irrigation (lavage)** is the washing out of a body cavity by a stream of water or other fluid that may or may not be medicated. Irrigation is performed for one or more of the following reasons:

- To clean the area, that is, to remove a foreign object or excessive secretions or discharge
- To apply heat or cold
- To apply a medication, such as an antiseptic
- To reduce inflammation
- To relieve discomfort

Surgical asepsis is required when there is a break in the skin (e.g., in a wound irrigation) or whenever a sterile body cavity

(e.g., the bladder) is entered. Some irrigations (e.g., a vaginal, rectal, or gastric irrigation) are often safely conducted using medical asepsis.

Different kinds of syringes are used for irrigations. The most common are the Asepto and the rubber bulb (Figure 35-60 ■). The syringes are often calibrated, permitting the nurse to determine the amount of irrigant being delivered at any given time.

The Asepto syringe is a plastic (or glass) syringe with a rubber bulb. Squeezing the air out of the bulb produces negative pressure, and fluid can be sucked into the syringe. When the bulb is squeezed again, the fluid is ejected from the syringe. Asepto syringes come in several sizes ranging from 30 mL (1 oz) to 120 mL (4 oz).

A

C

B

D

Figure 35-60 ■ Four types of syringes used for irrigations: *A,* Asepto; *B,* rubber bulb; *C,* piston syringe; *D,* Pomeroy.

The rubber bulb syringe is often used for irrigating the ears. Like the Asepto syringe, the rubber bulb syringe comes in a range of sizes.

Other syringes that can be used are the piston syringe, which has a tip to which a catheter can be attached, and the Pomeroy syringe. Catheters may be used for deep-wound irrigations and for some types of bladder irrigations. The Pomeroy syringe is a metal syringe commonly used for ear irrigations. A shield near the tip prevents the solution from spraying outward. Plastic squeezable bottles are also available for irrigations. These are commonly used for perineal irrigations and some wound irrigations.

The type, amount, temperature, and strength of the solution and the frequency of the irrigation are ordered by the primary care provider. Generally, normal saline at body temperature (37°C [98.6°F]) is used unless specified otherwise. The amount of solution used varies with the site and purpose of the irrigation. Guidelines for administering eye and ear irrigations are given in Skills 35-10 (eye) and 35-11 (ear).

CRITICAL THINKING CHECKPOINT

Mr. Ketron is a 20-year-old client who just returned to the nursing unit from surgery after undergoing an emergency appendectomy. He is awake and complaining of mild incisional pain. His dressing is dry and intact, and he has an intravenous infusion of lactated Ringer's solution running at 125 mL/hr. He is to receive Ancef (a cephalosporin antibiotic) 1 g intravenously every 4 hr until he is able to tolerate fluids, at which time he will be placed on oral Suprax (cefixime) 200 mg twice daily until discharged and for 1 week after returning home. He also has an order for morphine sulfate 2.5 mg to be given every 4 hours IVP as necessary for pain.

1. It is always possible that a person receiving antibiotic drugs may experience side effects or an allergic reaction. How does an allergic reaction differ from a drug side effect?

2. Predict the possible consequences of not obtaining a medication history from Mr. Ketron despite the fact that he will be receiving antibiotics and pain medication.

3. Mr. Ketron is complaining of pain and you have prepared his IVP morphine. What assessments will you make before giving the morphine?

4. What precautions should you take, if any, prior to administering Mr. Ketron's intravenous antibiotic medication?

5. Mr. Ketron will be placed on the oral antibiotic when he can tolerate food and oral fluids. What difference, if any, does it make if this drug is given before or after meals?

See Critical Thinking Possibilities in Appendix A.

CHAPTER 35 **REVIEW**

CHAPTER HIGHLIGHTS

- Federal drug legislation regulates the production, prescription, distribution, and administration of drugs.
- Nursing practice acts define limits on the nurse's responsibilities regarding medications.
- Medications have several names. Nurses need to know the generic and trade names of a medication and be aware of both its therapeutic and side effects.
- Adverse effects of medications include drug toxicity, drug allergy, drug tolerance, idiosyncratic effect, and drug interactions.
- Several factors other than the drug itself can affect its action. These include pregnancy; age; gender; cultural, ethnic, and genetic factors; diet; client environment; psychologic factors; illness and disease; and time of administration.
- Various routes are used to administer medications: oral, sublingual, buccal, parenteral, topical, or via a nasogastric or gastrostomy tube. When administering a medication, the nurse must ensure that it is appropriate for the route specified.
- Medication orders must include the client name, date and time the order is written, name of the medication, dosage, route, frequency of administration, and signature of the person writing the order. Nurses must question any unclear orders before implementing the order.
- Telephone or verbal orders must be cosigned by the primary care provider within a time specified by agency policy (usually 24 to 48 hours).
- Three systems of measurement are used in North America: the metric system, the apothecaries' system, and the household system. Weights and measures may need to be converted by the nurse within these three systems.
- Several formulas can be used to calculate dosages. Pediatric dosages are calculated by the child's weight or body surface area.
- Nurses must always assess a client's physical status before giving any medication and obtain a medication history.
- Medication reconciliation is another method that the nurse uses to ensure that clients receive the appropriate medications and dosages. Three important areas for medication reconciliation to occur are (a) on admission, (b) during shift reports, transfers, and with new medication orders, and (c) upon discharge.
- When administering medications the nurse observes specified "rights" to ensure accurate administration. When preparing medications, the nurse checks the medication container label against the medication administration record (MAR) three times.
- The nurse who prepares the medication administers it and must never leave a prepared medication unattended.

- The nurse always identifies the client appropriately before administering a medication and stays with the client until the medication is taken.
- Medications, once given, are documented as soon as possible after administration.
- Medications given parenterally act more quickly than those given orally or topically and must be prepared using sterile technique.
- When preparing two insulins to be mixed in the same syringe, a vial of unmodified insulin should never be contaminated with modified insulin.
- Proper site selection is essential for an intramuscular injection to prevent tissue, bone, and nerve damage. The nurse should always palpate anatomic landmarks when selecting a site.
- The Z-track method for intramuscular injection is recommended to prevent discomfort caused by leakage of irritating or staining medication into subcutaneous tissues.
- Clients receiving a series of injections should have the injection sites rotated.
- After use, needles should *not* be recapped but must be placed in puncture-resistant containers.
- Intravenous medications can be administered by various methods: in a large-volume infusion of intravenous fluid, by intermittent intravenous infusion, by volume-controlled infusion, by intravenous push (IVP) or bolus, or by intermittent venous access. In all of these methods the client has an existing intravenous line or an IV access site such as a heparin or saline lock.
- Topical medications are applied to the skin and mucous membranes primarily for their local effects, although some systemic effects may occur.
- A metered-dose inhaler (MDI) is a handheld nebulizer that can be used by clients to self-administer measured doses of an aerosol medication. To ensure correct delivery of the prescribed medication by MDIs, nurses need to instruct clients to use aerosol inhalers correctly.
- Irrigations of body cavities may be performed (a) to remove a foreign object or excessive secretions or discharge, (b) to apply heat or cold, (c) to apply a medication, such as an antiseptic, (d) to reduce inflammation, or (e) to relieve discomfort.
- Surgical asepsis for an irrigation is required when there is a break in the skin (e.g., in a wound irrigation), or whenever a sterile body cavity (e.g., the bladder) is entered.

TEST YOUR KNOWLEDGE

1. A client tells the nurse, "This pill is a different color than the one that I usually take at home." Which is the best response by the nurse?
   1. "Go ahead and take your medicine."
   2. "I will recheck your medication orders."
   3. "Maybe the doctor ordered a different medication."
   4. "I'll leave the pill here while I check with the doctor."

2. If the following medications are listed on a client's medication administration record (MAR), which one should the nurse question?
   1. Lasix 40 mg, po, STAT
   2. Ampicillin 500 mg, q 6 hr, IVPB
   3. Humulin L (Lente) insulin 36 u, sc, q am, ac
   4. Codeine q 4–6 hr, po, prn for pain

3. The primary care provider prescribed 5 mL of a medication to be given deep IM for a 40-year old female who is 5'7" tall and weighs 135 pounds. Which of the following is the most appropriate method of administration?
   1. A tuberculin syringe, #25–#27 gauge, 1/4- to 5/8-inch needle
   2. Two 3-mL syringes, #20–#23 gauge, 11/2-inch needle
   3. Two 2-mL syringes, #25 gauge, 5/8-inch needle
   4. Two 2-mL syringes, #20–#23 gauge, 1-inch needle

4. The nurse is to administer 0.75 mL of medication subcutaneously in the upper arm to a 50-year-old 300-pound client. The nurse can grasp approximately 2 inches of the client's tissue at the upper arm. Which of the following is the most appropriate for the nurse to use?
   1. A tuberculin syringe, #25-#27 gauge, 1/4- to 5/8-inch needle
   2. Two 3-mL syringes, #20-#23 gauge, 1 1/2-inch needle
   3. 2-mL syringe, #25 gauge, 5/8-inch needle
   4. 2-mL syringe, #20-#23 gauge, 1-inch needle

5. The nurse is to administer a tuberculin test to a 22-year-old male who is 6 feet tall and weighs 180 pounds. Which of the following is the most appropriate for the nurse to use?
   1. A tuberculin syringe, #25-#27 gauge, 1/4- to 5/8-inch needle
   2. Two 3-mL syringes, #20-#23 gauge, 1 1/2-inch needle
   3. 2-mL syringe, #25 gauge, 5/8-inch needle
   4. 2-mL syringe, #20-#23 gauge, 1-inch needle

6. The nurse is to administer 0.5 mL of a medication by IM injection to an elderly emaciated client. Which of the following is the most appropriate for the nurse to use?
   1. A tuberculin syringe, #25-#27 gauge, 1/4- to 5/8-inch needle
   2. Two 3-mL syringes, #20-#23 gauge, 1 1/2-inch needle
   3. 2-mL syringe, #25 gauge, 5/8-inch needle
   4. 2-mL syringe, #20-#23 gauge, 1-inch needle

7. An elderly client with renal insufficiency is to receive a cardiac medication. The nurse is most likely to administer which of the following?
   1. A decreased dosage
   2. The standard dosage
   3. An increased dosage
   4. Divided dosages

8. Proper administration of an otic medication to a two-year-old client includes which of the following?
   1. Pull the ear straight back
   2. Pull the ear down and back
   3. Pull the ear up and back
   4. Pull the ear straight upward

9. A primary care provider writes a prescription for 0.15 milligrams of digoxin intravenously every day. The medication is available in a concentration of 400 micrograms per mL. How many mL will the nurse administer? _____

10. A student nurse is preparing to administer insulin to a client with diabetes. Indicate the correct order for the administration of this medication:
    1. Cleanse the site with alcohol.
    2. Insert the needle quickly into the subcutaneous tissue.
    3. Mix the insulins.
    4. Assess the skin for the injection.
    5. Pinch the skin lightly.
    6. Inject the medication.
    7. Count to five.
    8. Remove the syringe.

Correct sequence:_____

See Answers to Test Your Knowledge in Appendix A ∞ .

EXPLORE MEDIALINK www.prenhall.com/berman

DVD-ROM
- Audio Glossary
- NCLEX Review
- Skills Checklist
- Animations:
    Drug Metabolization
    Agonist/Antagonist Mechanism of Action
    Injections
- Videos:
    Medical Drugs
    Metered-Dose Inhaler (MDI)
    Small Volume Nebulizer (SVN) Treatment

COMPANION WEBSITE
- Additional NCLEX Review
- Case Study: Preparing Medications
- Care Plan Activity: Client on Insulin
- Application Activity: Calculating Dosages
- Links to Resources

READINGS AND REFERENCES

SUGGESTED READINGS
Curry, L. C., Walker, C., Hogstel, M. O., & Burns, P. (2005). Teaching older adults to self-manage medications. Preventing adverse drug reactions. *Journal of Gerontological Nursing,* *31*(4), 32–42.
The authors point out that older adults use more prescription and over-the-counter medications than any other age group. This

article provides information to help the nurse teach older adults how to self-medicate safely.
Koschel, M. J. (2005). Sternal intraosseous infusions. Emergency vascular access in adults. *American Journal of Nursing, 105*(1), 66–68.
The author describes another vascular access for adults. Sternal intraosseous (IO) infusion is used in emergency situations when the client needs rapid fluid replacement and/or

medication administration and IV attempts have failed. This compelling article describes the insertion technique, post-insertion care, and discontinuation.
Manno, M. S. (2006). Preventing adverse drug events. *Nursing, 36*(3), 56–61.
The article points out that adverse drug events (ADEs) increase the cost of hospitalization by $2,200 to $3,200 per stay and prolong hospital

stays by 2 days on average. The author reviews causes of adverse drug events and the importance of building an organizational culture of client safety by learning from mistakes rather than placing blame.

Prows, C. A., & Prows, D. R. (2004). Medication selection by genotype. How genetics is changing drug prescribing and efficacy. *American Journal of Nursing, 104*(5), 60–70. *The authors provide helpful information about pharmacogenetics and nursing implications. The article also raises thoughtful medical and nursing implication questions that, as yet, have no answers.*

Schulmeister, L. (2005). Transdermal drug patches. Medicine with muscle. *Nursing, 35*(1), 48–52. *The number of available transdermal drug patches is increasing. This comprehensive article describes the benefits and the risks to their use. It includes important information for nurses to know and to teach their clients.*

RELATED RESEARCH

Cook, A. F., Hoas, H., Guttmannova, K., & Joyner, J. C. (2004). An error by any other name. *American Journal of Nursing, 104*(6), 32–43.

Hutin, Y., Hauri, A., Chiarello, L., Catlin, M., Stilwell, B., Ghebrehiwet, T., Garner, J., & the Injection Safety Best Practices Development Group. (2003). Best infection control practices for intradermal, subcutaneous, and intramuscular needle injections. *Bulletin of the World Health Organization, 81*(7), 491–500.

Zhan, L., & Chen, J. (2004). Medication practices among Chinese American older adults. A study of cultural influences. *Journal of Gerontological Nursing, 30*(4), 24–33.

REFERENCES

Abrams, A. C. (2004). *Clinical drug therapy: Rationales for nursing practice* (7th ed.). Philadelphia: Lippincott Williams & Wilkins.

Adams, M. P., Josephson, D. L., & Holland, L. N. (2005). *Pharmacology for nurses: A pathophysiologic approach.* Upper Saddle River, NJ: Pearson Prentice Hall.

American Diabetes Association. (2004). Insulin administration. *Diabetes Care, 27*(1), S106–S109.

Barr, D. H., & Thomas, C. H. (2005). Is aspiration necessary during intramuscular injection? *Advance online Editions for Nurses 7*(18), 27.

Bower, L. M. (2005). Is your patient's metered-dose inhaler technique up to snuff? *Nursing 35*(8), 50–51.

Bunce, M. (2003). Troubleshooting central lines. *RN, 66*(12), 28–34.

Grissinger, M., & Globus, N. J. (2004). Technology affects your risk of medication errors. *Nursing 34*(1), 36–42.

Institute for Healthcare Improvement (IHI). (n.d.). *Reconcile medications at all transition points.* Retrieved June 18, 2006 from http://www.ihi.org/IHI/Topics/PatientSafety/MedicationSystems/Changes/Reconcile+Medications+at+All+Transition+Points.htm

Joint Commission on Accreditation of Healthcare Organizations (JCAHO). (n.d.). *Official do not use abbreviations list.* Retrieved June 18, 2006, from http://www.jcaho.org/NR/rdonlyres/2329F8F5-6EC5-4E21-B932-54B2B7D53F00/0/06_dnu_list.pdf

Joint Commission on Accreditation of Healthcare Organizations (JCAHO). (2006). *2007 hospital/critical access hospital national patient safety goals.* Retrieved June 18, 2006, from http://www.jointcommission.org/PatientSafety/NationalPatientSafetyGoals/07_hap_cah_npsgs.htm

Karch, A. (2004). What's wrong with U? *American Journal of Nursing, 104*(6), 65–66.

Ketchum, K. Grass, C. A., & Padwojski, A. (2005). Medication reconciliation. *American Journal of Nursing, 105*(11), 78–85.

Lea, D. H. (2005). Tailoring drug therapy with pharmacogenetics. *Nursing, 35*(4), 22–23.

Manno, M. S., & Hayes, D. D. (2006). Best-practice interventions: How medication reconciliation saves lives. *Nursing, 36*(3), 63.

Munoz, C., & Hilgenberg, C. (2005). Ethnopharmacology. *American Journal of Nursing, 105*(8), 40–48.

Nicoll, L. H., & Hesby, A. (2002). Intramuscular injection: An integrative research review and guideline for evidence-based practice. *Applied Nursing Research, 16*(2), 149–162.

Pape, T. M., Guerra, D. M., Muzquiz, M., Bryant, J. B., Ingram, M., Schranner, B., et al. (2005). Innovative approaches to reducing nurses' distraction during medication administration. *Journal of Continuing Education in Nursing, 36*(3), 108–116.

Preston, S.T., & Hegadoren, K. (2004). Glass contamination in parenterally administered medication. *Journal of Advanced Nursing, 48*(3), 266–270.

Przybycien, P. (2005). *Safe meds.* St. Louis, MO: Elsevier Mosby.

Pullen, R. L. (2005). Administering medication by the z-track method. *Nursing 35*(7), 24.

Robbins, B., Rausch, K. J., Garcia, R. I., & Prestwood, K. W. (2004). Multicultural medication adherence: A comparative study. *Journal of Gerontological Nursing, 30*(7), 25–32.

Tarnow, K., & King, N. (2004). Intradermal injections: Traditional bevel up versus bevel down. *Applied Nursing Research, 17*(4), 275–282.

SELECTED BIBLIOGRAPHY

Bastable, S. B. (2003). *Nurse as educator* (2nd ed.). Boston: Jones & Bartlett.

Bindler, R. C., & Ball, J. W. (2003). *Clinical skills manual for pediatric nursing: Caring for children* (3rd ed.). Upper Saddle River, NJ: Prentice Hall.

Burke, K. G. (2005). The state of the science on safe medication administration symposium. *American Journal of Nursing, 105*(3), 73–78.

Cohen, H., Robinson, E. S., & Mandrack, M. (2003). Getting to the root of medication errors: Survey results. *Nursing, 33*(9), 36–45.

Cohen, M. R. (2005). Reconciling medications: Safeguarding transitions. *Nursing, 35*(7), 14.

Douglas, J., & Larrabee, S. (2003). Bring barcoding to the bedside. *Nursing Management, 34*(5), 36–40.

Greenway, K. (2004). Using the ventrogluteal site for intramuscular injection. *Nursing Standard, 18*(25), 39–42.

Hughes, R. G., & Edgerton, E. A. (2005). Reducing pediatric medication errors. *American Journal of Nursing, 105*(5), 79–91.

Kennedy, S. (2005). To err is not surprising. *American Journal of Nursing, 105*(6), 19.

Lafleur, K. J. (2004). Tackling med errors with technology. *RN, 67*(5), 29–35.

Macdonald, F. (2004). Iatrogenic prescribing in acute care: Learning from our mistakes. *Journal of Gerontological Nursing, 34, 20–25.*

McErlane, K. (2005). Keeping track of the patch. *American Journal of Nursing, 105*(6), 36–37.

Molony, S. L. (2003). Beers' criteria for potentially inappropriate medication use in the elderly. *Journal of Gerontological Nursing, 29*(11), 6–7.

Nelson, R. (2004). Needlestick injuries: Going but not gone? *American Journal of Nursing, 104*(11), 25–26.

Perry, J., & Jagger, J. (2005). Sharps safety update: "Are we there yet?" *Nursing, 35*(6), 17.

Perry, J., Robinson, E. S., & Jagger, J. (2004). Needle-stick and sharps-safety survey. *Nursing, 34*(4), 43–47.

Prettyman, J. (2005). Subcutaneous or intramuscular? Confronting a parenteral administration dilemma. *Medsurg Nursing, 14*(2), 93–99.

Pritchett & Hull. (n.d.). *JCAHO abbreviations to avoid.* Retrieved June 18, 2006, from, http://www.p-h.com/phcatalog/pnt_4.htm

Roark, D. C. (2004). Bar codes and drug administration. *American Journal of Nursing, 104*(1), 63–66.

Rushing, J. (2004). How to administer a subcutaneous injection. *Nursing, 34*(6), 32.

Schlenk, E. A., Dunbar-Jacob, J., & Engberg, S. (2004). Medication non-adherence among older adults. *Journal of Gerontological Nursing, 35, 33–43.*

Small, S. P. (2004). Preventing sciatic nerve injury from intramuscular injections: Literature review. *Journal of Advanced Nursing, 47*(3), 287–296.

Woods, A. (2003). How to use your medicine safely. *Nursing, 33*(12), 50–51.

Wooten, J., & Galavis, J. (2005). Polypharmacy: Keeping the elderly safe. *RN, 68*(8), 45–50.

CHAPTER 36

Skin Integrity and Wound Care

LEARNING OUTCOMES

After completing this chapter, you will be able to:

1. Describe factors affecting skin integrity.

2. Identify clients at risk for pressure ulcers.

3. Describe the four stages of pressure ulcer development.

4. Differentiate primary and secondary wound healing.

5. Describe the three phases of wound healing.

6. Identify three major types of wound exudate.

7. Identify the main complications of and factors that affect wound healing.

8. Identify assessment data pertinent to skin integrity, pressure sites, and wounds.

9. Identify nursing diagnoses associated with impaired skin integrity.

10. Identify essential aspects of planning care to maintain skin integrity and promote wound healing.

11. Discuss measures to prevent pressure ulcer formation.

12. Describe nursing strategies to treat pressure ulcers, promote wound healing, and prevent complications of wound healing.

13. Identify purposes of commonly used wound dressing materials and binders.

14. Identify essential steps of obtaining wound specimens, applying dressings, and irrigating a wound.

15. Identify physiologic responses to and purposes of heat and cold.

16. Describe methods of applying dry and moist heat and cold.

The skin is the largest organ in the body and serves a variety of important functions in maintaining health and protecting the individual from injury. Important nursing functions are maintaining skin integrity and promoting wound healing. Impaired skin integrity is not a frequent problem for most healthy people but is a threat to elders; to clients with restricted mobility, chronic illnesses, or trauma; and to those undergoing invasive health care procedures. To protect the skin and manage wounds effectively, the nurse must understand the factors affecting skin integrity, the physiology of wound healing, and specific measures that promote optimal skin conditions.

SKIN INTEGRITY

Intact skin refers to the presence of normal skin and skin layers uninterrupted by wounds. Chapter 30 ∞ provides details regarding physical examination of the integumentary system. The appearance of the skin and skin integrity are influenced by internal factors such as genetics, age, and the underlying health of the individual as well as external factors such as activity.

Genetics and heredity determine many aspects of a person's skin, including skin color, sensitivity to sunlight, and allergies. Age influences skin integrity in that the skin of both the very young and the very old is more fragile and susceptible to injury than that of most adults. Wounds tend to heal more rapidly in infants and children, however.

Many chronic illnesses and their treatments affect skin integrity. People with impaired peripheral arterial circulation may have skin on the legs that appears shiny, has lost its hair distribution, and damages easily. Some medications, corticosteroids for example, cause thinning of the skin and allow it to be much more readily harmed. Many medications increase sensitivity to sunlight and can predispose one to severe sunburns. Some of the most common ones that cause this damage are certain antibiotics, chemotherapy drugs for cancer, and some psychotherapeutic drugs. Poor nutrition alone can interfere with the appearance and function of normal skin.

TYPES OF WOUNDS

Body wounds are either intentional or unintentional. *Intentional* trauma occurs during therapy. Examples are operations or venipunctures. Although removing a tumor, for example, is therapeutic, the surgeon must cut into body tissues, thus traumatizing them. *Unintentional* wounds are accidental; for example, a person may fracture an arm in an automobile collision. If the tissues are traumatized without a break in the skin, the wound is closed. The wound is open when the skin or mucous membrane surface is broken.

Wounds may be described according to how they are acquired (see Table 36–1). They also can be described according to the likelihood and degree of wound contamination.

- *Clean wounds* are uninfected wounds in which minimal inflammation is encountered and the respiratory, alimentary, genital, and urinary tracts are not entered. Clean wounds are primarily closed wounds.
- *Clean-contaminated wounds* are surgical wounds in which the respiratory, alimentary, genital, or urinary tract has been entered. Such wounds show no evidence of infection.
- *Contaminated wounds* include open, fresh, accidental wounds and surgical wounds involving a major break in sterile technique or a large amount of spillage from the gastrointestinal tract. Contaminated wounds show evidence of inflammation.
- *Dirty* or *infected wounds* include wounds containing dead tissue and wounds with evidence of a clinical infection, such as purulent drainage.

Wounds, excluding pressure ulcers and burns, are classified by depth, that is, the tissue layers involved in the wound (see Box 36–1).

TABLE 36–1	**Types of Wounds**	
TYPE	**CAUSE**	**DESCRIPTION AND CHARACTERISTICS**
Incision	Sharp instrument (e.g., knife or scalpel)	Open wound; deep or shallow
Contusion	Blow from a blunt instrument	Closed wound, skin appears ecchymotic (bruised) because of damaged blood vessels
Abrasion	Surface scrape, either unintentional (e.g., scraped knee from a fall) or intentional (e.g., dermal abrasion to remove pockmarks)	Open wound involving the skin
Puncture	Penetration of the skin and often the underlying tissues by a sharp instrument, either intentional or unintentional	Open wound
Laceration	Tissues torn apart, often from accidents (e.g., with machinery)	Open wound; edges are often jagged
Penetrating wound	Penetration of the skin and the underlying tissues, usually unintentional (e.g., from a bullet or metal fragments)	Open wound

---

BOX 36–1   **Classifying Wounds by Depth**

- *Partial thickness:* Confined to the skin, that is, the dermis and epidermis; heal by regeneration
- *Full thickness:* Involving the dermis, epidermis, subcutaneous tissue, and possibly muscle and bone; require connective tissue repair

PRESSURE ULCERS

Pressure ulcers were previously called **decubitus ulcers,** *pressure sores,* or *bedsores.* A pressure ulcer is any lesion caused by unrelieved **pressure** (a compressing downward force on a body area) that results in damage to underlying tissue, as defined by the U.S. Public Health Service's Panel for the Prediction and Prevention of Pressure Ulcers in Adults (PPPPUA, 1992b).

Pressure ulcers are a problem in both acute care settings and long-term care settings, including homes. The best estimate of the incidence of pressure ulcers in hospital settings (the number of people who get pressure ulcers each year) between 2000 and 2004 was 7% to 9% (Whittington & Briones, 2004). *Healthy People 2010* has established the objective of reducing the prevalence of pressure ulcers in nursing homes (the number of people affected at any given time) by 50%—from 16/1,000 residents reported in 1997 to 8/1,000.

Etiology of Pressure Ulcers

Pressure ulcers are due to localized **ischemia,** a deficiency in the blood supply to the tissue. The tissue is compressed between two surfaces, usually the surface of the bed and the bony skeleton, with greater than 32 mm Hg pressure. When blood cannot reach the tissue, the cells are deprived of oxygen and nutrients, the waste products of metabolism accumulate in the cells, and the tissue consequently dies. Prolonged, unrelieved pressure also damages the small blood vessels.

After the skin has been compressed, it appears pale, as if the blood had been squeezed out of it. When pressure is relieved, the skin takes on a bright red flush, called **reactive hyperemia.** The flush is due to **vasodilation,** a process in which extra blood floods to the area to compensate for the preceding period of impeded blood flow. Reactive hyperemia usually lasts one-half to three-quarters as long as the duration of impeded blood flow to the area (PPPPUA, 1992a). If the redness disappears in that time, no tissue damage can be anticipated. If, however, the redness does not disappear, then tissue damage has occurred.

Risk Factors

Several factors contribute to the formation of pressure ulcers: immobility and inactivity, inadequate nutrition, fecal and urinary incontinence, decreased mental status, diminished sensation, excessive body heat, advanced age, and the presence of certain chronic conditions.

Friction and Shearing

Two other factors frequently act in conjunction with pressure to produce pressure ulcers: friction and shearing force. **Friction** is a force acting parallel to the skin surface. For example, sheets rubbing against skin create friction. Friction can abrade the skin, that is, remove the superficial layers, making it more prone to breakdown.

Shearing force is a combination of friction and pressure. It occurs commonly when a client assumes a Fowler's position in bed. In this position, the body tends to slide downward toward the foot of the bed. This downward movement is transmitted to the sacral bone and the deep tissues. At the same time, the skin over the sacrum tends not to move because of the adherence between the skin and the bed linens. The skin and superficial tissues are thus relatively unmoving in relation to the bed surface, whereas the deeper tissues are firmly attached to the skeleton and move downward. This causes a shearing force in the area where the deeper tissues and the superficial tissues meet. The force damages the blood vessels and tissues in this area.

Immobility

Immobility refers to a reduction in the amount and control of movement a person has. Normally people move when they experience discomfort due to pressure on an area of the body. Healthy people rarely exceed their tolerance to pressure. However, paralysis, extreme weakness, pain, or any cause of decreased activity can hinder a person's ability to change positions independently and relieve the pressure, even if the person can perceive the pressure.

Inadequate Nutrition

Prolonged inadequate nutrition causes weight loss, muscle atrophy, and the loss of subcutaneous tissue. These three reduce the amount of padding between the skin and the bones, thus increasing the risk of pressure ulcer development. More specifically, inadequate intake of protein, carbohydrates, fluids, zinc, and vitamin C contributes to pressure ulcer formation.

Hypoproteinemia (abnormally low protein content in the blood), due either to inadequate intake or abnormal loss, predisposes the client to dependent edema. Edema (the presence of excess interstitial fluid) makes skin more prone to injury by decreasing its elasticity, resilience, and vitality. Edema increases the distance between the capillaries and the cells, thereby slowing the diffusion of oxygen to the tissue cells and of metabolites away from the cells.

Fecal and Urinary Incontinence

Moisture from incontinence promotes skin **maceration** (tissue softened by prolonged wetting or soaking) and makes the epidermis more easily eroded and susceptible to injury. Digestive enzymes in feces, gastric tube drainage, and urea in urine also contribute to skin **excoriation** (area of loss of the superficial layers of the skin also known as *denuded* area). Any accumulation of secretions or excretions is irritating to the skin, harbors microorganisms, and makes an individual prone to skin breakdown and infection.

Decreased Mental Status

Individuals with a reduced level of awareness, for example, those who are unconscious, heavily sedated, or have dementia, are at risk for pressure ulcers because they are less able to recognize and respond to pain associated with prolonged pressure.

Diminished Sensation

Paralysis, stroke, or other neurologic disease may cause loss of sensation in a body area. Loss of sensation reduces a person's ability to respond to trauma, to injurious heat and cold, and to the tingling ("pins and needles") that signals loss of circulation. Sensory loss also impairs the body's ability to recognize and provide healing mechanisms for a wound.

Excessive Body Heat

Body heat is another factor in the development of pressure ulcers. An elevated body temperature increases the metabolic rate, thus increasing the cells' need for oxygen. This increased need is particularly severe in the cells of an area under pressure, which are already oxygen deficient. Severe infections with accompanying elevated body temperatures may affect the body's ability to deal with the effects of tissue compression.

Advanced Age

The aging process brings about several changes in the skin and its supporting structures, making the older person more prone to impaired skin integrity. These changes include the following:

- Loss of lean body mass
- Generalized thinning of the epidermis
- Decreased strength and elasticity of the skin due to changes in the collagen fibers of the dermis
- Increased dryness due to a decrease in the amount of oil produced by the sebaceous glands
- Diminished pain perception due to a reduction in the number of cutaneous end organs responsible for the sensation of pressure and light touch
- Diminished venous and arterial flow due to aging vascular walls

Chronic Medical Conditions

Certain chronic conditions such as diabetes and cardiovascular disease are risk factors for skin breakdown and delayed healing. These conditions compromise oxygen delivery to tissues by poor perfusion and thus cause poor and delayed healing and increase risk of pressure sores.

Other Factors

Other factors contributing to the formation of pressure ulcers are poor lifting and transferring techniques, incorrect positioning, hard support surfaces, and incorrect application of pressure-relieving devices.

Stages of Pressure Ulcers

The four recognized stages of pressure ulcers related to observable tissue damage are shown in Figure 36-1 ▪.

Risk Assessment Tools

Although clients may be at risk for developing a number of different alterations in skin integrity, the most common and most preventable are pressure ulcers. Several risk assessment tools are available that provide the nurse with systematic means of identifying clients at high risk for pressure ulcer development. The PPPPUA (1992a) has recommended that the tool include data collection in the areas of immobility, incontinence, nutrition, and level of consciousness.

In 1987, Bergstrom, Braden, Laguzza, and Holman published the Braden Scale for Predicting Pressure Sore Risk. Their scale consists of six subscales: sensory perception, moisture, activity, mobility, nutrition, and friction and shear (see Figure 36-2 ▪). A total of 23 points is possible. An adult who scores below 18 points is considered at risk (Folkedahl & Frantz, 2002b). For best results, nurses should be trained in proper use of the scale.

Norton's Pressure Area Risk Assessment Form Scale (Table 36–2) includes the categories of general physical condition, mental state, activity, mobility, and incontinence. A category of medications was added in 1987, resulting in a possible score of 24. Scores of 15 or 16 should be viewed as indicators, not predictors, of risk. The Braden and Norton tools should be used when the client first enters the health care agency and whenever the client's condition changes. In some long-term care facilities, a risk assessment scale such as the Braden or Norton scale is done on admission and then on a regular basis, usually weekly. This increases awareness of specific risk factors and serves as assessment data from which to plan goals and interventions to either maintain or improve skin integrity.

MediaLink

Client with Pressure Ulcer Care Plan Activity

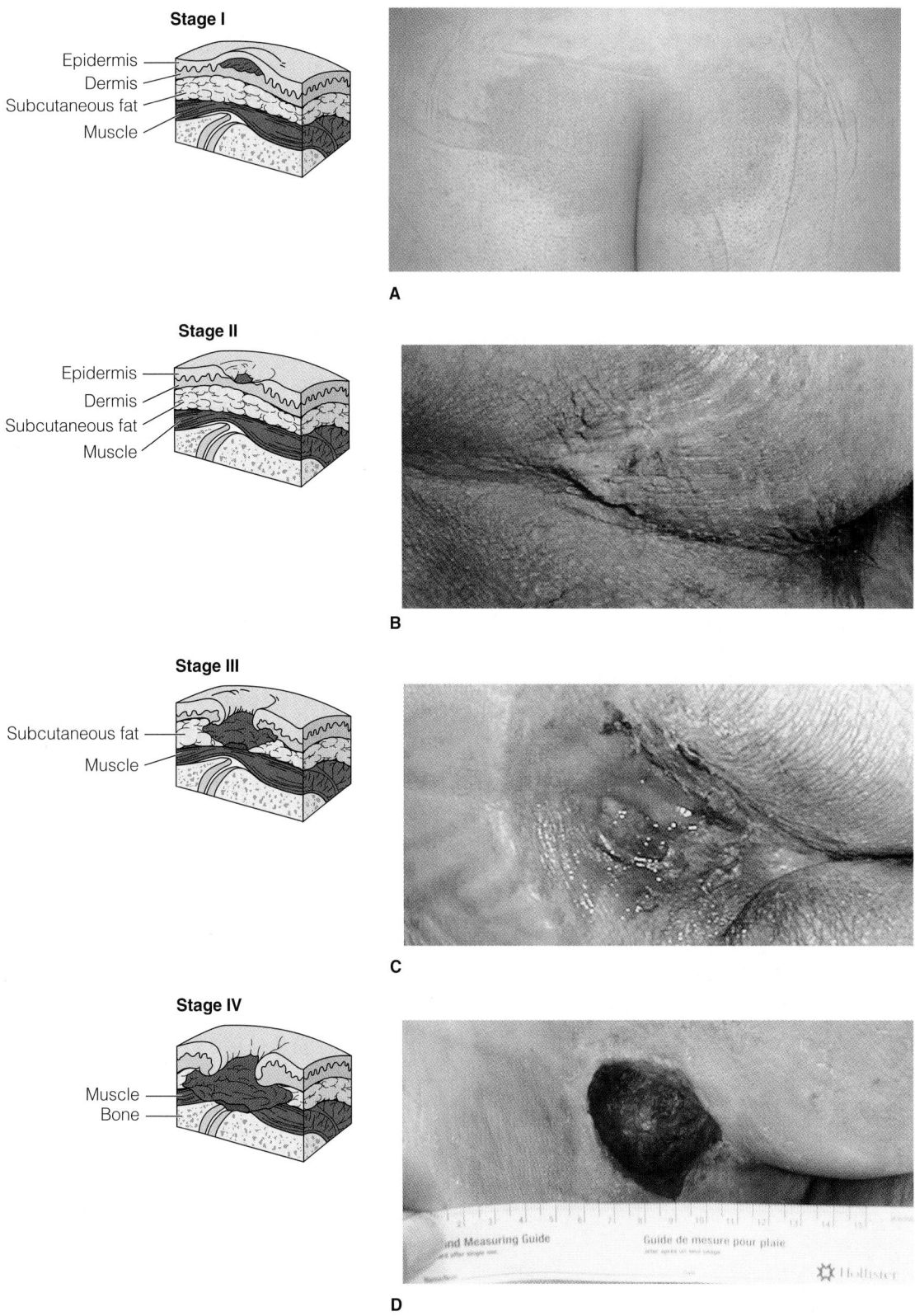

Figure 36-1 ■ Four stages of pressure ulcers. *A,* stage I: nonblanchable erythema signaling potential ulceration; *B,* stage II: partial-thickness skin loss (abrasion, blister, or shallow crater) involving the epidermis and possibly the dermis; *C,* stage III: full-thickness skin loss involving damage or necrosis of subcutaneous tissue that may extend down to, but not through, underlying fascia. The ulcer presents clinically as a deep crater with or without undermining of adjacent tissue; *D,* stage IV: full-thickness skin loss with tissue necrosis or damage to muscle, bone, or supporting structures, such as a tendon or joint capsule. Undermining and sinus tracts may also be present.

(Line art from "Clinical Practice Guideline, Pressure Ulcers in Adults: Prediction and Prevention," by U.S. Department of Health and Human Services, PPPPUA Pub. No. 92-0047, pp. 16–17, 1992, Rockville, MD: Public Health Service. Photos from Cory Patrick Hartley, RN.)

BRADEN SCALE FOR PREDICTING PRESSURE SORE RISK

Patient's Name _____ Evaluator's Name _____ Date of Assessment

SENSORY PERCEPTION

Ability to respond meaningfully to pressure-related discomfort

1. Completely Limited:
Unresponsive (does not moan, flinch, or grasp) to painful stimuli, due to diminished level of consciousness or sedation,
OR
limited ability to feel pain over most of body surface.

2. Very Limited:
Responds only to painful stimuli. Cannot communicate discomfort except by moaning or restlessness,
OR
has a sensory impairment which limits the ability to feel pain or discomfort over 1/2 of body.

3. Slightly Limited:
Responds to verbal commands but cannot always communicate discomfort or need to be turned,
OR
has some sensory impairment which limits ability to feel pain or discomfort in 1 or 2 extremities.

4. No Impairment:
Responds to verbal commands. Has no sensory deficit which would limit ability to feel or voice pain or discomfort.

MOISTURE

Degree to which skin is exposed to moisture

1. Constantly Moist:
Skin is kept moist almost constantly by perspiration, urine, etc. Dampness is detected every time patient is moved or turned.

2. Moist:
Skin is often but not always moist. Linen must be changed at least once a shift.

3. Occasionally Moist:
Skin is occasionally moist, requiring an extra linen change approximately once a day.

4. Rarely Moist:
Skin is usually dry; linen requires changing only at routine intervals.

ACTIVITY

Degree of physical activity

1. Bedfast:
Confined to bed.

2. Chairfast:
Ability to walk severely limited or nonexistent. Cannot bear own weight and/or must be assisted into chair or wheelchair.

3. Walks Occasionally:
Walks occasionally during day but for very short distances, with or without assistance. Spends majority of each shift in bed or chair.

4. Walks Frequently:
Walks outside the room at least twice a day and inside room at least once every 2 hours during waking hours.

MOBILITY

Ability to change and control body position

1. Completely Immobile:
Does not make even slight changes in body or extremity position without assistance.

2. Very Limited:
Makes occasional slight changes in body or extremity position but unable to make frequent or significant changes independently.

3. Slightly Limited:
Makes frequent though slight changes in body or extremity position independently.

4. No Limitations:
Makes major and frequent changes in position without assistance.

NUTRITION

Usual food intake pattern

1. Very Poor:
Never eats a complete meal. Rarely eats more than 1/3 of any food offered. Eats 2 servings or less of protein (meat or dairy products) per day. Takes fluids poorly. Does not take a liquid dietary supplement,
OR
is NPO and/or maintained on clear liquids or IV's for more than 5 days.

2. Probably Inadequate:
Rarely eats a complete meal and generally eats only about 1/2 of any food offered. Protein intake includes only 3 servings of meat or dairy products per day. Occasionally will take a dietary supplement,
OR
receives less than optimum amount of liquid diet or tube feeding.

3. Adequate:
Eats over half of most meals. Eats a total of 4 servings of protein (meat, dairy products) each day. Occasionally will refuse a meal, but will usually take a supplement if offered,
OR
is on a tube feeding or TPN regimen, which probably meets most of nutritional needs.

4. Excellent:
Eats most of every meal. Never refuses a meal. Usually eats a total of 4 or more servings of meat and dairy products. Occasionally eats between meals. Does not require supplementation.

FRICTION AND SHEAR

1. Problem:
Requires moderate to maximum assistance in moving. Complete lifting without sliding against sheets is impossible. Frequently slides down in bed or chair, requiring frequent repositioning with maximum assistance. Spasticity, contractures, or agitation leads to almost constant friction.

2. Potential Problem:
Moves feebly or requires minimum assistance. During a move skin probably slides to some extent against sheets, chair, restraints, or other devices. Maintains relatively good position in chair or bed most of the time but occasionally slides down.

3. No Apparent Problem:
Moves in bed and in chair independently and has sufficient muscle strength to lift up completely during move. Maintains good position in bed or chair at all times.

Total Score _____

Figure 36-2 ■ Braden Scale for Predicting Pressure Sore Risk.

(From "Clinical Practice Guideline, Pressure Ulcers in Adults: Prediction and Prevention," by U.S. Department of Health and Human Services, PPPPUA Pub No. 92-0047, pp. 16–17, 1992, Rockville, MD: Public Health Service. Copyright © Barbara Braden and Nancy Bergstrom, 1988. Reprinted with permission.)

Feature Integument Animation

MediaLink

Layers of the Skin Animation

MediaLink

TABLE 36–2	Norton's Pressure Area Risk Assessment Form (Scoring System)								
A. GENERAL PHYSICAL CONDITION		**B. MENTAL STATE**		**C. ACTIVITY**		**D. MOBILITY**		**E. INCONTINENCE**	
Good	4	Alert	4	Ambulatory	4	Full	4	Absent	4
Fair	3	Apathetic	3	Walks with help	3	Slightly limited	3	Occasional	3
Poor	2	Confused	2	Chairbound	2	Very limited	2	Usually urinary	2
Very bad	1	Stuporous	1	Bedfast	1	Immobile	1	Double	1

Note: Reprinted from *An Investigation of Geriatric Nursing Problems in Hospital,* by D. Norton, R. McLaren, and A. N. Exton-Smith, Copyright © 1975, with permission from Elsevier.

RESEARCH NOTE   Is a Chart Review or a Physical Exam the Better Method to Determine Pressure Ulcer Prevalence and Incidence in Acute Care?

A 6-year data review by Whittington and Briones was performed to determine if analysis of prevalence and incidence of pressure ulcers in acute care health care organizations (HCOs) was more accurate if a series of two physical examination surveys prevalence and incidence were conducted over a specified period of time or if a closed chart review was performed. A national prevalence and incidence study was launched March 1999 among 115 HCOs in 34 states. By the end of the study in 2004, 240 HCOs in 43 states contributed data. Each year the identical surveys were conducted. The data collection process during the studies included a chart review for evidence of documentation of a pressure ulcer on admission to the acute care setting.

The prevalence survey process required a physical examination of client's skin condition over the bony prominences. Five days following the prevalence examination the same groups of clients were reexamined on the same areas to determine if they acquired an assessable change in condition related to unrelieved pressure, resulting in a pressure ulcer.

IMPLICATIONS

The review found that 60% of the observed pressure ulcers were not documented on the nursing admission data collection forms. These data indicate that the frequently used method of conducting a chart review to obtain incidence data is far less accurate than verifying pressure ulcer status by clinical examination. A more accurate measure of incidence is the second observation of clients who did not have pressure ulcers in the prevalence study but who were observed to have one or more pressure ulcers on the day of the incidence study. In the study, 31,969 clients were assessed for prevalence data. Of those, 4,956 (16%) were found to have one or more pressure ulcers; most were stage I or II. No documentation of a pressure ulcer on admission could be found for 64% of clients who had evidence of a pressure ulcer during the prevalence study. Nurses need to be more diligent in assessing and recording pressure ulcer data.

Note: From "National Prevalence and Incidence Study: 6-Year Sequential Acute Care Data" by K. T. Whittington, and R. Briones, 2004, *Advances in Skin and Wound Care, 17,* pp. 490–494.

CLINICAL ALERT

The two validated assessment tools supported by the PPPPUA are the Braden scale and the Norton scale. ∎

The accompanying Practice Guidelines describe the principles of assessing common pressure sites.

WOUND HEALING

Healing is a quality of living tissue; it is also referred to as **regeneration** (renewal) of tissues. Healing can be considered in terms of *types of healing,* having to do with the caregiver's decision on whether to allow the wound to seal itself or to purposefully close the wound, and *phases of healing,* which refer to the steps in the body's natural processes of tissue repair. The phases are the same for all wounds, but the rate of healing depends on factors such as the type of healing, the location and size of the wound, and the health of the client.

Types of Wound Healing

There are two types of healing, influenced by the amount of tissue loss. **Primary intention healing** occurs where the tissue surfaces have been **approximated** (closed) and there is minimal or no tissue loss; it is characterized by the formation of minimal granulation tissue and scarring. It is also called *primary union* or *first intention healing.* An example of wound healing by primary intention is a closed surgical incision. Another example would be the use of tissue adhesive, a liquid "glue" that can be used to seal clean lacerations or incisions which may result in better appearing scars (Coulthard, Worthington, Esposito, van der Elst, & van Waes, 2005).

A wound that is extensive and involves considerable tissue loss, and in which the edges cannot or should not be approximated, heals by **secondary intention healing.** An example of wound healing by secondary intention is a pressure ulcer. Secondary intention healing differs from primary intention healing in three ways: (a) The repair time is longer, (b) the scarring is greater, and (c) the susceptibility to infection is greater.

Those wounds that are left open for 3 to 5 days to allow edema or infection to resolve or exudate to drain and are then closed with sutures, staples, or adhesive skin closures, heal by **tertiary intention.** This is also called delayed primary intention.

Phases of Wound Healing

Wound healing can be broken down into three phases: inflammatory, proliferative, and maturation or remodeling.

Inflammatory Phase

The *inflammatory phase* is initiated immediately after injury and lasts 3 to 6 days. Two major processes occur during this phase: hemostasis and phagocytosis.

PRACTICE GUIDELINES Assessing Common Pressure Sites

- Ensure the lighting is good, preferably natural or fluorescent, because incandescent lights can create a transilluminating effect.
- Regulate the environment before beginning the assessment so that the room is neither too hot nor too cold. Heat can cause the skin to flush; cold can cause the skin to blanch or become cyanotic.
- Inspect pressure areas (see Figure 36-3 ■) for discoloration. This can be caused by impaired blood circulation to the area. The pressure areas should have brisk capillary refill or blanch response when gently palpated with the end of a finger or thumb.

- Inspect pressure areas for abrasions and excoriations. An abrasion can occur when skin rubs against a sheet (e.g., when the client is pulled). Excoriations can occur when the skin has prolonged contact with body secretions or excretions or with dampness in skin folds.
- Palpate the surface temperature of the skin over the pressure areas (warm your hands first). Normally, the temperature is the same as that of the surrounding skin. Increased temperature is abnormal and may be due to inflammation or blood trapped in the area.
- Palpate over bony prominences and dependent body areas for the presence of edema, which feels spongy or boggy.

Figure 36-3 ■ Body pressure areas in *A,* supine position; *B,* lateral position; *C,* prone position; *D,* Fowler's position.

Hemostasis (the cessation of bleeding) results from vasoconstriction of the larger blood vessels in the affected area, retraction (drawing back) of injured blood vessels, the deposition of **fibrin** (connective tissue), and the formation of blood clots in the area. The blood clots, formed from blood platelets, provide a matrix of fibrin that becomes the framework for cell repair. A scab also forms on the surface of the wound. Consisting of clots and dead and dying tissue, this scab serves to aid hemostasis and inhibit contamination of the wound by microorganisms. Below the scab, epithelial cells migrate into the wound from the edges. The epithelial cells serve as a barrier between the body and the environment, preventing the entry of microorganisms.

The inflammatory phase also involves vascular and cellular responses intended to remove any foreign substances and dead and dying tissues. The blood supply to the wound increases, bringing with it oxygen and nutrients needed in the healing process. The area appears reddened and edematous as a result. Exudate of fluid and cell debris is a normal accumulation and helps cleanse the wound. Overproduction of this exudate and other factors can im-

pair wound healing, especially in chronic wounds (Hanson, Langemo, Thompson, Anderson, & Hunter, 2005).

During cell migration, leukocytes (specifically, neutrophils) move into the interstitial space. These are replaced about 24 hours after injury by macrophages, which arise from the blood monocytes. These macrophages engulf microorganisms and cellular debris by a process known as **phagocytosis.** The macrophages also secrete an angiogenesis factor (AGF), which stimulates the formation of epithelial buds at the end of injured blood vessels. The microcirculatory network that results sustains the healing process and the wound during its life. This inflammatory response is essential to healing. Measures that impair inflammation, such as steroid medications, can place the healing process at risk.

Proliferative Phase

The *proliferative phase,* the second phase in healing, extends from day 3 or 4 to about day 21 postinjury. Fibroblasts (connective tissue cells), which migrate into the wound starting about

MediaLink
Integumentary Repair Animation

24 hours after injury, begin to synthesize collagen. **Collagen** is a whitish protein substance that adds tensile strength to the wound. As the amount of collagen increases, so does the strength of the wound; thus the chance that the wound will remain closed progressively increases. If the wound is sutured, a raised "healing ridge" appears under the intact suture line. In a wound that is not sutured, the new collagen is often visible.

Capillaries grow across the wound, increasing the blood supply. Fibroblasts move from the bloodstream into the wound, depositing fibrin. As the capillary network develops, the tissue becomes a translucent red color. This tissue, called **granulation tissue,** is fragile and bleeds easily.

When the skin edges of a wound are not sutured, the area must be filled in with granulation tissue. When the granulation tissue matures, marginal epithelial cells migrate to it, proliferating over this connective tissue base to fill the wound. If the wound does not close by epithelialization, the area becomes covered with dried plasma proteins and dead cells. This is called **eschar.** Initially, wounds healing by secondary intention seep blood-tinged (serosanguineous) drainage. Later, if they are not covered by epithelial cells, they become covered with thick, gray, fibrinous tissue that is eventually converted into dense scar tissue.

Maturation Phase

The *maturation phase* begins about day 21 and can extend 1 or 2 years after the injury. Fibroblasts continue to synthesize collagen. The collagen fibers themselves, which were initially laid in a haphazard fashion, reorganize into a more orderly structure. During maturation, the wound is remodeled and contracted. The scar becomes stronger but the repaired area is never as strong as the original tissue. In some individuals, particularly dark-skinned persons, an abnormal amount of collagen is laid down. This can result in a hypertrophic scar, or **keloid.**

One method of documenting the progress of healing in pressure ulcers is to use the Pressure Ulcer Scale for Healing (PUSH) tool (National Pressure Ulcer Advisory Panel [NPUAP], 2003). This well-validated tool (Figure 36-4 ■) assigns scores to the ulcer length, width, amount of exudate, and tissue type. The change in the total score over time can be used as an indication of healing.

Types of Wound Exudate

Exudate is material, such as fluid and cells, that has escaped from blood vessels during the inflammatory process and is deposited in tissue or on tissue surfaces. The nature and amount of exudate vary according to the tissue involved, the intensity and duration of the inflammation, and the presence of microorganisms.

There are three major types of exudate: serous, purulent, and sanguineous (hemorrhagic). A **serous exudate** consists chiefly of serum (the clear portion of the blood) derived from blood and the serous membranes of the body, such as the peritoneum. It looks watery and has few cells. An example is the fluid in a blister from a burn.

A **purulent exudate** is thicker than serous exudate because of the presence of **pus,** which consists of leukocytes, liquefied

dead tissue debris, and dead and living bacteria. The process of pus formation is referred to as **suppuration,** and the bacteria that produce pus are called **pyogenic bacteria.** Not all microorganisms are pyogenic. Purulent exudates vary in color, some acquiring tinges of blue, green, or yellow. The color may depend on the causative organism.

A **sanguineous (hemorrhagic) exudate** consists of large amounts of red blood cells, indicating damage to capillaries that is severe enough to allow the escape of red blood cells from plasma. This type of exudate is frequently seen in open wounds. Mixed types of exudates are often observed. A **serosanguineous** (consisting of clear and blood-tinged drainage) exudate is commonly seen in surgical incisions. A *purosanguineous* discharge (consisting of pus and blood) is often seen in a new wound that is infected.

> ### CLINICAL ALERT
>
> A bright sanguineous exudate indicates fresh bleeding, whereas dark sanguineous exudate denotes older bleeding. ■

Complications of Wound Healing

Several untoward events can interfere with the healing of a wound. These include hemorrhage, infection, and dehiscence and evisceration.

Hemorrhage

Some escape of blood from a wound is normal. **Hemorrhage** (massive bleeding), however, is abnormal. A dislodged clot, a slipped stitch, or erosion of a blood vessel may cause severe bleeding.

Internal hemorrhage may be detected by swelling or distention in the area of the wound and, possibly, by sanguineous drainage from a surgical drain. Some clients will have a **hematoma,** a localized collection of blood underneath the skin that may appear as a reddish blue swelling (bruise). A large hematoma may be dangerous in that it places pressure on blood vessels and can thus obstruct blood flow.

The risk of hemorrhage is greatest during the first 48 hours after surgery. Hemorrhage is an emergency; the nurse should apply pressure dressings to the area and monitor the client's vital signs. In many instances, the client must be taken to the operating room for surgical intervention.

Infection

Contamination of a wound surface with microorganisms (colonization) is an inevitable result. Because the colonizing organisms compete with new cells for oxygen and nutrition, and because their by-products can interfere with a healthy surface condition, the presence of contamination can impair wound healing and lead to infection. When the microorganisms colonizing the wound multiply excessively or invade tissues, infection occurs. Infection suggested by the presence of a change in wound color, pain, or drainage is confirmed by performing a culture of the wound (see Chapter 34 ∞). Severe infection causes fever and elevated white blood cell count. Clients who are immunosuppressed, such

Pressure Ulcer Scale for Healing (PUSH)
PUSH Tool 3.0

Patient Name _____ Patient ID# _____

Ulcer Location _____ Date _____

Directions:

Observe and measure the pressure ulcer. Categorize the ulcer with respect to surface area, exudate, and type of wound tissue. Record a sub-score for each of these ulcer characteristics. Add the sub-scores to obtain the total score. A comparison of total scores measured over time provides an indication of the improvement or deterioration in pressure ulcer healing.

LENGTH X WIDTH (in cm2)	0	1	2	3	4	5	Sub-score
	0	< 0.3	0.3 – 0.6	0.7 – 1.0	1.1 – 2.0	2.1 – 3.0	
		6	7	8	9	10	
		3.1 – 4.0	4.1 – 8.0	8.1 – 12.0	12.1 – 24.0	> 24.0	
EXUDATE AMOUNT	0 None	1 Light	2 Moderate	3 Heavy			Sub-score
TISSUE TYPE	0 Closed	1 Epithelial Tissue	2 Granulation Tissue	3 Slough	4 Necrotic Tissue		Sub-score
							TOTAL SCORE

Length x Width: Measure the greatest length (head to toe) and the greatest width (side to side) using a centimeter ruler. Multiply these two measurements (length x width) to obtain an estimate of surface area in square centimeters (cm2). Caveat: Do not guess! Always use a centimeter ruler and always use the same method each time the ulcer is measured.

Exudate Amount: Estimate the amount of exudate (drainage) present after removal of the dressing and before applying any topical agent to the ulcer. Estimate the exudate (drainage) as none, light, moderate, or heavy.

Tissue Type: This refers to the types of tissue that are present in the wound (ulcer) bed. Score as a "4" if there is any necrotic tissue present. Score as a "3" if there is any amount of slough present and necrotic tissue is absent. Score as a "2" if the wound is clean and contains granulation tissue. A superficial wound that is reepithelializing is scored as a "1." When the wound is closed, score as a "0."

  4 – Necrotic Tissue (Eschar): black, brown, or tan tissue that adheres firmly to the wound bed or ulcer edges and may be either firmer or softer than surrounding skin.

  3 – Slough: yellow or white tissue that adheres to the ulcer bed in strings or thick clumps, or is mucinous.

  2 – Granulation Tissue: pink or beefy red tissue with a shiny, moist, granular appearance.

  1 – Epithelial Tissue: for superficial ulcers, new pink or shiny tissue (skin) that grows in from the edges or as islands on the ulcer surface.

  0 – Closed/Resurfaced: the wound is completely covered with epithelium (new skin).

Figure 36-4 ■ Pressure Ulcer Scale for Healing (PUSH) Tool.

as those with HIV or receiving myelosuppressive treatment for cancer, are especially susceptible to wound infections.

A wound can be infected with microorganisms at the time of injury, during surgery, or postoperatively. Wounds that occur as a result of injury (e.g., bullet and knife wounds) are most likely to be contaminated at the time of injury. Surgery involving the intestines can also result in infection from the microorganisms inside the intestine. Surgical infection is most likely to become apparent 2 to 11 days postoperatively.

Dehiscence with Possible Evisceration

Dehiscence is the partial or total rupturing of a sutured wound. Dehiscence usually involves an abdominal wound in which the layers below the skin also separate. **Evisceration** is the protrusion of the internal viscera through an incision. A number of factors, including obesity, poor nutrition, multiple trauma, failure of suturing, excessive coughing, vomiting, and dehydration, heighten a client's risk of wound dehiscence. Wound dehiscence is more likely to occur 4 to 5 days postoperatively before extensive collagen is deposited in the wound.

Sudden straining, such as coughing or sneezing, may precede dehiscence. It is not unusual for a client to feel that "something has given away." When dehiscence or evisceration occurs, the wound should be quickly supported by large sterile dressings soaked in sterile normal saline. Place the client in bed with knees bent to decrease pull on the incision. The surgeon must be notified because immediate surgical repair of the area may be necessary.

Factors Affecting Wound Healing

Characteristics of the individual such as age, nutritional status, lifestyle, and medications influence the speed of wound healing.

Developmental Considerations

Healthy children and adults often heal more quickly than elders, who are more likely to have chronic diseases that hinder healing. For example, reduced liver function can impair the synthesis of blood clotting factors. Box 36–2 lists factors inhibiting wound healing in elders.

BOX 36–2 Factors Inhibiting Wound Healing in Elders

- Vascular changes associated with aging, such as atherosclerosis and atrophy of capillaries in the skin, can impair blood flow to the wound.
- Collagen tissue is less flexible, which increases the risk of damage from pressure, friction, and shearing.
- Scar tissue is less elastic.
- Changes in the immune system may reduce the formation of the antibodies and monocytes necessary for wound healing.
- Nutritional deficiencies may reduce the numbers of red blood cells and leukocytes, thus impeding the delivery of oxygen and the inflammatory response essential for wound healing. Oxygen is needed for the synthesis of collagen and the formation of new epithelial cells.
- Having diabetes or cardiovascular disease increases the risk of delayed healing due to impaired oxygen delivery to these tissues.
- Cell renewal is slower, leading to delayed healing.

Nutrition

Wound healing places additional demands on the body. Clients require a diet rich in protein, carbohydrates, lipids, vitamins A and C, and minerals, such as iron, zinc, and copper. Malnourished clients may require time to improve their nutritional status before surgery, if this is possible. Obese clients are at increased risk of wound infection and slower healing because adipose tissue usually has a minimal blood supply.

Lifestyle

People who exercise regularly tend to have good circulation and because blood brings oxygen and nourishment to the wound, they are more likely to heal quickly. Smoking reduces the amount of functional hemoglobin in the blood, thus limiting the oxygen-carrying capacity of the blood, and constricts arterioles.

Medications

Anti-inflammatory drugs (e.g., steroids and aspirin) and antineoplastic agents interfere with healing. Prolonged use of antibiotics may make a person susceptible to wound infection by resistant organisms.

NURSING MANAGEMENT

Assessing

Assessment of Skin Integrity

The nurse conducts an examination of the integument as part of a routine assessment and during regular care. Removing barriers to assessment is very important. Antiembolic stockings, braces, or devices must be removed to assess the skin condition underneath.

NURSING HISTORY AND PHYSICAL ASSESSMENT. During the review of systems as part of the nursing history, information regarding skin diseases, previous bruising, general skin condition, skin lesions, and usual healing of sores is elicited. Inspection and palpation of the skin focus on determination of skin color distribution, skin turgor, presence of edema, and characteristics of any lesions that are present. Particular attention is paid to skin condition in areas most likely to break down: in skin folds such as under the breasts, in areas that are frequently moist such as the perineum, and in areas that receive extensive pressure such as the bony prominences. Refer to Chapter 30 ∞ for further detail regarding skin assessment.

Assessment of Wounds

Nurses commonly assess both untreated and treated wounds. Although a pressure ulcer can be categorized as an untreated or treated wound, the specific assessment of pressure ulcers is discussed separately.

UNTREATED WOUNDS. Untreated wounds usually are seen shortly after an injury (e.g., at the scene of an accident or in an emergency center). Assessment for these wounds is shown in the accompanying Practice Guidelines. Guidelines for care follow:

- Control severe bleeding by (a) applying direct pressure over the wound and (b) elevating the involved extremity.

- Prevent infection by (a) cleaning or flushing abrasions or lacerations with normal saline and (b) covering the wound with a clean dressing, if possible (a sterile dressing is preferred). When applying a dressing, wrap the wound tightly enough to apply pressure and approximate the wound edges, if possible. If the first layer of dressing becomes saturated with blood, apply a second layer. Do so without removing the first layer of dressing, because blood clots might be disturbed, resulting in more bleeding.
- Control swelling and pain by applying ice over the wound and surrounding tissues.
- If bleeding is severe or if internal bleeding is suspected, and if emergency equipment is available, assess the client for signs of shock (rapid thready pulse, cold clammy skin, pallor, lowered blood pressure).

TREATED WOUNDS. Treated wounds, or sutured wounds, are usually assessed to determine the progress of healing. These wounds may be inspected during changing of a dressing. If the wound itself cannot be directly inspected, the dressing is inspected and other data regarding the wound (e.g., the presence of pain) are assessed.

Assessment of a treated wound involves observation of its appearance, size, drainage, and the presence of swelling, pain, and status of drains or tubes. In some long-term facilities, home care situations, and outpatient clinics, photographs are taken weekly for a visual record of the progress of pressure ulcers and wounds. Other assessments are documented and dated along with the photograph. Details about these assessments and signs of healing for a surgical incision are discussed with surgical wounds in Chapter 37. ∞

Estimating the amount of wound drainage can be difficult. One recommendation is to describe the degree to which the dressing is saturated. Minimal drainage only stains the dressing, moderate drainage saturates the dressing without leakage prior to scheduled dressing changes, and heavy drainage overflows the dressing prior to scheduled changes (Brown, 2006). These terms, plus the description of the drainage and the amount and type of dressing material used, should be well understood by all care providers.

PRACTICE GUIDELINES
Assessing Untreated Wounds

- Assess the location and extent of tissue damage (e.g., partial thickness or full thickness). Measure the wound length, width, and depth.
- Inspect the wound for bleeding. The amount of bleeding varies according to the type of wound and location. Penetrating wounds may cause internal bleeding.
- Inspect the wound for foreign bodies (soil, broken glass, shreds of cloth, or other foreign substances).
- Assess associated injuries such as fractures, internal bleeding, spinal cord injuries, or head trauma.
- If the wound is contaminated with foreign material, determine when the client last had a tetanus toxoid injection. A tetanus immunization or booster may be necessary.

Sometimes, the wound reaches under the skin surface (called undermining). The edges of the wound around an open center may be raw or appear healed, but the undermining can result in a sinus tract or tunnel that extends the wound many centimeters beyond the main wound surface. To fully assess the size of the wound, the nurse gently explores the undermined area with a thin, flexible probe. Do not use a cotton-tipped swab since it can leave fibers behind in the wound. Once the end of the tract is reached, gently raise the probe so that the bulge created by the end can be seen and its length measured on the skin surface. Sinus tracts are often caused by infection and have significant drainage. They may be treated using antibiotics, irrigation, surgical incision to open and drain the tract, or vacuum therapy for large tracts.

PRESSURE ULCERS. When a pressure ulcer is present, the nurse notes the following:

- Location of the ulcer, related to a bony prominence
- Size of ulcer in centimeters (Measure length, width, and depth, beginning with length [head to toe] and then width [side to side]. To measure depth, insert a sterile applicator swab at the deepest part of the wound, and then measure it against a measuring guide.)
- Presence of undermining or sinus tracts, assessed as face on a clock, 12 o'clock as the client's head
- Stage of the ulcer (see Figure 36-1)
- Color of the wound bed and location of necrosis (dead tissue) or eschar
- Condition of the wound margins
- Integrity of surrounding skin
- Clinical signs of infection, such as redness, warmth, swelling, pain, odor, and exudate (note color of exudate)

Document the status of the client's skin and wounds on the standard agency form (see Figure 36-5 ■ for an example). It is important to be able to determine how these change over time.

LABORATORY DATA. Laboratory data can often support the nurse's clinical assessment of the wound's progress in healing. A decreased leukocyte count can delay healing and increase the possibility of infection. A hemoglobin level below normal range indicates poor oxygen delivery to the tissues. Blood coagulation studies are also significant. Prolonged coagulation times can result in excessive blood loss and prolonged clot absorption. Hypercoagulability can lead to intravascular clotting. Intra-arterial clotting can result in a deficient blood supply to the wound area. Serum protein analysis provides an indication of the body's nutritional reserves for rebuilding cells. Albumin is an important indicator of nutritional status. A value below 3.5 g/dL indicates poor nutrition and may increase the risk of poor healing and infection. Wound cultures can either confirm or rule out the presence of infection. Sensitivity studies are helpful in the selection of appropriate antibiotic therapy. The nurse obtains a wound culture whenever an infection is suspected.

Skill 36-1 provides guidelines to obtain a specimen of wound drainage.

Description of Pressure Ulcers & Classification

Stage I: Characterized by erythema that does not resolve within minutes of pressure relief. Skin remains intact.

Stage II: Partial thickness loss of skin involving the epidermis or dermis – may involve both. The ulcer is superficial and may present as a blister, abrasion, or shallow crater. Free of eschar.

Stage III: Full thickness loss which goes through the dermis to the subcutaneous tissue but does not extend through the underlying fascia. Appears as a crater and may include undermining.

Stage IV: Full thickness skin loss with extensive damage through the subcutaneous tissue to the fascia and may involve muscle layers, joint, and/or bone.

1 cm   2 cm   3 cm   4 cm   5 cm

- IDENTIFY LOCATION OF ALL PRESSURE ULCERS ABOVE BY NUMBERING (1, 2, 3): IF MORE THAN 3, USE ADDITIONAL SHEET.

- COMPLETE CHART BELOW FOR SITE #1, USE REVERSE SIDE FOR SITES 2 & 3.

Pressure relief methods in use:

❏ Low Airloss Bed

❏ Low Airloss Mattress Overlay

❏ Turning Q2h when pt. supine and Q1h if HOB↑

❏ Pressure Reducing Mattress Overlay

❏ Other _____

Date MD notified of ulcer:

_____

Patient Admitted On: _____

Date Sheet Initiated: _____

DOCUMENT WEEKLY AND P.R.N. SIGNIFICANT CHANGE IN ULCER'S APPEARANCE

SITE #1: LOCATION	DESCRIBE TREATMENT:			FREQUENCY:
DATE / TIME				
DIMENSIONS: LENGTH (in. cm.)				
WIDTH				
DEPTH				
ODOR (None or Foul)				
DESCRIBE DRAINAGE (Purulent, Serous, Serosanguinous) & AMOUNT (Scant, Moderate, Copious)				
STAGE (See Above)				
COMMENTARY: i.e. Describe tissue surrounding ulcer: is there undermining? % necrotic vs % granular, etc.				
NURSE				

Figure 36-5 ■ Wound/skin documentation sheet.

OBTAINING A WOUND DRAINAGE SPECIMEN FOR CULTURE

PURPOSES
- To identify the microorganisms potentially causing an infection and the antibiotics to which they are sensitive
- To evaluate the effectiveness of antibiotic therapy

ASSESSMENT
Assess
- Appearance of the wound and surrounding tissue. Check the character and amount of wound drainage.
- Client complaints of pain or discomfort at the wound site.
- Signs of infection such as fever, chills, or elevated white blood cell count (WBC).

PLANNING
Before obtaining a specimen of wound drainage, determine (a) whether the wound should be cleaned prior to obtaining the specimen and (b) whether the site from which to take the specimen has been specified.

Delegation
Obtaining a wound culture is an invasive procedure that requires the application of sterile technique, knowledge of wound healing, and potential problem solving to ensure client safety; therefore, the nurse needs to perform this skill and does not delegate it to unlicensed assistive personnel (UAP).

Equipment
- Personal protective equipment, goggles, and gown
- Clean gloves
- Sterile gloves
- Moisture-proof bag
- Sterile dressing set
- Normal saline and irrigating syringe
- Culture tube with swab and culture medium (aerobic and anaerobic tubes are available) and/or sterile syringe with needle for anaerobic culture
- Completed labels for each container
- Completed requisition to accompany the specimens to the laboratory

IMPLEMENTATION
Preparation
Check the medical orders to determine if the specimen is to be collected for an **aerobic** (growing only in the presence of oxygen) or **anaerobic** (growing only in the absence of oxygen) culture. Aerobic organisms are generally found on the surface of the wound, whereas anaerobic organisms would be found in deep wounds, tunnels, and cavities. Administer an analgesic 30 minutes before the procedure if the client is complaining of pain at the wound site.

Performance
1. Prior to performing the procedure, introduce self and verify the client's identity using agency protocol. Explain to the client what you are going to do, why it is necessary, and how he or she can cooperate. Discuss how the results will be used in planning further care or treatments.
2. Perform hand hygiene and observe appropriate infection control procedures (e.g., gloves).
3. Provide for client privacy.
4. Remove any moist outer dressings that cover the wound.
   - Put on clean gloves.
   - Remove the outer dressing, and observe any drainage on the dressing. Hold the dressing so that the client does not see the drainage. **Rationale:** *The appearance of the drainage could upset the client.*
   - Determine the amount of the drainage, for example, "one 2 × 2 gauze saturated with pale yellow drainage."
   - Discard the dressing in the moisture-proof bag. Handle it carefully so that the dressing does not touch the outside of the bag. **Rationale:** *Touching the outside of the bag will contaminate it.*
   - Remove your gloves and dispose of them properly.
5. Open the sterile dressing set using sterile technique (see Skill 31-3 ∞).
6. Assess the wound.
   - Put on sterile gloves (see Skill 31-4 ∞).
   - Assess the appearance of the tissues in and around the wound and the drainage. Infection can cause reddened tissues with a thick discharge, which may be foul smelling, whitish, or colored.
7. Cleanse the wound.
   - Using gauze swabs or irrigation (see Skill 36-2 later in this chapter) cleanse the wound with normal saline until all exudate has been removed.
   - After cleansing, apply a sterile gauze pad to the wound. **Rationale:** *This absorbs excess cleansing solution.*
   - If a topical antimicrobial ointment or cream is being used to treat the wound, use a swab to remove it. **Rationale:** *Residual antiseptic must be removed prior to culture.*
   - Remove and discard sterile gloves.
8. Obtain the aerobic culture.
   - Open a specimen tube and place the cap upside down on a firm, dry surface so that the inside will not become contaminated, or if the swab is attached to the lid, twist the cap to loosen the swab. Hold the tube in one hand and take out the swab in the other. ❶

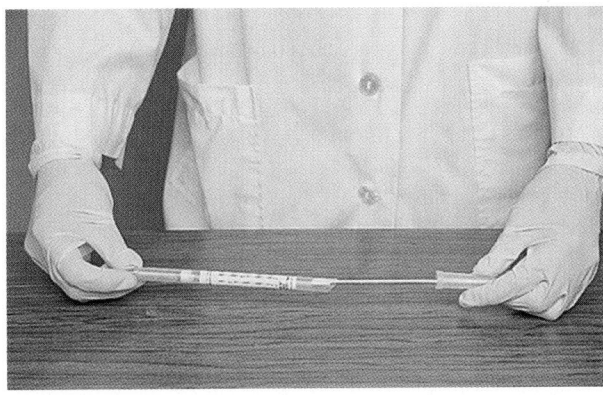

❶ A culturette tube for a wound specimen.

continued on page 916

OBTAINING A WOUND DRAINAGE SPECIMEN FOR CULTURE *continued*

- Rotate the swab back and forth over clean areas of granulation tissue from the sides or base of the wound. **Rationale:** *Microorganisms most likely to be responsible for a wound infection reside in viable tissue.*
- Do not use pus or pooled exudates to culture. **Rationale:** *These secretions contain a mixture of contaminants that are not the same as those causing the infection.*
- Avoid touching the swab to intact skin at the wound edges. **Rationale:** *This prevents the introduction of superficial skin organisms into the culture.*
- Return the swab to the culture tube, taking care not to touch the top or the outside of the tube. **Rationale:** *The outside of the container must remain free of pathogenic microorganisms to prevent their spread to others.*
- Crush the inner ampule containing the medium for organism growth at the bottom of the tube. **Rationale:** *This ensures that the swab with the specimen is surrounded by culture medium.*
- Twist the cap to secure.
- If a specimen is required from another site, repeat the steps. Specify the exact site (e.g., inferior drain site or lower aspect of incision) on the label of each container. Be sure to put each swab in the appropriately labeled tube.
9. Dress the wound.
 - Apply any ordered medication to the wound.
 - Cover the wound with a sterile wound dressing. See Table 36–5 for selecting a wound dressing.
10. Arrange for the specimen to be transported to the laboratory immediately. Be sure to include the completed requisition.

11. Document all relevant information.
 - Record on the client's chart the taking of the specimen and source.
 - Include the date and time; the appearance of the wound; the color, consistency, amount, and odor of any drainage; the type of culture collected; and any discomfort experienced by the client.

SAMPLE DOCUMENTATION

5/27/07 1000 Specimen from ® hip to lab for anaerobic culture. Pressure ulcer 3x3 cm, 6 mm deep, draining minimal amt. thick yellow. No odor. Skin around wound erythematous. Pain 0 on 0-10 scale. ———————— N. Jamaghani, RN

VARIATION: OBTAINING A SPECIMEN FOR ANAEROBIC CULTURE

- Insert a sterile 10-mL syringe (without needle) into the wound, and aspirate 1 to 5 mL of drainage into the syringe.
- Attach the needle to the syringe, and expel all air from the syringe and needle.
- Immediately inject the drainage into the anaerobic culture tube and cap the tube tightly.
or
- Use an anaerobic culture swab system in which the swab is immediately placed into a tube filled with an oxygen-free gas or gel environment.
- Label the tube or syringe appropriately.
- Send the tube or syringe of drainage to the laboratory immediately. Do not refrigerate the specimen.

EVALUATION
- Compare findings of wound assessment and drainage to previous assessments to determine any changes.
- Report the culture results to the primary care provider.
- Conduct appropriate follow-up such as administering antibiotics or modifying wound treatment as ordered.

Diagnosing

The NANDA nursing diagnoses (2007) that relate to clients who have skin wounds or who are at risk for skin breakdown are

- *Risk for Impaired Skin Integrity:* At risk for skin being adversely altered.
- *Impaired Skin Integrity:* Altered epidermis and/or dermis.
- *Impaired Tissue Integrity:* Damage to mucous membrane, corneal, integumentary, or subcutaneous tissues.

Impaired Skin Integrity commonly applies to pressure ulcers and to wounds extending through the epidermis but not through the dermis. *Impaired Tissue Integrity* applies to pressure ulcers and to wounds extending into subcutaneous tissue, muscle, or bone. Examples of clinical applications of these diagnoses using NANDA, NIC, and NOC designations are shown in Identifying Nursing Diagnoses, Outcomes, and Interventions.

Additional nursing diagnoses may be appropriate for clients with existing impaired skin or tissue integrity. Examples of these diagnoses include

- *Risk for Infection* if the skin impairment is severe, the client is immunosuppressed, or the wound is caused by trauma.

- *Pain* related to nerve involvement within the tissue impairment or as a consequence of procedures used to treat the wound.

Planning

The major goals for clients at *Risk for Impaired Skin Integrity* (pressure ulcer development) are to maintain skin integrity and to avoid potential associated risks. Clients with *Impaired Skin Integrity* need goals to demonstrate progressive wound healing and regain intact skin within a specified time frame (see Identifying Nursing Diagnoses, Outcomes, and Interventions).

Planning for Home Care

Increasingly, wound care is provided in the home rather than in health care facilities. The client and family assume much of the responsibility for assessing and treating existing wounds and for helping to prevent pressure ulcers. The accompanying Home Care Assessment feature outlines appropriate assessment for clients who have wounds or pressure ulcers or are at risk for developing pressure ulcers. In planning for client discharge, nurses are accountable for teaching the client and family wound preventive and care measures. See Client Teaching for a model.

IDENTIFYING NURSING DIAGNOSES, OUTCOMES, AND INTERVENTIONS
Clients At Risk for or With Impaired Skin Integrity

DATA CLUSTER Juanita Perez, an 85-year-old, is pale, emaciated, and listless. Weight 90 lb. is incontinent of urine and stool, and is bedridden.

NURSING DIAGNOSIS/ DEFINITION	SAMPLE DESIRED OUTCOMES*/ DEFINITION	INDICATORS	SELECTED INTERVENTIONS*/ DEFINITION	SAMPLE NIC ACTIVITIES
Risk for Impaired Skin Integrity related to incontinence and immobility/ *At risk for skin being adversely altered*	Tissue Integrity: Skin and Mucous Membranes [1101]/ *Structural intactness and normal physiological function of skin and mucous membranes*	Mildly compromised ■ Elasticity. None ■ Skin lesions	Positioning [0840]/*Deliberative placement of the patient or a body part to promote physiological and/or psychological well-being.* Pressure Ulcer Prevention [3540]/ *Prevention of pressure ulcers for an individual at high risk for developing them*	■ Explain to the client that she is going to be turned (and how often) ■ Position in proper body alignment ■ Place on an appropriate therapeutic mattress or bed ■ Document skin status at least each shift ■ Remove moisture from the skin caused by urinary and fecal incontinence ■ Apply protective barriers such as creams or pads to absorb excess moisture

DATA CLUSTER Matthew Brown, an obese 70-year-old hemiplegic, complains of discomfort in his left heel after attempting to move in bed. Superficial skin abrasion 1.2 cm in diameter present at base of left heel.

Impaired Skin Integrity (stage II pressure ulcer) related to friction/*Altered epidermis and/or dermis*	Wound Healing: Secondary Intention [1103]/*Extent of regeneration of cells and tissues in an open wound*	Substantial ■ Granulation ■ Decreased wound size	Pressure Ulcer Care [3520]/*Facilitation of healing in pressure ulcers*	■ Cleanse the skin around the ulcer with mild soap and water at least daily ■ Note characteristics of any drainage ■ Ensure adequate nutrition ■ Apply a transparent wound barrier ■ Use devices on the bed that protect the individual

*The NOC # for desired outcomes and the NIC # for nursing interventions are listed in brackets following the appropriate outcome or intervention. Outcomes, indicators, interventions, and activities selected are only a sample of those suggested by NOC and NIC and should be further individualized for each client.

HOME CARE ASSESSMENT
Wound Care and Prevention of Pressure Ulcers

CLIENT AND ENVIRONMENT
■ *Current level of knowledge:* Understanding of the cause of the wound or risk for developing a pressure ulcer; prevention or treatment strategies
■ *Self-care abilities for mobility:* Physical ability to change position, ambulate, and transfer including the use of assistive devices
■ *Self-care abilities for wound care:* Manual dexterity and visual acuity necessary to perform skin assessments and wound treatments
■ *Facilities:* Presence of running water, garbage, bathroom needed to perform wound care and contain potentially infectious materials
■ *Current level of nutrition:* Eating habits and preferences, laboratory values indicating need for teaching or other intervention

FAMILY
■ *Caregiver availability, skills, and responses:* Understanding of the cause of the wound or risk for developing a pressure ulcer; preven-

tion or treatment strategies; willingness to assist with wound care and actions to prevent pressure ulcers
■ *Family role changes and coping:* Effect on financial status, parenting and spousal roles, sexuality, social roles
■ *Alternate potential primary or respite caregivers:* For example, other family members, volunteers, church members, paid caregivers or housekeeping services; available community respite care (adult day care, senior centers, etc.)

COMMUNITY
■ *Resources:* Availability and familiarity with possible sources of assistance such as equipment and supply companies, organizations that offer medical supplies or financial assistance, home health agencies

A critical pathway can also be useful for planning client care at home (see the example below).

Implementing

Nursing interventions for maintaining skin integrity and wound care involve supporting wound healing, preventing pressure ul-

cers, treating pressure ulcers, dressing and cleaning wounds, applying heat and cold, and supporting and immobilizing wounds.

Supporting Wound Healing

The four major areas in which nurses can help clients develop optimal conditions for wound healing are maintaining moist

---

CLIENT TEACHING   Skin Integrity

MAINTAINING INTACT SKIN
- Discuss relationship between adequate nutrition (especially fluids, protein, vitamins B and C, iron, and calories) and healthy skin.
- Demonstrate appropriate positions for pressure relief.
- Establish a turning or repositioning schedule.
- Demonstrate application of appropriate skin protection agents and devices.
- Instruct to report persistent reddened areas.
- Identify potential sources of skin trauma and means of avoidance.

PROMOTING WOUND HEALING
- Discuss importance of adequate nutrition (especially fluids, protein, vitamins B and C, iron, and calories).

- Instruct in wound assessment and provide mechanism for documenting.
- Emphasize principles of asepsis, especially hand hygiene and proper methods of handling used dressings.
- Provide information about signs of wound infection and other complications to report.
- Reinforce appropriate aspects of pressure ulcer prevention.
- Demonstrate wound care techniques such as wound cleansing and dressing changing.
- Discuss pain control measures, if needed.

CRITICAL PATHWAY   Wound Management

ASSESSMENT DATA *Nursing Assessment for José Alonzo*

José Alonzo is a 42-year-old construction worker who was injured at work when a wheelbarrow filled with cement rolled into him and pushed him off a 4-foot ledge. He suffered several bruises and one 9-cm (3.5-in.) laceration on the anterior aspect of the lower left leg. The laceration was covered with a sterile compression dressing at the scene by paramedics. Prior to irrigation and cleansing with normal saline, the wound contained particles of cement and dirt. Marcella James, a nurse practitioner, sutured the wound with silk suture and discharged Mr. Alonzo. Mr. Alonzo is to return to the outpatient clinic

for suture removal in 10 days. He asks the nurse whether he can use an aloe herbal ointment on the wound and drink a healing herbal tea that his wife makes.

Physical Examination
Height: 177.8 cm (5'10")
Weight: 72.7 kg (160 lb)
Temperature: 37°C (98.6°F)
Pulse rate: 88 bpm
Respirations: 24/min
Blood pressure: 136/90 mm Hg

EXPECTED LENGTH OF TREATMENT: 7 to 10 Days

Outcomes	Client verbalizes understanding of teaching, including wound care, signs and symptoms to report, follow-up care.	At time of suture removal • Client is afebrile. • Client has a dry, clean wound with edges well approximated, healing by first intention.
	Date _____ Outpatient setting	Date _____ Daily for 10 days (Client activities)
Deficient Knowledge	Provide simple, brief instructions regarding injury and treatment. Encourage client to ask questions and seek assistance. Assess the client's knowledge about wound care. Review written instruction sheet for wound care with client and provide copy.	Follow written discharge teaching regarding wound care and dressing change. Call primary care provider with questions or problems and return to office in 10 days for suture removal.
Diet	Instruct client about foods high in protein and vitamin C and encourage adequate intake.	Diet high in protein and vitamin C. Cultural remedies that will not interfere with healing.
Wound care	Irrigate and clean the wound with normal saline. Surgical consultation for wound closure. Following wound closure, apply dry sterile dressing.	Change dressing daily and prn to keep dressing dry and clean. Inspect wound daily and report any signs and symptoms of infection (redness, pain, warmth, drainage, swelling, or fever).
Medications	Tetanus toxoid if indicated.	Only if ordered.

wound healing, providing sufficient nutrition and hydration, preventing wound infections, and proper positioning.

MOIST WOUND HEALING. The dressing and frequency of change should support moist wound bed conditions. Wound beds that are too dry or disturbed too often fail to heal.

NUTRITION AND FLUIDS. Clients should be assisted to take in at least 2,500 mL of fluids a day unless conditions contraindicate this amount. Although there is no evidence that excessive doses of vitamins or minerals enhance wound healing, adequate amounts are extremely important. The nurse should ensure that clients receive sufficient protein, vitamins C, A, B_1, and B_5, and zinc. Obtaining a registered dietitian consultation for wound healing nutrition is helpful for ensuring that correct supplementation needs are met.

PREVENTING INFECTION. There are two main aspects to controlling wound infection: preventing microorganisms from entering the wound, and preventing the transmission of bloodborne pathogens to or from the client to others. See Table 36–3, and see Chapter 31 ∞ for more information about infection control.

POSITIONING. To promote wound healing, clients must be positioned to keep pressure off the wound (sometimes referred to as *off-loading*). Changes of position and transfers can be accomplished without shear or friction damage. In addition to proper positioning, the client should be assisted to be as mobile as possible because activity enhances circulation. If the client cannot move independently, range-of-motion exercises and a turning schedule are implemented.

Preventing Pressure Ulcers

To reduce the likelihood of pressure ulcer development in all clients, the nurse employs a variety of preventive measures (i.e., skin hygiene and pressure relief devices) to maintain the skin integrity and instructs the client, support people, and caregivers in how to prevent pressure ulcers.

TABLE 36–3 Guidelines for Preventing Infection and the Transmission of Bloodborne Pathogens

Standard Precautions
- Wear gloves when touching blood and body fluids, mucous membranes, or nonintact skin of all clients, and when handling items or surfaces soiled with blood or body fluids.
- Wash hands thoroughly after removing gloves, and if contaminated with blood or body fluids.

Wound Care
- Wash hands before and after caring for wounds.
- Wear gloves, surgical masks, and protective eyewear as appropriate if procedures commonly cause droplets or splashing of blood or body fluids (e.g., wound irrigation).
- Touch an open or fresh surgical wound only when wearing sterile gloves or using a sterile instrument.
- Remove or change dressings over closed wounds when they become wet.

PROVIDING NUTRITION. Because an inadequate intake of calories, protein, vitamins, and iron is believed to be a risk factor for pressure ulcer development, nutritional supplements should be considered for nutritionally compromised clients. The diet should be similar to that which supports wound healing, as discussed earlier. Monitor weight regularly to help assess nutritional status. Pertinent lab work should also be monitored including lymphocyte count, protein (especially albumin), and hemoglobin.

MAINTAINING SKIN HYGIENE. Obtain baseline data using the established tool and then reassess the skin at least daily in the hospital and weekly at home. When bathing the client, the nurse should minimize the force and friction applied to the skin, using mild cleansing agents that minimize irritation and dryness and that do not disrupt the skin's "natural barriers." Also, avoid using hot water, which increases skin dryness and irritation. Nurses can minimize dryness by avoiding exposure to cold and low humidity. Dry skin is best treated with moisturizing lotions applied while the skin is moist after bathing. The client's skin should be kept clean and dry and free of irritation and maceration by urine, feces, sweat, or incomplete drying after a bath. Apply skin protection if indicated. Dimethicone-based creams or alcohol-free barrier films are available in liquid, spray, and moist wipe format and are very effective in preventing moisture or drainage from collecting on the skin. In most cases, the nurse can apply these without a primary care provider's order. Petroleum-based creams and ointments are no longer advised related to poor overall skin protection and interference with diaper/incontinence product absorption.

In addition, massage over bony prominences should be avoided. Traditionally, nurses have used massage to stimulate blood circulation, with the intention of preventing pressure ulcers. However, scientific evidence does not support this belief. In fact, vigorous massage may lead to deep tissue trauma (Folkedahl & Frantz, 2002a; NPUAP, 2001).

AVOIDING SKIN TRAUMA. Providing the client with a smooth, firm, and wrinkle-free foundation on which to sit or lie helps prevent skin trauma. To prevent injury due to friction and shearing forces, clients must be positioned, transferred, and turned correctly. For bedridden clients, shearing force can be reduced by elevating the head of the bed to no more than 30 degrees, if this position is not contraindicated by the client's condition. (For example, clients with respiratory disorders may find it easier to breathe in Fowler's position.) When the head of the bed is raised, the skin and superficial fascia stick to the bed linen while the deep fascia and skeleton slide down toward the bottom of the bed. As a result, blood vessels in the sacral area become twisted, and the tissues in the area can become ischemic and necrotic. Baby powder and cornstarch are never used as friction or moisture prevention. These powders create harmful abrasive grit damaging to tissues and are considered a respiratory hazard when airborne. Instead, use moisturizing creams and protective films, such as transparent dressings and alcohol-free barrier films.

Frequent shifts in position, even if only slight, effectively change pressure points. The client should shift weight 10 to 15 degrees every 15 to 30 minutes and, whenever possible, exercise or ambulate to stimulate blood circulation.

When lifting a client to change position, nurses should use a lifting device such as a trapeze rather than dragging the client across or up in bed. The friction that results from dragging the skin against a sheet can cause blisters and abrasions, which may contribute to more extensive tissue damage. Therefore, using devices that lift the client's weight off the bed surface is the method of choice.

Any at-risk client confined to bed—even when a special support mattress is used—should be repositioned at least every 2 hours, depending on the client's need, to allow another body surface to bear the weight. Six body positions can usually be used: prone, supine, right and left lateral (side-lying), and right and left Sims' positions. When a lateral position is used, the nurse should avoid positioning the client directly on the trochanter and instead position the client on a 30-degree angle. A written schedule should be established for turning and repositioning.

PROVIDING SUPPORTIVE DEVICES. In order for circulation to remain uncompromised, pressure on the bony prominences should remain below capillary pressure for as much time as possible through a combination of turning, positioning, and use of pressure-relieving surfaces. Mean capillary pressure can be estimated at 20 mm Hg although this varies. Although some research has been conducted evaluating the effectiveness of pressure-reducing support surfaces in preventing pressure ulcers in clients at low, intermediate, or high risk, the results are often inconclusive (Cullum, McInnes, Bell-Syer, & Legood, 2005). The nurse should review the manufacturer's product descriptions that report the amount of time that the pressure between the surface and the bony prominence is above or below specified levels and determine if this is adequate to protect a particular client.

For clients confined to bed, three types of support surfaces can be used to relieve pressure. The overlay mattress is applied on top of the standard bed mattress. A replacement mattress is used instead of the standard mattress; most are made of foam and gel combinations. Specialty beds replace hospital beds. They provide pressure relief, eliminate shearing and friction, and decrease moisture. Examples are high-air-loss beds, low-air-loss beds, and beds that provide kinetic therapy. Kinetic beds provide continuous passive motion or oscillation therapy, which is intended to counteract the effects of a client's immobility. Table 36–4 lists selected mechanical devices for reducing pressure on body parts.

When a client is confined to bed or to a chair, pressure-reducing devices, such as pillows made of foam, gel, air, or a combination of these, can be used. When the client is sitting, weight should be distributed over the entire seating surface so that pressure does not center on just one area. To protect a client's heels in bed, supports such as wedges or pillows can be used to raise the heels completely off the bed. Doughnut-type devices should not be used since they limit blood flow and can cause tissue damage to the areas in direct contact with the device.

Treating Pressure Ulcers

Pressure ulcers are a challenge for nurses because of the number of variables involved (e.g., risk factors, types of ulcers, and degrees of impairment) and the numerous treatment measures advocated. Existing and potential infections are the most serious complications of pressure ulcers. In treating pressure ulcers, nurses should follow the agency protocols and the primary care provider's orders, if any. Prompt treatment can prevent further tissue damage and pain and facilitate wound healing. See the accompanying Practice Guidelines regarding treating pressure ulcers.

THE RYB COLOR CODE. To guide wound care, the nurse can use the RYB color code of wounds. This concept is based on the color of an open wound—red, yellow, or black (RYB)—rather than the depth or size of a wound. On this scheme, the goals of wound care are to protect (cover) red, cleanse yellow, and debride black.

Wounds that are red are usually in the late regeneration phase of tissue repair (i.e., developing granulation tissue). They need to be protected to avoid disturbance to regenerating tissue. The nurse protects red wounds by (a) gentle cleansing (i.e., use of a noncytotoxic wound cleanser applied without pressure), (b) protecting periwound skin with alcohol-free barrier film, (c) filling dead space with hydrogel or alginate, (d) covering with an appropriate dressing such as transparent film, hydrocolloid dressing, or a clear absorbent acrylic dressing, and (e) changing the dressing as infrequently as possible.

Yellow wounds are characterized primarily by liquid to semiliquid "slough" that is often accompanied by purulent

---

PRACTICE GUIDELINES   Treating Pressure Ulcers

- Minimize direct pressure on the ulcer. Reposition the client at least every 2 hours. Make a schedule, and record position changes on the client's chart. Provide devices to minimize or float pressure areas.
- Clean the pressure ulcer with every dressing change. The method of cleaning depends on the stage of the ulcer, products available, and agency protocol. Skill 36-2 details the steps involved in irrigating a wound.

- Clean and dress the ulcer using surgical asepsis. Never use alcohol or hydrogen peroxide as they are cytotoxic to tissue beds.
- If the pressure ulcer is infected, obtain a sample of the drainage for culture and sensitivity to antibiotic agents (see Skill 36-1).
- Teach the client to move, even if only slightly, to relieve pressure.
- Provide range-of-motion (ROM) exercises and mobility out of bed as the client's condition permits.

TABLE 36–4 **Mechanical Devices for Reducing Pressure on Body Parts**

DEVICE	DESCRIPTION/COMMENTS
Gel flotation pads	Polyvinyl, silicone, or Silastic pads filled with a gelatinous substance similar to fat.
Pillows and wedges (foam, gel, air, fluid)	Supports positioning and offloads bone on bone contact.
Heel protectors (sheepskin boots, padded splints, off-loading inflatable boots, foam blocks)	Can raise or "float" a body part (e.g., heels) off the or surface. Prevent shearing and limit pressure on heel area. (Figure 36-6 ■).
Memory foam mattress/ chair pad	Polyurethane foam mattress distributes weight over bony areas evenly. Foam molds to the body.
Alternating pressure mattress	Composed of a number of cells in which the pressure alternately increases and decreases; uses a pump (see Figure 36-7 ■).
Water bed	Support surface filled with water. Water temperature can be controlled.
Static low-air-loss (LAL) bed	Consists of many air-filled cushions divided into four or five sections. Separate controls permit each section to be inflated to a different level of firmness; thus pressure can be reduced on bony prominences but increased under other body areas for support (see Figure 36-8 ■).
Active or second-generation LAL bed	Like the static LAL, but in addition gently pulsates or rotates from side to side, thus stimulating capillary blood flow and facilitating movement of pulmonary secretions.
Air-fluidized (AF) bed (static high-air-loss bed)	Forced temperature-controlled air is circulated around millions of tiny silicone-coated beads, producing a fluidlike movement. Provides uniform support to body contours. Decreases skin maceration by its drying effect. Moisture from the client penetrates the linens and soaks the beads. Air flow forces the beads away from the client and rapidly dries the sheet. A major disadvantage is that the head of the bed cannot be elevated. Some beds are a unique combination of air fluidized therapy and low air loss therapy on an articulating frame. These are used with patients who require head elevation (see Figure 36-9 ■).

Figure 36-6 ■ Heel protector.
(Courtesy of Gaymar Industries, Inc.)

Figure 36-7 ■ Alternating pressure mattress.
(Courtesy of Ease)

Figure 36-8 ■ Low-air-loss bed.
(KinAir MedSurg® Courtesy of KCI Licensing, Inc., San Antonio, TX).

Figure 36-9 ■ Low-air-loss and air-fluidized combo bed (Clinitron/Rite Hite).
Courtesy of Hill-Rom Services, Inc. Reprinted with permission. All rights reserved.

drainage or previous infection. The nurse cleanses yellow wounds to remove nonviable tissue. Methods used may include applying moist-to-moist normal saline dressings, irrigating the wound, using absorbent dressing materials such as impregnated hydrogel or alginate dressings, and consulting with the primary care provider about the need for a topical antimicrobial to minimize bacterial growth.

Black wounds are covered with thick necrotic tissue, or eschar. Black wounds require **debridement** (removal of the necrotic material). Removal of nonviable tissue from a wound must occur before the wound can be staged or heal. Debridement may be achieved in four different ways: sharp, mechanical, chemical, and autolytic. In *sharp debridement,* a scalpel or scissors is used to separate and remove dead tissue. In many settings, specially trained nurses (wound ostomy continence nurses [WOCNs]), physical therapists, and physician's assistants are permitted to perform sharp debridement. *Mechanical debridement* is accomplished through scrubbing force or moist-to-moist dressings. *Chemical debridement* is more selective than sharp or mechanical techniques. Collagenase enzyme agents such as papain-urea are currently most recommended for this use. In *autolytic debridement,* dressings that contain wound moisture, such as hydrocolloid and clear absorbent acrylic dressings, trap the wound drainage against the eschar. The body's own enzymes in the drainage break down the necrotic tissue. Although this method takes longer than the other three, it is the most selective and therefore causes the least damage to healthy surrounding and healing tissues. Recently, the use of fly larvae (maggots, *Phaenicia sericata*) has received increased attention. Larval therapy can be extremely effective in cleansing chronic wounds because the maggots secrete enzymes that break down necrotic tissue (while leaving healthy tissue untouched), eat bacteria, and decrease bacterial growth through the rise in surface pH that results from their presence (Sosin, 2005).

When the eschar is removed, the wound is treated as yellow, then red. When more than one color is present, the nurse treats the most serious color first, that is, black, then yellow, then red.

Dressing Wounds

Dressings are applied for the following purposes:

- To protect the wound from mechanical injury
- To protect the wound from microbial contamination
- To provide or maintain moist wound healing
- To provide thermal insulation
- To absorb drainage or debride a wound or both
- To prevent hemorrhage (when applied as a pressure dressing or with elastic bandages)
- To splint or immobilize the wound site and thereby facilitate healing and prevent injury

TYPES OF DRESSINGS. Various dressing materials are available to cover wounds. The type of dressing used depends on (a) the location, size, and type of the wound; (b) the amount of exudate; (c) whether the wound requires debridement or is infected; and (d) such considerations as frequency of dressing change, ease or difficulty of dressing application, and cost (Table 36–5).

Transparent Dressings. Transparent dressings are often applied to wounds including ulcerated or burned skin areas. These dressings offer several advantages:

- They act as temporary skin.
- They are nonporous, nonabsorbent, self-adhesive dressings that do not require changing as other dressings do. They are often left in place until healing has occurred or as long as they remain intact.
- Because they are transparent, the wound can be assessed through them.
- Because they are semi-occlusive, the wound remains moist and can retain a small amount of serous exudate, which promotes epithelial growth, hastens healing, and reduces the risk of infection.
- Because they are elastic, they can be placed over a joint without disrupting the client's mobility.
- They adhere only to the skin area around the wound and not to the wound itself because they keep the wound moist.
- They allow the client to shower or bathe without removing the dressing.

Hydrocolloid Dressings. Hydrocolloid dressings (see Table 36–5) are frequently used over pressure ulcers. These dressings offer several advantages:

- They last 3 to 7 days.
- They do not need a "cover" dressing and are water resistant, so the client can shower or bathe.
- They can be molded to uneven body surfaces.
- They act as temporary skin and provide an effective bacterial barrier.
- They decrease pain and thus reduce the need for analgesics.
- They absorb moderate drainage and therefore can be used on slowly draining wounds.
- They contain wound odor.

These dressings have certain limitations, however:

- They are occlusive, are opaque, and obscure wound visibility.
- They have a limited absorption capacity.
- They can facilitate anaerobic bacterial growth.
- They can soften and wrinkle at the edges with wear and movement.
- They can be difficult to remove and may leave a residue on the skin.

Because of these limitations, hydrocolloid dressings should not be used for infected wounds or those with deep tracts or *fistulas* (abnormal passage that develops between a hollow organ and the skin or between two hollow organs).

Securing Dressings. The nurse tapes the dressing over the wound, ensuring that the dressing covers the entire wound and does not become dislodged. The correct type of tape must be selected for the purpose. The nurse follows these steps:

1. Place the tape so that the dressing cannot be folded back to expose the wound. Place strips at the ends of the dressing, and space tapes evenly in the middle (see Figure 36-10 ■, *A*).

TABLE 36–5 Selected Types of Wound Dressings

DRESSING	DESCRIPTION	PURPOSE	INDICATIONS	EXAMPLES
Transparent film	Adhesive plastic, semipermeable, nonabsorbent dressings allow exchange of oxygen between the atmosphere and wound bed. They are impermeable to bacteria and water.	To provide protection against contamination and friction; to maintain a clean moist surface that facilitates cellular migration; to provide insulation by preventing fluid evaporation; and to facilitate wound assessment	IV dressing Central line dressing Superficial wounds Pressure ulcers Stage I	Tegaderm, Bioclusive. Op-Site
Impregnated nonadherent	Woven or nonwoven cotton or synthetic materials are impregnated with petrolatum, saline, zinc-saline, antimicrobials, or other agents. Require secondary dressings to secure them in place, retain moisture, and provide wound protection.	To cover, soothe, and protect partial- and full-thickness wounds without exudate	Postoperative dressing over staple/sutures Superficial burns	Adaptic, Carrasyn, Xeroform dressings
Hydrocolloids	Waterproof adhesive wafers, pastes, or powders. Wafers, designed to be worn for up to 7 days, consist of two layers. The inner adhesive layer has particles that absorb exudates and form a hydrated gel over the wound; the outer film provides an occlusive seal.	To absorb exudate; to produce a moist environment that facilitates healing but does not cause maceration of surrounding skin; to protect the wound from bacterial contamination, foreign debris, and urine or feces; and to prevent shearing	Pressure ulcers Stage II–IV Autolytic debridement of eschar Partial-thickness wounds	Tegasorb DuoDerm, Comfeel, Restore, Replicare
Clear absorbent acrylic	Transparent absorbent wafer designed to be worn 5–7 days. The acrylic layer absorbs exudates and evaporates the excess off the transparent membrane.	Maintains a transparent membrane for easy wound bed assessment, provides bacterial and shearing protection. Maintains moist wound healing. Can be used with alginates to provide packing to deeper wound beds.	Pressure ulcers Skin tears Venous stasis ulcers Surgical wounds Wounds undergoing chemical debridement agents	Tegaderm
Hydrogels	Glycerin or water-based nonadhesive jellylike sheets, granules, or gels are oxygen permeable, unless covered by a plastic film. Requires secondary occlusive dressing.	To liquefy necrotic tissue or slough, rehydrate the wound bed, and fill in dead space	Pressure ulcers Skin tears Partial-thickness wounds	Curosol, Tegaderm Hydrogel Elasto-Gel, Vigilon
Polyurethane foams	Nonadherent hydrocolloid dressings; these need to have their edges taped down or sealed. Require secondary dressings to obtain an occlusive environment. Surrounding skin must be protected to prevent maceration.	Absorbs up to heavy amounts of exudate; provides and maintains moist wound healing	Light to highly exudating wounds Pressure ulcers Skin tears Venous stasis ulcers Surgical wounds Wounds undergoing chemical debridement agents	Tegaderm Foam Lyofoam, Allevyn, Vigifoam, Flexzan
Alginates (exudate absorbers)	Nonadherent dressings of powder, beads or granules, ropes, sheets, or paste conform to the wound surface and absorb up to 20 times their weight in exudate; require a secondary dressing.	To provide a moist wound surface by interacting with exudate to form a gelatinous mass; to absorb exudate; to eliminate dead space or pack wounds; and to support debridement	Pressure ulcers Skin tears Venous stasis ulcers Surgical wounds Wounds undergoing chemical debridement agents	Debrisan, Sorbsan, Kaltostat, Algiderm

2. Ensure that the tape is long and wide enough to adhere to several inches of skin on each side of the dressing, but not so long or wide that the tape loosens with activity (see Figure 36-10 ■, *B*).
3. Place the tape in the opposite direction from the body action, for example, across a body joint or crease, not lengthwise (see Figure 36-11 ■).

Montgomery straps (tie tapes) are used for wounds requiring frequent dressing changes (see Figure 36-12 ■). These straps prevent skin irritation and discomfort caused by removing the adhesive each time the dressing is changed.

Medical tapes can cause injuries if used incorrectly. Blisters will form if too much tension is applied while placing the tape,

Figure 36-10 ■ The strips of tape should be placed at the ends of the dressing and must be sufficiently long and wide to secure the dressing. The tape should adhere to intact skin.

Figure 36-11 ■ Dressings over moving parts must remain secure in spite of the client's movement. Place the tape over a joint at a right angle to the direction the joint moves.

Figure 36-12 ■ Montgomery straps, or tie tapes, are used to secure large dressings that require frequent changing.

when edema has collected after the tape was placed, and when alcohol or benzoic-based prep solutions are used under the tape. Medical tape manufacturers issue safety guidelines for specific tape products. Before using medical tapes read the safety guidelines for indications of use and safe application and removal.

Cleaning Wounds

Wound cleaning involves the removal of debris (i.e., foreign materials, excess slough, necrotic tissue, bacteria, and other microorganisms). The choices of cleaning agent and method depend largely on agency protocol and the primary care provider's preference. Recommended guidelines for cleaning wounds are shown in the accompanying Practice Guidelines.

Commonly used methods to clean a surgical wound and drain site are shown in Chapter 37. ∞

WOUND IRRIGATION AND PACKING. An irrigation (lavage) is the washing or flushing out of an area. Sterile technique is required for a wound irrigation because there is a break in the skin integrity.

Using piston syringes instead of bulb syringes to irrigate a wound reduces the risk of aspirating drainage and provides safe, effective pressure. For deep wounds with small openings, a sterile straight catheter may also be necessary. Irrigation pressures should range from 4 to 15 pounds per square inch (psi). Below 4 psi, the irrigation may not be effective, and above 15 psi it may damage tissues. A 35-mL syringe with a 19-gauge needle or catheter provides approximately 8 psi (Bergstrom et al., 1994). Some providers advocate the use of a commercial oral water jet for wound cleansing. This can be effective if kept at the lowest setting that provides the desired pressure. Frequently used irrigation solutions are sterile normal saline, lactated Ringer's solution, and antibiotic solutions. Skill 36-2 details the steps involved in irrigating a wound.

Gauze **packing** using the damp-to-damp technique has been used to pack wounds that require debridement. In this technique, moist 4 × 4 non-cotton-filled gauzes are packed in the wound to absorb exudate but they are not allowed to dry before removal. However, newer advanced dressing materials have significant advantages over the use of gauze. See the accompanying Practice Guidelines for issues related to using damp-to-damp dressings.

Many of the techniques described here for dressing wounds may be combined depending on the specific type of wound. In addition, therapies are constantly being designed and evaluated.

PRACTICE GUIDELINES **Cleaning Wounds**

- Follow standard precautions for personal protection. Wear gloves, gown, goggles, and mask as indicated.
- Use solutions such as isotonic saline or wound cleansers to clean or irrigate wounds. If antimicrobial solutions are used, make sure they are well diluted.
- Microwave heating is not recommended. When possible, warm the solution to body temperature before use. *This prevents lowering the wound temperature, which slows the healing process. Microwave heating could cause the solution to become too hot.*
- If a wound is grossly contaminated by foreign material, bacteria, slough, or necrotic tissue, clean the wound at every dressing change. *Foreign bodies and devitalized tissue act as a focus for infection and can delay healing.*
- If a wound is clean, has little exudate, and reveals healthy granulation tissue, avoid repeated cleaning. *Unnecessary cleaning can delay wound healing by traumatizing newly produced, delicate*

tissues, reducing the surface temperature of the wound, and removing exudate which itself may have bactericidal properties.

- Use gauze squares. Avoid using cotton balls and other products that shed fibers onto the wound surface. *The fibers become embedded in granulation tissue and can act as foci for infection. They may also stimulate "foreign body" reactions, prolonging the inflammatory phase of healing and delaying the healing process.*
- Clean superficial noninfected wounds by irrigating them with normal saline. *The hydraulic pressure of an irrigating stream of fluid dislodges contaminating debris and reduces bacterial colonization.*
- *To retain wound moisture,* avoid drying a wound after cleaning it.
- Hold cleaning sponges with forceps or with a sterile gloved hand.
- Clean from the wound in an outward direction to avoid transferring organisms from the surrounding skin into the wound.
- Consider not cleaning the wound at all if it appears to be clean.

PRACTICE GUIDELINES **Issues Related to the Use of Damp Gauze Versus Advanced Dressings**

- To keep the gauze damp, it must be changed or remoistened with saline frequently. *If the gauze is allowed to dry out, removal results in pain and disruption of wound healing through drying of the surface and tissue adherence to the gauze.*
- A wound requires moisture and warmth for optimal healing. Evaporation of the saline causes wound cooling, vasoconstriction, and dehydration.
- Moistened gauze cannot prevent introduction of bacteria into the wound.
- Gauze is easy to use and can be manipulated to fit almost any wound.
- The diversity of advanced dressings may be confusing for clients and health care providers.

- Although gauze is much less expensive than advanced dressings (e.g., polymers, alginates, collagens), the cost per week can be higher due to the number of dressing changes required. Including the price of the dressing, gloves, saline, and tape, the materials cost for a gauze dressing change twice per day versus an advanced dressing three times per week is very similar. However, at approximately $100 per nurse home visit, the gauze dressing is almost five times as expensive.
- Wounds have been shown to heal twice as quickly with advanced dressings compared to gauze.

Conclusions: Practitioners should become familiar with the range and uses of advanced dressing materials. The selection of dressing materials must consider time, material cost, client comfort, and speed of wound healing.

IRRIGATING A WOUND

PURPOSES
- To clean the area
- To apply heat and hasten the healing process
- To apply an antimicrobial solution

ASSESSMENT
Assess

- The client's record to determine previous appearance and size of the wound

- The character of the exudate
- Presence of pain and the time of the last pain medication
- Clinical signs of systemic infection
- Allergies to the wound irrigation agent or tape

PLANNING
- Before irrigating a wound, determine (a) the type of irrigating solution to be used, (b) the frequency of irrigations, and (c) the temperature of the solution.
- If possible, schedule the irrigation at a time convenient for the client. Some irrigations require only a few minutes and others can take much longer.

Delegation

Due to the need for aseptic technique and assessment skills, wound irrigations are not delegated to UAP. However, UAP may observe the wound and dressing during usual care and must report abnormal findings to the nurse. Abnormal findings must be validated and interpreted by the nurse.

SKILL 36-2

continued on page 926

IRRIGATING A WOUND *continued*

Equipment
- Sterile dressing equipment and dressing materials
- Sterile irrigation set or individual supplies that include
  - Sterile syringe (e.g., a 30- to 60-mL syringe) with a catheter of an appropriate size (e.g., #18 or #19) or an irrigating (catheter) tip syringe
  - Sterile graduated container for irrigating solution
  - Basin for collecting the used irrigating solution
  - Moisture-proof sterile drape
- Moisture-proof bag

- Irrigating solution, usually 200 mL (6.5 oz) of solution warmed to body temperature, according to the agency's or primary care provider's choice
- Goggles, gown, and mask
- Clean gloves
- Sterile gloves

Although a wound may already be contaminated, sterile equipment is usually used during irrigation to prevent the possibility of adding new nonresident microorganisms to the site. In settings outside of hospitals, some reusable supplies such as irrigating syringes or basins may be cleaned and used again for a specific wound.

IMPLEMENTATION

Preparation
Check that the irrigating fluid is at the proper temperature.

Performance
1. Prior to performing the procedure, introduce self and verify the client's identity using agency protocol. Explain to the client what you are going to do, why it is necessary, and how he or she can cooperate. Discuss how the results will be used in planning further care or treatments.
2. Perform hand hygiene and observe appropriate infection control procedures.
3. Provide for client privacy.
4. Prepare the client.
   - Assist the client to a position in which the irrigating solution will flow by gravity from the upper end of the wound to the lower end and then into the basin.
   - Place the waterproof drape over the client and the bed.
   - Put on clean gloves and remove and discard the old dressing.
   - If indicated, clean the wound from the center of the wound outward, using circular strokes.
   - Use a separate swab for each stroke, and discard each swab after use. **Rationale:** *This prevents the introduction of microorganisms to other wound areas.*
   - Assess the wound and drainage.
   - Remove and discard clean gloves.
5. Prepare the equipment.
   - Open the sterile dressing set and supplies.
   - Pour the ordered solution into the solution container.
   - Position the basin below the wound to receive the irrigating fluid.
6. Irrigate the wound.
   - Instill a steady stream of irrigating solution into the wound. Make sure all areas of the wound are irrigated.
   - Use either a syringe with a catheter attached or with an irrigating tip to flush the wound. ❶
   - If you are using a catheter to reach tracks or crevices, insert the catheter into the wound until resistance is met. Do not force the catheter. **Rationale:** *Forcing the catheter can cause tissue damage.*

❶ Irrigating an open wound.
(Shirlee Synder)

   - Continue irrigating until the solution becomes clear (no exudate is present).
   - Dry the area around the wound. **Rationale:** *Moisture left on the skin promotes the growth of microorganisms and can cause skin irritation and breakdown.*
7. Assess and dress the wound.
   - Assess the appearance of the wound again, noting in particular the type and amount of exudate still present and the presence and extent of granulation tissue.
   - Using sterile technique, apply a dressing to the wound based on the amount of drainage expected (see Table 36–5).
8. Document the irrigation and the client's response in the client record using forms or checklists supplemented by narrative notes when appropriate. Many agencies use a designated wound/skin documentation sheet (see Figure 36-5).

SAMPLE DOCUMENTATION

6/5/07 1530 Midline abdominal wound 7 cm c̄ intact sutures except for center 3 cm. Open area draining moderate amt. thin serosang. Irrigated c̄ NS until clear. Redressed c̄ sterile technique. ———————————— *N. Jamaghani, RN*

EVALUATION
- Perform follow-up based on findings that deviate from expected or normal for the client. Relate findings to previous assessment data if available.

- Report significant deviations from normal to the primary care provider.

Figure 36-13 ■ Vacuum-assisted closure (VAC) system for wounds.

(V.A.C.® ATS Therapy System Courtesy of KCI Licensing, Inc., San Antonio, TX).

One example is *vacuum-assisted closure (VAC)*, which refers to the use of suction equipment to apply negative pressure to a variety of wound types. This therapy has been shown to speed tissue generation, reduce swelling around the wound, and enhance

wound healing by providing a moist and protected environment. Sterile foam sponges are placed into a clean wound and covered with a transparent adhesive drape, and then a hole is cut in the drape to allow insertion of the vacuum tubing (Figure 36-13 ■). For maximum effectiveness the vacuum is applied for almost 24 hours each day (Mendez-Eastman, 2005) and portable systems are available for ambulatory clients. VAC has also been shown to heal pressure ulcers better than alginate or hydrocolloid dressings (Smith, 2004).

Supporting and Immobilizing Wounds

Bandages and binders serve various purposes:

- Supporting a wound (e.g., a fractured bone)
- Immobilizing a wound (e.g., a strained shoulder)
- Applying pressure (e.g., elastic bandages on the lower extremities to improve venous blood flow)
- Securing a dressing (e.g., for an extensive abdominal surgical wound)
- Retaining warmth (e.g., a flannel bandage on a rheumatoid joint)

There are several types of bandages and binders and several ways in which they are applied. When correctly applied, they

LIFESPAN CONSIDERATIONS Pressure Ulcer and Wound Care

INFANTS
- The skin of infants is more fragile than that of older children and adults, and more susceptible to infection, shearing from friction, and burns.

CHILDREN
- Staphylococcus and fungus are two major infectious agents affecting the skin of children. Abrasions or small lacerations, commonly experienced by children, provide an entry in the skin for these organisms. Minor wounds should be cleansed with warm, soapy water, and covered with a sterile bandage. Children should be instructed not to touch the wound.
- With more serious skin lesions, remind the child not to touch the wound, drains, or dressing. Cover with an appropriate bandage that will remain intact during the child's usual activities. Cover a transparent dressing with opaque material if viewing the site is distressing to the child. Restrain only when all alternatives have been tried and when absolutely necessary.

- For younger children, demonstrate wound care on a doll. Reassure that the wound will not be permanent and that nothing will fall out of the body.

ELDERS
- Hold wrinkled skin taut during application of a transparent dressing. Obtain assistance if needed.
- Skin is more fragile and can easily tear with removal of tape (especially adhesive tape). Use paper tape and tape remover as indicated, keeping tape use to the minimum required. Use extreme caution during tape removal.
- Elders who are in long-term care facilities often have the following factors: immobility, malnutrition, and incontinence—all of which increase the risk for development of skin breakdown.
- Skin breakdown can occur as quickly as within 2 hours, so assessments should be done with each repositioning of the client.
- A thorough assessment of a client's heels should be done every shift. The skin can break down quickly from friction of movement in bed.

HOME CARE CONSIDERATIONS Wound Care

- Perform appropriate client teaching for promoting wound healing and maintenance of healthy skin.
- Instruct family about hygiene and medical asepsis; hand cleansing before and after dressing changes; and using a clean area for storage of dressing supplies.
- Instruct the client and family on where to obtain needed supplies. Be sensitive to the cost of dressings (e.g., transparent barriers are costly) and suggest less expensive alternatives if necessary. Be creative in the use of household items for padding pressure areas.

- Instruct the client and family in proper disposal of contaminated dressings. All contaminated items should be double bagged in moisture-proof bags.
- Verify how the client may bathe with the wound (i.e., does the wound need to be covered with a waterproof barrier or should it be cleansed in the shower?).
- Tap water may be used to cleanse wounds instead of normal saline (Fernandez, Griffiths, & Ussia, 2006).

PRACTICE GUIDELINES **Bandaging**

- Whenever possible, bandage the part in its normal position, with the joint slightly flexed *to avoid putting strain on the ligaments and the muscles of the joint.*
- Pad between skin surfaces and over bony prominences *to prevent friction from the bandage and consequent abrasion of the skin.*
- Always bandage body parts by working from the distal to the proximal end *to aid the return flow of venous blood.*
- Bandage with even pressure *to prevent interference with blood circulation.*
- Whenever possible, leave the end of the body part (e.g., the toe) exposed *so that you will be able to assess the adequacy of the blood circulation to the extremity.*
- Cover dressings with bandages at least 5 cm (2 in.) beyond the edges of the dressing *to prevent the dressing and wound from becoming contaminated.*

---

promote healing, provide comfort, and can prevent injury (see accompanying Practice Guidelines).

BANDAGES. A **bandage** is a strip of cloth used to wrap some part of the body. Bandages are available in various widths, most commonly 1.5 to 7.5 cm (0.5 to 3 in.). They are usually supplied in rolls for easy application to a body part.

Many types of materials are used for bandages. Gauze is one of the most commonly used, because it is light and porous and readily molds to the body. It is also relatively inexpensive, so it is generally discarded when soiled. Gauze is used to retain dressings on wounds and to bandage the fingers, hands, toes, and feet. It supports dressings and at the same time permits air to circulate; it can be impregnated with petroleum jelly or other medications for application to wounds.

Elasticized bandages are applied to provide pressure to an area. They are commonly used as tensor bandages or as partial stockings to provide support and improve the venous circulation in the legs.

PRACTICE GUIDELINES **Assessing before Applying Bandages or Binders**

- Inspect and palpate the area for swelling.
- Inspect for the presence of and status of wounds (open wounds will require a dressing before a bandage or binder is applied).
- Note the presence of drainage (amount, color, odor, viscosity).
- Inspect and palpate for adequacy of circulation (skin temperature, color, and sensation). Pale or cyanotic skin, cool temperature, tingling, and numbness can indicate impaired circulation.
- Ask the client about any pain experienced (location, intensity, onset, quality).
- Assess the ability of the client to reapply the bandage or binder when needed.
- Assess the capabilities of the client regarding activities of daily living (e.g., to eat, dress, comb hair, bathe) and assess the assistance required during the convalescence period.

The width of the bandage used depends on the size of the body part to be bandaged. For example, a 2.5-cm (1-in.) bandage is used for a finger, a 5-cm (2-in.) bandage for an arm, and a 7.5-cm or 10-cm (3-in. or 4-in.) bandage for a leg. Padding (e.g., abdominal pads and gauze squares) is frequently used to cover bony prominences (e.g., the elbow) or to separate skin surfaces (e.g., the fingers).

Before applying a bandage, the nurse needs to know its purpose and to assess the area requiring support (see accompanying Practice Guidelines). When bandages are used to secure dressings, the nurse wears gloves to prevent contact with body fluids.

BASIC TURNS FOR ROLLER BANDAGES. Applying bandages to various parts of the body involves one or more of five basic bandaging turns: circular, spiral, spiral reverse, recurrent, and figure-eight. *Circular* turns are used to anchor bandages and to terminate them. Circular turns usually are not applied directly over a wound because of the discomfort the bandage would cause.

Spiral turns are used to bandage parts of the body that are fairly uniform in circumference, for example, the upper arm or upper leg. *Spiral reverse* turns are used to bandage cylindrical parts of the body that are not uniform in circumference, for example, the lower leg or forearm. *Recurrent* turns are used to cover distal parts of the body, for example, the end of a finger, the skull, or the stump of an amputation. *Figure-eight* turns are used to bandage an elbow, knee, or ankle, because they permit some movement after application.

Circular Turns.

- Hold the bandage in your dominant hand, keeping the roll uppermost, and unroll the bandage about 8 cm (3 in.). This length of unrolled bandage allows good control for placement and tension.
- Apply the end of the bandage to the part of the body to be bandaged. Hold the end down with the thumb of the other hand (Figure 36-14 ■).
- Encircle the body part a few times or as often as needed, making sure that each layer overlaps one-half to two-thirds of the previous layer. This provides even support to the area.
- The bandage should be firm, but not too tight. Ask the client if the bandage feels comfortable. A tight bandage can interfere with blood circulation, whereas a loose bandage does not provide adequate protection.

Figure 36-14 ■ Starting a bandage with two circular turns.

Figure 36-15 ■ Applying spiral turns.

■ Secure the end of the bandage with tape or a safety pin over an uninjured area. Pins can cause discomfort when situated over an injured area.

Spiral Turns.
■ Make two circular turns. Two circular turns anchor the bandage.
■ Continue spiral turns at about a 30-degree angle, each turn overlapping the preceding one by two-thirds the width of the bandage (Figure 36-15 ■).
■ Terminate the bandage with two circular turns, and secure the end as described for circular turns.

Spiral Reverse Turns.
■ Anchor the bandage with two circular turns, and bring the bandage upward at about a 30-degree angle.
■ Place the thumb of your free hand on the upper edge of the bandage (Figure 36-16 ■, *A*). The thumb will hold the bandage while it is folded on itself.
■ Unroll the bandage about 15 cm (6 in.), and then turn your hand so that the bandage falls over itself (Figure 36-16 ■, *B*).
■ Continue the bandage around the limb, overlapping each previous turn by two-thirds the width of the bandage. Make each bandage turn at the same position on the limb so that the turns of the bandage will be aligned (Figure 36-16 ■, *C*).
■ Terminate the bandage with two circular turns, and secure the end as described for circular turns.

Recurrent Turns.
■ Anchor the bandage with two circular turns.
■ Fold the bandage back on itself, and bring it centrally over the distal end to be bandaged (Figure 36-17 ■).
■ Holding it with the other hand, bring the bandage back over the end to the right of the center bandage but overlapping it by two-thirds the width of the bandage.
■ Bring the bandage back on the left side, also overlapping the first turn by two-thirds the width of the bandage.
■ Continue this pattern of alternating right and left until the area is covered. Overlap the preceding turn by two-thirds the bandage width each time.
■ Terminate the bandage with two circular turns (Figure 36-18 ■). Secure the end appropriately.

Figure 36-17 ■ Starting a recurrent bandage.

Figure 36-18 ■ Completing a recurrent bandage.

A

B

Circular turns

Bandage folded over to make spiral reverse turn

C

Figure 36-16 ■ Applying spiral reverse turns.

Figure 36-19 ■ Applying a figure-eight bandage.

Figure 36-20 ■ Large arm sling.

Figure-Eight Turns.
■ Anchor the bandage with two circular turns.
■ Carry the bandage above the joint, around it, and then below it, making a figure-eight (Figure 36-19 ■).
■ Continue above and below the joint, overlapping the previous turn by two-thirds the width of the bandage.
■ Terminate the bandage above the joint with two circular turns, and then secure the end appropriately.

BINDERS. A **binder** is a type of bandage designed for a specific body part; for example, the triangular binder (sling) fits the arm. Binders are used to support large areas of the body, such as the abdomen, arm, or chest. Binders can be simple, inexpensive, and customizable by using plain material such as the triangular sling described below. Or, they can be of commercial design which are often easier to use, more expensive, and slightly less modifiable such as the hook-and-loop (Velcro) binder which is also described below.

Triangular Arm Sling.
■ Ask the client to flex the elbow to an 80-degree angle or less, depending on the purpose. The thumb should be facing upward or inward toward the body. *An 80-degree angle is sufficient to support the forearm, to prevent swelling of the hand, and to relieve pressure on the shoulder joint (e.g., to support the paralyzed arm of a stroke client whose shoulder might otherwise become dislocated). A more acute angle is preferred if there is swelling of the hand (see how to apply a sling for maximum hand elevation, below).*
■ Place one end of the unfolded triangular binder over the shoulder of the uninjured side so that the binder falls down the front of the chest of the client with the point of the triangle (apex) under the elbow of the injured side.
■ Take the upper corner, and carry it around the neck until it hangs over the shoulder on the injured side.
■ Bring the lower corner of the binder up over the arm to the shoulder of the injured side. Using a square knot, secure this corner to the upper corner at the side of the neck on the injured side (Figure 36-20 ■, A). *A square knot will not slip. Tying the knot at the side of the neck prevents pressure on the bony prominences of the vertebral column at the back of the neck.*

■ Make sure the wrist is supported, to maintain alignment.
■ Fold the sling neatly at the elbow, and secure it with safety pins or tape. It may be folded and fastened at the front (Figure 36-20 ■, B).
■ Remove the sling periodically to inspect the skin for indications of irritation, especially around the site of the knot.

Straight Abdominal Binder.
■ With the client in a supine position, place the binder smoothly under the body, with the upper border of the binder at the waist and the lower border at the level of the gluteal fold. *A binder placed over the waist interferes with respiration; one placed too low interferes with elimination and walking.*
■ Apply padding over the iliac crests if the client is thin.
■ Bring the ends around the client, overlap them, and secure them with pins or Velcro (Figure 36-21 ■). Place the top pin horizontally at the waist to allow for comfort when moving.

Securing Peritoneal Dressings. Previously, T-binders were used to secure dressings to the peritoneal area. T-binders have

Figure 36-21 ■ A straight abdominal binder.
(Patrick Watson)

LIFESPAN CONSIDERATIONS Applying Bandages and Binders

CHILDREN

- Allow the child to help with the procedure by holding supplies, opening boxes, counting turns, and so on.
- If a young client is apprehensive, demonstrate the procedure on a doll or stuffed animal.
- Encourage the child to decorate the bandage.
- Teach the caregivers to apply bandages and binders safely.

ELDERS

- Older clients may need extra support during the procedure, especially if arthritis, contractures, or tremors are present.
- Avoid constricting the client's circulation with a tight bandage or binder. Observe skin and bony prominences frequently for signs of impaired circulation. The risk for skin breakdown increases with age.

HOME CARE CONSIDERATIONS Applying Bandages and Binders

- Assess the client's or caregiver's knowledge level of reason for bandages or binders. Assess ability and willingness to perform the bandaging procedure.
- Ensure that the client has the proper supplies; assess for adequate and safe storage of supplies in the home, and ensure client knows how to obtain replacement supplies.
- The client should have two binders so that there is one to wear while the other is being washed. Bandages and binders should be washed inside a mesh laundry bag to keep them from becoming

twisted and to prevent Velcro or hooks from catching on other laundry.
- Instruct the client's caregiver on the importance of and how to
  1. Wash hands thoroughly before handling dressing supplies and applying the bandage.
  2. Report skin breakdown, redness, pain, or pallor of the affected area.
  3. Check for adequate peripheral circulation after applying the bandage.

---

been replaced with sanitary disposable garments that fit like briefs. Placing an appropriate sized abdominal pad or sanitary napkin in the garment allows the wound to be protected and drainage to be collected for either males or females.

Heat and Cold Applications

Heat and cold are applied to the body for local and systemic effects. Table 36–6 lists the physiologic effects of heat and cold.

LOCAL EFFECTS OF HEAT. Heat is an old remedy for aches and pains, and people often equate heat with comfort and relief. Heat causes vasodilation and increases blood flow to the affected area, bringing oxygen, nutrients, antibodies, and leukocytes.

Application of heat promotes soft tissue healing and increases suppuration. A possible disadvantage of heat is that it increases capillary permeability, which allows extracellular fluid and substances such as plasma proteins to pass through the capillary walls and may result in edema or an increase in preexisting edema. Heat is often used for clients with musculoskeletal problems such as joint stiffness from arthritis, contractures, and low back pain.

TABLE 36–6 Physiologic Effects of Heat and Cold

HEAT	COLD
Vasodilation	Vasoconstriction
Increases capillary permeability	Decreases capillary permeability
Increases cellular metabolism	Decreases cellular metabolism
Increases inflammation	Slows bacterial growth, decreases inflammation
Sedative effect	Local anesthetic effect

LOCAL EFFECTS OF COLD. Generally, the physiologic effects of cold are opposite to the effects of heat. Cold lowers the temperature of the skin and underlying tissues and causes **vasoconstriction.** Vasoconstriction reduces blood flow to the affected area and thus reduces the supply of oxygen and metabolites, decreases the removal of wastes, and produces skin pallor and coolness. Prolonged exposure to cold results in impaired circulation, cell deprivation, and subsequent damage to the tissues from lack of oxygen and nourishment. The signs of tissue damage due to cold are a bluish purple mottled appearance of the skin, numbness, and sometimes blisters and pain. Cold is most often used for sports injuries (e.g., sprains, strains, fractures) to limit postinjury swelling and bleeding.

SYSTEMIC EFFECTS OF HEAT AND COLD. Heat applied to a localized body area, particularly a large body area, may cause excessive peripheral vasodilation, which produces a drop in blood pressure. A significant drop in blood pressure can cause fainting. Clients who have heart or pulmonary disease and who have circulatory disturbances such as arteriosclerosis are more prone to this effect than healthy people are. With extensive cold applications and vasoconstriction, a client's blood pressure can increase because blood is shunted from the cutaneous circulation to the internal blood vessels. Shivering, a generalized effect of prolonged cold, is a normal response as the body attempts to warm itself.

THERMAL TOLERANCE. Various parts of the body differ in tolerance to heat and cold. The physiologic tolerance of individuals also varies (see Box 36–3). Specific conditions necessitate precautions in the use of hot or cold applications:

- *Neurosensory impairment.* People with sensory impairments are unable to perceive that heat is damaging the tissues and are at risk for burns or are unable to perceive discomfort from cold and prevent tissue injury.

BOX 36–3 Variables Affecting Physiologic Tolerance to Heat and Cold

Body part. The back of the hand and foot are not very temperature sensitive. In contrast, the inner aspect of the wrist and forearm, the neck, and the perineal area are temperature sensitive.

Size of the exposed body part. The larger the area exposed to heat and cold, the lower the tolerance.

Individual tolerance. The very young and the very old generally have the lowest tolerance. Persons who have neurosensory impairments may have a high tolerance, but the risk of injury is greater.

Length of exposure. People feel hot and cold applications most while the temperature is changing. After a period of time, tolerance increases.

Intactness of skin. Injured skin areas are more sensitive to temperature variations.

- *Impaired mental status.* People who are confused or have an altered level of consciousness need monitoring during applications to ensure safe therapy.
- *Impaired circulation.* People with peripheral vascular disease, diabetes, or congestive heart failure lack the normal ability to dissipate heat via the blood circulation, which puts them at risk for tissue damage with heat and cold applications.
- *Immediately after injury or surgery.* Heat increases bleeding and swelling.
- *Open wounds.* Cold can decrease blood flow to the wound, thereby inhibiting healing.

ADAPTATION OF THERMAL RECEPTORS. Heat and cold receptors adapt to temperature changes. When they are subjected to an abrupt change in temperature, the receptors are strongly stimulated initially. This strong stimulation declines rapidly during the first few seconds and then more slowly during the next half hour or more as the receptors adapt to the new temperature.

Nurses and clients need to understand this adaptive response when applying heat and cold. Clients may be tempted to change the temperature of a thermal application because of the change in thermal sensation following adaptation. Increasing the temperature of a hot application after adaptation can result in serious burns. Decreasing the temperature of a cold application can result in pain and serious impairment of circulation to the body part. Table 36–7 lists temperatures of hot and cold applications.

TABLE 36–7 Temperatures for Hot and Cold Applications

DESCRIPTION	TEMPERATURE	APPLICATION
Very cold	Below 15°C (59°F)	Ice bags
Cold	15–18°C (59–65°F)	Cold pack
Cool	18–27°C (65–80°F)	Cold compresses
Tepid	27–37°C (80–98°F)	Alcohol sponge bath
Warm	37–40°C (98–105°F)	Warm bath, aquathermia pads
Hot	40–46°C (105–115°F)	Hot soak, irrigations, hot compresses
Very hot	Above 46°C (above 115°F)	Hot water bags for adults

REBOUND PHENOMENON. The rebound phenomenon occurs at the time the maximum therapeutic effect of the hot or cold application is achieved and the opposite effect begins. For example, heat produces maximum vasodilation in 20 to 30 minutes; continuation of the application beyond 30 to 45 minutes brings tissue congestion, and the blood vessels then constrict for reasons unknown. If the heat application is continued, the client is at risk for burns because the constricted blood vessels are unable to dissipate the heat adequately via the blood circulation.

With cold applications, maximum vasoconstriction occurs when the involved skin reaches a temperature of 15°C (60°F). Below 15°C, vasodilation begins. This mechanism is protective: It helps to prevent freezing of body tissues normally exposed to cold, such as the nose and ears. It also explains the ruddiness of the skin of a person who has been walking in cold weather.

An understanding of the rebound phenomenon is essential for the nurse and client. Thermal applications must be halted before the rebound phenomenon begins.

Applying Heat and Cold

Heat can be applied to the body in both dry and moist forms. Dry heat is applied locally by means of a hot water bottle, aquathermia pad, disposable heat pack, or electric pad. Moist heat can be provided by compress, hot pack, soak, or sitz bath. Selected indications for the use of heat and cold are found in Table 36–8.

Dry cold is generally applied locally by means of a cold pack, ice bag, ice glove, or ice collar. Moist cold can be provided by compress or a cooling sponge bath.

For all local applications of heat or cold, the nurse needs to follow these guidelines:

- Determine the client's ability to tolerate the therapy.
- Identify conditions that might contraindicate treatment (e.g., bleeding, circulatory impairment).
- Explain the application to the client.
- Assess the skin area to which the heat or cold will be applied.
- Ask the client to report any discomfort.
- Return to the client 15 minutes after starting the heat or cold, and observe the local skin area for any untoward signs (e.g., redness). Stop the application if any problems occur.
- Remove the equipment at the designated time, and dispose of it appropriately.
- Examine the area to which the heat or cold was applied, and record the client's response.

For contraindications to the use of heat or cold, see Box 36–4.

HOT WATER BAG. A hot water bag or bottle has been a common source of dry heat used in the home. It is convenient and relatively inexpensive. However, because of the danger of burning from improper use, many agencies now use other devices.

The following temperatures of the water in the bag are considered safe in most situations and provide the desired effect: normal adult and child over 2 years, 46°C to 52°C (115°F to 125°F); debilitated or unconscious adult, or child under 2 years, 40.5°C to 46°C (105°F to 115°F).

TABLE 36–8 Selected Indications of Heat and Cold

INDICATION	EFFECT OF HEAT	EFFECT OF COLD
Muscle spasm	Relaxes muscles and increases their contractility.	Relaxes muscles and decreases muscle contractility.
Inflammation	Increases blood flow, softens exudates.	Vasoconstriction decreases capillary permeability, decreases blood flow, slows cellular metabolism.
Pain	Relieves pain, possibly by promoting muscle relaxation, increasing circulation, and promoting psychologic relaxation and a feeling of comfort; acts as a counterirritant.	Decreases pain by slowing nerve conduction rate and blocking nerve impulses; produces numbness, acts as a counterirritant, increases pain threshold.
Contracture	Reduces contracture and increases joint range of motion by allowing greater distention of muscles and connective tissue.	
Joint stiffness	Reduces joint stiffness by decreasing viscosity of synovial fluid and increasing tissue distensibility.	
Traumatic injury		Decreases bleeding by constricting blood vessels; decreases edema by reducing capillary permeability.

To apply a hot water bag

- Measure the temperature of the water using a bath thermometer.
- Fill the bag about two-thirds full.
- Expel the remaining air and secure the top. With the air removed, the bag can be molded to the body part.
- Dry the bag and hold it upside down to test for leakage.
- Wrap the bag in a towel or cover and place it on the body site.
- Remove after 30 minutes or in accordance with agency protocol.

AQUATHERMIA PAD.   The aquathermia or aquamatic pad (also referred to as a K-pad) is a pad constructed with tubes containing water. The pad is attached by tubing to an electrically powered control unit that has an opening for water and a temperature gauge (Figure 36-22 ■). Some aquathermia pads have an absorbent

Figure 36-22 ■ An aquathermia heating unit.

BOX 36–4   Contraindications to the Use of Heat and Cold

Determine the presence of any conditions contraindicating the use of heat:
- *The first 24 hours after traumatic injury.* Heat increases bleeding and swelling.
- *Active hemorrhage.* Heat causes vasodilation and increases bleeding.
- *Noninflammatory edema.* Heat increases capillary permeability and edema.
- *Localized malignant tumor.* Because heat accelerates cell metabolism and cell growth and increases circulation, it may accelerate metastases (secondary tumors).
- *Skin disorder that causes redness or blisters.* Heat can burn or cause further damage to the skin.

Determine the presence of any conditions contraindicating the use of cold:
- *Open wounds.* Cold can increase tissue damage by decreasing blood flow to an open wound.
- *Impaired circulation.* Cold can further impair nourishment of the tissues and cause tissue damage. In clients with Raynaud's disease, cold increases arterial spasm.
- *Allergy or hypersensitivity to cold.* Some clients have an allergy to cold that may be manifested by an inflammatory response, for ex-

ample, erythema, hives, swelling, joint pain, and occasional muscle spasm. Some react with a sudden increase in blood pressure, which can be hazardous if the person is hypersensitive.

Determine the presence of any conditions indicating the need for special precautions during heat and cold therapy:
- *Neurosensory impairment.* Persons with sensory impairments are unable to perceive that heat is damaging the tissues and are at risk for burns, or they are unable to perceive discomfort from cold and are unable to prevent tissue injury.
- *Impaired mental status.* Persons who are confused or have an altered level of consciousness need monitoring and supervision during applications to ensure safe therapy.
- *Impaired circulation.* Persons with peripheral vascular disease, diabetes, or congestive heart failure lack the normal ability to dissipate heat via the blood circulation, which puts them at risk for tissue damage with heat applications. Cold applications are contraindicated for these people.
- *Open wounds.* Tissues around an open wound are more sensitive to heat and cold.

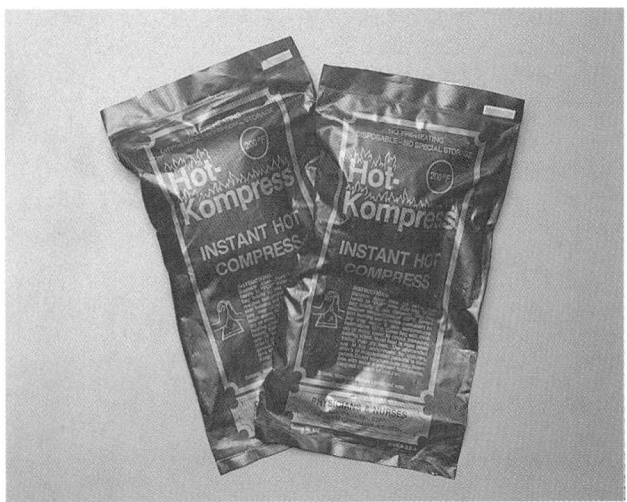

Figure 36-23 ■ Commercially prepared disposable hot packs.

surface through which moist heat can be applied. The other surface of the pad is waterproof. These pads are disposable.

To apply an aquathermia pad, the nurse carries out the following steps:

- Fill the reservoir of the unit two-thirds full of distilled water.
- Set the desired temperature. Check the manufacturer's instructions. Most units are set at 40.5°C (105°F) for adults.
- Cover the pad and plug in the unit. Some manufacturers suggest warming the pad before applying it.
- Apply the pad to the body part. The treatment is usually continued for 30 minutes. Check orders and agency protocol.

HOT AND COLD PACKS. Commercially prepared hot and cold packs (Figure 36-23 ■) provide heat or cold for a designated time. Directions on the package tell how to initiate the heating or cooling process, for example, by striking, squeezing, or kneading the pack.

ELECTRIC PADS. Electric pads provide a constant, even heat, are lightweight, and can be molded to a body part. Electric pads, however, can burn if the setting is too high. Some models have waterproof covers for use when the pad is placed over a moist dressing.

In applying electric pads, the nurse follows these guidelines:

- Do not insert sharp objects (e.g., pins) into the pad. The pin could damage a wire and cause an electric shock.
- Ensure that the body area is dry unless there is a waterproof cover on the pad. Electricity in the presence of water can cause a shock.
- Use pads with a preset heating switch so a client cannot increase the heat.
- Do not place the pad under the client. Heat will not dissipate, and the client may be burned.

ICE BAGS, ICE GLOVES, AND ICE COLLARS. Ice bags, ice gloves, and ice collars are filled either with ice chips or with an alcohol-based solution. They are applied to the body to provide cold to a localized area (e.g., a collar is often applied to

the throat following a tonsillectomy). Always wrap the container in a towel or cover.

COMPRESSES. Compresses can be either warm or cold. A **compress** is a moist gauze dressing applied to a wound. When hot compresses are ordered, the solution is heated to the temperature indicated by the order or according to agency protocol, for example, 40.5°C (105°F). When there is a break in the skin or when the body part (e.g., an eye) is vulnerable to microbial invasion, sterile technique is necessary; therefore, sterile gloves are needed to apply the compress and all materials must be sterile.

SOAK. A soak refers to immersing a body part (e.g., an arm) in a solution or to wrapping a part in gauze dressings and then saturating the dressing with a solution. Sterile technique is generally indicated for open wounds, such as a burn or an unhealed surgical incision. Determine agency protocol regarding the temperature of the solution. Hot soaks are frequently done to soften and remove encrusted secretions and dead tissue.

SITZ BATH. A **sitz bath,** or hip bath, is used to soak a client's pelvic area. The client sits in a special tub or chair and is usually immersed from the midthighs to the iliac crests or umbilicus. Special tubs or chairs are preferred because when the legs are also immersed, as in a regular bathtub, blood circulation to the perineum or pelvic area is decreased. Disposable sitz baths are also available.

The temperature of the water should be from 40°C to 43°C (105°F to 110°F), unless the client is unable to tolerate the heat. Determine agency protocol. Some sitz tubs have temperature indicators attached to the water taps. The duration of the bath is generally 15 to 20 minutes, depending on the client's health. To provide a sitz bath

- Assist the client into the tub. Provide support for the client's feet; a footstool can prevent pressure on the backs of the thighs.
- Provide a bath blanket for the client's shoulders, and eliminate drafts to prevent chilling.
- Observe the client closely during the bath for signs of faintness, dizziness, weakness, accelerated pulse rate, and pallor.
- Maintain the water temperature.
- Following the sitz bath, assist the client out of the tub. Help the client to dry.

COOLING SPONGE BATH. The purpose of a cooling sponge bath is to reduce a client's fever by promoting heat loss through conduction and vaporization. Cool sponge baths are used with extreme caution, and only for clients with very high temperatures such as over 40°C (104°F), because rapid skin temperature drop can cause chills that actually increase heat production. The bath is accompanied by antipyretic medication that acts to reset the hypothalamus set point. The temperatures for cooling sponge baths range from 18°C to 32°C (65°F to 93°F).

To provide a cooling sponge bath, the nurse should

- Sponge the face, arms, legs, back, and buttocks. The chest and abdomen are not usually sponged. Each area is sponged slowly and gently. Rubbing may increase heat production.

- Leave each area wet and cover with a damp towel.
- Place ice bags and cold packs, if used, or a cool cloth on the forehead for comfort and in each axilla and at the groin. These areas contain large superficial blood vessels that help the transfer of heat.
- Sponge one body part and then another. The sponge bath should take about 30 minutes. A bath given more quickly tends to increase the body's heat production by causing shivering.
- Discontinue the bath if the client becomes pale or cyanotic or shivers, or if the pulse becomes rapid or irregular.
- Reassess the vital signs at 15 minutes and after completing the sponge bath.

Evaluating

The goals established during the planning phase are evaluated according to specific desired outcomes also established in that phase (see Identifying Nursing Diagnoses, Outcomes, and Interventions earlier). To judge whether client outcomes have been achieved, the nurse uses data collected during care, such as skin status over bony prominences, nutritional and fluid intake, mental status, signs of healing if an ulcer is present, and so on. If outcomes are not achieved, the nurse should explore the reasons why:

- Has the client's physical condition changed?
- Were risk factors correctly identified?
- Were appropriate devices and techniques used?
- Did the client fail to comply with instructions about moving and turning? Why?
- Were appropriate pressure-relieving devices used, and were they applied correctly?
- Was the repositioning schedule adhered to?
- Are the client's nutritional and fluid intake adequate?
- Were appropriate measures used to control incontinence and protect the client's skin?
- Was the wound supported and immobilized effectively?
- Were stringent aseptic practices implemented when cleaning and changing dressings to prevent infection?
- Was the client receiving antineoplastic or anti-inflammatory medications that interfere with healing?
- Was nonviable tissue removed by autolytic, chemical, mechanical, or surgical debridement?
- Was the appropriate dressing applied to maintain moist wound healing?

CRITICAL THINKING CHECKPOINT

You have been assigned to care for Mr. Johns, a 74-year-old client being treated for a urinary tract disorder. Mr. Johns suffered a cerebrovascular accident (stroke) 6 months ago and has had difficulty ambulating and attending to his own needs because of right-sided weakness. While assessing Mr. Johns you note that he is thin for his height, is incontinent of foul-smelling urine, and has deeply reddened areas on his right hip, coccyx, and entire peritoneal area. Mr. Johns is alert and oriented to person, place, and time, but he has decreased sensation on his entire right side. He spends most of his time in bed or sitting at his bedside in a chair due to his difficulty with ambulation.

1. What data suggest that Mr. Johns is particularly vulnerable to pressure ulcer development?
2. What additional information do you need in order to use the Braden scale to determine Mr. Johns's potential for pressure ulcer development?
3. What independent measures can you take to protect Mr. Johns's skin from further breakdown?
4. Considering that Mr. Johns does not have any areas of skin breakdown, why is it important to institute treatment for pressure ulcers at this time?

See Critical Thinking Possibilities in Appendix A.

CHAPTER 36 **REVIEW**

CHAPTER HIGHLIGHTS

- Maintaining skin integrity is an important independent function of nursing.
- Wounds are described as intentional or unintentional, closed or open, and clean, clean-contaminated, contaminated, or dirty (infected). Wounds are also classified by depth as partial thickness or full thickness. In addition, wounds are classified according to how they are acquired, as incisions, contusions, abrasions, punctures, lacerations, and penetrating wounds.
- A pressure ulcer is any lesion caused by unrelieved pressure that results in damage to underlying tissues. Pressure ulcers usually occur over bony prominences.
- Two other factors that act in conjunction with pressure to produce a pressure ulcer are friction and shearing forces.
- Several factors increase the risk for the development of pressure ulcers: immobility and inactivity, inadequate nutrition, fecal and urinary incontinence, decreased mental status, diminished sensation, excessive body heat, and advanced age.
- Several risk assessment tools are available to identify clients at risk for pressure ulcer development. They include scoring systems to evaluate a person's degree of risk.
- There are four stages of pressure ulcers, which vary according to the degree of tissue damage.
- There are two types of wound healing, which are distinguished by the amount of tissue loss: primary intention healing and secondary intention healing.
- The wound-healing process has three phases: inflammatory, proliferative, and maturation.

- Major types of wound exudate are serous, purulent, and sanguineous (hemorrhagic). Exudate can be a combination of two or three of these types (e.g., serosanguineous). The process of pus formation is referred to as suppuration.
- The main complications of wound healing are hemorrhage, infection, dehiscence, and evisceration, each of which is identifiable by specific clinical signs and symptoms.
- Factors affecting wound healing include developmental stage, nutritional status, lifestyle, medications, underlying disease processes, and the presence of infection.
- Meticulous skin assessment of common pressure ulcer sites by the nurse is an important ongoing assessment activity for clients at risk.
- When a pressure ulcer is present, the nurse describes the ulcer in terms of location, size, depth, stage, color, status of wound bed and surrounding skin, and specific signs of infection, if present.
- Wound assessment is an ongoing process to evaluate healing. The nurse assesses wounds by visual inspection, palpation, measurements, and the sense of smell. Essential data for assessing wounds include wound appearance, size, exudate, swelling, pain, and the presence of tubes and drains.
- Laboratory data that may be used to assess the progress of wound healing include leukocyte count, hemoglobin, blood coagulation studies, serum protein analysis, and wound cultures. Nurses are usually responsible for obtaining specimens of wound drainage for culture.
- The NANDA nursing diagnoses *Risk for Impaired Skin Integrity,* *Impaired Skin Integrity,* and *Impaired Tissue Integrity* apply to clients at risk for developing and to those with pressure ulcers.
- Nursing diagnoses related to clients with wounds may include *Risk for Infection* and *Pain.*
- Major goals for clients at risk for developing pressure ulcers are to maintain skin integrity and to avoid potential associated risks.
- Nursing interventions to prevent the formation of pressure ulcers include conducting ongoing assessment of risk factors and skin status, providing skin care to maintain skin integrity, ensuring

adequate nutrition, implementing measures to avoid skin trauma, providing supportive devices, and client teaching.
- Treatment for pressure ulcers varies according to the stage of the ulcer and agency protocol.
- Major nursing responsibilities related to wound care include assisting the client in obtaining sufficient nutrition and fluids, preventing wound infections, and proper positioning.
- Wound care may involve cleaning/irrigating, protecting, filling/hydrating, and covering wounds; applying heat and cold; and applying bandages and binders.
- Various dressing materials are available to protect wounds, absorb exudate, and keep the wound bed moist, thus facilitating healing.
- Synthetic dressings have been developed for use with specific types of wounds. These include transparent adhesive films, impregnated nonadherent dressings, hydrocolloids, hydrogels, polyurethane foams, clear acrylic dressings, and alginates. The nurse must be aware of the specific purposes of each and their indications for use.
- The type of dressing used depends on (a) location, size, and type of the wound; (b) amount of exudate; (c) whether or not the wound requires debridement, is infected, or has sinus tracts; and (d) such considerations as frequency of dressing change, ease or difficulty of dressing applications, and cost.
- The RYB color code of wounds can assist nurses to provide appropriate nursing interventions for wounds that heal by secondary intention. In this scheme, the nurse protects red, cleanses yellow, and debrides black.
- Heat and cold produce specific local physiologic and systemic responses that account for their therapeutic effects.
- Various parts of the body differ in tolerance to heat and cold. The physiologic tolerance of individuals also varies. Specific conditions such as neurosensory and circulatory impairments necessitate precautions when applying heat or cold.
- When applying heat or cold, clients and nurses need to be aware of the effects of thermal receptor adaptation and the rebound phenomenon.

TEST YOUR KNOWLEDGE

1. Your client has a Braden scale score of 17. The appropriate nursing action is:
1. Assess the client again in 24 hours; the score is within normal limits.
2. Implement a turning schedule; the client is at increased risk of skin breakdown.
3. Apply a transparent wound barrier to major pressure sites; the client is at moderate risk of skin breakdown.
4. Request an order for a special low-air-loss bed; the client is at very high risk of skin breakdown.

2. Proper technique for performing a wound culture includes which of the following?
1. Cleansing the wound prior to obtaining the specimen
2. Swabbing for the specimen in the area with the largest collection of drainage
3. Removing crusts or scabs with sterile forceps and then culturing the site beneath
4. Waiting 8 hours following a dose of antibiotic to obtain the specimen

3. A client has a pressure ulcer with a shallow, partial skin thickness, eroded area but no necrotic areas. The nurse would treat the area with which of the following dressings?
1. Alginate
2. Dry gauze

3. Hydrocolloid
4. No dressing is indicated

4. Thirty (30) minutes after application is initiated, the client requests that the nurse leave the heating pad in place. The nurse explains to the client that:
1. Heat application for longer than 30 minutes can actually cause the opposite effect (constriction) of the one desired (dilation).
2. It will be acceptable to leave the pad in place if the temperature is reduced.
3. It will be acceptable to leave the pad in place for another 30 minutes if the site appears satisfactory when assessed.
4. It will be acceptable to leave the pad in place as long as it is moist heat.

5. Which statement, if made by the client or family member, would indicate the need for further teaching?
1. If a skin area gets red but then the red goes away after turning, I should report it to the nurse.
2. Putting foam pads under the heels or other bony areas can help decrease pressure.
3. If a person cannot turn himself or herself in bed, someone should help the person change position every 4 hours.
4. The skin should be washed with only warm water (not hot) and lotion put on while it is still a little wet.

6. Your client is only comfortable lying on the right or left side (not on the back or stomach). List four potential sites of pressure ulcers you must assess.

1.

2.

3.

4.

7. An appropriate nursing diagnosis for a client with large areas of skin excoriation resulting from scratching an allergic rash is:
1. *Risk for Impaired Skin Integrity.*
2. *Impaired Skin Integrity.*
3. *Impaired Tissue Integrity.*
4. *Risk for Infection.*

8. Which of the following are primary risk factors for pressure ulcers? Select all that apply.
1. Low-protein diet
2. Insomnia
3. Lengthy surgical procedures

4. Fever
5. Sleeping on a waterbed

9. Which of the following items are used to perform wound irrigation? Select all that apply.
1. Clean gloves
2. Sterile gloves
3. Refrigerated irrigating solution
4. 60-mL syringe

10. Which of the following indicates proper use of a triangle arm sling?
1. The elbow is kept flexed at 90 degrees or more.
2. The knot is placed on either side of the vertebrae of the neck.
3. The sling extends to just proximal of the hand.
4. Remove the sling every 2 hours to check for circulation and skin integrity.

See Answers to Test Your Knowledge in Appendix A.

EXPLORE MEDIALINK   www.prenhall.com/berman

DVD-ROM
- Audio Glossary
- NCLEX Review
- Skills Checklists
- Animations:
  Pressure Ulcers
  Feature Integument
  Layers of the Skin
  Integumentary Repair

COMPANION WEBSITE
- Additional NCLEX Review
- Case Study: Clients with Chronic Illnesses
- Care Plan Activity: Client with Pressure Ulcer
- Application Activity:
  Enterostomal Therapist
- Links to Resources

READINGS AND REFERENCES

SUGGESTED READINGS

Ayello, E. A., Dowsett, C., Schultz, G. S., Sibbald, G., Falanga, V., Harding, K., et al. (2004). Time heals all wounds. *Nursing, 34*(4), 36–42. *This comprehensive article uses the term TIME to stand for Tissue—nonviable or deficient, Infection or Inflammation, Moisture imbalance, and Edge of wound—nonadvancing or nonmigrating, to describe nonhealing wound assessment criteria. Photographs of wounds in various stages and conditions are included with detailed descriptions as is a review of wound-healing physiology. Clinical actions and expected outcomes are described for each of the TIME criteria.*

Van Rijswijk, L. (2004). Bridging the gap between research and practice: Moist dressings are better than dry ones. *American Journal of Nursing, 104*(2), 28–30. *This article describes several practices still common in nursing that are contrary to the research on effective wound care strategies. The author cites the abundance of different products available for wound care as one obstacle to evidence-based practice. The author also suggests the use of a multidisciplinary wound care protocol review committee as a strategy for overcoming the obstacle.*

RELATED RESEARCH

Defloor, T., & Grypdonck, M. F. (2005). Pressure ulcers, validation of two risk assessment scales. *Journal of Clinical Nursing, 14,* 373–382.

REFERENCES

Bergstrom, N., Allman, R. M., Alvarez, A. M., Bennett, M. A., Carlson, C. E., Frantz, R. A., et al. (1994). *Pressure Ulcer Treatment: Clinical Practice Guideline Number 15. Quick Reference Guide for Clinicians* (Publication No. 95-0653). Rockville, MD: Agency for Health Care Policy and Research, Public Health Service, U.S. Department of Health and Human Services.

Brown, G. (2006). Wound documentation: Managing risk. *Advances in Skin and Wound Care, 19,* 155–165.

Coulthard, P., Worthington, H., Esposito, M., van der Elst, M., & van Waes, O. J. F. (2005). Tissue adhesives for closure of surgical incisions. *The Cochrane Library* (ID #CD004287).

Cullum, N., McInnes, E., Bell-Syer, S. E. M., & Legood, R. (2005). Support surfaces for pressure ulcer prevention. *The Cochrane Library* (ID #CD001735).

Dochterman, J., & Bulechek, G. B. (Eds.). (2004). *Nursing interventions classification (NIC)* (4th ed.). St. Louis, MO: Mosby.

Fernandez, R., Griffiths, R., & Ussia, C. (2006). Water for wound cleansing (Cochrane Review). In *The Cochrane Library,* Issue 1, 2006. Oxford: Update Software.

Folkedahl, B. A., & Frantz, R. (2002a). *Prevention of pressure ulcers.* Iowa City, IA: University of Iowa Gerontological Nursing Interventions Research Center, Research Dissemination Core; 2002. Retrieved June 9, 2006, from http://www.guideline.gov/summary/summary. aspx?view_id=1&doc_id=3458&nbr=2684

Folkedahl, B. A., & Frantz, R. (2002b). *Treatment of pressure ulcers.* Iowa City; IA: University of Iowa Gerontological Nursing Interventions Research Center, Research Dissemination Core. Retrieved June 9, 2006, from http://www.guideline.gov/summary/summary. aspx?view_id=1&doc_id=3457&nbr=2683

Hanson, D., Langemo, D., Thompson, P., Anderson, J., & Hunter, S. (2005). Understanding wound fluid and the phases of healing. *Advances in Skin & Wound Care, 18,* 360–362.

Mendez-Eastman, S. (2005). Using negative-pressure for positive results. *Nursing, 35*(5), 48–50.

Moorhead, S., Johnson, M., & Maas, M. (Eds.). (2004). *Nursing outcomes classification (NOC)* (3rd ed.). St. Louis, MO: Mosby.

National Pressure Ulcer Advisory Panel. (2001). *Pressure ulcer prevention: RN competency-based curriculum.* Reston, VA: Author.

National Pressure Ulcer Advisory Panel. (2003). *PUSH Tool 3.0.* Retrieved June 9, 2006, from http://www.npuap.org/PDF/push3.pdf

NANDA International. (2007). *Nursing diagnoses: Definitions and classification 2007–2008.* Philadelphia: Author.

Norton, D., McLaren, R., & Exton-Smith, A. N. (1975). *An investigation of geriatric nursing problems in hospital.* Edinburgh, UK: Churchill Livingstone.

Panel for the Prediction and Prevention of Pressure Ulcers in Adults. (1992a). *Clinical practice guideline, pressure ulcers in adults: Prediction and prevention* (Publication No. 92–0047). Rockville, MD: Agency for Health Care Policy and Research, Public Health Service, U.S. Department of Health and Human Services.

Panel for the Prediction and Prevention of Pressure Ulcers in Adults. (1992b). *Pressure ulcers in adults: Prediction and prevention. Quick reference guide for clinicians* (AHCPR Publication No. 92-0050). Rockville, MD: Agency for Health Care Policy and Research, Public Health Service, U.S. Department of Health and Human Services.

Smith, N. (2004). The benefits of VAC therapy in the management of pressure ulcers. *British Journal of Nursing, 13,* 1359–60, 1362, 1364–5.

Sosin, J. (2005). Ancient remedy heals today's wounds. *Nursing Spectrum, 14*(6), 32–33.

U.S. Department of Health and Human Services. (2000). *Healthy people 2010: Understanding and improving health* (2nd ed.). Washington, DC: U.S. Government Printing Office.

Whittington, K. T., & Briones, R. (2004). National prevalence and incidence study, 6 year sequential acute care data. *Advances in Skin and Wound Care, 17,* 490–494.

SELECTED BIBLIOGRAPHY

Anderson, I. (2006). Debridement methods in wound care. *Nursing Standard, 20*(24), 65–66, 68, 70.

Ankrom, M. A., Bennett, R. G., Sprigle, S., Langemo, D., Black, J. M., Berlowitz, D. R., et al. (2005). Pressure related deep tissue injury under intact skin and the current pressure ulcer staging systems. *Advances in Skin and Wound Care, 18*(1), 35–42.

Baldwin, K. M. (2006). Damage control: Preventing and treating pressure ulcers. *Nursing Made Incredibly Easy, 4*(1), 12–15, 17–23, 25–27.

Baranoski, S., & Ayello, E. A. (2005). Wound & skin care. Using a wound assessment form. *Nursing, 35*(3), 14–15.

Braden, B. J., & Maklebust, J. (2005). Preventing pressure ulcers with the Braden Scale. *American Journal of Nursing, 105*(6), 70–72.

Duimel-Peeters, I. (2005). Preventing pressure ulcers with massage? *American Journal of Nursing, 105*(8), 31, 33.

Frantz, R. A., Tang, J. H., & Titler, M. G. (2004). Evidence-based protocol: Prevention of pressure ulcers. *Journal of Gerontological Nursing, 30*(5), 4–11.

Keefe, S. (2004). Healing severe wounds. *Advance for Nurses, 1*(12), 32, 40.

Langemo, D., & Hanson, D. (2005). Sizing up wounds accurately, *Nursing, 35*(4), 70–71.

Moz, T. (2004). Action Stat: Wound dehiscence and evisceration. *Nursing, 34*(5), 88.

Ousey, K. (2005). *Pressure area care.* Oxford, UK: Blackwell.

Sarvis, C. (2004). Wound and skin care: The role of bacterial toxins in wounds. *Nursing, 34*(7), 68.

Verdu, J. (2003). Can a decision tree help nurses to grade and treat pressure ulcers? *Journal of Wound Care, 12*(2), 45–50.

Whittington, K. T. (2005). Cost-saving wound assessments. *Advance for Nurses, 2*(2), 25–26.

Perioperative Nursing

LEARNING OUTCOMES

After completing this chapter, you will be able to:

1. Discuss various types of surgery according to degree of urgency, degree of risk, and purpose.

2. Describe the phases of the perioperative period.

3. Identify essential aspects of preoperative assessment.

4. Give examples of pertinent nursing diagnoses for surgical clients.

5. Identify nursing responsibilities in planning perioperative nursing care.

6. Describe essential preoperative teaching, including pain control, moving, leg exercises, and coughing and deep-breathing exercises.

7. Describe essential aspects of preparing a client for surgery, including skin preparation.

8. Compare various types of anesthesia.

9. Identify essential nursing assessments and interventions during the immediate postanesthetic phase.

10. Demonstrate ongoing nursing assessments and interventions for the postoperative client.

11. Identify potential postoperative complications and describe nursing interventions to prevent them.

12. Identify essential aspects of managing gastrointestinal suction.

13. Describe appropriate wound care for a postoperative client.

14. Evaluate the effectiveness of perioperative nursing interventions.

Surgery is a unique experience of a planned physical alteration encompassing three phases: preoperative, intraoperative, and postoperative. These three phases are together referred to as the **perioperative period.** Perioperative nursing is the delivery of nursing care through the framework of the nursing process. It also includes collaborating with members of the health care team, making nursing referrals, and delegating and supervising nursing care.

The **preoperative phase** begins when the decision to have surgery is made; it ends when the client is transferred to the operating table. The nursing activities associated with this phase include assessing the client, identifying potential or actual health problems, planning specific care based on the individual's needs, and providing preoperative teaching for the client, the family, and significant others.

The **intraoperative phase** begins when the client is transferred to the operating table and ends when the client is admitted to the postanesthesia care unit (PACU), also called the postanesthetic room or recovery room. The nursing activities related to this phase include a variety of specialized procedures designed to create and maintain a safe therapeutic environment for the client and the health care personnel. These activities include interventions that provide for the client's safety, maintaining an aseptic environment, ensuring proper functioning of equipment, and providing the surgical team with the instruments and supplies needed during the procedure.

The **postoperative phase** begins with the admission of the client to the postanesthesia area and ends when healing is complete. During the postoperative phase, nursing activities include assessing the client's response (physiologic and psychologic) to surgery, performing interventions to facilitate healing and prevent complications, teaching and providing support to the client and support people, and planning for home care. The goal is to assist the client to achieve the most optimal health status possible.

Perioperative nursing is practiced in hospital-based inpatient and outpatient surgical/laser/endoscopy suites, physician office-based surgical suites (outpatient), and/or freestanding outpatient/ambulatory surgical centers. Outpatient procedures do not require an overnight hospital stay. The client goes to the outpatient site the day of surgery, has the procedure, and leaves the same day.

The perioperative nurse's role is underscored by the nursing process and all the care activities inherent in that process regardless of the health care setting in which it is operationalized.

TYPES OF SURGERY

Surgical procedures are commonly grouped according to (a) purpose, (b) degree of urgency, and (c) degree of risk.

Purpose

Surgical procedures may be categorized according to their purpose (see Box 37–1).

Degree of Urgency

Surgery is classified by its urgency and necessity to preserve the client's life, body part, or body function. **Emergency surgery** is performed immediately to preserve function or the life of the client. Surgeries to control internal hemorrhage or repair a fracture are examples of emergency surgeries. **Elective surgery** is performed when surgical intervention is the preferred treatment for a condition that is not imminently life threatening (but may ultimately threaten life or well-being) or to improve the client's life. Examples of elective surgeries include cholecystectomy for chronic gallbladder disease, hip replacement surgery, and plastic surgery procedures such as breast reduction surgery.

Degree of Risk

Surgery is also classified as major or minor according to the degree of risk to the client. **Major surgery** involves a high degree of risk, for a variety of reasons: It may be complicated or prolonged, large losses of blood may occur, vital organs may be involved, or postoperative complications may be likely. Examples

BOX 37–1	**Purposes of Surgical Procedures**
Diagnostic	Confirms or establishes a diagnosis; for example, biopsy of a mass in a breast.
Palliative	Relieves or reduces pain or symptoms of a disease; it does not cure; for example, resection of nerve roots.
Ablative	Removes a diseased body part; for example, removal of a gallbladder (cholecystectomy).
Constructive	Restores function or appearance that has been lost or reduced; for example, breast implant.
Transplant	Replaces malfunctioning structures; for example, kidney transplant.

are organ transplant, open heart surgery, and removal of a kidney. In contrast, **minor surgery** normally involves little risk, produces few complications, and is often performed in an outpatient setting. Examples are breast biopsy, removal of tonsils, and knee surgery.

The degree of risk involved in a surgical procedure is affected by the client's age, general health, nutritional status, use of medications, and mental status.

Age

Neonates/infants and elder clients are greater surgical risks than children and adults. Age and developmental status affect a child's ability to cope with the physiologic and psychologic stresses of surgery. Neonates and infants have a higher metabolic rate and a different physiologic makeup than adults. These differences cause a substantially different response to a surgical procedure. For example, the blood volume in an infant is small, and fluid reserves are limited. This increases the risk of volume depletion during surgery resulting in inadequate oxygenation of body tissues. Because of the infant's relatively large body surface area and immature temperature regulatory mechanisms, the risk of hypothermia during surgery is significant. Other organ systems, such as the kidneys, liver, and immune system, also have not achieved maturity in infants, affecting their ability to metabolize and eliminate drugs and resist infection.

Toddlers and older children are better able to withstand surgery physiologically, but they often fear separation from their parents, strangers, bodily injury/mutilation, and death. The child's developmental level and age-appropriate communication are important in implementing the pediatric plan of care. The parent–child relationship, the parents' coping abilities, and the preoperative teaching and support will affect how well the child is able to deal with these surgical fears and the level of anxiety experienced.

The older adult (65 years and older) often has fewer physiologic reserves to meet the extra demands caused by surgery. The physiologic deficits of aging increase the surgical risk for the older adult. For example, because of a lower percentage of body water, decreased kidney function, and a decreased thirst response, elders are at greater risk for fluid and electrolyte imbalances. Many elders demonstrate changes in liver and kidney function, both of which can affect response to anesthesia and other medications that may be administered during the perioperative period. The older adult may be poorly nourished, which can impair healing. Declines in sensory function (hearing in particular) or the presence of dementia make it more difficult to understand directions and teaching. In addition, the elder is more likely to have a chronic disease, such as cardiovascular disease, chronic lung disease, or diabetes, that affects healing and responses to medication and surgery.

General Health

Surgery is least risky when the client's general health is good. Any infection or pathophysiology increases the risk. Of particular concern are upper respiratory tract infections, which together with a general anesthetic can adversely affect respiratory function. Where there is a high risk of infection, antibiotics may be administered parenterally within 1 hour of surgery and continued for 24 to 72 hours after surgery. This practice allows time for drugs to reach therapeutic levels in the tissues but does not permit bacterial resistance to develop. Common health problems that increase surgical risk and may lead to the decision to postpone or cancel surgery are listed in Box 37–2.

Nutritional Status

Adequate nutrition is required for normal tissue repair. Surgery increases the body's need for nutrients for the needed tissue healing and prevention of infection required during the postoperative period. Obesity and malnutrition increase surgical risk.

Obesity contributes to postoperative complications such as pneumonia, wound infections, and wound separation. Both obese and underweight clients are vulnerable to pressure ulcer formation due to positioning required for surgery. The perioperative nurse provides padding and other measures to protect the client's skin over pressure points during surgery.

Many vitamins and minerals are essential in wound healing (see Table 37–1). A malnourished client is at risk for delayed wound healing, wound infection, and fluid and electrolyte alterations. If a client has serious malnutrition, the surgery may be postponed to improve the nutritional status. If the surgery cannot be delayed, parenteral or enteral nutrition may be initiated.

BOX 37–2   Health Problems that Increase Surgical Risk

- Malnutrition can lead to delayed wound healing, infection, and reduced energy. Protein and vitamins are needed for wound healing; vitamin K is essential for blood clotting.
- Obesity leads to hypertension, impaired cardiac function, and impaired respiratory ventilation. Obese clients are also more likely to have delayed wound healing and wound infection because adipose tissue impedes blood circulation and its delivery of nutrients, antibodies, and enzymes required for wound healing.
- Cardiac conditions such as angina pectoris, recent myocardial infarction, hypertension, and heart failure weaken the heart. Well-controlled cardiac problems generally pose minimal operative risk.
- Blood coagulation disorders may lead to severe bleeding, hemorrhage, and subsequent shock.

- Upper respiratory tract infections or chronic obstructive lung diseases such as emphysema adversely affect pulmonary function, especially when exacerbated by the effects of general anesthesia. They also predispose the client to postoperative lung infections.
- Renal disease impairs regulation of the body's fluids and electrolytes and excretion of drugs and other toxins.
- Diabetes mellitus predisposes the client to wound infection and delayed healing.
- Liver disease (e.g., cirrhosis) impairs the liver's abilities to detoxify medications used during surgery, produce the prothrombin necessary for blood clotting, and metabolize nutrients essential for healing.
- Uncontrolled neurologic disease such as epilepsy may result in seizures during surgery or recovery.

TABLE 37–1 **Vitamins and Minerals Essential to Wound Healing**	
VITAMIN OR MINERAL	**FUNCTION**
Vitamin A	Promotes epithelialization and enhances collagen synthesis
Vitamin B complex	Cofactor of the enzyme system
Vitamin C (ascorbic acid)	Essential for collagen synthesis affecting wound tensile strength
Vitamin K	Essential in the synthesis of prothrombin and thus coagulation
Iron, zinc, and copper	Involved in collagen synthesis

Medications

The regular use of certain medications can increase surgical risk. Consider these examples:

- *Anticoagulants* increase blood coagulation time.
- *Tranquilizers* may interact with anesthetics, increasing the risk of respiratory depression.
- *Corticosteroids* may interfere with wound healing and increase the risk of infection.
- *Diuretics* may affect fluid and electrolyte balance.

Clients may be unaware of the potential adverse interactions of medications and may fail to report the use of medications for conditions unrelated to the indication for surgery. The astute nurse interviewer should question the client and family about the use of commonly prescribed medications, over-the-counter preparations, and any herbal remedies for specific conditions mentioned during the nursing history.

Mental Status

Disorders that affect cognitive function, such as mental illness, mental retardation, or developmental delay, affect the client's ability to understand and cope with the stresses of surgery. These clients also may require medication such as anticonvulsants or antipsychotic drugs that can interact with anesthetic and analgesic medications used during and after surgery.

Clients with dementia may have difficulty understanding proposed surgical procedures and may respond unpredictably to anesthetics. Manifestations of dementia such as confusion, disorientation, and agitation also may be aggravated by the change of environment in the hospital, interfering with the client's ability to cooperate with pre- and postoperative care.

Extreme anxiety also increases surgical risk and interferes with the client's ability to process information and respond appropriately to instructions. In some instances, professional counseling is indicated prior to surgery. It is also important to determine whether clients have coping skills and support systems to help them.

PREOPERATIVE PHASE
Preoperative Consent

Prior to any surgical procedure, informed consent is required from the client or legal guardian. Informed consent implies that the client has been informed and involved in decisions affecting his or her health. The surgeon is responsible for obtaining the informed consent by providing the following information to the client or legal guardian:

- The nature of and the reason for the surgery
- All available options and the risks associated with each option
- The risks of the surgical procedure and its potential outcomes
- Name and qualifications of the surgeon performing the procedure
- The right to refuse consent or later withdraw consent

The surgeon documents the informed consent conversation with the client or legal guardian in the preoperative progress note.

The surgical consent form, provided by the agency, protects the client from incorrect/unwanted procedures and the surgeon and agency from litigation related to unauthorized surgeries or uninformed clients. This consent form becomes part of the client's medical record and goes to the operating room with the client.

Although the surgeon maintains legal responsibility for ensuring that the client is giving informed consent, the nurse may witness the client's signature on the agency consent form. In doing so, the nurse ensures that the consent form is signed and serves as a witness to the signature, not to the fact that the client is informed. If the nurse assesses that the client does not understand the procedure to be performed, the surgeon is contacted and requested to speak with the client before surgery can proceed.

Informed consent is only possible when the client understands the provided information, that is, speaks the language and is conscious, mentally competent, and not sedated. Informed consent may not be given by a minor. Specific guidelines regarding consent for minors vary among the states. Nurses must be aware of their responsibilities regarding consent and of the particular hospital's policies (see Chapter 4). ∞

NURSING MANAGEMENT

Assessing

Preoperative assessment includes collecting and reviewing physical, psychologic, and social client data to determine the client's needs throughout the three perioperative phases. The perioperative nurse collects the data by interviewing the client in the presurgical care unit or by telephone prior to the day of surgery. When data cannot be collected directly, the perioperative nurse uses other data sources such as the nursing admission assessment. Although forms vary considerably among agencies, Box 37–3 summarizes essential preoperative information that should be included.

Physical Assessment

Preoperatively, the nurse performs a brief but complete physical assessment, paying particular attention to systems that could affect the client's response to anesthesia or surgery. A brief or "mini" mental status examination provides valuable baseline data for evaluating the client's mental status and alertness after surgery. It

BOX 37–3 **Preoperative Assessment Data**

- *Current health status.* Essential information includes general health status and the presence of any chronic diseases, such as diabetes or asthma, that may affect the client's response to surgery or anesthesia. Note any physical limitations that may affect the client's mobility or ability to communicate after surgery, as well as any prostheses such as hearing aids or contact lenses.
- *Allergies.* Include allergies to prescription and nonprescription drugs, food allergies, and allergies to tape, latex, soaps, or antiseptic agents. Some food allergies may indicate a potential reaction to drugs or substances used during surgery or diagnostic procedures; for example, an allergy to seafood alerts the nurse to a potential allergy to iodine-based dyes or soaps commonly used in hospitals.
- *Medications.* List all current medications (prescribed and OTC). It may be vital to maintain a blood level of some medications (e.g., anticonvulsants) throughout the surgical experience; others, such as anticoagulants or aspirin, increase the risks of surgery and anesthesia and need to be discontinued several days prior to surgery. It is important to include in the list any herbal remedies the client currently takes.
- *Previous surgeries.* Previous surgical experiences may influence the client's physical and psychologic responses to surgery or may reveal unexpected responses to anesthesia.
- *Mental status.* The client's mental status and ability to understand and respond appropriately can affect the entire perioperative experience. Note any developmental disabilities, mental illness, history of dementia, or excessive anxiety related to the procedure.
- *Understanding of the surgical procedure and anesthesia.* The client should have a good understanding of the planned procedure and what to expect during and after surgery as well as the expected outcome of the procedure.
- *Smoking.* Smokers may have more difficulty clearing respiratory secretions after surgery, increasing the risk of postoperative complications such as pneumonia and atelectasis and delayed wound healing.
- *Alcohol and other mind-altering substances.* Use of substances that affect the central nervous system, liver, or other body systems can affect the client's response to anesthesia and surgery, and postoperative recovery.
- *Coping.* Clients with a healthy self-concept who have successfully employed appropriate coping mechanisms in the past are better able to deal with the stressors associated with surgery.
- *Social resources.* Determine the availability of family or other caregivers as well as the client's social support network. These resources are important to the client's recovery, particularly for the client undergoing same-day or short-stay surgery.
- *Cultural and spiritual considerations.* Culture and spirituality influence the client's response to surgery; respecting cultural and spiritual beliefs and practices can reduce preoperative anxiety and improve recovery.

is also important to evaluate the client's ability to understand what is happening. For example, assessment of hearing and vision help guide perioperative teaching. Respiratory and cardiovascular assessments not only provide baseline data for evaluating the client's postoperative status but also may alert care providers to a problem (e.g., a respiratory infection or irregular pulse rate) that may affect the client's response to surgery and anesthesia. Other systems (gastrointestinal, genitourinary, and musculoskeletal) are examined to provide baseline data (see Chapter 30). ∞

Screening Tests

The surgeon and/or anesthesiologist orders preoperative diagnostic tests. Abnormalities may warrant treatment prior to surgery. The nurse's responsibility is to check the orders carefully, to see that they are carried out, and to ensure that the results are obtained and in the client's record prior to surgery. Table 37–2 lists routine preoperative screening tests. In addition to these routine tests, diagnostic tests directly related to the client's

TABLE 37–2 **Routine Preoperative Screening Tests**	
TEST	**RATIONALE**
Complete blood count (CBC)	RBCs, hemoglobin (Hgb), and hematocrit (Hct) are important to the oxygen-carrying capacity of the blood; WBCs are an indicator of immune function
Blood grouping and cross-matching	Determined in case blood transfusion is required during or after surgery
Serum electrolytes (Na^+, K^+, Ca^{2+}, Mg^{2+}, Cl^-, HCO_3^-)	To evaluate fluid and electrolyte status
Fasting blood glucose	High levels may indicate undiagnosed diabetes mellitus
Blood urea nitrogen (BUN) and creatinine	To evaluate renal function
ALT, AST, LDH, and bilirubin	To evaluate liver function
Serum albumin and total protein	To evaluate nutritional status
Urinalysis	To determine urine composition and possible abnormal components (e.g., protein or glucose) or infection
Chest x-ray	To evaluate respiratory status and heart size
Electrocardiogram (ECG) (all clients over 40 years of age and/or clients with preexisting cardiac conditions)	To identify preexisting cardiac problems or disease
Pregnancy test (all female clients of childbearing age)	To identify if the client is pregnant

disease are usually appropriate (e.g., gastroscopy to clarify the pathologic condition before gastric surgery).

Diagnosing

Nursing diagnoses that may be appropriate for the preoperative client include the following:

- *Deficient Knowledge* related to
  - A lack of education about the perioperative process
  - A lack of exposure to the specific perioperative experience
- *Anxiety* related to
  - Effects of surgery on ability to function in usual roles
  - Outcome of exploratory surgery for malignancy
  - Risk of death
  - Loss of control during anesthesia or waking up during anesthesia
  - Perceived inadequate postoperative analgesia
  - Change in health status and/or body image
- *Disturbed Sleep Pattern* related to
  - Hospital routines
  - Psychologic stress
- *Anticipatory Grieving* related to
  - Perceived loss of body part associated with planned surgery
- *Ineffective Coping* related to
  - Conflicting values (e.g., need for blood transfusion versus the religious values for a Jehovah's Witness)
  - Lack of clear outcomes of surgery
  - Unresolved past negative experience with surgery

Examples of clinical application of some of these diagnoses using NANDA, NIC, and NOC designations are shown in Identifying Nursing Diagnoses, Outcomes, and Interventions.

Planning

The overall goal in the preoperative period is to ensure that the client is mentally and physically prepared for surgery. Examples of nursing activities to meet this goal are discussed in the "Implementing" section that follows.

Planning should involve the client, the family, and/or significant others. Preoperative care planning and teaching interventions are usually done on an outpatient basis either in person or via a telephone interview by the perioperative nurse.

Examples of clinical application of NOC outcomes and NIC interventions are shown in Identifying Nursing Diagnoses, Outcomes, and Interventions.

Planning for Home Care

For the perioperative client, discharge planning begins before admission for the planned procedure. Early planning to meet the discharge needs of the client is particularly important for outpatient procedures, as generally these clients are discharged within hours after the procedure is performed.

Discharge planning incorporates an assessment of the client's, family's, and significant others' abilities and resources for care, their financial resources, and the need for referrals and home health services. However, the extent of discharge plan-

IDENTIFYING NURSING DIAGNOSES, OUTCOMES, AND INTERVENTIONS
The Preoperative Client

DATA CLUSTER Mr. Taylor, 62 years old, has disabling osteoarthritis and is scheduled for a total knee replacement tomorrow. This is his first surgical experience and he is asking many questions about what to expect before and after surgery. He says, "The more I know, the less anxious I feel."

NURSING DIAGNOSIS/ DEFINITION	SAMPLE DESIRED OUTCOME*/ DEFINITION	INDICATORS	SELECTED INTERVENTIONS/ DEFINITION	SAMPLE NIC ACTIVITIES
Deficient Knowledge (Surgery)/Absence or deficiency of cognitive information related to a specific topic	Knowledge: Treatment Procedure(s) [1814]/ *Extent of understanding conveyed about procedure(s) required as part of a treatment regimen*	Substantial: ■ Description of steps of procedure (e.g., preoperative process) ■ Description of treatment procedures (e.g., deep breathing and coughing, leg exercises)	Teaching: Preoperative [5610]/ *Assisting a patient to understand and mentally prepare for surgery and the postoperative recovery period*	■ Provide time for the client to ask questions and discuss concerns ■ Describe the preoperative routines (e.g., anesthesia, diet, tests/lab, voiding, IV therapy, family waiting area) as appropriate ■ Instruct the client on the technique of splinting his/her incision, coughing, and deep breathing ■ Evaluate the client's ability to return demonstrate leg exercise

*The NOC # for desired outcomes and the NIC # for nursing interventions are listed in brackets following the appropriate outcome or intervention. Outcomes, indicators, interventions, and activities selected are only a sample of those suggested by NOC and NIC and should be further individualized for each client.

ning and home care will vary significantly for clients having different types of surgery.

Implementing

The major nursing activity to ensure that the client is prepared for surgery is preoperative teaching.

Preoperative Teaching

Preoperative teaching is a vital part of nursing care. Studies have shown that preoperative teaching reduces clients' anxiety and postoperative complications and increases their satisfaction with the surgical experience. Good preoperative teaching also facilitates the client's successful and early return to work and other activities of daily living. Four dimensions of preoperative teaching have been identified as important to clients:

- *Information, including what will happen to the client, when, and what the client will experience, such as expected sensations and discomfort.* The nurse needs to listen carefully and attentively to the client to identify specific concerns and fears. Typical questions are: "What will happen during surgery? How will I feel after the operation? What will the surgeon find? How long will I be in the hospital?"
- *Psychosocial support to reduce anxiety.* The nurse provides support by actively listening and providing accurate information. It is important to rectify any misperceptions the client may have.
- *The roles of the client and support people in preoperative preparation, the surgical procedure, and during the postop-*

erative phase. Understanding his or her role during the perioperative experience increases the client's sense of control and reduces anxiety. This includes what will be expected of the client, desired behaviors, self-care activities, and what the client can do to facilitate recovery.

- *Skills training.* This includes moving, deep breathing, coughing, splinting incisions with the hands or a pillow, and using an incentive spirometer.

If the client is scheduled for outpatient surgery, preoperative teaching is often provided before the day of surgery using some combination of videos and verbal and written instructions. The client may have an appointment with the outpatient perioperative nurse (usually scheduled to coincide with preoperative diagnostic testing) to discuss preoperative concerns and implement the teaching plan. Written instructions are always provided to reinforce verbal teaching. Teaching is further reinforced on admission the day of surgery and before discharge from the postanesthesia unit. Preoperative instructions are summarized in Box 37–4.

When the client is a child, addressing the fears and anxieties of both the child and the family is vital. Parents need to know what to expect and to be able to express their concerns. Parents should be considered members of the perioperative team and allowed to participate in providing as much care as possible.

Skill 37-1 provides guidelines for teaching clients about moving, leg exercises, deep breathing, and coughing.

BOX 37–4 **Preoperative Instructions**

PREOPERATIVE REGIMEN
- Explain the need for preoperative tests (e.g., laboratory, x-ray, ECG).
- Discuss bowel preparation, if required.
- Discuss skin preparation, including operative area and preoperative bath or shower.
- Discuss preoperative medications, if ordered.
- Explain individual therapies ordered by the primary care provider, such as intravenous therapy, the insertion of a urinary catheter or nasogastric tube, use of a spirometer, or antiemboli stockings.
- Discuss the visit by the anesthetist.
- Explain the need to restrict food and oral fluids at least 8 hours before surgery.
- Provide a general timetable for perioperative events, including the time of surgery.
- Discuss the need to remove jewelry, makeup, and all prostheses (e.g., eyeglasses, hearing aids, complete or partial dentures, wig) immediately before surgery.
- Inform client about the preoperative holding area, and give the location of the waiting room for support people.
- Teach deep-breathing and coughing exercises, leg exercises, ways to turn and move (see Skill 37-1), and splinting techniques.
- Complete the preoperative checklist.

POSTOPERATIVE REGIMEN
- Discuss the postanesthesia recovery room's routines and emergency equipment.
- Review type and frequency of assessment activities.

- Discuss pain management.
- Explain usual activity restrictions and precautions related to getting up for the first time postoperatively.
- Describe usual dietary alterations.
- Discuss postoperative dressings and drains.
- Provide an explanation and tour of the intensive care unit if client is to be transferred there postoperatively.

OUTPATIENT SURGICAL CLIENTS
- Review all instructions in the preoperative and postoperative regimen.
  - Confirm place and time of surgery, including when to arrive (e.g., 1 to 1 1/2 hours before scheduled surgery) and where to register (e.g., reception desk).
- Discuss what to wear (e.g., clients having hand surgery should wear a garment with large sleeve openings to fit over a bulky dressing; all clients need to leave valuables at home).
- Explain the need for a responsible adult to drive or accompany the client home.
  - Discuss discharge criteria and how long the client should expect to stay postoperatively.
- Discuss medications, including specific preoperative medications and the client's current medication regimen.
- Communicate by telephone the evening before surgery to confirm time of surgery and arrival time.
- Communicate by telephone within 48 hours postoperatively to evaluate surgical outcomes and identify any problems or complications.

REAL WORLD PRACTICE

When teaching clients preoperatively about routines and expected behaviors, the nurse tries to incorporate all of the senses. Include experiences clients will have throughout the perioperative phase, as well as what they might expect to feel, hear, smell and taste from the time they are called to the OR until they return to their room. Discuss the bright lights, masks, and hair coverings that hospital personnel wear, operating room tables that feel hard and air that is cooler. The environment may smell of antiseptic solutions, noises will seem loud and monitor equipment beeps continuously. In the Post Anesthesia Unit (PACU), nurses will be calling out their name, asking them to take deep breaths, and checking to see if they are uncomfortable. Their mouths may feel dry and perhaps taste as if they've lost their toothbrush for a week. Dressings can feel tight, their throats may be sore, and their vision blurred. By describing sensory experiences, clients can have better outcomes, decreased pain and anxiety levels, and feel more satisfied because they know what to expect.

—*Mary Catherine Rawls, RN, MS, BC*
Dartmouth-Hitchcock Medical Center, Lebanon, NH

SKILL 37-1

TEACHING MOVING, LEG EXERCISES, DEEP BREATHING, AND COUGHING

PURPOSES

Moving

- To promote venous return
- To enhance lung expansion and mobilize secretions
- To stimulate gastrointestinal motility
- To facilitate early ambulation

Leg Exercises

- To promote venous return, thereby preventing thrombophlebitis and thrombus formation

Deep Breathing and Coughing

- To enhance lung expansion and mobilize secretions, thereby preventing atelectasis and pneumonia

ASSESSMENT

Assess

- Vital signs
- Discomfort
- Temperature and color of feet and legs
- Breath sounds
- Presence of dyspnea or cough
- Learning needs of the client
- Anxiety level of the client
- Client experience with previous surgeries and anesthesia

PLANNING

Before commencing to teach moving, leg exercises, deep-breathing exercises, and coughing, determine (a) the type of surgery, (b) the time of the surgery, (c) the name of the surgeon, (d) the preoperative orders, and (e) the agency's practices for preoperative care. Also, verify that the primary care provider has completed the medical history and physical examination and that the client or the family has signed the consent form.

Equipment

- Pillow
- Teaching materials (e.g., videotape, written materials) if available at the agency

Delegation

Assessment of the learning needs of the client and his or her support people and determining the teaching content and appropriate strategies for teaching requires application of professional knowledge and critical thinking. Preoperative teaching is conducted by the nurse and is not delegated to unlicensed assistive personnel (UAP). The UAP, however, can reinforce teaching, assist the client with the exercises, and report to the nurse if the client is unable to perform the exercises.

IMPLEMENTATION

Preparation

Ensure that potential distracters (e.g., pain, TV, visitors) to teaching are not present. Family and/or significant others should be included in the teaching plan, if appropriate.

Performance

1. Prior to performing the procedure, introduce self and verify the client's identity using agency protocol. Explain to the client what you are going to teach and the importance of the client's participation in the exercises he or she is going to be taught.
2. Perform hand hygiene and observe appropriate infection control procedures.
3. Provide for client privacy.
4. Show the client ways to turn in bed and to get out of bed.
   - Instruct a client who will have a right abdominal incision or a right-sided chest incision to turn to the left side of the bed and sit up as follows:

TEACHING MOVING, LEG EXERCISES, DEEP BREATHING, AND COUGHING *continued*

a. Flex the knees.

b. Splint the wound by holding the left arm and hand or a small pillow against the incision.

c. Turn to the left while pushing with the right foot and grasping a partial side rail on the left side of the bed with the right hand.

d. Come to a sitting position on the side of the bed by using the right arm and hand to push down against the mattress and swinging the feet over the edge of the bed.

- Teach a client with a left abdominal or left-sided chest incision to perform the same procedure but splint with the right arm and turn to the right.

- For clients with orthopedic surgery (e.g., hip surgery), use special aids, such as a trapeze, to assist with movement.

5. Teach the client the following three leg exercises:

- Alternate dorsiflexion and plantar flexion of the feet. **Rationale:** *This exercise is sometimes referred to as calf pumping, because it alternately contracts and relaxes the calf muscles, including the gastrocnemius muscles.* ❶

- Flex and extend the knees, and press the backs of the knees into the bed while dorsiflexing the feet. ❷ Instruct clients who cannot raise their legs to do isometric exercises that contract and relax the muscles.

- Raise and lower the legs alternately from the surface of the bed. Flex the knee of the stable leg and extend the knee of the moving leg. ❸ **Rationale:** *This exercise contracts and relaxes the quadriceps muscles.*

6. Demonstrate deep-breathing (diaphragmatic) exercises as follows.

- Place your hands palms down on the border of your rib cage, and inhale slowly and evenly through the nose until the greatest chest expansion is achieved. ❹

- Hold your breath for 2 to 3 seconds.
- Then exhale slowly through the mouth.
- Continue exhalation until maximum chest contraction has been achieved.

❷ Flexing and extending the knees.

❸ Raising and lowering the legs.

Anterior View

Quadriceps muscles

Vastus intermedius

Vastus lateralis

Vastus medialis
Rectus femoris

Gastrocnemius muscles

Posterior View

❶ Leg muscles: anterior and posterior views.

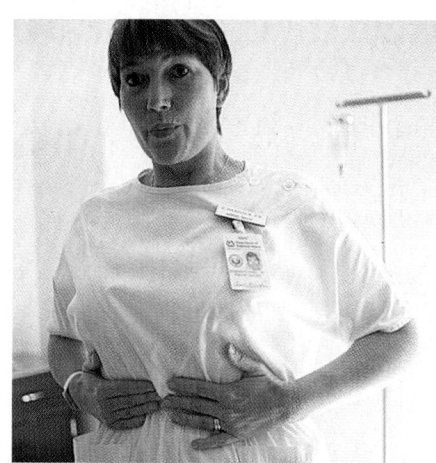

❹ Demonstrating deep breathing.

Photographer: Elena Dorfman

continued on page 948

TEACHING MOVING, LEG EXERCISES, DEEP BREATHING, AND COUGHING *continued*

7. Help the client perform deep-breathing exercises.
   - Ask the client to assume a sitting position.
   - Place the palms of your hands on the border of the client's rib cage to assess respiratory depth.
   - Ask the client to perform deep breathing, as described in step 6.
8. Instruct the client to cough voluntarily after five deep inhalations.
   - Ask the client to inhale deeply, hold the breath for a few seconds, and then cough once or twice.
   - Ensure that the client coughs deeply and does not just clear the throat.
9. If the incision will be painful when the client coughs, demonstrate techniques to splint the abdomen.
   - Show the client how to support the incision by placing the palms of the hands on either side of the incision site or directly over the incision site, holding the palm of one hand over the other. **Rationale:** *Coughing uses the abdominal and other accessory respiratory muscles. Splinting the incision may reduce pain while coughing if the incision is near any of these muscles.*
   - Show the client how to splint the abdomen with clasped hands and a firmly rolled pillow held against the client's abdomen. ❺
10. Inform the client about the expected frequency of these exercises.
    - Instruct the client to start the exercises as soon after surgery as possible.
    - Encourage clients to carry out deep breathing and coughing at least every 2 hours, taking a minimum of five breaths at each session. Note, however, that the number of breaths and frequency of deep breathing varies with the client's condition. People who are susceptible to pulmonary problems may need deep-breathing exercises every hour. People with chronic respiratory disease may need special breathing exercises (e.g.,

❺ Splinting an incision with a pillow while coughing.

Photographer: Elena Dorfman

pursed-lip breathing, abdominal breathing, exercises using various kinds of incentive spirometers). See Chapter 50. ∞

11. Document the teaching and all assessments. Some agencies may have a preoperative teaching flow sheet. Check agency policy.

SAMPLE DOCUMENTATION

3/19/2008 0900 Instructed how to splint abdomen while deep breathing and coughing. Able to perform correctly. Stated that he will use this technique after surgery.——— *A. Moore, RN*

EVALUATION

Document the outcome of the teaching plan such as:

- Client's demonstrated ability to perform moving, leg exercises, deep-breathing, and coughing exercises.
- Client's verbalization of key information presented.

LIFESPAN CONSIDERATIONS   **Preoperative Teaching**

CHILDREN

- Parents need to know what to expect and to be able to express their concerns.
- Separation from parents often is the child's greatest fear; the time of separation should be minimized and parents allowed to interact with the child both immediately preceding and following the surgery.
- Teaching/communicating with children (both timing and content) should be geared to the child's developmental level and cognitive abilities (e.g., "You will have a sore tummy").
- Play is an effective teaching tool with children (e.g., the child can put a bandage on an incision on a doll).

ELDERS

- Assess hearing ability to ensure the elder client hears the necessary information.
- Assess short-term memory. Presenting one focused idea at a time and repeating or reinforcing information may be necessary.

- Elders are at greater risk for postoperative complications, such as pneumonia. Reinforce moving and deep-breathing and coughing exercises.
- Assess potential postoperative needs at this time. Arrangements can be made preoperatively to obtain necessary items. Examples are medical equipment, such as walkers, raised toilet seats, and bed trapezes; Meals on Wheels; and help with transportation.
- If the elder client will need to be in extended care for a period of time after surgery, this is the time to initiate these plans.
- Assess the client for risk of pressure ulcer development postoperatively and be extra attentive to use of proper paddings and support devices to prevent injury during positioning and transfers in the operating room. Risks are
  - Older age.
  - Poor nutritional status.
  - History of diabetes or cardiovascular problems.
  - History of taking steroids, which cause increased bruising and skin breakdown.

HOME CARE CONSIDERATIONS Postoperative Instructions

Adults want information about activities they normally perform while they are recovering at home. This is important information for all surgical clients and particularly clients having the surgery as an outpatient. Discuss the following areas:

- *Food.* Eat small portions at first because anesthesia and pain medications slow gastric emptying.
- *Bowel movements.* Constipation occurs frequently as a result of decreased gastrointestinal mobility due to many causes (e.g., anesthesia, decreased activity, pain medications). Discuss strategies to prevent constipation.
- *Sexual activity.* Intimacy such as gentle hugging and kissing is allowed for clients when they feel like it. Full sexual intercourse cannot be resumed until wound soreness and tenderness is resolved, approximately 2 to 4 weeks. Check with the surgeon for gynecological procedures.

- *Wound care.* Discuss wound strength and care, including the signs and symptoms of infection and when to notify the surgeon.
- *Lifting.* Be specific about weight limits, if appropriate. Relate the weight limit to everyday items (e.g., a gallon of milk weighs approximately 8 pounds).
- *Pain.* Provide information about the client's pain medications. Ask the client to describe his or her daily activities, and discuss ways to avoid or reduce painful activities.
- *Bathing.* Check with the surgeon because some prefer the wound to be kept dry. There is no evidence that water on a closed wound is harmful or interferes with wound healing. If allowed, inform the client to shower, letting the warm water wash over the incision and gently pat the incision dry.
- *Activities.* Advise the client that he or she will tire easily and to plan short activities with frequent rest breaks.

Physical Preparation

Preoperative preparation includes the following areas: nutrition and fluids, elimination, hygiene, medications, rest, care of valuables and prostheses, special orders, and surgical skin preparation. In many agencies a preoperative checklist is used on the day of surgery. The nurse completes the agency's preoperative checklist following appropriate documenting procedures. It is essential that all pertinent records (laboratory records, x-ray films, consents) be available for perioperative personnel to refer to them and that all physical preparation is completed to ensure client safety.

NUTRITION AND FLUIDS. Adequate hydration and nutrition promote healing. Nurses need to identify and record any signs of malnutrition or fluid imbalance. If the client is on intravenous fluids or on measured fluid intake, nurses must ensure that the fluid intake and output is accurately measured and recorded.

The order "NPO after midnight" has been a long-standing tradition because it was believed that anesthestics depress gastrointestinal functioning and there was a danger the client would vomit and aspirate during the administration of a general anesthetic. Reevaluation and research, however, do not support this tradition. As a result, the American Society of Anesthesiology (ASA) revised its practice guidelines for preoperative fasting in healthy clients undergoing elective procedures. According to Crenshaw and Winslow (2002, p. 38), the revised guidelines allow for

- The consumption of clear liquids up to 2 hours before elective surgery requiring general anesthesia, regional anesthesia, or sedation-analgesia.
- A light breakfast (e.g., tea and toast) 6 hours before the procedure.
- A heavier meal 8 hours before surgery.

ELIMINATION. Enemas before surgery are no longer routine, but cleansing enemas may be ordered if bowel surgery is

planned. The enemas help prevent postoperative constipation and contamination of the surgical area (during surgery) by feces. After surgery involving the intestines, peristalsis often doesn't return for 24 to 48 hours.

Prior to surgery an in-and-out/straight catheterization or an indwelling Foley catheter may be ordered to ensure that the bladder remains empty. This helps prevent inadvertent injury to the bladder, particularly during pelvic surgery. If the client does not have a catheter, it is important to empty the bladder prior to receiving preoperative medications.

HYGIENE. In some settings, clients are asked to bathe or shower the evening or morning of surgery (or both). The purpose of hygienic measures is to reduce the risk of wound infection by reducing the amount of bacteria on the client's skin. The bath includes a shampoo whenever possible.

The client's nails should be trimmed and free of polish, and all cosmetics should be removed so that the nail beds, skin, and lips are visible when circulation is assessed during the perioperative phases.

Intraoperatively the client will be required to wear a surgical cap. The surgical cap contains the client's hair and any microorganisms on the hair and scalp.

Before going into the operating room the client should remove all hair pins and clips as they may cause pressure or accidental damage to the scalp when the client is unconscious. The client also removes personal clothing and puts on an operating room gown.

MEDICATIONS. The anesthetist or anesthesiologist may order routinely taken medications be held the day of surgery. In some settings preoperative medications are given to the client prior to going to the operating room. Commonly used preoperative medications include the following:

- *Sedatives* and *tranquilizers* such as secobarbital and diazepam (Valium) to reduce anxiety and ease anesthetic induction

- *Narcotic analgesics* such as morphine and meperidine (Demerol) to provide client sedation and reduce the required amount of anesthetic
- *Anticholinergics* such as atropine, scopolamine, and glycopyrrolate (Robinul) to reduce oral and pulmonary secretions and prevent laryngospasm
- *Histamine-receptor antihistamines* such as cimetidine (Tagamet) and ranitidine (Zantac) to reduce gastric fluid volume and gastric acidity
- *Neuroleptanalgesic* agents such as Innovar to induce general calmness and sleepiness

Preoperative medications must be given at a scheduled time or "on call," that is, when the operating room notifies the nurse to give the medication.

REST AND SLEEP. Nurses should do everything to help the client sleep the night before surgery. Often a sedative is ordered. Adequate rest helps the client manage the stress of surgery and helps healing.

VALUABLES. Valuables such as jewelry and money should be sent home with the client's family or significant other. If valuables/money cannot be sent home, they need to be labeled and placed in a locked storage area per the agency's policy. Removing jewelry also means removing body-piercing jewelry; there is a risk of injury from burns if an electrosurgical unit is used (Larkin, 2004). If a client wishes not to remove a wedding band, the nurse can tape it in place. Wedding bands must be removed, however, if there is danger of the fingers swelling after sur-

CULTURALLY COMPETENT CARE
Body Piercing

Body art (i.e., tattooing, piercing) has been practiced from ancient times to the present. Body piercing is considered one of the oldest forms of body art. The reasons for modern body piercing include making a fashion statement, observing a rite of passage, and creatively expressing oneself through highly visible piercing of the ears, nose, eyebrow, and navel. Piercings of the tongue, nipples, and genitals are of a more sexual expression or function. With the increasing number of people with body piercings, it is important for the perioperative nurse to deliver culturally sensitive care to clients with body piercings. Understanding the cultural and social meanings of body piercing helps provide cultural sensitivity while ensuring client safety.

The nurse needs to ensure that this jewelry is removed in addition to the more traditional jewelry. Safety issues that can occur if the body-piercing jewelry is not removed include alternate site burns when using electrosurgery, pressure injuries from the jewelry, dislocation and aspiration of the jewelry during tracheal intubation, and possible inability to insert a urinary catheter because of genitalia piercings.

The perioperative nurse may need to help the client remove the jewelry. It is important that the jewelry not be damaged or the client harmed (physically or psychologically) when removing the jewelry. Certain tools may need to be available for removal of the jewelry.

Note: Reprinted from *AORN Journal,* vol. 79, B. G. Larkin, "The Ins and Outs of Body Piercing," pp. 333–334. Copyright 2004, with permission from AORN, Inc.

gery. Situations warranting removal include surgery on or cast application to an arm, or a mastectomy that involves removal of the lymph nodes. (Mastectomies may cause edema of the arm and hand.)

PROSTHESES. All prostheses (artificial body parts, such as partial or complete dentures, contact lenses, artificial eyes, and artificial limbs) and eyeglasses, wigs, and false eyelashes must be removed before surgery. Hearing aids are often left in place and the operating room personnel notified.

In some hospitals, dentures are placed in a locked storage area; in others they are placed in labeled containers and kept at the client's bedside. Partial dentures can become dislodged and obstruct an unconscious client's breathing. The nurse also checks for the presence of chewing gum or loose teeth. Loose teeth are a common problem with 5- or 6-year-olds undergoing tonsillectomy because they can become dislodged and/or aspirated during anesthesia.

SPECIAL ORDERS. The nurse checks the surgeon's orders for special requirements (e.g., the insertion of a nasogastric tube prior to surgery, the administration of medications, such as insulin, or the application of antiemboli stockings). For the technique of inserting a nasogastric tube, see Skill 47-1 in Chapter 47. ∞

SKIN PREPARATION. In most agencies, skin preparation is carried out during the intraoperative phase. The surgical site is cleansed with an antimicrobial to remove soil and reduce the resident microbial count to subpathogenic levels.

SAFETY PROTOCOLS. The Joint Commission on Accreditation of Healthcare Organizations (JCAHO) established, effective July 2004, the Universal Protocol for Preventing Wrong Site, Wrong Procedure, Wrong Person Surgery (JCAHO, 2003; Steefel, 2004). This protocol involves three steps. The first step requires preoperative verification. Client verification used to be a one-time procedure. The protocol requires client verification at the time surgery is scheduled, during admission, and whenever the client is transferred to another caregiver.

The second step involves marking of the operative site in an unambiguous manner. The protocol does not specify the type of mark; however, JCAHO does require that the surgical site marking method be consistent throughout the facility and encourages client involvement. The facility chooses its own surgical site method (e.g., the client's initials, surgeon's initials, the word "YES"). An "X" is considered ambiguous and cannot be used for marking the site. The mark must be permanent and visible after the client has been prepped and draped for surgery.

The third step is called "time-out." Before surgery begins the surgical team takes a time-out to conduct a final verification of the correct client, procedure, and site. Any questions or concerns must be resolved before the procedure can begin.

VITAL SIGNS. Preoperatively assess and document vital signs for baseline data. Report any abnormal findings, such as elevated blood pressure or elevated temperature.

ANTIEMBOLI STOCKINGS. Antiemboli (elastic) stockings are firm elastic hose that compress the veins of the legs and thereby facilitate the return of venous blood to the heart. They also improve arterial circulation to the feet and prevent edema of the legs and feet. These stockings are frequently applied to surgical clients.

There are several types of stockings. One type extends from the foot to the knee and another from the foot to midthigh. These stockings usually have a partial foot that exposes the heel or toes so that extremity circulation can be assessed. Elastic stockings usually come in small, medium, and large sizes. Skill 37-2 details the steps required to apply antiemboli stockings.

APPLYING ANTIEMBOLI STOCKINGS

PURPOSES
- To facilitate venous return from the lower extremities
- To prevent venous stasis and venous thrombosis
- To reduce peripheral edema

ASSESSMENT
Assess both lower extremities for

- Rates, volumes, and rhythms of posterior tibial and dorsalis pedis pulses
- Skin color (note pallor, cyanosis, or other pigmentation)
- Skin temperature
- Presence of distended veins or edema
- Skin condition (e.g., thickened, shiny, taut)
- Homans' sign (pain in calf with passive dorsiflexion of the foot)

PLANNING
Before applying antiemboli stockings, determine any potential or present circulatory problems and the surgeon's orders involving the lower extremities.

Delegation
UAP frequently remove and apply antiemboli stockings as part of morning and evening hygiene care. The nurse should stress the importance of removing and reapplying the stockings and reporting any changes in the client's skin to the nurse.

Equipment
- Tape measure
- Clean antiemboli stockings of appropriate size and of the type ordered

IMPLEMENTATION
Preparation
Take measurements as needed to obtain the appropriate size stockings.

- Measure the length of both legs from the heel to the gluteal fold (for thigh-length stockings) or from the heel to the popliteal space (for knee-length stockings).
- Measure the circumference of each calf and each thigh at the widest point.
- Compare the measurements to the size chart to obtain stockings of correct size. Obtain two sizes if there is a significant difference. **Rationale:** *Stockings that are too large for the client do not place adequate pressure on the legs to facilitate venous return, and may bunch, increasing the risk of pressure and skin irritation. Stockings that are too small may impede blood flow to the feet and cause discomfort.*

Performance
1. Prior to performing the procedure, introduce self and verify the client's identity using agency protocol. Explain to the client what you are going to do, why it is necessary, and how he or she can cooperate.
2. Perform hand hygiene and observe other appropriate infection control procedures.
3. Provide for client privacy.
4. Select an appropriate time to apply the stockings.
   - Apply stockings in the morning, if possible, before the client arises. **Rationale:** *In sitting and standing positions, the veins can become distended so that edema occurs; the stockings should be applied before this happens.*
   - Assist the client who has been ambulating to lie down and elevate the legs for 15 to 30 minutes before applying the stockings. **Rationale:** *This facilitates venous return and reduces swelling.*
5. Prepare the client.
   - Assist the client to a lying position in bed.
   - Wash and dry the legs as needed.
6. Apply the stockings.
   - Reach inside the stocking from the top, and grasping the heel, turn the upper portion of the stocking inside out so the foot portion is inside the stocking leg. **Rationale:** *Firm elastic stockings are easier to fit over the foot and calf when inverted in this manner rather than bunching up the stocking.*
   - Ask the client to point his or her toes, then position the stocking on the client's foot. With the heel of the stocking down and stretching each side of the stocking, ease the stocking over the toes taking care to place the toe and heel portions of the stocking appropriately. ❶ **Rationale:** *Pointing the toes makes application easier.*

❶ Applying the inverted stocking over the toes.
Photographer: Elena Dorfman

continued on page 952

SKILL 37-2

APPLYING ANTIEMBOLI STOCKINGS *continued*

- Grasp the loose portion of the stocking at the ankle and gently pull the stocking over the leg, turning it right side out in the process. ❷
- Inspect the client's leg and stocking, smoothing any folds or creases. Ensure that the stocking is not rolled down or bunched at the top or ankle. **Rationale:** *Folds and creases can cause skin irritation under the stocking; bunching of the stocking can further impair venous return.*
- Remove the stockings for 30 minutes every 8 hours, inspecting the legs and skin while the stockings are off.
- Soiled stockings may be laundered by hand with warm water and mild soap. Hang to dry.

7. Document the procedure. Record the procedure, your assessment data, and when the stockings are removed and reapplied.

❷ Pulling the stocking snugly over the leg.
Photographer: Elena Dorfman

EVALUATION

- Remove antiembolism stockings one to three times a day for 30 minutes for skin care and inspection.
- Note the appearance of the legs and skin integrity, any edema, peripheral pulses, and skin color and temperature. Compare to previous assessment data.

- If complications occur, remove the stockings and report findings to the primary care provider.

LIFESPAN CONSIDERATIONS   Antiemboli Stockings

CHILDREN

- Antiemboli stockings are infrequently used on children.

ELDERS

- Because the elastic is quite strong in antiemboli stockings, the elder may need assistance with putting on the stockings. Clients with arthritis may need to have another person put the stockings on for them.
- Many elders have circulation problems and wear antiemboli stockings. It is important to check for wrinkles in the stockings and to

see if the stocking has rolled down or twisted. If so, correct immediately because the stockings must be evenly distributed over the limb to promote rather than hinder circulation.

- Stockings should be removed once each shift so that a thorough assessment can be made of the legs and feet. Redness and skin breakdown on the heels can occur quickly and go undetected if not thoroughly assessed on a regular basis.

HOME CARE CONSIDERATIONS   Antiemboli Stockings

- Teach the client or caregiver how to apply the antiemboli stockings.
- Stress the importance of no wrinkles or rolling down of the stockings and the rationale.
- Instruct the client or caregiver to remove the stockings daily and inspect the skin on the legs.

- Provide instructions about
  - Laundering the stockings.
  - The need for two pairs of stockings to allow for one pair to be worn while the other is being laundered.
  - Replacing the stockings when they lose their elasticity.

LIFESPAN CONSIDERATIONS   Postoperative Care

CHILDREN

- Infants and young children may not be able to state their level of pain postoperatively, may be physically active, and may appear not to have much pain. Use nonverbal signs such as crying, fussiness, refusal to eat, disturbed sleep, increased heart rate, increased blood pressure, and agitation to assess pain.

- Children are often undermedicated for pain postoperatively. Nurses should be alert to subtle signs of pain and provide medication in a timely manner. Well-controlled pain levels facilitate the healing process in children.
- Some recovery rooms/PACUs allow parents to be present when their child wakes from surgery. Having the parent at the bedside has been shown to calm the child and reduce parental anxiety.

LIFESPAN CONSIDERATIONS   Postoperative Care—*continued*

ELDERS

■ Elders have less efficient reserves and may take longer to recover postoperatively. Be attentive to vital signs, intake and output, and mental status and note significant changes.

■ Clients with dementia often experience an increase in confusion and agitation from the medications and anesthesia used during surgery. This poses a safety risk during the postoperative period and requires nursing staff to monitor these clients more frequently. It is important to maintain a calm, reassuring attitude. These

changes are often long-lasting, taking days or weeks to return to the preoperative level of cognition.

■ Elders may experience more fatigue and weakness after surgery. Encouraging activity is crucial, but it needs to be paced to prevent exhaustion.

■ When surgery is done on an outpatient basis, nurses should follow up with phone calls that evening and the next day to check on the client's condition and make sure that postoperative instructions were understood.

SEQUENTIAL COMPRESSION DEVICES. Clients who are undergoing surgery may benefit from a sequential compression device (SCD) to promote venous return from the legs. SCDs inflate and deflate plastic sleeves wrapped around the legs to promote venous flow. SCDs are discussed in Chapter 51 ∞ (see Skill 51-1).

Evaluating

The goals established during the planning phase are evaluated according to specific desired outcomes, also established in that phase. An example of client outcomes and related indicators was shown earlier in Identifying Nursing Diagnoses, Outcomes, and Interventions.

INTRAOPERATIVE PHASE

The intraoperative nurse uses the nursing process to design, coordinate, and deliver care to meet the identified needs of clients whose protective reflexes or self-care abilities are potentially compromised because they are having operative or other invasive procedures.

Types of Anesthesia

Anesthesia is classified as *general, regional,* or *local.* Anesthetic agents usually are administered by an anesthesiologist or a certified registered nurse anesthetist (CRNA). **General anesthesia** is the loss of all sensation and consciousness. Under general anesthesia, protective reflexes such as cough and gag reflexes are lost. A general anesthetic acts by blocking awareness centers in the brain so that amnesia (loss of memory), analgesia (insensibility to pain), hypnosis (artificial sleep), and relaxation (rendering a part of the body less tense) occur. General anesthetics are usually administered by intravenous infusion or by inhalation of gases through a mask or through an endotracheal tube inserted into the trachea.

General anesthesia has certain advantages. Because the client is unconscious rather than awake and anxious, respiration and cardiac function are readily regulated. Also, the anesthesia can be adjusted to the length of the operation and the client's age and physical status. Its chief disadvantage is that it depresses the respiratory and circulatory systems. Some clients become more anxious

about a general anesthetic than about the surgery itself. Often this is because they fear losing the capacity to control their own bodies.

Regional anesthesia is the temporary interruption of the transmission of nerve impulses to and from a specific area or region of the body. The client loses sensation in an area of the body but remains conscious. Several techniques are used.

■ **Topical (surface) anesthesia** is applied directly to the skin and mucous membranes, open skin surfaces, wounds, and burns. The most commonly used topical agents are lidocaine (Xylocaine) and benzocaine. Topical anesthetics are readily absorbed and act rapidly.

■ **Local anesthesia** (infiltration) is injected into a specific area and is used for minor surgical procedures such as suturing a small wound or performing a biopsy. Lidocaine or tetracaine 0.1% may be used.

■ A **nerve block** is a technique in which the anesthetic agent is injected into and around a nerve or small nerve group that supplies sensation to a small area of the body. Major blocks involve multiple nerves or a plexus (e.g., the brachial plexus anesthetizes the arm); minor blocks involve a single nerve (e.g., a facial nerve).

■ An **intravenous block (Bier block)** is used most often for procedures involving the arm, wrist, and hand. An occlusion tourniquet is applied to the extremity to prevent infiltration and absorption of the injected intravenous agent beyond the involved extremity.

■ **Spinal anesthesia** is also referred to as **subarachnoid block (SAB).** It requires a lumbar puncture through one of the interspaces between lumbar disc 2 (L_2) and the sacrum (S_1). An anesthetic agent is injected into the subarachnoid space surrounding the spinal cord. Spinal anesthesia is often categorized as a low, mid, or high spinal. Low spinals (saddle or caudal blocks) are primarily used for surgeries involving the perineal or rectal areas. Mid spinals (below the level of the umbilicus—T_{10}) can be used for hernia repairs or appendectomies, and high spinals (reaching the nipple line—T_4) can be used for surgeries such as cesarean sections.

■ **Epidural (peridural) anesthesia** is an injection of an anesthetic agent into the epidural space, the area inside the spinal column but outside the dura mater.

DRUG CAPSULE · *midazolam hydrochloride* (Versed)

THE CLIENT UNDERGOING ANESTHESIA

IV anesthetic agent used to induce general anesthesia. Commonly used prior to conscious sedation to produce anxiolytic, hypnotic, anticonvulsant, muscle relaxant, and amnesic effects.

NURSING RESPONSIBILITIES

■ Obtain baseline vital signs and level of consciousness before administration.

■ Monitor vital signs, level of consciousness, and oxygen saturation q 3–5 minutes intraoperatively and postoperatively. Notify primary care provider or CRNA if there are any changes.

■ Have resuscitative equipment readily available.

■ A too rapid IV administration or excessive dose increases the risk of respiratory depression/arrest.

■ Dosage must be individualized based on age, underlying disease, and desired effect. Too much or too little a dosage or improper administration may result in cerebral hypoxia, agitation, involuntary movement, hyperactivity, and/or combativeness.

Note: Prior to administering any medication, review all aspects with a current drug handbook or other reliable source.

Conscious sedation may be used alone or in conjunction with regional anesthesia for some diagnostic tests and surgical procedures. **Conscious sedation** refers to minimal depression of the level of consciousness in which the client retains the ability to maintain a patent airway and respond appropriately to commands. Intravenous narcotics such as morphine or fentanyl (Sublimaze) and antianxiety agents such as diazepam (Valium) or midazolam (Versed) are commonly used to induce and maintain conscious sedation. Conscious sedation increases the client's pain threshold and induces a degree of amnesia but allows for prompt reversal of its effects and a rapid return to normal activities of daily living. Procedures such as endoscopies, incision and drainage of abscesses, and even balloon angioplasty may be performed under conscious sedation.

NURSING MANAGEMENT

Assessing

On the client's admission to the surgical suite or procedure room, the perioperative nurse confirms the client's identity and assesses the client's physical and emotional status. The nurse verifies the information on the preoperative checklist and evaluates the client's knowledge about the surgery and events to follow. The client's response to preoperative medications is assessed, as well as the placement and patency of tubes such as IV lines, nasogastric tubes, and urinary catheters.

Assessment continues throughout surgery, as the anesthesiologist and/or the CRNA continuously monitor the client's vital signs (including blood pressure, heart rate, respiratory rate, and temperature), ECG, and oxygen saturation. Fluid intake and urinary output are monitored throughout surgery, and blood loss is estimated. In addition, arterial and venous pressures, pulmonary artery pressures, and laboratory values such as blood glucose, hemoglobin, hematocrit, serum electrolytes, and arterial blood gases may be evaluated during surgery. Continual assessment is necessary to rapidly identify adverse responses to surgery or anesthesia and intervene promptly to prevent complications.

Diagnosing

NANDA nursing diagnoses that may be appropriate for the intraoperative client include the following:

■ *Risk for Aspiration*
■ *Ineffective Protection*
■ *Impaired Skin Integrity*
■ *Risk for Perioperative Positioning Injury*
■ *Risk for Imbalanced Body Temperature*
■ *Ineffective Tissue Perfusion*
■ *Risk for Deficient Fluid Volume*

Planning

The overall goals of care in the intraoperative period are to maintain the client's safety and to maintain homeostasis. Examples of nursing activities to achieve these goals include the following:

■ Position the client appropriately for surgery.
■ Perform preoperative skin preparation.
■ Assist in preparing and maintaining the sterile field.
■ Open and dispense sterile supplies during surgery.
■ Provide medications and solutions for the sterile field.
■ Monitor and maintain a safe, aseptic environment.
■ Manage catheters, tubes, drains, and specimens.
■ Perform sponge, sharp, and instrument counts.
■ Document nursing care provided and the client's response to interventions.

Implementing

Intraoperative interventions are carried out by the circulating nurse and the scrub person. The **circulating nurse** coordinates activities and manages client care by continually assessing client safety, aseptic practice, and the environment (e.g., temperature, humidity, and lighting). The **scrub person** is usually a UAP but can be an RN or LPN. Their role is to assist the surgeons. They wear sterile gowns, gloves, caps, and eye protection. Their responsibilities include draping the client with sterile drapes and handling sterile instruments and supplies. The circulating nurse and scrub person are responsible for accounting of all sponges, needles, and instruments at the close of surgery. This precaution avoids leaving any foreign bodies inside the client.

Surgical Skin Preparation

Surgical skin preparation involves cleaning the surgical site, removing hair only if necessary, and applying an antimicrobial agent. In most surgery centers, skin preparation is done by surgery personnel near the time of surgery. The purpose of a surgical skin preparation is to reduce the risk of postoperative wound infection. This is done by

- Removing transient microbes from the skin.
- Reducing the resident microbial count to subpathogenic amounts in a short time and with the least amount of tissue irritation.
- Inhibiting rapid rebound growth of microbes.

The Association of Operating Room Nurses (AORN) recommends the following skin preparation practices to reduce the risk of postoperative wound infections:

- Clean the surgical site and surrounding areas. This can be accomplished before the surgical prep by having the client shower and shampoo or wash the surgical site before arriving in the surgical setting, or by washing the surgical site in the surgical setting immediately before applying an antimicrobial agent.
- Assess the surgical site before skin preparation. The nurse assesses the site for moles, warts, rashes, or other skin conditions such as pustules, abrasions, or exudate, and documents their presence before skin preparation.
- Remove hair from the surgical site only when necessary or according to the primary care provider's orders or institutional policies and procedures. Personnel skilled in hair removal should remove hair using techniques that preserve skin integrity. Electric clippers or a depilatory cream should be used to reduce the risk of traumatizing the skin during hair removal. If a depilatory is used, hypersensitivity testing is performed prior to applying it to the surgical site. Skin trauma and abrasions increase the risk of microorganisms colonizing the surgical site. If hair is to be removed, it is done as close to the time of surgery as possible and not in the vicinity of the sterile field to avoid dispersal of loose hair and potential contamination of the sterile field.
- Prepare the surgical site and surrounding area with an antimicrobial agent when indicated. A nontoxic antimicrobial agent with a broad range of germicidal action is used to inhibit the growth of microorganisms during and following the surgical procedure. The agent selected depends on the client's history of hypersensitivity reactions, the location of the surgical site, and the skin condition. The area prepared needs to be large enough to accommodate an extension of the incision and any potential drain sites or additional incisions if needed.
- Document surgical skin preparation in the client's record. Documentation should include the skin condition, including any growths, abrasions, or rashes; hair removal and the techniques used, if performed; the skin preparation, including cleansing and antimicrobial agent applied; who performed the preoperative skin preparation; and any adverse or hypersensitivity responses noted (Anonymous, 2002).

Positioning

The perioperative nurse, surgeon, and anesthesiologist/CRNA work as a team to minimize the risk of perioperative complications related to positioning (AORN, 2005).

The client's position should provide:

- Optimal visualization of and access to the surgical site.
- Optimal access to IV lines and monitoring devices.
- Protection of the client from harm (anatomical and physiological considerations).

Positioning is performed after anesthesia is induced and before surgical draping of the client. The client is lifted into position to prevent shearing forces on the skin from sliding or rolling. The exact position for the client depends on the operation, that is, the surgical approach. For example, a lithotomy position is usually used for vaginal surgery.

Positions on the operating table are maintained by straps, and body prominences are frequently padded. The position should consider normal joint range of motion and good body alignment, thereby avoiding strain or injury to muscles, bones, and ligaments.

CLINICAL ALERT

Be especially aware of the intraoperative position required for elders. Because elders are vulnerable to pressure ulcer formation, check the appropriate pressure points of that surgical position on the client. ■

Evaluating

The intraoperative nurse uses the goals developed during the planning stage (e.g., maintain client safety) and collects data to evaluate whether the desired outcomes have been achieved.

Documentation

The intraoperative nurse documents the perioperative plan of care including assessment, diagnosis, outcome identification, planning, implementation, and evaluation.

POSTOPERATIVE PHASE

Nursing during the postoperative phase is especially important for the client's recovery because anesthesia impairs the ability of clients to respond to environmental stimuli and to help themselves, although the degree of consciousness of clients will vary. Moreover, surgery itself traumatizes the body by disrupting protective mechanisms and homeostasis.

Immediate Postanesthetic Phase

Recovery/PACU nurses have specialized skills to care for clients recovering from anesthesia and surgery (Figure 37-1 ■). Once the health status has stabilized, the client is returned to the nursing unit or, in the case of an outpatient, to the outpatient surgery area before discharge. Assessment of the client in the immediate postanesthetic period is summarized in Box 37–5.

During the immediate postanesthetic stage, an unconscious client is positioned on the side, with the face slightly down. A pillow is not placed under the head. In this position, gravity keeps the tongue forward, preventing occlusion of the pharynx

ANATOMY & PHYSIOLOGY REVIEW   Client Positioning

The most common position for a client during a surgical procedure is the supine position. This position allows approach to the cranial, thoracic, and peritoneal body cavities as well as to all four extremities and the perineum. Proper body alignment and padding of potential pressure areas are essential to preventing client risk for injury during surgery.

The potential pressure areas are the occiput, scapula, olecranon, sacrum, coccyx, and calcaneus. The nursing intervention is to pad and protect bony prominences, pressure sites, and vulnerable nerves with pressure-reducing devices made of foam or gel. Proper positioning must provide optimal exposure to the surgical site as well as provide for client comfort and safety.

A

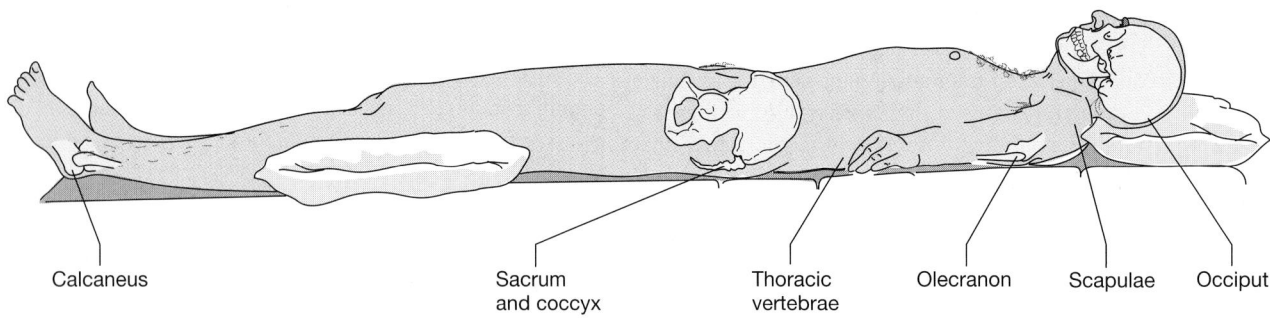

Calcaneus   Sacrum and coccyx   Thoracic vertebrae   Olecranon   Scapulae   Occiput

B

QUESTIONS

A 78-year-old male client scheduled for a colon resection is brought to the operating room. He weights 180 pounds and has type 2 diabetes and a history of arthritis in his hips and shoulders.

1. What baseline assessments would you gather before taking this client to the operating room?
2. What areas on this client are most likely to be injured as a result of poor positioning or inadequate padding?
3. What is the priority nursing diagnosis and outcome for this client?

and allowing drainage of mucus or vomitus out of the mouth rather than down the respiratory tree.

The nurse ensures maximum chest expansion by elevating the client's upper arm on a pillow. The upper arm is supported because the pressure of an arm against the chest reduces chest expansion potential. An artificial airway is maintained in place, and the client is suctioned as needed until cough and swallowing reflexes return. Generally the client spits out an oropharyngeal airway when coughing returns. Endotracheal tubes are not removed until clients are awake and able to maintain their own

airway. The client is then helped to turn, cough, and take deep breaths, provided that vital signs are stable. When spinal anesthesia is used, the client may be required to remain flat for a specified period. See Chapter 50 ∞ for information about artificial airways.

The return of the client's reflexes, such as swallowing and gagging, indicates that anesthesia is ending. Time of recovery from anesthesia varies with the kind of anesthetic agent used, its dosage, and the individual's response to it. Nurses should arouse clients by calling them by name, and in a normal tone of voice

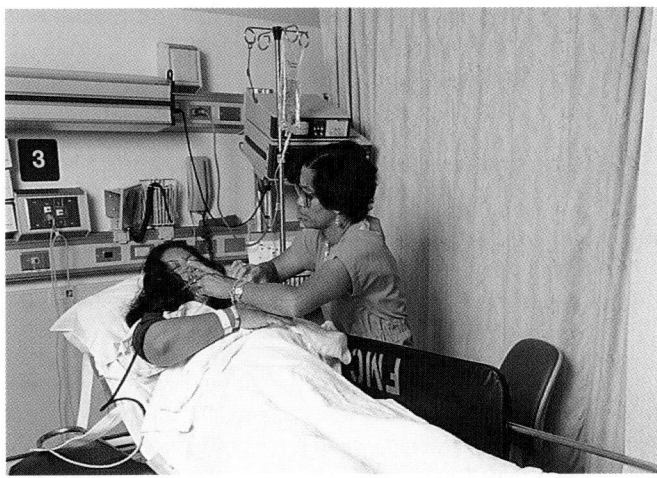

Figure 37-1 ■ PACU nurse provides constant assessment and care for clients recovering from anesthesia and surgery.

repeatedly telling them that the surgery is over and that they are in the PACU.

Once the health status has stabilized, the client is returned to the nursing unit or the outpatient surgery discharge area.

BOX 37–5 **Clinical Assessment**

IMMEDIATE POSTANESTHETIC PHASE

- Adequacy of airway
- Oxygen saturation
- Adequacy of ventilation
  - Respiratory rate, rhythm, and depth
  - Use of accessory muscles
  - Breath sounds
- Cardiovascular status
  - Heart rate and rhythm
  - Peripheral pulse amplitude and equality
  - Blood pressure
  - Capillary filling
- Level of consciousness
  - Not responding
  - Arousable with verbal stimuli
  - Fully awake
  - Oriented to time, person, and place
- Presence of protective reflexes (e.g., gag, cough)
- Activity, ability to move extremities
- Skin color (pink, pale, dusky, blotchy, cyanotic, jaundiced)
- Fluid status
  - Intake and output
  - Status of IV infusions (type of fluid, rate, amount in container, patency of tubing)
  - Signs of dehydration or fluid overload (see Chapter 52)
- Condition of operative site
  - Status of dressing
  - Drainage (amount, type, and color)
- Patency of and character and amount of drainage from catheters, tubes, and drains
- Discomfort (i.e., pain) (type, location, and severity), nausea, vomiting
- Safety (i.e., necessity for side rails, call bell within reach)

Clients are usually discharged from the PACU when

- They are conscious and oriented.
- They are able to maintain a clear airway and deep breathe and cough freely.
- Vital signs have been stable or consistent with preoperative vital signs for at least 30 minutes.
- Protective reflexes (e.g., gag, swallowing) are active.
- They are able to move all extremities.
- Intake and urinary output is adequate (at least 30 mL/hr).
- They are afebrile or a febrile condition has been attended to.
- Dressings are dry and intact; there is no overt drainage.

Preparing for Ongoing Care of the Postoperative Client

While the client is in the operating room, the client's bed and room are prepared for the postoperative phase. In some agencies, the client is brought back to the unit on a stretcher and transferred to the bed in the room. In other agencies, the client's bed is brought to the surgery suite, and the client is transferred there. In the latter situation, the bed needs to be made with clean linens as soon as the client goes to surgery so that it can be taken to the operating room when needed. In addition, the nurse must obtain and set up any special equipment, such as an intravenous pole, suction, oxygen equipment, and orthopedic appliances (e.g., traction). If these are not requested on the client's record, the nurse should consult with the perioperative nurse or surgeon.

NURSING MANAGEMENT

Assessing

As soon as the client returns to the nursing unit, the nurse conducts an initial assessment. The sequence of these activities varies with the situation. For example, the nurse may need to check the primary care provider's stat orders before conducting the initial assessment; in such a case, nursing interventions to implement the orders can be carried out at the same time as assessment.

The nurse consults the surgeon's postoperative orders to learn the following:

- Food and fluids permitted by mouth
- Intravenous solutions and intravenous medications
- Position in bed
- Medications ordered (e.g., analgesics, antibiotics)
- Laboratory tests
- Intake and output, which in some agencies are monitored for all postoperative clients
- Activity permitted, including ambulation.

The nurse also checks the PACU record for the following data:

- Operation performed
- Presence and location of any drains
- Anesthetic used
- Postoperative diagnosis
- Estimated blood loss
- Medications administered in the recovery room

Many hospitals have postoperative protocols for regular assessment of clients. In some agencies, assessments are made every 15 minutes until vital signs stabilize, every hour for the next 4 hours, then every 4 hours for the next 2 days. It is important that the assessments be made as often as the client's condition requires. The nurse assesses the following:

■ *Level of consciousness.* Assess orientation to time, place, and person. Most clients are fully conscious but drowsy when returned to their unit. Assess reaction to verbal stimuli and ability to move extremities.
■ *Vital signs.* Take the client's vital signs (pulse, respiration, blood pressure, and oxygen saturation level) every 15 minutes until stable or in accordance with agency protocol. Compare initial findings with PACU data. In addition, assess the client's lung sounds and assess for signs of common circulatory problems such as postoperative hypotension, hemorrhage, or shock. Hypovolemia due to fluid losses during surgery is a common cause of postoperative hypotension. Hemorrhage can result from insecure ligation of blood vessels or disruption of sutures. Massive hemorrhage or cardiac insufficiency can lead to shock postoperatively. Common postoperative complications with their manifestations and preventive measures are listed in Table 37–3.
■ *Skin color and temperature,* particularly that of the lips and nail beds. The color of the lips and nail beds is an indicator of **tissue perfusion** (passage of blood through the vessels). Pale, cyanotic, cool, and moist skin may be a sign of circulatory problems.

CLINICAL ALERT

Elders may not show the classic signs of infection (e.g., fever, tachycardia, increased WBC); instead there may be an abrupt change in their mental status. ■

■ *Comfort.* Assess pain with the client's vital signs and as needed between vital sign measurements. Assess the location and intensity of the pain. Do not assume that reported pain is incisional; other causes may include muscle strains, flatus, and angina. Ask the client to rate pain on a scale of 0 to 10, with 0 being no pain and 10 the worst pain imaginable. Evaluate the client for objective indicators of pain: pallor, perspiration, muscle tension, and reluctance to cough, move, or ambulate. Determine when and what analgesics were last administered, and assess the client for any side effects of medication such as nausea and vomiting.
■ *Fluid balance.* Assess the type and amount of intravenous fluids, flow rate, and infusion site. Monitor the client's fluid intake and output. In addition to watching for shock, assess the client for signs of circulatory overload, and monitor serum electrolytes. Anesthetics and surgery affect the hormones regulating fluid and electrolyte balance (aldosterone and anti-diuretic hormone in particular), placing the client at risk for decreased urine output and fluid and electrolyte imbalances.

■ *Dressing and bedclothes.* Inspect the client's dressings and bedclothes underneath the client. Excessive bloody drainage on dressings or on bedclothes, often appearing underneath the client, can indicate hemorrhage. The amount of drainage on dressings is recorded by describing the diameter of the stains or by denoting the number and type of dressings saturated with drainage.
■ *Drains and tubes.* Determine color, consistency, and amount of drainage from all tubes and drains. All tubes should be patent, and tubes and suction equipment should be functioning. Drainage bags must be hanging properly.

Document the client's time of arrival and all assessments. Many agencies have progress flow records for this purpose. Alter the frequency, parameters, and priorities to meet the individual needs of the client.

Diagnosing

Because surgery can involve many body systems both directly and indirectly and is a complex experience for the client, the nursing diagnoses focus on a wide variety of actual, potential, and collaborative problems.

Actual and potential NANDA diagnoses for the postoperative client include the following:

■ *Acute Pain*
■ *Risk for Infection*
■ *Risk for Injury*
■ *Risk for Deficient Fluid Volume*
■ *Ineffective Airway Clearance*
■ *Ineffective Breathing Pattern*
■ *Self-Care Deficit: Bathing/Hygiene, Dressing/Grooming, Toileting*
■ *Delayed Surgical Recovery*
■ *Disturbed Body Image*

Collaborative problems that may be experienced by the postoperative client are summarized in Table 37–3. Examples of clinical application of some of these diagnoses using NANDA, NIC, and NOC designations are shown in Identifying Nursing Diagnoses, Outcomes, and Interventions on page 961.

Planning

Postoperative care planning and discharge planning begin in the preoperative phase when preoperative teaching is implemented. Examples of clinical application of NOC outcomes and NIC interventions are shown in Identifying Nursing Diagnoses, Outcomes, and Interventions.

Planning for Home Care

To provide for continuity of care for the surgical client after discharge, the nurse needs to consider the client's needs for assistance with care in the home setting. Discharge planning for both the day-surgery client and the client who has been hospitalized for several days following surgery incorporates an assessment of the client's and family's abilities for self-care, financial resources, and the need for referrals and home health services.

TABLE 37–3 Potential Postoperative Problems

PROBLEM	DESCRIPTION	CAUSE	CLINICAL SIGNS	PREVENTIVE INTERVENTIONS
Respiratory				
Pneumonia	Inflammation of the alveoli	Infection, toxins, or irritants causing inflammatory process. Immobility and impaired ventilation result in atelectasis and promote growth of pathogens	Elevated temperature, cough, expectoration of blood-tinged or purulent sputum, dyspnea, chest pain	Deep-breathing exercises and coughing, moving in bed, early ambulation
Atelectasis	A condition in which alveoli collapse and are not ventilated	Mucous plugs blocking bronchial passageways, inadequate lung expansion, analgesics, immobility	Dyspnea, tachypnea, tachycardia; diaphoresis, anxiety; pleural pain, decreased chest wall movement; dull or absent breath sounds; decreased oxygen saturation (SpO$_2$)	Deep-breathing exercises and coughing, moving in bed, early ambulation
Pulmonary embolism	Blood clot that has moved to the lungs and blocks a pulmonary artery, thus obstructing blood flow to a portion of the lung	Stasis of venous blood from immobility, venous injury from fractures or during surgery, use of oral contraceptives high in estrogen, preexisting coagulation or circulatory disorder	Sudden chest pain, shortness of breath, cyanosis, shock (tachycardia, low blood pressure)	Turning, ambulation, antiemboli stockings, sequential compression devices
Circulatory				
Hypovolemia	Inadequate circulating blood volume	Fluid deficit, hemorrhage	Tachycardia, decreased urine output, decreased blood pressure	Early detection of signs; fluid and/or blood replacement
Hemorrhage	Internal or external bleeding	Disruption of sutures, insecure ligation of blood vessels	Overt bleeding (dressings saturated with bright blood; bright, free-flowing blood in drains or chest tubes), increased pain, increasing abdominal girth, swelling or bruising around incision	Early detection of signs
Hypovolemic shock	Inadequate tissue perfusion resulting from markedly reduced circulating blood volume	Severe hypovolemia from fluid deficit or hemorrhage	Rapid weak pulse, dyspnea, tachypnea; restlessness and anxiety; urine output less than 30 mL/hr; decreased blood pressure; cool, clammy skin, thirst, pallor	Maintain blood volume through adequate fluid replacement, prevent hemorrhage; early detection of signs
Thrombophlebitis	Inflammation of the veins, usually of the legs and associated with a blood clot	Slowed venous blood flow due to immobility or prolonged sitting; trauma to vein, resulting in inflammation and increased blood coagulability	Aching, cramping pain; affected area is swollen, red, and hot to touch; vein feels hard; discomfort in calf when foot is dorsiflexed or when client walks (Homans' sign)	Early ambulation, leg exercises, antiemboli stockings, SCDs, adequate fluid intake
Thrombus	Blood clot attached to wall of vein or artery (most commonly the leg veins)	As for thrombophlebitis for venous thrombi; disruption or inflammation of arterial wall for arterial thrombi	*Venous:* same as thrombophlebitis. *Arterial:* pain and pallor of affected extremity; decreased or absent peripheral pulses	*Venous:* same as thrombophlebitis. *Arterial:* maintain prescribed position; early detection of signs
Embolus	Foreign body or clot that has moved from its site of formation to another area of the body (e.g., the lungs, heart, or brain)	Venous or arterial thrombus; broken intravenous catheter, fat, or amniotic fluid	In venous system, usually becomes a pulmonary embolus (see pulmonary embolism); signs of arterial emboli may depend on the location	Turning, ambulation, leg exercises, sequential compression devices; careful maintenance of IV catheters

(continued)

TABLE 37–3 Potential Postoperative Problems—*continued*

PROBLEM	DESCRIPTION	CAUSE	CLINICAL SIGNS	PREVENTIVE INTERVENTIONS
Urinary				
Urinary retention	Inability to empty the bladder, with excessive accumulation of urine in the bladder	Depressed bladder muscle tone from narcotics and anesthetics; handling of tissues during surgery on adjacent organs (rectum, vagina)	Fluid intake larger than output; inability to void or frequent voiding of small amounts, bladder distention, suprapubic discomfort, restlessness	Monitoring of fluid intake and output, interventions to facilitate voiding, urinary catheterization as needed
Urinary tract infection	Inflammation of the bladder, ureters, or urethra	Immobilization and limited fluid intake, instrumentation of the urinary tract	Burning sensation when voiding, urgency, cloudy urine, lower abdominal pain	Adequate fluid intake, early ambulation, aseptic straight catheterization only as necessary, good perineal hygiene
Gastrointestinal				
Nausea and vomiting		Pain, abdominal distention, ingesting food or fluids before return of peristalsis, certain medications, anxiety	Complaints of feeling sick to the stomach, retching or gagging	IV fluids until peristalsis returns; then clear fluids, full fluids, and regular diet; antiemetic drugs if ordered; analgesics for pain
Constipation	Infrequent or no stool passage for abnormal length of time (e.g., within 48 hours after solid diet started)	Lack of dietary roughage, analgesics (decreased intestinal motility), immobility	Absence of stool elimination, abdominal distention, and discomfort	Adequate fluid intake, high-fiber diet, early ambulation
Tympanites	Retention of gases within the intestines	Slowed motility of the intestines due to handling of the bowel during surgery and the effects of anesthesia	Obvious abdominal distention, abdominal discomfort (gas pains), absence of bowel sounds	Early ambulation; avoid using a straw, provide ice chips or water at room temperature
Postoperative ileus	Intestinal obstruction characterized by lack of peristaltic activity	Handling the bowel during surgery, anesthesia, electrolyte imbalance, wound infection	Abdominal pain and distention; constipation; absent bowel sounds; vomiting	
Wound				
Wound infection	Inflammation and infection of incision or drain site	Poor aseptic technique; laboratory analysis of wound swab identifies causative microorganism	Purulent exudate, redness, tenderness, elevated body temperature, wound odor	Keep wound clean and dry, use surgical aseptic technique when changing dressings
Wound dehiscence	Separation of a suture line before the incision heals	Malnutrition (emaciation, obesity), poor circulation, excessive strain on suture line	Increased incision drainage, tissues underlying skin become visible along parts of the incision	Adequate nutrition, appropriate incisional support and avoidance of strain
Wound evisceration	Extrusion of internal organs and tissues through the incision	Same as for wound dehiscence	Opening of incision and visible protrusion of organs	Same as for wound dehiscence
Psychologic				
Postoperative depression	Mental disorder characterized by altered mood	Weakness, surprise nature of emergency surgery, news of malignancy, severely altered body image, other personal matter; may be a physiologic response to some surgeries	Anorexia, tearfulness, loss of ambition, withdrawal, rejection of others, feelings of dejection, sleep disturbances (insomnia or excessive sleeping)	Adequate rest, physical activity, opportunity to express anger and other negative feelings

IDENTIFYING NURSING DIAGNOSES, OUTCOMES, AND INTERVENTIONS
The Postoperative Client

DATA CLUSTER Mrs. Polk, 65 years old, was scheduled for a right total hip replacement and has returned to her room. Her VS are stable. She is NPO with an IV infusing at 100 cc/hr. Her right hip dressing is dry and intact. A Hemovac drain is in place and draining a small to moderate amount of bloody drainage. Her respirations are 30/min and shallow. Breath sounds are clear but diminished throughout. She is awake and c/o right hip pain which she rates as "8" on a 0–10 scale. She guards her right hip and flinches when someone touches her.

NURSING DIAGNOSIS/ DEFINITION	SAMPLE DESIRED OUTCOME*/ DEFINITION	INDICATORS	SELECTED INTERVENTIONS*/ DEFINITION	SAMPLE NIC ACTIVITIES
Acute Pain/Unpleasant sensory and emotional experience arising from actual or potential tissue damage (International Association for the Study of Pain); sudden or slow onset of any intensity from mild to severe with an anticipated or pre-dictable end and a dura-tion of less than 6 months	Pain Control [1605]/ *Personal actions to control pain*	Often demonstrated: <ul><li>Describes causal factors</li><li>Recognizes pain onset</li><li>Uses analgesics appropriately</li><li>Reports changes in pain symp-toms or sites to health care profes-sional</li><li>Reports pain controlled</li></ul>	Pain Management [1400]/*Alleviation of pain or a reduction in pain to a level of com-fort that is acceptable to the patient*	<ul><li>Perform a comprehensive assess-ment of pain to include location, characteristics, onset/duration, inten-sity or severity of pain and precipitat-ing factors</li><li>Assure client of attentive analgesic care</li><li>Consider cultural influences on pain response</li><li>Monitor client satisfaction with pain management at specified intervals</li></ul>
Ineffective Breathing Pattern/Inspiration and/ or expiration that does not provide adequate ventilation	Respiratory Status: Ventilation [0403]/ *Movement of air in and out of the lungs*	Not compromised: <ul><li>Respiratory rate in ex-pected range</li><li>Respiratory rhythm in ex-pected range</li><li>Ease of breathing</li></ul> No: <ul><li>Adventitious breath sounds</li></ul>	Respiratory Monitoring [3350]/*Collection and analysis of patient data to ensure airway patency and adequate gas exchange*	<ul><li>Monitor rate, rhythm, depth, and ef-fort of respirations</li><li>Auscultate breath sounds, noting ar-eas of decreased/absent ventilation and presence of adventitious sounds</li><li>Monitor client's ability to cough effectively</li></ul>
Risk for Infection/At increased risk for being invaded by pathogenic organisms	Wound Healing: Primary Intention [1102]/*Extent of regeneration of cells and tissues following intentional closure*	Extensive: <ul><li>Skin approximation</li></ul> No: <ul><li>Sanguineous drainage</li><li>Surrounding skin erythema</li></ul>	Infection Control [6540]/ *Minimizing the acquisition and transmission of infec-tious agents*	<ul><li>Wash hands before and after each client activity</li><li>Institute standard precautions</li><li>Ensure appropriate wound care technique</li></ul>

*The NOC # for desired outcomes and the NIC # for nursing interventions are listed in brackets following the appropriate outcome or intervention. Outcomes, indicators, inter-ventions, and activities selected are only a sample of those suggested by NOC and NIC and should be further individualized for each client.

1. *Absence of bleeding and the appearance of a clot binding the wound edges.* The wound edges are well approximated and bound by fibrin in the clot within the first few hours after surgical closure.
2. *Inflammation (redness and swelling) at the wound edges for 1 to 3 days.*
3. *Reduction in inflammation when the clot diminishes,* as granulation tissue starts to bridge the area. The wound is bridged and closed within 7 to 10 days. Increased inflammation associated with fever and drainage is indicative of wound infection; the wound edges then appear brightly inflamed and swollen.
4. *Scar formation.* Collagen synthesis starts 4 days after injury and continues for 6 months or longer.
5. *Diminished scar size over a period of months or years.* An increase in scar size indicates keloid formation.

See Chapter 36 ∞ for information about wound drainage, cleaning wounds, wound irrigation, hot and cold applications, and supporting and immobilizing wounds.

CLINICAL ALERT

Assess the client immediately if he or she reports a "giving" or "popping" sensation in the incisional area. The client may be experiencing dehiscence or evisceration of the wound. ■

SURGICAL DRESSINGS. Not all surgical dressings require changing. Sometimes surgeons in the operating room apply a dressing that remains in place until the sutures are removed, and no further dressings are required. In many situations, however, surgical dressings are changed regularly to prevent the growth of microorganisms.

In some instances a client may have a Penrose drain inserted (see the next section). In this situation the main surgical incision is considered cleaner than the surgical stab wound made for the drain insertion, because there is usually considerable drainage. The main incision is therefore cleaned first, and under no circumstances are materials that were used to clean the stab wound used subsequently to clean the main incision. In this way, the main incision is kept free of the microorganisms around the stab wound. Cleaning a wound and applying a sterile dressing are detailed in Skill 37-4.

WOUND DRAINS AND SUCTION. Surgical drains, for example a **Penrose drain,** are inserted to permit the drainage of excessive serosanguineous fluid and purulent material and to promote healing of underlying tissues. These drains may be inserted and sutured through the incision line, but they are most commonly inserted through stab wounds a few centimeters away from the incision line so that the incision itself may be kept dry. Without a drain, some wounds would heal on the surface and trap the discharge inside, and an abscess might form.

SKILL 37-4

CLEANING A SUTURED WOUND AND APPLYING A STERILE DRESSING

PURPOSES
- To promote wound healing by primary intention
- To prevent infection
- To assess the healing process
- To protect the wound from mechanical trauma

ASSESSMENT
Assess

- Client allergies to wound cleaning agents
- The appearance and size of the wound
- The amount and character of exudates
- Client complaints of discomfort
- The time of the last pain medication
- Signs of systemic infection (e.g., elevated body temperature, diaphoresis, malaise, leukocytosis)

PLANNING
Before changing a dressing, determine any specific orders about the wound or dressing.

Delegation

Cleaning a newly sutured wound, especially one with a drain, requires application of knowledge, problem solving, and aseptic technique. As a result, this procedure is not delegated to UAP. The nurse can ask the UAP to report soiled dressings that need to be changed or if a dressing has become loose and needs to be reinforced. The nurse is responsible for the assessment and evaluation of the wound.

Equipment
- Bath blanket (if necessary)
- Moisture-proof bag
- Mask (optional)
- Acetone or another solution (if necessary to loosen adhesive)
- Clean gloves
- Sterile gloves
- Sterile dressing set; if none is available, gather the following sterile items:
  - Drape or towel
  - Gauze squares
  - Container for the cleaning solution
  - Cleaning solution (e.g., normal saline)
  - Two pairs of forceps
  - Gauze dressings and surgipads
  - Applicators or tongue blades to apply ointments
- Additional supplies required for the particular dressing (e.g., extra gauze dressings and ointment, if ordered)
- Tape, tie tapes, or binder

CLEANING A SUTURED WOUND AND APPLYING A STERILE DRESSING *continued*

IMPLEMENTATION
Preparation
Prepare the client and assemble the equipment.

■ Acquire assistance for changing a dressing on a restless or confused adult. **Rationale:** *The person might move and contaminate the sterile field or the wound.*

■ Assist the client to a comfortable position in which the wound can be readily exposed. Expose only the wound area, using a bath blanket to cover the client, if necessary. **Rationale:** *Undue exposure is physically and psychologically distressing to most people.*

■ Make a cuff on the moisture-proof bag for disposal of the soiled dressings, and place the bag within reach. It can be taped to the bedclothes or bedside table. **Rationale:** *Making a cuff helps keep the outside of the bag free from contamination by the soiled dressings and prevents subsequent contamination of the nurse's hands or of sterile instrument tips when discarding dressing or sponges. Placement of the bag within reach prevents the nurse from reaching across the sterile field and the wound and potentially contaminating these areas.*

■ Put on a face mask, if required. **Rationale:** *Some agencies require that a mask be worn for surgical dressing changes to prevent contamination of the wound by droplet spray from the nurse's respiratory tract.*

Performance
1. Prior to performing the procedure, introduce self and verify the client's identity using agency protocol. Explain to the client what you are going to do, why it is necessary, and how he or she can cooperate. Discuss how the results will be used in planning further care or treatments.

2. Perform hand hygiene and observe other appropriate infection control procedures.

3. Provide for client privacy.

4. Remove binders and tape.
   ● Remove binders, if used, and place them aside. Untie tie tapes, if used. Montgomery straps (tie tapes) are commonly used for wounds requiring frequent dressing changes. ❶ **Rationale:** *These straps prevent skin irritation and discomfort caused by removing the adhesive each time the dressing is changed.*
   ● If adhesive tape was used, remove it by holding down the skin and pulling the tape gently but firmly toward the wound. **Rationale:** *Pressing down on the skin provides countertraction against the pulling motion. Tape is pulled toward the incision to prevent strain on the sutures or wound.*
   ● Use a solvent to loosen tape, if required. **Rationale:** *Moistening the tape with acetone or a similar solvent lessens the discomfort of removal, particularly from hairy surfaces.*

5. Remove and dispose of soiled dressings appropriately.
   ● Put on clean disposable gloves and remove the outer abdominal dressing or surgipad.
   ● Lift the outer dressing so that the underside is *away* from the client's face. **Rationale:** *The appearance and odor of the drainage may be upsetting to the client.*

● Place the soiled dressing in the moisture-proof bag without touching the outside of the bag. **Rationale:** *Contamination of the outside of the bag is avoided to prevent the spread of microorganisms to the nurse and subsequently to others.*
● Remove the under dressings, taking care not to dislodge any drains. If the gauze sticks to the drain, support the drain with one hand and remove the gauze with the other.
● Assess the location, type (color, consistency), and odor of wound drainage, and the number of gauzes saturated or the diameter of drainage collected on the dressings.
● Discard the soiled dressings in the bag as before.
● Remove gloves, dispose of them in the moisture-proof bag, and wash hands.

6. Set up the sterile supplies.
   ● Open the sterile dressing set, using surgical aseptic technique.
   ● Place the sterile drape beside the wound.
   ● Open the sterile cleaning solution and pour it over the gauze sponges in the plastic container.
   ● Put on sterile gloves.

7. Clean the wound, if indicated.
   ● Clean the wound, using your gloved hands or forceps and gauze swabs moistened with cleaning solution.
   ● If using forceps, keep the forceps tips lower than the handles at all times. **Rationale:** *This prevents their contamination by fluid traveling up to the handle and nurse's wrist and back to the tips.*
   ● Use the cleaning methods illustrated and described in ❷ or one recommended by agency protocol.
   ● Use a separate swab for each stroke and discard each swab after use. **Rationale:** *This prevents the introduction of microorganisms to other wound areas.*
   ● If a drain is present, clean it next, taking care to avoid reaching across the cleaned incision. Clean the skin around the

❶ Montgomery straps holding dressing.

continued on page 970

CLEANING A SUTURED WOUND AND APPLYING A STERILE DRESSING *continued*

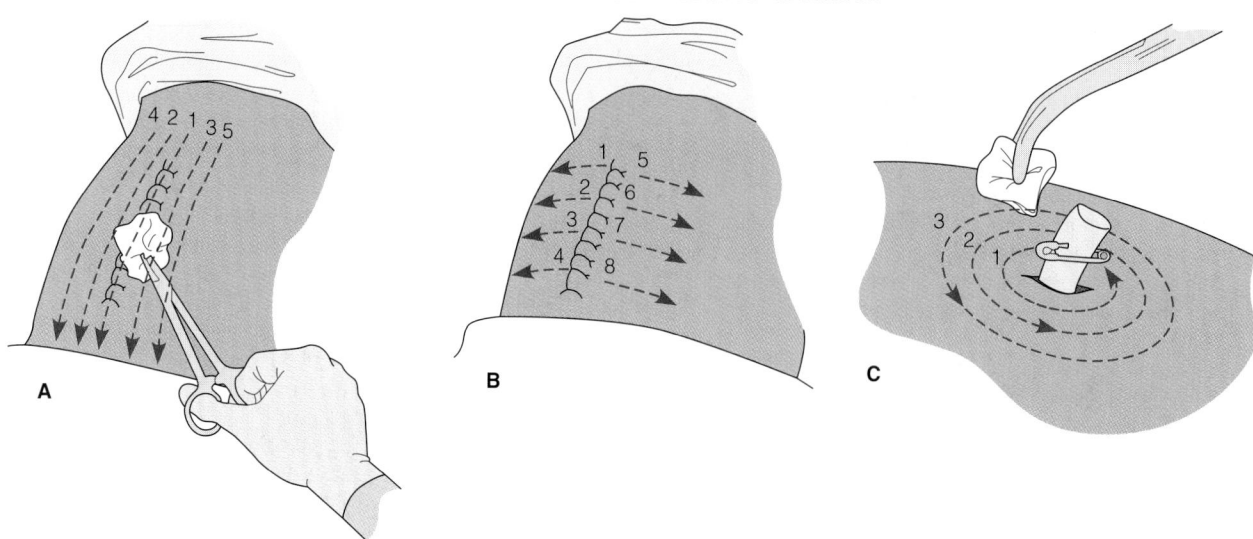

❷ Methods of cleaning surgical wounds: *A,* cleaning the wound from top to bottom, starting at the center; *B,* cleaning a wound outward from the incision; *C,* cleaning around a Penrose drain site. For all methods, a clean sterile swab is used for each stroke.

drain site by swabbing in half or full circles from around the drain site outward, using separate swabs for each wipe ❷ C.

- Support and hold the drain erect while cleaning around it. Clean as many times as necessary to remove the drainage.
- Dry the surrounding skin with dry gauze swabs as required. Do not dry the incision or wound itself. Moisture facilitates wound healing.

8. Apply dressings to the drain site and the incision.

- Place a precut 4 in. × 4 in. gauze snugly around the drain ❸, or open a 4 in. × 4 in. gauze to 4 in. × 8 in., fold it lengthwise to 2 in. × 8 in., and place the 2 in. × 8 in. gauze around the drain so that the ends overlap. **Rationale:** *This dressing absorbs the drainage and helps prevent it from excoriating the skin. Using precut gauze or folding it as described, instead of cutting the gauze, prevents any threads from coming loose and getting into the wound, where they could cause inflammation and provide a site for infection.*
- Apply the sterile dressings one at a time over the drain and the incision. Place the bulk of the dressings over the drain area and below the drain, depending on the client's usual position. **Rationale:** *Layers of dressings are placed for best absorption of drainage, which flows by gravity.*

❸ Precut gauze in place around a drain.

- Apply the final surgipad, remove gloves, and dispose of them. Secure the dressing with tape or ties.

9. Document the procedure and all nursing assessments.

SAMPLE DOCUMENTATION

3/21/2008 1100 Abdominal dressing changed. Small amount of sero-sanguinous drainage – size of a half dollar in middle of dressing. Incision approximated with slight redness at edges. Sutures intact. ————————————S. Jones, RN

EVALUATION

- Conduct appropriate follow-up, such as amount of granulation tissue or degree of healing; amount of drainage and its color, consistency, and odor; presence of inflammation; and degree of discomfort associated with the incision or drain site.
- Compare to previous findings, if available.
- Report significant deviations from normal to the primary care provider.

HOME CARE CONSIDERATIONS   **Cleaning a Sutured Wound**

Instruct caregivers to
- Provide pain medication approximately 30 minutes before the procedure if the wound care causes pain or discomfort.
- Wash hands thoroughly and dry prior to handling wound care supplies and providing wound care.
- Clean and wipe dry a flat surface for the sterile field.

HOME CARE CONSIDERATIONS **Cleaning a Sutured Wound—*continued***

- Keep pets out of the area when setting up for and performing sterile procedures.
- Acquire all needed supplies before starting a sterile procedure.
- Maintain sterile or clean technique as instructed.
- Handle all sterile supplies from the outside of the wrapper or the edges.
- Do not touch the parts of supplies or equipment that will touch the client.

- Avoid skin injury by using paper tape or Montgomery straps instead of adhesive tape.
- Report any increasing wound drainage, pain, or redness, increasing swelling, or opening or gaping of wound edges.
- Place any soiled dressing materials in a waterproof bag and dispose of it according to public health recommendations.

Figure 37-4 ■ Hemovac closed-wound drainage system.

A **closed-wound drainage system** consists of a drain connected to either an electric suction or a portable drainage suction, such as a Hemovac (Figure 37-4 ■) or Jackson-Pratt (Figure 37-5 ■). The closed system reduces the possible entry of microorganisms into the wound through the drain. The drainage tubes are sutured in place and connected to a reservoir. For example, the Jackson-Pratt drainage tube is connected to a reservoir that maintains constant low suction. These portable wound suctions also provide for accurate measurement of the drainage.

The surgeon inserts the wound drainage tube during surgery. Generally the suction is discontinued from 3 to 5 days postoperatively or when the drainage is minimal. Nurses are responsible for maintaining the wound suction, which hastens the healing process by draining excess exudate that might otherwise interfere with the formation of granulation tissue.

Closed-wound drainage systems have directions for use printed on the drainage container. When emptying the container, the nurse should wear gloves and avoid touching the drainage port (Figure 37-6 ■). To reestablish suction, the nurse places the container on a solid, flat surface with the port open. The palm of one hand presses the top and bottom together while the other hand cleanses the opening and plug with an alcohol swab (Figure 37-7 ■). Replace the drainage plug before releasing hand pressure to reestablish the vacuum necessary for the closed drainage system to work.

Figure 37-5 ■ Two Jackson-Pratt devices compressed to facilitate collection of exudates.

Figure 37-6 ■ Emptying drainage from Hemovac drainage system.

Home Care Considerations   Closed-Wound Drainage System

- Schedule regular nursing visits to teach wound care and to observe the drainage site.
- Teach the client or a caregiver to empty, measure, and record the drainage at least once daily.
- Instruct the caregiver to observe the wound daily for signs of infection, such as redness, edema, tenderness, or purulent drainage. The client's temperature should be measured twice daily. *Elevated temperature can indicate infection.*

- Ensure that the client has the proper supplies and knows how to obtain new items as needed.
- Notify the primary care provider of excess drainage, signs of infection, or occlusion of the tube.
- Determine when the primary care provider plans to remove the drain, and help the client keep the appointment.

Figure 37-7 ■ With one hand, press the top and bottom together. With the other hand, clean the opening and plug with an alcohol swab. Replace the plug before releasing hand.

SUTURES. A **suture** is a thread used to sew body tissues together. Sutures used to attach tissues beneath the skin are often made of an absorbable material that disappears in several days. Skin sutures, by contrast, are made of a variety of nonabsorbable materials, such as silk, cotton, linen, wire, nylon, and Dacron (polyester fiber). Silver wire clips or staples are also available. Usually skin sutures are removed 7 to 10 days after surgery.

There are various methods of suturing. Skin sutures can be broadly categorized as either interrupted (each stitch is tied and knotted separately) or continuous (one thread runs in a series of stitches and is tied only at the beginning and at the end of the run). Common methods of suturing are illustrated in Figure 37-8 ■).

Retention sutures are very large sutures used in addition to skin sutures for some incisions (Figure 37-9 ■). They attach underlying tissues of fat and muscle as well as skin and are used to support incisions in obese individuals or when healing may be prolonged. They are frequently left in place longer than skin sutures (14 to 21 days) but in some instances are removed at the same time as the skin sutures. To prevent these large sutures from irritating the incision, the surgeon may place rubber tubing over them or a roll of gauze under them extending down the incision line.

The primary care provider orders the removal of sutures. In some agencies, only primary care providers remove sutures; in others, registered nurses and nursing students with appropriate supervision may do so. Agency policies about removal of retention sutures vary. The nurse should verify whether they are to be removed and who may remove them.

Sterile technique and special suture scissors are used in suture removal. The scissors have a short, curved cutting tip that readily slides under the suture (Figure 37-10 ■). Wire clips or staples are removed with a special instrument that squeezes the center of the clip to remove it from the skin (Figure 37-11 ■). Guidelines for removing sutures and staples follow:

- Before removing skin sutures, verify (a) the orders for suture removal (in many instances, only *alternate* interrupted sutures are removed one day, and the remaining sutures are re-

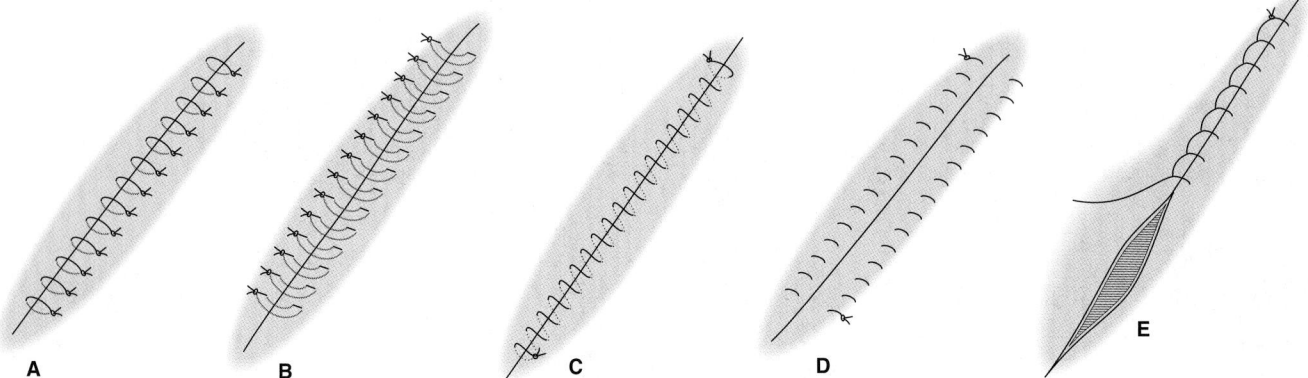

Figure 37-8 ■ Common sutures: *A,* plain interrupted; *B,* mattress interrupted; *C,* plain continuous; *D,* mattress continuous; *E,* blanket continuous.

Figure 37-9 ■ A surgical incision with retention sutures.

Photographer: Jenny Thomas

moved a day or two later) and (b) whether a dressing is to be applied following the suture removal. Some primary care providers prefer no dressing; others prefer a small, light gauze dressing to prevent friction by clothing.

■ Inform the client that suture removal may produce slight discomfort, such as a pulling or stinging sensation, but should not be painful.

■ Remove dressings and clean the incision in accordance with agency protocol. Cleaning the suture line with an antimicrobial solution before and after suture removal may help prevent infection.

Figure 37-10 ■ Suture scissors.

Figure 37-11 ■ Staple remover.

■ Put on sterile gloves.
■ Remove plain interrupted sutures as follows:
   a. Grasp the suture at the knot with a pair of forceps.
   b. Place the curved tip of the suture scissors under the suture as close to the skin as possible, either on the side opposite the knot (Figure 37-12 ■) or directly under the knot. Cut the suture. Sutures are cut as close to the skin as possible on one side of the visible part because the suture material that is visible to the eye is in contact with resident bacteria of the skin and must not be pulled beneath the skin during removal. Suture material that is beneath the skin is considered free from bacteria.
   c. With the forceps, pull the suture out in one piece. Inspect the suture carefully to make sure that all suture material is removed. Suture material left beneath the skin acts as a foreign body and causes inflammation.
■ Remove mattress interrupted sutures as follows:
   a. When possible, cut the visible part of the suture close to the skin at A and B in (Figure 37-13 ■), opposite the knot,

Figure 37-12 ■ Removing a plain interrupted skin suture.

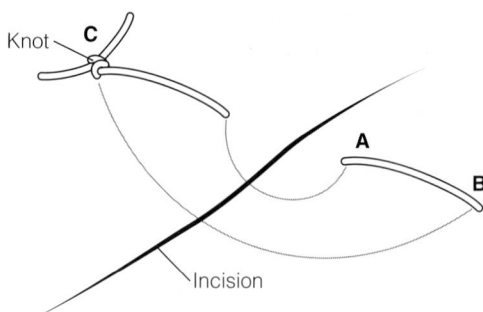

Figure 37-13 ■ Mattress interrupted sutures.

and remove this small visible piece. Discard it as described below. In some sutures, the visible part opposite the knot may be so small that it can be cut only once.

b. Grasp the knot (C) with forceps. Remove the remainder of the suture beneath the skin by pulling out in the direction of the knot.

■ Discard the suture onto a piece of sterile gauze or into the moisture-proof bag, being careful not to contaminate the forceps tips.

■ Continue to remove alternate sutures, that is, the third, fifth, seventh, and so forth. Alternate sutures are removed first so that remaining sutures keep the skin edges in close approximation and prevent any dehiscence from becoming large.

■ If no dehiscence occurs, remove the remaining sutures. If dehiscence does occur, do not remove the remaining sutures, and report the dehiscence to the nurse in charge.

■ If Steri-Strips are ordered by the primary care provider, apply them to the wound after removing the sutures or clips. Some primary care providers order Steri-Strip application to provide additional support to the healing wound.

■ Reapply a dressing, if indicated.

■ Document the suture removal; number of sutures removed; appearance of the incision; application of a dressing, Steri-Strips, or butterfly tapes (if appropriate); client teaching; and client tolerance of the procedure.

■ Remove staples as follows:

a. Remove dressings and clean the incision in accordance with agency protocol.

b. Place the lower tips of a sterile staple remover under the staple.

c. Squeeze the handles together until they are completely closed (Figure 37-14 ■). Pressing the handles together causes the staple to bend in the middle and pulls the edges of the staple out of the skin. Do not lift the staple remover when squeezing the handles.

d. When both ends of the staple are visible, gently move the staple away from the incision site.

e. Hold the staple remover over a disposable container, release the staple remover handles, and release the staple.

Figure 37-14 ■ Removing surgical clips or staples.

HOME CARE CONSIDERATIONS
Removing Sutures or Staples

■ Perform the procedure in a well-lighted, private area of the home.

■ Instruct the client to observe the incision daily and call the health care provider if increased redness, drainage, or open areas are observed.

■ Provide instructions and supplies for care of the incision, and tell the client when to shower for the first time.

■ Assess the client's ability to keep the incision clean and protected at home.

Home Care Teaching

To ensure continuity of care and restoration of the client's health, nurses must meet the learning needs of clients and their support people. Teaching should focus on actions to maintain comfort, to promote healing and restore wellness, and to make use of appropriate community agencies and other sources of help.

MAINTAINING COMFORT

■ Instruct the client to use pain medications as ordered, not allowing pain to become severe before taking the prescribed dose.

■ If not contraindicated, discuss the use of over-the-counter analgesics such as aspirin or acetaminophen as postoperative pain becomes less severe or if the client is reluctant to use prescription drugs due to side effects.

■ Teach the client to avoid using alcohol or other central nervous system depressants while taking narcotic analgesics.

■ Discuss the importance of gradually resuming activities, avoiding overexertion.

- Emphasize the importance of paying attention to increasing pain or discomfort. Instruct the client to contact the primary care provider if pain increases after a period of decreasing discomfort.
- Teach the client to use nonpharmacologic measures to help manage pain, such as conscious relaxation, distraction, meditation, or visualization.

PROMOTING HEALING

- If indicated, teach the client how to change wound dressings and perform wound care.
- Emphasize the importance of hygiene and hand washing to prevent infections.
- Instruct the client to report promptly to the primary care provider any increasing redness, swelling, pain, or discharge from the incision or drain sites.
- Discuss any prescribed activity restrictions such as avoiding lifting.
- Discuss the importance of keeping follow-up appointments to monitor healing and recovery after surgery.

RESTORING WELLNESS

- Discuss the relationship of increasing activities to restoring wellness and promoting a sense of well-being.
- Teach the client that surgery and stressors can depress immune function and to avoid exposure to illness (e.g., crowded areas and people with upper respiratory illnesses) whenever possible.
- Emphasize the importance of adequate rest for healing and immune function.
- If appropriate, discuss lifestyle changes to promote wellness, such as smoking cessation, increasing activity level, reducing stress, and consuming a healthy diet high in fruits, vegetables, and whole grains with adequate protein to promote healing.

COMMUNITY AGENCIES AND OTHER SOURCES OF HELP

- Provide information about where durable medical equipment can be purchased, rented, or obtained free of charge; how to access home health and other services; and where to obtain supplies such as dressings or nutritional supplements.
- Suggest additional sources of information, such as the National Rehabilitation Information Center, Reach to Recovery, and United Ostomy Association.

REFERRALS. THE NURSE NEEDS TO CONSIDER APPROPRIATE REFERRALS FOR THE CLIENT, SUCH AS

- Home health agencies for wound care and assessment and for assistance with ADLs if necessary.
- Community social services for assistance in obtaining medical and assistive equipment.
- Respiratory, physical, or occupational therapy services as indicated.

Evaluating

Using the goals developed during the planning stage, the nurse collects data to evaluate whether the identified goals and desired outcomes have been achieved. Examples of client outcomes and related indicators are shown in the earlier Identifying Nursing Diagnoses, Outcomes, and Interventions boxes.

If the desired outcomes are not achieved, the nurse and client, and support people, if appropriate, need to explore the reasons before modifying the care plan. For example, if the outcome "Pain control" is not met, questions to be considered include:

- What is the client's perception of the problem?
- Does the client understand how to use PCA?
- Is the prescribed analgesic dose adequate for the client?
- Is the client allowing pain to become intense prior to requesting medication or using PCA?
- Where is the client's pain? Could it be due to a problem unrelated to surgery (e.g., chronic arthritis, anginal pain)?
- Is there evidence of a complication that could cause increased pain (an infection, abscess, or hematoma)?

CRITICAL THINKING CHECKPOINT

Mr. Teng is a 77-year-old client with a history of chronic obstructive pulmonary disease. Currently his respiratory condition is being controlled with medications and he is free of infection. He has just been transferred to the postanesthesia care unit following a hernia repair performed under spinal anesthesia. His blood pressure is 132/88, pulse 84, respirations 28, and tympanic temperature 36.5°C (97.8°F). He is awake and stable.

1. What factors place Mr. Teng at increased risk for the development of complications during and after surgery?

2. Speculate about why Mr. Teng's surgeon and anesthesiologist decided to perform Mr. Teng's surgery under regional anesthesia as opposed to general anesthesia.

3. What preparations were taken during the preoperative period to protect Mr. Teng from possible complications during and after his surgery?

4. How will Mr. Teng's postoperative assessments differ from a person who received general anesthesia?

5. What postoperative precautions are especially important to Mr. Teng in view of his chronic lung condition?

See Critical Thinking Possibilities in Appendix A.

CHAPTER 37 **REVIEW**

CHAPTER HIGHLIGHTS

- Surgery is a unique experience that creates stress and necessitates physical and psychologic changes.
- The perioperative period includes three phases: preoperative, intraoperative, and postoperative.
- Surgical procedures are categorized by degree of urgency, purpose, and degree of risk.
- Factors such as age, general health, nutritional status, medication use, and mental status affect a client's risk during surgery.
- Clients must agree to surgery via informed consent and sign a consent form.
- Nursing history and physical assessment data are important sources for planning preoperative and postoperative care.
- The overall goal of nursing care during the preoperative phase is to prepare the client mentally and physically for surgery.
- Preoperative teaching includes situational information and psychosocial support, the role of the client throughout the perioperative period, expected sensations and discomfort, and training for the postoperative period.
- Preoperative teaching should include moving, leg exercises, and coughing and deep-breathing exercises. Many aspects of preoperative teaching are intended to prevent postoperative complications.
- Physical preparation includes the following areas: nutrition and fluids, elimination, hygiene, rest, medications, care of valuables and prostheses, special orders, and surgical skin preparation.
- Antiemboli stockings or sequential compression devices may be ordered for some clients to facilitate venous return.
- A preoperative checklist provides a guide to and documentation of a client's preparation before surgery.
- Maintaining the client's safety is the overall goal of nursing care during the intraoperative phase.
- Anesthesia may be general or regional. Regional anesthesia includes topical, local, nerve block, intravenous block, spinal anesthesia (subarachnoid block), and epidural.

- A surgical skin preparation should be carried out as close to the time of surgery as possible and is commonly performed during the intraoperative phase.
- Positioning of the client during surgery is important to reduce the risk of tissue and nerve damage.
- Immediate postanesthetic care focuses on assessment and monitoring parameters to prevent complications from anesthesia or surgery.
- Initial and ongoing assessment of the postoperative client includes level of consciousness, vital signs, oxygen saturation, skin color and temperature, comfort, fluid balance, dressings, drains, and tubes.
- The overall goals of nursing care during the postoperative period are to promote comfort and healing, restore the highest possible level of wellness, and prevent associated risks such as infection or respiratory and cardiovascular complications.
- Ongoing postoperative nursing interventions include (a) managing pain, (b) appropriate positioning, (c) encouraging incentive spirometry and deep-breathing and coughing exercises, (d) promoting leg exercises and early ambulation, (e) maintaining adequate hydration and nutritional status, (f) promoting urinary elimination, (g) continuing gastrointestinal suction, and (h) providing wound care.
- Surgical aseptic technique (sterile technique) is used when changing dressings on surgical wounds to promote healing and reduce the risk of infection.
- Penrose drains and Hemovac drainage systems are examples of drains that may be placed in or near surgical wounds to promote drainage of excess serosanguineous or purulent exudate.
- Sutures, wire clips, or staples are used to approximate skin and underlying tissues after surgery. These are generally removed 7 to 10 days after surgery.

TEST YOUR KNOWLEDGE

1. Which of the following tests is the best resource for determing the status of a client's preoperative liver function?
   1. Serum electrolytes
   2. Blood urea nitrogen (BUN), creatinine
   3. Alanine amino transferase (ALT), aspirate amino transferase (AST), bilirubin
   4. Serum albumin

2. A client who is having a mastectomy expresses sadness about losing her breast. Based on this information, the nurse would identify that the client is at risk for which nursing diagnosis?
   1. *Body Image Disturbance*
   2. *Anticipatory Grieving*
   3. *Fear*
   4. *Ineffective Coping*

3. Which of the following statements by the client indicates that the preoperative teaching regarding gallbladder surgery has been effective?
   1. "I cannot eat or drink anything after midnight."
   2. "I'm not going to cough after surgery because it might open my incision."
   3. "I might have a stroke if I stop taking my anticoagulant."
   4. "The nurse showed me how to contract and relax my calf muscles."

4. The nurse assesses a postoperative client who has a rapid, weak pulse; urine output less than 30 mL/hr; and decreased blood pressure. The client's skin is cool and clammy. What complication should the nurse suspect?
   1. Thrombophlebitis
   2. Hypovolemic shock
   3. Aspiration pneumonia
   4. Wound dehiscence

5. The client is most likely to require the greatest amount of analgesia for pain during which of the following time periods?
   1. Immediately after surgery
   2. 4 hours after surgery
   3. 12 to 36 hours after surgery
   4. 48 to 60 hours after surgery

6. A postop client who had abdominal surgery is holding a pillow against his abdomen during deep breathing and coughing. What term does the nurse use to describe this technique?

   _____

7. A semi-conscious client in the post-anesthesia care unit (PACU) is experiencing dyspnea (difficulty breathing). Which of the following immediate actions should the nurse perform first?
   1. Place a pillow under the client's head.
   2. Remove the oropharyngeal airway.
   3. Apply oxygen by mask.
   4. Reposition the client to keep the tongue forward.

8. The client's postop orders state "diet as tolerated." The client has been NPO. The nurse will advance the client's diet to clear liquids based on which of the following assessments? Select all that apply.
 1. No complaints of nausea or vomiting
 2. Pain level is maintained at a rating of 2–3/10
 3. States passing flatus
 4. Ambulates with minimal assistance
 5. Expresses feeling "hungry"

9. The overall goal of nursing care during the intraoperative phase is the client's _____.

10. The nurse plans to remove the client's sutures. Which of the following actions demonstrate appropriate standards of care? Select all that apply.
 1. Use clean technique.
 2. Grasp the suture at the knot with a pair of forceps.
 3. Place the curved tip of the suture scissors under the suture as close to the skin as possible.
 4. Pull the suture material that is visible beneath the skin during removal.
 5. Remove alternate sutures first.

See Answers to Test Your Knowledge in Appendix A.

EXPLORE MEDIALINK www.prenhall.com/berman

DVD-ROM
- Audio Glossary
- NCLEX Review
- Skills Checklist
- End of Unit Concept Map Activity
- Animation: Diazepam
- Video: Role of Scrub Nurse

COMPANION WEBSITE
- Additional NCLEX Review
- Case Study: Clients Having Surgical Procedures
- Care Plan Activity: Coronary Artery Bypass Procedure
- Application Activities:
  Developing Operative Care Policies
  Preadmission Testing
- Links to Resources

READINGS AND REFERENCES

SUGGESTED READINGS
Dunn, D. (2005). Preventing perioperative complications in special populations. *Nursing, 35*(11), 36–43.
 The author provides practical guidelines for providing perioperative nursing care for children and obese adults.
Dunn, D. (2006). Age-smart care. Preventing perioperative complications in older adults. *Nursing Made Incredibly Easy, 4*(3), 30–39.
 The author reviews how advancing age affects the older adult's surgical risks and makes communication difficult. This is an important review of the older adult's special needs at the time of surgery.

RELATED RESEARCH
Bernier, M. J., Sanares, D. C., Owen, S. V., & Newhouse, P. L. (2003). Preoperative teaching received and valued in a day surgery setting. *AORN Journal, 77*(3), 563–582.
Oetker-Black, S. L., Jones, S., Estok, P., Ryan, M., Gale, N., & Parker, C. (2003). Preoperative teaching and hysterectomy outcomes. *AORN Journal, 77*(6), 1215–1231.
Rassin, M., Gutman, Y., & Silner, D. (2004). Developing a computer game to prepare children for surgery. *AORN Journal, 80*(6), 1095–1102.
Tranmer, J. E., & Parry, M. (2004). Enhancing postoperative recovery of cardiac surgery patients: A randomized clinical trial of an advanced practice nursing intervention. *Western Journal of Nursing Research, 26*(4), 515.
Yellen, E. (2003). The influence of nurse-sensitive variables on patient satisfaction. *AORN Journal, 78*(5), 783–793.

REFERENCES
Anonymous. (2002). Recommended practices for skin preparation of patients. *AORN Journal, 75*(1), 184–187.
Association of Operating Room Nurses. (2005). Recommended practices for positioning the patient in the perioperative practice setting. *2005 standards, recommended practices, and guidelines.* Denver, CO: Author.

Crenshaw, J. T., & Winslow, E. H. (2002). Preoperative fasting: Old habits die hard. *American Journal of Nursing, 102*(5), 36–44.
Dochterman, J., & Bulechek, G. (Eds.). (2004). *Nursing interventions classification (NIC)* (4th ed.). St. Louis, MO: Mosby.
Joint Commission on Accreditation of Healthcare Organizations. (2003). *Universal protocol for preventing wrong site, wrong procedure, wrong person surgery.* Retrieved July 12, 2006, from http://www.jointcommission.org/NR/rdonlyres/E3C600EB-043B-4E86-B04E-CA4A89AD5433/0/universal_protocol.pdf
Larkin, B. G. (2004). The ins and outs of body piercing. *AORN Journal, 79*(2), 333–342.
Moorhead, S., Johnson, M., & Maas, M. (Eds.). (2004). *Nursing outcomes classification (NOC)* (3rd ed.). St. Louis, MO: Mosby.
NANDA International. (2007). *NANDA nursing diagnoses: Definitions & classification 2007–2008.* Philadelphia: Author.
Sherwood, G. D., McNeil, J. A., Starck, P. L., & Disnard, G. (2003). Changing acute pain management outcomes in surgical patients. *AORN Journal, 77*(2), 374–393.
Steefel, L. (2004). Marks of safety. Preop safety protocols help teams check blind spots that will prevent surgical errors. *Nurse Week MountainWest Edition, 5*(20), 17–18.

SELECTED BIBLIOGRAPHY
Amella, E. J. (2006). Presentation of illness in older adults. *AORN Journal, 83*(2), 373–391.
American Society of PeriAnesthesia Nurses. (2006). *Standards, recommended practices and guidelines.* Denver, CO: Author.
Anonymous. (2005). AORN guidance statement: Preoperative patient care in the ambulatory surgery setting. *AORN Journal, 81*(4), 871–878.
Anonymous. (2005). AORN guidance statement: Postoperative patient care in the ambulatory surgery setting. *AORN Journal, 81*(4), 881–888.
Cofer, M. J. (2005). Unwelcome companion to older patients: Postoperative delirium. *Nursing, 35*(1), 32hn1–32hn3.

Connor, R. (2001). *Ambulatory surgery principles and practices: Standards and recommended practices for ambulatory surgery* (2nd ed.). Denver, CO: AORN.
Ebersole, P., Hess, P., & Luggen, A. (2004). *Towards healthy aging: Human needs and nursing response* (6th ed.). St. Louis, MO: Mosby.
Golembiewski, J., & O'Brien, D. (2003). Morphine and hydromorphone for post-operative analgesia: Focus on safety. *Journal of PeriAnesthesia Nursing, 18*(2), 120–122.
Halliday, A. B. (2006). Shades of sedation. *Nursing, 36*(4), 36–41.
Her, C., & Culhane-Pera, K. A. (2004). Culturally responsive care for Hmong patients. *Postgraduate Medicine, 116*(6), 39–45.
Meeker, M. H., & Rothrock, J. C. (2003). *Alexander's care of the patient in surgery* (12th ed.). St. Louis, MO: Mosby.
Meltzer, B. (2003). Seven keys to fast-track anesthesia. *Outpatient Surgery, IV*(3), 52–62.
Meyer, M., & Driscoll, E. (2004). Perioperative surgery in the twenty-first century. *AORN Journal, 80*(4), 725–733.
Millsaps, C. C. (2006). Pay attention to patient positioning! *RN, 69*(1), 59–63.
Moz, T. (2004). Wound dehiscence and evisceration. *Nursing, 34*(5), 88.
Murphy, E. K. (2004). Negligence cases concerning positioning injuries. *AORN Journal, 30*(2), 311–314.
Pullen, R. (2003). Removing sutures and staples. *Nursing , 33*(10), 18.
Seal, L., & Paul-Cheadle, D. (2004). A systems approach to preoperative surgical patient skin preparation. *American Journal of Infection Control, 32*(2), 57–62.
Squires, A. (2003). Documenting surgical incision site care. *Nursing, 33*(1), 74.
Tittle, M., McMillan, S., & Hagan, S. (2003). Validating the Brief Pain Inventory for use with surgical patients with cancer. *Oncology Nursing Forum, 30*(2), 325–330.
Warnock, K. (2003). Preventing surgical errors: The role of the surgical technologist. *Surgical Technologist, 35*(6), 15–29.

UNIT 9

Promoting Psychosocial Health

Vital to the art of providing effective and appropriate nursing care is the nurse's ability to convey understanding, sensitivity, and compassion to the client who has a negative self-concept or who confronts a stressful life event. The nurse recognizes the impact of low self-esteem, loss, or other stressors on the individual client as well as on the family and support persons. By providing a supportive environment in which to express feelings, by listening attentively, and offering comfort, the nurse helps those affected to develop a healthy self-image or cope with stress and to transcend the experience of loss.

CHAPTER 38

Sensory Perception

LEARNING OUTCOMES

After completing this chapter, you will be able to:

1. Discuss anatomic and physiologic components of the sensory-perception process.

2. Describe factors influencing sensory function.

3. Identify clinical signs and symptoms of sensory overload and deprivation.

4. Describe essential components in assessing a client's sensory-perception function.

5. Discuss factors that place a client at risk for sensory disturbances.

6. Develop nursing diagnoses and outcome criteria for clients with impaired sensory function.

7. Discuss nursing interventions to promote and maintain sensory function.

8. Identify strategies to promote and maintain orientation to person, place, time, and situation for the client with acute confusion/delirium.

9. Promote structured sensory stimulation for the unconscious client.

An individual's senses are essential for growth, development, and survival. Sensory stimuli give meaning to events in the environment. Any alteration in people's sensory functions can affect their ability to function within the environment. For example, many clients have impaired sensory functions that put them at risk in the health care setting; nurses can help them find ways to function safely in this often confusing environment.

COMPONENTS OF THE SENSORY EXPERIENCE

The sensory process involves two components: reception and perception. **Sensory reception** is the process of receiving stimuli or data. These stimuli are either external or internal to the body. External stimuli are **visual** (sight), **auditory** (hearing), **olfactory** (smell), **tactile** (touch), and **gustatory** (taste). Gustatory stimuli can be internal as well. Other types of internal stimuli are kinesthetic or visceral. **Kinesthetic** refers to awareness of the position and movement of body parts. For example, a person walking is aware of which leg is forward. A related sense is **stereognosis,** the ability to perceive and understand an object through touch by its size, shape, and texture. For example, a person holding a tennis ball is aware of its size, round shape, and soft surface without seeing it. **Visceral** refers to any large organ within the body. Visceral organs may produce stimuli that make a person aware of them (e.g., a full stomach). **Sensory perception** involves the conscious organization and translation of the data or stimuli into meaningful information.

For an individual to be aware of the surroundings, four aspects of the sensory process must be present: a stimulus, a receptor, impulse conduction, and perception.

- *Stimulus.* This is an agent or act that stimulates a nerve receptor.
- *Receptor.* A nerve cell acts as a receptor by converting the stimulus to a nerve impulse. Most receptors are specific, that is, sensitive to only one type of stimulus, such as visual, auditory, or touch.
- *Impulse conduction.* The impulse travels along nerve pathways to the spinal cord or directly to the brain (see Figure 38-1 ■). For example, auditory impulses travel to the organ of Corti in the inner ear. From there the impulses travel along the eighth cranial nerve to the temporal lobe of the brain.
- *Perception.* Perception, or awareness and interpretation of stimuli, takes place in the brain, where specialized

Radiations to cerebral cortex

Visual impulses

Reticular formation

Ascending general sensory tracts (touch, pain, temperature)

Auditory impulses

Descending motor projections to spinal cord

Figure 38-1 ■ The nerve impulses run along the ascending sensory tracts to reach the reticular activating system (RAS); then certain impulses reach the cerebral cortex where they are perceived.

(From *Human Anatomy & Physiology,* 7th ed., by Elaine N. Marieb and Katja Hoehn. Copyright © 2007 (p. 455) by Benjamin Cummings Publishing Company. Reprinted by permission of Pearson Education, Inc.)

brain cells interpret the nature and the quality of the sensory stimuli. The level of consciousness affects the perception of the stimuli.

Arousal Mechanism

For the person to receive and interpret stimuli, the brain must be alert. The *reticular activating system* (RAS) in the brain stem is thought to mediate the arousal mechanism. There are two components of the reticular activating system, the *reticular excitatory area* (REA) and the *reticular inhibitory area* (RIA). The REA is responsible for stimulus arousal and wakefulness.

People have their own zone of optimum arousal, the level at which the person feels comfortable. **Sensoristasis** is the term used to describe when a person is in optimal arousal. Beyond this comfort zone people must adapt to the increased or decreased sensory stimuli. An absence of stimuli from the RAS to the cerebrum results in the brain's becoming inactive or useless.

The brain has the capacity to adapt to sensory stimuli. For example, a person living in a city may not notice traffic noise that someone from a rural area finds loud and disturbing. Not all sensory stimuli are acted upon; some are stored by the memory to be used at a later date. Cognition is cerebral functioning. It involves

TABLE 38–1	**States of Awareness**
STATE	**DESCRIPTION**
Full consciousness	Alert; oriented to time, place, person; understands verbal and written words
Disoriented	Not oriented to time, place, or person
Confused	Reduced awareness, easily bewildered; poor memory, misinterprets stimuli; impaired judgment
Somnolent	Extreme drowsiness but will respond to stimuli
Semicomatose	Can be aroused by extreme or repeated stimuli
Coma*	Will not respond to verbal stimuli

*See Glasgow Coma Scale, Table 30–10 in Chapter 30. ∞

such processes as conscious thought, reality orientation, problem solving, judgment, and comprehension.

Awareness is the ability to perceive environmental stimuli and body reactions and to respond appropriately through thought and action. The normal, alert person can assimilate many kinds of information at one time. There are several states of awareness (see Table 38–1).

SENSORY ALTERATIONS

People become accustomed to certain sensory stimuli, and when these change markedly the individual may experience discomfort. For example, when clients enter a hospital they usually experience stimuli that differ in quantity and quality from those to which they are accustomed. These changes may cause clients to become confused and disoriented (see Table 38–1).

Nurses are aware of the behaviors that often result from different stimuli. They now pay more attention to color, sound, privacy, and social interaction for clients so that the stimuli more closely resemble those in the home environment. Factors that contribute to alterations in behavior include sensory deprivation, sensory overload, and sensory deficits.

Sensory Deprivation

Sensory deprivation is generally thought of as a decrease in or lack of meaningful stimuli. When a person experiences sensory deprivation, the balance in the reticular activating system is disturbed. The RAS is unable to maintain normal stimulation to the cerebral cortex. Because of this reduced stimulation, a person becomes more acutely aware of the remaining stimuli and often perceives these in a distorted manner. Thus the person often experiences alterations in perception, cognition, and emotion. The Clinical Manifestations box at the top of this page lists clinical signs of sensory deprivation.

Sensory Overload

Sensory overload generally occurs when a person is unable to process or manage the amount or intensity of sensory stimuli. Three factors contribute to sensory overload:

- Increased quantity or quality of internal stimuli, such as pain, dyspnea, anxiety

CLINICAL MANIFESTATIONS
SENSORY DEPRIVATION

- Excessive yawning, drowsiness, sleeping
- Decreased attention span, difficulty concentrating, decreased problem solving
- Impaired memory
- Periodic disorientation, general confusion, or nocturnal confusion
- Preoccupation with somatic complaints, such as palpitations
- Hallucinations or delusions
- Crying, annoyance over small matters, depression
- Apathy, emotional lability

- Increased quantity or quality of external stimuli, such as a noisy health care setting, intrusive diagnostic studies, contacts with many strangers
- Inability to disregard stimuli selectively, perhaps as a result of nervous system disturbances or medications that stimulate the arousal mechanism

Sensory overload can prevent the brain from ignoring or responding to specific stimuli. Because of the many stimuli, the individual has difficulty perceiving the environment in a way that makes sense. As a result the individual's thoughts race in many directions and restlessness occurs. The person usually feels overwhelmed and does not feel in control. It is important for nurses to remember that sights and sounds that are familiar to them often represent overload to clients. People who have sensory overload may appear fatigued. They often cannot internalize new information and experience cognitive overload as a result of everything that is happening to them. Such factors as pain, lack of sleep, and worry can also contribute to sensory overload. See Clinical Manifestations below for common signs of sensory overload.

Sensory Deficits

A **sensory deficit** is impaired reception, perception, or both, of one or more of the senses. Blindness and deafness are sensory deficits. When only one sense is affected, other senses may become more acute to compensate for the loss. However, sudden loss of eyesight can result in disorientation.

When the loss of sensory function is gradual, individuals often develop behaviors to compensate for the loss; sometimes these behaviors are unconscious. For example, a person with gradual hearing loss in the right ear may unconsciously turn the left ear toward a speaker. When the loss is sudden, however, compensatory behavior often takes days or weeks to develop.

CLINICAL MANIFESTATIONS
SENSORY OVERLOAD

- Complaints of fatigue, sleeplessness
- Irritability, anxiety, restlessness
- Periodic or general disorientation
- Reduced problem-solving ability and task performance
- Increased muscle tension
- Scattered attention and racing thoughts

Visceral Effectors A & P Review Animation

MediaLink

Some neurologic diseases cause changes in the kinesthetic sense and tactile perceptions. Diseases of the inner ear, for example, can cause loss of kinesthetic sense.

Clients with sensory deficits are at risk for both sensory deprivation and sensory overload. Persons with visual problems may be unable to read, watch television, or recognize nurses by sight. An unfamiliar environment can add to their confusion. Blind people often have highly structured home environments, and the diversity and unfamiliarity of the hospital environment can create sensory overload. At the same time, impaired vision often results in an inability to move around readily or socialize with others.

FACTORS AFFECTING SENSORY FUNCTION

A number of factors affect the amount and quality of sensory stimulation, including a person's developmental stage, culture, level of stress, medications and illness, and lifestyle.

Developmental Stage

Perception of sensation is critical to the intellectual, social, and physical development of infants and children. Infants learn to recognize the face of the mother or caregiver and establish bonding essential to later emotional development. Young children respond to music by singing and dancing as they begin to interact with their peers in groups. As children grow, they learn to interpret visual and auditory signals when preparing to cross the street. Adults have many learned responses to sensory cues. The sudden loss or impairment of any sense, therefore, has a profound effect on both the child and the adult.

Normal physiologic changes in older adults put them at higher risk for altered sensory function. The diminishing of sensory perception that may come with chronic disease or aging is generally gradual. For example, hearing loss is the third most common condition reported by the elderly. Approximately 40% to 45% of people over age 65 and more than 83% over the age of 70 have a hearing impairment (Gordon-Salant, 2005).

Culture

An individual's culture often determines the amount of stimulation that a person considers usual or "normal." For example, a child reared in a big-city Latino neighborhood where extended families share responsibilities for all the children may be accustomed to more stimulation than a child reared in a European American suburb of scattered single-family homes. In addition, the normal amount of stimulation associated with ethnic origin, religious affiliation, and income level, for example, also affects the amount of stimulation an individual desires and believes to be meaningful. A sudden change in cultural surroundings experienced by immigrants or visitors to a new country, especially where there are differences in language, dress, and cultural behaviors, may also result in sensory overload or cultural shock.

Cultural deprivation, or **cultural care deprivation,** is a lack of culturally assistive, supportive, or facilitative acts. It is important that nurses be sensitive to what stimulation is culturally ac-

ceptable to a client. For example, in some cultures touching is comforting, whereas in others it is offensive. Some clients find the presence of cultural or religious symbols reassuring and their absence a source of anxiety. Nurses should encourage clients who want to have culturally related symbols present and to follow practices with which they are comfortable, provided that these practices do not endanger health.

Stress

During times of increased stress, people may find their senses already overloaded and thus seek to decrease sensory stimulation. For example, a client dealing with physical illness, pain, hospitalization, and diagnostic tests may wish to have only close support people visit. In addition, the client may need the nurse's help to decrease unnecessary stimuli (e.g., noise) as much as possible. On the other hand, clients may seek sensory stimulation during times of low stress.

Medications and Illness

Certain medications can alter an individual's awareness of environmental stimuli. Narcotics and sedatives, for example, can decrease awareness of stimuli. Some antidepressants can alter perceptions of stimuli. Anyone taking several medications concurrently may show alterations in sensory function; elders are especially at risk and need to be monitored carefully. Certain medications, if taken over a long period of time, become ototoxic, injuring the auditory nerve and causing hearing loss that may be irreversible. Some of these medications are aspirin, furosemide (Lasix), the aminoglycosides, and certain drugs given for cancer chemotherapy.

Certain diseases, such as atherosclerosis, restrict blood flow to the receptor organs and the brain, thereby decreasing awareness and slowing responses. Uncontrolled diabetes mellitus can impair vision and is a leading cause of blindness in the United States. Some central nervous system diseases cause varying degrees of paralysis and sensory loss.

Lifestyle and Personality

Lifestyle influences the quality and quantity of stimulation to which an individual is accustomed. A client who is employed in a large company may be accustomed to many diverse stimuli, whereas a client who is self-employed and works in the home is exposed to fewer, less diverse stimuli. People's personalities also differ in terms of the quantity and quality of stimuli with which they are comfortable. Some people delight in constantly changing stimuli and excitement, whereas others prefer a more structured life with few changes.

 NURSING MANAGEMENT

Assessing

Nursing assessment of sensory-perceptual functioning includes six components: (a) nursing history, (b) mental status examination, (c) physical examination, (d) identification of clients at risk, (e) the client's environment, and (f) social support network.

Nursing History

During the nursing history the nurse assesses present sensory perceptions, usual functioning, sensory deficits, and potential problems. In some instances, significant others can provide data the client cannot. For example, support people may reveal signs of recent changes in the client's hearing ability, such as inattention to others, recent mood swings, difficulty following clear instructions, frequent requests to have something repeated, and unusually loud radio or television volumes. Examples of interview questions to elicit data about the client's sensory-perceptual functioning are shown in the accompanying Assessment Interview.

ASSESSMENT INTERVIEW
Sensory-Perceptual Functioning

VISUAL
- How would you rate your vision (excellent, good, fair, or poor)?
- Do you wear eyeglasses or contact lenses?
- Describe any recent changes in your vision.
- Do you have any difficulty seeing near or far objects?
- Do you have any difficulty seeing at night? Have you ever experienced blurred vision, double vision, spots moving in front of your eyes, blind spots, light sensitivity, flashing lights, or halos around objects?
- When did you last visit an eye doctor?

AUDITORY
- How would you rate your hearing (excellent, good, fair, or poor)?
- Do you wear a hearing aid?
- Describe any recent changes in your hearing.
- Can you locate the direction of sounds and distinguish various voices?
- Do you experience any dizziness or vertigo? Do you experience any ringing, buzzing, humming, crackling noises, or fullness in the ears?

GUSTATORY
- Have you experienced any changes in taste (e.g., difficulty in differentiating sweet, sour, salty, and bitter tastes)?
- Do you enjoy the taste of foods as you did previously?

OLFACTORY
- Have you experienced any changes in smell?
- Do things (foods, flowers, perfumes, and so on) smell the same as previously?
- Can you distinguish foods by their odors and tell when something is burning?
- Have you experienced any changes in appetite? (Changes in appetite may be related to an impaired sense of smell.)

TACTILE
- Are you experiencing any pain or discomfort?
- Have you experienced any decrease in your ability to perceive heat, cold, or pain in your limbs?
- Do you have any numbness or tingling in your extremities?

KINESTHETIC
- Have you noticed any difficulty in perceiving the position of parts of your body?

Mental Status

Mental status is critical to any evaluation of the sensory-perceptual process. Usually data on mental status including level of consciousness, orientation, memory, and attention span can be obtained during the nursing history (see Chapter 30 ∞). It is important to note that sensory alterations can cause changes in cognitive functioning (Wahl & Heyl, 2003).

Physical Examination

Physical assessment determines whether the senses are impaired. During the physical examination the nurse assesses vision and hearing, and the olfactory, gustatory, tactile, and kinesthetic senses. The examination should reveal the client's specific visual and hearing abilities; perception of heat, cold, light touch, and pain in the limbs; and awareness of the position of the body parts. Specific sensory tests include the following:

- Visual acuity, using a Snellen chart or other reading material such as a newspaper, and visual fields
- Hearing acuity, by observing the client's conversation with others and by performing the whisper test and the Weber and Rinne tuning fork tests
- Olfactory sense, by identifying specific aromas
- Gustatory sense, by identifying three tastes such as lemon, salt, and sugar
- Tactile sense, by testing light touch, sharp and dull sensation, two-point discrimination, hot and cold sensation, vibration sense, position sense, and stereognosis

These tests are described in detail in Chapter 30 ∞ . The nurse should also determine whether sensory adaptive devices that the client uses, such as eyeglasses or hearing aids, function properly.

Clients at Risk for Sensory Deprivation or Overload

Clients at risk for sensory-perceptual alterations need to be identified to ensure that preventive measures can be initiated. Box 38–1 describes clients at risk.

Client Environment

The nurse assesses the client's environment for quantity, quality, and type of stimuli. The client's environment may produce insufficient stimuli, placing the client at risk for sensory deprivation, or excessive stimuli, placing the client at risk for sensory overload. Nonstimulating environments include those that (a) severely restrict physical activity and (b) limit social contact with family and friends. Because appropriate or meaningful stimuli decrease the incidence of sensory deprivation, the nurse must consider the client's health care environment for the presence of the following stimuli:

- Radio or other auditory device (e.g., cassette or CD player), television
- Clock or calendar
- Reading material (or toys for children)
- Number and compatibility of roommates
- Number of visitors

BOX 38–1   **Clients at Risk for Sensory Deprivation and Overload**

Sensory Deprivation: Clients who
- are confined in a nonstimulating or monotonous environment in the home or health care agency
- have impaired vision or hearing
- have mobility restrictions such as quadriplegia or paraplegia with bed rest, traction apparatus
- are unable to process stimuli (e.g., clients who have brain damage or who are taking medications that affect the central nervous system)
- have emotional disorders (e.g., depression) and withdraw within themselves
- have limited social contact with family and friends (e.g., clients from a different culture)

Sensory Overload: Clients who
- have pain or discomfort
- are acutely ill and have been admitted to an acute care facility
- are being closely monitored in an intensive care unit (ICU) (Figure 38-2 ■) and have intrusive tubes such as IVs, catheters, or nasogastric or endotracheal tubes
- have decreased cognitive ability (e.g., head injury)

Figure 38-2 ■ A client in an ICU may experience sensory overload.

In the client's home, the nurse may also note the presence of a video/DVD recorder, pets, bright colors, adequate lighting, and so on.

To assess a health care environment that produces excessive stimuli, the nurse considers, for example, bright lights, noise, therapeutic measures, and frequency of assessments and procedures.

CLINICAL ALERT

Are you aware of the noise level around you or the noise level you create while providing nursing care? The standard of 45 decibels (dB) for rest and sleep is often not met. For example, studies have shown that sounds in critical care units range from 60 to 83 dB, thereby suggesting sensory overload. ■

Social Support Network

The degree of isolation a person feels is significantly influenced by the quality and quantity of support from family members and friends. The nurse assesses (a) whether the client lives alone, (b) who visits and when, and (c) any signs indicating social deprivation, such as withdrawal from contact with others to avoid embarrassment or dependence on others, negative self-image, reports of lack of meaningful communication with others, and absence of opportunities to discuss fears or concerns that facilitate coping mechanisms.

Diagnosing

The North American Nursing Diagnosis Association (NANDA International, 2007) includes the following diagnostic labels for sensory perception alterations:

- *Disturbed Sensory Perception (Specify: Visual, Auditory, Kinesthetic, Gustatory, Tactile, Olfactory):* Change in the amount or patterning of incoming stimuli accompanied by a diminished, exaggerated, distorted, or impaired response to such stimuli (NANDA International, 2005, p. 172). This diag-

nostic label is used to describe clients whose perception has been altered by physiologic factors such as pain, sleep deprivation, immobility, and excessive or decreased meaningful environmental stimuli (Carpenito-Moyet, 2006, p. 696).

Other diagnostic labels that can relate to sensory perception alterations include

- *Acute Confusion:* Abrupt onset of a cluster of global, transient changes and disturbances in attention, cognition, psychomotor activity level of consciousness, and/or sleep/wake cycle (NANDA International, 2005, p. 38).
- *Chronic Confusion:* Irreversible, long-standing, and/or progressive deterioration of intellect and personality characterized by decreased ability to interpret environmental stimuli; and decreased capacity for intellectual thought processes; and manifested by disturbances of memory, orientation, and behavior (NANDA International, 2005, p. 39).
- *Impaired Memory:* Inability to remember or recall bits of information or behavior skills. Impaired memory may be attributed to pathophysiological or situational causes that are either temporary or permanent (NANDA International, 2005, p. 116).

CLINICAL ALERT

It is easy to confuse the two nursing diagnoses *Disturbed Sensory Perception* and *Disturbed Thought Processes.* You may find it helpful to remember that the diagnosis *Disturbed Sensory Perception* refers to sensory input—the person's ability to accurately interpret stimuli. In contrast, when a person's cognitive abilities (because of mental disorders, i.e., dementia) interfere with the ability to interpret stimuli accurately, the diagnosis is more likely *Disturbed Thought Processes.* Double-check your assessment data to see if the primary problem is one of sensory input or cognitive ability. ■

Examples of clinical application of some of these diagnoses using NANDA, Nursing Interventions Classification (NIC), and Nursing Outcomes Classification (NOC) designations are shown in Identifying Nursing Diagnoses, Outcomes, and Interventions.

Sensory-Perception Problem as the Etiology

Depending on the data obtained, alterations in sensory-perception function may affect other areas of human functioning and indicate other diagnoses. In these instances the sensory-perception problem becomes the etiology.

Examples of nursing diagnoses for which sensory-perception disturbances are the etiology include the following:

- *Risk for Injury* related to sensory-perception disturbance (specify). For example,
  a. Visual impairment (e.g., decreased depth perception)
  b. Reduced tactile sensation secondary to neurologic or circulatory alterations
  c. Decreased sense of smell
  d. Hearing impairment
  e. Decreased kinesthetic sense
- *Impaired Home Maintenance* related to sensory-perception disturbance (declining visual abilities)
- *Risk for Impaired Skin Integrity* related to sensory-perception disturbance (altered tactile sensation)
- *Impaired Verbal Communication* related to sensory-perception disturbance (specify). For example,
  a. Altered level of consciousness
  b. Hearing impairment
  c. Sensory overload
  d. Sensory deprivation
- *Self Care Deficit: Bathing/Hygiene* related to sensory-perception disturbance (specify). For example,
  a. Visual impairment
  b. Diminished kinesthetic sense
  c. Inability to perceive body part or spatial relationship
- *Social Isolation* related to sensory-perception disturbance (specify). For example,
  a. Impaired vision
  b. Impaired hearing

Planning

Planning includes goals associated with the care of clients independent of setting and those specific to the home environment.

Planning Independent of Setting

The overall outcome criteria for clients with sensory-perception alterations are to

- Prevent injury.
- Maintain the function of existing senses.
- Develop an effective communication mechanism.
- Prevent sensory overload or deprivation.
- Reduce social isolation.
- Perform activities of daily living independently and safely.

The NIC developed by the Iowa Intervention Project can be a guide when planning care (Dochterman & Bulechek, 2004).

Appropriate nursing activities may be selected from the following nursing interventions:

- Cognitive Stimulation
- Communication Enhancement: Hearing Deficit
- Communication Enhancement: Visual Deficit
- Nutrition Management
- Environmental Management
- Fall Prevention
- Body Mechanics Promotion
- Peripheral Sensation Management
- Emotional Support
- Surveillance: Safety

Examples of clinical application of NOC outcomes and NIC interventions are shown in Identifying Nursing Diagnoses, Outcomes, and Interventions.

Planning for Home Care

To provide for continuity of care, the nurse must consider the client's needs for assistance with care in the home or residential treatment setting. Some clients with severe alterations in sensory-perception functioning may be discharged to an assisted living facility that provides the specific support the client requires. Discharge planning incorporates a reassessment of the client's abilities for self-care, the availability and skills of support people, financial resources, and the need for referrals and home health services. See the accompanying Home Care Assessment for sensory-perception alterations and confusion. A major aspect of discharge planning involves the instructional needs of the client and family. The next section provides strategies to support visual and auditory function and maintain a safe environment for clients.

Implementing

Nurses can assist clients with sensory alterations by promoting healthy sensory function, by adjusting environmental stimuli, and by helping clients to manage acute sensory deficits.

HOME CARE ASSESSMENT
Sensory Perception Disturbances

CLIENT AND ENVIRONMENT

- *Self-care abilities:* Ability to care for self while adapting to sensory impairment
- *Safety:* Physical safety of client's environment including lighting, noise, access, lack of clutter or obstructions, use of stairs, assistive devices with respect to sensory impairment, such as flashing fire alarms or telephones for hearing impaired
- *Level of knowledge:* Assistive devices available; ways to maximize use of other senses; local, regional, or national organizations that may provide education, training, support, or other assistance, such as the National Braille Association, Guide Dogs for the Blind, the National Association of the Deaf
- *Resources:* Availability of family, friends, community assistance such as senior centers, transportation and religious or cultural organizations

IDENTIFYING NURSING DIAGNOSES, OUTCOMES, AND INTERVENTIONS
Clients with Sensory Perception Disturbances

DATA CLUSTER Anthony Broom, a 52-year-old lawyer, has multiple sclerosis. Muscle strength and tactile sensation have declined during the past 2 years. He uses a motorized wheelchair to move about. He reports loss of sensation in his lower limbs and fingers and inability to discern temperature differences. His wife assists with bathing and grooming.

NURSING DIAGNOSIS/ DEFINITION	SAMPLE DESIRED OUTCOMES*/ DEFINITION	INDICATORS	SELECTED INTERVENTIONS*/ DEFINITION	SAMPLE NIC ACTIVITIES
Risk for Injury/At risk of injury as a result of environmental conditions interacting with the individual's adaptive and defensive resources	Risk Control [1902]/*Personal actions to prevent, eliminate or reduce modifiable health threats*	Often demonstrated: ■ Acknowledges risk factors ■ Monitors environmental risk factors ■ Develops effective risk control strategies	Risk Identification [6610]/*Analysis of potential risk factors, determination of health risks, and prioritization of risk reduction strategies for an individual or group*	■ Institute routine risk assessment, using reliable and valid instruments ■ Determine past and current level of functioning ■ Identify individual's usual coping strategies ■ Determine presence/absence of basic living needs ■ Identify agency resources to assist in decreasing risk factors

DATA CLUSTER Emma Robertson, an 84-year-old widow, lives alone in her apartment. She can hear words spoken clearly and close to the left ear but cannot hear any sounds with the right ear. She says she spends her time listening to the television and radio (at loud volume). She tends to speak loudly and shout when talking with others, and nods and smiles when others speak. Her daughter, who visits, says she refuses to wear a hearing aid. (Ms. Robertson says it doesn't help and is uncomfortable.) Her daughter has recently noted that her mother has become withdrawn, appears absorbed in her own thoughts, and talks and laughs to herself.

Disturbed Sensory Perception (Auditory)/Change in the amount or patterning of incoming stimuli accompanied by a diminished, exaggerated, distorted, or impaired response to such stimuli	Hearing Compensation Behavior [1610]/*Personal actions to identify, monitor and compensate for hearing loss*	Often demonstrated: ■ Positions self to advantage hearing ■ Reminds others to use techniques that advantage hearing ■ Uses hearing assistive devices (e.g., light on telephone, fire alarm, door bell)	Communication Enhancement: Hearing Deficit [4974]/*Assistance in accepting and learning alternate methods for living with diminished hearing*	■ Facilitate appointment for hearing examination, as appropriate ■ Teach that sounds will be experienced differently with the use of a hearing aid ■ Move closer to less affected ear ■ Obtain attention through touch
Impaired Verbal Communication/Decreased, delayed or absent ability to receive, process, transmit, and use a system of symbols	Communication: Receptive [0904]/*Reception and interpretation of verbal and/or non-verbal messages*	Mildly compromised: ■ Interpretation of spoken language ■ Acknowledgment of messages received	As above	As above plus: ■ Keep hearing aid clean ■ Face the client directly; speak slowly, clearly, and concisely ■ Use simple words and short sentences ■ Use paper, pencil or computer communication when necessary

*The NOC # for desired outcomes and the NIC # for nursing interventions are listed in brackets following the appropriate outcome or intervention. Outcomes, indicators, interventions, and activities selected are only a sample of those suggested by NOC and NIC and should be further individualized for each client.

Promoting Healthy Sensory Function

Detecting sensory problems early is one step toward preventing serious problems. The arousal mechanism for sensation is normally present at birth; however, it is undifferentiated. The special senses are also present at birth, although some changes in function occur during the growth process.

Early screening to detect problems in the visual and hearing functions is essential. All infants should be screened for hearing loss by 1 month of age, preferably before hospital discharge. Infants identified with a hearing loss should get follow-up evaluation before 3 months; those who are deaf or hard of hearing should be enrolled in an intervention program by 6 months of age (Centers for Disease Control and Prevention, 2004). In addition, children with chronic ear infections and people who live or work in an environment where there is a high noise level should receive routine auditory testing. Women who are considering pregnancy should be advised of the importance of testing for syphilis and rubella, which can cause hearing impairments in newborns. Periodic vision screening of all newborns and children is recommended to detect congenital blindness, strabismus, and refractive errors. A child's visual acuity develops during early childhood. Children often have 20/20 vision by 6 years of age (Ball & Bindler, 2006, p. 251).

Healthy sensory function can be promoted with environmental stimuli that provide appropriate sensory input. This input should vary and be neither excessive nor too limited. As many senses as possible should be stimulated. Various colors, sounds, textures, smells, and body positions can provide various sensations. Nurses can teach parents to stimulate infants and children, and teach family members to stimulate an elderly person and others in the home with sensory deficits. Social activities often help stimulate the mind and the senses.

Nurses should also teach clients at risk of sensory loss how to prevent or reduce the loss and should teach general health measures, such as getting regular eye examinations and controlling chronic diseases such as diabetes (see Client Teaching).

ENSURING CLIENT SAFETY. Nurses must implement safety precautions in health care settings for clients with sensory deficits. Examples of precautions include, keeping the bed in the lowest position and placing the call light within reach.

Adjusting Environmental Stimuli

The client functions best when the environment is somewhat similar to that of the individual's ordinary daily life. Sometimes nurses need to take steps to adjust the client's environment to prevent either sensory overload or sensory deprivation.

PREVENTING SENSORY OVERLOAD. For clients who are at risk of overstimulation, nurses should reduce the number and type of environmental stimuli. The nurse can counteract sensory overload by blocking stimuli and by helping the client organize the stimuli and alter responses to the stimuli.

Dark glasses with UV protection can partially block light rays, and a window shade or drape can reduce visual stimulation. Earplugs reduce auditory stimuli, as do soft background music and earphones. The odor from a draining wound can be minimized by keeping the dressing dry and clean and applying a liquid deodorant on a gauze near the wound.

Another method of blocking stimuli is to reduce novelty and surprise and provide rest intervals free of interruptions. Sometimes the number of visitors and the length of visits must be restricted. Also, if the nurse carries out several nursing measures together, the client can have a scheduled quiet period before the next activity.

By explaining sounds in the environment, the nurse can help the client organize them mentally: A bell signals a change of shift; a beep, an IV alarm. When clients understand their meaning, stimuli are frequently less confusing and more easily ignored. People can also learn through practice and feedback to alter their responses to the stimuli. Clients can employ relaxation techniques to reduce anxiety and stress despite continual sensory stimulation (see Chapter 42 ∞). Box 38–2 provides nursing measures for clients with sensory overload.

PREVENTING SENSORY DEPRIVATION. For clients who are at risk for sensory deprivation, nurses can increase environmental stimuli in a number of ways. For example, newspapers, books, music, and television can stimulate the visual and au-

---

CLIENT TEACHING   Preventing Sensory Disturbances

- Have regular health examinations.
- Have regular eye examinations as recommended by the primary care provider to screen for eye problems. For clients ages 40 and over, a medical eye examination is generally recommended every 3 to 5 years, or every 1 to 2 years if there is a family history of glaucoma.
- Seek early medical attention (a) if signs suggesting visual impairment arise, for example, failure to react to light, or reduced eye contact from an infant; (b) if the child complains of an earache or has an ear infection; and (c) for persistent eye redness, discharge or increased tearing, growths on or near the eye, pupil asymmetry or other irregularity, or any pain or discomfort.
- Obtain regular immunizations of children against diseases capable of causing hearing loss (e.g., rubella, mumps, and measles).

- Avoid giving infants and toddlers toys with long pointed handles and keep pointed instruments (e.g., scissors and screwdrivers) out of reach. Supervise preschoolers when they use scissors.
- Make sure that toddlers do not walk or run with a pointed object in hand; teach preschoolers to walk carefully when carrying such objects as sticks or toy weapons.
- Teach school-age children and adolescents the proper use of sports equipment (e.g., hockey sticks) and power tools.
- Wear protective eye goggles when using power tools, riding motorcycles, spraying chemicals, and so on.
- Wear ear protectors when working in an environment with high noise levels or brief loud impulse noises (e.g., blasting).
- Wear dark glasses with UV protection to avoid damage from ultraviolet rays and never look directly into the sun.

BOX 38–2 Preventing Sensory Overload

- Minimize unnecessary light, noise, and distraction. Provide dark glasses and earplugs as needed.
- Control pain as indicated at the level desired by the client, on a scale of 0 to 10.
- Introduce yourself by name, and address the client by name.
- Provide orienting cues, such as clocks, calendars, equipment, and furniture in the room.
- Provide a private room.
- Limit visitors.
- Plan care to allow for uninterrupted periods for rest or sleep.
- Schedule a routine of care so the client knows when and what to expect (post the schedule for the client wherever possible).
- Speak in a low tone of voice and in an unhurried manner.
- Provide new information gradually to enable the client to process the meaning. When providing information, ask the client to repeat it so that there are no misunderstandings.
- Describe any tests and procedures to the client beforehand.
- Reduce noxious odors. Empty a commode or bedpan immediately after use, keep wounds clean and covered, use a room deodorizer when indicated, and provide good ventilation.
- Take time to discuss the client's problems and to correct misinterpretations.
- Assist the client with stress-reducing techniques.

BOX 38–3 Preventing Sensory Deprivation

- Encourage the client to use eyeglasses and hearing aids.
- Address the client by name and touch the client while speaking if this is not culturally offensive.
- Communicate frequently with the client and maintain meaningful interactions (e.g., discuss current events).
- Provide a telephone, radio and/or TV, clock, and calendar.
- Provide murals, pictures, sculptures, and wall hangings. Many libraries and museums will lend artwork free of charge, or a local school may provide art projects developed by their students.
- Have family and friends bring freshly cut flowers and plants.
- Consider having a resident pet such as fish, a cat, or a bird or make arrangements for pets to visit on a regular basis.
- Include different textured objects to feel such as a sheepskin pillow, silk scarf, soft blanket, or other inanimate object.
- Increase tactile stimulation through physical care measures such as back massages, hair care, and foot soaks.
- Encourage social interaction through activity groups or visits by family and friends.
- Encourage the use of crossword puzzles or games to stimulate mental function.
- Encourage environment changes such as a walk through a mall, or for an immobilized client, sitting near a window or at a place on the nursing unit where the client can watch local traffic.
- Encourage the use of self-stimulation techniques such as singing, humming, whistling, or reciting.

ditory senses. Providing objects that are pleasant to touch, such as a pet to stroke, can provide tactile and interactive stimulation. Clocks that differentiate night from day by color can help orient a client to time. The olfactory sense can be stimulated by the presence of fresh flowers or plants.

Arrangements should also be made for people to visit and talk with the client regularly. Many church and community groups provide visitors to "shut-ins," that is, people who are confined to their homes or who reside in nursing homes. Box 38–3 provides measures to prevent sensory deprivation.

Managing Acute Sensory Deficits

When assisting clients who have a sensory deficit, the nurse needs to (a) encourage the use of sensory aids to support residual sensory function, (b) promote the use of other senses, (c) communicate effectively, and (d) ensure client safety.

Sensory Aids

Many sensory aids are available for clients who have visual and hearing deficits. Examples are listed in Box 38–4. Sensory aids can be used in the health care setting as well as in the home. In all situations, the assistance of support people needs to be enlisted whenever possible to help the client deal with the deficit.

Promoting the Use of Other Senses

When one sense is lost, the nurse can teach the client to use other senses to supplement the loss. This stimulation is similar to that provided to prevent sensory deprivation, discussed earlier. However, the type of stimulation needs to be adapted in accordance with the client's specific deficit. For example, for the visually impaired client, stimulation of hearing, taste, smell, and touch can be encouraged. A radio, audiotapes of music or

books, clocks that chime, music boxes, and wind chimes can be used for auditory stimulation. Diets that include a variety of flavors, temperatures, and textures can be planned to stimulate the taste buds. Taking sips of water between foods and eating foods

BOX 38–4 Sensory Aids for Visual and Hearing Deficits

VISUAL
- Eyeglasses of the correct prescription, clean and in good repair
- Adequate room lighting, including night-lights
- Sunglasses or shades on windows to reduce glare
- Bright contrasting colors in the environment
- Magnifying glass
- Phone dialer with large numbers
- Clock and wristwatch with large numbers
- Color code or texture code on stoves, washer, medicine containers, and so on
- Colored or raised rims on dishes
- Reading material with large print
- Braille or recorded books
- Seeing-eye dog

HEARING
- Hearing aid in good order
- Lip reading
- Sign language
- Amplified telephones
- Telecommunication device for the deaf (TDD)
- Amplified telephone ringers and doorbells
- Flashing alarm clocks
- Flashing smoke detectors

separately can emphasize the taste sensation. Fresh flowers, scented candles (safely used), room fragrances, brewing coffee, and baking can stimulate the sense of smell. Clients can also be encouraged to remember pleasant or familiar odors such as the perfume of sweet peas. Measures such as providing a hug, massage, hair brushing, grooming, different textures in clothing and upholstery fabrics, and pets can be used to stimulate touch receptors.

Communicating Effectively

Communication with clients who have sensory deficits should convey respect, enhance the person's self-esteem, and ensure the exchange of correct information. A person with a hearing impairment has to concentrate more than other people and therefore tires more readily. Fatigue compounded by an illness can further reduce the person's ability to hear. A person with a visual impairment is unable to observe most nonverbal cues during communication and relies largely on the spoken word and tone of voice. Guidelines for communicating with people who are visually or hearing impaired are shown in Box 38–5.

Impaired Vision

For clients with visual impairments, nurses need to do the following in a health care setting:

- Orient the client to the arrangement of room furnishings and maintain an uncluttered environment.
- Keep pathways clear and do not rearrange furniture without orienting the client. Ensure that housekeeping personnel are informed about this.
- Organize self-care articles within the client's reach and orient the client to his or her location.
- Keep the call light within easy reach and place the bed in the low position.

CULTURALLY COMPETENT CARE
Vision Impairment and Older Adults

The most common vision diseases affecting older adults are macular degeneration, glaucoma, cataract, and diabetic retinopathy.

- Age-related macular degeneration (ARMD) is the most common cause of new cases of vision impairment in people older than 65. It is the leading cause of vision impairment in adults 75 and older. The prevalence of ARMD is the same for African Americans and Caucasians up to age 75, with rates higher for Caucasians after 75.
- African Americans are 3 to 4 times more likely to have open-angle glaucoma.
- People of Asian descent and Eskimos are more likely to have closed-angle glaucoma.
- Diabetic retinopathy is more prevalent among African Americans, Hispanics, and Native Americans, than among Caucasians.

Note: From "The Prevalence and Consequences of Vision Impairment in Later Life," by A. Horowitz, 2004, *Topics in Geriatric Rehabilitation, 20*(3), pp. 185–195. Reprinted with permission.

- Assist with ambulation by standing at the client's side, walking about 1 foot ahead, and allowing the person to grasp your arm. Confirm whether the client prefers grasping your arm with the dominant or nondominant hand.

Research has established an association between vision impairment and greater disability in activities of daily living (e.g., bathing, dressing, eating) and instrumental tasks (e.g., shopping, housekeeping) (Horowitz, 2004). Studies have also shown that visual impairment increases the risk of depression among older adults living in the community (Horowitz, 2003, 2004). Explanations for this relationship vary. One explanation is that vision loss leads to increased disability which leads to depression. Another

---

BOX 38–5 Communicating with Clients Who Have a Visual or Hearing Deficit

VISUAL DEFICIT
- Always announce your presence when entering the client's room and identify yourself by name.
- Stay in the client's field of vision if the client has a partial vision loss.
- Speak in a warm and pleasant tone of voice. Some people tend to speak louder than necessary when talking to a blind person.
- Always explain what you are about to do before touching the person.
- Explain the sounds in the environment.
- Indicate when the conversation has ended and when you are leaving the room.

HEARING DEFICIT
- Before initiating conversation, convey your presence by moving to a position where you can be seen or by gently touching the person.
- Decrease background noises (e.g., television) before speaking.
- Talk at a moderate rate and in a normal tone of voice. Shouting does not make your voice more distinct and in some instances makes understanding more difficult.
- Address the person directly. Do not turn away in the middle of a remark or story. Make sure the person can see your face easily and that it is well lighted.

- Avoid talking when you have something in your mouth, such as chewing gum. Avoid covering your mouth with your hand.
- Keep your voice at about the same volume throughout each sentence, without dropping the voice at the end of each sentence.
- Always speak as clearly and accurately as possible. Articulate consonants with particular care.
- Do not "overarticulate"; mouthing or overdoing articulation is just as troublesome as mumbling. Pantomime or write ideas, or use sign language or finger spelling as appropriate.
- Use longer phrases, which tend to be easier to understand than short ones. For example, "Would you like a drink of water?" presents much less difficulty than "Would you like a drink?" Word choice is important: "Fifteen cents" and "fifty cents" may be confused, but "half a dollar" is clear.
- Pronounce every name with care. Make a reference to the name for easier understanding, for example, "Joan, the girl from the office" or "Sears, the big downtown store."
- Change to a new subject at a slower rate, making sure that the person follows the change to the new subject. A key word or two at the beginning of a new topic is a good indicator.

DRUG CAPSULE   *travoprost* (Travatan)

CLIENT TAKING MEDICATION FOR GLAUCOMA

Travoprost is an anti-glaucoma drug that decreases intraocular pressure in open-angle glaucoma

NURSING RESPONSIBILITIES

- Assess eye for inflammation, exudate, and pain.
- Note iris color.

CLIENT AND FAMILY TEACHING

- Use once daily as directed.
- Do not let the tip of the dropper touch any part of the eye.
- It may be used with other eye products to lower intraocular pressure. If more than one medication, administer 5 minutes apart.

- Inform of risk of darkening of the iris, eyelashes, or skin around the eye.
- Do not administer while wearing contact lenses. Remove contact lens and wait 15 minutes after instilling eyedrop before reinserting contact lens.
- Discard the container within 6 weeks of removing it from the sealed pouch.

Note: Prior to administering any medication, review all aspects with a current drug handbook or other reliable source.

ANATOMY & PHYSIOLOGY REVIEW   Glaucoma

Glaucoma is a group of diseases of the eye caused by increased intraocular pressure that can lead to optic nerve damage and eventual vision loss (see Part D). Review Part A for the normal anatomy of the eye.

A clear liquid, the aqueous humor, circulates inside the front portion of the eye nourishing the lens and cornea. To maintain a normal level of pressure in the eye, the body constantly produces a small amount of aqueous humor and an equal amount flows out of the eye through a drainage system at the junction of the iris and the cornea (Halvorson, 2005, p. 42). It is at this angle that the fluid passes through a trabecular meshwork and drains into the Canal of Schlemm and enters into the bloodstream in the back of the eye.

In acute open-angle glaucoma, the anterior chamber angle remains open but drainage of the aqueous humor through the Canal of Schlemm is impaired. This causes a slow rise of the intraocular pressure. The eye's drainage angle becomes less efficient as a person ages and the risk of developing chronic open-angle glaucoma increases. The cause is unknown.

In acute closed-angle glaucoma, the drainage angle narrows and closes or becomes blocked by the iris. The intraocular pressure can rise quickly and cause an acute attack.

A

A, The normal anatomy of the eye.

ANATOMY & PHYSIOLOGY REVIEW Glaucoma—*continued*

Lens

Slowly rising intraocular pressure

Anterior chamber
Cornea
Flow of aqueous humor
Normal anterior chamber angle
Canal of Schlemm
Trabecular meshwork

Congestion in trabecular meshwork reduces flow through Canal of Schlemm.

B

Lens

Rapidly rising intraocular pressure

Anterior chamber
Cornea

Closed anterior chamber angle

Trabecular meshwork and Canal of Schlemm blocked, preventing outflow of aqueous humor.

C

D

B, Open-angle (chronic) glaucoma. *C*, Closed-angle (acute) glaucoma. *D*, Narrowing of the optical fields is a typical symptom of untreated glaucoma.

QUESTIONS
1. Review Part B. Describe the angle between the iris and the cornea: _____
2. Review Part C. Describe the angle between the iris and the cornea: _____
3. Open-angle glaucoma is represented by which figure? _____
4. Closed-angle glaucoma is represented by which figure? _____
5. The increasing fluid pressure pushes against what important part of the eye with the resulting damage leading to vision loss? _____

See Appendix A for answers. ∞

explanation states that loss of vision causes fear—a fear of losing one's autonomy and becoming dependent on another or others. Visual loss also affects how a person obtains information (e.g., reading the newspaper). In addition, reading is often a leisure activity and its loss can affect a person's quality of life. It is important for the nurse to be aware of and assess for signs of depression and intervene as appropriate if an older adult is experiencing depression as a result of a visual impairment.

Impaired Hearing

Clients with hearing impairments who are unable to hear the alarms of IV pumps and cardiac monitors need to be assessed frequently. They can be taught to use their visual sense to identify kinks in the IV tubing or a loose ECG lead, and so on. For home safety, clients with impaired hearing need to obtain devices that either amplify sounds or respond with flashing lights to sounds such as a doorbell or smoke detector, a baby crying, or a burglar alarm. The sounds of doorbells and alarm clocks may be amplified or changed to a lower frequency or buzzerlike sound. These devices can be obtained from hearing aid dealers, telephone companies, and appliance stores.

An important consequence of a decline in hearing as a person ages is difficulty understanding speech. Factors that influence this difficulty are the environment, rate of speech, and

RESEARCH NOTE Can Assistance Have a Negative Influence on the Well-Being of Adults Who Are Visually Impaired?

Adults who are visually impaired need assistance from friends and family. Recently it has been observed that this need for assistance can have a negative as well as positive influence on the provider and the receiver. The researchers studied the receivers. This group of receivers were young and middle-aged adults who became visually impaired at the age of 18 years or older. All were working adults.

Overprotection was the major problem for the visually impaired. They reported that they were prevented from learning because their support systems would not stop intervening during the learning process. For example, one receiver was willing and able to learn to use a cane but the supporter continued to guide.

IMPLICATIONS

The role of the nurse is to be aware of the problem and to intervene as needed. Although this study was limited in the number of clients, it should increase the awareness of the nurse and nursing student to the problem of overprotection. The client's full potential may be severely limited by the support system. It is essential that the nurse understand and appreciate that the support system believes that they are working in the best interest of the client. Positive nursing interventions such as applauding the support given, encouraging a letting go, and encouraging the client to take positive forward actions will benefit both the client and the support system.

Note: Adapted from V. R. Cimarolli and K. Boerner, "Social Support and Well-being in Adults Who Are Visually Impaired," *Journal of Visual Impairment & Blindness, 99*(9), pp. 521–534, copyright © 2005, by AFB Press, American Foundation for the Blind. All rights reserved.

presence of an accent. Environments that are noisy and reverberant (echoing, hollow sounds) cause difficulty for elderly listeners. Elderly adults with a hearing loss have difficulty understanding fast speech. Research indicates that the older adult's ability to process the fast verbal information is slower and that rapid speech allows for less time for the older adult to recognize the acoustic or auditory cues of the speech (Gordon-Salant, 2005). A person who speaks with an accent can also affect speech understanding by the older person. Non-native English speakers may vary their pronunciation of syllables and/or words, making it challenging for the older adult.

Impaired Olfactory Sense

Clients with an impaired sense of smell need to be taught about the dangers of cleaning with chemicals such as ammonia. Because a gas leak can go undetected, clients need to keep gas stoves and heaters in good working order. Strong chemicals such as ammonia used in confined spaces such as a bathroom may affect the client before they are smelled. Food poisoning is a concern with clients who have difficulty detecting spoiled meat or dairy products. These clients need to carefully inspect food for freshness (check its color and texture) and check expiration dates on food packages.

Impaired Tactile Sense

Clients with an impaired sense of touch may not be aware of hot temperatures, which can cause burns, or pressure on bony

prominences, which can produce pressure ulcers. Clients with decreased sensation to temperature should have the temperature adjusted on their hot water heater and test water temperature with a thermometer before bathing. Clients with decreased sensation to pressure must change their position frequently.

The Confused Client

Confusion can occur in clients of all ages, but it is most commonly seen in older people. The terms *acute confusion* and *delirium* are used interchangeably by most health professionals, with nurses tending to favor the use of *acute confusion* and physicians using the term *delirium* (McCurren & Cronin, 2003, p. 319). Delirium occurs in 6% to 30% of the general hospital population and 7% to 52% of postsurgical clients (Edwards, 2003, p. 347). Delirium in the intensive care unit (ICU) setting is a common problem and has been described as sundown syndrome, ICU psychosis, and ICU syndrome. Unfortunately, delirium is unrecognized or misdiagnosed by both the physician and the nurse in up to two-thirds of cases (Hanley, 2004, p. 218).

There are numerous reasons for the older adult being at risk for delirium when hospitalized. They often have other chronic medical problems (e.g., dementia, chronic obstructive pulmonary disease, hypertension, stroke) that place them at risk. Many elders take numerous medications with anticholinergics,

RESEARCH NOTE What Is the Impact of Hearing Loss on the Quality of Life for Older Adults?

The researchers investigated the impact of hearing loss on communication, activities of daily living (ADLs), instrumental activities of daily living (IADLs) and health-related quality of life issues in a large population (i.e., 2,800) of older adults ranging from 57 to 97 years of age. Standardized audiometric testing procedures and self-reported surveys were used.

The study resulted in the following findings:

- Fifty-two percent of the participants self-reported having problems with communication.
- Severity of hearing loss was associated with reduced functioning of ADLs and IADLs. The researchers noted that hearing loss was not a direct cause of ADL functioning (e.g., toileting, ambulation) but an indication that hearing loss accompanies the general decline of aging. On the other hand, the IADLs (e.g., shopping, managing finances, preparing meals, and talking on the telephone) are directly affected by hearing loss as communication is needed for IADL activities.
- Severity of hearing loss and self-report of communication problems were associated with reduced quality of life.

IMPLICATIONS

Hearing loss is often dismissed as not being important or as a part of the aging process. It is important to realize how it can affect quality of life for the older person. Identifying hearing loss, supplying adaptive equipment, and teaching coping strategies may have a positive effect on quality of life for older adults.

Note: From "The Impact of Hearing Loss on Quality of Life in Older Adults," by D. Dalton, K. Cruickshanks, B. Klein, R. Klein, T. Wiley, and D. Nondahl, *The Gerontologist,* 2003.

TABLE 38–2 Differentiating between Delirium and Dementia

CHARACTERISTIC	DELIRIUM	DEMENTIA
Distinguishing feature	Acute, fluctuating change in mental status.	Memory impairment.
Onset	Sudden, acute onset.	Slow, insidious.
Duration	Temporary. May last hours to days.	Chronic, gradual, irreversible.
Time of day	Worsens at night.	No change with time of day.
Sleep–wake cycles	Disturbed. Cycles often reversed.	Disturbed. Fragmented. Awakens often during the night.
Alertness	Fluctuates. May be alert and oriented during the day but become confused and disoriented at night.	Generally normal.
Thinking	Disorganized, distorted. Impaired attention. Alterations in memory.	Judgment impaired. Difficulty with abstraction and word finding.
Delusions/hallucinations	May have visual, auditory, and tactile hallucinations. Misinterpretation of real sensory experiences.	Delusions. Usually no hallucinations.
Causative and risk factors	Cerebral and cardiovascular disease, infections, reduced hearing and vision, environmental change, stress, sleep deprivation, polypharmacy, dehydration.	Alzheimer's disease. Multiple infarct dementia.

narcotics, and sedatives often increasing the risk for delirium. Undertreating pain can also contribute to the risk. Many elders have a vision or hearing loss. All of these risks plus the unfamiliar surroundings and routine of a hospital, possible sleep deprivation, stress, and sensory overload compound the older adult's risk for developing delirium.

Confusion often presents with subtle symptoms, but an attempt should be made to differentiate between **acute confusion (delirium)** and chronic confusion (*dementia*). Delirium is often called acute confusion; it has an abrupt onset and a cause which, when treated, reverses the confusion. Dementia is often called chronic confusion with symptoms that are gradual and irreversible (e.g., Alzheimer's disease). It is often difficult to differentiate between the two conditions, but it is important to treat causes, if possible, in order to be able to reverse the condition. See Table 38–2. Clients who are confused often know something is wrong and want help. Box 38–6 lists nursing interventions to help promote a therapeutic environment for the client with acute confusion/delirium (see Figure 38-3 ■).

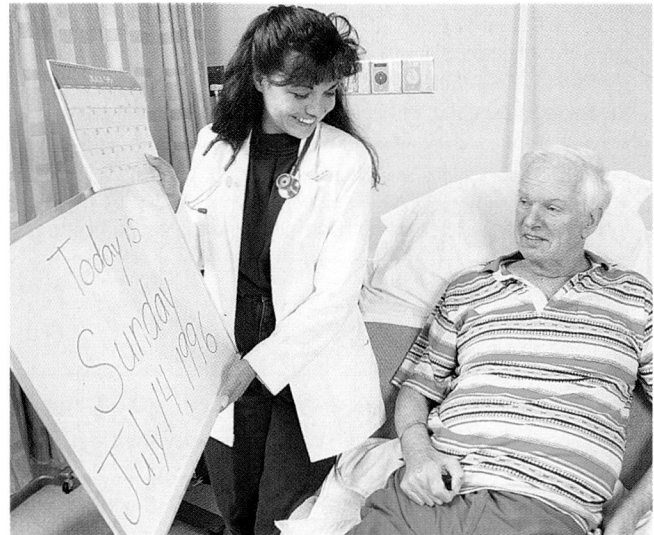

Figure 38-3 ■ Promoting orientation to time and date is essential for clients who are confused or have a memory loss.

BOX 38–6 Promoting a Therapeutic Environment for a Client with Acute Confusion/Delirium

- Wear a readable name tag.
- Address the person by name and introduce yourself frequently: "Good morning, Mr. Richards. I am Betty Brown. I will be your nurse today."
- Identify time and place as indicated: "Today is December 5, and it is 8:00 in the morning."
- Ask the client, "Where are you?" and orient the client to place (e.g., nursing home) if indicated.
- Place a calendar and clock in the client's room. Mark holidays with ribbons, pins, or other means.
- Speak clearly and calmly to the client, allowing time for your words to be processed and for the client to give a response.
- Encourage family to visit frequently except if this activity causes the client to become hyperactive.
- Provide clear, concise explanations of each treatment procedure or task.

- Eliminate unnecessary noise.
- Reinforce reality by interpreting unfamiliar sounds, sights, and smells; correct any misconceptions of events or situations.
- Schedule activities (e.g., meals, bath, activity and rest periods, treatments) at the same time each day to provide a sense of security. If possible, assign the same caregivers.
- Provide adequate sleep.
- Keep glasses and hearing aid within reach.
- Ensure adequate pain management.
- Keep familiar items in the client's environment (e.g., photographs), and keep the environment uncluttered. A disorganized, cluttered environment increases confusion.
- Keep room well lit during waking hours.

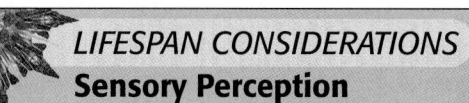
CULTURALLY COMPETENT CARE   Hmong Elders

In the 1970s the Hmong arrived in the United States as taking advantage of resettlement opportunities. The largest numbers of Hmong live in California, Minnesota, and Wisconsin.

Spiritual beliefs join their beliefs related to health and illness. The Hmong of Laos believe that a person has multiple souls and that health results from the souls living in harmony. Spiritual illness results when one or more of the souls leave the physical body. Healing ceremonies are performed to call and retrieve the lost soul(s).

In Laos, Hmong elders are treated with great respect. Others consult the elders because they have acquired wisdom and insight from their experiences. Many older Hmong in the United States do not speak English, and an interpreter will be needed. Avoiding di-

rect eye contact and speaking in a calm, caring manner will facilitate communication.

Among the Hmong who practice traditional beliefs, confusion and memory impairment of an older adult may be treated with herbal teas and a spiritual ceremony conducted by a shaman. Hmong families living in the United States may seek out both their traditional healers and Western medicine health professionals to help the older adult(s) in their family. Nurses need to honor traditional beliefs while providing Western medical care.

Note: From "Chronic Confusion and Memory Impairment in Hmong Elders," by L. A. Gerdner, S. V. Xiong, and D. Cha, 2006, *Journal of Gerontological Nursing, 32*(3), pp. 23–31. Copyright © 2006 SLACK, Inc. Reprinted with permission.

The Unconscious Client

The number of people surviving with traumatic brain injury is increasing, and most experience some form of coma and significant deficits. Coma is a deep state of unconsciousness that lasts for a period more than 2 to 4 weeks following a traumatic brain injury (Gerber, 2005, p. 98). Previously, the client would be medically stablilized and approximately 6 months later transferred to a rehabilitation setting for coma stimulation. It is thought that unconscious clients suffer from sensory deprivation because they are in a cold, sterile environment, immobilized, and without the usual stimulation humans need (Gerber, 2005, p. 104). As a result, the

current trend is to begin a coma stimulation program earlier, while the client is in the acute care setting. Coma stimulation consists of providing sensory stimulation to promote brain recovery by waking up the reticular activating system (RAS). Box 38–7 provides examples of sensory stimulation that a nurse and/or family member may provide for the unconscious client. It is important that the stimulation be delivered in a quiet environment (to prevent sensory overload) and done slowly to allow time for a response to occur. Sensory stimulation sessions are of a certain time duration (e.g., 30 to 45 minutes), and the number of sessions will vary in a 12-hour day. It is also important to provide the client with sleep/rest periods that alternate with the structured sensory stimulation sessions.

BOX 38–7   Promoting Sensory Stimulation for the Unconscious Client

AUDITORY
- Introduce yourself to the client.
- Orient the client to time, month, year, location, and what happened.
- Inform client beforehand the care to be provided.
- Read literature aloud to the client.
- Play a tape recording of a familiar voice.
- Converse directly to the client.

VISUAL
- Sit client upright in a chair or bed (provides normal visual orientation).

OLFACTORY
- Provide aromatic stimuli that may include client's favorites (e.g., coffee, lemon, cologne or perfume).

GUSTATORY
- Provide mouth care using mint-flavored cleaning agent.
- Place different tastes on tongue.

TACTILE
- Incorporate during bath activities (e.g., temperature and texture of washcloth, back massage, brushing hair, rubbing lotion on extremities).

KINESTHETIC
- Perform range-of-motion exercises.
- Change client's position.

Note: From C. Gerber, "Understanding and Managing Coma Stimulation: Are We Doing Everything We Can?", *Critical Care Nursing Quarterly, 2005* vol. 28, issue number 2, pp. 94–108. Copyright © 2005 Lippincott, Williams & Wilkins. Reprinted with permission.

LIFESPAN CONSIDERATIONS
Sensory Perception

CHILDREN

Newborns should be screened for hearing loss prior to hospital discharge. Universal screening of all newborns is mandated in at least 30 states, and in all states screening is done for children who are at high risk (e.g., have a history of infection during gestation, or are born with anomalies of the head or face). If a hearing loss is detected early, treatment can begin early and complications such as speech loss can be prevented. If an infant is found to have a hearing loss, it is recommended that treatment begin before 6 months of age (Joint Committee on Infant Hearing, 2000).

ELDERS

Normal changes of aging often result in varying degrees of impairments in sensory perception of the senses—hearing, vision, smell, taste, and touch. Diseases and conditions that are more common in elders and which also alter sensory perception are diabetes, strokes, and other neurologic disorders such as Parkinson's disease. Nursing interventions need to be very specific and individualized and may be directed to either increase or decrease sensory stimuli.

The goals of nursing care should be focused on maintaining safety and communication with clients who have these impairments. Clients with dementia may have problems that fit more appropriately under "altered thought processes," but the goals should be similar—to maximize their potential, maintain their quality of life and dignity, and at the same time, be aware of safety and communication issues.

Evaluating

Using the measurable desired outcomes developed during the planning stage as a guide, the nurse collects data needed to judge whether client goals and outcomes have been achieved.

Examples of client outcomes and related indicators are shown in the earlier Identifying Nursing Diagnoses, Outcomes, and Interventions and in the Nursing Care Plan. If outcomes are not achieved, the nurse and client, and support people if appropriate, need to explore the reasons before modifying the care plan.

NURSING CARE PLAN Sensory-Perception Disturbance

ASSESSMENT DATA	NURSING DIAGNOSIS	DESIRED OUTCOMES*
Nursing Assessment Julia Hagstrom is an 80-year-old widow who has recently become a resident of an extended care facility. Just prior to her admission she underwent surgery for the removal of cataracts and also experienced more difficulty with hearing. Her children were concerned about her physical safety and lack of socialization and urged her to enter a nursing home. Mrs. Hagstrom had cared for herself independently for 15 years in her own home. Three days after admission the nurse finds the client somewhat confused and disoriented to place, and time. She appears restless and withdrawn. She states, "I'm afraid of all of these strange creatures in this orphanage."	*Disturbed Sensory Perception (Sensory Overload)* related to change in environment, and hearing loss (as evidenced by disorientation to time and place; restlessness; and altered behavior)	**Cognitive Orientation** [0901] as evidenced by not compromised: ■ Identifies significant other(s) ■ Identifies current place ■ Identifies correct season **Hearing Compensation Behavior** [1610] as evidenced by often demonstrated: ■ Positions self to advantage hearing ■ Reminds others to use techniques that advantage hearing ■ Eliminates background noise ■ Uses hearing supportive devices

Physical Examination

Diagnostic Data

Height: 160 cm (5'3")
Weight: 55.3 kg (122 lb)
Temperature: 37°C (98.6°F)
Pulse: 72 BPM
Respirations: 18/minute
Blood Pressure: 128/74 mm Hg
Rinne test: negative

Chest x-ray, CBC, and urinalysis all negative

NURSING INTERVENTIONS*/SELECTED ACTIVITIES	RATIONALE
Reality Orientation [4820]	
Provide a consistent physical environment and a daily routine.	*Routine eliminates the element of surprise, overstimulation, and further confusion.*
Provide access to familiar objects, when possible.	*Familiarity helps reduce confusion.*
Provide a low-stimulation environment for Mrs. Hagstrom because disorientation may be increased by overstimulation.	*A disruption in the quality or quantity of incoming stimuli can affect a person's cognitive status. Sensory overload blocks out meaningful stimuli.*
Provide for adequate rest, sleep, and daytime naps.	*Reduces overstimulation and fatigue, which may be contributing factors to confusion.*
Use a calm and unhurried approach when interacting with Mrs. Hagstrom.	*Promotes communication that enhances the person's sense of dignity.*
Speak to the client in a slow, distinct manner with appropriate volume.	*The client who has difficulty hearing will be better able to lip read and comprehend speech.*
Engage Mrs. Hagstrom in concrete "here and now" activities (that is, ADLs) that focus on something outside the self that is concrete and reality oriented.	*Assists the individual to differentiate between own thoughts and reality.*

NURSING CARE PLAN Sensory-Perception Disturbance *continued*

NURSING INTERVENTIONS*/SELECTED ACTIVITIES	RATIONALE
Communication Enhancement: Hearing Deficit [4974]	
■ Facilitate use of hearing aids, as appropriate.	*Hearing can be enhanced if the volume is appropriate and the hearing aid is consistently used.*
■ Listen attentively.	*Effective listening is essential in a nurse–client relationship. Poor listening skills can undermine trust and block therapeutic communication.*
■ Use simple words and short sentences, as appropriate.	*Using simple terms and short sentences facilitates understanding and minimizes anxiety.*
■ Obtain Mrs. Hagstrom's attention through touch.	*Gaining the attention of a client with a hearing impairment is an essential first step toward effective communication. However, the client's personal space should be respected and permission to touch should be obtained.*

EVALUATION

Outcomes met. Mrs. Hagstrom identifies her primary nurse by sight and name on the third day. She is aware that Christmas is 3 weeks away and is anxious to go shopping with the group. Her daughter has brought new batteries for her hearing aid, which she wears during the day.

The NOC # for desired outcomes and the NIC # for nursing interventions are listed in brackets following the appropriate outcome or intervention. Outcomes, interventions, and activities selected are only a sample of those suggested by NOC and NIC and should be further individualized for each client.

CRITICAL THINKING CHECKPOINT

Mrs. Dodd is a 51-year-old client who is being cared for in the critical care unit following an automobile accident in which she suffered extensive traumatic injuries. Mrs. Dodd is connected to several monitoring devices, has an intubation tube and ventilator to assist her with respirations, and is receiving various pain and other medications.

1. Identify factors that place Mrs. Dodd at risk for the development of sensory deprivation or overload.

2. What assessment findings would alert you to Mrs. Dodd's experiencing sensory overload as opposed to sensory deprivation?
3. How can you intervene to help Mrs. Dodd during this stressful event?
4. How might the care of a client in the home setting differ from the care of a client such as Mrs. Dodd who is receiving care in a critical care unit?

See Critical Thinking Possibilities in Appendix A.

CONCEPT MAP **Sensory-Perception Disturbance**

JH
89 y.o. female
widow

→ assess →

- Lived independently in own home for 15 years
- Recent removal of cataracts
- Experiencing more difficulty hearing
- Children concerned about her safety and lack of socialization and urged her to enter a nursing home
- Confused

- Disoriented to place & time
- Restless
- Withdrawn
- Stated "I'm afraid of all these strange creatures in this orphanage"
- VS: WNL
- CXR, CBC, U/A: negative

↓ generate nursing diagnosis

Disturbed Sensory-Perception (sensory overload) r/t change in environment and hearing loss

outcome ↓   outcome ↓

Outcome met:
- Able to identify her nurse by name
- Aware that Christmas is 3 weeks away
- Anxious to go shopping with the group
- Wears hearing aid during the day

← Evaluation —

Cognitive Orientation aeb not compromised:
- Identifies others, current place, correct season

Hearing Compensation Behavior aeb often demonstrated:
- Positions self to advantage hearing
- Reminds others to use techniques that advantage hearing
- Eliminates background noise
- Uses hearing aid

— Evaluation →

Outcome met:
- Wears hearing aid during the day

nursing intervention ↓

Reality Orientation

activity ↓   activity ↓   activity ↓   activity

Provide consistent physical environment and daily routine

Provide access to familiar objects

Use calm unhurried approach

Provide a low-stimulus environment

Provide or adequate rest and sleep

Speak slowly and distinctly

nursing intervention ↓

Communication Enhancement: Hearing Deficit

activity ↓   activity ↓   activity ↓   activity ↓

Listen attentively

Facilitate use of hearing aid

Obtain attention through touch

Use simple words, short sentences

CHAPTER 38 **REVIEW**

CHAPTER HIGHLIGHTS

- The sensory experience consists of two components: sensory reception and sensory perception.
- Sensory stimuli can be either external or internal. Visual, auditory, olfactory, tactile, and gustatory stimuli orient a person to the external environment. Kinesthetic and visceral stimuli orient the person to the internal environment. Kinesthetic stimuli make the person aware of the position and movement of body parts.
- Sensory perception involves the awareness and interpretation of stimuli into meaningful information. This process occurs in the cerebral cortex.
- The reticular activating system (RAS), with its many ascending and descending connections to other areas of the brain, monitors and regulates incoming stimuli. The RAS maintains, enhances, or inhibits cortical arousal.
- The normal, alert person can assimilate many kinds of information at one time and respond appropriately through thought and action.
- Sensory deprivation occurs when a person receives decreased sensory input or monotonous or meaningless sensory input.
- Sensory overload occurs when a person experiences excessive sensory input and is unable to process or manage the stimuli. The person feels overwhelmed and not in control.
- Responses to both sensory deprivation and sensory overload include perceptual changes (e.g., mild distortions or hallucinations), cognitive changes (e.g., decreased concentration and problem-solving ability), and affective changes (e.g., apathy, anxiety, anger, depression, and rapid mood swings).
- Clients at risk for sensory deprivation include (a) those who are homebound or institutionalized, (b) those on bed rest or isolation precautions, (c) those with sensory deficits, (d) those who come from a different culture, (e) those with certain affective disorders or disturbances of the nervous system, and (f) those on certain medications that affect the central nervous system.
- Clients at risk for sensory overload include (a) those in pain, (b) those in intensive care units, (c) those with intrusive and uncomfortable monitoring or treatment equipment, and (d) those with disturbances of the nervous system.

- Factors affecting sensory stimulation include developmental stage, culture, stress, medications, illness, and lifestyle and personality.
- Assessment for sensory-perception disturbances includes (a) a nursing history to identify sensory deficits, (b) physical examination, (c) mental status, (d) identification of clients at risk, (e) immediate environment, and (f) presence of clinical signs of sensory deprivation or overload.
- NANDA nursing diagnoses related to a client's sensory-perception impairments are *Sensory Perception Disturbances: Visual, Auditory, Gustatory, Olfactory, Tactile, Kinesthetic; Acute Confusion; Chronic Confusion; Impaired Memory; Social Isolation; Impaired Verbal Communication; Risk for Impaired Skin Integrity; Self-Care Deficit: Bathing/Hygiene; Impaired Home Maintenance;* and *Risk for Injury.*
- Goals for persons with sensory-perception disturbances include (a) maintaining or promoting the function of existing senses, (b) maintaining or improving communication, (c) preventing injury, (d) avoiding sensory deprivation or overload, (e) reducing social isolation, and (f) maintaining or restoring ability to function safely in the environment and to perform self-care.
- Interventions to prevent or modify sensory deprivation, sensory overload, and sensory deficits include promoting healthy sensory function, adjusting environmental stimuli, and managing sensory deficits.
- Clients with sensory deficits need instruction about sensory aids available to support residual sensory function, ways to promote the use of other senses, and methods to ensure safety from bodily harm.
- Nurses and support persons need to devise and implement effective communication mechanisms for clients who have visual and hearing impairments.
- Clients with acute confusion/delirium need care that is directed to promoting their orientation to time, place, person, and situation.
- Nurses need to promote structured sensory stimulation for the unconscious client.

TEST YOUR KNOWLEDGE

1. Which client is at greatest risk for experiencing sensory overload?
   1. A 40-year-old client in isolation with no family
   2. A 28-year-old quadriplegic client in a private room
   3. A 16-year-old listening to loud music
   4. An 80-year-old client admitted for emergency surgery

2. An alert 80-year-old client is transferred to a long-term care facility. On the second night he becomes confused and agitated. What is the most appropriate nursing diagnosis?
   1. *Chronic Confusion*
   2. *Impaired Memory*
   3. *Disturbed Sensory Perception*
   4. *Disturbed Thought Processes*

3. The nursing diagnosis *Risk for Impaired Skin Integrity* related to sensory-perception disturbance would best fit a client who:
   1. Cut foot by stepping on broken glass
   2. Uses a wheelchair due to paraplegia

   3. Wears glasses because of poor vision
   4. Is legally blind and smokes in bed

4. Which of the following statements indicates the client needs a sensory aid in the home?
   1. "I tripped over that throw rug again."
   2. "I can't hear the doorbell."
   3. "My eyesight is good if I wear my glasses."
   4. "I can hear the TV if I turn it up high."

5. A hospitalized client is disoriented and believes she is in a train station. Which of the following is the most appropriate response by the nurse?
   1. "You wouldn't be getting a bath at the train station."
   2. "Let's finish your bath before the train arrives."
   3. "Don't you know where you are?"
   4. "It may seem like a train station sometimes, but this is Valley Hospital."

6. A client with impaired vision is admitted to the hospital. Which interventions are most appropriate to meet the client's needs? Select all that apply.
1. Identify yourself by name.
2. Decrease background noise before speaking.
3. Stay in the client's field of vision.
4. Explain the sounds in the environment.
5. Keep your voice at the same level throughout the conversation.

7. A client is exhibiting signs and symptoms of acute confusion/delirium. The nurse implements which of the following strategies to promote a therapeutic environment?
1. Keep lights in the room dimmed to reduce stimulation.
2. Keep the environmental noise level high to increase stimulation.
3. Keep the room organized and clean.
4. Use restraints for client safety.

8. A client is at risk for sensory deprivation. Which of the following clinical signs are most likely to contribute? Select all that apply.
1. Sleeplessness
2. Decreased attention span
3. Irritability
4. Excessive sleeping
5. Crying, depression

9. The nurse is assessing for sensory function. Match the assessment tool to the specific sense it will be testing.

Identifying taste	1. Visual
Stereognosis	2. Hearing
Snellen chart	3. Tactile
Identifying aromas	4. Olfactory
Tuning fork	5. Gustatory

10. An 85-year-old client has impaired hearing. When creating the care plan, which of the following should have the highest priority?
1. Obtaining an amplified telephone
2. Teaching the importance of changing his position
3. Providing reading material with large print
4. Checking expiration dates on food packages

See Answers to Test Your Knowledge in Appendix A *.*

EXPLORE MEDIALINK www.prenhall.com/berman

DVD-ROM
▪ Audio Glossary
▪ NCLEX Review
▪ Skills Review
▪ Animations:
    Visceral Effectors A & P Review
    Components of a Reflex Arc
    Meninges of the Brain A & P Review
    The Ear A & P Review
    The Eye A & P Review

COMPANION WEBSITE
▪ Additional NCLEX Review
▪ Case Study: Clients with Altered Sensory Perception
▪ Care Plan Activity: The Confused and Agitated Client
▪ Application Activity: Client with Second-Degree Burns
▪ Links to Resources

READINGS AND REFERENCES

SUGGESTED READINGS

Ball, J., & Haight, B. K. (2005). Creating a multisensory environment for dementia: The goals of a Snoezelen® room. *Journal of Gerontological Nursing, 31*(10), 4–10.
A multisensory room is an innovative approach to provide a variety of sensory experiences that can increase the quality of life for a person with dementia. This article describes the theoretical basis, philosophy, goal, and procedure for setting up a multisensory environment.

McCurren, C., & Cronin, S. N. (2003). Delirium: Elders tell their stories and guide nursing practice. *Medsurg Nursing, 12*(5), 318–323.
This phenomenologic study provides great insight into the elder's "lived experience" of delirium. Reading their stories increases the reader's awareness of the potential for delirium or acute confusion occurring in the acute care setting. It also underscores the importance of explanations and therapeutic communication.

Smith, M., & Buckwalter, K. (2005). Behaviors associated with dementia: Whether resisting care or exhibiting apathy, an older adult with

dementia is attempting communication. Nurses and other caregivers must learn to "hear" this language. *American Journal of Nursing, 105*(7), 40–52.
This article reviews common types of dementia, principles of care, nursing interventions relating to sensory enhancement and socialization, and tips for nurses by health care setting.

Wahl, H., & Heyl, V. (2003). Connection between vision, hearing, and cognitive function. *Generations, 27*(1), 39–47.
Vision, hearing, and cognitive function are closely associated and all are related to higher cortical functions. This article discusses the need to assess the relationship between these functions and to be aware that cognitive function may be altered as the result of diminished vision and/or hearing. Changes in these senses alter the lifestyle of the client by affecting the client's ability to perform self-care activities such as taking medications, shopping, and paying bills. Teaching is essential to assist the client and his or her family/friends to adjust to the changes.

RELATED RESEARCH

Allen, N. H., Burns, A., Newton, V., Hickson, F., Ramsden, R., Rogers, J., et al. (2003). The effects of improving hearing in dementia. *Age and Ageing, 32*(2), 189–193.

Connolly, J. L., Carron, J. D., & Roark, S. D. (2005). Universal newborn hearing screening: Are we achieving the Joint Committee on Infant Hearing (JCIH) objectives? *Laryngoscope, 115*(2), 232–236.

Crews, J. E., & Campbell, V. A. (2004). Vision impairment and hearing loss among community-dwelling older Americans: Implications for health and functioning. *American Journal of Public Health, 94*(5), 823–829.

Pankow, L., Luchins, D., Studebaker, J., & Chettleburgh, D. (2004). Evaluation of a vision rehabilitation program for older adults with visual impairment. *Topics in Geriatric Rehabilitation, 20*(3), 223–232.

Pitkala, K. H., Laurila, J. V., Strandberg, T. E., & Tilvis, R. S. (2006). Multicomponent geriatric intervention for elderly inpatients with delirium: A randomized, controlled trial. *Journal of Gerontology, 61A*(2), 176–181.

Wahl, H., Becker, S., Burmedi, D., & Schilling, O. (2004). The role of primary and secondary control in adaptation to age-related vision loss: A study of older adults with macular degeneration. *Pschology and Aging, 19*(1), 235–239.

REFERENCES
Ball, J. W., & Bindler, R. C. (2006). *Child health nursing*. Upper Saddle River, NJ: Pearson Prentice Hall.
Carpenito-Moyet, L. J. (2006). *Nursing diagnosis: Application to clinical practice* (11th ed.). Philadelphia: Lippincott Williams & Wilkins.
Centers for Disease Control and Prevention, Developmental Disabilities. (2004). *Hearing loss: Screening*. Retrieved June 28, 2006, from http://www.cdc.gov/ncbddd/dd/ddhi.htm
Cimarolli, V. R., & Boerner, K. (2005). Social support and well-being in adults who are visually impaired. *Journal of Visual Impairment & Blindness, 99*(9), 521–534.
Dalton, D. S., Cruickshanks, K. J., Klein, B. E., Klein, R., Wiley, T. L., & Nondahl, D. M. (2003). The impact of hearing loss on quality of life in older adults. *Gerontologist, 43*(5), 661–668.
Dochterman, J. M., & Bulechek, G. M. (Eds.). (2004). *Nursing interventions classification (NIC)* (4th ed.). St. Louis, MO: Mosby.
Edwards, N. (2003). Differentiating the three D's: Delirium, dementia, and depression. *Medsurg Nursing, 12*(6), 347–357.
Gerber, C. (2005). Understanding and managing coma stimulation: Are we doing everything we can? *Critical Care Nursing Quarterly, 28*(2), 94–108.
Gerdner, L. A., Xiong, S. V., & Cha, D. (2006). Chronic confusion and memory impairment in Hmong elders. *Journal of Gerontological Nursing, 32*(3), 23–31.
Gordon-Salant, S. (2005). Hearing loss and aging: New research findings and clinical implications. *Journal of Rehabilitation Research & Development, 42*(4), 9–24.

Halvorson, P. (2005). The silent thief. *RN, 68*(3), 41–45.
Hanley, C. (2004). Delirium in the acute care setting. *Medsurg Nursing, 13*(4), 217–225.
Horowitz, A. (2003). Depression and vision and hearing impairment in later life. *Generations, 27*(1), 32–38.
Horowitz, A. (2004). The prevalence and consequences of vision impairment in later life. *Topics in Geriatric Rehabilitation, 20*(3), 185–195.
Joint Committee on Infant Hearing. (2000). Joint Committee on Infant Hearing year 2000 position statement: Principles and guidelines for early hearing detection and intervention programs. *Pediatrics, 106*(4), 798–817.
Marieb, E., & Hoehn, K. (2007). *Anatomy and physiology* (7th ed.). San Francisco: Pearson Benjamin Cummings.
Moorhead, S., Johnson, M., & Maas, M. (2004). *Nursing outcomes classification (NOC)* (3rd ed.). St. Louis, MO: Mosby.
NANDA International. (2005). *NANDA nursing diagnoses: Definitions and classification 2005–2006*. Philadelphia: Author.
NANDA International. (2007). *NANDA nursing diagnoses: Definitions and classification 2007–2008*. Philadelphia: Author.

SELECTED BIBLIOGRAPHY
Arditi, A. (2005). Enhancing the visual environment for older and visually impaired persons. *Alzheimer's Care Quarterly, 6*(4), 294–299.
Arnold, E. (2005). Sorting out the 3 D's: Delirium, dementia, depression: Learn how to sift through overlapping signs and symptoms so you can help improve an older patient's quality of life. *Holistic Nursing Practice, 19*(3), 99.
Bakker, R. (2003). Sensory loss, dementia, and environments. *Generations, 27*(1), 46–51.

Boyd-Monk, H. (2005). The eyes have it: Understanding problems of the aging eye. *Nursing Made Incredibly Easy, 3*(5), 34–45.
Celik, S., Oztekin, D., Akyolcu, N., & Issever, H. (2005). Sleep disturbance: The patient care activities applied at the night shift in the intensive care unit. *Journal of Clinical Nursing, 14*(1), 102–106.
Cohen, A. S., & Ayello, E. A. (2005). Diabetes has taken a toll on your patient's vision—how can you help? *Nursing, 35*(5), 44–47.
Ebersole, P., & Hess, P. (2003). *Toward healthy aging: Human needs and nursing response*. New York: Elsevier.
Eliopoulos, C. (2004). *Gerontological nursing* (6th ed.). Philadelphia: Lippincott.
Hertz, J., Koren, M., Rossetti, J., Monroe, D., Berent, G., & Plonczynski, D. (2005). Collaboration to promote best practices in care of older adults. *Medsurg Nursing, 14*(5), 311–315.
Marshall, M. C., & Soucy, M. D. (2003). Delirium in the intensive care unit. *Critical Care Nursing Quarterly, 26*(3), 172–178.
Munson, B. L. (2006). Now, listen up! Understanding hearing loss and deafness. *Nursing Made Incredibly Easy, 4*(2), 38–47.
Pullen, R. L. (2006). Spin control: Caring for a patient with inner ear disease. *Nursing, 36*(5), 48–51.
Ricketts, T. A. (2005). Directional hearing aids: Then and now. *Journal of Rehabilitation Research and Development, 42*(4), 133–145.
Spires, R. (2006). How you can help when older eyes fail. *RN, 69*(2), 38–43.
Twedell, D. (2005). Delirium. *Journal of Continuing Education in Nursing, 36*(3), 102–103.
Wold, G. H. (2003). *Basic geriatric nursing* (3rd ed.). New York: Elsevier.
Zeng, F. (2004). Trends in cochlear implants. *Trends in Amplification, 8*(1), 1–34.

CHAPTER 39

Self-Concept

LEARNING OUTCOMES

After completing this chapter, you will be able to:

1. Identify four dimensions of self-concept.

2. Give Erikson's explanation of the effects of psychosocial tasks on self-concept and self-esteem.

3. Describe the four components of self-concept.

4. Identify common stressors affecting self-concept and coping strategies.

5. Describe the essential aspects of assessing role relationships.

6. Identify nursing diagnoses related to altered self-concept.

7. Describe nursing interventions designed to achieve identified outcomes for clients with altered self-concept.

8. Describe ways to enhance client self-esteem.

Self-concept is one's mental image of oneself. A positive self-concept is essential to a person's mental and physical health. Individuals with a positive self-concept are better able to develop and maintain interpersonal relationships and resist psychologic and physical illness. An individual possessing a strong self-concept should be better able to accept or adapt to changes that may occur over the life span. How one views oneself affects one's interaction with others.

Nurses have a responsibility to assess clients for a negative self-concept and to identify the possible causes in order to help them develop a more positive view of themselves. Individuals who have a poor self-concept may express feelings of worthlessness, self-dislike, or even self-hatred. They may feel sad or hopeless, and may state they lack energy to perform even the simplest of tasks.

SELF-CONCEPT

Self-concept involves all of the self-perceptions—appearance, values, and beliefs—that influence behavior and are referred to when using the words *I* or *me.* Self-concept is a complex idea that influences the following:

- How one thinks, talks, and acts
- How one sees and treats another person
- Choices one makes
- Ability to give and receive love
- Ability to take action and to change things

There are four dimensions of self-concept:

- *Self-knowledge:* the knowledge that one has about oneself, including insights into one's abilities, nature, and limitations
- *Self-expectation:* what one expects of oneself; may be a realistic or unrealistic expectation
- *Social self:* how a person is perceived by others and society
- *Social evaluation:* the appraisal of oneself in relationship to others, events, or situations

People who value "how I perceive me" above "how others perceive me" can be termed *me-centered.* They try hard to live up to their own expectations and compete only with themselves, not others. In contrast, strongly *other-centered* people have a high need for approval from others and try hard to live up to the expectations of others, comparing, competing, and evaluating themselves in relation to others. They tend not to deal with their personal shortcomings, are unable to assert themselves, and fear disapproval. The positive self-concept, therefore, is me-centered and is formed with minimal reference to others' opinions.

Assessing and promoting a positive self-concept is not limited to the nurse acting on the client. A nurse's own self-concept is also important. Nurses who understand the different dimensions of themselves are better able to understand the needs, desires, feelings, and conflicts of their clients. Nurses who feel positive about themselves are more likely to help clients meet their needs.

Self-awareness refers to the relationship between one's perception of himself or herself and others' perceptions of him or her. Thus, a nurse who is very self-aware has perceptions that are very congruent. Becoming more self-aware is a process that requires time and energy and is never complete. One important component of the process is introspection, which involves the nurse considering his or her own beliefs, attitudes, motivations, strengths, and limitations (Donnelly, 2004). In addition to using individual reflective exercises, the nurse gains insight into the self through working with other nurses who serve as mentors and by taking seriously and acting on the feedback obtained during regular performance reviews.

Once the nurse has developed a clear understanding and awareness of self, the nurse can respect and avoid projecting his or her own beliefs onto others. While in the caregiver role, the self-aware nurse is able to suspend judgment and focus on the needs of the client, even if they differ from those of the nurse. When conflicts arise, the nurse can analyze his or her reactions through introspection and by asking

- "What is there in me that produces this kind of reaction in the client?"
- "Why do I react this way (fear, anger, anxiety, annoyance, worry)?"
- "Can I change the way I respond to this situation to affect the client's reaction in a helpful way?"

FORMATION OF SELF-CONCEPT

A person is not born with a self-concept; rather, it develops as a result of social interactions with others. Chapter 20 ∞ discusses the development of self-concept, including Erikson's stages of development, Piaget's cognitive developmental stages, and Havighurst's developmental tasks.

According to Erikson (1963), throughout life people face developmental tasks associated with eight psychosocial stages that provide a theoretical framework. The success with which a

TABLE 39–1 Examples of Behaviors Associated with Erikson's Stages of Psychosocial Development

STAGE: DEVELOPMENTAL TASKS	BEHAVIORS INDICATING POSITIVE RESOLUTION	BEHAVIORS INDICATING NEGATIVE RESOLUTION
Infancy: trust vs. mistrust	Requesting assistance and expecting to receive it Expressing belief of another person Sharing time, opinions, and experiences	Restricting conversation to superficialities Refusing to provide a person with personal information Being unable to accept assistance
Toddlerhood: autonomy vs. shame and doubt	Accepting the rules of a group but also expressing disagreement when it is felt Expressing one's own opinion Easily accepting deferment of a wish fulfillment	Failing to express needs Not expressing one's own opinion when opposed Overconcern about being clean
Early childhood: initiative vs. guilt	Starting projects eagerly Expressing curiosity about many things Demonstrating original thought	Imitating others rather than developing independent ideas Apologizing and being very embarrassed over small mistakes Verbalizing fear about starting a new project
Early school years: industry vs. inferiority	Completing a task once it has been started Working well with others Using time effectively	Not completing tasks started Not assisting with the work of others Not organizing work
Adolescence: identity vs. role confusion	Asserting independence Planning realistically for future roles Establishing close interpersonal relationships	Failing to assume responsibility for directing one's own behavior Accepting the values of others without question Failing to set goals in life
Early adulthood: intimacy vs. isolation	Establishing a close, intimate relationship with another person Making a commitment to that relationship, even in times of stress and sacrifice Accepting sexual behavior as desirable	Remaining alone Avoiding close interpersonal relationships
Middle-aged adults: generativity vs. stagnation	Being willing to share with another person Guiding others Establishing a priority of needs, recognizing both self and others	Talking about oneself instead of listening to others Showing concern for oneself in spite of the needs of others Being unable to accept interdependence
Older adults: integrity vs. despair	Using past experience to assist others Maintaining productivity in some areas Accepting limitations	Crying and being apathetic Not accepting changes Demanding unnecessary assistance and attention from others

person copes with these developmental tasks largely determines the development of self-concept. Difficulty in coping results in self-concept problems at the time and, often, later in life. Table 39–1 lists examples of behaviors indicating successful and unsuccessful resolution of these developmental tasks.

There are three broad steps in the development of one's self-concept:

- The infant learns that the physical self is separate and different from the environment.
- The child internalizes others' attitudes toward self.
- The child and adult internalize the standards of society.

The term **global self** refers to the collective beliefs and images one holds about oneself. It is the most complete description that individuals can give of themselves at any one time. It is also a person's frame of reference for experiencing and viewing the world. Some of these beliefs and images represent statements of fact, for example, "I am a woman"; "I am a father"; "I am short." Others refer to less tangible aspects of self, for instance, "I am competent"; "I am shy."

Each separate image and belief one holds about oneself has a bearing on self-concept. However, self-concept is not simply a sum of its parts. The various images and beliefs people hold about themselves are not given equal weight and prominence. Each person's self-concept is like a piece of art. At the center of the art are the beliefs and images that are most vital to the person's identity. They constitute **core self-concept.** For example: "I am very smart/of average intelligence"; "I am male/female." Images and beliefs that are less important to the person are on the periphery. For example: "I am left-/right-handed"; "I am athletic/unathletic."

People are thought to base their self-concept on how they perceive and evaluate themselves in these areas:

- Vocational performance
- Intellectual functioning
- Personal appearance and physical attractiveness
- Sexual attractiveness and performance
- Being liked by others
- Ability to cope with and resolve problems
- Independence
- Particular talents

Self-concept in these areas also extends to the choices people make and perceptions they have about their health. Persons with strong positive self-concept about appearance are likely to value healthy behaviors and take action to maintain the health of their skin, hair, and body tone, for example. Persons with negative self-concepts may be less proactive about health promotion and illness prevention activities.

Maintaining and evaluating one's self-concept is an ongoing process. Events or situations may change the level of self-concept over time. Having a basic self-concept includes how we see ourselves and how we are seen by others. There is also the **ideal self,** which is how we should be or would prefer to be. The ideal self is the individual's perception of how one should behave based on certain personal standards, aspirations, goals, and values. Sometimes this ideal self is realistic; sometimes it is not. When perceived self is close to ideal self, people do not wish to be much different from what they believe they already are. A discrepancy between ideal self and perceived self can be an incentive to self-improvement. However, when the discrepancy is great, low self-esteem can result.

Nurses, like other adults, view themselves based on both internal and external inputs acquired over many years. The ability to appraise one's own strengths, the desire to follow in the steps of role models, and the feedback received from colleagues and clients are some of the influences on the nurse's self-concept.

COMPONENTS OF SELF-CONCEPT

There are four components of self-concept: personal identity, body image, role performance, and self-esteem.

Personal Identity

Personal identity is the conscious sense of individuality and uniqueness that is continually evolving throughout life. People often view their identity in terms of name, sex, age, race, ethnic origin or culture, occupation or roles, talents, and other situational characteristics (e.g., marital status and education).

Personal identity also includes beliefs and values, personality, and character. For instance, is the person outgoing, friendly, reserved, generous, selfish? Personal identity thus encompasses both the tangible and factual, such as name and sex, and the intangible, such as values and beliefs. Identity is what distinguishes self from others.

A person with a strong sense of identity has integrated body image, role performance, and self-esteem into a complete self-concept. This sense of identity provides a person with a feeling of continuity and a unity of personality. Furthermore, the individual sees himself or herself as a unique person.

Body Image

The image of physical self, or **body image,** is how a person perceives the size, appearance, and functioning of the body and its parts. Body image has both cognitive and affective aspects. The cognitive is the knowledge of the material body; the affective includes the sensations of the body, such as pain, pleasure, fatigue, and physical movement. Body image is the sum of these

Figure 39-1 ■ Body image is the sum of a person's conscious and unconscious attitudes about his or her body.

attitudes, conscious and unconscious, that a person has toward his or her body.

Body image includes clothing, makeup, hairstyle, jewelry, and other things intimately connected to the person (Figure 39-1 ■). It also includes body prostheses, such as artificial limbs, dentures, and hairpieces, as well as devices required for functioning, such as wheelchairs, canes, and eyeglasses. Past as well as present perceptions and how the body has evolved over time are part of one's body image.

A person's body image develops partly from others' attitudes and responses to that person's body and partly from the individual's own exploration of the body. For example, body image develops in infancy as the parents or caregivers respond to the child with smiles, holding, and touching, and as the child explores its own body sensations during breast-feeding, thumb sucking, and the bath. Cultural and societal values also influence a person's body image.

The various information and entertainment media have played a part over the years in how individuals view themselves and others. During adolescence, concerns related to body image are of paramount concern. The "ideal" person portrayed by the media is really an unrealistic goal for many.

If a person's body image closely resembles one's body ideal, the individual is more likely to think positively about the physical and nonphysical components of the self. The body ideal is greatly influenced by cultural standards. For example, currently in North America the fit, well-toned body is admired.

Another aspect of body image is the understanding that different parts of the body have different values for different people. For example, large breasts may be highly important to one woman and unimportant to another, or the occurrence of gray hair may be traumatic to one person and barely noticed by another.

A person with a healthy body image will normally show concern for both health and appearance. This person will seek help if ill and will include health-promoting practices in daily activities. A person who has an unhealthy body image is likely to be overly concerned about minor illness and to neglect activities like sleep and a healthy diet that are important to health.

The individual who has a body image disturbance may hide or not look at or touch a body part that is significantly changed in structure by illness or trauma. Some individuals may also express feelings of helplessness, hopelessness, powerlessness, and vulnerability, and may exhibit self-destructive behavior such as over- or undereating or suicide attempts.

Role Performance

Throughout life people undergo numerous role changes. A **role** is a set of expectations about how the person occupying one position behaves. **Role performance** relates what a person in a particular role does to the behaviors expected of that role. **Role mastery** means that the person's behaviors meet social expectations. Expectations, or standards of behavior of a role, are set by society, a cultural group, or a smaller group to which a person belongs. Each person usually has several roles, such as husband, parent, brother, son, employee, friend, nurse, and church member. Some roles are assumed for only limited periods, such as client, student, and ill person. **Role development** involves socialization into a particular role. For example, nursing students are socialized into nursing through exposure to their instructors, clinical experience, classes, laboratory simulations, and seminars.

To act appropriately, people need to know who they are in relation to others and what society expects for the positions they hold. **Role ambiguity** occurs when expectations are unclear, and people do not know what to do or how to do it and are unable to predict the reactions of others to their behavior. Failure to master a role creates frustration and feelings of inadequacy, often with consequent lowered self-esteem.

Self-concept is also affected by role strain and role conflicts. People undergoing **role strain** are frustrated because they feel or are made to feel inadequate or unsuited to a role. Role strain is often associated with sex role stereotypes. For example, women in occupations traditionally held by men might be treated as having less knowledge and competence than men in the same roles.

Role conflicts arise from opposing or incompatible expectations. In an interpersonal conflict, people have different expectations about a particular role. For example, a grandparent may have different expectations than the mother about how she should care for her children. In an interrole conflict, one person's or group's role expectations differ from the expectations

of another person or group. For example, a woman who has little flexibility in her full-time job schedule has a role conflict if her husband expects her to handle all child care problems. In a person-role conflict, role expectations violate the beliefs or values of the role occupant. For example, a nurse in a family planning clinic may be expected to advise couples about birth control methods that are not consistent with the nurse's belief system regarding prevention or management of unwanted pregnancy. Role conflict can lead to tension, decrease in self-esteem, and embarrassment if needs for achievement, independence, and recognition are unmet.

CLINICAL ALERT

If Maslow's level of love and belonging needs are met, the needs for self-esteem are next higher on the hierarchy. When the need for self-esteem is satisfied, the individual strives for self-actualization. ■

Self-Esteem

Self-esteem is one's judgment of one's own worth, that is, how that person's standards and performances compare to others and to one's ideal self. If a person's self-esteem does not match with the ideal self, then low self-concept results.

There are two types of self-esteem: global and specific. **Global self-esteem** is how much one likes oneself as a whole. **Specific self-esteem** is how much one approves of a certain part of oneself. Global self-esteem is influenced by specific self-esteem. For example, if a man values his looks, then how he looks will strongly affect his global self-esteem. By contrast, if a man places little value on his cooking skills, then how well or badly he cooks will have little influence on his global self-esteem.

Self-esteem is derived from self and others. In infancy, self-esteem is related to the caregiver's evaluations and acceptances. Later the child's self-esteem is affected by competition with others. As an adult, a person who has high self-esteem has feelings of significance, of competence, of the ability to cope with life, and of control over one's destiny.

The foundation for self-esteem is established during early life experiences, usually within the family structure. However, an adult's level of overall self-esteem may change markedly from day to day and moment to moment. Severe stress—for example, stress related to prolonged illness or unemployment—can substantially lower a person's self-esteem. In health care, persons who believe that their condition is viewed negatively by society may have lower self-esteem (Berge & Ranney, 2005). People frequently focus on their negative aspects and spend less time on their positive aspects. It is important that both strengths and weaknesses be identified.

FACTORS THAT AFFECT SELF-CONCEPT

Many factors affect a person's self-concept. Major factors are stage of development, family and culture, stressors, resources, history of success and failure, and illness.

RESEARCH NOTE Can Assertiveness Training Improve Nursing Students' Self-Esteem?

These researchers' objective was to evaluate a training program on nursing and medical students' assertiveness, self-esteem, and inter-personal communication satisfaction. They followed 69 participants who had been identified as having low assertiveness assigned to either an experimental or comparison group. Participants in the experimental group received assertiveness training once a week. Data were collected before and after training and again one month after the end of the training. The assertiveness and self-esteem of the experimental group were significantly improved in nursing and medical students after assertiveness training, although interpersonal communication satisfaction of the experimental group was not significantly improved after the training program.

IMPLICATIONS

This study shows that it is possible to improve both self-esteem and assertiveness through educational intervention if the initial level of assertiveness is low. It is unknown for how long the improvement might last. The details regarding the training, and the meaning of the failure to improve satisfaction with communication, need to be evaluated for influence of culture. Communication styles differ significantly among ethnic groups and it is important to determine whether the ethnicity of health care providers is similar to or different from that of the dominant society (see Chapter 18 ∞).

Note: From "Evaluation of an Assertiveness Training Program on Nursing and Medical Students' Assertiveness, Self Esteem, and Interpersonal Communication Satisfaction," by Y. Lin, I. Shiah, T. Lai, K. Wang, and K. Chou, 2004, *Nurse Education Today, 24*(8), pp. 656–665.

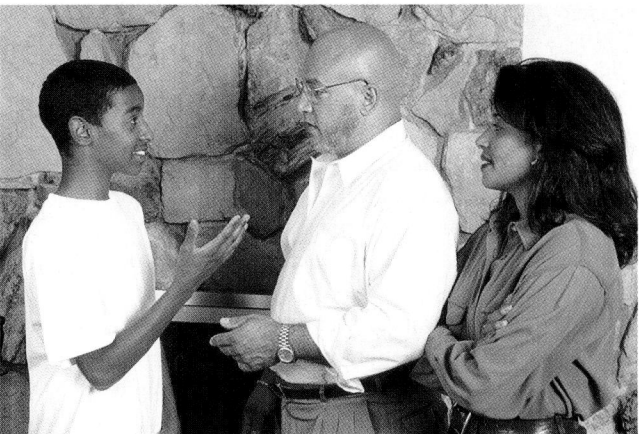

Figure 39-2 ■ A child is often pulled in opposite directions by family and peer expectations.
(Jonathan Nourak/PhotoEdit.)

Resources

An individual's resources are internal and external. Examples of internal resources include confidence and values, whereas external resources include support network, sufficient finances, and organizations. Generally the greater the number of resources a person has and uses, the more positive the effect on the self-concept.

History of Success and Failure

People who have a history of failures come to see themselves as failures, whereas people with a history of successes will have a more positive self-concept. Likewise, persons with a positive self-concept tend to find contentment in their level of success while a negative self-concept can lead to viewing one's life situation as negative.

Stage of Development

As an individual develops, the conditions that affect the self-concept change. For example, an infant requires a supportive, caring environment, while a child requires freedom to explore and learn. Elders' self-concept is based on their experiences in progressing through life's stages.

Family and Culture

A young child's values are largely influenced by the family and culture. Later on, peers influence the child and thereby affect the sense of self. When the child is confronted by differing expectations from family, culture, and peers, the child's sense of self is often confused (Figure 39-2 ■). For example, a child may realize that his parents expect he will not drink alcohol and that he will attend religious services each Saturday evening. At the same time, his peers drink beer and encourage him to spend Saturday evenings with them.

Stressors

Stressors can strengthen the self-concept as an individual copes successfully with problems. On the other hand, overwhelming stressors can cause maladaptive responses including substance abuse, withdrawal, and anxiety. The ability of a person to handle stressors will largely depend on personal resources.

REAL WORLD PRACTICE

Some new nurses may appear more timid, less confident, and more nervous than other new nurses. If you are the more nervous type, know your limitations, but do not be afraid of them. Be aware of all the assets you bring to the bedside. Maybe you are able to listen or sympathize well with the client or family.

Code situations, rare bedside procedures, or certain diagnoses are nerve racking to everyone. Don't worry! You will notice your nervousness decrease as you gain experience. When you are constantly having new experiences you learn to trust that you will know what to do. Part of being a "good" nurse is being able to problem solve. If you don't know the answer to something, don't panic, because you can guarantee that you won't know everything. Instead, trouble-shoot or look at your protocols. If you need help, ask for it. Nursing should be a team effort. One thing that helped me gain confidence was writing down new information. I learned from my mistakes, and from other nurses and other health care personnel. Now, I can look back and see how far I have come since I first started out as a nurse.

— *Teresa Hsieh, BSN, RN*
Children's Memorial Hospital, Chicago, IL

Illness

Illness and trauma can also affect the self-concept. A woman who has a mastectomy may see herself as less attractive, and the loss may affect how she acts and values herself. People respond to stressors such as illness and alterations in function related to aging in a variety of ways. Acceptance, denial, withdrawal, and depression are common reactions.

It is sometimes difficult to determine the direction of the relationship between self-concept and health. Some research has shown that persons with a positive self-concept may enhance their health because they are more likely to follow the health care plan (Burkhart & Rayens, 2005). Other research shows that health conditions, including psychosocial situations such as loss and grieving, have an impact on self-concept (see Montpetit, Bisconti, & Bergeman, 2004). Thus, self-concept and health-related behavior are intertwined.

 NURSING MANAGEMENT

Assessing

A thorough assessment includes a psychosocial assessment of the client and the family or support person because this provides clues to actual or potential problems. The nurse assessing self-concept focuses on the four components: (a) personal identity, (b) body image, (c) role performance, and (d) self-esteem.

Before conducting a psychosocial assessment, the nurse must establish trust and a working relationship with the client. Guidelines for conducting a psychosocial assessment include the following:

- Create a quiet, private environment.
- Minimize interruptions if possible.
- Maintain appropriate eye contact.
- Sit at eye level with the client.
- Demonstrate an interest in the client's concerns.
- Indicate acceptance of the client by not criticizing, frowning, or demonstrating shock.
- Ask open-ended questions to encourage the client to talk rather than close-ended questions that tend to block free sharing.
- Avoid asking more personal questions than are actually needed.
- Minimize writing detailed notes during the interview because this can create client concern that confidential material is being "recorded" as well as interfere with your ability to focus on what the client is saying.
- Determine whether the family can provide additional information.
- Maintain confidentiality.
- Be aware of your own biases and discomforts that could influence the assessment.
- Consider how the client's behavior is influenced by culture.

It is also important that the nurse identify any stressors that may affect aspects of the self-concept. See Box 39–1 for examples

---

CULTURALLY COMPETENT CARE
Assessing Self-Concept

It is the nurse's responsibility to use therapeutic communication and to remain sensitive to the effect that cultural influences will have on the client's behaviors and needs. Cultural background is not only assessed directly but is also considered as a factor in the areas of self-perception, role relationships, major stressors, and coping strategies. In the area of behaviors that may suggest low self-esteem, nurses need to ask themselves the following question: Is this really a behavior that would suggest a low self-esteem or is it part of the cultural behavior(s) of the client? In addition, might the client be experiencing cultural dissonance, a situation in which there are conflicting beliefs and attitudes between the client's culture and the one in which the client is living?

of stressors that may place a client at risk for problems with self-concept.

When stressors are identified, the nurse needs to determine how the client perceives the stressor. A positive, growth-oriented perception of stressful events reinforces self-worth; a negative, hopeless, defeatist perception leads to decreased self-esteem. The nurse should also identify the client's coping style and

---

BOX 39–1 Stressors Affecting Self-Concept

IDENTITY STRESSORS
- Change in physical appearance (e.g., facial wrinkles)
- Declining physical, mental, or sensory abilities
- Inability to achieve goals
- Relationship concerns
- Sexuality concerns
- Unrealistic ideal self

BODY IMAGE STRESSORS
- Loss of body parts (e.g., amputation, mastectomy, hysterectomy)
- Loss of body functions (e.g., from stroke, spinal cord injury, neuromuscular disease, arthritis, declining mental or sensory abilities)
- Disfigurement (e.g., through pregnancy, severe burns, facial blemishes, colostomy, tracheostomy)
- Unrealistic body ideal (e.g., a muscular configuration that cannot be achieved)

SELF-ESTEEM STRESSORS
- Lack of positive feedback from significant others
- Repeated failures
- Unrealistic expectations
- Abusive relationship
- Loss of financial security

ROLE STRESSORS
- Loss of parent, spouse, child, or close friend
- Change or loss of job or other significant role
- Divorce
- Illness
- Ambiguous or conflicting role expectations
- Inability to meet role expectations

determine whether this style is effective by asking the client such questions as these:

- When you have a problem or face a stressful situation, how do you usually deal with it?
- Do these methods work?

Personal Identity

When assessing self-concept, the information the nurse first needs is about the client's personal identity. This involves who the client believes he or she is. See the accompanying Assessment Interview for examples of questions to ask.

Body Image

If there are indications of a body image disturbance, the nurse should assess the client carefully for possible functional or physical problems. The disturbance may be a result of a present deformity or malfunction or an anticipated one. In addition to the stated responses about the problem, it is important to assess related behavior. See the accompanying Assessment Interview for examples of questions to ask about body image.

Role Performance

The nurse assesses the client's satisfactions and dissatisfactions associated with role responsibilities and relationships: family roles, work roles, student roles, and social roles. Family roles are especially important to people because family relationships are particularly close. Relationships can be supportive and growth producing or, at the opposite extreme, highly stressful if there is violence or abuse. Assessment of family role relationships may begin with structural aspects such as the number in the family group, ages, and residence location. To obtain data related to the client's family relationships and satisfaction or dissatisfaction with work roles and social roles, the nurse might ask some of the questions shown in the accompanying Assessment Interview. Keep in mind, however, that questions need to be tailored to the individuals and their culture, age, and situation.

ASSESSMENT INTERVIEW
Personal Identity

- How would you describe your personal characteristics? *or,* How do you see yourself as a person?
- How do others describe you as a person?
- What do you like about yourself?
- What do you do well?
- What are your personal strengths, talents, and abilities?
- What would you change about yourself if you could?
- Does it bother you a great deal if you think someone doesn't like you?

ASSESSMENT INTERVIEW
Body Image

- Is there any part of your body you would like to change?
- Are you comfortable discussing your surgery?
- Do you feel different or inferior to others?
- How do you feel about your appearance?
- What changes in your body do you expect following your surgery?
- How have significant others in your life reacted to changes in your body?

Self-Esteem

A nurse can ask the following questions to determine a client's self-esteem:

- Are you satisfied with your life?
- How do you feel about yourself?
- Are you accomplishing what you want?
- What goals in life are important to you?

It is important for the nurse to determine the client's cultural background first in order to not misinterpret specific behaviors. The following behaviors might reflect low self-esteem or may be misinterpreted due to the client's cultural background:

- Avoids eye contact.
- Stoops in posture and moves slowly.
- Is poorly groomed and has an unkempt appearance.
- Is hesitant or halting in speech.
- Is overly critical of self (e.g., "I'm no good," "I'm ugly," or "People don't like me.").

ASSESSMENT INTERVIEW
Role Performance

FAMILY RELATIONSHIPS

- Tell me about your family.
- What is home like?
- How is your relationship with your spouse/partner/significant other (if appropriate)?
- What are your relationships like with your other relatives?
- How are important decisions made in your family?
- What are your responsibilities in the family?
- How well do you feel you accomplish what is expected of you?
- What about your role or responsibilities would you like changed?
- Are you proud of your family members?
- Do you feel your family members are proud of you?

WORK ROLES AND SOCIAL ROLES

- Do you like your work?
- How do you get along at work?
- What about your work would you like to change if you could?
- How do you spend your free time?
- Are you involved in any community groups?
- Are you most comfortable alone, with one other person, or in a group?
- Who is most important to you?
- Whom do you seek out for help?

MediaLink A Change in Attitude Application

- May be overly critical of others.
- Is unable to accept positive remarks about self.
- Apologizes frequently.
- Verbalizes feelings of hopelessness, helplessness, and powerlessness, such as "I really don't care what happens," "I'll do whatever anyone wants," "Whatever is destined will happen."

Diagnosing

Three of the NANDA nursing diagnostic labels relating specifically to the domain of self-perception and the classes

of self-concept, self-esteem, and body image include the following:

- *Disturbed Body Image*
- *Ineffective Role Performance*
- *Chronic Low Self-Esteem.*

Examples of clinical applications of these diagnoses using NANDA, NIC, and NOC designations are shown in Identifying Nursing Diagnoses, Outcomes, and Interventions.

IDENTIFYING NURSING DIAGNOSES, OUTCOMES, AND INTERVENTIONS
Clients with Self-Concept and Role Problems

DATA CLUSTER Frank Sawyers had a permanent colostomy 7 days ago for cancer of the sigmoid colon. When the nurse was changing the colostomy appliance, Frank said, "I am really repulsed by this." He avoided looking at the stoma and put his arm over his eyes.

NURSING DIAGNOSIS/ DEFINITION	SAMPLE DESIRED OUTCOMES*/ DEFINITION	INDICATORS	SELECTED INTERVENTIONS*/ DEFINITION	SAMPLE NIC ACTIVITIES
Disturbed Body Image/ Confusion in mental picture of one's physical self	Body Image [1200]/ *Perception of own appearance and body functions*	Often positive - Willingness to touch affected body part - Adjustment to changes in body function	Body Image Enhancement [522]/*Improving a patient's conscious and unconscious perceptions and attitudes toward his/her body* Self-Care Assistance [1800]/*Assisting another to perform activities of daily living*	- Assist patient to discuss changes caused by illness/surgery - Assist patient in identifying parts of his body that have positive perceptions associated with them - Facilitate contact with individuals with similar changes in body image - Encourage independence but intervene when patient is unable to perform

DATA CLUSTER Sophie Ferraro, a 73-year-old with right-sided (dominant) hemiplegia, says, "Although the Rehabilitation Center taught me so much about how to manage in my home, my poor husband has to do a lot to help me with cooking meals and cleaning the house."

Ineffective Role Performance/ Patterns of behavior and self-expression that do not match the environmental context, norms, and expectations	Caregiver–Patient Relationship [2204]/ *Positive interactions and connections between the caregiver and the care recipient*	Not compromised - Effective communication - Companionship - Collaborative problem solving	Role Enhancement [5370]/*Assisting a patient, significant other, and/or family to improve relationships by clarifying and supplementing specific role relationships*	- Assist patient to identify positive strategies for managing role changes - Facilitate discussion of expectations between patient and significant other in reciprocal role

DATA CLUSTER George Kawazi, a first-year college student, is studying liberal arts and the sciences. George states that even though he attends all his classes and studies every day and on weekends, his grades do not please his father, who expects straight A's. "I've always had trouble measuring up to Father's expectations. He never thought I was as good as my older brother."

Chronic Low Self-Esteem/Long-standing negative self-evaluation/feelings about self or self-capabilities	Self-Esteem [1205]/*Personal judgment of self-worth*	Often positive - Acceptance of self-limitations - Willingness to confront others - Description of success in school	Self-Esteem Enhancement [5400]/*Assisting a patient to increase his/her personal judgment of self-worth*	Determine patient's confidence in own judgment - Reinforce strengths the patient identifies - Assist in setting realistic goals - Explore previous experiences of success

*The NOC # for desired outcomes and the NIC # for nursing interventions are listed in brackets following the appropriate outcome or intervention. Outcomes, indicators, interventions, and activities selected are only a sample of those suggested by NOC and NIC and should be further individualized for each client.

Additional nursing diagnoses that may apply to clients with problems of self-concept include the following:

- *Disturbed Personal Identity*
- *Anxiety* related to changed physical appearance (e.g., amputation, mastectomy)
- *Impaired Adjustment* to changed physical functioning or appearance
- *Ineffective Coping* with role change related to death of spouse
- *Grieving* or *Complicated Grieving* related to change in physical appearance
- *Hopelessness*
- *Powerlessness*
- *Parental Role Conflict*
- *Readiness for Enhanced Self-Concept*
- *Disturbed Sleep Pattern*
- *Social Isolation*
- *Spiritual Distress*
- *Disturbed Thought Processes*

Planning

The nurse develops plans in collaboration with the client and support people when possible, according to the client's state of health, level of anxiety, resources, coping mechanisms, and sociocultural and religious affiliation. The nurse who has little experience in intervening with clients with altered self-concept may wish to consult with a more experienced nurse to develop effective plans. The nurse and client set goals to enhance the client's self-concept.

The goals established will vary according to the diagnoses and defining characteristics related to each individual. Examples of desired outcomes, interventions, and activities are shown in Identifying Nursing Diagnoses, Outcomes, and Interventions. Specific nursing orders associated with each of these activities can be selected to meet the individual needs of the client.

A critical pathway may also be used as a plan of care. See the Critical Pathway for an example of a plan of care for a client undergoing a total mastectomy.

Implementing

Nursing interventions to promote a positive self-concept include helping a client to identify areas of strength. In addition, for clients who have an altered self-concept, nurses should establish a therapeutic relationship and assist clients to evaluate themselves and make behavioral changes.

Identifying Areas of Strength

Healthy people often perceive their problems and weaknesses more easily than their assets and strengths. People with low self-esteem tend to focus even more on their limitations and to be aware of fewer strengths and many more problems. When a client has difficulty identifying personality strengths and assets, the nurse provides the client with a set of guidelines or a framework for identifying personality strengths (Box 39–2).

Nurses can employ the following specific strategies to reinforce strengths:

BOX 39–2 Framework for Identifying Personality Strengths

Note past, present, and anticipated future participation in
- Hobbies and crafts.
- Expressive arts such as writing, painting, sketching, or music appreciation.
- Sports and outdoor activities, including spectator sports.
- Education, training, and related areas (including self-education).
- Work, vocation, job, or position.

In addition, determine
- Sense of humor and the ability to laugh at oneself and take kidding.
- Health status including healthy aspects of body function and good health maintenance practices.
- Special aptitudes such as sales or mechanical ability; a "green thumb"; ability to recognize and enjoy beauty; ability to solve problems; a liking for adventure or pioneering; having perseverance and the drive needed to get things done.
- Relationship strengths including the ability to make people feel comfortable, the capacity to enjoy being with people, being aware of people's needs and feelings, and being able to listen.
- Emotional strengths including the capacity to give and receive warmth, affection, and love; the ability to "take" anger and to feel and express a wide range of emotions; and the capacity for empathy.
- Spiritual strengths such as religious faith or love of God, membership and participation in church and related activities.

- Stress positive thinking rather than self-negation.
- Notice and verbally reinforce client strengths.
- Encourage the setting of attainable goals.
- Acknowledge goals that have been attained.
- Provide honest, positive feedback.

Enhancing Self-Esteem

Nurses assisting clients who have an altered self-concept must establish a therapeutic relationship. To do this the nurse must have self-awareness and effective communication skills. The following nursing techniques may help clients analyze the problem and enhance the self-concept:

- Encourage clients to appraise the situation and express their feelings.
- Encourage clients to ask questions.
- Provide accurate information.
- Become aware of distortions, inappropriate or unrealistic standards, and faulty labels in clients' speech.
- Explore clients' positive qualities and strengths.
- Encourage clients to express positive self-evaluation more than negative self-evaluation.
- Avoid criticism.
- Teach clients to substitute negative self-talk ("I can't walk to the store anymore") with positive self-talk ("I can walk half a block each morning"). Negative self-talk reinforces a negative self-concept.

Certain strategies vary depending on the age of the client (see Lifespan Considerations on page 1013).

MediaLink Client Who Lost His Job Care Plan Activity

CRITICAL PATHWAY Client Following Total Mastectomy

	Date_____ First 24 hours postoperative	Date_____ 48 hours postoperative	Date_____ 3 days postoperative
Daily Outcomes	Client will • Be afebrile. • Have clean, dry dressing. • Recover from anesthesia as evidenced by vital signs returning to baseline; being awake, alert, and oriented. • Verbalize understanding and demonstrate cooperation with turning, coughing, deep breathing, and splinting. • Tolerate ordered diet without nausea and vomiting. • Verbalize control of incisional pain. • Verbalize ability to cope.	Client will • Be afebrile. • Have clean, dry wound with edges well approximated, healing by first intention. • Demonstrate cooperation with turning, coughing, deep breathing, and splinting. • Tolerate ordered diet without nausea and vomiting. • Ambulate 4 times per day in hallway. • Verbalize control of incisional pain. • Verbalize beginning ability to cope with changes in body image. • Verbalize beginning understanding of home care instructions.	Client will • Be afebrile. • Have clean, dry wound with edges well approximated, healing by first intention. • Manage pain with oral medications and/or nonpharmacologic measures. • Be independent in self-care. • Be fully ambulatory. • Have resumed preadmission urine and bowel elimination pattern. • Verbalize home care instructions. • Tolerate usual diet. • Verbalize ability to cope with changes in body image and ongoing stressors. • Demonstrate progressive upper extremity exercises that include external rotation and abduction of the affected shoulder when the stitches are removed 7 to 10 days after surgery.
Tests and Treatments	Vital signs and O_2 saturation, neurovascular assessment, dressing and wound drainage assessment q15min × 4; q30min × 4; q1h × 4 and then q4h if stable. NO BLOOD PRESSURES OR VENIPUNCTURE ON AFFECTED ARM. Assess respiratory status q4h and prn. Incentive spirometer q2h. Intake and output q shift. Assess voiding—if unable to void, try suggestive voiding techniques or catheterize q8h or prn.	Vital signs and dressing and wound drainage assessment q4h. NO BLOOD PRESSURES OR VENIPUNCTURE ON AFFECTED ARM. Assess respiratory status q4h. Incentive spirometer q2h until fully ambulatory. Intake and output q shift.	Vital signs and dressing and wound drainage assessment q4h–8h. NO BLOOD PRESSURES OR VENIPUNCTURE ON AFFECTED ARM. Assess respiratory status q4h–8h. Assess wound and apply dry sterile dressing q day and prn.
Knowledge	Orient to room and surroundings. Provide simple, brief instructions. Review preoperative preparation, including hospital and specific postoperative care: turning, coughing, deep breathing, incentive spirometer, mobilization, intravenous infusions, pain management.	Review plan of care and importance of early mobilization. Begin discharge teaching regarding wound care/dressing change, diet, and activity. Review written discharge instructions with client and support person.	Complete discharge teaching to include wound care, diet, follow-up care, signs and symptoms to report, activity, and medication (frequency, dose, route, and side effects). Provide client with written discharge instructions including upper arm and shoulder exercises for affected arm.
Activity	Provide safety precautions. Ambulate 4 times in room. Encourage finger, wrist, and elbow movement and use of affected arm for ADLs and personal hygiene.	Fully ambulatory in room. Walk in hall 4 to 6 times per day. Encourage finger, wrist, and elbow movement and use of affected arm for ADLs and personal hygiene. Instruct client in progressive upper arm exercises.	Fully ambulatory. Encourage finger, wrist, and elbow movement and use of affected arm for ADLs and personal hygiene. Reinforce instructions regarding progressive exercises.
Medications	IV/PCA analgesics. IV antibiotics. IV fluids.	PO or IV/PCA analgesics. IV antibiotics. Intermittent IV device.	PO analgesics. Discontinue IV device.

CRITICAL PATHWAY   Client Following Total Mastectomy—*continued*

	Date_____ First 24 hours postoperative	Date_____ 48 hours postoperative	Date_____ 3 days postoperative
Body Image	Establish a trusting relationship with client. Encourage client and significant others to verbalize their feelings about the mastectomy. Listen to client and significant others and show interest and concerns. Allow the client to respond to loss of body part and changed body image with grieving behaviors. Support the client's strengths and assist her to look at herself in totality.	Maintain trusting relationship with client. Encourage client and significant others to verbalize their feelings about the mastectomy. Listen to client and significant others and show interest and concern. Allow the client to respond to loss of body part and changed body image with grieving behaviors. Support the client's strengths and assist her to look at herself in totality.	Provide opportunities to verbalize ongoing concerns regarding changes in body image and self-concept. Encourage and provide opportunities for self-care of wound and dressing. Provide opportunity for client to meet with volunteer from Reach to Recovery. Assist client to obtain temporary breast prosthesis. Answer questions and provide information on breast reconstruction.
Psychosocial	Assess coping status. Use active listening. Provide a nonthreatening environment. Determine support people and resources available to the client. Assess responses of support people. Allow for client's input regarding sequence of care. Be supportive of client's effective coping behaviors.	Assess coping status. Use active listening. Provide a nonthreatening environment. Determine support people and resources available to the client. Assess responses of support people. Allow for client's input regarding sequence of care. Be supportive of client's effective coping behaviors. Review progress toward discharge goals.	Assess coping status. Use active listening. Provide a nonthreatening environment. Determine support people and resources available to the client. Assess responses of support people. Allow for client's input regarding sequence of care. Be supportive of client's effective coping behaviors.
Transfer/ Discharge Plans	Determine discharge needs with client and support people. Begin home care instructions.	Finalize discharge plans.	Complete discharge instructions.

LIFESPAN CONSIDERATIONS   Enhancing Self-Esteem

CHILDREN

■ Children build strong self-esteem if they develop five basic attitudes: (a) security and trust, (b) identity, (c) belonging, (d) purpose, and (e) personal competence.

• Security and trust are developed early in life; infants should not be left "to cry it out," for example, but should learn that they can rely on their parents to meet their needs promptly and consistently. With older children, trust and security are strengthened when adults spend time with them: listening, playing, reading, or just being there. Both emotional and physical contact, such as a hug, convey warmth and caring.

• Identity is developed when children are allowed to explore and experiment with the world around them and to express themselves as unique individuals in that world. They should be given opportunities to "practice" who they are. Preschoolers, for example, love to dress themselves and should be allowed to wear outlandish outfits (within limits of weather and safety) if they choose. Teenagers who try new hair colors and styles, some of which may "offend" their parents, are engaging in a crucial developmental step.

• Belonging is essential for all humans, and having a sense that others in your social network care about you, want you there, and benefit by your contribution is important to healthy self-esteem. Children gain this sense of belonging by being included in activities, by being praised for their efforts and achievements, and by being valued by parents, siblings, caregivers, and other adults. Parents should make an effort to "catch their children doing well" and praise them for it (e.g., "I like the way you share with your brother"). Children should also hear that they are valued just for being themselves (e.g., "I like doing things with you. Remember when we went to the park? Wasn't that fun?").

• Purpose and belonging are closely related. Children need opportunities to participate in the family and their community in order to discover what they can best contribute based on their strengths and skills. One mother, for example, stated "Leo (age 4) is our actor. He is wonderful with costumes and can make any of us smile when he starts his routine." Leo may never become an actor, but he knows he makes a significant contribution to his family's well-being. He brings them joy.

(continued)

LIFESPAN CONSIDERATIONS   Enhancing Self-Esteem—*continued*

- Personal competence grows as children identify and refine their skill sets. Children develop competence as they confront and solve problems, face challenges, expand their thinking, and are asked to do more than they think they can do. Adults must, however, provide children with support, guidance, appropriate assistance, and constructive feedback (including praise) in order to prevent the child from being overwhelmed. Too much frustration or uncertainty can lead to giving up, avoidance, lying, bullying, and other antisocial behaviors. If adults help children to accomplish goals that are important to them, children are more likely to develop a sense of personal competence and independence.
- Key ingredients for helping children develop high self-esteem are love, acceptance, firmness, consistency, and the establishment of expectations. Such qualities provide children with a safe, loving, supportive, and predictable world in which to live.

ADOLESCENTS

- Provide increasing levels of responsibility. Adolescents need to experience successes and failures and the consequences of their own behavior.
- Encourage discussion about issues including problems and mistakes.
- Show appreciation for effort and contributions. Emphasize the process, not just the result.
- Ask for their opinions and suggestions.
- Encourage participation in decision making in areas that affect the adolescent. Show confidence in the teen's judgments.
- Avoid comparison with or ridicule or punishment in front of others.
- Assist in the creation of realistic goals and standards.
- Adolescents often engage in volunteer activities in their schools or communities, helping them to identify their strengths and find meaning in their activities. Knowing that they have a purpose and make a difference gives children strong self-esteem.

ADULTS

- Explore the meaning of self-esteem and how his or her self-esteem has influenced past behaviors and actions (and can influence present and future plans and decisions).
- Assist the client in assessing the internal and external forces contributing to or retarding his or her self-esteem.
- Act in ways that demonstrate belief that the person can cope with the realities and demands of life and is worthy of experiencing joy and happiness.
- Avoid comparisons with other people.
- Discourage statements about the self that are negative.
- Encourage the use of affirmations to enhance self-esteem: statements such as "I like myself" or "I am a valuable person."
- Encourage associations with positive, supportive people.
- Make positive statements about the person's past successes (major or minor).

- Assist the person to make a list of his or her positive qualities and to review this list often.
- Suggest the person do things for others. Making a positive contribution enhances positive feelings of self-worth.

ELDERS

Elders who become increasingly dependent can develop low self-esteem. Old age is frequently accompanied by changes such as reduced income, decline in physical health, loss of friends and family, and retirement. In addition to those actions listed above for use with adults, nurses can use the following techniques to help elders enhance their self-esteem:

- Encourage clients to participate in planning their own care.
- Listen carefully to their concerns.
- Assist clients to identify and use their own strengths.
- Encourage them to participate in activities in which they can be successful.
- Communicate that the client is valued. Use the client's name and ask for advice.
- Encourage elders to stay connected with their memories. Reminiscing by writing or recording an autobiography or storytelling are excellent ways to do this.
- For elders who are in hospitals or nursing homes, make sure that they are always shown respect and dignity and are provided privacy.
- Encourage creative activities to tap their resources. Examples are music, art, storytelling, quilting, and photography.
- Work with clients to establish goals in small steps that are achievable—this, in itself, can bolster self-esteem.

WEAVING THE TAPESTRY OF LIFE

The mainstays of the tapestry of life are the powers in one's life—self-esteem, love of life and humanity, and closeness to and recognition of the Godlife in oneself and others.

The weavings that form the patterns in one's life are experiences, knowledge and dreams. Beauty can be seen throughout, but strength of the fabric increases with age as the tapestry displays interweavings and integration of these special qualities.

As time goes on, aging is often accompanied by a fragileness of the physical body and an increased number of inevitable losses—emotional and social, as well as physical. This is when the integration of those special fibers—strengthening qualities—becomes so crucial to the overall quality of life of the individual.

When these strengths are displayed in the tapestry of life, the individual is not only given a feeling of self-worth and self-love, but the tapestry is a beautiful gift for all who behold it and are somehow touched by it.

Grace Miller

Evaluating

To determine whether client outcomes have been achieved, the nurse uses data collected during interactions with the client and significant others (see earlier Identifying Nursing Diagnoses, Outcomes, and Interventions). If outcomes are not achieved, the nurse should explore the reasons, considering questions such as the following:

- Have old situations recurred, triggering feelings or behaviors associated with low self-esteem?
- Have new stressful situations occurred with which the client feels unable to cope, resulting in continuing or recurrent low self-esteem?
- Are new or additional roles causing increased stress in adapting?
- Are significant others supporting the client adequately in attempts to improve self-esteem?

- Did the client follow through on referrals to appropriate agencies? Did the agencies provide the expected services?
- Were the client's expectations too high in relation to the time needed for successful resolution of self-esteem problems?

The nurse, client, and significant others need to understand that to change beliefs, feelings, and behaviors affecting self-esteem requires time and ongoing effort. Unlike many physical problems (e.g., wounds) where healing can be quickly observed, improving one's self-concept can be a continuing concern and is not so easily evaluated. New crises can cause clients to doubt themselves and revert to former feelings of inadequacy. People can learn from each new situation and gain new strategies for feeling satisfied with themselves.

CRITICAL THINKING CHECKPOINT

Craig is a 20-year-old male college student who was involved in an automobile crash 3 days ago, suffering a traumatic amputation of his left lower leg. Craig's mother has remained with him since the crash and is very supportive. His father is grief stricken and having difficulty dealing with Craig's condition because Craig was captain of his college basketball team and had aspirations of becoming a professional athlete. Craig's condition is stable and he is being placed into a rehabilitation program immediately. Soon, he will be fitted for a leg prosthesis. Usually an outgoing individual, Craig is somber and nontalkative. He does not look at his leg when dressings are being changed and he refuses to discuss his rehabilitation program.

1. Given Craig's age, speculate about whether Craig's self-concept is at risk for being adversely affected by his disability.
2. What data suggest that Craig's self-esteem is, or is at risk for being, negatively affected by his amputation?
3. What factors are likely to affect Craig's adaptation to his amputation and rehabilitation?
4. How would your interventions differ for a client with the same condition who was 70 years old?
5. What other groups of clients, in addition to those with amputations, are at risk for the development of altered self-esteem or body image?

See Critical Thinking Possibilities in Appendix A. ∞

CHAPTER 39 **REVIEW**

CHAPTER HIGHLIGHTS

- A positive self-concept is essential to a person's physical and psychologic well-being.
- A person's self-perception can differ from the person's perception of how others see him or her and from the ideal self, that is, how the person would like to be.
- Interactions with significant others create the conditions that influence self-concept throughout life.
- When individuals are able to conceptualize the self, they begin a lifelong process of deciding whether and to what extent they are valuable and worthy.
- Individuals who grow up in families whose members value each other are likely to feel good about themselves.
- Factors affecting self-concept include development, family and culture, stressors, resources, history of success and failure, and illness.

- The nurse assesses four areas of self-concept: personal identity, body image, self-esteem, and role performance and relationships.
- Because a positive self-concept is basic to health, one of the nurse's major responsibilities is to assist clients whose self-concept is disturbed to develop a more positive and realistic image of themselves.
- A trusting client–nurse relationship is essential for the effective assessment of a client's self-concept, for providing help and support, and for motivating client behavior change.

TEST YOUR KNOWLEDGE

1. Sally is 5'7", weighs 105 lb, and believes she's fat. Which of the following most represents this perception?
   1. Altered body image
   2. Altered personal identity
   3. Excessive self-expectation
   4. Altered core self-concept

2. Students juggling the responsibilities of work, school, and family are most likely to experience which of the following?
   1. Role ambiguity
   2. Role strain
   3. Role conflict
   4. Role enhancement

3. An appropriate desired outcome for clients with situational low self-esteem includes which of the following?
   1. Restored self-esteem
   2. Consistently verbalizes self-acceptance
   3. Teaches adaptive skills
   4. Describes preoccupation with altered self

4. An 89-year-old client states, "I'm a lost cause. I can't even stand long enough to cook my own meals anymore." Which of the following is the most appropriate response?
1. "That must be difficult. What things are you still able to do?"
2. "Well, that is to be expected at your age."
3. "Do you have someone else who can cook for you?"
4. "Are you a good cook?"

5. An adult who has failed to satisfactorily resolve the developmental task of adolescence—identity versus confusion—is most likely to show which behavior?
1. Asserts independence
2. Is unable to express personal desires
3. Has difficulty working as a member of a team
4. Goes along with the crowd in all activities

6. During an annual performance review, which statement by the nurse indicates the area of self-awareness?
1. "I rarely make any medication errors."
2. "I am willing to mentor new nurses."
3. "My client satisfaction reports agree that I am friendly and helpful."
4. "All of my clients have recovered quickly from their health problems."

7. When asked to describe herself, a client newly diagnosed with a chronic illness describes only those roles involving others (e.g., wife, mother, medical assistant) and no personal hobbies or interests. In planning her care, the nurse should include which of the following?
1. How her treatment will affect her ability to perform those roles
2. How to set goals for her to develop personal hobbies or interests
3. That the family must be present while the treatment plan is being developed
4. That she will need psychologic counseling for role performance in addition to her medical treatment

8. You are caring for a client who has a nursing diagnosis of *Chronic Low Self-Esteem*. Which behaviors are consistent with this diagnosis? (Select all that apply.)
1. Confronts authority
2. Verbalizes own weaknesses
3. Is unable to perform consistent with his/her family role (e.g., mother, father)
4. Sets unrealistic goals
5. Has difficulty making positive observations about self
6. Has difficulty sleeping

9. Which of the following interventions are appropriate for a client with low/poor self-concept? (Select all that apply.)
1. Encourage the client to compare self with others.
2. Suggest the client not say negative things about self.
3. Suggest the client say positive things about self.
4. Recommend the client avoid situations of having to care for others.
5. Communicate very low-level expectations of the client's behavior.

10. Self-concept may vary according to a variety of conditions affecting the individual. The nurse recognizes that even appropriate nursing interventions are least likely to alter which of the following?
1. Resources
2. Self-knowledge
3. Core self-concept
4. Social self

See Answers to Test Your Knowledge in Appendix A.

EXPLORE MEDIALINK www.prenhall.com/berman

DVD-ROM
- Audio Glossary
- NCLEX Review

COMPANION WEBSITE
- Additional NCLEX Review
- Case Study: Refusal to Accept a Medical Diagnosis
- Care Plan Activity: Client Who Lost His Job
- Application Activity: A Change in Attitude
- Links to Resources

READINGS AND REFERENCES

SUGGESTED READINGS
Larner, S. (2005). Common psychological challenges for patients with newly acquired disability. *Nursing Standard, 19*(28), 33–39.
A client's attitude to a newly acquired disability is often the determining factor in successful rehabilitation. This attitude is determined by his or her perceived ability to manage symptoms, deal with hospital procedures, form and maintain relationships, and manage his or her feelings about the disability. This article describes seven common psychological challenges that clients experience with a newly acquired disability or during recovery from major illness. Strategies are outlined to assist clients to come to terms with their disability and to cope more effectively during rehabilitation.

RELATED RESEARCH
Benjamin, O., & Kamin-Shaaltiel, S. (2004). It's not because I'm fat: Perceived overweight and anger avoidance in marriage. *Health Care for Women International, 25,* 853–871.
Limb, M. K. (2004). An evaluation survey of self concept issues in adult clients undergoing limb reconstruction procedures. *Journal of Orthopaedic Nursing, 8*(1), 34–40.

REFERENCES
Berge, M., & Ranney, M. (2005). Self esteem and stigma among persons with schizophrenia: Implications for mental health. *Journal of Long Term Home Health Care, 6,* 139–144.
Burkhart, P. V., & Rayens, M. K. (2005). Self-concept and health locus of control: Factors related to children's adherence to recommended asthma regimen. *Pediatric Nursing, 31,* 404–409.

Dochterman, J., & Bulechek, G. B. (Eds.). (2004). *Nursing interventions classification (NIC)* (4th ed.). St. Louis, MO: Mosby.

Donnelly, G. (2004). Thinking about feeling: The value of introspection. *Holistic Nursing Practice, 18,* 275.

Erikson, E. H. (1963). *Childhood and society* (2nd ed.). New York: Norton.

Lin, Y., Shiah, I., Chang, Y., Lai, T., Wang, K., & Chou, K. (2004). Evaluation of an assertiveness training program on nursing and medical students' assertiveness, self esteem, and interpersonal communication satisfaction. *Nurse Education Today, 24*(8), 656–665.

Montpetit, M., Bisconti, T., & Bergeman, C. (2004). Self-concept in bereavement: Evidence for structural change. *Gerontologist, 44,* 572–573.

Moorhead, S., Johnson, M., & Maas, M. (Eds.). (2004). *Nursing outcomes classification (NOC)* (3rd ed.). St. Louis, MO: Mosby.

NANDA International. (2007). *NANDA nursing diagnoses: Definitions and classification 2007–2008*. Philadelphia: Author.

SELECTED BIBLIOGRAPHY

Boston Women's Health Book Collective. (2005). *Our bodies, our selves: A new edition for a new era.* New York: Touchstone.

Gordon, A. (2004). Maintaining an older person's concept of self. *Nursing and Residential Care, 6,* 536–538.

Heidrich, S. M., & Wells, T. J. (2004). Effects of urinary incontinence, psychological well being and distress in older community dwelling women. *Journal of Gerontological Nursing, 30*(5), 47–54.

Patterson, C. (2006). Measuring changes in self-concept: A qualitative evaluation of outcome questionnaires in people having acupuncture for their chronic health problems. *BMC Complementary and Alternative Medicine, 6*(7), 1–11.

Stewart, J. (2004). *Self-esteem*. John D. and Catherine T. MacArthur Research Network on Socioeconomic Status and Health. Retrieved June 14, 2006, from http://www.macses. ucsf.edu/Research/Psychosocial/notebook/ selfesteem.html

CHAPTER 40

Sexuality

LEARNING OUTCOMES

After completing this chapter, you will be able to:

1. Describe sexual development and concerns across the life span.

2. Define sexual health.

3. Discuss the varieties of sexuality.

4. Give examples of how the family, culture, religion, and personal ethics influence one's sexuality.

5. Describe physiologic changes in males and females during the sexual response cycle.

6. Identify the forms of male and female sexual dysfunction.

7. Identify basic sexual questions the nurse should ask during client assessment.

8. Formulate nursing diagnoses and interventions for the client experiencing sexual problems.

9. Recognize health promotion teaching related to reproductive structures.

All humans are sexual beings. Regardless of gender, age, race, socioeconomic status, religious beliefs, physical and mental health, or other demographic factors, we express our sexuality in a variety of ways throughout our lives.

Human sexuality is difficult to define. Sexuality is an individually expressed and highly personal phenomenon whose meaning evolves from life experiences. Physiologic, psychosocial, and cultural factors influence a person's sexuality and lead to the wide range of attitudes and behaviors seen in humans. There are no normal, universal sexual behaviors. Satisfying or "normal" sexual expression can generally be described as whatever behaviors give pleasure and satisfaction to those adults involved, without threat of coercion or injury to self or others. What constitutes "normal" sexual expression, however, varies among cultures and religions.

DEVELOPMENT OF SEXUALITY

The development of sexuality begins with conception and continues throughout the life span. Table 40–1 outlines characteristics of sexual development through the life span, with nursing interventions and teaching guidelines for each developmental stage.

Birth to 12 Years

The ability of the human body to experience a sexual response is present before birth. As evidenced by ultrasound, males have erections several months before birth. They continue to experience erections after birth. Since females have vaginal lubrication at birth, it is assumed that lubrication also occurs prior to birth. When babies find their fingers and toes, they also find their genitals. They seem to experience a pleasurable sensation from the touch but one would not call this a sexual experience. By the age of 3 more purposeful masturbation begins and the orgasmic response is quite common, although males do not ejaculate until after puberty. By age 2 1/2 or 3, children know what gender they are and have beginning awareness of genital differences between males and females.

Around age 9 or 10, the first physical changes of puberty begin—the development of breast buds in girls and the growth of pubic hair. As the adrenal glands mature they produce more testosterone and estradiol, which contributes to the first experiences of sexual attraction to another person. Girls need to be taught about **menstruation** (monthly uterine bleeding) and related self-care.

Adolescence

During early adolescence (12 to 13 years), primary and secondary sex characteristics continue to develop, necessitating more information about body changes. For boys, the testes and scrotum increase in size, the skin over the scrotum becomes darker, pubic hair grows, and axillary sweating begins. Development of the genitals to adult size takes about 5 to 6 years. For girls, the pelvis and hips broaden, the breast tissue develops (see page 630 in Chapter 30 ∞), pubic hair grows, axillary sweating begins, and vaginal secretions become milky and change from an alkaline to an acid pH.

Although it is difficult to apply statistical data on large populations to local populations, it is generally accepted that sexual experimentation is currently occurring at ages younger than in previous decades. One study showed first sexual experience reported occurring within ages 10 to 16 for one-third of the sample of almost 10,000 young adults (Kaestle, Halpern, Miller, & Ford, 2005).

Teenagers may have irregular menstruation initially, which can lead to embarrassment because of stained clothing. They can be taught to be aware of subtle signs of impending menstruation, such as tender breasts, water retention or bloating, or the appearance of skin eruptions or pimples. Girls should also be counseled regarding the variety of feminine hygiene products available (e.g., sanitary pads and tampons) so that they can make intelligent choices. Parents and nurses should advise teenage girls to wash their hands thoroughly before inserting a tampon, to change tampons frequently, to alternate them with sanitary pads, and to use pads at night. These measures will help to decrease infection, including the risk of "toxic shock," a particular type of *Staphylococcus aureus* infection. Thorough cleaning of the genital area and wiping from front to back will also decrease infection and prevent odors.

Dysmenorrhea (painful menstruation) is prevalent among adolescent females. Cramping, lower abdominal pain radiating to the back and upper thighs, nausea, vomiting, diarrhea, and headaches may occur for a few hours up to 3 days. Dysmenorrhea results from powerful uterine contractions, which cause ischemia and, in turn, cramping pain. The symptoms of

TABLE 40–1 Sexual Development throughout Life

STAGE	CHARACTERISTICS	NURSING INTERVENTIONS AND TEACHING GUIDELINES
Infancy Birth to 18 months	Given gender assignment of male or female. Differentiates self from others gradually. External genitals are sensitive to touch. Male infants have penile erections; females, vaginal lubrication.	Self-manipulation of the genitals is normal. Caregivers need to recognize these behaviors as common in children.
Toddler 1–3 years	Continues to develop gender identity. Able to identify own gender.	Body exploration and genital fondling is normal. Use names for body parts. Children from single-parent homes should have contact with adults of both sexes.
Preschooler 4–5 years	Becomes increasingly aware of self. Explores own and playmates' body parts. Learns correct names for body parts. Learns to control feelings and behavior. Focuses love on parent of the other sex.	Answer questions about "where babies come from" honestly and simply. Parental overreaction to exploration of genitals and masturbation can lead to feelings that sex is "bad."
School Age 6–12 years	Has strong identification with parent of same gender. Tends to have friends of the same gender. Has increasing awareness of self. Increased modesty, desire for privacy. Continues self-stimulating behavior. Learns the role and concepts of own gender as part of the total self-concept. At about 8 or 9 years becomes concerned about specific sex behaviors and often approaches parents with explicit concerns about sexuality and reproduction.	Provide parents and children with opportunities to express their concerns and ask questions regarding sex. Answer all questions with factual data and perhaps follow up with appropriate books and other material. Advise parents to discuss basic information about sexual intercourse, menstruation, and reproduction with children at about 10 years of age. Give children reading material and then discuss it with them.
Adolescence 12–18 years	Primary and secondary sex characteristics develop. Menarche usually takes place. Develops relationships with interested partners. Masturbation is common. May participate in sexual activity. May experiment with homosexual relationships. Are at risk for pregnancy and sexually transmitted diseases.	Adolescents require information about body changes. Peer groups have great importance at this time and assist in forming gender roles. Dating helps adolescents prepare for adult roles. Parents influence values and beliefs regarding behavior. Teenagers require information about contraceptive measures and precautions to take in regard to STIs.
Young Adulthood 18–40 years	Sexual activity is common. Establishes own lifestyle and values. Homosexual identity usually established by mid-20s. Many couples share financial obligations and household tasks.	Young adults often require information about measures to prevent unwanted pregnancies (i.e., abstinence or contraceptive devices). Require information to prevent STIs. Regular communication is required to understand partner's sexual needs and to work through problems and stresses.
Middle Adulthood 40–65 years	Men and women experience decreased hormone production. The menopause occurs in women, usually anywhere between 40 and 55 years. The climacteric occurs gradually in men. Quality rather than the number of sexual experiences becomes important. Individuals establish independent moral and ethical standards.	Women and men may need help adjusting to new roles. People may require counseling to help them reevaluate and direct their energies. Encourage couples to look at the positive aspects of this time of life.

TABLE 40–1	**Sexual Development throughout Life—***continued*	
STAGE **Late Adulthood**	**CHARACTERISTICS**	**NURSING INTERVENTIONS** **AND TEACHING GUIDELINES**
65 years and over	Interest in sexual activity often continues. Sexual activity may be less frequent. Women's vaginal secretions diminish, and breasts atrophy. Men produce fewer sperm and need more time to achieve an erection and to ejaculate.	Elders often continue to be sexually active. Couples may require counseling about adapting their affection and sexual needs to physical limitations.

dysmenorrhea are treated with bed rest, administration of analgesics such as aspirin, application of heat to the abdomen, certain exercises such as abdominal muscle strengthening, biofeedback, and nonsteroidal anti-inflammatory medications, such as ibuprofen. Masturbation to orgasm also eases cramping through the associated uterine contractions and increased blood flow.

All adolescents want to know about sexual behaviors but are often uneasy about discussing these concerns with their parents. Nurses, the schools, and the family need to provide accurate information. During the nursing assessment, teenagers should be asked directly what they know about sex, contraception, and reproduction. Sometimes a lot of the teenager's information is based on popular myths and little, if any, on fact. The nurse should discuss factual information about sex, sexual actions and their consequences, the individual's right to make a decision regarding ways to express oneself sexually, and the responsibilities of each person with respect to sexual activity. See Table 40–2.

Sexually transmitted infections (STIs) are the most common bacterial infections among adolescents. Teens need education about these diseases, preventive measures, and early treatment. The Clinical Manifestations feature lists the common types and symptoms of STIs for which teenagers should seek medical care. The nurse should also inform teens about the various methods of birth control: abstinence, pills, timed-release transdermal patches and implants, diaphragms, intrauterine devices, the rhythm method, and condoms to prevent an unplanned pregnancy. These are discussed later in this chapter.

Young and Middle Adulthood

In young adulthood, many people begin to form intimate relationships with long-term implications. These relationships may take the form of dating, cohabitation, or marriage. Note, however, that some people do not form intimate relationships until late adulthood and that some never form these types of relationships.

Young adult men and women are often concerned about normal sexual response, for both themselves and their partners. In heterosexual relationships, problems may arise because of basic differences in male and female expectations and responses. Gay and lesbian couples often fare better in this respect. Couples need to communicate their needs to one another early in their courtship so that a successful intimate relationship can develop and grow. Young adults should also be aware that because sexual needs and responses may change, each partner should listen and respond to the needs of the other.

During middle adulthood both men and women experience decreased hormone production, causing the climacteric, usually called menopause in women. These events often affect the individual's sexual self-concept, body image, and sexual identity. See Chapter 23 ∞ for further information on menopause.

MediaLink — Oogenesis and Spermatogenesis Terms and Definitions Animation

TABLE 40–2	**Common Sexual Misconceptions**
MISCONCEPTION	**FACT**
Nearly all men over 70 years old have erectile dysfunction.	Sexual ability is not lost due to age. Changes are commonly due to disease or medication.
Masturbation causes certain mental instabilities.	Masturbation is a common and healthy behavior.
Sexual activity weakens a person.	There is no evidence that sexual activity weakens a person.
Women who have experienced orgasm are more likely to become pregnant.	Conceiving is not related to experiencing orgasm.
Nice girls shouldn't feel entitled to their own sexual satisfaction.	As women become more comfortable with their own sexuality, they advocate for their own sexual fulfillment.
A large penis provides greater sexual satisfaction to women than a small penis.	There is no evidence that a large penis provides greater satisfaction.
Alcohol is a sexual stimulant.	Alcohol is a relaxant and central nervous system depressant. Chronic alcoholism is associated with erectile dysfunction.
Intercourse during menstruation is dangerous (i.e., it will cause vaginal tissue damage).	There is no physiologic basis for abstinence during menses.
The face-to-face coital position is the moral or proper one.	The position that offers the most pleasure and is acceptable to both partners is the correct one.

CLINICAL MANIFESTATIONS   SEXUALLY TRANSMITTED INFECTIONS

Infection	Male	Female
Gonorrhea	Painful urination; urethritis with watery white discharge, which may become purulent.	May be asymptomatic; or vaginal discharge, pain, and urinary frequency may be present.
Syphilis	Chancre, usually on glans penis, which is painless and heals in 4–6 weeks; secondary symptoms—skin eruptions, low-grade fever, inflammation of lymph glands—in 6 weeks to 6 months after chancre heals.	Chancre on cervix or other genital areas, which heals in 4–6 weeks; symptoms same as for male.
Genital warts (condyloma acuminatum)	The infection is caused by the human papilloma virus (HPV). Single lesions or clusters of lesions growing beneath or on the foreskin, at external meatus, or on the glans penis. On dry skin areas, lesions are hard and yellow-gray. On moist areas, lesions are pink or red and soft with a cauliflower-like appearance.	Certain strains of HPV have been linked to cervical cancer. Lesions appear at the bottom part of the vaginal opening, on the perineum, the vaginal lips, inner walls of the vagina, and the cervix.
Chlamydial urethritis	Urinary frequency; watery, mucoid urethral discharge.	Commonly a carrier; vaginal discharge, dysuria, urinary frequency.
Trichomoniasis	Slight itching; moisture on top of penis; slight, early morning urethral discharge. Many males are asymptomatic.	Itching and redness of vulva and skin inside thighs; copious watery, frothy vaginal discharge.
Candidiasis	Itching, irritation, discharge, plaque of cheesy material under foreskin.	Red and excoriated vulva; intense itching of vaginal and vulvar tissues; thick, white, cheesy or curd-like discharge.
Acquired immune deficiency syndrome (AIDS)	Symptoms can appear anytime from several months to several years after acquiring the virus. The person has reduced immunity to other diseases. Symptoms include any of the following for which there is no other explanation: persistent heavy night sweats; extreme fatigue; severe weight loss; enlarged lymph glands in neck, axillae, or groin; persistent diarrhea; skin rashes; blurred vision or chronic headache; harsh, dry cough; thick gray-white coating on tongue or throat.	
Herpes genitalis (herpes simplex of the genitals)	Primary herpes involves the presence of painful sores or large, discrete vesicles that last for weeks; vesicles rupture. Recurrent herpes is itchy rather than painful; it lasts for a few hours to 10 days.	

Older Adulthood

Elders may define sexuality far more broadly and include in their definition such things as touching, hugging, romantic gestures (e.g., giving or receiving roses), comfort, warmth, dressing up, joy, spirituality, and beauty. Interest in sexual activity is not lost as people age. For men, however, more time is needed to achieve an erection and to ejaculate (the erection may last longer than at a younger age); more direct genital stimulation is required to achieve an erection; the volume of ejaculated fluid decreases; and the intensity of contractions with orgasm may decrease. The refractory period after orgasm is longer.

Older women remain capable of multiple orgasms and may, in fact, experience an increase in sexual desire after menopause; vaginal lubrication and elasticity decrease with menopause and decreased estrogen, and phases of the sexual response cycle may take longer to occur. There is a possibility of pain during sexual activity and intercourse (dyspareunia) related to vaginal dryness or chronic health conditions (e.g., diabetes or arthritis). Lack of privacy may be a concern for older adults who live with family or in a rehabilitation or nursing home facility.

Many products are available to assist older adults with enhancing their sexual experiences. These range from simple lu-

LIFESPAN CONSIDERATIONS

ELDERS

It's nice when grown people whisper to each other under the covers. Their ecstasy is more leaf-sigh than bray and the body is the vehicle, not the point. They reach, grown people, for something beyond, way beyond and way, way down underneath tissue. . . . They are inward toward each other.

This quote is from the book *Jazz* by Toni Morrison, 1993 winner of the Nobel Prize in Literature. It is an excellent portrayal of sexuality of most elders. Their sexuality does not change as they get older, but their expression of it does. When they are comfortable with themselves, they can still relate to each other in a meaningful way. Sex-related changes of aging are outlined elsewhere in this chapter, as well as a discussion of other contributing factors for problems related to sexual functioning. Nurses who are sensitive to these changes and challenges to elders can be of great help in developing interventions that can help decrease the problem, and at the same time, help elders maintain their dignity and positive self-worth.

Note: From *Jazz* (p. 228), by T. Morrison, 1992, New York: Alfred A. Knopf, Inc. Reprinted with permission from International Creative Management, Inc. Copyright © 1992 by Toni Morrison.

bricants to surgically implanted devices that enable penile erections. Although older adults' technique may require modification, the nurse should never assume that they are less interested or motivated to have an active sex life.

SEXUAL HEALTH

Sexual health is an individual and constantly changing phenomenon falling within the wide range of human sexual thoughts, feelings, needs, and desires. For most people, sexual health is not considered until its absence or an impairment is noticed. A person's degree of sexual health is best determined by that individual, sometimes with the assistance of a qualified professional. The World Health Organization defined **sexual health** in 1975 as "the integration of the somatic, emotional, intellectual, and social aspects of sexual being, in ways that are positively enriching and that enhance personality, communication, and love" (p. 6). This definition recognizes the biologic, psychologic, and sociocultural dimensions of sexuality. Characteristics of sexual health are listed in Box 40–1.

Components of Sexual Health

Five critical components of sexual health are sexual self-concept, body image, gender identity, gender role behavior, and freedoms and responsibilities.

One's **sexual self-concept** (how one values oneself as a sexual being) determines with whom one will have sex, the gender and kinds of people a person is attracted to, and the values about when, where, with whom, and how one expresses sexuality. A positive sexual self-concept enables people to form intimate relationships throughout life. A negative sexual self-concept may impede the formation of relationships.

Body image, a central part of the sense of self, is constantly changing. Pregnancy, aging, trauma, disease, and therapies can alter an individual's appearance and function, which can affect body image. How a person feels about his or her body is related to one's sexuality. People who feel good about their bodies are likely to be comfortable with and enjoy sexual activity. People who have a poor body image may respond negatively to sexual arousal. A major influence on body image for women is the media focus on physical attractiveness and large breasts. Likewise, many men worry about penis size. The myth that "larger is better," particularly if it is erect and has staying power, is pervasive in North America. A person's body image can suffer when unable to achieve these expectations.

Gender identity is one's self-image as a female or male. More than just the biologic component, it also includes social and cultural norms. Gender identity is the result of a long series of developmental events that may or may not conform to one's apparent biologic sex. Once gender identity is established, it cannot be easily changed.

Gender-role behavior is the outward expression of a person's sense of maleness or femaleness as well as the expression of what is perceived as gender-appropriate behavior. Each society defines its roles for males and females; boys are given reinforcement for behaving in a "masculine" way, and girls receive reinforcement for exhibiting "feminine" behaviors.

Physical structure, variations in the internal sense of what is male or female, family values, and cultural values all influence gender-role behavior. In North America, expected adult male roles include breadwinner, heterosexual lover, father, and athlete. Expected male behaviors include wearing trousers, demonstrating physical strength, and expressing feelings in a controlled fashion. Women are expected to express their emotions more freely and to be gentler in their physical responses; they also have a broader choice of clothing than men do.

Androgyny, or flexibility in gender roles, is the belief that most characteristics and behaviors are human qualities that should not be limited to one specific gender or the other. Being androgynous does not mean being sexually neutral or imply anything about one's sexual orientation. Rather, it describes the degree of flexibility a person has regarding gender-stereotypic behaviors. Adults who can behave flexibly regarding their sexual roles may be able to adapt better than those who adopt rigid stereotyped gender roles.

Sexual health includes both *freedoms* and *responsibilities.* Sexually healthy people engage in activities that are freely chosen, including both self-pleasuring and shared-pleasuring activities. Individuals also have freedom of their sexual thoughts, feelings, and fantasies. Sexually healthy people are ethically motivated to exercise behavioral, emotional, economic, and social responsibility for themselves ("Vision of Sexual Health," 2004).

VARIETIES OF SEXUALITY

There are many varieties of sexuality. There is a tremendous range of variation in how people experience and express their sexuality. There are also many differences in the priority people place on sexuality in their lives. Sexual varieties include sexual orientation, gender identity, erotic preferences, and sexual lifestyles.

Sexual Orientation

One's attraction to people of the same sex, other sex, or both sexes is referred to as **sexual orientation.** Sexual orientation lies

---

BOX 40–1 Characteristics of Sexual Health

- Knowledge about sexuality and sexual behavior
- Ability to express one's full sexual potential, excluding all forms of sexual coercion, exploitation, and abuse
- Ability to make autonomous decisions about one's sexual life within a context of personal and social ethics
- Experience of sexual pleasure as a source of physical, psychologic, cognitive, and spiritual well-being
- Capability to express sexuality through communication, touch, emotional expression, and love
- Right to make free and responsible reproductive choices
- Ability to access sexual health care for the prevention and treatment of all sexual concerns, problems, and disorders

Note: From *Declaration of Sexual Rights,* by the World Association of Sexology, 1999, Adopted at the 14th World Congress of Sexology, Hong Kong and People's Republic of China. Reprinted with permission from the World Association for Sexual Health (WAS). All rights reserved.

along a continuum with a wide range between the two extremes of exclusively heterosexual attraction and exclusively homosexual attraction. Individuals who are attracted to people of both genders are referred to as *bisexuals.*

The origins of sexual orientation are still not well understood. Some biologic theories describe sexual orientation in terms of the genetic composition of the individual. Psychologic theories stress the role of early learning experiences and cognitive processes. Other theories acknowledge the confluence of genetics and the environment in the development of sexual orientation.

Estimates of the percentage of the population with a homosexual orientation vary, although the usual figure is 5% to 10% of men and 2% to 4% of women (McCammon, Knox, & Schacht, 2004). Because these individuals grow up acutely aware of the discrimination they face in North America, many do not disclose their sexual orientation; thus actual figures are not available.

Gender Identity

Western culture is deeply committed to the idea that there are only two sexes. Biologically speaking, however, there are many gradations running from female to male; this is known as **transgenderism.** In some cases gender is clear, in other cases there is a blending of both genders within the same individual, and in some it is unclear.

Intersex

About 1 in every 2,000 babies is born with an **intersex** condition in which there are contradictions among chromosomal gender, gonadal gender, internal organs, and external genital appearance. The gender of such an infant is ambiguous. What this means is that an intersexed person has some parts usually associated with males and some parts usually associated with females. Intersex anatomy may not be apparent at birth. Sometimes it is undetected until puberty, until the person is identified as an infertile adult, or until the person dies and is autopsied. For more information, see the Intersex Society of North America.

Transsexuals

The medical profession considers **transsexuals** to have a condition called *gender dysphoria* (strong and persistent feelings of discomfort with one's assigned gender) or *gender identity disorder.* For the transsexual person, sexual anatomy is not consistent with gender identity. Those who are born physically male but are emotionally and psychologically female are called male-to-female (MTF) transsexuals. Those who are born female but are emotionally and psychologically male are called female-to-male (FTM) transsexuals.

Most transsexuals report that they have felt gender dysphoria since early childhood. They often suffer for many years and try to hide the situation from family and friends for fear of being considered "crazy." Being transgendered puts women and men at extreme risk of being:

- Ridiculed and humiliated.
- In constant jeopardy over getting and keeping a job.
- Evicted without cause from restaurants and stores.
- Denied housing.
- Refused medical treatment, even to save a life (Lips, 2005).

As self-understanding and acceptance increase, many transsexuals live part or full time as members of the other sex. Cross-dressing (dressing in the clothing of the other sex) not only makes their outward appearance consistent with their inner identity and gender role, but also increases their comfort with themselves. Their sexual orientation may be heterosexual, homosexual, or bisexual.

Cross-Dressers

Cross-dressers are typically males who cross-dress to express the feminine side of their personality. In most instances cross-dressers are not interested in permanently altering their bodies through surgical means, especially since the majority of them are comfortable with their original birth identity and behavior in their public and professional lives.

Cross-dressing is a conscious choice and may occur at home or in public settings. The frequency of the activity ranges from rarely to often. It is not unusual for cross-dressers to have a female name to go with the female personality and wardrobe. Cross-dressing occurs more frequently in cultures where males are expected to be strong, independent, and unemotional protectors. If the social climate is considered to be one with rigid gender roles, some men may need to express their gentleness and dependence by creating a separate world and female persona within that social climate (Barnett & Rivers, 2004).

Erotic Preferences

Over a lifetime, sexual fantasies and single-partner sex are the most common sexual outlets for women and men, single and coupled persons, and heterosexual, gay/lesbian, and bisexual persons. **Masturbation** is the ongoing love affair that each of us has with ourselves throughout our lifetime. It is the way we discover our erotic feelings and learn about our sexual response. Mutual masturbation can provide sexual pleasuring and intimacy without hurrying to genital interaction before both partners are ready. Masturbation shared with a partner is a safe alternative to unprotected genital sex.

Male-to-female or female-to-female **oral–genital sex** is known technically as *cunnilingus.* This involves kissing, licking, or sucking of the female genitals including the mons pubis, vulva, clitoris, labia, and vagina. *Fellatio* is oral stimulation of the penis by licking and sucking. *Sixty-nine* is simultaneous oral–genital stimulation by two persons. Preconceptions and myths are a major deterrent for those who have not tried oral sex. However, like most sexual practices, oral–genital sex is not completely free of the potential for STI transmission, and safe sex practices must be used.

Anal stimulation can be a source of sexual pleasure because the anus has a rich nerve supply. Stimulation may be applied with fingers, mouth, or sex toys such as vibrators. The anus is surrounded by strong muscles, and the rectum contains no natural lubrication. Thus inserting a finger or penis in the rectum requires relaxation and water-soluble lubricant.

A common form of sexual activity for heterosexual couples is **genital intercourse.** Penile–vaginal intercourse (coitus) can be both physically and emotionally satisfying. There are varieties of positions for this kind of intercourse; the most common is lying face to face (with female or male on top). Side-lying, standing, sitting, and rear-entry positions are also used. Side-lying, female-on-top, and rear-entry positions facilitate clitoral stimulation, either by penile or manual contact. The choice of intercourse positions and activities depends on physical comfort and beliefs, values, and attitudes about different practices.

During intercourse, the man moves the penis back and forth along the vaginal walls by rhythmic thrusting movements of his hips. At the same time the woman may move her own body to match the partner's hip movements. Movements continue until orgasm is achieved by one or both partners. Simultaneous orgasm can be difficult to achieve. After coitus, caressing, hugging, and kissing can increase the shared intimacy and should be encouraged.

The other form of genital intercourse is *anal intercourse,* during which the penis is inserted into the anus and rectum of the partner. Anal intercourse is commonly practiced by gay men, but a number of heterosexual couples engage in it as well. Positions for anal intercourse are similar to those for penile–vaginal intercourse, with minor differences due to the position of the anus.

Current practice dictates the use of a condom in both forms of intercourse to prevent the transmission of disease. Because anorectal tissue is not self-lubricating, a lubricant must be used on the condom. Also, since normal bacterial flora from the bowel can produce infection in other parts of the body, the used condom should be removed and another applied before inserting the penis into other body orifices.

There are many other varieties of sexuality that are beyond the scope of this chapter. These include several or many partners, nudism, swinging, group sex, fetishism, sexual sadism, and sexual masochism.

FACTORS INFLUENCING SEXUALITY

Many factors influence a person's sexuality. Discussed here are family, culture, religion, and personal expectations and ethics.

Family

For the majority of us, the family is the earliest and most enduring social relationship. Families are the fabric of our day-to-day lives and shape the quality of our lives by influencing our outlooks on life, our motivations, our strategies for achievement, and our styles for coping with adversity. It is within our families that we develop our gender identity, body image, sexual self-concept, and capacity for intimacy. Through family interactions we learn about relationships and gender roles and our expectations of others and ourselves.

From earliest beginnings, children observe their parents and model themselves after these role models. If parents are able to share affection with one another and other family members, children will most likely become adults who are able to give and receive affection. If parents seldom hug, hold hands, or kiss each other, their children may become adults who are very un-

comfortable with romantic touch. If family gender role behavior is very rigid, arguments and hurt feelings will abound if a person from this system is partnered with a person who grew up in an androgynous family system. Family messages about sex range from "sex is so shameful it shouldn't be talked about" to "sex is a joyful part of adult relationships." The following are some common sexual messages children get from their families:

- Sex is dirty.
- Premarital sex is sinful.
- Good girls don't do it.
- Masturbation is disgusting.
- Men should be the sexual experts.
- Sex is mainly for procreating.
- Bodies, including genitals, are beautiful.
- Sex should be fun for both women and men.
- Sexual thoughts and feelings are natural.
- Masturbation is a common, pleasurable activity.
- There is great variety in sexual behaviors.

Culture

Sexuality is regulated by the individual's culture. For example, culture influences the sexual nature of dress, rules about marriage, expectations of role behavior and social responsibilities, and specific sex practices. Societal attitudes vary widely. Attitudes about childhood sexual play with self or children of the same gender or other gender may be restrictive or permissive. Premarital and extramarital sex and homosexuality may be unacceptable or tolerated. Polygamy (several marriage partners) or monogamy (one marriage partner) may be the norm. Gender role behavior also varies from culture to culture. Culture is so much a part of everyday life that it is taken for granted. We tend to assume that others share our own perspective, including those for whom we provide care. It is impossible to provide sensitive nursing care if we believe that our own culture is more important than, and preferable to, any other culture.

Cultures differ with regard to which body parts they find to be erotic. In some cultures, legs are erotic and breasts are not. Body weight may also be a determinant of sexual attractiveness. There is a great deal of pressure in American culture to be very thin. Women who would be considered to be obese in America are found highly attractive in other cultures. The degree of public nudity ranges from women's entire bodies and faces being covered in Islamic societies to complete nudity in some cultures in New Guinea and Australia.

Female circumcision, also known as female genital mutilation, female ritual cutting (FRC), or *female genital cutting* (FGC), is a dangerous practice in parts of Africa. Some of the cultural beliefs behind the practice include the following: female genitals are offensive to men, if not removed the clitoris will become the size of a penis, the labia get in the way of intercourse, the cutting enhances fertility, and it prepares the woman for childbirth. Removal of the clitoris may or may not be accompanied by removal of the labia and closure of the vaginal entrance except for a small opening. Long-term medical complications include urinary incontinence, chronic urinary tract infections, vaginal scarring, pain syndromes, infertility, and sexual dysfunctions. FGC is illegal in several African and European countries and in Canada and the United States. In 1980, the World Health Organization and the United Nations Children's Fund (UNICEF) unanimously recommended that all forms of female circumcision be abolished (Elwood, 2005).

Male circumcision is controversial. The American Academy of Pediatrics Committee on the Fetus and Newborn stated in 1971 that there were no valid medical indications for circumcision for newborns. The Academy's current policy is that "Existing scientific evidence demonstrates potential medical benefits of newborn male circumcision; however, these data are not sufficient to recommend routine neonatal circumcision" (American Academy of Pediatrics Task Force on Circumcision, 1999). They support informed decision making on the part of parents. The change of rate of circumcisions is variably reported. Some studies show an increase (Nelson, Dunn, Wan, & Wei, 2005), while the U.S. National Center for Health Statistics (2005) indicates little change in the overall rate of about 65% in the past 20 years. All studies show highest rates in the Midwest segment of the country (81%) and lowest rates in the West (37%).

Religion

Religion influences sexual expression. It provides guidelines for sexual behavior and acceptable circumstances for the behavior, as well as prohibited sexual behavior and the consequences of breaking the sexual rules. The guidelines or rules may be detailed and rigid or broad and flexible. For example, some religions view forms of sexual expression other than male–female intercourse as unnatural and hold virginity before marriage to be the rule.

Many religious values conflict with the more flexible values of society that have developed during the last few decades (often labeled the "sexual revolution"), such as the acceptance of premarital sex, unwed parenthood, homosexuality, and abortion. These conflicts create marked anxiety and potential sexual dysfunctions in some individuals. See Chapter 41 ∞ for additional information about religious values.

Personal Expectations and Ethics

Although ethics is integral to religion, ethical thought and ethical approaches to sexuality can be viewed separately from religion. Cultures have developed written or unwritten codes of conduct based on ethical principles. Personal expectations concerning sexual behavior come from these cultural norms. What one person or culture views as bizarre, perverted, or wrong may be completely natural and right to another. Examples include values regarding masturbation, oral or anal intercourse, and cross-dressing. Many people accept a variety of sexual expressions if they are performed by consenting adults, are practiced in private, and are not harmful. Couples need to explore and communicate clearly about various types of acceptable sexual expression to prevent domination of sexual decision making by one member of the couple. To assess a few of your personal values, complete the statements in Box 40–2.

BOX 40–2 **Assessing Personal Sexual Values**
■ I believe sexual satisfaction is . . .
■ When I think of my parents having sex, I . . .
■ If I were to care for a transgendered client I would . . .
■ When I think about lesbians, gays, and bisexuals, I . . .
■ Masturbation is . . .
■ My beliefs about oral sex are . . .

SEXUAL RESPONSE CYCLE

Commonly occurring phases of the human sexual response follow a similar sequence in both females and males regardless of sexual orientation. It does not matter if the motive for being sexually active is true love or passionate lust. Table 40–3 provides a summary of the physiologic changes associated with each of the phases of the cycle.

The response cycle starts in the brain, with conscious sexual desires called the **desire phase.** Sexually arousing stimuli, often called erotic stimuli, may be real or symbolic. Sight, hearing, smell, touch, and imagination (sexual fantasy) can all invoke sexual arousal. Sexual desire fluctuates within each person and varies from person to person. If people suppress or block out conscious sexual desires, they may not experience any physiologic response. Although psychologic issues are the more common causes of lack of sexual desire, medications, drugs, and hormone imbalances can also interfere.

The **excitement phase** involves two primary physiologic changes (see Figure 40-1 ■). *Vasocongestion* is an increase in the blood flow to various body parts resulting in erection of the penis and clitoris and swelling of the labia, testes, and breasts. Vasocongestion stimulates sensory receptors within these body parts that in turn transmit messages to the conscious brain where they are usually interpreted as pleasurable sensations. When

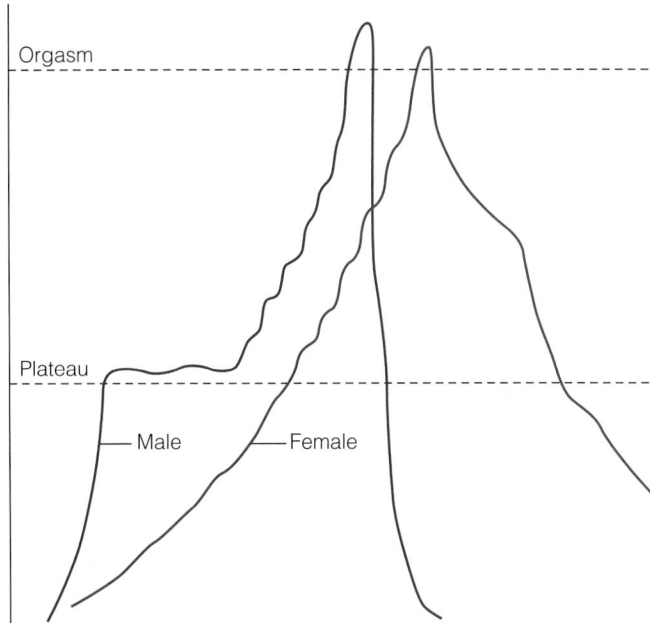

Figure 40-1 ■ Phases of the sexual response cycle.

TABLE 40–3 Physiologic Changes Associated with the Sexual Response Cycle

PHASE OF THE SEXUAL RESPONSE CYCLE	SIGNS PRESENT IN BOTH SEXES	SIGNS PRESENT IN MALES ONLY	SIGNS PRESENT IN FEMALES ONLY
Excitement/Plateau	Muscle tension increases as excitement increases. Sex flush, usually on chest. Nipple erection.	Penile erection; glans size increases as excitement increases. Appearance of a few drops of lubricant, which may contain sperm.	Erection of the clitoris. Vaginal lubrication. Labia may increase 2 to 3 times in size. Breasts enlarge. Inner two-thirds of vagina widens and lengthens; outer third swells and narrows. Uterus elevates.
Orgasmic	Respirations may increase to 40 breaths per minute. Involuntary spasms of muscle groups throughout the body. Diminished sensory awareness. Involuntary contractions of the anal sphincter. Peak heart rate (110–180 BPM), respiratory rate (40/min or greater), and blood pressure (systolic 30–80 mm Hg and diastolic 20–50 mm Hg above normal).	Rhythmic, expulsive contractions of the penis at 0.8-sec intervals. Emission of seminal fluid into the prostatic urethra from contraction of the vas deferens and accessory organs (stage 1 of the expulsive process). Closing of the internal bladder sphincter just before ejaculation to prevent retrograde ejaculation into bladder. Orgasm may occur without ejaculation. Ejaculation of semen through the penile urethra and expulsion from the urethral meatus. The force of ejaculation varies from man to man and at different times but diminishes after the first two to three contractions (stage 2 of the expulsive process).	Approximately 5–12 contractions in the orgasmic platform at 0.8-sec intervals. Contraction of the muscles of the pelvic floor and the uterine muscles. Varied pattern of orgasms, including minor surges and contractions, multiple orgasms, or a simple intense orgasm similar to that of the male.
Resolution	Reversal of vasocongestion in 10–30 min; disappearance of all signs of myotonia within 5 min. Genitals and breasts return to their preexcitement states. Sex flush disappears in reverse order of appearance. Heart rate, respiratory rate, and blood pressure return to normal. Other reactions include sleepiness, relaxation, and emotional outbursts such as crying or laughing.	A refractory period during which the body will not respond to sexual stimulation; varies, depending on age and other factors, from a few moments to hours or days.	

stimulation is continued, vasocongestion increases until it either is released by orgasm or fades away. Likewise, *myotonia,* an increase of tension in muscles, may increase until released by orgasm, or it may also simply fade away.

The **orgasmic phase** is the involuntary climax of sexual tension, accompanied by physiologic and psychologic release. This phase is considered the measurable peak of the sexual experience. Although the entire body is involved, the major focus of the orgasm is felt in the pelvic region. Male orgasms usually last 10 to 30 seconds while female orgasms last 10 to 50 seconds. Men usually have an *ejaculation* and expel semen as part of their orgasm. Before puberty and in later years, males experience orgasms without ejaculation.

The **resolution phase,** the period of return to the unaroused state, may last 10 to 15 minutes after orgasm, or longer if there is no orgasm. This phase in females is quite varied as some women experience multiple successive orgasms followed by a longer period of resolution.

ALTERED SEXUAL FUNCTION

The ability to engage in sexual behavior is of great importance to most people. Many individuals experience transient problems with their ability to respond to sexual stimulation or to maintain the response. A smaller percentage of people experience problems that are lifelong in duration. The problems may be generalized to all sexual interactions and settings, or they may be situational, occurring in a specific setting or with specific types of sexual activity. It is often difficult to sort out the multiple factors contributing to an individual's or a couple's sexual problems. Generally a number of past and current factors are involved.

Past and Current Factors

Sociocultural factors interfering in sexual function include a very restrictive upbringing accompanied by inadequate sex education. Rigid gender role socialization may inhibit exploration of sexual activities, positions, toys, and other lovemaking behaviors. If people's religious affiliations believe that sex is only for procreation, there may be great difficulty in celebrating the pleasure and fun of a loving sexual relationship. Another factor may be parental punishment for normally exploring one's genitals or for normal childhood sex play. In our current culture, the pressures of family and work often leave couples with too little time and not enough energy to enjoy sex.

Psychologic factors may include negative feelings, such as guilt, anxiety, or fear, that interfere with the ability to experience pleasure and joy. Some people experience guilt when they simply enjoy sex or when they participate in what they label "unusual" sexual activities, or guilt regarding the choice of the partner. Adults who have been sexually abused at any time of their lives may experience overwhelming anxiety when faced with the decision to engage in sex. Fears may include pregnancy, sexually transmitted infections, or pain. Because vulnerability and intimacy are inherent in most sexual relationships, fear of these may lead to an avoidance of sex. Fear of failure in sexual performance often becomes a vicious cycle; that is, fear of failure creates actual failure, which in turn produces more fear. Spectatoring is the detached appraisal of sexual performance or the body during a sexual act: "Am I going to lose my erection?" "Am I going to have an orgasm this time?" "My stomach is too flabby." "When did his thighs get that fat?" Depressed people lose interest in sexual activity and often experience a complete loss of sexual desire and fulfillment.

Cognitive factors include the internalization of negative expectations and beliefs. Those with low self-esteem may not understand how another person could value and love them and also find them sexually attractive. For those who have not yet accepted their sexual orientation or gender identity, this cognitive conflict may interfere with sexual relationships.

Sexual problems may also be symptomatic of *relationship* problems. Conflict and anger with one's partner are not conducive to positive sexual interaction. Some persons lose the physical attraction to another or feel more attracted to someone else.

Lack of intimacy and feeling like a sex object inhibit the feeling of communion and connection that is an important part of making love. Another factor is expecting one's partner to read one's mind about sexual needs. Failure to communicate may result in one or both partners not knowing how to please the other. Unless the partners experiment, sex may, in time, become boring. Disagreements in sexual frequency and/or sexual activities may lead to further relationship conflict.

Health factors can interfere with people's expression of sexuality. Physical changes brought on by illness, injury, or surgery may inhibit full sexual expression. Throughout your program of nursing education, you will learn about the sexual side effects of a number of diseases such as heart disease, diabetes mellitus, joint disease, cancer, and mental disorders. You will also study the impact of surgeries such as hysterectomy, prostate surgery, and radical surgeries that alter a person's body image. Spinal cord injuries, traumatic amputations, or disfiguring accidents negatively affect sexual functioning. The presence of an STI in one partner induces fear of transmission in the other, often resulting in abstinence of sexual contact. In some situations, the presence of an STI is unknown and transmission occurs.

Many prescription medications have side effects that affect sexual functioning beyond those intended for that purpose. Most frequently, the impact is negative, but sometimes there is a positive impact. Table 40–4 provides an overview of the effects of medications on sexual function. For example, antidepressants may slow ejaculation. This may be a problem for the man who finds himself suddenly feeling unable to ejaculate. If the man is suffering from rapid ejaculation, however, the antidepressant may "cure" this problem. Some street drugs such as marijuana, amphetamines, and cocaine enhance sexual functioning. Others, such as opioids and anabolic steroids, interfere with sexual functioning.

Sexual Desire Disorders

For most people, sexual desire varies from day to day as well as over the years. Some people, however, report a deficiency in or absence of sexual fantasies and persistently low interest or a total lack of interest in sexual activity; these clients suffer from **hypoactive sexual desire disorder.** If both individuals in a relationship are similarly uninterested in sex, there really is no problem. More typically, there is a disparity of sexual needs, and the person with the greater desire becomes dissatisfied with the sexual relationship. The key issue in the relationship is not frequency but rather the dovetailing of partners' needs.

Sexual aversion disorder is a severe distaste for sexual activity or the thought of sexual activity, which then leads to a phobic avoidance of sex. It occurs in both women and men. Intense emotional dread of an impending sexual interaction also can trigger the physiologic symptoms of anxiety: sweating, increased heart rate, and extreme muscle tension. The person then stops the sexual interaction or prevents it from even beginning. The most common cause of sexual aversion disorder is childhood sexual abuse or adult rape. The severe trauma can lead to a phobic response to sexual activity (McCammon et al., 2004).

Sexual Arousal Disorders

Sexual arousal refers to the physiologic responses and subjective sense of excitement experienced during sexual activity. Lack of lubrication and failure to attain or maintain an erection are the major disorders of the arousal phase. In **female sexual arousal disorder,** the lack of vaginal lubrication causes discomfort or pain during sexual intercourse. The diagnosis of **male erectile disorder** is usually made when the man has erection problems during 25% or more of his sexual interac-

TABLE 40–4 Effects of Medications on Sexual Function

MEDICATION	POSSIBLE EFFECTS*
Alcohol	Moderate amounts: increased sexual functioning; chronic use: decreased sexual desire, orgasmic dysfunction, and erectile dysfunction
Alpha-blockers	Inability to ejaculate
Amphetamines	Increased sex drive, delayed orgasm
Amyl nitrate	Reported enhanced orgasm; vasodilation, fainting
Anabolic steroids	Decreased sex drive, shrinking of testicles and infertility in men
Antianxiety agents	Decreased sexual desire; orgasmic dysfunction in women; delayed ejaculation
Anticonvulsants	Decreased sexual desire; reduced sexual response
Antidepressants	Decreased sexual desire; orgasmic delay or dysfunction in women; delayed or failed ejaculation; painful erection
Antihistamines	Decreased vaginal lubrication; decreased desire
Antihypertensives	Decreased sexual desire; erectile failure; ejaculation dysfunction
Antipsychotics	Decreased sexual desire; orgasmic dysfunction in women; delayed ejaculation; ejaculatory failure
Barbiturates	In low doses, increased sexual pleasure; in large doses, decreased sexual desire, orgasmic dysfunction, and erectile dysfunction
Beta-blockers	Decreased sexual desire
Cardiotonics	Decreased sexual desire
Cocaine	Increased intensity of sexual experience; with chronic use, decreased sexual desire and sexual dysfunction
Diuretics	Decreased vaginal lubrication; decreased sexual desire; erectile dysfunction
Marijuana	As above for cocaine, but prolonged use reduces testosterone levels and reduces sperm production
Narcotics	Inhibited sexual desire and response; erectile and ejaculatory dysfunctions

Nurses and clients must familiarize themselves with the specific medication prescribed or used, because effects vary in each category of drug.

tions. Some men cannot attain a full erection, and others lose their erection prior to orgasm. The term commonly applied to this condition, *impotency,* implies that the man is feeble, inadequate, and incompetent. The accurate term is *erectile dysfunction (ED)*, which is objectively descriptive and not judgmental. Arousal disorder may also be diagnosed even when lubrication and erection are adequate if individuals re-

port a persistent or recurring lack of subjective sexual excitement or pleasure.

Orgasmic Disorders

The term commonly applied in the past to women who did not experience orgasm, *frigid*, implied that the woman was totally incapable of responding sexually. The more accurate and objective

---

DRUG CAPSULE phosphodiesterase type 5 (PDE5) inhibitor

sildenafil citrate (Viagra); *tadalafil* (Cialis); *vardenafil* (Levitra)

THE CLIENT TAKING MEDICATION FOR ERECTILE DYSFUNCTION (ED)

In erectile dysfunction (ED) the sexually stimulated penis does not achieve or maintain an erection, often due to restricted blood flow to the penis. These medications inhibit the breakdown of the enzymes and products that allow the muscle relaxation which, in turn, facilitates adequate blood flow to the penis. Thus, the medications do not enhance sexual desire or cure the ED but allow the stimulated penis to obtain and sustain an erection.

NURSING RESPONSIBILITIES

- ED medications are contraindicated for men with uncontrolled high or low blood pressure, stroke, renal or liver problems, vision loss, or bleeding disorders.
- Men with an anatomically deformed penis should consult with the primary care provider prior to taking these medications.
- Medications come in different dose strengths and may require adjustment.

CLIENT AND FAMILY TEACHING

- General safety in using these medications is the same as for engaging in sexual activity overall. The risk of adverse outcomes of sexual activity after taking these medications is not increased.

- Explain that men who take medications that are nitrates—those that are prescribed (e.g., nitroglycerin) or those that are recreational (e.g., amyl nitrate—"poppers")—should not take these medications.
- The client should, take the medication about 1 hour prior to sexual activity (up to 4 hours prior) and not more than once per day.
- Teach side effects to immediately report to the primary care provider: loss of vision, or erection that lasts more than 4 hours.
- Other common side effects may include headache, muscle pain, flushing, or stuffy nose.
- These medications do not prevent pregnancy or STIs.

Note: Prior to administering any medication, review all aspects with a current drug handbook or other reliable source.

Erectile Dysfunction Video

MediaLink

term is **female orgasmic disorder,** which simply means that the sexual response stops before orgasm occurs. *Preorgasmic* women have never experienced an orgasm. Studies indicate that 10% to 15% of women are preorgasmic, and another 20% to 22% report irregular orgasms. Compounding the orgasmic difficulty is the associated anxiety. In the preoccupation with orgasm, the real goal of being sexual—mutual pleasuring and intimacy—is lost, and the interchange becomes one of anxiety, frustration, and anger (McCammon et al., 2004).

Some men suffer from **male orgasmic disorder.** Men with this disorder can maintain an erection for long periods (an hour or more) but have extreme difficulty ejaculating, referred to as *retarded ejaculation.* In heterosexual intercourse, the difficulty may be limited to ejaculation in the vagina. Some men ejaculate after self-stimulation or manual or oral stimulation by the partner, whereas others have great difficulty ejaculating with any type of stimulation. This disorder is much less common than rapid ejaculation.

Rapid ejaculation is one of the most common sexual dysfunctions among men. There are many definitions, with descriptions ranging from ejaculating before being touched, ejaculating before penetration, ejaculating with one internal thrust, to ejaculating within a minute or two of penetration. A more helpful description is the absence of voluntary control of ejaculation. The problem is best self-defined as when a man is concerned about his ejaculatory control, or the couple agrees that ejaculation is too rapid for mutual satisfaction.

Sexual Pain Disorders

Both women and men can experience **dyspareunia,** pain during or immediately after intercourse. It is associated with many physiologic causes, especially those that inhibit lubrication. Thus skin irritations, vaginal infections, estrogen deficiencies, and use of medications that dry vaginal secretions can cause women to experience discomfort with intercourse.

Pelvic disorders, such as infections, lesions, endometriosis, scar tissue, or tumors, can result in painful intercourse. Similarly, in males, infection or inflammation of the glans penis or other genitourinary organs can cause pain with intercourse. Also, some contraceptive foams, creams, sponges, or latex products can irritate either the vagina or penis.

Vaginismus is the involuntary spasm of the outer one-third of the vaginal muscles, making penetration of the vagina painful and sometimes impossible. The woman often experiences desire, excitement, and orgasm with stimulation of the external sexual structures. Attempts at intercourse, however, elicit the involuntary spasm. She may have similar difficulty undergoing pelvic exams and inserting tampons or a diaphragm.

Vulvodynia is constant, unremitting burning that is localized to the vulva with an acute onset. The girl or woman has problems in sitting, standing, and sleeping related to the intensity of pain. **Vestibulitis** causes severe pain only on touch or attempted vaginal entry. Half of the women with vestibulitis report lifelong dyspareunia. Women with either of these disorders report a negative impact on their sexual functioning and partner relationship, as well as their self-esteem and mental health (Metzger, 2004).

Problems with Satisfaction

Some people experience sexual desire, arousal, and orgasm and yet feel dissatisfied with their sexual relationships. These sexual problems are more commonly related to the emotional tone of the relationship than to the physiologic response. Since giving and receiving pleasure in a mutually intimate relationship are the primary goals of sex for most people, **dissatisfaction problems** may be more disturbing than other types of sexual dysfunctions.

At times, satisfaction problems may be situational. For example, one partner may choose an inconvenient time, or a partner may feel anxious and therefore cannot experience much pleasure or joy. Some people describe their problems as related to lack of extragenital satisfaction. These people describe how much they miss and continue to need all the touching and caressing of their earlier lovemaking experiences. Unfortunately, people who have been relating sexually for a long time often become genitally focused and neglect the rest of the body. One or both partners may feel touch starved, long for more extragenital loving, and become dissatisfied with sex.

Satisfaction problems are often related to relationship difficulties. The inability to communicate effectively in other relationship areas frequently results in sexual frustration. Partners who are angry with each other and make love without resolving the conflict may feel unhappy about the relationship despite having experienced arousal and orgasm. Couples who define their relationship in terms of rigid, unequal power and gender roles may have difficulty negotiating and compromising about sexual issues. Not infrequently, the person with the least amount of power feels helpless and dissatisfied with the sexual interchanges.

Lack of intimacy or a feeling of connectedness is understandably related to satisfaction problems. If one has sex with a stranger, the body may function well, but there is often a sense of something missing after the sexual experience. Making love to one person while feeling more attracted to or in love with another person can result in feelings of emptiness or disconnection. Even couples in a committed relationship may complain of lack of intimacy. Dissatisfaction issues include lack of romance, love, tenderness, and nurturance. Fulfillment of sexuality, then, depends on the ability to relate with a partner in an intimate and mutually pleasing manner that is compatible with values and chosen lifestyle.

NURSING MANAGEMENT

Assessing

Because sexuality and sexual functioning are aspects of health and well-being, they are a part of nursing care and need to be assessed. Clients are often hesitant to introduce the topic of sex with their primary health care providers. They may be too embarrassed, they may think that they should not have sexual problems in our liberated times, or they may think they are too old or too young to have these problems. When health care professionals do not introduce the topic, these individuals are unrecognized and unserved.

Information about a client's sexual health status should always be an integral part of a nursing assessment. The amount and kind of data collected depend on the context of the assessment, that is, the client's reason for seeking health care and how the client's sexuality interacts with other problems.

Generally, the nurse conducts a sexual history on the following categories of clients:

- Those receiving care for pregnancy, infertility, contraception, or an STI
- Those whose illness or therapy will affect sexual functioning (e.g., clients with diabetes, gynecologic problems, or heart disease)
- Those currently experiencing a sexual problem

Nursing History

Including a sexual history as part of the general nursing history is important for some clients and not important for other clients. It is critical, however, to introduce the topic of sexuality to all clients in order to give them permission to bring up any concerns or problems. All nursing histories should at least include a question such as "Have there been any changes in your sexual functioning that might be related to your illness or the medications you take?" Nurses might also facilitate communication by saying, "As a nurse, I'm concerned about all aspects of your health. People often have questions about sexual matters, both when they are well and when they are ill. When I take your history, sexual concerns are included to help plan a comprehensive treatment approach."

It is critical that nurses not make assumptions about clients because assumptions interfere with accurate history taking. If you assume that all people do all things, you will be more open to clients than if you make assumptions about who is and who is not sexually active and how. Imposing personal values on others is detrimental to the nurse–client relationship.

Interviewing a client regarding sexual health may be uncomfortable for some nurses (and for the client). Nurses must be

ASSESSMENT INTERVIEW · Sexual Health History

- Are you currently sexually active? With men, women, or both?
- With one or more than one partner?
- Describe the positive and negative aspects of your sexual functioning.
- Do you have difficulty with sexual desire? Arousal? Orgasm? Satisfaction?
- Do you experience any pain with sexual interaction?
- If there are problems, how have they influenced how you feel about yourself? How have they affected your partner? How have they affected the relationship?
- Do you expect your sexual functioning to be altered because of your illness?
- What are your partner's concerns about your future sexual functioning?
- Do you have any other sexual questions or concerns that I have not addressed?

aware of their own feelings and beliefs so that they can prepare approaches for gathering data and creating the nursing care plan. The nurse sets aside personal values about sexual practices and uses a culturally competent, nonjudgmental, nonthreatening, and reassuring approach. It is extremely important to create an atmosphere that facilitates open communication and comfort for the client. Remind the client that all personal health information is handled in a confidential manner. Also see Chapter 5 ∞ for a review of values clarification and Chapter 11 ∞ for more information on the health history.

The accompanying Assessment Interview: Sexual Health History provides questions that nurses may ask as part of the health history. These questions typically are asked in the assessment process after a rapport has been established.

RESEARCH NOTE · How Is Sexual Orientation Related to Sexual Health Risks in Homeless Adolescents?

In this study, 248 homeless males and 177 homeless females (total 425 teens) were surveyed regarding their sexual health risks and protective resources. Previous studies grouped gay, lesbian, and bisexual (GLB) youth in a single category of sexual minorities. The purpose of this study was to compare similarities and differences between GLB youth and heterosexual youth in the homeless population. A further goal was to determine if there were differences between the gay, lesbian, and bisexual subgroups.

Heterosexual youth were more likely to be homeless because of their parents' disapproval of their drug/alcohol use. Gay and lesbian youth were more likely to be homeless because of their parents' disapproval of their sexual orientation, and bisexual youth identified physical abuse at home as the cause of their homelessness. GLB youth reported higher incidence rates for all sexually transmitted infections. The order of childhood sexual abuse history is as follows: gay/lesbian, 77.6%; bisexual, 62.5%; and heterosexual, 37.1%. There was no sig-

nificant relationship between sexual orientation and receiving immunizations for hepatitis B. There were no significant differences between the use of condoms or the measure of risky sexual behaviors.

IMPLICATIONS

Nurses must ensure that their histories and assessments do not presume heterosexuality. An example of this is: "Are you sexually active? If so, with males, females, or both?" Youth who are homeless as the result of disapproval and abuse have difficulty trusting adults. Nurses must be nonjudgmental and ensure confidentiality for these young people.

Note: From "Sexual Health Risks and Protective Resources in Gay, Lesbian, Bisexual, and Heterosexual Homeless Youth," by L. Rew, T. A. Whittaker, M. A. Taylor-Seehafer, and L. R. Smith, 2005, *Journal for Specialists in Pediatric Nursing, 10*(1), pp. 11–19.

Physical Examination

Physical examination of the female genitals and reproductive tract and the male genitals is part of a routine physical examination in some agencies. Check agency protocol. See Chapter 30 ∞ for details of the examination. If the client has not been examined in the past year or if data from the recent nursing history indicate a need, the nurse performs a physical examination. Nursing history data indicating the need for a physical examination include the following:

- Suspicion of infertility, pregnancy, or an STI
- Reports of discharge, presence of a lump or sore, or change in color, size, and shape of a genital organ
- Changes in urinary function
- Need for Papanicolaou test
- Request for birth control

Identifying Clients at Risk

Clients at risk for altered sexual patterns include those experiencing the following:

- Altered body structure or function due to trauma, pregnancy, recent childbirth, anatomic abnormalities of the genitals, or a variety of diseases
- Physical, psychosocial, emotional, or sexual abuse; sexual assault
- Disfiguring conditions, such as burns, skin conditions, birthmarks, scars (e.g., mastectomy), and ostomies
- Specific medication therapy that causes sexual problems (see Table 40–4)
- Temporary or long-term impaired physical ability to perform grooming and maintain sexual attractiveness
- Value conflicts between personal beliefs and religious doctrine
- Loss of a partner
- Lack of knowledge or misinformation about sexual functioning and expression

Diagnosing

The NANDA nursing diagnoses relating specifically to sexuality include the following:

- *Ineffective Sexuality Pattern*
- *Sexual Dysfunction.*

Examples of clinical applications of these diagnoses using NANDA, NIC, and NOC designations are shown in Identifying Nursing Diagnoses, Outcomes, and Interventions.

Sexual problems can also be the etiology of other diagnoses, including the following:

- *Deficient Knowledge* (e.g., about conception, STIs, contraception, or normal sexual changes over the life span) related to misinformation and sexual myths
- *Pain* related to inadequate vaginal lubrication or effects of genital surgery
- *Anxiety* related to loss of sexual desire or functioning
- *Fear* related to history of sexual abuse or dyspareunia
- *Disturbed Body Image* (e.g., mastectomy) related to perceived sexual rejection by spouse

Planning

Overall goals to meet clients' sexual needs include the following:

- Maintain, restore, or improve sexual health.
- Increase knowledge of sexuality and sexual health.
- Prevent the occurrence or spread of STIs.
- Prevent unwanted pregnancy.
- Increase satisfaction with the level of sexual functioning.
- Improve sexual self-concept.

Examples of specific desired outcomes related to some of these goals are provided in Identifying Nursing Diagnoses, Outcomes, and Interventions. Nursing interventions to promote sexual health and function focus largely on the nurse's teaching role. For example, clients need to be taught about normal sexual function, the effects of medications on sexual function, preventing sexually transmitted diseases, and performing breast and testicular self-examinations. In addition to teaching, nurses can do the following to help clients maintain a healthy sexual self-concept:

- Provide privacy during intimate body care.
- Involve the client's partner in physical care.
- Give attention to the client's appearance and dress.
- Give clients privacy to meet their sexual needs alone or with a partner within physically safe limits.

Remember that clients' comfort in discussing sex-related topics and being examined is culturally influenced. For example, Latina women prefer to establish a comfortable rapport with providers by discussing casual topics before discussing intimate issues (Katz, 2003). Culture and age interact in determining some sexual practices. For example, one study showed that sexually active African American adolescents with demanding mothers were more likely to use condoms, and sexually active white adolescents with demanding mothers were less likely to use condoms (Cox, 2006). Asian American adolescents receive very little sex education from their parents since this is a culturally unmentionable subject. However, although they believe themselves to be at low risk, Asian American women have among the highest rates of certain STIs (Kao, 2006). Thus, planning for these clients must include using culturally sensitive communication techniques implemented with both clients and culturally appropriate family members.

Implementing

The interventions the nurse selects are based on the data obtained from the client and the identified nursing diagnoses. Many interventions are directed at providing information about sexual health and counseling for altered sexual function.

Nurses require six basic skills to help clients in the area of sexuality:

- Self-knowledge and comfort with their own sexuality
- Acceptance of sexuality as an important area for nursing intervention and a willingness to work with clients who express their sexuality in a variety of ways
- Knowledge of sexual growth and development throughout the life cycle

IDENTIFYING NURSING DIAGNOSES, OUTCOMES, AND INTERVENTIONS
Clients with Sexuality Problems

DATA CLUSTER Marsha Ogilvy, 55 years old, reports vaginal burning and pain whenever she and her husband have intercourse. Her last menses was 14 months ago. She says her husband is concerned about the lack of her usual response to lovemaking.

NURSING DIAGNOSIS/ DEFINITION	SAMPLE DESIRED OUTCOMES*/ *DEFINITION*	INDICATORS	SELECTED INTERVENTIONS*/ *DEFINITION*	SAMPLE NIC ACTIVITIES
Sexual Dysfunction/The state in which an individual experiences a change in sexual function during the sexual response phases of desire, excitation, and/or orgasm, which is viewed as unsatisfying, unrewarding, or inadequate	Physical Aging [0113]/*Normal physical changes that occur with the natural aging process*	No deviation from normal range ■ Sexual functioning	Health Education [5510]/*Developing and providing instruction and learning experiences to facilitate voluntary adaptation of behavior conducive to health in individuals, families, groups, or communities*	■ Determine current health knowledge and lifestyle behaviors of individual and family ■ Incorporate strategies to enhance the client's self-esteem ■ Teach strategies that can be used to minimize client's discomfort

DATA CLUSTER Larry Stogryn, 52 years old, has a history of hypertension for which he has been taking an antihypertensive. He says he has lost interest in sex in the past few months, and when he does have sex, he has trouble keeping an erection.

Ineffective Sexuality Patterns/Expression of concern regarding own sexuality	Sexual Functioning [0119]/*Integration of physical, socioemotional, and intellectual aspects of sexual expression*	Often demonstrated ■ Sustained penile erection ■ Performs sexually with assistive device as needed ■ Adapts sexual technique as needed	Sexual Counseling [5248]/*Use of an interactive helping process focusing on the need to make adjustments in sexual practice or enhance coping with a sexual event/disorder*	■ Discuss the effect of medication on sexuality ■ Discuss any alternative forms of sexual expression that might be acceptable to the client ■ Provide referral to other members of the health care team as appropriate, such as primary care provider to explore alternative blood pressure medications or use of medications for erectile dysfunction such as sildenafil citrate (Viagra); urologist for consideration of prosthesis, penile injections, and other interventions

*The NOC # for desired outcomes and the NIC # for nursing interventions are listed in brackets following the appropriate outcome or intervention. Outcomes, indicators, interventions, and activities selected are only a sample of those suggested by NOC and NIC and should be further individualized for each client.

■ Knowledge of basic sexuality, including how certain health problems and treatments may affect sexuality and sexual function and which interventions facilitate sexual expression and functioning
■ Therapeutic communication skills
■ Ability to recognize the need for all clients and family members to have the topic of sexuality introduced not only in written or audiovisual materials but also in a verbal discussion.

CLINICAL ALERT

As a result of culture, age, gender, and personal characteristics, not every nurse will be comfortable discussing sex with every client. However, it is the nurse's responsibility to ensure that someone introduces the topic with the client. ■

Providing Sexual Health Teaching

Providing education for sexual health is an important component of nursing implementation. Many sexual problems exist because of sexual ignorance; many others can be prevented with effective sexual health teaching. Examples of important areas of teaching are sex education (including self-examination) and responsible sexual behavior.

SEX EDUCATION. Nurses can assist clients to understand their anatomy and how their body functions. For example, understanding the anatomy of the genitals may help women learn how their body responds to sexual stimulation. Both men and women need to learn the kind of stimulation that is pleasing and causes arousal. The importance of open communication between partners should also be encouraged. Women may also benefit from learning Kegel exercises. These exercises involve contraction and relaxation of the pubococcygeal muscle, the muscle that contracts when a person prevents urine flow. The benefits of Kegel exercises include increased pelvic floor muscle tone; increased vaginal lubrication during sexual arousal; increased sensation during intercourse; increased genital sensitivity; stronger gripping of the base of the penis; earlier postpartum recovery of the pelvic floor muscle; and increased flexibility of episiotomy scars (Berman & Berman, 2005). The steps to perform Kegel exercises are discussed in Chapter 48 ∞ because these exercises are also used in bladder retraining.

Details about physiologic changes that occur during major developmental crises should be provided as part of general health care. For example, the nurse needs to discuss the effects of puberty, pregnancy, menopause, and the male climacteric on sexual function. When clients experience illness or surgery that may alter sexual function, the nurse needs to discuss effects of treatment (e.g., medications) and any changes that need to be undertaken to ensure safe sex (e.g., position changes or a safe time to resume sexual intercourse after a heart attack).

Parents often need assistance to learn ways to answer questions and what information to provide for their children starting in the preschool years. Parents need to be the primary educators of children at an early age; however, peers, teachers, media, and toys also teach about sexual issues.

Although there is an increasing awareness today of sexuality and sexual functioning, some people still hold certain myths and misconceptions about sexuality. Many of these are handed down in families and are part of the beliefs in a particular culture. It is highly important that nurses learn about the beliefs clients hold and provide up-to-date information. The website of the Sexuality Information and Education Council of the United States has a wealth of information on various aspects of sexuality.

TEACHING SELF-EXAMINATION. Monthly breast self-examination (BSE) for women and monthly testicular self-examination (TSE) for men can play an important role in early detection of disease, resulting in a greater chance of cure and less complex treatment. Clients need to be assured that most lumps discovered are not cancerous, but it is essential that all lumps or other detected abnormalities be checked by the client's primary care provider for accurate diagnosis. All nursing history assessments of clients need to include the client's understanding and practice of BSE or TSE. Self-examination involves both inspection and palpation procedures and should be conducted once a month.

Although 99% of the more than 200,000 new breast cancers in the United States each year occur in women (Jemal et al., 2005), men with an increased risk of breast cancer due to high estrogen levels or strong family history of breast cancer should also learn BSE (Smith, Cokkinides, & Eyre, 2006). For BSE a regular time is best—such as 1 week following menstruation, when breast tenderness and fullness caused by fluid retention have subsided, or on the same day of the month for men or postmenopausal women. People who examine themselves regularly become familiar with the shape and texture of their breasts. The steps of BSE are very similar to those used when the nurse performs breast examination (see Skill 30-14 in the Health Assessment chapter ∞). For specific techniques of breast self-examination, see Client Teaching.

Testicular cancer occurs in more than 8,000 American men each year (Jemal et al., 2005). Starting at age 15, monthly self-exams of the testicles are an effective way for men to get to know this area of their body and thus detect testicular cancer at an early and very curable stage. The best time for TSE is after a warm bath or shower when the scrotal sac is relaxed. For spe-

---

CLIENT TEACHING   Breast Self-Examination

INSPECTION BEFORE A MIRROR

Look for any change in size or shape; lumps or thickenings; any rashes or other skin irritations; dimpled or puckered skin; any discharge or change in the nipples (e.g., position or asymmetry). Inspect the breasts in all of the following positions:

- Stand and face the mirror with your arms relaxed at your sides or hands resting on the hips; then turn to the right and the left for a side view (look for any flattening in the side view).
- Bend forward from the waist with arms raised over the head.
- Stand straight with the arms raised over the head and move the arms slowly up and down at the sides. (Look for free movement of the breasts over the chest wall.)
- Press your hands firmly together at chin level while the elbows are raised to shoulder level.

PALPATION: LYING POSITION

- Place a pillow under your right shoulder and place the right hand behind your head. This position distributes breast tissue more evenly on the chest.
- Use the finger pads (tips) of the three middle fingers (held together) on your left hand to feel for lumps.

- Press the breast tissue against the chest wall firmly enough to know how your breast feels. A ridge of firm tissue in the lower curve of each breast is normal.
- Use small circular motions systematically all the way around the breast as many times as necessary until the entire breast is covered. (Review Figures 4-6 in Skill 30-14 (pages 629–630) in Chapter 30 ∞ for patterns that the client may use.)
- Bring your arm down to your side and feel under your armpit, where breast tissue is also located.
- Repeat the exam on your left breast, using the finger pads of your right hand.

PALPATION: STANDING OR SITTING

- Repeat the examination of both breasts while upright with one arm behind your head. This position makes it easier to check the area where a large percentage of breast cancers are found, the upper outer part of the breast and toward the armpit.
- *Optional:* Do the upright BSE in the shower. Soapy hands glide more easily over wet skin. Report any changes to your health care provider promptly.

CLIENT TEACHING Testicular Self-Examination

- Choose one day of each month (e.g., the first or last day of each month) to examine yourself.
- Examine yourself when you are taking a warm shower or bath.
- Support the testicle underneath with one hand. Place the fingers of the other hand under the testicle and the thumb on top (this may be easier to do if the leg on that side is raised).
- Roll each testicle between the thumb and fingers of your hand, feeling for lumps, thickening, or a hardening in consistency (Figure 40-2 ■). The testes should feel smooth.
- Palpate the epididymis, a cordlike structure on the top and back of the testicle. The epididymis feels soft and not as smooth as a testicle.
- Locate the spermatic cord, or vas deferens, which extends upward from the scrotum toward the base of the penis. It should feel firm and smooth.
- Using a mirror, inspect your testicles for swelling, any enlargement, or lumps in the skin of the testicle.

- Report any lumps or other changes to your health care provider promptly.

Figure 40-2 ■ Rolling the testicle between the thumb and fingers.

---

cific techniques of self-examination, see the Client Teaching feature.

CLINICAL ALERT

It may be wise for both male and female nurses to request permission from a parent or guardian before teaching testicular self-examination to teenage boys. Although the nurse need not touch the boy during the teaching, the boy must touch himself during TSE and parents may prefer the nurse not instruct him to do so. ■

RESPONSIBLE SEXUAL BEHAVIOR. Responsible sexual behavior involves the prevention of sexually transmitted diseases, the prevention of unwanted pregnancy, and the avoidance of sexual harassment or abuse.

STI Prevention. The prevention of STIs is an essential part of sexual health teaching (Figure 40-3 ■). Increases in these diseases are due to two factors: (a) changing sexual morality that has permitted increased sexual activity and (b) an increase in the

number of sexual partners. Because the term *sexually transmitted disease* elicits feelings of guilt, shame, and fear, people frequently do not seek medical help as early as they should. Clients need education about these diseases, preventive measures, and early treatment. Many STIs can be treated quickly and effectively. Others may have serious consequences. For example, women may develop pelvic inflammatory disease (PID) resulting in damage to the reproductive structures and possible infertility. AIDS has no cure. The anxiety about AIDS transmission has caused many individuals to alter their sexual behavior, such as using a condom during intercourse.

The Clinical Manifestations feature, earlier in this chapter, lists common signs of STIs for which people should seek medical care. Methods for decreasing exposure to STIs are described in the Client Teaching feature.

Figure 40-3 ■ Adolescents require age-appropriate teaching about sexuality and sexually transmitted diseases.
(Will Hart/PhotoEdit.)

CLIENT TEACHING Preventing Transmission of STIs and HIV

- Limit the number of sexual partners.
- Use condoms in nonmonogamous and homosexual relationships or other relationships that have the potential for STI transmission.
- Follow safe sex practices during oral sex including the use of a latex dental dam during cunnilingus to prevent STI transmission.
- Talk openly with sexual partners about how to have "safer sex" and be honest about any history of an STI.
- Abstain from high-risk sexual activity with a partner known to have or suspected of having an STI.
- Report to a health care facility for examination whenever in doubt about possible exposure or when signs of an STI are evident.
- When an STI is diagnosed, notify all partners and encourage them to seek treatment.
- Avoid transfusions of banked blood or blood products. Use autologous transfusions (donation of own blood before surgery) for elective surgery whenever possible.

Figure 40-4 ■ Methods of contraception.

Prevention of Unwanted Pregnancies. Prevention of unwanted pregnancies must be addressed not only with adolescents but also with couples who are planning the time of births and want to space children and limit family size. Nurses need to be familiar with various contraceptive methods and their advantages, disadvantages, contraindications, effectiveness, safety, and cost (Figure 40-4 ■). The various methods are outlined in Box 40–3. It is beyond the scope of this text to discuss contraceptives in detail.

Counseling for Altered Sexual Function

One technique nurses can use to help clients with altered sexual function is the PLISSIT model, developed by Annon (1974) for this purpose. The model involves four progressive levels represented by the acronym PLISSIT:

P   Permission giving
LI   Limited information
SS   Specific suggestions
IT   Intensive therapy

BOX 40–3   Methods of Contraception

- Abstinence
- Withdrawal of the penis before ejaculation (coitus interruptus)
- Fertility awareness (identification of the days of the month when conception is most likely to occur and abstaining during that time)
- Mechanical barriers: vaginal diaphragm, cervical cap, condom (*Note:* There are three types of condom materials: latex, lambskin, and polyurethane. All are equally effective at preventing pregnancy. Latex condoms are the least expensive. Lambskin pore size does not protect against STIs as well as the others. Polyurethane condoms are recommended if contact with latex should be avoided. Polyurethane is the material used in female condoms.)
- Chemical barriers: insertion of spermicidal foams, creams, jellies, or suppositories into the vagina before intercourse
- Intrauterine devices (IUDs)
- Hormonal: oral contraceptives (birth control pills), subdermal implants of synthetic progestin, transdermal patches (*Note:* Certain antibiotics decrease the effectiveness of oral contraceptives and patches. Women on these antibiotics must use an alternative method of contraception until their antibiotic treatment is completed. Other drug interactions can occur with implants.)
- Surgical sterilization: tubal ligation and vasectomy
- Abortion

At each level, the nurse provides additional guidance and information to the client and therefore requires more specialized and specific knowledge and skill. All professional nurses should be able to function at the first three levels. At the levels of limited information, specific suggestions, and intensive therapy, the nurse can also refer the client to a health care provider more skilled to assist the client with the particular issues identified during the first level.

PERMISSION GIVING. Clients may feel that they need permission to be sexual beings, to ask questions, to show affection, and to express themselves sexually. Giving permission means that the nurse by attitude or word lets the client know that sexual thoughts, fantasies, and behaviors between informed consenting adults are allowed. Giving permission begins when the nurse acknowledges the client's spoken and unspoken sexual concerns and conveys the attitude that sexual concerns and needs are important to health and recovery.

For example, the nurse might ask a client recuperating from a heart attack the following questions:

> "Now that you're recuperating and you've had some time to sort out your feelings, have you thought about how your heart attack might alter your sex life?"
> "Have you and your partner discussed how you both feel about it?"

LIMITED INFORMATION. Clients need accurate but concise information. The nurse might explain what is normal; how some medical conditions, treatments, injuries, or surgeries may affect sexuality and sexual functioning; or how aging may affect sexuality and functioning.

Continuing with the preceding example, the nurse shares information and informs the client about how the heart attack might affect the client's sex life, including the following:

> "Your heart attack will not change your sexual responsiveness. Most people can resume intercourse in 4 to 6 weeks, but this should be confirmed by your doctor. If you can climb a flight of stairs without having chest pain you should be able to resume having sex since it takes about the same amount of energy."
> "Many postcoronary clients fear sexual intercourse because of the physical exertion associated with it. However, your prescribed program of progressive physical activity will also increase your tolerance for sexual activity."

Many clients recuperating from childbirth, for example, or specific illness or disease (e.g., heart attack) need instruction about safe sexual activities and the effects that therapy may have on sexual functioning. The following topics need to be considered:

- When sexual activity is safe
- Specific sexual activities that are unsafe, and why
- Adaptations needed for resuming a satisfactory sexual life
- The side effects of prescribed medications on sexual functioning, and the need to notify the primary care provider for possible dose or medication adjustment should problems develop

SPECIFIC SUGGESTIONS. At this level, the nurse requires specialized knowledge and skill about how sexuality and functioning may be affected by a disease process or therapy and what interventions might be effective. The nurse offers suggestions to help the client adapt sexual activity to promote optimal functioning, such as what measures might be used to alleviate vaginal dryness, safe positions for intercourse following a total hip replacement, safe and unsafe sexual practices following a heart attack, and ways to handle ostomy appliances, urinary catheters, casts, or other devices (e.g., prostheses) during sexual activity. Similarly, nurses who work on a cardiac unit need specialized knowledge about sexual readjustment during cardiac rehabilitation, and nurses working with clients with spinal cord injuries need information about the sexual consequences of spinal injuries at various levels.

Using the example of the client recuperating from a heart attack, the nurse may offer the following suggestion:

> "Many people express concern about the stress of certain positions for intercourse, but you may use whatever position is comfortable for you and your partner, or try side-lying or partner-on-top positions."

INTENSIVE THERAPY. At this level of intervention, nurses must have specialized preparation and knowledge of sexual and gender identity disorders. Nurses who function in the sex therapist role should meet the qualifications for practice identified by the American Association of Sexuality Educators, Counselors, and Therapists (AASECT), which differentiate sex counseling from sex therapy. *Sex counseling* helps clients incorporate their sexual knowledge into satisfying lifestyles and socially responsible behavior. *Sex therapy* is a highly specialized, in-depth treatment to help clients resolve serious sexual problems. AASECT publishes a national directory of professionals certified to provide sex education, counseling, or therapy.

Dealing with Inappropriate Sexual Behavior

Nurses, both male and female, may encounter a variety of sexually inappropriate behaviors for a number of reasons. The behavior may be either aggressive or nonaggressive. Clients may act out sexually by

- Exposing themselves.
- Asking the nurse to provide intimate physical care, such as bathing genital areas, when they are capable of doing this themselves.
- Touching or grabbing the nurse's genitals or buttocks.
- Making blatant sexual statements to the nurse.
- Offering the nurse sex.
- Whistling; making comments about the nurse's attractiveness or desirability.
- Making sexual comments to another client in the same room or to visitors about the "sexy" nurse or what they would like to do sexually with the nurse.

Possible reasons for this inappropriate behavior are

- Fear or anxiety over future ability to function sexually.
- Unmet needs for intimacy and sexual closeness because of hospitalization, injury, illness, treatment, lack of a partner, or lack of privacy.
- Misinterpretation of the nurse's behavior as sexual or provocative.
- Need for reassurance that they are still sexual beings and still sexually attractive.
- Need for attention.
- Confusion: Neurologic impairment or trauma can lead clients to use profane sexual language, engage in masturbation, expose themselves, or inappropriately touch or grab at the nurse.
- Need to control: Clients may be experiencing loss of control over their lives because of hospitalization, injury, or illness.
- Need for power.
- Belief that flirtatious behavior is expected due to media portrayal of nurses as sexy, available, and experienced.

Before implementing any nursing interventions, the nurse should first ensure that the behavior is inappropriate and not an attempt to communicate a physical need. For example, clients may expose themselves if they are febrile, pull at the penis if a catheter is uncomfortable or irritating, or reach for the nurse if unable to communicate verbally. Nursing strategies to deal with inappropriate sexual behavior are listed in Box 40–4.

BOX 40–4 Nursing Strategies for Inappropriate Sexual Behavior

- Communicate that the behavior is not acceptable by saying, for example, "I really do not like the things you are saying," or "I see you are not dressed. I will be back in 10 minutes and will help you with breakfast when you get your clothes on."
- Tell the client how the behavior makes you feel: "When you act like that toward me, I am very uncomfortable. It embarrasses me and makes it hard for me to give you the kind of nursing care you need."
- Identify the behavior you expect: "Please call me by my name, not 'honey,'" or "I expect you to keep yourself covered when I am in the room. If you are feeling hot or something is uncomfortable, let me know, and I will try to make you more comfortable."
- Set firm limits: Take the client's hand and move it away, use direct eye contact, and say, "Don't do that!"

- Try to refocus clients from the inappropriate behavior to their real concerns and fears; offer to discuss sexuality concerns: "All morning you have been making very personal sexual comments about yourself. Sometimes people talk like that when they are concerned about the sexual part of their life and how their illness will affect them. Are there things that you have questions about or would like to talk about?"
- Report the incident to your nursing instructor, charge nurse, or clinical nurse specialist. Discuss the incident, your feelings, and possible interventions.
- Assign a nurse who will confront the behavior and relate to the client in a consistent manner.
- Clarify the consequences of continued inappropriate behavior (avoidance, withdrawal of services, no chance to help resolve underlying concerns of client).

CRITICAL THINKING CHECKPOINT

Mr. Curry is a 50-year-old African American male with diabetes who suffered a heart attack 3 weeks ago. He is doing well and is in a cardiac rehabilitation program. His diabetes is controlled with diet, and his only medications consist of a daily aspirin and an antihypertensive medication. During a routine checkup you inquire how he is feeling and whether he is doing well on his medications. Reluctantly, he admits that he is having some sexual problems. You encourage further discussion of the matter by displaying interest and explaining that it is okay for him to share his concerns with you. Mr. Curry states that he is having some difficulty achieving erections, but is more con-

cerned that he will have another heart attack if he engages in sexual activities.

1. Speculate about Mr. Curry's reluctance to discuss his sexual concerns.
2. What factors influence nurses' abilities to discuss sexual concerns with their clients?
3. What is the relationship between health and sexual function?
4. How can you best intervene to help Mr. Curry?

See Critical Thinking Possibilities in Appendix A.

CHAPTER 40 **REVIEW**

CHAPTER HIGHLIGHTS

- Sexuality is important in developing self-identity, interpersonal relationships, intimacy, and love.
- There is a tremendous range of variation in how people express their sexuality including sexual orientation, gender identity, erotic preferences, and sexual lifestyles.
- Factors that affect sexuality include developmental level, family, culture, religious values, personal expectations and ethics, disease processes, medications, and relationship problems.
- Sexual problems include desire disorders, arousal disorders, orgasmic disorders, problems with satisfaction, and sexual pain disorders.
- Assessing risk for or actual sexual problems is part of the initial nursing assessment. Assessment should also be carried out when clients or support people present cues that problems exist or when clients have an illness that could cause sexual problems.
- Nurses assess attitudes toward sexuality, including factors that affect attitudes and behaviors.
- Before assisting clients with sexual problems, nurses must acquire accurate information about sexuality, identify and accept their own

sexual values and behaviors as well as those of others, and be comfortable acquiring and disseminating information about sexuality.
- Nursing diagnoses for clients with sexual problems are related to many contributing factors, including altered body structure or function, lack of knowledge or misinformation about sexual matters, physical or psychologic abuse, value conflicts, and loss or lack of a partner.
- Nursing interventions focus largely on teaching clients about sexual function and sexuality, responsible sexual behavior that includes the prevention of STIs and unwanted pregnancies, and self-examination of the breasts and testicles.
- Counseling clients with altered sexual functions can be facilitated by using the PLISSIT model: permission giving (P), limited information (LI), and specific suggestions (SS). Intensive therapy (IT) requires intervention by clinical nurse specialists or sex therapists.

TEST YOUR KNOWLEDGE

1. Clients are least likely to introduce the topic of sex with health care providers for which of the following reasons?
   1. They assume that health care providers know little about sexual functioning.
   2. Most clients have few, if any, questions or problems.
   3. Female clients prefer to discuss problems with female health care providers.
   4. They are too embarrassed to introduce the topic of sex.

2. A nurse receives information that a client is a transsexual. Appropriate care is based on the knowledge that which of the following is most representative of this client?
   1. Gonadal gender, internal organs, and external genitals are contradictory.
   2. Sexual anatomy is not consistent with gender identity.
   3. Sexual attraction is to individuals of both genders.
   4. Gender identity is altered by acute psychosis.

3. In conducting client teaching the nurse bases content on knowing that which of the following is true regarding masturbation?
   1. People who masturbate are psychologically disturbed.
   2. Teenage masturbation interferes with academic achievement.
   3. Most people do not masturbate past the teenage years.
   4. Masturbation is a way people learn about their sexual response.

4. A male client is beginning an antidepressant medication. Which of the following should be included in the teaching?
   1. "Your partner will be pleased because your sexual functioning is going to improve."
   2. "You may find that your desire for sex will decrease while on this medication."
   3. "Retrograde ejaculation is a common problem when taking antidepressants."
   4. "Your skin will probably become supersensitive to touch, so you may need to change your activity during sex."

5. A client who had a hysterectomy 3 days ago, says to the nurse, "I no longer feel like a real woman." What is the best response?
   1. "Don't worry about that. The feeling will probably go away."
   2. "You should talk to your doctor about how you feel."
   3. "I don't blame you. I would feel like half a woman also."
   4. "I hear your concern. Tell me more about your feelings."

6. Because a client reports having dyspareunia, it is most appropriate to ask which of the following questions?
   1. "Have you talked with your partner about this discomfort?"
   2. "Have you had these spasms since you became sexually active?"
   3. "Do you have pain before your period begins?"
   4. "Do your breasts swell large enough to need a larger bra?"

7. Including at least some sexual health history questions would be most relevant for clients taking:
   1. Anti-inflammatories (such as aspirin or ibuprofen).
   2. Hypnotics (sleeping pills).
   3. Antihypertensives (blood pressure medications).
   4. Antihistamines (cold medications).

8. A nurse informs a client who is 8½ months pregnant that it is best to abstain from intercourse until after the birth of the baby. This communication is most representative of which component of the PLISSIT model?
   1. Permission giving (P)
   2. Limited information (LI)
   3. Specific suggestions (SS)
   4. Intensive therapy (IT)

9. A 75-year-old male client reports decreased frequency of sexual intercourse although he does not express dissatisfaction or difficulty. He seems a little embarrassed by the discussion but is engaged and asks some questions. An appropriate nursing diagnosis would be which of the following?
   1. *Sexual Dysfunction*
   2. *Disturbed Body Image*
   3. *Sedentary Lifestyle*
   4. *Readiness for Enhanced Knowledge*

10. Which of the following outcomes may indicate the need for referral to a more highly skilled therapist?
   1. The client verbalizes methods of modifying sexual activity according to physical limitations.
   2. The client requests the phone number of a sex education support group.
   3. Suggestions given by the nurse are ineffective in reaching the desired goals.
   4. The client reports experimenting with new sexual activities.

See Answers to Test Your Knowledge in Appendix A.

EXPLORE MEDIALINK www.prenhall.com/berman

DVD-ROM
- Audio Glossary
- NCLEX Review
- Animations:
    Spermatogenesis
    Oogenesis and Spermatogenesis
    Oogenesis and Spermatogenesis A & P Review
    Oogenesis and Spermatogenesis Terms and Definitions
    Female Reproductive System A & P Review
    Female Reproductive System Terms & Definitions
    Male Reproductive System A & P Review
    Male Reproductive System Terms & Definitions
    Ovulation A & P Review
- Videos:
    Gender Identity
    Erectile Dysfunction

COMPANION WEBSITE
- Additional NCLEX Review
- Case Study: Client in a Motor Vehicle Crash
- Care Plan Activity: Client with a Mastectomy
- Application Activities:
    Society for Human Sexuality
    Campus Health Promotion
- Links to Resources

READINGS AND REFERENCES

SUGGESTED READINGS
Lewis, J. H., Rosen, R., Goldstein, I., & the Consensus Panel on Health Care Clinician Management of Erectile Dysfunction. (2003). Erectile dysfunction: A panel's recommendations for management. *American Journal of Nursing, 102*(10), 48–57.
This extensive article describes the team's results describing the pathophysiology, assessment, diagnosis, and treatment of ED. It includes a brief survey instrument for self-assessment of ED by the client.

Mick, J., Hughes, M., & Cohen, M. Z. (2004). Using the BETTER model to assess sexuality. *Clinical Journal of Oncology Nursing, 8,* 84–86.
Although the PLISSIT model is used broadly in nursing, it is not the only tool. This article describes an additional instrument based on the 6-step BETTER model.

RELATED RESEARCH
Katz, A. (2005). The sounds of silence: Sexuality information for cancer patients. *Journal of Clinical Oncology, 23,* 238–241.

van Daalen, C. (2005). Girls' experiences in physical education, competition, evaluation, & degradation. *Journal of School Nursing, 21*(2), 115–121.

REFERENCES
American Academy of Pediatrics Task Force on Circumcision. (1999). Circumcision policy statement. *Pediatrics, 103,* 686–693.
Annon, J. (1974). *The behavioral treatment of sexual problems. Vol. 1. Brief therapy.* New York: Harper & Row.

Barnett, R., & Rivers, C. (2004). *Same difference.* New York: Basic Books.

Berman, L., & Berman, J. (2005). *Secrets of the sexually satisfied woman: Ten keys to unlocking ultimate pleasure.* New York: Hyperion Press.

Cox, M. F. (2006). Racial differences in parenting dimensions and adolescent condom use at sexual debut. *Public Health Nursing, 23*(1), 2–10.

Dochterman, J., & Bulechek, G. B. (Eds.). (2004). *Nursing interventions classification (NIC)* (4th ed.). St. Louis, MO: Mosby.

Elwood, A. (2005). Female genital cutting, `circumcision' and mutilation. *Contemporary Sexuality, 39*(1), i–vii.

Jemal, A., Tiwari, R. C., Murray, T., Ghafoor, A., Samuels, A., Ward, E., et al. (2005). Cancer statistics, 2004. *CA: A Cancer Journal for Clinicians, 54,* 8–29, 57–59.

Kaestle, C. E., Halpern, C. T., Miller, W. C., & Ford, C. A. (2005). Young age at first sexual intercourse and sexually transmitted infections in adolescents and young adults. *American Journal of Epidemiology, 161,* 774–780.

Kao, T. S. (2006). Sexual health education disparities in Asian American adolescents. *Journal for Specialists in Pediatric Nursing, 11,* 57–60.

Katz, A. (2003). Culturally competent care. "Where I come from, we don't talk about that": Exploring sexuality & culture among Blacks, Asians and Hispanics. *AWHONN-Lifelines, 6*(6), 533–536.

Lips, H. M. (2005). *Sex and gender* (5th ed.). Columbus, OH: McGraw-Hill.

McCammon, S. L., Knox, D., & Schacht, C. (2004). *Choices in sexuality* (2nd ed.). Cincinnati, OH: Atomic Dog Publishing.

Metzger, D. A. (2004). New advances in the diagnosis and treatment of vulvar/vestibular pain disorders. *Conference proceedings: Women's Sexual Health.* The Berman Center and Northwestern University, Feinberg School of Medicine, Department of Obstetrics and Gynecology, Chicago.

Moorhead, S., Johnson, M., & Maas, M. (Eds.). (2004). *Nursing outcomes classification (NOC)* (3rd ed.). St. Louis, MO: Mosby.

Morrison, T. (1992). *Jazz.* New York: Alfred A. Knopf.

NANDA International. (2007). *NANDA nursing diagnoses: Definitions and classification 2007–2008.* Philadelphia: Author.

Nelson, C. P., Dunn, R., Wan, J., & Wei, J. T. (2005). The increasing incidence of newborn circumcision: Data from the nationwide inpatient sample. *Journal of Urology, 173,* 978–981.

Rew, L., Whittaker, T. A., Taylor-Seehafer, M. A., & Smith, L. R. (2005). Sexual health risks and protective resources in gay, lesbian, bisexual, and heterosexual homeless youth. *Journal for Specialists in Pediatric Nursing, 10*(1), 11–19.

Smith, R. A., Cokkinides, V., & Eyre, H. J. (2006). American Cancer Society recommendations for the early detection of cancer, 2006. *CA: A Cancer Journal for Clinicians, 56,* 11–25.

U.S. National Center for Health Statistics. (2005). *Trends in circumcisions among newborns.* Retrieved July 10, 2006, from http://www.cdc.gov/nchs/products/pubs/pubd/hestats/circumcisions/circumcisions.htm

Vision of sexual health. (2004). *Contemporary Sexuality, 38*(7), 1–5.

World Association of Sexology. (1999). *Declaration of sexual rights.* Adopted at the 14th World Congress of Sexology, Hong Kong and People's Republic of China.

World Health Organization. (1975). *Education and treatment in human sexuality: The training of health professionals.* Geneva: Author.

SELECTED BIBLIOGRAPHY

Butler, S. S. (2004). Gay, lesbian, bisexual, and transgender (GLBT) elders: The challenges and resilience of this marginalized group. *Journal of Human Behavior in the Social Environment, 9*(4), 25–44.

Cornog, M. (2003). *The BIG book of masturbation.* San Francisco: Down There Press.

Elson, J. (2004). *Am I still a woman? Hysterectomy and gender identity.* Philadelphia: Temple University Press.

Givson, M. C. (2004). Sexual health: The neglected component of care. *Perspectives, 27*(4), 5–7.

Hammoud, M. M., White, C. B., & Fetters, M. D. (2005). Opening cultural doors: Providing culturally sensitive healthcare to Arab American and American Muslim patients. *American Journal of Obstetrics and Gynecology, 193,* 1307–1311.

Higgins, A., Barker, P., & Begley, C. M. (2004). Hypersexuality and dementia: Dealing with inappropriate sexual expression. *British Journal of Nursing, 13,* 1330–1334.

Joannides, P. (2004). *The guide to getting it on* (3rd ed.). West Hollywood, CA: Goofy Foot Press.

Katz, A. (2005). Sexually speaking. Sexuality and hysterectomy: Finding the right words: Responding to patients' concerns about the potential effects of surgery. *American Journal of Nursing, 105*(12), 65–68.

Katz, A. (2005). Cultural diversity. "Caregiving" is cultural. *Journal of Professional Nursing, 21,* 139–140.

Katz, A. (2005). Sexually speaking. Do ask, do tell: Why do so many nurses avoid the topic of sexuality? *American Journal of Nursing, 105*(7), 66–68.

Kaufman, M., Silverberg, C., & Odette, F. (2003). *The ultimate guide to sex and disability: For all of us who live with disabilities, chronic pain and illness.* San Francisco: Cleis Press.

Lund-Nielsen, B., Muller, K., & Adamsen, L. (2005). Malignant wounds in women with breast cancer: Feminine and sexual perspectives. *Journal of Clinical Nursing, 14,* 56–64.

Snow, J. (2004). *How it feels to have a gay or lesbian parent.* Binghamton, NY: Haworth Press.

Spirituality

LEARNING OUTCOMES

After completing this chapter, you will be able to:

1. Define the concepts of spirituality and religion as they relate to nursing and health care.

2. Identify characteristics of spiritual health.

3. Identify factors associated with spiritual distress and manifestations of it.

4. Describe the spiritual development of the individual across the life span.

5. Describe the influence of spiritual and religious beliefs about diet, dress, prayer and meditation, and birth and death on health care.

6. Assess the spiritual needs of clients and plan nursing care to assist clients with spiritual needs.

7. Describe nursing interventions to support clients' spiritual beliefs and religious practices.

8. Identify desired outcomes for evaluating the client's spiritual health.

Because nurses provide holistic care, they care not only for the physical body and mind, but also for the client's spirit. Meeting the client's spiritual needs can decrease suffering and aid in physical and mental healing. To implement spiritual care, nurses need to be skilled in establishing trusting nurse–client relationships. Such spiritual caregiving skill requires that the nurse possess a healthy spiritual self-awareness. This personal spirituality, inevitably, influences nursing care. In particular, this spiritual self-awareness will help the nurse to identify and be empathic toward the spiritual concerns of clients.

In addition to spiritual self-awareness, nurses need some awareness of the diverse spiritual beliefs and practices that their clients may possess. Because spiritual beliefs and practices are coping resources for persons, understanding how such beliefs and practices help or hinder a client's health is vital. A client's experience with what is seen as sacred or divine is complex and individual. Thus, each client needs to be approached in light of these unique needs. In addition to distressing spiritual or religious needs, many clients have spiritual strengths that the nurse can nurture. Whether the client presents with a need to relieve spiritual distress or to enhance spiritual health, nurses can implement spiritual care therapeutics that promote spiritual and emotional health, help with coping and adjustment, or assist one to face a more peaceful death.

SPIRITUALITY DESCRIBED

Spirituality, faith, and religion are separate entities, yet the words are often used interchangeably. The word *spiritual* derives from the Latin word *spiritus,* which means "to blow" or "to breathe," and has come to connote that which gives life or essence to being human. **Spirituality** refers to that part of being human that seeks meaningfulness through intra-, inter-, and transpersonal connection (Reed, 1992). Spirituality generally

involves a belief in a relationship with some higher power, creative force, divine being, or infinite source of energy. For example, a person may believe in "God," "Allah," the "Great Spirit," or a "Higher Power." Spirituality includes the following aspects (Martsolf & Mickley, 1998):

- Meaning (having purpose, making sense of life)
- Value (having cherished beliefs and standards)
- Transcendence (appreciating a dimension that is beyond the self)
- Connecting (relating to others, nature, Ultimate Other)
- Becoming (which involves reflection, allowing life to unfold, and knowing who one is)

Words or concepts reflective of spirituality, such as faith, courage, cheer, and hope, may be used in ordinary speech when discussing spirituality.

Spirituality can be described by measuring it, so to speak, on a "spirit titer" (Jourard, 1971). One's spirit titer is influenced by numerous factors, such as life experiences, coping skills, social supports, and individual belief systems. Individuals experience multiple changes and losses over their life span, and if their spirit titer is low they may become dis-spirited, or depressed. If they have a high spirit titer, they will lean toward being inspired and becoming an inspiration to others in spite of hardships they experience (Figure 41-1 ■). Nurses need to direct their goals and planning to assist clients in attaining and maintaining a high spirit titer.

Spiritual Needs

Just as everybody has a spiritual dimension, all clients have needs that reflect their spirituality. These needs are often accentuated by an illness or other health crisis. Clients who have well-defined spiritual beliefs may find that their beliefs are

Figure 41-1 ■ Spirit titer.

challenged by their health situation, or may cling to their beliefs more firmly and appreciatively. Clients who have no defined beliefs may suddenly come face to face with challenging questions such as "why me?" and others related to the meaning and purpose of life. Nurses need to be sensitive to indications of the client's spiritual needs and respond appropriately, as discussed later. Examples of spiritual needs are listed in Box 41–1.

Spiritual Well-Being

Spiritual health, or **spiritual well-being,** is manifested by a feeling of being "generally alive, purposeful, and fulfilled" (Ellison, 1983, p. 332). According to Pilch (1998), spiritual wellness is "a way of living, a lifestyle that views and lives life as purposeful and pleasurable, that seeks out life-sustaining and life-enriching options to be chosen freely at every opportunity, and that sinks its roots deeply into spiritual values and/or specific religious beliefs" (p. 31). Spiritual health, as defined by the Nursing Outcomes Classification project (Moorhead, Johnson, & Maas, 2004, p. 519) is the "connectedness with self, others, higher power, all life, nature and the universe that transcends and empowers the self." Indicators of spiritual health are shown in Box 41–2.

People nurture or enhance their spirituality in many ways. Some focus on development of the inner self; others focus on the expression of their spiritual energy with others or the outer world. Relating to one's inner self or soul may be achieved by conducting an inner dialogue with a higher power or with oneself through prayer or meditation, by analyzing dreams, by communing with nature, or by experiencing the inspiration of art (e.g., drama, music, dance). The expression of a person's spiritual energy to others is manifested in loving relationships with

BOX 41–1 **Examples of Spiritual Needs**

Needs related to the self:
- need for meaning and purpose
- need to express creativity
- need for hope
- need to transcend life challenges
- need for personal dignity
- need for gratitude
- need for vision
- need to prepare for and accept death

Needs related to others:
- need to forgive others
- need to cope with loss of loved ones

Needs related to the Ultimate Other:
- need to be certain there is a God or Ultimate Power in the universe
- need to believe that God is loving, and personally present
- need to worship

Needs among and within groups:
- need to contribute or improve one's community
- need to be respected and valued
- need to know what and when to give and take

Note: From *Spiritual Care: Nursing Theory, Research, and Practice* by E. J. Taylor, 2002, Upper Saddle River, NJ: Prentice Hall. Reprinted by permission of Pearson Education, Inc., Upper Saddle River, New Jersey.

BOX 41–2 **Indicators of Spiritual Health**

Uncompromised. . .
- faith
- hope
- meaning and purpose in life
- achievement of spiritual world
- feelings of peacefulness
- ability to love
- ability to forgive
- ability to pray
- ability to worship
- spiritual experiences
- participation in spiritual rites and passages
- participation in meditation
- participation in spiritual reading
- interaction with spiritual leaders
- expression through song/music
- expression through art
- expression through writing
- connectedness with inner-self
- connectedness with others
- interaction with others to share thoughts, feelings, and beliefs

Note: Reprinted from *Iowa Intervention Project: Nursing Outcome Classification* by S. Moorhead, M. Johnson, & M. Maas. Copyright © 2004, with permission from Elsevier.

and service to others, joy and laughter, participation in religious services and associated fellowship gatherings and activities, and expression of compassion, empathy, forgiveness, and hope. Nurses who attend to their own spirituality are better able to work with clients who have spiritual needs (Taylor, 2005). Therefore, it is important to be comfortable with one's own spirituality.

Spiritual Distress

Spiritual distress refers to a challenge to the spiritual well-being or to the belief system that provides strength, hope, and meaning to life. Some factors that may be associated with or contribute to a person's spiritual distress include physiologic problems, treatment-related concerns, and situational concerns. Physiologic problems include having a medical diagnosis of a terminal or debilitating disease, experiencing pain, experiencing the loss of a body part or function, or experiencing a miscarriage or stillbirth. Treatment-related factors include recommendation for blood transfusions, abortion, surgery, dietary restrictions, amputation of a body part, or isolation. Situational factors include the death or illness of a significant other, inability to practice one's spiritual rituals, or feelings of embarrassment when practicing them (Carpenito-Moyet, 2006).

NANDA International (2007) offers the following as defining characteristics of spiritual distress:

- Expresses lack of hope, meaning and purpose in life, forgiveness of self
- Expresses being abandoned by or having anger toward God
- Refuses interaction with friends, family
- Sudden changes in spiritual practices
- Requests to see a religious leader
- No interest in nature, reading spiritual literature

MediaLink Emotional, Social, and Spiritual Needs Video

No list could be complete, however, considering the complexity and variability of people and their spiritual dimensions.

RELATED CONCEPTS

Because spirituality is a reflection of an inner experience that is expressed individually, it includes as many representations as there are human beings. Concepts related to spirituality include religion, faith, hope, transcendence, and forgiveness.

Religion

Religion is an organized system of beliefs and practices. It offers a way of spiritual expression that provides guidance for believers in responding to life's questions and challenges. According to Vardey (1996, p. xv), the organized religions offer (a) a sense of community bound by common beliefs; (b) the collective study of scripture (the Torah, Bible, Koran, or others); (c) the performance of ritual; (d) the use of disciplines and practices, commandments, and sacraments; and (e) ways of taking care of the person's spirit (such as fasting, prayer, and meditation). Many traditional religious practices and rituals are related to such life events as birth, transition from childhood to adulthood, marriage, illness, and death (Figure 41-2 ■). Religious rules of conduct, typically influenced concurrently by culture, may also apply to matters of daily life such as dress, food, social interaction, menstruation, and sexual relationships.

Religious development of an individual refers to the acceptance of specific beliefs, values, rules of conduct, and rituals. Religious development may or may not parallel spiritual development. For example, a person may follow certain religious practices and yet not internalize the symbolic meaning behind the practices. Often religious development undergirds and enhances spirituality by providing a system of belief that can suggest areas of growth to the believer. For example, the daily prayers of the Muslims bring the believers into direct relationship with the profound questions of life several times per day.

Figure 41-2 ■ Hospital chaplains minister to clients and their families.

An **agnostic** is a person who doubts the existence of God or a supreme being or believes the existence of God has not been proved. An **atheist** is one without belief in a God. **Monotheism** is the belief in the existence of one God, while **polytheism** is the belief in more than one god.

Faith

Faith is to believe in or be committed to something or someone. Fowler (1981) described faith as being present in both religious and nonreligious people. Faith gives life meaning, providing the individual with strength in times of difficulty. For the client who is ill, faith—whether in a higher authority (e.g., God, Allah, Jehovah), in oneself, in the health care team, or in a combination of all—provides strength and hope.

Hope

Hope is a concept that incorporates spirituality. Stephenson (1991) suggested this definition: "a process of anticipation that involves the interaction of thinking, acting, feeling, and relating, and is directed toward a future fulfillment that is personally meaningful" (p. 1459). In the absence of hope, the client gives up, losing spirit, and illness is likely to progress more rapidly.

Transcendence

The term **transcendence** is often used interchangeably with self-transcendence, which Coward (1990) defined as: "the capacity to reach out beyond oneself, to extend oneself beyond personal concerns and to take on broader life perspectives, activities, and purposes" (p. 162). Transcendence is also thought to involve a person's recognition that there is something other or greater than the self and a seeking and valuing of that greater other, whether it is an ultimate being, force, or value.

Forgiveness

The concept of forgiveness is receiving increased attention among health care professionals. For many clients, illness or disability bring a sense of shame or guilt. The health problem is interpreted as a punishment for past sins (e.g., "Having sex before I got married is why I have breast cancer"). Clients facing imminent death may seek forgiveness from others as well as from God. Mickley and Cowles's (2001) research suggested that nurses can play a pivotal role in assisting clients to understand the process of forgiveness and to persevere through it.

SPIRITUAL DEVELOPMENT

Just as individuals develop physically, cognitively, and morally, they also develop spiritually. Several theologians have identified specific linear stages through which individuals may progress while maturing spiritually. Westerhoff (1976), for example, described faith as a way of behaving that evolves from a faith guided by parents and others during infancy and childhood to an owned faith that is internalized in adulthood and serves as

TABLE 41–1	**Stages of Spiritual Development**
DEVELOPMENTAL STAGE	**CHARACTERISTICS**
0–3 years	Neonates and toddlers are acquiring fundamental spiritual qualities of trust, mutuality, courage, hope, and love. Transition to next stage of faith begins when child's language and thought begin to allow use of symbolism.
3–7 years	Fantasy-filled, imitative phase when child can be influenced by examples, moods, actions. Child relates intuitively to ultimate conditions of existence through stories and images, the fusion of facts and feelings. Make-believe is experienced as reality (Santa Claus, God as grandfather in the sky).
7–12 years, even into adulthood	Child attempting to sort fantasy from fact by demanding proofs or demonstrations of reality. Stories are important for finding meaning and organizing experience. Child accepts stories and beliefs literally. Ability to learn the beliefs and practices of the culture, religion.
Adolescence	Experience of the world now beyond the family unit and spiritual beliefs can aid understanding of extended environment. Generally conform to the beliefs of those around them; begin to examine beliefs objectively, especially in late adolescence.
Young adulthood	Development of a self-identity and worldview differentiated from those of others. The individual forms independent commitments, lifestyle, beliefs, and attitudes. Begins to develop personal meaning for symbols of religion and faith.
Mid-adulthood	Newfound appreciation for the past; increased respect for inner voice; more awareness of myths, prejudices, and images that exist because of social background. Attempts to reconcile contradictions in mind and experience and to remain open to others' truths.
Mid- to late adulthood	Able to believe in, and live with a sense of participation in, a nonexclusive community. May work to resolve social, political, economic, or ideological problems in society. Able to embrace life, yet hold it loosely. (Martin Luther King, Jr., Mahatma Gandhi, and Mother Teresa illustrate this stage.)

Note: Adapted from content from *Stages of Faith Development: The Psychology of Human Development and the Quest for Meaning,* by James W. Fowler. Copyright © 1981, by James W. Fowler. Reprinted with permission of HarperCollins Publishers.

a directive for action. Table 41–1 describes some of the aspects of spiritual development and healthful religious behaviors during different life stages.

SPIRITUAL PRACTICES AFFECTING NURSING CARE

Clients frequently identify religious practices such as prayer as important strategies for coping with illness (Mauk & Schmidt, 2004; Taylor, 2003b). The most common practices affecting the nursing care of clients include holy days, sacred writings, sacred symbols, prayer, meditation, and those associated with diet, nutrition, healing, dress, birth, and death.

It is possible for nurses to unethically impose personal spiritual beliefs on clients, whose circumstances inherently leave them vulnerable. Observing guidelines for ethical conduct in spiritual caregiving is essential. The following guidelines for nurses were offered by Winslow and Winslow (2003):

- First seek a basic understanding of clients' spiritual needs, resources, and preferences (i.e., assess).
- Follow the client's expressed wishes regarding spiritual care.
- Do not prescribe or urge clients to adopt certain spiritual beliefs or practices, and do not pressure them to relinquish such beliefs or practices.
- Strive to understand personal spirituality and how it influences caregiving.
- Provide spiritual care in a way that is consonant with personal beliefs.

CLINICAL ALERT

While some clients are eager for nurses' overt offers of "spiritual care," others may be uncertain or opposed to such offers (Taylor, 2003a). Clients often confuse religiosity with spirituality; this may contribute to their uncertainty about receiving spiritual care from nurses. Observing and using the client's language for spirituality (e.g., "being at peace" or "faith"), as well as large measures of sensitivity and respect, will help nurses to converse therapeutically with clients to provide spiritual care. ■

Holy Days

A **holy day** is a day set aside for special religious observance, and all the world religions observe certain holy days. For example, Christians observe Easter and Christmas, Jews observe Yom Kippur and Passover, Buddhists observe the birthday of the Buddha, Muslims observe the month-long holy period of Ramadan, and Hindus observe Mahashivarathri, a celebration of Lord Shiva. Many religions require fasting, extended prayer, and reflection or ritual observances on sacred (or high holy) days. Believers who are seriously ill are often exempted from such requirements.

The concept of the Sabbath is common to both Christians and Jews, in response to the biblical commandment "Remember the Sabbath day to keep it holy." Most Christians observe the Sabbath on Sunday, whereas Jews and sabbatarian Christians (e.g., Seventh-Day Adventists) observe Saturday as their Sabbath. Clients who are devout in their religious practices may want to avoid any special treatments or other intrusions on their day of rest and reflection.

Muslims follow the practice of prayer fives times a day, and the Muslim client may need assistance to maintain this commitment. In addition, Muslims traditionally gather on Friday at noon to worship and learn about their faith. Both Hindus and Buddhists practice meditation, and the nurse may create a quiet time for them to meditate.

Solemn religious observances throughout the year may be referred to as *high holy days* and may include fasting, reflection, and prayer. Examples of such holy days are Rosh Hashanah and Yom Kippur (Jewish), Good Friday (Christian), and the month-long Ramadan (Islam). Many hospitals and health organizations facilitate ritual observances for clients and staff on holy days. Because many religions follow calendars other than the Gregorian calendar, a multifaith calendar can be used to identify the holy days of the various religious groups (Griffith, 1996).

Sacred Writings

Each religion has sacred and authoritative scriptures that provide guidance for its adherents' beliefs and behaviors; in addition, sacred writings frequently tell instructive stories of the religion's leaders, kings, and heroes. In most religions, these scriptures are thought to be the word of the Supreme Being as written down by prophets or other human representatives. Christians rely on the Bible, Jews on the Torah and Talmud, and Muslims on the Koran; Hindus have several holy texts, or Vedas, and Buddhists value the teachings of the Tripitakas. Scriptures generally set forth religious law in the form of admonitions and rules for living (e.g., the Ten Commandments). This religious law may be interpreted in various ways by subgroups of a religion's adherents and may affect a client's willingness to accept treatment suggestions; for example, blood transfusions are in conflict with the religious admonitions of Jehovah's Witnesses.

People often gain strength and hope from reading religious writings when they are ill or in crisis. Examples of scriptural stories that may give comfort to clients are Job's suffering, in both the Jewish and Christian scriptures, and Jesus's healing of people who were physically or mentally ill, in the New Testament.

Sacred Symbols

Sacred symbols include jewelry, medals, amulets, icons, totems, or body ornamentation (e.g., tattoos) that carry religious or spiritual significance. They may be worn to pronounce one's faith, to remind the practitioner of the faith, to provide spiritual protection, or to be a source of comfort or strength. People may wear religious medals at all times, and they may wish to wear them when they are undergoing diagnostic studies, medical treatment, or surgery. People who are Roman Catholic may carry a rosary for prayer; a person who is Muslim may carry a mala, or string of prayer beads (Figure 41-3 ■).

People may have religious icons or statues in their home, car, or place of work as a personal reminder of their faith or as part of a personal place of worship or meditation. Hospitalized clients or long-term care residents may wish to have their spiritual icons or statues with them as a source of comfort.

Figure 41-3 ■ Clients may bring objects to the hospital to use in prayer or other religious rituals. Caregivers should respect such objects, because they usually have great significance for clients.

Prayer and Meditation

Prayer is a spiritual practice; for many, it is also a religious practice. An encyclopedia of religion defines **prayer** simply as "human communication with divine and spiritual entities" (Gill, 1987, p. 489). Some argue that because prayer requires a belief in a divine or spiritual entity not all people pray, while others consider prayer a universal phenomenon that does not require such belief. Ulanov and Ulanov (1983), for example, proposed that everyone prays: "People pray whether or not they call it prayer. We pray every time we ask for help, understanding, or strength, in or out of religion . . . who and what we are speak out of us. . . . To pray is to listen to and hear this self who is speaking" (p. 1). Prayer is intention plus love, often communicated with "the Absolute," according to Dossey (1999); that is, prayer is a loving wish or thought for oneself or another, and not an invocation of positive or negative forms of magic.

There are different types of prayer experience. Poloma and Gallup (1991) categorized prayer experiences as follows:

■ Ritual (e.g., Hail Mary, memorized prayers that can be repeated)
■ Petitionary (e.g., "God, cure me!" or intercessory prayers when one is requesting something of the divine)

- Colloquial (i.e., conversational prayers)
- Meditational (e.g., moments of silence focused on nothing, a meaningful phrase, or a certain aspect of the divine)

While meditational and colloquial prayer experiences have been found to be associated with spiritual well-being and quality of life in healthy adults, ritual and petitionary prayer experiences may be most comforting and appropriate for those who are ill.

Some religions have prescribed prayers that are printed in a prayer book, such as the Anglican/Episcopal *Book of Common Prayer* or the Catholic *Missal.* Some religious prayers are attributed to the source of faith; for example, the Lord's Prayer for Christians is attributed to Jesus, and the first sutra for Muslims is attributed to Mohammed.

Some religions require daily prayers or dictate specific times for prayer and worship: the five daily prayers, or Salat, of the Muslims (performed while facing east toward Mecca at dawn, noon, midafternoon, sunset, and evening), the daily Kaddish of the Jews, or the seven canonical prayers of the Roman Catholics. People who are ill may want to continue or increase their prayer practices (Moschella, Pressman, Pressman, & Weissman, 1997). They may need uninterrupted quiet time during which they have their prayer books, rosaries, malas, or other icons available to them.

Meditation is the act of focusing one's thoughts or engaging in self-reflection or contemplation. Some people believe that, through deep meditation, one can influence or control physical and psychologic functioning and the course of illness.

Beliefs Affecting Diet and Nutrition

Many religions have proscriptions regarding diet. There may be rules about which foods and beverages are allowed and which are prohibited. For example, Orthodox Jews are not to eat shellfish or pork, and Muslims are not to drink alcoholic beverages or eat pork. Members of the Church of Jesus Christ of Latter-Day Saints (Mormons) are not to drink caffeinated or alcoholic beverages. Older Catholics may choose not to eat meat on Fridays because it was proscribed in years past. Buddhists and Hindus are generally vegetarian, not wanting to take life to support life. Religious law may also dictate how food is prepared; for example, many Jewish people require **kosher** food, which is food prepared according to Jewish law.

Some solemn religious observances are marked by fasting, which is the abstinence from food for a specified period of time. Some religions also restrict beverages; others allow drinking of water or other sustaining beverages on fast days. Examples of religions that observe fasting include Islam, Judaism, and Catholicism. During the month of Ramadan, devout Muslims eat no food and avoid beverages during daylight hours; the fast is broken after sunset. Members of Jewish synagogues fast on Yom Kippur, and devout Catholics may fast on Good Friday. Most religions lift the fasting requirements for seriously ill believers for whom fasting may be a detriment to health (e.g., diabetic clients). Some religions may exempt nursing mothers or menstruating women from fasting requirements.

It is important that health care providers prescribe diet plans with an awareness of the client's dietary and fasting beliefs.

Beliefs Related to Healing

Clients may have religious beliefs that attribute illness to a spiritual disruption. Healing for such clients may appear to be unrelated to current treatment practices. The nurse needs to assess the client's beliefs and, if possible, include some aspects of healing that are part of the client's belief system in the planning of care.

Beliefs Related to Dress

Many religions have laws or traditions that dictate dress. For example, Orthodox and Conservative Jewish men believe that it is important to have their heads covered at all times and therefore wear yarmulkes. Orthodox Jewish women cover their hair with a wig or scarf as a sign of respect to God. Many Muslim women also cover their hair in accordance with their particular ethnic or national background. Mormons may wear temple undergarments in compliance with religious law.

Some religions require that women dress in a conservative manner, which may include wearing sleeves and modestly cut tops, and skirts that cover the knees. Some religions, for example, Islam, may require that the body (torso, arms, and legs) be covered. Hindu women accustomed to wearing saris prefer to cover all of the body except arms and feet (Figure 41-4 ■). Hospital gowns may make women wishing to comply with religious dress codes uneasy and uncomfortable. Clients may be

Figure 41-4 ■ Hindu women dressed in saris.

(Charlie Westerman/Getty Images.)

especially disconcerted when undergoing diagnostic tests or treatments, such as mammography, that require body parts to be bared.

Beliefs Related to Birth

For all religions the birth of a child is an important event giving cause for celebration. Many religions have specific ritual ceremonies that consecrate the new child to God. When a Muslim child is born, "someone recites the call to prayer in the infant's ear." On the seventh day after birth, the child is named, and a tuft of hair is shaved from the head (Denny, 1993, p. 682).

In the Christian faith, baptism and christening ceremonies may take place after the birth of a child to confirm that the "infant [was] born into a Christian family as part of the organism of the church" (Frankiel, 1993, p. 556). Christian parents of seriously ill infants may want baptism performed at birth by the nurse or primary care provider, if a chaplain or clergy person is not present.

In the Jewish religion, the ritual circumcision conducted on male children on the eighth day after birth is an expression of the religious bond between the prophet Abraham, his descendants, and their God. Following the ritual circumcision by the trained person, called a *mohel,* the child is named. Girls are named in the synagogue on the Sabbath after the birth (Fishbane, 1993).

When nurses are aware of the religious needs of families and their infants, they can assist families in fulfilling their religious obligations. This is especially important when the newborn infant is seriously ill or in danger of dying because some people believe that if religious obligations are not fulfilled the infant will not be accepted into the community of the faithful after death.

Beliefs Related to Death

Spiritual and religious beliefs play a significant role in the believer's approach to death just as they do in other major life events. Many believe that the person who dies transcends this life for a better place or state of being.

Some religions have special rituals surrounding dying and death that must be observed by the faithful. Observance of these rituals provides comfort to the dying person and their loved ones. Some rituals are carried out while the person is still alive, and can include special prayers, singing or chants, and reading of sacred scriptures. Roman Catholic priests perform the Sacrament of the Sick (previously referred to as the Last Rites) when clients are very ill or near death. Muslims who are dying want their body or head turned toward Mecca (Denny, 1993).

Jews have a tradition of burial within 24 hours following death, except on the Sabbath, and they "sit Shiva" (gather to pay respects), draping any mirrors in black to ensure that guests are focused on memory of the deceased rather than on themselves. Tibetan Buddhists read the *Tibetan Book of the Dead* within 7 days of the death to release the soul of the deceased from the Bardos, or nether worlds. Hindus cremate the body within 24 hours to release the soul from any earthly attachment.

Griffith (1996) suggested that during a terminal illness the client and family should be queried about observances or rituals

that follow death. Some religions require that the body of the deceased be touched only by members of that faith. In both the Muslim (Denny, 1993) and the Jewish (Fishbane, 1993) religions, believers may require that a ritual bath be done after death by a family member or by a ritual burial society. Religious symbols or objects should be treated with respect and kept with the body (Griffith, 1996). The nurse can support the family of the deceased by providing an environment conducive to the performance of their traditional death rituals.

CLINICAL ALERT

Before sharing personal beliefs or practices, a nurse must consider questions such as the following:

- For what purpose am I sharing my beliefs or practices? By doing so, am I meeting my needs or my client's?
- Is my spiritual care reflecting a spiritual assessment?
- Am I preying on a vulnerable client?
- Am I offering my beliefs or practices in a manner that allows my client comfortably to refuse?
- Does my spiritual care hurt or contribute to a therapeutic relationship with the client? ■

SPIRITUAL HEALTH AND THE NURSING PROCESS

The nursing process, which includes assessing, diagnosing, planning, implementing, and evaluating, can be applied to the area of spiritual health.

 NURSING MANAGEMENT

Assessing

Data about a client's spiritual beliefs are obtained from the client's general history (religious preferences or orientation); through a nursing history; and by clinical observations of the client's behavior, verbalizations, mood, and so on. Nurses should never assume that a client follows all the practices of the client's stated religion.

Nursing History

The Joint Commission on Accreditation of Healthcare Organizations (2000) mandates that each client admitted to an institution's care must be assessed for spiritual beliefs and practices. Several experts (Cole, Benore, & Pargament, 2004; Koenig, 2002; Massey, Fitchett, & Roberts, 2004; Taylor, 2002) recommend a two-tiered approach to spiritual assessment. All clients can be asked a general question or two (e.g., "What spiritual beliefs or practices are important to you now while you live with illness?" "How would you like your health care team to support you spiritually?"). Only those who manifest some type of unhealthful spiritual need or are at risk for spiritual distress need be subjected to a more thorough spiritual assessment. Even this assessment can be streamlined to hone in on the particular spiritual concern present.

- Are any particular religious practices important to you? If so, could you please tell me about them?
- How will being sick interfere with your religious practices?
- How is your faith helpful to you? In what ways is it important to you right now?
- In what ways can I support your spirit? For example, would you like me to read your prayer book to you?
- Would you like a visit from your spiritual counselor or the hospital chaplain?
- What are your hopes and your sources of strength right now? What comforts you during hard times?

Although the nurse will continually be assessing, the initial spiritual assessment is best taken at the end of the assessment process, or following the psychosocial assessment, after the nurse has developed a relationship with the client and/or support person. A nurse who has demonstrated sensitivity and personal warmth, earning some rapport, will be more successful during a spiritual assessment.

The questions provided in the accompanying Assessment Interview may be suitable. Remembering an acronym such as FICA can also help the nurse to ask appropriate questions:

> F (faith or beliefs)—for example, What spiritual beliefs are most important to you?
> I (implications or influence)—for example, How is your faith affecting the way you cope now?
> C (community)—for example, Is there a group of like-minded believers with which you regularly meet?
> A (address)—for example, How would you like your health care team to support you spiritually? (Dameron, 2005; Massey et al., 2004).

Clinical Assessment

Cues to spiritual and religious preferences, strengths, concerns, or distress may be revealed by one or more of the following (Taylor, 2002):

1. *Environment.* Does the client have a Bible, Torah, Koran, other prayer book, devotional literature, religious medals, a rosary, cross, Star of David, or religious get-well cards in the room? Does a church send altar flowers or Sunday bulletins?
2. *Behavior.* Does the client appear to pray before meals or at other times or read religious literature? Does the client have nightmares and sleep disturbances or express anger at religious representatives or at a deity?
3. *Verbalization.* Does the client mention God or a higher power, prayer, faith, the church, synagogue, temple, a spiritual or religious leader, or religious topics? Does the client ask about a visit from the clergy? Does the client express fear of death, concern with the meaning of life, inner conflict about religious beliefs, concern about a relationship with the deity, questions about the meaning of existence or

the meaning of suffering, or about the moral or ethical implications of therapy?
4. *Affect and attitude.* Does the client appear lonely, depressed, angry, anxious, agitated, apathetic, or preoccupied?
5. *Interpersonal relationships.* Who visits? How does the client respond to visitors? Does a minister come? How does the client relate to other clients and nursing personnel?

See also specific manifestations of spiritual health and spiritual distress on page 1043.

Diagnosing

In diagnosing spiritual health, the nurse may find that spiritual problems provide the diagnostic label, or that spiritual distress is the etiology of the problem.

Spiritual Issues as the Diagnostic Label

The North American Nursing Diagnosis Association (NANDA International, 2007) recognizes three diagnoses related to spirituality:

- *Spiritual Distress* is "impaired ability to experience and integrate meaning and purpose in life through a person's connectedness with self, others, art, music, literature, nature, or a power greater than oneself" (p. 186). See Identifying Nursing Diagnoses, Outcomes, and Interventions for a clinical illustration of this diagnosis.
- *Readiness for Enhanced Spiritual Well-Being* recognizes that spiritual well-being is the "ability to experience and integrate meaning and purpose in life through a person's connectedness with self, others, art, music, literature, nature, or a power greater than oneself" (p. 189). This wellness diagnosis describing spiritual health acknowledges that some people respond to adversity with an increased sensitivity to spirituality or spiritual maturation.
- *Risk for Spiritual Distress* is defined by NANDA (2005) as being "at risk for an impaired ability to experience and integrate meaning and purpose in life through a person's connectedness with self, other persons, art, music, literature, nature, and/or a power greater than oneself" (p. 188). This diagnosis may be appropriate for a client who presently shows no indication of this disruption of spirit yet may if a nurse fails to intervene.

Religious Issues as the Diagnostic Label

Recently, NANDA International accepted three new nursing diagnoses that reflect client religious issues. These include the following (Burkhart, 2005, p. 10):

> *Impaired Religiosity* "Impaired ability to exercise reliance on religious beliefs and/or participate in rituals of a particular faith tradition"
> *Risk for Impaired Religiosity* "At risk for an impaired ability to exercise reliance on religious beliefs and/or participate in rituals of a particular faith tradition"
> *Readiness for Enhanced Religiosity* "Ability to increase reliance on religious beliefs and/or participate in rituals of a particular faith tradition"

MediaLink

Supporting a Client's Spiritual Practices Case Study

Spiritual or Religious Distress as the Etiology

Spiritual distress may affect other areas of functioning and indicate other diagnoses. In these instances, spiritual distress becomes the etiology. Examples include the following:

- *Fear* related to apprehension about soul's future after death and unpreparedness for death
- *Chronic* or *Situational Low Self-Esteem* related to failure to live within the precepts of one's faith
- *Disturbed Sleep Pattern* related to spiritual distress
- *Ineffective Coping* related to feelings of abandonment by God and loss of religious faith
- *Decisional Conflict* related to conflict between treatment plan and religious beliefs

Planning

In the planning phase, the nurse identifies interventions to help the client achieve the overall goal of maintaining or restoring spiritual well-being so that spiritual strength, serenity, and satisfaction are realized (see Identifying Nursing Diagnoses, Outcomes, and Interventions).

Planning in relation to spiritual needs should be designed to do one or more of the following:

- Help the client fulfill religious obligations.
- Help the client draw on and use inner resources more effectively to meet the present situation.
- Help the client maintain or establish a dynamic, personal relationship with a supreme being in the face of unpleasant circumstances.
- Help the client find meaning in existence and the present situation.
- Promote a sense of hope.
- Provide spiritual resources otherwise unavailable.

Implementing

Numerous nursing actions are available to help clients meet their spiritual needs (Cole et al., 2004; Mauk & Schmidt, 2004; Taylor, 2002). Spiritual care includes actions as diverse as rec-

IDENTIFYING NURSING DIAGNOSES, OUTCOMES, AND INTERVENTIONS
Clients with Spiritual Distress

DATA CLUSTER Marilyn Eckhardt, 72 years old, is crying, fingering her rosary, and voicing concern that she has not seen her priest for confession since being admitted to the hospital. She states that she is afraid to die without confessing her sins. She also states that she does not want to see the hospital chaplain, but rather her own priest, whose parish is about 30 miles away. The hospital record indicates that Ms. Eckhardt is Roman Catholic.

NURSING DIAGNOSIS/ DEFINITION	SAMPLE DESIRED OUTCOME*/ DEFINITION	INDICATORS	SELECTED INTERVENTIONS*/ DEFINITION	SAMPLE NIC ACTIVITIES
Spiritual Distress related to inability to practice spiritual ritual (confession with parish priest)/*Impaired ability to experience and integrate meaning and purpose in life through a person's connectedness with self, others, art, music, literature, nature, or a power greater than oneself*	Spiritual Health [2001]/*Personal expressions of connectedness with self, others, higher power, all life, nature, and the universe that transcend and empower the self*	Mildly Compromised: ■ Interaction with spiritual leaders ■ Participation in spiritual rites and passages ■ Ability to pray	Spiritual Support [5420]/*Assisting the client to feel balance and connection with a greater power*	■ Refer to spiritual advisor of client's choice ■ Encourage chapel service attendance, if desired ■ Encourage the use of spiritual resources, if desired ■ Provide desired spiritual articles, according to client preferences

DATA CLUSTER John Ames, 42 years old, is in a terminal state with an AIDS-related condition. He has become withdrawn but states to the nurse, "What have I done that God has punished me so?" The nurse observes religious literature on his bedside cabinet.

Spiritual Distress related to crisis of illness and impending death/*Impaired ability to experience and integrate meaning and purpose in life through a person's connectedness with self, others, art, music, literature, nature, or a power greater than oneself*	Dignified Life Closure [1307]/ *Personal actions to maintain control during approaching end of life*	Sometimes: ■ Discusses spiritual experiences ■ Discusses spiritual concerns ■ Shares feelings about dying	Spiritual Support [5420]/ *Assisting the client to feel balance and connection with a greater power*	■ Be available to listen to client's feelings ■ Be open to client's feelings about illness and death ■ Use values clarification techniques to help client clarify beliefs and values, as appropriate ■ Encourage the use of spiritual resources, if desired

*The NOC # for desired outcomes and the NIC # for nursing interventions are listed in brackets following the appropriate outcome or intervention. Outcomes, indicators, interventions, and activities selected are only a sample of those suggested by NOC and NIC and should be further individualized for each client.

ognizing and validating inner resources of an individual, such as coping methods, humor, motivation, self-determination, positive attitude, and optimism. It can also include assisting the client to leave a legacy by storytelling and/or recording life stories for family and friends, and encouraging creative expression through art, music, and writing. (This keeps the imagination alive and serves to regenerate the body, mind, and spirit.) Fostering ways for clients to keep in touch with nature and maintain a sense of wonder are also forms of spiritual care. Recognizing the seasons, the emergence of flowers in spring, the phases of the moon, the migrations of birds, and the unchanging stars provides examples of orderliness in the universe, even in the midst of chaos and loss. A client with a good measure of spiritual health will find hope, meaning, purpose, and value in existence. Although nursing therapeutics that enhance spiritual health are diverse, some of the most common and most desired include (a) providing presence, (b) supporting religious practices, (c) assisting clients with prayer, and (d) referring clients for spiritual counseling (Taylor & Mamier, 2005).

Providing Presence

Presencing, which is defined as being present, being there, or just being with a client, is a term that identifies one of the competencies incorporated by expert nurses (Zerwekh, 1997). Pettigrew (1990) identified four distinguishing features of presencing:

- Giving of self in the present moment
- Being available with all of the self
- Listening, with full awareness of the privilege of doing so
- Being there in a way that is meaningful to another person

Fredriksson (1999) noted that presencing is a "gift of self" given by the nurse who maintains an attitude of attentiveness toward the client. Thus, nurses who listen attentively to clients yet fail to give of self (i.e., inwardly "make room") diminish their effectiveness.

There are multiple levels of presencing. Osterman and Schwartz-Barcott (1996) identified four ways of being present for clients:

- Presence (when a nurse is physically present but not focused on the client)
- Partial presence (when a nurse is physically present and attending to some task on the client's behalf but not relating to the client on any but the most superficial level)
- Full presence (when a nurse is mentally, emotionally, and physically present; intentionally focusing on the client)
- Transcendent presence (when a nurse is physically, mentally, emotionally, and spiritually present for a client; involves a transpersonal and transforming experience)

Presencing is often the best and sometimes the only intervention to support a client who suffers under circumstances that medical interventions cannot address. When a client is helpless, powerless, and vulnerable, a nurse's presencing can be most beneficial. Rather than worrying about saying or doing "the right thing," nurses should focus on being fully present (Taylor, 2002).

Supporting Religious Practices

During the assessment of the client, the nurse will have obtained specific information about the client's religious preference and practices. Nurses need to consider specific religious practices that will affect nursing care, such as the client's beliefs about birth, death, dress, diet, prayer, sacred symbols, sacred writings, and holy days as discussed earlier in this chapter. See Practice Guidelines for ways the nurse can help clients to continue their usual spiritual practices. Box 41–3 provides health-related information about specific religions.

Assisting Clients with Prayer

Prayer involves a sense of love and connection, as well as a reaching out. It has many health benefits and healing properties (Dossey, 1996). It offers a means for someone to talk to, a mechanism for expressing care, and a sense of serenity and connection with something greater.

Clients may choose to participate in private prayer or want group prayer with family, friends, or clergy. In such situations the nurse's major responsibility is to ensure a quiet environment

---

PRACTICE GUIDELINES **Supporting Religious Practices**

- Create a trusting relationship with the client so that any religious concerns or practices can be openly discussed and addressed.
- If unsure of client religious needs, ask how nurses can assist in having these needs met. Avoid relying on personal assumptions when caring for clients.
- Do not discuss personal spiritual beliefs with a client unless the client requests it. Be sure to assess whether such self-disclosure contributes to a therapeutic nurse–client relationship.
- Inform clients and family caregivers about spiritual support available at your institution (e.g., chapel or meditation room, chaplain services).
- Allow time and privacy for, and provide comfort measures prior to, private worship, prayer, meditation, reading, or other spiritual activities.
- Respect and ensure safety of the client's religious articles (e.g., icons, amulets, clothing, jewelry).

- If desired by client, facilitate clergy or spiritual care specialist visitation. Collaborate with chaplain (if available).
- Prepare client's environment for spiritual rituals or clergy visitations as needed (e.g., have chair near bedside for clergy, create private space).
- Make arrangements with dietitian so that dietary needs can be met. If institution cannot accommodate client's needs, ask family to bring food. (Most religions have some recommendations about diet, such as espousing vegetarianism, rejecting alcohol.)
- Acquaint yourself with the religions, spiritual practices, and cultures of the area in which you are working.
- Remember the difference between facilitating/supporting a client's religious practice and participating in it yourself.
- Ask another nurse to assist you if a particular religious practice makes you uncomfortable.
- All spiritual interventions must be done within agency guidelines.

and privacy. Nursing care may need to be adjusted to accommodate periods for prayer.

Illness can interfere with some clients' ability to pray (Taylor, 2003a). Feelings such as anxiety, fear, guilt, grief, despair, and isolation can produce barriers to relationships in general and to the relationship the person has with the Divine. In these instances the client may ask the nurse to pray with him or her. Prayers with clients should only be done when there is mutual agreement between the clients and those praying with them. Nurses who are unaccustomed to praying aloud or in public may find it helpful to have a formal prayer or a scriptural passage readily available. Because prayer can evoke deep feelings, the nurse needs to spend time with the

client following a prayer to enable the client to express these feelings. Practice Guidelines provide clinical suggestions for praying with clients.

Referring Clients for Spiritual Counseling

There are times when spiritual care is best referred to other members of the health care team. Referrals can be made for hospitalized clients and their families through the hospital chaplain's office if one is available. Nurses in home and community health settings can identify spiritual resources by checking directories of community service agencies, telephone directories, or religious directories that describe available spiritual counselors and the services provided through the religious commu-

---

BOX 41–3   Health-Related Information about Specific Religions: A Sampler

Amish, Mennonite—Likely will not have insurance coverage; rely on religious community for support.

Anglicans, Episcopalians, Roman Catholics—Appreciate receiving Eucharist (Holy Communion), a ritual of ingesting bread and wine (or grape juice) led by clergy or lay leaders to commemorate death of Jesus. Forehead may be marked by priest with ashes on Ash Wednesday (40 days before Easter); no need to wash off. Lenten season (Ash Wednesday to Easter) may involve some degree of abstention from food.

Buddhist—May be vegetarian. Facilitate meditation (may desire incense, visual focal point, use breathing or chanting, etc.).

Christian Scientist—Typically oppose Western medical interventions, relying instead on lay and professional Christian Science practitioners.

Hindu—Most eat no beef; many are vegetarian. Cleanliness highly valued. Many food preferences (e.g., foods fresh or cooked in oil).

Jehovah's Witnesses—Abstain from most blood products; need to discuss alternative treatments such as blood conservation strategies, autologous techniques, hematopoietic agents, nonblood volume expanders, and so on; contact local Jehovah's Witness hospital liaison committee.

Jews—Some observe kosher diet to varying degrees (e.g., avoid pork and shellfish, do not mix dairy and meat). Sabbath observance varies (e.g., Orthodox Jews avoid traveling in vehicles, writing, turning on electric appliances and lights, etc.).

Latter-Day Saints (LDS or Mormons)—Avoid alcohol, caffeine, smoking. Prefer to wear temple undergarments. Arrange for priestly blessing if requested.

Muslim—Respect modesty, avoid nakedness. Provide same-gender nurse if possible. Support prayers five times daily (may need to assist with ritual washing and positioning beforehand). Allow for family and imam (religious leader) to follow Islamic guidelines for burial when client dies. Eat no pork. Children, pregnant, elderly, and sick exempt from daytime fast during month of Ramadan.

Roman Catholics—Sacrament of the Sick (previously known as Last Rites) appropriate for the ill. Be aware that some may think rite means they are dying.

Seventh-Day Adventists—Avoid unnecessary treatments on Saturday (Sabbath). Sabbath begins Friday sundown, ends Saturday sundown. Adventists prefer restful, spirit-nurturing, family activities on Sabbaths. Likely to be vegetarian and abstain from caffeinated beverages. Do not smoke or drink alcohol.

RESEARCH NOTE   Spiritual Care Nursing: What Do Cancer Clients and Family Caregivers Want?

A convenience sample of 156 adult cancer clients and 68 family caregivers self-completed the Nurse Spiritual Therapeutics Scale, which measured how much these clients would want a nurse to provide different spiritual care therapeutics—for example, how much they would want a nurse to help them have quiet time or space, listen to them talk about spiritual concerns, ask them about religious practices, arrange for a minister or chaplain to visit, pray, and so forth.

Findings from these data indicated that while some cancer clients and family members are eager for a nurse to provide some spiritual care "therapeutics," others do not want it. Therapeutics that did not involve much intimacy, are traditional, and are not overtly religious are those most desired by clients. To illustrate, these participants *most wanted* the nurse to provide

- humor,
- private prayer,
- and help to find quiet time or space.

Least wanted therapeutics included instruction about writing or drawing their spirituality, discussion about the difficulties of praying when sick, and help with understanding dreams. No differences were observed between client and family member preferences. A modest, positive correlation was also found between frequency of attending religious services and greater desire for nurse-provided spiritual care.

IMPLICATIONS

The researchers concluded that nurses must be sensitive to providing spiritual care in ways that are welcomed by clients.

Note: From "Spiritual Care Nursing: What Cancer Patients and Family Caregivers Want," by E. J. Taylor and I. Mamier, 2005, *Journal of Advanced Nursing. 49(3),* pp. 260–267.Copyright © 2005 Blackwell Publishing. Reprinted with permission.

PRACTICE GUIDELINES   Praying with Clients

- Clients' preferences for prayer reflect their personalities. That is, introverts may prefer being alone to pray, and their prayers will reflect their capacity for introspection. In contrast, extroverts' prayers may revolve around their relationships with others and be expressed in creative, verbal ways. Similarly, a prayer of a feeling type of client may be emotion filled, whereas the prayer of a thinking-type client may be based on ideas and logic. Structure prayer interventions accordingly.
- When assessing whether a client would like you to pray, ask to pray in a way that allows both of you to feel comfortable if the answer is no. ("Some people tell me prayer helps them to cope with rough times like this. Would you feel comfortable if I prayed with you?")
- Assess how the client approaches the addressee of prayer. For example, a Baptist may pray to Jesus, whereas a Jew would pray directly to God, or Yahweh. This assessment can usually be made while listening to a client talk about religious beliefs.
- Before praying, assess what they would like for you to pray. Listen carefully. The answer may provide greater insight into their fears and concerns.
- Personalize the prayer. Present your client's name and personal concerns to the Divine.
- Prayer can be used to summarize a conversation. This lets the client know you have heard what was said. It may also help the client to view circumstances more objectively.
- Prayer may be the springboard to further discussion or catharsis. Stay with the client after a prayer until there has been time for conversation.
- Follow a prayer with nonverbal communication (e.g., eye contact or touch) to convey "See, I am me, a person, and you are you, and we have returned from our brief journey inward."

- Remember some clients would like to pray aloud with you, just as you may with them. This can be a beautiful experience that nurtures both the client and nurse. It allows the client to reciprocate caring.
- Be mindful of one difference between magic and prayer. Magic invokes a greater power for personal gain. Prayer allows the greater power to do the greater good ("Thy will be done").
- Praying with a client may not involve verbalization. You may feel it will be more comfortable or appropriate if you remain quiet and fully present, praying silently.
- Facilitate the clients' prayer practices. Schedule time for them when they will be undisturbed, palliate distressing symptoms that interfere with praying, help with articles that accompany prayers (e.g., rosaries, prayer garments, books of prayers), and so on.
- In times of distress, a client or loved one may not be able to construct a prayer spontaneously. You may want to teach a centering prayer that is very brief (e.g., "Lord, have mercy/ healing"). Nurses can discuss with care recipients what prayer would benefit them most and encourage them to use it while alone. These prayers may be more beneficial when they are framed in a positive sense. To illustrate, "Jesus loves me" or "The Lord has mercy."
- Encourage clients to think (privately or with you) about what prayer means to them. Offer questions like these: Why do you pray? What do you expect from your praying? Are these expectations appropriate? How content are you with your prayer experiences? Is there a yearning for something more in your prayer experience?

Note: From "Caring for the Spirit," by E. J. Taylor. In *Psychosocial Dimensions of Oncology Nursing Care,* by C. C. Burke (Ed.), 1998, pp. 55–75. Pittsburgh, PA: Oncology Nursing Press. Adapted with permission.

PRACTICE GUIDELINES   When Nurse–Client Spiritual Values Conflict: Steps to Resolution

- Assess spiritual or religious assumptions or beliefs that determine the client's approach to explaining illness and responding to it. For example, What do you think has caused your illness [or distressed your spirit]? What do you think your sickness does to you [spiritually]? How does it work? What do you think are the best things to do for your illness [or spiritual health]? What [spiritual] concerns has your illness caused you? What do you do about them?
- Explain simply to the client your beliefs about the cause (or meaning) and how best to respond to (or cope with) this illness.
- Openly compare with the client how these beliefs differ.
- Objectively discuss how your different religious and cultural backgrounds contribute to these contrasting beliefs.

- Encourage the client to ask questions about your model.
- Support client beliefs and practices that are healthful (from your perspective).
- Accommodate for client beliefs and practices that are neither helpful nor harmful.
- Change and provide alternatives for client beliefs and practices that are harmful without trying to change the underlying belief system, if possible. Engage family member(s) or client's clergy as therapeutic allies.

Note: From "Spirituality, Culture, and Cancer Care," by E. J. Taylor, 2001, *Seminars in Oncology Nursing, 17,* pp. 197–205. Adapted with permission.

nity. Many religious counselors will provide assistance to members of their faith who are not members of their specific religious community. For example, a priest may attend a client in the hospital or at home even though the person is not a member of the priest's parish.

Referrals may be necessary when the nurse makes a diagnosis of spiritual distress. In this situation the nurse and religious counselor can work together to meet the client's needs. One situation the nurse may encounter is client refusal of necessary medical intervention because of religious tenets. In this case the nurse encourages the client, primary care provider, and spiritual adviser to discuss the conflict and consider alternative methods of therapy. The nurse's major role is to provide information the client needs to make an informed decision, and to support the client's decision. See the Practice Guidelines on page 1053.

Evaluating

Using the measurable desired outcomes developed during the planning stage, the nurse collects data needed to judge whether client goals and outcomes have been achieved. See the accompanying Nursing Care Plan.

LIFESPAN CONSIDERATIONS Spiritual Development

CHILDREN

The development of spirituality in children parallels their cognitive and psychosocial development. As children mature, they are increasingly capable of understanding spiritual matters, stating spiritual beliefs, and incorporating spirituality into their lives.

A developing spirituality includes:

- A sense of wholeness, having internal resources and identity.
- Being attached to others, being a part of a greater, even transcendent world.
- Having a sense of meaning and purpose in one's life.
- Being able to express hope, even in the face of fear, uncertainty, and serious illness (Howden, 1992).

Nurses should help ill children and their parents identify and express these qualities. This can be done by actively listening, by offering opportunities to practice religious rituals, and by providing materials for nonverbal expression (e.g., painting, play, music).

ELDERS

Many elders frequently use and highly value religious coping strategies such as prayer. Evidence shows spiritual well-being to be directly correlated with mental health and less medical illness among elders (Koenig, 2002). It is, therefore, important to address the spiritual issues of elders. Elders may be especially concerned about living a purposeful life, about maintaining loving relationships to avoid social isolation, and about preparing for a good death. Nursing care for elders that attends to such spiritual issues includes:

- Supporting meaning-making activities (e.g., conducting a life review or reminiscence therapy; allowing the client to weave together the strands of lived life; encouraging the client to become dedicated to some social, political, religious, or artistic cause; supporting the client to leave a legacy or do an altruistic deed). Such activities provide elders with a sense of purpose for their life and assist them to make sense of the life that they have lived.
- Allowing open discussions about suffering and dying, encouraging client disclosure by asking open-ended questions, and providing responses that are respectful and compassionate. Do not avoid discomforting topics and questions elders raise by imposing positivity, giving "pat" answers, and otherwise minimizing or avoiding their spiritual pain.
- As appropriate, supporting elders to reframe the "losses" of aging as "liberations." For example, elders possess great wisdom and are in a season of life that promotes spiritual growth.

Elders with dementia present special circumstances for spiritual caregiving. Nurses can help those with early stages of dementia to focus on the positives, the "haves" rather than the losses. Allowing elders with dementia to tell their stories allows them to maintain some identity (amidst a disease that threatens the very sense of self), and allows the nurse a window into their world. Elders with dementia can also worship and express their hope and creativity through various art forms (e.g., movement, painting, music). It is also possible for them to experience the compassion of others when they feel their caring touch or hear their soothing voice.

CRITICAL THINKING CHECKPOINT

Terry is a 32-year-old male who received several pints of blood following an automobile crash 10 years ago. Five years ago he was diagnosed with acquired immune deficiency syndrome (AIDS) and is now in the hospital with pneumonia and severe diarrhea. He is very ill and very discouraged. While you are caring for Terry, he comments, "I might as well die right now because I'm not going to get well. My folks were Methodist, but I guess I'm being punished because I'm not very religious."

1. Terry stated that he was "not very religious." Does that mean that he is not spiritual? Explain.
2. What data suggest that Terry may be experiencing spiritual distress?
3. How might illness affect one's spiritual beliefs? Religious beliefs?
4. How might a spiritual assessment be of benefit to both you and Terry?

See Critical Thinking Possibilities in Appendix A.

NURSING CARE PLAN   Spiritual Distress

ASSESSMENT DATA	NURSING DIAGNOSIS	DESIRED OUTCOMES**

Nursing Assessment

Mrs. Sally Horton is a 60-year-old hospitalized homemaker who is recovering from a right radical mastectomy. Her primary care provider told her yesterday that due to metastases of the cancer, her prognosis is poor. This morning her nurse finds her tearful, stating she slept poorly and has no appetite. She asks the nurse, "Why has God done this to me? Perhaps it's because I have sinned in my life. I've not gone to church or spoken to a minister in several years. Is there a chapel in the hospital where I could go and pray? I'm terribly afraid of dying and what awaits me."

Physical Examination

Height: 165.1 cm (5' 5")
Weight: 54.0 kg (199 lb)
Temperature: 36.6°C (98°F)
Pulse: 88 BPM
Respirations: 22/minute
Blood Pressure: 146/86 mm Hg

Large surgical dressing right chest wall and axillary region, dry and intact. Slight edema right hand and arm.

Diagnostic Data

RBC: 3.5×10^6/mL
Hgb: 10.5 g/L
Hct: 35%

Spiritual Distress related to feelings of guilt and alienation from God as evidenced by questioning why "God has done this"; inquiries about praying in a chapel; insomnia; no appetite

Spiritual Health [2001] as evidenced by
- Interacts with spiritual leader of her religion
- Uses a type of spiritual experience that provides her comfort
- Connects with others to share thoughts, feelings, and beliefs

NURSING INTERVENTIONS*/SELECTED ACTIVITIES	RATIONALE

Spiritual Support [5420]

Be open to Mrs. Horton's feelings about illness and death.	*Encourages expression of inner fears and concerns and teaches the client the value of confronting issues.*
Assist her to properly express and relieve anger in appropriate ways.	*Anger can be a source of energy and its release a source of freedom when expressed in a constructive manner.*
Observe and listen empathetically to her communication.	*The nature of spiritual care may directly affect the speed and quality of recovery and/or redefining hope and finding meaning in death.*
Encourage the use of spiritual resources, if desired.	*Spiritual needs may sometimes be overlooked or ignored. Recognizing and respecting the individual's spiritual needs is an important advocacy role for nurses.*

Coping Enhancement [5230]

Create an accepting, nonjudgmental atmosphere.	*Establishes rapport and the therapeutic relationship, which promotes communication and open expression.*
Encourage verbalization of feelings, perceptions, and fears. Allow time for grieving.	*Being with the person who is suffering gives meaning to his or her experience.*
Encourage her to list values that guide behavior in times of tragedy.	*Helps the client clarify values and beliefs by reflecting on past behaviors. Experience is a major source for values development.*

EVALUATION

Outcome met. Mrs. Horton has been visited on several occasions by her minister. She reads scripture each day and has found consolation in reading the Book of Psalms. She states "God is merciful and will help me bear my suffering."

The NOC # for desired outcomes and the NIC # for nursing interventions are listed in brackets following the appropriate outcome or intervention. Outcomes, indicators, interventions, and activities selected are only a sample of those suggested by NOC and NIC and should be further individualized for each client..

CONCEPT MAP Spiritual Distress

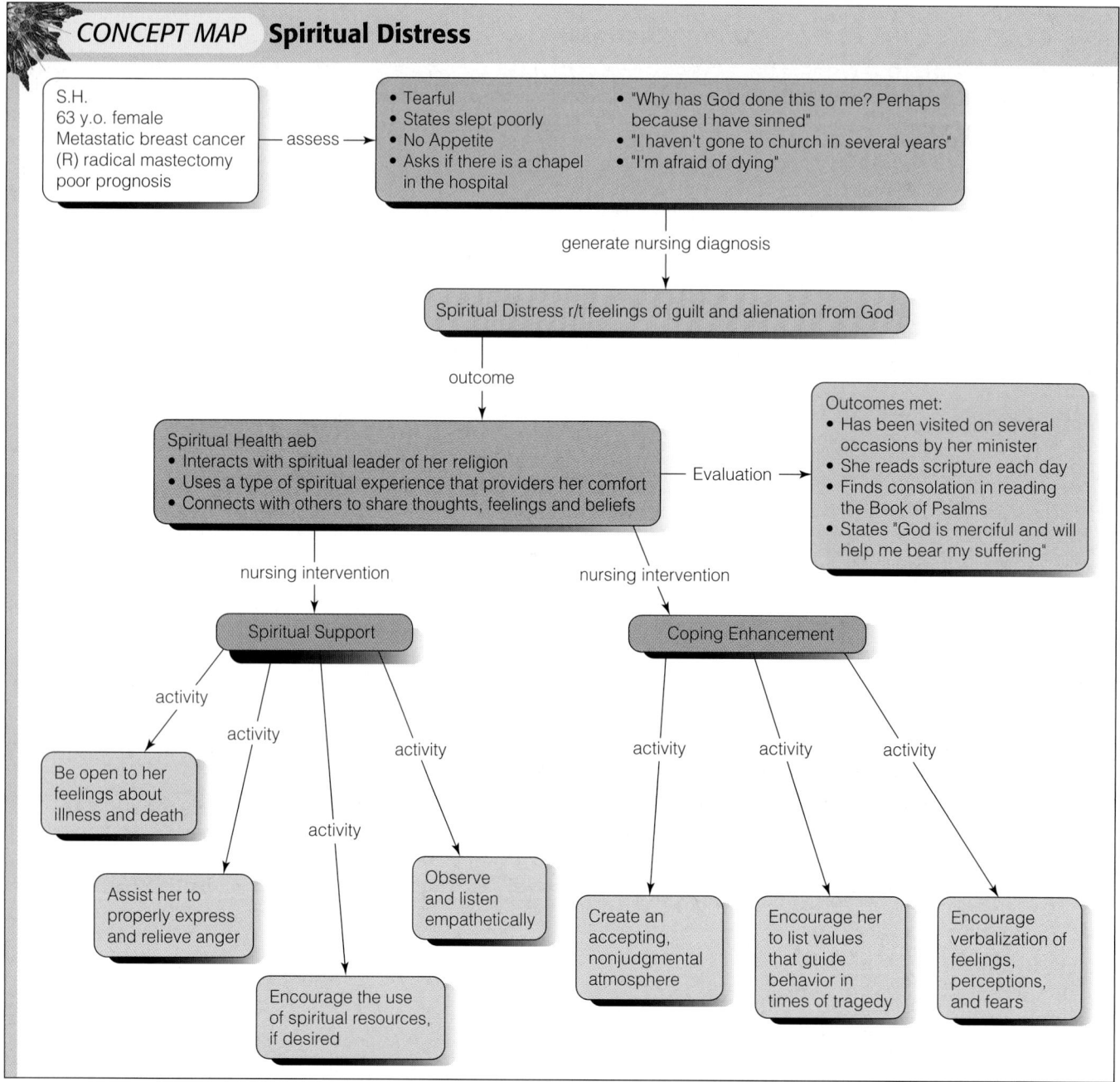

S.H.
63 y.o. female
Metastatic breast cancer
(R) radical mastectomy
poor prognosis

→ assess →

- Tearful
- States slept poorly
- No Appetite
- Asks if there is a chapel in the hospital
- "Why has God done this to me? Perhaps because I have sinned"
- "I haven't gone to church in several years"
- "I'm afraid of dying"

generate nursing diagnosis

Spiritual Distress r/t feelings of guilt and alienation from God

outcome

Spiritual Health aeb
- Interacts with spiritual leader of her religion
- Uses a type of spiritual experience that providers her comfort
- Connects with others to share thoughts, feelings and beliefs

Evaluation

Outcomes met:
- Has been visited on several occasions by her minister
- She reads scripture each day
- Finds consolation in reading the Book of Psalms
- States "God is merciful and will help me bear my suffering"

nursing intervention

Spiritual Support

activity — Be open to her feelings about illness and death

activity — Assist her to properly express and relieve anger

activity — Encourage the use of spiritual resources, if desired

activity — Observe and listen empathetically

nursing intervention

Coping Enhancement

activity — Create an accepting, nonjudgmental atmosphere

activity — Encourage her to list values that guide behavior in times of tragedy

activity — Encourage verbalization of feelings, perceptions, and fears

CHAPTER 41 REVIEW

CHAPTER HIGHLIGHTS

- To implement spiritual care, nurses need to be skilled in establishing a trusting nurse–client relationship.
- Clients have a right to receive care that respects their individual spiritual and religious values.
- Nurses must follow ethical guidelines for providing spiritual care, and not impose personal beliefs or practices on clients.
- Nurses need to be aware of their own spiritual beliefs in order to be comfortable assisting others.

- The spiritual needs of clients and support persons often come into focus at a time of illness. Spiritual beliefs can help people accept illness and plan for what lies ahead.
- Spiritual distress refers to a disturbance in or a challenge to a person's belief or value system that provides strength, hope, and

meaning to life. Possible factors in spiritual distress include physiologic problems, treatment-related concerns, and situational concerns. Spiritual distress may be reflected in a number of behaviors, including depression, anxiety, verbalizations of unworthiness, and fear of death.

- Nurses can support clients' religious practices if they understand needs related to holy days, sacred writings, sacred symbols, prayer and meditation, dietary practices, dress requirements or prohibitions, healing, birth rituals, and death rituals.

- Spiritual assessment can follow a two-tiered approach. While all clients should be screened for spiritual needs, only those who indicate needs require a pertinent, in-depth assessment. The initial spiritual assessment should collect information not only about spiritual beliefs and practices affecting health, but also about how the client desires spiritual care from the health care team.

- Nursing interventions that promote spiritual health include offering one's presence, supporting the client's religious practices, praying with a client, and referring the client to a religious counselor.

TEST YOUR KNOWLEDGE

1. When planning care for an elder residing in your skilled nursing facility who is searching to make life meaningful, which nursing action would be most beneficial?
   1. Assess for depression.
   2. Diagnose and document that the client has "spiritual distress."
   3. Keep the client busy with social activities.
   4. Explore with the client their desired legacy.

2. A client's wife asks the nurse to pray for her. What would be the best initial response for a nurse who believes in prayer?
   1. "May I call the chaplain to come and pray with you?"
   2. "I know your faith is important to you. It is to me, too."
   3. "What should I pray for?"
   4. "Isn't it wonderful that we have a God with whom we can share our concerns?"

3. A client is experiencing severe pain that cannot be controlled by analgesics. An appropriate intervention is full presencing, which involves which of the following?
   1. Physical presence
   2. Physical presence with mental awareness of the client
   3. Physical, mental, and emotional presence
   4. Physical, mental, emotional, and spiritual presence

4. A client reports, "Cancer was the best thing that happened to me! It is making me appreciate life so much more." This statement fits best with which NANDA diagnosis?
   1. *Spiritual Distress*
   2. *Risk for Spiritual Distress*
   3. *Readiness for Enhanced Spiritual Well-Being*
   4. *Cognitive Denial*

5. A dying client states, "Part of what makes dying hard is that I don't know for sure where I'm going. Nurse, what do you believe happens in the hereafter?" Which ethical guideline should guide your response?
   1. Never share personal spiritual beliefs.
   2. Share all spiritual beliefs, favoring none.
   3. Share only your beliefs.
   4. First assess client beliefs.

6. Research evidence that supports providing spiritual care to elders suggests that:
   1. Elders are not very religious, but are very spiritual.
   2. Elders who are more religious have more illness.

   3. Spiritual health and mental health are correlated.
   4. Increased spiritual well-being is found among elders with depression.

7. A client in the emergency department, who needs red blood cells, is a Jehovah's Witness who believes it would be medical rape for the nurse to give the prescribed blood transfusion. Which of the following statements would most likely lead to a resolution for this conflict?
   1. You must accept the transfusion or else leave.
   2. Don't worry, you can ask for pardon after taking the blood.
   3. May I please call a representative of your religion so that I can understand your position better?
   4. I understand your position; I'll be here with you as you die.

8. An 88-year-old woman has just been admitted to a skilled nursing facility. She tells the nurse that she has been a Sunday School teacher and volunteers for many of her church's projects. Which of the following NANDA diagnoses is most appropriate?
   1. *Risk for Spiritual Distress*
   2. *Risk for Impaired Religiosity*
   3. *Readiness for Enhanced Spiritual Well-Being*
   4. *Impaired Religiosity*

9. Which of the following is an appropriate spiritual screening or assessment question?
   1. "Tell me more about your religion."
   2. "How can we support your spiritual beliefs and practices?"
   3. "How has your prayer experience been affected by your illness?"
   4. "What do you see as the purpose or mission for your life?"

10. The mother of a pediatric client status, "I can't understand why God would allow this to happen to my innocent child!" Which NANDA diagnosis is most accurate?
    1. *Spiritual Distress* related to search for meaning of child's illness
    2. *Impaired Religiosity* related to anger at God
    3. *Ineffective Coping* related to anger
    4. *Risk for Spiritual Distress* related to threatened sense of hope

See Answers to Test Your Knowledge in Appendix A.

EXPLORE MEDIALINK www.prenhall.com/berman

DVD-ROM
- Audio Glossary
- NCLEX Review
- Video: Emotional, Social, and Spiritual Needs

COMPANION WEBSITE
- Additional NCLEX Review
- Case Study: Supporting a Client's Spiritual Practices
- Care Plan Activity: Care of a Paralyzed Client
- Application Activities:
  Researching Atheism
  Spirituality, Health, and Holistic Nursing
- Links to Resources

READINGS AND REFERENCES

SUGGESTED READINGS

Andrews, M. M., & Hanson, P. A. (2003). Religion, culture, and nursing. In M. M. Andrews & J. S. Boyle (Eds.), *Transcultural concepts in nursing care* (4th ed., pp. 432–502). Philadelphia: Lippincott.
The authors discuss religious practices, holy days, sacraments, beliefs related to healing, and beliefs of major world religions about diet, medications, medical treatment, and surgical procedures. Andrews and Hanson also discuss health issues that may be controversial within the religious group, the religious support system for ill believers, and religion-specific issues related to death and dying.

Burkhardt, M. A., & Nagai-Jacobson, M. G. (2002). *Spirituality: Living our connectedness.* Albany, NY: Delmar.
These nurse authors write thoroughly about ways health care professionals can heal themselves through nurturing their own spirituality. They discuss numerous approaches to spiritual self-care.

Carson, V. B., & Koenig, H. G. (2004). *Spiritual caregiving: Healthcare as ministry.* Philadelphia: Templeton Foundation Press.
This book is authored by a nurse and physician. The description of spiritual caregiving is peppered with anecdotes from clinicians. A thorough listing of resources is provided in the appendices.

Sorajjakool, S., & Lamberton, H. (Eds.). (2004). *Spirituality, health, and wholeness: An introductory guide for health care professionals.* New York: Haworth Press.
Although most contributors to this volume are trained in psychology, theology, and chaplaincy, this book is very useful to nurses wanting a more in-depth look at selected aspects of spiritual caregiving. Chapters address such diverse topics as mirthful laughter, a theology of wholeness, working with difficult clients, racial discrimination in health care, spiritual care basic principles, and spiritually coping with trauma.

Taylor, E. J. (2002). *Spiritual care: Nursing theory, research, and practice.* Upper Saddle River, NJ: Prentice Hall.
This nurse author describes in practical terms how nurses can nurture spiritual health in their clients. Based on theory and research, she discusses conducting spiritual assessments; documentation and diagnosis of spiritual concerns; how to assist clients in transforming tragedy; how to support spiritual rituals like prayer; and how to nurture spirituality with journal writing, art, dream analysis, empathic listening, and more.

RELATED RESEARCH

Halstead, M. T., & Hull, M. (2001). Struggling with paradoxes: The process of spiritual development in women with cancer. *Oncology Nursing Forum, 28,* 1534–1544.

Knestrick, J., & Lohri-Posey, B. (2005). Spirituality and health: Perceptions of older women in a rural senior high rise. *Journal of Gerontological Nursing, 31*(10), 44–50.

Kociszewski, C. (2004). Spiritual care: A phenomenologic study of critical care nurses. *Heart & Lung, 33,* 401–411.

Taylor, E. J., & Outlaw, F. H. (2002). Use of prayer among persons with cancer. *Holistic Nursing Practice, 16*(3), 46–60.

Van Leeuwen, R., & Cusveller, B. (2004). Nursing competencies for spiritual care. *Journal of Advanced Nursing, 48,* 234–246.

REFERENCES

Burkhardt, M. A. (1989). Spirituality: An analysis of the concept. *Holistic Nursing Practice, 3*(3), 69–77.

Burkhart, L. (2005). A click away: Documenting spiritual care. *Journal of Christian Nursing, 22*(1), 6–12.

Carpenito-Moyet, L. J. (2006). *Nursing diagnosis: Application to clinical practice* (11th ed.). Philadelphia: Lippincott.

Cole, B., Benore, E., & Pargament, K. I. (2004). Spirituality and coping with trauma. In S. Sorajjakool & H. Lamberton (Eds.), *Spirituality, health, and wholeness* (pp. 49–76). New York: Haworth Press.

Coward, D. D. (1990). The lived experience of self-transcendence in women with advanced breast cancer. *Nursing Science Quarterly, 3*(4), 162–169.

Dameron, C. M. (2005). Spiritual assessment made easy... with acronyms! *Journal of Christian Nursing, 22*(1), 14–16.

Denny, F. M. (1993). Islam and the Muslim community. In H. Byron Earhart (Ed.), *Religious traditions of the world* (pp. 603–713). New York: HarperSanFrancisco.

Dochterman, J. M., & Bulechek, G. M. (Eds.). (2004). *Nursing interventions classification (NIC)* (4th ed.). St. Louis, MO: Mosby.

Dossey, L. (1996). *Prayer is good medicine. How to reap the benefits of prayer.* New York: HarperCollins.

Dossey, L. (1999). Healing and the nonlocal mind: Interview by Bonnie Horrigan. *Alternative Therapies in Health and Medicine, 5*(6), 85–93.

Ellison, C. W. (1983, April). Spiritual well-being: Conceptualization and measurement. *Journal of Psychology and Theology, 11,* 330–340.

Fishbane, M. (1993). Judaism: Revelation and traditions. In H. Byron Earhart (Ed.), *Religious traditions of the world* (pp. 373–484). New York: HarperSanFrancisco.

Fowler, J. W. (1981). *Stages of faith development: The psychology of human development and the quest for meaning.* San Francisco: Harper & Row.

Frankiel, S. S. (1993). Christianity: A way of salvation. In H. Byron Earhart (Ed.), *Religious traditions of the world* (pp. 484–601). New York: HarperSanFrancisco.

Fredriksson, L. (1999). Modes of relating in a caring conversation: A research synthesis on presence, touch, and listening. *Journal of Advanced Nursing, 30,* 1167–1176.

Gill, S. D. (1987). Prayer. In M. Eliade (Ed.), *The encyclopedia of religion* (pp. 489–492). New York: Macmillan.

Griffith, J. K. (1996). *The religious aspects of nursing care.* Vancouver, BC: Author.

Howden, J. W. (1992). *Development and psychometric characteristics of the Spirituality Assessment Scale.* Unpublished doctoral dissertation, Texas Women's University, Denton.

Joint Commission on Accreditation of Healthcare Organizations. (2000). *Hospital accreditation standards.* Oakbrook, IL: Author.

Jourard, S. (1971). *The transparent self.* London: D. Van Nostrand.

Koenig, H. G. (2002). *Spirituality in patient care: Why, how, when, and what.* Radnor, PA: Templeton Press.

Martsolf, D. S., & Mickley, J. R. (1998). The concept of spirituality in nursing theories: Differing world-views and extent of focus. *Journal of Advanced Nursing, 27,* 294–303.

Massey, K., Fitchett, G., & Roberts, P. A. (2004). In K. L. Mauk & N. K. Schmidt (Eds.), *Spiritual care in nursing practice. Assessment and diagnosis in spiritual care* (Chapter 14, pp. 209–242). Philadelphia: Lippincott Williams & Wilkins.

Mauk, K. L., & Schmidt, N. K. (2004). *Spiritual care in nursing practice.* Philadelphia: Lippincott Williams & Wilkins.

Mickley, J. R., & Cowles, K. (2001). Ameliorating the tension: Use of forgiveness for healing. *Oncology Nursing Forum, 28,* 31–38.

Moorhead, S., Johnson, M., & Maas, M. (2004). *Iowa intervention project: Nursing outcome classification.* St. Louis, MO: Mosby.

Moschella, V. D., Pressman, K. R., Pressman, P., & Weissman, D. E. (1997). The problem of theodicy and religious responses to cancer. *Journal of Religion & Health, 36*(1), 17–20.

NANDA International. (2007). *NANDA nursing diagnoses: Definitions and classification 2007–2008.* Philadelphia: Author.

Osterman, P., & Schwartz-Barcott, D. (1996). Presence: Four ways of being there. *Nursing Forum, 31*(2), 23–30.

Pettigrew, J. (1990). Intensive nursing care: The ministry of presence. *Critical Care Nursing Clinics of North America, 2,* 503–508.

Pilch, J. J. (1998, May/June). Wellness spirituality. *Health Values, 12,* 28–31.

Poloma, M. M., & Gallup, G. H., Jr. (1991). *Varieties of prayer: A survey report.* Philadelphia: Trinity Press International.

Reed, P. G. (1992). An emerging paradigm for the investigation of spirituality in nursing. *Research in Nursing and Health, 15,* 349–357.

Stephenson, C. (1991). The concept of hope revisited for nursing. *Journal of Advances in Nursing, 16,* 1456–1461.

Taylor, E. J. (1998). Caring for the spirit. In C. C. Burke (Ed.), *Psychosocial dimensions of oncology nursing care.* Pittsburgh: Oncology Nursing Press.

Taylor, E. J. (2001). Spirituality, culture, and cancer care. *Seminars in Oncology Nursing, 17*(3), 197–205.

Taylor, E. J. (2002). *Spiritual care: Nursing theory, research, and practice.* Upper Saddle River, NJ: Prentice Hall.

Taylor, E. J. (2003a). Nurses caring for the spirit: Patients with cancer and family caregiver expectations. *Oncology Nursing Forum, 30,* 585–594.

Taylor, E. J. (2003b). Prayer's clinical issues and implications. *Holistic Nursing Practice, 17*(4), 179–188.

Taylor, E. J. (2005). What have we learned from spiritual care research? *Journal of Christian Nursing, 22*(1), 22–28.

Taylor, E. J., & Mamier, I. (2005). Spiritual care nursing: what cancer patients and family caregivers want. *Journal of Advanced Nursing, 49*(3), 260–267.

Ulanov, A., & Ulanov, B. (1983). *Primary speech: A psychology of prayer.* Atlanta, GA: John Knox Press. (Classic.)

Vardey, L. (1996). *God in all worlds.* Toronto: Vintage Canada.

Westerhoff, J. (1976). *Will our children have faith?* New York: Seabury Press.

Winslow, G. R., & Winslow, B. W. (2003). Examining the ethics of praying with patients. *Holistic Nursing Practice, 17*(4), 170–177.

Zerwekh, J. V. (1997). The practice of presencing. *Seminars in Oncology Nursing, 13,* 260–262.

SELECTED BIBLIOGRAPHY

Butcher, H. K., & McGonigal-Kenney, M. (2005). Depression & dispiritedness in later life. *American Journal of Nursing, 105*(12), 52–61.

Murray, C. K. (1998). Say a little prayer. *Nursing, 28*(6), 55.

Plotnikoff, G. A. (2000). Should medicine reach out to the spirit? Understanding a patient's spiritual foundation can guide appropriate care. *Postgraduate Medicine, 108*(6), 19–21.

Sherwood, G. D. (2000). The power of nurse-client encounters: Interpreting spiritual themes. *Journal of Holistic Nursing, 18*(2), 159–175.

Sulmasy, D. P. (2001). Addressing the religious and spiritual needs of dying patients. *Western Journal of Medicine, 175*(4), 251–254.

Taylor, E. J., Outlaw, F. H., Bernardo, T., & Roy, A. (1999). Spiritual conflicts associated with praying about cancer. *Psycho-Oncology, 8,* 386–414.

Van Dover, L. J., & Bacon, J. M. (2001). Spiritual care in nursing practice: A close-up view. *Nursing Forum, 36*(3), 18–28.

CHAPTER 42

Stress and Coping

LEARNING OUTCOMES

After completing this chapter, you will be able to:

1. Differentiate the concepts of stress as a stimulus, as a response, and as a transaction.

2. Describe the three stages of Selye's general adaptation syndrome.

3. Identify physiologic, psychologic, and cognitive indicators of stress.

4. Differentiate four levels of anxiety.

5. Identify behaviors related to specific ego defense mechanisms.

6. Discuss types of coping and coping strategies.

7. Identify essential aspects of assessing a client's stress and coping patterns.

8. Identify nursing diagnoses related to stress.

9. Describe interventions to help clients minimize and manage stress.

Stress is a universal phenomenon. All people experience it. Parents refer to the stress of raising children, working people talk of the stress of their jobs, and students at all levels talk of the stress of school. Stress can result from both positive and negative experiences. For example, a bride preparing for her wedding, a graduate preparing to start a new job, and a husband concerned about caring for his wife and family following a diagnosis of cancer all experience stress reactions.

The concept of stress is important because it provides a way of understanding the person as a being who responds in totality (mind, body, and spirit) to a variety of changes that take place in daily life.

CONCEPT OF STRESS

Stress is a condition in which the person experiences changes in the normal balanced state. A **stressor** is any event or stimulus that causes an individual to experience stress. When a person faces stressors, responses are referred to as *coping strategies, coping responses,* or *coping mechanisms.*

Sources of Stress

There are many sources of stress. They can be broadly classified as internal or external stressors, or developmental or situational stressors. *Internal stressors* originate within a person, for example, infection or feelings of depression. *External stressors* originate outside the individual, for example, a move to another city, a death in the family, or pressure from peers. *Developmental stressors* occur at predictable times throughout an individual's life (Table 42–1). *Situational stressors* are unpredictable and may occur at any time during life. Situational stress may be positive or negative. The following are examples of this type of stress:

- Death of a family member
- Marriage or divorce
- Birth of a child
- New job
- Illness

The degree to which any of these events has positive or negative effects can depend to some extent on an individual's developmental stage. For example, the death of a parent may be more stressful for a 12-year-old than for a 40-year-old.

TABLE 42–1 Selected Stressors Associated with Developmental Stages

DEVELOPMENTAL STAGE	STRESSORS
Child	Beginning school Establishing peer relationships Peer competition
Adolescent	Changing physique Relationships involving sexual attraction Exploring independence Choosing a career
Young adult	Marriage Leaving home Managing a home Getting started in an occupation Continuing one's education Children
Middle adult	Physical changes of aging Maintaining social status and standard of living Helping teenage children to become independent Aging parents
Older adult	Decreasing physical abilities and health Changes in residence Retirement and reduced income Death of spouse and friends

Effects of Stress

Stress can have physical, emotional, intellectual, social, and spiritual consequences. Usually the effects are mixed, because stress affects the whole person. Physically, stress can threaten a person's physiologic homeostasis. Emotionally, stress can produce negative or nonconstructive feelings about the self. Intellectually, stress can influence a person's perceptual and problem-solving abilities. Socially, stress can alter a person's relationships with others. Spiritually, stress can challenge one's beliefs and values. Many conditions have been linked to stress (Figure 42-1 ■).

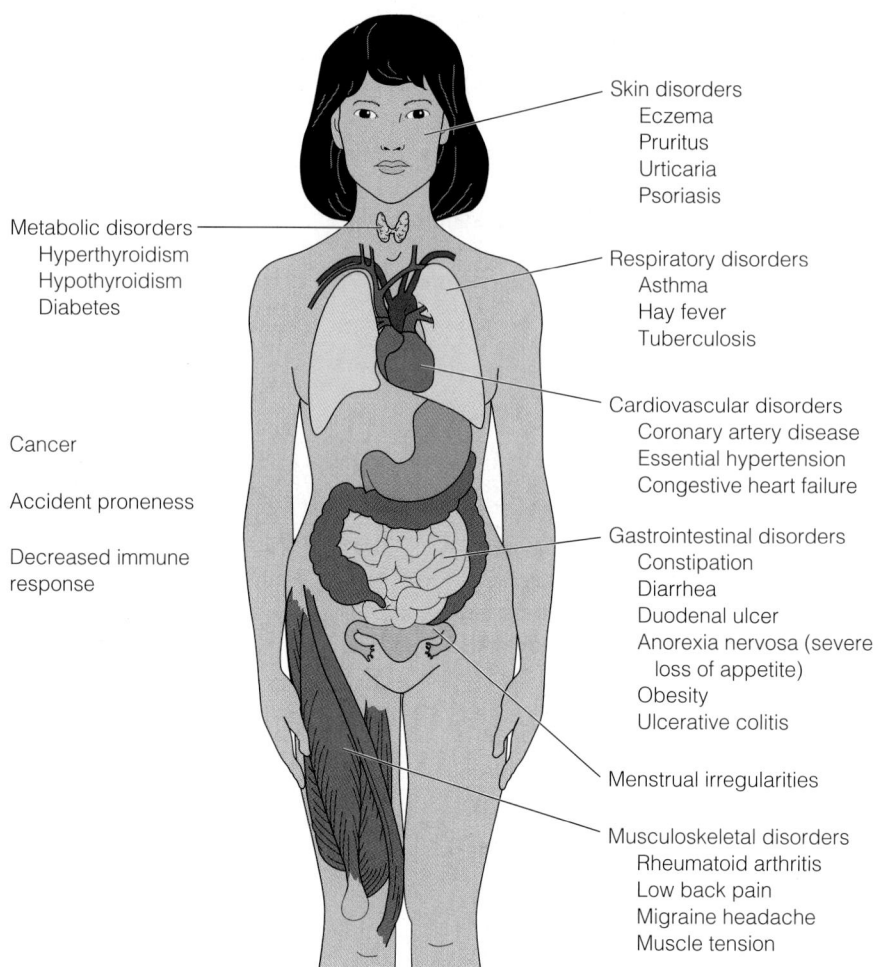

Figure 42-1 ■ Some disorders that can be caused or aggravated by stress.

(From *Health and Wellness: A Holistic Approach*, 9th ed. (p. 46), by G. Edlin and E. Golanty, 2007, Boston: Jones & Bartlett. Adapted with permission.)

MODELS OF STRESS

Models of stress assist nurses to identify the stressor in a particular situation and to predict the individual's responses. Nurses can use these models to assist clients in strengthening healthy coping responses and in adjusting unhealthy, unproductive responses. Three main models of stress are stimulus based, response based, and transaction based.

Stimulus-Based Models

In **stimulus-based stress models,** stress is defined as a stimulus, a life event, or a set of circumstances that arouses physiologic and/or psychologic reactions that may increase the individual's vulnerability to illness. In their classic work, Holmes and Rahe (1967) assigned a numerical value to 43 life changes or events. The most recent version of that scale includes 77 items (Miller & Rahe, 1997), and a shortened version (54 items, full stress and coping inventory competed in 15 minutes) was created more recently (Rahe & Tolles, 2002). The scale of stressful life events is used to document a person's relatively recent experiences, such as divorce, pregnancy, and retirement. In this view, both positive and negative events are considered stressful.

Similar scales have since been developed, but all scales should be used with caution because the degree of stress an event presents is highly individual. For example, a divorce may be highly traumatic to one person and cause relatively little anxiety to another. In addition, many scales have not been tested for age, socioeconomic status, or cultural sensitivity.

Response-Based Models

Stress may also be considered as a response. This definition was developed and described by Selye (1956, 1976) as "the nonspecific response of the body to any kind of demand made upon it" (1976, p. 1).

Selye's stress response is characterized by a chain or pattern of physiologic events called the **general adaptation syndrome (GAS)** or *stress syndrome*. To differentiate the cause of stress from the response to stress, Selye (1976) used the term *stressor* to denote any factor that produces stress and disturbs the body's equilibrium. Because stress is a state of the body, it can be observed only by the changes it produces in the body. This response of the body, the stress syndrome or GAS, occurs with the release of certain adaptive hormones and subsequent changes in the structure and chemical composition of the body. Parts of the body particularly

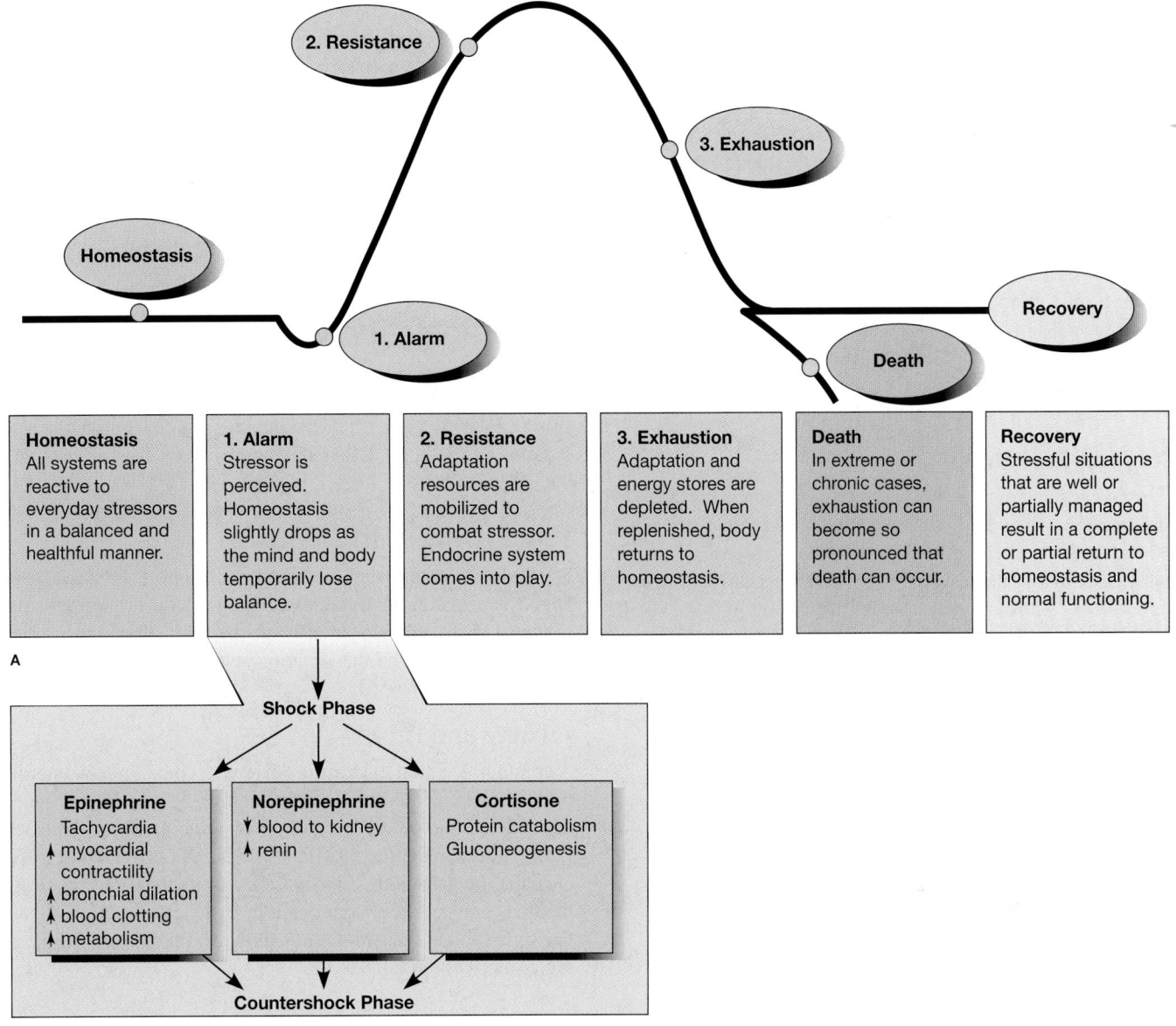

Figure 42-2 ■ The three stages of adaptation to stress: The alarm reaction, the stage of resistance, and the stage of exhaustion.

(*Note:* "A" is from *Wellness: Concepts and Application,* 6th ed. (p. 298), by D. J. Anspaugh, M. Hamrick, and F. D. Rosato, 2005, New York: McGraw-Hill. Reprinted with permission.)

affected by stress are the gastrointestinal tract, the adrenal glands, and the lymphatic structures. With prolonged stress, the adrenal glands enlarge considerably; the lymphatic structures, such as the thymus, spleen, and lymph nodes, atrophy (shrink); and deep ulcers appear in the lining of the stomach.

In addition to adapting globally, the body can also react locally; that is, one organ or a part of the body reacts alone. This is referred to as the **local adaptation syndrome (LAS).** One example of the LAS is inflammation. Selye (1976) proposed that both the GAS and the LAS have three stages: alarm reaction, resistance, and exhaustion (see Figure 42-2 ■).

Alarm Reaction

The initial reaction of the body is the **alarm reaction,** which alerts the body's defenses. Selye (1976) divided this stage into two parts: the shock phase and the countershock phase.

During the **shock phase** (Figure 42-2, *B*), the stressor may be perceived consciously or unconsciously by the person. Stressors stimulate the sympathetic nervous system, which in turn stimulates the hypothalamus. The hypothalamus releases corticotropin-releasing hormone (CRH), which stimulates the anterior pituitary gland to release adrenocorticotropic hormone (ACTH). During times of stress, the adrenal medulla secretes epinephrine and norepinephrine in response to sympathetic stimulation. Significant body responses to epinephrine include the following:

1. Increased myocardial contractility, which increases cardiac output and blood flow to active muscles
2. Bronchial dilation, which allows increased oxygen intake
3. Increased blood clotting
4. Increased cellular metabolism

5. Increased fat mobilization to make energy available and to synthesize other compounds needed by the body

The principal effect of norepinephrine is decreased blood to the kidneys and increased secretion of renin. Renin is an enzyme that hydrolyzes one of the blood proteins to produce angiotensin. Angiotensin tends to increase the blood pressure by constricting arterioles. The sum of all of these adrenal hormonal effects permits the person to perform far more strenuous physical activity than would otherwise be possible. The person is then ready for "fight or flight." This primary response is short-lived, lasting from 1 minute to 24 hours.

The second part of the alarm reaction is called the **countershock phase.** During this time, the changes produced in the body during the shock phase are reversed. Thus, a person is best mobilized to react during the shock phase of the alarm reaction.

Stage of Resistance

The second stage in the GAS and LAS syndromes, the **stage of resistance,** is when the body's adaptation takes place. In other words, the body attempts to cope with the stressor and to limit the stressor to the smallest area of the body that can deal with it.

Stage of Exhaustion

During the third stage, the **stage of exhaustion,** the adaptation that the body made during the second stage cannot be maintained. This means that the ways used to cope with the stressor have been exhausted. If adaptation has not overcome the stressor, the stress effects may spread to the entire body. At the end of this stage, the body may either rest and return to normal, or death may be the ultimate consequence. The end of this stage depends largely on the adaptive energy resources of the individual, the severity of the stressor, and the external adaptive resources that are provided, such as oxygen.

Transaction-Based Models

Transactional theories of stress are based on the work of Lazarus (1966), who stated that the stimulus theory and the response theory do not consider individual differences. Neither theory explains which factors lead some people and not others to respond effectively nor interprets why some people are able to adapt for longer periods than are others.

Although Lazarus recognizes that certain environmental demands and pressures produce stress in substantial numbers of people, he emphasizes that people and groups differ in their sensitivity and vulnerability to certain types of events, as well as in their interpretations and reactions. For example, in terms of illness, one person may respond with denial, another with anxiety, and still another with depression. To explain variations among individuals under comparable conditions, the Lazarus model takes into account cognitive processes that intervene between the encounter and the reaction, and the factors that affect the nature of this process. In contrast to Selye, who focuses on physiologic responses, Lazarus includes mental and psychologic components or responses as part of his concept of stress.

The Lazarus **transactional stress theory** encompasses a set of cognitive, affective, and adaptive (coping) responses that arise out of person–environment transactions. The person and the en-

vironment are inseparable; each affects and is affected by the other. Stress "refers to any event in which environmental demands, internal demands, or both tax or exceed the adaptive resources of an individual, social system, or tissue system" (Monat & Lazarus, 1991, p. 3). The individual responds to perceived environmental changes by adaptive or coping responses.

INDICATORS OF STRESS

Indicators of an individual's stress may be physiologic, psychologic, or cognitive.

Physiologic Indicators

Responses to stress vary depending on the individual's perception of events. The physiologic signs and symptoms of stress result from activation of the sympathetic and neuroendocrine systems of the body. Clinical Manifestations lists physiologic indicators of stress.

Psychologic Indicators

Psychologic manifestations of stress include anxiety, fear, anger, depression, and unconscious ego defense mechanisms. Some of these coping patterns are helpful; others are a hindrance, depending on the situation and the length of time they are used or experienced.

Anxiety and Fear

A common reaction to stress is **anxiety,** a state of mental uneasiness, apprehension, dread, or foreboding or a feeling of helplessness related to an impending or anticipated unidentified threat to self or significant relationships. Anxiety can be experienced at the conscious, subconscious, or unconscious level. As many as one-fourth of Americans experience an anxiety disorder sometime in their lifetime, over half of which are debilitating (Antai-Otong, 2003).

CLINICAL MANIFESTATIONS **STRESS**

- Pupils dilate to increase visual perception when serious threats to the body arise.
- Sweat production (diaphoresis) increases to control elevated body heat due to increased metabolism.
- Heart rate and cardiac output increase to transport nutrients and by-products of metabolism more efficiently.
- Skin is pallid because of constriction of peripheral blood vessels, an effect of norepinephrine.
- Sodium and water retention increase due to release of mineralocorticoids, which increases blood volume.
- Rate and depth of respirations increase because of dilation of the bronchioles, promoting hyperventilation.
- Urinary output decreases.
- Mouth may be dry.
- Peristalsis of the intestines decreases, resulting in possible constipation and flatus.
- For serious threats, mental alertness improves.
- Muscle tension increases to prepare for rapid motor activity or defense.
- Blood sugar increases because of release of glucocorticoids and gluconeogenesis.

Anxiety may be manifested on four levels:

1. Mild anxiety produces a slight arousal state that enhances perception, learning, and productive abilities. Most healthy people experience mild anxiety, perhaps as a feeling of mild restlessness that prompts a person to seek information and ask questions.
2. Moderate anxiety increases the arousal state to a point where the person expresses feelings of tension, nervousness, or concern. Perceptual abilities are narrowed. Attention is focused more on a particular aspect of a situation than on peripheral activities.
3. Severe anxiety consumes most of the person's energies and requires intervention. Perception is further decreased. The person, unable to focus on what is really happening, focuses on only one specific detail of the situation generating the anxiety.
4. Panic is an overpowering, frightening level of anxiety causing the person to lose control. It is less frequently experienced than other levels of anxiety. The perception of a panicked person can be affected to the degree that the person distorts events.

Table 42–2 lists indicators of these levels.

Fear is an emotion or feeling of apprehension aroused by impending or seeming danger, pain, or another perceived threat. The fear may be in response to something that has already occurred, in response to an immediate or current threat, or in response to something the person believes will happen. The object of fear may or may not be based in reality. For example, the beginning nursing student may be fearful in anticipation of the first experience in a client care setting. The student may fear that the client will not want to be cared for by the student or that the student might inadvertently harm the client.

Anxiety and fear differ in four ways:

- The source of anxiety may not be identifiable; the source of fear is identifiable.
- Anxiety is related to the future, that is, to an anticipated event. Fear is related to the present.
- Anxiety is vague, whereas fear is definite.
- Anxiety is the result of psychologic or emotional conflict; fear is the result of a discrete physical or psychologic entity.

CLINICAL ALERT

Mild or moderate anxiety motivates goal-directed behavior. In this sense, anxiety is an effective coping strategy. For example, mild anxiety motivates students to study. Excessive anxiety, however, often has destructive effects. ■

Anger

Anger is an emotional state consisting of a subjective feeling of animosity or strong displeasure. People may feel guilty when they feel anger because they have been taught that to feel angry is wrong. However, anger can be expressed in a nonalienating verbal manner; it is then considered a positive emotion and a sign of emotional maturity because growth and beneficial interactions result from it.

A verbal expression of anger can be considered a signal to others of one's internal psychologic discomfort and a call for assistance to deal with perceived stress. In contrast, hostility is usually marked by overt antagonism and harmful or destructive behavior; aggression is an unprovoked attack or a hostile, injurious, or destructive action or outlook; and violence is the exertion of physical force to injure or abuse. Verbally expressed anger differs from hostility, aggression, and violence, but it can lead to destructiveness and violence if the anger persists unabated.

TABLE 42–2 Indicators of Levels of Anxiety

CATEGORY	LEVEL OF ANXIETY			
	MILD	**MODERATE**	**SEVERE**	**PANIC**
Verbalization changes	Increased questioning	Voice tremors and pitch changes	Communication difficult to understand	Communication may not be understandable
Motor activity changes	Mild restlessness	Tremors, facial twitches, and shakiness	Increased motor activity, inability to relax	Increased motor activity, agitation
	Sleeplessness	Increased muscle tension	Fearful facial expression	Unpredictable responses
Perception and attention changes	Feelings of increased arousal and alertness	Narrowed focus of attention	Inability to focus or concentrate	Trembling, poor motor coordination
		Able to focus but selectively inattentive	Easily distracted	Perception distorted or exaggerated
	Uses learning to adapt	Learning slightly impaired	Learning severely impaired	Unable to learn or function
Respiratory and circulatory changes	None	Slightly increased respiratory and heart rates	Tachycardia, hyperventilation	Dyspnea, palpitations, choking, chest pain, or pressure
Other changes	None	Mild gastric symptoms (e.g., "butterflies in the stomach")	Headache, dizziness, nausea	Feeling of impending doom
				Paresthesia, sweating

Note: From *Nursing Diagnosis: Application to Clinical Practice,* 11th ed. (pp. 97–109), by L. J. Carpenito-Moyet, 2006, Philadelphia: Lippincott; *Mental Health Nursing,* 5th ed. (p. 273), by K. L. Fontaine and J. S. Fletcher, 2003, Upper Saddle River, NJ: Prentice Hall. Adapted with permission.

DRUG CAPSULE   selective serotonin reuptake inhibitor (SSRI)   *sertraline HCl* (Zoloft)

THE CLIENT TAKING ANTI-ANXIETY MEDICATION

Sertraline is approved to treat depression, social anxiety disorder, posttraumatic stress disorder (PTSD), panic disorder, obsessive-compulsive disorder (OCD), and premenstrual dysphoric disorder (PMDD) in adults over age 18. It is also approved for OCD in children and adolescents age 6 to 17 years. It prevents serotonin from being reabsorbed by the sending nerve cells so that more serotonin is available for acceptance by the receiving nerve cells.

NURSING RESPONSIBILITIES

- Sertraline may be given with or without meals but with sufficient water. The concentrate must be diluted after measurement.
- Setraline is available as oral concentrate or tablets. It is taken once per day.
- This medication should not be taken if the client is already taking monoamine oxidase inhibitors (MAOI) or pimozide. Use with caution in clients taking anticoagulant medications. Always check the list of client medications for possible interactions.
- Adverse effects may include dry mouth, insomnia, sexual side effects, diarrhea, nausea, and sleepiness.
- There is a warning from the U.S. Food and Drug Administration (FDA) on all materials related to antidepressants due to an increased risk of suicidal thoughts and behavior from 2% to 4% in people under age 18. This risk must be balanced with the medical need. Those starting medication should be watched closely for suicidal thoughts, worsening of depression, or unusual changes in behavior.

- This is an expensive medication. It can cost more than $2.50 per day. Explore insurance and other forms of the client's ability to manage this cost.

CLIENT AND FAMILY TEACHING

- This medication is not habit forming and does not cause weight gain (as do some medications prescribed for similar purposes).
- Do not stop taking this medication without consulting the primary care provider. Some symptoms might start to improve within 1 to 2 weeks, but it could take up to 8 weeks, depending on the person. Treatment may last 6 months to 1 year.
- Sertraline comes in different dose strengths, and the primary care provider may need to adjust the dosage to find the correct amount.
- Avoid alcohol while taking sertraline.
- Take at the same time every day.
- Store at room temperature.
- Use caution when driving, operating machinery, or performing other hazardous activities. Sertraline may cause dizziness or drowsiness.

Note: Prior to administering any medication, review all aspects with a current drug handbook or other reliable source.

A clearly expressed verbal communication of anger, when the angry person tells the other person about the anger and carefully identifies the source, is constructive. This clarity of communication gets the anger out into the open so that the other person can deal with it and help to alleviate it. The angry person "gets it off the chest" and prevents an emotional buildup.

Depression

Depression is a common reaction to events that seem overwhelming or negative. **Depression,** an extreme feeling of sadness, despair, dejection, lack of worth, or emptiness, affects millions of Americans a year. The signs and symptoms of depression and the severity of the problem vary with the client and the significance of the precipitating event. Emotional symptoms can include feelings of tiredness, sadness, emptiness, or numbness. Behavioral signs of depression include irritability, inability to concentrate, difficulty making decisions, loss of sexual desire, crying, sleep disturbance, and social withdrawal. Physical signs of depression may include loss of appetite, weight loss, constipation, headache, and dizziness. Many people experience short periods of depression in response to overwhelming stressful events, such as the death of a loved one or loss of a job; prolonged depression, however, is a cause for concern and may require treatment.

Ego Defense Mechanisms

Ego defense mechanisms are unconscious psychologic adaptive mechanisms or, according to Sigmund Freud (1946), mental

mechanisms that develop as the personality attempts to defend itself, establish compromises among conflicting impulses, and calm inner tensions. Defense mechanisms are the unconscious mind working to protect the person from anxiety. They can be considered precursors to conscious cognitive coping mechanisms that will ultimately solve the problem. Like some verbal and motor responses, defense mechanisms release tension. Table 42–3 describes these mechanisms and lists examples of their adaptive and maladaptive use.

Cognitive Indicators

Cognitive indicators of stress are thinking responses that include problem solving, structuring, self-control or self-discipline, suppression, and fantasy. *Problem solving* involves thinking through the threatening situation, using specific steps to arrive at a solution. The person assesses the situation or problem, analyzes or defines it, chooses alternatives, carries out the selected alternative, and evaluates whether the solution was successful.

Structuring is the arrangement or manipulation of a situation so that threatening events do not occur. For example, a nurse can structure or control an interview with a client by asking only direct, closed questions. Structuring can be productive in certain situations. A person who schedules a dental examination semi-annually to prevent severe dental disease is using productive structuring.

Self-control (discipline) is assuming a manner and facial expression that convey a sense of being in control or in charge. When self-control prevents panic and harmful or nonproductive

TABLE 42–3 Defense Mechanisms

DEFENSE MECHANISM	EXAMPLE(S)	USE/PURPOSE
Compensation Covering up weaknesses by emphasizing a more desirable trait or by overachievement in a more comfortable area.	A high school student too small to play football becomes the star long-distance runner for the track team.	Allows a person to overcome weakness and achieve success.
Denial An attempt to screen or ignore unacceptable realities by refusing to acknowledge them.	A woman, though told her father has metastatic cancer, continues to plan a family reunion 18 months in advance.	Temporarily isolates a person from the full impact of a traumatic situation.
Displacement The transferring or discharging of emotional reactions from one object or person to another object or person.	A husband and wife are fighting, and the husband becomes so angry he hits a door instead of his wife.	Allows for feelings to be expressed through or to less dangerous objects or people.
Identification An attempt to manage anxiety by imitating the behavior of someone feared or respected.	A student nurse imitates the nurturing behavior she observes one of her instructors using with clients.	Helps a person avoid self-devaluation.
Intellectualization A mechanism by which an emotional response that normally would accompany an uncomfortable or painful incident is evaded by the use of rational explanations that remove from the incident any personal significance and feelings.	The pain over a parent's sudden death is reduced by saying, "He wouldn't have wanted to live with a disability."	Protects a person from pain and traumatic events.
Introjection A form of identification that allows for the acceptance of others' norms and values into oneself, even when contrary to one's previous assumptions.	A 7-year-old tells his little sister, "Don't talk to strangers." He has introjected this value from the instructions of parents and teachers.	Helps a person avoid social retaliation and punishment; particularly important for the child's development of superego.
Minimization Not acknowledging the significance of one's behavior.	A person says, "Don't believe everything my wife tells you. I wasn't so drunk I couldn't drive."	Allows a person to decrease responsibility for own behavior.
Projection A process in which blame is attached to others or the environment for unacceptable desires, thoughts, shortcomings, and mistakes.	A mother is told her child must repeat a grade in school, and she blames this on the teacher's poor instruction. A husband forgets to pay a bill and blames his wife for not giving it to him earlier.	Allows a person to deny the existence of shortcomings and mistakes; protects self-image.
Rationalization Justification of certain behaviors by faulty logic and ascribing motives that are socially acceptable but did not in fact inspire the behavior.	A mother spanks her toddler too hard and says it was all right because he couldn't feel it through the diapers anyway.	Helps a person cope with the inability to meet goals or certain standards.
Reaction formation A mechanism that causes people to act exactly opposite to the way they feel.	An executive resents his bosses for calling in a consulting firm to make recommendations for change in his department but verbalizes complete support of the idea and is exceedingly polite and cooperative.	Aids in reinforcing repression by allowing feelings to be acted out in a more acceptable way.
Regression Resorting to an earlier, more comfortable level of functioning that is characteristically less demanding and responsible.	An adult throws a temper tantrum when he does not get his own way. A critically ill client allows the nurse to bathe and feed him.	Allows a person to return to a point in development when nurturing and dependency were needed and accepted with comfort.
Repression An unconscious mechanism by which threatening thoughts, feelings, and desires are kept from becoming conscious; the repressed material is denied entry into consciousness.	A teenager, seeing his best friend killed in a car accident, becomes amnesic about the circumstances surrounding the accident.	Protects a person from a traumatic experience until he or she has the resources to cope.
Sublimation Displacement of energy associated with more primitive sexual or aggressive drives into socially acceptable activities.	A person with excessive sexual drives invests psychic energy into a well-defined religious value system.	Protects a person from behaving in irrational, impulsive ways.
Substitution The replacement of a highly valued, unacceptable, or unavailable object by a less valuable, acceptable, or available object.	A woman wants to marry a man exactly like her dead father and settles for someone who looks a little bit like him.	Helps a person achieve goals and minimizes frustration and disappointment.
Undoing An action or words designed to cancel some disapproved thoughts, impulses, or acts in which the person relieves guilt by making reparation.	A father spanks his child and the next evening brings home a present for him. A teacher writes an exam that is far too easy, then constructs a grading curve that makes it difficult to earn a high grade.	Allows a person to appease guilty feelings and atone for mistakes.

Note: From Mental Health Nursing, 5th ed. (pp. 11–12), by K. L. Fontaine and J. S. Fletcher, 2003, Upper Saddle River, NJ: Prentice Hall. Reprinted with permission.

actions in a threatening situation, it is a helpful response that conveys strength. Self-control carried to an extreme, however, can delay problem solving and prevent a person from receiving the support of others, who may perceive the person as handling the situation well, as cold, or as unconcerned.

Suppression is consciously and willfully putting a thought or feeling out of mind: "I won't deal with that today. I'll do it tomorrow." This response relieves stress temporarily but does not solve the problem. A man who keeps ignoring a toothache, pushing it out of his mind because he fears the pain of having a filling, will not obtain relief of his symptoms.

Fantasy or *daydreaming* is likened to make-believe. Unfulfilled wishes and desires are imagined as fulfilled, or a threatening experience is reworked or replayed so that it ends differently from reality. Experiences can be relived, everyday problems solved, and plans for the future made. The outcome of current problems may also be fantasized. For example, a client who is awaiting the results of a breast biopsy may fantasize the surgeon as saying, "You do not have cancer." Fantasy responses can be helpful if they lead to problem solving. For example, the client awaiting breast biopsy results might say to herself, "Even if the doctor says, 'You have cancer,' as long as he also says it can be treated, I can accept that." Fantasies can be destructive and nonproductive if a person uses them to excess and retreats from reality.

COPING

Coping may be described as dealing with change—successfully or unsuccessfully. A **coping strategy (coping mechanism)** is a natural or learned way of responding to a changing environment or specific problem or situation. According to Folkman and Lazarus (1991), coping is "the cognitive and behavioral effort to manage specific external and/or internal demands that are appraised as taxing or exceeding the resources of the person" (p. 210).

Two types of coping strategies have been described: problem-focused and emotion-focused coping. *Problem-focused coping* refers to efforts to improve a situation by making changes or taking some action. *Emotion-focused coping* includes thoughts and actions that relieve emotional distress. Emotion-focused coping does not improve the situation, but the person often feels better. Both types of strategies usually occur together (Lazarus, 2000).

Coping strategies are also viewed as long term or short term. *Long-term coping strategies* can be constructive and realistic. For example, in certain situations, talking with others and trying to find out more about the situation are long-term strategies. Other long-term strategies include a change in lifestyle patterns such as eating a healthy diet, exercising regularly, balancing leisure time with working, or using problem solving in decision making instead of anger or other nonconstructive responses.

Short-term coping strategies can reduce stress to a tolerable limit temporarily but are ineffective ways to permanently deal with reality. They may even have a destructive or detrimental effect on the person. Examples of short-term strategies are using alcoholic beverages or drugs, daydreaming and fantasizing, relying on the belief that everything will work out, and giving in to others to avoid anger.

Coping strategies vary among individuals and are often related to the individual's perception of the stressful event. Three approaches to coping with stress are to alter the stressor, adapt to the stressor, or avoid the stressor. A person's coping strategies often change with a reappraisal of a situation. There is never only one way to cope. Some people choose avoidance; others confront a situation as a means of coping. Still others seek information or rely on religious beliefs.

Coping can be adaptive or maladaptive. *Adaptive coping* helps the person to deal effectively with stressful events and minimizes distress associated with them. *Maladaptive coping* can result in unnecessary distress for the person and others associated with the person or stressful event. In nursing literature, effective and ineffective coping are often differentiated. *Effective coping* results in adaptation; *ineffective coping* results in maladaptation.

Although the coping behavior may not always seem appropriate, the nurse needs to remember that coping is always purposeful. The effectiveness of an individual's coping is influenced by a number of factors, including

- The number, duration, and intensity of the stressors.
- Past experiences of the individual.
- Support systems available to the individual.
- Personal qualities of the person.

If the duration of the stressors is extended beyond the coping powers of the individual, that person becomes exhausted and may develop increased susceptibility to health problems. Reaction to long-term stress is seen in family members who undertake the care of a person in the home for a long period. This stress is called **caregiver burden** and produces responses such as chronic fatigue, sleeping difficulties, and high blood pressure. Prolonged stress can also result in mental illness. As coping strategies or defense mechanisms become ineffective, the individual may have interpersonal problems, work difficulties, and a significant decrease in abilities to meet basic human needs (see Table 42–4).

TABLE 42-4 Examples of the Negative Effects of Stress on Basic Human Needs

NEEDS	EFFECTS
Physiologic	Altered elimination pattern Change in appetite Altered sleep pattern
Safety and security	Expresses nervousness and feelings of being threatened Focuses on stressors, inattention to safety measures
Love and belonging	Isolated and withdrawn Becomes overly dependent Blames others for own problems
Self-esteem	Fails to socialize with others Becomes a workaholic Draws attention to self
Self-actualization	Preoccupied with own problems Shows lack of control Unable to accept reality

RESEARCH NOTE How Might Clients', Their Caregivers', and Their Health Care Professionals' View of Needs and Support Influence Caregiver Burden?

Caregiver burden is an increasing problem, with clients surviving longer and more care tasks falling to informal caregivers. Fifty-seven clients with advanced cancer, 45 of their caregivers, and 40 of their health professionals were included in the study. Caregivers and clients consistently identified higher levels of available support for the client than health care professionals, with caregivers identifying higher levels of support than clients. Caregivers also identified more client unmet needs than health care professionals, who in turn identified more than clients. Unmet needs decreased over the 6-month time period of the study.

IMPLICATIONS

These results suggest that health care professionals underestimate available support to clients, and both clients and health care professionals underestimate clients' unmet needs in comparison to caregivers. Caregivers' reports of clients' unmet needs are important to consider as they were associated with high levels of caregiver burden, including poorer caregiver health. Health care professionals should encourage opportunities for caregivers to discuss their views of the ongoing needs of clients with advanced cancer.

Note: From "The Relationship between Available Support, Unmet Needs and Caregiver Burden in Patients with Advanced Cancer and Their Carers," by L. Sharpe, P. Butow, C. Smith, D. McConnell, and S. Clarke, 2005, *Psycho-Oncology, 14*, pp. 102–114.

NURSING MANAGEMENT

Assessing

Nursing assessment of a client's stress and coping patterns includes (a) nursing history and (b) physical examination of the client for indicators of stress (e.g., nail biting, nervousness, weight changes) or stress-related health problems (e.g., hypertension, dyspnea). When obtaining the nursing history, the nurse poses questions about client-perceived stressors or stressful incidents, manifestations of stress, and past and present coping strategies. During the physical examination, the nurse observes for verbal, motor, cognitive, or other physical manifestations of stress. Remember, however, that clinical signs and symptoms may not occur when cognitive coping is effective.

In addition, the nurse should be aware of expected developmental transitions (predictable tasks that must be accomplished if the person is to grow psychologically as well as physically; see Chapters 20 to 23 ∞). Persons go through different developmental stages from infancy to old age when certain tasks are expected to be completed or resolved. When these tasks are carried over and not resolved, stress increases as they become older. For example, if an infant does not learn to trust those around him during infancy, this mistrust may accompany him through life, influencing his relationships and possibly being the root of dysfunction, stress, and ineffective

ASSESSMENT INTERVIEW Stress and Coping Patterns

- On a scale of 1 to 10, where 1 is "very minor" and 10 is "extreme," how would you rate the stress you are experiencing in the following areas?
  a. Home
  b. Work or school
  c. Finance
  d. Recent illness or loss of loved one
  e. Your health
  f. Family responsibilities
  g. Relationships with friends
  h. Relationship with parents or children
  i. Relationship with partner
  j. Recent hospitalization
  k. Other (specify)
- How long have you been dealing with these stressors?
- How do you usually handle stressful situations? If the client does not adequately describe, prompt with the following:
  a. Cry
  b. Get angry
  c. Talk to someone (Who?)
  d. Withdraw from the situation
  e. Control others or situation
  f. Go for a walk or perform physical exercise
  g. Try to arrive at a solution
  h. Pray
  i. Laugh, joke, or use some other expression of humor
  j. Meditate or use some other relaxation technique such as yoga or guided imagery
- How well does your usual coping strategy work?

coping. This knowledge helps the nurse identify additional stressors that are present and the client's response to them (see Table 42–1). Questions to elicit data about the client's stress and coping patterns are shown in the accompanying Assessment Interview.

Diagnosing

NANDA diagnostic labels related to stress, adaptation, and coping include (in alphabetical order)

- *Anxiety:* Vague, uneasy feeling of discomfort or dread accompanied by an autonomic response (the source often nonspecific or unknown to the individual); a feeling of apprehension caused by the anticipation of danger. It is an alerting signal that warns of impending danger and enables the individual to take measures to deal with a threat.
- *Caregiver Role Strain:* Difficulty in performing the caregiver role.
- *Compromised Family Coping:* Usually supportive primary person (family member or close friend) provides insufficient, ineffective, or compromised support, comfort, assistance, or encouragement that may be needed by the client to manage or master adaptive tasks related to his or her health challenge.

MediaLink Becoming Parents Case Study

- *Decisional Conflict (Specify):* Uncertainty about course of action to be taken when the choice among competing actions involves risk, loss, or challenge to personal life values.
- *Defensive Coping:* Repeated projection of falsely positive self-evaluation based on a self-protective pattern that defends against underlying perceived threats to positive self-regard.
- *Disabled Family Coping:* Behavior of significant person (family member or other primary person) that disables his/her capacities and the client's capacities to effectively address tasks essential to either person's adaption to the health challenge.
- *Fear:* Response to perceived threat that is consciously recognized as a danger.
- *Impaired Adjustment:* Inability to modify lifestyle/behavior in a manner consistent with a change in health status.

- *Ineffective Coping:* Inability to form a valid appraisal of the stressors, inadequate choices of practiced responses, and/or inability to use resources.
- *Ineffective Denial:* Conscious or unconscious attempt to disavow the knowledge or meaning of an event to reduce anxiety/fear, but leading to the detriment of health.
- *Post-Trauma Syndrome:* Sustained maladaptive response to a traumatic, overwhelming event.
- *Relocation Stress Syndrome:* Physiologic and/or psychosocial disturbance following transfer from one environment to another.

Examples of clinical applications of these diagnoses using NANDA, NIC, and NOC designations are shown in Identifying Nursing Diagnoses, Outcomes, and Interventions.

IDENTIFYING NURSING DIAGNOSES, OUTCOMES, AND INTERVENTIONS
Clients With Stress and Coping Challenges

DATA CLUSTER   Darryl Johnson, a 67-year-old accountant, was diagnosed with a heart attack. "I'm scared about this. My dad died of a heart attack when he was 68 years old. But, I don't think I can give up smoking, take up exercising, and change my diet."

NURSING DIAGNOSIS/ DEFINITION	SAMPLE DESIRED OUTCOMES*/ *DEFINITION*	INDICATORS	SELECTED INTERVENTIONS*/ *DEFINITION*	SAMPLE NIC ACTIVITIES
Impaired Adjustment/ Inability to modify lifestyle behavior in a manner consistent with a change in health status	Psychosocial Adjustment: Life Change [1305]/*Adaptive psychosocial response of an individual to a significant life change*	Substantial ■ Recognition of reality of current health situation ■ Demonstration of positive self-regard ■ Clarification of values	Counseling [5240]/ *Use of an interactive helping process focusing on the needs, problems, or feelings of the patient and significant others to enhance or support coping, problem-solving, and interpersonal relationships*	■ Demonstrate empathy, warmth, and genuineness ■ Provide factual information as appropriate ■ Use techniques of reflection and clarification to facilitate expression of feelings

DATA CLUSTER   Sonia Park, 33-year-old mother of three, returned to work after 8 years at home. "I'm so tired since I started work. I'm not keeping up with housekeeping the way I should, and I'm not spending as much time with the kids. I'm too tired to shop and go to my son's baseball game. Everyone is helping out and not complaining, but I just keep thinking they wish I still baked cookies and played more with them. I'm sure not sleeping well, and I'm having awful headaches."

Decisional Conflict (Work Versus Home Responsibilities Causing Emotional and Physical Stress)/ *Uncertainty about a course of action to be taken when the choice among competing actions involves risk, loss, or challenge to personal life values*	Decision Making [0906]/*Ability to make judgments and choose between two or more alternatives*	Often demonstrated ■ Identifies alternatives ■ Identifies resources necessary to support each alternative ■ Chooses among alternatives	Decision-Making Support [5250]/ *Providing information and support for a patient who is making a decision regarding health care*	■ Inform her of alternative views or solutions ■ Help her identify advantages and disadvantages to each alternative ■ Facilitate her articulation of goals

*The NOC # for desired outcomes and the NIC # for nursing interventions are listed in brackets following the appropriate outcome or intervention. Outcomes, indicators, interventions, and activities selected are only a sample of those suggested by NOC and NIC and should be further individualized for each client.

Planning

The nurse develops plans in collaboration with the client and significant support people when possible, according to the client's state of health (e.g., ability to return to work), level of anxiety, support resources, coping mechanisms, and sociocultural and religious affiliation. The nurse with little experience intervening with clients undergoing stress may wish to consult with a more experienced nurse to develop effective plans. The nurse and client set goals to change the existing client responses to the stressor or stressors.

The overall client goals for persons experiencing stress-related responses are to

- Decrease or resolve anxiety.
- Increase ability to manage or cope with stressful events or circumstances.
- Improve role performance.

Examples of clinical applications of NOC outcomes and NIC interventions are shown in Identifying Nursing Diagnoses, Outcomes, and Interventions. A sample nursing care plan and concept map using NIC interventions and selected activities are shown on pages 1075–1076.

Planning for Home Care

Clients who are experiencing stress may require ongoing nursing support or referral to community agencies that can provide support to meet client needs and enhance client coping. The determination of how much and what type of planning and home care follow-up is needed is based in great part on the nurse's knowledge of how the client and family have coped with previous stressors and the nature of the present stressor. The Home Care Assessment feature describes data to be gathered for home care or follow-up assessment.

Implementing

Although stress is part of daily life, it is also highly individual; a situation that to one person is a major stressor may not affect another. Some methods to help reduce stress will be effective for one person; other methods will be appropriate for a different person. A nurse who is sensitive to clients' needs and reactions can choose those methods of intervention that will be most effective for each individual.

Encouraging Health Promotion Strategies

Several health promotion strategies are often appropriate as interventions for clients with stress-related nursing diagnoses. Among these are physical exercise, optimal nutrition, adequate rest and sleep, and time management.

EXERCISE. Regular exercise promotes both physical and emotional health. Physiologic benefits include improved muscle tone, increased cardiopulmonary function, and weight control. Psychologic benefits include relief of tension, a feeling of well-being, and relaxation. In 2005, the federal Dietary Guidelines Advisory Committee recommended 30 minutes of daily exercise (United States Department of Agriculture, 2005).

HOME CARE ASSESSMENT
Stress and Coping

CLIENT

- Knowledge: Client's understanding of the nature of the stressors
- Current coping strategies: Effectiveness of current coping strategies and willingness to learn new stress management techniques
- Self-care abilities: Physical, emotional, social, and financial ability to minimize associated stressors
- Role expectations: Client's perception of the need to return to prior roles and possible stressors associated with these roles

FAMILY

- Knowledge: Family members' and significant others' understanding of the nature of the client's stressors and their own relationship with client stressors
- Family coping strategies: Effectiveness of family members' and significant others' coping strategies and willingness to learn new stress management techniques
- Role expectations: Family members' and significant others' perception of the need for the client to return to family and work roles
- Support people's availability and skills: Family members' and significant others' sensitivity to the client's emotional and physical needs and ability to provide a supportive environment

COMMUNITY

- Resources: Availability of and familiarity with possible sources of assistance for stress management such as massage therapists, religious or spiritual centers, physical care providers, support groups, and so on

---

NUTRITION. Optimal nutrition is essential for health and in increasing the body's resistance to stress. To minimize the negative effects of stress (e.g., irritability, hyperactivity, anxiety), people need to avoid excesses of caffeine, salt, sugar, and fat, and deficiencies in vitamins and minerals. Guidelines for a well-balanced, healthy diet are detailed in Chapter 47. ∞

CLINICAL ALERT

Many persons have "comfort foods"— things they like to eat that actually make them feel better emotionally. ∎

SLEEP. Sleep restores the body's energy levels and is an essential aspect of stress management. To ensure adequate sleep, clients may need help to attain comfort (such as pain management) and to learn techniques that promote peace of mind and relaxation. (See "Using Relaxation Techniques" on page 1072.)

TIME MANAGEMENT. People who manage their time effectively usually experience less stress because they feel more in control of their circumstances. Clients who feel overwhelmed often need help to prioritize tasks and to consider whether modifications can be made to decrease role demands. Working mothers, for example, may need to consider delegating tasks to family members or hiring part-time help. Controlling the demands of others is also an important aspect of effective time management because requests made by others cannot always be met. Clients may need to learn to develop an awareness of which requests they can meet without undue stress, which ones can be negotiated, and which ones need to be declined. Feelings of control can be enhanced when clients schedule a daily or weekly period of time to deal with specific tasks. Time management must address both what is important to the client and what can realistically be achieved. For example, clients need to consider whether a clean house and time spent with the children can both be accomplished satisfactorily and, if not, which is more important. Clients who are feeling overwhelmed need to reexamine the "should do," "ought to do," and "must do" situations in their lives and develop realistic self-expectations.

Minimizing Anxiety

Nurses carry out measures to minimize clients' anxiety and stress. For example, nurses encourage clients to take deep breaths before an injection, explain procedures before they are implemented including sensations likely to be experienced during the procedure, administer a massage to help the client relax, and offer support to clients and families during times of illness. The nurse recognizes that quick action may be necessary to avoid the contagious nature of anxiety. That is, the anxious feeling of one person tends to make others around him or her also anxious. This can include family members, other clients nearby, or health care providers. General guidelines for helping clients who are stressed and feeling anxious are outlined in Box 42–1.

Mediating Anger

Often nurses find clients' anger difficult to handle. Caring for the client who is angry is difficult for two reasons:

- Clients seldom state, "I feel angry or frustrated," or indicate the reason for their anger. Instead, they may refuse treatment, become verbally abusive or demanding, threaten violence, or become overly critical. Their complaints rarely reflect the cause of their anger.
- Anger from clients can elicit fear and anger in the nurse, who may respond in a manner that intensifies the client's anger, even to the point of violence. Nurses tend to respond in a way that reduces their own stress rather than the client's stress.

Fontaine and Fletcher (2003) recommend the following strategies for dealing with clients' anger:

- Know and understand your own response to the feelings and expressions of anger.
- Accept the client's right to be angry; feelings are real and cannot be discounted or ignored.
- Try to understand the meaning of the client's anger.
- Ask the client what contributed to the anger.
- Help the client "own" the anger—do not assume responsibility for her or his feelings.
- Let clients talk about their anger.
- Listen to the client, and act as calmly as possible.

BOX 42–1   Minimizing Stress and Anxiety

- Listen attentively; try to understand the client's perspective on the situation.
- Provide an atmosphere of warmth and trust; convey a sense of caring and empathy.
- Determine if it is appropriate to encourage clients' participation in the plan of care; give them choices about some aspects of care but do not overwhelm them with choices.
- Stay with clients as needed to promote safety and feelings of security and to reduce fear.
- Control the environment to minimize additional stressors such as reducing noise, limiting the number of persons in the room, and providing care by the same nurse as much as possible.
- Implement suicide precautions if indicated.
- Communicate in short, clear sentences.
- Help clients to
  a. Determine situations that precipitate anxiety and identify signs of anxiety.
  b. Verbalize feelings, perceptions, and fears as appropriate. Some cultures discourage the expression of feelings.
  c. Identify personal strengths.
  d. Recognize usual coping patterns and differentiate positive from negative coping mechanisms.
  e. Identify new strategies for managing stress (e.g., exercise, massage, progressive relaxation).
  f. Identify available support systems.
- Teach clients about
  a. The importance of adequate exercise, a balanced diet, and rest and sleep to energize the body and enhance coping abilities.
  b. Support groups available such as Alcoholics Anonymous, Weight Watchers or Overeaters Anonymous, and parenting and child abuse support groups.
  c. Educational programs available such as time management, assertiveness training, and meditation groups.

- After the interaction is completed, take time to process your feelings and your responses to the client with your colleagues (pp. 28–29).

Always ensure the safety of the client and others. Know the agency procedures to call for assistance from other staff or security personnel if you believe someone (including yourself) is in danger.

CLINICAL ALERT

A nurse who is concerned for his or her own safety while working with an angry client should withdraw from the situation or obtain support from another individual. ■

Using Relaxation Techniques

Several relaxation techniques can be used to quiet the mind, release tension, and counteract the fight or flight responses of GAS discussed earlier in this chapter. Nurses can teach these techniques to clients. Nurses should also encourage clients to use these techniques when they encounter stressful health situations. Examples of these situations are (a) during childbirth, (b) postoperatively to cope with pain, and (c) before and during a painful procedure. Many agencies now have relaxation tapes available that the client can borrow or purchase. Some clients make their own recordings. Specific relaxation techniques are discussed in Chapter 19 ∞ and include the following:

- Breathing exercises
- Massage
- Progressive relaxation
- Imagery
- Biofeedback
- Yoga
- Meditation
- Therapeutic touch
- Music therapy
- Humor and laughter

Crisis Intervention

A *crisis* is an acute, time-limited state of disequilibrium resulting from situational, developmental, or societal sources of stress. A person in crisis is temporarily unable to cope with or adapt to the stressor by using previous methods of problem solving. People in crisis generally have a distorted perception of the event and do not have adequate situational support or coping mechanisms. Common characteristics of crises are shown in Box 42–2.

Crisis intervention is a short-term helping process of assisting clients to (a) work through a crisis to its resolution and (b) restore their precrisis level of functioning. It is a process that includes not only the client in crisis but also various members of the client's support network. Crisis intervention is not the specialty of any one professional group. People who intervene in crises come from the fields of nursing, medicine, psychology, social work, and theology. Police officers, teachers, school guidance counselors, and rescue workers, among others, are often on the spot in moments of crisis.

Because a state of disequilibrium is so uncomfortable, a crisis is self-limiting. However, a person experiencing a crisis alone is more vulnerable to unsuccessful negotiation than is a person working through a crisis with help. Working with an-

---

BOX 42–2 Common Characteristics of Crises

- All crises are experienced as sudden. The person is usually not aware of a warning signal, even if others could "see it coming." The individual or family may feel that they had little or no preparation for the event or trauma.
- The crisis is often experienced as ultimately life threatening, whether this perception is realistic or not.
- Communication with significant others is often decreased or cut off.
- There may be perceived or real displacement from familiar surroundings or loved ones.

All crises have an aspect of loss, whether actual or perceived. The losses can include an object, a person, a hope, a dream, or any significant factor for that individual.

---

other person increases the likelihood that the person in crisis will resolve it in a positive way. Often a state of crisis offers the individual or family great potential for growth and change.

The traditional steps of the nursing process correspond closely to the steps of crisis intervention. In assessment, the nurse or helper must focus on the person and the problem, collecting data about the client, the client's coping style, the precipitating event, the situational supports, the client's perception of the crisis, and the client's ability to handle the problem. This information is the basis for later decisions about how and when to intervene and whom to call. An individual's perception of the event and personal response will determine the nursing diagnoses. The most common nursing diagnoses for people in crisis are similar to those cited earlier in this chapter. In addition, diagnoses such as *Risk for Self Directed Violence, Risk for Other Directed Violence, Rape Trauma Syndrome,* and *Hopelessness* may be appropriate.

Effective planning for crisis intervention must be based on careful assessment and developed in active collaboration with the person in crisis and the significant people in that person's life.

Implementation involves crisis counseling and home crisis visits. **Crisis counseling** focuses on solving immediate problems and it involves individuals, groups, or families. Crisis intervention centers rely heavily on telephone counseling by volunteers who have professional consultation available to them. Also known as hotlines and often available around the clock, they allow callers to remain anonymous. The volunteers usually work within a protocol that indicates what information they need from the client to assess the crisis. Their goal is to plan steps to provide immediate relief and then long-term follow-up if necessary.

Crisis home visits are made when telephone counseling does not suffice or when the crisis workers need to obtain additional information by direct observation or to reach a client who is unobtainable by telephone. Home visits are appropriate when crisis workers need to initiate contacts rather than waiting for clients to come to them; for example, when a telephone caller is assessed to be highly suicidal or when a concerned neighbor, primary care provider, or clergy member informs the agency of clients in potential crisis.

Stress Management for Nurses

Nurses, like clients, are susceptible to experiencing anxiety and stress. Nursing practice involves many stressors related to both clients and the work environment—understaffing, increasing severity of client illnesses, adjusting to various work shifts, being expected to assume responsibilities for which one is not prepared, inadequate support from supervisors and peers, visiting homes that are depressing, caring for dying clients, and so on. Although most nurses cope effectively with the physical and emotional demands of nursing, in some situations nurses become overwhelmed and develop **burnout,** a complex syndrome of behaviors that can be likened to the exhaustion stage of the general adaptation syndrome. The nurse with burnout manifests physical and emotional depletion, a negative attitude and self-concept, and feelings of helplessness and hopelessness.

Nurses can prevent burnout by using the techniques to manage stress discussed for clients. Nurses must first recognize their stress and become attuned to such responses as feelings of being overwhelmed, fatigue, angry outbursts, physical illness, and increases in coffee drinking, smoking, or substance abuse. Once attuned to stress and personal reactions, it is necessary to identify which situations produce the most pronounced reactions so that steps may be taken to reduce the stress. Suggestions include:

■ Plan a daily relaxation program with meaningful quiet times to reduce tension (e.g., read, listen to music, soak in a tub, or meditate).

■ Establish a regular exercise program to direct energy outward.

■ Study assertiveness techniques to overcome feelings of powerlessness in relationships with others. Learn to say no.

■ Learn to accept failures—your own and others—and make it a constructive learning experience. Recognize that most people do the best they can. Learn to ask for help, to show your feelings with colleagues, and to support your colleagues in times of need.

■ Accept what cannot be changed. There are certain limitations in every situation. Get involved in constructive change efforts if organizational policies and procedures cause stress.

■ Develop collegial support groups to deal with feelings and anxieties generated in the work setting.

■ Participate in professional organizations to address workplace issues.

■ Seek counseling if indicated to help clarify concerns.

Evaluating

Using the desired outcomes developed during the planning stage as a guide, the nurse collects data needed to determine whether client goals and outcomes have been achieved. Examples of client goals and related outcomes are shown in Identifying Nursing Diagnoses, Outcomes, and Interventions earlier and in the accompanying Nursing Care Plan.

If outcomes are not achieved, the nurse, client, and support people, if appropriate, need to explore the reasons before modifying the care plan. Questions such as the following need to be considered:

■ How does the client perceive the problem?
■ Is there an underlying problem that has not been identified?
■ Have new stressors occurred that interfere with successful coping?
■ Were existing coping strategies sufficient to meet intended outcomes?
■ How does the client perceive the effectiveness of new coping strategies?
■ Did the client implement new coping strategies properly?
■ Did the client access and use available resources?
■ Have family members and significant others provided effective support?

LIFESPAN CONSIDERATIONS Stress and Coping

INFANTS AND CHILDREN

■ Children's perceptions of and responses to stress are dependent on their developmental stage. Infants sense stressors in their environment and respond in a diffuse way, often crying and clinging. Toddlers and preschool-age children may be frightened and react by withdrawing or losing control. School-age children and adolescents are more capable of thinking about incidents that cause stress (e.g., a catastrophic accident) and talking about it with adults.

■ Temperament is a factor that influences how children respond to stress. An outgoing, low-sensitivity child, for example, is less likely than a timid, intense child to be upset by a family move to a different state.

■ Anxiety disorders are the most common psychiatric disorders in children but are frequently unrecognized (Antai-Otong, 2003).

■ As children grow, they are able to develop more coping skills to manage stressful situations. Nurses have an important role in teaching parents to recognize stress in their children and to help their children cope.

MIDDLE-AGED ADULTS

■ Middle-aged adults are often called the "sandwich generation." They find themselves caring for children and grandchildren and often caring for aging parents at the same time. When these activities become time and energy consuming, there is often not enough time left for attention to self. Nurses need to be aware of this and assist in suggesting resources and effective planning to ease the strain.

ELDERS

■ Elders experience many losses and changes in their lives. They may be incremental and, over time, become stressful and possibly overwhelming. Changes in health, decreased functional ability and independence, need for relocation, loss of family and friends, and becoming a caregiver for a spouse or friend are a few of the stresses often experienced by elders. Many of them have survived significant challenges in their earlier lives and have learned effective coping skills. Nurses can help them plan, evaluate their strategies, and learn new strategies, if needed. Informal and formal social supports are very important in learning to successfully live with these changes and stress.

■ Some effective coping methods for elders are exercise, learning different relaxation techniques, participation in activities, adequate nutrition and rest, and engaging in expressive creative activities, such as art, music, and journaling. Referral to community resources and supports should be done when appropriate. It is most important to see elders as unique individuals, with unique past experiences and very specific needs as they age.

NURSING CARE PLAN Ineffective Coping

ASSESSMENT DATA	NURSING DIAGNOSIS	DESIRED OUTCOMES*
Nursing Assessment Ruby Smithson is a 55-year-old mother of four children who is hospitalized with breast cancer. She is scheduled for a modified radical mastectomy. Ruby was relatively healthy until she found a lump in her right breast 1 week ago. She and her husband are extremely anxious about the surgery. Ruby confides to the admitting nurse that "I can't stand the idea of having one of my breasts cut off; I don't know how I'm going to be able to even look at myself." Mr. Smithson informs the nurse that Ruby has been abusing alcohol since her diagnosis and neglecting her responsibilities as a mother. She is tearful and doesn't see how she will be able to continue her work as a dress designer.	*Ineffective Coping* related to personal vulnerability secondary to mastectomy (as evidenced by verbalization of inability to cope, substance abuse, inability to meet role expectations)	**Coping** [1302], as evidenced by often demonstrating ability to ■ Identify effective and ineffective coping patterns ■ Verbalize sense of control ■ Report decrease in negative feelings ■ Modify lifestyle as needed **Social Support** [1504], as evidenced by substantial reports of ■ Willingness to call on others for help ■ Emotional assistance provided by others

Physical Examination

Height: 164 cm (5'5")
Weight: 58 kg (158 lb)
Temperature: 37°C (98.6°F)
Pulse rate: 88 BPM
Respirations: 16/minute
Blood pressure: 142/88 mm Hg

Diagnostic Data

Chest x-ray negative, CBC, and urinalysis within normal limits

NURSING INTERVENTIONS*/SELECTED ACTIVITIES	RATIONALE
Coping Enhancement [5230]	
Provide an atmosphere of acceptance.	*Establishing rapport is essential to a therapeutic relationship and supports the client in self-reflection. Recognizing problems and sharing feelings is best brought about in an atmosphere of warmth and trust.*
Provide factual information concerning the diagnosis, treatment, and prognosis.	*Factual information serves as a foundation for Ruby to explore feelings and alternative coping strategies. Stressed clients often misunderstand facts and require frequent clarification so that appropriate conclusions can be drawn. Having valid information helps relieve stress.*
Appraise Ruby's adjustment to changes in body image.	*Alteration in body image may be a major issue for Ruby and should be explored to facilitate therapeutic intervention. Coping strategies often change with a reappraisal of the situation.*
Arrange situations that encourage her autonomy. Give her as many opportunities as possible to make decisions/choices for herself.	*Enhances a sense of control, personal achievement, and self-esteem.*
Explore with her previous methods of dealing with life problems.	*Present and past coping status assists both Ruby and her husband in capitalizing on successful methods, identifying ineffective strategies, and developing new skills more appropriate to the present situation. Also determines risk for inflicting self-harm.*
Encourage verbalization of feelings, perceptions, and fears.	*Open, nonthreatening discussions facilitate the identification of causative and contributing factors.*
Encourage Ruby to identify her own strengths and abilities.	*Assists Ruby to develop appropriate strategies for coping based on personal strengths and previous experiences. Improves self-concept and sense of ability to manage stress.*

NURSING CARE PLAN **Ineffective Coping** *continued*

NURSING INTERVENTIONS/SELECTED ACTIVITIES*	RATIONALE
Encourage Ruby to realistically describe changes in her role.	*Individuals experiencing stress may have unrealistic perceptions or reality distortions. Helping Ruby clearly describe her role would be beneficial in developing realistic goals for role achievement.*
Foster constructive outlets for anger and hostility.	*Assists the individual in channeling potentially harmful emotions and physical energy into constructive behavior.*

Support System Enhancement [5440]

Observe the degree of family support.	*Assessing family interaction serves as a basis for identifying Ruby's support systems or lack thereof.*
Determine barriers to using support systems.	*Although adequate support systems may be available, Ruby may not be using them or may be using them ineffectively.*
Involve husband, family, and friends in the care and planning.	*Supporting Ruby in acknowledging changes in her appearance conveys acceptance and provides a foundation for her to begin to adjust.*
Discuss with concerned others how they can help.	*Family and friends are often willing but unsure how to help. Identifying specific strategies such as praise and encouragement during rehabilitation and healing will promote acceptance of change.*
Refer Ruby to a community-based breast cancer support group.	*Community support is beneficial in helping to meet unresolved needs, decreasing feelings of social isolation, and facilitating a positive self-image.*

EVALUATION

The coping outcome was not met. Following surgery, Ruby was withdrawn. During bathing, she would not assist and turned her head away when the dressing was removed. She refused to learn how to manage the wound drain or to discuss her feelings or plans for the future. Because clients having a mastectomy are often only hospitalized for a few days, it may be that she requires more time to reach the desired outcome. Continue to offer information and demonstrate availability for when she is ready to verbalize feelings. Social support outcome partly met. Ruby allows her husband to provide direct care and emotional support for her. A social worker was consulted and discharge was delayed for 24 hours. Ruby has agreed that the social worker can contact a breast cancer support group and ask the group to call her.

*The NOC # for desired outcomes and the NIC # for nursing interventions are listed in brackets following the appropriate outcome or intervention. Outcomes, indicators, interventions, and activities selected are only a sample of those suggested by NOC and NIC and should be further individualized for each client.

APPLYING CRITICAL THINKING

1. If Ruby had been able to choose a lumpectomy rather than a mastectomy (less visible, smaller, potentially less "meaningful" tissue removal), would the nursing diagnosis and expected outcomes remain the same? Why or why not?
2. Does Ruby's situation reflect more of a stimulus-based model or a response-based model? Why?
3. While working with Ruby, she becomes very angry and says to you "You don't understand. You've never had to go through this." How would you respond?

4. Based on the evaluation above, do you believe that Ruby is in crisis? What factors led to your decision? How does your view change the modifications indicated in her care plan?
5. Give one example of how Ruby might use the defense mechanisms described on page 1067. Explain whether this is adaptive or maladaptive.

See Critical Thinking Possibilities in Appendix A.

CONCEPT MAP For Ineffective Coping

R.S.
55 y.o. female
Medical DX:
Breast cancer

→ assess →

- Lump detected 1 week ago. Very anxious, tearful
- Husband reports alcohol abuse and ineffective mothering since Dx

- Height: 164 cm (5'5")
- Weight: 58 kg (158 lb)
- T37C (98.6°F), P:88, R:16, BP142/88
- Chest x-ray negative, CBC, and urinalysis with normal limits

generate nursing diagnosis ↓

Ineffective Coping r/t personal vulnerability secondary to mastectomy (as evidenced by verbalization of inability to cope, substance abuse, inability to meet role expectations)

outcome ↓   outcome ↓

Social Support aeb substantial reports of
- Willingness to call on others for help
- Emotional assistance provided by others

Coping aeb often demonstrating ability to
- Identify effective and ineffective coping patterns
- Verbalize sense of control
- Report decrease in negative feelings
- Modify lifestyle as needed

nursing intervention ↓   nursing intervention ↓

Support System Enhancement

Coping Enhancement

activity → Observe degree of family support

activity → Determine barriers to using support systems

activity → Involve husband, family and friends in the care and planning

activity → Discuss with concerned others how they can help

activity → Refer to a community-based breast cancer support group

Provide factual information concerning the diagnosis, treatment, and prognosis

Arrange situations that encourage her autonomy

Provide an atmosphere of acceptance

Explore with her previous methods of dealing with life problems

Appraise adjustment to change in body image

Encourage verbalization of feelings, perceptions, and fears

Encourage to identify her own strengths and abilities

Encourage to realistically describe changes in her role

Foster constructive outlets for anger and hostility

evaluation ↓   evaluation ↓

Outcome partly met
- Allows husband to provide direct care and emotional support
- Social worker consulted; discharge delayed 24 hours

Outcome not met
- Following surgery was withdrawn. Did not assist with bathing, turned head away when dressing removed
- Refused to learn to manage wound drain or discuss feelings or plans for the future

CHAPTER 42 **REVIEW**

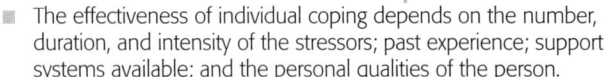

CHAPTER HIGHLIGHTS

- Stress is a state of physiologic and psychologic tension that affects the whole person—physically, emotionally, intellectually, socially, and spiritually.
- Models view stress as a stimulus, stress as a response, and stress as a transaction.
- General adaptation syndrome (GAS) is a multisystem response to stress and involves three steps: alarm reaction, stage of resistance, and stage of exhaustion.
- Local adaptation syndrome (LAS) is a localized physiologic response that also expresses the three stages of GAS. An example of LAS is the inflammatory response.
- There are physiologic, psychologic, and cognitive indicators of stress. Physiologic indicators are the result of increased activity of the sympathetic and neuroendocrine systems.
- Common psychologic indicators are anxiety, fear, anger, and depression. Anxiety, the most common response, has four levels: mild, moderate, severe, and panic. Ego defense mechanisms such as denial, rationalization, compensation, and sublimation protect individuals from anxiety.
- Cognitive indicators or thinking responses to stress include problem solving, structuring, self-control (discipline), suppression, and fantasy.
- Coping strategies to deal with stress vary significantly among individuals. Strategies may be problem focused or emotion focused, long term or short term, and effective or ineffective.
- The effectiveness of individual coping depends on the number, duration, and intensity of the stressors; past experience; support systems available; and the personal qualities of the person.
- Prolonged stress and ineffective coping interfere with the meeting of basic needs and can affect physical and mental health.
- Nursing assessment of a client experiencing stress involves a nursing history to identify perceptions of and duration of stressors and coping strategies and also a physical examination for physical indicators of stress.
- Nursing interventions for clients who are stressed are aimed at encouraging health promotion strategies (exercise, healthy diet, adequate rest, and time management), minimizing anxiety, mediating anger, teaching about specific relaxation techniques, and implementing crisis interventions as needed.
- Because nursing practice involves many stressors related to both clients and the work environment, nurses are susceptible to anxiety and burnout. Like clients, they need to implement stress reduction measures.

TEST YOUR KNOWLEDGE

1. After the death of several long-term clients, which of the following actions indicates the nurse is demonstrating ineffective coping?
   1. The nurse talks at length to her partner about the deaths.
   2. The nurse keeps busy with other actions and doesn't think about the deaths for several days.
   3. The nurse offers to work extra shifts for several weeks.
   4. Several nurses schedule a group session with the agency clergy to discuss the deaths.

2. The nurse helps a 50-year-old diabetic client who is to begin giving insulin injections identify previously successful coping strategies that may be useful in the current situation. Which of the following stressors is closely related to the new stressor?
   1. Interviewing for a new job
   2. Death of a pet while the person was a teenager
   3. The person's partner filing for a divorce
   4. Starting to wear eyeglasses at age 30

3. Two people have been in a motor vehicle crash and have similar injuries. According to the transaction-based model, their degree of stress from the crash would be
   1. Based on previous experience and personal characteristics
   2. Extremely similar since they had the same stimulus
   3. The identical physiologic alarm reaction
   4. Different depending on their external resources and support levels

4. A client who was informed of a cancer diagnosis assures the nurse he is fine. Which of the following is the most indicative physical evidence to the nurse of the client's stress?
   1. Constricted pupils
   2. Dilated peripheral blood vessels (flush)
   3. Hyperventilation
   4. Decreased heart rate

5. Immediately after the parents of a hospitalized child are informed that the child has leukemia, the father responds by continuing his usual work schedule, rarely visiting, and asking when the child can return to school. Of the following, which is the **least** likely to be an appropriate nursing diagnosis at this time?
   1. *Ineffective Denial*
   2. *Caregiver Role Strain*
   3. *Fear*
   4. *Compromised Family Coping*

6. The nurse has recently changed jobs to work with young adults and recocognizes that sources of stress common to that population include which of the following? (Select all that apply.)
   1. Marriage
   2. Aging parents
   3. Starting a new job
   4. Leaving the parental home
   5. Decreased physical abilities
   6. Changing body structure

7. A middle-aged male client is experiencing job-related stress associated with the fear of layoff, resulting in his accepting projects that require a great deal of travel. Which of the following would be the most important health promotion strategy for this client?
   1. Exercise
   2. Sleep
   3. Nutrition
   4. Time management

8. The first time the nurse enters the client's room, the client is on the phone. Immediately, the client slams down the phone, sweeps everything off the overbed table, and demands that the nurse perform several duties "this very minute." Which of the following would be the most appropriate response for the nurse?

1. Tell the client "I will return" and then leave the room.
2. Tell the client no care will be given until the screaming ends.
3. Begin providing needed care calmly and quietly.
4. Allow the client to complete venting, then respond calmly.

See Answers to Test Your Knowledge in Appendix A.

EXPLORE MEDIALINK www.prenhall.com/berman

DVD-ROM
- Audio Glossary
- NCLEX Review
- Animation: Reuptake Inhibitor

COMPANION WEBSITE
- Additional NCLEX Review
- Case Study: Becoming Parents
- Care Plan Activity: Client Going Through a Divorce
- Application Activities:
  - Resources for Stress Management
  - School Nursing Care of Teenagers
- Links to Resources

READINGS AND REFERENCES

SUGGESTED READINGS

Santos, S. R., Carroll, C. A., Cox, K. S., Teasley, S. L., Simon, S. D., Bainbridge, L., et al. (2003). Baby boomer nurses bearing the burden of care: A four site study of stress, strain, and coping for inpatient registered nurses. *Journal of Nursing Administration, 33,* 243–250.
This study describes stress, strain, and coping (as influenced by age) across hospital types for inpatient registered nurses. The researchers found evidence to support the need for focused interventions to address challenges of specific types of stressors and age group needs. Baby Boomer nurses (born between 1946 and 1964) had significantly worse scores than other age groups, specifically with the stress and strain subscales of role overload, role insufficiency, role ambiguity, role boundary, and interpersonal strain.

RELATED RESEARCH

De Jong, M. J., Moser, D. K., An, K., & Chung, M. L. (2004). Anxiety is not manifested by elevated heart rate and blood pressure in acutely ill cardiac patients. *European Journal of Cardiovascular Nursing, 3,* 247–253.

Dracup, K., Evangelista, L. S., Doering, L., Tullman, D., Moser, D. K., & Hamilton, M. (2004). Emotional well being in spouses of patients with advanced heart failure. *Heart and Lung, 33,* 354–361.

REFERENCES

Anspaugh, D. J., Hamrick, M., & Rosato, F. D. (2005). *Wellness: Concepts and applications* (6th ed.). New York: McGraw-Hill.

Antai-Otong, D. (2003). Anxiety disorders: Helping your patient conquer her fears. *Nursing, 33*(12), 36–41.

Carpenito-Moyet, L. J. (2006). *Nursing diagnosis: Application to clinical practice* (11th ed.). Philadelphia: Lippincott.

Dochterman, J., & Bulechek, G. B. (Eds.). (2004). *Nursing interventions classification (NIC)* (4th ed.). St. Louis, MO: Mosby.

Edlin, G., & Golanty, E. (2007). *Health and wellness: A holistic approach* (9th ed.). Boston: Jones & Bartlett.

Folkman, S., & Lazarus, R. S. (1991). Coping and emotion. In A. Monat & R. S. Lazarus (Eds.), *Stress and coping* (3rd ed.). New York: Columbia University Press.

Fontaine, K. L., & Fletcher, J. S. (2003). *Mental health nursing* (5th ed.). Upper Saddle River, NJ: Prentice Hall.

Freud, S. (1946). *The ego and the mechanisms of defense.* New York: International Universities Press.

Holmes, T. H., & Rahe, R. H. (1967). The social readjustment rating scale. *Journal of Psychosomatic Research, 11,* 213–218.

Lazarus, R. S. (1966). *Psychological stress and the coping process.* New York: McGraw-Hill.

Lazarus, R. S. (2000). Toward better research on stress and coping. *American Psychologist, 55,* 665–673.

Miller, M. A., & Rahe, R. H. (1997). Life changes scaling for the 1990s. *Journal of Psychosomatic Research, 43,* 279–292.

Monat, A., & Lazarus, R. S. (Eds.). (1991). *Stress and coping* (3rd ed.). New York: Columbia University Press.

Moorhead, S., Johnson, M., & Maas, M. (Eds.). (2004). *Nursing outcomes classification (NOC)* (3rd ed.). St. Louis, MO: Mosby.

NANDA International. (2007). *NANDA nursing diagnoses: Definitions and classification 2007–2008.* Philadelphia: Author.

Rahe, R. H., & Tolles, R. L. (2002). The brief stress and coping inventory: A useful stress management instrument. *International Journal of Stress Management, 9,* 61–70.

Selye, H. (1956). *The stress of life.* New York: McGraw-Hill.

Selye, H. (1976). *The stress of life* (revised ed.). New York: McGraw-Hill.

Sharpe, L., Butow, P., Smith, C., McConnell, D., & Clarke, S. (2005).The relationship between available support, unmet needs and caregiver burden in patients with advanced cancer and their carers. *Psycho-Oncology, 14,* 102–114.

United States Department of Agriculture. (2005). *Nutrition and your health: Dietary guidelines for Americans.* Retrieved June 18, 2006, from http://www.health.gov/dietaryguidelines/ dga2000/document/aim.htm#physical_top

SELECTED BIBLIOGRAPHY

Cooke, M., Chaboyer, W., & Hiratos, M. A. (2005). Music and its effect on anxiety in short waiting periods: A critical appraisal. *Journal of Clinical Nursing, 14,* 145–155.

Cote, J. K., & Pepler, C. (2005). Cognitive coping intervention for acutely ill HIV positive men. *Journal of Clinical Nursing, 14,* 321–326.

Cox, S. (2004). Curing fixer-pleaser syndrome. *Nursing, 34*(5), 64.

Larner, S. (2005). Common psychological challenges for patients with newly acquired disability. *Nursing Standard, 19*(28), 33–39.

LeSergent, C. M., & Haney, C. J. (2005). Rural hospital nurse's stressors and coping strategies: A survey. *International Journal of Nursing Studies, 42,* 315–324.

Lyons, K. S., Stewart, B. J., Archbold, P. G., Carter, J. H., & Perrin, N. A. (2004). Pessimism and optimism as early warning signs for compromised health for caregivers of patients with Parkinson's disease. *Nursing Research, 53,* 354–362.

Mitchell, M. L., & Courtney, M. (2004). Reducing family members' anxiety and uncertainty in illness around transfer from intensive care, an intervention study. *Intensive and Critical Care Nursing, 20,* 223–231.

Wanzer, M., Booth-Butterfield, M. M., & Booth-Butterfield, S. (2005). "If we didn't use humor, we'd cry": Humorous coping communication in health care settings. *Journal of Health Communication, 10,* 105–125.

CHAPTER 43

Loss, Grieving, and Death

LEARNING OUTCOMES

After completing this chapter, you will be able to:

1. Describe types and sources of losses.
2. Discuss selected frameworks for identifying stages of grieving.
3. Identify clinical symptoms of grief.
4. Discuss factors affecting a grief response.
5. Identify measures that facilitate the grieving process.
6. List clinical signs of impending and actual death.
7. Describe helping clients die with dignity.
8. Describe the role of the nurse in working with families or caregivers of dying clients.
9. Describe nursing measures for care of the body after death.

KEY TERMS

actual loss, *1082*	**end-of-life care,** *1095*	**mourning,** *1082*
algor mortis, *1096*	**grief,** *1082*	**mutual pretense,** *1092*
anticipatory grief, *1082*	**heart-lung death,** *1091*	**open awareness,** *1092*
anticipatory loss, *1082*	**higher brain death,** *1091*	**palliative care,** *1095*
bereavement, *1082*	**hospice,** *1094*	**perceived loss,** *1082*
cerebral death, *1091*	**livor mortis,** *1097*	**rigor mortis,** *1096*
closed awareness, *1092*	**loss,** *1081*	**shroud,** *1097*
complicated grief, *1083*	**mortician,** *1097*	**undertaker,** *1097*

Everyone experiences loss, grieving, and death at some time during his or her life. People may suffer the loss of valued relationships through life changes, such as moving from one city to another, separation, divorce, or the death of a parent, spouse, or friend. People may grieve changing life roles as they watch grown children leave home or they retire from their lifelong work. The loss of valued material objects through theft or natural disaster can evoke feelings of grief and loss. When people's lives are affected by civil or national strife, they may grieve the loss of valued ideals such as safety, freedom, or democracy.

In the clinical setting, the nurse encounters clients who may be experiencing grief related to declining health, loss of a body part, terminal illness, or the impending death of self or a significant other. The nurse may also work with clients in community settings who are grieving losses related to personal crisis (e.g., divorce, separation) or disaster (war, earthquakes, terrorism, or hurricanes). Therefore, it is important for the nurse to understand the significance of loss and develop the ability to assist clients as they work through the grieving process.

Nurses may interact with dying clients and their families or caregivers in a variety of settings, from a fetal demise (death of an unborn child), to the adolescent victim of an accident, to the elderly client who finally succumbs to a chronic illness. Nurses must recognize the various influences on the dying process—legal, ethical, religious and spiritual, biologic, personal—and be prepared to provide sensitive, skilled, and supportive care to all those affected.

LOSS AND GRIEF

Loss is an actual or potential situation in which something that is valued is changed or no longer available. People can experience the loss of body image, a significant other, a sense of well-being, a job, personal possessions, or beliefs. Illness and hospitalization often produce losses.

Death is a fundamental loss, both for the dying person and for those who survive. Although death is inevitable, it can stimulate people to grow in their understanding of themselves and others. Death can be viewed as the dying person's final opportunity to experience life in ways that bring significance and fulfillment. People experiencing loss often search for the meaning of the event, and it is generally accepted that finding meaning is needed in order for healing to occur. However, persons can be well adjusted without searching for meaning, and even those who find meaning may not see it as an end point but rather an ongoing process.

R EAL WORLD PRACTICE

Taking care of a client who is dying and dealing with the client's family is one of the hardest jobs in nursing. You will never forget your first "Code Blue." Some clients and their families will stay with you forever. Figuring out how to deal with clients and their families during such an emotional time is a challenge and is very individualized, as we all bring with us our own life experiences, spirituality, and values.

If I could share one thing I have learned over the years, it would be this: Don't be afraid to cry with the family. We all have to figure out how much space we need emotionally to do our job and function appropriately, especially in emergency situations. Yet, to ignore our own emotions sometimes makes us appear as if we don't care, that the sadness of the situation has no effect on us. Whether we like it or not, those family members will remember us for a very long time. I have shed tears in front of parents and families. I have hugged them. I have cried openly with them when I have cared for their child long enough to have formed a relation-

ship with them. The tears oftentimes were cathartic, and the simple act of sharing the sadness made all the difference to the family.

As nurses we need to be professional, but we can be professional and show our human side simultaneously. Years ago I cared for a baby who was born with a congenital heart defect that required surgery. It was Mom's first baby. The mom insisted on staying with her baby day after day, despite my urges to take care of herself and get some sleep. The baby was in our ICU for about a month and died. I cried with that mom many times. I knew why she couldn't leave her baby. She knew he wasn't going to make it and didn't want him to be alone. I get Christmas cards from Mom to this day. She and her husband went on to have two more beautiful children. I count myself lucky to have been a part of the first baby's life and know that I am a positive part of Mom's memories as well.

—Sherrie Hatch, BSN, RN, CCRN,
UC Davis Medical Center, Sacramento, CA

Types and Sources of Loss

There are two general types of loss, actual and perceived. An **actual loss** can be recognized by others. A **perceived loss** is experienced by one person but cannot be verified by others. Psychologic losses are often perceived losses in that they are not directly verifiable. For example, a woman who leaves her employment to care for her children at home may perceive a loss of independence and freedom. Both losses can be anticipatory. An **anticipatory loss** is experienced before the loss actually occurs. For example, a woman whose husband is dying may experience actual loss in anticipation of his death.

Loss can be viewed as situational or developmental. The loss of one's job, the death of a child, or the loss of functional ability because of acute illness or injury are *situational losses.* Losses that occur in the process of normal development—such as the departure of grown children from the home, retirement from a career, and the death of aged parents—are *developmental losses* that can to some extent be anticipated and prepared for.

There are many sources of loss: (a) loss of an aspect of oneself—a body part, a physiologic function, or a psychologic attribute; (b) loss of an object external to oneself; (c) separation from an accustomed environment; and (d) loss of a loved or valued person.

Aspect of Self

The loss of an aspect of self changes a person's body image, even though the loss may not be obvious. A face scarred from a burn is generally obvious to people; loss of part of the stomach or loss of ability to feel emotion may not be as obvious. The degree to which these losses affect a person largely depends on the integrity of the person's body image.

During old age, changes occur in physical and mental capabilities. Again the self-image is vulnerable. Old age is the stage in life when people may experience many losses: of employment, of usual activities, of independence, of health, of friends, and of family.

External Objects

Loss of external objects includes (a) loss of inanimate objects that have importance to the person, such as the loss of money or the burning down of a family's house; and (b) loss of animate (live) objects such as pets that provide love and companionship.

Familiar Environment

Separation from an environment and people who provide security can result in a sense of loss. The 6-year-old is likely to feel loss when first leaving the home environment to attend school. The university student who moves away from home for the first time also experiences a sense of loss.

Loved Ones

The loss of a loved one or valued person through illness, divorce, separation, or death can be very disturbing. In some illnesses (such as Alzheimer's dementia), a person may undergo personality changes that make friends and family feel they have lost that person.

The death of a loved one is a permanent and complete loss. In contemporary American society, people may be uncomfortable talking about death and being around people who are dying. There is a tendency to consider using extraordinary measures to prolong and preserve life.

Grief, Bereavement, and Mourning

Grief is the total response to the emotional experience related to loss. Grief is manifested in thoughts, feelings, and behaviors associated with overwhelming distress or sorrow. **Bereavement** is the subjective response experienced by the surviving loved ones after the death of a person with whom they have shared a significant relationship. **Mourning** is the behavioral process through which grief is eventually resolved or altered; it is often influenced by culture, spiritual beliefs, and custom. Grief and mourning are experienced not only by the person who faces the death of a loved one but also by the person who suffers other kinds of losses. Grieving is essential for good mental and physical health. It permits the individual to cope with the loss gradually and to accept it as part of reality. Grief is a social process; it is best shared and carried out with the assistance of others.

Working through one's grief is important because bereavement may have potentially devastating effects on health. Among the symptoms that can accompany grief are anxiety, depression, weight loss, difficulties in swallowing, vomiting, fatigue, headaches, dizziness, fainting, blurred vision, skin rashes, excessive sweating, menstrual disturbances, palpitations, chest pain, and dyspnea. The bereaved may also experience alterations in libido, concentration, and patterns of eating, sleeping, activity, and communication.

Although bereavement can threaten health, a positive resolution of the grieving process can enrich the individual with new insights, values, challenges, openness, and sensitivity. For some, the pain of loss, though diminished, recurs for the rest of their lives.

Types of Grief Responses

A normal grief reaction may be abbreviated or anticipatory. *Abbreviated grief* is brief but genuinely felt. This can occur when the lost object is not significantly important to the grieving person or may have been replaced immediately by another, equally esteemed object. **Anticipatory grief** is experienced in advance of the event such as the wife who grieves before her ailing husband dies. A young girl may grieve in advance of an operation that will leave a scar on her body. Because many of the normal symptoms of grief will have already been expressed in anticipation, the reaction when the loss actually occurs is sometimes quite abbreviated.

Disenfranchised grief occurs when a person is unable to acknowledge the loss to other persons. Situations in which this may occur often relate to a socially unacceptable loss that cannot be spoken about, such as suicide, abortion, or giving a child up for adoption. Other examples include losses of relationships that are socially unsanctioned and may not be known to other people (such as homosexuality or extramarital relationships).

Unhealthy grief—that is, pathologic or **complicated grief**—exists when the strategies to cope with the loss are maladaptive. Many factors can contribute to complicated grief, including a prior traumatic loss, family or cultural barriers to the emotional expression of grief, sudden death, strained relationships between the survivor and the deceased, and lack of adequate support for the survivor (Egan & Arnold, 2003).

Complicated grief may take several different forms. *Unresolved or chronic grief* is extended in length and severity. The same signs are expressed as with normal grief, but the bereaved may also have difficulty expressing the grief, may deny the loss, or may grieve beyond the expected time. With *inhibited grief,* many of the normal symptoms of grief are suppressed, and other effects, including somatic, are experienced instead. *Delayed grief* occurs when feelings are purposely or subconsciously suppressed until a much later time. A survivor who appears to be using dangerous activities as a method to lessen the pain of grieving may be experiencing *exaggerated grief.*

Complicated grief after a death may be inferred from the following data or observations:

- The client fails to grieve; for example, a husband does not cry at, or absents himself from, his wife's funeral.
- The client avoids visiting the grave and refuses to participate in memorial services, even though these practices are a part of the client's culture.
- The client becomes recurrently symptomatic on the anniversary of a loss or during holidays.
- The client develops persistent guilt and lowered self-esteem.
- Even after a prolonged period, the client continues to search for the lost person. Some may consider suicide to effect reunion.

- A relatively minor event triggers symptoms of grief.
- Even after a period of time, the client is unable to discuss the deceased with composure; for example, the client's voice cracks and quivers, and eyes become moist.
- After the normal period of grief, the client experiences physical symptoms similar to those of the person who died.
- The client's relationships with friends and relatives worsen following the death.

Many factors contribute to unresolved grief after a death:

- Ambivalence (intense feelings, both positive and negative) toward the lost person
- A perceived need to be brave and in control; fear of losing control in front of others
- Endurance of multiple losses, such as the loss of an entire family, which the bereaved finds too overwhelming to contemplate
- Extremely high emotional value invested in the dead person; failure to grieve in this instance helps the bereaved avoid the reality of the loss
- Uncertainty about the loss—for example, when a loved one is "missing in action"
- Lack of support systems

Stages of Grieving

Many authors have described stages or phases of grieving, perhaps the most well known of them being Kübler-Ross (1969), who described five stages: denial, anger, bargaining, depression, and acceptance (Table 43–1). Engel (1964) identified six stages of grieving: shock and disbelief, developing

TABLE 43–1	**Client Responses and Nursing Implications in Kübler-Ross's Stages of Grieving**	
STAGE	**BEHAVIORAL RESPONSES**	**NURSING IMPLICATIONS**
Denial	Refuses to believe that loss is happening. Is unready to deal with practical problems, such as prosthesis after the loss of a leg. May assume artificial cheerfulness to prolong denial.	Verbally support client but do not reinforce denial. Examine your own behavior to ensure that you do not share in client's denial.
Anger	Client or family may direct anger at nurse or staff about matters that normally would not bother them.	Help client understand that anger is a normal response to feelings of loss and powerlessness. Avoid withdrawal or retaliation; do not take anger personally. Deal with needs underlying any angry reaction. Provide structure and continuity to promote feelings of security. Allow clients as much control as possible over their lives.
Bargaining	Seeks to bargain to avoid loss. May express feelings of guilt or fear of punishment for past sins, real or imagined.	Listen attentively, and encourage client to talk to relieve guilt and irrational fear. If appropriate, offer spiritual support.
Depression	Grieves over what has happened and what cannot be. May talk freely (e.g., reviewing past losses such as money or job), or may withdraw.	Allow client to express sadness. Communicate nonverbally by sitting quietly without expecting conversation. Convey caring by touch.
Acceptance	Comes to terms with loss. May have decreased interest in surroundings and support people. May wish to begin making plans (e.g., will, prosthesis, altered living arrangements).	Help family and friends understand client's decreased need to socialize. Encourage client to participate as much as possible in the treatment program.

TABLE 43-2 **Engel's Stages of Grieving**	
STAGE	**BEHAVIORAL RESPONSES**
Shock and disbelief	Refuses to accept loss. Has stunned feelings. Accepts the situation intellectually, but denies it emotionally.
Developing awareness	Reality of loss begins to penetrate consciousness. Anger may be directed at agency, nurses, or others.
Restitution	Conducts rituals of mourning (e.g., funeral).
Resolving the loss	Attempts to deal with painful void. Still unable to accept new love object to replace lost person or object. May accept more dependent relationship with support person. Thinks over and talks about memories of the lost object.
Idealization	Produces image of lost object that is almost devoid of undesirable features. Represses all negative and hostile feelings toward lost object. May feel guilty and remorseful about past inconsiderate or unkind acts to lost person. Unconsciously internalizes admired qualities of lost object. Reminders of lost object evoke fewer feelings of sadness. Reinvests feelings in others.
Outcome	Behavior influenced by several factors: importance of lost object as source of support, degree of dependence on relationship, degree of ambivalence toward lost object, number and nature of other relationships, and number and nature of previous grief experiences (which tend to be cumulative).

Note: From "Grief and Grieving," by G. L. Engel, 1964, *American Journal of Nursing, 64*(9), pp. 93–98. Copyright © Lippincott, Williams & Wilkins, 1964. Adapted with permission.

awareness, restitution, resolving the loss, idealization, and outcome (Table 43–2). Sanders (1998) described five phases of bereavement: shock, awareness, conservation/withdrawal, healing, and renewal (Table 43–3).

Martocchio (1985) described five clusters of grief—shock and disbelief; yearning and protest; anguish, disorganization, and despair; identification in bereavement; and reorganization and restitution—and maintained that there is no single correct way, nor a correct timetable, by which a person progresses through the grief process. Whether a person can succeed in integrating the loss and how this is accomplished are related to that person's individual development and personal makeup. In addition, individuals responding to the very same loss cannot be expected to follow the same pattern or schedule in resolving their grief, even while they support each other.

Rando (1991, 1993, 2000) has written extensively on the subject of grief, describing three categories of responses: avoidance, confrontation, and accommodation. Avoidance is similar to Kübler-Ross's phases of denial, anger, and bargaining and Engel's phase of shock and disbelief. Confrontation is the most upsetting phase for the grieving person facing the loss. Accommodation is the phase in which the person begins to resume more usual activities, feels better, and places the loss in perspective.

Manifestations of Grief

The nurse assesses the grieving client or family members following a loss to determine the phase or stage of grieving. Physiologically, the body responds to a current or anticipated loss with a stress reaction. The nurse can assess the clinical signs of this response. See Chapter 42. ∞

Manifestations of grief that would be considered normal include verbalization of the loss, crying, sleep disturbance, loss of appetite, and difficulty concentrating. Complicated grieving may be characterized by extended time of denial, depression, severe physiologic symptoms, or suicidal thoughts.

Factors Influencing the Loss and Grief Responses

A number of factors affect a person's response to a loss or death. These factors include age, significance of the loss, culture, spiritual beliefs, gender, socioeconomic status, support systems, and the cause of the loss or death. Nurses can learn general concepts about the influence of these factors of the grieving experience, but the constellation of these factors and their significance will vary from individual to individual.

Age

Age affects a person's understanding of and reaction to loss. With familiarity, people usually increase their understanding and acceptance of life, loss, and death.

People do not usually experience the loss of loved ones at regular intervals. As a result, preparation for these experiences is difficult. Coping with other of life's losses, such as the loss of a pet, the loss of a friend, and the loss of youth or a job, can help people anticipate the more severe loss of death of loved ones by teaching them successful coping strategies.

CHILDHOOD. Children differ from adults not only in their understanding of loss and death but also in how they are affected by the loss of others. The loss of a parent or other significant person can threaten the child's ability to develop, and regression sometimes results. Assisting the child with the grief experience includes helping the child regain the normal continuity and pace of emotional development.

Some adults may assume that children do not have the same need as an adult to grieve the loss of others. In situations of cri-

TABLE 43–3 Sander's Phases of Bereavement

PHASE	DESCRIPTION	BEHAVIORAL RESPONSES
Shock	Survivors are left with feelings of confusion, unreality, and disbelief that the loss has occurred. They are often unable to process the normal thought sequences. Phase may last from a few minutes to many days.	Disbelief Confusion Restlessness Feelings of unreality Regression and helplessness State of alarm Physical symptoms: dryness of mouth and throat, sighing, weeping, loss of muscular control, uncontrolled trembling, sleep disturbance, and loss of appetite Psychologic symptoms: preoccupation with thoughts of the deceased and psychologic distancing
Awareness of loss	Friends and family resume normal activities. The bereaved experience the full significance of their loss.	Separation anxiety Conflicts Acting out emotional expectations Prolonged stress Physical symptoms: crying and sleep disturbance Psychologic symptoms: anger, guilt, frustration, shame, oversensitivity, disbelief and denial, dreaming, sense of presence of the deceased, and fear of death
Conservation/withdrawal	During this phase, survivors feel a need to be alone to conserve and replenish both physical and emotional energy. The social support available to the bereaved has decreased, and they may experience despair and helplessness.	Physical symptoms: weakness, fatigue, need for more sleep, and a weakened immune system Psychologic symptoms: withdrawal, obsessional review, grief work, and ultimately a renewal of hope
Healing: the turning point	During this phase, the bereaved move from distress about living without their loved one to learning to live more independently.	Assuming control Identity restructuring Relinquishing roles, such as spouse, child, or parent Physical symptoms: increased energy, sleep restoration, immune system restoration, and physical healing Psychologic symptoms: forgiving, forgetting, searching for meaning, and hope
Renewal	In this phase, survivors move on to a new self-awareness, an acceptance of responsibility for self, and learning to live without the loved one.	Functional stability Revitalization Assumption of responsibility for self-care needs Psychologic symptoms: loneliness, anniversary reactions, and a reaching out to others

Note: From *Grief: The Mourning After: Dealing with Adult Bereavement,* 2nd ed., by C. M. Sanders, copyright ©1998, New York: John Wiley & Sons. Reprinted with permission of John Wiley & Sons, Inc.

sis and loss, children are sometimes pushed aside or protected from the pain. They can feel afraid, abandoned, and lonely. Careful work with bereaved children is especially necessary because experiencing a loss in childhood can have serious effects later in life (Figure 43-1 ■).

EARLY AND MIDDLE ADULTHOOD. As people grow, they come to experience loss as part of normal development. By middle age, for example, the loss of a parent through death seems a more normal occurrence compared to the death of a younger person. Coping with the death of an aged parent has even been viewed as an essential developmental task of the middle-aged adult.

The middle-aged adult can experience losses other than death. For example, losses resulting from impaired health or body function and losses of various role functions can be difficult for the middle-aged adult. How the middle-aged adult responds to such losses is influenced by previous experiences with loss, the person's sense of self-esteem, and the strength and availability of support.

Figure 43-1 ■ Children experience the same emotions of grief as adults.
David Young-Wolff/PhotoEdit

LATE ADULTHOOD. Losses experienced by older adults include loss of health, mobility, independence, and work role. Limited income and the need to change one's living accommodations can also lead to feelings of loss and grieving.

For older adults, the loss through death of a longtime mate is profound. Although individuals differ in their ability to deal with such a loss, research suggests that health problems for widows and widowers increase following the death of the spouse (Caserta, Lund, & Obray, 2004). Because the majority of deaths occur among elderly people, and because the number of elderly people is increasing in North America, nurses will need to be especially alert to the potential problems of older grieving adults.

Significance of the Loss

The significance of a loss depends on the perceptions of the individual experiencing the loss. One person may experience a great sense of loss over a divorce; another may find it only mildly disrupting. A number of factors affect the significance of the loss:

- Importance of the lost person, object, or function
- Degree of change required because of the loss
- The person's beliefs and values

For older people who have already encountered many losses, an anticipated loss such as their own death may not be viewed as highly negative, and they may be apathetic about it instead of reactive. More than fearing death, some may fear loss of control or becoming a burden.

Culture

Culture influences an individual's reaction to loss. How grief is expressed is often determined by the customs of the culture. Unless an extended family structure exists, grief is handled by the nuclear family. The death of a family member in a typical nuclear family leaves a great void because the same few individuals fill most of the roles. In cultures where several generations and extended family members either reside in the same household or are physically close, the impact of a family member's death may be softened because the roles of the deceased are quickly filled by other relatives.

Some persons have adopted the belief that grief is a private matter to be endured internally. Therefore, feelings tend to be repressed and may remain unidentified. People who have been socialized to "be strong" and "make the best of the situation" may not express deep feelings or personal concerns when they experience a serious loss.

Some cultural groups value social support and the expression of loss. In some groups, expressions of grief through wailing, crying, physical prostration, and other outward demonstrations are acceptable and encouraged. Other groups may frown on this demonstration as a loss of control, favoring a more quiet and stoic expression of grief. In cultural groups where strong kinship ties are maintained, physical and emotional support and assistance are provided by family members.

Spiritual Beliefs

Spiritual beliefs and practices greatly influence both a person's reaction to loss and subsequent behavior. Most religious groups have practices related to dying, and these are often important to the client and support people. To provide support at a time of death, nurses need to understand the client's particular beliefs and practices.

Gender

The gender roles into which many people are socialized in the United States and Canada affect their reactions at times of loss. Men are frequently expected to "be strong" and show very little emotion during grief, whereas it is acceptable for women to show grief by crying. Often when a wife dies, the husband, who is the chief mourner, is expected to repress his own emotions and to comfort sons and daughters in their grieving.

Gender roles also affect the significance of body image changes to clients. A man might consider his facial scar to be "macho," but a woman might consider hers ugly. Thus the woman, but not the man, would see the change as a loss.

Socioeconomic Status

The socioeconomic status of an individual often affects the support system available at the time of a loss. A pension plan or insurance, for example, can offer a widowed or disabled person a choice of ways to deal with a loss; a person who is confronted with both severe loss and economic hardship may not be able to cope with either.

Support System

The people closest to the grieving individual are often the first to recognize and provide needed emotional, physical, and functional assistance. However, because many people are uncomfortable or inexperienced in dealing with losses, the usual support people may instead withdraw from the grieving individual. In addition, support may be available when the loss is first recognized, but as the support people return to their usual activities, the need for ongoing support may be unmet. Sometimes, the grieving individual is unable or unready to accept support when it is offered.

Cause of Loss or Death

Individual and societal views on the cause of a loss or death may significantly influence the grief response. Some diseases are considered "clean," such as cardiovascular disorders, and engender compassion, whereas others may be viewed as repulsive and less unfortunate. A loss or death that is beyond the control of those involved may be more acceptable than one that is preventable, such as a drunk driving accident. Injuries or deaths occurring during respected activities, such as "in the line of duty," are considered honorable, whereas those occurring during illicit activities may be considered the individual's just rewards.

NURSING MANAGEMENT

Assessing

Nursing assessment of the client experiencing a loss includes three major components: (a) nursing history, (b) assessment of personal coping resources, and (c) physical assessment. During the routine

ASSESSMENT INTERVIEW   Loss and Grieving

PREVIOUS LOSSES

- Have you ever lost someone or something very important to you?
- Have you or your family ever moved to a new home or location?
- What was it like for you when you first started school? Moved away from home? Got a job? Retired?
- Are you physically able to do all the things you used to do?
- Has anyone important or close to you died?
- Do you think there will be any losses in your life in the near future?

If there has been previous grieving:

- Tell me about (the loss). What was losing _____ like for you?
- Did you have trouble sleeping? Eating? Concentrating?
- What kinds of things did you do to make yourself feel better when something like that happened?
- Did you observe any spiritual or cultural practices when you had a loss like that?
- Whom did you turn to if you were very upset about (the loss)?
- How long did it take you to feel more like yourself again and go back to your usual activities?

If there is a current loss:

- What have you been told about (the loss)? Is there anything else you would like to know or don't understand?
- What changes do you think this (illness, surgery, problem) will cause in your life? What do you think it will be like without (the lost object)?
- Have you ever experienced a loss like this before?
- Can you think of anything good that might come out of this?
- What kind of help do you think you will need? Who is going to be helping you with this loss?
- Are there any people or organizations in your community that might be able to help?

CURRENT GRIEVING

- Are you having trouble sleeping? Eating? Concentrating? Breathing?
- Do you have any pain or other new physical problems?
- What are you doing to help you deal with this loss?
- Are you taking any drugs or medications to help you cope with this loss?

---

health assessment of every client, the nurse poses questions regarding previous and current losses. The nature of the loss and the significance of such losses to the client must be explored.

If there is a current or recent loss, greater detail is needed in the assessment. Because clients do not always associate physical ailments with emotional responses such as grief, the nurse may need to probe to identify possible loss-related stresses. If the client reports significant losses, it is important to examine how the client usually copes with loss and what resources are available to assist the client in coping. Data regarding general health status; other personal stressors; cultural and spiritual traditions, rituals, and beliefs related to loss and grieving; and the person's support network will be needed in order to determine a plan of care (see the Assessment Interview). In assessing the client's response to a current loss, the nurse may identify complicated grief best treated by a health care professional who is expert in assisting such clients. If the nursing assessment reveals severe physical or psychologic signs and symptoms, the client should be referred to an appropriate care provider.

Diagnosing

Nursing diagnoses (NANDA International, 2007) relating specifically to grieving include the following:

- *Grieving:* A normal complex process that includes emotional, physical, spiritual, social, and intellectual responses and behaviors by which individuals, families, and communities incorporate an actual, anticipated, or perceived loss into their daily lives.
- *Complicated Grieving:* a disorder that occurs after the death of a significant other, in which the experience of distress accompanying bereavement fails to follow normative expectations and manifests in functional impairment. *Risk for Complicated Grieving* replaced *Risk for Dysfunctional Grieving* in 2007 which had been added as a new diagnosis in 2005.

Other nursing diagnoses may include

- *Interrupted Family Processes* if the loss has such impact on the individual and family that usual effective roles and interactions are negatively affected.
- *Risk-prone Health Behavior* if the client has great difficulty placing the loss in appropriate perspective to his or her other life activities.
- *Risk for Loneliness* related to the loss of relationships with others.

Examples of clinical applications of some of these diagnoses using NANDA, NIC, and NOC designations are shown in Identifying Nursing Diagnoses, Outcomes, and Interventions.

Planning

The overall goals for clients who are grieving the loss of body function or a body part are to adjust to the changed ability and to redirect both physical and emotional energy into rehabilitation. The goals for clients who are grieving the loss of a loved one or thing are to remember them without feeling intense pain and to redirect emotional energy into one's own life and adjust to the actual or impending loss.

Examples of clinical applications of NOC outcomes and NIC interventions are shown in Identifying Nursing Diagnoses, Outcomes, and Interventions.

Planning for Home Care

Clients who have sustained or anticipate a loss may require ongoing nursing care to assist them in adapting to the loss. The determination of how much and what type of home care follow-up is needed is based in great part on the nurse's knowledge of how the client and family have coped with previous losses. In preparation for home care, the nurse reassesses the client's abilities and needs. The Home Care Assessment on page 1088 describes data to gather for home care or follow-up assessment.

IDENTIFYING NURSING DIAGNOSES, OUTCOMES, AND INTERVENTIONS
Clients Who Are Grieving

DATA CLUSTER Teresa Jimenez's son Ramon, age 15, has cystic fibrosis of the lungs. Mother and son are waiting for an appropriate donor for a heart-lung transplant. She says, "We've been called to the transplant unit twice, but things didn't work out. Ramon gets his hopes all geared up, and then he's deflated. I can't eat or sleep worrying. I don't know what I'll do if he doesn't get that transplant. He's all I've got since my husband left us six years ago."

NURSING DIAGNOSIS/ DEFINITION	SAMPLE DESIRED OUTCOMES*/ DEFINITION	INDICATORS	SELECTED INTERVENTIONS*/ DEFINITION	SAMPLE NIC ACTIVITIES
Grieving/A normal complex process that includes emotional, physical, spiritual, social, and intellectual responses and behaviors by which individuals, families, and communities incorporate an actual, anticipated, or perceived loss into their daily lives	Grief Resolution [1304]/Adjustment to actual or impending loss	Often demonstrated: ▪ Maintains living environment ▪ Seeks social support ▪ Progresses through stages of grief	Grief Work Facilitation [5290]/Assistance with the resolution of a significant loss	▪ Encourage discussion of previous loss experiences (e.g., husband leaving) ▪ Communicate acceptance of discussing loss ▪ Identify sources of community support ▪ Reinforce progress made in the grieving process

DATA CLUSTER Tom Bauer's wife died 14 months ago of a ruptured aortic aneurysm at age 59. He lives alone, has no children, and refuses to see friends. He reports frequent headaches, inability to concentrate at work, little interest in food, and early morning insomnia. These symptoms increase at the time of his wife's birthday and their anniversary. He says, "I still can't find it in myself to visit her grave. There are times when I'd just like to die and be with her."

Complicated Grieving/ A disorder that occurs after the death of a significant other, in which the experience of distress accompanying bereavement fails to follow normative expectations and manifests in functional impairment.	Concentration [0905]/ Ability to focus on a specific stimulus	Mildly compromised: ▪ Maintains attention ▪ Maintains focus without being distracted	Mood Management [5330]/Providing for safety, stabilization, recovery, and maintenance of a patient who is experiencing dysfunctionally depressed or elevated mood	▪ Determine whether he presents safety risk to self ▪ Assist him to maintain a normal cycle of sleep/wakefulness ▪ Provide opportunity for physical activity ▪ Teach decision-making skills ▪ Provide or refer for psychotherapy when appropriate ▪ Assist him to consciously monitor mood

*The NOC # for desired outcomes and the NIC # for nursing interventions are listed in brackets following the appropriate outcome or intervention. Outcomes, indicators, interventions, and activities selected are only a sample of those suggested by NOC and NIC and should be further individualized for each client.

Implementing

The skills most relevant to situations of loss and grief are attentive listening, silence, open and closed questioning, paraphrasing, clarifying and reflecting feelings, and summarizing.

Less helpful to clients are responses that give advice and evaluation, those that interpret and analyze, and those that give unwarranted reassurance. To ensure effective communication, the nurse must make an accurate assessment of what is appropriate for the client.

HOME CARE ASSESSMENT   Grieving

CLIENT

- *Knowledge:* Client's understanding of the implications of the loss
- *Self-care abilities:* Skill in caring for self based on any physical abilities that may have been altered by the loss
- *Current coping:* Stage in the grieving or bereavement process
- *Current manifestations of the grief response:* Adaptive or maladaptive signs and symptoms; cultural or spiritually based behaviors
- *Role expectations:* Client's perception of the need to return to work or family roles

FAMILY

- *Knowledge:* Various family members' perception of the loss
- *Support people's availability and skills:* Sensitivity to the client's emotional and physical needs; ability to provide an accepting environment
- *Role expectations:* Family perception of client's need to return to work or family roles

COMMUNITY

- *Resources:* Availability and familiarity with possible sources of assistance such as grief support groups, religious or spiritual centers, counseling services, physical care providers

Communication with grieving clients needs to be relevant to their stage of grief. Whether the client is angry or depressed affects how the client hears messages and how the nurse interprets the client's statements.

In addition to using effective communication skills, the nurse implements a plan to provide client and family teaching and to help the client work through the stages of grief.

Facilitating Grief Work

■ Explore and respect the client's and family's ethnic, cultural, religious, and personal values in their expressions of grief.
■ Teach the client or family what to expect in the grief process, such as that certain thoughts and feelings are normal (acceptable) and that labile emotions, feelings of sadness, guilt, anger, fear, and loneliness will stabilize or lessen over time. Knowing what to expect may lessen the intensity of some reactions.
■ Encourage the client to express and share grief with support people. Sharing feelings reinforces relationships and facilitates the grief process.
■ Teach family members to encourage the client's expression of grief, not to push the client to move on or enforce his or her own expectations of appropriate reactions. If the client is a child, encourage family members to be truthful and to allow the child to participate in the grieving activities of others.
■ Encourage the client to resume normal activities on a schedule that promotes physical and psychologic health. Some clients may try to return to normal activities too quickly. However, a prolonged delay in return may indicate complicated grieving.

Providing Emotional Support

■ Use silence and personal presence along with techniques of therapeutic communication. These techniques enhance exploration of feelings and let clients know that the nurse acknowledges their feelings.
■ Acknowledge the grief of the client's family and significant others. Family support persons are part of the grieving client's world.

■ Offer choices that promote client autonomy. Clients need to have a sense of some control over their own lives at a time when much control may not be possible.
■ Provide appropriate information regarding how to access community resources: clergy, support groups, and counseling services.
■ Suggest additional sources of information and help such as
   a. Grief Recovery Institute.
   b. Partnership of Caring: America's Voice for the Dying.
   c. American Association of Retired Persons.
   d. Compassionate Friends (for those who have lost a child).

Examples of nursing actions appropriate for clients in various stages of the grief process are shown in the Concept Map.

Evaluating

Evaluating the effectiveness of nursing care of the grieving client is difficult because of the long-term nature of the life transition. Criteria for evaluation must be based on goals set by the client and family.

Client goals and related desired outcomes for a grieving client will depend on the characteristics of the loss and the client. Examples of client goals and related outcomes are shown in the accompanying Identifying Nursing Diagnoses, Outcomes, and Interventions.

If outcomes are not achieved, the nurse needs to explore why the plan was unsuccessful. Such exploration begins with reassessing the client in case the nursing diagnoses were inappropriate. Examples of questions guiding the exploration include

■ Do the client's grieving behaviors indicate dysfunctional grieving or another nursing diagnosis?
■ Is the expected outcome unrealistic for the given time frame?
■ Does the client have additional stressors previously not considered that are affecting grief resolution?
■ Have nursing orders been implemented consistently, compassionately, and genuinely?

RESEARCH NOTE   Is There a Better Way to Treat Complicated Grief?

This study compared standard treatment for complicated grief—interpersonal psychotherapy (IPT)—with a new method, complicated grief treatment (CGT). The research was prompted by recognition that complicated grief is a debilitating disorder associated with important negative health consequences, but the results of existing treatments for it have been disappointing. A total of 83 women and 12 men aged 18 to 85 years recruited from a university-based psychiatric research clinic as well as a satellite clinic in a low-income African American community were randomly assigned to receive IPT (n = 46) or CGT (n = 49). Each participant received 16 sessions over about 19 weeks time. IPT focuses on restoring effective interpersonal functioning of the grieving person. CGT has greater emphasis on reviewing the loss, coping with depression, and facing difficult situations. Both treatments produced improvement in complicated grief symptoms. The improvement was statistically significantly better and faster for CGT than for IPT.

IMPLICATIONS

The "gold standard" in research is the randomized clinical trial. This study is reported to be the first of its kind to examine the population of persons experiencing complicated grief. Although CGT was more effective than the standard, it still only achieved results in half the participants. Thus, the study provides evidence that one treatment may be more beneficial than another, but much more research is needed to identify truly effective treatment for a broad population. The nurse may use these results to recommend that clients experiencing complicated grief may achieve greater resolution of symptoms with CGT if IPT has not been successful.

Note: From "Treatment of Complicated Grief: A Randomized Controlled Trial," by K. Shear, E. Frank, P. R. Houck, and C. F. Reynolds, 2005, *Journal of the American Medical Association, 293*, pp. 2601–2608.

DYING AND DEATH

The concept of death is developed over time, as the person grows, experiences various losses, and thinks about concrete and abstract concepts. In general, humans move from a childhood belief in death as a temporary state, to adulthood in which death is accepted as very real but also very frightening, to older adulthood in which death may be viewed as more desirable than living with a poor quality of life. Table 43–4 describes some of the specific beliefs common to different age groups. The nurse's knowledge of these developmental stages helps in understanding some of the client's responses to a life-threatening situation.

Responses to Dying and Death

The reaction of any person to another person's impending or real death, or to the potential reality of his or her own death, depends on all the factors regarding loss and the development of the concept of death. In spite of the individual variations in a person's views about the cause of death, spiritual beliefs, availability of support systems, or any other factor, responses tend to cluster in the phases described by theorists (see Tables 43–1 to 43–3).

Both the client who is dying and the family members grieve as they recognize the loss. Defining characteristics for the nursing diagnosis of *Grieving* include denial, guilt, anger, despair, feelings of worthlessness, crying, and inability to concentrate. They may extend to thoughts of suicide, delusions, and hallucinations. *Fear,* the feeling of disruption that is related to an identifiable source (in this case someone's death), may also be present. Many of the characteristics seen in a fearful person are similar to those of grieving and include crying, immobility, increased pulse and respirations, dry mouth, anorexia, difficulty

sleeping, and nightmares. *Hopelessness* occurs when the person perceives no solutions to a problem—when the death becomes inevitable and the person is unable to see how to move beyond the death. The nurse may observe apathy, pessimism, and inability to make decisions. A person who does perceive a solution to the problem but does not believe that it is possible to implement the solution may be said to experience *Powerlessness*. This loss of control may be manifested by anger, violence, acting out, or depression and passive behavior.

CLINICAL ALERT

Persons who have experienced the deaths of multiple significant others, such as members of the AIDS community, do not necessarily feel the loss or grieve any more or less than those who have experienced fewer deaths. ■

Caregivers, both professionals and support persons, also respond to the impending death. The NANDA diagnosis *Risk for Caregiver Role Strain* may be applied to this group. The ongoing responsibilities for providing physical, economic, psychologic, and social support to a dying person can create extreme stress for the provider. Often, the length of time between a terminal diagnosis and when death will occur is unknown and the people supporting the dying person become fatigued and depressed. There may be anger due to loss of time and resources for personal activities or attention to other people. Within a family that usually functions effectively, death of a member may result in *Interrupted Family Processes*. In this situation, the family may be unable to meet the physical, emotional, or spiritual needs of the members and may have difficulty communicating and problem solving.

TABLE 43–4	**Development of the Concept of Death**
AGE	**BELIEFS/ATTITUDES**
Infancy to 5 years	Does not understand concept of death.
	Infant's sense of separation forms basis for later understanding of loss and death.
	Believes death is reversible, a temporary departure, or sleep.
	Emphasizes immobility and inactivity as attributes of death.
5 to 9 years	Understands that death is final.
	Believes own death can be avoided.
	Associates death with aggression or violence.
	Believes wishes or unrelated actions can be responsible for death.
9 to 12 years	Understands death as the inevitable end of life.
	Begins to understand own mortality, expressed as interest in afterlife or as fear of death.
12 to 18 years	Fears a lingering death.
	May fantasize that death can be defied, acting out defiance through reckless behaviors (e.g., dangerous driving, substance abuse).
	Seldom thinks about death, but views it in religious and philosophic terms.
	May seem to reach "adult" perception of death but be emotionally unable to accept it.
	May still hold concepts from previous developmental stages.
18 to 45 years	Has attitude toward death influenced by religious and cultural beliefs.
45 to 65 years	Accepts own mortality.
	Encounters death of parents and some peers.
	Experiences peaks of death anxiety.
	Death anxiety diminishes with emotional well-being.
65+ years	Fears prolonged illness.
	Encounters death of family members and peers.
	Sees death as having multiple meanings (e.g., freedom from pain, reunion with already deceased family members).

Professional caregivers, including nurses, may experience role strain due to repeated interactions with dying clients and their families. Although most nurses who work in oncology, hospice, intensive care, emergency, or other areas where client deaths are common have chosen such assignments, there can still be a sense of failure when clients die. Just as there must be support systems for grieving clients, there must also be support systems for grieving health care professionals.

Some people may think of death as the worst occurrence in life and do their best to avoid thinking or talking about death—especially their own. Nurses are not immune to such attitudes. They need to take time to analyze their own feelings about death before they can effectively help others with a terminal illness. Nurses who are uncomfortable with dying clients tend to impede the clients' attempts to discuss dying and death in these ways:

- Change the subject (e.g., "Let's think of something more cheerful" or "You shouldn't say things like that").
- Offer false reassurance (e.g., "You are doing very well").
- Deny what is happening (e.g., "You don't really mean that" or "You're going to live until you're a hundred").
- Be fatalistic (e.g., "Everyone dies sooner or later" or "What's meant to be, will be").
- Block discussion (e.g., "I don't think things are really that bad") and convey an attitude that stops further discussion of the subject.
- Be aloof and distant or avoid the client.
- "Manage" the client's care and make the client feel increasingly dependent and powerless.

Caring for the dying and the bereaved is one of the nurse's most complex and challenging responsibilities, bringing into play all the skills needed for holistic physiologic and psychosocial care. To be effective, nurses must come to grips with their own attitudes toward loss, death, and dying, because these attitudes will directly affect their ability to provide care.

Definitions and Signs of Death

The traditional clinical signs of death were cessation of the apical pulse, respirations, and blood pressure, also referred to as **heart-lung death.** However, since the advent of artificial means to maintain respirations and blood circulation, identifying death is more difficult. In 1968, the World Medical Assembly adopted the following guidelines for physicians as indications of death:

- Total lack of response to external stimuli
- No muscular movement, especially breathing
- No reflexes
- Flat encephalogram (brain waves)

In instances of artificial support, absence of brain waves for at least 24 hours is an indication of death. Only then can a physician pronounce death, and only after this pronouncement can life-support systems be shut off.

Another definition of death is **cerebral death** or **higher brain death,** which occurs when the higher brain center, the cerebral cortex, is irreversibly destroyed. In this case, there is "a clinical syndrome characterized by the permanent loss of cerebral and

brainstem function, manifested by absence of responsiveness to external stimuli, absence of cephalic reflexes, and apnea. An isoelectric electroencephalogram for at least 30 minutes in the absence of hypothermia and poisoning by central nervous system depressants supports the diagnosis" (Stedman's Medical Dictionary, 2005). People who support this definition of death believe the cerebral cortex, which holds the capacity for thought, voluntary action, and movement, is the individual.

Death-Related Religious and Cultural Practices

Various cultural and religious traditions and practices associated with death, dying, and the grieving process help people cope with these experiences. Nurses are often present through the dying process and at the moment of death. Knowledge of the client's religious and cultural heritage helps nurses provide individualized care to clients and their families, even though they may not participate in the rituals associated with death.

In many cultures, people prefer a peaceful death at home rather than in the hospital. Members of some ethnic groups may request that health professionals not reveal the prognosis to dying clients. They believe the person's last days should be free of worry. People in other cultures prefer that a family member (preferably a male in some cultures) be told the diagnosis so that the client can be tactfully informed by a family member in gradual stages or not be told at all. Nurses also need to determine whom to call, and when, as the impending death draws near.

Beliefs and attitudes about death, its cause, and the soul also vary among cultures. Unnatural deaths, or "bad deaths," are sometimes distinguished from "good deaths." In addition, the death of a person who has behaved well in life may be considered less threatening based on the belief that the person will be reincarnated into a good life.

Beliefs about preparation of the body, autopsy, organ donation, cremation, and prolonging life are closely allied to the person's religion. Autopsy, for example, may be prohibited, opposed, or discouraged by Eastern Orthodox religions, Muslims, Jehovah's Witnesses, and Orthodox Jews. Some religions prohibit the removal of body parts or dictate that all body parts be given appropriate burial. Organ donation is prohibited by Jehovah's Witnesses and Muslims, whereas Buddhists in America consider it an act of mercy and encourage it. Cremation is discouraged, opposed, or prohibited by the Mormon, Eastern Orthodox, Islamic, and Roman Catholic faiths. Hindus, in contrast, prefer cremation and cast the ashes in a holy river. Prolongation of life is generally encouraged; however, some religions, such as Christian Science, are unlikely to recommend medical means to prolong life, and the Jewish faith generally opposes prolonging life after irreversible brain damage. In hopeless illness, Buddhists may permit euthanasia.

Nurses also need to be knowledgeable about the client's death-related rituals, such as last rites, chanting at the bedside, and other practices, such as special procedures for washing, dressing, positioning, shrouding, and attending the dead. For example, certain cultures retain their native customs in which family members of the same sex wash and prepare the body for burial and cremation. Muslims also customarily turn the body toward Mecca. In several religions, the body cannot be left unattended until burial and persons may be hired to sit with the body if family members do not perform this duty. Nurses need to ask family members about their preference and verify who will carry out these activities. Burial clothes and other cultural or religious items are often important symbols for the funeral. For example, Mormons are often dressed in their "temple clothes." Some Native Americans may be dressed in elaborate apparel and jewelry and wrapped in new blankets with money. The nurse must ensure that any ritual items present in the health care agency be returned to the family or to the funeral home.

 NURSING MANAGEMENT

Assessing

To gather a complete database that allows accurate analysis and identification of appropriate nursing diagnoses for dying clients and their families, the nurse first needs to recognize the states of awareness manifested by the client and family members.

In cases of terminal illness, the state of awareness shared by the dying person and the family affects the nurse's ability to communicate freely with clients and other health care team members and to assist in the grieving process. Three types of awareness that have been described are closed awareness, mutual pretense, and open awareness (Glaser & Strauss, 1965).

In **closed awareness,** the client is not made aware of impending death. The family may choose this because they do not completely understand why the client is ill or they believe the client will recover. The primary care provider may believe it is best not to communicate a diagnosis or prognosis to the client. Nursing personnel are confronted with an ethical problem in this situation. See Chapter 5 ∞ for further information on ethical dilemmas.

With **mutual pretense,** the client, family, and health personnel know that the prognosis is terminal but do not talk about it and make an effort not to raise the subject. Sometimes the client refrains from discussing death to protect the family from distress. The client may also sense discomfort on the part of health personnel and therefore not bring up the subject. Mutual pretense permits the client a degree of privacy and dignity, but it places a heavy burden on the dying person, who then has no one in whom to confide.

With **open awareness,** the client and others know about the impending death and feel comfortable discussing it, even though it is difficult. This awareness provides the client an opportunity to finalize affairs and even participate in planning funeral arrangements.

Not all people are comfortable with open awareness. Some believe that terminal clients acquire knowledge of their condition even if they are not directly informed. Others believe that clients remain unaware of their condition until the end. It is difficult, however, to distinguish what clients know from what they are willing to accept or acknowledge.

Nursing care and support for the dying client and family include making an accurate assessment of the physiologic signs of

CLINICAL MANIFESTATIONS IMPENDING CLINICAL DEATH

LOSS OF MUSCLE TONE

- Relaxation of the facial muscles (e.g., the jaw may sag)
- Difficulty speaking
- Difficulty swallowing and gradual loss of the gag reflex
- Decreased activity of the gastrointestinal tract, with subsequent nausea, accumulation of flatus, abdominal distention, and retention of feces, especially if narcotics or tranquilizers are being administered
- Possible urinary and rectal incontinence due to decreased sphincter control
- Diminished body movement

SLOWING OF THE CIRCULATION

- Diminished sensation
- Mottling and cyanosis of the extremities
- Cold skin, first in the feet and later in the hands, ears, and nose (the client, however, may feel warm if there is a fever)
- Slower and weaker pulse
- Decreased blood pressure

CHANGES IN RESPIRATIONS

- Rapid, shallow, irregular, or abnormally slow respirations
- Noisy breathing, referred to as the death rattle, due to collecting of mucus in the throat
- Mouth breathing, dry oral mucous membranes

SENSORY IMPAIRMENT

- Blurred vision
- Impaired senses of taste and smell

approaching death. In addition to signs related to the client's specific disease, certain other physical signs are indicative of impending death. The four main characteristic changes are loss of muscle tone, slowing of the circulation, changes in respirations, and sensory impairment. Clinical Manifestations lists indications of impending clinical death.

Various consciousness levels may exist just before death. Some clients are alert, whereas others are drowsy, stuporous, or comatose. Hearing is thought to be the last sense lost.

As death approaches, the nurse assists the family and other significant people to prepare. Depending in part on knowledge of the person's state of awareness, the nurse asks questions that help identify ways to provide support during the period before and after death. In particular, the nurse needs to know what the family expects to happen when the person dies so accurate information can be given at the appropriate depth. See the Assessment Interview for sample interview questions. When the family members know what to expect, they may be better able to support the dying person and others who are grieving. In addition, they may be able to make certain decisions about events surrounding the death such as whether they will want to view the body after death.

Diagnosing

A range of nursing diagnoses, addressing both physiologic and psychosocial needs, can be applied to the dying client, depending on the assessment data. Diagnoses that may be particularly

ASSESSMENT INTERVIEW   The Family of the Dying Client

Ask the spouse, partner, or significant others:
- Have you ever been close to someone who was dying before?
- What have you been told about what may happen when death occurs?
- Do you have questions about what may happen at the time of death?
- How do you think you would like to say goodbye?
- How are you taking care of yourself during these times?
- Whom can you turn to for help at this time?
- Is there anyone you would like us to contact now or when the death occurs?

appropriate for the dying client are *Fear, Hopelessness,* and *Powerlessness.* In addition, *Risk for Caregiver Role Strain* and *Interrupted Family Processes* are not uncommon diagnoses for caregivers and family members.

Examples of clinical applications of some of these diagnoses using NANDA, NIC, and NOC designations are shown in Identifying Nursing Diagnoses, Outcomes, and Interventions.

Planning

Major goals for dying clients are (a) maintaining physiologic and psychologic comfort and (b) achieving a dignified and peaceful death, which includes maintaining personal control and accepting declining health status. When planning care with these clients, the Dying Person's Bill of Rights (Box 43–1) can be a useful guide.

Examples of clinical applications of NOC outcomes and NIC interventions are shown in Identifying Nursing Diagnoses, Outcomes, and Interventions.

Planning for Home Care

People facing death may need help accepting that they have to depend on others. Some dying clients require only minimal care; others need continuous attention and services. People need

IDENTIFYING NURSING DIAGNOSES, OUTCOMES, AND INTERVENTIONS
Clients Who Are Dying

DATA CLUSTER   Keisha Washington, who has multiple sclerosis and is paralyzed from the neck down, has appealed for someone to help her commit suicide. Her mind and speaking ability appear unimpaired. "I don't want to end up like my sister, who also had MS and had severe pain and became blind and mute before she died."

NURSING DIAGNOSIS/ DEFINITION	SAMPLE DESIRED OUTCOMES*/ *DEFINITION*	INDICATORS	SELECTED INTERVENTIONS*/ *DEFINITION*	SAMPLE NIC ACTIVITIES
Hopelessness/Subjective state in which an individual sees limited or no alternatives or personal choices available and is unable to mobilize energy on own behalf	Quality of Life [2000]/*Extent of positive perception of current life circumstances*	Moderately satisfied: • Ability to cope • Pervasive mood	Hope Instillation [5310]/*Facilitation of the development of a positive outlook in a given situation*	• Assist Keisha to identify areas of hope in life • Expand her repertoire of coping mechanisms • Facilitate her reliving and savoring past achievements and experiences • Provide her opportunity to be involved with support groups

DATA CLUSTER   John Yee, age 63, has metastatic carcinoma of the bowel. He has noticed a rapid deterioration in energy in the past week and feels bloated and nauseated. He has become increasingly jaundiced and says, "I know I haven't long to live. Nothing I do will help. Why can't they just give me a big dose of morphine and get it over with?"

Powerlessness/Perception that one's own action will not significantly affect an outcome; a perceived lack of control over a current situation or immediate happening	Participation: Health Care Decisions [1606]/ *Personal involvement in selecting and evaluating health care options to achieve desired outcome*	Sometimes demonstrated: • Seeks information • Defines available options • Identifies available support for achieving desired outcomes	Teaching: Individual [5606]/*Planning, implementation, and evaluation of a teaching program designed to address a patient's particular needs*	• Determine John's motivation to learn specific information about death • Set realistic goals with him • Select appropriate learning materials • Document the content taught, materials provided, and John's understanding of the information

*The NOC # for desired outcomes and the NIC # for nursing interventions are listed in brackets following the appropriate outcome or intervention. Outcomes, indicators, interventions, and activities selected are only a sample of those suggested by NOC and NIC and should be further individualized for each client.

BOX 43–1   The Dying Person's Bill of Rights

I have the right to be treated as a living human being until I die.

I have the right to maintain a sense of hopefulness however changing its focus may be.

I have the right to express my feelings and emotions about my approaching death in my own way.

I have the right to participate in decisions concerning my care.

I have the right to expect continuing medical and nursing attention even though cure goals must be changed to comfort goals.

I have the right not to die alone.

I have the right to be free from pain.

I have the right to have my questions answered honestly.

I have the right not to be deceived.

I have the right to have help from and for my family in accepting my death.

I have the right to die in peace and with dignity.

I have the right to retain my individuality and not be judged for my decisions which may be contrary to the beliefs of others.

I have the right to be cared for by caring, sensitive, knowledgeable people who will attempt to understand my needs and will be able to gain some satisfaction in helping me face my death.

Note: From "The Dying Person's Bill of Rights," by A. J. Barbus, 1975, created at the workshop *The Terminally Ill Patient and the Helping Person*, Lansing, MI: South Western Michigan Inservice Education Council.

---

help, well in advance of death, in planning for the period of dependence. They need to consider what will happen and how and where they would like to die.

A major factor in determining whether a person will die in a health care facility or at home is the availability of willing and able caregivers. If the dying person wishes to be at home, and family or others can provide care to maintain symptom control, the nurse should facilitate a referral to outpatient hospice services. Hospice staff and nurses will then conduct a full assessment of the home and care providers' skills.

Implementing

The major nursing responsibility for clients who are dying is to assist the client to a peaceful death. More specific responsibilities are the following:

- To minimize loneliness, fear, and depression
- To maintain the client's sense of security, self-confidence, dignity, and self-worth
- To help the client accept losses
- To provide physical comfort

Helping Clients Die with Dignity

Nurses need to ensure that the client is treated with dignity, that is, with honor and respect. Dying clients often feel they have lost control over their lives and over life itself. Helping clients die with dignity involves maintaining their humanity, consistent with their values, beliefs, and culture. By introducing options available to the client and significant others, nurses can restore and support feelings of control. Some choices that clients can make are the location of care (e.g., hospital, home, or hospice facility), times of appointments with health professionals, activity schedule, use of health resources, and times of visits from relatives and friends.

Clients want to be able to manage the events preceding death so they can die peacefully. Nurses can help clients to determine their own physical, psychologic, and social priorities. Dying people often strive for self-fulfillment more than for self-preservation, and may need to find meaning in continuing to live while suffering. Part of the nurse's challenge, then, is to support the client's will and hope.

Although it is natural for people to be uncomfortable discussing death, steps can be taken to make such discussions eas-

ier for both the nurse and the client. Strategies include the following:

- Identify your personal feelings about death and how they may influence interactions with clients. Acknowledge personal fears about death, and discuss them with a friend or colleague.
- Focus on the client's needs. The client's fears and beliefs may be different from the nurse's. It is important that the nurse avoid imposing personal fears and beliefs on the client or family.
- Talk to the client or the family about how the client usually copes with stress. Clients will use their usual coping strategies for dealing with impending death. For example, if they are usually quiet and reflective, they will become more quiet and withdrawn when facing terminal illness.
- Establish a communication relationship that shows concern for and commitment to the client. Communication strategies that let the client know you are available to talk about death include the following:
  a. Describe what you see, for example, "You seem sad. Would you like to talk about what's happening to you?"
  b. Clarify your concern, for example, "I'd like to know better how you feel and how I may help you."
  c. Acknowledge the client's struggle, for example, "It must be difficult to feel so uncomfortable. I would like to help you be more comfortable."
  d. Provide a caring touch. Holding the client's hand or offering a comforting massage can encourage the client to verbalize feelings.
- Determine what the client knows about the illness and prognosis.
- Respond with honesty and directness to the client's questions about death.
- Make time to be available to the client to provide support, listen, and respond.

Hospice and Palliative Care

The hospice movement was founded by the physician Cecily Saunders (who died in 2005) in London, England, in 1967. It was later extended to the United States by Sylvia Lack, also a medical doctor. **Hospice** care focuses on support and care of the dying person and family, with the goal of facilitating a peaceful and dignified death. Hospice care is based on holistic concepts, emphasizes care to improve quality of life rather than cure, supports the client and family through the dying process, and supports the family through bereavement. Assessing the needs of the client's family is just as important as caring for the client who is receiving hospice care. The condition of the client usually deteriorates, and attention needs to be focused on the caregivers to ensure that they are receiving support and resources as these changes occur. If the hospice team meets regularly, these needs can be discussed and interventions initiated. Physical needs are usually apparent, but emotional and behavioral signs are often more subtle. A good assessment and ongoing evaluation can help indicate when modifications or changes are needed.

The principles of hospice care can be carried out in a variety of settings, the most common being home and the hospital (or nursing home)-based unit. Services focus on symptom control and pain management. Commonly, clients are eligible for hospice care or hospice insurance benefits when certified by a physician to be likely to die within 6 months. Hospice care is always provided by a team of both health professionals and nonprofessionals to ensure a full range of care services. The National Hospice and Palliative Care Organization reports that over 1 million Americans access hospice services each year.

Palliative care, as described by the World Health Organization,

is an approach that improves the quality of life of clients and their families facing the problem associated with life-threatening illness, through the prevention and relief of suffering by means of early identification and impeccable assessment and treatment of pain and other problems, physical, psychosocial and spiritual. Palliative care:

- provides relief from pain and other distressing symptoms;
- affirms life and regards dying as a normal process;
- intends neither to hasten nor postpone death;
- integrates the psychological and spiritual aspects of client care;
- offers a support system to help clients live as actively as possible until death;
- offers a support system to help the family cope during the client's illness and in their own bereavement;
- uses a team approach to address the needs of clients and their families, including bereavement counselling, if indicated;
- will enhance quality of life, and may also positively influence the course of illness;
- is applicable early in the course of illness, in conjunction with other therapies that are intended to prolong life, such as chemotherapy or radiation therapy, and includes those investigations needed to better understand and manage distressing clinical complications (n.d.).

This care may differ from hospice in that the client is not necessarily believed to be imminently dying. Both hospice and palliative care can include **end-of-life care,** that is, the care provided in the final weeks before death.

There are more than 9,000 nurses in the United States who are nationally certified in hospice and palliative care (National Board for Certification of Hospice and Palliative Nurses, 2006). Beginning in 2005, advanced hospice and palliative care certification is also available for master's prepared nurses.

Meeting the Physiologic Needs of the Dying Client

The physiologic needs of people who are dying are related to a slowing of body processes and to homeostatic imbalances. Interventions include providing personal hygiene measures; controlling pain; relieving respiratory difficulties; assisting with movement, nutrition, hydration, and elimination; and providing measures related to sensory changes (also see Table 43–5).

Pain control is essential to enable clients to maintain some quality in their life and their daily activities, including eating, moving, and sleeping. Many drugs have been used to control the pain associated with terminal illness: morphine, heroin, methadone, and alcohol. Usually the primary care provider determines the dosage, but the client's opinion should be considered; the client is the one ultimately aware of personal pain tolerance and fluctuations of internal states. Because primary care providers usually prescribe dosage ranges for pain medication, nurses use their own judgment as to the amount and frequency of pain medication in providing client relief. Because of decreased blood circulation, if analgesics cannot be administered orally, they are given by intravenous infusion, sublingually, or rectally, rather than subcutaneously or intramuscularly. Clients on narcotic pain medications also require implementation of a protocol to treat opioid-induced constipation. See Chapter 46 ∞ for more on pain management.

Providing Spiritual Support

Spiritual support is of great importance in dealing with death. Although not all clients identify with a specific religious faith or belief, most have a need for meaning in their lives, particularly as they experience a terminal illness.

The nurse has a responsibility to ensure that the client's spiritual needs are attended to, either through direct intervention or by arranging access to individuals who can provide spiritual care. Nurses need to be aware of their own comfort with spiritual issues and be clear about their own ability to interact supportively with the client. Nurses have a responsibility to not impose their own religious or spiritual beliefs on a client but to respond to the client in relation to the client's own background and needs. Communication skills are most important in helping the client articulate needs and in developing a sense of caring and trust.

Specific interventions may include facilitating expressions of feeling, prayer, meditation, reading, and discussion with appropriate clergy or a spiritual adviser. It is important for nurses to establish an effective interdisciplinary relationship with spiritual support specialists. For a further discussion of spiritual issues, see Chapter 41. ∞

Supporting the Family

The most important aspects of providing support to the family members of a dying client involve using therapeutic communication to facilitate their expression of feelings. When nothing can reverse the inevitable dying process, the nurse can provide an empathetic and caring presence. The nurse also serves as a teacher, explaining what is happening and what the family can

TABLE 43–5   **Physiologic Needs of Dying Persons**

PROBLEM	NURSING CARE
Airway clearance	Fowler's position: conscious clients Throat suctioning: conscious clients Lateral position: unconscious clients Nasal oxygen for hypoxic clients Anticholinergic medications may be indicated to help dry secretions
Air hunger	Open windows or use a fan to circulate air Morphine may be indicated in an acute episode
Bathing/hygiene	Frequent baths and linen changes if diaphoretic Mouth care as needed for dry mouth Liberal use of moisturizing creams and lotions for dry skin Moisture-barrier skin preparations for incontinent clients
Physical mobility	Assist client out of bed periodically, if able Regularly change client's position Support client's position with pillows, blanket rolls, or towels as needed Elevate client's legs when sitting up Implement pressure ulcer prevention program and use pressure-relieving surfaces as indicated
Nutrition	Antiemetics or a small amount of an alcoholic beverage to stimulate appetite Encourage liquid foods as tolerated
Constipation	Dietary fiber as tolerated Stool softeners or laxatives as needed
Urinary elimination	Skin care in response to incontinence of urine or feces Bedpan, urinal, or commode chair within easy reach Call light within reach for assistance onto bedpan or commode Absorbent pads placed under incontinent client; linen changed as often as needed Catheterization, if necessary Keep room as clean and odor-free as possible
Sensory/perceptual changes	Check preference for light or dark room Hearing is not diminished; speak clearly and do not whisper Touch is diminished, but client will feel pressure of touch Implement pain management protocol if indicated

expect. Due to the stress of moving through the grieving process, family members may not absorb what they are told and may need to have information provided repeatedly. The nurse must have a calm and patient demeanor.

CLINICAL ALERT

People may use a variety of terms instead of the word *died*. Serious examples include *passed away, gone to a better place, lost*, or *free from suffering.* Humorous examples include *bought the farm, kicked the bucket,* or *croaked.* ■

Family members should be encouraged to participate in the physical care of the dying person as much as they wish to and are able. The nurse can suggest they assist with bathing, speak or read to the client, and hold hands. The nurse must not, however, have specific expectations for family members' participation. Those who feel unable to care for or be with the dying person also require support from the nurse and from other family members. They should be shown an appropriate waiting area if they wish to remain nearby.

Sometimes, it seems as if the client is "holding on," possibly out of concern for the family not being ready. It may be therapeutic for both the client and the family for the family to verbally give permission to the client to "let go," to die when he or she is ready. This is a painful process, and the nurse must be pre-

pared to encourage and support the family through saying their last good-byes.

After the client dies, the family should be encouraged to view the body, because this has been shown to facilitate the grieving process (Rich, 2005). They may wish to clip a lock of hair as a remembrance. Children should be included in the events surrounding the death if they wish to.

Postmortem Care

Rigor mortis is the stiffening of the body that occurs about 2 to 4 hours after death. It results from a lack of adenosine triphosphate (ATP), which causes the muscles to contract, which in turn immobilizes the joints. Rigor mortis starts in the involuntary muscles (heart, bladder, and so on), then progresses to the head, neck, and trunk, and finally reaches the extremities.

Because the deceased person's family often wants to view the body, and because it is important that the deceased appear natural and comfortable, nurses need to position the body, place dentures in the mouth, and close the eyes and mouth before rigor mortis sets in. Rigor mortis usually leaves the body about 96 hours after death.

Algor mortis is the gradual decrease of the body's temperature after death. When blood circulation terminates and the hypothalamus ceases to function, body temperature falls about 1°C (1.8°F) per hour until it reaches room temperature. Simultaneously, the skin loses its elasticity and can easily be broken when removing dressings and adhesive tape.

After blood circulation has ceased, the red blood cells break down, releasing hemoglobin, which discolors the surrounding tissues. This discoloration, referred to as **livor mortis,** appears in the lowermost or dependent areas of the body.

Tissues after death become soft and eventually liquefied by bacterial fermentation. The hotter the temperature, the more rapid the change. Therefore, bodies are often stored in cool places to delay this process. Embalming prevents the process through injection of chemicals into the body to destroy the bacteria.

Nursing personnel may be responsible for care of a body after death. Postmortem care should be carried out according to the policy of the hospital or agency. Because care of the body may be influenced by religious law, the nurse should check the client's religion and make every attempt to comply. If the deceased's family or friends wish to view the body, it is important to make the environment as clean and pleasant as possible and to make the body appear natural and comfortable. All equipment, soiled linen, and supplies should be removed from the bedside. Some agencies require that all tubes in the body remain in place; in other agencies, tubes may be cut to within 2.5 cm (1 in.) of the skin and taped in place; in others, all tubes may be removed.

Normally the body is placed in a supine position with the arms either at the sides, palms down, or across the abdomen. One pillow is placed under the head and shoulders to prevent blood from discoloring the face by settling in it. The eyelids are closed and held in place for a few seconds so they remain closed. Dentures are usually inserted to help give the face a natural appearance. The mouth is then closed.

Soiled areas of the body are washed; however, a complete bath is not necessary, because the body will be washed by the **mortician** (also referred to as an **undertaker**), a person trained in care of the dead. Absorbent pads are placed under the buttocks to take up any feces and urine released because of relaxation of the sphincter muscles. A clean gown is placed on the client, and the hair is brushed and combed. All jewelry is removed, except a wedding band in some instances, which is taped to the finger. The top bed linens are adjusted neatly to cover the client to the shoulders. Soft lighting and chairs are provided for the family.

In the hospital, after the body has been viewed by the family, the deceased's wrist identification tag is left on and additional identification tags are applied. The body is wrapped in a **shroud,** a large piece of plastic or cotton material used to enclose a body after death. Identification is then applied to the outside of the shroud. The body is taken to the morgue if arrangements have not been made to have a mortician pick it up from the client's room. Nurses have a duty to handle the deceased with dignity and to label the corpse appropriately. Mishandling can cause emotional distress to survivors. Mislabeling can create legal problems if the body is inappropriately identified and prepared incorrectly for burial or a funeral.

Evaluating

To evaluate the achievement of client goals, the nurse collects data in accordance with the desired outcomes established in the planning phase. Evaluation activities may include the following:

- Listening to the client's reports of feeling in control of the environment surrounding death, such as control over pain relief, visitation of family and support people, or treatment plans
- Observing the client's relationship with significant others
- Listening to the client's thoughts and feelings related to hopelessness or powerlessness

Examples of desired outcomes for dying clients are shown in Identifying Nursing Diagnoses, Outcomes, and Interventions on page 1093. Some of the special needs of elders and their families during death and dying are found in Lifespan Considerations.

LIFESPAN CONSIDERATIONS **Responses to Death**

CHILDREN

- Children's response to death or loss depends on the messages they get from adults and others around them as well as their understanding of death. When adults are able to cope effectively with a death, they are more likely to be able to support children through the process.
- As children develop, they will "reprocess" their grieving around a loss or death. Preschoolers who have lost a parent, for example, often reconceptualize their understanding of that loss when they reach school age and adolescence and have greater cognitive and emotional skills. The same process occurs with parents who have lost a child to death; as the years pass and the child "would have been in first grade," for example, parents must cope with the added dimensions of the loss.

ELDERS

Elders who are dying often have a need to know that their lives had meaning. An excellent way to assure them of this is to make audiotapes or videotapes of them telling stories of their lives. This gives the client a sense of value and worth and also lets him or her know that family members and friends will also benefit from it. Doing this with children and grandchildren often eases communication and support during this difficult time.

Caregivers of a dying person need ongoing support and ongoing teaching as the client's condition changes. Some of these needs are teaching

- ways to feed the client when swallowing becomes difficult.
- ways to transfer and reposition the client safely.
- ways to communicate if verbalization becomes more difficult.
- nonpharmacological methods of pain control.
- comfort measures, such as frequent oral care and frequent repositioning.

CRITICAL THINKING CHECKPOINT

Mrs. Govinda, 75, was admitted to the hospital after repeated episodes of pneumonia. Despite aggressive antibiotic therapy, her condition rapidly deteriorated and she died unexpectedly 1 week after being admitted to the hospital. Mrs. Govinda's oldest son, who lived nearby and frequently cared for his mother, arranged for the funeral and visited with relatives. He misses his mother and cries occasionally but managed to return to work the following week. The youngest son had difficulty attending the funeral, has been unable to sleep or eat, cannot concentrate at work, and cannot believe that his mother is dead. The middle son did not weep at the funeral and had little to say to his brothers or other relatives. He returned home to another state but has remained distant. He is back to work but feels very fatigued and apathetic.

1. From the data provided, describe the phase of bereavement being experienced by each of the three surviving sons.
2. What factors may have affected how each of the brothers reacted to the death of their mother?
3. What cues, other than physical signs, might have indicated that Mrs. Govinda was dying, even though her death was unexpected?
4. With the diagnosis of pneumonia, a respiratory infection, what physiological (palliative) needs might she have had?
5. How might your own feelings about death affect the care you provide to the dying client?

See Critical Thinking Possibilities in Appendix A.

CONCEPT MAP **The Grieving Client**

Denial Stage

Example Behavior

Wife of dying client states: "Next year, we are going to move to a warmer climate."

Possible nursing intervention → Nurse; "Have you thought about what might happen if he does not get well again?"

Possible nursing intervention → Provide accurate explanation of the clients condition, e.g., "His heart is no longer able to keep his blood pressure up."

Possible nursing intervention → Ensure other persons are available to provide support to the wife (clergy, family).

Anger Stage

Example Behavior

Teenage girl with a spinal cord injury yells at all caregivers.

Possible nursing intervention → Anticipate her anger and portray a calm demeanor.

Possible nursing intervention → Reassure her that her reactions are part of the process of learning to accept her loss.

Possible nursing intervention → Encourage her to talk about her feelings: "You are really angry. Tell me about it."

Idealization Stage

Example Behavior

The son of an 89-year-old mother who has just died tells everyone he sees about how wonderful she always was and what a terrible son he was to her.

Possible nursing intervention → Remind him that all persons have both good and bad in them.

Shock Stage

Example Behavior

Parents of a stillborn baby cry continously, cannot eat, experience chest pains.

Possible nursing intervention → Use silence and presence to demonstrate acceptance.

Possible nursing intervention → Consider requesting medical treatment if their own health beomes at risk.

Note: All nursing actions must be individualized to the client and the stage of the grieving process.

CHAPTER 43 **REVIEW**

CHAPTER HIGHLIGHTS

- Nurses help clients deal with all kinds of losses, including loss of body image, loss of a loved one, loss of a sense of well-being, and loss of a job.
- Loss, especially loss of a loved one or a valued body part, can be viewed as either a situational or a developmental loss and as either an actual or a perceived loss (both of which can be anticipatory).
- Grieving is a normal, subjective emotional response to loss; it is essential for mental and physical health. Grieving allows the bereaved person to cope with loss gradually and to accept it as part of reality.
- Knowledge of different stages or phases of grieving and factors that influence the loss reaction can help the nurse understand the responses and needs of clients.
- How an individual deals with loss is closely related to the individual's stage of development, personal resources, and social support system.

- Caring for the dying and the bereaved is one of the nurse's most complex and challenging responsibilities.
- Nurses' attitudes about death and dying directly affect their ability to provide care.
- Nurses must consider the entire family as requiring care in situations involving loss, especially death.
- Dying clients require open communication, physical help, and emotional and spiritual support to ensure a peaceful and dignified death. They need to maintain a sense of control in managing the events preceding death.

TEST YOUR KNOWLEDGE

1. Which of the following may be considered normal or "healthy" types of grief? Select all that apply.
1. Abbreviated grief
2. Anticipatory grief
3. Disenfranchised grief
4. Complicated grief
5. Unresolved grief
6. Inhibited grief

2. A client's family tells the nurse that their culture does not permit a dead person to be left alone before burial. Hospital policy states that after 6:00 PM when mortuaries are closed, bodies are to be stored in the hospital morgue refrigerator until the next day. How would the nurse best manage this situation?
1. Gently explain the policy to the family and then implement it.
2. Inquire of the nursing supervisor how an exception to the policy could be made.
3. Call the client's primary care provider for advice.
4. Move the deceased to an empty room and assign an aide to stay with the body.

3. The shift changed while the nursing staff was waiting for the adult children of a deceased client to arrive. The oncoming nurse has never met the family. Which of the following greetings is most appropriate?
1. "I'm very sorry for your loss."
2. "I'll take you in to view the body."
3. "I didn't know your father but I am sure he was a wonderful person."
4. "How long will you want to stay with your father?"

4. At which age does a child begin to accept that he or she will someday die?
1. Less than 5 years old
2. 5–9 years old
3. 9–12 years old
4. 12–18 years old

5. An 82-year-old man has been told by his primary care provider that it is no longer safe for him to drive a car. Which statement by the client would indicate beginning positive adaptation to this loss?
1. "I told the doctor I would stop driving, but I am not going to yet."
2. "I always knew this day would come, but I hoped it wouldn't be now."
3. "What does he know? I'm a better driver than he will ever be."
4. "Well, at least I have friends and family who can take me places."

6. When asked to sign the permission form for surgical removal of a large but noncancerous lesion on her face, the client begins to cry. Which of the following is the most appropriate response?
1. "Tell me what it means to you to have this surgery."
2. "You must be very glad to be having this lesion removed."
3. "I cry when I am happy or relieved sometimes, too."
4. "Isn't it wonderful that the lesion is not cancer?"

7. A nursing care plan includes the desired outcome of "quality of life" for a client with a chronic degenerative illness who is likely to live for many more years. Which of the following is one example that would indicate the outcome has been met?
1. The client demonstrates having adequate financial resources to pay for health care for many more years.
2. The client spends the majority of his or her time in spiritual reflection.
3. The client has no signs or symptoms of preventative complications of the illness.
4. The client verbalizes satisfaction with current relationships with other persons.

8. The nurse is caring for a family in a shelter two days following the loss of their home due to a fire. The fire caused minor burns to several members of the family but no life-threatening conditions. Which of the following is the *most* important assessment data for the nurse to gather at this time?

1. Availability of insurance coverage for rebuilding the house
2. Family members' understanding of the extent of their physical injuries
3. Psychological support resources available from friends or other sources
4. Family members' grief responses and coping behaviors

See Answers to Test Your Knowledge in Appendix A. ∞

EXPLORE MEDIALINK www.prenhall.com/berman

DVD-ROM
▦ Audio Glossary
▦ NCLEX Review
▦ End of Unit Concept Map Activity
▦ Video: Terminally Ill Clients

COMPANION WEBSITE
▦ Additional NCLEX Review
▦ Case Study: Helping a Family Accept a Terminal Illness
▦ Care Plan Activity: Client with an Arm Amputation
▦ Application Activities:
    Dealing with a Pet Loss
    Care of a Grieving Parent
▦ Links to Resources

READINGS AND REFERENCES

SUGGESTED READINGS
American Nurses Association publishes position statements on topics of critical importance to nurses related to death and dying. *Assisted suicide.* Retrieved June 24, 2006, from http://nursingworld.org/readroom/position/ethics/etsuic.htm *Pain management and control of distressing symptoms in dying patients.* Retrieved June 24, 2006, from http://nursingworld.org/readroom/position/ethics/etpain.htm. *Active euthanasia.* Retrieved June 24, 2006, from http://nursingworld.org/readroom/position/ethics/eteuth.htm *Nursing and the Patient Self-Determination Acts.* Retrieved June 24, 2006, from http://nursingworld.org/readroom/position/ethics/etsdet.htm

Lorenz, K., Lynn, J., Morton, S. C., Dy, S., Mularski, R., Shugarman, L., et al. (2004). *End-of-life care and outcomes.* Summary, Evidence Report/Technology Assessment: No. 110. AHRQ Publication No. 05-E004-1. Rockville, MD: Agency for Healthcare Research and Quality. Retrieved June 24, 2006, from http://www.ahrq.gov/clinic/epcsums/eolsum.htm *This literature review identified a large and diverse body of literature reflecting the tremendous growth and importance of the field of end-of-life care over the last decade. Evidence supported the association of satisfaction and quality of care with pain management, communication, practical support, and enhanced caregiving. Evidence also supported the effectiveness of interventions to improve satisfaction, ameliorate pain, relieve depression in cancer, provide nonpharmacologic interventions for behavioral problems in dementia, and foster continuity in care. Opportunities for future research to strengthen the evidence base for end-of-life care are included.*

Pitorak, E. F. (2003). Care at the time of death. *American Journal of Nursing, 103*(7), 42–52. *This article describes clearly and with helpful hints the process of dying and appropriate nursing care. Signs, symptoms, and interventions are identified by system and supported by research findings.*

RELATED RESEARCH
Moules, N. J., Simonson, K., Prins, M., Angus, P., & Bell, J. M. (2004). Making room for grief: Walking backwards and living forward. *Nursing Inquiry, 11,* 99–107.
Pevey, C. (2005). Patient speaking: Hospice patients discuss their care. *American Journal of Hospice and Palliative Medicine, 22,* 129–133.
Teno, J. M., Clarridge, B. R., Casey, V., Welch, L. C., Wetle, T., Shield, R., et al. (2004). Family perspectives on end-of-life care at the last place of care. *Journal of the American Medical Association, 291,* 88–93.

REFERENCES
Barbus, A. J. (1975). *The dying person's bill of rights.* Created at the workshop *The terminally ill patient and the helping person,* Lansing, MI, South Western Michigan Inservice Education Council.
Caserta, M. S., Lund, D. A., & Obray, S. J. (2004). Promoting self-care and daily living skills among older widows and widowers: Evidence from the Pathfinders demonstration project. *OMEGA: The Journal of Death and Dying, 49,* 217–236.
Dochterman, J., & Bulechek, G. B. (Eds.). (2004). *Nursing interventions classification (NIC)* (4th ed.). St. Louis, MO: Mosby.
Egan, K. A., & Arnold, R. L. (2003). Grief and bereavement care. *American Journal of Nursing, 103*(9), 42–53.
Engel, G. L. (1964). Grief and grieving. *American Journal of Nursing, 64,* 93–98.
Glaser, B., & Strauss, A. (1965). *Awareness of dying.* Chicago: Aldine.
Kübler-Ross, E. (1969). *On death and dying.* New York: Macmillan.
Martocchio, B. C. (1985). Grief and bereavement: Healing through hurt. *Nursing Clinics of North America, 20,* 327–341.
Moorhead, S., Johnson, M., & Maas, M. (Eds.). (2004). *Nursing outcomes classification (NOC)* (3rd ed.). St. Louis, MO: Mosby.
NANDA International. (2007). *NANDA nursing diagnoses: Definitions and classification 2007–2008.* Philadelphia: Author.

National Board for Certification of Hospice and Palliative Nurses. (2006). Certificants. Retrieved June 24, 2006, from http://www.nbchpn.org/Certificants_List.asp?Cert=CHPN
Rando, T. A. (1991). *How to go on living when someone you love dies.* New York: Bantam.
Rando, T. A. (1993). *Treatment of complicated mourning.* Champaign, IL: Research Press.
Rando, T. A. (2000). *Clinical dimensions of anticipatory mourning: Theory and practice in working with the dying, their loved ones, and their caregivers.* Champaign, IL: Research Press.
Rich, S. (2005). Providing quality end-of-life care. *Journal of Cardiovascular Nursing, 20,* 141–145.
Sanders, C. M. (1998). *Grief: The mourning after: Dealing with adult bereavement* (2nd ed.). New York: John Wiley & Sons.
Shear, K., Frank, E., Houck, P. R., & Reynolds, C. F. (2005). Treatment of complicated grief: A randomized controlled trial. *Journal of the American Medical Association, 293,* 2601–2608.
Stedman's medical dictionary for the health professions and nursing (5th ed.). (2005). Philadelphia: Lippincott Williams & Wilkins.
World Health Organization. (n.d.). *WHO definition of palliative care.* Retrieved June 24, 2006, from http://www.who.int/cancer/palliative/definition/en/

SELECTED BIBLIOGRAPHY
Clements, P. T., & Stenerson, H. J. (2004). Surviving sudden loss: When life, death, and technology collide. *Journal of Vascular Nursing, 22,* 134–137.
Dobbins, E. H. (2005). Helping your patient to a "good death." *Nursing, 35*(2), 43–45.
Dunne, K. (2004). Grief and its manifestations. *Nursing Standard, 18*(45), 45–53.
Ferrell, B. R., & Coyle, N. (Eds.). (2006). *Textbook of palliative care nursing* (2nd ed.). Oxford, England: Oxford University Press.
Furman, J. (2004). Healing the mind and spirit as the body fails. *Nursing, 34*(4), 50–51.
Griffie, J., Nelson-Marten, P., & Muchka, S. (2004). Acknowledging the 'elephant': Communication in palliative care. *American Journal of Nursing, 104*(1), 48–57.

Hoffmann, R. L. (2005). The evolution of hospice in America: Nursing's role in the movement. *Journal of Gerontological Nursing, 31*, 26–34.

Kübler-Ross, E. (1974). *Questions and answers on death and dying.* New York: Macmillan.

Kübler-Ross, E. (1975). *Death: The final stage of growth.* Englewood Cliffs, NJ: Prentice Hall.

Kübler-Ross, E. (1978). *To live until we say good-bye.* Englewood Cliffs, NJ: Prentice Hall.

Lunney, J. R., Lynn, J., Foley, D. J., Lipson, S., & Guralnik, J. M. (2003). Patterns of functional decline at the end of life. *Journal of the American Medical Association, 289*, 2387–2392.

Mathes, M. M. (2004). Assisted suicide and nursing ethics. *Medsurg Nursing, 13*, 261–264.

Matzo, M., & Sherman, D. W. (Eds.). (2005). *Palliative care nursing: Quality care to the end of life* (2nd ed.). New York: Springer.

Mazanec, P., & Tyler, M. K. (2003). Cultural considerations in end-of-life care. *American Journal of Nursing, 103*(3), 50–58.

McClement, S. E., Chochinov, H. M., Hack, T. F., Kristjanson, L. J., & Harlos, M. (2004). Dignity-conserving care: Application of research findings to practice. *International Journal of Palliative Nursing, 10*, 173–179.

National Consensus Project for Quality Palliative Care. (2004). *Clinical practice guidelines for quality palliative care.* Retrieved June 24, 2006, from http://www. nationalconsensus project.org/ Guidelines_Download.asp

Resnik, D. (2005). *Dying declarations: Notes from a hospice volunteer.* Binghamton, NY: Haworth Press.

Scanlon, C. (2003). Ethical concerns in end-of-life care. *American Journal of Nursing, 103*(1), 48–55.

Sheehan, D. K., & Schirm, V. (2003). End-of-life care of older adults: Debunking some common misconceptions about dying in old age. *American Journal of Nursing, 103*(11), 48–58.

Virani, R., & Sofer, D. (2003). Improving the quality of end-of-life care. *American Journal of Nursing, 103*(5), 52–61.

Westley, C., & Briggs, L. A. (2004). Using the stages of change model to improve communication about advance care planning. *Nursing Forum, 39*(3), 5–12.

Promoting Physiologic Health

The human body consists of a complex network of intricate and interacting systems. Drawing on a comprehensive knowledge base, nurses are cognizant of a host of factors that influence physical health as they provide care to support optimal physiologic function. Efforts to restore, maintain, or improve function include measures that address a client's need for nourishment, comfort, and activity.

CHAPTER 44

Activity and Exercise

LEARNING OUTCOMES

After completing this chapter, you will be able to:

1. Describe four basic elements of normal movement.

2. Differentiate isotonic, isometric, isokinetic, aerobic, and anaerobic exercise.

3. Compare the effects of exercise and immobility on body systems.

4. Identify factors influencing a person's body alignment and activity.

5. Assess activity-exercise pattern, alignment, mobility capabilities and limitations, activity tolerance, and potential problems related to immobility.

6. Develop nursing diagnoses and outcomes related to activity, exercise, and mobility problems.

7. Use safe practices when positioning, moving, lifting, and ambulating clients.

KEY TERMS

active ROM exercises, *1146*
activity-exercise pattern, *1106*
activity tolerance, *1107*
aerobic exercise, *1112*
ambulation, *1147*
anabolism, *1120*
anaerobic exercise, *1112*
ankylosed, *1118*
anorexia, *1120*
atrophy, *1118*
basal metabolic rate, *1120*
base of support, *1106*
bed rest, *1117*
calculi, *1120*
catabolism, *1120*
center of gravity, *1106*
contracture, *1118*
crepitation, *1124*
dorsal position, *1132*
dorsal recumbent position, *1132*
embolus, *1119*
exercise, *1107*
flaccid, *1117*

foot drop, *1118*
Fowler's position, *1131*
functional strength, *1107*
gait, *1122*
high Fowler's position, *1131*
hypertrophy, *1113*
individualized exercise
  prescription, *1116*
isokinetic (resistive)
  exercise, *1112*
isometric (static or setting)
  exercise, *1112*
isotonic (dynamic) exercise, *1107*
lateral position, *1133*
line of gravity, *1106*
logrolling, *1138*
lordosis, *1122*
low Fowler's position, *1131*
metabolism, *1119*
mobility, *1106*
orthopneic position, *1132*
orthostatic hypotension, *1118*
osteoporosis, *1116*

pace, *1124*
paresis, *1117*
passive ROM
  exercises, *1146*
physical activity, *1107*
prone position, *1132*
proprioception, *1107*
range of motion (ROM), *1107*
relaxation response, *1115*
semi-Fowler's position, *1131*
Sims' position, *1133*
spastic, *1117*
supine position, *1132*
thrombophlebitis, *1119*
thrombus, *1119*
tripod (triangle) position, *1154*
urinary incontinence, *1120*
urinary reflux, *1121*
urinary retention, *1120*
urinary stasis, *1120*
Valsalva maneuver, *1118*
vital capacity, *1119*

Whether we engage our diaphragm muscle to improve oxygenation and immune function, walk a labyrinth to achieve greater peace of mind, or practice yoga while lying in bed, our ability to move is an essential aspect of our well-being. Psychophysiologic self-regulation and overall health are affected by our activities. In ancient times, individuals such as Hippocrates and Aristotle understood the importance of activity and exercise. Hippocrates argued strongly that "All parts of the body . . . if used in moderation . . . become thereby healthy, well developed and age more slowly, but if unused and left idle, they become liable to disease, defective in growth, and age quickly" (Freeman, 2004). At the 2005–2006 North American Nursing Diagnosis Association (NANDA) Conference, the new diagnosis *Sedentary Lifestyle* was approved, underscoring the role of exercise and activity as an essential component of health.

Many *Healthy People 2010* objectives pertain to exercise and activity, for example: increase the proportion of people who engage in moderate physical activity for at least 30 minutes a day; increase the proportion of adults and children who perform physical activities that enhance and maintain muscle strength, endurance, and flexibility; increase the proportion of work sites offering employer-sponsored physical activity and fitness programs; reduce activity limitation due to chronic back conditions; and reduce the number of overweight people (Edelman & Mandle, 2006).

A strong, well-developed body of research evidence supports the role of exercise in improving the health status of individuals with cardiovascular disease, pulmonary dysfunction, disabilities of aging, and depression. Integrating well-researched exercise protocols with conventional nursing and medical approaches will result in optimal treatment of these common disorders. Evidence shows that exercise can prevent and even reverse many of the chronic diseases experienced by aging adults. A growing body of research supports the preventive and therapeutic effects of exercise for individuals with diabetes, cancer, arthritis, chronic fatigue syndrome, fibromyalgia, menopause, urinary incontinence, and HIV/AIDS (Freeman, 2004; Micozzi, 2006).

According to researchers at Harvard's School of Public Health (HSPH), a mixture of healthy eating and regular physical activity is the best form of health promotion and maintenance. Current trends that are unhealthy include dieting without exercise, and exercising only when it's time to lose weight. Regular physical activity is important for everyone, and a sedentary lifestyle increases the chances of becoming overweight as well as developing a number of chronic diseases, including heart disease, stroke, certain cancers, type 2 diabetes, arthritis, osteoporosis, depression, and anxiety (Harvard School of Public Health, 2006).

Recent data from the large Nurses' Health Study conducted through HSPH suggest that weight and exercise are both important predictors of longevity (Hu et al., 2004). During 24 years of data collection, mortality rates have been lowest for women who are both lean *and* active, moderate for women who are one or the other, and highest for women who are obese *and* sedentary. Indeed, there is growing evidence that exercise and activity are *the most important* behaviors in which we can engage for developing and maintaining health.

An **activity-exercise pattern** refers to a person's routine of exercise, activity, leisure, and recreation. It includes (a) activities of daily living (ADLs) that require energy expenditure such as hygiene, dressing, cooking, shopping, eating, working, and home maintenance, and (b) the type, quality, and quantity of exercise, including sports.

Mobility, the ability to move freely, easily, rhythmically, and purposefully in the environment, is an essential part of living. People must move to protect themselves from trauma and to meet their basic needs. Mobility is vital to independence; a fully immobilized person is as vulnerable and dependent as an infant.

People often define their health and physical fitness by their activity because mental well-being and the effectiveness of body functioning depend largely on their mobility status. For example, when a person is upright, the lungs expand more easily, intestinal activity (peristalsis) is more effective, and the kidneys are able to empty completely. In addition, motion is essential for proper functioning of bones and muscles.

The ability to move without pain also influences self-esteem and body image. For most people, self-esteem depends on a sense of independence and a feeling of usefulness or being needed. People with mobility impairments may feel helpless and burdensome to others, and their ability to work and earn a living may be compromised. Painful mobility makes coping even more difficult. Body image can be altered by paralysis, amputations, or any motor impairment. The reaction of others to impaired mobility can also alter self-esteem and body image significantly.

For those with impaired mobility, movement must be fostered to the full extent of capability to facilitate a satisfying life. For example, many persons who have impairments or use wheelchairs participate in athletics to experience the joys of competition and fitness. Many individuals with paralysis can use a hand control to enter and drive adapted vans or use their mouth to manipulate a paintbrush and create art. No matter what their level of mobility, they must be encouraged to breathe fully, engage their abdominal muscles, and move as much as possible to prevent the physical and psychoemotional hazards of immobility.

NORMAL MOVEMENT

Normal movement and stability are the result of an intact musculoskeletal system, an intact nervous system, and intact inner ear structures responsible for equilibrium. Body movement requires coordinated muscle activity and neurologic integration. It involves four basic elements: body alignment (posture), joint mobility, balance, and coordinated movement.

Alignment and Posture

Proper body alignment and posture bring body parts into position in a manner that promotes optimal balance and maximal body function whether the client is standing, sitting, or lying down. A person maintains balance as long as the **line of gravity** (an imaginary vertical line drawn through the body's center of gravity) passes through the **center of gravity** (the point at which all of the body's mass is centered) and the **base of support** (the foundation on which the body rests). In humans, the

Figure 44-1 ■ The center of gravity and the line of gravity influence standing alignment.

usual line of gravity begins at the top of the head and falls between the shoulders, through the trunk, slightly anterior to the sacrum, and between the weight-bearing joints and base of support (Figure 44-1 ■).

When the body is well aligned, strain on the joints, muscles, tendons, or ligaments is minimized and internal structures and organs are supported. Proper body alignment enhances lung expansion and promotes efficient circulatory, renal, and gastrointestinal functions. A person's posture is one criterion for assessing general health, physical fitness, and attractiveness. Posture reflects the mood, self-esteem, and personality of an individual, and vice versa.

Abdominal and skeletal muscles function almost continuously, making tiny adjustments that enable an erect or seated posture despite the endless downward pull of gravity. The extensor muscles, often referred to as the *antigravity muscles,* carry the major load as they keep the body upright.

Joint Mobility

Joints are the functional units of the musculoskeletal system. The bones of the skeleton articulate at the joints, and most of the skeletal muscles attach to the two bones at the joint. These muscles are categorized according to the type of joint movement they produce on contraction. Muscles are therefore called flexors, extensors, internal rotators, and the like. The flexor muscles are stronger than the extensor muscles. Thus, when a person is inactive, the joints are pulled into a flexed (bent) position. If this tendency is not counteracted with exercise and position

TABLE 44–1	**Types of Joint Movements**
MOVEMENT	**ACTION**
Flexion	Decreasing the angle of the joint (e.g., bending the elbow)
Extension	Increasing the angle of the joint (e.g., straightening the arm at the elbow)
Hyperextension	Further extension or straightening of a joint (e.g., bending the head backward)
Abduction	Movement of the bone away from the midline of the body
Adduction	Movement of the bone toward the midline of the body
Rotation	Movement of the bone around its central axis
Circumduction	Movement of the distal part of the bone in a circle while the proximal end remains fixed
Eversion	Turning the sole of the foot outward by moving the ankle joint
Inversion	Turning the sole of the foot inward by moving the ankle joint
Pronation	Moving the bones of the forearm so that the palm of the hand faces downward when held in front of the body
Supination	Moving the bones of the forearm so that the palm of the hand faces upward when held in front of the body

changes, the muscles permanently shorten, and the joint becomes fixed in a flexed position (contracture). Types of joint movement are shown in Table 44–1.

The **range of motion (ROM)** of a joint is the maximum movement that is possible for that joint. Joint range of motion varies from individual to individual and is determined by genetic makeup, developmental patterns, the presence or absence of disease, and the amount of physical activity in which the person normally engages. Table 44–2 shows the various joint movements and the usual ranges of motion.

Balance

The mechanisms involved in maintaining balance and posture are complex and involve informational inputs from the labyrinth (inner ear), from vision (vestibulo-ocular input), and from stretch receptors of muscles and tendons (vestibulospinal input). Mechanisms of equilibrium (sense of balance) respond, frequently without our awareness, to various head movements. The labyrinth consists of the cochlea, vestibule, and semicircular canals. The cochlea is concerned with hearing, and the vestibule and semicircular canals with equilibrium. Under normal conditions the equilibrium receptors in the semicircular canals and vestibule, collectively called the vestibular apparatus, send signals to the brain that initiate reflexes needed to make required changes in position. The receptors, hairlike cells, respond to displacement of the head in any direction. When the head moves, the fluid flow within the vestibule and semicircular canals stimulates sensory hair cells. Information from these balance receptors goes directly to reflex centers in the brain stem rather than to the cerebral cortex as with other special senses. This enables fast reflexive responses to body imbalance. **Proprioception** is

the term used to describe awareness of posture, movement, and changes in equilibrium and the knowledge of position, weight, and resistance of objects in relation to the body.

Coordinated Movement

Balanced, smooth, purposeful movement is the result of proper functioning of the cerebral cortex, cerebellum, and basal ganglia. The cerebral cortex initiates voluntary motor activity, the cerebellum coordinates the motor activities of movement, and the basal ganglia maintain posture. The cerebral cortex operates movements, not muscles. The cortex, for example, may direct the arm to pick up a cup of coffee. The cerebellum, which operates below the level of consciousness, blends and coordinates the muscles involved in voluntary movement. It does not direct the movement but translates the "instructions" from the cerebral cortex into detailed actions by the many different muscles in the hand, arm, and shoulder. When a client's cerebellum is injured, movements become clumsy, unsure, and uncoordinated.

EXERCISE

The U.S. Department of Health and Human Services defines exercise and physical activity as follows (Edelman & Mandle, 2006):

- **Physical activity** is bodily movement produced by skeletal muscle contraction that increases energy expenditure.
- **Exercise** is a type of physical activity defined as a planned, structured, and repetitive bodily movement performed to improve or maintain one or more components of physical fitness.

People participate in exercise programs to decrease risk factors for cardiovascular disease and to increase their health and well-being. **Activity tolerance** is the type and amount of exercise or daily living activities an individual is able to perform without experiencing adverse effects. **Functional strength** is another goal of exercise, and defined as the ability of the body to perform work.

Types of Exercise

Exercise involves the active contraction and relaxation of muscles. Exercises can be classified according to the type of muscle contraction (isotonic, isometric, or isokinetic) and according to the source of energy (aerobic or anaerobic).

Isotonic (dynamic) exercises are those in which the muscle shortens to produce muscle contraction and active movement. Most physical conditioning exercises—running, walking, swimming, cycling, and other such activities—are isotonic, as are ADLs and active ROM exercises (those initiated by the client). Examples of isotonic bed exercises are pushing or pulling against a stationary object, using a trapeze to lift the body off the bed, lifting the buttocks off the bed by pushing with the hands against the mattress, and pushing the body to a sitting position.

Isotonic exercises increase muscle tone, mass, and strength and maintain joint flexibility and circulation. During isotonic

TABLE 44–2 Selected Joint Movements and Example of Corresponding Activity of Daily Living (ADL)

BODY PART—TYPE OF JOINT/MOVEMENT	NORMAL RANGE AND EXAMPLE OF CORRESPONDING ADL	ILLUSTRATION	
Neck—Pivot Joint			
Flexion. Move the head from the upright midline position forward, so that the chin rests on the chest (Figure 44-2 ■).	45° from midline Example: Nodding head "yes"	Figure 44-2	
Extension. Move the head from the flexed position to the upright position (Figure 44-2).	45° from midline Example: Nodding head "yes"		
Hyperextension. Move the head from the upright position back as far as possible (Figure 44-2).	45° from midline	Figure 44-3	
Lateral flexion. Move the head laterally to the right and left shoulders (Figure 44-3 ■).	40° from midline		
Rotation. Turn the face as far as possible to the right and left (Figure 44-4 ■).	70° from midline Example: Shaking head "no"	Figure 44-4	
Shoulder—Ball-and-Socket Joint			
Flexion. Raise each arm from a position by the side forward and upward to a position beside the head (Figure 44-5 ■).	180° from the side Example: Reaching to turn on overhead light	Figure 44-5	
Extension. Move each arm from a vertical position beside the head forward and down to a resting position at the side of the body (Figure 44-5).	180° from vertical position beside the head		
Hyperextension. Move each arm from a resting side position to behind the body (Figure 44-5).	50° from side position		
Abduction. Move each arm laterally from a resting position at the sides to a side position above the head, palm of the hand away from the head (Figure 44-6 ■).	180° Example: Reaching to bedside stand on same side of bed as arm	Figure 44-6	
Adduction (anterior). Move each arm from a position at the sides across the front of the body as far as possible (Figure 44-6). The elbow may be straight or bent.	50° Example: Reaching across body toward opposite side of bed		
Circumduction. Move each arm forward, up, back, and down in a full circle (Figure 44-7 ■).	360°	Figure 44-7	
External rotation. With each arm held out to the side at shoulder level and the elbow bent to a right angle, fingers pointing down, move the arm upward so that the fingers point up (Figure 44-8 ■).	90° Example: Reaching over opposite shoulder to scratch upper back	Figure 44-8	
Internal rotation. With each arm held out to the side at shoulder level and the elbow bent to a right angle, fingers pointing up, bring the arm forward and down so that the fingers point down (Figure 44-8).	90° Example: Reaching to scratch same side lower back		

BODY PART—TYPE OF JOINT/MOVEMENT	NORMAL RANGE AND EXAMPLE OF CORRESPONDING ADL	ILLUSTRATION
Elbow—Hinge Joint		
Flexion. Bring each lower arm forward and upward so that the hand is at the shoulder (Figure 44-9 ■).	150° Example: Eating, bathing, shaving	Figure 44-9
Extension. Bring each lower arm forward and downward, straightening the arm (Figure 44-9).	150° Example: Eating, bathing, shaving	
Rotation for supination. Turn each hand and forearm so that the palm is facing upward (Figure 44-10 ■).	70° to 90°	Figure 44-10
Rotation for pronation. Turn each hand and forearm so that the palm is facing downward (Figure 44-10).	70° to 90°	
Wrist—Condyloid Joint		
Flexion. Bring the fingers of each hand toward the inner aspect of the forearm (Figure 44-11 ■).	80° to 90° Example: Eating, bathing, shaving, writing	Figure 44-11
Extension. Straighten each hand to the same plane as the arm (Figure 44-11).	80° to 90° Example: Eating, bathing, shaving	
Hyperextension. Bend the fingers of each hand back as far as possible (Figure 44-12 ■).	70° to 90°	Figure 44-12
Radial flexion (abduction). Bend each wrist laterally toward the thumb side with hand supinated (Figure 44-13 ■).	0° to 20°	Figure 44-13
Ulnar flexion (adduction). Bend each wrist laterally toward the fifth finger with the hand supinated (Figure 44-13).	30° to 50°	
Hand and Fingers: Metacarpophalangeal Joints— Condyloid; Interphalangeal Joints—Hinge		
Flexion. Make a fist with each hand (Figure 44-14 ■).	90° Example: Squeezing, gripping, writing	Figure 44-14
Extension. Straighten the fingers of each hand (Figure 44-14).	90°	
Hyperextension. Bend the fingers of each hand back as far as possible (Figure 44-14).	30°	
Abduction. Spread the fingers of each hand apart (Figure 44-15 ■).	20°	Figure 44-15
Adduction. Bring the fingers of each hand together (Figure 44-15).	20° Example: Writing, gripping, eating, many hobbies involving fine motor coordination (e.g., art, music)	
Thumb—Saddle Joint		
Flexion. Move each thumb across the palmar surface of the hand toward the fifth finger (Figure 44-16 ■).	90°	Figure 44-16
Extension. Move each thumb away from the hand (Figure 44-16).	90°	
Abduction. Extend each thumb laterally (Figure 44-17 ■).	30°	Figure 44-17
Adduction. Move each thumb back to the hand (Figure 44-17).	30°	

continued on page 1110

BODY PART—TYPE OF JOINT/MOVEMENT	NORMAL RANGE AND EXAMPLE OF CORRESPONDING ADL	ILLUSTRATION
Thumb—Saddle Joint—continued		
Opposition. Touch each thumb to the top of each finger of the same hand. The thumb joint movements involved are abduction, rotation, and flexion (Figure 44-18 ■).		Figure 44-18
Hip—Ball-and-Socket Joint		
Flexion. Move each leg forward and upward. The knee may be extended or flexed (Figure 44-19 ■).	Knee extended, 90°; knee flexed, 120° Example: Walking, leg lifts in front of the body	Figure 44-19
Extension. Move each leg back beside the other (Figure 44-20 ■)	90° to 120° Example: Walking, lining the leg up with the body	Figure 44-20
Hyperextension. Move each leg back behind the body (Figure 44-20).	30° to 50° Example: Walking; lying on side, reach the leg behind the body	
Abduction. Move each leg out to the side (Figure 44-21 ■).	45° to 50° Example: Moving leg away from body	Figure 44-21
Adduction. Move each leg back to the other leg and beyond in front of it (Figure 44-21).	20° to 30° beyond other leg Example: Moving leg over the other leg toward the middle of the body	
Circumduction. Move each leg backward, up, to the side, and down in a circle (Figure 44-22 ■).	360° Example: Leg circles clockwise and counterclockwise	Figure 44-22
Internal rotation. Turn each foot and leg inward so that the toes point as far as possible toward the other leg (Figure 44-23 ■).	45°	Figure 44-23
External rotation. Turn each foot and leg outward so that the toes point as far as possible away from the other leg (Figure 44-23).	45°	
Knee—Hinge Joint		
Flexion. Bend each leg, bringing the heel toward the back of the thigh (Figure 44-24 ■).	120° to 130° Example: Knee bends, walking	Figure 44-24

TABLE 44–2 Selected Joint Movements and Example of Corresponding Activity of Daily Living (ADL)

BODY PART—TYPE OF JOINT/MOVEMENT	NORMAL RANGE AND EXAMPLE OF CORRESPONDING ADL	ILLUSTRATION
Knee—Hinge Joint **Extension.** Straighten each leg, returning the foot to its position beside the other foot (Figure 44-24).	120° to 130° Example: Straightening leg from bent position, walking	
Ankle—Hinge Joint **Extension (plantar flexion).** Point the toes of each foot downward (Figure 44-25 ■). **Flexion (dorsiflexion).** Point the toes of each foot upward (Figure 44–25).	20° Example: Pressing toes away from face, walking 45° to 50° Example: Pulling toes toward face, walking	Figure 44-25
Foot—Gliding **Eversion.** Turn the sole of each foot laterally (Figure 44-26 ■). **Inversion.** Turn the sole of each foot medially (Figure 44-26).	5° Example: Foot circles clockwise and counterclockwise 5° Example: Foot circles clockwise and counterclockwise Example: Walking , wiggling toes	Figure 44-26
Toes: Interphalangeal Joints—Hinge; Metatarsophalangeal Joints—Hinge; Intertarsal Joints—Gliding **Flexion.** Curl the toe joints of each foot downward (Figure 44-27 ■). **Extension.** Straighten the toes of each foot (Figure 44-27).	35° to 60° 35° to 60°	Figure 44-27
Trunk—Gliding Joint **Flexion.** Bend the trunk toward the toes (Figure 44-28 ■). **Extension.** Straighten the trunk from a flexed position (Figure 44-28). **Hyperextension.** Bend the trunk backward (Figure 44-28). **Lateral flexion.** Bend the trunk to the right and to the left (Figure 44-29 ■). **Rotation.** Turn the upper part of the body from side to side (Figure 44-30 ■).	70° to 90° Example: Touching toes 20° to 30° Example: Gentle supported back bend with hands on buttocks 35° on each side Example: Gently allow right hand to slide down right side of thigh, repeat on left side 30° to 45° Example: Gently swing torso right and left, maintaining forward hip alignment	Figure 44-28 Figure 44-29 Figure 44-30

the International Osteoporosis Foundation emphasized the equal importance of weight-bearing exercise and diet for maintaining bone strength.

Cardiovascular System

The American Heart Association's most recent guidelines for primary prevention of stroke and cardiovascular disease (Freeman, 2004) place great emphasis on physical activity. Adequate moderate-intensity exercise (40% to 60% of maximum capacity such as walking a mile in 15 to 20 minutes) increases the heart rate, the strength of heart muscle contraction, and the blood supply to the heart and muscles through increased cardiac output. In two studies with male participants, levels of "good" (high-density lipoprotein [HDL]) cholesterol were increased through regular endurance (walking/jogging) exercise. Exercise also promotes heart health by mediating the harmful effects of stress. The types of exercise that will provide cardiac benefit vary. They include aerobic exercise such as walking and cycling (Freeman, 2004). Research evidence for modalities that were formerly considered outside of mainstream health care support the benefits of yoga practice on cardiovascular health. Statistically significant effects include lowering systolic and diastolic blood pressure, improved oxygen uptake, improved heart rate variability, improved circulation, and self-reported stress reduction (Fontaine, 2005; Freeman, 2004; McCaffrey, Ruknui, Hatthakit, & Kasetsomboon, 2005).

Respiratory System

Ventilation (air circulating into and out of the lungs) and oxygen intake increase during exercise, thereby improving gas exchange. More toxins are eliminated with deeper breathing, and problem solving and emotional stability are enhanced due to increased oxygen to the brain. Adequate exercise also prevents pooling of secretions in the bronchi and bronchioles, decreasing breathing effort and risk of infection (Freeman, 2004). Attention to exercising muscles of respiration (by deep breathing) throughout activity as well as rest enhances oxygenation (improving stamina) and circulation of lymph (improving immune function). A strong body of evidence supports the use of lower extremity exercise forms (e.g., walking, treadmill, stationary bike, stair climbing) for treating individuals with chronic obstructive pulmonary disease (COPD) (Freeman, 2004). Research reports citing the benefits of yogic breathing and postures for persons with asthma are increasing in the literature (Fontaine, 2005; Freeman, 2004; Micozzi, 2006).

Gastrointestinal System

Exercise improves the appetite and increases gastrointestinal tract tone, facilitating peristalsis. Activities such as rowing, swimming, walking, and sit-ups work the abdominal muscles and can help relieve constipation (Fontaine, 2005). Abdominal compressive exercise, such as with twisting and forward bending yoga postures, has been shown to improve symptoms of irritable bowel syndrome (Fontaine, 2005; Micozzi, 2006).

Metabolic/Endocrine System

Exercise elevates the metabolic rate, thus increasing the production of body heat and waste products and calorie use. During strenuous exercise, the metabolic rate can increase to as much as 20 times the normal rate. This elevation lasts after exercise is completed. Exercise increases the use of triglycerides and fatty acids, resulting in a reduced level of serum triglycerides and cholesterol. Weight loss and exercise stabilize blood sugar and make cells more responsive to insulin. The Diabetes Prevention Program, a large 3-year study, showed that even a modest 5% decrease in body weight (about 10 pounds in most participants) achieved through exercise and dietary modification reduced the risk of diabetes by a striking 58%. In those over 60 years of age, the reduction was 71% (Freeman, 2004).

Urinary System

As adequate exercise promotes efficient blood flow, the body excretes wastes more effectively. In addition, stasis (stagnation) of urine in the bladder is usually prevented.

Immune System

As respiratory and musculoskeletal effort increase with exercise and as gravity is enlisted with postural changes, lymph fluid is more efficiently pumped from tissues into lymph capillaries and vessels throughout the body. Circulation through lymph nodes where destruction of pathogens and removal of foreign antigens can occur is also improved. Research in the elderly has shown benefits of moderate exercise on natural killer cell function, circulating T-cell function, and cytokine production, potentially increasing resistance to viral infections and preventing formation of malignant cells (Freeman, 2004).

While moderate exercise seems to enhance immunity, strenuous exercise may reduce immune function, leaving a window of opportunity for infection during the recovery phase. Adequate rest is important after vigorous training to allow the body to recover (Edelman & Mandle, 2006).

Psychoneurologic System

Mental or affective disorders such as depression or chronic stress may affect a person's desire to move. The depressed person may lack enthusiasm for taking part in any activity and may even lack energy for usual hygiene practices. Lack of visible energy is seen in a slumped posture with head bowed. Chronic stress can deplete the body's energy reserves to the point that fatigue discourages the desire to exercise, even though exercise can energize the person and facilitate coping. By contrast, individuals with eating disorders may exercise excessively in an effort to prevent weight gain.

A strong and growing body of evidence supports the role of exercise in elevating mood and relieving stress and anxiety across the life span. Solid data examining relationships between both aerobic and nonaerobic styles of exercise support the use of this modality to relieve symptoms of depression. The mechanism of action is thought to be a result of one or more of the following: exercise increases levels of metabolites for neurotransmitters such as norepinephrine and serotonin; exercise releases endogenous opioids, thus increasing levels of endorphins; exercise increases levels of oxygen to the brain and other body systems, inducing euphoria; and through muscular exertion (especially with movement modalities such as yoga and t'ai chi) the body releases stored stress associated with accumulated emotional demands. Regular exercise also improves quality of sleep for most individuals (Freeman, 2004).

By eliciting the **relaxation response** (RR), exercise is beneficial for counteracting some of the harmful effects of stress on the body and mind. First described by Dr. Herbert Benson, the RR is a healthful physiologic state that can be elicited through deep relaxation breathing with emphasis on a prolonged exhalation phase (Edelman & Mandle, 2006). Emphasis on the exhalation recruits parasympathetic nervous system response, the "rest and digest" reflex. Progressive muscle relaxation techniques involve contracting and then releasing groups of muscles throughout the body until all parts of the body feel relaxed. These movements are subtle and, along with relaxation breathing, can be done by almost anyone at any time, regardless of mobility or fitness status, providing potent stress relief and neurocardiovascular health benefits.

Cognitive Function

Current research supports the positive effects of exercise on cognitive functioning, in particular decision-making and problem-solving processes, planning, and paying attention. Physical exertion induces cells in the brain to strengthen and build neuronal connections. Research evidence demonstrates that athletic older adults have denser brains than their inactive counterparts (Freeman, 2004). Brain Gym (educational kinesiology) is a series of easy, mostly cross-lateral movements that enhance right- and left-brain integration thus improving mood, learning, problem solving, and performance in persons of all ages. These contralateral movements have been shown to help individuals with attention deficit disorder (ADD), attention deficit/hyperactivity disorder (ADHD), learning disorders, and mood disorders.

Spiritual Health

Jackson (2003) found that a program of Pilates and yoga-style exercise significantly enhanced students' experiences of mind-bodyspirit connection and relationship with God. The emphasis on breathing in both Pilates and yoga is thought to soothe the nervous and cardiorespiratory systems, promoting relaxation and preparedness for contemplative experience. Recitation of a word or phrase (mantra) and rosary prayer were both found to powerfully enhance and synchronize cardiovascular rhythms because of the resulting decrease in respiratory rate. Slow breathing enhances heart rate variability and baroreflex sensitivity, both beneficial for those with heart disease (Micozzi, 2006).

Slowly walking a labyrinth (a circular mandala) can induce a meditative state, decreasing heart and respiratory rates, lowering blood pressure, and reducing incidents of chronic pain and insomnia (Fontaine, 2005; Zielinski, 2004). Many hospitals, hospices, and churches have labyrinths in garden and atrium spaces. Canvas labyrinths can be purchased and spread out on large surfaces such as a gymnasium. Even using a finger to slowly and mindfully trace and retrace a path to the center and back out of the mandala pictured in Figure 44-34 ■ can serve as a contemplative activity that will trigger slowed heart and respiratory rates.

Figure 44-34 ■ Mandala in the floor of Chartres Cathedral, France.

FACTORS AFFECTING BODY ALIGNMENT AND ACTIVITY

A number of factors affect an individual's body alignment, mobility, and daily activity level. These include growth and development, nutrition, personal values and attitudes, certain external factors, and prescribed limitations.

Growth and Development

A person's age and musculoskeletal and nervous system development affect posture, body proportions, body mass, body movements, and reflexes. Newborn movements are reflexive and random. All extremities are generally flexed but can be passively moved through a full range of motion. As the neurologic system matures, control over movement progresses during the first year. Gross motor development precedes fine motor skills. Gross motor development occurs in a head-to-toe fashion, that is, progression from head control, to crawling, to pulling up to a standing position, to standing, and to walking, usually after the first birthday. The contralateral motion of crawling, however brief, is an important building block for walking. Initially, walking involves a wide stance and unsteady gait, thus the term *toddler*. From ages 1 to 5 years, both gross and fine motor skills are refined. For example, preschoolers master riding a tricycle, dancing, running, jumping, using crayons to draw, fastening or using zippers, and brushing their teeth. Immobility can impair the social and motor development of young children.

From 6 to 12 years, refinement of motor skills continues and exercise patterns for later life are generally determined. Many schools provide physical education and competitive sports programs to enhance physical activity. Posture in school-age children is usually excellent. In adolescence, growth spurts and behaviors such as carrying heavy book bags on one shoulder and extended computer use may result in postural changes that often persist into adulthood.

Adults between 20 and 40 years of age generally have few physical changes affecting mobility, with the exception of pregnant women. Pregnancy alters center of gravity and affects balance. The most recent recommendations from the American College of Obstetricians and Gynecologists (Edelman & Mandle, 2006) suggest that healthy pregnant women *should* exercise according to recommendations for the general population (30 minutes or more of moderate exercise on most if not all days of the week). This reflects a philosophical change from the 1994 recommendations that stated, "pregnant women *can* exercise." In addition, the report indicates that exercise can prevent gestational diabetes, even in very obese clients. This report cited the need to evaluate safety and limitations for women with heart and/or lung disease and orthopedic conditions. Additional studies support the long-term benefits of exercise during pregnancy to control excess weight gain, thus preventing long-term obesity after delivery. Leaner babies may also be at lower risk for obesity later in life.

As age advances, muscle tone and bone density decrease, joints lose flexibility, reaction time slows, and bone mass decreases, particularly in women who have osteoporosis. **Osteoporosis** is a condition in which the bones become brittle and fragile due to calcium depletion. Osteoporosis is common in older women and primarily affects the weight-bearing joints of the lower extremities and the anterior aspects of spinal bones, causing compression fractures of the vertebrae and hip fractures. All of these changes affect older adults' posture, gait, and balance. Posture becomes forward leaning and stooped, which shifts the center of gravity forward. To compensate for this shift, the knees flex slightly for support and the base of support is widened. Gait becomes wide based, short stepped, and shuffling.

A strong body of research supports the benefits of regular activity for elders to maintain and regain strength, flexibility, cardiovascular fitness, and bone density. Other health benefits are well documented, including reduction in falls, mood stabilization, and diabetes management (Burke & Laramie, 2004).

Nutrition

Both undernutrition and overnutrition can influence body alignment and mobility. Poorly nourished people may have muscle weakness and fatigue. Vitamin D deficiency causes bone deformity during growth. Inadequate calcium intake and vitamin D synthesis and intake increase the risk of osteoporosis. Obesity can distort movement and stress joints, adversely affecting posture, balance, and joint health.

The Institute of Medicine (IOM) cites properly balanced nutrition and exercise as important for preventing cancers and chronic disease. The IOM recommends that adults get 45% to 65% of calories from complex carbohydrates, 20% to 35% from healthy fats, and 10% to 35% from protein. Total caloric needs should be adjusted for weight, height, gender, and *levels of physical activity*.

Personal Values and Attitudes

Whether people value regular exercise is often the result of family influences. In families that incorporate regular exercise in their daily routine or spend time together in activities, children learn to value physical activity. Sedentary families, on the other hand, participate in sports only as spectators, and this lifestyle is often transmitted to their children. With the increase in TV, computer, and video activities, youth are increasingly sedentary with attendant declines in health. Values about physical appearance also influence some people's participation in regular exercise. People who value a muscular build or physical attractiveness may participate in regular exercise programs to produce the appearance they desire.

Choice of physical activity or type of exercise is also influenced by values. Choices may be influenced by geographic location and cultural role expectations. For many, thinking of exercise more as "recreational movement," "enhancement of well-being," and "an essential part of daily self-care" may help overcome perceptions that exercise is drudgery. Options include informal and fun activities such as dancing to music. Motivational states influence our behavior and choices, and vary widely from day to day. To design **individualized exercise prescriptions** that tailor exercise mode and dose and address these varying states with each person will ensure greater adherence to an exercise program (Burke & Laramie, 2004; Edelman & Mandle, 2006). Prescriptions should include frequency of the activity, intensity, and time (the FIT model). In those who are building toward a fitness goal, these parameters will change over time to increase the client's level of conditioning (Burke & Laramie, 2004).

Nurses must assess each client for potentially motivating factors such as the following: degree of fun or challenge of any given activity; use of music; opportunities for socializing and group cohesion and having an exercise partner; positive sensations of the exercise experience; pleasurable feelings associated with increased stress reduction; increased energy and fitness; mastering the activity; goal setting and progress; daily logs or weekly written schedules; competition with oneself or others; promotion of a sense of accomplishment; weight management; emphasis on self-talk about how exercise will prevent fatigue, depression, weight gain, or anxiety; and the need to explore less intense and challenging, noncompetitive activities (Keele-Smith & Leon, 2003).

Nurses, taking into account motivation to participate, medical conditions and level of fitness, and safety issues, can use individualized exercise prescriptions to encourage exercise and activity in all of their clients. Clients who experience orthostatic hypotension, impaired equilibrium, and gait disturbance should begin exercising in supervised environments. For example, a frail or sedentary person may need to begin with a prescription that emphasizes stretching, strengthening, and development of balance rather than aerobic training. For apparently active and healthy people, the prescription can immediately include moderate aerobic conditioning, strength training, and stretching (Burke & Laramie, 2004).

External Factors

Many external factors affect a person's mobility. Excessively high temperatures and high humidity discourage activity, whereas comfortable temperatures and low humidity are conducive to activity. Proper hydration needs vary according to the individual, health status, activity levels, and environment. The IOM recommends that men consume 3 liters (12 cups) of beverage a day, and women 2.2 liters (about 9 cups). Quality water is the best fluid to replace loss incurred through metabolic processes and exercise. Drinking 1 to 2 cups of water is usually adequate for shorter bouts of exercise. For longer bouts such as marathons, drinking 2 cups of water 2 hours prior to the event and then replacing fluids with a sports drink that contains sodium during and after can be beneficial.

The availability of recreational facilities also influences activity; for example, lack of money may prohibit a client from joining an exercise club or gymnasium. Neighborhood safety promotes outdoor activity, whereas an unsafe environment discourages people from going outdoors. Adolescents, in particular, may spend many hours sitting at computers, watching television, or playing video games rather than engaging in physical activities.

Prescribed Limitations

Limitations to movement may be medically prescribed for some health problems. To promote healing, devices such as casts, braces, splints, and traction are often used to immobilize body parts. Clients who are short of breath may be advised not to walk up stairs. Bed rest may be the therapeutic choice for certain clients, for example, to relieve edema, to reduce metabolic and oxygen needs, to promote tissue repair, or to decrease pain.

The term **bed rest** varies in meaning to some extent. In some agencies bed rest means strict confinement to bed or "complete" bed rest. Others may allow the client to use a bedside commode or have bathroom privileges. Nurses need to familiarize themselves with the meaning of bed rest in their practice setting. In any case, the effects of limiting activity are immediate and negative. For example, with complete bed rest involving the limiting of all exercise, muscle strength atrophies at approximately 3% per day (Freeman, 2004). The ability to perform basic ADLs is rapidly lost under these conditions. There is rarely a need for complete bed rest (NANDA, 2005).

EFFECTS OF IMMOBILITY

Mobility and activity tolerance are affected by any disorder that impairs the ability of the nervous system, musculoskeletal system, cardiovascular system, respiratory system, and vestibular apparatus. Congenital problems such as hip dysplasia, spina bifida, cerebral palsy, and the muscular dystrophies affect motor functioning. Disorders of the nervous system such as Parkinson's disease, multiple sclerosis, central nervous system tumors, cerebrovascular accidents (strokes), infectious processes (e.g., meningitis), and head and spinal cord injuries can leave muscle groups weakened, paralyzed (**paresis**), **spastic** (with too much muscle tone), or **flaccid** (without muscle tone). Musculoskeletal disorders affecting mobility include strains, sprains, fractures, joint dislocations, amputations, and joint replacements. Inner ear infections and dizziness can impair balance. Many other acute and chronic illnesses that limit the supply of oxygen and nutrients needed for muscle contraction and movement can seriously affect activity tolerance. Examples include chronic obstructive lung disease, anemia, congestive heart failure, and angina.

Individuals who have inactive lifestyles or who are faced with inactivity because of illness or injury are at risk for many problems that can affect major body systems. Whether immobility causes any problems often depends on the duration of the inactivity, the client's health status, and the client's sensory awareness. The most obvious signs of prolonged immobility are often manifested in the musculoskeletal system, and the deconditioning effects can be observed even after a matter of days. Clients experience a significant decrease in muscular strength and agility whenever they do not maintain a moderate amount of physical activity. In addition, immobility adversely affects the cardiovascular, respiratory, metabolic, urinary, and psychoneurologic systems. Nurses need to understand these effects and encourage client movement as much as possible. Early ambulation after illness or surgery is an essential measure to prevent complications.

CLINICAL ALERT

A review of 39 studies on effects of bed rest in clients with 15 different disorders revealed that bed rest for treatment of medical conditions is associated with worse outcomes than early mobilization. In general, there are few indications for bed rest, and bed rest may delay recovery or actually harm clients (NANDA, 2005). ■

Figure 44-35 ■ Plantar flexion contracture (foot drop).

Musculoskeletal System

- *Disuse osteoporosis.* Without the stress of weight-bearing activity, the bones demineralize. They are depleted chiefly of calcium, which gives the bones strength and density. Regardless of the amount of calcium in a person's diet, the demineralization process, known as *osteoporosis,* continues with immobility. The bones become spongy and may gradually deform and fracture easily.
- *Disuse atrophy.* Unused muscles **atrophy** (decrease in size), losing most of their strength and normal function.
- *Contractures.* When the muscle fibers are not able to shorten and lengthen, eventually a **contracture** (permanent shortening of the muscle) forms, limiting joint mobility. This process eventually involves the tendons, ligaments, and joint capsules; it is irreversible except by surgical intervention. Joint deformities such as **foot drop** (Figure 44-35 ■), wrist drop, and external hip rotation occur when a stronger muscle dominates the opposite muscle.
- *Stiffness and pain in the joints.* Without movement, the collagen (connective) tissues at the joint become **ankylosed** (permanently immobile). In addition, as the bones demineralize, excess calcium may deposit in the joints, contributing to stiffness and pain.

Cardiovascular System

- *Diminished cardiac reserve.* Decreased mobility creates an imbalance in the autonomic nervous system, resulting in a preponderance of sympathetic activity over cholinergic activity that increases heart rate. Rapid heart rate reduces diastolic pressure, coronary blood flow, and the capacity of the heart to respond to any metabolic demands above the basal levels. Because of this diminished cardiac reserve, the immobilized person may experience tachycardia with even minimal exertion.
- *Increased use of the Valsalva maneuver.* The **Valsalva maneuver** refers to holding the breath and straining against a closed glottis. For example, clients tend to hold their breath when attempting to move up in a bed or sit on a bedpan. This builds up sufficient pressure on the large veins in the thorax to interfere with the return blood flow to the heart and coronary arteries. When the client exhales and the glottis again opens, pressure is suddenly released, and a surge of blood flows to the heart. Cardiac arrhythmias can result if the client has cardiac disease.
- *Orthostatic (postural) hypotension.* **Orthostatic hypotension** is a common result of immobilization. Under normal conditions, sympathetic nervous system activity causes

automatic vasoconstriction in the blood vessels in the lower half of the body when a mobile person changes from a horizontal to a vertical posture. Vasoconstriction prevents pooling of the blood in the legs and effectively maintains central blood pressure to ensure adequate perfusion of the heart and brain. During any prolonged immobility, this reflex becomes dormant. When the immobile person attempts to sit or stand, this reconstricting mechanism fails to function properly in spite of increased adrenalin output. The blood pools in the lower extremities, and central blood pressure drops. Cerebral perfusion is seriously compromised, and the person feels dizzy or light-headed and may even faint. This sequence is usually accompanied by a sudden and marked increase in heart rate, the body's effort to protect the brain from an inadequate blood supply.

- *Venous vasodilation and stasis.* The skeletal muscles of an active person contract with each movement, compressing the blood vessels in those muscles and helping to pump the blood back to the heart against gravity. The tiny valves in the leg veins aid in venous return to the heart by preventing backward flow of blood and pooling. In an immobile person, the skeletal muscles do not contract sufficiently, and the muscles atrophy. The skeletal muscles can no longer assist in pumping blood back to the heart against gravity. Blood pools in the leg veins, causing vasodilation and engorgement. The valves in the veins can no longer work effectively to prevent backward flow of blood and pooling (Figure 44-36 ■). This phenomenon is known as incompetent valves. As the blood continues to pool in the veins, its greater volume increases venous blood pressure, which can become much higher than that exerted by the tissues surrounding the vessel.
- *Dependent edema.* When the venous pressure is sufficiently great, some of the serous part of the blood is forced

Figure 44-36 ■ Leg veins: *A,* in a mobile person; *B,* in an immobile person.

out of the blood vessel into the interstitial spaces surrounding the blood vessel, causing edema. Edema is most common in parts of the body positioned below the heart. Dependent edema is most likely to occur around the sacrum or heels of a client who sits up in bed or in the feet and lower legs of a client who sits in a chair. Edema further impedes venous return of blood to the heart, causing more pooling and more edema. Edematous tissue is uncomfortable and more susceptible to injury than normal tissue.

■ *Thrombus formation.* Three factors collectively predispose a client to the formation of a **thrombophlebitis** (a clot that is loosely attached to an inflamed vein wall): impaired venous return to the heart, hypercoagulability of the blood (sometimes caused by medications such as oral contraceptives), and injury to a vessel wall.

A **thrombus** (clot) is particularly dangerous if it breaks loose from the vein wall to enter the general circulation as an **embolus** (an object that has moved from its place of origin, causing obstruction to circulation elsewhere). Large emboli that enter the pulmonary circulation may occlude the vessels that nourish the lungs to cause an infarcted (dead) area of the lung. If the infarcted area is large, pulmonary function may be seriously compromised, or death may ensue. Emboli traveling to the coronary vessels or brain can produce a similarly dangerous outcome.

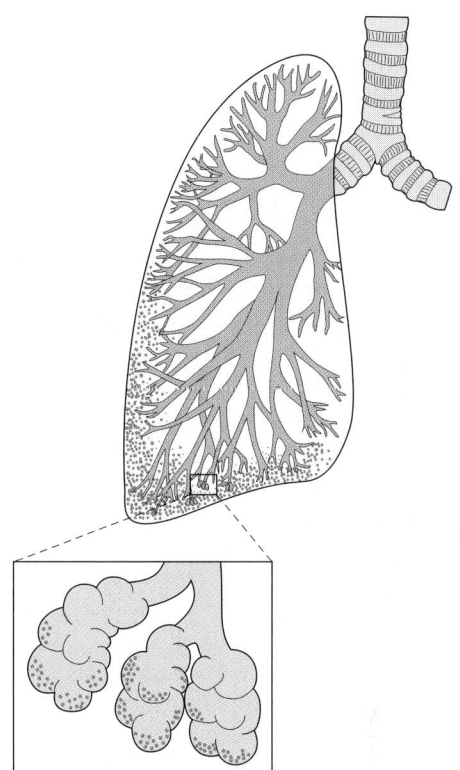

Figure 44-37 ■ Pooling of secretions in the lungs of an immobile person.

CLINICAL ALERT

Prolonged inactivity (such as bed rest or sleeping during a long plane ride) in combination with oral contraceptive use can lead to dangerous clot formation in deep leg veins, even in otherwise healthy young women. Smoking increases this risk. Regular movement, stretching, and keeping legs uncrossed are recommended. Monitor for tenderness, redness or discoloration, warmth, and/or swelling in the legs. ■

Respiratory System

■ *Decreased respiratory movement.* In a recumbent, immobile client, ventilation of the lungs is passively altered. The body presses against the rigid bed and curtails chest movement. The abdominal organs push against the diaphragm, restricting lung movement and making it difficult to expand the lungs fully. An immobile recumbent person rarely sighs, partly because overall muscle atrophy also affects the respiratory muscles and partly because there is no stimulus of activity. Without these periodic stretching movements, the cartilaginous intercostal joints may become fixed in an expiratory phase of respiration, further limiting the potential for maximal ventilation. These changes produce shallow respirations and reduce **vital capacity** (the maximum amount of air that can be exhaled after a maximum inhalation).

■ *Pooling of respiratory secretions.* Secretions of the respiratory tract are normally expelled by changing positions or posture and by coughing. Inactivity allows secretions to pool by gravity (Figure 44-37 ■), interfering with the normal diffusion of oxygen and carbon dioxide in the alveoli. The ability to cough up secretions may also be

hindered by loss of respiratory muscle tone, dehydration (which thickens secretions), or sedatives that depress the cough reflex. Poor oxygenation and retention of carbon dioxide in the blood can, if allowed to continue, predispose the person to respiratory acidosis, a potentially lethal disorder.

■ *Atelectasis.* When ventilation is decreased, pooled secretions may accumulate in a dependent area of a bronchiole and effectively block it. Because of changes in regional blood flow, bed rest decreases the amount of surfactant produced. (Surfactant enables the alveoli to remain open.) The combination of decreased surfactant and blockage of a bronchiole with mucus can cause atelectasis (the collapse of a lobe or of an entire lung) distal to the mucous blockage. Immobile elderly, postoperative clients are at greatest risk of atelectasis.

■ *Hypostatic pneumonia.* Pooled secretions provide excellent media for bacterial growth. Under these conditions, a minor upper respiratory infection can evolve rapidly into a severe infection of the lower respiratory tract. Pneumonia caused by static respiratory secretions can severely impair oxygen–carbon dioxide exchange in the alveoli and is a fairly common cause of death among weakened, immobile persons, especially heavy smokers.

Metabolic System

■ *Decreased metabolic rate.* **Metabolism** refers to the sum of all the physical and chemical processes by which living substance is formed and maintained and by which energy is made available for use by the body. The **basal metabolic rate** is the minimal energy expended for the maintenance of these processes, expressed in calories per hour per square meter of body surface. In immobile clients, the basal metabolic rate and gastrointestinal motility and secretions of various digestive glands decrease as the energy requirements of the body decrease.

- *Negative nitrogen balance.* In an active person, a balance exists between protein synthesis (**anabolism**) and protein breakdown (**catabolism**). Immobility creates a marked imbalance, and the catabolic processes exceed the anabolic processes. Catabolized muscle mass releases nitrogen. Over time, more nitrogen is excreted than is ingested, producing a negative nitrogen balance. The negative nitrogen balance represents a depletion of protein stores that are essential for building muscle issue and for wound healing.

- *Anorexia.* Loss of appetite (**anorexia**) occurs because of the decreased metabolic rate and the increased catabolism that accompany immobility. Reduced caloric intake is usually a response to the decreased energy requirements of the inactive person. If protein intake is reduced, the nitrogen imbalance may become more pronounced, sometimes so severely that malnutrition ensues.

- *Negative calcium balance.* A negative calcium balance occurs as a direct result of immobility. Greater amounts of calcium are extracted from bone than can be replaced. The absence of weight bearing and of stress on the musculoskeletal structures is the direct cause of the calcium loss from bones. Weight bearing and stress are also required for calcium to be replaced in bone.

Urinary System

- *Urinary stasis.* In a mobile person, gravity plays an important role in the emptying of the kidneys and the bladder. The shape and position of the kidneys and active kidney contractions are important in completely emptying the urine from the calyces, renal pelvis, and ureters (Figure 44-38 ■ A). The shape and position of the urinary bladder (the detrusor muscle) and active bladder contractions are also important in achieving complete emptying (Figure 44-39 ■ A).

Figure 44-38 ■ Pooling of urine in the kidney: *A,* The client is in an upright position. *B,* The client is in a back-lying position.

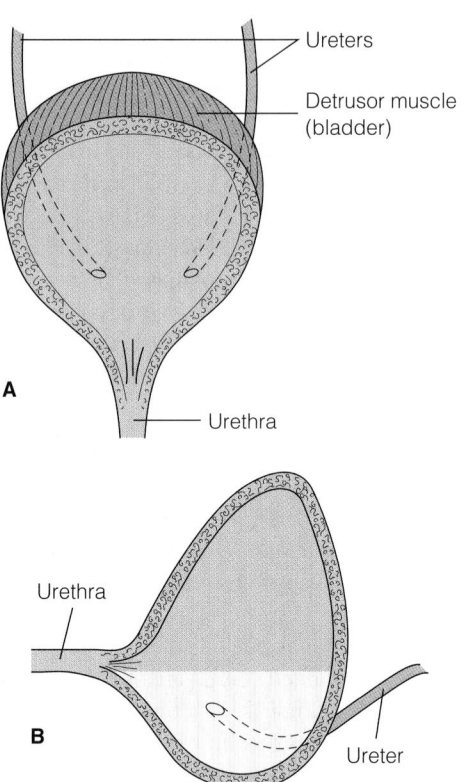

Figure 44-39 ■ Pooling of urine in the urinary bladder: *A,* The client is in an upright position. *B,* The client is in a back-lying position.

When the person remains in a horizontal position, gravity impedes the emptying of urine from the kidneys and the urinary bladder. To urinate, the person who is supine (in a back-lying position) must push upward, against gravity (Figures 44-38 ■ B, and 44-39 ■, B). The renal pelvis may fill with urine before it is pushed into the ureters. Emptying is not as complete, and **urinary stasis** (stoppage or slowdown of flow) occurs after a few days of bed rest. Because of the overall decrease in muscle tone during immobilization, including the tone of the detrusor muscle, bladder emptying is further compromised.

- *Renal calculi.* In a mobile person, calcium in the urine remains dissolved because calcium and citric acid are balanced in appropriately acidic urine. With immobility and the resulting excessive amounts of calcium in the urine, this balance is no longer maintained. The urine becomes more alkaline, and the calcium salts precipitate out as crystals to form renal **calculi** (stones). In an immobile person in a horizontal position, the renal pelvis filled with stagnant, alkaline urine is an ideal location for calculi to form. The stones usually develop in the renal pelvis and pass through the ureters into the bladder. As the stones pass along the long, narrow ureters, they cause extreme pain and bleeding and can sometimes obstruct the urinary tract.

- *Urinary retention.* The immobile person may suffer from **urinary retention** (accumulation of urine in the bladder), bladder distention, and occasionally **urinary incontinence** (involuntary urination). The decreased muscle tone of the urinary bladder inhibits its ability to empty completely. In addition, the discomfort of using a bedpan or urinal, the embarrassment and lack of privacy associated with this function, and the unnatural position for urination combine to make it difficult for the client to relax the perineal muscles sufficiently to urinate while lying in bed.

When urination is not possible, the bladder gradually becomes distended with urine. The bladder may stretch excessively, eventually inhibiting the urge to void. When bladder distention is considerable, some involuntary urinary "dribbling" may occur (retention with overflow). This does not relieve the urinary distention, because most of the stagnant urine remains in the bladder.

■ *Urinary infection.* Static urine provides an excellent medium for bacterial growth. The flushing action of normal, frequent urination is absent, and urinary distention often causes minute tears in the bladder mucosa, allowing infectious organisms to enter. The increased alkalinity of the urine caused by the hypercalcuria supports bacterial growth. The organism most commonly causing urinary tract infections is *Escherichia coli,* which normally resides in the colon. The normally sterile urinary tract may be contaminated by improper perineal care, the use of an indwelling urinary catheter, or occasionally **urinary reflux** (backward flow). During reflux, contaminated urine from an overly distended bladder backs up into the renal pelvis to contaminate the kidney pelvis as well.

Gastrointestinal System

Constipation is a frequent problem for immobilized people because of decreased peristalsis and colon motility. The overall skeletal muscle weakness affects the abdominal and perineal muscles used in defecation. When the stool becomes very hard, more strength is required to expel it. The immobile person may lack this strength.

The bedfast person's unnatural and uncomfortable position on the bedpan does not facilitate elimination. The backward-leaning posture does not promote effective use of the muscles used in defecation. Some people are reluctant to use the bedpan in the presence of others. The embarrassment, lack of privacy, dependence on others to assist with the bedpan, and disruption of normal bowel habits may cause the individual to postpone or ignore the urge for elimination. Repeated postponement eventually suppresses the urge and weakens the defecation reflex.

Some persons may make excessive use of the Valsalva maneuver by straining at stool in an attempt to expel the hard stool. This effort dangerously increases intra-abdominal and intrathoracic pressures and places undue stress on the heart and circulatory system.

Integumentary System

■ *Reduced skin turgor.* The skin can atrophy as a result of prolonged immobility. Shifts in body fluids between the fluid compartments can affect the consistency and health of the dermis and subcutaneous tissues in dependent parts of the body, eventually causing a gradual loss in skin elasticity.

■ *Skin breakdown.* Normal blood circulation relies on muscle activity. Immobility impedes circulation and diminishes the supply of nutrients to specific areas. As a result, skin breakdown and formation of pressure (decubitus) ulcers can occur.

Psychoneurologic System

Due to a decline in production of mood-elevating substances such as endorphins, people experience negative effects on mood when unable to engage in physical activity. People who are unable to carry out the usual activities related to their roles (e.g., as breadwinner, husband, mother, or athlete) become aware of an increased dependence on others. These factors lower the person's self-esteem. Frustration and the decrease in self-esteem may in turn provoke exaggerated emotional reactions. Emotional reactions vary considerably. Some individuals become apathetic and withdrawn, some regress, and some become angry and aggressive.

Because the immobilized person's participation in life becomes much narrower and the variety of stimuli decreases, the person's perception of time intervals deteriorates. Problem-solving and decision-making abilities may deteriorate as a result of lack of intellectual stimulation and the stress of the illness and immobility. In addition, the loss of control over events can cause anxiety.

NURSING MANAGEMENT

Assessing

Assessment relative to a client's activity and exercise should be routinely addressed and includes a nursing history and a physical examination of body alignment, gait, appearance and movement of joints, capabilities and limitations for movement, muscle mass and strength, activity tolerance, problems related to immobility, and physical fitness.

The nurse collects information from the client, from other nurses, and from the client's records. The examination and history are important sources of information about disabilities affecting the client's mobility and activity status, such as contractures, edema, pain in the extremities, or generalized fatigue.

Nursing History

An activity and exercise history is usually part of the comprehensive nursing history. Examples of interview questions to elicit these data are shown in the accompanying Assessment Interview. If the client indicates a recent pattern change or difficulties with mobility, a more detailed history is required. This detailed history should include the specific nature of the problem, when it first began, its frequency, its causes if known, how the problem affects daily living, what the client is doing to cope with the problem, and whether these methods have been effective.

Physical Examination

Conduct of the physical examination focusing on activity and exercise emphasizes body alignment, gait, appearance and

ASSESSMENT INTERVIEW Activity and Exercise

DAILY ACTIVITY LEVEL

- What activities do you carry out during a routine day?
- Are you able to carry out the following tasks independently?
  a. Eating
  b. Dressing/grooming
  c. Bathing
  d. Toileting
  e. Ambulating
  f. Using a wheelchair
  g. Transferring in and out of bed, bath, and car
  h. Cooking
  i. House cleaning
  j. Shopping
- Where problems exist in your ability to carry out such tasks:
  a. Would you rate yourself as partially or totally dependent?
  b. How is the task achieved (by family, friend, agency, or use of specialized equipment)?

ACTIVITY TOLERANCE

- What types of activities make you tired?

- Do you ever experience dizziness, shortness of breath, marked increase in respiratory rate, or other problems following mild or moderate activity?

EXERCISE

- What type of exercise do you carry out to enhance your physical fitness?
- What is the frequency and length of this exercise session?
- Do you believe exercise is beneficial to your health? Explain.

FACTORS AFFECTING MOBILITY

- Environmental factors. Do stairs, lack of railings or other assistive devices, or an unsafe neighborhood impede your mobility or exercise regimen?
- Health problems. Do any of the following health problems affect your muscle strength or endurance: heart disease, lung disease, stroke, cancer, neuromuscular problems, musculoskeletal problems, visual or mental impairments, trauma, or pain?
- Financial factors. Are your finances adequate to obtain equipment or other aids that you require to enhance your mobility?

movement of joints, capabilities and limitations for movement, muscle mass and strength, and activity tolerance.

BODY ALIGNMENT. Assessment of body alignment includes an inspection of the client while the client stands. The purpose of body alignment assessment is to identify

- Normal developmental variations in posture.
- Posture and learning needs to maintain good posture.
- Factors contributing to poor posture, such as fatigue or low self-esteem.
- Muscle weakness or other motor impairments.

To assess alignment, the nurse inspects the client from lateral (Figure 44-40 ■, A), anterior, and posterior perspectives. From the anterior and posterior views, the nurse should observe whether

- The shoulders and hips are level.
- The toes point forward.
- The spine is straight, not curved to either side.

The "slumped" posture (Figure 44-40 ■, B) is the most common problem that occurs when people stand. The neck is flexed far forward, the abdomen protrudes, the pelvis is thrust forward to create **lordosis** (an exaggerated anterior/inward curvature of the lumbar spine), and the knees are hyperextended. Low back pain and fatigue occur quickly in people with poor posture.

GAIT. The characteristic pattern of a person's **gait** (walk) is assessed to determine the client's mobility and risk for injury due to falling. Two phases of normal gait are stance and swing (Figure 44-41 ■). When one leg is in the swing phase, the other is in the stance phase. In the *stance phase*, (a) the heel of one foot strikes the ground, and (b) body weight is spread over the ball of that foot while the other heel pushes off and leaves the ground. In the *swing phase*, the leg from behind moves in front of the body.

The nurse assesses gait as the client walks into the room or asks the client to walk a distance of 10 feet down a hallway and observes for the following:

- Chin is level, gaze is straight ahead, sternum is lifted, and shoulders are down and back, relaxed away from the ears.
- Heel strikes the ground before the toe. It is here, where both feet are taking some body weight, that the spine is most rotated.
- Feet are dorsiflexed in the swing phase.

A   **B**

Figure 44-40 ■ A standing person with A, good trunk alignment; B, poor trunk alignment. The arrows indicate the direction in which the pelvis is tilted.

ANATOMY & PHYSIOLOGY REVIEW   Upper and Lower Body Integration and the Spine's Role in Locomotion

It is important to be aware of the connection between the upper and lower body in terms of function, comfort, and mobility. The iliopsoas muscles (hip flexors) allow us to stand upright and are crucial for spinal alignment and locomotion. Prolonged sitting and inactivity can shorten these muscles, compromising mobility, function, and comfort in the back, hips, and legs. The shoulder blades and surrounding muscles are a major part of the shoulder girdle and allow the arms to be in relationship with the back. Muscular imbalance in the shoulder girdle will cause dysfunctional movement patterns throughout the body, including the spine. Balanced strength in the pelvic muscles enhances back stability and alignment of the feet and legs. Muscular imbalance in the pelvis will also cause dysfunctional movement patterns throughout the body, including the cervical and thoracic spine. All of these considerations affect total body alignment, comfort, and gait. Proper alignment and function lead to greater efficiency of movement and conservation of energy (Young, 2003).

It is theorized that gait originates in the spine rather than in the legs. This "spinal engine" theory (developed by S. A. Gracovetsky) rejects the notion that locomotion is a function of leg movement with the trunk being passively carried along. Rather, motion in the spine and surrounding tissues precedes that of the legs, comprising the basic engine of locomotion. The contralateral swinging of each leg with the opposite arm (e.g., the right arm swings forward with the left leg and vice versa) constitutes the rhythm of a normal gait with free motion in the shoulders and hips. The coordinated and fluid connection between upper and lower body motion indicates overall balance, energy efficiency, and comfort in movement.

Nursing Implications: Nurses should keep upper–lower body connection and spinal rotation in mind when evaluating gait, and encourage clients to walk with flowing contralateral movement between upper and lower limbs and a loose, rhythmic swing in the hips (Rice et al., 2004; Young, 2003).

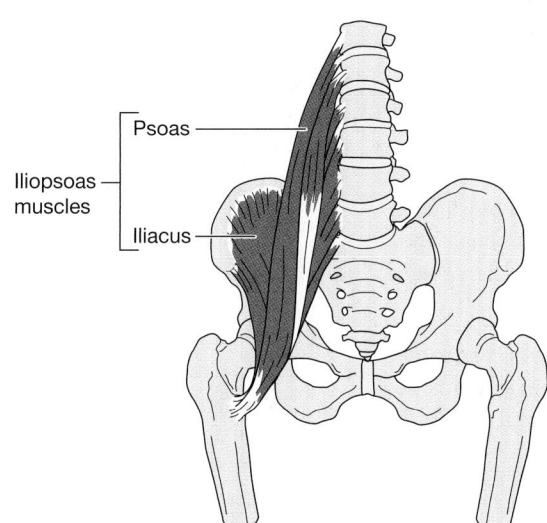

The iliopsoas muscle is frequently regarded as a single muscle because it is a blending of two muscles, the psoas and the iliacus. The psoas originates on the lumbar vertebrae and attaches to the femur. The iliacus originates on the pelvic crest and attaches on the femur. The connection between the spine and legs is evident when visualizing the iliopsoas muscles.

Spinal rotation precedes locomotion.

QUESTIONS

1. Why might someone with a foot or knee problem develop low back pain?
2. Why is contralateral movement of the upper and lower limbs important in a fluid, balanced gait?

Swing phase   Stance phase   Swing phase
begins   completed

Figure 44-41 ■ The stance and swing phases of a normal gait.

- Arm opposite the swing-through foot moves forward at the same time.
- Gait is smooth, coordinated, and rhythmic, with even weight borne on each foot. Hips gently sway with spinal rotation; the body moves forward smoothly, stopping and starting with ease.

The nurse may also assess **pace** (the number of steps taken per minute), which often slows with age and disability. A normal walking pace is 70 to 100 steps per minute. The pace of an older person may slow to about 40 steps per minute.

The nurse should also note the client's need for a prosthesis or assistive device, such as a cane or walker. For a client who uses assistive aids, the nurse assesses gait without the device and compares the assisted and unassisted gaits.

APPEARANCE AND MOVEMENT OF JOINTS.

Physical examination of the joints involves inspection, palpation, assessment of range of active motion, and if active motion is not possible, assessment of range of passive motion. The nurse should assess the following:

- Any joint swelling or redness, which could indicate the presence of an injury or an inflammation.
- Any deformity, such as a bony enlargement or contracture, and symmetry of involvement.
- The muscle development associated with each joint and the relative size and symmetry of the muscles on each side of the body.
- Any reported or palpable tenderness.
- **Crepitation** (palpable or audible crackling or grating sensation produced by joint motion and frequently experienced in joints that have suffered repeated trauma over time).
- Increased temperature over the joint. Palpate the joint using the backs of the fingers and compare the temperature with that of the symmetric joint.
- Degree of joint movement. Ask the client to move selected body parts as shown in Table 44–2. If indicated, measure the extent of

movement with a goniometer, a device that measures the angle of the joint in degrees. See Figure ❶ in Skill 30-16, page 641.

Assessment of range of motion should not be unduly fatiguing, and the joint movements need to be performed smoothly, slowly, and rhythmically. No joint should be forced. Uneven, jerky movement and forcing can injure the joint and its surrounding muscles and ligaments.

CAPABILITIES AND LIMITATIONS FOR MOVEMENT.

The nurse needs to obtain data that may indicate hindrances or restrictions to the client's movement and the need for assistance, including the following:

- How the client's illness influences the ability to move and whether the client's health contraindicates any exertion, position, or movement.
- Encumbrances to movement, such as an intravenous line in place or a heavy cast.
- Mental alertness and ability to follow directions. Check whether the client is receiving medications that hinder the ability to walk safely. Narcotics, sedatives, tranquilizers, and some antihistamines cause drowsiness, dizziness, weakness, and orthostatic hypotension.
- Balance and coordination.
- Presence of orthostatic hypotension before transfers. Specifically, assess for any increase in pulse rate, marked fall in blood pressure, dizziness, light-headedness, and dimming of vision when the client moves from a supine to a vertical posture.
- Degree of comfort. People who have pain may not want to move and may require an analgesic before they are moved.
- Vision. Is it adequate to prevent falls?

The nurse also assesses the amount of assistance the client requires for the following:

- Moving in the bed. In particular, observe for the amount of assistance the client requires for turning
  a. From a supine position to a lateral position.
  b. From a lateral position on one side to a lateral position on the other.
  c. From a supine position to a sitting position in bed.
- Rising from a lying position to a sitting position on the edge of the bed. Healthy people can normally rise without support from the arms.
- Rising from a chair to a standing position. Normally this can be done without pushing with the arms.
- Coordination and balance. Determine the client's abilities to hold the body erect, to bear weight and keep balance in a standing position on both legs or only one, to take steps, and to push off from a chair or bed.

MUSCLE MASS AND STRENGTH.

Before the client undertakes a change in position or attempts to ambulate, it is essential that the nurse assess the client's strength and ability to move. Providing appropriate assistance lowers the risk of muscle strain and body injury to both the client and nurse. Assessment of upper extremity strength is especially important for clients who use ambulation aids, such as walkers and crutches. For information on how to determine muscle mass and strength in lower and upper extremities, see Chapter 30. ∞

ACTIVITY TOLERANCE. By determining an appropriate activity level for a client, the nurse can predict whether the client has the strength and endurance to participate in activities that require similar expenditures of energy. This assessment is useful in encouraging increasing independence in people who (a) have a cardiovascular or respiratory disability, (b) have been completely immobilized for a prolonged period, (c) have decreased muscle mass or a musculoskeletal disorder, (d) have experienced inadequate sleep, (e) have experienced pain, or (f) are depressed, anxious, or unmotivated.

The most useful measures in predicting activity tolerance are heart rate, strength, and rhythm; respiratory rate, depth, and rhythm; and blood pressure. These data are obtained at the following times:

- Before the activity starts (baseline data), while the client is at rest
- During the activity
- Immediately after the activity stops
- Three minutes after the activity has stopped and the client has rested

The activity should be stopped immediately in the event of any physiologic change indicating the activity is too strenuous or prolonged for the client. These changes include the following:

- Sudden facial pallor
- Feelings of dizziness or weakness
- Change in level of consciousness
- Heart rate or respiratory rate that significantly exceeds baseline or preestablished levels
- Change in heart or respiratory rhythm from regular to irregular
- Weakening of the pulse
- Dyspnea, shortness of breath, or chest pain
- Diastolic blood pressure change of 10 mm Hg or more

If, however, the client tolerates the activity well, and if the client's heart rate returns to baseline levels within 5 minutes after the activity ceases, the activity is considered safe. This activity, then, can serve as a standard for predicting the client's tolerance for similar activities.

PROBLEMS RELATED TO IMMOBILITY. When collecting data pertaining to the problems of immobility, the nurse uses the assessment methods of inspection, palpation, and auscultation; checks results of laboratory tests; and takes measurements, including body weight, fluid intake, and fluid output. Specific techniques for assessing immobility problems and abnormal assessment findings related to the complications of immobility are listed in Table 44–3.

It is extremely important to obtain and record baseline assessment data soon after the client first becomes immobile. These baseline data serve as the standard against which all data collected throughout the period of immobilization are compared.

Because a major nursing responsibility is to prevent the complications of immobility, the nurse needs to identify clients at risk of developing such complications before problems arise.

Clients at risk include those who (a) are poorly nourished; (b) have decreased sensitivity to pain, temperature, or pressure; (c) have existing cardiovascular, pulmonary, or neuromuscular problems; and (d) have an altered level of consciousness.

Diagnosing

Mobility problems may be appropriate as the diagnostic label or as the etiology for other nursing diagnoses.

NANDA includes the following nursing diagnostic labels for activity and exercise problems:

- *Activity Intolerance:* Insufficient physiological or psychological energy to endure or complete required or desired daily activities. Four levels that can be used after the diagnostic label include:
  Level I: Walk, regular pace, on level ground indefinitely; climb one flight of stairs or more but more short of breath than normally.
  Level II: Walk one city block or 500 feet on level ground; climb one flight slowly without stopping.
  Level III: Walk no more than 50 feet on level ground without stopping; unable to climb one flight of stairs without stopping.
  Level IV: Dyspnea and fatigue at rest.
- *Risk for Activity Intolerance:* At risk for experiencing insufficient physiological or psychological energy to endure or complete required or desired daily activities.
- *Impaired Physical Mobility:* Limitation in independent, purposeful physical movement of the body or of one or more extremities.
  More specific versions of this diagnosis are
  Impaired Bed Mobility.
  Impaired Walking.
  Impaired Wheelchair Mobility.
  Impaired Transfer Ability.
- *Sedentary Lifestyle:* Reports a habit of life that is characterized by a low physical activity level.
- *Risk for Disuse Syndrome:* At risk for deterioration of body systems as the result of prescribed or unavoidable musculoskeletal inactivity.

A clinical example of this nursing diagnosis is shown in the Nursing Care Plan and the Concept Map on pages 1158–1159.

Depending on the data obtained, problems with mobility often affect other areas of human functioning and indicate other diagnoses. In these instances, the mobility problem becomes the etiology. Examples in which *Impaired Physical Mobility* is the etiology follow. The etiology needs to be described more explicitly in terms such as reduced ROM, neuromuscular impairment or musculoskeletal impairment of upper and lower extremities, or joint pain.

- *Fear* (of falling)
- *Ineffective Coping*
- *Low Self-Esteem*
- *Powerlessness*
- *Risk for Falls*
- *Self–Care Deficit*

TABLE 44–3 **Assessing Problems of Immobility**	
ASSESSMENT	**PROBLEM**
Musculoskeletal System	
Measure arm and leg circumferences	Decreased circumference due to decreased muscle mass
Palpate and observe body joints	Stiffness or pain in joints
Take goniometric measurements of joint ROM	Decreased joint ROM, joint contractures
Cardiovascular System	
Auscultate the heart	Increased heart rate
Measure blood pressure	Orthostatic hypotension
Palpate and observe sacrum, legs, and feet	Peripheral dependent edema, increased peripheral vein engorgement
Palpate peripheral pulses	Weak peripheral pulses
Measure calf muscle circumferences	Edema
Observe calf muscle for redness, tenderness, and swelling	Thrombophlebitis
Respiratory System	
Observe chest movements	Asymmetric chest movements, dyspnea
Auscultate chest	Diminished breath sounds, crackles, wheezes, and increased respiratory rate
Metabolic System	
Measure height and weight	Weight loss due to muscle atrophy and loss of subcutaneous fat
Palpate skin	Generalized edema due to low blood protein levels
Urinary System	
Measure fluid intake and output	Dehydration
Inspect urine	Cloudy, dark urine; high specific gravity
Palpate urinary bladder	Distended urinary bladder due to urinary retention
Gastrointestinal System	
Observe stool	Hard, dry, small stool
Auscultate bowel sounds	Decreased bowel sounds due to decreased intestinal motility
Integumentary System	
Inspect skin	Break in skin integrity
Psychoneurologic System	
Observe behaviors, affect, and cognition	Anger, flat affect, crying, confusion, anxiety, decline in cognitive function,
Monitor developmental skills in children	or vegetative signs such as sleep and appetite disturbances warrant further evaluation

When problems associated with prolonged immobility arise, many other diagnoses may be necessary. Examples include, but are not limited to, the following:

- *Ineffective Airway Clearance* if there is stasis of pulmonary secretions
- *Risk for Infection* if there is stasis of urinary or pulmonary secretions
- *Risk for Injury* if orthostatic hypotension is present
- *Risk for Disturbed Sleep Pattern* if there is a lack of daytime physical activity
- *Risk for Situational Low Self-Esteem* if there is functional impairment and/or role disturbance

Planning

When planning for desired outcomes, Nursing Outcomes Classification (NOC) labels that pertain to exercise and activity can be helpful and include the following: activity tolerance; anxiety level and self-control; body image; body positioning; bowel elimination; caregiver physical health; coordinated movement; depression self-control; diabetes self-management; endurance;

fall prevention behavior; immobility consequences, both physiological and psycho-cognitive; joint movement; mobility; mood equilibrium; personal well-being; physical fitness; play participation; quality of life; respiratory status, ventilation and gas exchange; role performance; self-care; sleep; stress level; and weight control (Moorhead, Johnson, & Maas, 2004).

Positioning, transferring, and ambulating clients are almost always independent nursing functions. The primary care practitioner usually orders specific body positions only after surgery, anesthesia, or trauma involving the nervous and musculoskeletal systems. All clients should have an activity order written by their primary care practitioner when they are admitted to the agency for care.

As part of planning, the nurse is responsible for identifying those clients who need assistance with body alignment and determining the degree of assistance they need. The nurse must be sensitive to the client's need to function as independently as possible yet provide assistance when the client needs it.

Most clients require some nursing guidance and assistance to learn about, achieve, and maintain proper body mechanics. The nurse should also plan to teach clients applicable skills. For example, a client with a back injury needs to learn how to get out of bed safely and comfortably, a client with an injured leg needs to learn how to transfer from bed to wheelchair safely, and a client with a newly acquired walker needs to learn how to use it safely. Nurses often teach family members or caregivers safe moving, lifting, and transfer techniques in the home setting.

The goals established for clients will vary according to the diagnosis and defining characteristics related to each individual. Examples of overall goals for clients with actual or potential problems related to mobility or activity follow.

The client will have

- Increased tolerance for physical activity.
- Restored or improved capability to ambulate and/or participate in ADLs.
- Absence of injury from falling or improper use of body mechanics.
- Enhanced physical fitness.
- Absence of any complications associated with immobility.
- Improved social, emotional, and intellectual well-being.

Examples of desired outcomes, interventions, and activities are provided in the Nursing Care Plan and Concept Map on pages 1158–1159.

Planning for Home Care

Clients who have been hospitalized for activity or mobility problems often need continued care in the home. In preparation for discharge, the nurse needs to determine the client's actual and potential health problems, strengths, and resources. The accompanying Home Care Assessment describes the specific assessment data required before establishing a discharge plan for clients with mobility or activity problems. A major aspect of discharge planning involves instructional needs of the client and family. See Client Teaching features throughout this chapter.

Implementing

Nurses can initiate and apply a wide variety of exercise and activity interventions as needed to address a multitude of client concerns. Nursing Interventions Classification (NIC) labels that pertain to exercise and activity include the following: activity therapy; calming technique; cardiac care; rehabilitation; cognitive stimulation; constipation management; distraction; exercise promotion (strength and stretching); exercise therapy (ambulation, balance, joint mobility, muscle control); fall prevention; health education; infection prevention; memory training; mood management; pelvic muscle exercise; pressure ulcer prevention; progressive muscle relaxation; recreation therapy; religious ritual enhancement; self-care assistance; self-esteem enhancement; simple relaxation therapy; sleep enhancement; spiritual growth facilitation; sports-injury prevention; teaching: prescribed activity/exercise; therapeutic play; and weight management and weight reduction (Dochterman & Bulechek, 2004).

Nursing strategies to maintain or promote body alignment and mobility involve positioning clients appropriately, moving and turning clients in bed, transferring clients, providing ROM exercises, ambulating clients with or without mechanical aids, and strategies to prevent the complications of immobility.

HOME CARE ASSESSMENT
Mobility and Activity Problems

CLIENT AND ENVIRONMENT

- Capabilities or tolerance for required and desired activities: Self-care (feeding, bathing, toileting, dressing, grooming, home maintenance, shopping, cooking); recreational activities
- Mobility aids required: Cane, walker, crutches, wheelchair, transfer boards
- Equipment required if immobilized: Special bed, side rails, pressure-reducing mattress
- Current level of knowledge: Body mechanics for use of mobility aids; specific exercises prescribed
- Home mobility hazard appraisal: Adequacy of lighting; presence of handrails; safety of pathways and stairs; congested areas; unanchored rugs, mats, or electrical cords, and any other obstacles to safe movement; structural adjustments needed for wheelchair access

FAMILY OR CAREGIVER

- Caregiver availability, skills, and willingness to assist: Assess learning needs and develop appropriate teaching plan, primary people able to assist client with self-care, movement, shopping, and so on; physical and emotional status to assist with care
- Family role changes and coping: Effect on financial status, parenting and spousal roles, social roles
- Availability of caregiver support: Other support people available for occasional duties such as shopping, transportation, housekeeping, cooking, budgeting; refer to community agencies for respite care, where appropriate

COMMUNITY

- Resources: Availability and familiarity with sources of medical equipment, financial assistance, homemaker services, hygienic care; Meals on Wheels; spiritual counselors and visitors; sources of respite for caregiver

Whenever positioning, moving, lifting, and ambulating clients, nurses must use proper body mechanics to avoid musculoskeletal strain and injury.

Using Body Mechanics

Body mechanics is the term used to describe the efficient, coordinated, and safe use of the body to move objects and carry out the activities of daily living. Until recently, it was thought that using good body mechanics reduced energy requirements, fatigue, and risk of injury for both nurses and clients, especially during lifting, transferring, and repositioning. In reality, 35 years of body mechanics (ergonomics) research show that:

- Training nurses in body mechanics alone will not prevent job-related injuries.
- Back belts are likely **not** effective in reducing back injury.
- Nurses who are physically fit are at no less risk of injury.
- The average nurse should not lift more than 51 pounds and only under very controlled circumstances.
- Long-term benefits of proper equipment (e.g., mechanical lifts) far outweigh costs related to injuries.

CLIENT TEACHING   Home Care Activity and Exercise

MAINTAINING MUSCULOSKELETAL FUNCTION

- Teach the systematic performance of passive or assistive ROM exercises to maintain joint mobility.
- Demonstrate, as appropriate, the proper way to perform isotonic, isometric, or isokinetic exercises to maintain muscle mass and tone (collaborate with the physical therapist about these). Incorporate ADLs into exercise program if appropriate.
- Provide a written schedule for the type, frequency, and duration of exercises; encourage the use of a progress graph or chart to facilitate adherence with the therapy.
- Offer an ambulation schedule.
- Instruct in the availability of assistive ambulatory devices and correct use of them.
- Discuss pain control measures required before exercise.

PREVENTING INJURY

- Provide assistive devices for moving and transferring, whenever possible, and teach safe transfer and ambulation techniques.
- Discuss safety measures to avoid falls (e.g., locking wheelchairs, wearing appropriate footwear, using rubber tips on crutches, keeping the environment safe, and using mechanical aids such as raised toilet seat, grab bars, urinal, and bedpan or commode to facilitate toileting).

- Teach the use of proper body mechanics, especially for those times when assistive equipment is not used.
- Teach ways to prevent postural hypotension.

MANAGING ENERGY TO PREVENT FATIGUE

- Discuss activity and rest patterns and develop a plan as indicated; intersperse rest periods with activity periods.
- Discuss ways to minimize fatigue such as performing activities more slowly and for shorter periods, resting more often, and using more assistance as required.
- Provide information about available resources to help with ADLs and home maintenance management.
- Teach ways to increase energy (e.g., increasing intake of high-energy foods, ensuring adequate rest and sleep, controlling pain, sharing feelings with a trusted listener).
- Teach techniques to monitor activity tolerance as appropriate.

REFERRALS

- Provide appropriate information about accessing community resources: home care agencies, physical and occupational therapy agencies, local YMCAs and other agencies that provide structured exercise and movement programs, and sources of adaptive equipment.

- Staff will use equipment when they participate in the decision-making process for purchasing the equipment (American Nurses Association, n.d.).

Even with careful attentions to body mechanics, nursing is ranked as the sixth most at-risk occupation for back injuries. In fact, results from several studies indicate that 52% of nurses complain of chronic back pain; 12% leave the profession because of back pain; 20% transfer to a different work setting due to back pain; 12% consider leaving the profession; 38% suffer work-related back pain severe enough to require leave of absence; and 25% reported changing jobs due to neck, shoulder, and back problems (American Nurses Association, n.d.). The development of assistive client handling equipment and devices has rendered strict "manual" client handling unnecessary. It is also thought to provide greater client safety, dignity, and comfort. Costs of equipment appear to be less than the costs of work-related injury (Nelson, Fragala, & Menzel, 2003). The equipment recommendations include full sling mechanical lift devices for totally dependent or extensive assistance level clients; full sling, stand assist lift, or full sling mechanical lifts for dependent lifts from the floor; and transfer or gait belts for client-assisted lifts from the floor.

Until all work settings provide safe environments in which nurses have the equipment they need, content pertaining to body mechanics will be included here. Readers are encouraged to support "No Manual Lift" and "No Solo Lift" policies in their workplaces, and to become involved in legislation and equipment purchase initiatives. Nurses must participate in this shift in ergonomic awareness, and are encouraged to visit the American Nurses Association website to read more about the "Handle with Care" campaign to prevent workplace injuries.

When a person moves, the center of gravity shifts continuously in the direction of the moving body parts. Balance depends on the interrelationship of the center of gravity, the line of gravity, and the base of support. The closer the line of gravity is to the center of the base of support, the greater the person's stability (Figure 44-42 ■ A). Conversely, the closer the line of gravity is to the edge of the base of support, the more precarious the balance (Figure 44-42 ■ B). If the line of gravity falls outside the base of support, the person falls (Figure 44-42 ■ C).

CLINICAL ALERT

The American Federation of State, County, and Municipal Employees (AFSCME) reports that back injuries are caused by force, repetition, and awkward positions. The most common injuries among health care workers are low back pain, herniated discs, strained muscles, pulled and/or torn ligaments, and disc degradation (AFSCME, 2002). ■

The broader the base of support and the lower the center of gravity, the greater the stability and balance. Body balance, therefore, can be greatly enhanced by (a) widening the base of support and (b) lowering the center of gravity, bringing it closer to the base of support. The base of support is easily widened by spreading the feet farther apart. The center of gravity is readily lowered by flexing the hips and knees until a squatting position is achieved. The importance of these alterations cannot be overemphasized for nurses.

Two movements to avoid because of their potential for causing back injury are twisting (rotation) of the thoracolumbar spine and acute flexion of the back with hips and knees straight (stooping). Undesirable twisting of the back can be prevented

- Center of gravity
- Line of gravity
- Base of support

A   **B**   **C**

Figure 44-42 ■ *A,* Balance is maintained when the line of gravity falls close to the base of support. *B,* Balance is precarious when the line of gravity falls at the edge of the base of support. *C,* Balance cannot be maintained when the line of gravity falls outside the base of support.

by squarely facing the direction of movement, whether pushing, pulling, or sliding, and moving the object directly toward or away from one's center of gravity.

LIFTING. It is important to remember that nurses should not lift more than 51 pounds without assistance from proper equipment and/or other persons. Types of assistive equipment include partial standing lifts, permanently mounted ceiling lifts, and horizontal air-transfer mattresses (E-Z Lift, E-Z Lift Assist, and the Slipp® Patient Mover are examples of such devices). See Figures 44-43 ■ and 44-44 ■. At times it may be necessary to lift under less than ideal circumstances. It is always wise to use proper body mechanics, even though they do not guarantee freedom from injury.

When a person lifts or carries an object, for example, a suitcase, the weight of the object becomes part of the person's body weight. This weight affects the location of the person's center of gravity, which is displaced in the direction of the added weight. To counteract this potential imbalance, body parts (e.g., arm and trunk) move in a direction away from the weight. In this way, the center of gravity is maintained over the base of support. By holding the lifted object as close as possible to the body's center of gravity, the lifter avoids undue displacement of the center of gravity and achieves greater stability.

People can lift more weight when they use a lever than when they do not. In the body, the bones of the skeleton act as levers, a joint is a fulcrum (fixed point about which a lever moves), and the muscles exert the force (Figure 44-45 ■). Use of the arms as levers is often applied in clinical practice when the nurse needs to raise a client's head off the bed, for example, or give back care to a client in traction.

Figure 44-43 ■ EZ Lift is an electric client lift that functions to lift clients from bed, chair, toilet, and floor.

(EZ Way, Inc.)

Figure 44-44 ■ The Slipp® Patient Mover is a client-moving device that reduces the nurse's exposure to back injuries and maximizes client comfort.

(Wright Products, Inc.)

Figure 44-45 ■ Using the arm as a lever.

Because lifting involves movement against gravity, the nurse must use the major muscle groups of the thighs, knees, upper and lower arms, abdomen, and pelvis to prevent back strain. The nurse can increase overall muscle strength by synchronized use of as many muscle groups as possible during an activity. For instance, when the arms are used in an activity, dividing the work between the arms and legs helps prevent back strain.

Another technique based on the principle of leverage can be used when lifting objects from the floor to waist level. In this technique, the back and knees are flexed until the load is at thigh level, at which point the knees remain flexed to provide thrust as the back begins to straighten (Figure 44-46 ■). This technique provides for balance, leverage, and synchronized use of muscles, which help avoid back pain and injury. When one lifts an object to knee level, the shoulder and arm muscles pull, the abdominal and lumbar muscles contract for leverage and pull, and the thigh and leg muscles exert the upward thrust to bring the object off the floor. When one lifts an object from midthigh to waist level, essentially the leg and thigh muscle groups provide force, but the back and lumbar muscles remain contracted.

Figure 44-46 ■ Lifting heavy objects from the floor to waist level. *A,* Stand close to the load and flex the back and the knees, lowering the body to grasp the load. *B,* Begin lifting with the back flexed, and gradually straighten the knees so that the leg muscles bear most of the burden. *C,* To hold or walk with the object, maintain a less flexed but not a completely straight position.

In all positions, it is important to maintain a distance of at least 30 cm (12 in.) between the feet and to keep the load close to the body, especially when it is at knee level. Before attempting the lift, the nurse must ensure that there are no hazards on the floor, that there is a clear path for moving the object, and that the nurse's base of support is secure.

PULLING AND PUSHING. When pulling or pushing an object, a person maintains balance with least effort when the base of support is enlarged in the direction in which the movement is to be produced or opposed. For example, when pushing an object, a person can enlarge the base of support by moving the front foot forward. When pulling an object, a person can enlarge the base of support by (a) moving the rear leg back if the person is facing the object or (b) moving the front foot forward if the person is facing away from the object. It is easier and safer to pull an object toward one's own center of gravity than to push it away, because a person can exert more control of the object's movement when pulling it.

CLINICAL ALERT

Lateral-assist devices such as horizontal air transfer mattresses and transfer chairs are essential equipment for most client care areas to prevent acute and chronic back pain and disability. Observing principles of body mechanics is recommended even when using assistive equipment, as any lifting and forceful movement is potentially injurious, especially when repeated over time. ■

PIVOTING. Pivoting is a technique in which the body is turned in a way that avoids twisting of the spine. To pivot, place one foot ahead of the other, raise the heels very slightly, and put the body weight on the balls of the feet. When the weight is off the heels, the frictional surface is decreased and the knees are not twisted when turning. Keeping the body aligned, turn (pivot) about 90 degrees in the desired direction. The foot that was forward will now be behind.

Preventing Back Injury

Many factors increase the potential for lower back injuries. A major contributor is habitually poor standing and sitting posture, which produces lordosis. Overweight individuals who carry their extra weight over their abdomen, pregnant women, and women who consistently wear high-heeled shoes are at risk because of the exaggerated lumbar curvature these situations produce. Sedentary persons are at greater risk because of weak back and abdominal muscles.

Guidelines for preventing back injuries are presented in Client Teaching.

Positioning Clients

Positioning a client in good body alignment and changing the position regularly (every 2 hours) and systematically are essential aspects of nursing practice. Clients who can move easily automatically reposition themselves for comfort. Such people generally require minimal positioning assistance from nurses, other than guidance about ways to maintain body alignment and to exercise their joints. However, people who are weak, frail, in pain,

CLIENT TEACHING   Preventing Back Injuries

- Understand that the use of body mechanics will not necessarily prevent injury if manually handling a load greater than 51 pounds without the use of assistive devices.
- Avoid lifting anything greater than 51 pounds. Use assistive equipment, get help from co-workers, and participate in the purchasing/ordering process of appropriate assistive equipment for your work setting.
- Become consciously aware of your posture and body mechanics.
- When standing for a period of time, periodically move legs and hips, and flex one hip and knee and rest your foot on an object if possible.
- When sitting, keep your knees slightly higher than your hips.
- Use a firm mattress and soft pillow that provide good body support at natural body curvatures.

- Exercise regularly to maintain overall physical condition and regulate weight; include exercises that strengthen the pelvic, abdominal, and spinal muscles.
- Avoid movements that cause pain or require spinal flexion with straight legs (e.g., toe-touching and sit-ups) or spinal rotation (twisting).
- When moving an object, spread your feet apart to provide a wide base of support.
- When lifting an object, distribute the weight between large muscles of the legs and arms, limiting the load to 15 to 25 pounds held at elbow height.
- Wear comfortable low-heeled shoes that provide good foot support and reduce the risk of slipping, stumbling, or turning your ankle.

paralyzed, or unconscious rely on nurses to provide or assist with position changes. For all clients, it is important to assess the skin and provide skin care before and after a position change.

Any position, correct or incorrect, can be detrimental if maintained for a prolonged period. Frequent change of position helps to prevent muscle discomfort, undue pressure resulting in pressure ulcers, damage to superficial nerves and blood vessels, and contractures. Position changes also maintain muscle tone and stimulate postural reflexes.

When the client is not able to move independently or assist with moving, the preferred method is to use appropriate assistive equipment, as well as to have two or more people move or turn the client. Appropriate assistance reduces the risk of muscle strain and body injury to both the client and nurse, and is likely to protect the dignity and comfort of the client.

When positioning clients in bed, the nurse can do a number of things to ensure proper alignment and promote client comfort and safety:

- Make sure the mattress is firm and level yet has enough give to fill in and support natural body curvatures. A sagging mattress, a mattress that is too soft, or an underfilled waterbed used over a prolonged period can contribute to the development of hip flexion contractures and low back strain and pain. Bed boards made of plywood and placed beneath a sagging mattress are increasingly recommended for clients who have back problems or are prone to them. Some bed boards are hinged across the middle so that they will bend as the head of the bed is raised. It is particularly important in the home setting to inspect the mattress for support.
- Ensure that the bed is clean and dry. Wrinkled or damp sheets increase the risk of pressure ulcer formation. Make sure extremities can move freely whenever possible. For example, the top bedclothes need to be loose enough for clients to move their feet.
  - Place support devices in specified areas according to the client's position. Box 44-1 lists commonly used support devices. Use only those support devices needed to maintain alignment and to prevent stress on the client's muscles and joints. If the person is capable of movement, too

many devices limit mobility and increase the potential for muscle weakness and atrophy.
- Avoid placing one body part, particularly one with bony prominences, directly on top of another body part. Excessive pressure can damage veins and predispose the client to thrombus formation. Pressure against the popliteal space may damage nerves and blood vessels in this area. Pillows can provide needed cushioning.
- Plan a systematic 24-hour schedule for position changes.

Sometimes a person who appears well aligned may be experiencing real discomfort. Both appearance, in relation to alignment criteria, and comfort are important in achieving effective alignment.

FOWLER'S POSITION. **Fowler's position,** or a semisitting position, is a bed position in which the head and trunk are raised 45 to 90 degrees. In **low Fowler's** or **semi-Fowler's position** (Figure 44-47 ■), the head and trunk are raised 15 to 45 degrees; in **high Fowler's position,** the head and trunk are raised

BOX 44-1   Support Devices

- Pillows. Different sizes are available. Used for support or elevation of a body part (e.g., an arm). Specially designed dense pillows can be used to elevate the upper body.
- Mattresses. There are two types of mattresses: ones that fit on the bed frame (e.g., standard bed mattress) and mattresses that fit on the standard bed mattress (e.g., egg crate mattress). Mattresses should be periodically rotated and evenly supportive.
- Bed boards. The boards are usually made of wood and are placed under the mattress to provide support.
- Chair beds. These beds can be placed into the position of a chair for clients who cannot move from the bed but require a sitting position.
- Foot boot. These are made of a variety of substances. They usually have a firm exterior and padding of foam to protect the skin. They provide support to the feet in a natural position and keep the weight of covers off the toes. Clients who are able to sit may benefit from high-top shoes to maintain foot alignment.
- Footboard. A flat panel often made of plastic or wood. It keeps the feet in dorsiflexion to prevent plantar flexion.

TABLE 44–4 Fowler's Position

UNSUPPORTED POSITION	PROBLEM TO BE PREVENTED	CORRECTIVE MEASURE*
Bed-sitting position with upper part of body elevated 30–90° commencing at hips	Posterior flexion of lumbar curvature	Pillow at lower back (lumbar region) to support lumbar region
Head rests on bed surface	Hyperextension of neck	Pillows to support head, neck, and upper back
Arms fall at sides	Shoulder muscle strain, possible dislocation of shoulders, edema of hands and arms with flaccid paralysis, flexion contracture of the wrist	Pillow under forearms to eliminate pull on shoulder and assist venous blood flow from hands and lower arms
Legs lie flat and straight on lower bed surface	Hyperextension of knees	Small pillow under thighs to flex knees
Heels rest on bed surface	Pressure on heels	Pillow under lower legs
Feet are in plantar flexion	Plantar flexion of feet (foot drop)	Footboard to provide support for dorsal flexion

*The amount of correction depends on the needs of the individual client.

Figure 44-47 ■ Low Fowler's (semi-Fowler's) position (supported). Note that arm support is omitted in this instance. The amount of support depends on the needs of the individual client.

90 degrees (see Table 44–4). In this position, the knees may or may not be flexed.

Fowler's position is the position of choice for people who have difficulty breathing and for some people with heart problems. When the client is in this position, gravity pulls the diaphragm downward, allowing greater chest expansion and lung ventilation.

A common error nurses make when aligning clients in Fowler's position is placing an overly large pillow or more than one pillow behind the client's head. This promotes the development of neck flexion contractures. If a client desires several head pillows, the nurse should encourage the client to rest without a pillow for several hours each day to extend the neck fully and counteract the effects of poor neck alignment.

ORTHOPNEIC POSITION. In the **orthopneic position,** the client sits either in bed or on the side of the bed with an overbed table across the lap (Figure 44-48 ■). This position facilitates respiration by allowing maximum chest expansion. It is particularly helpful to clients who have problems exhaling, because they can press the lower part of the chest against the edge of the overbed table.

DORSAL RECUMBENT POSITION. In the **dorsal recumbent** (back-lying) **position** (Figure 44-49 ■), the client's head and shoulders are slightly elevated on a small pillow. In some agencies, the terms *dorsal recumbent* and *supine* are used interchangeably; strictly speaking, however, in the **supine** or **dorsal position** the head and shoulders are not elevated. In both positions, the client's forearms may be elevated on pillows or placed

Figure 44-48 ■ Orthopneic position.

Figure 44-49 ■ Dorsal recumbent position (supported).

at the client's sides. Supports are similar in both positions, except for the head pillow (see Table 44–5). The dorsal recumbent position is used to provide comfort and to facilitate healing following certain surgeries or anesthetics (e.g., spinal).

PRONE POSITION. In the **prone position,** the client lies on the abdomen with the head turned to one side (Figure 44-50 ■). The hips are not flexed. Both children and adults often sleep in this position, sometimes with one or both arms flexed over their heads. It is the only bed position that allows full extension of the hip and knee joints. When used periodically, the prone position helps to prevent flexion contractures of the hips and knees, thereby counteracting a problem caused by all

Figure 44-50 ■ Prone position (supported).

TABLE 44–5 **Dorsal Recumbent Position**		
UNSUPPORTED POSITION	**PROBLEM TO BE PREVENTED**	**CORRECTIVE MEASURE***
Head is flat on bed surface	Hyperextension of neck in thick-chested person	Pillow of suitable thickness under head and shoulders if necessary for alignment
Lumbar curvature of spine is apparent	Posterior flexion of lumbar curvature	Roll or small pillow under lumbar curvature
Legs may be externally rotated	External rotation of legs	Roll or sandbag placed laterally to trochanter of femur (optional)
Legs are extended	Hyperextension of knees	Small pillow under thigh to flex knee slightly
Feet assume plantar flexion position	Plantar flexion (foot drop)	Footboard or rolled pillow to support feet in dorsal flexion
Heels on bed surface	Pressure on heels	Pillow under lower legs

*The amount of correction depends on the needs of the individual client.

other bed positions. The prone position also promotes drainage from the mouth and is especially useful for unconscious clients or those clients recovering from surgery of the mouth or throat (see Table 44–6).

The prone position poses some distinct disadvantages. The pull of gravity on the trunk produces a marked lordosis in most people, and the neck is rotated laterally to a significant degree. For this reason, the prone position may not be recommended for people with problems of the cervical or lumbar spine. This position also causes plantar flexion. Some clients with cardiac or respiratory problems find the prone position confining and suffocating because chest expansion is inhibited during respirations. *The prone position should be used only when the client's back is correctly aligned, only for short periods, and only for people with no evidence of spinal abnormalities.*

LATERAL POSITION. In the **lateral** (side-lying) **position** (Figure 44-51 ■), the person lies on one side of the body. Flexing the top hip and knee and placing this leg in front of the body creates a wider, triangular base of support and achieves greater stability. The greater the flexion of the top hip and knee, the greater the stability and balance in this position. This flexion reduces lordosis and promotes good back alignment. For this reason, the lateral position is good for resting and sleeping clients. The lateral position helps to relieve pressure on the sacrum and heels in people who sit for much of the day or who are confined to bed and rest in Fowler's or dorsal recumbent positions much of the time. In the lateral position,

Figure 44-51 ■ Lateral position (supported).

most of the body's weight is borne by the lateral aspect of the lower scapula, the lateral aspect of the ilium, and the greater trochanter of the femur. People who have sensory or motor deficits on one side of the body usually find that lying on the uninvolved side is more comfortable (see Table 44–7).

SIMS' POSITION. In **Sims'** (semiprone) **position** (Figure 44-52 ■), the client assumes a posture halfway between the lateral and the prone positions. The lower arm is positioned behind the client, and the upper arm is flexed at the shoulder and the elbow. Both legs are flexed in front of the client. The upper leg is more acutely flexed at both the hip and the knee than is the lower one.

Sims' position may be used for unconscious clients because it facilitates drainage from the mouth and prevents aspiration of fluids. It is also used for paralyzed clients because it reduces pressure over the sacrum and greater trochanter of the hip. It is often used for clients receiving enemas and occasionally for clients undergoing examinations or treatments of the perineal area. Many people, especially pregnant women, find Sims' position comfortable for sleeping. People with sensory or motor

TABLE 44–6 **Prone Position**		
UNSUPPORTED POSITION	**PROBLEM TO BE PREVENTED**	**CORRECTIVE MEASURE***
Head is turned to side and neck is slightly flexed	Flexion or hyperextension of neck	Small pillow under head unless contraindicated because of promotion of mucous drainage from mouth
Body lies flat on abdomen accentuating lumbar curvature	Hyperextension of lumbar curvature; difficulty breathing; pressure on breasts (women); pressure on genitals (men)	Small pillow or roll under abdomen just below diaphragm
Toes rest on bed surface; feet are in plantar flexion	Plantar flexion (foot drop)	Allow feet to fall naturally over end of mattress, or support lower legs on a pillow so that toes do not touch the bed

*The amount of correction depends on the needs of the individual client.

TABLE 44–7   Lateral Position

UNSUPPORTED POSITION	PROBLEM TO BE PREVENTED	CORRECTIVE MEASURE*
Body is turned to side, both arms in front of body, weight resting primarily on lateral aspects of scapula and ilium	Lateral flexion and fatigue of sternocleidomastoid muscles	Pillow under head and neck to provide good alignment
Upper arm and shoulder are rotated internally and adducted	Internal rotation and adduction of shoulder and subsequent limited function; impaired chest expansion	Pillow under upper arm to place it in good alignment; lower arm should be flexed comfortably
Upper thigh and leg are rotated internally and adducted	Internal rotation and adduction of femur; twisting of the spine	Pillow under leg and thigh to place them in good alignment; shoulders and hips should be aligned

The amount of correction depends on the needs of the individual client.

Figure 44-52 ■ Sims' position (supported).

deficits on one side of the body usually find that lying on the uninvolved side is more comfortable (see Table 44–8).

Moving and Turning Clients in Bed

Although healthy people usually take for granted that they can change body position and go from one place to another with little effort, ill people may have difficulty moving, even in bed. How much assistance clients require depends on their own ability to move and their health status. Nurses should be sensitive to both the need of people to function independently and their need for assistance to move.

When a nurse assists a person to move, correct body mechanics need to be employed so that the nurse is not injured. Correct body alignment for the client must also be maintained so that undue stress is not placed on the musculoskeletal system.

Actions and rationales applicable to moving and lifting clients include these:

- Before moving a client, assess the degree of exertion permitted, the client's physical abilities (e.g., muscle strength, presence of paralysis) and ability to assist with the move, ability to understand instructions, degree of comfort or discomfort when moving, client's weight, presence of orthostatic hypotension (particularly important when client will be standing), and your own strength and ability to move the client.
- If indicated, use pain relief modalities or medication prior to moving the client.
- Prepare any needed assistive devices and supportive equipment (e.g., pillows, trochanter roll).
- Plan around encumbrances to movement such as an IV or heavy cast.
- Be alert to the effects of any medications the client takes that may impair alertness, balance, strength, or mobility.
- Obtain required assistance from other persons.
- Explain the procedure to the client and listen to any suggestions the client or support people have.
- Provide privacy.
- Wash hands.
- Raise the height of the bed *to bring the client close to your center of gravity.*
- Lock the wheels on the bed, and raise the rail on the side of the bed opposite you *to ensure client safety.*

TABLE 44–8   Sims' (Semiprone) Position

UNSUPPORTED POSITION	PROBLEM TO BE PREVENTED	CORRECTIVE MEASURE*
Head rests on bed surface; weight is borne by lateral aspects of cranial and facial bones	Lateral flexion of neck	Pillow supports head, maintaining it in good alignment unless drainage from the mouth is required
Upper shoulder and arm are internally rotated	Internal rotation of shoulder and arm; pressure on chest, restricting expansion during breathing	Pillow under upper arm to prevent internal rotation
Upper leg and thigh are adducted and internally rotated	Internal rotation and adduction of hip and leg	Pillow under upper leg to support it in alignment
Feet assume plantar flexion	Foot drop	Sandbags to support feet in dorsal flexion

The amount of correction depends on the needs of the individual client.

- Face in the direction of the movement *to prevent spinal twisting.*
- Assume a broad stance *to increase stability and provide balance.*
- Lean your trunk forward, and flex your hips, knees, and ankles *to lower your center of gravity, increase stability, and ensure use of large muscle groups during movements.*
- Tighten your gluteal, abdominal, leg, and arm muscles *to prepare them for action and prevent injury.*
- Rock from the front leg to the back leg when pulling or from the back leg to the front leg when pushing *to overcome inertia, counteract the client's weight, and help attain a balanced, smooth motion.*

After moving the client, determine and document the client's comfort (presence of anxiety, dizziness, or pain), body alignment, tolerance of the activity (e.g., check pulse rate, blood pressure), ability to assist, use of support devices, and safety precautions required (e.g., side rails).

See Skills 44-1 through 44-4 on moving and turning clients in bed and helping them sit up on the edge of the bed.

Note: The Assessment, Planning, Delegation, and Equipment sections as listed in Skill 44-1 are the same for each of these four procedures and are not repeated. The Evaluation section at the end of Skill 44-4 is also the same for all four procedures and, hence, is not repeated.

MOVING A CLIENT UP IN BED

SKILL 44-1

ASSESSMENT
Before moving a client, assess the following:

- The client's physical abilities (e.g., muscle strength, presence of paralysis)
- Ability to understand instructions
- Degree of comfort or discomfort when moving. If needed, administer analgesics or perform other pain relief measures (see Chapter 46 ∞).
- Client's weight
- The availability of equipment and other personnel to assist you

PLANNING
Review the client record to determine if previous nurses have recorded information about the client's ability to move. Use proper assistive equipment and additional personnel whenever needed.

> **Delegation**
> The skills of moving and turning clients in bed can be delegated to unlicensed assistive personnel (UAP). The nurse should make sure that any needed equipment and additional personnel are available to reduce risk of injury to the health care personnel. Emphasize the need for the UAP to report changes in the client's condition that require assessment and intervention by the nurse.

Equipment
- Assistive devices such as overhead trapeze, pull and/or turn sheet, and transfer or sliding bar

Purposes
- Clients who have slid down in bed from the Fowler's position or been pulled down by traction often need assistance to move up in bed.

IMPLEMENTATION
Preparation
Determine:

- Assistive devices that will be required.
- Encumbrances to movement such as an IV or a heavy cast on one leg.
- Medications the client is receiving, because certain medications may hamper movement or alertness of the client.
- Assistance required from other health care personnel.

Performance
1. Prior to performing the procedure, introduce self and verify the client's identity using agency protocol. Explain to the client what you are going to do, why it is necessary, and how he or she can cooperate. Listen to any suggestions made by the client or support people. Discuss how the results will be used in planning further care or treatments.
2. Perform hand hygiene and observe other appropriate infection control procedures.
3. Provide for client privacy.
4. Adjust the bed and the client's position.
   - Adjust the head of the bed to a flat position or as low as the client can tolerate. Moving the client upward against gravity requires more force and can cause back strain.
   - Raise the bed to the height of your center of gravity.
   - Lock the wheels on the bed and raise the rail on the side of the bed opposite you.
   - Remove all pillows, then place one against the head of the bed. **Rationale:** *This pillow protects the client's head from inadvertent injury against the top of the bed during the upward move.*
5. Elicit the client's help in lessening your workload.
   - Ask the client to flex the hips and knees and position the feet so that they can be used effectively for pushing. **Rationale:** *Flexing the hips and knees keeps the entire lower leg off the bed surface preventing friction during movement, and ensures use of the large muscle groups in the client's legs when pushing, thus increasing the force of movement.*
   - Ask the client to
     a. Grasp the head of the bed with both hands and pull during the move
     or
     b. Raise the upper part of the body on the elbows and push with the hands and forearms during the move
     or
     c. Grasp the overhead trapeze with both hands and lift and pull during the move. **Rationale:** *Client assistance provides additional power to overcome inertia and friction*

continued on page 1136

SKILL 44-1

MOVING A CLIENT UP IN BED *continued*

during the move. These actions also keep the client's arms partially off the bed surface, reducing friction during movement, and make use of the large muscle groups of the client's arms to increase the force during movement.

6. Position yourself appropriately, and move the client.

- Face the direction of the movement, and then assume a broad stance with the foot nearest the bed behind the forward foot and weight on the forward foot. Lean your trunk forward from the hips. Flex hips, knees, and ankles.
- Place your near arm under the client's thighs. ❶ **Rationale:** *This supports the heaviest part of the body (the buttocks).* Push down on the mattress with the far arm. **Rationale:** *The far arm acts as a lever during the move.*
- Tighten your gluteal, abdominal, leg, and arm muscles and rock from the back leg to the front leg and back again. Then, shift your weight to the front leg as the client pushes with the heels and pulls with the arms so that the client moves toward the head of the bed.

7. Ensure client comfort.

- Elevate the head of the bed and provide appropriate support devices for the client's new position.
- See the sections on positioning clients earlier in this chapter.

Variation: A Client Who Has Limited Strength of the Upper Extremities

- Assist the client to flex the hips and knees as in step 5 previously. Place the client's arms across the chest. **Rationale:** *This keeps them off the bed surface and minimizes friction during movement.* Ask the client to flex the neck during the move and keep the head off the bed surface.

❶ Moving a client up in bed.

- Position yourself as in step 6 and place one arm under the client's back and shoulders and the other arm under the client's thighs. **Rationale:** *This placement of the arms distributes the client's weight and supports the heaviest part of the body (the buttocks).* Shift your weight as in step 6.

Variation: Two Nurses Using a Hand–Forearm Interlock

Two people are required to move clients who are unable to assist because of their condition or weight. Using the technique described in step 6, with the second staff member on the opposite side of the bed, both of you interlock your forearms ❷ under the client's thighs and shoulders and lift the client up in bed.

Variation: Two Nurses Using A Turn Sheet

Two nurses can use a turn sheet to move a client up in bed. **Rationale:** *A turn sheet distributes the client's weight more evenly, decreases friction, and exerts a more even force on the client during the move. In addition, it prevents injury of the client's skin, because the friction created between two sheets when one is moved is less than that created by the client's body moving over the sheet.*

- Place a drawsheet or a full sheet folded in half under the client, extending from the shoulders to the thighs. Each person rolls up or fanfolds the turn sheet close to the client's body on either side.
- Both individuals grasp the sheet close to the shoulders and buttocks of the client. **Rationale:** *This draws the weight closer to the nurse's center of gravity and increases the nurse's balance and stability, permitting a smoother movement.* Follow the method of moving clients with limited upper extremity strength as described earlier.

8. Document all relevant information.

Record:
- Time and change of position moved from and position moved to.
- Any signs of pressure areas.
- Use of support devices.
- Ability of client to assist in moving and turning.
- Response of client to moving and turning (e.g., anxiety, discomfort, dizziness).

❷ Two nurses using a hand–forearm interlock.

TURNING A CLIENT TO THE LATERAL OR PRONE POSITION IN BED

PURPOSES
■ Movement to the lateral (side-lying) position may be necessary when placing a bedpan beneath the client, when changing the client's bed linen, or when repositioning the client.

IMPLEMENTATION

Preparation
Determine:
■ Assistive devices that will be required.
■ Encumbrances to movement such as an IV or a heavy cast on one leg.
■ Medications the client is receiving, because certain medications may hamper movement or alertness of the client.
■ Assistance required from other health care personnel.

Performance
1. Prior to performing the procedure, introduce self and verify the client's identity using agency protocol. Explain to the client what you are going to do, why it is necessary, and how he or she can cooperate. Discuss how the results will be used in planning further care or treatments.
2. Perform hand hygiene and observe other appropriate infection control procedures.
3. Provide for client privacy.
4. Position yourself and the client appropriately before performing the move.
   ● Move the client closer to the side of the bed opposite the side the client will face when turned. **Rationale:** *This ensures that the client will be positioned safely in the center of the bed after turning.* Use a pull sheet beneath the client's trunk and thighs to pull the client to the side of the bed. Roll up the sheet as close as possible to the client's body and pull the client to the side of the bed. Adjust the client's head and reposition the legs appropriately.
   ● While standing on the side of the bed nearest the client, place the client's near arm across the chest. Abduct the client's far shoulder slightly from the side of the body and externally rotate the shoulder (Figure 44-8 on page 1108). **Rationale:** *Pulling the one arm forward facilitates the turning motion. Pulling the other arm away from the body and externally rotating the shoulder prevents that arm from being caught beneath the client's body during the roll.*
   ● Place the client's near ankle and foot across the far ankle and foot. **Rationale:** *This facilitates the turning motion. Making these preparations on the side of the bed closest to the client helps prevent unnecessary reaching.*
   ● Raise the side rail next to the client before going to the other side of the bed. **Rationale:** *This ensures that the client, who is close to the edge of the mattress, will not fall.*
   ● Position yourself on the side of the bed toward which the client will turn, directly in line with the client's waistline and as close to the bed as possible.
   ● Lean your trunk forward from the hips. Flex your hips, knees, and ankles. Assume a broad stance with one foot forward and the weight placed on this forward foot.
5. Pull or roll the client toward you to the lateral position.
   ● Place one hand on the client's far hip and the other hand on the client's far shoulder. ❶ **Rationale:** *This position of the hands supports the client at the two heaviest parts of the body, providing greater control in movement during the roll.*

A

B

❶ Moving a client to a lateral position.

   ● Tighten your gluteal, abdominal, leg, and arm muscles; rock backward, shifting your weight from the forward to the backward foot, and roll the client onto the side of the body to face you. **Rationale:** *Turning the client toward you promotes the client's sense of security.*
   ● Position the client on his or her side with arms and legs positioned and supported properly (see Table 44–7).

Variation: Turning the Client to a Prone Position
To turn a client to the prone position, follow the preceding steps, with two exceptions:
   ● Instead of abducting the far arm, keep the client's arm alongside the body for the client to roll over. **Rationale:** *Keeping the arm alongside the body prevents it from being pinned under the client when the client is rolled.*
   ● Roll the client completely onto the abdomen. **Rationale:** *It is essential to move the client as close as possible to the edge of the bed before the turn so that the client will be lying on the center of the bed after rolling. Never pull a client across the bed while the client is in the prone position.* **Rationale:** *Doing so can injure a woman's breasts or a man's genitals.*
6. Document all relevant information.
   Record:
   ● Time and change of position moved from and position moved to.
   ● Any signs of pressure areas.
   ● Use of support devices.
   ● Ability of client to assist in moving and turning.
   ● Response of client to moving and turning (e.g., anxiety, discomfort, dizziness).

LOGROLLING A CLIENT

PURPOSES

- **Logrolling** is a technique used to turn a client whose body must at all times be kept in straight alignment (like a log). An example is the client with a spinal injury. Considerable care must be taken to prevent additional injury. This technique requires two nurses or, if the client is large, three nurses. For the client who has a cervical injury, one nurse must maintain the client's head and neck alignment.

IMPLEMENTATION

Preparation

Determine:

- Assistive devices that will be required.
- Encumbrances to movement such as an IV or a heavy cast on one leg.
- Medications the client is receiving, because certain medications may hamper movement or alertness of the client.
- Assistance required from other health care personnel.

Performance

1. Prior to performing the procedure, introduce self and verify the client's identity using agency protocol. Explain to the client what you are going to do, why it is necessary, and how he or she can cooperate. Discuss how the results will be used in planning further care or treatments.
2. Perform hand hygiene and observe other appropriate infection control procedures.
3. Provide for client privacy.
4. Position yourselves and the client appropriately before the move.
   - Stand on the same side of the bed, and assume a broad stance with one foot ahead of the other.
   - Place the client's arms across the chest. **Rationale:** *Doing so ensures that they will not be injured or become trapped under the body when the body is turned.*
   - Lean your trunk, and flex your hips, knees, and ankles.
   - Place your arms under the client as shown in ❶ or ❷, depending on the client's size. **Rationale:** *Each staff member then has a major weight area of the client centered between the arms.*
   - Tighten your gluteal, abdominal, leg, and arm muscles.
5. Pull the client to the side of the bed.
   - One nurse counts: One, two, three, go. Then, at the same time, all staff members pull the client to the side of the bed by shifting their weight to the back foot. **Rationale:** *Moving the client in unison maintains the client's body alignment.*
   - Elevate the side rail on this side of the bed. **Rationale:** *This prevents the client from falling while lying so close to the edge of the bed.*

❶ Correct arm placement for moving a client to the side of the bed: two nurses.

❷ Correct arm placement for moving a client to the side of the bed: three nurses.

❸ Correct hand placement for logrolling a client.

6. Move to the other side of the bed, and place supportive devices for the client when turned.
   - Place a pillow where it will support the client's head after the turn. **Rationale:** *The pillow prevents lateral flexion of the neck and ensures alignment of the cervical spine.*
   - Place one or two pillows between the client's legs to support the upper leg when the client is turned. **Rationale:** *This pillow prevents adduction of the upper leg and keeps the legs parallel and aligned.*
7. Roll and position the client in proper alignment.
   - All nurses flex their hips, knees, and ankles and assume a broad stance with one foot forward.
   - All nurses reach over the client and place hands as shown in. ❸ **Rationale:** *Doing so centers a major weight area of the client between each nurse's arms.*
   - One nurse counts: One, two, three, go. Then, at the same time, all nurses roll the client to a lateral position.
   - Support the client's head, back, and upper and lower extremities with pillows.
   - Raise the side rails and place the call bell within the client's reach.

Variation: Using a Turn or Lift Sheet

- Use a turn sheet to facilitate logrolling. First, stand with another nurse on the same side of the bed. Assume a broad stance with one foot forward, and grasp half of the fanfolded or rolled edge of the turn sheet. On a signal, pull the client toward both of you. ❹
- Before turning the client, place pillow supports for the head and legs, as described in step 6. This helps maintain the client's alignment when turning. Then, go to the other side of the bed (farthest from the client), and assume a stable stance. Reaching over the client, grasp the far edges of the turn sheet, and roll the client toward you. ❺ The second nurse (behind the client) helps turn the client and provides pillow supports to ensure good alignment in the lateral position.
8. Document all relevant information.
   Record:
   - Time and change of position moved from and position moved to.
   - Any signs of pressure areas.
   - Use of support devices.
   - Ability of client to assist in moving and turning.
   - Response of client to moving and turning (e.g., anxiety, discomfort, dizziness).

LOGROLLING A CLIENT *continued*

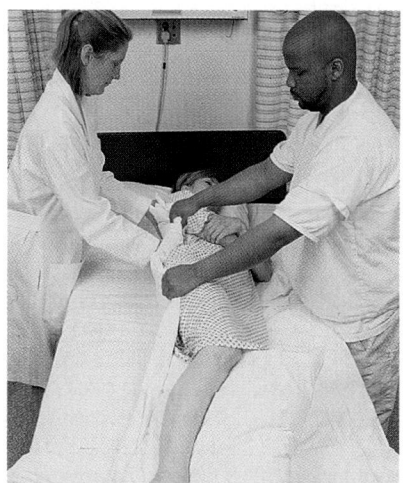

④ Using a turn sheet, the nurses pull the sheet with the client on it to the edge of the bed.

⑤ The nurse on the right uses the far edge of the sheet to roll the client toward him; the nurse on the left remains behind the client and assists with turning.

ASSISTING THE CLIENT TO SIT ON THE SIDE OF THE BED (DANGLING)

PURPOSES
■ The client assumes a sitting position on the edge of the bed before walking, moving to a chair or wheelchair, eating, or performing other activities.

IMPLEMENTATION
Preparation
Determine:

■ Assistive devices that will be required.
■ Encumbrances to movement such as an IV or a heavy cast on one leg.
■ Medications the client is receiving, because certain medications may hamper movement or alertness of the client.
■ Assistance required from other health care personnel.

Performance
1. Prior to performing the procedure, introduce self and verify the client's identity using agency protocol. Explain to the client what you are going to do, why it is necessary, and how he or she can cooperate. Discuss how the results will be used in planning further care or treatments.
2. Perform hand hygiene and observe other appropriate infection control procedures.
3. Provide for client privacy.
4. Position yourself and the client appropriately before performing the move.
   • Assist the client to a lateral position facing you.
   • Raise the head of the bed slowly to its highest position. **Rationale:** *This decreases the distance that the client needs to move to sit up on the side of the bed.*
   • Position the client's feet and lower legs at the edge of the bed. **Rationale:** *This enables the client's feet to move easily off the bed during the movement, and the client is aided by gravity into a sitting position.*

• Stand beside the client's hips and face the far corner of the bottom of the bed (the angle in which movement will occur). Assume a broad stance, placing the foot nearest the client forward. Lean your trunk forward from the hips. Flex your hips, knees, and ankles. ①

① Assisting a client to a sitting position on the edge of the bed.

continued on page 1140

SKILL 44-4

ASSISTING THE CLIENT TO SIT ON THE SIDE OF THE BED (DANGLING) *continued*

5. Move the client to a sitting position.
   - Place one arm around the client's shoulders and the other arm beneath both of the client's thighs near the knees. **Rationale:** *Supporting the client's shoulders prevents the client from falling backward during the movement. Supporting the client's thighs reduces friction of the thighs against the bed surface during the move and increases the force of the movement.*
   - Tighten your gluteal, abdominal, leg, and arm muscles.
   - Lift the client's thighs slightly. **Rationale:** *This reduces the friction of the client's thighs and the nurse's arm against the bed surface.*
   - Pivot on the balls of your feet in the desired direction facing the foot of the bed while pulling the client's feet and legs off the bed (Figure ❶, B). **Rationale:** *Pivoting prevents twisting of the nurse's spine. The weight of the client's legs swinging downward increases downward movement of the lower body and helps make the client's upper body vertical.*
   - Keep supporting the client until the client is well balanced and comfortable. **Rationale:** *This movement may cause some clients to faint.*
   - Assess vital signs (e.g., pulse, respirations, and blood pressure) as indicated by the client's health status.

Variation: Teaching a Client How to Sit on the Side of the Bed Independently

A client who has had recent abdominal surgery or who is weak may have too much abdominal pain or too little strength to sit straight up in bed. This person can be taught to assume a dangle position without assistance. Instruct the client to:

   - Roll to the side and lift the far leg over the near leg.
   - Grasp the mattress edge with the lower arm and push the fist of the upper arm into the mattress. ❷

A

B

❷ Moving to a sitting position independently.

   - Push up with the arms as the heels and legs slide over the mattress edge.
   - Maintain the sitting position by pushing both fists into the mattress behind and to the sides of the buttocks.

6. Document all relevant information.
   Record:
   - Ability of client to assist in moving and turning.
   - Response of client to moving and turning (e.g., anxiety, discomfort, dizziness).

EVALUATION

- Check the skin integrity of the pressure areas from the previous position. Relate findings to previous assessment data if available. Conduct follow-up assessment for previous and/or new skin breakdown areas.
- Check for proper alignment after the position change. Do a visual check and ask the client for a comfort assessment.

- Determine that all required safety precautions (e.g., side rails) are in place.
- Determine client's tolerance of the activity (e.g., vital signs before and after dangling), particularly the first time the client changes position.
- Report significant changes to the primary care practitioner.

LIFESPAN CONSIDERATIONS Positioning, Moving, and Turning Clients

INFANTS

- Position infants on their back for sleep, even after feeding. There is little risk of regurgitation and choking, and the rate of sudden infant death syndrome (SIDS) is significantly lower in infants who sleep on their backs.
- The skin of newborns can be fragile and may be abraded or torn (sheared) if the infant is pulled across a bed.

CHILDREN

- Carefully inspect the dependent skin surfaces of all infants and children confined to bed at least three times in each 24-hour period.

ELDERS

- In clients who have had cerebrovascular accidents (strokes), there is a risk of shoulder displacement on the paralyzed side from improper moving or repositioning techniques. Use care when moving, positioning in bed, and transferring. Pillows or foam devices are helpful to support the affected arm and shoulder and prevent injury.
- Decreased subcutaneous fat and thinning of the skin place elders at risk for skin breakdown. Repositioning approximately every 2 hours (more or less, depending on the unique needs of the individual client) helps reduce pressure on bony prominences and avoid tissue trauma.

HOME CARE CONSIDERATIONS   Positioning, Moving, and Turning Clients

- Assess the height of the bed and the person's leg length to ensure that self-movement in and out of the bed are smooth.
- When making a home visit, it is particularly important to inspect the mattress for support. A sagging mattress, a mattress that is too soft, or an underfilled waterbed used over a prolonged period can contribute to the development of hip flexion contractures and low back strain and pain. Bed boards made of plywood and placed beneath a sagging mattress are increasingly recommended for clients who have back problems or are prone to them.
- Assess the caregivers' knowledge and application of body mechanics to prevent injury.
- Demonstrate how to turn and position the client in bed. Observe the caregiver performing a return demonstration. Re-evaluate

- this technique periodically to reinforce correct application of body mechanics.
- Teach caregivers the basic principles of body alignment and how to check for proper alignment after the client has been changed to a new position.
- Warn caregivers of the dangers of lifting and repositioning and encourage the use of assistive devices and a "no solo lift" policy.
- Teach the caregiver to check the client's skin for redness and integrity after repositioning the client. Stress the importance of informing the nurse about the length of time skin redness remains over pressure areas after the person has been repositioned. Emphasize that reddened areas should not be massaged as it may lead to tissue trauma.

Transferring Clients

Many clients require some assistance in transferring between bed and chair or wheelchair, between wheelchair and toilet, and between bed and stretcher. Before transferring any client, however, the nurse must determine the client's physical and mental capabilities to participate in the transfer technique. In addition, the nurse must analyze and organize the activity. General guidelines for transfer techniques include these:

- Plan what to do and how to do it. Determine the space in which the transfer is maneuvered (bathrooms, for instance, are usually cramped); the number of assistants (one or two) needed to accomplish the transfer safely; the skill and strength of the nurse(s); and the client's capabilities.
- Obtain essential equipment before starting (e.g., transfer belt, wheelchair), and check its function.
- Remove obstacles from the area used for the transfer.
- Explain the transfer to the client, including what the client should do.

- Explain the transfer to the nursing personnel who are helping; specify who will give directions (one person needs to be in charge).
- Always support or hold the client rather than the equipment and ensure the client's safety and dignity.
- During the transfer, explain step by step what the client should do, for example, "Move your right foot forward."
- Make a written plan of the transfer, including the client's tolerance (e.g., pulse and respiratory rates).

Because wheelchairs and stretchers are unstable, they can predispose the client to falls and injury. Guidelines for the safe use of wheelchairs and stretchers are shown in the accompanying Practice Guidelines.

Transfer (walking) belts provide the greatest safety. The nurse grasps the belt to control movement of the client during the transfer. Hospitals and nursing homes should require that personnel use the transfer belt to ambulate or move clients. See Skill 44-5 for transferring a client between a bed and a chair, and Skill 44-6 for transferring a client between a bed and a stretcher. The Evaluation section at the end of Skill 44-6 also applies to Skill 44-5.

PRACTICE GUIDELINES   Wheelchair Safety

- Always lock the brakes on both wheels of the wheelchair when the client transfers in or out of it.
- Raise the footplates before transferring the client into the wheelchair.
- Lower the footplates after the transfer, and place the client's feet on them.
- Ensure the client is positioned well back in the seat of the wheelchair.
- Use seat belts that fasten behind the wheelchair to protect confused clients from falls. *Note:* Seat belts are a form of restraint and must be used in accordance with policies and procedures that apply to the use of restraints (see Chapter 32). ∞

- Back the wheelchair into or out of an elevator, rear large wheels first.
- Place your body between the wheelchair and the bottom of an incline.

CLINICAL ALERT

Air, foam, and gel cushions that distribute weight evenly (**not** doughnut-type cushions) are essential for clients confined to a wheelchair and must be checked frequently to ensure they are intact. Strict continence management is also important for preventing skin breakdown. Maintaining tire pressure will prevent added resistance and energy expenditure. Periodically monitor the client's upper extremities for pain and overuse syndromes. ∎

PRACTICE GUIDELINES   Safe Use of Stretchers

- Lock the wheels of the bed and stretcher before the client transfers in or out of them.
- Fasten safety straps across the client on a stretcher, and raise the side rails.
- Never leave a client unattended on a stretcher unless the wheels are locked and the side rails are raised on both sides and/or the safety straps are securely fastened across the client.
- Always push a stretcher from the end where the client's head is positioned. This position protects the client's head in the event of a collision.

- If the stretcher has two swivel wheels and two stationary wheels:
  a. Always position the client's head at the end with the stationary wheels and
  b. Push the stretcher from the end with the stationary wheels. The stretcher is maneuvered more easily when pushed from this end.
- Maneuver the stretcher when entering the elevator so that the client's head goes in first.

SKILL 44-5

TRANSFERRING BETWEEN BED AND CHAIR

PURPOSES
- A client may need to be transferred between the bed and a wheelchair or chair, the bed and the commode, or a wheelchair and the toilet. There are numerous variations in the technique.

Which variation the nurse selects depends on factors related to the client, the environment, and the health care provider that are assessed prior to beginning the transfer.

ASSESSMENT
Before transferring a client, assess the following:

- The client's body size
- Ability to follow instructions
- Activity tolerance
- Muscle strength
- Joint mobility
- Presence of paralysis

- Level of comfort
- Presence of orthostatic hypotension
- The technique with which the client is familiar
- The space in which the transfer will need to be maneuvered (bathrooms, for example, are usually cramped)
- The number of assistants (one or two) needed to accomplish the transfer safely
- The skill and strength of the nurse(s)

PLANNING
Review the client record to determine if previous nurses have recorded information about the client's ability to transfer. Implement pain-relief measures so that they are effective when the transfer begins.

Delegation
The skill of transferring a client can be delegated to UAP who have demonstrated safe transfer technique for the involved client. It is important for the nurse to assess the client's capabilities and communicate specific information about what the UAP should report back to the nurse.

Equipment
- Robe or appropriate clothing
- Slippers or shoes with nonskid soles
- Transfer (walking) belt
- Chair, commode, wheelchair, or stretcher as appropriate to client need
- Sliding board

IMPLEMENTATION
Preparation
- Plan what to do and how to do it.
- Obtain essential equipment before starting (e.g., transfer belt, wheelchair), and check that it is functioning correctly.
- Remove obstacles from the area used for the transfer.

Performance
1. Prior to performing the procedure, introduce self and verify the client's identity using agency protocol. Explain the transfer process to the client. During the transfer, explain step by step what the client should do, for example, "Move your right foot forward."
2. Perform hand hygiene and observe other appropriate infection control procedures.
3. Provide for client privacy.

4. Position the equipment appropriately.
   - Lower the bed to its lowest position so that the client's feet will rest flat on the floor. Lock the wheels of the bed.
   - Place the wheelchair parallel to the bed as close to the bed as possible. ❶ Put the wheelchair on the side of the bed that allows the client to move toward his or her stronger side. Lock the wheels of the wheelchair and raise the footplate.
5. Prepare and assess the client.
   - Assist the client to a sitting position on the side of the bed (see Skill 44-4).
   - Assess the client for orthostatic hypotension before moving the client from the bed.
   - Assist the client in putting on a bathrobe and nonskid slippers or shoes.
   - Place a transfer belt snugly around the client's waist. Check to be certain that the belt is securely fastened.

TRANSFERRING BETWEEN BED AND CHAIR *continued*

❶ The wheelchair is placed parallel to the bed as close to the bed as possible. Note that placement of the nurse's feet mirrors that of the client's feet.

6. Give explicit instructions to the client.

   Ask the client to:

   - Move forward and sit on the edge of the bed. **Rationale:** *This brings the client's center of gravity closer to the nurse's.*
   - Lean forward slightly from the hips. **Rationale:** *This brings the client's center of gravity more directly over the base of support and positions the head and trunk in the direction of the movement.*
   - Place the foot of the stronger leg beneath the edge of the bed and put the other foot forward. **Rationale:** *In this way, the client can use the stronger leg muscles to stand and power the movement. A broader base of support makes the client more stable during the transfer.*
   - Place the client's hands on the bed surface or on your shoulders so that the client can push while standing. **Rationale:** *This provides additional force for the movement and reduces the potential for strain on the nurse's back. The client should not grasp your neck for support.* **Rationale:** *Doing so can injure the nurse.*

7. Position yourself correctly.

   - Stand directly in front of the client. Lean the trunk forward from the hips. Flex the hips, knees, and ankles. Assume a broad stance, placing one foot forward and one back. Mirror the placement of the client's feet, if possible. **Rationale:** *This helps prevent loss of balance during the transfer.*
   - Encircle the client's waist with your arms, and grasp the transfer belt at the client's back ❷ with thumbs pointing downward. **Rationale:** *The belt provides a secure handle for holding on to the client and controlling the movement. Downward placement of the thumbs prevents potential wrist injury as the nurse lifts. By supporting the client in this manner, you keep the client from tilting backward during the transfer.*
   - Tighten your gluteal, abdominal, leg, and arm muscles.

8. Assist the client to stand, and then move together toward the wheelchair.

   - On the count of three, ask the client to push with the back foot, rock to the forward foot, and extend (straighten) the joints of the lower extremities. Push or pull up with the hands, while pushing with the forward foot, rock to the back

❷ Using a transfer (walking) belt.

   foot, extend the joints of the lower extremities, and pull the client (directly toward your center of gravity) into a standing position.

   - Support the client in an upright standing position for a few moments. **Rationale:** *This allows the nurse and the client to extend the joints and provides the nurse with an opportunity to ensure that the client is stable before moving away from the bed.*
   - Together, pivot or take a few steps toward the wheelchair.

9. Assist the client to sit.

   - Ask the client to:
     a. Back up to the wheelchair and place the legs against the seat. **Rationale:** *Having the client place the legs against the wheelchair seat minimizes the risk of the client falling when sitting down.*
     b. Place the foot of the stronger leg slightly behind the other. **Rationale:** *This supports body weight during the movement.*
     c. Keep the other foot forward. **Rationale:** *This provides a broad base of support.*
     d. Place both hands on the wheelchair arms or on your shoulders. **Rationale:** *This increases stability and lessens the strain on the nurse.*
   - Stand directly in front of the client. Place one foot forward and one back.
   - Tighten your grasp on the transfer belt, and tighten your gluteal, abdominal, leg, and arm muscles.
   - On the count of three, have the client shift the body weight by rocking to the back foot. Lower the body onto the edge of the wheelchair seat by flexing the joints of the legs and arms. Place some body weight on the arms, while shifting your body weight by stepping back with the forward foot and pivoting toward the chair while lowering the client onto the wheelchair seat.

10. Ensure client safety.

    - Ask the client to push back into the wheelchair seat. **Rationale:** *Sitting well back on the seat provides a broader base of support and greater stability and minimizes the risk of falling from the wheelchair. A wheelchair can topple*

continued on page 1144

TRANSFERRING BETWEEN BED AND CHAIR *continued*

forward when the client sits on the edge of the seat and leans far forward.
- Lower the footplates, and place the client's feet on them.
- Apply a seat belt as required.

Variation: Angling the Wheelchair

For clients who have difficulty walking, place the wheelchair at a 45-degree angle to the bed. **Rationale:** *This enables the client to pivot into the chair and lessens the amount of body rotation required.*

Variation: Transferring Without a Belt

- For clients who need minimal assistance, place the hands against the sides of the client's chest (not at the axillae) during the transfer. For clients who require more assistance, reach through the client's axillae and place the hands on the client's scapulae during the transfer. Avoid placing hands or pressure on the axillae, especially for clients who have upper extremity paralysis or paresis.
- Follow the steps described previously.

Variation: Transferring With a Belt and Two Nurses

- When the client is able to stand, position yourselves on both sides of the client, facing the same direction as the client. Flex your hips, knees, and ankle. Grasp the client's transfer belt with the hand closest to the client, and with the other hand support the client's elbows.

- Coordinating your efforts, all three of you stand simultaneously, pivot, and move to the wheelchair. Reverse the process to lower the client onto the wheelchair seat.

Variation: Transferring a Client With an Injured Lower Extremity

When the client has an injured lower extremity, movement should always occur toward the client's unaffected (strong) side. For example, if the client's right leg is injured and the client is sitting on the edge of the bed preparing to transfer to a wheelchair, position the wheelchair on the client's left side. In this way, the client can use the unaffected leg most effectively and safely.

Variation: Using A Sliding Board

- For clients who cannot stand, use a sliding board to help them move without nursing assistance. This method not only promotes clients' sense of independence but also preserves your energy.

11. Document relevant information:
    - Client's ability to bear weight and pivot
    - Number of staff needed for transfer
    - Length of time up in chair
    - Client response to transfer and being up in chair or wheelchair

---

TRANSFERRING BETWEEN BED AND STRETCHER

PURPOSES
- The stretcher, or gurney, is used to transfer supine clients from one location to another. Whenever the client is capable of accomplishing the transfer from bed to stretcher independently, either by lifting onto it or by rolling onto it, the client should be encouraged to do so. If the client cannot move onto the stretcher independently, at least two nurses are needed to assist with the transfer; more are needed if the client is totally helpless or is heavy.

ASSESSMENT
Before transferring a client, assess the following:
- The client's body size
- Ability to follow instructions
- Activity tolerance
- Level of comfort
- The space in which the transfer is maneuvered
- The number of assistants (one or two others) needed to accomplish the transfer safely
- The skill and strength of the nurses

PLANNING
Review the client record to determine if previous nurses have recorded information about how the client tolerated similar transfers. If indicated, implement pain-relief measures so that they are effective when the transfer begins.

Delegation
The skill of transferring a client can be delegated to UAP who have demonstrated good body mechanics and safe transfer technique for the involved client. It is important for the nurse to assess the client's capabilities and communicate specific information about what the UAP should report to the nurse.

Equipment
- Stretcher
- Optional: sliding board

IMPLEMENTATION
Preparation
Obtain the necessary equipment and nursing personnel to assist in the transfer.

Performance
1. Prior to performing the procedure, introduce self and verify the client's identity using agency protocol. Explain to the client what you are going to do, why it is necessary, and how he or she can

TRANSFERRING BETWEEN BED AND STRETCHER *continued*

cooperate. Explain the transfer to the nursing personnel who are helping and specify who will give directions (one person needs to be in charge).

2. Wash hands and observe other appropriate infection control procedures.

3. Provide for client privacy.

4. Adjust the client's bed in preparation for the transfer.
   - Lower the head of the bed until it is flat or as low as the client can tolerate.
   - Raise the bed so that it is slightly higher than the surface of the stretcher. **Rationale:** *It is easier for the client to move down a slant.*
   - Ensure that the wheels on the bed are locked.
   - Pull the drawsheet out from both sides of the bed.

5. Move the client to the edge of the bed and position the stretcher.
   - Roll the drawsheet as close to the client's side as possible.
   - Pull the client to the edge of the bed and cover the client with a sheet or bath blanket to maintain comfort.
   - Place the stretcher parallel to the bed next to the client and lock the stretcher wheels.
   - Fill the gap that exists between the bed and the stretcher loosely with the bath blankets (optional).

6. Transfer the client securely to the stretcher.
   - In unison with the other staff members, press your body tightly against the stretcher. **Rationale:** *This prevents the stretcher from moving.*
   - Roll the pull sheet tightly against the client. **Rationale:** *This achieves better control over client movement.*

   - Flex your hips and pull the client on the pull sheet in unison directly toward you and onto the stretcher. **Rationale:** *Pulling downward requires less force than pulling along a flat surface.*
   - Ask the client to flex the neck during the move, if possible, and place the arms across the chest. **Rationale:** *This prevents injury to these body parts.*

7. Ensure client comfort and safety.
   - Make the client comfortable, unlock the stretcher wheels, and move the stretcher away from the bed.
   - Immediately raise the stretcher side rails and/or fasten the safety straps across the client. **Rationale:** *Because the stretcher is high and narrow, the client is in danger of falling unless these safety precautions are taken.*

Variation: Using A Transfer Board

The transfer board is a lacquered or smooth polyethylene board measuring 45 to 55 cm (18 to 22 in.) by 182 cm (72 in.) with handholds along its edges. Transfer mattresses are also available, as are mechanical assistive devices. It is imperative to have enough people assisting with the transfer to prevent injury to staff as well as clients. Turn the client to a lateral position away from you, position the board close to the client's back, and roll the client onto the board. Pull the client and board across the bed to the stretcher. Safety belts may be placed over the chest, abdomen, and legs.

8. Document relevant information:
   - Equipment used
   - Number of people needed for transfer
   - Destination if reason for transfer is transport from one location to another

EVALUATION

- Compare client capabilities such as weight-bearing, pivoting ability, and strength and control to previous transfers.
- Report any significant deviations from normal to the primary care practitioner.

- Note use of appropriate safety measures (e.g., transfer belt, locking wheels of bed and wheelchair) by UAP during transfer process.

LIFESPAN CONSIDERATIONS Transferring Clients

INFANTS

- The infant who is lying down, on the side or supine, can be placed in either a bassinet or crib for transport. If the bassinet has a bottom shelf, it can be used for carrying the IV pump or monitor.

CHILDREN

- The toddler should be transported in a high-top crib with the side rails up and the protective top in place. Stretchers should not be used because the mobile toddler may roll or fall off.

ELDERS

- Since conditions of elders can change from day to day, always assess the situation to ensure that you have the right equipment and enough people to assist when transferring a client.

- Use special caution with older clients to prevent skin tears or bruising during a transfer or when using a hydraulic lift.
- Write the method used to transfer each client—equipment used, best position, and number of people needed to assist in transfer. This can be part of the care plan and also be available in the client's room as a guide to all personnel caring for the client.
- Avoid sudden position changes. They can cause orthostatic hypotension and increase the risk of fainting and falls.

Using a Hydraulic Lift

Hydraulic lifts, such as the Hoyer lift, are an example of assistive equipment to take the place of manual lifts and transfers. The lift can be used in transferring the client between the bed and a wheelchair, the bed and the bathtub, and the bed and a stretcher. The Hoyer lift consists of a base on casters, a hydraulic mechanical pump, a mast boom, and a sling (Figure 44-53 ■). The sling may consist of a one-piece or two-piece canvas seat. The one-piece seat stretches from the client's head to the knees. The two-piece seat has one canvas strap to support the client's buttocks and thighs and a second strap extending up to the axillae to support the back. It is important to be familiar with the model used and the practices that accompany use. Before using the lift, the nurse ensures that it is in working order and that the hooks, chains, straps, and canvas seat are in good repair. Most agencies recommend that two nurses operate a lift. Check agency policy.

Providing ROM Exercises

When people are ill, they may need to perform ROM exercises until they can regain their normal activity levels. **Active ROM exercises** are isotonic exercises in which the client moves each joint in the body through its complete range of movement, maximally stretching all muscle groups within each plane over the

Figure 44-53 ■ A one-piece seat hydraulic lift.

joint. These exercises maintain or increase muscle strength and endurance and help to maintain cardiorespiratory function in an immobilized client. They also prevent deterioration of joint capsules, ankylosis, and contractures.

Full ROM does not occur spontaneously in the immobilized individual who independently achieves ADLs, moves about in bed, transfers between bed and wheelchair or chair, or ambulates a short distance, because only a few muscle groups are maximally stretched during these activities. Although the client may successfully achieve some active ROM movements of the upper extremities while combing the hair, bathing, and dressing, the immobilized client is very unlikely to achieve any active ROM movements of the lower extremities when these are not used in the normal functions of standing and walking about. For this reason, most clients who use a wheelchair and many ambulatory clients need active ROM exercises until they regain their normal activity levels.

At first, the nurse may need to teach the client to perform the needed ROM exercises; eventually, the client may be able to accomplish these independently. Instructions for the client performing active ROM exercises are shown in the accompanying Client Teaching feature.

During **passive ROM exercises,** another person moves each of the client's joints through its complete range of movement, maximally stretching all muscle groups within each plane over each joint. Because the client does not contract the muscles, passive ROM exercises are of no value in maintaining muscle strength but are useful in maintaining joint flexibility. For this reason, passive ROM exercises should be performed only when the client is unable to accomplish the movements actively.

Passive ROM exercises should be accomplished for each movement of the arms, legs, and neck that the client is unable to achieve actively. As with active ROM exercises, passive ROM exercises should be accomplished to the point of slight resistance, but not beyond, and never to the point of discomfort. The movements should be systematic, and the same sequence should be followed during each exercise session. Each exercise should consist of three repetitions, and the series of exercises should be done twice daily. Performing one series of exercises along with the bath is helpful. Passive ROM exercises are accomplished most effectively when the client lies supine in bed. General guidelines for providing passive exercises are shown in the accompanying Practice Guidelines.

During active-assistive ROM exercises, the client uses a stronger, opposite arm or leg to move each of the joints of a limb incapable of active motion. The client learns to support and move the weak arm or leg with the strong arm or leg as far as possible. Then the nurse continues the movement passively to its maximal degree. This activity increases active movement on the strong side of the client's body and maintains joint flexibility on the weak side.

Such exercise is especially useful for stroke client's who have had a stroke and are hemiplegic (paralyzed on one-half of the body).

CLINICAL ALERT

Clients who require passive ROM exercises after a disability should have a goal of progressing to active-assistive ROM exercises and, finally, to active ROM exercises. ■

Ambulating Clients

Ambulation (the act of walking) is a function that most people take for granted. However, when people are ill they are often confined to bed and are thus nonambulatory. The longer clients are in bed, the more difficulty they have walking.

Even 1 or 2 days of bed rest can make a person feel weak, unsteady, and shaky when first getting out of bed. A client who has

---

PRACTICE GUIDELINES   Providing Passive ROM Exercises

- Ensure that the client understands the reason for doing ROM exercises.
- If there is a possibility of hand swelling, make sure rings are removed.
- Clothe the client in a loose gown, and cover the body with a bath blanket.
- Use correct body mechanics when providing ROM exercise to avoid muscle strain or injury to both yourself and the client.
- Position the bed at an appropriate height.
- Expose only the limb being exercised to avoid embarrassing the client.
- Support the client's limbs above and below the joint as needed to prevent muscle strain or injury (Figure 44-54 ■). This may also be done by cupping joints in the palm of your hand or cradling limbs along your forearm (Figure 44-55 ■). If a joint is painful (e.g., arthritic), support the limb in the muscular areas above and below the joint.
- Use a firm, comfortable grip when handling the limb.
- Move the body parts smoothly, slowly, and rhythmically. Jerky movements cause discomfort and, possibly, injury. Fast movements can cause spasticity (sudden, prolonged involuntary muscle contraction) or rigidity (stiffness or inflexibility).
- Avoid moving or forcing a body part beyond the existing range of motion. Muscle strain, pain, and injury can result. This is particularly important for people with flaccid (limp) paralysis, whose muscles can be stretched and joints dislocated without their awareness.
- If muscle spasticity occurs during movement, stop the movement temporarily, but continue to apply slow, gentle pressure on the part until the muscle relaxes; then proceed with the motion.

- If a contracture is present, apply slow firm pressure, without causing pain, to stretch the muscle fibers.
- If rigidity occurs, apply pressure against the rigidity, and continue the exercise slowly.
- Teach client's caregiver the purposes and technique of performing passive ROM at home if appropriate.
- Avoid hypertension of joints in elders if joints are arthritic.
- Use the exercises as an opportunity to also assess skin condition.

Figure 44-54 ■ Supporting a limb above and below the joint for passive exercise.

Figure 44-55 ■ Holding limbs for support during passive exercise: *A,* cupping; *B,* cradling.

RESEARCH NOTE **What Effect Does Mind-Body Exercise Have on Cognition and Quality of Life?**

Researchers wanted to explore if there might be benefits of mind–body exercise techniques such as yoga because such modalities involve an active attentional or *mindfulness* component. A total of 135 healthy men and women 65 to 85 years of age were randomly assigned to 6 months of one of the following: hatha yoga class (once/week with independent home practice), walking exercise class (once/week with independent home practice), or a wait-list control group. The researchers collected before and after assessments of cognitive measures, mood states, fatigue, health-related quality of life, and physical measures. Results indicated no effects from either of the active interventions on cognitive function (possibly due to the high baseline level of cognitive functioning in this group of participants). The yoga intervention produced significant improvements in physical measures (strength and flexibility) as well as quality of life measures

related to well-being, energy, and fatigue as compared to walking exercise and wait-list controls.

IMPLICATIONS

This study, and others like it, highlights benefits of mind–body types of exercise for improving physical functioning and mood in older adults. While the participants in this study did not show improvement in cognitive function, a strong body of evidence supports the use of exercise for improving cognitive function (Freeman, 2004). Nurses can recommend yoga as a tool for maintaining and improving health in older adults.

Note: From *Alternative Therapies in Health and Medicine*, by B. Oken, D. Zajdel, S. Kishiyama. Copyright 2006 by Innovision Communications. Reproduced with permission of Innovision Communications in the format Textbook via Copyright Clearance Center.

had surgery, is elderly, or has been immobilized for a longer time will feel more pronounced weakness. The potential problems of immobility are far less likely to occur when clients become ambulatory as soon as possible. The nurse can assist clients to prepare for ambulation by helping them become as independent as possible while in bed. Nurses should encourage clients to perform ADLs, maintain good body alignment, and carry out active ROM exercises to the maximum degree possible yet within the limitations imposed by their illness and recovery program.

PREAMBULATORY EXERCISES. Clients who have been in bed for long periods often need a plan of muscle tone exercises to strengthen the muscles used for walking before attempting to walk. One of the most important muscle groups is the quadriceps femoris, which extends the knee and flexes the thigh. This group is also important for elevating the legs, for example, for walking upstairs. These exercises are frequently called quadriceps drills or sets. To strengthen these muscles, the client consciously tenses them, drawing the kneecap upward and inward. The client pushes the popliteal space of the knee against the bed surface, relaxing the heels on the bed surface (Figure 44-56 ■). On the count of 1, the muscles are tensed; they are held during the counts of 2, 3, 4; and they are relaxed at the count of 5. The exercise should be done within the client's tolerance, that is, without fatiguing the muscles. Carried out several times an hour during waking hours, this simple exercise significantly strengthens the muscles used for walking.

Figure 44-56 ■ Tensing the quadriceps femoris muscles before ambulation.

ASSISTING CLIENTS TO AMBULATE. Clients who have been immobilized for even a few days may require assistance with ambulation. The amount of assistance will depend on the client's condition, including age, health status, and length of inactivity. Assistance may mean walking alongside the client while providing physical support (see Skill 44-7) or providing instruction to the client about the use of assistive devices such as a cane, walker, or crutches.

Some clients experience postural (orthostatic) hypotension on assuming a vertical position from a lying position and may need information about ways to control this problem (see Client Teaching). The client may exhibit some or all of the following symptoms: pallor, diaphoresis, nausea, tachycardia, and dizziness. If any of these are present, the client should be assisted to a supine position in bed and closely assessed.

CLIENT TEACHING **Controlling Postural Hypotension**

- Rest with the head of the bed elevated 8 to 12 inches. This position makes the position change on rising less severe.
- Avoid sudden changes in position. Arise from bed in three stages:
  a. Sit up in bed for 1 minute.
  b. Sit on the side of the bed with legs dangling for 1 minute.
  c. Stand with care, holding onto the edge of the bed or another nonmovable object for 1 minute.
- Never bend down all the way to the floor or stand up too quickly after stooping.
- Postpone activities such as shaving and hair grooming for at least 1 hour after rising.
- Wear elastic stockings at night to inhibit venous pooling in the legs.

- Be aware that the symptoms of hypotension are most severe at the following times:
  a. 30 to 60 minutes after a heavy meal
  b. 1 to 2 hours after taking an antihypertension medication
- Get out of a hot bath very slowly, because high temperatures can lead to venous pooling.
- Use a rocking chair to improve circulation in the lower extremities. Even mild leg conditioning can strengthen muscle tone and enhance circulation.
- Refrain from any strenuous activity that results in holding the breath and bearing down. This Valsalva maneuver slows the heart rate, leading to subsequent lowering of blood pressure.

ASSISTING THE CLIENT TO AMBULATE

PURPOSE

- To provide a safe condition for the client to walk with whatever support is needed.

ASSESSMENT

Assess the following:

- Length of time in bed and time up previously
- Baseline vital signs
- Range of motion of joints needed for ambulating (e.g., hips, knees, ankles)
- Muscle strength of lower extremities
- Need for ambulation aids (e.g., cane, walker, crutches)

- Client's intake of medications (e.g., narcotics, sedatives, tranquilizers, and antihistamines) that may cause drowsiness, dizziness, weakness, and orthostatic hypotension and seriously hinder the client's ability to walk safely
- Presence of joint inflammation, fractures, muscle weakness, or other conditions that impair physical mobility
- Ability to understand directions
- Level of comfort

PLANNING

Implement pain-relief measures so that they are effective when the transfer begins.

The amount of assistance needed while ambulating will depend on the client's condition, for example, age, health status, length of inactivity, and emotional readiness. Review any previous experiences with ambulation and the success of such efforts. Plan the length of the walk with the client, in light of the nursing or primary care practitioner's orders. Be prepared to shorten the walk according to the person's activity tolerance.

Delegation

Ambulation of clients is frequently delegated to UAP. However, the nurse should conduct an initial assessment of the client's abilities in order to direct other personnel in providing appropriate assistance. Any unusual events that arise from assisting the client in ambulation must be validated and interpreted by the nurse.

Equipment

- Transfer belt if the client is known to be unsteady
- Wheelchair for following client, or chairs along the route if the client needs to rest

IMPLEMENTATION

Preparation

Be certain that others are available to assist you if needed. Also, plan the route of ambulation that has the fewest hazards.

Performance

1. Prior to performing the procedure, introduce self and verify the client's identity using agency protocol. Explain to the client how you are going to assist, why ambulation is necessary, and how he or she can cooperate. Discuss how this activity relates to the overall plan of care.

2. Perform hand hygiene and observe appropriate infection control procedures.

3. Ensure that the client is appropriately dressed to walk and has shoes or slippers with nonskid soles.

4. Prepare the client for ambulation.
   - Apply elastic (antiemboli) stockings as required.
   - Assist the client to sit on the edge of the bed.
   - Assess the client carefully for signs and symptoms of orthostatic hypotension (dizziness, light-headedness, or a sudden increase in heart rate) prior to leaving the bedside.
   - Assist the client to stand by the side of the bed until he or she feels secure.

5. Ensure client safety while assisting the client to ambulate.
   - Encourage the client to ambulate independently if he or she is able, but walk beside the client's weak side, if appropriate.
   - Remain physically close to the client in case assistance is needed at any point.
   - Use a transfer or walking belt if the client is slightly weak and unstable. Make sure the belt is pulled snugly around the client's waist and fastened securely. Grasp the belt at the client's back, and walk behind and slightly to one side of the client. ❶
   - If it is the client's first time out of bed following surgery, injury, or an extended period of immobility, or if the client is

❶ Using a transfer (walking) belt to support the client.

quite weak or unstable, have an assistant follow you and the client with a wheelchair in the event that it is needed quickly.
   - If the client is moderately weak and unstable, walk on the client's weaker side and interlock your forearm with the client's closest forearm. Encourage the client to press the forearm against your hip or waist for stability if desired. In addition, have the client wear a transfer or walking belt. **Rationale:** *You can quickly grab the belt and prevent a fall if the client feels faint.*
   - If the client is very weak and unstable, place your near arm around the client's waist, and with your other arm support the client's near arm at the elbow. Walk on the client's stronger side. Again, have the client wear a transfer or walking belt in case of an emergency. Encourage the client to assume a normal walking stance and gait as much as possible.

continued on page 1150

ASSISTING THE CLIENT TO AMBULATE *continued*

6. Protect the client who begins to fall while ambulating.
   - If a client begins to experience the signs and symptoms of orthostatic hypotension or extreme weakness, quickly assist the client into a nearby wheelchair or other chair, and help the client to lower the head between the knees.
   - Stay with the client. **Rationale:** *A client who faints while in this position could fall head first out of the chair.*
   - When the weakness subsides, assist the client back to bed.
   - If a chair is not close by, assist the client to a horizontal position on the floor before fainting occurs. ❷
     a. Assume a broad stance with one foot in front of the other. **Rationale:** *A broad stance widens your base of support. Placing one foot behind the other allows you to rock backward and use the femoral muscles when supporting the client's weight and lowering the center of gravity (see the next step), thus preventing back strain.*
     b. Bring the client backward so that your body supports the person. **Rationale:** *Clients who faint or start to fall usually pitch slightly forward because of the momentum of ambulating. Bringing the client's weight backward against your body allows gradual movement to the floor without injury to the client.*
     c. Allow the client to slide down your leg, and lower the person gently to the floor, making sure the client's head does not hit any objects.

Variation: Two Nurses

   - After the client stands, assume a position with one nurse at either side. Grasp the inferior aspect of the client's upper arm with your nearest hand and the client's lower arm or hand with your other hand. ❸ **Rationale:** *This provides a secure grip for each nurse.*
   - *Optional:* Place a walking belt around the client's waist. Each nurse grasps the side handle with the near hand and the lower aspect of the client's upper arm with the other hand.
   - Walk in unison with the client, using a smooth, even gait, at the same speed and with steps the same size as the client's. **Rationale:** *This gives the client a greater feeling of security.*
   - If the client starts to fall and cannot regain strength or balance, slip your arms under the client's axillae, grasp the client's hands, and lower the person gently to the floor or to a nearby chair. ❹ **Rationale:** *Placing the nurse's arms under the client's axillae evenly balances the client's weight between the two nurses, preventing injury to both the nurses and the client.*

7. Document distance and duration of ambulation in the client record using forms or checklists supplemented by narrative notes when appropriate. Include description of the client's gait (including body alignment) when walking; pace; activity tolerance when walking (e.g., pulse rate, facial color, any shortness of breath, feelings of dizziness, or weakness); degree of support required; and respiratory rate and blood pressure after initial ambulation to compare with baseline data.

EVALUATION

▪ Establish a plan for continued ambulation based on expected or normal ability for the client.

❷ Lowering a fainting client to the floor.

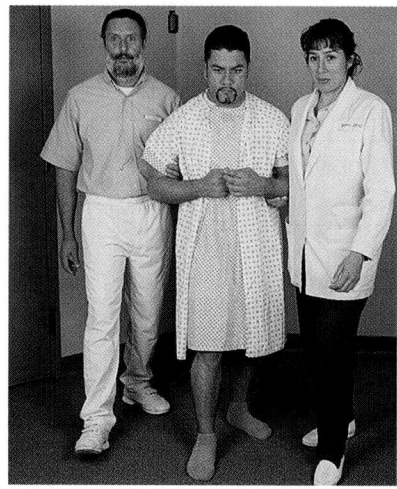

❸ Two nurses supporting an ambulatory client.

❹ Two nurses lowering a fainting client to the floor.

LIFESPAN CONSIDERATIONS **Assisting the Client to Ambulate**

CHILDREN

- Children and adolescents who have suffered a sports injury (e.g., sprained ankle) may want to be more active than they should be. A cast, splint, or boot may be put in place to limit activity and assist in healing. Teach the child the importance of appropriate activity, and the use of assistive devices (e.g., crutches) if necessary. Help them focus on what they *can* do rather than what they cannot do (e.g., "You can stand at he free-throw line and shoot baskets").

ELDERS

- Inquire how the client has ambulated previously and modify assistance accordingly.
- Take into account a decrease in speed, strength, resistance to fatigue, reaction time, and coordination due to a decrease in nerve conduction.
- Be cautious when using a transfer belt with a client with osteoporosis. Too much pressure from the belt can increase the risk of vertebral compression fractures.

- If assistive devices such as a walker or cane are used, make sure clients are supervised in the beginning to learn the proper method of using them. Crutches may be much more difficult for elders due to decreased upper body strength.
- Be alert to signs of activity intolerance, especially in elders with cardiac and lung problems.
- Set small goals and increase slowly to build endurance, strength, and flexibility.
- Be aware of any fall risks the elder may have, such as the following:
  - Effects of medications
  - Neurological disorders
  - Environmental hazards
  - Orthostatic hypotension
  - In elders, the body's responses return to normal more slowly. For instance, an increase in heart rate from exercise may stay elevated for hours before returning to normal.

HOME CARE CONSIDERATIONS
Assisting the Client to Ambulate

- When making a home visit, assess carefully for safety issues for ambulation. Counsel the client and family about unfastened rugs, slippery floors, and loose objects on the floors.
- Check the surroundings for adequate supports such as railings and grab bars.
- Recommend that nonskid strips be placed on outside steps and inside stairs that are not carpeted.

Using Mechanical Aids for Walking

Mechanical aids for ambulation include canes, walkers, and crutches.

CANES. Two types of canes are used today: the standard straight-legged cane and the quad cane, which has four feet and provides the most support (Figure 44-57 ■). Cane tips should have rubber caps to improve traction and prevent slipping. The standard cane is 91 cm (36 in.) long; some aluminum canes can be adjusted from 56 to 97 cm (22 to 38 in.). The length should permit the elbow to be slightly flexed. Clients may use either one or two canes, depending on how much support they require.

WALKERS. Walkers are mechanical devices for ambulatory clients who need more support than a cane provides. Walkers come in many different shapes and sizes, with devices suited to individual needs. The standard type is made of polished aluminum. It has four legs with rubber tips and plastic hand grips (Figure 44-60 ■). Many walkers have adjustable legs.

The standard walker needs to be picked up to be used. The client therefore requires partial strength in both hands and wrists, strong elbow extensors, and strong shoulder depressors.

The client also needs the ability to bear at least partial weight on both legs.

Four-wheeled and two-wheeled models of walkers (roller walkers) do not need to be picked up to be moved, but they are less stable than the standard walker is. They are used by clients who are too weak or unstable to pick up and move the walker with each step. Some roller walkers have a seat at the back so the client can sit down to rest when desired. An adaptation of

Figure 44-57 ■ A quad cane.

CLIENT TEACHING   Using Canes

- Hold the cane with the hand on the stronger side of the body to provide maximum support and appropriate body alignment when walking.
- Position the tip of a standard cane (and the nearest tip of other canes) about 15 cm (6 in.) to the side and 15 cm (6 in.) in front of the near foot, so that the elbow is slightly flexed.

WHEN MAXIMUM SUPPORT IS REQUIRED

- Move the cane forward about 30 cm (1 ft), or a distance that is comfortable while the body weight is borne by both legs (Figure 44-58 ■, A).
- Then move the affected (weak) leg forward to the cane while the weight is borne by the cane and stronger leg (Figure 44-58 ■, B).

- Next, move the unaffected (stronger) leg forward ahead of the cane and weak leg while the weight is borne by the cane and weak leg (Figure 44-58, C).
- Repeat the steps. This pattern of moving provides at least two points of support on the floor at all times.

AS YOU BECOME STRONGER AND REQUIRE LESS SUPPORT

- Move the cane and weak leg forward at the same time, while the weight is borne by the stronger leg (Figure 44-59 ■, A).
- Move the stronger leg forward, while the weight is borne by the cane and the weak leg (Figure 44-59 ■, B).

Figure 44-58 ■ Steps involved in using a cane to provide maximum support.

 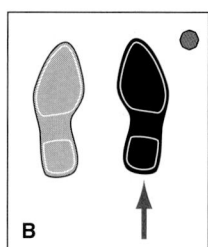

Figure 44-59 ■ Steps involved in using a cane when less than maximum support is required.

the standard and four-wheeled walker is one that has two tips and two wheels. This type provides more stability than the four-wheeled model yet still permits the client to keep the walker in contact with the ground all the time. The client tilts the walker toward the body, lifting the tips while the wheels remain on the ground, and then pushes the walker forward.

The nurse may need to adjust the height of a client's walker so that the hand bar is just below the client's waist and the client's elbows are slightly flexed. This position helps the client assume a more normal stance. A walker that is too low causes the client to stoop; one that is too high makes the client stretch and reach.

CRUTCHES. Crutches may be a temporary need for some people and a permanent one for others. Sometimes clients are discouraged when they attempt crutch walking. Clients confined to bed are often unaware of weakness that becomes apparent when they try to stand or walk. Clients realize that they can no longer take balance for granted when they must cope with the weight of a heavy cast or a paralyzed limb. Frequently, progress may be slower than the client anticipated.

Encouragement from the nurse and the setting of realistic goals are especially important.

There are several kinds of crutches. The most frequently used are the underarm crutch, or axillary crutch with hand bars,

CLIENT TEACHING   Using Walkers

WHEN MAXIMUM SUPPORT IS REQUIRED

- Move the walker ahead about 15 cm (6 in.) while your body weight is borne by both legs.
- Then move the right foot up to the walker while your body weight is borne by the left leg and both arms.
- Next, move the left foot up to the right foot while your body weight is borne by the right leg and both arms.

IF ONE LEG IS WEAKER THAN THE OTHER

- Move the walker and the weak leg ahead together about 15 cm (6 in.) while your weight is borne by the stronger leg.
- Then move the stronger leg ahead while your weight is borne by the affected leg and both arms.

A

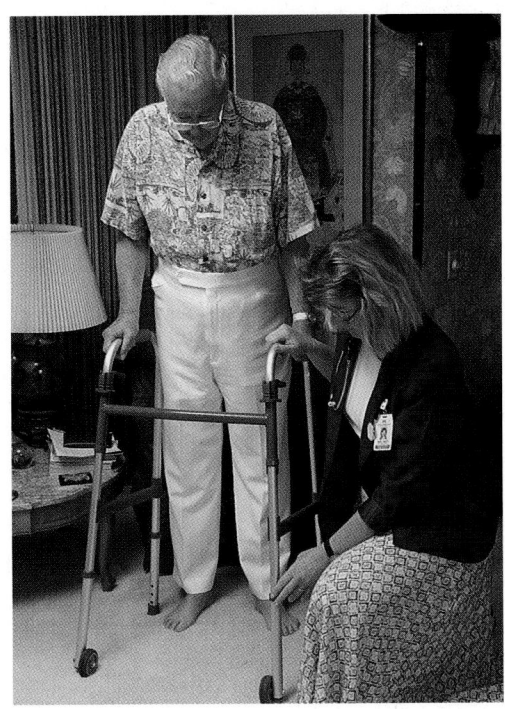

B

Figure 44-60 ■ *A*, standard walker. *B*, Two-wheeled walker.

and the Lofstrand crutch, which extends only to the forearm (Figure 44-61 ■). On the Lofstrand crutch, the metal cuff around the forearm and the metal bar stabilize the wrists and thus make walking safer and easier. The platform, or elbow extensor, crutch also has a cuff for the upper arm (Figure 44-61). All crutches require suction tips, usually made of rubber, which help to prevent slipping on a floor surface.

Figure 44-61 ■ Types of crutches: axillary, Lofstrand, and platform.

In crutch walking, the client's weight is borne by the muscles of the shoulder girdle and the upper extremities. Before beginning crutch walking, exercises that strengthen the upper arms and hands are recommended.

CLIENT TEACHING   Using Crutches

- Follow the plan of exercises developed for you to strengthen your arm muscles before beginning crutch walking.
- Have a health care professional establish the correct length for your crutches and the correct placement of the handpieces. Crutches that are too long force your shoulders upward and make it difficult for you to push your body off the ground. Crutches that are too short will make you hunch over and develop an improper body stance.
- The weight of your body should be borne by the arms rather than the axillae (armpits). Continual pressure on the axillae can injure the radial nerve and eventually cause crutch palsy, a weakness of the muscles of the forearm, wrist, and hand.
- Maintain an erect posture as much as possible to prevent strain on muscles and joints and to maintain balance.
- Each step taken with crutches should be a comfortable distance for you. It is wise to start with a small rather than large step.
- Inspect the crutch tips regularly, and replace them if worn.
- Keep the crutch tips dry and clean to maintain their surface friction. If the tips become wet, dry them well before use.
- Wear a shoe with a low heel that grips the floor. Rubber soles decrease the chances of slipping. Adjust shoelaces so they cannot come untied or reach the floor where they might catch on the crutches. Consider shoes with alternative forms of closure (e.g., Velcro), especially if you cannot easily bend to tie laces. Slip-on shoes are acceptable only if they are snug and the heel does not come loose when the foot is bent.

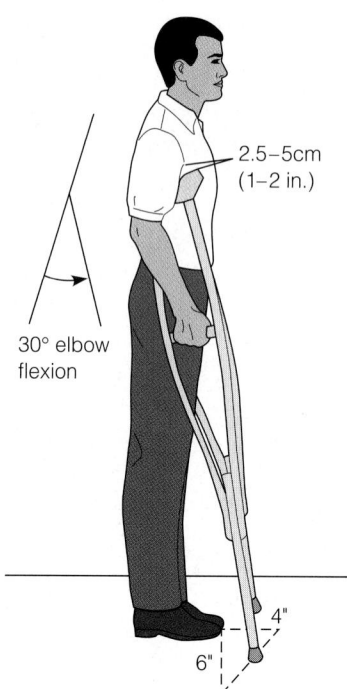

Figure 44-62 ■ The standing position for measuring the correct length for crutches.

Measuring Clients for Crutches. When nurses measure clients for axillary crutches, it is most important to obtain the correct length for the crutches and the correct placement of the hand piece. There are two methods of measuring crutch length:

1. The client lies in a supine position and the nurse measures from the anterior fold of the axilla to the heel of the foot and adds 2.5 cm (1 in.).
2. The client stands erect and positions the crutch as shown in Figure 44-62 ■. The nurse makes sure the shoulder rest of the crutch is at least three finger widths, that is, 2.5 to 5 cm (1 to 2 in.), below the axilla.

To determine the correct placement of the hand bar:

1. The client stands upright and supports the body weight by the hand grips of the crutches.
2. The nurse measures the angle of elbow flexion. It should be about 30 degrees. A goniometer (Figure ➊ in Skill 30-16) may be used to verify the correct angle.

Crutch Gaits. The crutch gait is the gait a person assumes on crutches by alternating body weight on one or both legs and the crutches. Five standard crutch gaits are the four-point gait, three-point gait, two-point gait, swing-to gait, and swing-through gait. The gait used depends on the following individual factors: (a) the ability to take steps, (b) the ability to bear weight and keep balance in a standing position on both legs or only one, and (c) the ability to hold the body erect.

Clients also need instruction about how to get into and out of chairs and go up and down stairs safely. All of these crutch skills are best taught before the client is discharged and preferably before the client has surgery.

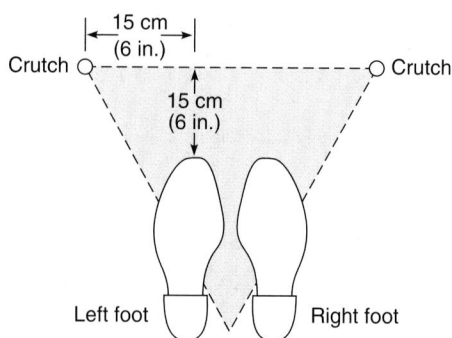

Figure 44-63 ■ The tripod position.

Crutch Stance (Tripod Position). Before crutch walking is attempted, the client needs to learn facts about posture and balance. The proper standing position with crutches is called the **tripod (triangle) position** (Figure 44-63 ■). The crutches are placed about 15 cm (6 in.) in front of the feet and out laterally about 15 cm (6 in.), creating a wide base of support. The feet are slightly apart. A tall person requires a wider base than a short person does. Hips and knees are extended, the back is straight, and the head is held straight and high. There should be no hunch to the shoulders and thus no weight borne by the axillae. The elbows are extended sufficiently to allow weight bearing on the hands. If the client is unsteady, the nurse places a walking belt around the client's waist and grasps the belt from above, not from below. A fall can be prevented more effectively if the belt is held from above.

Four-Point Alternate Gait. This is the most elementary and safest gait, providing at least three points of support at all times, but it requires coordination. Clients can use it when walking in crowds because it does not require much space. To use this gait, the client needs to be able to bear weight on both legs (Figure 44-64 ■, reading from bottom to top). The nurse asks the client to

1. Move the right crutch ahead a suitable distance, such as 10 to 15 cm (4 to 6 in.).
2. Move the left front foot forward, preferably to the level of the left crutch.
3. Move the left crutch forward.
4. Move the right foot forward.

Three-Point Gait. To use this gait, the client must be able to bear the entire body weight on the unaffected leg. The two crutches and the unaffected leg bear weight alternately (Figure 44-65 ■, reading from bottom to top). The nurse asks the client to

1. Move both crutches and the weaker leg forward.
2. Move the stronger leg forward.

Two-Point Alternate Gait. This gait is faster than the four-point gait. It requires more balance because only two points support the body at one time; it also requires at least partial weight bearing on each foot. In this gait, arm movements with the crutches are similar to the arm movements during normal walking (Figure 44-66 ■, reading from bottom to top). The nurse asks the client to

1. Move the left crutch and the right foot forward together.
2. Move the right crutch and the left foot ahead together.

Swing-To Gait. The swing gaits are used by clients with paralysis of the legs and hips. Prolonged use of these gaits results in

Figure 44-64 ■ The four-point alternate crutch gait.

Figure 44-65 ■ The three-point crutch gait.

atrophy of the unused muscles. The swing-to gait is the easier of these two gaits. The nurse asks the client to

1. Move both crutches ahead together (Figure 44-67 ■, *A*).
2. Lift body weight by the arms and swing to the crutches (Figure 44-67 ■, *B*).

Swing-Through Gait. This gait requires considerable skill, strength, and coordination. The nurse asks the client to

1. Move both crutches forward together (Figure 44-68 ■, *A*).
2. Lift body weight by the arms and swing through and beyond the crutch (Figure 44-68 ■, *B*).

Getting into a Chair. Chairs that have armrests and are secure or braced against a wall are essential for clients using crutches. For this procedure, the nurse instructs the client to

1. Stand with the back of the unaffected leg centered against the chair. The chair helps support the client during the next steps.
2. Transfer the crutches to the hand on the affected side and hold the crutches by the hand bars. The client grasps the arm of the chair with the hand on the unaffected side (Figure 44-69 ■). This allows the client to support the body weight on the arms and the unaffected leg.
3. Lean forward, flex the knees and hips, and lower into the chair.

Step 2
Right crutch
and left limb advance

Step 1
Left crutch and
right limb advance

Tripod position

Figure 44-66 ■ The two-point alternate crutch gait.

Getting Out of a Chair. For this procedure, the nurse instructs the client to

1. Move forward to the edge of the chair and place the unaffected leg slightly under or at the edge of the chair. This position helps the client stand up from the chair and

Figure 44-67 ■ The swing-to crutch gait.

Figure 44-68 ■ The swing-through crutch gait.

achieve balance, since the unaffected leg is supported against the edge of the chair.
2. Grasp the crutches by the hand bars in the hand on the affected side, and grasp the arm of the chair by the hand on the unaffected side. The body weight is placed on the crutches and the hand on the armrest to support the unaffected leg when the client rises to stand.
3. Push down on the crutches and the chair armrest while elevating the body out of the chair.
4. Assume the tripod position before moving.

Going Up Stairs. For this procedure, the nurse stands behind the client and slightly to the affected side if needed. The nurse instructs the client to

1. Assume the tripod position at the bottom of the stairs.
2. Transfer the body weight to the crutches and move the unaffected leg onto the step (Figure 44-70 ■).
3. Transfer the body weight to the unaffected leg on the step and move the crutches and affected leg up to the step. The affected leg is always supported by the crutches.
4. Repeat steps 2 and 3 until the client reaches the top of the stairs.

Going Down Stairs. For this procedure, the nurse stands one step below the client on the affected side if needed. The nurse instructs the client to

1. Assume the tripod position at the top of the stairs.
2. Shift the body weight to the unaffected leg, and move the crutches and affected leg down onto the next step (Figure 44-71 ■).
3. Transfer the body weight to the crutches, and move the unaffected leg to that step. The affected leg is always supported by the crutches.
4. Repeat steps 2 and 3 until the client reaches the bottom of the stairs.

Figure 44-69 ■ A client using crutches getting into a chair.

Figure 44-71 ■ Descending stairs: moving the crutches and affected leg to the next step.

Figure 44-70 ■ Climbing stairs: placing weight on the crutches while first moving the unaffected leg onto a step.

Evaluating

The goals established during the planning phase are evaluated according to specific desired outcomes, also established in that phase. Examples of these are shown in the accompanying Nursing Care Plan.

If outcomes are not achieved, the nurse, client, and support person if appropriate need to explore the reasons before modifying the care plan. For example, the following questions may be considered if an immobilized client fails to maintain muscle mass and tone and joint mobility:

■ Has the client's physical or mental condition changed motivation to perform required exercise?
■ Were appropriate range-of-motion exercises implemented?
■ Was the client encouraged to participate in self-care activities as much as possible?
■ Was the client encouraged to make as many decisions as possible when developing a daily activity plan and to express concerns?
■ Did the nurse provide appropriate supervision and monitoring?
■ Was the client's diet adequate to provide appropriate nourishment for energy requirements?

MediaLink Activity and Exercise Care Plan Activity

NURSING CARE PLAN Risk for Disuse Syndrome

ASSESSMENT DATA	NURSING DIAGNOSIS	DESIRED OUTCOMES*

Nursing Assessment

Peter Chan, a 69-year-old, unmarried accountant being treated for congestive heart failure, states he has dyspnea with mild activity. ("I cannot climb a flight of stairs without stopping and resting and become breathless even when walking on level ground.") Prefers the orthopneic position. He works at home and sits at a table for most of the day.

Physical Examination

Height: 178 cm (5'10")
Weight: 102 kg (225 lb)
Temperature: 37.8°C (100.4°F)
Pulse rate: 94 BPM
Respirations: 20/minute
Blood pressure: 174/92 mm Hg
Rales present in both lungs.
Respirations slightly labored.
Color pale.
3+ (5 mm) edema both feet and ankles

Diagnostic Data

CBC, and urinalysis within normal limits.

CXR reveals an enlarged heart.

Risk for Disuse Syndrome related to decreased activity resulting from inadequate balance between oxygen supply and demand associated with decreased cardiac output and obesity.

Immobility Consequences: Physiological [0204], as evidenced by no
- Pressure ulcers
- Decreased muscle strength

Immobility Consequences: Psycho-cognitive [0205], as evidenced by no
- Apathy
- Sleep disturbances
- Negative body image

Mobility [0208], as evidenced by mildly compromised
- Walking
- Balance

NURSING INTERVENTIONS*/SELECTED ACTIVITIES	RATIONALE

Positioning [0840]

Position to alleviate dyspnea, e.g., high Fowler's.	*Clients with increased pulmonary secretions are able to breathe better when upright because abdominal organs are lower and there is greater room for lung and diaphragmatic excursion.*
Provide support to edematous areas, e.g., elevate feet on foot stool when sitting.	*Elevating the dependent area assists with decreasing tissue pressure and promoting fluid return to the venous system and the heart.*
Encourage active range of motion exercises.	*Active ROM helps keep muscles in current strength and promotes circulation. Mild activity also helps burn unneeded calories.*

Exercise Therapy: Muscle Control [0226]

Collaborate with physical, occupational, and recreational therapists in developing and executing an individually tailored exercise program.	*This client will need a multidisciplinary approach to his care. Each member contributes from his or her area of expertise. Research supports efficacy of individually tailored exercise plans. Factors such as having an exercise partner, using music, and type of activity can motivate client and enhance adherence to the plan over time.*
Offer options, explain rationale for type of exercise and protocol to client, and allow him to make choices that appeal to him and that address his needs.	*If the client understands what the reasons are for activity, he can make good choices.*
Provide step-by-step cuing for each motor activity during exercise or ADLs.	*As-needed reminders help the client recall what to do next.*
Use visual aids to facilitate learning how to perform exercises.	*Some people have better visual memory than auditory memory.*

EVALUATION

Outcomes met. Mr. Chan did not develop any skin breakdown or other evidence of the complications of immobility to date. However, since the risk factors remain, the care plan will be ongoing.

*The NOC # for desired outcomes and the NIC # for nursing interventions are listed in brackets following the appropriate outcome or intervention. Outcomes, indicators, interventions, and activities selected are only a sample of those suggested by NOC and NIC and should be further individualized for each client.

APPLYING CRITICAL THINKING

NURSING CARE PLAN **Risk for Disuse Syndrome** *(continued)*

1. What assessment findings alert you that Mr. Chan is developing problems associated with his current state of decreased mobility?

2. Mr. Chan may benefit from using a walker to assist with ambulation at home. What teaching should be done in regard to use of a walker?

3. The care plan does not address one of Mr. Chan's risk factors—obesity. Would you add this to the plan?

4. What assumptions has the nurse made in assigning the desired outcome of "Immobility Consequences: Psycho-Cognitive"?

5. How are the choices of outcomes influenced by the cause of his nursing diagnosis (a chronic illness)?

See Critical Thinking Possibilities in Appendix A.

CONCEPT MAP   Client at Risk for Disuse Syndrome

PC
69 y.o. male
CHF

— assess →

- Unmarried accountant: works at home c/o dyspnea on exertion
- Height: 178 cm (5' 10")
- Weight: 102 kg (225 lb)
- Temperature: 37.8°C (100.4°F)
- Pulse rate: 94 BPM
- Respirations: 20/minute
- Blood pressure: 174/92 mm Hg
- CBC and urinalysis within normal limits
- CXR shows enlarged heart

generate nursing diagnosis

Risk for Disuse Syndrome r/t decreased activity resulting from inadequate balance between oxygen supply & demand associated with decreased CO and obesity

outcome

outcome

Outcomes met:
- Did not develop any skin breakdown or other evidence of the complication of immobility to date

← evaluation —

Immobility Consequences: Physiological aeb no:
- Pressure ulcers
- Decreased muscle strength

Mobility aeb mildly compromised:
- Walking
- Balance

— evaluation →

Outcomes met:
- Did not develop any compromised muscle function
- However, since the risk factors remain, the care plan will be ongoing

nursing intervention

nursing intervention

Positioning

Exercise Therapy-Muscle Control

activity

activity

activity

activity

activity

activity

activity

Position to alleviate dyspnea (e.g., high Fowler's)

Provide support to edematous areas, e.g., elevate feet on foot stool when sitting

Encourage active range-of-motion exercises

Use visual aids to facilitate learning how to perform exercises

Provide step-by-step cuing for each motor activity during exercise or ADLs

Explain rationale for type of exercise and protocol to client

Collaborate with physical occupational, and recreational therapists in developing and executing exercise program

CHAPTER 44 REVIEW

CHAPTER HIGHLIGHTS

- The ability to move freely, easily, and purposefully in the environment is essential for people to meet their basic needs.
- Exercise and activity are essential components for maintaining and regaining health and wellness.
- Research on exercise has demonstrated it to be an excellent strategy for preventing and treating some cardiovascular and pulmonary diseases, mood disorders, diseases of aging, diabetes, and immune diseases.
- Purposeful coordinated movement of the body relies on the integrated functioning of the musculoskeletal system, the nervous system, and the vestibular apparatus of the inner ear.
- Body movement involves four basic elements: body alignment, joint mobility, balance, and coordinated movement.
- People maintain alignment and balance when the line of gravity passes through the center of gravity and the base of support.
- The broader the base of support and the lower the center of gravity, the greater the stability and balance achieved.
- Exercise is physical activity performed to maintain muscle tone and joint mobility, to enhance physiologic functioning of body systems, and to improve physical fitness. Activity tolerance is the type and amount of exercise or daily living activities an individual is able to perform without experiencing adverse effects. Functional strength is the ability to do work.
- Exercise is classified as either isotonic, isometric, or isokinetic and as either aerobic or anaerobic.
- Many factors influence body alignment and activity. These include growth and development, physical health, mental health, personal values and attitudes, medications, and prescribed limitations to movement.
- Immobility affects almost every body organ and system adversely; complications also include psychosocial problems. Exercise, by contrast, provides many benefits to the same body organs and systems, and can actually be used to prevent and treat many disease processes.
- Problems of immobility include disuse osteoporosis and atrophy; contractures; diminished cardiac reserve; orthostatic hypotension; venous stasis, edema, and thrombus formation; decreased respiratory movement and pooling of secretions; decreased metabolic rate and negative nitrogen balance; urinary stasis, retention, infection, and calculi; constipation; and varying emotional reactions.
- Complete bed rest is almost never required, and is usually dangerous due to the hazards of immobility. A risk-benefit assessment and ongoing assessment of rationale for complete bed rest is essential.
- The nurse has responsibilities (a) to determine root causes of immobility and address these whenever possible (with the client) with the goal of getting the client moving as much and as soon as possible, (b) to prevent the complications of immobility and reduce the severity of any problems resulting from immobility, and (c) to partner with the client and appropriate support persons to design individualized exercise programs for clients that promote wellness.

- Assessment relative to a client's activity and exercise includes a nursing history and physical examination of body alignment, gait, joint appearance and movement, capabilities and limitations for movement, muscle mass and strength, activity tolerance, and problems related to immobility.
- An activity and exercise history includes daily activity level, activity tolerance, type and frequency of exercise, and factors affecting mobility.
- NANDA nursing diagnoses that relate to activity and mobility problems include *Activity Intolerance, Risk for Activity Intolerance, Impaired Physical Mobility,* and *Risk for Disuse Syndrome.* Other relevant diagnoses are *Self-Care Deficit, Risk for Injury, Fear* (of falling), *Powerlessness, Low Self-Esteem, Ineffective Coping,* and, if the client is immobilized, many other potential problems such as *Ineffective Airway Clearance* and *Risk for Infection.*
- Body mechanics is the efficient, coordinated, and safe use of the body to move objects and carry out the activities of daily living.
- Nurses must use good body mechanics in their daily work and especially when moving and turning clients in bed and assisting clients to make transfers. Proper body mechanics do not ensure protection from injury, however, and nurses and caregivers are encouraged to avoid manual lifting and repositioning of clients. At the very least, they should avoid solo lifting, repositioning, and transferring.
- Positioning a client in good body alignment and changing the position regularly and systematically are essential aspects of nursing practice.
- Before positioning dependent clients, the nurse should plan a systematic 24-hour schedule for position changes, including positions that provide for full extension of the neck, hips, and knees. The nurse also uses appropriate supportive devices to maintain alignment and prevent strain on the client's muscles and joints.
- Before moving, turning, or transferring a client, the nurse must consider the client's health status and degree of exertion permitted, physical ability to assist, ability to comprehend instruction, degree of discomfort, client's weight, and whether to use assistive devices or another caregiver to assist.
- Assistance from others or the use of mechanical lifting aids is essential for most all nonpediatric clients.
- Safety measures must always be employed when the nurse uses a wheelchair or stretcher to move and transfer clients.
- Ambulating techniques that facilitate normal walking gait yet provide needed supports are most effective. The nurse can assist clients to prepare for ambulation by helping them become as independent as possible while in bed.
- Preambulatory exercises that strengthen the muscles for walking are essential for clients who have been immobilized for a prolonged period.
- Clients need specific instructions about appropriate use of canes, walkers, and crutches.

TEST YOUR KNOWLEDGE

1. To increase stability during client transfer, the nurse increases the base of support by performing which of the following?
   1. Leaning slightly backward
   2. Spacing the feet farther apart
   3. Tensing the abdominal muscles
   4. Bending the knees

2. Isotonic exercises such as walking are intended to achieve which of the following? Select all that apply.
   1. Increase muscle tone and improve circulation
   2. Increase blood pressure
   3. Increase muscle mass and strength
   4. Decrease heart rate and cardiac output
   5. Maintain joint range of motion

3. Five minutes after the client's first postoperative exercise, the client's vital signs have not yet returned to baseline. An appropriate nursing diagnosis might be
   1. *Activity Intolerance.*
   2. *Risk for Activity Intolerance.*
   3. *Impaired Physical Mobility.*
   4. *Risk for Disuse Syndrome.*

4. Which of the following statements from a client with one weak leg regarding use of crutches when using stairs indicates a need for increased teaching?
   1. "Going up, the strong leg goes first, then the weaker leg with both crutches."
   2. "Going down, the weaker leg goes first with both crutches, then the strong leg."
   3. "The weaker leg always goes first with both crutches."
   4. "A cane or single crutch may be used instead of both crutches if held on the weaker side."

5. Which of the following drugs seem to be implicated most frequently as contributing to falls and fractures in the elderly?
   1. Sinemet
   2. Benzodiazepines
   3. Elavil
   4. Lasix

6. When assessing a client's gait, nurses should look for and encourage which of the following?
   1. The spine rotates, initiating locomotion.
   2. Gaze is slightly downward.

   3. Toes strike the ground before the heel.
   4. Arm on the same side as the swing-through foot moves forward at the same time.

7. Performance of activities of daily living (ADLs) and active range of motion (ROM) exercises can be accomplished simultaneously as illustrated by which of the following? Select all that apply.
   1. Elbow flexion with eating and bathing
   2. Elbow extension with shaving and eating
   3. Wrist hyperextension with writing
   4. Thumb ROM with eating and writing
   5. Hip flexion with walking

8. Because the client weighs 250 pounds, the nurse should provide the unlicensed assistive personnel (UAP) with instructions that reflect an awareness of workplace injury. Which of the following is most appropriate?
   1. "Using proper body mechanics will prevent you from injuring yourself."
   2. "You are physically fit and at lesser risk for injury when transferring the client."
   3. "Use the mechanical lift and another person to transfer the client from the bed to the chair."
   4. "Use the back belt to avoid hurting your back."

9. The client is ambulating for the first time after surgery. The client tells the nurse, "I feel faint." The best action by the nurse includes which of the following?
   1. Find another nurse for help.
   2. Return the client to her room as quickly as possible.
   3. Tell the client to take rapid, shallow breaths.
   4. Assist the client to a nearby chair.

10. The nurse is performing an assessment of an immobilized client. Which of the following assessments causes the nurse to take action?
   1. Heart rate 86
   2. Reddened area on sacrum
   3. Nonproductive cough
   4. Urine output of 50 mL/hour

See Answers to Test Your Knowledge in Appendix A.

EXPLORE MEDIALINK www.prenhall.com/berman

DVD-ROM
- Audio Glossary
- NCLEX Review
- Skills Checklists
- Animations:
    A & P Review
    Classification of Joints
    Movement of Joints
    Muscle Contraction
    Muscles

COMPANION WEBSITE
- Additional NCLEX Review
- Case Study: Client with Mobility Problems
- Care Plan Activity: Activity and Exercise
- Application Activity: Exercise for Seniors
- Links to Resources

READINGS AND REFERENCES

SUGGESTED READINGS

American Nurses Association (ANA) website. This website provides helpful information about ANA's *"Handle with Care"* campaign to promote the issue of safe patient handling and the prevention of musculoskeletal disorder among nurses in the United States. Retrieved July 3, 2006, from, http://www.nursingworld.org/handlewithcare/factsheet.htm

RELATED RESEARCH

Robitaille, Y., Laforest, S., Fournier, M., Gauvin, L., Parisien, M., Corriveau, H., et al. (2005). Moving forward in fall prevention: An intervention to improve balance among older adults in real-world settings. *American Journal of Public Health, 95*(11), 2049–2056.

REFERENCES

American Federation of State, County, and Municipal Employees. (2002). *Preventing back injuries in health care.* Retrieved July 3, 2006, from http://www.afscme.org/health/faq-back.htm

American Nurses Association. (n.d.). *Handle with care fact sheet.* Retrieved July 3, 2006, from http://www.nursingworld.org/handlewithcare/factsheet.htm

Borg, G. (1998). *Borg's perceived exertion and pain scales.* Champaign, IL: Human Kinetics.

Burke, M., & Laramie, J. (2004). *Primary care of the older adult: A multidisciplinary approach* (2nd ed.). Philadelphia: Mosby/Elsevier.

Cummings, R., & Couteur, D. (2003). Benzodiazepines and risk of hip fractures in older people: A review of the evidence. *CNS Drugs, 17*(11), 825–837.

Dochterman, J., & Bulechek, G. M. (Eds.). (2004). *Nursing interventions classification (NIC)* (4th ed.). St. Louis, MO: Mosby.

Edelman, C., & Mandle, C. (2006). *Health promotion throughout the lifespan* (6th ed.). Philadelphia: Mosby/Elsevier.

Fontaine, K. (2005). *Complementary and alternative therapies for nursing practice* (2nd ed.). Upper Saddle River, NJ: Pearson/Prentice Hall.

Freeman, L. (2004). *Mosby's complementary & alternative medicine: A research-based approach* (2nd ed.). Philadelphia: Mosby/Elsevier.

French, D., Campbell, R., Spehar, A., & Angaran, D. (2004). Benzodiazepines and injury: A risk adjusted model. *Pharmacoepidemiology and Drug Safety, 14*(1), 17–24.

Harvard School of Public Health. (2006). *Exercise.* Retrieved July 4, 2006, from http://www.hsph.harvard.edu/nutritionsource/Exercise.htm

Hu, F. B., Willett, W. C., Li, T., Stampfer, M. J., Colditz, G. A., & Manson, J. E. (2004). Adiposity as compared with physical activity in predicting mortality among women. *New England Journal of Medicine, 351*(26), 2649–2703.

International Osteoporosis Foundation. (2005). *Invest in your bones. Move it or lose it.* Retrieved July 3, 2006, from http://www.osteofound.org/publications/move_it_or_lose_it.html

Jackson, C. (2003). Movement, breathing and Christian meditation: Catalysts for spiritual growth. *International Journal of Healing and Caring On-Line, 3*(2), 1–24.

Keele-Smith, R., & Leon, T. (2003). Evaluation of individually tailored interventions on exercise adherence. *Western Journal of Nursing Research, 25*(6), 623–640.

Liu, B. (2003). Relationship between antidepressants and the risk of falls. *Geriatrics and Aging, 6*(7), 45–47.

McCaffrey, R., Ruknui, P., Hatthakit, U., & Kasetsomboon, P. (2005). The effects of yoga on hypertensive persons in Thailand. *Holistic Nursing Practice, 19*(4), 173–180.

Micozzi, M. (2006). *Fundamentals of complementary and alternative medicine* (3rd ed.). Philadelphia: Mosby/Elsevier.

Moorhead, S., Johnson, M., & Maas, M. (Eds.). (2004). *Nursing outcomes classification (NOC)* (3rd ed.). St. Louis, MO: Mosby.

NANDA International. (2005). *Nursing diagnoses: Definitions and classification 2005–2006.* Philadelphia: author.

NANDA International. (2007). *Nursing diagnoses: Definitions and classification 2007–2008.* Philadelphia: Author.

Nelson, A., Fragala, G., & Menzel, N. (2003). Myths and facts about back injuries in nursing. *American Journal of Nursing, 103*(2), 32–40.

Oken, B., Zajdel, D., Kishiyama, S., Flegal, K., Dehen, C., Haas, M., et al. (2006). Randomized, controlled, six-month trial of yoga in healthy seniors: Effects on cognition and quality of life. *Alternative Therapies, 12*(1), 40–47.

Rice, J., Kaliszer, M., Walsh, M., Jenkinson, A., & O'Brien, T. (2004). Movements at the low back during normal walking. *Clinical Anatomy, 17*(8), 662–666.

Wilson, B., Shannon, M., & Stang, C. (2006). *Nurse's drug guide 2006.* Upper Saddle River, NJ: Prentice Hall.

Young, M. (2003). *A review on postural realignment and its muscular and neural components.* Retrieved July 3, 2006, from www.elitetrack.com/posture.pdf

Zielinski, K. (2004). The healing power of the labyrinth. *Real Living with Multiple Sclerosis, 11*(8), 6–7.

SELECTED BIBLIOGRAPHY

Ackley, B., & Ladwig, G. (2004). *Nursing diagnosis handbook: A guide to planning care* (6th ed.). Philadelphia: Mosby/Elsevier.

Blocks, M. (2005). Practical solutions for safe patient handling. *Nursing, 35*(10), 44–45.

Centers for Disease Control and Prevention. (n.d.). *Introducing the youth media campaign.* Retrieved July 3, 2006, from http://www.cdc.gov/youthcampaign/index.htm

Clements, P. T., DeRanieri, J. T., Clark, K., Manno, M. S., & Kuhn, D. W. (2005). Workplace violence and corporate policy for health care settings. *Nursing Economics, 23*(3), 119–124.

Converso, A., & Murphy, C. (2004). Winning the battle against back injuries. *RN, 67*(2), 52–57.

Doenges, M. E., Moorhouse, M. F., & Geissler-Murr, A. C. (2005). *Nursing diagnosis manual: Planning, individualizing and documenting client care.* Philadelphia: F. A. Davis.

Morgan, R., Virnig, B., Duque, M., Abdel-Moty, E., & DeVito, C. (2004). Low-intensity exercise and reduction of the risk for falls among at-risk elders. *Journals of Gerontology Series A: Biological and Medical Sciences, 59,* M 1062–M 1067.

Nelson, A., Owen, B., Lloyd, J. D., Fragala, G., Matz, M. W., Amato, M., et al. (2003). Safe patient handling & movement. *American Journal of Nursing, 103*(3), 32–43.

Powers, S., & Dodd, S. (2003). *Total fitness and wellness.* New York: Benjamin Cummings.

Sleep

LEARNING OUTCOMES

After completing this chapter, you will be able to:

1. Explain the functions and the physiology of sleep.

2. Identify the characteristics of the sleep states: NREM and REM sleep.

3. Describe variations in sleep patterns throughout the life span.

4. Identify factors that affect normal sleep.

5. Describe common sleep disorders.

6. Identify the components of a sleep pattern assessment.

7. Develop nursing diagnoses, outcomes, and nursing interventions related to sleep problems.

8. Describe interventions that promote normal sleep.

Sleep is a basic human need; it is a universal biological process common to all people. Humans spend about one-third of their lives asleep. We require sleep for many reasons: to cope with daily stresses, to prevent fatigue, to conserve energy, to restore the mind and body, and to enjoy life more fully. Sleep enhances daytime functioning. It is vital for not only optimal psychological functioning but also physiological functioning as the rate of healing of damaged tissue is greatest during sleep (Robinson, Weitzel, & Henderson, 2005, p. 263). Sleep is an important factor in a person's quality of life. And yet, a 2006 report from the Institute of Medicine (IOM) states that sleep disorders and sleep deprivation is an unmet public health problem. It is estimated that 50 million to 70 million Americans suffer from a chronic disorder of sleep and wakefulness that hinders daily functioning and adversely affects health (IOM, 2006, p. 24). Numerous *Sleep in America* polls by the National Sleep Foundation reflect that Americans, from infants to elders, need more sleep.

Furthermore, many members of the general public and health professionals are unaware of the consequences of chronic sleep loss (e.g., increased risk of hypertension, diabetes, obesity, depression, heart attack, and stroke). Almost 20% of all serious car crash injuries are associated with driver sleepiness (IOM, 2006, p. 25). As a result, the IOM report made a number of recommendations, including: (a) increasing financial investments in interdisciplinary **somnology** (the study of sleep) and sleep medicine research training; (b) increasing public awareness by establishing a multimedia public education campaign; (c) increasing education and training of health care professionals in somnology and sleep medicine; (d) developing new technologies for the diagnosis and treatment of sleep disorders; and (e) monitoring the American population's sleep patterns and the prevalence and health outcomes associated with sleep disorders (IOM, 2006).

PHYSIOLOGY OF SLEEP

Historically, sleep was considered a state of unconsciousness. More recently, **sleep** has come to be considered an altered state of consciousness in which the individual's perception of and reaction to the environment are decreased. Sleep is characterized by minimal physical activity, variable levels of consciousness, changes in the body's physiologic processes, and decreased responsiveness to external stimuli. Some environmental stimuli, such as a smoke detector alarm, will usually awaken a sleeper, whereas many other noises will not. It appears that individuals respond to meaningful stimuli while sleeping and selectively disregard nonmeaningful stimuli. For example, a mother may respond to her baby's crying but not to the crying of another baby.

The cyclic nature of sleep is thought to be controlled by centers located in the lower part of the brain. Neurons within the reticular formation, located in the brain stem, integrate sensory information from the peripheral nervous system and relay the information to the cerebral cortex (see Anatomy & Physiology Review). The upper part of the reticular formation consists of a network of ascending nerve fibers called the reticular activating system (RAS), which is involved with the sleep–wake cycle. An intact cerebral cortex and reticular formation are necessary for the regulation of sleep and waking states.

Neurotransmitters, located within neurons in the brain, affect the sleep–wake cycles. For example, serotonin is thought to lessen the response to sensory stimulation and gamma-aminobutyric acid (GABA) to shut off the activity in the neurons of the reticular activating system. Another key factor to sleep is exposure to darkness. Darkness and preparing for sleep causes a decrease in stimulation of the RAS. During this time, the pineal gland in the brain begins to actively secrete the natural hormone melatonin, and the person feels less alert. During sleep, the growth hormone is secreted and cortisol is inhibited.

With the beginning of daylight, melatonin is at its lowest level in the body and the stimulating hormone, cortisol, is at its highest. Wakefulness is also associated with high levels of acetylcholine, dopamine, and noradrenaline. Acetylcholine is released in the reticular formation, dopamine in the midbrain, and noradrenaline in the pons. These neurotransmitters are localized within the reticular formation and influence cerebral cortical arousal.

Circadian Rhythms

Biological rhythms exist in plants, animals, and humans. In humans, these are controlled from within the body and synchronized with environmental factors, such as light and darkness. The most familiar biological rhythm is the circadian rhythm. The term *circadian* is from the Latin *circa dies,* meaning "about a day." Although sleep and waking cycles are the best known of the circadian rhythms, body temperature, blood pressure, and many other physiologic functions also follow a circadian pattern.

Sleep is a complex biological rhythm. When a person's biological clock coincides with the sleep–wake cycles, the person is said to be in circadian synchronization; that is, the person is awake when the body temperature is highest, and asleep when the body temperature is lowest. Circadian regularity begins to develop by the sixth week of life, and by 3 to 6 months most infants have a regular sleep–wake cycle.

ANATOMY & PHYSIOLOGY REVIEW **Reticular Activating System**

Nerve impulses from the senses reach the reticular activating system (RAS), which is in the reticular formation (located in the brain stem) with projections to the hypothalamus and cerebral cortex. The nerve fibers in the RAS relay impulses to the cerebral cortex for perception by the person.

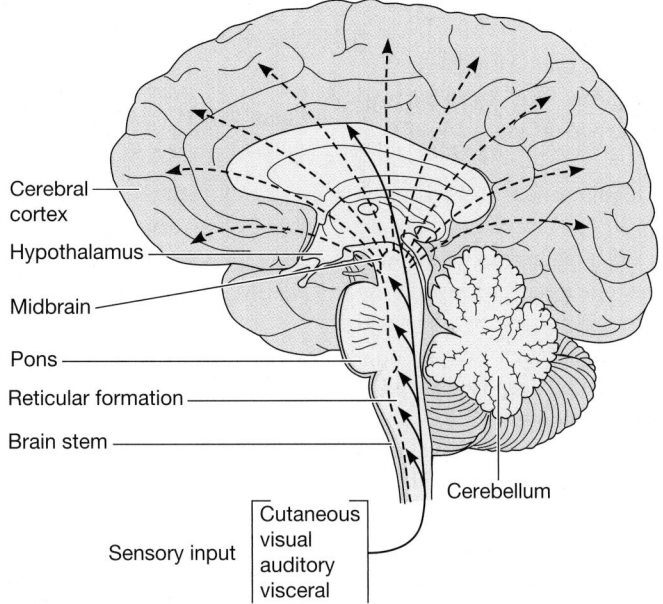

Cerebral cortex

Hypothalamus

Midbrain

Pons

Reticular formation

Brain stem

Cerebellum

Sensory input

Cutaneous
visual
auditory
visceral

The reticular formation in the brain stem.

QUESTIONS
1. How would you describe activity of the RAS in preparation for and during sleep?
2. What happens physiologically when your alarm clock wakes you in the morning?
3. What areas of the brain are affected by head trauma or stroke and affect an individual's level of alertness?

Types of Sleep

Sleep architecture refers to the basic organization of normal sleep. There are two types of sleep: **NREM** (non-rapid-eye-movement) **sleep** and **REM** (rapid-eye-movement) **sleep.** During sleep, NREM and REM sleep alternate in cycles. Irregular cycling and/or absent sleep stages are associated with sleep disorders (IOM, 2006, p. 42).

NREM Sleep

NREM sleep occurs when activity in the RAS is inhibited. About 75% to 80% of sleep during a night is NREM sleep. NREM sleep is divided into four stages, each associated with distinct brain activity and physiology. *Stage I* is the stage of very light sleep and lasts only a few minutes. During this stage, the person feels drowsy and relaxed, the eyes roll from side to side, and the heart and respiratory rates drop slightly. The sleeper can be readily awakened and may deny that he or she was sleeping.

Stage II is the stage of light sleep during which body processes continue to slow down. The eyes are generally still, the heart and respiratory rates decrease slightly, and body temperature falls. Stage II lasts only about 10 to 15 minutes but constitutes 44% to 55% of total sleep (IOM, 2006, p. 44). An individual in stage II requires more intense stimuli than in stage I to awaken.

Stages III and IV are the deepest stages of sleep, differing only in the percentage of delta waves recorded during a 30-second period. During *deep sleep* or *delta sleep,* the sleeper's heart and respiratory rates drop 20% to 30% below those exhibited during waking hours. The sleeper is difficult to arouse. The person is not disturbed by sensory stimuli, the skeletal muscles are very relaxed, reflexes are diminished, and snoring is most likely to occur. Even swallowing and saliva production are reduced during delta sleep (Orr, 2000). These stages are essential for restoring energy and releasing important growth hormones. See Box 45–1.

BOX 45–1 Physiologic Changes during NREM Sleep

- Arterial blood pressure falls.
- Pulse rate decreases.
- Peripheral blood vessels dilate.
- Cardiac output decreases.
- Skeletal muscles relax.
- Basal metabolic rate decreases 10% to 30%.
- Growth hormone levels peak.
- Intracranial pressure decreases.

REM Sleep

REM sleep usually recurs about every 90 minutes and lasts 5 to 30 minutes. Most dreams take place during REM sleep but usually will not be remembered unless the person arouses briefly at the end of the REM period.

During REM sleep, the brain is highly active, and brain metabolism may increase as much as 20%. For example, during REM sleep, levels of acetylcholine and dopamine increase, with the highest levels of acetylcholine release occurring during REM sleep. Since both of these neurotransmitters are associated with cortical activation, it makes sense that their levels would be high during dreaming sleep. This type of sleep is also called paradoxical sleep because electroencephalogram (EEG) activity resembles that of wakefulness. Distinctive eye movements occur, voluntary muscle tone is dramatically decreased, and deep tendon reflexes are absent. In this phase, the sleeper may be difficult to arouse or may wake spontaneously, gastric secretions increase, and heart and respiratory rates often are irregular. It is thought that the regions of the brain that are used in learning, thinking, and organizing information are stimulated during REM sleep.

Sleep Cycles

During a sleep cycle, people typically pass through NREM and REM sleep, the complete cycle usually lasting about 90 to 110 minutes in adults. In the first sleep cycle, a sleeper usually passes through all of the first three NREM stages in a total of about 20 to 30 minutes. Then, stage IV may last about 30 minutes. After stage IV NREM, the sleep passes back through stages III and II over about 20 minutes. Thereafter, the first REM stage occurs, lasting about 10 minutes, completing the first sleep cycle. It is not unusual for the first REM period to be very brief or even skipped entirely. The healthy adult sleeper usually experiences four to six cycles of sleep during 7 to 8 hours (see Figure 45-1 ■). The sleeper who is awakened during any stage must begin anew at stage I NREM sleep and proceed through all the stages to REM sleep.

The duration of NREM stages and REM sleep varies throughout the sleep period. During the early part of the night, the deep sleep periods are longer. As the night progresses, the sleeper spends less time in stages III and IV of NREM sleep.

Figure 45-1 ■ Time spent in REM and non-REM stages of sleep in an adult.

REM sleep increases and dreams tend to lengthen. Before sleep ends, periods of near wakefulness occur, and stages I and II NREM sleep and REM sleep predominate.

FUNCTIONS OF SLEEP

The effects of sleep on the body are not completely understood. Sleep exerts physiologic effects on both the nervous system and other body structures. Sleep in some way restores normal levels of activity and normal balance among parts of the nervous system. Sleep is also necessary for protein synthesis, which allows repair processes to occur.

The role of sleep in psychological well-being is best noticed by the deterioration in mental functioning related to sleep loss. Persons with inadequate amounts of sleep tend to become emotionally irritable, have poor concentration, and experience difficulty making decisions.

NORMAL SLEEP PATTERNS AND REQUIREMENTS

Although it used to be believed that maintaining a regular sleep–wake rhythm is more important than the number of hours actually slept, recent research has shown that sleep deprivation is associated with significant cognitive and health problems. Although reestablishing the sleep–wake rhythm (e.g., after the disruption of surgery) is an important aspect of nursing, it is not appropriate to curtail or decrease daytime napping in hospitalized clients.

Newborns

Newborns sleep 16 to 18 hours a day, on an irregular schedule with periods of 1 to 3 hours spent awake. Unlike older children and adults, newborns enter REM sleep (called active sleep during the newborn period) immediately. Rapid eye movements are observable through closed lids, and the body movements and irregular respirations may be observed. NREM sleep (also called quiet sleep during the newborn period) is characterized by regular respirations, closed eyes, and the absence of body and eye movements. Newborns spend nearly 50% of their time in each of these states, and the sleep cycle is about 50 minutes.

It is best to put newborns to bed when they are sleepy but not asleep. Newborns can be encouraged to sleep less during the day by exposing them to light and by playing more with them during the day hours. As evening approaches, the environment can be less bright and quieter with less activity (National Sleep Foundation, n.d.d).

Infants

At first, infants awaken every 3 or 4 hours, eat, and then go back to sleep. Periods of wakefulness gradually increase during the first months. By 6 months, most infants sleep through the night (from midnight to 5 AM) and begin to establish a pattern of daytime naps. At the end of the first year, an infant usually takes two naps per day and should get about 14 to 15 hours of sleep in 24 hours.

About half of the infant's sleep time is spent in light sleep. During light sleep, the infant exhibits a great deal of activity, such as movement, gurgles, and coughing. Parents need to make sure that infants are truly awake before picking them up for feeding and changing. Putting infants to bed when they are drowsy but not asleep helps them to become "self-soothers." This means that they fall asleep independently and if they do awake at night, they can put themselves back to sleep. Infants who become used to parental assistance at bedtime may become "signalers" and cry for their parents to help them return to sleep at night (National Sleep Foundation, n.d.a).

Toddlers

Between 12 and 14 hours of sleep are recommended for children 1 to 3 years of age. Most still need an afternoon nap, but the need for midmorning naps gradually decreases. The toddler may exhibit a great deal of resistance to going to bed and may awaken during the night. Nighttime fears and nightmares are also common. A security object such as a blanket or stuffed animal may help. Parents need assurance that if the child has had adequate attention from them during the day, maintaining a daily sleep schedule and consistent bedtime routine will promote good sleep habits for the entire family.

Preschoolers

The preschool child (3 to 5 years of age) requires 11 to 13 hours of sleep per night, particularly if the child is in preschool. Sleep needs fluctuate in relation to activity and growth spurts. Many children of this age dislike bedtime and resist by requesting another story, game, or television program. The 4- to 5-year-old may become restless and irritable if sleep requirements are not met.

Parents can help children who resist bedtime by maintaining a regular and consistent sleep schedule. It also helps to have a relaxing bedtime routine that ends in the child's room. Preschool children wake up frequently at night, and they may be afraid of the dark or experience night terrors or nightmares. Often limiting or eliminating TV will reduce the number of nightmares.

School-Age Children

The school-age child (5 to 12 years of age) needs 10 to 11 hours of sleep, but most receive less because of increasing demands

---

RESEARCH NOTE Are There Barriers to Following the Back-to-Sleep Recommendations for Infants?

Research has shown that placing infants to sleep in the supine position decreases the risk of SIDS. The Back-to-Sleep educational initiative resulted in many more caregivers placing their infants in the supine position for sleep. The incidence of SIDS has decreased by 50%. In spite of this overall decrease, racial differences in the incidence of SIDS continue with African American infants having a higher incidence of SIDS than Caucasian and Latino infants. Previous studies found that it was more common for African American caregivers to place their infants in the prone position for sleep. Other factors associated with placing the infant in the prone position included having a grandmother living in the home, young age of the mother, and having previous child-rearing experience.

The researchers wanted to determine new barriers and more information about previously identified barriers that interfere with adherence to the Back-to-Sleep recommendations among inner-city caregivers, primarily African Americans. They conducted a qualitative research study using focus groups. Forty-nine caregivers participated, with 86% being African American, 6% Hispanic, 4% white, and 4% other.

Four themes were identified:

1. Safety. All were concerned about the safety of their infants while they slept, which prompted some of the participants to bring their infants into their beds for closer observation. Many believed that the infant would choke if placed in the supine position.
2. Comfort. Many of the participants made their decision about the position of the infant based on their perception of whether the baby seemed comfortable. Some felt that the infant looked more comfortable on its side or stomach and the baby slept longer in that position. Some felt that the infant seemed more comfortable close to them and had the infant sleep in bed with them.
3. Advice. Participants trusted the advice of older female family members with previous child-rearing experience. They also trusted their own instincts and their previous experience. Some did not trust health care providers as a reliable source of advice, especially about the care of infants. They recommended that advice from health professionals be delivered in a certain way: "Don't tell us. . . . Tell us why."
4. Knowledge. Some of the participants believed that SIDS could only happen if the infant slept in a crib (SIDS is sometimes called crib death) and, as a result, did not place their infant in a crib. Some doubted the existence of SIDS and others referred to religious beliefs (e.g., "it's an act of God . . . there is no way to really stop it").

IMPLICATIONS

The generalizability of this study is limited because the data were collected in only two cities. However, the study did identify barriers to following the Back-to-Sleep recommendations. Nurses need to assess a caregiver's knowledge about SIDS and use effective teaching strategies that will enhance the trust of the caregiver.

Note: Reprinted from "Barriers to Following the Back-to-Sleep Recommendations: Insights from Focus Groups with Inner-City Caregivers," by E. R. Colson, L. K. McCabe, K. Fox, S. Levenson, T. Colton, G. Lister, et al., 2005, *Ambulatory Pediatrics, 5*(6), 349–354. Copyright © 2005 with permission from the Ambulatory Pediatric Association.

(e.g., homework, sports, social activities). They may also be spending more time at the computer and watching TV. Some may be drinking caffeinated beverages. All of these activities can lead to difficulty falling asleep and fewer hours of sleep. Nurses can teach parents and school-age children about healthy sleep habits. A regular and consistent sleep schedule and bedtime routine need to be continued.

CLINICAL ALERT

Children who have a TV and/or computer in their bedroom are more likely to get less sleep. ■

Adolescents

Adolescents (12 to 18 years of age) require 9 to 10 hours of sleep each night; however, few actually get that much sleep (IOM, 2006, p. 56). The National Sleep Foundation's 2006 *Sleep in America* poll found that teens are sleepy at times and places where they should be fully awake—at school, at home, and on the road. This can result in lower grades, negative moods (e.g., unhappy, sad, tense), and increased potential for car accidents. Interestingly, while more than half of the adolescents knew they were not getting enough sleep, 90% of the parents believed their adolescent was getting enough sleep. Nurses can teach parents to recognize signs and symptoms that indicate their teen is not getting enough sleep. See Clinical Manifestations.

As children reach adolescence, their circadian rhythms tend to shift. Research in the 1990s found that later sleep and wake patterns among adolescents are biologically determined; the natural tendency for teenagers is to stay up late at night and wake up later in the morning (National Sleep Foundation, n.d.a).

CLINICAL MANIFESTATIONS
SLEEP DEPRIVATION AND
SLEEP PROBLEMS IN TEENS

The teen:
■ Has difficulty waking in the morning for school and yawns frequently throughout the day.
■ Is continuously late for class and has trouble getting out the door in the morning.
■ Can't seem to get through the day without drinking caffeinated beverages like coffee or cola.
■ Is having difficulty in school, or a teacher notices that he or she falls asleep in class periodically.
■ Is irritable, is anxious, and gets angry easily on days when he or she gets less sleep.
■ Runs from one activity to the next—he or she participates in extra-curricular activities, has a job, and stays up late doing homework every night, cutting into sleep time.
■ Takes naps during the week for more than 45 minutes and "sleeps in" for 2 hours or longer on the weekends than during the week.

Note: From "Parents of Teens: Recognize the Signs & Symptoms of Sleep Deprivation and Sleep Problems," by National Sleep Foundation (n.d.e). Retrieved July 2, 2006, from http://www.sleepfoundation.org/_content/hottopics/teensigns.pdf. Used with permission of the National Sleep Foundation. For further information, please visit http://www.sleepfoundation.org.

Figure 45-2 ■ Many adolescents do not get enough sleep.
(Patrick Watson)

Many schools, however, start at 7 AM which is in conflict with the adolescent's sleep patterns and needs and contributes to their sleep deprivation (Figure 45-2 ■). As a result, some members of Congress have introduced resolutions to encourage schools and school districts to reconsider the early school start times.

During adolescence, boys begin to experience **nocturnal emissions** (orgasm and emission of semen during sleep), known as "wet dreams," several times each month. Boys need to be informed about this normal development to prevent embarrassment and fear.

Adults

Most healthy adults need 7 to 9 hours of sleep a night (National Sleep Foundation, n.d.b). However, there is individual variation as some adults may be able to function well (e.g., without sleepiness or drowsiness) with 6 hours of sleep and others may need 10 hours to function optimally. Signs that may indicate that a person is not getting enough sleep include falling asleep or becoming drowsy during a task that is not fatiguing (e.g., listening to a boring or monotonous presentation), not being able to concentrate or remember information, and being unreasonably irritable with others.

The National Sleep Foundation (n.d.b) reports that certain adults are particularly vulnerable for not getting enough sleep: students, shift workers, travelers, and persons suffering from acute stress, depression, or chronic pain. Adults working long hours or multiple jobs may find their sleep less refreshing. Also, the sleep habits of children have an impact on the adults caring for them. Parents and caregivers whose children get the least amount of sleep are twice as likely to say they sleep less than 6 hours a night (National Sleep Foundation, n.d.b). Parents of infants lose the most sleep—nearly an hour on a typical night. Women may experience more disrupted sleep during pregnancy, menses, and the perimenopausal period.

Nurses need to teach adults the importance of obtaining sufficient sleep and tips on how to promote sleep that results in the client waking up feeling restored or refreshed. See the Client Teaching box later in this chapter.

Elders

A hallmark change with age is a tendency toward earlier bedtime and wake times. Older adults (65 to 75 years) usually awaken 1.3 hours earlier and go to bed approximately 1 hour earlier than younger adults (ages 20 to 30). Elders may show an increase in disturbed sleep that can create a negative impact on their quality of life, mood, and alertness. Although the ability to sleep becomes more difficult, the need to sleep does not decrease with age (IOM, 2006, pp. 57–59).

The National Sleep Foundation's 2003 *Sleep in America* poll was the first poll to look at the sleep habits of Americans between the ages of 55 and 84. It found that older adults are sleeping 7 to 9 hours on both weeknights and weekends. Of interest, however, was the striking relationship between the elder individual's health and quality of life and the person's sleep quantity and quality. The poll found that the better the health of older adults, the more likely they are to sleep well. And, conversely, the more diagnosed medical conditions, the more likely they were to report sleep problems (National Sleep Foundation, n.d.c). Elders who have several medical conditions and complain of having sleeping problems should discuss this with their primary care provider. The elder may have a major sleep disorder that is complicating treatment of the other conditions. It is important for the nurse to teach about the connection between sleep, health, and aging. See the Client Teaching box about sleep promotion later in this chapter.

Some elderly clients with dementia may experience *sundown syndrome*. Although not a sleep disorder directly, it refers to a pattern of symptoms (e.g., agitation, anxiety, aggression, and sometimes delusions) that occur in the late afternoon (thus the name). These symptoms can last through the night, further disrupting sleep (Arnold, 2004).

FACTORS AFFECTING SLEEP

Both the quality and the quantity of sleep are affected by a number of factors. *Sleep quality* is a subjective characteristic and is often determined by whether a person wakes up feeling energetic or not. *Quantity of sleep* is the total time the individual sleeps.

Illness

Illness that causes pain or physical distress (e.g., arthritis, back pain) can result in sleep problems. People who are ill require

---

LIFESPAN CONSIDERATIONS   Sleep Disturbances

CHILDREN

Learning to sleep alone without the parent's help is a skill that all children need to master. Regular bedtime routines and rituals such as reading a book help children learn this skill and can prevent sleep disturbance. Some sleep disturbances seen in children include the following:

- Trained night feeder. Infants who are fed during the night, who are fed until they fall asleep and then put in bed, or who have a bottle left with them in their bed learn to expect and demand middle-of-the-night feedings. Infants who are growing well do not need night feeding after about 4 months of age. Infants who are failing to thrive may need feeding at night.
- Sleep refusal. Many toddlers and young children are resistant to settling down to sleep. This sleep refusal may be due to not being tired, anxiety about separation from the parent, stress (e.g., a recent move), lack of a regular sleep routine, the child's temperament, or changes in sleep arrangements (e.g., move from a crib to a "big" bed).
- Night terrors. Night terrors are partial awakenings from non-REM, stage III or IV sleep. They are usually seen in children 3 to 6 years of age. The child may sleepwalk, or may sit up in bed screaming and thrashing about. They usually cannot be wakened, but should be protected from injury, helped back to bed, and soothed back to sleep. Baby-sitters should be alerted to the possibility of a night terror occurring. Children do not remember the incident the next day, and there is no indication of a neurological or emotional problem. Excessive fatigue and a full bladder may contribute to the problem. Having the child take an afternoon nap and empty the bladder before going to sleep at night may be helpful.

ADULTS

- New jobs, pregnancy, and babies are common examples that often disrupt the sleep of a young adult.

- The sleep patterns of middle-aged adults can be disrupted by taking care of elderly parents and/or chronically ill partners in the home.
- See the Client Teaching box on page 1177 for healthy sleep tips for the adult.

ELDERS

The quality of sleep is often diminished in elders. Some of the leading factors that often are influential in sleep disturbances include the following:

- Side effects of medications
- Gastric reflux disease
- Respiratory and circulatory disorders, which may cause breathing problems or discomfort
- Pain from arthritis, increased stiffness, or impaired immobility
- Nocturia
- Depression
- Loss of life partner and/or close friends
- Confusion related to delirium or dementia

Interventions to promote sleep and rest can help enhance the rejuvenation and renewal that sleep provides. The following interventions can help promote sleep:

- Reduce or eliminate the consumption of caffeine and nicotine.
- Be sure their environment is warm and safe, especially if they get out of bed during the night.
- Provide comfort measures, such as analgesics if indicated, and proper positioning.
- Enhance the sense of safety and security by checking on clients frequently and making sure that the call light is within reach.
- If lack of sleep is caused by medications or certain health conditions, interventions should focus on resolving the underlying problem.
- Evaluate the situation and find out what the rest and sleep disturbances mean to the client. They may not perceive sleeplessness to be a serious problem, but will just do other activities and sleep when tired.

more sleep than normal, and the normal rhythm of sleep and wakefulness is often disturbed. People deprived of REM sleep subsequently spend more sleep time than normal in this stage.

Respiratory conditions can disturb an individual's sleep. Shortness of breath often makes sleep difficult, and people who have nasal congestion or sinus drainage may have trouble breathing and hence may find it difficult to sleep.

People who have gastric or duodenal ulcers may find their sleep disturbed because of pain, often a result of the increased gastric secretions that occur during REM sleep.

Certain endocrine disturbances can also affect sleep. Hyperthyroidism lengthens presleep time, making it difficult for a client to fall asleep. Hypothyroidism, conversely, decreases stage IV sleep. Women with low levels of estrogen often report excessive fatigue. In addition, they may experience sleep disruptions due, in part, to the discomfort associated with hot flashes or night sweats that can occur with reduced estrogen levels.

Elevated body temperatures can cause some reduction in delta sleep and REM sleep.

The need to urinate during the night also disrupts sleep, and people who awaken at night to urinate sometimes have difficulty getting back to sleep.

Environment

Environment can promote or hinder sleep. Any change—for example, noise in the environment—can inhibit sleep. The absence of usual stimuli or the presence of unfamiliar stimuli can prevent people from sleeping. Hospital environments can be quite noisy, and special care needs to be taken to reduce noise in the hallways and nursing care units. In fact, some hospitals have instituted "quiet times" in the afternoon on nursing units where the lights are lowered and activity and noise are purposefully decreased so clients can rest or nap.

Discomfort from environmental temperature (e.g., too hot or cold) and lack of ventilation can affect sleep. Light levels can be another factor. A person accustomed to darkness while sleeping may find it difficult to sleep in the light. Another influence includes the comfort and size of the bed. A person's partner who has different sleep habits, snores, or has other sleep difficulties may become a problem for the person also.

Lifestyle

Following an irregular morning and nighttime schedule can affect sleep. Moderate exercise in the morning or early afternoon usually is conducive to sleep, but exercise late in the day can delay sleep. The person's ability to relax before retiring is an important factor affecting the ability to fall asleep. It is best, therefore, to avoid doing homework or office work before or after getting into bed.

Night shift workers frequently obtain less sleep than other workers and have difficulty falling asleep after getting off work. Wearing dark wrap-around sunglasses during the drive home and light-blocking shades can minimize the alerting effects of exposure to daylight, thus making it easier to fall asleep when body temperature is rising.

Emotional Stress

Stress is considered by most sleep experts to be the number one cause of short-term sleeping difficulties (National Sleep Foundation, n.d.b). A person preoccupied with personal problems

---

RESEARCH NOTE   Can Clients Sleep in a Hospital?

Nurses know the importance of sleep. However, the researchers believe that sleep has been undervalued by nursing practice. For example, noise is a major disturbance in the hospital setting, making it difficult for clients to sleep. Clients are often awakened early for obtaining lab specimens, weights, assessments, and medication administration. Using a conceptual model developed by Dreher, the researchers implemented a nonpharmacological intervention to promote sleep on a 36-bed medical unit.

Guided by a nurse manager, clinical nurse IV, and gerontological clinical nurse specialist, the certified nursing assistants (CNAs) completed an educational program about how to implement nonpharmacological interventions that promote sleep. The program used "sleep baskets" which held materials needed for the interventions and a list of possible interventions to help remind the CNA (e.g., back rub, warm drink, aromatherapy, a warmed blanket, relaxation music, earplugs, and closed doors).

In preparation for bedtime, the CNA used the sleep basket and asked the client to select sleep interventions. In addition, other noise reduction strategies were used. Staff were reminded to use "quiet voices" after 10 PM and to avoid hallway discussions on the night shift. Doors to client rooms were closed when bedtime routines were completed (unless the client required close monitoring). And, the intercom was not used at night.

To evaluate the effectiveness of the project, the CNA who used a sleep basket on the evening shift completed a form as to which interventions were performed. The next morning, the day CNA asked the client to rate the quality and quantity of sleep, to identify which interventions were the most helpful, and if the nonpharmacological interventions helped them sleep. During the evaluation period, 40 clients (average age of 75) were evaluated. The warmed blanket was their favorite intervention. Seventy-five percent of the clients stated that the interventions helped them sleep, and 60% rated their sleep quality as "good."

IMPLICATIONS

Project interventions appear helpful for sleep improvement, especially during the retiring phase of sleep. The researchers state that the program is now being used on four nursing units. Nurses and CNAs are more aware of clients who have had an exhausting day and try to help these clients take a 45-minute nap by posting signs that say: "Do not disturb. Client napping between the hours of _____ and _____."

Note: From "The Sh-h-h-h Project. Nonpharmacological Interventions" by S. B. Robinson, T. Weitzel, & L. Henderson. (2005). *Holistic Nursing Practice, 19*(6), 263–266. Copyright Lippincott, Williams & Wilkins. Reprinted with permission.

(e.g., school- or job-related pressures, family or marriage problems) may be unable to relax sufficiently to get to sleep. Anxiety increases the norepinephrine blood levels through stimulation of the sympathetic nervous system. This chemical change results in less deep sleep and REM sleep and more stage changes and awakenings.

Stimulants and Alcohol

Caffeine-containing beverages act as stimulants of the central nervous system. Drinking beverages containing caffeine in the afternoon or evening may interfere with sleep. People who drink an excessive amount of alcohol often find their sleep disturbed. Alcohol disrupts REM sleep, although it may hasten the onset of sleep. While making up for lost REM sleep after some of the effects of the alcohol have worn off, people often experience nightmares. The alcohol-tolerant person may be unable to sleep well and become irritable as a result.

Diet

Weight gain has been associated with reduced total sleep time as well as broken sleep and earlier awakening. Weight loss, on the other hand, seems to be associated with an increase in total sleep time and less broken sleep. Dietary L-tryptophan—found, for example, in cheese and milk—may induce sleep, a fact that might explain why warm milk helps some people get to sleep.

Smoking

Nicotine has a stimulating effect on the body, and smokers often have more difficulty falling asleep than nonsmokers do. Smokers are usually easily aroused and often describe themselves as light sleepers. By refraining from smoking after the evening meal, the person usually sleeps better; moreover, many former smokers report that their sleeping patterns improved once they stopped smoking.

Motivation

Motivation can increase alertness in some situations (e.g., a tired person can probably stay alert while attending an interesting concert or surfing the Web late at night). Motivation alone, however, is usually not sufficient to overcome the normal circadian drive to sleep during the night. Nor is motivation sufficient to overcome sleepiness due to insufficient sleep. Boredom alone is not sufficient to cause sleepiness, but when insufficient sleep combines with boredom, sleep is likely to occur.

Medications

Some medications affect the quality of sleep. Most hypnotics can interfere with deep sleep and suppress REM sleep. Beta-blockers have been known to cause insomnia and nightmares. Narcotics, such as meperidine hydrochloride (Demerol) and morphine, are known to suppress REM sleep and to cause frequent awakenings and drowsiness. Tranquilizers interfere with REM sleep. Although antidepressants suppress REM sleep, this effect is considered a therapeutic action. In fact, selectively depriving a depressed client of REM sleep will result in an immediate but transient improvement in mood. Clients accustomed to taking hypnotic medications and antidepressants may experience a REM rebound (increased REM sleep) when these medications are discontinued. Warning clients to expect a period of more intense dreams when these medications are discontinued may reduce their anxiety about this symptom. Boxes 45–2 and 45–3 list drugs that can disrupt sleep or cause excessive daytime sleepiness.

COMMON SLEEP DISORDERS

A knowledge of common sleep disorders can help nurses assess the sleep complaints of their clients and, when appropriate, make a referral to a specialist in sleep disorders medicine. Although sleep

---

RESEARCH NOTE Are Shortened Sleep Durations Contributing to the Growing Epidemic of Obesity?

Previous studies have shown that sleep deprivation results in decreased leptin levels and increased ghrelin levels (two hormones involved in the regulation of appetite and hunger), markedly elevated hunger and appetite ratings, and cravings for sweet, starch, and salty snacks. Sleep loss has also been linked to changes in decreased glucose tolerance and altered insulin responses to glucose challenges in healthy individuals.

To determine if the number of hours of sleep was associated with obesity and weight gain, the researchers used data from 9,588 adults who participated in the 1982–1984, 1987, and 1992 Epidemiologic Follow-up Studies of the First National Health and Nutrition Examination Survey (NHANES I). After controlling for depression, physical activity, education, ethnicity, alcohol consumption, cigarette smoking, gender, waking during the night, daytime sleepiness, and age, a longitudinal and cross-sectional analysis showed that participants who obtained less than 7 hours sleep were significantly more likely to be obese or overweight. Subjects obtaining 5 hours of sleep were 60% more likely to be obese, and subjects obtaining 6 hours of sleep per night were 27% more likely

to be obese than subjects obtaining 7 hours of sleep. Males who averaged over 9 hours of sleep per night, and females who averaged 8 hours of sleep per night were also more likely to be obese than those who averaged only 7 hours of sleep per night.

IMPLICATIONS

This very large study suggests that short sleep durations may be a contributing factor to the current epidemic of obesity in the country. The researchers acknowledge that the longer sleep times associated with obesity may relate to the presence of a pre-existing sleep disorder (e.g., sleep apnea), something that subjects were not screened for when the study began in 1982. The optimal sleep duration for adults, based on this study and others, appears to be 7 hours.

Note: From *Sleep* by J. E. Gangwisch, D. Malaspina, B. Boden-Albala, and S. B. Heymsfield. Copyright 2005 by *American Academy of Sleep Medicine.* Reproduced with permission of *American Academy of Sleep Medicine* in the format Textbook via Copyright Clearance Center.

These drugs may disrupt REM sleep, delay onset of sleep, or decrease sleep time:

- Alcohol
- Amphetamines
- Antidepressants
- Beta-blockers
- Bronchodilators
- Caffeine
- Decongestants
- Narcotics
- Steroids

CLINICAL MANIFESTATIONS INSOMNIA

- Difficulty falling asleep
- Waking up frequently during the night
- Difficulty returning to sleep
- Waking up too early in the morning
- Unrefreshing sleep
- Daytime sleepiness
- Difficulty concentrating
- Irritability

Note: From "Insomnia Symptoms" by National Sleep Foundation, 2005b. Retrieved July 2, 2006, from http://www.sleepfoundation.forg/sleeptionary/index.php?id=19&subsection=symptoms. Used with permission of the National Sleep Foundation. For further information, please visit http://www.sleepfoundation.org

disorders are typically categorized for the purpose of research as dysomnias, parasomnias, and disorders associated with medical or psychiatric illness, it is usually more appropriate for clinicians to focus on the client's symptoms (e.g., insomnia, excessive sleepiness, and abnormal events) occurring during sleep (parasomnias).

Insomnia

Insomnia is described as the inability to fall asleep or remain asleep. Persons with insomnia awaken not feeling rested.

Insomnia is the most common sleep complaint in America. Acute insomnia lasts one to several nights and is often caused by personal stressors and/or worry. If the insomnia persists for longer than a month, it is considered chronic insomnia. More often, people experience chronic-intermittent insomnia, which means difficulty sleeping for a few nights, followed by a few nights of adequate sleep before the problem returns (National Sleep Foundation, 2005a). See Clinical Manifestations for symptoms of insomnia. The two main risk factors of insomnia are older age and female gender (IOM, 2006, p. 91). Women suffer sleep loss in connection with hormonal changes (e.g., menstruation, pregnancy, and menopause). The incidence of insomnia increases with age, but it is thought that this is caused by some other medical condition.

Treatment for insomnia frequently requires the client to develop new behavior patterns that induce sleep and maintain sleep. Examples of behavioral treatments include the following:

- Stimulus control: creating a sleep environment that promotes sleep
- Cognitive therapy: learning to develop positive thoughts and beliefs about sleep
- Sleep restriction: following a program that limits time in bed in order to get to sleep and stay asleep throughout the night (National Sleep Foundation, 2005a).

These drugs may be associated with excessive daytime sleepiness:

- Antidepressants
- Antihistamines
- Beta-blockers
- Narcotics

The long-term efficacy of hypnotic medications is questionable. Such medications do not deal with the cause of the problem, and their prolonged use can create drug dependencies. Although antihistamines such as diphenhydramine (Benadryl) are thought to be safer for elderly clients than hypnotics, their side effects (i.e., atropine-like effects, dizziness, sedation, and hypotension) make them extremely hazardous. In fact, antihistamines should not be recommended for any client with a history of asthma, increased intraocular pressure, hyperthyroidism, cardiovascular disease, or hypertension.

Excessive Daytime Sleepiness

Clients may experience excessive daytime sleepiness as a result of hypersomnia, narcolepsy, sleep apnea, and insufficient sleep.

Hypersomnia

Hypersomnia refers to conditions where the affected individual obtains sufficient sleep at night but still cannot stay awake during the day. Hypersomnia can be caused by medical conditions, for example, central nervous system damage and certain kidney, liver, or metabolic disorders, such as diabetic acidosis and hypothyroidism. Rarely does hypersomnia have a psychological origin.

Narcolepsy

Narcolepsy is a disorder of excessive daytime sleepiness caused by the lack of the chemical hypocretin in the area of the central nervous system that regulates sleep. Clients with narcolepsy have sleep attacks or excessive daytime sleepiness, and their sleep at night usually begins with a sleep-onset REM period (dreaming sleep occurs within the first 15 minutes of falling asleep). The majority of clients also have cataplexy or the sudden onset of muscle weakness or paralysis in association with strong emotion, sleep paralysis (transient paralysis when falling asleep or waking up), hypnagogic hallucinations (visual, auditory, or tactile hallucinations at sleep onset or when waking up), and/or fragmented nighttime sleep. Their fragmented nocturnal sleep is not the cause of their excessive daytime sleepiness; many clients, particularly younger clients, have sound restorative nocturnal sleep but still cannot stay awake during the daytime. Onset of symptoms tends to occur between ages 15 and 30, and symptom severity usually stabilizes within the first 5 years of onset. Central nervous system stimulants such as methylphenidate (Ritalin) or amphetamines have been used to reduce excessive daytime sleepiness. Antidepressants, both older MAO inhibitors and the newer sertonergic antidepressants, are usually quite effective for controlling cataplexy. In 1999, the U.S. Food and Drug Administration (FDA), approved modafinil (Provigil) for control of excessive daytime sleepiness in narcoleptic clients. Although its exact mechanism of action is unknown, it has fewer side effects, and a lower potential for abuse. A second drug, sodium oxybate (Xyrem), approved in 2002 for the treatment of cataplexy, has also been shown to reduce excessive daytime sleepiness in clients with narcolepsy. Because Xyrem is difficult to administer (it is only available as a liquid and taken at bedtime and then again 2.5 to 4 hours after sleep onset) and its use is tightly controlled by the FDA, only those clients whose symptoms are not controlled by other medications are usually offered Xyrem. Only one pharmacy in the United States is allowed to dispense Xyrem. As a result, clients need to allow adequate time for obtaining their medications from the central pharmacy.

> **CLINICAL ALERT**
>
> Sodium oxybate is also known as gamma hydroxybutyrate or GHB—one of the drugs frequently associated with "date rapes." ■

Sleep Apnea

Sleep apnea is characterized by frequent short breathing pauses during sleep. Although all individuals have occasional periods of apnea during sleep, more than five apneic episodes or five breathing pauses longer than 10 seconds/hour is considered abnormal and should be evaluated by a sleep medicine specialist. Symptoms suggestive of sleep apnea include loud snoring, frequent nocturnal awakenings, excessive daytime sleepiness, difficulties falling asleep at night, morning headaches, memory and cognitive problems, and irritability. Although sleep apnea is most frequently diagnosed in men and postmenopausal women, it may occur during childhood.

The periods of apnea, which last from 10 seconds to 2 minutes, occur during REM or NREM sleep. Frequency of episodes ranges from 50 to 600 per night. Because these apneic pauses are usually associated with an arousal, clients frequently report that their sleep is nonrestorative and that they regularly fall asleep when engaging in sedentary activities during the day.

Three common types of sleep apnea are obstructive apnea, central apnea, and mixed apnea. Obstructive apnea occurs when the structures of the pharynx or oral cavity block the flow of air. The person continues to try to breathe; that is, the chest and abdominal muscles move. The movements of the diaphragm become stronger and stronger until the obstruction is removed. Enlarged tonsils and adenoids, a deviated nasal septum, nasal polyps, and obesity predispose the client to obstructive apnea. An episode of obstructive sleep apnea usually begins with snoring; thereafter, breathing ceases, followed by marked snorting as breathing resumes. Toward the end of each apneic episode, increased carbon dioxide levels in the blood cause the client to wake.

Central apnea is thought to involve a defect in the respiratory center of the brain. All actions involved in breathing, such as chest movement and airflow, cease. Clients who have brain stem injuries and muscular dystrophy, for example, often have central sleep apnea. At this time, there is no available treatment. Mixed apnea is a combination of central apnea and obstructive apnea.

Treatment for sleep apnea is directed at the cause of the apnea. For example, enlarged tonsils may be removed. Other surgical procedures, including laser removal of excess tissue in the pharynx, reduce or eliminate snoring and may be effective in relieving the apnea. In other cases, the use of a nasal continuous positive airway pressure (CPAP) device at night is effective in maintaining an open airway. Weight loss may also help decrease the severity of symptoms.

Sleep apnea profoundly affects a person's work or school performance. In addition, prolonged sleep apnea can cause a sharp rise in blood pressure and may lead to cardiac arrest. Over time, apneic episodes can cause cardiac arrhythmias, pulmonary hypertension, and subsequent left-sided heart failure.

> **CLINICAL ALERT**
>
> Partners of clients with sleep apnea may become aware of the problem because they hear snoring that stops during the apneic period and then restarts. Surgical removal of tonsils or other tissue in the pharynx, if not the cause of the sleep apnea, can actually worsen the situation by removing the snoring and, thus, the warning that apnea is occurring. ■

Insufficient Sleep

Healthy individuals who obtain less sleep than they need will experience sleepiness and fatigue during the daytime hours. Depending on the severity and chronicity of this voluntary, albeit unintentional sleep deprivation, individuals may develop attention and concentration deficits, reduced vigilance, distractibility, reduced motivation, fatigue, malaise, and occasionally diplopia and dry mouth. The cause of these symptoms may or may not be attributed to insufficient sleep, since many Americans believe that 6.8 hours of sleep is sufficient to maintain optimal daytime performance. In fact, the sleep times of Americans have decreased dramatically over the past decade, with adults averaging only 6.8 hours of sleep on weekdays and 7.4 hours on weekends. All age groups, not just adults and adolescents, are getting less than the recommended amounts of sleep. Even 4 to 5-year-old children now average less than 9.5 hours of sleep, approximately 1.5 to 2.5 hours less than recommended.

Although the effects of obtaining less than optimal amounts of sleep are generally considered benign, there is growing evidence that insufficient sleep can have significant deleterious effects. Staying awake 19 consecutive hours produces the same impairments in reaction times and cognitive function as a blood alcohol level of 0.05, and staying awake for 24 consecutive hours has the same effects on reaction times and cognitive function as being legally drunk (with a blood alcohol level of 0.1). Nurses who report reduced hours of sleep are more likely to make an error, to have difficulty staying awake on duty, and to have difficulty staying awake while driving home from work than those who obtained more sleep.

When clients report obtaining more sleep on weekends or days off, it usually indicates that they are not obtaining sufficient sleep.

BOX 45–4   Parasomnias

- *Bruxism.* Usually occurring during stage II NREM sleep, this clenching and grinding of the teeth can eventually erode dental crowns, cause teeth to come loose, and lead to deterioration of the temporomandibular joint and TMJ syndrome.
- *Enuresis.* Bed-wetting during sleep can occur in children over 3 years old. More males than females are affected. It often occurs 1 to 2 hours after falling asleep, when rousing from NREM stages III and IV.
- *Periodic limb movements (PLMs) disorder.* In this condition, the legs jerk twice or three times per minute during sleep. It is most common among elders. This kicking motion can wake the client and result in poor sleep. The condition may be treated with medications such as those otherwise used for Parkinson's disease. PLMs differ from restless leg syndrome (RLS), which occurs whenever the person is at rest, not just at night when sleeping. RLS may occur during pregnancy or be due to other medical problems that can be treated.
- *Sleeptalking.* Talking during sleep occurs during NREM sleep before REM sleep. It rarely presents a problem to the person unless it becomes troublesome to others.
- *Somnambulism.* Somnambulism (sleepwalking) occurs during stages III and IV of NREM sleep. It is episodic and usually occurs 1 to 2 hours after falling asleep. Sleepwalkers tend not to notice dangers (e.g., stairs) and often need to be protected from injury.

Convincing the client to obtain more sleep may be difficult, but it can result in the resolution of their daytime symptoms.

Parasomnias

A **parasomnia** is behavior that may interfere with sleep and may even occur during sleep. The *International Classification of Sleep Disorders* (American Sleep Disorders Association, 2005) subdivides parasomnias into arousal disorders (e.g., sleepwalking, sleep terrors), sleep–wake transition disorders (e.g., sleep talking), parasomnias associated with REM sleep (e.g., nightmares), and others (e.g., bruxism). Box 45–4 describes examples of parasomnias.

NURSING MANAGEMENT

Assessing

A complete assessment of a client's sleep difficulty includes a sleep history, health history, physical exam, and, if warranted, a sleep diary and diagnostic studies. Only nurse practitioners with specialized training should investigate a complaint of excessive daytime sleepiness, investigate a sleep complaint lasting more than 6 months, or order and interpret diagnostic studies. All nurses, however, can take a brief sleep history and educate their clients about normal sleep.

Sleep History

A brief sleep history, which is usually part of the comprehensive nursing history, should be obtained for all clients entering a health care facility. It should, however, be deferred or omitted if the client is critically ill. Key questions to ask include the following:

- When do you usually go to sleep? And when do you wake up? Do you nap? If so, when? If the client is a child, it is also

important to ask about bedtime rituals. This information provides the nurse with information about the client's usual sleep duration and preferred sleep times, and allows for the incorporation of the client's preferences in the plan of care.

- Do you have any problems with your sleep? Has anyone ever told you that you snore loudly or thrash around a lot at night? Are you able to stay awake at work, when driving, or engaging in your usual activities?

  These questions elicit information about sleep complaints including the possibility of excessive daytime sleepiness. Loud snoring suggests the possibility of obstructive sleep apnea, and any client replying yes to this question should be referred to a specialist in sleep disorders medicine. Referrals should also be made if clients indicate they have difficulty staying awake during the day or that their movements disturb the sleep of their bed partners.

- Do you take any prescribed medications, over-the-counter medications, or herbal remedies to help you sleep? Or to stay awake?

  This information alerts the nurse to the use of prescription hypnotics and stimulants as well as the use of over-the-counter sleep aids and herbal remedies.

- Is there anything else I need to know about your sleep?

  This allows the client to voice any concerns or bring up topics that the nurse may not have asked about.

If the client is being admitted to a long-term care facility, it is also appropriate to ask about preferred room temperature, lighting (complete darkness versus using a night-light), and preferred bedtime routine.

A more detailed assessment is required if the client indicates any difficulty sleeping, difficulty remaining awake during the day, and/or recent changes in sleep pattern. This detailed history should explore the exact nature of the problem and its cause, when it first began and its frequency, how it affects daily living, what the client is doing to cope with the problem, and whether these methods have been effective. Questions the nurse might ask the client with a sleeping disturbance are shown in the accompanying Assessment Interview.

Health History

A health history is obtained to rule out medical or psychiatric causes of the client's difficulty sleeping. It is important to note that the presence of a medical or psychiatric illness (e.g., depression, Parkinson's disease, Alzheimer's disease, arthritis, or other disorders) does not preclude the possibility that a second problem (e.g., obstructive sleep apnea) may be contributing to the difficulty sleeping. Since medications can frequently cause or exacerbate sleep disturbances, information should be obtained about all of the prescribed and nonprescription medications, including herbal remedies that a client consumes.

Physical Examination

Rarely are sleep abnormalities noted during the physical exam unless the client has obstructive sleep apnea or some other health problem. Common findings among clients with sleep apnea include an enlarged and reddened uvula and soft palate, enlarged tonsils and adenoids (in children), obesity (in adults), and in male clients a neck size greater than 17.5 inches. Occasionally a deviated septum may be noted, but it is rarely the cause of obstructive sleep apnea.

Sleep Diary

A sleep specialist may ask clients to keep a sleep diary or log for 1 to 2 weeks in order to get a more complete picture of their sleep complaints. A sleep diary may include all or selected aspects of the following information that pertain to the client's specific problem:

■ Time of (a) going to bed, (b) trying to fall asleep, (c) falling asleep (approximate time), (d) any instances of waking up and duration of these periods, (e) waking up in the morning, and (f) any naps and their duration

■ Activities performed 2 to 3 hours before bedtime (type, duration, and time)

■ Consumption of caffeinated beverages and alcohol and amounts of those beverages

■ Any prescribed medications, over-the-counter medications, and herbal remedies taken during the day

■ Bedtime rituals before sleep

■ Any difficulties remaining awake during the day and times when difficulties occurred

■ Any worries that the client believes may affect sleep

■ Factors that the client believes have a positive or negative effect on sleep

If the client is a child, the sleep diary or log may be completed by a parent.

Diagnostic Studies

Sleep is measured objectively in a sleep disorder laboratory by **polysomnography:** An **electroencephalogram (EEG), electromyogram (EMG),** and **electro-oculogram (EOG)** are recorded simultaneously. Electrodes are placed on the scalp to record brain waves (EEG), on the outer canthus of each eye to record eye movement (EOG), and on the chin muscles to record the structural electromyogram (EMG). The electrodes transmit electric energy from the cerebral cortex and muscles of the face to pens that record the brain waves and muscle activity on graph paper. Respiratory effort and airflow, ECG, leg movements, and oxygen saturation are also monitored. Oxygen saturation is determined by monitoring with a pulse oximeter, a light-sensitive electric cell that attaches to the ear or a finger. Oxygen saturation and ECG assessments are of particular importance if sleep apnea is suspected. Through polysomnography, the client's activity (movements, struggling, noisy respirations) during sleep can be assessed. Such activity of which the client is unaware may be the cause of arousal during sleep.

Diagnosing

Insomnia, the NANDA (2007) diagnosis given to clients with sleep problems, is usually made more explicit with descriptions such as "difficulty falling asleep" or "difficulty staying asleep;" for example, *Insomnia* (delayed onset of sleep) related to overstimulation prior to bedtime.

Various factors or etiologies may be involved and must be specified for the individual. These include physical discomfort or pain; anxiety about actual or anticipated loss of a loved one, loss of a job, loss of life due to serious disease process, or worry about a family member's behavior or illness; frequent changes in sleep time due to shift work or overtime; and changes in sleep environment or bedtime rituals (e.g., noisy environment, alcohol or other drug dependency, drug withdrawal, misuse of sedatives prescribed for insomnia, and effects of medications such as steroids or stimulants). Examples of clinical applications of this diagnosis using NANDA, NIC, and NOC designations are shown in Identifying Nursing Diagnoses, Outcomes, and Interventions.

Sleep pattern disturbances may also be stated as the etiology of another diagnosis, in which case the nursing interventions are

IDENTIFYING NURSING DIAGNOSES, OUTCOMES, AND INTERVENTIONS
Clients with Sleep Problems

DATA CLUSTER Gillian Marks, 51, states she has had a problem falling asleep since her mastectomy 2 months ago. Says fears of prognosis become prominent when she is not active and busy. Has tried reading or watching TV but neither make her sleepy or relaxed. Appears agitated and restless.

NURSING DIAGNOSIS/ DEFINITION	SAMPLE DESIRED OUTCOMES*/ DEFINITION	INDICATORS	SELECTED INTERVENTIONS*/ DEFINITION	SAMPLE NIC ACTIVITIES
Insomnia/A disruption in amount and quality of sleep that impairs functioning	Personal Well-Being [2002]/Extent of positive perception of one's own health status and life circumstances	Very satisfied with • Ability to relax • Ability to express emotions	Coping Enhancement [5230]/Assisting a patient to adapt to perceived stressors, changes, or threats that interfere with meeting life demands and roles	• Appraise adjustment to changes in body image • Explore previous methods of dealing with life problems • Encourage verbalization of feelings, perceptions, and fears • Instruct on the use of relaxation techniques

DATA CLUSTER Thomas Strep states that a recent shortage of paramedics has resulted in extensive overtime and frequent "double shifts" and rotations from his usual two weekly 7–3 and 3–7 shifts. States, "All I want to do is go to sleep when I get home, but I can't. I guess I'm too riled up."

Sleep Deprivation/ Prolonged periods of time without sleep (sustained natural, periodic suspension of relative consciousness)	Rest [0003]/Quantity and pattern of diminished activity for mental and physical rejuvenation	Not compromised • Amount of rest • Rest pattern • Mentally rested	Progressive Muscle Relaxation [1460]/ Facilitating the tensing and releasing of successive muscle groups while attending to the resulting differences in sensation Simple Guided Imagery [6000]/ Purposeful use of imagination to achieve relaxation and/or direct attention away from undesirable sensations	• Choose quiet, comfortable setting • Have the client tense, for 5 to 10 seconds, each of 8 to 16 major muscle groups • Instruct client to focus on the sensations in the muscles when tensed and when relaxed • Discuss an image the client has experienced that is pleasurable and relaxing, such as lying on a beach, watching a snowfall, floating on a raft • Choose a scene that involves as many of the senses as possible • Have the client travel mentally to the scene and report how it smells, looks, feels, etc. • Assist the client to develop a method of ending the imagery such as counting while breathing deeply

*The NOC # for desired outcomes and the NIC # for nursing interventions are listed in brackets following the appropriate outcome or intervention. Outcomes, indicators, interventions, and activities selected are only a sample of those suggested by NOC and NIC and should be further individualized for each client.

directed toward the sleep disturbance itself. Examples include the following:

■ *Risk for Injury* related to somnambulism
■ *Ineffective Coping* related to insufficient quality and quantity of sleep
■ *Fatigue* related to insufficient sleep
■ *Risk for Impaired Gas Exchange* related to sleep apnea
■ *Deficient Knowledge* (Nonprescription remedies for sleep) related to misinformation
■ *Anxiety* related to sleep apnea and/or the diagnosis of a sleep disorder
■ *Activity Intolerance* related to sleep deprivation or excessive daytime sleepiness

Planning

The major goal for clients with sleep disturbances is to maintain (or develop) a sleeping pattern that provides sufficient energy for daily activities. Other goals may relate to enhancing the client's feeling of well-being or improving the quality and quantity of the client's sleep. The nurse plans specific nursing interventions to reach the goal based on the etiology of each nursing diagnosis. These interventions may include reducing environmental distractions, promoting bedtime rituals, providing comfort measures, scheduling nursing care to provide for uninterrupted sleep periods, and teaching stress reduction, relaxation techniques, or good sleep hygiene.

Examples of NOC outcomes and NIC interventions to assist clients with sleep disturbances are shown in Identifying Nursing Diagnoses, Outcomes, and Interventions. Specific nursing activities associated with each of these interventions can be selected to meet the individual needs of the client. See the Nursing Care Plan and Concept Map at the end of the chapter.

Implementing

Sleep hygiene is a term referring to interventions used to promote sleep. Nursing interventions to enhance the quantity and quality of clients' sleep involve largely nonpharmacologic measures. These involve health teaching about sleep habits, support of bedtime rituals, the provision of a restful environment, specific measures to promote comfort and relaxation, and appropriate use of hypnotic medications.

For hospitalized clients, sleep problems are often related to the hospital environment or their illness. Assisting the client to sleep in such instances can be challenging to a nurse, often involving scheduling activities, administering analgesics, and providing a supportive environment. Explanations and a supportive relationship are essential for the fearful or anxious client. Different types of hypnotics may be prescribed depending on the type of sleep problem (e.g., difficulties falling asleep or difficulties maintaining sleep). Drugs with longer half-lives are often prescribed for difficulties maintaining sleep, but must be used with caution in the elderly.

Client Teaching

Healthy individuals need to learn the importance of sleep in maintaining active and productive lifestyles. They need to learn (a) the conditions that promote sleep and those that interfere with sleep, (b) safe use of sleep medications, (c) effects of other prescribed medications on sleep, and (d) effects of their disease states on sleep. Client teaching for promoting sleep is shown in Client Teaching.

Supporting Bedtime Rituals

Most people are accustomed to bedtime rituals or presleep routines that are conducive to comfort and relaxation. Altering or eliminating such routines can affect a client's sleep. Common prebedtime activities of adults include listening to music, reading, taking a soothing bath, and praying. Children need to be socialized into a presleep routine such as a bedtime story, holding onto a favorite toy or blanket, and kissing everyone goodnight. Sleep is also usually preceded by hygienic routines, such as washing the face and hands (or bathing), brushing the teeth, and voiding.

In institutional settings, nurses can provide similar bedtime rituals—assisting with a hand and face wash, providing a massage or hot drink, plumping of pillows, and providing extra blankets as needed. Conversing about accomplishments of the day or enjoyable events such as visits from friends can also help to relax clients and bring peace of mind.

Creating a Restful Environment

All people need a sleeping environment with minimal noise, a comfortable room temperature, appropriate ventilation, and appropriate lighting. Although most people prefer a darkened environment, a low light source may provide comfort for children or those in a strange environment. Infants and children need a

---

CLIENT TEACHING   Promoting Sleep

SLEEP PATTERN

- If you have difficulty falling asleep or staying asleep, it is important to establish a regular bedtime and wake-up time for all days of the week to enhance your biological rhythm. A short daytime nap (e.g., 15 to 30 minutes), particularly among elders, can be restorative and not interfere with nighttime sleep. A younger person with insomnia should not nap.
- Establish a regular, relaxing bedtime routine before sleep such as reading, listening to soft music, taking a warm bath, or doing some other quiet activity you enjoy.
- Avoid dealing with office work or family problems before bedtime.
- Get adequate exercise during the day to reduce stress, but avoid excessive physical exertion at least 3 hours before bedtime.
- Use the bed for sleep or sexual activity, so that you associate it with sleep. Take work material, computers, and TVs out of the bedroom. Lying awake, tossing and turning, will strengthen the association between wakefulness and lying in bed (many people with insomnia report falling asleep in a chair or in front of the TV but having trouble falling asleep in bed).
- When you are unable to sleep, get out of bed, go into another room, and pursue some relaxing activity until you feel drowsy.

ENVIRONMENT

- Create a sleep-conducive environment that is dark, quiet, comfortable, and cool.

- Keep noise to a minimum; block out extraneous noise as necessary with white noise from a fan, air conditioner, or white noise machine. Music is not recommended as studies have shown that music will promote wakefulness (it is interesting and people will pay attention to it).
- Sleep on a comfortable mattress and pillows.

DIET

- Avoid heavy meals 2 to 3 hours before bedtime.
- Avoid alcohol and caffeine-containing foods and beverages (e.g., coffee, tea, chocolate) at least 4 hours before bedtime. Caffeine can interfere with sleep. Both caffeine and alcohol act as diuretics, creating the need to void during sleep time.
- If a bedtime snack is necessary, consume only light carbohydrates or a milk drink. Heavy or spicy foods can cause gastrointestinal upsets that disturb sleep.

MEDICATIONS

- Use sleeping medications only as a last resort. Use over-the-counter medications sparingly because many contain antihistamines that cause daytime drowsiness.
- Take analgesics before bedtime to relieve aches and pains.
- Consult with your health care provider about adjusting other medications that may cause insomnia.

6. A college student was referred to the campus health service because of difficulty staying awake in class. Of the following items, what should be included in the nurse's assessment? Select all that apply.
   1. Amount of sleep he usually obtains during the week and on weekends
   2. How much alcohol he usually consumes
   3. Onset and duration of symptoms
   4. Whether or not his classes are boring

7. During a yearly physical, a 52-year-old male client mentions that his wife frequently complains about his snoring. During the physical exam, the nurse notes that his neck size is 18 inches, his soft palate and uvula are reddened and swollen, and he is overweight. The most appropriate nursing intervention for this client is to:
   1. Recommend that he and his wife sleep in separate bedrooms so that his snoring does not disturb his wife.
   2. Refer him to a dietitian for a weight loss program.
   3. Caution him not to drink or take sleeping pills since they may make his snoring worse.
   4. Refer him to a sleep disorders center for evaluation and treatment of his symptoms.

8. A new nursing graduate's first job requires 12-hour night shifts. Which of the following strategies will make it easier for the graduate to sleep during the day and remain awake at night?
   1. Wear dark wrap-around sunglasses when driving home in the morning, and sleep in a darkened bedroom.
   2. Exercise on the way home to avoid having to stand around waiting for equipment at the gym.
   3. Drink several cups of strong coffee or 16 oz of caffeinated soda when beginning the shift.
   4. Try to stay in a brightly lit area when working at night.

9. The nurse is answering questions after a presentation on sleep at a local senior citizens center. A woman in her late 70s asks for an opinion about the advisability of allowing her husband to nap for 15 to 20 minutes each afternoon. The nurse's best response would be which of the following?
   1. "Taking an afternoon nap will interfere with his being able to sleep at night. If he's tired in the afternoon, see if you can interest him in some type of stimulating activity to keep him awake."
   2. "He shouldn't need to take an afternoon nap if he's getting enough sleep at night."
   3. "Unless your husband has trouble falling asleep at night, a brief afternoon nap is fine."
   4. "Encourage him to consume coffee or some other caffeinated beverage at lunch to prevent drowsiness in the afternoon."

10. During admission to a hospital unit, the client tells the nurse that her sleep tends to be very light and that it is difficult for her to get back to sleep if she's awakened at night. Which of the following interventions should the nurse implement? Select all that apply.
    1. Remind colleagues to keep their conversation in the halls to a minimum at night.
    2. Encourage the client's family members to bring in a radio to play soft music at night.
    3. Avoid scheduling medications and procedures including vital signs between 11 PM and 6 AM.
    4. Encourage the client to ask family members to bring in a fan to provide white noise.

See Answers to Test Your Knowledge in Appendix A. ∞

EXPLORE MEDIALINK   www.prenhall.com/berman

DVD-ROM
▨ Audio Glossary
▨ NCLEX Review
▨ Video: Sleep Apnea

COMPANION WEBSITE
▨ Additional NCLEX Review
▨ Case Study: Client with Difficulty Falling Asleep
▨ Care Plan Activity: Client with a Sleep Disorder
▨ Application Activity: Diagnosing Sleep Apnea
▨ Links to Resources

READINGS AND REFERENCES

SUGGESTED READINGS
Griffiths, M. F., & Peerson, A. (2005). Risk factors for chronic insomnia following hospitalization. *Journal of Advanced Nursing, 49,* 245–253.
The researchers evaluated the sleep of 86 clients prior to elective cardiac and orthopedic procedures and 3 months after their discharge. Prior to surgery, 10% of the participants reported symptoms of insomnia (quite similar to the prevalence of insomnia in adults). Afterwards, 19% of the participants reported insomnia.
Lower, J., Bonsack, C., & Guion, J. (2003). Peace and quiet. *Nursing Management, 34*(4), 40A – 40D.
The authors reviewed factors that make it difficult for clients to rest in hospitals and steps that are needed to help provide a healing
environment (e.g., uninterrupted sleep, massage, music). They describe their vision, implementation, and outcomes of providing quiet time between 2 and 4 PM for clients in two ICUs.*
Tranmer, J. E., Minard, J. Fox, L. A., & Rebelo, L. (2003). The sleep of medical and surgical clients. *Clinical Nursing Research, 12,* 159–173.
The researchers surveyed 56 surgical clients and 54 medical clients about their sleep during a 3-day period. Surgical clients reported receiving more care during the night than medical clients, although the intensity of care decreased as the postop period lengthened. Medical clients were more likely than surgical clients to receive sedative or hypnotic medications. Most clients reported
receiving some type of analgesic at night and having their sleep interrupted at least once for vital signs, venipuncture, or dressing changes. Pain, noise, and environmental factors were frequency cited as causes of disturbed sleep.*

RELATED RESEARCH
Carter, P. A., & Action, G. J. (2006). Personality and coping: Predictors of depression and sleep problems among caregivers of individuals who have cancer. *Journal of Gerontological Nursing, 32*(2), 45–53.
Dorsey, C. M., Lee, K. A., & Scharf, M. B. (2004). Effect of zolpidem on sleep in women with perimenopausal and postmenopausal insomnia: A 4-week, randomized, multicenter, double-blind, placebo-controlled study. *Clinical Therapeutics. 26,* 1578–1586.

Huth, M. M., Zink, K. A., & van Horn, N. R. (2005). The effects of massage therapy in improving outcomes for youth with cystic fibrosis: An evidence review. *Pediatric Nursing, 31,* 328–333.

McNamara, M. E., Burnham, D. C., Smith, C., & Carroll, D. L. (2003). The effects of back massage before diagnostic cardiac catheterization. *Alternative Therapies, 9*(1), 50–57.

Melancon, B., & Miller, L. H. (2005). Massage therapy versus traditional therapy for low back pain relief: Implications for holistic nursing practice. *Holistic Nursing Practice, 19*(3), 116–119.

Millman, R. P. (2005). Excessive sleepiness in adolescents and young adults: Causes, consequences, and treatment strategies. *Pediatrics, 115*(6), 1774–1786.

Mok, E., & Woo, C. P. (2004). The effects of slow stroke back massage on anxiety and shoulder pain in older stroke patients. *Complementary Therapy in Nursing and Midwifery, 10,* 209–216.

National Center on Sleep Disorders Research (n.d.). *2003 national sleep disorders research plan.* Retrieved July 4, 2006, from http://www.nhlbi.nih.gov/health/prof/sleep/res_plan/

Taras, H., & Potts-Datema, W. (2005). Sleep and student performance at school. *The Journal of School Health, 75*(7), 248–254.

REFERENCES

American Sleep Disorders Association. (2005). *The international classification of sleep disorders: Diagnostic and coding manual.* Lawrence, KS: Allen Press.

Arnold, E. (2004). Sorting out the 3 D's: Delirium, dementia, and depression. *Nursing, 34*(6), 36–42.

Colson, E. R., McCabe, L. K., Fox, K., Levenson, S., Colton, T., Lister, G., & Corwin, M. J. (2005). Barriers to following the back-to-sleep recommendations: Insights from focus groups with inner-city caregivers. *Ambulatory Pediatrics, 5*(6), 349–354.

Dochterman, J. M., & Bulechek, G. M. (Eds.). (2004). *Nursing interventions classification (NIC)* (4th ed.). St. Louis, MO: Mosby.

Gangwisch, J. E., Malaspina, D., Boden-Albala, B., & Heymsfield, S. B. (2005). Inadequate sleep as a risk factor for obesity: Analysis of the NHANES I. *Sleep, 28,* 1289–1296.

Institute of Medicine (IOM). (2006). *Sleep disorders and sleep deprivation: An unmet public health problem.* Washington, DC: Author.

Moorhead, S., Johnson, M., & Maas, M. (Eds.). (2004). *Nursing outcomes classification (NOC)* (3rd ed.). St. Louis, MO: Mosby.

NANDA International. (2007). *NANDA nursing diagnoses: Definitions and classification 2007–2008.* Philadelphia: Author.

National Sleep Foundation. (n.d.a). *A look at the school start times debate.* Retrieved June 29, 2006, from http://www.sleepfoundation.org/hottopics/index.php?secid=18&id=206

National Sleep Foundation. (n.d.b). *ABCs of ZZZZ—When you can't sleep.* Retrieved June 29, 2006, from http://www.sleepfoundation.org/sleeplibrary/index.php?secid=id=53

National Sleep Foundation. (n.d.c). *Aging gracefully and sleeping well.* Retrieved June 29, 2006, from http://www.sleepfoundation.org/hottopics/index.php?secid=12&id=225

National Sleep Foundation. (n.d.d). *Children's sleep habits.* Retrieved June 29, 2006, from http://www.sleepfoundation.org/hottopics/index.php?secid=11&id=39

National Sleep Foundation. (n.d.e). *Parents of teens: Recognize the signs and symptoms of sleep deprivation and sleep problems.* Retrieved July 2, 2006, from http://www.sleepfoundation.org/_content/hottopics/teensigns.pdf

National Sleep Foundation. (2005a). *Insomnia.* Retrieved June 29, 2006, from http://www.sleepfoundation.org/sleeptionary/index.php?id=19.

National Sleep Foundation. (2005b). *Insomnia symptoms.* Retrieved July 2, 2006, from http://www.sleepfoundation.org/sleeptionary/index.php?id=19&subsection=symptoms

National Sleep Foundation. (2006). *National Sleep Foundation 2006 Sleep in America poll highlights and key findings.* Retrieved July 4, 2006, from http://www.sleepfoundation.org/_content/hottopics/Highlights_facts_06.pdf

Orr, W. C. (2000). Editorial: Sleep and functional bowel disorders: Can bad bowels cause bad dreams? *American Journal of Gastroenterology, 95,* 1118–1121.

Robinson, S. B., Weitzel, T., & Henderson, L. (2005). The sh-h-h-h project. Nonpharmacological interventions. *Holistic Nursing Practice, 19*(6), 263–266.

Vitiello, M. V. (1999). Effective treatments for age-related sleep disturbances. *Geriatrics, 54,* 47–52.

SELECTED BIBLIOGRAPHY

Bephage, G. (2005). Promoting quality sleep in older people: The nursing care role. *British Journal of Nursing, 14*(4), 205–210.

Carlson, B. W., & Mascarella, J. J. (2005). Changes in sleep patterns in COPD. *American Journal of Nursing, 103*(12), 71–74.

Cmiel, C. A., Gasser, D. M., Oliphant, L. M., & Neveau, A. J. (2004). Noise control: A nursing team's approach to sleep promotion. *American Journal of Nursing, 104*(2), 40–48.

Cole, C., & Richards, K. C. (2006). Sleep in persons with dementia: Increasing quality of life by managing sleep disorders. *Journal of Gerontological Nursing, 32*(3), 48–53.

Dulak, S. B. (2005). Dangerous bedfellows. *RN, 68*(4), 33–37.

Hoffman, S. (2003). Sleep in older adults. *Geriatric Nursing, 24,* 210–216.

Honkus, V. L. (2003). Sleep deprivation in critical care units. *Critical Care Nursing Quarterly, 26*(3), 179–189.

Hughes, R. G., & Rogers, A. E. (2004). Are you tired? Sleep deprivation compromises nurses' health—and jeopardizes patients. *American Journal of Nursing, 104,* 36–37.

Joanna Briggs Institute. (2004). Strategies to manage sleep in residents of aged care facilities. *Best Practice. Evidence Based Practice Information Sheets for Health Professionals, 8*(3), 1–5.

Kennedy, M. (2004). Back to sleep. Many nurses don't follow the recommended sleep guidelines for infants. *American Journal of Nursing, 104*(6), 17.

Kreiger, A. C., & Redeker, N. S. (2002). Obstructive sleep apnea syndrome: Its relationship with hypertension. *Journal of Cardiovascular Nursing, 17,* 1–11.

Maindonald, E. (2005). Helping parents reduce the risk of SIDS. *Nursing, 35*(7), 50–53.

Mauk, K. L. (2005). Promoting sound sleep habits in older adults. *Nursing, 35*(2), 22,25.

McKibbin, C. L., Ancoli-Isreal, S., Dimsdale, J., Archuleta, C., von Kanel, R., Mills, P., et al. (2005). Sleep in spousal caregivers of people with Alzheimer's disease. *Sleep, 28,* 1245–1250.

Nagel, C. L., Markie, M. B., Richards, K. C., & Taylor, J. L. (2003). Sleep promotion in hospitalized elders. *Medsurg Nursing, 12*(5), 279–289.

Quillen, T. F. (2005). Sounding the alarm for narcolepsy. *Nursing, 35*(6), 74–75.

Rogers, A. E., & Dreher, H. M. (2002). Narcolepsy. *Nursing Clinics of North America, 37,* 1–18.

Smith, B. K. (2004). Test your stamina for workplace fatigue. *Nursing Management, 35*(10), 38–40.

Smyth, C. (2003). The Pittsburgh sleep quality index. *Medsurg Nursing, 12*(4), 261–262.

Thompson, D. G. (2005). Safe sleep practices for hospitalized infants. *Pediatric Nursing, 31*(5), 400–403.

Westley, C. (2004). Sleep: Geriatric self-learning module. *Medsurg Nursing, 13*(5), 291–295.

Williams, J. (2004). Gerontologic nurse practitioner care guidelines: Sleep in the elderly. *Geriatric Nursing, 25,* 310–312.

Yantis, M. A. (2002). Obstructive sleep apnea. *American Journal of Nursing, 102*(6), 83, 85.

CHAPTER 46

Pain Management

LEARNING OUTCOMES

After completing this chapter, you will be able to:

1. Discriminate between physiological and neuropathic pain categories.

2. Describe the four processes involved in nociception and how pain interventions can work during each process.

3. Describe how the physical, mental, spirtual, and social aspects of pain contribute to concepts such as pain tolerance, suffering, and pain behavior.

4. Describe the gate control theory and its application to nursing care.

5. Identify subjective and objective data to collect and analyze when assessing pain.

6. Identify examples of nursing diagnoses for clients with pain.

7. Individualize a pain treatment plan based on clinical and personal goals, while setting objective outcome criteria by which to evaluate a client's response to interventions for pain.

8. Compare and contrast barriers to effective pain management affecting nurses and clients.

9. Differentiate tolerance, dependence, and addiction.

10. Describe pharmacologic interventions for pain.

11. Describe the World Health Organization's ladder step approach developed for cancer pain control.

12. Give an example of rational polypharmacy described by the American Pain Society.

13. Identify risks and benefits of various analgesic delivery routes and analgesic delivery technologies.

14. Describe nonpharmacologic pain control interventions.

15. List three nonpharmacologic interventions directed at each of the following: the body, the mind, the spirit, and social interactions.

Pain is an unpleasant and highly personal experience that may be imperceptible to others, while consuming all parts of the person's life. The widely agreed-upon definition of **pain** is "an unpleasant sensory and emotional experience associated with actual or potential tissue damage, or described in terms of such damage" (American Pain Society [APS], 2003; Gordon, 2002). Three parts of this definition have important implications for nurses. First, pain is a physical *and* emotional experience, not all in the body or all in the mind. Second, it is in response to actual *or* potential tissue damage, so there may not be abnormal lab or radiographic reports despite real pain. Finally, pain is described in terms of such damage. This final component is aligned with McCaffery's often quoted definition of pain, "Pain is whatever the experiencing person says it is, existing whenever he says it does" (McCaffery & Pasero, 1999, p. 17). Given that some clients are reluctant to disclose the presence of pain unless prompted, nurses will not know of the client's pain until they assess for it. Additionally, it is clear that even nonverbal clients (e.g., preverbal children, intubated clients, the cognitively impaired) experience pain that demands nursing assessment and treatment even if clients are unable to "describe in terms" the nature of their discomfort.

Epidemiological studies estimate that most people have experienced pain in the last month, and between one-third and one-half of adults live with some form of chronic pain (APS, 1999; Elliott, Smith, Penny, Smith, & Chambers, 1999) with the prevalence higher among the older populations (Reyes-Gibby, Aday, & Cleeland, 2002). Approximately 25 million Americans live with persistent pain described as "very severe," causing them to be unable to work or independently perform activities of daily living (APS, 1999). Severe or persistent pain affects all body systems, causing potentially serious health problems while increasing the risk of complications, delays in healing, and an accelerated progression of fatal illnesses (Arnstein, 2003). Even if the original cause of the pain heals, the changes in the nervous system resulting from suboptimal pain manage-

ment can result in the development of incurable chronic pain (Arnstein, 1997; Katz, Jackson, Kavanagh, & Sandler, 1996). Persistent pain also contributes to insomnia, weight gain, constipation, hypertension, deconditioning, chronic stress, and depression (Dodd et al., 2001; Monteiro-Cruz & Mattos-Pimenta, 2001; Wilson, Eriksson, D'Eon, Mikail, & Emery, 2002). These effects interfere with work, recreation, domestic activities, and personal care activities to the point that leads many sufferers to question if life is worth living (Hitchcock, Ferrell, & McCaffery, 1994). Effective pain management is an important aspect of nursing care to promote healing, prevent complications, reduce suffering, and prevent the development of incurable pain states.

Pain is more than a symptom of a problem; it is a high-priority problem in itself. Pain presents both physiologic and psychologic dangers to health and recovery. Severe pain is viewed as an emergency situation deserving attention and prompt professional treatment.

THE NATURE OF PAIN

Although pain is a universal experience, the nature of the experience is unique to the individual based, in part, on the type of pain experienced, the psychosocial context or meaning, and the response needed. Adding to the complexity, pain may be a physiological warning system alerting the nurse to a problem or unmet need demanding attention; or it may be a diseased, malfunctioning segment of the nervous system. Advances in the understanding of physiological mechanisms may someday replace the currently used categories of acute pain or chronic pain. In addition to the underlying mechanisms, nurses attuned to a holistic view of care need to consider how these physiological signals affect the mind, body, spirit, and social interactions. In this section, a review is included of the scientific, theoretical, and clinical concepts that form the foundation of knowledge needed by nurses to assess and treat clients with pain in a holistic, comprehensive fashion.

Types of Pain

Pain may be described in terms of location, duration, intensity, and etiology.

Location

Classifications of pain based on where it is in the body (e.g., headache, backache, chest pain) may be useful in determining the client's underlying problems or needs; or it may be problematic given that most clients don't fit neatly into one of the categories. For example, categorizing a head pain as a headache can be difficult as the International Headache Society recognizes 300 different types of headaches; many have similar clinical presentations, but different clinical needs (IHS, 2004). Location of pain is, however, a very important component to note. For example, if after knee surgery, a client reports moderately severe chest pain, the nurse must act immediately to further evaluate and treat this discomfort. The ability to discriminate between cardiac and noncardiac chest pain challenges even expert clinicians, but the fact that chest pain is evaluated and treated differently than knee pain in this client is understandable. Complicating the categorization of pain by location is the fact that some pains radiate (spread or extend) to other areas (e.g., low back to legs). Also pain may be **referred** (appear to arise in different areas) to other parts of the body. For example, cardiac pain may be felt in the shoulder or left arm, with or without chest pain. **Visceral pain** (pain arising from organs or hollow viscera) often presents this way, being perceived in an area remote from the organ causing the pain (Figure 46-1 ■).

Duration

When pain lasts only through the expected recovery period, it is described as **acute pain,** whether it has a sudden or slow onset and regardless of the intensity. **Chronic pain,** on the other hand, is prolonged, usually recurring or persisting over 6 months or longer, and interferes with functioning. Acute and chronic pain result in different physiologic and behavioral responses, as shown in Table 46–1. Although experts may disagree on whether the cutoff point for chronic pain should be 1, 3, or 6 months after onset, or expected healing time, NANDA specifies the accepted nursing diagnosis of *Chronic Pain* to be mild to severe, constant or recurring, without an anticipated or predictable end and a duration of greater than 6 months (Ackley & Ladwig, 2006).

The categories differentiating chronic cancer (malignant) pain from chronic nonmalignant pain have also been problematic. **Cancer pain** may result from the direct effects of the disease and its treatment, or it may be unrelated to the disease and its treatment in individuals with cancer. Over the years, other diagnoses have been included in the "malignant pain" category, such as HIV/AIDS or burn pain, which tend to be treated more aggressively than "nonmalignant pain."

Intensity

To avoid ambiguity, categorizing pain according to intensity (mild, moderate, severe) or the underlying physiology (somatic, visceral, neuropathic) has emerged as a useful way to identify types of pain. Serlin, Mendoza, Nakamura, Edwards, and Cleeland (1995) conducted a large-scale international study that

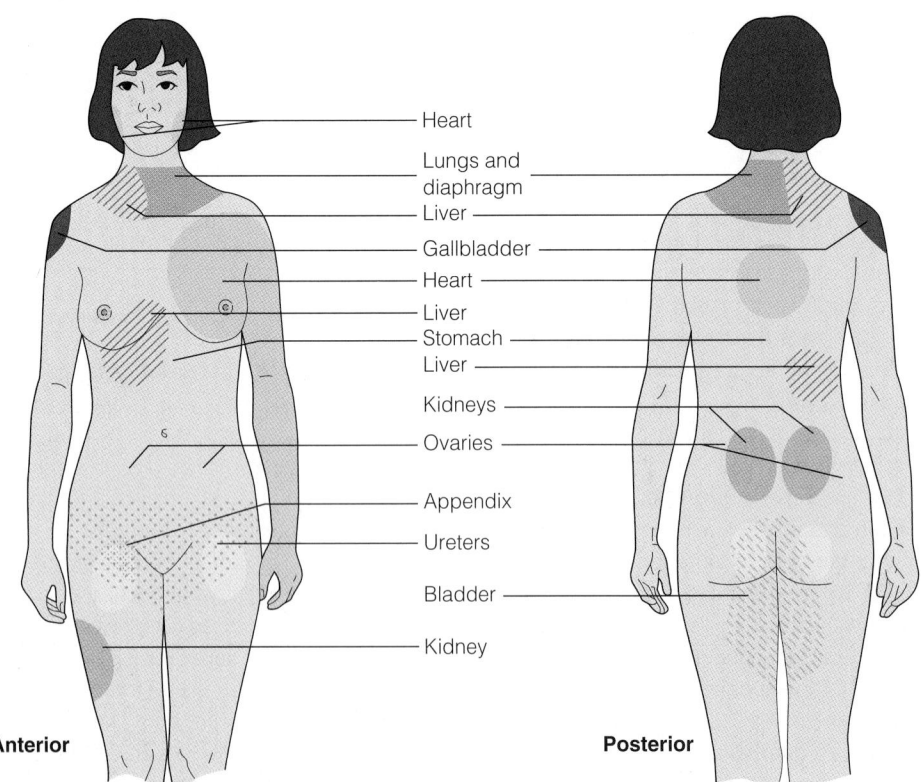

Heart
Lungs and diaphragm
Liver
Gallbladder
Heart
Liver
Stomach
Liver
Kidneys
Ovaries
Appendix
Ureters
Bladder
Kidney

Anterior

Posterior

Figure 46-1 ■ Common sites of referred pain from various body organs.

TABLE 46–1 Comparison of Acute and Chronic Pain

ACUTE PAIN	CHRONIC PAIN
Mild to severe	Mild to severe
Sympathetic nervous system responses:	Parasympathetic nervous system responses:
Increased pulse rate	Vital signs normal
Increased respiratory rate	
Elevated blood pressure	
Diaphoresis	Dry, warm skin
Dilated pupils	Pupils normal or dilated
Related to tissue injury; resolves with healing	Continues beyond healing
Client appears restless and anxious	Client appears depressed and withdrawn
Client reports pain	Client often does not mention pain unless asked
Client exhibits behavior indicative of pain: crying, rubbing area, holding area	Pain behavior often absent

confirmed earlier classifications of pain by intensity using a standard 0 (no pain) to 10 (worst possible pain) scale. Linking the rating to health and functioning scores, pain in the 1–3 range is deemed **mild pain,** a rating of 4–6 is **moderate pain,** and pain reaching 7–10 is ranked **severe pain** and is associated with the worst outcomes.

Etiology

Designating types of pain by etiology can be done under the broad categories of physiological pain and neuropathic pain. **Physiological pain** is experienced when an intact, properly functioning nervous system sends signals that tissues are damaged, requiring attention and proper care. For example, the pain experienced following a cut or broken bone alerts the person to avoid further damage until it is properly healed. Once stabilized or healed, the pain goes away; thus this pain is transient. There may also be persistent forms of physiological pain. For example, a person who has lost the protective cartilage in joints will have pain when they stress those joints, as the bone-to-bone contact damages tissues. This common form of arthritis produces pain in millions of sufferers, some of whom have intermittent pain whereas others have constant pain that persists for years.

Subcategories of physiological pain include somatic or visceral. **Somatic pain** originates in the skin, muscles, bone, or connective tissue. The sharp sensation of a paper cut or aching of a sprained ankle are common examples of somatic pain. Visceral pain results from activation of pain receptors in the organs and/or hollow viscera. Visceral pain tends to be poorly located, and may have a cramping, throbbing, pressing, or aching quality. Often visceral pain is associated with feeling sick (e.g., sweating, nausea, or vomiting) as in the examples of labor pain, angina pectoris, or irritable bowel.

Neuropathic pain is experienced by people who have damaged or malfunctioning nerves. The nerves may be abnormal due to illness (e.g., postherpetic neuralgia, diabetic peripheral neuropathy), injury (e.g., phantom limb pain, spinal cord injury pain), or undetermined reasons.

Subtypes of neuropathic pain are being developed based on the part of the nervous system believed to be damaged (Pasero, 2004). **Peripheral neuropathic pain** (e.g., phantom limb pain, postherpetic neuralgia, carpal tunnel syndrome) follows damage and/or sensitization of peripheral nerves. **Central neuropathic pain** (e.g., spinal cord injury pain, poststroke pain, multiple sclerosis pain) results from malfunctioning nerves in the central nervous system. **Sympathetically maintained pain** occurs occasionally when abnormal connections between pain fibers and the sympathetic nervous system perpetuate problems with both the pain and sympathetically controlled functions (e.g., edema, temperature and blood flow regulation). Neuropathic pain is typically chronic; it is described as burning, "electric-shock," and/or tingling, dull, and aching. Episodes of sharp, shooting pain can also be experienced (Herr, 2004). Neuropathic pain tends to be difficult to treat. Unfortunately, evidence suggests that in some instances, neuropathic pain results from a failure to treat pain effectively during the perioperative period (Manais, Bucknall, & Botti, 2005).

Common pain syndromes are briefly described in Clinical Manifestations.

Concepts Associated with Pain

There are some concepts that are useful for nurses to know to better understand and treat pain. It is useful to differentiate pain threshold from pain tolerance. **Pain threshold** is the least amount of stimuli that is needed for a person to label a sensation as pain. Threshold studies are typically conducted in a laboratory with many controls and measured amounts of stimuli (typically electrically generated). Pain threshold may vary slightly from person to person, and may be related to age, gender, or race, but it changes little in the same individual over time. **Pain tolerance** is the maximum amount of painful stimuli that a person is willing to withstand without seeking avoidance of the pain or relief. Pain tolerance does vary considerably from person to person, even within the same person at different times and in different circumstances. For example, a woman may tolerate a considerable amount of labor pain because she does not want to alter her level of alertness or the vitality of her baby. She likely would not tolerate a fraction of that pain during a routine dental procedure before demanding medicine or running out of the office.

Some other concepts that are useful to know relate to abnormal pain conditions. Hyperalgesia, allodynia, hyperpathia, and dysesthesia are conditions of abnormal pain processing that may signal the development of neuropathic processes, which if caught early may be reversed, yet if ignored, may lead to the development of incurable pain syndromes. **Hyperalgesia** and **hyperpathia** are terms that may be used interchangeably to denote a heightened response to a painful stimuli (e.g., severe pain response to a paper cut). This is differentiated from **allodynia** where nonpainful stimuli (e.g., contact with linen, water, or wind) produce pain, and from **dysesthesia,** which is

CLINICAL MANIFESTATIONS
COMMON PAIN SYNDROMES

- *Postherpetic neuralgia.* A case of herpes zoster (shingles) typically erupts decades after a primary infection (chickenpox) during a period of stress or compromised immune functioning. After the painful unilateral vesicular rash fades, burning or electric-shock pain in the area may persist for months or years. Advancing age is a risk factor for persistent postherpetic neuralgia, which currently affects 2 million Americans.
- *Phantom pain.* Phantom sensations, the feeling that a lost body part is present, occurs in most people after amputation. For many, this sensation is painful and it may occur spontaneously, or is evoked (e.g., using a poor-fitting prosthesis). When the amputation involves a limb, it is termed *phantom limb pain,* whereas following breast surgery, it is called *postmastectomy pain.* If the limb was painful or mangled before the amputation, that is commonly the sensation that is experienced (unless the discomfort is completely relieved prior to surgery).
- *Trigeminal neuralgia.* This is an intense stablike pain that is distributed by one or more branches of the trigeminal nerve (fifth cranial). The pain is usually experienced on parts of the face and head. It is so severe that it produces facial muscle spasms.
- *Headache.* An estimated 40% of the worldwide population suffers at least one severe, disabling headache per year. This commonly occurring painful condition can be caused by either intracranial or extracranial problems, serious or benign conditions. To establish a plan to prevent or treat headache, the nurse needs to assess the quality, location, onset, duration, and frequency of the pain, as well as any signs and symptoms that precede the headache.
- *Low back pain.* Approximately 80% of Americans suffer from low back pain at some time during their life. It accounts for 11 million visits to physicians annually, affecting men and women alike, and results in over 100 million lost workdays annually (Guo, Tanaka, Halperin, Cameron, 1999). Although 50% of people who develop low back pain will achieve a near-complete recovery within 2 weeks, half develop recurrent and/or chronic back pain with 5% of cases becoming severe, persistent, and debilitating (van Tulder, & Koes, 2004). These 5% with persistent pain account for 75% of the estimated $100 billion the United States spends annually in low back pain.
- *Fibromyalgia.* An estimated 5 million Americans suffer from a condition known as fibromyalgia, a chronic disorder characterized by widespread musculoskeletal pain, fatigue, and multiple tender points. "Tender points" refers to tenderness that occurs in precise, localized areas, particularly in the neck, spine, shoulders, and hips. People with this syndrome may also experience sleep disturbances, morning stiffness, irritable bowel syndrome, anxiety, and other symptoms. Although the symptoms present as muscle pain, stiffness, and weakness, it is considered by many to be a problem of abnormal CNS functioning, particularly as it relates to the way nerves process pain.

BOX 46–1   Concepts Associated with Pain

Acute pain: Pain that is directly related to tissue injury and resolves when tissue heals.
Cancer pain: Pain associated with the disease, treatment, or some other factor in individuals with cancer.
Chronic pain: Pain that persists beyond 6 months secondary to chronic disorders or nerve malfunctions that produce ongoing pain after healing is complete.
Intractable pain: A pain state (generally severe) for which there is no cure possible after accepted medical evaluation and treatments have been implemented. The focus of treatment turns from cure to pain reduction, functional improvement, and the enhancement of quality of life.
Neuropathic pain: Pain that is related to damaged or malfunctioning nervous tissue in the peripheral and/or central nervous system.
Nociceptive pain: Pain that is directly related to tissue damage. May be somatic (e.g., damage to skin, muscle bone) or visceral (e.g., damage to organs).
Pain threshold: The process of recognizing, defining, and responding to pain.
Pain tolerance: The most pain an individual is willing or able to tolerate before taking evasive actions.

The following states indicate abnormal nerve functioning, and the associated cause needs to be identified/treated (as soon as possible) before irreversible damage occurs.

Allodynia: Sensation of pain from a stimulus that normally does not produce pain, e.g., light touch.
Dysesthesia: An unpleasant abnormal sensation that can be either spontaneous or evoked.
Hyperalgesia: Increased sensation of pain in response to a normally painful stimulus.

The following concepts are important reasons to prevent pain or treat it as soon as possible to prevent the amplification, spread, and persistence of pain.

Sensitization: An increased sensitivity of a receptor after repeated activation by noxious stimuli.
Windup: Progressive increase in excitability and sensitivity of spinal cord neurons, leading to persistent, increased pain.

an unpleasant abnormal sensation. Dysesthesia mimics or imitates the pathology of a central neuropathic pain disorder, such as the pain that follows a stroke or spinal cord injury. See Box 46–1 for a review of concepts associated with pain.

PHYSIOLOGY OF PAIN

How pain is transmitted and perceived is complex, in part because of the nature of the fully integrated, constantly changing structure of the central nervous system, and the symphony of chemical mediators, only a fraction of which are understood. The extent to which pain is perceived depends on the interaction between the body's analgesia system and the nervous system's transmission and the mind's interpretation of stimuli and its meaning.

Nociception

The peripheral nervous system includes primary sensory neurons specialized to detect mechanical, thermal, or chemical conditions associated with potential tissue damage. The signals, when these nociceptors are activated, must be transduced and transmitted to the spine and brain where the signals are modified before they are ultimately understood and "felt." The physiologic processes related to pain perception are described as **nociception.** Four physiologic processes are involved in nociception: transduction, transmission, perception, and modulation (Paice, 2002).

TABLE 46–2 Types of Pain Stimuli

STIMULUS TYPE	PHYSIOLOGIC BASIS OF PAIN
Mechanical	
1. Trauma to body tissues (e.g., surgery)	Tissue damage; direct irritation of the pain receptors; inflammation
2. Alterations in body tissues (e.g., edema)	Pressure on pain receptors
3. Blockage of a body duct	Distention of the lumen of the duct
4. Tumor	Pressure on pain receptors; irritation of nerve endings
5. Muscle spasm	Stimulation of pain receptors (also see chemical stimuli)
Thermal	
Extreme heat or cold (e.g., burns)	Tissue destruction; stimulation of thermosensitive pain receptors
Chemical	
1. Tissue ischemia (e.g., blocked coronary artery)	Stimulation of pain receptors because of accumulated lactic acid (and other chemicals, such as bradykinin and enzymes) in tissues
2. Muscle spasm	Tissue ischemia secondary to mechanical stimulation (see above)

Transduction

Specialized pain receptors or **nociceptors** can be excited by mechanical, thermal, or chemical stimuli (see Table 46–2). During the transduction phase, noxious stimuli (with the potential to injure tissue) trigger the release of biochemical mediators (e.g., prostaglandins, bradykinin, serotonin, histamine, substance P) that sensitize nociceptors. Noxious or painful stimulation also causes movement of ions across cell membranes, which excites nociceptors. Pain medications can work during this phase by blocking the production of prostaglandin (e.g., ibuprofen or aspirin) or by decreasing the movement of ions across the cell membrane (e.g., local anesthetic). Another example is the topical analgesic capsaicin (Zostrix), which depletes the accumulation of substance P and blocks transduction.

Transmission

The second process of nociception, transmission of pain, includes three segments (McCaffery & Pasero, 1999). During the first segment, the pain impulse travels from the peripheral nerve fibers to the spinal cord. Substance P serves as a neurotransmitter, enhancing the movement of impulses across the nerve synapse from the primary afferent neuron to the second-order neuron in the dorsal horn of the spinal cord (Figure 46-2 ■). Two types of nociceptor fibers cause this transmission to the dorsal horn of the spinal cord: unmyelinated C fibers, which transmit dull, aching pain, and thin A-delta fibers, which transmit sharp, localized pain. In the dorsal horn, the pain signal is modified by modulating factors (e.g., excitatory amino acids or endorphins) before the amplified or dampened signal travels via spinothalamic tracts. The second segment is transmission from the spinal cord, and ascension, via spinothalamic tracts, to the brain stem and thalamus (Figure 46-3 ■). The third segment involves transmission of signals between the thalamus to the somatic sensory cortex where pain perception occurs.

Pain control can take place during this second process of transmission. For example, opioids (narcotic analgesics) block the release of neurotransmitters, particularly substance P, which stops the pain at the spinal level. Capsaicin may also deplete substance P that could inhibit the transmission of pain signals.

Modulation

Often described as the "descending system," this third process occurs when neurons in the thalamus and brain stem send signals back down to the dorsal horn of the spinal cord (Paice, 2002, p. 75). These descending fibers release substances such as endogenous opioids, serotonin, and norepinephrine, which can inhibit (dampen) the ascending noxious (painful) impulses in the dorsal horn. In contrast, excitatory amino acids (e.g., glutamate, N-methyl-D-aspartate [NMDA]), and the upregulation of excitatory glial cells can facilitate (amplify) these pain signals. The effects of excitatory amino acids and glial cells tend to persist, while the effects of the inhibitory neurotransmitters tend to be short-lived as they are reabsorbed into the nerves. Tricyclic antidepressants block the reuptake of norepinephrine and serotonin; or NMDA antagonists (e.g., ketamine, dextromethorphan) may be used to help diminish the signals of pain.

Perception

The final process, perception, is when the client becomes conscious of the pain. Pain perception is the sum of complex activities in the central nervous system that may shape the character and intensity of pain perceived and ascribe meaning to the pain. The psychosocial context of the situation and the meaning of the

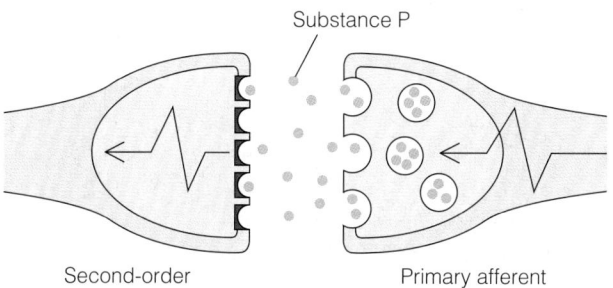

Figure 46-2 ■ Substance P assists the transmission of impulses across the synapse from the primary afferent neuron to a second-order neuron in the spinothalamic tract.

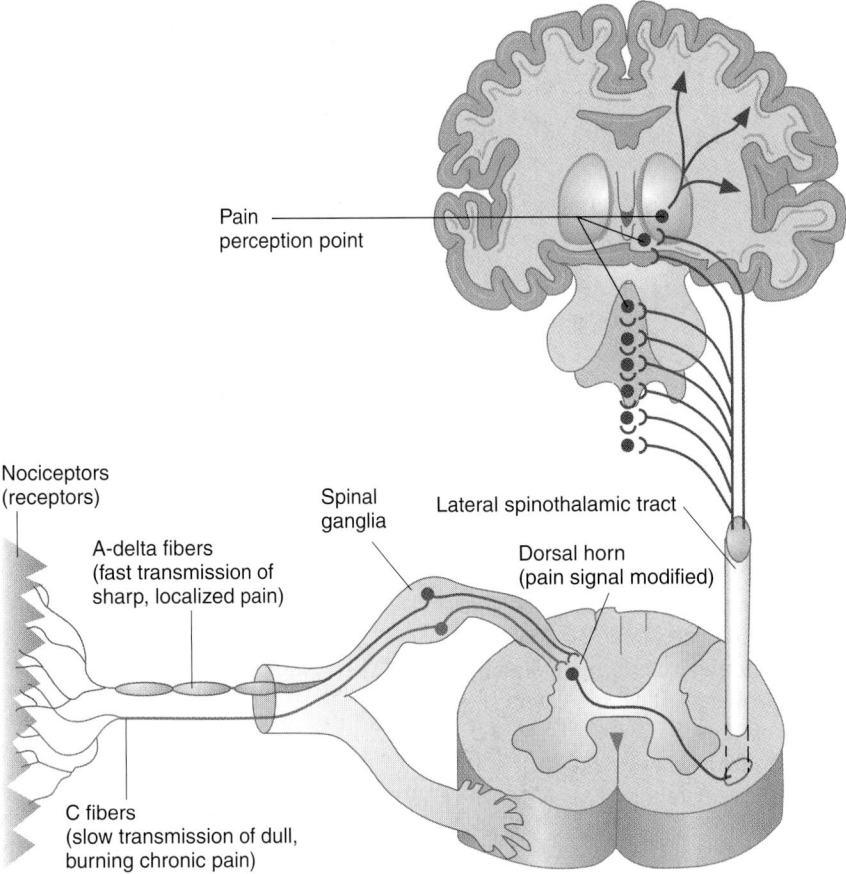

Figure 46-3 ■ Physiology of pain perception.

pain based on past experiences and future hopes/dreams help to shape the behavioral response that follows.

Gate Control Theory

According to Melzack and Wall's gate control theory (1965), small-diameter (A-delta, or C) peripheral nerve fibers carry signals of noxious stimuli to the dorsal horn, where these signals are modified when they are exposed to the substantia gelatinosa (the mileu in the central nervous system) that may be imbalanced in an excitatory or inhibitory direction. Ion channels on the pre- and postsynaptic membranes serve as gates that, when open, permit positively charged ions to rush into the second order neuron, sparking an electrical impulse and sending signals of pain to the thalamus.

Peripherally, large-diameter (A-delta) nerve fibers, which typically send messages of touch, or warm or cold temperatures, have an inhibitory effect on the substantia gelatinosa, and may activate descending mechanisms that can lessen the intensity of pain perceived or inhibit the transmission of those pain impulses—that is, close the (ion) gates (Figure 46-4 ■).

Higher centers in the brain, especially those associated with affect and motivation, are capable of modifying the substantia gelatinosa and influence the opening or closing of the gates. For example, if a little girl is playing with a ball that rolls under the couch, and in the process of retrieving it her hand gets stuck and pinched (the A-delta fibers are activated), the anxiety of not knowing what to do, combined with the negative impact on mo-

tivation (not being able to play with the ball), excites the substantia gelatinosa and facilitates opening the gates transmitting messages of pinching pain. When her mother comes and frees her and "kisses her boo-boo," the A-delta fibers are activated by

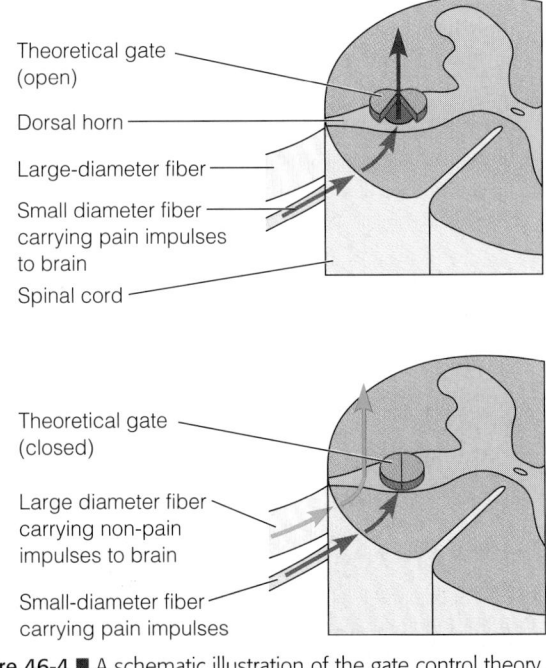

Figure 46-4 ■ A schematic illustration of the gate control theory.

the light touch, moisture, and warmth of the kiss. The girl feels love and is motivated to please her mother, all of which combine to calm the substantia gelatinosa and close the gates, inhibiting the transmission of further pain. Clinically, nurses can use this model to stop nociceptor firing (treat the underlying cause), apply topical therapies (e.g., heat, ice, electrical stimulation, or massage), and address the client's mood (e.g., reduce fear, anxiety, and anger) and goals (e.g., client education, anticipatory guidance).

Responses to Pain

The body's response to pain is a complex process rather than a specific action. It has both physiologic and psychosocial aspects. Initially the sympathetic nervous system responds, resulting in the fight-or-flight response, with a noticeable increase in pulse and blood pressure. The person may hold his or her breath, or have short, shallow breathing. There may also be some reflexive movements as the person withdraws from the painful stimuli (Figure 46-5 ■). Over a matter of minutes, or hours, the pulse and blood pressure return to baseline despite the persistance of pain. Contrary to the adaptation noted in vital signs, the pain fibers themselves adapt very little and become sensitized in a way that intensifies, prolongs, and/or spreads the pain.

Unrelieved pain has been noted to have a potentially harmful effect on the person's well-being. Pain interferes with sleep, affects appetite, and lowers the quality of life for clients and their family members. A natural response to pain is to stop activity, tense muscles, and withdraw from the pain-provoking activities. This reduced mobility may produce muscle atrophy and

painful spasm, putting the person at risk of complications related to immobility and/or cardiopulmonary deconditioning. Uncontrolled pain impairs immune function, which slows healing and increases susceptibility to infections and dermal ulcers. The short, shallow breathing that accompanies pain produces atelectasis, lowers circulating oxygen levels, and increases cardiac workload. Undertreated pain also increases morbidity and mortality for a wide variety of conditions, including speeding metastasis of cancer and extending cardiac damage during a heart attack (Page, Ben-Eliyahu, Yirmiya, & Liebeskind, 1993; Puntillo & Weiss, 1994). The physical stress and emotional distress of severe or prolonged pain can contribute to the development of a wide variety of physical and emotional disorders.

Persistent, severe pain changes the nervous system in a way that intensifies, spreads, and prolongs the pain, risking the development of incurable chronic pain syndromes. Beginning at 24 hours, persistent unrelieved severe pain changes the structure and function of the nervous system in such a way that prolongs and intensifies the pain experience. A windup phenomenon occurs, tipping the balance in the substantia gelatinosa heavily in the direction of excitation, and establishing new nerve growth, including the development of reverberating loops, which further prolong, spread, and intensify the noxious stimuli (Arnstein, 1997). The pain threshold is lowered and the cells are said to be sensitized. Sensitization of the central nervous system is reflected by spontaneous neuron firing, reduced thresholds or increased responsiveness to afferent inputs, prolonged after-discharges to repeated stimulation, and the expansion of the peripheral receptive field of dorsal horn neurons. A similar process can occur in the peripheral nerves, when sensitized, normally innocuous stimuli (e.g., light touch) may be perceived as painful. Thus to prevent the development of persistent pain and promote overall health and well-being, the nurse must act to promote optimal and expedient pain control.

Factors Affecting the Pain Experience

Numerous factors can affect a person's perception of and reaction to pain. These include the person's ethnic and cultural values, developmental stage, environment and support people, previous pain experiences, and the meaning of the current pain.

Ethnic and Cultural Values

Ethnic background and cultural heritage have long been recognized as factors that influence both a person's reaction to pain and the expression of that pain. Behavior related to pain is a part of the socialization process. For example, individuals in one culture may have learned to be expressive about pain, whereas individuals from another culture may have learned to keep those feelings to themselves and not bother others.

Although there appears to be little variation in pain threshold, cultural background can affect the level of pain that an individual is willing to tolerate. In some Middle Eastern and African cultures, self-infliction of pain is a sign of mourning or grief. In other groups, pain may be anticipated as part of the ritualistic practices, and therefore tolerance of pain signifies strength and endurance. Additionally, there are significant variations in the expression of pain. Studies have shown that

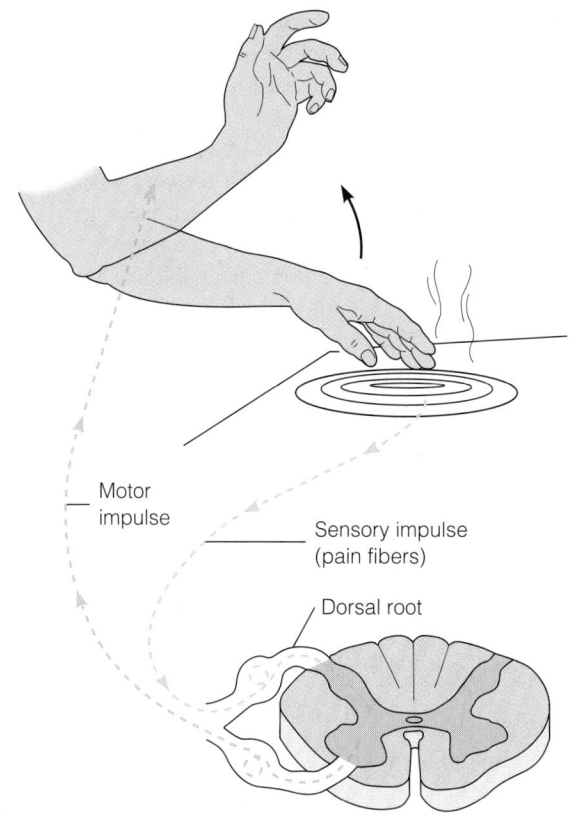

Motor impulse

Sensory impulse (pain fibers)

Dorsal root

Figure 46-5 ■ Proprioceptive reflex to a pain stimulus.

CULTURALLY COMPETENT CARE
Transcultural Differences in Responses to Pain

Expressions of pain vary from culture to culture and may vary from person to person *within* a culture.

AFRICAN AMERICANS

- Some believe pain and suffering is a part of life and is to be endured.
- Some may deny or avoid dealing with the pain till it becomes unbearable.
- Some believe that prayer and laying on of hands will free a person from suffering and pain.

MEXICAN AMERICANS

- May tend to view pain as a part of life and as an indicator of the seriousness of an illness.
- Some believe that enduring pain is a sign of strength.

PUERTO RICANS

- Many tend to be loud and outspoken in their expressions of pain. This is a socially learned way to cope and it is important for the nurse to not judge or disapprove.

ASIAN AMERICANS

- Chinese culture values silence. As a result, some clients may be quiet when in pain because they do not want to cause dishonor to themselves and their family.
- Japanese may have a stoic (minimal verbal and nonverbal expressions) response to pain. They may even refuse pain medication.
- Filipino clients may believe that pain is "God's will". Some elderly Filipino clients may refuse pain medication..

NATIVE AMERICANS

- In general, Native Americans are quiet, less expressive verbally and nonverbally and may tolerate a high level of pain. They tend to not request pain medication and may tolerate pain until they are physically disabled.

ARAB AMERICANS

- Pain responses are considered private and reserved for immediate family, not with health professionals. As a result, this may lead to conflicting perceptions between the family members and the nurse regarding the effectiveness of the client's pain relief.

Note: From *Transcultural Communication in Nursing*, 2nd ed., by C. Munoz & J. Luckmann, 2005, Clifton Park: Delmar Learning and *Transcultural Concepts in Nursing Care*, 4th ed., by M. M. Andrews & J. S. Boyle, 2003, Philadelphia: Lippincott Williams & Wilkins.

individuals of northern European descent tend to be more stoic and less expressive of their pain than individuals from southern European backgrounds.

Nurses must realize they have their own attitudes and expectations about pain. Andrews and Boyle (2003) pointed out that health care has been dominated by white Anglo-Saxon Protestants and most nurses have been influenced by these values and beliefs. For example, nurses may place a higher value on silent suffering or self-control in response to pain. Nurses expect people to be objective about pain and to be able to provide a detailed description of the pain. Nurses who deny, refute, or downplay the pain they observe in others may be culturally incompetent (unaware and emotionally apathetic toward others' viewpoints). To become culturally competent, nurses must become knowledgeable about differences in the meaning of and appropriate responses to pain. They must be sympathetic to concerns and develop the skills needed to address pain in a culturally sensitive way.

Developmental Stage

The age and developmental stage of a client is an important variable that will influence both the reaction to and the expression of pain. Age variations and related nursing interventions are presented in Table 46–3.

The field of pain management for infants and children has grown significantly. It is now accepted that anatomic, physiologic, and biochemical elements necessary for pain transmission are present in newborns, regardless of their gestational age. The American Academy of Pediatrics and the Canadian Paediatric Society (2000) recommend that environmental, nonpharmacologic, *and* pharmacologic interventions be used to prevent, reduce, or eliminate pain in neonates. Physiologic indicators may vary in infants, so behavioral observation is recommended for pain assessment (Ball & Bindler, 2003). Children may be less able than an adult to articulate their experience or needs related to pain, which may result in their pain being undertreated. However, children as young as 3 years can accurately report the location and intensity of their pain if it is evaluated properly.

With puberty comes the emergence of some pain syndromes, particularly for women. Unfortunately, women are overrepresented in a large number of painful disorders, including headaches, fibromyalgia, lupus, and menstrual-related disorders. Men are more vulnerable to pain related to their occupational or risk-taking patterns, including burn pain, posttrauma pain, and pain related to HIV/AIDS. A needless disparity is that the very young, the very old, women, and ethnic minorities are undertreated for their pain more frequently than their adult male counterparts.

Studies have shown that chronic pain affects 25% to 50% of older clients living in the community and 45% to 80% of those in nursing homes (American Geriatrics Society [AGS], 1998). With the number of older persons in our society increasing dramatically, by 2030, nurses will be caring for elders in all settings of care in greater numbers.

Elders constitute the largest group of individuals seeking health care services. The prevalence of pain in the older population is generally higher due to both acute and chronic disease conditions. Pain threshold does not appear to change with aging, although the effect of analgesics may increase due to physiologic changes related to drug metabolism and excretion (Stanley, Blair, & Beare, 2005).

Environment and Support People

A strange environment such as a hospital, with its noises, lights, and activity, can compound pain. In addition, the lonely person who is without a support network may perceive pain as severe, whereas the person who has supportive people around may per-

TABLE 46–3 Age Variations in the Pain Experience

AGE GROUP	PAIN PERCEPTION AND BEHAVIOR	SELECTED NURSING INTERVENTIONS
Infant	Perceives pain.	Give a glucose pacifier.
	Responds to pain with increased sensitivity.	Use tactile stimulation. Play music or tapes of a heartbeat.
	Older infant tries to avoid pain; for example, turns away and physically resists.	
Toddler and preschooler	Develops the ability to describe pain and its intensity and location.	Distract the child with toys, books, pictures. Involve the child in blowing bubbles as a way of "blowing away the pain."
	Often responds with crying and anger because child perceives pain as a threat to security.	Appeal to the child's belief in magic by using a "magic" blanket or glove to take away pain.
	Reasoning with child at this stage is not always successful.	Hold the child to provide comfort.
	May consider pain a punishment.	Explore misconceptions about pain.
	Feels sad.	
	May learn there are gender differences in pain expression.	
	Tends to hold someone accountable for the pain.	
School-age child	Tries to be brave when facing pain.	Use imagery to turn off "pain switches."
	Rationalizes in an attempt to explain the pain.	Provide a behavioral rehearsal of what to expect and how it will look and feel.
	Responsive to explanations.	Provide support and nurturing.
	Can usually identify the location and describe the pain.	
	With persistent pain, may regress to an earlier stage of development.	
Adolescent	May be slow to acknowledge pain.	Provide opportunities to discuss pain.
	Recognizing pain or "giving in" may be considered weakness.	Provide privacy.
	Wants to appear brave in front of peers and not report pain.	Present choices for dealing with pain. Encourage music or TV for distraction.
Adult	Behaviors exhibited when experiencing pain may be gender-based behaviors learned as a child.	Deal with any misconceptions about pain.
	May ignore pain because to admit it is perceived as a sign of weakness or failure.	Focus on the client's control in dealing with the pain.
	Fear of what pain means may prevent some adults from taking action.	Allay fears and anxiety when possible.
Elder	May have multiple conditions presenting with vague symptoms.	Thorough history and assessment is essential.
	May perceive pain as part of the aging process.	Spend time with the client and listen carefully.
	May have decreased sensations or perceptions of the pain.	
	Lethargy, anorexia, and fatigue may be indicators of pain.	
	May withhold complaints of pain because of fear of the treatment, of any lifestyle changes that may be involved, or of becoming dependent.	Clarify misconceptions.
		Encourage independence whenever possible.
	May describe pain differently, that is, as "ache," "hurt," or "discomfort."	
	May consider it unacceptable to admit or show pain.	

ceive less pain. Some people prefer to withdraw when they are in pain, whereas others prefer the distraction of people and activity around them. Family caregivers can be a significant support for a person in pain. With the increase in outpatient and home care, families are assuming an increased responsibility for the management of pain. Education related to the assessment and management of pain can positively affect the perceived quality of life for both clients and their caregivers (McCaffery & Pasero, 1999).

Expectations of significant others can affect a person's perceptions of and responses to pain. In some situations, for example, girls may be permitted to express pain more openly than boys. Family role can also affect how a person perceives or responds to pain. For instance, a single mother supporting three children may ignore pain because of her need to stay on the job. The presence of support people often changes a client's reaction to pain. For example, toddlers often tolerate pain more readily when supportive parents or nurses are nearby.

LIFESPAN CONSIDERATIONS Pain

CHILDREN

Children continue to receive inadequate medication to treat their pain. This may be due to nurses' lack of knowledge about how to evaluate pain in children. The pain of infants and young children who cannot verbalize well is particularly difficult to assess. Nurses will benefit from learning how to use pain assessment tools and by being alert to the possibility that children may be experiencing significant levels of pain, even if they do not appear to be (Simons & MacDonald, 2004).

ELDERS

The presentation of pain may vary in elders for a variety of reasons. Changes in nerve structure and functioning, or vascular changes with aging may cause a variation in the pain sensation. Sometimes the pain is heightened in those whose nervous systems have been sensitized from previous unresolved pain; whereas other times significant tissue damage (e.g., silent heart attack) may occur without pain being experienced. In some situations, pain presents itself with atypical symptoms, such as confusion, restlessness, or irritability. This is especially true in clients with dementia who have a difficult time understanding and verbalizing what they are feeling.

Maintaining optimal function is especially crucial for a high quality of life in elders. If pain is not effectively controlled, the following areas are often affected in their daily lives:

- Activity tolerance
- Mobility
- Ability to socialize
- Sleep disturbance
- Ability to perform activities of daily living
- Ability to remain as independent as possible

All efforts, pharmacologic and nonpharmacologic, should be used to help provide pain reduction, while maintaining or enhancing functional ability. Involvement of the client and family is important when working with the primary care provider, pharmacist, and nurse to plan which treatment is most appropriate and most acceptable to the client.

The principle "start low and go slow" is especially important when ordering dosages and pain medications for elders. Typically, the starting dose of medicines for older adults is reduced by 25% to 50%, and then titrated for effect. Decreased renal and liver function may prolong the duration of action, but it also increases the risk of toxicity from pain medications in older clients. In particular, risk of silent gastrointestinal bleeding and renal damage from nonsteroidal anti-inflammatory drugs (NSAIDs) increases, so dosages and lab work need to be carefully monitored related to hematocrit and renal function (liver function is monitored with acetaminophen). Comorbid conditions may also affect medication selection in elders, as clients with gastric ulcers, hypertension, or the combination of asthma and nasal polyps should not receive NSAIDs. Elders with chronic obstructive pulmonary disease (COPD) must have their respiratory rate carefully monitored when placed on an opioid pain reliever, especially at night when respirations slow and the risk of oxygen desaturation is high.

Past Pain Experiences

Previous pain experiences alter a client's sensitivity to pain. People who have personally experienced pain or who have been exposed to the suffering of someone close are often more threatened by anticipated pain than people without a pain experience. In addition, the success or lack of success of pain relief measures influences a person's expectations for relief and future response to interventions. For example, a person who has tried several nondrug pain relief measures without success may have little hope about the helpfulness of nursing interventions and may demand medication as the only thing that helps the pain.

Meaning of Pain

Some clients may accept pain more readily than others, depending on the circumstances and the client's interpretation of its significance. A client who associates the pain with a positive outcome may withstand the pain amazingly well. For example, a woman giving birth to a child or an athlete undergoing knee surgery to prolong his career may tolerate pain better because of the benefit associated with it. These clients may view the pain as a temporary inconvenience rather than a potential threat or disruption to daily life.

By contrast, clients with unrelenting chronic pain may suffer more intensely. Chronic pain affects the body, mind, spirit, and social relationships in an undesirable way. Physically, the pain limits functioning and contributes to the disuse or deconditioning alluded to previously. For many, the change in activities of daily living (e.g., eating, sleeping, toileting) also takes a toll. The side effects of the many medications used to try to control

the pain also place a heavy burden on the body. Mentally, individuals with chronic pain change their outlook, becoming more pessimistic, often to the point of helplessness and hopelessness. Mood often becomes impaired when pain persists, because the sadness of being unable to do important or enjoyable activities combines with self-doubts and learned helplessness to produce depression. Anxiety, worry, and uncertainty about coping with the pain may escalate emotionally, to the point of panic. Spiritually, pain may be viewed in a variety of ways. It may be perceived as a punishment for wrongdoing, a betrayal by the higher power, a test of fortitude, or a threat to the essense of who the person is. Pain may be a source of spiritual distress, or it may be a source of strength and enlightenment. Socially, pain often strains valued relationships, in part because of the impaired ability to fulfill role expectations.

NURSING MANAGEMENT

Assessing

Accurate pain assessment is essential for effective pain management. Many health facilities are making pain assessment the **fifth vital sign.** The strategy of linking pain assessment to routine vital sign assessment and documentation represents a push to make pain assessment a routine aspect of care for all clients. Given the highly subjective and individually unique nature of pain, a comprehensive assessment of the pain experience (physiologic, psychologic, behavioral, emotional, and sociocultural) provides the necessary foundation for optimal pain control.

The extent and frequency of the pain assessment varies according to the situation and the organizational policy. For clients experiencing acute, severe pain, the nurse may focus only on location, quality, and severity, and provide interventions to control the pain before conducting a more detailed evaluation. Clients with less severe or chronic pain can usually provide a more detailed description of the experience. As the fifth vital sign, pain should be screened for every time vital signs are evaluated. A simple screening question such as, "Are you experiencing any discomfort right now?" will usually suffice. For example, in the initial postoperative period, vital signs are taken as frequently as every 15 minutes. Screening for pain this frequently is justifiable as there is a high incidence of pain in the perioperative period. Local, regional, or general anesthesia may be wearing off, or if severe pain is reported, the medication administered postoperatively is frequently administered via the intravenous route and has a peak effect noted within 15 minutes.

Major barriers to better pain control for both nurses and clients relate to inadequate assessment of pain and fear of treatment-related problems (Horbury, Henderson, & Bromely, 2005). Given that many people will not voice their pain unless asked about it, pain assessments must be initiated by the nurse. Some of the many reasons clients may be reluctant to report pain are listed in Box 46–2. Because the words *pain* or *complain* may have emotional or sociocultural meaning attached, it is better to ask, "do you have any discomforts to report?" rather than "do you have any complaints of pain?" It is also essential that nurses listen to and believe the client's perceptions of pain. Believing the person's perceptions is crucial in establishing the sense of trust needed to develop a therapeutic relationship.

Pain assessments consist of two major components: (a) a pain history to obtain facts from the client and (b) direct observation of behaviors, physical signs of tissue damage, and secondary physiologic responses of the client. The goal of assessment is to gain an objective understanding of a subjective experience. Box 46–3 provides one example of a helpful mnemonic to make a complete pain assessment.

BOX 46–2 Why Clients May Be Reluctant to Report Pain

- Unwillingness to trouble staff who are perceived as busy
- Don't want to be labeled as a "complainer" or "bad"
- Fear of the injectable route of analgesic administration—especially children
- Belief that unrelieved pain is expected—normal part of recovery or aging
- Belief that others will think they are weak if they express pain
- Difficulty or inability to communicate their discomfort
- Concern about risks associated with opioid drugs (e.g., addiction)
- Concern about unwanted side effects, especially of opioid drugs
- Concern that use of drugs now will render the drug inefficient later in life
- Fear that reporting pain will lead to further tests and expenses
- Belief that nothing can be done to control pain
- Belief that enduring pain and suffering may lead to spiritual enlightenment

---

BOX 46–3 Mnemonic for Pain Assessment: COLDERR

Character: describe the sensation (e.g., sharp, aching, burning),
Onset: when it started, how it has changed,
Location: where it hurts (all locations),
Duration: constant versus intermittent in nature,
Exacerbation: factors that make it worse,
Relief: factors that make it better (medications and other factors), and
Radiation: pattern of shooting/spreading/location of pain away from its origin.

Note: Reprinted from "Optimizing Perioperative Pain Management," 2002, by P. M. Arnstein. *AORN Journal, 76*(5), 812–818. Copyright © 2002 with permission of Elsevier.

Pain History

While taking pain histories, the nurse must provide an opportunity for clients to express in their own words how they view the pain and the situation. This will help the nurse understand what the pain means to the client and how the client is coping with it. Remember that each person's pain experience is unique and that the client is the best interpreter of the pain experience. This history should be geared to the specific client. For example, questions asked of an accident victim would be different from those asked of a postoperative client or one suffering from chronic pain. The initial pain assessment for someone in severe acute pain may consist of only a few questions before intervention occurs. In addition, the nurse may focus on the following:

- Previous pain treatment and effectiveness
- When and what analgesics were last taken
- Other medications being taken
- Allergies to medications

For the person with chronic pain, the nurse may focus on the client's coping mechanisms, effectiveness of current pain management, and ways in which the pain has affected the client's body, thoughts and feelings, activities, and relationships.

Data that should be obtained in a comprehensive pain history include pain location, intensity, quality, patterns, precipitating factors, alleviating factors, associated symptoms, effect on ADLs, past pain experiences, meaning of the pain to the person, coping resources, and affective responses. Questions to elicit these data are shown in the Assessment Interview.

LOCATION. To ascertain the specific location of the pain, ask the individual to point to the site of the discomfort. A chart consisting of drawings of the body can assist in identifying pain locations. The client marks the location of pain on the chart. This tool can be especially effective with clients who have more than one source of pain. A client who has multiple pains of different character can use symbols to draw the distribution of different pain types (e.g., circle aching areas, mark areas where shock-like pain is felt with an X).

When assessing the location of a child's pain, the nurse needs to understand the child's vocabulary. For example, "tummy" might refer either to the abdomen or to part of the chest. Asking

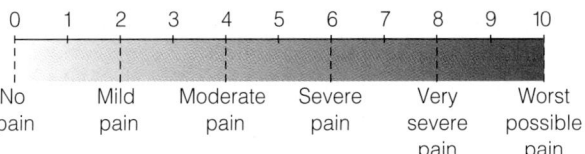

Figure 46-6 ■ An 11-point pain intensity scale with word modifiers.

ASSESSMENT INTERVIEW
Pain History

- Location: Where is your discomfort?
- Quality: Tell me what your discomfort feels like.
- Intensity: On a scale of 0 to 10, with "0" representing no pain (substitute the word they use, e.g., no burning) and 10 representing the worst possible pain (e.g., burning sensation), how would you rate the degree of discomfort you are having right now?
- Pattern
  a. Time of onset: When did or does the pain start?
  b. Duration: How long have you had it, or how long does it usually last?
  c. Constancy: Do you have pain-free periods? When? And for how long?
- Precipitating factors: What triggers the pain or makes it worse?
- Alleviating factors: What measures or methods have you found helpful in lessening or relieving the pain? What pain medications do you use?
- Associated symptoms: Do you have any other symptoms (e.g., nausea, dizziness, blurred vision, shortness of breath) before, during, or after your pain?
- Effects on ADLs: How does the pain affect your daily life (e.g., eating, working, sleeping, and social and recreational activities)?
- Past pain experiences: Tell me about past pain experiences you have had and what was done to relieve the pain.
- Meaning of pain: What does having this pain mean to you? Does it signal something about the future or past? What worries or scares you the most about your pain?
- Coping resources: What do you usually do to help you deal with pain?
- Affective response: How does the pain make you feel? Anxious? Depressed? Frightened? Tired? Burdensome?

(0–10) rating scale is shown in Figure 46-6 ■. The inclusion of word modifiers on the scale can assist some clients who find it difficult to apply a number level to their pain. For example, after ruling out "0" and "10" (neither no pain nor the worst possible pain), a nurse can ask the client if it is mild (2), mild to moderate (4), moderate to severe (6), or severe (8).

Another way to evaluate the intensity of pain for clients who are unable to use the numeric rating scales is to determine the extent of pain awareness and degree of interference with functioning. For example, 0 = no pain, 2 = awareness of pain only when paying attention to it, 4 = can ignore pain and do things, 6 = can't ignore pain, interferes with functioning, 8 = impairs ability to function or concentrate, and 10 = intense incapacitating pain. It is believed that the degree that pain interferes with functioning is a good marker for the severity of pain, especially for those with chronic pain.

CLINICAL ALERT

Perception is reality. The client's self-report of pain is what must be used to determine pain intensity. The nurse is obligated to record the pain intensity as reported by the client. By challenging the believability of the client's report, the nurse is undermining the therapeutic relationship and preventing the fulfillment of advocacy and helping people with pain, which is called for in the ANA 2005 Scope and Standards of Practice in Pain Management Nursing. ■

---

the child to point to the pain helps clarify the child's word usage to identify location. The use of figure drawings can assist in identifying pain locations. Parents can also be helpful in interpreting the meaning of a child's words.

When documenting pain location the nurse may use various body landmarks. Further clarification is possible with the use of terms such as *proximal*, *distal*, *medial*, *lateral*, and *diffuse.*

PAIN INTENSITY OR RATING SCALES. The single most important indicator of the existence and intensity of pain is the client's report of pain. In practice, however, McCaffery, Ferrell, and Pasero (2000) found that nurses tend to use less reliable measures for assessing pain. The top factors identified by nurses were culturally influenced (e.g., facial expressions, verbalization, request for relief). In addition, studies have shown that health care providers may underrate or overrate the pain intensity (Bergh & Sjostrom, 1999). The use of pain intensity scales is an easy and reliable method of determining the client's pain intensity. Such scales provide consistency for nurses to communicate with the client and other health care providers. To avoid confusion, scales should use a 0 to 10 range with 0 indicating "no pain" and the highest number indicating the "worst pain possible" for that individual. An 11-point

When noting pain intensity it is important to determine any related factors that may be affecting the pain. When the intensity changes, the nurse needs to consider the possible cause. For example, the abrupt cessation of acute abdominal pain may indicate a ruptured appendix. Several factors affect the perception of intensity: (a) the amount of distraction, or the client's concentration on another event; (b) the client's state of consciousness; (c) the level of activity; and (d) the client's expectations.

Not all clients can understand or relate to numerical pain intensity scales. These include preverbal children, elderly clients with impairments in cognition or communication, and people who do not speak English. For these clients the Wong-Baker FACES Rating Scale (Figure 46-7 ■) may be easier to use (Wong, Hockenberry-Eaton, Wilson, Winkelstein, & Schwartz, 2001). The face scale includes a number scale in relation to each expression so that the pain intensity can be documented.

When clients are unable to verbalize their pain for reasons of age, mental capacity, medical interventions, or other reasons, nurses need to accurately assess the intensity of each client's pain and the effectiveness of the pain management interventions. For these clients, the nurse must rely on observation of behavior.

0	1	2	3	4	5
NO HURT	HURTS LITTLE BIT	HURTS LITTLE MORE	HURTS EVEN MORE	HURTS WHOLE LOT	HURTS WORST

Explain to the person that each face is for a person who feels happy because he has no pain (hurt) or sad because he has some or a lot of pain. Face 0 is very happy because he doesn't hurt at all. Face 1 hurts just a little bit. Face 2 hurts a little more. Face 3 hurts even more. Face 4 hurts a whole lot. Face 5 hurts as much as you can imagine, although you don't have to be crying to feel this bad. Ask the person to choose the face that best describes how he is feeling.

Rating scale is recommended for persons age 3 years and older.

Brief word instructions: Point to each face using the words to describe the pain intensity. Ask the child to choose the face that best describes own pain and record the appropriate number.

Figure 46-7 ■ The Wong-Baker FACES Rating Scale.

(*Note:* From *Wong's Essentials of Pediatric Nursing,* 6th ed. (p.1301), by D. L. Wong, M. Hockenberry-Eaton, D. Wilson, M. L. Winkelstein, and P. Schwartz, 2001, St. Louis, MO: Mosby. Copyright by Mosby, Inc. Reprinted with permission.)

Several validated behavioral pain rating scales can be used in specific populations. The FLACC scale has been validated in children 2 months to 7 years old and rates pain behaviors manifested in Facial expressions, Leg movement, Activity, Cry, and Consolability measures that yield a 0 to 10 score (Merkel, Voepel-Lewis, Shayevitz, & Malviyga, 1997). Warden, Hurley, and Volicer (2003) tested a similar behavioral measure for elders with dementia, which quantified respirations, vocalizations, facial expressions, body language, and consolability. Given the diversity of pain and behaviors among clients spanning a broad range of age and physical and mental capabilities, it is unrealistic to believe a single pain assessment tool can be applied across all populations. As an organization committed to improving the way pain is evaluated and treated, the American Society for Pain Management Nursing (ASPMN) has assembled a team of nurse experts to develop a position paper on assessing pain in the nonverbal patient.

For effective use of pain rating scales, clients need not only to understand the use of the scale but also to be educated about how the information will be used to determine changes in their condition and the effectiveness of pain management interventions. Clients should also be asked to indicate what level of comfort is acceptable so that they can perform specific activities (Acello, 2000). To align the client's goals and expectations with reality, it is important to note that acute pain can typically be cut by 50% and chronic pain can be cut by 25%. To ensure that optimal pain management is achieved, the client works together with professionals toward established goals of pain reduction and functional improvement.

The use of a pain rating scale together with a pain flow sheet (Figure 46-8 ■) has been shown to be effective in improving pain management (McCaffery & Pasero, 1999). Documentation can be completed by the nurse, the client, or a caregiver and can be used in acute, outpatient, and home care settings.

PAIN QUALITY. Descriptive adjectives help people communicate the quality of pain. A headache may be described as "unbearable" or an abdominal pain as "piercing like a knife." The astute clinician can glean subtle clinical clues from the quality of the pain described; thus it is important to record the description verbatim. Some of the commonly used pain descriptors are listed in Table 46–4. Note that the term "unbearable" is listed as an affective term and "piercing" is a sensory term. Both pains are real physical conditions signaling an underlying condition,

TABLE 46–4 Commonly Used Pain Descriptors

TERM	SENSORY WORDS	AFFECTIVE WORDS
Pain	Searing	Unbearable
	Scalding	Killing
	Sharp	Intense
	Piercing	Torturing
	Drilling	Agonizing
	Wrenching	Terrifying
	Shooting	Exhausting
	Burning	Suffocating
	Crushing	Frightful
	Penetrating	Punishing
		Miserable
Hurt	Hurting	Heavy
	Pricking	
	Pressing	Throbbing
	Tender	
Ache	Numb	Annoying
	Cold	Nagging
	Flickering	Tiring
	Radiating	Troublesome
	Dull	Gnawing
	Sore	Uncomfortable
	Aching	Sickening
	Cramping	Tender

SR-1420 (6/00)

Sunrise Hospital and Medical Center & Sunrise Children's Hospital
Pain Management Flow Sheet

Patient's stated pain level goal: _____

*Monitoring Guidelines outlined on back of form

Mode of Administration

A-PO opioid and nonopioid medications
B-PCA Infuser Basal with Patient Control
C-Continuous Infusion
D-Epidural Infuser Continuous Basal Only
E-Epidural Infuser Basal & Patient Control
F-Intermittent IV/IM Injection
G-Transdermal opioids
H-On-QPump
I-Per Rectum

Level of Pain Assessment Scales

Faces Pain Rating Scale

0 · · · 2 · · · 4 · · · 6 · · · 8 · · · 10

1-10 Pain Scale

0 - - - - - - - - - - - 10

No pain or pain relieved   Worst pain imaginable

0-10 Sum Scale

A. Vocal
0 = Positive/ETT
1 = Whimpers
2 = Crying
3 = Screaming

C. Facial
0 = Smiling
1 = Neutral
2 = Frown/grimace
3 = Clenched teeth

B. Body Movement
0 = Moves easily
1 = Neutral shifting
2 = Tense/flailing limbs

D. Touching (localizing)
0 = Notouching
1 = Reaching/patting
2 = Grabbing

Location of Pain:

A = No pain
B-Z = Use letters to mark location of pain on graph

Frequency of Pain:
O = Occasional   F = Frequent   C = Constant

Type of Pain
A = Burning   D = Sharp   G = Isolated
B = Stabbing   E = Shooting   H = Other
C = Radiating   F = Dull

Arousal Score:
0 = Alert   1 = Medically sedated/ETT
2 = Drowsy   3 = Somnolent
                       4 = Asleep

Non-Pharmacologic Interventions L
C = Cold   P = Pacifier
D = Distraction   PO = Positioning
H = Heat   R = Relaxation
HO = Holding   RO = Rocking
I = Imagery   S = Security/Object
M = Massage   T = TensUnit
MU = Music   0 = Other

Analgesia Order:
1 = Increase in dosage/rate
2 = Decrease in doseage/rate
3 = Extra bolus
4 = PRN medication for break-through pain
5 = Discontinue

Reason for Analgesia Order:
1 = Unrelieved pain
2 = Decreased arousal/neuroscore
3 = Side effects (Seebelow)
4 = Discontinue therapy/change to oral route
5 = Adverse drug reactions
(Document all adverse drug reactions in Nsg notes and complete an ADR report)

Side Effects: 0 = None
A = Anxiety   N = Nausea
C = Confused   R = Respiratory Depression
Co = Constipation   U = Urinary Rentention
I = Itching   V = Vomiting

Sensory Function   Epidural Only
0 = Moves all extremities well
1 = Unable to move all extremities well

Motor Function   Epidural Only
0 = Able to feel tactile pressure
1 = Unable to feel tactile pressure

Neuro Score: Epidural Only
0 = No numbness, no weakness
1 = Medically sedated/ETT
2 = Numbness with out weakness
3 = Numbness and weakness

Catheter Site: Epidural Only
1 = No redness, drainage, inflammation or swelling
2 = Red, inflamed
3 = Visable clear drainage
4 = Visable purulent drainage
5 = Visable serosanguinous/sanguinous drainage
6 = Swelling

Catheter Integrity Upon Removal: Epidural Only
1 = Catheter tip visually intact
2 = Catheter NOT visually intact-See Nsg Notes

Date												
Time												
Initials												
Mode of Admin												
Level of Pain												
Location of Pain												
Frequency of Pain												
Type of Pain												
Arousal Score												
Non-Pharm. Intervent.												
Analgesia Order												
Reason for Order												
Side Effects												
Adverse Effects (Y/N)												
Sensory Function **Epidural Only**												
Motor Function **Epidural Only**												
Neuro Score **Epidural Only**												
Catheter Site **Epidural Only**												
Cath Integrity **Epidural Only**												
O₂ Saturation												
Respirations												
Pulse												
Blood Pressure												
See Nursing Notes (Y/N)												

Initials	Signature

Patient Identification Label

Right   Left   Left   Right

Figure 46-8 ■ Pain Management Flow Sheet.

(Courtesy of Aptille Ciaverella, RN, and Lori Townsend, RN, at Sunrise Hospital and Medical Center and Sunrise Children's Hospital, Las Vegas, Nevada.)

but the affective description "unbearable" suggests that there is a coexisting emotional distress that needs to be addressed as well. Pain described as burning or shock-like tends to be neuropathic in origin and may be responsive to anticonvulsants (e.g., gabapentin), with or without an opioid (e.g., morphine).

PATTERN. The pattern of pain includes time of onset, duration, and recurrence or intervals without pain. The nurse therefore determines when the pain began; how long the pain lasts; whether it recurs and, if so, the length of the interval without pain; and when the pain last occurred. Attention to the pattern of pain helps the nurse anticipate and meet the needs of the client, as well as recognize patterns of grave concern (e.g., chest pain only on exertion).

PRECIPITATING FACTORS. Certain activities sometimes precede pain. For example, physical exertion may precede chest pain, or abdominal pain may occur after eating. These observations can help prevent pain and determine its cause. Environmental factors such as extreme cold or heat and extremes of humidity can affect some types of pain. For example, people with rheumatic conditions have worse pain on cold, damp days or just before a large storm. Physical and emotional stressors can also precipitate pain. Strong emotions can trigger a migraine headache or an episode of chest pain. Extreme physical exertion can trigger muscle spasms in the neck, shoulders, or back.

ALLEVIATING FACTORS. Nurses must ask clients to describe anything that they have done to alleviate the pain (e.g., home remedies such as herbal teas, medications, rest, applications of heat or cold, prayer, or distractions like TV). It is important to explore the effect any of these measures had on the pain, whether or not relief was obtained, or whether the pain became worse.

ASSOCIATED SYMPTOMS. Also included in the clinical appraisal of pain are associated symptoms such as nausea, vomiting, dizziness, and diarrhea. These symptoms may relate to the onset of the pain or they may result from the presence of the pain.

EFFECT ON ACTIVITIES OF DAILY LIVING (ADL). Knowing how ADLs are affected by pain helps the nurse understand the client's perspective on the pain's severity. The nurse asks the client to describe how the pain has affected the following aspects of life:

- Sleep
- Appetite
- Concentration
- Work/school
- Interpersonal relationships
- Marital relations/sex
- Home activities
- Driving/walking
- Leisure activities
- Emotional status (mood, irritability, depression, anxiety)

A rating scale of none, a little, or a great deal, or another range can be used to determine the degree of alteration.

COPING RESOURCES. Each individual will exhibit personal ways of coping with pain. Strategies may relate to earlier pain experiences or the specific meaning of the pain; some may reflect religious or cultural influences. Nurses can encourage and support the client's use of methods known to have helped in modifying pain, unless they are specifically contraindicated. Strategies may include seeking quiet and solitude, learning about their condition, pursuing interesting or exciting activities (for distraction), prayer (or other meaningful rituals), or social (from family, friends, support groups, etc.).

AFFECTIVE RESPONSES. Affective responses vary according to the situation, the degree and duration of pain, the interpretation of it, and many other factors. The nurse needs to explore the client's feelings of anxiety, fear, exhaustion, depression, or a sense of failure. Because many people with chronic pain become depressed and potentially suicidal, it may also be necessary to assess the client's suicide risk. In such situations, the nurse needs to ask the client, "Do you ever feel so bad that you want to die? Have you considered harming yourself or others recently?" Hitchcock, Ferrell, and McCaffery (1994) found that about half of the people with chronic pain surveyed have thought, at least at one time, they'd be better off dead. This may be reassuring to those who answered affirmatively to the first question. The vast majority of chronic pain sufferers, however, are not actively suicidal and do not have a specific, lethal plan. For those who express suicidal intent, nurses need to be familiar with state regulations, organizational policies, and resources available to guide practice in this area.

RESEARCH NOTE **Is There a Relationship between Pain Control and Satisfaction with Care?**

It has been suggested from prior research that there are health benefits for maintaining pain below the midpoint on pain scales (e.g., less than 5 on a 0–10 scale), but that client satisfaction does not always correlate to pain. This study was conducted to identify factors associated with the client's satisfaction with pain relief. A total of 207 subjects were enrolled in a clinical trial preoperatively to examine their patterns of pain control and related satisfaction with care. Clients who were "very satisfied" with pain control had pain intensity levels that averaged around 3, whereas those who were "somewhat satisfied" had pain of 4 on the 0–10 scale. Those having pain at or above the midpoint 5 were not satisfied.

IMPLICATIONS

This adds to the evidence that reducing pain below the midpoint of a pain scale is the target professionals should strive to achieve for overall health and well-being, as well as client satisfaction.

Note: Reprinted from *The Journal of Pain,* vol. 6, M. P. Jensen, S. A. Martin, and R. Cheung, pp. 400–406, Copyright 2005, with permission from Elsevier.

HOME CARE ASSESSMENT
Pain

CLIENT

■ Level of knowledge: Pharmacologic and nonpharmacologic pain relief measures selected; adverse effects and measures to counteract these effects; warning signs to report to primary care provider

■ Self-care abilities for analgesic administration: Ability to use analgesics appropriately (e.g., to prepare correct dosages of analgesics and adhere to scheduled administration); physical dexterity to take pills or to administer intravenous medications and to store medications safely; and ability to obtain prescriptions or over-the-counter medications at the pharmacy

FAMILY

■ Caregiver availability, skills, and willingness: Primary and secondary persons able and willing to assist with pain management; shopping if the client has restricted activity; ability to comprehend selected therapies (e.g., infusion pumps, imagery, massage, positioning, and relaxation techniques) and perform them or assist the client with them as needed

■ Family role changes and coping: Effect on financial status, parenting and spousal roles, sexuality, social roles

COMMUNITY

■ Resources: Availability of and familiarity with resources such as supplies, home health aid, or financial assistance

When the client's pattern and level of pain can be anticipated or is already known, regular or scheduled administration of analgesics can provide a steady serum level. With acute pain, this may be possible in the first 24 to 48 hours following surgery when the client is likely to have pain requiring opioid analgesics. Frequency of administration can be adjusted to prevent pain from recurring. When persistent, continuous pain exists, analgesics should be given around the clock (ATC), with addi-

tional as-needed (prn) doses available (Herr, 2002). Nonpharmacologic interventions should also be regularly scheduled. The additional advantage of scheduling measures is that the client spends less time in pain and does not experience as much anxiety or fear of the pain recurring, or the helplessness of not knowing what to do when pain flares.

Planning for Home Care

In preparation for discharge, the nurse needs to determine the client's and family's needs, strengths, and resources. The accompanying Home Care Assessment describes the specific assessment data required when establishing a discharge plan. Using the assessment data, the nurse tailors a teaching plan for the client and family.

Implementing

Pain management is the alleviation of pain or a reduction in pain to a level of comfort that is acceptable to the client. It includes two basic types of nursing interventions: pharmacologic and nonpharmacologic. Nursing management of pain consists of both independent and collaborative nursing actions. In general, noninvasive measures may be performed as an independent nursing function, whereas administration of analgesic medication generally requires a medical order from a primary care provider. However, because many analgesics are ordered to be administered on an "as needed" (prn) basis, the decision to administer the prescribed medication is frequently the nurse's, often requiring judgment as to the dose and the time of administration. Recent changes to the way range orders are written provide a little more structure than in the past; however, professional nursing judgment remains a key factor in relieving pain by determining which medication in what dosage would best meet the client's comfort needs (Gordon et al., 2005).

Generally speaking, a combination of strategies is best for the client in pain. Sometimes strategies need to be tried and changed

CLIENT TEACHING   Monitoring Pain in the Home Setting

■ Teach client to keep a pain diary to monitor pain onset, activity before pain, pain intensity, use of analgesics or other relief measures, and so on.

■ Instruct client to contact a health care professional if planned pain control measures are ineffective.

PAIN CONTROL

■ Teach the use of preferred and selected nonpharmacologic techniques such as relaxation, guided imagery, distraction, music therapy, massage, and so on.

■ Discuss the actions, side effects, dosages, and frequency of administration of prescribed analgesics.

■ Suggest ways to handle side effects of medications.

■ Provide accurate information about tolerance, physical dependence, and addiction if opioid analgesics are prescribed and these topics are of concern.

■ Instruct the client to use pain control measures before the pain becomes severe.

■ Inform the client of the effects of untreated pain.

■ Demonstrate and have the client or caregiver return demonstrate appropriate skills to administer analgesics (e.g., skin patches, injections, infusion pumps, or patient-controlled analgesia). If a home infusion pump is being used, caregivers need to be able to
  a. Demonstrate stopping and starting the pump.
  b. Change the medication cartridge and tubing.
  c. Adjust the delivery dose.
  d. Demonstrate site care.
  e. Identify signs indicating the need to change an injection site.
  f. Describe care of the pump and insertion site when the client is ambulatory, bathing, sleeping, or traveling.
  g. Perform problem solving for pumps when alarms are activated.
  h. Change the battery.

RESOURCES

■ Provide appropriate information about how to access community resources, home care agencies, and associations that offer self-help groups and educational materials.

PRACTICE GUIDELINES   Individualizing Care for Clients with Pain

■ Establish a trusting relationship. Convey your concern, and acknowledge that you believe that the client is experiencing pain. A trusting relationship promotes expression of the client's thoughts and feelings and enhances effectiveness of planned pain therapies.

■ Consider the client's ability and willingness to participate actively in pain relief measures. Clients who are excessively fatigued, sedated, or have altered levels of consciousness are less able to participate actively. For example, a client with an altered level of consciousness or altered thought processes cannot safely or effectively use patient-controlled analgesia. In contrast, a fatigued client may express a willingness to use pain relief measures that require little effort, such as listening to music or performing relaxation techniques.

■ Use a variety of pain relief measures. It is thought that using more than one measure has an additive, if not synergistic, effect in relieving pain. Two types of relief measures that should be part of any pain treatment plan are active (relief strategies that are self-initiated) and passive (relief strategies that require the assistance of others). Establishing rapport and client teaching are necessary components of all therapeutic encounters and may be implicit or explicit in the care plan. Because a client's pain may vary throughout a 24-hour period, different types of pain relief or preemptive interventions may be scheduled (e.g., medication 1 hour before dressing change, relaxation techniques with pleasant imagery after bedtime medication).

■ Provide measures to relieve pain before it becomes severe. For example, providing an analgesic before the onset of pain is preferable to waiting for the client to complain of pain, when a larger dose may be required.

■ Use pain-relieving measures that the client believes are effective. It has been recognized that clients are the authorities about their own pain. Thus, incorporating the client's preferred methods of relieving their pain into the treatment plan should be seriously considered.

■ The selection of pain relief measures should be aligned with the client's report of the severity of the pain. If a client reports mild pain, an analgesic such as aspirin may be indicated, whereas a client who reports severe pain often requires a more potent relief measure. Telling a client to ignore the pain (e.g., through distraction techniques) when he or she is reporting severe pain is an example of a misalignment of the pain severity and intervention selected.

■ If a pain relief measure is ineffective, encourage the client to try it again before abandoning it. Medications may need repeated doses to saturate plasma proteins before sufficient "free drug" is available to work on the intended target. Many nonpharmacologic measures require practice before they are effective.

■ Maintain an unbiased attitude (open mind) about what may relieve the pain. New ways to relieve pain are continually being developed. It is not always possible to explain the effectiveness of particular pain relief measures; however, using approaches the client believes will work should be considered.

■ Keep trying. Do not ignore a client because pain persists despite failed attempts to alleviate the discomfort. In these circumstances, reassess the pain and consider other relief measures.

■ Prevent harm to the client. Pain therapy should not increase discomfort or harm the client. Some pain relief measures may have adverse untoward effects, such as fatigue, but they should not disable the client.

■ Educate the client and caregivers about pain. Clients and support people need to be informed about possible causes of pain, precipitating and alleviating factors, and alternatives to drug therapy. Misconceptions also need to be corrected.

CULTURALLY COMPETENT CARE
Clients in Pain

Nurses are in a position of power as they decide whether to believe the client's subjective report of pain. It is, therefore, important to develop an effective, positive relationship with the client, a relationship that incorporates caring behaviors.

■ Respect clients as individuals by
  • Recognizing that clients can hold different beliefs about pain.
  • Inquiring about the client's beliefs and ways of coping with pain.

■ Respect the client's response to pain by
  • Recognizing that clients have the right to respond to pain in the way they learned is appropriate.
  • Recognizing that expressions of pain vary widely and no expression is good or bad.

■ Never stereotype a person on the basis of culture. Expressions of pain vary between cultures and within cultures.

Note: From *Transcultural Concepts in Nursing Care,* 4th ed. (pp. 409–411), by M. M. Andrews and J. S. Boyle, 2003, Philadelphia: Lippincott Williams & Wilkins. Copyright Lippincott, Williams & Wilkins. Reprinted with permission.

until the client obtains effective pain relief. See the Practice Guidelines for individualizing care for clients with pain.

Barriers to Pain Management

Misconceptions and biases can affect pain management. These may involve attitudes of the nurse or the client as well as knowledge deficits. Clients respond to pain experiences based on their culture, personal experiences, and the meaning the pain has for them. For many people, pain is expected and accepted as a normal aspect of illness. Clients and families may lack knowledge of the adverse effects of pain and may have misinformation regarding the use of analgesics. Clients may not report pain because they expect nothing can be done, they think it is not severe enough, or they feel it would distract or prejudice the health care provider. Other common misconceptions are shown in Table 46–5. Another barrier to effective pain management is the fear of becoming addicted, especially when long-term opioid use is prescribed. This fear is often held by both nurses and clients. It is important that all individuals know the difference between tolerance, dependence, and addiction (see Box 46–4). Pseudoaddiction is a condition that results from the undertreatment of pain where the client

TABLE 46–5 Common Misconceptions about Pain

MISCONCEPTION	CORRECTION
Clients experience severe pain only when they have had major surgery.	Even after minor surgery, clients can experience intense pain.
The nurse or other health care professionals are the authorities about a client's pain.	The person who experiences the pain is the only authority about its existence and nature.
Administering analgesics regularly for pain will lead to addiction.	Clients are unlikely to become addicted to an analgesic provided to treat pain.
The amount of tissue damage is directly related to the amount of pain.	Pain is a subjective experience, and the intensity and duration of pain vary considerably among individuals.
Visible physiologic or behavioral signs accompany pain and can be used to verify its existence.	Even with severe pain, periods of physiologic and behavioral adaptation can occur.

may become focused on obtaining medications, may "clock watch," and may otherwise seem inappropriately "drug seeking." Even behaviors such as illicit drug use and deception can occur in the client's efforts to obtain pain relief. Pseudoaddiction can be distinguished from true addiction in that the behaviors resolve when the pain is treated effectively.

Key Strategies in Pain Management

Key strategies to reduce pain include acknowledging and accepting the client's pain, assisting support persons, reducing misconceptions about pain, reducing fear and anxiety, and preventing pain.

ACKNOWLEDGING AND ACCEPTING CLIENT'S PAIN. According to the professional standards of conduct, nurses have a duty to ask clients about their pain and to believe their reports of discomfort. Challenging the client's report of discomfort undermines the environment of trust that is an essential component in the therapeutic relationship. Consider these four ways of communicating this belief:

1. Acknowledge the possibility of the pain. "Many people with your condition are bothered by leg pain. Are you experiencing any leg discomfort? What does it feel like? How concerned/upset are you about it?"
2. Listen attentively to what the client says about the pain, restating your understanding of the reported discomfort.

Adding an empathetic statement like, "I'm sorry you are hurting, it must be very upsetting. I want to help you feel better" lets the client know you believe the pain is real and intend to help.
3. Convey that you need to ask about the pain because, despite some similarities, everybody's experience is unique, for example, "Many people with your condition report having some discomforts. Do you have any pain or other discomforts now?"
4. Attend to the client's needs promptly. It is unconscionable to believe the client's report of pain and then do nothing. After determining the client has pain, discuss options and plan actions for providing relief.

CLINICAL ALERT

So what if you are fooled by a client's self-report of pain? Evidence suggests 5% of people reporting pain are dishonest and seeking some secondary gain. By believing everyone, you will not shortchange the 95% of people who so desperately need to have help controlling their pain, providing them with competent, compassionate, and appropriate nursing care based on the best available information. ■

ASSISTING SUPPORT PERSONS. Support persons often need assistance to respond in a helpful manner to the person experiencing pain. Nurses can help by giving them accurate information about the pain and providing opportunities for them to

BOX 46–4 Definitions

The American Academy of Pain Medicine, the American Pain Society, and the American Society of Addiction Medicine recognize the following definitions and recommend their use.

ADDICTION
Addiction is a primary, chronic, neurobiologic disease, with genetic, psychosocial, and environmental factors influencing its development and manifestations. It is characterized by behaviors that include one or more of the following: impaired control over drug use, compulsive use, craving, and continued use despite harm.

PHYSICAL DEPENDENCE
Physical dependence is a state of adaptation that is manifested by a drug class specific withdrawal syndrome that can be produced by abrupt ces-

sation, rapid dose reduction, decreasing blood level of the drug, and/or administration of an antagonist.

TOLERANCE
Tolerance is a state of adaptation in which exposure to a drug induces changes that result in a diminution of one or more of the drug's effects over time.

Note: From "Definitions Related to the Use of Opioids for the Treatment of Pain," *A Consensus Document from the American Academy of Pain Medicine, the American Pain Society, and the American Society of Addiction Medicine,* 2006, American Academy of Pain Medicine, American Pain Society, and the American Society of Addiction Medicine. Retrieved August 20, 2006, from http://www.ampainsoc.org/advocacy/opioids2.htm

REAL WORLD REFLECTION

THE STORY

My client this evening was a 17-year-old girl with end stage renal disease requiring dialysis three times a week. She was currently in the Pediatric ICU with severe, uncontrollable hypertension (HTN). When I showed up to observe the dialysis treatment the client was undergoing a series of tests and was connected to an ECG monitor. Nitroprusside was being administered IV to control her HTN. She was complaining of severe headache and nausea.

Approximately one hour into treatment, the client became inconsolable and began crying, complaining of severe headaches and her nausea progressed to vomiting. She had already been given an antiemetic for vomiting and Tylenol for pain but neither appeared to be working. Dilaudid was ordered for the pain and appeared to provide some relief. The client indicated her pain was at a 7 level after the dilaudid was administered. I provided her with cool washcloths while the primary ICU nurse gave her a scalp massage. The combination appeared to be working; she stopped crying and settled into an uneasy rest.

STUDENT REFLECTION

What I learned from this experience is that medication alone cannot always ease the client's pain. Where I previously may have felt that medications were the panacea to all client complaints, this experience reinforced the need to treat the entire client.

This is probably the first time I realized that pain medications are not always 100% effective. Also, I don't know why, but it seems I always think the client is overstating their pain or making up symptoms in order to receive pain medication. Maybe this is the result of watching too many ER episodes. My primary nurse brought me back to reality in this instance by asking if I had ever experienced a headache bad enough to make me vomit. With this perspective I could now somewhat relate to what the client must be experiencing.

FACULTY REFLECTION

Scott made two important discoveries. One is that pain is personal, complex, and multidimensional. Because it is so complex, we should not be surprised when a pain medication alone cannot relieve its intensity. It is also important to recognize what conclusions we formulate when a client's pain is not relieved with medication. Can you think of other factors that might be contributing to this patient's experience of pain? Are there other pain relief interventions you as a nurse could institute?

—*Student: Scott Eddy,*
Faculty member: Deb Filer, PhD, RN

discuss their emotional reactions, which may include anger, fear, frustration, and feelings of inadequacy. Teaching the support persons about the disease and medications (including warning signs to report) and nondrug pain-relieving techniques they can help with (e.g., massage, application of ice, coached relaxation techniques) may diminish their feelings of helplessness and strengthen their relationship. Support persons also may need the nurse's understanding, reassurance, and perhaps access to resources that will help them cope as they add the caregiver role to an already stressful life circumstance.

REDUCING MISCONCEPTIONS ABOUT PAIN. Reducing a client's misconceptions about the pain and its treatment will remove one of the barriers to optimal pain relief. The nurse should explain to the client that pain is a highly individual experience and that it is only the client who really experiences the pain, although others can understand and empathize. Misconceptions are also dealt with when the nurse and client discuss the context of pain control as part of the healing process. For example, a client may refuse pain medicine out of concern for addiction, explaining that the pain is more tolerable as long as he or she remains totally still. This misconception overstates the risk of addiction (estimated at < 5% of clients without a history of substance abuse when treated for acute pain) while underestimating the risks associated with immobility (atelectasis, muscle atrophy, decubitus ulcers, infections, etc.).

RESEARCH NOTE   Have Previous Professional Barriers to Pain Control Been Overcome?

Despite successful research and clinical approaches suggesting that pain can be better managed, much pain goes unrelieved. Continuing education programs that are implemented to influence the desired change in status have been poorly attended. A questionnaire with client vignettes was distributed to clinical nurses to identify underlying beliefs and intentions regarding pain management. The analysis of 221 questionnaires suggested that nurses may be reluctant to accept the client's self-report of pain and administer opioids in the absence of objective signs of pain. This is consistent with findings of similar studies a decade earlier that identified poor assessment and exaggerated concerns over the risk of pain relievers as major "professional" barriers to better pain control.

IMPLICATIONS

Given the failure of traditional methods of in-service or continuing education to change these underlying attitudes and practice patterns, new innovative approaches are needed to help nurses believe (1) that the client's verbal report of pain is a more reliable indicator of pain than physical signs or pain behaviors (e.g., facial grimace); and (2) that in the absence of oversedation or respiratory depression, opioids can be given more frequently or in higher doses for better pain control.

Note: From "Influences of Patient Behavior on Clinical Nurses' Pain Assessment: Implications for Continuing Education," by C. Horbury, A. Henderson, and B. Bromley, 2005, *Journal of Continuing Education in Nursing, 36*(1), pp. 18–24. Copyright © 2005 SLACK, Inc. Reprinted with permission.

PRACTICE GUIDELINES Strategies for Holding Colleagues Accountable for Believing Clients and Managing Pain

What do we do if the health care team does not respond positively to the client's report of pain?

- Speak up! Inappropriate professional behavior will persist if not challenged. If necessary, file an "incident" or "variance" report for persistent patterns or egregious violations of standards of care. These types of behaviors (ignoring reports of pain, failing to treat or mistreating people with pain) are not only unethical, but legally indefensible (Shapiro, 1996).
- Clarify that the sensation of pain is subjective and that professionals have a duty to believe clients' reports of their symptoms.
- Cite recommendations from evidence-based clinical practice guidelines (e.g., American Pain Society, Agency for Health Care Policy and Research), JCAHO standards, organization-specific documents (e.g., mission statement, patient bill of rights, practice standards), or relevant research/quality reports. As necessary, distribute or post with key passages highlighted.
- Involve key committees, managers, and administrators in studying and addressing the problem from a cost, quality, competency, and credentialing perspective.

CLINICAL ALERT

Emphasize to the client that at times, treatment may need to balance the demands of providing pain reduction with functional improvement. Too much pain medicine might impair alertness or gait; too much pain impairs alertness and ability to move. Thus a client may have to tolerate mild pain in order to do what is necessary to maximize functioning and recovery (e.g., cough, deep breathe, and walk). ■

REDUCING FEAR AND ANXIETY. It is important to help relieve strong emotions capable of amplifying pain (e.g., anxiety, anger, and fear). When clients have no opportunity to talk about their pain and associated fears, their perceptions and re-

actions to the pain can be intensified. Often, these emotions are related to uncertainty about the future, feeling mistreated in the past, or having unmet expectations. By providing accurate information, the nurse can also reduce many of the client's fears or anxiety, while clarifying expectations can minimize frustration and anger. Specifically, client education about the range of pain that is considered normal for the condition as well as the types of discomforts that signal a potential for problems will help alleviate this fear and uncertainty.

PREVENTING PAIN. A preventive approach to pain management involves the provision of measures to treat the pain before it occurs or before it becomes severe. **Preemptive analgesia** is the administration of analgesics prior to an invasive or operative procedure in order to treat pain before it occurs. For example, treating clients preoperatively with local infiltration of an anesthetic or parenteral administration of an opioid can reduce postoperative pain. Nurses can also use a preemptive approach by providing an analgesic around the clock (ATC), and supplementing with as needed prn doses prior to painful procedures (e.g., dressing changes, physical therapy). This strategy prevents the windup and sensitization described earlier that spreads, intensifies, and prolongs pain.

Pharmacologic Pain Management

Pharmacologic pain management involves the use of opioids (narcotics), nonpioids/nonsteroidal anti-inflammatory drugs (NSAIDs), and coanalgesic drugs (see Box 46–5). The principles of modern analgesic use are built on a foundation established by the World Health Organization (WHO) three-step approach to treating cancer pain (Figure 46-9 ■). This approach focuses on aligning the proper analgesic with the intensity of pain. This approach has evolved into what is currently termed "rational polypharmacy," which demands that health professionals be aware of all ingredients of medications that alleviate pain and use combinations to reduce the need for high doses of any one medication, and to maximize pain control with a minimum of side effects or toxicity. These multidrug strategies, combined with multimodal therapy (use of nondrug approaches

BOX 46–5 Categories and Examples of Analgesics

NONOPIOID ANALGESICS/NSAIDS
- Acetaminophen (Tylenol, Datril)
- Acetylsalicylic acid (aspirin)
- Choline magnesium trisalicylate (Trilisate)
- Diclofenac sodium (Voltaren)
- Ibuprofen (Motrin, Advil)
- Indomethacin sodium trihydrate (Indocin)
- Naproxen (Naprosyn), naproxen sodium (Anaprox)
- Celecoxib (Celebrex)
- Piroxicam (Feldene)
- Meloxicam (Mobic)

MIXED OR WEAK OPIOID ANALGESICS
- Butorphanol (Stadol)
- Hydrocodone (Lortab, Vicodin)

- Codeine (Tylenol No. 3, Empirin No. 3)
- Tramadol (Ultram, Ultracet)
- Propoxyphene napsylate (Darvon-N, Darvocet-N)

STRONG OPIOID ANALGESICS
- Fentanyl citrate (Sublimaze, transdermal patches)
- Hydromorphone hydrochloride (Dilaudid)
- Meperidine hydrochloride (Demerol)
- Morphine sulfate (morphine)
- Methadone (Dolophiné)

COANALGESICS
- Tricyclic antidepressants (nortriptyline)
- Anticonvulsants (gabapentin)
- Topical local anesthetic (Lidoderm)
- Hydroxyzine (Vistaril)

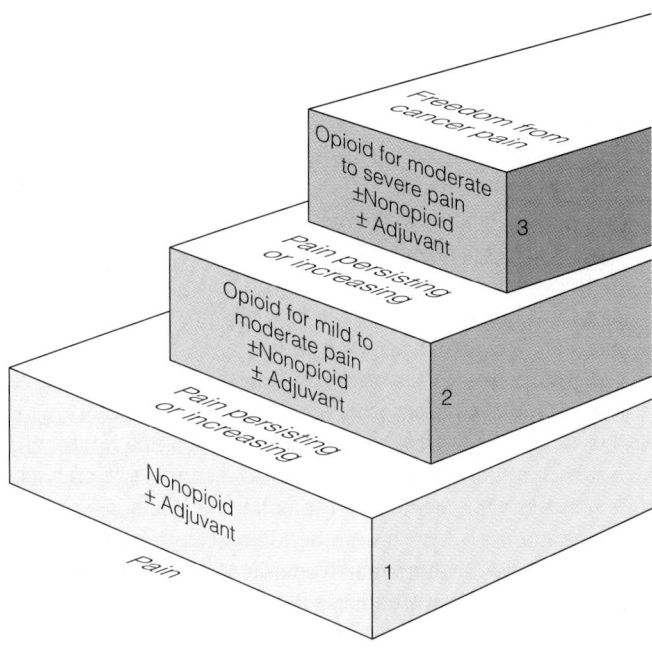

Figure 46-9 ■ The WHO three-step analgesic ladder.

(*Note:* From *Cancer Pain Relief*, 2nd ed., by World Health Organization, 1996, Geneva: Author. © Copyright World Health Organization (WHO), 2006. All rights reserved.)

like heat/relaxation) "may permit opioid dose reduction and improve patient outcomes" (APS, 2003, p. 34).

WORLD HEALTH ORGANIZATION (WHO) THREE-STEP APPROACH.

For clients with mild pain (1–3 on a 0–10 scale), step 1 of the analgesic ladder, nonopioid analgesics (with or without a coanalgesic) is the appropriate starting point. If the client has mild pain that persists or increases despite using full doses of step 1 medications, or if the pain is moderate (4–6 on a 0–10 scale), then a step 2 regimen is appropriate. At the second step, a weak opioid (e.g., codeine, tramadol, pentazocine) or a combination of opioid and nonopioid medicine (e.g., oxycodone with acetaminophen, hydrocodone with ibuprofen) is provided with or without coanalgesic medications. If the client has moderate pain that persists or increases despite using full doses of step 2 medications, or if the pain is severe (7–10 on a 0–10 scale), then a step 3 regimen is medically indicated. At the third step, strong opiates (e.g., morphine, hydromorphone, fentanyl) are administered and titrated in around-the-clock scheduled doses until the pain is relieved or dose-limiting respiratory depression occurs.

CLINICAL ALERT

Combining opioid and nonopioid analgesics is frequently overlooked. Each has different side effects, mechanisms of action, and toxicity profile. Alternating the two or giving them at the same time creates no danger and often produces a synergistic rather than merely additive effect. ■

NONOPIOIDS/NSAIDS.

Nonopioids include acetaminophen and **nonsteroidal anti-inflammatory drugs (NSAIDs)** such as ibuprofen or aspirin. NSAIDs have anti-inflammatory, analgesic, and antipyretic effects, whereas acetaminophen has only analgesic and antipyretic effects. The anti-inflammatory action relieves pain by interfering with the cyclooxygenase (COX) chemical cascade that is activated by damaged tissue. The COX chemical reactions produce prostaglandins and other inflammatory chemicals that cause a firing of nociceptive fibers. The COX-1 specific isoforms are found in platelets, the gastrointestinal (GI) tract, kidneys, and most other tissue, and are believed to be the cause of the well-known side effects of NSAIDs (GI bleed, diminished renal blood flow, inhibited clotting, etc.).

In the 1990s a second isoform (COX-2) was found and believed to be specific only for pain and inflammation. The resulting new "safer" (COX-2 selective) NSAIDs were tested, approved, and widely used. These drugs demonstrated significantly less GI bleeding, but uncommon cardiovascular events and rare skin problems in susceptible individuals prompted the U.S. Food and Drug Administration (FDA) to request a withdrawal of rofecoxib (Vioxx) in 2004 and a few months later to have valdecoxib (Bextra) also withdrawn from the marketplace. On April 6 and 7 of 2005, a memorandum and a public health advisory (respectively) were issued from the FDA warning consumers of the increased risk of serious cardiovascular events from the use of NSAIDs, both COX-2 selective and nonselective products. All prescription NSAIDs now must carry the strong "black box" warning of the risks of using these drugs. Even nonprescription NSAIDs (e.g., aspirin, ibuprofen, naproxen) must be relabeled to warn consumers of the potential dangers of using those products (FDA, 2005).

Individual drugs in this category vary little in their analgesic potency, but do vary in their anti-inflammatory properties, metabolism, excretion, and side effects. These drugs have a ceiling effect and a narrow therapeutic index. The *ceiling effect* means that once the maximum analgesic benefit is achieved, more drug will not produce more analgesia; however, more toxicity may occur. The *narrow therapeutic index* indicates that there's not much margin for safety between the dose that produces a desired effect and the dose that may produce a toxic, even lethal effect. The most common side effect of nonopioid analgesics is gastrointestinal, such as heartburn or indigestion. These effects can become toxic or lethal when silent GI bleeding occurs. Given the interference with platelet aggregation, a small stomach ulcer can bleed a lot, making it a potentially life-threatening condition. Clients should be taught to take NSAIDs with food and a full glass of water, and be routinely monitored by a health professional if they take these preparations daily for more than a couple of weeks.

Acetaminophen (Tylenol), on the other hand, has a different mechanism of action and side effect/toxicity profile. It does not affect platelet function and rarely causes GI distress, ulcers, or kidney, skin, or cardiovascular problems. It was not included in the public health advisory issued by the FDA; however, hepatotoxicity, and possible renal toxicity, does occur with high doses or with long-term use. Generally, 10 grams of acetaminophen is considered a lethal dose, with 6 grams per day causing measurable liver damage. It is recommended that otherwise young and healthy people limit their acetaminophen consumption to less than 4 grams per day, with susceptible (e.g., elderly, those with

BOX 46–6 Consumption Parameters for Common Pain Medications Containing Acetaminophen

Medication	Total Daily Tablet Limit (2.5–4 Grams Acetaminophen)*
Tylenol No. 3	8–12 tablets
Percocet	8–12 tablets
Lortab	5–8 tablets
Vicodin	5–8 tablets
Tylox	5–8 tablets
Darvocet-N 100	3–6 tablets
Vicodin ES (750 mg)	3–5 tablets

*Clients at risk for toxicity (e.g., elderly, liver disease, alcohol consumption, cardiac disease, pulmonary disease) to consume at low end of the range.

a history of alcoholism, dehydration, or liver disease) individuals limiting their consumption to 2.4 grams per day or less. Given that acetaminophen is so well tolerated, it is often a hidden ingredient in over-the-counter (OTC) remedies (e.g., pain, fever, allergy, cough and cold preparations), so clients must be instructed to read the ingredient list of all OTC medicines they take. Box 46–6 provides consumption parameters for medications that contain acetaminophen. Table 46–6 lists common misconceptions about nonopioids.

OPIOIDS. There are three primary types of opioids:

1. *Full agonists.* These pure opioid drugs bind tightly to mu receptor sites, producing maximum pain inhibition, an agonist effect. A full **agonist analgesic** includes morphine (e.g., Kadian, MS Contin), oxycodone (e.g., Percocet, OxyContin), and hydromorphone (e.g. Dilaudid, Pal-ladone). There is no ceiling on the level of analgesia from these drugs; their dose can be steadily increased to relieve pain. There is also no maximum daily dose limit unless they are in compound with a nonopioid analgesic drug like acetaminophen, which has a daily maximum limit of 2,400 to 4,000 mg.

2. *Mixed agonists-antagonists.* **Agonist-antagonist analgesic** drugs can act like opioids and relieve pain (agonist effect) when given to a client who has not taken any pure opioids. However, they can block or inactivate other opioid analgesics when given to a client who has been taking pure opioids (antagonist effect). These drugs include dezocine (Dalgan), pentazocine hydrochloride (Talwin), butorphanol tartrate (Stadol), and nalbuphine hydrochloride (Nubain). They block the mu receptor site and activate a kappa receptor site. If a client has been receiving a mu agonist (e.g., morphine, Percocet, or Vicodin for pain) daily for more than a couple of weeks, the administration of a mixed agonist-antagonist may result in an immediate and severe withdrawal reaction. These drugs also have a ceiling effect that limits the dose. They are not recommended for use with terminally ill clients. In the opioid naïve client with acute pain (e.g., migraine headache), these agents have a favorable effect and low side effect burden.

3. *Partial agonists.* Partial agonists have a ceiling effect in contrast to a full agonist. These drugs such as buprenorphine (Buprenex) block the mu receptors or are neutral at that receptor but bind at a kappa receptor site. This drug has good analgesic potency and is emerging as an alternative to methadone for opioid maintenance/narcotic treatment programs. The safety and favorable side effect profile make it an increasingly popular choice.

TABLE 46–6 Misconceptions about Nonopioids

MISCONCEPTION	CORRECTION
Regular daily use of NSAIDs is much safer than taking opioids.	Side effects from long-term use of NSAIDs are considerably more severe and life threatening than the side effects from daily doses of oral morphine or other opioids. The most common side effect from long-term use of opioids is constipation, whereas NSAIDs can cause gastric ulcers, increased bleeding time, and renal insufficiency. Acetaminophen can cause hepatotoxicity.
A nonopioid should not be given at the same time as an opioid.	It is safe to administer a nonopioid and opioid at the same time. Giving a dose of nonopioid at the same time as a dose of opioid poses no more danger than giving the doses at different times. In fact, many opioids are compounded with a nonopioid (e.g., Percocet [oxycodone and acetaminophen]).
Administering antacids with NSAIDs is an effective method of reducing gastric distress.	Administering antacids with NSAIDs can lessen distress but may be counterproductive. Antacids reduce the absorption and therefore the effectiveness of the NSAID by releasing the drug in the stomach rather than in the small intestine where absorption occurs.
Nonopioids are not useful analgesics for severe pain.	Nonopioids alone are rarely sufficient to relieve severe pain, but they are an important part in the total analgesic plan. One of the basic principles of analgesic therapy is: Whenever pain is severe enough to require an opioid, adding a nonopioid should be considered.
Gastric distress (e.g., abdominal pain) is indicative of NSAID-induced gastric ulceration.	Most clients with gastric lesions have no symptoms until bleeding or perforation occurs.

Note: Reprinted from *Pain: Clinical Manual,* 2nd ed., by M. McCaffery and C. Pasero, 1999, St. Louis, MO: Mosby. Copyright © 1999, Mosby, Inc. with permission from Elsevier.

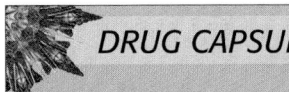

DRUG CAPSULE Narcotic Analgesic

oxycodone (OxyContin)
oxycodone/acetaminophen (Percocet)
oxycodone/aspirin (Percodan)

THE CLIENT WITH PAIN

Opioids relieve moderate to severe pain by inhibiting the release of substance P in both central and peripheral nerves, reducing the perception of pain, producing sedation, and decreasing the emotional stress of pain.

Oxycodone is a semisynthetic derivative of codeine. It is a Schedule II controlled substance. It is often administered as a combination drug with acetaminophen or aspirin.

NURSING RESPONSIBILITIES

- Assess pain prior to and 60 minutes after administration.
- Assess bowel function to prevent constipation.
- Keep track of the total amount of acetaminophen or aspirin the client is receiving when taking a combination drug. The maximum daily dose of acetaminophen is 4,000 mg.

CLIENT AND FAMILY TEACHING

- Take with food to decrease GI upset.
- Avoid crushing or chewing long-acting tablets (e.g., OxyContin).
- Avoid alcohol or other CNS depressants.
- Explain that the medication may cause dizziness, and instruct to make position changes slowly.
- Instruct that constipation is a common side effect. Discuss preventive measures.
- Take only as prescribed.

Note: Prior to administering any medication, review all aspects with a current drug handbook or other reliable source.

Weak or Mixed Opioid Analgesics. These include drugs that are weak opioids (e.g., propoxyphene, codeine, tramadol); mixed agonist-antagonist drugs; or combination opioids with nonopioid (NSAIDs) analgesics compounds. These medicines are generally 2 to 4 times more potent that nonopioids alone, and have some of the risks of both drug classes. With a rare exception, these are controlled substances and must be ordered by a physician or nurse practitioner, adhering to applicable federal and state laws. These drugs also have a ceiling effect and a maximum daily dose limit. There are advantages to giving combination drugs, such as lowering the amount of any one medicine needed in a 24-hour period, thus reducing the potential for side effects or toxicity; however, nurses need to be familiar with each medication and be aware of daily dose limits of the ingredients as well as the potential to receive duplicate medications for different clinical indications (e.g., Tylenol in the mixed drug, Tylenol for fever, and Tylenol in the headache preparation).

Among the weak opioids, there is a narrow therapeutic index. Codeine at doses of 30 to 60 mg produces dose-limiting gastrointestinal distress in many people. Propoxyphene produces a by-product that irritates nerves and muscles, and tramadol lowers seizure threshold. The mixed agonist-antagonist drugs have some properties of naloxone (Narcan), and thus in individuals who have been on opioids for a period of time, these drugs can cause a serious withdrawal reaction. Therefore, mixed agonist-antagonist medications (Talwin, Stadol, Nubain, etc.) may be a first opioid tried, but the client is not switched from another opioid to these preparations.

Strong Opioid Analgesics. Pure agonist opioid analgesics include opium derivatives, such as morphine, hydromorphone, oxycodone, fentanyl, and methadone (APS, 2003). *Opioid* is the pharmacologic class of pain relievers, many of which are "scheduled" as a controlled substance (narcotic) due to the potential for misuse. Pure agonist opioids relieve pain primarily by binding to mu receptors in the peripheral and central nervous systems. In addition to pain reduction, changes in mood may make the person

feel more comfortable even though the pain persists. As the most potent class of pain relievers, these drugs are indicated for severe pain, or when other medications have failed to control moderately severe or worse pain. Among this class, meperidine (Demerol) has received a lot of attention in recent years as a medication to avoid because of its short half-life, toxic metabolite, and potential to induce seizures with repeated doses.

Opioid Side Effects. When administering any analgesic, the nurse must review side effects. Side effects of the opioids typically include respiratory depression, sedation, nausea/vomiting, urinary retention, blurred vision, sexual dysfunction, and constipation. The most concerning adverse effect of opioids is respiratory depression (e.g., 8 per minute or less), which usually occurs early in therapy among opioid naïve clients; with dose escalation; or in clients with drug–drug or drug–disease interactions. Clinically, the client will appear overly sedated, and respirations will be slow and deep with periods of apnea. The nurse needs to assess a client's level of alertness and respiratory rate for baseline data before administering narcotics. See the sedation rating scale in Box 46–7. Often clients will manifest an increase in sedation *before* they manifest a decrease in respiratory rate and depth. Early recognition of an increasing level of sedation or respiratory depression will enable the nurse to implement appropriate measures promptly (e.g., pulse oximetry monitoring, obtaining an order to decrease the opioid dosage).

BOX 46–7 Sedation Scale

S = Sleep, easy to arouse
1 = Awake and alert
2 = Slightly drowsy, easily aroused
3 = Frequently drowsy, arousable, drifts off to sleep during conversation
4 = Somnolent, minimal or no response to physical stimulation

Note: Reprinted from *Pain: Clinical Manual,* 2nd ed. (p. 267), by M. McCaffery and C. Pasero, 1999, St. Louis, MO: Mosby. Copyright © 1999, Mosby, Inc. with permission from Elsevier.

BOX 46–8 Common Opioid Side Effects, Preventive, and Treatment Measures

CONSTIPATION
- Increase fluid intake (e.g., 6 to 8 glasses daily).
- Increase fiber and bulk-forming agents to the diet (e.g., fresh fruits and vegetables). Increasing exercise is often ineffective in controlling this type of constipation.
- Administer daily stool softeners combined with a mild laxative (e.g., Senokot-S) as a first line of prevention against constipation for clients on opioid maintenance therapy.
- Stimulants (bisacodyl), osmotic laxatives (lactulose, sorbitol, and polyethylene glycol), enemas (tap water and sodium phosphate), and even prokinetic agents (metoclopramide) may be needed for refractory cases of constipation (Kurz & Sessler, 2003).

NAUSEA AND VOMITING
- Inform client that tolerance to this emetic effect generally develops after several days of opiate therapy.
- Provide an antiemetic (antihistamines [e.g., Vistaril, Phenergan], antimuscarinics [e.g., cyclizine, hyoscine], and dopamine receptor antagonists [e.g., Haldol]) as indicated.
- Change the dose or analgesic agent as indicated.

SEDATION
- Inform client that tolerance usually develops over 3 to 5 days.
- Consider the administration of a stimulant (e.g., Dexedrine or Ritalin) or an alternative route of administration (e.g., epidural) for clients with persistent pain and sedation.

- Observe client for evidence of respiratory depression that may occur with sedation.

RESPIRATORY DEPRESSION
- Administer an opioid antagonist, such as naloxone hydrochloride (Narcan), cautiously by diluting 1 ampule in 10 mL of saline and then administering 1 cc per minute until the respirations are ≥ 10/min. Make provisions for repeat administration, continuous infusion, or a longer acting version of a reversal agent as the half-life of naloxone is considerably shorter than most opioids being reversed.
- Stop, change, or slow the administration of opioids until respirations are restored.

PRURITUS
- Apply cool packs, lotion, and diversional activity.
- Administer an antihistamine (e.g., diphenhydramine hydrochloride [Benadryl]).
- Inform the client that tolerance also develops to pruritus.

URINARY RETENTION
- May need to catheterize client, or change or lower the analgesic dose.
- Administer narcotic antagonist (naloxone hydrochloride [Narcan]) or longer acting reversal agent (methylnaltrexone is pending FDA approval). Extreme caution is urged with the use of Narcan.

Box 46–8 provides suggested measures to prevent and treat side effects of opioid analgesics.

CLINICAL ALERT

Constipation is an almost universal adverse effect of opioid use. All clients should receive prophylactic stimulant laxative therapy, unless contraindicated. Stool softeners are not useful alone, but are a good choice when combined with a stimulant laxative (e.g, Senokot-S). If those products are ineffective, a regimen of cathartic laxatives (e.g., bisacodyl), followed by more aggressive forms of treatment (e.g., osmotic laxatives, enema, manual disimpaction) may be necessary. ■

Older clients are particularly sensitive to the analgesic properties of opioids and may require less medication, or medication administered at less frequent intervals, than younger clients. This sensitivity may be related to reduced or delayed excretion of the drug in elderly clients. As such, the clinical pearl of "start low (25%–50% dose reduction) and go (titrate) slow" is often followed in the older population (AGS, 2002).

CLINICAL ALERT

Assessing for sedation and respiratory status is critical during the first 12 to 24 hours after starting opioid therapy. The most critical period is during the peak effect of the first dose (15 minutes if administered IV; first hour after IM, oral, or rectal route). An exception is with opioids administered via the spinal route. Respiratory depression may increase over time with epidural infusions and with intrathecal analgesia; respiratory depression may manifest 24 hours after the spinal injection even after the analgesic effect has worn off. In general, the longer the client receives opioids, the wider the safety margin as the client develops a tolerance to the sedative and respiratory depressive effects of the drug. ■

EQUIANALGESIC DOSING. The term **equianalgesia** refers to the relative potency of various opioid analgesics compared to a standard dose of parenteral morphine. This tool helps professionals individualize the analgesic regimen by guiding the adjustment of medication, dose, time interval, and route of administration. An equianalgesic chart can be used to help provide doses of approximately equal ability to relieve pain. The two basic techniques for calculating doses based on equianalgesic equivalents are ratio and cross-multiplication methods. For example, with the ratio technique, it is known that the oral:IV morphine ratio is 3:1, meaning IV morphine is 3 times more potent than oral morphine. Thus, a client who has required 100 mg of IV morphine per day will require 300 mg of oral morphine per day to control the same level of pain. If a different client who had an opioid requirement of 40 mg IV morphine per day were to be switched to oral Dilaudid, the equianalgesia chart informs us that 10 mg IV morphine is equivalent to 7.5 mg hydromorphone (Dilaudid). Using the cross-multiplication technique (X represents unknown dose), the following steps are calculated:

- 10 mg IV morphine = 7.5 mg oral hydromorphone
- 40 mg IV morphine = X mg hydromorphone
  - Cross-multiply
    - $10X = 7.5 \times 40$
    - $10X = 300$
    - $X = 30$

- Thus 30 mg oral hydromorphone per day would provide equivalent analgesia to 40 mg of parenteral morphine per day. The hydromorphone dose is then divided based on the duration of action of the available preparations (extended-release Palladone every 12 hours or Dilaudid every 4 hours).

CLINICAL ALERT

Many health care professionals underestimate the effectiveness of ordinary aspirin and acetaminophen. The ordinary dose of aspirin or acetaminophen relieves as much pain as 1.5 mg of parenteral morphine, whereas standard doses of mixed analgesics (e.g., Tylenol No. 3 or Percocet) are approximately equivalent to 2.5 to 5 mg of morphine. ∎

COANALGESICS. A **coanalgesic** agent (formerly known as an adjuvant) is a medication that is not classified as a pain medication. However, coanalgesics have properties that may reduce pain alone or in combination with other analgesics, relieve other discomforts, potentiate the effect of pain medications, or reduce the pain medication's side effects. Examples of coanalgesics that relieve pain are antidepressants (support the function of the pain-modulating system); anticonvulsants (stabilize nerve membranes, reducing excitability and spontaneous firing); and local anesthetics (block the transmission of pain signals). Anxiolytics, sedatives, and antispasmodics are examples of medicines that relieve other discomforts; however, they do not alleviate pain and thus should be used in addition to rather than instead of analgesics. Examples of medications used to reduce the side effects of analgesics include stimulants, laxatives, and antiemetics.

Coanalgesics appear to be particularly beneficial for the management of neuropathic pain. Tricyclic antidepressant drugs seem to be particularly useful for central neuropathic pain, which often manifests as pain with a burning, unusual, or stinging quality. Anticonvulsant drugs, such as gabapentin seem particularly useful for peripheral neuropathic conditions that often present with a stabbing, shooting, or electrical-shock quality. Local anesthetics such as the Lidoderm patch also alleviate neuropathic as well as other types of pain, and are particularly useful for clients with the skin sensitivity known as allodynia. There is a growing scientific and clinical basis for the use of these medications in relieving pain, especially for persistent pain that is not relieved by the analgesic classes of medication alone.

Administration of Placebos

A **placebo** is "any medication or procedure, including surgery, that produces an effect in a client because of its implicit or explicit intent and not because of its specific physical or chemical properties" (McCaffery & Pasero, 1999). *Placebos* often take the form of sugar pills, saline injections, minuscule doses of drugs, or sham procedures designed to be void of any known therapeutic value. In contrast, the *placebo effect* is a perceptible, measurable, and desirable consequence which exceeds the anticipated biological changes and may occur as a result of interpersonal factors such as the presence of a caring person or a healing intent (Arnstein, 2003). Some professionals try to justify the use of placebos to elicit the desirable placebo effect or in a misguided attempt to determine if the client's pain is "real." The use of placebos, outside the context of an approved research study, is deceptive and represents fraudulent and unethical treatment. The American Society for Pain Management Nursing

(2005) and other professional organizations have published position papers that adamantly oppose the use of placebos without consent.

Routes for Opiate Delivery

Opioids have traditionally been administered by oral, subcutaneous, intramuscular, and intravenous routes. In addition, newer methods of delivering opiates have been developed to circumvent potential obstacles that occur with these traditional routes. Examples are transnasal, transmucosal, and transdermal drug therapy, continuous subcutaneous infusions, and intraspinal infusion.

ORAL. Oral administration of opiates remains the preferred route of delivery because of ease of administration. Given the duration of action of most opiates is approximately 4 hours, people with chronic pain have had to awaken during the night to medicate themselves for pain. To circumvent this problem, long-acting or sustained-release forms of morphine with a duration of 8 or more hours have been developed. Two examples of long-acting morphine are MS Contin and Oramorph SR. Clients receiving long-acting morphine may also need prn "rescue" doses of immediate-release analgesics such as short-acting oral transmucosal fentanyl citrate (Actiq) for acute breakthrough pain (Rhiner & Kedziera, 1999). As a transmucosal agent, it immediately enters the bloodstream and begins to work. Another method of oral opiate delivery is high-concentration liquid morphine. This formulation enables clients who can swallow only small amounts to continue taking the drug orally.

NASAL. Transnasal administration has the advantage of rapid action of the medication because of direct absorption through the vascular nasal mucosa. A commonly used agent is a mixed agonist-antagonist butorphanol (Stadol) for acute migraine headaches. Treating migraine headaches via the nasal route of administration is particularly beneficial because of the nausea, vomiting, and gastroparesis that occurs with that condition, making oral medications relatively contraindicated.

TRANSDERMAL. Transdermal drug therapy is advantageous in that it delivers a relatively stable plasma drug level and is noninvasive. Fentanyl (Duragesic) is an opioid currently available as a skin patch with various dosages. It provides drug delivery for up to 72 hours. The transdermal route is distinguished from the topical route, in that the effects of the medications are systemic after the medication is absorbed, whereas topical medications placed on the skin (e.g., Lidoderm, capsaicin, or Aspercreme) work locally at the point they are placed on the body.

RECTAL. Several nonopiate and opiate medicines are now available in suppository form. The rectal route is particularly useful for clients who have dysphagia (difficulty swallowing) or nausea and vomiting. It is best to use commercially available rectal preparations, or have them compounded by a licensed compound pharmacist. Occasionally, nurses modify oral medications for rectal use. This practice is outside the scope of nursing practice and may be lethal in the event that a sustained-release analgesic is crushed, thus disarming the safety matrix that prevents an overdose.

SUBCUTANEOUS. Although the subcutaneous (SC) route has been used extensively to deliver opioids, another technique uses subcutaneous catheters and infusion pumps to provide continuous subcutaneous infusion (CSCI) of narcotics. CSCI is particularly helpful for clients (a) whose pain is poorly controlled by oral medications, (b) who are experiencing dysphagia or gastrointestinal obstruction, or (c) who have a need for prolonged use of parenteral narcotics. CSCI involves the use of a small, light, battery-operated pump that administers the drug through a 23- or 25-gauge butterfly needle. The needle can be inserted into the anterior chest, the subclavicular region, the abdominal wall, the outer aspects of the upper arms, or the thighs. Client mobility is maintained with the application of a shoulder bag or holster to hold the pump (Figure 46-10 ■). The frequency of site change ranges from 3 to 7 days.

Because family caregivers must operate the pump and also change and care for the injection site, the nurse needs to provide appropriate instruction. Caregivers need to be able to

- Describe the basic parts and symbols of the system.
- Identify ways to determine whether the pump is working.
- Change the battery.
- Change the medication.
- Demonstrate stopping and starting the pump.
- Demonstrate tubing care, site care, and changing of the injection site.
- Identify signs indicating the need to change an injection site.
- Describe general care of the pump when the client is ambulatory, bathing, sleeping, or traveling.
- Identify actions to take to solve problems when the alarm signals.

INTRAMUSCULAR. The intramuscular (IM) route should be avoided if possible because of variable absorption, unpredictable onset of action and peak effect, as well as the tissue damage that may result, even if properly administered. Regardless of precautions taken, there is pain involved with ad-

Figure 46-10 ■ Subcutaneous infusion needle placement. Figure shows sites for SC infusion needle placement, which may be attached to an ambulatory infusion pump. Other sites to consider include upper arms and thighs. Sites should be rotated.

(*Note:* From *Pain: Clinical Manual,* 2nd ed. (p. 211), by M. McCaffery and C. Pasero, 1999, St. Louis, MO: Mosby, Copyright 1999, Mosby, Inc. Reprinted with permission from Elsevier Science.)

ministration, and there may be damage to nerves or blood vessels punctured by the needle, or necrosis of muscle and/or subcutaneous tissue may result from a toxic combination of medicines (e.g., Demerol with Phenergan, or Vistaril).

INTRAVENOUS. The intravenous (IV) route provides rapid and effective pain relief with few side effects. However, just as the onsent of pain relief occurs in 5 to 10 minutes, so can adverse effects, like repiratory depression. The analgesic can be administered by IV bolus or by slow continuous infusion. Caution is needed to prevent the introduction of air or bacteria into the tubing, and to prevent introducing medications that are incompatible with other medications dissolved in the intravenous solution.

INTRASPINAL. An increasingly popular method of delivery is the infusion of opiates into the epidural or intrathecal (subarachnoid) space (Figure 46-11 ■). Analgesics administered via the intraspinal route are delivered adjacent to the opiate receptors in the dorsal horn of the spinal cord. Two commonly used medications are morphine sulfate and fentanyl. All medicines administered via the intraspinal route need to be sterile and preservative-free (preservatives are neurotoxic). The major benefit of intraspinal drug therapy is superior analgesia with less medication used. The epidural space is most commonly used because the dura mater acts as a protective barrier against infection, including meningitis, and there is less risk of developing a "spinal headache." Intraspinal catheters are not in constant contact with blood, and thus an infusion can be stopped and restarted later without concern that the catheter has become clotted off.

Intrathecal administration delivers medication directly into the cerebrospinal fluid (CSF) that bathes and nourishes the spinal cord. Medicines quickly and efficiently bind to the opioid receptor sites in the dorsal horn when administered in this way, speeding the onset and peak effect, while prolonging the duration of action of the analgesic. An example of how the route of administration affects the relative potency of opiates is as follows: A client who needs 300 mg of oral morphine per day to control pain will need 100 mg of parenteral morphine, 10 mg of epidural morphine, and only 1 mg of intrathecal morphine in a 24-hour period. Very little drug is absorbed by blood vessels into the systemic circulation. In fact the drug must circulate through the CSF to be excreted. As a result, there may be a delayed onset (24 hours after the administration) of respiratory depression, as medication that has left the spinal opioid sites travels through the brain to be eliminated.

In contrast, the epidural space is separated from the spinal cord by the dura mater, which acts as a barrier to drug diffusion. In addition, it is filled with fatty tissue and an extensive venous system. With this diffusion delay, some medications (especially fat-soluble medications like fentanyl) from the epidural space enter the systemic circulation via the venous plexus. Thus a higher dose of opiate is required to create the desired effect, which can produce side effects of itching, urinary retention, and/or respiratory depression. Often, a mixture of an opioid (e.g., fentanyl) and a local anesthetic (e.g., bupivacaine) are combined to lower the dose of opioid needed. As a result, there

Figure 46-11 ■ Placement of intraspinal catheter in the epidural space.

may be an increase in fall risk for some clients who develop muscular weakness in their legs or orthostatic hypotention in response to the local anesthetic.

Intraspinal analgesia can be administered by three modes of operation:

1. *Bolus.* A single or repeated bolus dose(s) may be provided. When clients have spinal anesthesia (e.g., during a cesarean section), a bolus of 1 mg intrathecal morphine can provide significant pain control for up to 24 hours. For shorter acting medications, an epidural catheter may be intact and accessed by a qualified health professional (e.g., anesthesiologist or nurse anesthetist) to administer bolus doses on an "as needed" basis. Check your state regulations and agency policy regarding who can provide these bolus doses, how they are documented, and the postbolus monitoring procedures.
2. *Continuous infusion administered by pump.* The pump may be external (for acute or chronic pain) or surgically implanted (for chronic pain) to provide a continuous infusion of pain relievers into the epidural or intrathecal space.
3. *Continuous plus intermittent bolus.* With this mode of operation, the client receives a continuous infusion with bolus "rescue" doses administered for breakthrough pain. Often a pump with *patient-controlled epidural analgesia (PCEA)* capabilities is used for this mode of operation. This is similar to patient-controlled analgesia (detailed later) in which a basal rate may or may not be used to meet the client's anticipated analgesic need, with the client's ability to request an incremental dose at set intervals by pressing a button. PCEA is often used to manage acute postoperative pain, chronic pain, and intractable cancer pain. The "walking epidurals" used for women in labor are typically PCEA devices that are programmed in the bolus mode without a continuous infusion (basal rate) set.

The anesthesiologist or nurse anesthetist inserts a needle into the intrathecal or epidural space (typically in the lumbar region) and threads a catheter through the needle to the desired level. The catheter is connected to tubing that is then positioned along the spine and over the client's shoulder for the nurse to access. The entire catheter and tubing are taped securely to prevent dislodgment. Often an occlusive, transparent dressing is placed over the insertion site for easy identification of catheter displacement or local inflammation. Temporary catheters, used for short-term acute pain management, are usually placed at the lumbar or thoracic vertebral level and often removed after 2 to 4 days. Permanent catheters, for clients with chronic pain, may be tunneled subcutaneously through the skin and exit at the client's side or be connected to a pump implanted in the abdomen. Tunneling of the catheter reduces the risk of infection and displacement of the catheter. After the catheter is inserted, the nurse is responsible for monitoring the infusion and assessing the client per institutional policy. Nursing care of clients with intraspinal infusions is summarized in Table 46–7.

There are misconceptions, either overstating or ignoring the risks of spinal analgesia. This is in part due to the importance of the technique of the professional inserting the catheter, which varies considerably. In general, clients receiving epidural analgesia do not need to be monitored in an intensive care setting, but they do need vigilant assessment of their pain, neurological and respiratory status, and the insertion site frequently during the course of therapy.

CLINICAL ALERT

As a precaution, have naloxone (Narcan), sodium chloride 0.9% diluent, and injection equipment on hand for each client receiving an opioid-containing epidural infusion. ■

TABLE 46–7   Nursing Interventions for Clients Receiving Analgesics through an Epidural Catheter

NURSING GOALS	INTERVENTIONS
Maintain client safety	Label the tubing, the infusion bag, and the front of the pump with tape marked EPIDURAL to prevent confusion with similar-looking IV lines. Post sign above client's bed indicating epidural is in place. Secure all connections with tape. If there is no continuous infusion, apply tape over all injection ports on the epidural line to avoid the injection of substances intended for IV administration into the epidural catheter. Do not use alcohol in any care of catheter or insertion site as it can be neurotoxic. Ensure that any solution injected or infused intraspinally is sterile, preservative-free, and safe for intraspinal administration.
Maintain catheter placement	Secure temporary catheters with tape. When bolus doses are used, gently aspirate prior to medication administration to determine catheter has not migrated into the subarachnoid space. (Expect <1 mL of fluid return in syringe.) Assist client in repositioning or moving out of bed. Teach client to avoid tugging on the catheter. Assess insertion site for leakage with each bolus dose or at least every 8–12 hours.
Prevent infection	Use strict aseptic techniques with all epidural-related procedures. Maintain sterile occlusive dressing over insertion site. Assess insertion site for signs of infection. Assess for increasing diffuse back pain or tenderness and/or paresthesia on intraspinal injection because these are cardinal signs of intraspinal infection (McCaffery & Pasero, 1999, p. 234).
Maintain urinary and bowel function	Monitor intake and output. Assess for bowel and bladder distention.
Prevent respiratory depression	Assess sedation level and respiratory status q1h for the first 24 hours and thereafter q4h. Do not administer other opioids or central nervous system depressants unless ordered. Keep an ampule of naloxone hydrochloride (0.4 mg) at the bedside. Notify the clinician in charge if the respiratory rate falls below 8 per minute or if the client is difficult to rouse.

REAL WORLD PRACTICE

Mrs. Black was an end stage renal disease client who had been on hemodialysis for many years. She was also dealing with neuropathy pain stemming from her diabetes. After receiving a new diagnosis of colon cancer with spinal metastasis, spinal cord compression, and increased nerve pain in both legs, Mrs. Black and her family wanted pain relief as her life neared its end. The evening nurse initiated a morphine PCA at 2 mg per hour basal rate with injections of 1 mg when the client had jolts of nerve pain. She would push the button before turning, since it precipitated the jolts of pain. Mrs. Black and her family had decided on a No Code Blue status and comfort care.

As Mrs. Black became more sedated due to the dialysis being terminated, she was unable to push the button on her PCA. The daughters decided that they should push the button for their mother when she had jolts of pain during turning throughout the night.

When I arrived on duty the next morning, I introduced myself to Mrs. Black and her family. I told them that my goal for the day was to get her comfortable and that because of hospital policy only the client should push the button on the PCA. I explained that we could titrate the morphine basal rate, which would deliver more constant pain relief, and that I would like to add Ativan in combination with the morphine to help the nerve pain and the jolts of pain. By the end of my shift, we had the morphine running at 5 mg per hour and used the Ativan twice, especially before turning. When the family noticed any signs of moaning or agitation, they would notify the nurse for a dose of Ativan. Mrs. Black was comfortable and we achieved our goal.

Mrs. Black died the next day with her family at her side in comfort due to combination drug therapy.

—Ann M. Ohmann RNC, OCN,
St Cloud Hospital, MN

CONTINUOUS LOCAL ANESTHETICS. Continuous subcutaneous administration of long-acting local anesthetics into or near the surgical site is a technique being used to provide postoperative pain control. This technique has been used for a variety of surgical procedures, including knee arthroplasty, abdominal hysterectomy, hernia repair, and mastectomy. Nursing interventions for the client with infusion of a continuous local anesthetic include:

- Conduct pain assessment and documentation every 2 to 4 hours while the client is awake.
- Check the dressing every shift for intactness. The dressing is not usually changed in order to avoid dislodging the catheter. Contact the primary care provider if the dressing becomes loose.
- Check the site of the catheter. It should be clean and dry.
- Assess the client for signs of local anesthetic toxicity (e.g., cardiac arrhythmias, dizziness; ringing in the ears; a metallic taste; tingling or numbness of the lips, gums, or tongue) or neurological deficit distal to the catheter insertion site.
- Notify the primary care provider of signs of local anesthetic toxicity or neurological deficit. If detected early, prompt treatment can be initiated and serious complications avoided.

Patient-Controlled Analgesia

Patient-controlled analgesia (PCA) is an interactive method of pain management that permits clients to treat their pain by self-administering doses of analgesics. The oral route for PCA is most common, but the subcutaneous, intravenous, and epidural routes are increasingly being used. The PCA mode of therapy minimizes the roller-coaster effect of peaks of sedation and valleys of pain that occur with the traditional method of prn dosing. With the parenteral routes, the client administers a predetermined dose of a narcotic by an electronic infusion pump. This allows the client to maintain a more constant level of relief yet need less medication for pain relief. Patient-controlled analgesias can be effectively used for clients with acute pain related to a surgical incision, traumatic injury, or labor and delivery, and for chronic pain as with cancer.

In some settings PCAs are used even if the client is unable to initiate a dose by pushing the button, as long as a caregiver is willing to accept the responsibility (for example, when the client is an infant or toddler or is physically or cognitively impaired). This has been termed *PCA by proxy* and has been the subject of concern for the client's safety. In December 2004, the Joint Commission on Accreditation of Healthcare Organizations (JCAHO) published "sentinel events" pointing toward serious toxic reactions, even deaths associated with this practice. Fifteen of 460 PCA-related deaths in America were directly related to this practice. In general, in the absence of a strict protocol and vigilant monitoring, this practice should be avoided, with even stronger recommendations to prohibit this practice (JCAHO, 2004).

The prescriber orders the analgesic dose, route, and frequency, with the client administering the medication. Whether in an acute hospital setting, an ambulatory clinic, or with home care, the nurse is responsible for the initial instruction regarding use of the PCA and for the ongoing monitoring of the therapy. The client's pain, ability to understand, and use of the device must be assessed at regular intervals, and analgesic use is documented in the client's record.

Patient-controlled analgesia pumps are designed with built-in safety mechanisms to prevent client overdosage, abusive use, and narcotic theft. The most significant adverse effects are respiratory depression and hypotension; however, they occur rarely. Although PCA pumps vary in design, they all have similar protective features. The line of the PCA pump, a syringe-type pump, is usually introduced into the injection port of a primary IV fluid line (Figure 46-12 ■). When clients want a dose of analgesic, they can push a

Figure 46-13 ■ The older child is able to regulate a PCA pump.

button attached to the infusion pump and the preset dose is delivered (Figure 46-13 ■). A programmable lockout interval (usually 6 to 15 minutes) follows the dose, during which an additional dose cannot be given even if the client activates the button. It is also possible to program the maximum dose that can be delivered over a period of hours (usually 4). Many pumps are capable of delivering a basal rate (continuous infusion), with or without additional PCA doses available.

Nonpharmacologic Pain Management

Nonpharmacologic pain management consists of a variety of physical, cognitive-behavioral, and lifestyle pain management strategies that target the body, mind, spirit, and social interactions (see Table 46–8). Physical modalities include cutaneous

Figure 46-12 ■ PCA line introduced into the injection port of a primary line.

Primary (maintenance) IV fluid

PCA pump

Y-connector site for PCA tubing and primary line

CLIENT TEACHING
Client Self-Management of Pain

Choose a time to teach the client about pain management when the pain is controlled so that the client is able to focus on the teaching.

Teaching the client about self-management of pain can include the following:

■ Demonstrate the operation of the PCA pump and explain that the client can safely push the button without fear of overmedicating. Sometimes it helps clients who are reluctant to repeatedly push the button to know that they must dose themselves (i.e., push the button) 5 to 10 times to receive the same amount of medication (10 mg morphine equivalent) they would receive in a standard "shot."

■ Describe the use of the pain scale and encourage the client to respond in order to demonstrate understanding.

■ Explore a variety of nondrug pain relief techniques that the client is willing to learn and use to promote pain relief and optimize functioning.

■ Explain to the client the need to notify staff when ambulation is desired (e.g., for bathroom use) if applicable.

LIFESPAN CONSIDERATIONS
PCA Pump

CHILDREN
■ Include the parents in teaching.
■ Assess the child's ability to use the client control button.

ELDERS
■ Carefully monitor for drug side effects.
■ Use cautiously for individuals with impaired pulmonary or renal function.
■ Assess the client's cognitive and physical ability to use the client control button.

HOME CARE CONSIDERATIONS
PCA Pump

■ Monitor for signs and symptoms of oversedation such as excessive drowsiness, slowed respiratory rate, or change in mental state.
■ Do not adjust settings without consulting with the appropriate primary care provider.
■ Tape to the back of the pump the following emergency contact numbers: emergency medical services, primary care provider, home care agency, and pump manufacturer.

TABLE 46–8 Nonpharmacologic Interventions for Pain Control

TARGET DOMAIN OF PAIN CONTROL	INTERVENTION
Body	Reducing pain triggers, promoting comfort
	Massage
	Applying heat or ice
	Electric stimulation (TENS)
	Positioning, bracing (selective immobilization)
	Acupressure
	Diet, nutritional supplements
	Exercise, pacing activities
	Invasive interventions (e.g., blocks)
	Sleep hygiene
Mind	Relaxation, imagery
	Self-hypnosis
	Pain diary, journal writing
	Distracting attention
	Repatterning thinking
	Attitude adjustment
	Reducing fear, anxiety, stress
	Reducing sadness, helplessness
	Information about pain
Spirit	Prayer, meditation
	Self-reflection re: life and pain
	Meaningful rituals
	Energy work (e.g., therapeutic touch, Reiki)
	Spiritual healing
Social interactions	Functional restoration
	Improved communication
	Family therapy
	Problem solving
	Vocational training
	Volunteering
	Support groups

stimulation, ice or heat, immobilization or therapeutic exercises, transcutaneous electrical nerve stimulation (TENS), and acupuncture. Mind–body (cognitive-behavioral) interventions include distracting activities, relaxation techniques, imagery, meditation, biofeedback, hypnosis, cognitive-reframing, emotional counseling, and spiritually-directed approaches such as therapeutic touch or Reiki. Lifestyle management approaches include symptom monitoring, stress management, exercise, nutrition, pacing activities, disability management, and other approaches needed by many clients with persistent pain that has drastically changed their life. For further information on selected mind–body interventions and acupuncture, see Chapter 19. ∞ This discussion is limited to selected physical and cognitive-behavioral interventions.

PHYSICAL INTERVENTIONS. The goals of physical intervention include providing comfort, altering physiologic responses to reduce pain perception, and optimizing functioning.

CUTANEOUS STIMULATION. Cutaneous stimulation can provide effective temporary pain relief. It distracts the client and focuses attention on the tactile stimuli, away from the painful sensations, thus reducing pain perception. Cutaneous stimulation is also believed to interfere with the transmission and perception of pain by stimulating the large-diameter A-beta sensory nerve fibers that activate the descending mechanisms that can reduce the intensity of pain, activate the endorphin system of pain control, and thus diminish conscious awareness of pain. Selected cutaneous stimulation techniques include the following:

■ Massage
■ Application of heat or cold
■ Acupressure
■ Contralateral stimulation

Cutaneous stimulation can be applied directly to the painful area, proximal to the pain or distal to the pain (along the nerve path or dermatome), and contralateral (exact location, opposite side of the body) to the pain. Cutaneous stimulation is contraindicated in areas of skin breakdown or impaired neurological functioning.

Massage. Massage is a comfort measure that can aid relaxation, decrease muscle tension, and may ease anxiety because the physical contact communicates caring. It can also decrease pain intensity by increasing superficial circulation to the area. Massage can involve the back and neck, hands and arms, or feet. The use of ointments or liniments may provide localized pain relief with joint or muscle pain. Massage is contraindicated in areas of skin breakdown, suspected clots, or infections. See Skill 46-1.

PROVIDING A BACK MASSAGE

Effleurage is a type of massage consisting of long, slow, gliding strokes. Research demonstrates that back massage can enhance client comfort and relaxation and have a positive effect on cardiovascular parameters such as blood pressure, heart rate, and respiratory rate (McNamara, Burnham, Smith, & Carroll, 2003).

PURPOSES
- To relieve muscle tension
- To decrease pain intensity
- To promote physical and mental relaxation

ASSESSMENT
Assess the following:

- Behaviors indicating potential need for a back massage, such as a complaint of stiffness, muscle tension in the back or shoulders, or difficulty sleeping related to tenseness or anxiety

- Whether the client is willing to have a massage, because some individuals may not enjoy a massage
- Contraindications for back massage (e.g., impaired skin integrity, back surgery, vertebral, or rib fracture)

PLANNING
Ensure that you have the full amount of time available for the massage. Although the actual technique may require only about 5 minutes, the entire process should be conducted in a calm and unhurried manner.

Delegation
The nurse can delegate this skill to UAP; however, the nurse should first assess for any contraindications and client willingness.

Equipment
- Lotion
- Towel for excess lotion

IMPLEMENTATION
Preparation
Determine (a) previous assessments of the skin, (b) special lotions to be used, and (c) positions contraindicated for the client. Arrange for a quiet environment with no interruptions to promote maximum effect of the back massage.

Performance
1. Prior to performing the procedure, introduce self and verify the client's identity using agency protocol. Explain to the client what you are going to do, why it is necessary, and how he or she can cooperate. Encourage the client to give you feedback as to the amount of pressure you are using during the back rub.
2. Perform hand hygiene.
3. Provide for client privacy.
4. Prepare the client.
   - Assist the client to move to the near side of the bed within your reach and adjust the bed to a comfortable working height *to prevent back strain.*
   - Establish which position the client prefers. The prone position is recommended for a back rub. The side-lying position can be used if a client cannot assume the prone position.
   - Expose the back from the shoulders to the inferior sacral area. Cover the remainder of the body *to prevent chilling and minimize exposure.*
5. Massage the back.
   - Pour a small amount of lotion onto the palms of your hands and hold it for a minute. The lotion bottle can also be placed in a bath basin filled with warm water. **Rationale:** *Back rub preparations tend to feel uncomfortably cold to people. Warming the solution facilitates client comfort.*
   - Using your palm, begin in the sacral area using smooth, circular strokes.

❶ One suggested pattern for a back massage.

   - Move your hands up the center of the back and then over both scapulae.
   - Massage in a circular motion over the scapulae.
   - Move your hands down the sides of the back.
   - Massage the areas over the right and left iliac crests. ❶
   - Apply firm, continuous pressure without breaking contact with the client's skin.
   - Repeat above for 3 to 5 minutes, obtaining more lotion as necessary.
   - While massaging the back, assess for skin redness and areas of decreased circulation.
   - Pat dry any excess lotion with a towel.

continued on page 1220

PROVIDING A BACK MASSAGE *continued*

6. Document that a back rub was performed and the client's response. Record any unusual findings.

SAMPLE DOCUMENTATION

6/22/2007 1400 c/o aching, intermittent back pain. Wincing and grimacing when attempting to move in bed. Rates pain at 4–5 on 0–10 scale. States uses massage to help relieve pain when

at home. Percocet given. Back massaged. Stated the massage helped him "to relax." Lights dimmed and door to room closed.
———————————————————D. Aubrey, RN

1430 Rates pain at 1–2/10. States feels "much more comfortable." Moving in bed with ease.————————D. Aubrey, RN

EVALUATION
Compare the client's current response to his or her previous response. Is there a positive client outcome such as increased relaxation and decrease in pain and anxiety because of the back massage?

Heat and Cold Applications. A warm bath, heating pads, ice bags, ice massage, hot or cold compresses, and warm or cold sitz baths in general relieve pain and promote healing of injured tissues (see Chapter 36 ∞).

Acupressure. Acupressure developed from the ancient Chinese healing system of acupuncture. The therapist applies finger pressure to points that correspond to many of the points used in acupuncture (see Chapter 19 ∞).

Contralateral Stimulation. Contralateral stimulation can be accomplished by stimulating the skin in an area opposite to the painful area (e.g, stimulating the left knee if the pain is in the right knee). The contralateral area may be scratched for itching, massaged for cramps, or treated with cold packs or analgesic ointments. This method is particularly useful when the painful area cannot be touched because it is hypersensitive, when it is inaccessible by a cast or bandages, or when the pain is felt in a missing part (phantom pain).

IMMOBILIZATION/BRACING. Immobilizing or restricting the movement of a painful body part (e.g., arthritic joint, traumatized limb) may help to manage episodes of acute pain. Splints or supportive devices should hold joints in the position of optimal function and should be removed regularly in accordance with agency protocol to provide range-of-motion (ROM) exercises. Prolonged immobilization can result in joint contracture, muscle atrophy, and cardiovascular problems. Therefore, clients should be encouraged to participate in self-care activities and remain as active as possible, with frequent ROM exercises.

TRANSCUTANEOUS ELECTRICAL NERVE STIMULATION. **Transcutaneous electrical nerve stimulation (TENS)** is a method of applying low-voltage electrical stimulation directly over identified pain areas, at an acupressure point, along peripheral nerve areas that innervate the pain area, or along the spinal column. The TENS unit consists of a portable, battery-operated device with lead wire and electrode pads that are applied to the chosen area of skin (Figure 46-14 ■). Cutaneous stimulation from the TENS unit is thought to activate large-diameter fibers that modulate the transmission of the nociceptive impulse in the peripheral and central nervous system (closing the pain "gate"), resulting in pain re-

Figure 46-14 ■ A transcutaneous electric nerve stimulator.

lief. This stimulation may also cause a release of endorphins from the CNS centers. The use of TENS is contraindicated for clients with pacemakers or arrhythmias, or in areas of skin breakdown. It is generally not used on the head or over the chest.

COGNITIVE-BEHAVIORAL INTERVENTIONS. The goals of cognitive-behavioral interventions include providing comfort, altering psychologic responses to reduce pain perception, and optimizing functioning. Selected cognitive-behavioral interventions include distraction, eliciting the relaxation response, repatterning thinking, and facilitating coping with emotions.

Distraction. Distraction draws the person's attention away from the pain and lessens the perception of pain. In some instances, distraction can make a client completely unaware of pain. Distraction makes the person unaware of the pain only for the amount of time and to the extent that the distracting activity holds his or her "undivided" attention. For example, a client recovering from surgery may feel no pain while watching a football game on television, yet feel pain again during commercials or when the game is over. Different types of distractions are shown in Box 46–9. Using multiple forms of distraction simultaneously adds value to the activity. For example, listening to music can be distracting; however, the value can be added by tapping to the music, singing along, or playing along on a musical instrument.

BOX 46–9 Types of Distraction

VISUAL DISTRACTION
- Reading or watching TV
- Watching a baseball game
- Guided imagery

AUDITORY DISTRACTION
- Humor
- Listening to music

TACTILE DISTRACTION
- Slow, rhythmic breathing
- Massage
- Holding or stroking a pet or toy

INTELLECTUAL DISTRACTION
- Crossword puzzles
- Card games (e.g., bridge)
- Hobbies (e.g., stamp collecting, writing a story)

Eliciting the Relaxation Response. Stress increases pain, in part by increasing muscle tension, activating the sympathetic nervous system, and putting the client at risk for stress-related types of pain (e.g., tension headaches). The relaxation response decreases and counteracts the harmful effects of stress, including the effect it has on physical, cognitive, and emotional functioning. Eliciting this response requires more than simply helping a person relax; rather it involves a structured technique designed to focus the mind and relax muscle groups. Basic techniques with helpful scripts are detailed by McCaffery and Pasero (1999), with common techniques including progressive relaxation, breath-focus relaxation, and meditation. The nurse can coach the client, urge self-directed meditation, or provide an audiotaped guide to help elicit the relaxation response. Many clients can achieve the desired state after a few attempts, but mastery of this skill requires daily practice over a few weeks. In general, relaxation techniques by themselves do not have remarkable pain-relieving properties; however, they can reduce pain that may have been exacerbated by stress. Some clients may become more consciously aware of their pain while practicing relaxation techniques before they have learned mastery of controlling "mind chatter" and remaining mentally focused.

Once the client has mastered the basic skills for eliciting the relaxation response, techniques of imagery or self-hypnosis can be used. Both imagery and hypnosis begin with attaining a deep state of relaxation and are capable of altering the experience of pain; for example, having the client replace the pain with a feeling of pleasant numbness (Arnstein, 2004). Additional posthypnotic suggestions can then be made, linking these pleasant numb sensations to coping efforts used during the day (e.g., "every time you stop to take a slow, deep, diaphragmatic breath, you will feel this pleasant numbness instead of pain").

Repatterning Unhelpful Thinking. Some people harbor strong self-doubts, unrealistic expectations (e.g., "I just want someone to make the pain go away"), rumination (e.g., "I keep thinking about my pain and the person who did this to me"), helplessness (e.g., "I can't do anything"), and magnification (e.g., "my life is ruined, I'll never be a good parent because of my pain"). These cognitive patterns have been identified as important contributors to treatment failures, the intensification of pain, disability, and depression (Arnstein, Caudil, Mandle, Norris, & Beasley, 1999; DeGood & Kiernan, 1997). Nurses can help by challenging the truthfulness and helpfulness of these thoughts, and replacing them with realistic and confidence-building ones that are particularly powerful predictors of more effective coping, better clinical outcomes, and improved quality of life (Caudill, 2002).

Facilitating Coping. Nurses can help by intervening with clients who are anxious, are sad, or express overly pessimistic or helpless points of view. Awareness of the client's misperceptions or unrealistic expectations also helps the professional avoid a common cause of therapeutic failure. Therapeutic communication with an emphasis on listening, providing encouragement, teaching self-management skills, sharing vicarious experiences, and persuading them to act on their own behalf are strategies that enhance coping. Helping clients to better communicate with the professional staff, family members, and friends can also promote coping. Counseling from trained professionals may be indicated for those clients with severe emotional distress, but must be offered to them in a sensitive way that does not convey the notion that pain is "in their head."

Selected Spiritual Interventions. The spiritual dimension encompasses a person's innermost concerns and values, including the ascribed purpose, meaning, and driving force in his or her life. It may include rituals that help the individual become part of a community, or feel a bond with the universe that is not necessarily religious in nature. For those who express their spirituality in a religious context, it is appropriate to offer prayer, intercessory prayer (being prayed for by others), or access to meaningful rituals. For some clients, a caring presence, attentive listening, and facilitating the process of acceptance can help reduce spiritual distress, whereas other clients benefit from manipulation of energy patterns (e.g., therapeutic touch).

Through improved spiritual insights, individuals with pain can find meaning in what seems incomprehensible and learn to cope with the intolerable. This process often begins by making peace with their past, being spiritually aware in the present, and making a commitment to go forward with life despite the pain (St. Marie & Arnold, 2002). By shifting awareness from within to external sources of power, pain sufferers can transcend the limits of their pain to find new energy and a renewed sense of purpose.

Nonpharmacologic Invasive Therapies

A **nerve block** is a chemical interruption of a nerve pathway, effected by injecting a local anesthetic into the nerve. Nerve blocks are widely used during dental work. The injected drug blocks nerve pathways from the painful tooth, thus stopping the transmission of pain impulses to the brain. Nerve blocks are often used to relieve the pain of whiplash injury, lower back disorders, bursitis, and cancer. With the intention of quieting "pain

LIFESPAN CONSIDERATIONS Pain Management

INFANTS

- Giving an infant, particularly a very-low-birth-weight infant, a water and sucrose solution administered through a pacifier provides some evidence of pain reduction during procedures that may be painful, but should not be a substitute for anesthetic or analgesic medications.

CHILDREN

- Distract the child with toys, books, or pictures.
- Hold the child to console and promote comfort.
- Explore misconceptions about pain and correct in understandable "concrete" terms. Be aware of how your explanations may be misunderstood. For example, telling a child they won't hurt during surgery because they will be "put to sleep" will be very upsetting to a child who knows of an animal that was "put to sleep."

- Children can use their imagination during guided imagery. Ask the child to imagine a "pain switch" (even give it a color) and to visualize turning the switch off in the area where there is pain. A "magic glove" or "magic blanket" is an imaginary object that the child applies on areas of the body (e.g., hand, thigh, back, hip) to lessen discomfort.

ELDERS

- Promote the client's use of pain control measures that have worked in the past for them.
- Spend time with the client and listen carefully.
- Clarify misconceptions. Encourage independence whenever possible.
- Carefully review the treatment plan to avoid drug–drug, food–drug, or disease–drug interactions.

---

generators" (irritable nerves that cause the pain), a combination of a long-acting local anesthetic and a steroid is injected adjacent to the problem nerve (e.g., lumbar epidural steroid injections, joint injections). The local anesthetic should provide relief for several hours, before the effect of the steroid begins a day or two later. Often a series of three injections are scheduled weeks or months apart. Each subsequent injection should result in a longer duration of pain relief. No more than three injections per year are recommended because of the mineral-robbing effect steroids have on bones in the area. For longer lasting results after a nerve block has worked, more permanent blocks may be attempted. The "permanent" blocks involve damaging nerves with alcohol, phenol, or radio frequency (heat). These nerve-killing procedures are controversial as nerve fibers often regenerate and the pain returns in a significant proportion of clients.

Pain conduction pathways can be interrupted surgically. Because this disruption is permanent, surgery is performed only as a last resort, generally for intractable pain. Several surgical procedures may be performed. A **cordotomy** obliterates pain. Temperature sensation below the level of the spinothalamic portion of the anterolateral tract is severed. This procedure is usually done for pain in the legs and trunk. **Rhizotomy** interrupts the anterior or posterior nerve root between the ganglion and the cord. Interruption of anterior motor nerve roots stops spasmodic movements that accompany paraplegia. Interruption of posterior sensory nerve roots eliminates pain in areas innervated by that specific nerve root. Rhizotomies are generally performed on cervical nerve roots to alleviate pain of the head and neck from cancer or neuralgia, and increasingly they use radio frequency technologies.

In **neurectomy,** peripheral or cranial nerves are interrupted to alleviate localized pain, such as pain in the lower leg or foot arising from a vascular occlusion. In a **sympathectomy,** pathways of the sympathetic division of the autonomic nervous system are severed. This procedure eliminates vasospasm, improves peripheral blood supply, and thus is effective in treating painful vascular disorders such as Raynaud's disease.

Spinal cord stimulation (SCS) is used with persistent pain that has not been controlled with less invasive therapies. SCS involves the insertion of an electrode (may be a single channel or multichannel device) adjacent to the spinal cord in the epidural space. The electrode(s) is attached to an impulse-generator (external or implanted) that sends electric impulses to the spinal cord to control pain. The client is awake during the insertion procedure to aid in the optimal placement of the electrodes.

Evaluating

The goals established in the planning phase are evaluated according to specific desired outcomes, also established in that phase (see the Identifying Nursing Diagnoses, Outcomes, and Interventions box earlier in this chapter). To assist in the evaluation process, flow sheet records or a client diary may be helpful. A weekly log or diary can be structured in a similar fashion for the individual client. For example, columns including day, time, onset of pain, activity before pain, pain relief measure, and duration of pain can be devised to help the client and nurse determine the effectiveness of pain relief strategies.

HOME CARE CONSIDERATIONS
Pain Management

- Teach the client to keep a pain diary to monitor pain onset, activity before pain, pain intensity, use of analgesics, or other relief measures.
- Instruct the client to contact a health care professional if planned pain control measures are ineffective.
- Teach the use of preferred and selected nonpharmacologic techniques such as relaxation, guided imagery, distraction, music therapy, and massage.
- Instruct the client to use pain control measures before the pain becomes severe.
- Inform the client of the effects of untreated pain.
- Provide appropriate information about how to access community resources, home care agencies, and associations that offer self-help groups and educational materials.

CLINICAL ALERT

The statement "Please tell me how I can best help you control your pain" sends a couple of subtle messages that are an important part of treatment planning and evaluation of care. First, it places the ownership and responsibility for controlling pain on the client. Second, it acknowledges that the client may be the best judge of what is needed, respecting the cultural meaning of pain and acceptable ways of expressing/controlling pain. Third, it establishes the nurse's role in helping the client be more comfortable and in control of his or her condition. ■

If outcomes are not achieved, the nurse and client need to explore the reasons before modifying the care plan. The nurse might consider the following questions:

■ Is adequate analgesic being given? Would the client benefit from a change in dose or in the time interval between doses?

■ Were the client's beliefs, expectations, and values about pain therapy considered?

■ Did the client understate the pain experience for some reason?

■ Were appropriate instructions provided to allay misconceptions about pain management?

■ Did the client and support people understand the instructions about pain management techniques?

■ Is the client receiving adequate support for both physical pain and emotional distress?

■ Has the client's physical condition changed, necessitating modifications in interventions?

■ Should selected intervention strategies be reevaluated?

See the Nursing Care Plan and the Concept Map.

CRITICAL THINKING CHECKPOINT

Mrs. Lundahl underwent abdominal surgery approximately 6 hours ago. She has a 15-cm midline incision that is covered with a dry and intact surgical dressing. Upon assessing Mrs. Lundahl you note that she is perspiring, lying in a rigid position, holding her abdomen, and grimacing. Her blood pressure is 150/90, heart rate 100, and respiratory rate 32. When asked to rate her pain on a scale of 0 to 10, Mrs. Lundahl rates her pain as 5 as long as she remains perfectly still. There is a sharp area of pain at her incision; however, the most bothersome pain is crampy and dull, like she was "kicked in the stomach" with severe exacerbations that come in unpredictable waves.

1. What conclusions, if any, can be drawn about Mrs. Lundahl's pain status?
2. Does Mrs. Lundahl's rating her pain as 5 mean that she is not experiencing pain severe enough to warrant intervention?
3. What type of pain is Mrs. Lundahl experiencing?
4. What interventions, in addition to pain medication, may be useful in reducing Mrs. Lundahl's pain?
5. How will you know if your interventions have been effective in reducing Mrs. Lundahl's pain?

See Critical Thinking Possibilities in Appendix A.

NURSING CARE PLAN   Acute Pain

ASSESSMENT DATA	NURSING DIAGNOSIS	DESIRED OUTCOMES*
Nursing Assessment Mr. C. is a 57-year-old businessman who was admitted to the surgical unit for treatment of a possible strangulated inguinal hernia. Two days ago he had a partial bowel resection. Postoperative orders include NPO, intravenous infusion of D51/2 NS at 125 cc/hr left arm, nasogastric tube to low intermittent suction. Mr. C. is in a dorsal recumbent (supine) position and is attempting to draw up his legs. He appears restless and is complaining of abdominal pain (7 on a scale of 0–10).	*Acute Pain* related to tissue injury secondary to surgical intervention (as evidenced by restlessness; pallor; elevated pulse, respirations, and systolic blood pressure; dilated pupils; and report of 7/10 abdominal pain)	**Pain Control** [1605] as evidenced by often demonstrating ability to ■ Use analgesics appropriately ■ Use nonanalgesic relief measures ■ Report uncontrolled symptoms to health care professional **Pain Level** [2102] As evidenced by mild to no ■ Reported pain ■ Protective body positioning ■ Restlessness ■ Pupil dilation ■ Perspiration ■ Change in BP, HR, R from normal baseline data
Physical Examination **Diagnostic Data** Height: 188 cm (6′ 3″) Chest x-ray and urinalysis neg- Weight: 90.0 kg (200 lb) ative, WBC 12,000 Temperature: 37°C (98.6°F) Pulse: 90 BPM Respirations: 24/minute Blood pressure: 158/82 mm Hg Skin pale and moist, pupils dilated. Midline abdominal incision, sutures dry and intact.		

continued on page 1224

NURSING CARE PLAN **Acute Pain** *continued*

NURSING INTERVENTIONS*/SELECTED ACTIVITIES	RATIONALE
Pain Management [1400]	
Perform a comprehensive assessment of pain to include location, characteristics, onset, duration, frequency, quality, intensity or severity, and precipitating factors of pain.	*Pain is a subjective experience and must be described by the client in order to plan effective treatment.*
Consider cultural influences on pain response (e.g., cultural beliefs about pain may result in a stoic attitude).	*Each person experiences and expresses pain in an individual manner using a variety of sociocultural adaptation techniques.*
Reduce or eliminate factors that precipitate or increase Mr. C.'s pain experience (e.g., fear, fatigue, monotony, and lack of knowledge).	*Personal factors can influence pain and pain tolerance. Factors that may be precipitating or augmenting pain should be reduced or eliminated to enhance the overall pain management program.*
Teach the use of nonpharmacologic techniques (e.g., relaxation, guided imagery, music therapy, distraction, and massage) before, after, and if possible during painful activities; before pain occurs or increases; and along with other pain relief measures.	*The use of noninvasive pain relief measures can increase the release of endorphins and enhance the therapeutic effects of pain relief medications.*
Provide Mr. C. optimal pain relief with prescribed analgesics.	*Each client has a right to expect maximum pain relief. Optimal pain relief using analgesics includes determining the preferred route, drug, dosage, and frequency for each individual. Medications ordered on a prn basis should be offered to the client at the interval when the next dose is available.*
Medicate before an activity to increase participation, but evaluate the hazard of sedation.	*Turning and ambulation activities will be enhanced if pain is controlled or tolerable. Assessing level of sedation should precede the activity to ensure necessary safety precautions are put in place.*
Evaluate the effectiveness of the pain control measures used through ongoing assessment of Mr. C.'s pain experience.	*Research shows that the most common reason for unrelieved pain is failure to routinely assess pain and pain relief. Many clients silently tolerate pain if not specifically asked about it.*
Analgesic Administration [2210]	
Check the medical order for drug, dose, and frequency of analgesic prescribed.	*Ensures that the nurse has the right drug, right route, right dosage, right client, right frequency.*
Determine analgesic selections (narcotic, nonnarcotic, or NSAID) based on type and severity of pain.	*Various types of pain (e.g., acute, chronic, neuropathic, nociceptive) require different analgesic approaches. Some types of pain respond to nonopioid drugs alone, while others can be relieved by combining a low-dose opioid with a nonopioid.*
Institute safety precautions as appropriate if Mr. C. receives narcotic analgesics.	*Side effects of opioid narcotics include drowsiness and sedation.*
Instruct Mr. C. to request prn pain medication before the pain is severe.	*Severe pain is more difficult to control and increases the client's anxiety and fatigue. The preventive approach to pain management can reduce the total 24-hour analgesic dose.*
Evaluate the effectiveness of analgesic at regular, frequent intervals after each administration and especially after the initial doses, also observing for any signs and symptoms of untoward effects (e.g., respiratory depression, nausea and vomiting, dry mouth, and constipation).	*The analgesic dose may not be adequate to raise the client's pain threshold or may be causing intolerable or dangerous side effects or both. Ongoing evaluation will assist in making necessary adjustments for effective pain management.*
Document Mr. C.'s response to analgesics and any untoward effects.	*Documentation facilitates pain management by communicating effective and noneffective pain management strategies to the entire health care team.*
Implement actions to decrease untoward effects of analgesics (e.g., constipation and gastric irritation).	*Constipation is a common side effect of opioid narcotics, and a treatment plan to prevent occurrence should be instituted at the beginning of analgesic therapy. For Mr. C., constipation could result from his primary condition or his analgesia. Assess for overall GI functioning, possible complications of surgery (e.g., ileus), as well as opioid-induced constipation or NSAID-induced gastritis.*

NURSING CARE PLAN **Acute Pain** *continued*

NURSING INTERVENTIONS/SELECTED ACTIVITIES*	RATIONALE
Simple Relaxation Therapy [6040]	
Consider Mr. C.'s willingness and ability to participate, preference, past experiences, and contraindications before selecting a specific relaxation strategy.	*The client must feel comfortable trying a different approach to pain management. To avoid ineffective strategies, the client should be involved in the planning process.*
Elicit behaviors that are conditioned to produce relaxation, such as deep breathing, yawning, abdominal breathing, or peaceful imaging.	*Relaxation techniques help reduce skeletal muscle tension, which will reduce the intensity of the pain.*
Create a quiet, nondisruptive environment with dim lights and comfortable temperature when possible.	*Comfort and a quiet atmosphere promote a relaxed feeling and permit the client to focus on the relaxation technique rather than external distraction.*
Individualize the content of the relaxation intervention (e.g., by asking for suggestions about what Mr. C. enjoys or finds relaxing).	*Each person may find different images or approaches to relaxation more helpful than others. The nurse should have a variety of relaxation scripts or audiovisual aids to help clients find the best one for them.*
Demonstrate and practice the relaxation technique with Mr. C.	*Return demonstrations by the participant provide an opportunity for the nurse to evaluate the effectiveness of teaching sessions.*
Evaluate and document his response to relaxation therapy.	*Conveys to the health care team effective strategies in reducing or eliminating pain.*

EVALUATION

Outcomes partially met. The client verbalizes pain and discomfort, requesting analgesics at onset of pain. States "the pain is a 2" (on a scale of 0–10) 30 minutes after a parenteral analgesic administration. Requests analgesic 30 minutes before ambulation. States willingness to try relaxation techniques; however, has not attempted to do so.

The NOC # for desired outcomes and the NIC # for nursing interventions are listed in brackets following the appropriate outcome or intervention. Outcomes, indicators, interventions, and activities selected are only a sample of those suggested by NOC and NIC and should be further individualized for each client.

APPLYING CRITICAL THINKING

1. Is there any other assessment data you would want to gather to help plan Mr. C.'s pain management?
2. Mr. C. does not have a PCA. What nursing interventions are important?
3. What kind of data would you gather prior to having a discussion with the primary care provider about options for improving pain control in this client?

See Critical Thinking Possibilities in Appendix A. ∞

CONCEPT MAP **Acute Pain**

LC
57 y.o. male
Strangulated inguinal
hernia --> partial bowel
obstruction --> second
day postop

→ assess →

- 6' 3", 200 lb
- C/o abdominal pain (7/10)
- Restless
- Legs drawn up to chest
- Pupils dilated
- Midline abd incision with
  sutures dry and intact
- HR = 90
- BP = 158/82
- Resp = 24
- Skin pale, moist
- CXR and UA negative
- WBC 12,000

generate nursing diagnosis

Acute Pain r/t tissue injury secondary to surgical intervention

outcome   outcome

Outcomes partially
met:
- Requests
  analgesic
  30 minutes
  before
  ambulation
- Willing to try
  relaxation
  techniques but
  has not done so
  to date

← evaluation ←

Pain Control aeb often
demonstrating ability to:
- Use analgesics
  appropriately
- Use non-analgesic
  relief measures
- Report uncontrolled
  symptoms to health
  care professional

Pain Level aeb mild
to no:
- Reported pain
- Protective body
  positioning
- Restlessness
- Pupil dilation
- Perspiration
- Change in BP, HR,
  R from normal
  baseline data

← evaluation →

Outcomes partially
met:
- Verbalizes pain
  and discomfort
- States pain is
  2/10 30 minutes
  after analgesic
- No protective
  body positioning
- No pupil dilation

nursing intervention   nursing intervention   nursing intervention

Analgesic Administration   Simple Relaxation Therapy   Pain Management

activity   activity   activity   activity   activity   activity   activity

Evaluate
effectiveness
of analgesic

Demonstrate and
practice relaxation
techniques

Pain
Assessment

Consider
cultural
influences

Determine type
of analgesic
based on pain
assessment

Instruct to
request
analgesic at
onset of pain

Check willingness
to use relaxation
strategies

Reduce or
eliminate factors
that increase
the pain

CHAPTER 46 **REVIEW**

CHAPTER HIGHLIGHTS

- Pain is a subjective sensation to which no two people respond in the same way. It can directly impair health and prolong recovery from surgery, disease, and trauma.
- Types of pain may be described in terms of location, duration, intensity, and etiology.
- Pain threshold is generally similar in all people, but pain tolerance and response vary considerably.
- The physiologic processes related to pain perception are described as nociception. Four processes are involved in nociception: transduction, transmission, modulation, and perception.
- For nociceptive pain to be perceived, nociceptors must be stimulated. Three types of pain stimuli are mechanical, thermal, and chemical.
- According to the gate control theory, peripheral nerve fibers carrying pain to the spinal cord can have their input modified at the spinal cord level before transmission to the brain. This theory is the basis of many pain intervention strategies.
- Numerous factors influence a person's perception and reaction to pain: ethnic and cultural values, developmental stage, environment and support people, past pain experiences, and meaning of pain.
- Pain is subjective, and the most reliable indicator of the presence or intensity of pain is the client's self-report. Pain assessment is the fifth vital sign. Assessment of a client who is experiencing pain should include a comprehensive pain history.
- Although the nursing diagnosis given to clients suffering pain is *Acute Pain* or *Chronic Pain,* the pain itself may be the etiology of many other nursing diagnoses.
- Overall client goals include preventing, modifying, or eliminating pain so that the client is able to partly or completely resume usual daily activities and to cope more effectively with the pain experience.
- When planning, nurses need to choose pain relief measures appropriate for the client.
- Key strategies to reduce pain include acknowledging and accepting the client's pain, assisting support persons, reducing

misconceptions about pain, reducing fear and anxiety, and preventing pain.
- Pain management includes two basic types of nursing interventions: pharmacologic and nonpharmacologic.
- Pharmacologic interventions, ordered by the physician (or nurse practitioner), include the use of opioids, nonopioids/NSAIDs, and coanalgesic drugs.
- The World Health Organization recommends a three-step ladder approach to manage chronic cancer pain. This model establishes the pharmacologic foundation upon which other types of pain are managed.
- Placebos fail to relieve pain for many people. Deceptive use of placebos is unethical practice.
- Analgesic medication can be delivered through a variety of routes and methods to meet the specific needs of the client. These routes include oral, transmucosal, nasal, rectal, transdermal, topical, subcutaneous, intramuscular, intravenous, intraspinal, and continuous local anesthetics.
- Patient-controlled analgesia enables the client to exercise control and treat the pain by self-administering doses of analgesics.
- Physical modalities of nonpharmacologic pain interventions include such cutaneous stimulation as hot and cold applications, massage, acupressure, and contralateral stimulation; transcutaneous electrical nerve stimulation (TENS); and immobilization/bracing.
- Cognitive-behavioral interventions include distraction techniques, eliciting the relaxation response, repatterning unhelpful thinking, facilitating coping, and selected spiritual interventions.
- Evaluation of the client's pain therapy includes the response of the client, the changes in the pain, and the client's perceptions of the effectiveness of the therapy. Ongoing verbal or written feedback from the client and family is integral to this process.

TEST YOUR KNOWLEDGE

1. During the transduction phase of nociception, which method of pain control is most effective?
1. Tricyclic antidepressants
2. Opioids
3. Ibuprofen
4. Distraction

2. When a client has arrived to the nursing unit from surgery, the nurse is most likely to give priority to which of the following assessments?
1. Vital signs
2. Pain intensity
3. Location of pain
4. Pain history

3. A client who describes his pain as 6 on a scale of 1 to 10 is classified as having which of the following?
1. Mild pain
2. Mild to moderate pain
3. Moderate to severe pain
4. Very severe pain

4. A client who had abdominal surgery 4 hours ago is receiving a continuous epidural infusion of an analgesic. Which of the

following observations indicates the nurse should monitor the client closely?
1. Drowsy; drifts off to sleep before completing a sentence
2. Respirations = 18/minute
3. Drowsy; easily aroused
4. Pain rating 1–2/10

5. The client has an order of morphine 2.5 to 5.0 mg IV every 4 hours. He received 2.5 mg IV 4 hours ago for pain rated at 3 on a scale of 0 to 10. He is now watching TV and visiting with family members. When you ask about his pain, he rates it as a 5. His VS are stable. What nursing intervention is the most appropriate?
1. Give morphine 3.5 mg IV and inform him to continue watching TV because it is a distraction from the pain.
2. Give 2.5 mg of morphine IV to avoid the client becoming addicted.
3. Give nothing at this time because he is not exhibiting any signs of pain.
4. Give morphine 5.0 mg IV and reassess in 20 minutes.

6. During an admission nursing assessment, a client with diabetes describes his leg pain as a "dull, burning sensation." The nurse recognizes this description to be characteristic of which type of pain?
   1. Physiological
   2. Somatic
   3. Visceral
   4. Neuropathic

7. Which of the following interventions, when implemented by the nurse, would apply the gate control theory of pain? Select all that apply.
   1. Oral analgesics around the clock (ATC)
   2. Massage
   3. Patient-controlled analgesia (PCA)
   4. Heat or cold application
   5. Teaching

8. Which statement best reflects the nurse's assessment of the fifth vital sign?
   1. "Do you have any complaints?"
   2. "Are you experiencing any discomfort right now?"
   3. "Is there anything I can do for you now?"
   4. "Do you have any complaints of pain?"

9. When planning care for pain control of older clients, the nurse should apply which of the following principles? Select all that apply.
   1. Pain is a natural outcome of the aging process.
   2. Pain perception increases with age.
   3. The client may deny pain.
   4. The nurse should avoid use of narcotics.
   5. The client may describe pain as an "ache" or "discomfort."

10. A client recovering from abdominal surgery refuses analgesia, saying that he is "fine, as long as he doesn't move." Which of the following nursing diagnoses should be a priority?
    1. *Deficient Knowledge* (pain control measures)
    2. *Ineffective Health Maintenance*
    3. *Risk for Ineffective Airway Clearance*
    4. *Impaired Physical Mobility*

See Answers to Test Your Knowledge in Appendix A.

EXPLORE MEDIALINK www.prenhall.com/berman

DVD-ROM
- Audio Glossary
- NCLEX Review
- Skill Checklist
- Video: Pain Management
- Animations
  - Refex Arc
  - Morphine
  - Naproxen

COMPANION WEBSITE
- Additional NCLEX Review
- Case Study: Client with Stomach Cancer
- Care Plan Activity: Treating Chronic Back Pain
- Application Activities:
  - The Mayday Pain Project
  - Resources for Arthritis
- Links to Resources

READINGS AND REFERENCES

SUGGESTED READINGS

McCaffery, M., Grimm, M. A., Pasero, C., Ferrell, B., & Uman, G. C. (2005). *Pain Management Nursing, 6*(4), 122–132.
Nurses frequently label clients as "drug seeking." This term is poorly defined. The authors discuss their development of a survey to identify what nurses think the term means, to explore how nurses regard the use of the term, and to identify if there were any differences in responses between general nurses, emergency department nurses, and pain management nurses. In addition to providing the results of the survey, the authors also discuss the effects of using stigmatizing terms such as "drug seeking" in clinical practice.

Schaffer, S. D., & Yucha, C. B. (2004). Relaxation & pain management. *American Journal of Nursing, 104*(8), 75–82.
The authors provide valuable information on how to teach the relaxation response in order to assist with pain management. The article also provides research study evidence of the effect of relaxation on pain.

RELATED RESEARCH

Cleeland, C. S., Portenoy, R. K., Rue, M., Mendoza, T. R., Weller, E., Payne, R., et al., (2005). Does an oral analgesic protocol improve pain control for patients with cancer? An intergroup study coordinated by the Eastern Cooperative

Oncology Group. *Annals of Oncology, 16* (6),972–980.

Huth, M. M., Broome, M. E., & Good, M. (2004). Imagery reduces children's post-operative pain. *Pain, 110*(1–2), 439–448.

Melancon, B., & Miller, L. H. (2005). Massage therapy versus traditional therapy for low back pain relief: Implications for holistic nursing practice. *Holistic Nursing Practice, 19*(3), 116–120.

Molony, S. L., Kobayashi, M., Holleran, E., & Mezey, M. (2005). Assessing pain as a fifth vital sign in long-term care facilities: Recommendations from the field. *Journal of Gerontological Nursing, 31*(3), 16–24.

REFERENCES

Acello, B. (2000). Meeting JCAHO standards for pain control. *Nursing, 30*(3), 52–54.

Ackley, B. J., & Ladwig, G. B. (2006). *Nursing diagnosis handbook* (7th ed.). St. Louis, MO: Mosby Elsevier.

American Academy of Pain Medicine, American Pain Society, and the American Society of Addiction Medicine. (2006). *Definitions related to the use of opioids for the treatment of pain: A consensus document from the American Academy of Pain Medicine, the American Pain Society, and the American Society of Addiction Medicine*. Author. Retrieved August 20, 2006, from http:// www.ampaoinsoc.org/advocacy/opioids2.htm

American Academy of Pediatrics & Canadian Paediatric Society. (2000). Prevention and management of pain and stress in the neonate. *Pediatrics, 105*(2), 454–461.

American Geriatrics Society (AGS) Clinical Practice Guidelines. (1998). The management of chronic pain in older persons. *Journal of the American Geriatrics Society, 46*, 635–651.

American Geriatrics Society (AGS). (2002). The management of persistent pain in older persons. *Journal of the American Geriatrics Society, 50* (6 Suppl.), S205–24.

American Pain Society (APS). (1999). *Chronic pain in America: Roadblocks to relief.* Retrieved June 22, 2006, from http:// www.ampainsoc.org/whatsnew/toc_road.htm

American Pain Society (APS). (2003). *Principles of analgesic use in the treatment of acute pain and cancer pain* (5th ed.). Glenview, IL: Author.

American Society for Pain Management Nursing. (2005). *Position paper: Use of placebos in pain management.* Retrieved June 22, 2006, from http://aspmn.org/pdfs/ Use%20of%20Placebos.pdf

Andrews, M. M., & Boyle, J. S. (2003). *Transcultural concepts in nursing care* (4th ed.). Philadelphia: Lippincott Williams & Wilkins.

Arnstein, P. M. (1997). The neuroplastic phenomenon: A physiologic link between chronic pain and learning. *Journal of Neuroscience Nursing, 29*(3), 179–186.

Arnstein, P. M. (2002). Optimizing perioperative pain management. *AORN Journal, 76*(5), 812–818.

Arnstein, P. M. (2003). Comprehensive assessment and management of chronic pain. *Nursing Clinics of North America, 38,* 403–417.

Arnstein, P. M. (2004). Chronic neuropathic pain: Issues in patient education. *Pain Management Nursing, 5*(4), Suppl., 34–41.

Arnstein, P., Caudill, M., Mandle, C. L., Norris, A., & Beasley, R. (1999). Self efficacy as a mediator of the relationship between pain intensity, disability and depression in chronic pain patients. *Pain, 80*(3), 483–491.

Ball, J. W., & Bindler, R. C. (2003). *Pediatric nursing: Caring for children* (3rd ed.). Upper Saddle River, NJ: Prentice Hall.

Bergh, I., & Sjostrom, B. (1999). A comparative study of nurses' and elderly patients' ratings of pain and pain tolerance. *Journal of Gerontological Nursing, 25*(5), 30–36.

Caudill, M. A. (2002). *Managing pain before it manages you* (revised ed.). New York: Guilford Press.

DeGood, D. E., & Kiernan, B. D. (1997). Pain related cognitions as predictors of pain treatment outcomes. *Advances in Medical Psychotherapy, 9,* 73–90.

Dochterman, J. M., & Bulechek, G. M. (Eds.). (2004). *Nursing interventions classification (NIC)* (4th ed.). St. Louis, MO: Mosby.

Dodd, M., Janson, S., Facione, N., Faucett, J., Froelicher, E. S., Humphreys, J., et al. (2001). Advancing the science of symptom management. *Journal of Advanced Nursing, 33*(5), 668–676.

Ebersole, P., Hess, P., Touhy, T., & Jett, K. (2005). *Gerontological nursing & healthy aging* (2nd ed.). St. Louis, MO: Elsevier Mosby.

Elliott, A. M., Smith, B. H., Penny, K. I., Smith, W. C., & Chambers, W. A. (1999). The epidemiology of chronic pain in the community. *Lancet, 354,* 1248–1252.

FDA: U.S. Food and Drug Administration. (2005). *FDA Public Health Advisory: FDA announces important changes and additional warnings for COX-2 selective and non-selective non-steroidal anti-inflammatory drugs (NSAIDs).* Retrieved June 22, 2006, from http://www.fda.gov/cder/drug/advisory/COX2.htm

Gordon, M. (2002). *The manual of nursing diagnosis* (10th ed.). St. Louis, MO: Mosby.

Gordon, D., Dahl, J., Phillips, P., Frandsen, J., Cowley, C., Foster, R., et al. (2005). The use of 'as-needed' range order for opioid analgesics in the management of acute pain: A consensus statement of the American Society for Pain Management Nursing and the American Pain Society. *Home Healthcare Nurse, 23*(6), 388–396.

Guo, H. R., Tanaka, S., Halperin, W. E., & Cameron, L. L. (1999). Back pain prevalence in US industry and estimates of lost workdays. *American Journal of Public Health, 89*(7), 1029–1035.

Herr, K. (2002). Chronic pain in the older patient: Management strategies. *Journal of Gerontological Nursing, 28*(2), 28–34.

Herr, K. (2004). Neuropathic pain: A guide to comprehensive assessment. *Pain Management Nursing, 5*(4), Suppl., 1, 9–8.

Hitchcock, L. S., Ferrell, B. R., & McCaffery, M. (1994). The experience of chronic non-malignant pain. *Journal of Pain and Symptom Management, 9*(5), 312–318.

Horbury, C., Henderson, A., & Bromely, B. (2005). Influences of patient behavior on clinical nurses' pain assessment; Implications for continuing education. *Journal of Continuing Education in Nursing, 36*(1), 18–24.

International Headache Society (IHS). (2004). The international classification of headache disorders (2nd ed.). *Cephalalgia: International Journal of Headache Disorders, 24* (Suppl. 1), 1–150.

Katz, J., Jackson, M., Kavanagh, B. P., & Sandler, A. N. (1996). Acute pain after thoracic surgery predicts long-term post-thoracotomy pain. *Clinical Journal of Pain, 12,* 50–55.

Kurz, A., & Sessler, D. I. (2003). Opioid-induced bowel dysfunction: Pathophysiology and potential new therapies. *Drugs, 63*(7), 649–671.

Jensen, M. P., Martin, S. A., & Cheung, R. (2005). The meaning of pain relief in a clinical trial. *Journal of Pain, 6*(6), 400–406.

Joint Commission on Accreditation of Healthcare Organizations (JCAHO). (2004). *Patient controlled analgesia by proxy. Sentinel event alert.* Issue 33. Retrieved June 21, 2006, from http://www.jointcommission.org/Sentinel Events/SentinelEventAlert/sea_33.htm

Manais, E., Bucknall, T., & Botti, M. (2005). Nursing strategies for managing pain in the postoperative setting. *Pain Management Nursing, 6*(1), 18–29.

McCaffery, M., Ferrell, B. R., & Pasero, C. (2000). Nurses' personal opinions about patients' pain and their effect on recorded assessments and titration of opioid doses. *Pain Management Nursing, 1*(3), 79–87.

McCaffery, M., & Pasero, C. (1999). *Pain: Clinical manual* (2nd ed.). St. Louis, MO: Mosby.

McNamara, M. E., Burnham, D. C., Smith, C., & Carroll, D. L. (2003). The effects of back massage before diagnostic cardiac catheterization. *Alternative Therapies in Health and Medicine, 9*(1), 50–57.

Melzack, R., & Wall, P. D. (1965). Pain mechanisms: A new theory. *Science, 150,* 971–979.

Merkel, S. I., Voepel-Lewis, T., Shayevitz, J. R., & Malviya, S. (1997). The FLACC: A behavioral scale for scoring postoperative pain in young children. *Pediatric Nursing, 23*(3), 293–297.

Monteiro-Cruz, D. A. L., & Mattos-Pimenta, C. A. (2001). Chronic pain: Nursing diagnosis or syndrome? *Nursing Diagnosis, 12*(4), 117–127.

Moorhead, S., Johnson, M., & Maas, M. (Eds.). (2004). *Nursing outcomes classification (NOC)* (3rd ed.). St. Louis, MO: Mosby.

Munoz, C., & Luckmann, J. (2005). *Transcultural communication in nursing* (2nd ed.). Clifton Park, NY: Delmar Learning.

NANDA International. (2007). *NANDA nursing diagnoses: Definitions and classification 2007–2008.* Philadelphia: Author.

Page, G. G., Ben-Eliyahu, S., Yirmiya, R., & Liebeskind, J. C. (1993). Morphine attenuates surgery-induced enhancement of metastatic colonization in rats. *Pain, 54*(1), 21–28.

Paice, J. A. (2002). Controlling pain. Understanding nociceptive pain. *Nursing, 32*(3), 74–75.

Pasero, C. (2004). Pathophysiology of neuropathic pain. *Pain Management Nursing, 5,* 4, (Suppl. 1), 3–8.

Puntillo, K. A., & Weiss, S. J. (1994). Pain: Its mediators and associated morbidity in critically ill cardiovascular surgical patients. *Nursing Research, 43,* 31–36.

Purnell, L. D., & Paulanka, B. J. (2005). *Guide to culturally competent health care.* Philadelphia: F. A. Davis.

Reyes-Gibby, C. C., Aday, L., & Cleeland, C. (2002). Impact of pain on self-rated health in community-dwelling older adults. *Pain, 95,* 75–82.

Rhiner, M., & Kedziera, P. (1999). Managing breakthrough pain: A new approach. *American Journal of Nursing, 99*(3), Suppl. 3–12.

Serlin, R. C., Mendoza, T.R., Nakamura, Y., Edwards, K. R., & Cleeland, C. S. (1995). When is cancer pain mild, moderate or severe? Grading pain severity by its interference with function. *Pain, 61,* 277–284.

Shapiro, R. S. (1996). Health care providers' liability exposure for inappropriate pain management. *Journal of Law and Medical Ethics, 24*(4), 360–364.

Simons, J. M., & MacDonald, L. M. (2004). Pain assessment tools: Children's nurses' views. *Journal of Child Health Care, 8*(4), 264–278.

St. Marie, B., & Arnold, S. (2002). *When your pain flares up.* Minneapolis, MN: Fairview Press.

Stanley, M., Blair, K. A., & Beare, P. G. (2005). *Gerontological nursing: Promoting successful aging with older adults* (3rd ed.). Philadelphia: F. A. Davis.

Van Tudler, M., & Koes, B. (2004). Low back pain (acute). *Clinical Evidence, 12,* 1643–1658.

Warden, V., Hurley, A. C., & Volicer, L. (2003). Development and psychometric evaluation for the pain assessment in advanced dementia (PAINAD) scale. *Journal of the American Medical Directors Association, 4*(1), 9–15.

Wilson, K. G., Eriksson, M. Y., D'Eon, J. L., Mikail, S. F., & Emery, P. C. (2002). Major depression and insomnia in chronic pain. *Clinical Journal of Pain, 18*(2), 77–83.

Wong, D. L., Hockenberry-Eaton, M., Wilson, D., Winkelstein, M. L., & Schwartz, P. (2001). *Essentials of pediatric nursing* (6th ed.). St. Louis, MO: Mosby.

World Health Organization. (1996). *Cancer pain relief* (2nd ed.). Geneva, Switzerland: Author.

SELECTED BIBLIOGRAPHY

Agency for Health Care Policy and Research (AHCPR). (1994). *Acute low back problems in adults. Clinical Practice Guideline No.14.* AHCPR Publication No. 94-0592. Rockville, MD: U.S. Department of Health and Human Services.

American Nurses Association. (2005). *Scope and standards of practice: pain management nursing.* Silver Spring, MD: NursingBooks.org.

American Society for Pain Management Nursing (ASPMN). (n.d.). *A position statement on the use of "as-needed" range orders for opioid analgesics in the management of acute pain.* Retrieved on June 22, 2006, from http://www.aspmn.org/pdfs/As%20Needed%20Range%20Orders.pdf

Arnstein, P. M. (2004). Chronic neuropathic pain: Issues in patient education. *Pain Management Nursing, 5,* 4, (Suppl. 1), 34–41.

Arnstein, P. (2006). Placebo: No relief for Ms. Mahoney's pain. *American Journal of Nursing, 106*(2), 54–57.

Bines, A., & Paice, J. A. (2005). Are your pain management skills up-to-date? *Nursing, 35*(1), 36–37.

D'Arcy, Y. (2004). Assessing pain in patients who can't communicate. *Nursing, 34*(10), 27.

D'Arcy, Y. (2004). Using regional blockade for adjunct pain relief. *Nursing, 34*(11), 74–75.

D'Arcy, Y. (2005). Pain management standards, the law, and you. *Nursing, 35*(4), 17.

D'Arcy, Y. (2005). Liposomes: A new way to deliver pain medications. *Nursing, 35*(7), 17.

D'Arcy, Y. (2006). Hot topics in pain management: Using NSAIDs safely. *Nursing, 36*(2), 22–23.

Ernst, E. (2003). Massage treatment for back pain. *British Medical Journal, 326*(7389), 562–564.

Gordon, D. B., & Love, G. (2004). Pharmacologic management of neuropathic pain. *Pain Management Nursing, 5* (4, Suppl. 1), 19–33.

Grace, P. J. (2006). The clinical use of placebos. *American Journal of Nursing, 106*(2), 58–61.

Hutchison, R. (2004). COX-2-selective NSAIDs. A review and comparison with nonselective NSAIDs. *American Journal of Nursing, 104*(3), 52–54.

Keller, D. L. (2006). Pain relievers. *RN, 69*(4), 22–25.

Lafleur, K. J. (2004). Taking the fifth (vital sign). *RN, 67*(7), 30–36.

Lane, P. (2004). Assessing pain in patients with advanced dementia. *Nursing, 34*(8), 17.

Long, C. O. (2005). Seeking out pain-management resources. *Nursing, 35*(1), 74–75.

Marders, J. (2004). PCA by proxy: Too much of a good thing. *Nursing, 34*(4), 24.

Mather, D. (2004). A low-tech approach to pain relief. *RN, 67*(3), 41–42.

McCaffery, M., & Arnstein, P. (2006). The debate over placebos in pain management. *American Journal of Nursing, 106*(2), 62–65.

McCaffery, M., & Pasero, C. (2003). Breakthrough pain: It's common in patients with chronic pain. *American Journal of Nursing, 103*(4), 83–85.

Murauski, J. D., & Gonzalez, K. R. (2002). Peripheral nerve blocks for postoperative analgesia. *AORN Journal, 75* (1), 136–147.

Nguyen, M., Ugarte, C., Fuller, I., Haas, G., & Portenoy, R. K. (2005). Access to care for chronic pain: Racial and ethnic differences. *Journal of Pain, 6*(5), 301–314.

Noah, V. (2003). PCA by proxy: Minimizing the risks. *Nursing, 103*(12), 17.

Pasero, C. (2003). Lidocaine patch 5%: How to use a topical method of controlling localized pain. *American Journal of Nursing, 103*(9), 75–78.

Pasero, C. (2004). Pain relief for neonates. *American Journal of Nursing, 104,*(5), 44–47.

Pasero, C., & McCaffery, M. (2004). Controlled-release oxycodone: It's worth considering when treating around-the-clock pain. *American Journal of Nursing, 104*(1), 30–32.

Pasero, C., & McCaffery, M. (2005). Ketamine: Low doses may provide relief for some painful conditions. *American Journal of Nursing, 105*(4), 60–64.

Pasero, C., & McCaffery, M. (2005). Authorized and unauthorized use of PCA pumps. *American Journal of Nursing, 105*(7), 30–32.

Pasero, C., & McCaffery, M. (2005). No self-report means no pain-intensity rating. *American Journal of Nursing, 105*(10), 50–53.

Schwartz, A. J. (2006). Learning the essentials of epidural anesthesia. *Nursing, 36*(1), 44–49.

Siedlecki, S. (2004). Assessing chronic pain. *Nursing, 34*(5), 17.

Spagrud, L. J., Piira, T., & vonBaeyer, C. L. (2003). Children's self-report of pain intensity. *American Journal of Nursing, 103*(12), 62–64.

vanDijk, M., Peters, W. B., vanDeventer, P., & Tibboel, D. (2005). The COMFORT behavior scale: A tool for assessing pain and sedation in infants. *American Journal of Nursing, 105*(1), 33–36.

Yezierski, R. P., Radson, E., & Vanderah, T. W. (2004). Understanding chronic pain. *Nursing, 34*(4), 22–23.

Nutrition

CHAPTER

47

LEARNING OUTCOMES

After completing this chapter, you will be able to:

1. Identify essential nutrients and their dietary sources.

2. Describe normal digestion, absorption, and metabolism of carbohydrates, proteins, and lipids.

3. Explain essential aspects of energy balance.

4. Discuss body weight and body mass standards.

5. Identify factors influencing nutrition.

6. Identify developmental nutritional considerations.

7. Evaluate a diet using a food guide pyramid.

8. Discuss essential components and purposes of nutritional assessment and nutritional screening.

9. Identify risk factors for and clinical signs of malnutrition.

10. Describe nursing interventions to promote optimal nutrition.

11. Discuss nursing interventions to treat clients with nutritional problems.

12. Perform the skills of inserting enteral tubes, administering feedings and medications through enteral tubes, and removing enteral tubes.

13. Plan, implement, and evaluate nursing care associated with nursing diagnoses related to nutritional problems.

KEY TERMS

Nutrition is the sum of all the interactions between an organism and the food it consumes. In other words, nutrition is what a person eats and how the body uses it. **Nutrients** are organic and inorganic substances found in foods that are required for body functioning. Adequate food intake consists of a balance of nutrients: water, carbohydrates, proteins, fats, vitamins, and minerals. Foods differ greatly in their **nutritive value** (the nutrient content of a specified amount of food), and no one food provides all essential nutrients. Nutrients have three major functions: providing energy for body processes and movement, providing structural material for body tissues, and regulating body processes.

ESSENTIAL NUTRIENTS

The body's most basic nutrient need is water. Because every cell requires a continuous supply of fuel, the most important nutritional need, after water, is for nutrients that provide fuel, or energy. The energy-providing nutrients are carbohydrates, fats, and proteins. Hunger compels people to eat enough energy-providing nutrients to satisfy their energy needs. Carbohydrates, fats, and protein are referred to as **macronutrients,** because they are needed in large amounts (e.g., hundreds of grams) to provide energy. **Micronutrients,** vitamins and minerals, are those required in small amounts (e.g., milligrams or micrograms) to metabolize the energy-providing nutrients.

Carbohydrates

Carbohydrates are composed of the elements carbon (C), hydrogen (H), and oxygen (O) and are of two basic types: simple carbohydrates (sugars) and complex carbohydrates (starches and fiber). As with all nutrients, carbohydrates must be ingested, digested, and metabolized.

Types of Carbohydrates

SUGARS. Sugars, the simplest of all carbohydrates, are water soluble and are produced naturally by both plants and animals. Sugars may be **monosaccharides** (single molecules) or **disaccharides** (double molecules). Of the three monosaccharides (glucose, fructose, and galactose), glucose is by far the most abundant simple sugar.

Most sugars are produced naturally by plants, especially fruits, sugar cane, and sugar beets. However, other sugars are from an animal source. For example, lactose, a combination of glucose and galactose, is found in animal milk. Processed or refined sugars (e.g., table sugar, molasses, and corn syrup) have been extracted and concentrated from natural sources.

STARCHES. Starches are the insoluble, nonsweet forms of carbohydrate. They are **polysaccharides;** that is, they are composed of branched chains of dozens, sometimes hundreds, of glucose molecules. Like sugars, nearly all starches exist naturally in plants, such as grains, legumes, and potatoes. Other foods, such as cereals, breads, flour, and puddings, are processed from starches.

FIBER. Fiber, a complex carbohydrate derived from plants, supplies roughage, or bulk, to the diet. However, fiber cannot be digested by humans. This complex carbohydrate satisfies the appetite and helps the digestive tract to function effectively and eliminate waste. Fiber is present in the outer layer of grains, bran, and in the skin, seeds, and pulp of many vegetables and fruits.

Natural sources of carbohydrates also supply vital nutrients, such as protein, vitamins, and minerals that are not found in processed foods. Processed carbohydrate foods are relatively low in nutrients in relation to the large number of calories they contain and thus are often referred to as "empty calories." For example, alcoholic beverages may contain significant amounts of carbohydrate, but they are empty calories. Therefore, it is important that carbohydrate intake include natural foods.

Carbohydrate Digestion

Major enzymes of carbohydrate digestion include ptyalin (salivary amylase), pancreatic amylase, and the disaccharidases: maltase, sucrase, and lactase. **Enzymes** are biologic catalysts that speed up chemical reactions. The desired end products of carbohydrate digestion are monosaccharides. Some simple sugars are already monosaccharides and require no digestion. Essentially, all monosaccharides are absorbed by the small intestine in healthy people.

Carbohydrate Metabolism

Carbohydrate metabolism is a major source of body energy. After the body breaks carbohydrates down into glucose, some glucose continues to circulate in the blood to maintain blood levels and to provide a readily available source of energy. The remainder is either used as energy or stored. Insulin, a hormone secreted by the pancreas, enhances the transport of glucose into cells.

STORAGE AND CONVERSION. Carbohydrates are stored either as glycogen or as fat. **Glycogen** is a large polymer (compound molecule) of glucose. The process of glycogen formation is called **glycogenesis.** Almost all body cells are capable of storing glycogen; however, most is stored in the liver and skeletal muscles, where it is available for conversion back into glucose. Glucose that cannot be stored as glycogen is converted to fat.

Proteins

Amino acids, organic molecules made up primarily of carbon, hydrogen, oxygen, and nitrogen, combine to form proteins. Every cell in the body contains some protein, and about three-quarters of body solids are proteins.

Amino acids are categorized as essential or nonessential. **Essential amino acids** are those that cannot be manufactured in the body and must be supplied as part of the protein ingested in the diet. Nine essential amino acids—histidine, isoleucine, leucine, lysine, methionine, phenylalanine, tryptophan, threonine, and valine—are necessary for tissue growth and maintenance. A tenth, arginine, appears to have a role in the immune system.

Nonessential amino acids are those that the body can manufacture. The body takes amino acids derived from the diet and reconstructs new ones from their basic elements. Nonessential amino acids include alanine, aspartic acid, cystine, glutamic acid, glycine, hydroxyproline, proline, serine, and tyrosine.

Proteins may be complete or incomplete. **Complete proteins** contain all of the essential amino acids plus many nonessential ones. Most animal proteins, including meats, poultry, fish, dairy products, and eggs, are complete proteins. Some animal proteins, however, contain less than the required amount of one or more essential amino acids and therefore cannot alone support continued growth. These proteins are sometimes referred to as **partially complete proteins.** Examples are gelatin, which has small amounts of tryptophan, and the milk protein casein, which has only a little arginine.

Incomplete proteins lack one or more essential amino acids (most commonly lysine, methionine, or tryptophan) and are usually derived from vegetables. If, however, an appropriate mixture of plant proteins is provided in the diet, a balanced ratio of essential amino acids can be achieved. For example, a combination of corn (low in tryptophan and lysine) and beans (low in methionine) is a complete protein. Such combinations of two or more vegetables are called *complementary proteins.* Another way to take full advantage of vegetable proteins is to eat them with a small amount of animal protein. Spaghetti with cheese, rice with pork, noodles with tuna, and cereal with milk are just a few examples of combining vegetable and animal proteins.

Protein Digestion

Digestion of protein foods begins in the mouth, where the enzyme *pepsin* breaks protein down into smaller units. However, most protein is digested in the small intestine. The pancreas secretes the proteolytic enzymes trypsin, chymotrypsin, and carboxypeptidase; glands in the intestinal wall secrete aminopeptidase and dipeptidase. These enzymes break protein down into smaller molecules and eventually into amino acids.

Storage

Amino acids are absorbed by active transport through the small intestine into the portal blood circulation. The liver uses some amino acids to synthesize specific proteins (e.g., liver cells and the plasma proteins albumin, globulin, and fibrinogen). Plasma proteins are a storage medium that can rapidly be converted back into amino acids.

Other amino acids are transported to tissues and cells throughout the body where they are used to make protein for cell structures. In a sense, protein is stored as body tissue. The body cannot actually store excess amino acids for future use. However, a limited amount is available in the "metabolic pool" that exists because of the constant breakdown and buildup of the protein in body tissues.

Protein Metabolism

Protein metabolism includes three activities: **anabolism** (building tissue), **catabolism** (breaking down tissue), and nitrogen balance.

ANABOLISM. All body cells synthesize proteins from amino acids. The types of proteins formed depend on the characteristics of the cell and are controlled by its genes.

CATABOLISM. Because a cell can accumulate only a limited amount of protein, excess amino acids are degraded for energy or converted to fat. Protein degradation occurs primarily in the liver.

NITROGEN BALANCE. Because nitrogen is the element that distinguishes protein from lipids and carbohydrates, nitrogen balance reflects the status of protein nutrition in the body. **Nitrogen balance** is a measure of the degree of protein anabolism and catabolism; it is the net result of intake and loss of nitrogen. When nitrogen intake equals nitrogen output, a state of nitrogen balance exists.

Lipids

Lipids are organic substances that are greasy and insoluble in water but soluble in alcohol or ether. **Fats** are lipids that are solid at room temperature; **oils** are lipids that are liquid at room temperature. In common use, the terms *fats* and *lipids* are used interchangeably. Lipids have the same elements (carbon, hydrogen, and oxygen) as carbohydrates, but they contain a higher proportion of hydrogen.

Fatty acids, made up of carbon chains and hydrogen, are the basic structural units of most lipids. Fatty acids are described as saturated or unsaturated, according to the relative number of hydrogen atoms they contain. **Saturated fatty acids** are those in which all carbon atoms are filled to capacity (i.e., saturated) with hydrogen; an example is butyric acid, found in butter. An **unsaturated fatty acid** is one that could accommodate more hydrogen atoms than it currently does. It has at least two carbon atoms that are not attached to a hydrogen atom; instead, there is a double bond between the two carbon atoms. Fatty acids with one double bond are called **monounsaturated fatty acids;** those with more than one double bond (or many carbons not bonded to a hydrogen atom) are **polyunsaturated fatty acids.** An example of a polyunsaturated fatty acid is linoleic acid, found in vegetable oil.

Based on their chemical structure, lipids are classified as simple or compound. **Glycerides,** the simple lipids, are the most common form of lipids. They consist of a glycerol molecule with up to three fatty acids attached. **Triglycerides** (which have three fatty acids) account for more than 90% of the lipids in food and in the body. Triglycerides may contain saturated or unsaturated fatty acids. Saturated triglycerides are found in animal products, such as butter, and are usually solid at room temperature. Unsaturated triglycerides are usually liquid at room temperature and are found in plant products, such as olive oil and corn oil.

Cholesterol is a fatlike substance that is both produced by the body and found in foods of animal origin. Most of the body's cholesterol is synthesized in the liver; however, some is absorbed from the diet (e.g., from milk, egg yolk, and organ meats). Cholesterol is needed to create bile acids and to synthesize steroid hormones. Along with phospholipids, large quantities of cholesterol are present in cell membranes as well as other cell structures.

Lipid Digestion

Although chemical digestion of lipids begins in the stomach, they are digested mainly in the small intestine, primarily by bile, pancreatic lipase, and enteric lipase, an intestinal enzyme. The end products of lipid digestion are glycerol, fatty acids, and cholesterol. These are immediately reassembled inside the intestinal cells into triglycerides and cholesterol esters (cholesterol with a fatty acid attached to it), which are not water soluble. For these reassembled products to be transported and used, the small intestine and the liver must convert them into soluble compounds called lipoproteins. **Lipoproteins** are made up of various lipids and a protein.

Lipid Metabolism

Converting fat into usable energy occurs through the use of the enzyme hormone-sensitive lipase that breaks down triglycerides in adipose cells, releasing glycerol and fatty acids into the blood. A pound of fat provides 3,500 kilocalories. Fasting persons will obtain most of their calories from fat metabolism, but some amount of carbohydrate or protein must also be used because the brain, nerves, and red blood cells require glucose. Only the glycerol molecules in fat can be converted to glucose. A typical triglyceride has 50 carbon atoms, of which the one glycerol molecule represents only three carbons (Rolfes, Pinna, & Whitney, 2006).

Micronutrients

A **vitamin** is an organic compound that cannot be manufactured by the body and is needed in small quantities to catalyze metabolic processes. Thus, when vitamins are lacking in the diet, metabolic deficits result. Vitamins are generally classified as fat soluble or water soluble. **Water-soluble vitamins** include C and the B-complex vitamins: B_1 (thiamine), B_2 (riboflavin), B_3 (niacin or nicotinic acid), B_6 (pyridoxine), B_9 (folic acid), B_{12} (cobalamin), pantothenic acid, and biotin. The body cannot store water-soluble vitamins; thus, people must get a daily supply in the diet. Water-soluble vitamins can be affected by food processing, storage, and preparation.

Fat-soluble vitamins include A, D, E, and K. The body can store these vitamins, although there is a limit to the amounts of vitamins E and K the body can store. Therefore, a daily supply of fat-soluble vitamins is not absolutely necessary. Vitamin content is highest in fresh foods that are consumed as soon as possible after harvest.

Minerals are found in organic compounds, as inorganic compounds, and as free ions. Calcium and phosphorus make up 80% of all mineral elements in the body. The two categories of minerals are macrominerals and microminerals. **Macrominerals** are those that people require daily in amounts over 100 mg. They include calcium, phosphorus, sodium, potassium, magnesium, chloride, and sulfur. **Microminerals** are those that people require daily in amounts less than 100 mg. They include iron, zinc, manganese, iodine, fluoride, copper, cobalt, chromium, and selenium.

Common problems associated with the mineral nutrients are iron deficiency resulting in anemia, and osteoporosis resulting from loss of bone calcium. Additional information about major

MediaLink

Lipids Animation

minerals associated with the body's fluid and electrolyte balance is given in Chapter 52. ∞

ENERGY BALANCE

Energy balance is the relationship between the energy derived from food and the energy used by the body. The body obtains energy in the form of calories from carbohydrates, protein, fat, and alcohol. The body uses energy for voluntary activities such as walking and talking and for involuntary activities such as breathing and secreting enzymes. A person's energy balance is determined by comparing his or her energy intake with energy output.

Energy Intake

The amount of energy that nutrients or foods supply to the body is their **caloric value.** A **calorie (c, cal, kcal)** is a unit of heat energy. A **small calorie** is the amount of heat required to raise the temperature of 1 gram of water 1 degree Celsius. This unit of measure is used in chemistry and physics. A **large calorie (Calorie, kilocalorie [Kcal])** is the amount of heat energy required to raise the temperature of 1 gram of water 15 to 16 degrees Celsius and is the unit used in nutrition (although it is not universally capitalized). It was recommended in 1970 that the unit kilojoule (kJ), a metric measurement, replace the kilocalorie.

However, to date, the United States and Canada have not made the change. A **kilojoule (kJ)** is the amount of work energy required when a force of 1 newton (N) moves 1 kilogram of weight 1 meter distance.

One Calorie (Kcal) equals 4.18 kilojoules. The energy liberated from the metabolism of food has been determined to be:

- 4 Calories/gram (17 kJ) of carbohydrates.
- 4 Calories/gram (17 kJ) of protein.
- 9 Calories/gram (38 kJ) of fat.
- 7 Calories/gram (29 kJ) of alcohol.

Energy Output

Metabolism refers to all biochemical and physiologic processes by which the body grows and maintains itself. Metabolic rate is normally expressed in terms of the rate of heat liberated during these chemical reactions. The **basal metabolic rate (BMR)** is the rate at which the body metabolizes food to maintain the energy requirements of a person who is awake and at rest. The energy in food maintains the basal metabolic rate of the body and provides energy for activities such as running and walking.

Resting energy expenditure (REE) is the amount of energy required to maintain basic body functions; in other words, the calories required to maintain life. The REE of healthy persons

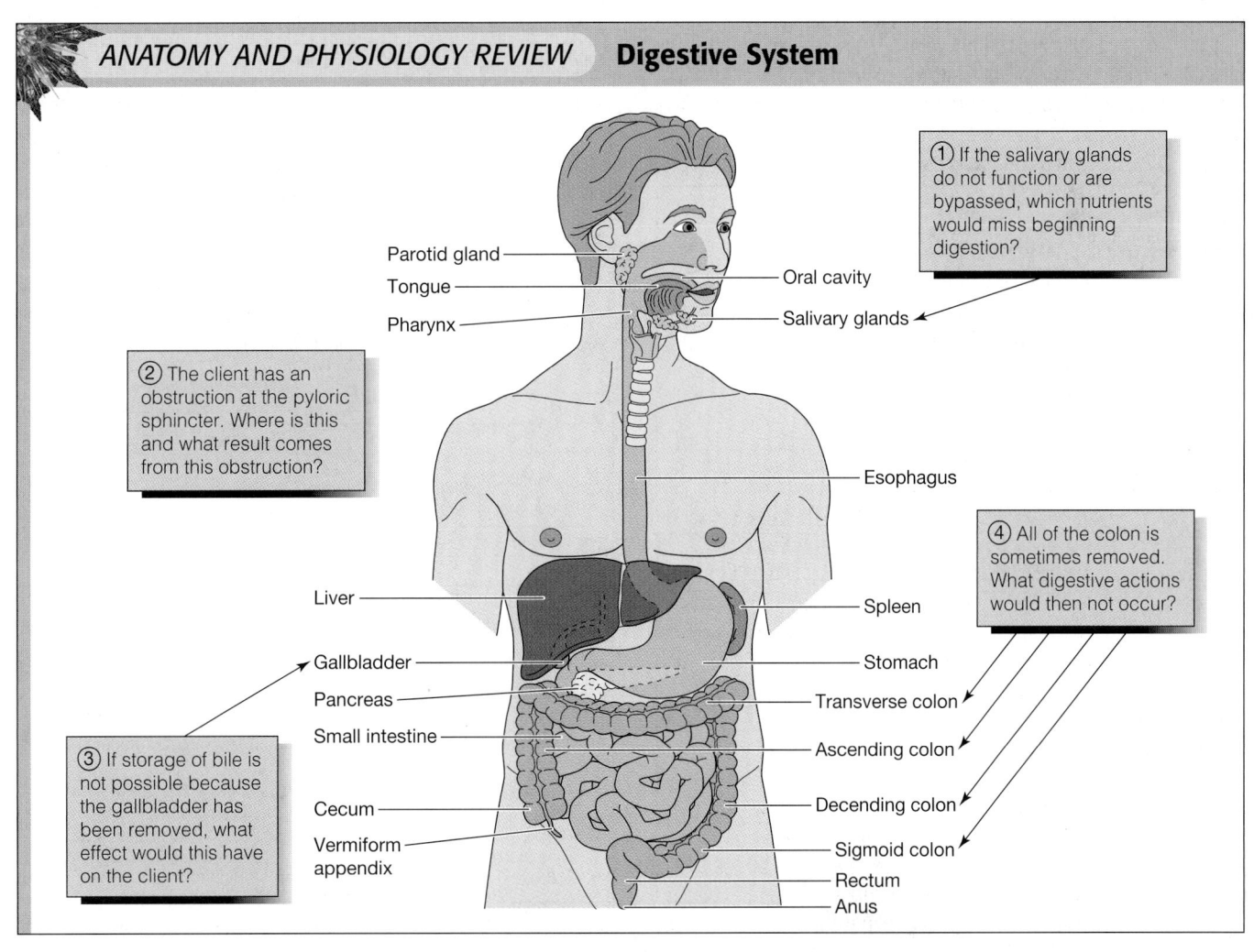

ANATOMY AND PHYSIOLOGY REVIEW   **Digestive System**

① If the salivary glands do not function or are bypassed, which nutrients would miss beginning digestion?

② The client has an obstruction at the pyloric sphincter. Where is this and what result comes from this obstruction?

③ If storage of bile is not possible because the gallbladder has been removed, what effect would this have on the client?

④ All of the colon is sometimes removed. What digestive actions would then not occur?

Parotid gland
Tongue
Pharynx
Oral cavity
Salivary glands
Esophagus
Liver
Spleen
Gallbladder
Stomach
Pancreas
Transverse colon
Small intestine
Ascending colon
Decending colon
Cecum
Sigmoid colon
Vermiform appendix
Rectum
Anus

is generally about 1 cal/kg of body weight/hr for men and 0.9 cal/kg/hr for women although there is great variation among individuals. BMR is calculated by measuring the REE in the early morning, 12 hours after eating.

The actual daily expenditure of energy depends on the degree of activity of the individual. Some activities require many times the REE. Examples of approximate real caloric expenditures compared to the REE are as follows:

Light housework	210%
Walking steadily	350%
Heavy housework	400%
Laboring	500%
Average jogging/cycling/energetic swimming	700%

BODY WEIGHT AND BODY MASS STANDARDS

Maintaining a healthy or ideal body weight requires a balance between the expenditure of energy and the intake of nutrients. Generally, when energy requirements of an individual equate with the daily caloric intake, the body weight remains stable. **Ideal body weight (IBW)** is the optimal weight recommended for optimal health. To determine an individual's approximate IBW, the nurse can consult standardized tables or can quickly calculate a value using the Rule of 5 for women and the Rule of 6 for men (see Box 47–1). Many standardized tables and formulas were developed many years ago and are based on limited samples (Pai & Paloucek, 2000). The nurse should use great caution in suggesting that these weights apply to all clients.

BOX 47–1 Approximating Ideal Body Weight

Rule of 5 for females:

    100 lb for 5 ft of height
    + 5 lb for each inch over 5 ft
    ±10% for body-frame size*

Rule of 6 for males:

    106 lb for 5 ft of height
    + 6 lb for each inch over 5 ft
    ±10% for body-frame size*

---

*Determine body-frame size by measuring the client's wrist circumference and applying to the table below. Add 10% for large body-frame size, and subtract 10% for small body-frame size.

	Female Wrist Measurements			Male Wrist Measurements
	Height less than 5' 2" (less than 155 cm)	Height 5' 2" – 5' 5" (155 cm – 163 cm)	Height more than 5' 5" (more than 163 cm)	Height more than 5' 5" (More than 163 cm)
Small	Less than 5.5" (140 mm)	Less than 6.0" (152 mm)	Less than 6.25" (159 mm)	5.5" – 6.5" (140 – 165 mm)
Medium	5.5" – 5.75" (140 – 146 mm)	6" – 6.25" (152 – 159 mm)	6.25" – 6.5" (159 – 165 mm)	6.5" – 7.5" (165 – 191 mm)
Large	More than 5.75" (146 mm)	More than 6.25" (159 mm)	More than 6.5" (165 mm)	More than 7.5" (191 mm)

Many health professionals consider the body mass index to be a more reliable indicator of a person's healthy weight. For people older than 18 years, the **body mass index (BMI)** is an indicator of changes in body fat stores and whether a person's weight is appropriate for height, and may provide a useful estimate of malnutrition. However, the results must be used with caution in people who have fluid retention (e.g., ascites or edema), athletes, or elders. To calculate the BMI:

1. Measure the person's height in meters, e.g., 1.7 m (1 meter = 3.3 ft, or 39.6 in)
2. Measure the weight in kilograms, e.g., 72 kg (1 kg = 2.2 pounds)
3. Calculate the BMI using the following formula

$$BMI = \frac{\text{Weight in kilograms}}{(\text{Height in meters})^2}$$

or

$$\frac{72 \text{ kilograms}}{1.7 \times 1.7 \text{ (meters)}^2} = 24.9$$

Box 47–2 provides an interpretation of the results.

Another measure of body mass is percent body fat. Because BMI uses only height and weight, it can give misleading results for certain groups of clients such as athletes, the frail elderly, and children. Percent of body fat can be measured by underwater weighing and dual-energy x-ray absorptiometry (DEXA), but these methods are time consuming and expensive. Other indirect, but more practical measures include waist circumference (see Box 47–2), skinfold testing, and near-infrared interactance.

Bioelectrical impedance analysis (BIA) is used by some modern weight scales and is considered one of the most accurate methods of body fat determination (Kyle et al., 2004). The speed with which an electrical signal passes through the body is influenced by the amount of water in the body. The more mus-

---

BOX 47–2 Classification of Overweight and Obesity by BMI, Waist Circumference, and Associated Disease Risks*

	BMI (kg/m²)	Obesity Class	Disease Risk* Relative to Normal Weight and Waist Circumference	
			Men 102 cm (40 in) or less Women 88 cm (35 in) or less	Men > 102 cm (40 in) Women > 88 cm (35 in)
Underweight	< 18.5		-	-
Normal+	18.5 – 24.9		-	-
Overweight	25.0 – 29.9		Increased	High
Obesity	30.0 – 34.9	I	High	Very high
	35.0 – 39.9	II	Very high	Very high
Extreme obesity	40.0 +	III	Extremely high	Extremely high

* Disease risk for type 2 diabetes, hypertension, and cardiovascular disease.

+ Increased waist circumference can also be a marker for increased risk even in persons of normal weight.

Note: From *Clinical Guidelines on the Identification, Evaluation, and Treatment of Overweight and Obesity in Adults: The Evidence Report,* by the National Heart, Lung, and Blood Institute, 1998, p. xvii, Washington, DC: U.S. Department of Health & Human Services. Retrieved June 25, 2006, from http://www.nhlbi.nih.gov/guidelines/obesity/ob_gdlns.htm

cle, the more water the body can hold, and the easier it is for current to pass through it. The more fat, the more resistance to the current. Height, age, gender, and weight or other physical characteristics such as body type, physical activity level, and ethnicity are used with the impedance data to determine percent body fat. BIA is safe and it does not hurt.

FACTORS AFFECTING NUTRITION

Although the nutritional content of food is an important consideration when planning a diet, an individual's food preferences and habits are often a major factor affecting actual food intake. Habits about eating are influenced by developmental considerations, gender, ethnicity and culture, beliefs about food, personal preferences, religious practices, lifestyle, economics, medications and therapy, health, alcohol consumption, advertising, and psychologic factors.

Development

People in rapid periods of growth (i.e., infancy and adolescence) have increased needs for nutrients. Elders, on the other hand, need fewer calories and dietary changes in view of the risk of coronary heart disease, osteoporosis, and hypertension.

Gender

Nutrient requirements are different for men and women because of body composition and reproductive functions. The larger muscle mass of men translates into a greater need for calories and proteins. Because of menstruation, women require more iron than men do prior to menopause. Pregnant and lactating women have increased caloric and fluid needs.

Ethnicity and Culture

Ethnicity often determines food preferences. Traditional foods (e.g., rice for Asians, pasta for Italians, curry for Indians) are eaten long after other customs are abandoned.

Nurses should not use a "good food, bad food" approach, but rather should realize that variations of intake are acceptable under different circumstances. The only "universally" accepted guidelines are (a) to eat a wide variety of foods to furnish adequate nutrients and (b) to eat moderately to maintain correct body weight. Food preference probably differs as much among individuals of the same cultural background as it does generally between cultures. Not all Italians like pizza, for example, and many undoubtedly enjoy Mexican food.

Beliefs about Food

Beliefs about effects of foods on health and well-being can affect food choices. Many people acquire their beliefs about food from television, magazines, and other media. For example, some people are reducing their intake of animal fats in response to evidence that excessive consumption of animal fats is a major risk factor in vascular disease, including heart attack and stroke (Sauvaget, Nagano, Hayashi, & Yamada, 2004).

Food fads that involve nontraditional food practices are relatively common. A **fad** is a widespread but short-lived in-

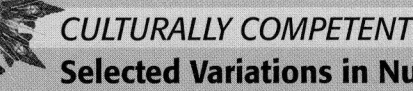

CULTURALLY COMPETENT CARE
Selected Variations in Nutritional Practices and Preferences Among Different Cultures

AFRICAN AMERICAN HERITAGE
- Gifts of food are common and should never be rejected.
- Diets are often high in fat, cholesterol, and sodium.
- Being overweight is viewed as positive.
- Most persons are lactose intolerant.

ARAB HERITAGE
- Many spices and herbs are used such as cinnamon, allspice, cloves, mint, ginger, and garlic.
- Meats are often skewer roasted or slow simmered; most common are lamb and chicken.
- Bread is served at every meal.
- Muslims do not eat pork, and all meats must be cooked well done.
- Food is eaten (and clients fed) with the right hand.
- Beverages are drunk after the meal, not during.
- Muslims fast during daylight hours during the month of Ramadan (may fall at a slightly different time each year on non-Muslim calendars).

CHINESE HERITAGE
- Foods are served at meals in a specific order.
- Each region in China has its own traditional diet.
- Traditional Chinese may not want ice in their drinks.
- Foods are chosen to balance *yin* and *yang* in order to avoid indigestion.

JEWISH HERITAGE
- Dietary laws govern killing, preparation, and eating of foods.
- Meat and milk are not eaten at the same time; dairy substitutes (e.g., margarine) are permitted.
- Pork is one meat that is forbidden to eat.
- All blood must be drained from meats.
- Always wash hands before eating.

MEXICAN HERITAGE
- Rice, beans, and tortillas are core, essential foods.
- Many persons are lactose intolerant. Leafy green vegetables and stews with bones provide calcium.
- Being overweight is viewed as positive.
- Sweet fruit drinks, including adding sugar to juice, are popular.
- The main meal of the day is at noontime.
- Foods are chosen according to *hot* and *cold* theory.

NAVAJO HERITAGE
- Rites of passage and ceremonies are celebrated with food.
- Herbs are used to treat many illnesses.
- Sheep are the major source of meat.
- Squash and corn are major vegetables.
- Most persons are lactose intolerant.

terest or a practice followed with considerable zeal. It may be based either on the belief that certain foods have special powers or on the notion that certain foods are harmful. Examples of some food fads are given in Box 47–3. Food fads appeal to

---

BOX 47–3   Examples of Food Fads and Myths

- Large amounts of yogurt and vitamin E retards aging.
- Honey is healthier than sugar, more readily digested, and a cure for the common cold.
- Eating cabbage and onions turn breast milk sour.
- Raw eggs, rare lean beef, and oysters increase sexual potency or fertility.
- Organic foods are always healthier than those exposed to pesticides.
- Stomach enzymes cannot work on vegetables and fish at the same time and therefore these foods should not be eaten together.

---

the individual seeking a miracle cure for a disease, the person who desires superior health, or one who wants to delay aging. Some fad diets are harmless, but others are potentially dangerous (Daniels, 2004). Determining the needs a fad diet fills for the client enables the nurse both to support these needs and to suggest a more nutritious diet.

Personal Preferences

People develop likes and dislikes based on associations with a typical food. A child who loves to visit his grandparents may love pickled crabapples because they are served in the grandparents' home. Another child who dislikes a very strict aunt grows up to dislike the chicken casserole she often prepares. People often carry such preferences into adulthood.

Individual likes and dislikes can also be related to familiarity. Children often say they dislike a food before they sample it. Some adults are very adventuresome and eager to try new foods. Others prefer to eat the same foods repeatedly. Preferences in the tastes, smells, flavors (blends of taste and smell), temperatures, colors, shapes, and sizes of food influence a person's food choices. For example, some people may prefer sweet and sour tastes to bitter or salty tastes. Textures play a great role in food preferences. Some people prefer crisp food to limp food, firm to soft, tender to tough, smooth to lumpy, or dry to soggy.

Religious Practices

Religious practice also affects diet. Some Roman Catholics avoid meat on certain days, and some Protestant faiths prohibit meat, tea, coffee, or alcohol. Both Orthodox Judaism and Islam prohibit pork. Orthodox Jews observe kosher customs, eating certain foods only if they are inspected by a rabbi and prepared according to dietary laws. The nurse must plan care with consideration of such religious dietary practices.

Lifestyle

Certain lifestyles are linked to food-related behaviors. People who are always in a hurry probably buy convenience grocery items or eat restaurant meals. People who spend many hours at home may take time to prepare more meals "from scratch." Individual differences also influence lifestyle patterns (e.g., cooking skills, concern about health). Some people work at different times, such as evening or night shifts. They might need to adapt their eating habits to this and also make changes in their medication schedules if they are related to food intake.

Muscular activity affects metabolic rate more than any other factor; the more strenuous the activity, the greater the stimulation of the metabolism. Mental activity, which requires only about 4 Kcal per hour, provides very little metabolic stimulation.

Economics

What, how much, and how often a person eats are frequently affected by socioeconomic status. For example, people with limited income, including some elders, may not be able to afford meat and fresh vegetables. In contrast, people with higher incomes may purchase more proteins and fats and fewer complex carbohydrates. Not all persons have the financial resources for extensive food preparation and storage facilities. The nurse should not assume that clients have their own stove, refrigerator, or freezer. In some low-income areas, food costs at small local grocery stores can be significantly higher than at large chain stores farther away.

Medications and Therapy

The effects of drugs on nutrition vary considerably. They may alter appetite, disturb taste perception, or interfere with nutrient absorption or excretion. Nurses need to be aware of the nutritional effects of specific drugs when evaluating a client for nutritional problems. The nursing history interview should include questions about the medications the client is taking. Conversely, nutrients can affect drug utilization. Some nutrients can decrease drug absorption; others enhance absorption. For example, the calcium in milk hinders absorption of the antibiotic tetracycline but enhances the absorption of the antibiotic erythromycin. Elders are at particular risk for drug–food interactions due to the number of medications they may take, age-related physiologic changes affecting medication actions (e.g., decrease in lean-to-fat ratio, decrease in renal or hepatic function), and disease-restricted diets (Leibovitch, Deamer, & Sanderson, 2004). Selected drug and nutrient interactions are shown in Table 47–1.

Therapies (e.g., chemotherapy and radiation) prescribed for certain diseases may also adversely affect eating patterns and nutrition. Normal cells of the bone marrow and the gastrointestinal mucosa are naturally very active and particularly susceptible to antineoplastic agents. Oral ulcers, intestinal bleeding, or diarrhea resulting from the toxicity of antineoplastic agents used in chemotherapy can seriously diminish a person's nutritional status.

The effects of radiotherapy depend on the area that is treated. For example, radiotherapy of the head and neck may cause decreased salivation, taste distortions, and swallowing difficulties; radiotherapy of the abdomen and pelvis may cause malabsorption, nausea, vomiting, and diarrhea. Many clients feel profound fatigue and anorexia (loss of appetite).

Health

An individual's health status greatly affects eating habits and nutritional status. The lack of teeth, ill-fitting dentures, or a sore mouth makes chewing food difficult. Difficulty swallowing (**dysphagia**) due to a painfully inflamed throat or a stricture of the esophagus can prevent a person from obtaining adequate

TABLE 47–1 Selected Drug–Nutrient Interactions

DRUG	EFFECT ON NUTRITION
Acetylsalicylic acid	Decreases serum folate and folacin nutrition Increases excretion of vitamin C, thiamine, potassium, amino acids, and glucose May cause nausea and gastritis
Antacids containing aluminum or magnesium hydroxide	Decrease absorption of phosphate and vitamin A Inactivate thiamine May cause deficiency of calcium and vitamin D Increase excretion of sodium, potassium, chloride, calcium, magnesium, zinc, and riboflavin
Thiazide diuretics	May cause anorexia, nausea, vomiting, diarrhea, or constipation Decrease absorption of vitamin B_{12} May cause diarrhea, nausea, or vomiting
Potassium chloride	Increases excretion of potassium, magnesium, and calcium May cause anorexia, nausea, or vomiting Is incompatible with protein hydrolysates
Laxatives	May cause calcium and potassium depletion Mineral oil and phenolphthalein (Ex-Lax) decrease absorption of vitamins A, D, E, and K
Antihypertensives	Hydralazine (Apresoline) may cause anorexia, vomiting, nausea, and constipation Methyldopa (Aldomet) increases need for vitamin B_{12} and folate May cause dry mouth, nausea, vomiting, diarrhea, and constipation
Anti-inflammatory agents	Colchicine decreases absorption of vitamin B_{12}, carotene, fat, lactose, sodium, potassium, protein, and cholesterol Prednisone decreases absorption of calcium and phosphorus
Antidepressants	Amitriptyline (Elavil) increases food intake (large amounts may suppress intake)
Antineoplastics	Can cause nausea, vomiting, anorexia, malabsorption, and diarrhea
NUTRIENT	**EFFECT ON DRUGS**
Grapefruit	Can cause toxicity when taken with a variety of medications including cisapride, carbamazepine, diazepam, cyclosporine, saquinavir, verapamil, nifedipine, amiodarone, terfenadine, lovastatin (Dahan & Altman, 2004)
Vitamin K	Can decrease the effectiveness of warfarin (Coumadin)
Tyramine (found in aged cheeses, tap beer, dried sausages, fermented soy, sauerkraut)	In combination with monoamine oxidase inhibitor (MAOI) medications, e.g., phenelzine (Nardil), tranylcypromine (Parnate), isocarboxazid (Marplan), isoniazid, linezolid, creates sudden increase in epinephrine leading to headaches, increased pulse and blood pressure, and possible death
Milk	Interferes with absorption of tetracycline antibiotics

nourishment. Disease processes and surgery of the gastrointestinal tract can affect digestion, absorption, metabolism, and excretion of essential nutrients. Gastrointestinal and other diseases also create nausea, vomiting, and diarrhea, all of which can adversely affect a person's appetite and nutritional status. Gallstones, which can block the flow of bile, are a common cause of impaired lipid digestion. Metabolic processes can be impaired by diseases of the liver. Diseases of the pancreas can affect glucose metabolism or fat digestion.

Between 30 million and 50 million Americans have lactose intolerance, a shortage of the enzyme lactase which is needed to break down the sugar in milk. Certain populations are more widely affected: As many as 80% of African Americans, 80% to 100% of American Indians, and 90% to 100% of Asian Americans are lactose intolerant (National Institute of Diabetes and Digestive and Kidney Diseases, 2006).

Alcohol Consumption

The calories contained in alcoholic drinks include both those of the alcohol itself and of the juices or other beverages added to the drink. In total, these can constitute large numbers of calories, for example, 150 calories for a regular 12-ounce beer, and 160 calories for a "screwdriver" (1.5 ounces vodka plus 4 ounces orange juice). Drinking alcohol can lead to weight gain through the addition of these calories to the regular diet plus the effect of alcohol on fat metabolism. A small amount of the alcohol is converted directly to fat. However, the greater effect is that the remainder of the alcohol is converted into acetate by the liver. The acetate released to the bloodstream is used for energy instead of fat and the fat is then stored.

Excessive alcohol use contributes to nutritional deficiencies in a number of ways. Alcohol may replace food in a person's diet, and it can depress the appetite. Excessive alcohol can have a toxic effect on the intestinal mucosa, thereby decreasing the absorption of nutrients. The need for vitamin B increases, because it is used in alcohol metabolism. Alcohol can impair the storage of nutrients and increase nutrient catabolism and excretion.

A number of studies have shown some health benefits of moderate alcohol consumption. Examples include reduced risk of cardiovascular disease. However, analysis of the literature indicates that there are many flaws in the research and it is too early to make recommendations for clients (Masters, 2005).

Advertising

Food producers try to persuade people to change from the product they currently use to the brand of the producer. Popular actors and actresses are often used to influence television viewers' or radio listeners' choices. Advertising is thought to influence people's food choices and eating patterns to a certain extent. Of note is that such products as alcoholic beverages, coffee, frozen foods, and soft drinks are more heavily advertised than such products as bread, vegetables, and fruits. Convenience foods (frozen or packaged and easy to prepare) and take-out (fast) foods are heavily advertised. Children's television show commercials often promote snack foods, candy, soda, and sugared cereals over fresh, healthy foods. Australia, Canada, Sweden, and Great Britain have adopted regulations prohibiting food advertising on programs targeting audiences of young children (American Psychological Association, 2004).

There has been an increase in advertising that targets elders in particular and encourages use of herbs and supplements. Some products are nutritionally safe whereas others are not and can cause interactions with medications they might be taking or cause unexpected side effects. The cost of some of these supplements is also usually high, is generally not covered by health insurance, and may take money that the person could spend for healthier food.

Psychologic Factors

Although some people overeat when stressed, depressed, or lonely, others eat very little under the same conditions. Anorexia and weight loss can indicate severe stress or depression. Anorexia nervosa and bulimia are severe psychophysiologic conditions seen most frequently in female adolescents.

NUTRITIONAL VARIATIONS THROUGHOUT THE LIFE CYCLE

Nutritional requirements vary throughout the life cycle. Guidelines follow for the major developmental stages.

Neonate to 1 Year

The neonate's fluid and nutritional needs are met by breast milk or formula. Fluid needs of infants are proportionately greater than those of adults because of a higher metabolic rate, immature kidneys, and greater water losses through the skin and the lungs. The last is largely due to rapid respirations. Therefore, fluid balance is a critical factor. Under normal environmental conditions, infants do not need additional water; however, neonates in very warm environments may require additional fluids.

The total daily nutritional requirement of the newborn is about 80 to 100 mL of breast milk or formula per kilogram of body weight. The newborn infant's stomach capacity is about 90 mL, and feedings are required every 2 1/2 to 4 hours.

The newborn infant is usually fed "on demand." **Demand feeding** means that the child is fed when hungry. This method tends to decrease the problem of overfeeding or underfeeding the infant. The newborn who is hungry usually cries and exhibits tension in the entire body. During feeding, the infant sucks readily and needs burping after each ounce of formula or after 5 minutes of breast-feeding. Parents should be warned that infant bottles should never be propped up for feeding. There is a real danger that aspiration or choking could result.

Infants demonstrate satisfaction by slowing their sucking activity or by falling asleep. Once satisfaction has been demonstrated, infants should not be coaxed into finishing the feeding. This could lead to discomfort or overfeeding. When feeding is completed, healthy infants can be placed in a supine position for sleep during the first 6 months of life to reduce the risk of sudden infant death syndrome, or SIDS.

Regurgitation, or spitting up, during or after a feeding is a common occurrence during the first year. Although this may be of concern to parents, it does not usually result in nutritional deficiency. Demonstration of adequate weight gain should reassure parents that the infant is receiving adequate nutrition.

The addition of solid food to the diet usually takes place between 4 and 6 months of age. Six-month-old infants can consume solid food more readily because they can sit up, can hold a spoon, and have decreased sucking and tongue protrusion reflexes. Solid foods (strained or pureed) are generally introduced in the following order: cereals (rice), fruits, vegetables (yellow before green), and strained meats. Foods are introduced one at a time, usually with only one new food introduced every 5 days to ensure that the infant tolerates the food and demonstrates no allergy to it. This sequence can vary according to cultural preferences. With the eruption of teeth at about 7 to 9 months, the infant is ready to chew and can begin to experience different textures of food. At this time, the infant enjoys finger foods, such as skinless fruit cut into small pieces to prevent choking, dry cereal, or toast.

Because honey can contain spores of *Clostridium botulinum* and this has been a source of infection (and death) for infants, children less than 12 months old should not be fed honey. According to the Centers for Disease Control (2005), honey is safe for persons 1 year of age and older.

At about 6 months of age, infants require iron supplementation to prevent **iron deficiency anemia.** Iron deficiency anemia is a form of **anemia** (decrease in red blood cells) caused by inadequate supply of iron for synthesis of hemoglobin. Cow's milk is low in iron and, thus, iron-fortified cereals or formulas are usually recommended by 6 months of age and are continued until the child reaches 18 months.

Weaning from the breast or bottle to the cup takes place gradually and is usually achieved by 12 to 24 months of age. It is recommended that infants be breast-fed until 1 year of age (American Academy of Pediatrics, 2005). Some infants have difficulty giving up the bottle, particularly at naptime or bedtime. Parents should be warned that having the bottle in bed can lead to **bottle mouth syndrome.** The term describes decay of the teeth caused by constant contact with sweet liquid from the bottle. Some dentists advocate brushing or cleaning the infant's teeth to prevent bottle mouth syndrome, especially for the infant who requires a bottle only at naptime or bedtime. Weaning from the bottle can be facilitated by diluting the formula with water increasingly until the infant is drinking plain water. By the age of 1, most infants can be completely fed on table food, and milk intake is about 20 ounces per day.

Toddler

Because of a maturing gastrointestinal tract, toddlers can eat most foods and adjust to three meals each day. Toddlers' fine motor skills are sufficiently well developed for them to learn how to feed themselves. Before the age of 20 months, most toddlers require help with glasses and cups because their wrist control is limited. By age 3, when most of the deciduous teeth have emerged, the toddler is able to bite and chew adult table food.

Developing independence may be exhibited through the toddler's refusal of certain foods. Meals should be short because of the toddler's brief attention span and environmental distractions. Often toddlers display their liking of rituals by eating foods in a certain order, cutting foods a specific way, or accompanying certain foods with a particular drink.

The toddler is less likely to have fluid imbalances than the infant. The toddler's gastrointestinal function is more mature, and the percentage of fluid body weight is lower. A healthy toddler weighing 15 kg (33 lb) needs about 1,250 mL of fluid per 24 hours.

During the toddler stage, the caloric requirement is 900 to 1,800 Kcal per day. From 1 to 2 years of age, the toddler may be eating a combination of prepared toddler foods and some table foods. Parents should be instructed to read labels carefully and be aware that table foods offer more variety and are less expensive and more nutritious than prepared toddler foods. The need for adequate iron, calcium, and vitamins C and A, which are common toddler deficiencies, should also be discussed.

The following suggestions may help parents meet the child's nutritional needs and promote effective parent–child interactions: (a) Make mealtime a pleasant time by avoiding tensions at the table and discussions of bad behavior; (b) offer a variety of simple, attractive foods in small portions, and avoid meals that combine foods into one dish, such as a stew; (c) do not use food as a reward or punish a child who does not eat; (d) schedule meals, sleep, and snack times that will allow for optimum appetite and behavior; and (e) avoid the routine use of sweet desserts.

Preschooler

The preschooler eats adult foods. Parents should become informed about the diet of their child in day-care or preschool settings so that they can be sure of meeting the child's total nutritional needs. Children at this age are very active and may rush through meals to return to playing. The 4-year-old still requires parents' help in cutting meat and may spill milk when pouring from a large container. Parents also need to teach the preschooler how to use utensils and should provide them with the opportunity to practice (e.g., buttering bread). However, 4- and 5-year-olds often use their fingers to pick food up. Table manners are marginal at best. Active children often require snacks between meals. Cheese, fruits, yogurt, raw vegetables, and milk are good choices. Children at this age may enjoy helping in the kitchen, and both girls and boys should be encouraged to do so.

The preschooler is even less susceptible than the toddler to fluid imbalances. The average 5-year-old weighing 20 kg (45 lb) requires at least 75 mL of liquid per kilogram of body weight per day, or 1,500 mL every 24 hours.

School-Age Child

Nutrition continues to be a high priority for growing children. School-age children require a balanced diet including 2,400 Kcal per day. School-age children eat three meals a day and one or two nutritious snacks. Children need a protein-rich food at breakfast to sustain the prolonged physical and mental effort required at school. Children who skip breakfast become inattentive and restless by late morning and have decreased problem-solving ability. Undernourished children become fatigued easily and face a greater risk of infection, resulting in frequent absences from school.

The average healthy 8-year-old weighing 30 kg (66 lb) requires about 1,750 mL of fluid per day. Many school-age children have only one meal a day with their family, at dinner. Mealtime should be a social time enjoyed by all, and parents should refrain from discussing a child's poor eating habits at this time. Parents should be aware that children learn many of their food habits by observing their parents. Eating a balanced diet should be the norm for both parent and child.

The school-age child generally eats lunch at school. The child may bring lunch from home or buy lunch at the school. Many dietary problems stem from this independence in food choices. The children may trade their food, not eat lunch at all, or buy sweets or junk food with their lunch money. Parents should discuss with the child the foods that they should eat and continue to provide a balanced diet in the home setting.

Poor eating habits may result in obesity. Childhood obesity is an increasing problem. More than 18% of children ages 6 to 11 are overweight (at or above the 95% for BMI) as are more than 17% of adolescents ages 12 to 19 (Ogden et al., 2006). Obesity in school-age children tends to result in adult obesity and all the related health risks. It is both caused by and results in decreased activity as well as psychosocial problems. Obese children may be ridiculed and discriminated against by peers. Such behavior reinforces low self-esteem. The goal of treatment for overweight children is to reduce weight gain, allowing their weight to increase more slowly than their height. Counseling and teaching parents should include the following:

- Reviewing the child's eating habits, including snacks
- Altering meal content
- Using rewards other than food
- Promoting regular exercise

Adolescent

The adolescent's need for nutrients and calories increases, particularly during the growth spurt. In particular, the need for protein, calcium, vitamin D, iron, and B vitamins increases during adolescence. An adequate diet for an adolescent is 1 quart of milk per day as well as appropriate amounts of meat, vegetables, fruits, breads, and cereals. Calcium intake during adolescent years (1,200 to 1,500 mg/day) may help decrease osteoporosis (a decrease in bone density) in later life (Schettler & Gustafson, 2004).

Many parents may observe that teenagers, particularly boys, seem to be eating all the time. Teenagers have active lifestyles and irregular eating patterns. They tend to diet or snack frequently, often eating high-calorie foods such as doughnuts, soft drinks, ice cream, and fast foods. Parents and nurses can promote better lifelong eating habits by encouraging teenagers to eat healthy snacks. Parents can provide healthy snacks such as

MediaLink

Anorexia Video

MediaLink

Bulimia Video

fruits and cheese and at the same time limit the amount of "junk food" available in the home. The teenager's food choices relate to physical, social, and emotional factors and impulses and may not be influenced by teaching. Nurses need to advise parents that adolescents must take responsibility for their decisions in many areas of life, and parents should avoid conflicts that relate to food.

Common problems related to nutrition and self-esteem among adolescents include obesity, anorexia nervosa, and bulimia. Obesity is a common problem of the preadolescent period and continues to be a problem in the adolescent period. Many obese adolescents feel ugly and socially unacceptable. Depression is not unusual among obese adolescents. Treatment of obesity in this age group includes education on nutrition as well as assessment of psychosocial problems that may produce overeating.

Under social pressure to be slim, some adolescents severely limit their food intake to a level significantly below that required to meet the demands of normal growth. In some instances, the adolescent may develop an eating disorder, such as anorexia or bulimia. Anorexia nervosa and bulimia are severe psychophysiologic conditions usually seen in adolescent girls and young women. These are considered to be disorders related to the need for control. **Anorexia nervosa** is characterized by a prolonged inability or refusal to eat, rapid weight loss, and emaciation in persons who continue to believe they are fat. Anorexics may also induce vomiting and use laxatives and diuretics to remain thin. **Bulimia** is an uncontrollable compulsion to consume enormous amounts of food (binge) and then expel it by

self-induced vomiting or by taking laxatives (purge). These illnesses are most effectively treated in the early stages by psychotherapy. Hospitalization may be necessary when the effects of starvation become life threatening.

Young Adult

The nutritional habits established during young adulthood often lay the foundation for the patterns maintained throughout a person's life. Many young adults are aware of the food groups but may not be knowledgeable about how many servings of each group they need or how much a serving constitutes. The nurse should provide the young adult client with resources such as a chart or list that contains the foods and the amounts needed in each category.

Young adult females need to maintain adequate iron intake. A substantial number of women do not ingest sufficient dietary iron each day. To prevent iron deficiency anemia, menstruating females should ingest 18 mg of iron daily. The nurse should instruct the female client to include iron-rich foods, such as organ meats (liver and kidneys), eggs, fish, poultry, leafy vegetables, and dried fruits, in her daily diet (see Major Food Sources of Iron on page 1244).

Calcium is needed in young adulthood to maintain bones and help decrease the chances of developing osteoporosis in later life. Along with calcium, the person must have adequate vitamin D, necessary for the calcium to enter the bloodstream. Vitamin D is made in the skin on exposure to the sun. If the person does not get sufficient sun exposure (15 minutes three times each week), supplements may be indicated.

DRUG CAPSULE Mineral   *ferrous sulfate* (Slow-Fe, Feosol)

THE CLIENT WITH IRON DEFICIENCY ANEMIA

Immediate and timed-release forms are available.

Iron is required for the formation of red blood cells. When iron stores are low, the body cannot produce enough red blood cells and anemia can develop. Symptoms of iron deficiency anemia include fatigue, listlessness, anorexia, and pallor. Although iron deficiency anemia is not the only kind of anemia, it is possibly the most common and one of the easiest to treat.

NURSING RESPONSIBILITIES

- Administer on an empty stomach, 1 hour before or 2 hours after meals, with a full glass of water. If the client experiences gastric upset, administer with or after food. Immediate release is administered up to three times per day.
- Administer at least 2 hours apart from antacids, ciprofloxacin, tetracycline, and several other medications. Consult a drug handbook for possible drug interactions.
- Liquid forms should be diluted in a glass of water or juice and sipped through a straw to prevent staining of the teeth.
- Shake suspension forms well before each use; take with a full glass of water.
- Iron comes in different dose strengths and may require adjustment for optimal effect.

CLIENT AND FAMILY TEACHING

- Take the medication on an empty stomach, 1 hour before or 2 hours after meals, with a full glass of water. If upset stomach occurs, take with or after food, but not with coffee, tea, eggs, or milk because these decrease absorption. Do not lie down for 30 minutes after taking the tablet or capsule.
- Sustained-release capsules and tablets must be swallowed whole. Do not crush or chew them because side effects may be increased.
- Common side effects may include nausea, stomach cramps, vomiting, and constipation. These should decrease within a few days even while continuing the iron.
- Stools will turn green-black, and this is normal.
- Do not stop taking the medication, even if you feel stronger.
- Do not take iron without consulting the primary care provider if you have a history of intestinal problems.
- Store at room temperature, away from moisture and sunlight. Keep away from children. Accidental overdose can be fatal.

Note: Prior to administering any medication, review all aspects with a current drug handbook or other reliable source.

Obesity may occur during the young adult years as the active teen becomes the sedentary adult but does not decrease caloric intake. The overweight or obese young adult is at risk for hypertension, a major health problem for this age group.

Hypertension and obesity are two of more than 40 risk factors that have been identified in the development of cardiovascular (CV) disease. Preventing these risk factors and lowering the risk of CV disease are critical. Low-fat and/or low-cholesterol diets play a significant role in both the prevention and treatment of CV disease.

Middle-Aged Adult

The middle-aged adult should continue to eat a healthy diet, following the recommended portions of the food groups, with special attention to protein, calcium, and limiting cholesterol and caloric intake. Two or three liters of fluid should be included in the daily diet. Postmenopausal women need to ingest sufficient calcium and vitamin D to reduce osteoporosis, and antioxidants such as vitamins A, C, and E may be helpful in reducing the risks of heart disease in women. Although iron supplements are no longer needed, the amount in a multivitamin is not harmful and may be beneficial for postmenopausal women taking estrogen supplements (Maurer et al., 2005).

Middle-aged adults who gain weight may not be aware of some common facts about this age period. Decreased metabolic activity and decreased physical activity mean a decrease in caloric need. The nurse's role in nutritional health promotion is to counsel clients to prevent obesity by reducing caloric intake and participating in regular exercise. Clients should also be warned that being overweight is a risk factor for many chronic diseases, such as diabetes and hypertension, and for problems of mobility, such as arthritis.

For the client who requires additional management resources, a variety of programs is frequently available. Most programs use behavior modification techniques and group support to assist clients in reaching their goals. Clients should seek medical advice before considering any major changes in their diets.

During late middle age, gastric juice secretions and free acid gradually decline. As a result, some individuals may complain of "heartburn" (acid indigestion) or an increase in belching. They may determine that certain foods disagree with them. Clients should be advised to develop sensible eating habits and avoid fried or fatty foods.

Elders

The older adult requires the same basic nutrition as the younger adult. However, fewer calories are needed by elders because of the lower metabolic rate and the decrease in physical activity.

Some elders may need more carbohydrates for fiber and bulk, but most nutrient requirements remain relatively unchanged. Such physical changes as tooth loss and impaired sense of taste and smell may affect eating habits. Decreased saliva and gastric juice secretion may also affect a person's nutrition.

Psychosocial factors may also contribute to nutritional problems. Some elders who live alone do not want to cook for themselves or eat alone. As a result, they may adopt poor dietary habits. Other factors, such as lack of transportation, poor access to stores, and inability to prepare the food also affect nutritional status. Loss of spouse, anxiety, depression, dependence on others, and lowered income all affect eating habits (see Table 47–2). Guidelines for the inclusion of high-nutrient foods that are compatible with the nutritional needs of elders are summarized in Client Teaching and in the Nutritional Reference Guide on pages 1244-1245. Also see Lifespan Considerations on page 1246.

TABLE 47–2 Problems Associated with Nutrition in Older Adults

PROBLEMS	NURSING INTERVENTIONS
Difficulty chewing	Encourage regular visits to the dentist to have dentures repaired, refitted, or replaced. Chop fruits and vegetables finely; shred green, leafy vegetables; select ground meat, poultry, or fish.
Lowered glucose tolerance	Eat more complex carbohydrates (e.g., breads, cereals, rice, pasta, potatoes, and legumes) rather than sugar-rich foods.
Decreased social interaction, loneliness	Promote appropriate social interaction at meals, when possible. Encourage the client and spouse to take an interest in food preparation and serving, perhaps as an activity they can do together. Encourage family or caregivers to present the food at a dining table with place mats, table cloths, and napkins to trigger eating associations for the elder. If food preparation is not possible, suggest community resources, such as Meals on Wheels. Suggest picnics in the yard or inviting friends over for meals.
Loss of appetite and senses of smell and taste	Eat essential, nutrient-dense foods first; follow with desserts and low-nutrient-density foods. Review dietary restrictions, and find ways to make meals appealing within these guidelines. Eat small meals frequently instead of three large meals a day.
Limited income	Suggest using generic brands and coupons. Substitute milk, dairy products, and beans for meat. Avoid convenience foods if able to cook. Buy foods that are on sale and freeze for future use. Suggest community resources and nutrition programs.
Difficulty sleeping at night	Have the major meal at noon instead of in the evening. Avoid tea, coffee, or other stimulants in the evening.

CLIENT TEACHING Nutrition for Elders

- *Include each group on the Food Pyramid.* For example, a 65-year-old female who performs less than 30 minutes of exercise per day requires 1,600 Kcalories consisting of the following:

Grains	5 ounces
Vegetables	2 cups
Fruits	1.5 cups
Milk, yogurt, and cheese	3 cups
Meat and beans	5 ounces

- *Reduce caloric intake.* Caloric needs generally decrease in elders often because of decreased activity. Elders need to consume nutrient-dense foods and avoid foods that are high in calories but have few nutrients.
- *Reduce fat consumption.* Use leaner cuts of meat, and limit portions to 4 to 6 oz per day. (But be sure intake of meat is sufficient, because elders often consume inadequate amounts of these foods.) Broil, boil, or bake foods instead of frying them. Use low-fat milk and cheese; limit intake of butter, margarine, and salad dressings.
- *Reduce consumption of empty calories.* Substitute fruit or puddings made with low-fat milk in place of pastry, cookies, and rich desserts.
- *Reduce sodium consumption for clients who have hypertension or other cardiac problems.* Avoid canned soups, ketchup, and mustard. Avoid salted, smoked, cured, and pickled meats (e.g., ham and bacon), poultry, and fish. Do not add salt when cooking foods or at the table.
- *Ensure adequate calcium intake (at least 800 mg) to prevent bone loss.* Milk, cheese, yogurt, cream soups, puddings, and frozen milk products are good sources. See the Major Food Sources of Calcium table.
- *Ensure adequate vitamin D intake.* Vitamin D is essential to maintain calcium homeostasis. Include some milk, because other dairy products are not usually fortified with vitamin D. If milk cannot be tolerated because of a lactose deficiency, provide vitamin supplements.
- *Ensure adequate iron intake.* Iron intake in older people may be compromised by such factors as increased incidence of gastrointestinal disturbance, chronic diarrhea, regular aspirin use, and possible reduction in meat consumption. See the Major Food Sources of Iron table.
- *Consume fiber-rich foods to prevent constipation and minimize use of laxatives.* See the Fiber-Rich Foods table on page 1245. Because fiber-rich foods provide bulk and a feeling of fullness, they help people control their appetites and lose weight.

NUTRITIONAL REFERENCE GUIDE Major Food Sources of Calcium

Foods	Household Measure	Calcium (mg)	Foods	Household Measure	Calcium (mg)
Dairy Products			**Fish, Meat, and Poultry**		
Cheese, cheddar	1 oz	213	Salmon (canned)	1 oz	91
Cheese, cottage, 4% milk fat	1 oz	27	Sardines	1 oz	124
Cheese, processed	1 oz (1 slice)	198	Shellfish	1 oz	35
Cheese, Swiss	1 oz	262	**Vegetables**		
Custard	1/2 cup	148	Beet greens	1/2 cup	72
Ice cream	1/2 cup	97	Broccoli (cooked)	1 medium stalk	158
Milk, nonfat dry (reconstituted)	1 cup	240	Greens, collards	1/2 cup	179
Milk, skim (1% fat)	1 cup	296	Okra	10 pods	98
Milk, whole	1 cup	288	**Fruits**		
Yogurt	1 cup	295	Blackberries	1 cup	46
			Dates	10	45
			Orange	1 medium	54
			Rhubarb (sweetened)	1/2 cup	105

NATIONAL REFERENCE GUIDE Major Food Sources of Iron

Foods	Household Measure	Iron (mg)	Foods	Household Measure	Iron (mg)
Meat, Fish, Poultry			**Vegetables and Fruits**		
Beef (ground)	3 oz	3.2	Beet greens	2/3 cup	1.9
Beef liver	3 oz	5.1	Chick peas	1/2 cup	3
Beef heart	3 1/2 oz	5.9	Dates (pitted)	1/2 cup	3
Beef kidneys	3 1/2 oz	7.4	Kidney beans	1/2 cup	3
Chicken (breast)	3 oz	1.3	Prune juice	1/2 cup	4.1
Oysters	5 to 8 medium	5.5	Raisins	2/3 cup	3.5
Scallops	3 1/2 oz	3.0	Soybeans	3 1/2 oz	2.8
Shrimp	3 1/2 oz	3.1	Spinach		
Tuna (canned)	3 oz	1.5	Raw	1/2 cup	2
			Cooked	1/2 cup	2.2

NATIONAL REFERENCE GUIDE Major Food Sources of Iron (continued)

Foods	Household Measure	Iron (mg)	Foods	Household Measure	Iron (mg)
Grain Products			**Other**		
Bread			Corn syrup	1/3 cup	4.1
White	1 slice	0.6	Eggs	2 medium	2.3
Whole-wheat	1 slice	0.8	Molasses	1 T	0.9
Cereal (bran flakes)	1 oz	5.3	Peanuts	2/3 cup	2.1
Cereal (oat flakes)	1 oz	5.4	Tofu (soybean curd)	1/2 cup	1.9
Enriched pasta	1/2 cup	2.0			
Spaghetti (enriched)	1/2 cup	0.3			

NUTRITIONAL REFERENCE GUIDE
Fiber-Rich Foods

Food	Portion	Insoluble Dietary Fiber Content (g)
Apple	1 medium	3.3
Banana	1	2.1
Beans, green	1/2 cup	1.8–2.2
Broccoli	1 cup	4.8
Cereal, all bran	1/3 cup	7.8
Cereal, bran flakes	1 cup	6.8
Fresh pear	1 medium	4.2
Kidney beans	1/2 cup	5.6
Lima beans	1/2 cup	3.2
Peas	1 cup	5.0

NUTRITIONAL REFERENCE GUIDE
Types of Vegetarian Diets

Kind	Description
Vegan	Strict vegetarians; avoid all foods of animal origin.
Lacto-ovo-vegetarian	Use dairy products and eggs but avoid eating flesh.
Lacto-vegetarian	Use dairy products but avoid eating flesh and eggs.
Ovo-vegetarian	Use eggs but avoid dairy products and flesh.
Pesco-vegetarian	Use dairy products, eggs, and fish but avoid all other meat products.
Partial vegetarian (semivegetarian)	Avoid selected meats (e.g., red meat).
Fruitarian	Use only fresh (raw) fruits, juices, nuts, honey, and/or olive oil.
Macrobiotic vegetarian	Progress through 10 dietary stages from a widely inclusive selection to a restrictive selection.

NUTRITIONAL REFERENCE TO GUIDE Daily Food Guide—Based on an 1,800 to 2,000-Calorie Diet

Food Groups and Servings per Day	Foods and Sizes of Servings	Major Nutrients
Grains 6 to 7 oz, at least half whole grains	1 oz = 1 slice bread, 1 cup ready-to-eat cereal, or 1/2 cup of the following: cooked cereal, cornmeal, grits, spaghetti, macaroni, noodles, popcorn, tortillas, or rice	Complex carbohydrate; thiamine; niacin; iron; some protein; fiber

Vegetable Group
2.5 to 3 oz
  a. 3 cups/week dark green vegetables
  b. 2 cups/week orange vegetables
  c. 3 cups/week legumes
  d. 3 cups/week starchy vegetables
	1 oz = 2 cups raw leafy vegetables; 1 cup other fresh, frozen, or canned vegetables; 1 cup fresh, frozen, or canned juice	Carbohydrate; vitamin C; vitamin A; iron; folacin; calcium; fiber (naturally low in fat)

Fruit Group 1.5 to 2 cups	1 cup = 1 medium apple, banana, or orange; 1 cup of raw, cooked, or canned fruit; 1 cup of fruit juice; 1/2 cup of dried fruit	Vitamins A and C; potassium; folacin; fiber (naturally low in sodium)
Meat and Beans 5 to 6 oz	1 oz = 1 egg; 1/4 cup cooked dry legumes; 3 oz tofu; 2 T peanut butter; 1/2 oz nuts or seeds; 1 oz lean beef, pork, lamb, veal, poultry, or fish (no bone)	Protein; vitamin B; iron; zinc; niacin; fats (in meats, nuts, and seeds)
Milk, Yogurt, and Cheese 3 cups (Choose skim and low-fat products.)	1 cup = 8 oz milk or yogurt, 1 1/2 oz natural cheese, 2 oz processed cheese food	Protein; fat; vitamins A and D; riboflavin; B$_{12}$; calcium; phosphorus
Oils 5 to 6 tsp	Plant and fish oils (liquid at room temperature) Foods high in oil (e.g., nuts, olives, avocados, mayonnaise, margarine)	Fat

LIFESPAN CONSIDERATIONS Nutrition

CHILDREN

- Children learn eating habits from their parents. It is the parents' responsibility to be good nutritional role models, both in terms of what they eat and how they incorporate food into their lifestyle.
- During the preschool and early school-age years children learn life-long eating habits. It is the parents' responsibility to provide the child with adequate amounts of nutritious foods in an environment that is relaxed and comfortable for eating. It is the child's responsibility to decide what and how much of the nutritious foods to eat. Parents should be counseled that eating can become a source of conflict if the parent tries to tell the child what and how much to eat, or if the child tries to tell the parent what foods should be eaten. Children's access to "junk food" should be limited, but completely forbidding a food may also create conflict.
- Although adolescents who are vegetarians are at risk for some nutritional deficits, the diet of adolescents who eat eggs, milk products, and, on occasion, non-red meat is more healthful than that of their red-meat-eating peers (Haddad & Tanzman, 2003).

ELDERS

Most elders take several medications as a result of having an increase in the number of chronic illnesses. Considerations for potential problems include:

- Some foods interact adversely or decrease the effectiveness of certain medications, such as foods high in vitamin K and the anticoagulant Coumadin. Elders should not change their diet significantly

without consulting the health care provider since drug dosage may have been based on the elder's previous dietary intake.

- Some medications increase appetite, such as glucocorticoids.
- Some medications decrease appetite by their actions or by causing an unpleasant taste.
- Certain tablets should not be crushed to be given by mouth or by gastric tubes, such as enteric-coated or slow-release medications.

Conditions such as neuromuscular disorders and dementia can make it difficult for elders to eat or to be fed. Safety should always be a priority concern with attention paid to prevent aspiration. All health care personnel and family caregivers should be taught proper techniques to reduce this risk. Effective techniques include:

- Use the chin-tuck method when feeding clients with dysphagia. Having them flex the head toward the chest when swallowing decreases the risk of aspiration into the lungs.
- Use foods of prescribed consistency. Many elders can swallow foods with thicker consistency more easily than thin liquids.
- Try to focus on food preferences—the family can help provide this information.
- Try to maintain mealtime as a positive social occasion with conversations and extra attention to having a pleasant environment.

Economic factors may influence elders' nutritional status if they cannot afford food, especially if a prescribed diet requires expensive supplements. Inexpensive or convenience foods such as canned soups are often high in fat and sodium.

STANDARDS FOR A HEALTHY DIET

Various daily food guides have been developed to help healthy people meet the daily requirements of essential nutrients and to facilitate meal planning. Food group plans emphasize the general types or groups of foods rather than the specific foods, because related foods are similar in composition and often have similar nutrient values. For example, all grains, whether wheat or oats, are significant sources of carbohydrate, iron, and the B vitamin thiamine. Daily food guides that are currently used include *Dietary Guidelines for Americans* and the Food Guide Pyramids.

Dietary Guidelines for Americans

This guide is published by the U.S. Department of Agriculture (USDA) every 5 years, and the 2005 revision contains recommendations for food choices to help reduce calorie consumption and increase physical activity. Key points of the dietary guidelines follow:

- Consume nutrient-dense foods within caloric needs.
- Maintain weight in a healthy range.
- Engage in regular physical activity.
- Consume recommended amounts of fruit, vegetables, whole grains, and milk each day.
- Keep total fat intake within 20% to 35% of total calories and less than 10% from saturated fatty acids. (See also Client Teaching for ways to reduce fat intake.)

- Consume less than 2,300 mg of sodium per day and add potassium-rich foods.
- If you drink alcohol, do so in moderation (one drink per day for women and two drinks per day for men).

CLIENT TEACHING
Reducing Dietary Fat

- Cook meat by grilling, baking, broiling, or microwaving rather than frying.
- Substitute popcorn or pretzels for such snacks as potato chips, cheese puffs, and corn chips.
- Read labels. Some crackers, for example, are high in fat; others are not.
- Limit desserts high in fat, such as candy, ice cream, cake, and cookies.
- Substitute hard candies for chocolate bars.
- Use skim or reduced-fat milk instead of whole milk, for drinking as well as in recipes.
- Use less butter or margarine on breads.
- Remove fat from meat and skin from chicken before cooking.
- Eat less meat; eat more fish.
- Use less dressing, or use low-fat dressings, on salads.
- Eat plant sources of protein (e.g., kidney, lima, and navy beans).
- Use nuts as a source of protein, but since they are high in fat, use to replace meat rather than in addition.

These dietary recommendations are intended to help achieve the nutritional goals stated in *Healthy People 2010*. In that report, the U.S. surgeon general identified 25 specific nutritional objectives, such as the following (U.S. Department of Health and Human Services, 2000):

- Reduce the incidence of overweight adults (target = 15%) and children (target = 5%).
- Reduce growth retardation among low-income children aged 5 and younger to less than 5%.
- Increase the proportion of persons aged 2 years and older who consume no more than 30% of calories from total fat to 75%.
- Increase the proportion of persons aged 2 years and older who consume no more than 2,400 mg of sodium daily to 65%.

The Food Guide Pyramid

The Food Guide Pyramid is a graphic aid that was developed by the USDA as a guide in making daily food choices. Previously, one pyramid was intended for use by all persons. In 2005, the USDA issued a new pyramid in a food guidance system on the Internet to allow people to customize their pyramid based on a variety of characteristics. On the new pyramid, the food groups—grains, vegetables, fruits, milk, and meat and beans—are drawn from the base of the pyramid to the apex. This indicates that activity, moderation, personalization, proportionality, variety, and gradual improvement are the keys to good nutrition (see Figure 47-1 ■).

There are many variations of the standard food pyramid, not all of which have been modified following issuance of the new general pyramid. Examples include the pyramid for young children (Figure 47-2 ■) and the pyramid for elders (Figure 47-3 ■). There are pyramids or other shaped diagrams of food guides for many countries, and Georgia State University has translated the original pyramid into more than 37 languages.

Using and following this guide does not guarantee that a person will consume the necessary levels of all essential nutrients. For example, someone who chooses cooked and low-fiber fruits and vegetables might have an inadequate intake of dietary fiber even though the recommended number of servings is eaten. However, the food guide is easy to follow, and people who eat

Anatomy of MyPyramid

One size doesn't fit all

USDA's new MyPyramid symbolizes a personalized approach to healthy eating and physical activity. The symbol has been designed to be simple. It has been developed to remind consumers to make healthy food choices and to be active every day. The different parts of the symbol are described below.

Activity
Activity is represented by the steps and the person climbing them, as a reminder of the importance of daily physical activity.

Moderation
Moderation is represented by the narrowing of each food group from bottom to top. The wider base stands for foods with little or no solid fats or added sugars. These should be selected more often. The narrower top area stands for foods containing more added sugars and solid fats. The more active you are, the more of these foods can fit into your diet.

Personalization
Personalization is shown by the person on the steps, the slogan, and the URL. Find the kinds and amounts of food to eat each day at MyPyramid.gov.

Proportionality
Proportionality is shown by the different widths of the food group bands. The widths suggest how much food a person should choose from each group. The widths are just a general guide, not exact proportions. Check the Web site for how much is right for you.

Variety
Variety is symbolized by the 6 color bands representing the 5 food groups of the Pyramid and oils. This illustrates that foods from all groups are needed each day for good health.

Gradual Improvement
Gradual improvement is encouraged by the slogan. It suggests that individuals can benefit from taking small steps to improve their diet and lifestyle each day.

MyPyramid.gov
STEPS TO A HEALTHIER YOU

U.S. Department of Agriculture
Center for Nutrition Policy
and Promotion
April 2005 CNPP-16

USDA is an equal opportunity provider and employer.

| GRAINS | VEGETABLES | FRUITS | OILS | MILK | MEAT & BEANS |

Figure 47-1 ■ The Food Guide Pyramid.

(*Note:* From U.S. Department of Agriculture and U.S. Department of Health and Human Services, 2005.)

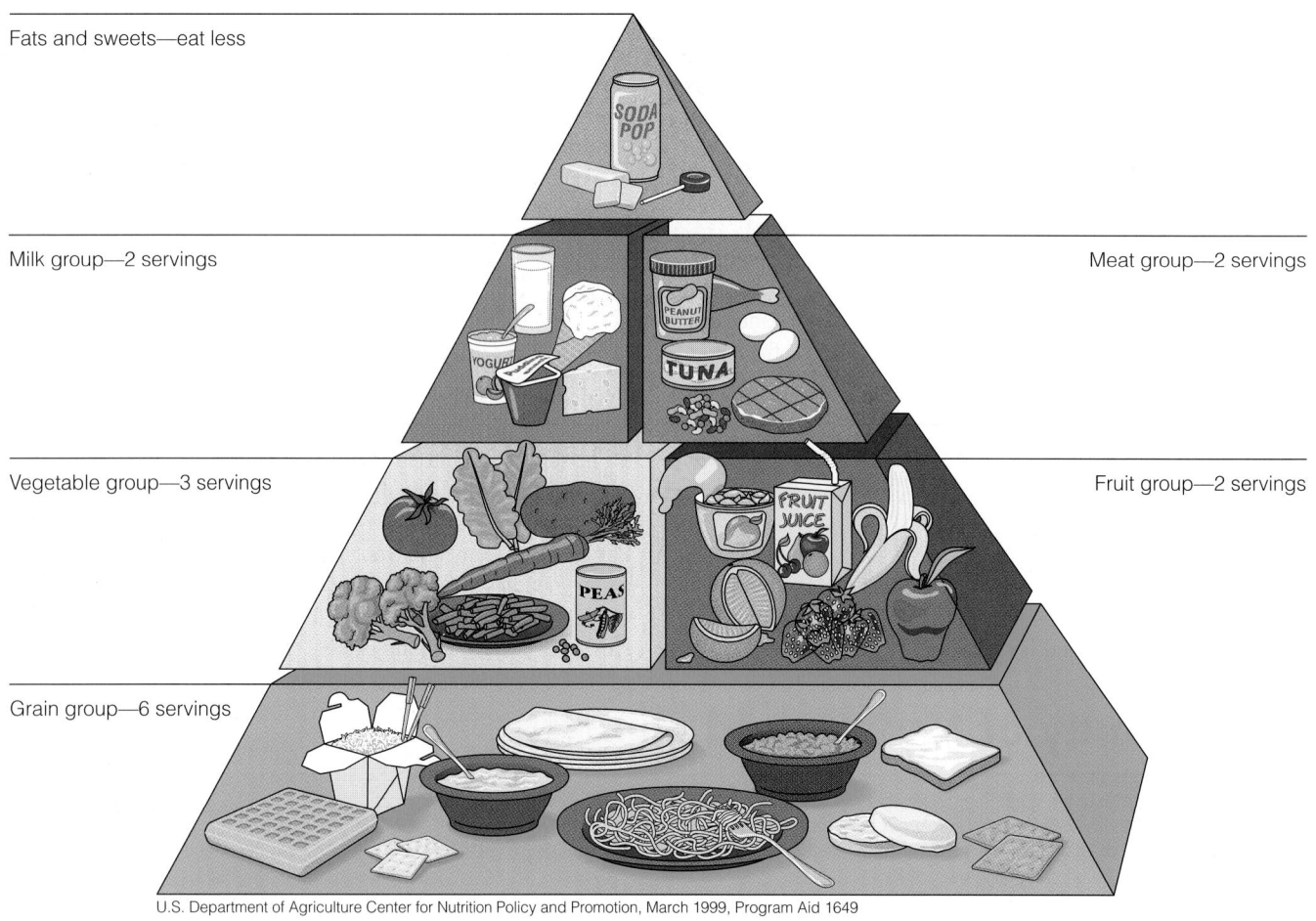

Fats and sweets—eat less

Milk group—2 servings

Meat group—2 servings

Vegetable group—3 servings

Fruit group—2 servings

Grain group—6 servings

U.S. Department of Agriculture Center for Nutrition Policy and Promotion, March 1999, Program Aid 1649

WHAT COUNTS AS ONE SERVING

GRAIN GROUP
1 slice of bread
1/2 cup of cooked rice or pasta
1/2 cup of cooked cereal
1 ounce of ready-to-eat cereal

VEGETABLE GROUP
1/2 cup of chopped raw
    or cooked vegetables
1 cup of raw leafy vegetables

FRUIT GROUP
1 piece of fruit or melon wedge
3/4 cup of juice
1/2 cup of canned fruit
1/4 cup of dried fruit

MILK GROUP
1 cup of milk or yogurt
2 ounces of cheese

MEAT GROUP
2 to 3 ounces of cooked lean
    meat, poultry, or fish

1/2 cup of cooked dry beans, or
1 egg counts as 1 ounce of lean
meat. 2 tablespoons of peanut
butter count as 1 ounce of
meat.

FATS AND SWEETS
Limit calories from these.

Four- to 6-year-olds can eat these serving sizes. Offer 2- to 3-year-olds less, except for milk.
Two- to 6 year-old children need a total of 2 servings from the milk group each day.

Figure 47-2 ■ Food guide pyramid for young children.
(*Note:* From U.S. Department of Agriculture and U.S. Department of Health and Human Services, 1999.)

a variety of foods from each group, in the suggested amounts, are likely to come close to recommended nutrient levels. The Food Guide Pyramid does not address fluid intake or provide guidelines about combination foods (such as chili, which contains meat, beans, and a vegetable) or about convenience foods (such as hamburgers, milk shakes, and pizzas), which are a large part of the North American diet, although a chart with some of this information is found on the website.

Recommended Dietary Intake

The Committee on the Scientific Evaluation of Dietary Reference Intakes of the Institute of Medicine publishes the Dietary Reference Intakes (DRIs) tables, which contain four sets of reference values: estimated average requirements (EARs), recommended dietary allowances (RDAs), adequate intakes (AIs), and tolerable upper intake levels (ULs). Definitions of these terms are found in Box 47–4 on page 1250. The values for

TUFTS

Food Guide Pyramid for Older Adults

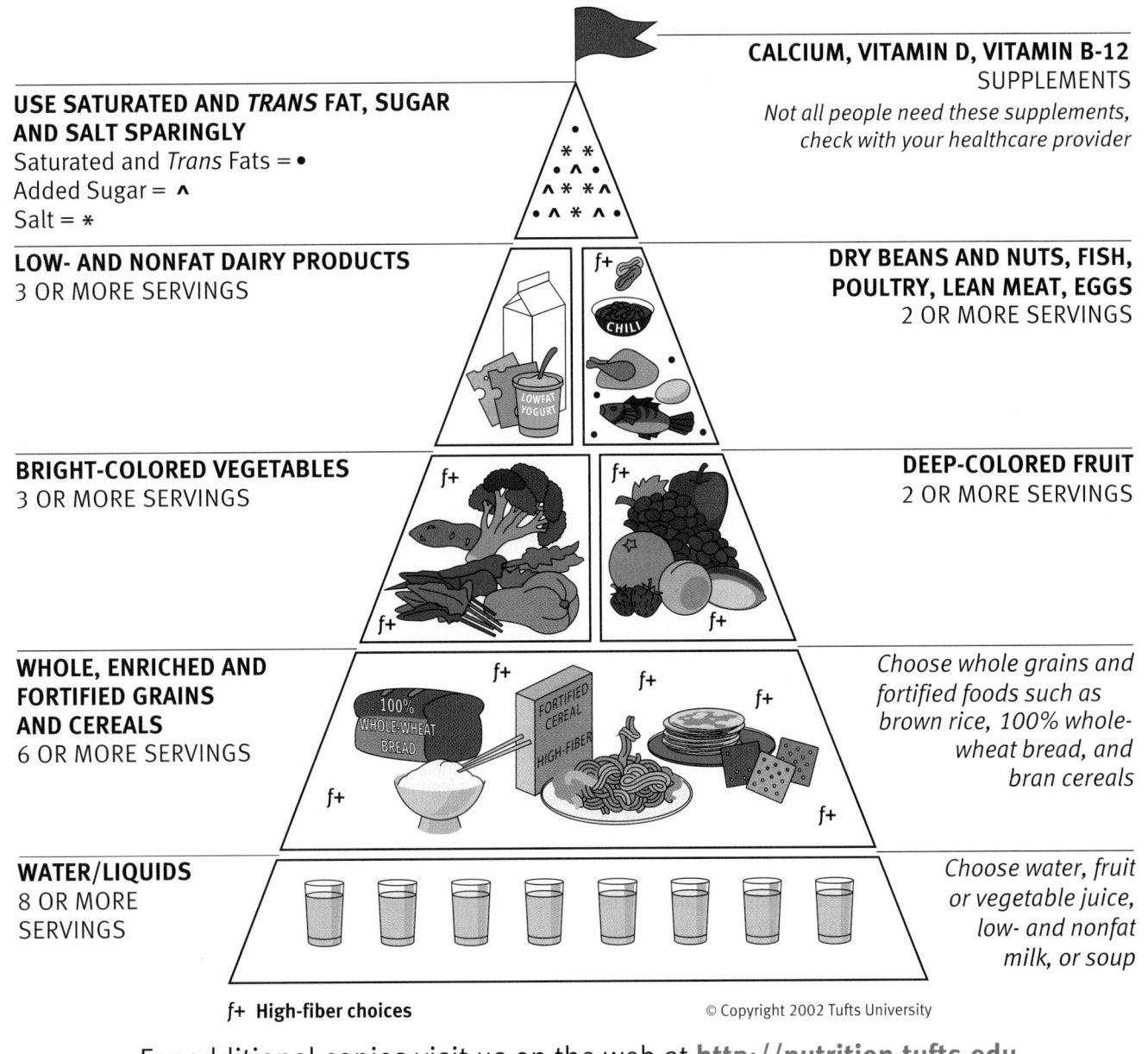

CALCIUM, VITAMIN D, VITAMIN B-12
SUPPLEMENTS
*Not all people need these supplements,
check with your healthcare provider*

**USE SATURATED AND *TRANS* FAT, SUGAR
AND SALT SPARINGLY**
Saturated and *Trans* Fats = •
Added Sugar = ∧
Salt = *

LOW- AND NONFAT DAIRY PRODUCTS
3 OR MORE SERVINGS

**DRY BEANS AND NUTS, FISH,
POULTRY, LEAN MEAT, EGGS**
2 OR MORE SERVINGS

BRIGHT-COLORED VEGETABLES
3 OR MORE SERVINGS

DEEP-COLORED FRUIT
2 OR MORE SERVINGS

**WHOLE, ENRICHED AND
FORTIFIED GRAINS
AND CEREALS**
6 OR MORE SERVINGS

*Choose whole grains and
fortified foods such as
brown rice, 100% whole-
wheat bread, and
bran cereals*

WATER/LIQUIDS
8 OR MORE
SERVINGS

*Choose water, fruit
or vegetable juice,
low- and nonfat
milk, or soup*

f+ **High-fiber choices**

© Copyright 2002 Tufts University

For additional copies visit us on the web at **http://nutrition.tufts.edu**

Figure 47-3 ■ A modified food guide pyramid for people older than 70 years of age.

RDAs and AIs in the tables are modified for different age groups and according to gender. The Canadian Department of National Health and Welfare also adopted the DRIs in 2003. The effect of illness or injury (increasing the need for nutrients) and the variability among individuals within any given subgroup are not taken into account in the DRIs.

Consumers most commonly learn recommended dietary intake information from the U.S. Food and Drug Administration (FDA) nutrition labels called Nutrition Facts. Food labeling is required for most prepared foods, such as breads, cereals, canned and frozen foods, snacks, desserts, and drinks. Nutrition labeling for raw produce (fruits and vegetables) and fish is storage of energy in the form of adipose tissue. As the amount of stored fat increases, the individual becomes overweight or obese. A person is said to be **overweight** when BMI is between 25 and 29.9 kg/m² and **obese** when BMI is >30 kg/m² (National Heart, Lung, and Blood Institute, 1998).

Excess body weight increases the stress on body organs and predisposes people to chronic health problems such as hypertension and diabetes mellitus. Obesity that interferes with mobility or breathing is referred to as morbid obesity. Obese people may also manifest undernourishment in important nutrients (e.g., essential vitamins or minerals) even though excess calories are ingested.

Undernutrition refers to an intake of nutrients insufficient to meet daily energy requirements because of inadequate food intake or improper digestion and absorption of food. An inadequate food intake may be caused by the inability to acquire and prepare food, inadequate knowledge about essential nutrients and a balanced diet, discomfort during or after eating, dysphagia, anorexia, nausea, vomiting, and so on. Improper digestion and absorption of nutrients may be caused by an inadequate production of hormones or enzymes or by medical conditions resulting in inflammation or obstruction of the gastrointestinal tract.

Inadequate nutrition is associated with marked weight loss, generalized weakness, altered functional abilities, delayed wound healing, increased susceptibility to infection, decreased immunocompetence, impaired pulmonary function, and prolonged length of hospitalization. In response to undernutrition, carbohydrate reserves, stored as liver and muscle glycogen, are mobilized. However, these reserves can only meet energy requirements for a short time (e.g., 24 hours) and then body protein is mobilized.

Protein-calorie malnutrition (PCM), once associated with the manifestation of undernutrition seen in starving children of third world countries, is now recognized as a significant problem of clients with long-term deficiencies in caloric intake (e.g., those with cancer and chronic disease). Characteristics of PCM are depressed visceral proteins (e.g., albumin), weight loss, and visible muscle and fat wasting.

Protein stores in the body are generally divided into two compartments: somatic and visceral. Somatic protein consists largely of skeletal muscle mass; it is assessed most commonly by conducting anthropometric measurements such as the mid-arm circumference (MAC) and the mid-arm muscle circumference (MAMC). (See the "Anthropometric Measurements" section on page 1258.) Visceral protein includes plasma protein, hemoglobin, several clotting factors, hormones, and antibodies. It is usually assessed by measuring serum protein levels such as albumin and transferrin, discussed in the "Laboratory Data" section of "Assessing," which follows.

NURSING MANAGEMENT

Assessing

The purpose of a nutritional assessment is to identify clients at risk for malnutrition and those with poor nutritional status. In most health care facilities, the responsibility for nutritional assessment and support is shared by the primary care provider, the dietitian, and the nurse. Because a comprehensive nutritional assessment is time consuming and expensive, various levels and types of assessment are available. Generally, nurses perform a nutritional screen. A comprehensive nutritional assessment is often performed by a nutritionist or a dietitian, and the primary care provider. Components of a nutritional assessment are shown in Table 47–3 and may be remembered as ABCD data: anthropometric, biochemical, clinical, and dietary.

Nutritional Screening

A nutritional screen is an assessment performed to identify clients at risk for malnutrition or those who are malnourished. Clients who are found to be at moderate or high risk are followed with a comprehensive assessment by a dietitian (see Box 47–6). Medicare standards for nursing homes require that any

TABLE 47–3 **Components of a Nutritional Assessment**		
	SCREENING DATA	**ADDITIONAL IN-DEPTH DATA**
Anthropometric Data	■ Height ■ Weight ■ Ideal body weight ■ Usual body weight ■ Body mass index	■ Triceps skinfold (TSF) ■ Mid-arm circumference (MAC) ■ Mid-arm muscle circumference (MAMC)
Biochemical Data	■ Hemoglobin ■ Serum albumin ■ Total lymphocyte count	■ Serum transferrin level ■ Urinary urea nitrogen ■ Urinary creatinine excretion
Clinical	■ Skin ■ Hair and nails ■ Mucous membranes ■ Activity level	■ Hair analysis ■ Neurological testing
Dietary Data	■ 24-hour food recall ■ Food frequency record	■ Selective food frequency record ■ Food diary ■ Diet history

BOX 47–6   Summary of Risk Factors for Nutritional Problems

DIET HISTORY
- Chewing or swallowing difficulties (including ill-fitting dentures, dental caries, and missing teeth)
- Inadequate food budget
- Inadequate food intake
- Inadequate food preparation facilities
- Inadequate food storage facilities
- Intravenous fluids (other than total parenteral nutrition for 10 or more days)
- Living and eating alone
- No intake for 10 or more days
- Physical disabilities
- Restricted or fad diets

MEDICAL HISTORY
- Adolescent pregnancy or closely spaced pregnancies
- Alcohol or substance abuse
- Catabolic or hypermetabolic condition: burns, trauma
- Chronic illness: end-stage renal disease, liver disease, HIV, pulmonary disease (COPD), cancer
- Dental problems: difficulty chewing, ill-fitting dentures

- Fluid and electrolyte imbalance
- Gastrointestinal problems: anorexia, dysphagia, nausea, vomiting, diarrhea, constipation
- Neurologic or cognitive impairment
- Oral and gastrointestinal surgery
- Unintentional weight loss or gain of 10% within 6 months

MEDICATION HISTORY*
- Antacid
- Antidepressants
- Antihypertensives
- Anti-inflammatory agents
- Antineoplastic agents
- Aspirin
- Digitalis
- Diuretics (thiazides)
- Laxatives
- Potassium chloride

*The potential effects of some medications on nutrition are shown in Table 47–1 on page 1239.

resident whose percent of meals eaten falls below 75% receive a full nutritional assessment by a nurse.

Nurses carry out nutritional screens through routine nursing histories and physical examinations. Custom-designed screens for a particular population (e.g., elders and pregnant women) and specific disorders (e.g., cardiac disease) are available.

Screening tools such as the Patient-Generated Subjective Global Assessment (PG-SGA) and the Nutrition Screening Initiative (NSI) can be incorporated into the nursing history. The PG-SGA is a method of classifying clients as either well nourished, moderately malnourished, or severely malnourished based on a dietary history and physical examination. It was established primarily for use with cancer patients but has been widely tested and is appropriate for both inpatient and outpatient

clients with various diagnoses (Green & Watson, 2005). A version of the instrument (Figure 47-5 ■ on pages 1254–1255) can be completed and analyzed online by the client without a health care provider.

The NSI is an ongoing project of the American Academy of Family Physicians, the American Dietetic Association, the National Council on Aging, and other organizations to promote nutrition screening and improved nutritional care for elders. The NSI estimates that approximately half of hospitalized, nursing home, and home care elders are malnourished. The NSI screens elders using a nutrition checklist that contains nine warning signs of conditions that can interfere with good nutrition (see Box 47–7). Elders can also complete the tool online and have a risk score calculated. The booklet *A Physician's*

BOX 47–7   Nutritional Screening Tool

Read the statement. Circle the number in the Yes column for those that apply to you. Total your nutritional assessment.

Nutritional Assessment Statements	Yes
I have an illness or condition that made me change the kind or amount of food I eat.	2
I eat fewer than two meals per day.	3
I eat few fruits, vegetables, or milk products.	2
I have three or more drinks of beer, liquor, or wine almost every day.	2
I have tooth or mouth problems that make it hard for me to eat.	2
I do not always have enough money to buy the food I need.	4
I eat alone most of the time.	1
I take three or more different prescribed or over-the-counter drugs a day.	1

Without wanting to, I have lost or gained 10 pounds in the last 6 months.	2
I am not always physically able to shop, cook, or feed myself.	2
Total	

If you scored 0–2: Good! Recheck your nutritional score in 6 months.

If you scored 3–5: You are at moderate nutritional risk. See what can be done to improve your eating habits and lifestyle. Recheck your score in 3 months.

If you scored 6 or above: You are at high nutritional risk. Take this checklist to your doctor, nurse practitioner, or home health nurse. Ask for help to improve your nutritional health.

Note: From *Determine Your Nutritional Health*, by the Nutrition Screening Initiative, 2003, Washington, DC: National Council on Aging. Reprinted with permission by the Nutrition Screening Initiative, a project of the American Dietetic Association, funded in part by a grant from Ross Products Division, Abbott Laboratories, Inc.

Patient ID Information

Scored Patient-Generated Subjective Global Assessment (PG-SGA)
History (Boxes 1–4 are designed to be completed by the patient.)

1. Weight *(See Worksheet 1)*

In summary of my current and recent weight:

I currently weigh about _____ pounds
I am about _____ feet _____ tall

One month ago I weighed about _____ pounds
Six months ago I weighed about _____ pounds

During the past two weeks my weight has:

☐ decreased $_{(1)}$ ☐ not changed $_{(0)}$ ☐ increased $_{(0)}$

Box 1 ☐

2. Food Intake: As compared to my normal intake, I would rate my food intake during the past month as:
☐ unchanged $_{(0)}$
☐ more than usual $_{(0)}$
☐ less than usual $_{(1)}$
   I am now taking:
   ☐ *normal food* but less than normal amount $_{(1)}$
   ☐ little solid food $_{(2)}$
   ☐ only liquids $_{(3)}$
   ☐ only nutritonal supplements $_{(3)}$
   ☐ very little of anything $_{(4)}$
   ☐ only tube feedings or only nutrition by vein $_{(0)}$

Box 2 ☐

3. Symptoms: I have had the following problems that have kept me from eating enough during the past two weeks (check all that apply):
☐ no problems eating $_{(0)}$

☐ no appetite, just did not feel like eating $_{(3)}$

☐ nausea $_{(1)}$ ☐ vomiting $_{(3)}$
☐ constipation $_{(1)}$ ☐ diarrhea $_{(3)}$
☐ mouth sores $_{(2)}$ ☐ dry mouth $_{(1)}$
☐ things taste funny or have no taste $_{(1)}$ ☐ smells bother me $_{(1)}$
☐ problems swallowing $_{(2)}$ ☐ feel full quickly $_{(1)}$
☐ pain; where? $_{(3)}$_____
☐ other** $_{(1)}$_____

** Examples: depression, money, or dental problems

Box 3 ☐

4. Activities and Function: Over the past month, I would generally rate my activity as:

☐ normal with no limitations $_{(0)}$

☐ not my normal self, but able to be up and about with fairly normal activities $_{(1)}$

☐ not feeling up to most things, but in bed or chair less than half the day $_{(2)}$

☐ able to do little activity and spend most of the day in bed or chair $_{(3)}$

☐ pretty much bedridden, rarely out of bed $_{(3)}$

Box 4 ☐

Additive Score of the Boxes 1–4 ☐ A

The remainder of this form will be completed by your doctor, nurse, or therapist. Thank you.

5. Disease and its relation to nutritional requirements *(See Worksheet 2)*

All relevant diagnoses (specify) _____

Primary disease stage (circle if known or appropriate)   I   II   III   IV   Other _____

Age _____

Numerical score from Worksheet 2 ☐ B

6. Metabolic Demand *(See Worksheet 3)*

Numerical score from Worksheet 3 ☐ C

7. Physical *(See Worksheet 4)*

Numerical score from Worksheet 4 ☐ D

Global Assessment *(See Worksheet 5)*
☐ Well-nourished or anabolic (SGA-A)
☐ Moderate or suspected malnutrition (SGA-B)
☐ Severely malnourished (SGA-C)

Total PG-SGA score

(Total numerical score of A+B+C+D above) ☐
(See triage recommendations below)

Clinician Signature _____ RD RN PA MD DO Other ___   Date _____

Nutritional Triage Recommendations: Additive score is used to define specific nutritional interventions including patient & family education, symptom management including pharmacologic intervention, and appropriate nutrient intervention (food, nutritional supplements, enteral, or parenteral triage). First line nutrition intervention includes optimal symptom management.

0–1 No intervention required at this time. Re-assessment on routine and regular basis during treatment.

2–3 Patient & family education by dietitian, nurse, or other clinician with pharmacologic intervention as indicated by symptom survey (Box 3) and laboratory values as appropriate.

4–8 Requires intervention by dietitian, in conjunction with nurse or physician as indicated by symptoms survey (Box 3).

≥ 9 Indicates a critical need for improved symptom management and/or nutrient intervention options.

Figure 47-5 ■ Scored Patient-Generated Subjective Global Assessment (PG-SGA).

Worksheets for PG-SGA Scoring

**Boxes 1–4 of the PG-SGA are designed to be completed by the patient. The PG-SGA numerical score is determined using
1) the parenthetical points noted in boxes 1–4 and 2) the worksheets below for items not marked with parenthetical points. Scores for
boxes 1 and 3 are additive within each box and scores for boxes 2 and 4 are based on the highest scored item checked off by the patient.**

Worksheet 1 — Scoring Weight (Wt) Loss

To determine score, use 1 month weight data if available. Use 6 month
data only if there is no 1 month weight data. Use points below to score
weight change and add one extra point if patient has lost weight during the
past 2 weeks. Enter total point score in Box 1 of the PG-SGA.

Wt loss in 1 month	Points	Wt loss in 6 months
10% or greater	4	20% or greater
5–9.9%	3	10–19.9%
3–4.9%	2	6–9.9%
2–2.9%	1	2–5.9%
0–1.9%	0	0–1.9%

Score for Worksheet 1 ☐
Record in Box 1

Worksheet 2 — Scoring Criteria for Condition

Score is derived by adding 1 point for each of the conditions listed below
that pertain to the patient.

Category Points

Cancer	1
AIDS	1
Pulmonary or cardiac cachexia	1
Presence of decubitus, open wound, or fistula	1
Presence of trauma	1
Age greater than 65 years	1

Score for Worksheet 2 = ☐
Record in Box B

Worksheet 3 — Scoring Metabolic Stress

Score for metabolic stress is determined by a number of variables known to increase protein & calorie needs. The score is additive so that a patient who has a fever
of > 102 degrees (3 points) and is on 10 mg of prednisone chronically (2 points) would have an additive score for this section of 5 points.

Stress	none (0)	low (1)	moderate (2)	high (3)
Fever	no fever	>99 and <101	≥101 and <102	≥102
Fever duration	no fever	<72 hrs	72 hrs	> 72 hrs
Corticosteroids	no corticosteroids	low dose (<10mg prednisone equivalents/day)	moderate dose (≥10 and <30mg prednisone equivalents/day)	high dose steroids (≥30mg prednisone equivalents/day)

Score for Worksheet 3 = ☐
Record in Box C

Worksheet 4 — Physical Examination

Physical exam includes a subjective evaluation of 3 aspects of body composition: fat, muscle, & fluid status. Since this is subjective, each aspect of the exam is
rated for degree of deficit. Muscle deficit impacts point score more than fat deficit. Definition of categories: 0 = no deficit, 1+ = mild deficit, 2+ = moderate
deficit, 3+ = severe deficit. Rating of deficit in these categories are *not* additive but are used to clinically assess the degree of deficit (or presence of excess fluid).

Fat Stores:

orbital fat pads	0	1+	2+	3+
triceps skin fold	0	1+	2+	3+
fat overlying lower ribs	0	1+	2+	3+
Global fat deficit rating	**0**	**1+**	**2+**	**3+**

Fluid Status:

ankle edema	0	1+	2+	3+
sacral edema	0	1+	2+	3+
ascites	0	1+	2+	3+
Global fluid status rating	**0**	**1+**	**2+**	**3+**

Muscle Status:

temples (temporalis muscle)	0	1+	2+	3+
clavicles (pectoralis & deltoids)	0	1+	2+	3+
shoulders (deltoids)	0	1+	2+	3+
interosseous muscles	0	1+	2+	3+
scapula (latissimus dorsi, trapezius, deltoids)	0	1+	2+	3+
thigh (quadriceps)	0	1+	2+	3+
calf (gastrocnemius)	0	1+	2+	3+
Global muscle status rating	**0**	**1+**	**2+**	**3+**

Point score for the physical exam is determined by the overall
subjective rating of total body deficit.

No deficit	score = 0 points
Mild deficit	score = 1 point
Moderate deficit	score = 2 points
Severe deficit	score = 3 points

Score for Worksheet 4 = ☐
Record in Box D

Worksheet 5 — PG-SGA Global Assessment Categories

	Stage A	Stage B	Stage C
Category	Well-nourished	Moderately malnourished or suspected malnutrition	Severely malnourished
Weight	No wt loss **OR** Recent non-fluid wt gain	~5% wt loss within 1 month (or 10% in 6 months) **OR** No wt stabilization or wt gain (i.e., continued wt loss)	> 5% wt loss in 1 month (or >10% in 6 months) **OR** No wt stabilization or wt gain (i.e., continued wt loss)
Nutrient Intake	No deficit **OR** Significant recent improvement	Definite decrease in intake	Severe deficit in intake
Nutrition Impact Symptoms	None **OR** Significant recent improvement allowing adequate intake	Presence of nutrition impact symptoms (Box 3 of PG-SGA)	Presence of nutrition impact symptoms (Box 3 of PG-SGA)
Functioning	No deficit **OR** Significant recent improvement	Moderate functional deficit **OR** Recent deterioration	Severe functional deficit **OR** recent significant deterioration
Physical Exam	No deficit **OR** Chronic deficit but with recent clinical improvement	Evidence of mild to moderate loss of SQ fat &/or muscle mass &/or muscle tone on palpation	Obvious signs of malnutrition (e.g., severe loss of SQ tissues, possible edema)

Global PG-SGA rating (A, B, or C) = ☐

Figure 47-5 ■ *continued*

Guide to Nutrition in Chronic Disease Management for Older Adults contains information for primary care providers and handouts for clients and is also available online.

Nursing History

As mentioned earlier, nurses obtain considerable nutrition-related data in the routine admission nursing history. Data include but are not limited to the following:

- Age, sex, and activity level
- Difficulty eating (e.g., impaired chewing or swallowing)
- Condition of the mouth, teeth, and presence of dentures
- Changes in appetite
- Changes in weight
- Physical disabilities that affect purchasing, preparing, and eating food
- Cultural and religious beliefs that affect food choices
- Living arrangements (e.g., living alone) and economic status

- General health status and medical condition
- Medication history

Physical Examination

Physical examination reveals some nutritional deficiencies and excesses in addition to obvious weight changes. Assessment focuses on rapidly proliferating tissues such as skin, hair, nails, eyes, and mucosa but also includes a systematic review comparable to any routine physical examination. See Clinical Manifestations and Figure 47-6 ■ for signs associated with malnutrition. These signs must be viewed as suggestive of malnutrition because the signs are nonspecific. For example, red conjunctiva may indicate an infection rather than a nutritional deficit, and dry, dull hair may be related to excessive exposure to the sun rather than severe protein-energy malnutrition. To confirm malnutrition, clinical findings need to be substantiated with laboratory tests and dietary data.

A

B

C

D

Figure 47-6 ■ Examples of nutritional deficiencies. *A,* Dull, sparse hair from protein deficiency. *B,* Inflammation of the corners of the mouth from riboflavin deficiency. *C,* Inflammation of the tongue from niacin, B₆ or riboflavin deficiency. *D,* Spongy bleeding gums from vitamin C deficiency.

(*A* and *B* from Centers for Disease Control and Prevention (CDC), *C* from Custom Medical Stock Photo, Inc., *D* from Pearson Education/PH College)

CLINICAL MANIFESTATIONS **MALNUTRITION**

Area of Examination (possible cause)	Signs Associated with Malnutrition
General appearance and vitality	Apathetic, listless, looks tired, easily fatigued
Weight	Overweight or underweight
Skin	Dry, flaky, or scaly; pale or pigmented; presence of petechiae or bruises; lack of subcutaneous fat; edema
Nails	Brittle, pale, ridged, or spoon shaped (iron)
Hair	Dry, dull, sparse, loss of color, brittle (see Figure 47-6, A)
Eyes	Pale or red conjunctiva, dryness, soft cornea, dull cornea, night blindness (vitamin A deficiency)
Lips	Swollen, red cracks at side of mouth, vertical fissures (B vitamins) (see Figure 47-6, B)
Tongue	Swollen, beefy red or magenta colored (B vitamins); smooth appearance (B vitamins deficiency); decrease or increase in size (see Figure 47-6, C)
Gums	Spongy, swollen, inflamed; bleed easily (vitamin C deficiency) (see Figure 47-6, D)
Muscles	Underdeveloped, flaccid, wasted, soft
Gastrointestinal system	Anorexia, indigestion, diarrhea, constipation, enlarged liver, protruding abdomen
Nervous system	Decreased reflexes, sensory loss, burning and tingling of hands and feet (B vitamins), mental confusion or irritability

Calculating Percentage of Weight Loss

Accurate assessment of the client's height, current body weight (CBW), and usual body weight (UBW) is essential. Although the client's CBW can be compared with an ideal body weight discussed earlier, the IBW is based on healthy people and does not account for changes in the client's body composition that ac-

company illness or reflect any changes in weight. The client's UBW better indicates weight change and the possibility of malnutrition. Calculation and interpretation of the percent of deviation from UBW and the percent of weight loss are shown in Box 47-8. An important aspect of weight assessment, obtained in the nursing history, is a description of weight change. The nurse should describe any weight loss or gain, the duration of the change, and whether the weight change was intentional or unintentional.

Dietary History

A dietary history includes data about the client's usual eating patterns and habits; food preferences, allergies, and intolerances; frequency, types, and quantities of foods consumed; and social, economic, ethnic, or religious factors influencing nutrition. Factors may include, but are not limited to, living and eating companions, ability to purchase and prepare food, availability of refrigeration and cooking facilities, income, and effect of religion and ethnicity on food choices.

Four possible methods for collecting dietary data are a 24-hour food recall, a food frequency record, a food diary, and a diet history.

For a **24-hour food recall,** the nurse asks the client to recall all the food and beverages the client consumes during a typical 24-hour period when at home. The data obtained are then generally evaluated according to the Food Guide Pyramid to judge overall adequacy.

A **food frequency record** is a checklist that indicates how often general food groups or specific foods are eaten. Frequency may be categorized as times/day, times/week, times/month, or frequently, seldom, never. This record, like the 24-hour food recall, provides information about the types of foods eaten but not the quantities. When specific foods or nutrients are suspected of being deficient or excessive, the health care professional may use a selective food frequency that focuses, for example, on fat, fruit, vegetable, and fiber intake.

A **food diary** is a detailed record of measured amounts (portion sizes) of all food and fluids a client consumes during a specified period, usually 3 to 7 days.

A **diet history** is a comprehensive time-consuming assessment of a client's food intake that involves an extensive interview by a nutritionist or dietitian. It includes characteristics of foods usually eaten as well as the frequency and amount of food consumed. Thus, it may include a 24-hour recall, a food frequency record, and a food diary. Medical and psychosocial

---

BOX 47-8 **Calculating and Interpreting the Percent of Deviation from Usual Body Weight and the Percent of Weight Loss**

Calculating Percent of Usual Body Weight		Calculating Percent of Weight Loss	
% usual body weight = $\dfrac{\text{Current weight}}{\text{Usual body weight}} \times 100$		% weight loss = $\dfrac{\text{Usual weight} - \text{current weight}}{\text{Usual weight}} \times 100$	
Mild malnutrition	85–90%	**Significant Weight Loss**	**Severe Weight Loss**
Moderate malnutrition	75–84%	5% over 1 mo	> 5% over 1 mo
Severe malnutrition	Less than 74%	7.5% over 3 mo	> 7.5% over 3 mo
		10% over 6 mo	> 10% over 6 mo

factors are also assessed to evaluate their impact on nutritional requirements, food habits, and choices. Data obtained are analyzed by computer and translated into caloric and nutrient intake. Results are compared with the DRIs that are appropriate for the client's age, sex, and condition.

Anthropometric Measurements

Anthropometric measurements are noninvasive techniques that aim to quantify body composition. A **skinfold measurement** is performed to determine fat stores. The most common site for measurement is the triceps skinfold (TSF). The fold of skin measured includes subcutaneous tissue but not the underlying muscle. It is measured in millimeters using special calipers. To measure the TSF, locate the midpoint of the upper arm (halfway between the acromion process and the olecranon process), then grasp the skin on the back of the upper arm along the long axis of the humerus (Figure 47-7 ■). Placing the calipers 1 cm (0.4 in.) below the nurse's fingers, measure the thickness of the fold to the nearest millimeter.

The **mid-arm circumference (MAC)** is a measure of fat, muscle, and skeleton. To measure the MAC, ask the client to sit or stand with the arm hanging freely and the forearm flexed to horizontal. Measure the circumference at the midpoint of the arm, recording the measurement in centimeters, to the nearest millimeter (e.g., 24.6 cm) (Figure 47-8 ■).

The **mid-arm muscle circumference (MAMC)** is then calculated by using reference tables or by using a formula that incorporates the TSF and the MAC. The MAMC is an estimate of lean body mass, or skeletal muscle reserves. If tables are not available, the nurse uses the following formula to calculate the MAMC from the triceps skinfold and MAC direct measurements:

$$\text{MAMC cm} = \frac{\text{MAC (cm)} - 3.143\ \text{TSF (mm)}}{10}$$

Standard values for anthropometric measurements for adults are shown in Table 47–4.

Changes in anthropometric measurements often occur slowly and reflect chronic rather than acute changes in nutritional status. They are, therefore, used to monitor the client's

Figure 47-8 ■ Measuring the mid-arm circumference.
(Patrick Watson)

progress for months to years rather than days to weeks. Ideally, initial and subsequent measurements need to be taken by the same clinician. In addition, measurements obtained need to be interpreted with caution. Fluctuations in hydration status that often occur during illness can influence the accuracy of results. In addition, normal standards often do not account for normal changes in body composition such as those that occur with aging.

Laboratory Data

Laboratory tests provide objective data to the nutritional assessment, but because many factors can influence these tests, no single test specifically predicts nutritional risk or measures the presence or degree of a nutritional problem. The tests most commonly used are serum proteins, urinary urea nitrogen and creatinine, and total lymphocyte count.

SERUM PROTEINS. Serum protein levels provide an estimate of visceral protein stores. Tests commonly include hemoglobin, albumin, transferrin, and total iron-binding capacity. A low hemoglobin level may be evidence of iron deficiency anemia. However, abnormal blood loss or a pathologic process such as gastrointestinal cancer must be ruled out before iron deficiency related to diet is confirmed.

Albumin, which accounts for more than 50% of the total serum proteins, is one of the most common visceral proteins evaluated as part of the nutritional assessment. Because there is so much albumin in the body and because it is not broken down very quickly (i.e., it has a long half-life of 18–20 days), albumin

TABLE 47–4 Standard Values for Anthropometric Measurements for Adults

MEASUREMENT	MALE	FEMALE
Triceps skinfold (mm)	12	20
Mid-arm circumference (cm)	32	28
Mid-arm muscle circumference (cm²)	54	30

Note: From *The Merck Manual of Diagnosis and Therapy*, 18th ed., M. H. Beers and R. Berkow (Eds.), 2006. Copyright John Wiley & Sons. Reprinted with permission.

Figure 47-7 ■ Measuring the triceps skinfold.

concentrations change slowly. Thus, a low serum albumin level is a useful indicator of prolonged protein depletion rather than acute or short-term changes in nutritional status. However, many conditions besides malnutrition can depress albumin concentration, such as altered liver function, hydration status, and losses from open wounds and burns.

Transferrin is a protein that binds and carries iron from the intestine through the serum. Because it has a shorter half-life than albumin (8–9 days), transferrin is likely to respond more quickly to protein depletion than albumin. Serum transferrin can be measured directly or by a total iron-binding capacity (TIBC) test, which indicates the amount of iron in the blood to which transferrin can bind. Transferrin levels below normal indicate protein loss, iron deficiency anemia, pregnancy, hepatitis, or liver dysfunction. An increase in TIBC can indicate iron deficiency; a decrease, anemia.

Prealbumin, also referred to as thyroxine-binding albumin and transthyretin, has the shortest half-life and smallest body pool, and is, therefore, the most responsive serum protein to rapid changes in nutritional status. It is now considered the "gold standard" for assessing for possible protein malnutrition (Kuszajewski & Clontz, 2005). It should be measured twice a week: prealbumin levels of 15 to 35 mg/dL are normal, below 15 indicates clients at risk, and below 11 indicates that aggressive nutritional intervention is needed.

URINARY TESTS. Urinary urea nitrogen and urinary creatinine are measures of protein catabolism and the state of nitrogen balance. **Urea,** the chief end product of amino acid metabolism, is formed from ammonia detoxified by the liver, circulated in the blood, and transported to the kidneys for excretion in urine. Urea concentrations in the blood and urine, therefore, directly reflect the intake and breakdown of dietary protein, the rate of urea production in the liver, and the rate of urea removal by the kidneys.

The state of nitrogen balance is determined by comparing the nitrogen intake (grams of protein) to the nitrogen output over a 24-hour period. A positive nitrogen balance exists when intake exceeds nitrogen output; a negative nitrogen balance occurs when output exceeds nitrogen intake. Protein intake must be accurately recorded and kidney function must be normal to ensure the validity of a urinary urea nitrogen test.

Urinary creatinine reflects a person's total muscle mass because creatinine is the chief end product of the creatine produced when energy is released during skeletal muscle metabolism. The rate of creatinine formation is directly proportional to the total muscle mass. Creatinine is removed from the bloodstream by the kidneys and excreted in the urine at a rate that closely parallels its formation. The greater the muscle mass, the greater the excretion of creatinine. As skeletal muscle atrophies during malnutrition, creatinine excretion decreases. Standards for creatinine excretion are developed based on gender and height. Urinary creatinine is also influenced by protein intake, exercise, age, renal function, and thyroid function.

TOTAL LYMPHOCYTE COUNT. Certain nutrient deficiencies and forms of PCM can depress the immune system. The total number of lymphocytes decreases as protein depletion occurs.

Diagnosing

NANDA (2007) includes the following diagnostic labels for nutritional problems:

- *Imbalanced Nutrition: More Than Body Requirements*
- *Imbalanced Nutrition: Less Than Body Requirements*
- *Readiness for Enhanced Nutrition*
- *Risk for Imbalanced Nutrition: More Than Body Requirements*

Clinical examples of assessment data clusters and related nursing diagnoses are shown in Identifying Nursing Diagnoses, Outcomes, and Interventions.

Many other NANDA nursing diagnoses may apply to certain individuals, because nutritional problems often affect other areas of human functioning. In this case, the nutritional diagnostic label may be used as the etiology of other diagnoses. Examples include

- *Activity Intolerance* related to inadequate intake of iron-rich foods resulting in iron-deficiency anemia.
- *Constipation* related to inadequate fluid intake and fiber intake.
- *Low Self-Esteem* related to obesity.
- *Risk for Infection* related to immunosuppression secondary to insufficient protein intake.

Planning

Major goals for clients with or at risk for nutritional problems include

- Maintain or restore optimal nutritional status.
- Promote healthy nutritional practices.
- Prevent complications associated with malnutrition.
- Decrease weight.
- Regain specified weight.

Examples of NOC outcomes and NIC interventions related to some of these goals are shown in Identifying Nursing Diagnoses, Outcomes, and Interventions. Specific nursing activities associated with each of these interventions can be selected to meet the individual needs of the client. See the Nursing Care Plan and Concept Map at the end of this chapter.

Planning for Home Care

To provide for continuity of care, the nurse must consider the client's need for assistance with nutrition. Some clients will need help with eating, purchasing food, and preparing meals; others will need instructions about enteral and parenteral nutrition therapy.

Home care planning incorporates an assessment of the client and family's abilities for self-care, financial resources, and the need for referrals and home health services. The Home Care Assessment box outlines a home care assessment about nutritional problems and needs. A major aspect of discharge planning involves instructional needs of the client and family (see Home Care Assessment and Client Teaching).

Implementing

Nursing interventions to promote optimal nutrition for hospitalized clients are often provided in collaboration with the primary

IDENTIFYING NURSING DIAGNOSES, OUTCOMES, AND INTERVENTIONS
Clients with Nutritional Disorders

DATA CLUSTER Mark Malakoff, 71 years old, has chronic obstructive lung disease. His wife died 2 years ago. He says, "I'm not interested in food. Even if I were, I don't have the energy to cook. It's too much bother to fix meals for just me." He is 5' 10" (178 cm) tall and weighs 135 lb (61.2 kg). His TSF is 9.2 mm; MAMC is 20.4 mm; UBW is 155 lb (70.5 kg). Dietary assessment indicates that he eats mostly bread, cereal, whole milk, and canned fish and meats. He eats almost no fruits and vegetables.

NURSING DIAGNOSIS/ DEFINITION	SAMPLE DESIRED OUTCOMES*/ DEFINITION	INDICATORS	SELECTED INTERVENTIONS*/ DEFINITION	SAMPLE NIC ACTIVITIES
Imbalanced Nutrition: Less Than Body Requirements/Intake of nutrients insufficient to meet metabolic needs	Nutritional Status: Nutrient Intake [1009]/*Adequacy of usual pattern of nutrient intake*	Substantially adequate ▪ Caloric intake ▪ Vitamin intake	Nutrition Therapy [1120]/*Administration of food and fluids to support metabolic processes of a client who is malnourished or at high risk of becoming malnourished*	▪ Determine food preferences with consideration of cultural and religious preferences ▪ Determine—in collaboration with the dietitian—the number of calories and type of nutrients needed ▪ Provide needed nourishment within limits of prescribed diet ▪ Structure the environment to create a pleasant and relaxing atmosphere ▪ Arrange for appropriate referrals to community resources that provide meals

DATA CLUSTER Rose Rosenthal, a 27-year-old taxi dispatcher, says that her parents, who are both pastry cooks, are "fat." "I love Dad's doughnuts and often bring some to work to munch on through the day. I hate exercise, but at this rate, I'm going to have to do something, or I'll end up looking like Mum and Dad." Height, 5' 1" (155 cm); weight 130 lb (58.5 kg).

Risk for Imbalanced Nutrition: More Than Body Requirements/At risk for an intake of nutrients that exceeds metabolic needs	Weight: Body Mass [1006]/*Extent to which body weight, muscle, and fat are congruent to height, frame, gender, and age*	Mild deviation from expected range ▪ Weight ▪ Waist/hip circumference ratio	Nutritional Monitoring [1160]/*Collection and analysis of patient data to prevent or minimize malnourishment*	▪ Weigh client at specified intervals ▪ Monitor type and amount of usual exercise ▪ Monitor environment where eating occurs ▪ Determine if client requires nutrition education

*The NOC # for desired outcomes and the NIC # for nursing interventions are listed in brackets following the appropriate outcome or intervention. Outcomes, indicators, interventions, and activities selected are only a sample of those suggested by NOC and NIC and should be further individualized for each client.

care provider who writes the diet orders and the dietitian who informs clients about special diets. The nurse reinforces this instruction and, in addition, creates an atmosphere that encourages eating, provides assistance with eating, monitors the client's appetite and food intake, administers enteral and parenteral feedings, and consults with the primary care provider and dietitian about nutritional problems that arise.

In the community setting, the nurse's role is largely educational. For example, nurses promote optimal nutrition at health fairs, in schools, at prenatal classes, and with well or ill clients and support people in their homes. In the home setting, nurses also initiate nutritional screens, refer clients at risk to appropriate resources, instruct clients about enteral and parenteral feedings, and offer nutrition counseling as needed. Nutrition counseling involves more than simply providing information. The nurse must help clients integrate diet changes into their lifestyle and provide strategies to motivate them to change their eating habits.

Assisting with Special Diets

Alterations in the client's diet are often needed to treat a disease process such as diabetes mellitus, to prepare for a special examination or surgery, to increase or decrease weight, to restore nutritional deficits, or to allow an organ to rest and promote healing. Diets are modified in one or more of the following aspects: texture, kilocalories, specific nutrients, seasonings, or consistency.

Hospitalized clients who do not have special needs eat the regular (standard or house) diet, a balanced diet that supplies the metabolic requirements of a sedentary person (about 2,000 Kcal). Most agencies offer clients a daily menu from which to select their meals for the next day; others provide standard meals to each client on the general diet. Certain foods (e.g., cabbage, which tends to produce flatus, and highly seasoned and fried foods, which are difficult for some people to digest) are usually omitted from the regular diet.

CLIENT/ENVIRONMENT

■ Self-care abilities: Assess ability to feed self, to purchase food, and to prepare meals.

■ Adaptive feeding aids required: Determine need for special drinking cups, plates, or feeding utensils.

■ Instructional needs: Consider nutritional requirements (e.g., Food Guide Pyramid, dietary guidelines, special diet), adaptive aids available, recommended lifestyle variations, and management of enteral/parenteral nutrition.

■ Physical environment: Assess adequacy of water, electricity, refrigeration, and telephone facilities; and presence of clean, secure area to store and set up enteral/parenteral equipment as needed.

FAMILY

■ Caregiver availability, skills, and willingness: Primary and secondary persons able to assist with food purchase, meal preparation, and feeding and able to comprehend and administer special diets or enteral/parenteral nutrition required.

■ Family role changes and coping: Effect on parenting and spousal roles, financial resources, and social roles.

■ Alternate potential primary or respite caregivers: For example, other family members, volunteers, church members, paid caregivers, or housekeeping services; available community respite care (adult day care, senior centers) and so on.

COMMUNITY

■ Current knowledge, use, and experience with community resources: Nutritional counseling services; home health agencies for enteral/parenteral nutrition support; dietitian or nutritionist for planning appropriate meals for prescribed diet, ways to include ethnic food preferences into the diet, and providing written meal plans; medical equipment and supply companies; financial assistance services; and support and educational services such as

● Weight management programs (e.g., Weight Watchers).

● National Center for Nutrition and Dietetics for information on all nutrition topics.

● National Eating Disorder Information Center.

● Meals on Wheels.

■ Instruct clients about the content of a healthy diet based on the Food Guide Pyramid and *Dietary Guidelines for Americans.*

■ Encourage clients, particularly older clients, to reduce dietary fat (see Client Teaching on reducing dietary fat, page 1246).

■ Instruct strict vegetarians about proper protein complementation and additional vitamin and mineral supplementation.

■ Discuss foods high in specific nutrients required such as protein, iron, calcium, vitamin C, and fiber.

■ Discuss importance of properly fitted dentures and dental care.

■ Discuss safe food preparation and preservation techniques as appropriate.

DIETARY ALTERATIONS

■ Explain the purpose of the diet.

■ Discuss allowed and excluded foods.

■ Explain the importance of reading food labels when selecting packaged foods.

■ Include family or significant others.

■ Reinforce information provided by the dietitian or nutritionist as appropriate.

■ Discuss herbs and spices as alternatives to salt and substitutes for sugar.

FOR OVERWEIGHT CLIENTS

■ Discuss physiologic, psychologic, and lifestyle factors that predispose to weight gain.

■ Provide information about desired weight range and recommended calorie intake.

■ Discuss principles of a well-balanced diet and high- and low-calorie foods.

■ Encourage intake of low-calorie, caffeine-free beverages and plenty of water.

■ Discuss ways to adapt eating practices by using smaller plates, taking smaller servings, chewing each bite a specified number of times, and putting fork down between bites.

■ Discuss ways to control the desire to eat by taking a walk, drinking a glass of water, or doing slow deep-breathing exercises.

■ Discuss the importance of exercise and help the client plan an exercise program.

■ Discuss stress reduction techniques.

■ Provide information about available community resources (e.g., weight-loss groups, dietary counseling, exercise programs, self-help groups).

FOR UNDERWEIGHT CLIENTS

■ Discuss factors contributing to inadequate nutrition and weight loss.

■ Discuss recommended calorie intake and desired weight range.

■ Provide information about the content of a balanced diet.

■ Provide information about ways to increase calorie intake (e.g., high-protein or high-calorie foods and supplements).

■ Discuss ways to manage, minimize, or alter the factors contributing to malnourishment.

■ If appropriate, discuss ways to purchase low-cost nutritious foods.

■ Provide information about community agencies that can assist in providing food (e.g., Meals on Wheels).

PREVENTING FOODBORNE ILLNESS

■ Reinforce hygienic handling of food and dishes.

● Wash hands before preparing foods.

● Wash hands and all dishes and utensils with hot water and soap after contact with raw meats.

● Defrost frozen foods in the refrigerator.

● Cook beef, poultry, and eggs thoroughly. Use a cooking thermometer.

● Refrigerate leftovers promptly (at 40°F [5°C] or less) and keep no more than 3 to 5 days.

● Wash or peel raw fruits and vegetables.

● Do not use foods from containers that have been damaged or have opened seals.

● Follow the rules "keep hot foods hot and cold foods cold" and "when in doubt, throw it out."

■ Recommend the client consider a preventive vaccination for hepatitis A.

■ Instruct clients to seek medical attention for prolonged vomiting, fever, abdominal pain, or severe diarrhea following a meal.

A variation of the regular diet is the light diet, designed for postoperative and other clients who are not ready for the regular diet. Foods in the light diet are plainly cooked and fat is usually minimized, as are bran and foods containing a great deal of fiber.

Diets that are modified in consistency are often given to clients before and after surgery or to promote healing in clients with gastrointestinal distress. These diets include clear liquid, full liquid, soft, and diet as tolerated. In some agencies, gastrointestinal surgery clients are not permitted red-colored liquids or candy since, if vomited, the color may be confused with blood.

CLEAR LIQUID DIET. This diet is limited to water, tea, coffee, clear broths, ginger ale, or other carbonated beverages, strained and clear juices, and plain gelatin. Note that "clear" does not necessarily mean "colorless." This diet provides the client with fluid and carbohydrate (in the form of sugar) but does not supply adequate protein, fat, vitamins, minerals, or calories. It is a short-term diet (24–36 hours) provided for clients after certain surgeries or in the acute stages of infection, particularly of the gastrointestinal tract. The major objectives of this diet are to relieve thirst, prevent dehydration, and minimize stimulation of the gastrointestinal tract. Examples of foods allowed in clear liquid diets are shown in Box 47–9.

FULL LIQUID DIET. This diet contains only liquids or foods that turn to liquid at body temperature, such as ice cream (see Box 47–9). Full liquid diets are often eaten by clients who have gastrointestinal disturbances or are otherwise unable to tolerate solid or semisolid foods. This diet is not recommended for long-term use because it is low in iron, protein, and calories. In addition, its cholesterol content is high because of the amount of milk offered. Clients who must receive only liquids for long periods are usually given a nutritionally balanced oral supplement, such as Ensure or Sustacal. The full liquid diet is monotonous and difficult for clients to accept. Planning six or more feedings per day may encourage a more adequate intake.

SOFT DIET. The soft diet is easily chewed and digested. It is often ordered for clients who have difficulty chewing and

swallowing. It is a low-residue (low-fiber) diet containing very few uncooked foods; however, restrictions vary among agencies and according to individual tolerance. Examples of foods that can be included in a soft or semisoft diet are shown in Box 47–9. The **pureed diet** is a modification of the soft diet. Liquid may be added to the food, which is then blended to a semisolid consistency.

DIET AS TOLERATED. Diet as tolerated is ordered when the client's appetite, ability to eat, and tolerance for certain foods may change. For example, on the first postoperative day a client may be given a clear liquid diet. If no nausea occurs, normal intestinal motility has returned as evidenced by active bowel sounds and client reports passing gas, and the client feels like eating, the diet may be advanced to a full liquid, light, or regular diet.

MODIFICATION FOR DISEASE. Many special diets may be prescribed to meet requirements for disease process or altered metabolism. For example, a client with diabetes mellitus may need a diet recommended by the American Diabetes Association, an obese client may need a calorie restricted diet, a cardiac client may need sodium and cholesterol restrictions, and a client with allergies will need a hypoallergenic diet.

Some clients must follow certain diets (e.g., the diabetic diet) for a lifetime. If the diet is long term, the client must understand the diet and also develop a healthy, positive attitude toward it. Assisting clients and support persons with special diets is a function shared by the dietitian or nutritionist and the nurse. The dietitian informs the client and support persons about the specific foods allowed and not allowed and assists the client with meal planning. The nurse reinforces this instruction, assists the client to make changes, and evaluates the client's responses.

DYSPHAGIA. Some clients may have no difficulty with choosing a healthy diet, but be at risk for nutritional problems due to dysphagia. These clients may have inadequate solid or fluid intake, be unable to swallow their medications, or aspirate food or fluids into the lungs—causing pneumonia. Clients at risk for dysphagia in-

BOX 47–9 Examples of Foods for Clear Liquid, Full Liquid, and Soft Diets

Clear Liquid	*Full Liquid*	*Soft*
Coffee, regular and decaffeinated	All foods on clear liquid diet plus:	All foods on full and clear liquid diets, plus:
Tea	Milk and milk drinks	Meat: All lean, tender meat, fish, or poultry (chopped, shredded); spaghetti sauce with ground meat over pasta
Carbonated beverages	Puddings, custards	Meat alternatives: Scrambled eggs, omelet, poached eggs; cottage cheese and other mild cheese
Bouillon, fat-free broth	Ice cream, sherbet	Vegetables: Mashed potatoes, sweet potatoes, or squash; vegetables in cream or cheese sauce; other cooked vegetables as tolerated (e.g., spinach, cauliflower, asparagus tips), chopped and mashed as needed; avocado
Clear fruit juices (apple, cranberry, grape)	Vegetable juices	
Other fruit juices, strained	Refined or strained cereals (e.g., cream of rice)	Fruits: Cooked or canned fruits; bananas, grapefruit and orange sections without membranes, applesauce
Popsicles	Cream, butter, margarine	Breads and cereals: Enriched rice, barley, pasta; all breads; cooked cereals (e.g., oatmeal)
Gelatin	Eggs (in custard and pudding)	
Sugar, honey	Smooth peanut butter	Desserts: Soft cake, bread pudding
Hard candy	Yogurt	

clude elders, those who have experienced a stroke, cancer patients who have had radiation therapy to the head and neck, and others with cranial nerve dysfunction. Nurses may be the first persons to detect dysphagia and are in an excellent position to recommend further evaluation; implement specialized feeding techniques and diets; and work with clients, family members, and other health care professionals to develop a plan to assist the client with difficulties. If the client condition suggests dysphagia, the nurse should review the history in detail; interview the client or family; assess the mouth, throat, and chest; and observe the client swallowing. Presence of the gag reflex, often thought to indicate that the client can swallow safely, has not been shown to be a reliable indicator (Zagaria, 2005). Confirmation of the tendency for food to divert to the trachea is best done through x-ray.

A multidisciplinary group has developed the National Dysphagia Diet (NDD), which delineates standards of food textures (American Dietetic Association, 2003). The four levels of liquid foods are thin, nectar-like, honey-like, and spoon-thick liquids. The four levels of semisolid/solid foods are pureed, mechanically altered, advanced/mechanically soft, and regular/general. In consultation with the dietitian, occupational therapist, swallowing specialist, speech-language pathologist, and/or primary care provider, these levels can be used to determine a consistent approach to a particular client's dysphagia. For example, a mechanically soft diet may result in lower pneumonia rates than a pureed diet in stroke patients with a history of aspiration pneumonia. Early detection and intervention can prevent the adverse outcomes of dysphagia in most clients.

All dietary instructions must be individually designed to meet the client's intellectual ability, motivation level, lifestyle, culture, and economic status. Both nutritionists and dietitians help to adapt a diet to suit the client. Simple verbal instructions need to be given and reinforced with written material. Family and support persons must be included in the dietary instruction.

Stimulating the Appetite

Physical illness, unfamiliar or unpalatable food, environmental and psychologic factors, and physical discomfort or pain may depress the appetites of many clients. A short-term decrease in food intake usually is not a problem for adults; over time, however, it leads to weight loss, decreased strength and stamina, and other nutritional problems. A decreased food intake is often accompanied by a decrease in fluid intake, which may cause fluid and electrolyte problems. Stimulating a person's appetite requires the nurse to determine the reason for the lack of appetite and then deal with the problem. Some general interventions for improving the client's appetite are summarized in Box 47–10.

Assisting Clients with Meals

Because clients in health care agencies are frequently confined to their beds, meals are brought to the client. The client receives a tray that has been assembled in a central kitchen. Nursing personnel may be responsible for giving out and collecting the trays; however, in most settings this is done by dietary personnel. Long-term care facilities and some hospitals serve meals to mobile clients in a special dining area. Guidelines for providing meals to clients are summarized in Box 47–11.

BOX 47–10 **Improving Appetite**

- Provide familiar food that the person likes. Often the relatives of clients are pleased to bring food from home but may need some guidance about special diet requirements.
- Select small portions so as not to discourage the anorexic client.
- Avoid unpleasant or uncomfortable treatments immediately before or after a meal.
- Provide a tidy, clean environment that is free of unpleasant sights and odors. A soiled dressing, a used bedpan, an uncovered irrigation set, or even used dishes can negatively affect the appetite.
- Encourage or provide oral hygiene before mealtime. This improves the client's ability to taste.
- Relieve illness symptoms that depress appetite before mealtime; for example, give an analgesic for pain or an antipyretic for a fever or allow rest for fatigue.
- Reduce psychologic stress. A lack of understanding of therapy, the anticipation of an operation, and fear of the unknown can cause anorexia. Often, the nurse can help by discussing feelings with the client, giving information and assistance, and allaying fears.

Two groups of people frequently require help with their meals: elders who are weakened; and persons with disabilities, such as blind clients, those who must remain in a back-lying position, or those who cannot use their hands. The client's nursing care plan will indicate that assistance is required with meals.

The nurse must be sensitive to clients' feelings of embarrassment, resentment, and loss of autonomy. Whenever possible, the nurse should help incapacitated clients feed themselves rather than feed them. Some clients become depressed because they require help and because they believe they are burdensome to busy nursing personnel. Although feeding a client is time consuming, nurses should try to appear unhurried and convey that they have ample time. Sitting at the bedside is one way to convey this impression. If the client is to be fed by unlicensed assistive personnel, the nurse must ensure that the same standards are met.

When feeding a client, ask in which order the client would like to eat the food. If the client cannot see, tell the client which food is being given. Always allow ample time for the client to chew and swallow the food before offering more. Also, provide fluids as requested, or, if the client is unable to communicate, offer fluids after every three or four mouthfuls of solid food. It is important to make the time a pleasant one, choosing topics of conversation that are of interest to clients who want to talk.

Although normal utensils should be used whenever possible, special utensils may be needed to assist a client to eat. For clients who have difficulty drinking from a cup or glass, a straw often permits them to obtain liquids with less effort and less spillage. Special drinking cups are also available. One model has a spout; another is specially designed to permit drinking with less tipping of the cup than is normally required.

Many adaptive feeding aids are available to help clients maintain independence. A standard eating utensil with a built-up or widened handle helps clients who cannot grasp objects easily. Utensils with wide handles can be purchased, or a regular eating utensil can be modified by taping foam around the

MediaLink Client Experiencing Loss of Appetite Care Plan Activity

BOX 47–11 Providing Client Meals

- Offer the client assistance with hand washing and oral hygiene before a meal.
- If it is permitted, assist the client to a comfortable position in bed or in a chair, whichever is appropriate.
- Clear the overbed table so that there is space for the tray. If the client must remain in a lying position in bed, arrange the overbed table close to the bedside so that the client can see and reach the food.
- Check each tray for the client's name, the type of diet, and completeness. Do not leave an incorrect diet for a client to eat.
- Assist the client as required (e.g., remove the food covers, butter the bread, pour the tea, and cut the meat).
- For a blind person, identify the placement of the food as you would describe the time on a clock (Figure 47-9 ■). For instance, the nurse might say, "The potatoes are at eight o'clock, the chicken at 12 o'clock, and the green beans at 4 o'clock."
- After the client has completed the meal, observe how much and what the client has eaten and the amount of fluid taken. Use a standard tool to estimate the amount eaten in relation to a typical meal. For example, if served a donut and hot chocolate for breakfast, although the client may have eaten all of these, they certainly do not represent 100% of a nutritious breakfast.
- If the client is on a special diet or is having problems eating, record the amount of food eaten and any pain, fatigue, or nausea experienced.
- If the client is not eating, document this so that changes can be made, such as rescheduling the meals, providing smaller, more frequent meals, or obtaining special self-feeding aids.

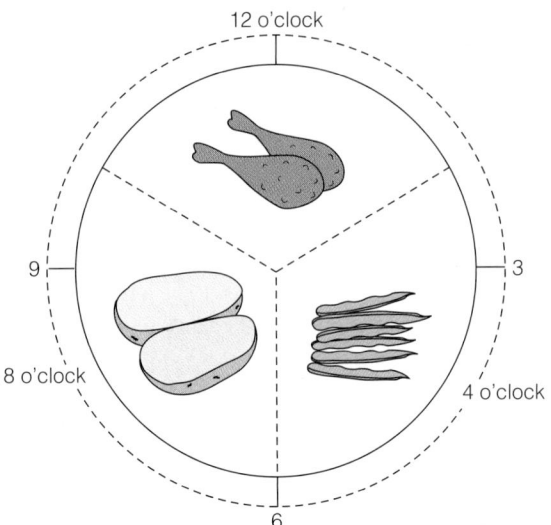

Figure 47-9 ■ For a client who is blind, the nurse can use the clock system to describe the location of food on the plate.

handle. The foam increases friction and thus steadies the client's grasp. Handles may be bent or angled to compensate for limited motion. Collars or bands that prevent the utensil from being dropped can be attached to the end of the handle and fit over the client's hand. Clients requiring pureed or liquid diets are sometimes fed with a feeding syringe.

Plates with rims and plastic or metal plate guards enable the client to pick up the food by first pushing it against this raised edge. A suction cup or damp sponge or cloth may be placed under the dish to keep it from moving while the client is eating.

No-spill mugs and two-handled drinking cups are especially useful for persons with impaired hand coordination. Stretch terry cloth and knitted or crocheted glass covers enable the client to keep a secure grasp on a glass. Lidded tip-proof glasses are also available. Figures 47-10 ■ and 47-11 ■ show some of these aids.

Special Community Nutritional Services

In many places, community programs have been developed to help special groups meet nutritional needs. For elders who can-

---

RESEARCH NOTE   Do the Beliefs of Nursing Assistants Influence the Way They Feed Nursing Home Residents?

Since almost half of nursing home residents require some assistance with eating, the role of the certified nursing assistant (CNA), who performs the majority of the feeding of residents, is significant. The author proposed a conceptual framework incorporating the variables of CNA knowledge, experience, and values forming CNA beliefs with resident characteristics and institutional factors to accomplish resident feedings goals (nutrition, safety, and dignity). Twenty female CNAs from four nursing homes were interviewed and asked to sort statements related to feeding residents by how much they agreed or disagreed.

The research showed two distinct groups of CNAs: social feeders who believed socializing with the residents during feeding was as important as nutrition, and technical feeders who believed that feeding time was focused on ensuring that the resident ate adequately. Both groups valued the other but their beliefs strongly influenced their different techniques. Technical feeders tended to push eating on the res-

ident, whereas social feeders were more accepting if the resident did not wish to eat.

IMPLICATIONS

The study had a very small sample and included primarily very experienced CNAs. Thus, the findings may not be applicable to CNAs with different characteristics. Also, the study did not investigate the actual impact of the feeding type on the resident's nutritional status or possible adverse impact of the feeding (e.g., malnutrition or aspiration). However, it suggests that the belief system of the CNA has an important impact on the way they feed the residents. These are important implications for education, training, and support of CNAs in nursing homes.

Note: From "Feeding Beliefs of Certified Nurse Assistants in the Nursing Home: A Factor Influencing Practice," by C. A. Pelletier, 2005, *Journal of Gerontological Nursing, 31*(7), pp. 5–10.

Figure 47-10 ■ Left to right: glass holder, cup with hole for nose, two-handled cup holder.

not prepare meals or leave their homes, ready-to-eat meals or frozen dinners are delivered to the home by local organizations. Meals on Wheels is one such well-known organization. For people who can prepare meals but have physical disabilities and are unable to shop for groceries, there are grocery delivery services.

For the poor in the United States, the USDA funds a food stamp program. People with low incomes can use stamps to purchase food at any approved grocery store. The value of the food stamps provided depends on the size and income of the family.

Enteral Nutrition

An alternative feeding method to ensure adequate nutrition includes **enteral** (through the gastrointestinal system) methods. Enteral nutrition (EN), also referred to as total enteral nutrition (TEN), is provided when the client is unable to ingest foods or the upper gastrointestinal tract is impaired and the transport of food to the small intestine is interrupted. Enteral feedings are administered through nasogastric and small-bore feeding tubes, or through gastrostomy or jejunostomy tubes.

ENTERAL ACCESS DEVICES. Enteral access is achieved by means of nasogastric or nasointestinal (nasoenteric) tubes, or gastrostomy or jejunostomy tubes.

A **nasogastric tube** is inserted through one of the nostrils, down the nasopharynx, and into the alimentary tract. Traditional firm, large-bore nasogastric tubes (i.e., those larger than 12 Fr in diameter) are placed in the stomach. Examples are the Levin tube, a flexible rubber or plastic, single-lumen tube with holes near the tip, and the Salem sump tube, with a double lumen (Figure 47-12 ■). The larger lumen of the Salem sump tube allows delivery of liquids to the stomach or removal of gastric contents. When the Salem tube is used for suction of gastric contents, the smaller vent lumen (the proximal port is often referred to as the *blue pigtail*) allows for an inflow of atmospheric air, which prevents a vacuum if the gastric tube adheres to the wall of the stomach. Irritation of the gastric mucosa is thereby avoided. Softer, more flexible and less irritating small-bore tubes (smaller than 12 Fr in diameter) are frequently used (Figure 47-13 ■).

A

B

Figure 47-12 ■ *A,* Single-lumen Levin tube. *B,* Double-lumen Salem sump tube with filter on air vent port and connector on suction port.

Figure 47-11 ■ Dinner plate with guard attached and lipped plate facilitate scooping; wide-handled spoon and knife facilitate grip.

Figure 47-13 ■ Nasoenteric feeding tubes. *A,* 12 Fr 36 in.; *B,* 8 Fr opaque, 45 in., stylet, weighted tip. Note that both have a Y-port connector to permit irrigation and medication administration without disconnecting feeding device.
(Courtesy of Ross Products Division of Abbott Laboratories, Columbus, Ohio.)

Nasogastric tubes are used for feeding clients who have adequate gastric emptying, and who require short-term feedings. They are not advised for feeding clients without intact gag and cough reflexes since the risk of accidental placement of the tube into the lungs is much higher in those clients. These reflexes are present if a tongue depressor advanced to the back of the throat elicits retching or coughing responses. Skill 47-1 provides guidelines for inserting a nasogastric tube. Skill 47-2 outlines the steps for removing a nasogastric tube.

Although the focus of this chapter is nutrition, nasogastric tubes may be inserted for reasons other than to provide a route for feeding the client, including these:

■ To prevent nausea, vomiting, and gastric distention following surgery. In this case, the tube is attached to a suction source.
■ To remove stomach contents for laboratory analysis.

■ To lavage (wash) the stomach in cases of poisoning or overdose of medications.

A **nasoenteric (or nasointestinal) tube,** a longer tube than the nasogastric tube (at least 40 inches for an adult) is inserted through one nostril down into the upper small intestine. Some agencies may require specially trained nurses or primary care providers for this procedure. Nasoenteric tubes are used for clients who are at risk for aspiration. Clients at risk for aspiration are those who manifest the following:

■ Decreased level of consciousness
■ Poor cough or gag reflexes
■ Endotracheal intubation
■ Recent extubation
■ Inability to cooperate with the procedure
■ Restlessness or agitation

SKILL 47-1

INSERTING A NASOGASTRIC TUBE

PURPOSES
■ To administer tube feedings and medications to clients unable to eat by mouth or swallow a sufficient diet without aspirating food or fluids into the lungs

■ To establish a means for suctioning stomach contents to prevent gastric distention, nausea, and vomiting
■ To remove stomach contents for laboratory analysis
■ To lavage (wash) the stomach in case of poisoning or overdose of medications

ASSESSMENT
Assess the following:

■ Check for history of nasal surgery or deviated septum. Assess patency of nares.

■ Determine presence of gag reflex.
■ Assess mental status or ability to cooperate with procedure.

PLANNING
Before inserting a nasogastric tube, determine the size of tube to be inserted and whether the tube is to be attached to suction.

Delegation
Insertion of a nasogastric tube is an invasive procedure requiring application of knowledge (e.g., anatomy and physiology, risk factors) and problem solving. In some agencies, only health care providers with advanced training are permitted to insert nasogastric tubes that require use of a stylet. Delegation of this skill to unlicensed assistive personnel (UAP) is not appropriate. The UAP, however, can assist with the oral hygiene needs of a client with a nasogastric tube.

Equipment
■ Large- or small-bore tube (nonlatex preferred)
■ Nonallergenic adhesive tape, 2.5 cm (1 in.) wide
■ Clean gloves
■ Water-soluble lubricant
■ Facial tissues
■ Glass of water and drinking straw
■ 20- to 50-mL syringe with an adapter
■ Basin
■ pH test strip or meter
■ Bilirubin dipstick
■ Stethoscope

INSERTING A NASOGASTRIC TUBE *continued*

- Disposable pad or towel
- Clamp or plug (optional)
- Antireflux valve for air vent if Salem sump tube is used

- Suction apparatus
- Safety pin and elastic band
- CO_2 detector (optional)

IMPLEMENTATION
Preparation
Assist the client to a high Fowler's position if his or her health condition permits, and support the head on a pillow. **Rationale:** *It is often easier to swallow in this position and gravity helps the passage of the tube.* Place a towel or disposable pad across the chest.

Performance
1. Prior to performing the insertion, introduce self and verify the client's identity using agency protocol. Explain to the client what you are going to do, why it is necessary, and how he or she can cooperate. The passage of a gastric tube is unpleasant because the gag reflex is activated during insertion. Establish a method for the client to indicate distress and a desire for you to pause the insertion. Raising a finger or hand is often used for this.
2. Perform hand hygiene and observe other appropriate infection control procedures (e.g., clean gloves).
3. Provide for client privacy.
4. Assess the client's nares.
   - Ask the client to hyperextend the head, and, using a flashlight, observe the intactness of the tissues of the nostrils, including any irritations or abrasions.
   - Examine the nares for any obstructions or deformities by asking the client to breathe through one nostril while occluding the other.
   - Select the nostril that has the greater airflow.
5. Prepare the tube.
   - If a small-bore tube is being used, ensure stylet or guidewire is secured in position. **Rationale:** *An improperly positioned stylet or guidewire can traumatize the nasopharynx, esophagus, and stomach.*
6. Determine how far to insert the tube.
   - Use the tube to mark off the distance from the tip of the client's nose to the tip of the earlobe and then from the tip of the earlobe to the tip of the xiphoid. ❶ **Rationale:** *This length approximates the distance from the nares to the stomach. This distance varies among individuals.*

   - Mark this length with adhesive tape if the tube does not have markings.
7. Insert the tube.
   - Put on gloves.
   - Lubricate the tip of the tube well with water-soluble lubricant or water to ease insertion. **Rationale:** *A water-soluble lubricant dissolves if the tube accidentally enters the lungs. An oil-based lubricant, such as petroleum jelly, will not dissolve and could cause respiratory complications if it enters the lungs.*
   - Insert the tube, with its natural curve toward the client, into the selected nostril. Ask the client to hyperextend the neck, and gently advance the tube toward the nasopharynx. **Rationale:** *Hyperextension of the neck reduces the curvature of the nasopharyngeal junction.*
   - Direct the tube along the floor of the nostril and toward the ear on that side. **Rationale:** *Directing the tube along the floor avoids the projections (turbinates) along the lateral wall.*
   - Slight pressure and a twisting motion are sometimes required to pass the tube into the nasopharynx, and some client's eyes may water at this point. **Rationale:** *Tears are a natural body response.* Provide the client with tissues as needed.
   - If the tube meets resistance, withdraw it, relubricate it, and insert it in the other nostril. **Rationale:** *The tube should never be forced against resistance because of the danger of injury.*
   - Once the tube reaches the oropharynx (throat), the client will feel the tube in the throat and may gag and retch. Ask the client to tilt the head forward, and encourage the client to drink and swallow. **Rationale:** *Tilting the head forward facilitates passage of the tube into the posterior pharynx and esophagus rather than into the larynx; swallowing moves the epiglottis over the opening to the larynx.* ❷

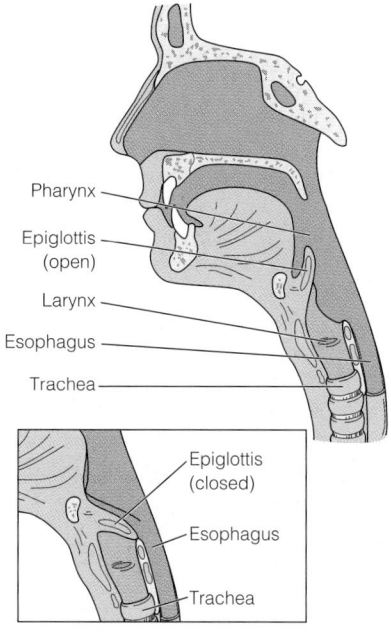

❶ Measuring the appropriate length to insert a nasogastric tube.

❷ Swallowing closes the epiglottis.

continued on page 1268

INSERTING A NASOGASTRIC TUBE *continued*

- If the client gags, stop passing the tube momentarily. Have the client rest, take a few breaths, and take sips of water to calm the gag reflex.
- In cooperation with the client, pass the tube 5 to 10 cm (2 to 4 in.) with each swallow, until the indicated length is inserted.
- If the client continues to gag and the tube does not advance with each swallow, withdraw it slightly, and inspect the throat by looking through the mouth. **Rationale:** *The tube may be coiled in the throat.* If so, withdraw it until it is straight, and try again to insert it.
- If a CO_2 detector is used, after the tube has been advanced approximately 30 cm (12 in.), draw air through the detector. Any change in color of the detector indicates placement of the tube in the respiratory tract. Immediately withdraw the tube and reinsert.

8. Ascertain correct placement of the tube.
   - Aspirate stomach contents, and check the pH, which should be acidic. **Rationale:** *Testing pH is a reliable way to determine location of a feeding tube. Gastric contents are commonly pH 1 to 5; 6 or greater would indicate the contents are from lower in the intestinal tract or in the respiratory tract. Some researchers suggest that a pH of greater than 5 should be followed by further confirmation of tube location* (Huffman, Jarczyk, O'Brien, Pieper, & Bayne, 2004).
   - Aspirate can also be tested for bilirubin. Bilirubin levels in the lungs should be almost zero, while levels in the stomach will be approximately 1.5 mg/dL and in the intestine over 10 mg/dL.
   - Almost all nasogastric tubes are radiopaque, and position can be confirmed by x-ray. Check agency policy. If a small-bore tube is used, leave the stylet or guidewire in place until correct position is verified by x-ray. If the stylet has been removed, never reinsert it while the tube is in place. **Rationale:** *The stylet is sharp and could pierce the tube and injure the client or cut off the tube end.*
   - Place a stethoscope over the client's epigastrium and inject 10 to 30 mL of air into the tube while listening for a whooshing sound. Although still one of the methods used, do not use this method as the *primary* method for determining placement of the feeding tube *because it does not guarantee tube position.*
   - If the signs indicate placement in the lungs, remove the tube and begin again.
   - If the signs do not indicate placement in the lungs or stomach, advance the tube 5 cm (2 in.), and repeat the tests.

9. Secure the tube by taping it to the bridge of the client's nose.
   - If the client has oily skin, wipe the nose first with alcohol to defat the skin.
   - Cut 7.5 cm (3 in.) of tape, and split it lengthwise at one end, leaving a 2.5-cm (1-in.) tab at the end.
   - Place the tape over the bridge of the client's nose, and bring the split ends either under and around the tubing, or under the tubing and back up over the nose. ❸ **Rationale:** *Taping in this manner prevents the tube from pressing against and irritating the edge of the nostril.*

10. Once correct position has been determined, attach the tube to a suction source or feeding apparatus as ordered, or clamp the end of the tubing.

❸ Taping a nasogastric tube to the bridge of the nose.

11. Secure the tube to the client's gown.
    - Loop an elastic band around the end of the tubing, and attach the elastic band to the gown with a safety pin.
      or
    - Attach a piece of adhesive tape to the tube, and pin the tape to the gown. **Rationale:** *The tube is attached to prevent it from dangling and pulling.*

If a Salem sump tube is used, attach the antireflux valve to the vent port (if used) and position the port above the client's waist *so gastric contents do not flow into the vent lumen.*

12. Document relevant information: the insertion of the tube, the means by which correct placement was determined, and client responses (e.g., discomfort or abdominal distention).

13. Establish a plan for providing daily nasogastric tube care.
    - Inspect the nostril for discharge and irritation.
    - Clean the nostril and tube with moistened, cotton-tipped applicators.
    - Apply water-soluble lubricant to the nostril if it appears dry or encrusted.
    - Change the adhesive tape as required.
    - Give frequent mouth care. Due to the presence of the tube, the client may breathe through the mouth.

14. If suction is applied, ensure that the patency of both the nasogastric and suction tubes is maintained.
    - Irrigations of the tube may be required at regular intervals. In some agencies, irrigations must be ordered by the primary care provider.
    - If a Salem sump tube is used, follow agency policies for irrigating the vent lumen with air to maintain patency of the suctioning lumen. Often, a sucking sound can be heard from the vent port if it is patent.
    - Keep accurate records of the client's fluid intake and output, and record the amount and characteristics of the drainage.

15. Document the type of tube inserted, date and time of tube insertion, type of suction used, color and amount of gastric contents, and the client's tolerance of the procedure.

SAMPLE DOCUMENTATION

11/5/06 1030 #8 Fr feeding tube inserted c̄ difficulty through R nare c̄ stylet in place. To x-ray to check placement. Radiologist reports tube tip in stomach. Stylet removed. Aspirate pH 4. Tube secured to nose. Pt. verbalizes understanding of need to not pull on tube. ————————————L. Traynor, RN

EVALUATION

Conduct appropriate follow-up, such as degree of client comfort, client tolerance of the nasogastric tube, correct placement of nasogastric tube in stomach, client understanding of restrictions, color and amount of gastric contents if attached to suction, or stomach contents aspirated.

REMOVING A NASOGASTRIC TUBE

ASSESSMENT

Assess

- For the presence of bowel sounds.
- For the absence of nausea or vomiting when tube is clamped.

PLANNING

Delegation

Due to the need for assessment of client status, the skill of removing a nasogastric tube is not delegated to UAP.

Equipment

- Disposable pad or towel
- Tissues
- Clean gloves
- 50-mL syringe (optional)
- Plastic trash bag

IMPLEMENTATION

Preparation

- Confirm the primary care provider's order to remove the tube.
- Assist the client to a sitting position if health permits.
- Place the disposable pad or towel across the client's chest to collect any spillage of secretions from the tube.
- Provide tissues to the client to wipe the nose and mouth after tube removal.

Performance

1. Prior to performing the removal, introduce self and verify the client's identity using agency protocol. Explain to the client what you are going to do, why it is necessary, and how he or she can cooperate. Discuss how the results will be used in planning further care or treatments.
2. Perform hand hygiene and observe other appropriate infection control procedures (e.g., clean gloves).
3. Provide for client privacy.
4. Detach the tube.
   - Disconnect the nasogastric tube from the suction apparatus, if present.
   - Unpin the tube from the client's gown.
   - Remove the adhesive tape securing the tube to the nose.
5. Remove the nasogastric tube.
   - Put on clean gloves.
   - (Optional) Instill 50 mL of air into the tube. **Rationale:** *This clears the tube of any contents such as feeding or gastric drainage.*
   - Ask the client to take a deep breath and to hold it. **Rationale:** *This closes the glottis, thereby preventing accidental aspiration of any gastric contents.*
   - Pinch the tube with the gloved hand. **Rationale:** *Pinching the tube prevents any contents inside the tube from draining into the client's throat.*
   - Smoothly, withdraw the tube.
   - Place the tube in the plastic bag. **Rationale:** *Placing the tube immediately into the bag prevents the transference of microorganisms from the tube to other articles or people.*
   - Observe the intactness of the tube.
6. Ensure client comfort.
   - Provide mouth care if desired.
   - Assist the client as required to blow the nose. **Rationale:** *Excessive secretions may have accumulated in the nasal passages.*
7. Dispose of the equipment appropriately.
   - Place the pad, bag with tube, and gloves in the receptacle designated by the agency. **Rationale:** *Correct disposal prevents the transmission of microorganisms.*
8. Document all relevant information.
   - Record the removal of the tube, the amount and appearance of any drainage if connected to suction, and any relevant assessments of the client.

SAMPLE DOCUMENTATION

11/8/06 1500 NG tube removed intact s̄ difficulty. Oral & nasal care given. No bleeding or excoriation noted. Pt. states is hungry & thirsty. 60 mL apple juice given. No c/o nausea.

—L. Traynor, RN

EVALUATION

- Perform a follow-up examination, such as presence of bowel sounds, absence of nausea or vomiting when tube is removed, and intactness of tissues of the nares.
- Relate findings to previous assessment data if available.
- Report significant deviations from normal to the primary care provider.

Gastrostomy and **jejunostomy** devices are used for long-term nutritional support, generally more than 6 to 8 weeks. Tubes are placed surgically or by laparoscopy through the abdominal wall into the stomach (gastrostomy, Figure 47-14 ■) or into the jejunum (jejunostomy, Figure 47-15 ■). A **percutaneous endoscopic gastrostomy (PEG)** or **percutaneous endoscopic jejunostomy (PEJ)** is created by using an endoscope to visualize the inside of the stomach, making a puncture through the skin and subcutaneous tissues

of the abdomen into the stomach, and inserting the PEG or PEJ catheter through the puncture.

The surgical opening is sutured tightly around the tube or catheter to prevent leakage. Care of this opening before it heals requires surgical asepsis. The catheter has an external bumper and an internal inflatable retention balloon to maintain placement. When the tract is established (about 1 month), the tube or catheter can be removed and reinserted for each

Figure 47-14 ■ Percutaneous endoscopic gastrostomy (PEG) tube.

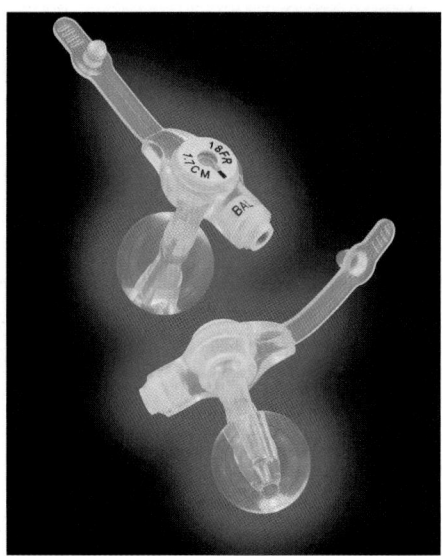

Figure 47-16 ■ Low profile gastrostomy feeding tube.

(© 2002 Kimberly-Clark Worldwide, Inc.)

feeding. Alternatively, a skin-level tube can be used that remains in place (Figure 47-16 ■). A feeding set is attached when needed.

TESTING FEEDING TUBE PLACEMENT. Before feedings are introduced, tube placement is confirmed by radiography, particularly when a small-bore tube has been inserted or when the client is at risk for aspiration. After placement is confirmed, the nurse marks the tube with indelible ink or tape at its exit point from the nose and documents the length of visible tubing for baseline data. The nurse is responsible, however, for verifying tube placement (i.e., gastrointestinal placement versus respiratory placement) before each intermittent feeding and at regular intervals (e.g., at least once per shift) when continuous feedings are being administered.

Methods nurses use to check tube placement include the following:

1. Aspirate gastrointestinal secretions. Small-bore tubes offer more resistance during aspirations than large-bore tubes and are more likely to collapse when negative pressure is applied. Gastric secretions tend to be a grassy-green, off-white, or tan color; intestinal fluid is stained with bile and has a golden yellow or brownish green color.

2. Measure the pH of aspirated fluid. This is the recommended method to determine tube placement. Testing the pH of aspirates can help distinguish gastric from respiratory and intestinal placement (Metheny & Meert, 2004) as follows:

   ● Gastric aspirates tend to be acidic and have a pH of 1 to 4 but may be as high as 6 if the client is receiving medications that control gastric acid.
   ● Small intestine aspirates generally have a pH equal to or higher than 6.

LIFESPAN CONSIDERATIONS
Inserting a Nasogastric Tube

INFANTS AND YOUNG CHILDREN

■ Restraints may be necessary during tube insertion and throughout therapy. *Restraints will prevent accidental dislodging of the tube.*

■ Place the infant in an infant seat or position the infant with a rolled towel or pillow under the head and shoulders.

■ When assessing the nares, obstruct one of the infant's nares and feel for air passage from the other. If the nasal passageway is very small or is obstructed, an orogastric tube may be more appropriate.

■ Measure appropriate nasogastric tube length from the nose to the tip of the earlobe and then to the point midway between the umbilicus and the xiphoid process.

■ If an orogastric tube is used, measure from the tip of the earlobe to the corner of the mouth to the xiphoid process.

■ Do not hyperextend or hyperflex an infant's neck. *Hyperextension or hyperflexion of the neck could occlude the airway.*

■ Tape the tube to the area between the end of the nares and the upper lip as well as to the cheek.

Figure 47-15 ■ Percutaneous endoscopic jejunostomy (PEJ) tube.

- Respiratory secretions are more alkaline with values of 7 or higher. However, there is a slight possibility of respiratory placement when the pH reading is as low as 6. Therefore, when pH readings are 6 or higher, radiographic confirmation of tube location needs to be considered, especially in clients with diminished cough and gag reflexes.

3. Auscultate the epigastrium while injecting 5 to 20 mL of air. Air injected into the stomach produces whooshing, gurgling, or bubbling sounds over the epigastrium and the upper left quadrant. Accuracy of this method in predicting placement is less reliable than pH testing.

4. Confirm length of tube insertion with the insertion mark. If more of the tube is now exposed, the position of the tip should be questioned.

Currently, the most effective method appears to be radiographic verification of tube placement. Repeated x-ray studies, however, are not feasible in terms of cost. More research is required to devise effective alternatives, especially for placement of small-bore tubes. In the meantime, nurses should (a) ensure initial radiographic verification of small-bore tubes, (b) aspirate contents when possible and check their acidity, (c) closely observe the client for signs of obvious distress, and (d) consider tube dislodgment after episodes of coughing, sneezing, and vomiting.

ENTERAL FEEDINGS. The type and frequency of feedings and amounts to be administered are ordered by the primary care provider. Liquid feeding mixtures are available commercially or may be prepared by the dietary department in accordance with the primary care provider's orders. A standard formula provides 1 Kcal per milliliter of solution with protein, fat, carbohydrate, minerals, and vitamins in specified proportions.

Enteral feedings can be given intermittently or continuously. Intermittent feedings are the administration of 300 to 500 mL of enteral formula several times per day. The stomach is the preferred site for these feedings, which are usually administered over at least 30 minutes. Bolus intermittent feedings are those that use a syringe to deliver the formula into the stomach. Because the formula is delivered rapidly by this method, it is not usually recommended but may be used in long-term situations if the client tolerates it. These feedings must be given only into the stomach; the client must be monitored closely for distention and aspiration.

Continuous feedings are generally administered over a 24-hour period using an infusion pump (often referred to as a kangaroo pump) that guarantees a constant flow rate (Figure 47-17 ■). Continuous feedings are essential when feedings are administered in the small bowel. They are also used when smaller bore gastric tubes are in place or when gravity flow is insufficient to instill the feeding.

Cyclic feedings are continuous feedings that are administered in less than 24 hours (e.g., 12 to 16 hours). These feedings, often administered at night, allow the client to attempt to eat regular meals through the day. Because nocturnal feedings may

Figure 47-17 ■ An enteric feeding pump.

use higher nutrient densities and higher infusion rates than the standard continuous feeding, particular attention needs to be given to monitoring fluid status and circulating volume.

Enteral feedings are administered to clients through open or closed systems. Open systems use an open-top container or a syringe for administration. Enteral feedings for use with open systems are provided in flip-top cans or powdered formulas that are reconstituted with sterile water. Sterile water, rather than tap water, reduces the risk of microbial contamination. Open systems should have no more than 8 to 12 hours of formula poured at one time. At the completion of this time, remaining formula should be discarded and the container rinsed before new formula is poured. The bag and tubing should be replaced every 24 hours (Rolfes et al., 2006). Closed systems consist of a prefilled container that is spiked with enteral tubing and attached to the enteral access device. Prefilled containers can hang safely for 48 hours if sterile technique is used.

Skill 47-3 provides the essential steps involved in administering a tube feeding, and Skill 47-4 indicates the steps involved in administering a gastrostomy or jejunostomy tube feeding.

ADMINISTERING A TUBE FEEDING

PURPOSES
- To restore or maintain nutritional status
- To administer medications

ASSESSMENT
Assess

- For any clinical signs of malnutrition or dehydration.
- For allergies to any food in the feeding. If the client is lactose intolerant, check the tube feeding formula. Notify the primary care provider if any incompatibilities exist.

- For the presence of bowel sounds.
- For any problems that suggest lack of tolerance of previous feedings (e.g., delayed gastric emptying, abdominal distention, diarrhea, cramping, or constipation).

PLANNING

Before commencing a tube feeding, determine the type, amount, and frequency of feedings and tolerance of previous feedings.

Delegation

Administering a tube feeding requires application of knowledge and problem solving and it is not usually delegated to UAP. Some agencies, however, may allow a trained UAP to administer a feeding. In this case, it is the responsibility of the nurse to assess tube placement and determine that the tube is patent. The nurse should reinforce major points, such as making sure the client is sitting upright, and instruct the UAP to report any difficulty administering the feeding or any complaints voiced by the client.

Equipment
- Correct type and amount of feeding solution
- 60-mL catheter-tip syringe
- Emesis basin

- Clean gloves
- pH test strip or meter
- Large syringe or calibrated plastic feeding bag with label and tubing that can be attached to the feeding tube or prefilled bottle with a drip chamber, tubing, and a flow-regulator clamp
- Measuring container from which to pour the feeding (if using open system)
- Water (60 mL unless otherwise specified) at room temperature
- Feeding pump as required

CLINICAL ALERT

Do not add colored food dye to tube feedings. Previously, blue dye was often added to assist in recognition of aspiration. However, the FDA reports cases of many adverse reactions to the dye, including toxicity and death. ■

IMPLEMENTATION
Preparation

Assist the client to a Fowler's position (at least 30 degrees elevation) in bed or a sitting position in a chair, the normal position for eating. If a sitting position is contraindicated, a slightly elevated right side-lying position is acceptable. **Rationale:** *These positions enhance the gravitational flow of the solution and prevent aspiration of fluid into the lungs.*

Performance

1. Prior to performing the feeding, introduce self and verify the client's identity using agency protocol. Explain to the client what you are going to do, why it is necessary, and how he or she can cooperate. Inform the client that the feeding should not cause any discomfort but may cause a feeling of fullness.
2. Perform hand hygiene and observe appropriate infection control procedures (e.g., clean gloves).
3. Provide privacy for this procedure if the client desires it. Tube feedings are embarrassing to some people.
4. Assess tube placement.
   - Attach the syringe to the open end of the tube and aspirate. Check the pH.
   - Allow 1 hour to elapse before testing the pH if the client has received a medication.
   - Use a pH meter rather than pH paper if the client is receiving a continuous feeding. Follow agency policy if the pH is or greater 6.
5. Assess residual feeding contents.
   - If the tube is placed in the stomach, aspirate all contents and measure the amount before administering the feeding.

Rationale: *This is done to evaluate absorption of the last feeding; that is, whether undigested formula from a previous feeding remains. If the tube is in the small intestine, residual contents cannot be aspirated.*

- If 100 mL (or more than half the last feeding) is withdrawn, check with the nurse in charge or refer to agency policy before proceeding. The precise amount is usually determined by the primary care provider's order or by agency policy. **Rationale:** *At some agencies, a feeding is delayed when the specified amount or more of formula remains in the stomach.*

or
- Reinstill the gastric contents into the stomach if this is the agency policy or primary care provider's order. **Rationale:** *Removal of the contents could disturb the client's electrolyte balance.*
- If the client is on a continuous feeding, check the gastric residual every 4 to 6 hours or according to agency protocol.

6. Administer the feeding.
   - Before administering feeding:
     Check the expiration date of the feeding.
     Warm the feeding to room temperature. **Rationale:** *An excessively cold feeding may cause abdominal cramps.*
   - When an open system is used, clean the top of the feeding container with alcohol before opening it. **Rationale:** *This minimizes the risk of contaminants entering the feeding syringe or feeding bag.*

Feeding Bag (Open System)
- Hang the labeled bag from an infusion pole about 30 cm (12 in.) above the tube's point of insertion into the client.

ADMINISTERING A TUBE FEEDING *continued*

- Clamp the tubing and add the formula to the bag.
- Open the clamp, run the formula through the tubing, and reclamp the tube. **Rationale:** *The formula will displace the air in the tubing, thus preventing the instillation of excess air into the client's stomach or intestine.*
- Attach the bag to the feeding tube ❶ and regulate the drip by adjusting the clamp to the drop factor on the bag (e.g., 20 drops/mL) if not placed on a pump.

Syringe (Open System)

- Remove the plunger from the syringe and connect the syringe to a pinched or clamped nasogastric tube. **Rationale:** *Pinching or clamping the tube prevents excess air from entering the stomach and causing distention.*
- Add the feeding to the syringe barrel. ❷
- Permit the feeding to flow in slowly at the prescribed rate. Raise or lower the syringe to adjust the flow as needed. Pinch or clamp the tubing to stop the flow for a minute if the client experiences discomfort. **Rationale:** *Quickly administered feedings can cause flatus, cramps, and/or vomiting.*

Prefilled Bottle With Drip Chamber (Closed System)

- Remove the screw-on cap from the container and attach the administration set with the drip chamber and tubing. ❸
- Close the clamp on the tubing.
- Hang the container on an intravenous pole about 30 cm (12 in.) above the tube's insertion point into the client. **Rationale:** *At this height, the formula should run at a safe rate into the stomach or intestine.*
- Squeeze the drip chamber to fill it to one-third to one-half of its capacity.
- Open the tubing clamp, run the formula through the tubing, and reclamp the tube. **Rationale:** *The formula will displace the air in the tubing, thus preventing the instillation of excess air.*
- Attach the feeding set tubing to the feeding tube and regulate the drip rate to deliver the feeding over the desired length of time or attach to a feeding pump.

7. If another bottle is not to be immediately hung, flush the feeding tube before all of the formula has run through the tubing.
   - Instill 50 to 100 mL of water through the feeding tube or medication port. **Rationale:** *Water flushes the lumen of the tube, preventing future blockage by sticky formula.*
   - Be sure to add the water before the feeding solution has drained from the neck of a syringe or from the tubing of an administration set. **Rationale:** *Adding the water before the syringe or tubing is empty prevents the instillation of air into the stomach or intestine and thus prevents unnecessary distention.*

8. Clamp the feeding tube.
   - Clamp the feeding tube before all of the water is instilled. **Rationale:** *Clamping prevents leakage and air from entering the tube if done before water is instilled.*

9. Ensure client comfort and safety.
   - Secure the tubing to the client's gown. **Rationale:** *This minimizes pulling of the tube, thus preventing discomfort and dislodgment.*
- Ask the client to remain sitting upright in Fowler's position or in a slightly elevated right lateral position for at least 30 minutes. **Rationale:** *These positions facilitate digestion and movement of*

❶ Using a calibrated plastic bag to administer a tube feeding.

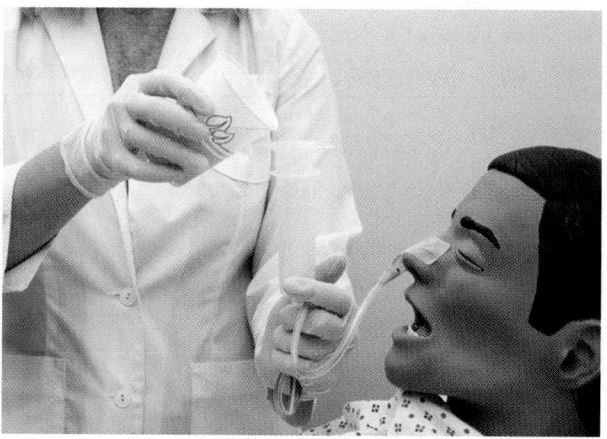

❷ Using the barrel of a syringe to administer a tube feeding.

❸ Feeding set tubing with drip chamber. (Ross Products Division, Abbott Laboratories. Used with permission.)

continued on page 1274

ADMINISTERING A TUBE FEEDING *continued*

the feeding from the stomach along the alimentary tract, and prevent the potential aspiration of the feeding into the lungs.

- Check the agency's policy on the frequency of changing the nasogastric tube and the use of smaller lumen tubes if a large-bore tube is in place. **Rationale:** *These measures prevent irritation and erosion of the pharyngeal and esophageal mucous membranes.*

10. Dispose of equipment appropriately.
    - If the equipment is to be reused, wash it thoroughly with soap and water so that it is ready for reuse.
    - Change the equipment every 24 hours or according to agency policy.

11. Document all relevant information.
    - Document the feeding, including amount and kind of solution taken, duration of the feeding, and assessments of the client.
    - Record the volume of the feeding and water administered on the client's intake and output record.

    SAMPLE DOCUMENTATION

    11/5/06 1330 Aspirated 20 mL pale yellow fluid from NG tube, pH 5. Pt. in Fowler's position. 1 L room-temperature ordered formula begun @ 60 mL/hour on pump. No nausea reported. ————— L. Traynor, RN

12. Monitor the client for possible problems.
    - Carefully assess clients receiving tube feedings for problems.
    - To prevent dehydration, give the client supplemental water in addition to the prescribed tube feeding as ordered.

Variation: Continuous-Drip Feeding

- Clamp the tubing at least every 4 to 6 hours, or as indicated by agency protocol or the manufacturer, and aspirate and measure the gastric contents. Then flush the tubing with 30 to 50 mL of water. **Rationale:** *This determines adequate absorption and verifies correct placement of the tube.* If placement of a small-bore tube is questionable, a repeat x-ray should be done.
- Determine agency protocol regarding withholding a feeding. Many agencies withhold the feeding if more than 75 to 100 mL of feeding is aspirated.
- To prevent spoilage or bacterial contamination, do not allow the feeding solution to hang longer than 4 to 8 hours. Check agency policy or manufacturer's recommendations regarding time limits.
- Follow agency policy regarding how frequently to change the feeding bag and tubing. Changing the feeding bag and tubing every 24 hours reduces the risk of contamination.

EVALUATION

Perform a follow-up examination of the following:

- Tolerance of feeding (e.g., nausea, cramping)
- Bowel sounds
- Regurgitation and feelings of fullness after feedings
- Weight gain or loss

- Fecal elimination pattern (e.g., diarrhea, flatulence, constipation)
- Skin turgor
- Urine output and specific gravity
- Glucose and acetone in urine

Relate findings to previous assessment data if available. Report significant deviations from normal to the primary care provider.

ADMINISTERING A GASTROSTOMY OR JEJUNOSTOMY FEEDING

PURPOSES
See Skill 47-3.

ASSESSMENT
See Skill 47-3.

PLANNING
Before commencing a gastrostomy or jejunostomy feeding, determine the type and amount of feeding to be instilled, frequency of feedings, and any pertinent information about previous feedings (e.g., the positioning in which the client best tolerates the feeding).

Delegation
See Skill 47-3.

Equipment
- Correct amount of feeding solution
- Graduated container and tubing with clamp to hold the feeding
- 60-mL catheter-tip syringe

For a Tube that Remains in Place
- Mild soap and water
- Clean gloves
- Petrolatum, zinc oxide ointment, or other skin protectant
- Precut 4-in. × 4-in. gauze squares
- Uncut 4-in. × 4-in. gauze squares

For Tube Insertion
- Clean gloves
- Moisture-proof bag
- Water-soluble lubricant
- Feeding tube (if needed)

IMPLEMENTATION
Preparation
See Skill 47-3.

Performance
1. Prior to performing the feeding, introduce self and verify the client's identity using agency protocol. Explain to the client what

ADMINISTERING A GASTROSTOMY OR JEJUNOSTOMY FEEDING *continued*

you are going to do, why it is necessary, and how he or she can cooperate. Discuss how the results will be used in planning further care or treatments.

2. Perform hand hygiene and observe other appropriate infection control procedures (e.g., clean gloves).
3. Provide for client privacy.
4. Assess and prepare the client.
   See Skill 47-3.
5. Insert a feeding tube, if one is not already in place.
   - Wearing gloves, remove the dressing. Then discard the dressing and gloves in the moisture-proof bag.
   - Apply new clean gloves.
   - Lubricate the end of the tube, and insert it into the ostomy opening 10 to 15 cm (4 to 6 in.).
6. Check the location and patency of a tube that is already in place.
   - Determine correct placement of the tube by aspirating secretions and checking the pH.
   - Follow agency policy for amount of residual formula. This may include withholding the feeding, rechecking in 3 to 4 hours, or notifying the primary care provider if a large residual remains.
   - For continuous feedings, check the residual every 4 to 6 hours and hold feedings according to agency policy.
   - Remove the syringe plunger. Pour 15 to 30 mL of water into the syringe, remove the tube clamp, and allow the water to flow into the tube. **Rationale:** *This determines the patency of the tube. If water flows freely, the tube is patent.*
   - If the water does not flow freely, notify the nurse in charge and/or primary care provider.
7. Administer the feeding.
   - Hold the barrel of the syringe 7 to 15 cm (3 to 6 in.) above the ostomy opening.
   - Slowly pour the solution into the syringe and allow it to flow through the tube by gravity.
   - Just before all the formula has run through and the syringe is empty, add 30 mL of water. **Rationale:** *Water flushes the tube and preserves its patency.*

- If the tube is to remain in place, hold it upright, remove the syringe, and then clamp or plug the tube to prevent leakage.
- If a catheter was inserted for the feeding, remove it.

8. Ensure client comfort and safety.
   - After the feeding, ask the client to remain in the sitting position or a slightly elevated right lateral position for at least 30 minutes. **Rationale:** *This minimizes the risk of aspiration.*
   - Assess status of peristomal skin. **Rationale:** *Gastric or jejunal drainage contains digestive enzymes that can irritate the skin.* Document any redness and broken skin areas.
   - Check orders about cleaning the peristomal skin, applying a skin protectant, and applying appropriate dressings. Generally, the peristomal skin is washed with mild soap and water at least once daily. The tube may be rotated between thumb and forefinger to release any sticking and promote tract formation. Petrolatum, zinc oxide ointment, or other skin protectant may be applied around the stoma, and precut 4-in. × 4-in. gauze squares may be placed around the tube. The precut squares are then covered with regular 4-in. × 4-in. gauze squares, and the tube is coiled over them.
   - Observe for common complications of enteral feedings: aspiration, hyperglycemia, abdominal distention, diarrhea, and fecal impaction. Report findings to primary care provider. Often, a change in formula or rate of administration can correct problems.
   - When appropriate, teach the client how to administer feedings and when to notify the health care provider concerning problems.
9. Document all assessments and interventions.

SAMPLE DOCUMENTATION

1/24/07 2045 No fluid aspirated from gastrostomy tube. Pt. in Fowler's position. 30 mL water flowed freely by gravity through tube. 250 mL room-temperature Ensure formula given over 20 minutes. No complaints of discomfort. ————*L. Traynor, RN*

EVALUATION
See Skill 47-3.

LIFESPAN CONSIDERATIONS Administering a Tube Feeding

INFANTS
- Feeding tubes may be reinserted at each feeding to prevent irritation of the mucous membrane, nasal airway obstruction, and stomach perforation that may occur if the tube is left in place continuously. Check agency practice.

CHILDREN
- Position a small child or infant in your lap, provide a pacifier, and hold and cuddle the child during feedings. This promotes comfort, supports the normal sucking instinct of the infant, and facilitates digestion.

ELDERS
- Physiologic changes associated with aging may make the elder more vulnerable to complications associated with enteral feedings.

Decreased gastric emptying may necessitate checking frequently for gastric residual. Diarrhea from administering the feeding too fast or at too high a concentration may cause dehydration. If the feeding has a high concentration of glucose, assess for hyperglycemia because with aging, the body has a decreased ability to handle increased glucose levels.
- Conditions such as hiatal hernia and diabetes mellitus may cause the stomach to empty more slowly. This increases the risk of aspiration in a client receiving a tube feeding. Checking for gastric residual more frequently can help document this if it is an ongoing problem. Changing the formula or the rate of administration, repositioning the client, or obtaining a primary care provider's order for a medication to increase stomach emptying may resolve this problem.

HOME CARE CONSIDERATIONS Administering a Tube Feeding

- Teach and provide the client or caregiver the rationale for how to assess for tube placement using pH measurement before administering the feeding. Instruct regarding actions to take if the pH is greater than 6.
- Provide instructions and rationale for care of the tube and insertion site.

- Discuss strategies for hanging formula containers if an IV pole is unavailable or inconvenient.
- Plan for optimal timing of feedings to allow for daily activities. Many clients can tolerate having the majority of their feedings run during sleep so they are free from the equipment during the day.
- Teach signs and symptoms to report to the doctor or home health nurse.

Before administering a tube feeding, the nurse must determine any food allergies of the client and assess tolerance to previous feedings. Table 47–5 lists essential assessments to conduct before administering tube feedings. The nurse must also check the expiration date on a commercially prepared formula or the preparation date and time of agency-prepared solution, discarding any formula that has passed the expiration date or that was prepared more than 24 hours previously.

Feedings are usually administered at room temperature unless the order specifies otherwise. The nurse warms the specified amount of solution in a basin of warm water or leaves it to stand for a while until it reaches room temperature. Because a formula that is warmed can grow microorganisms, it should not hang longer than the manufacturer recommends. Continuous-feeding formulas should be kept cold; excessive heat coagulates feedings of milk and egg, and hot liquids can irritate the mucous membranes. However, excessively cold feedings can reduce the flow of digestive juices by causing vasoconstriction and may cause cramps. Guidelines for teaching clients and families regarding administration of tube feedings in the home are found in the Client Teaching box.

Managing Clogged Feeding Tubes

Even if feeding tubes are flushed with water before and after feedings and medications, they can still become clogged. This can occur when the feeding container runs dry, solid medication is not adequately crushed, or medications are mixed with formula. Even the important practice of aspirating to check residual volume increases the incidence of clogging (Reising & Neal, 2005). To avoid the necessity of removing the tube and reinserting a new tube, both prevention and intervention strategies must be used.

To prevent clogged feeding tubes, flush liberally (at least 30 mL water) before, between, and after each separate medication is instilled, using a 60-mL piston syringe. The larger the barrel of the syringe, the less the pressure exerted. Too great a pressure can rupture the tube—especially small-bore feeding tubes. Do not add medications to formula or to each other.

Many strategies have been used to try to unclog feeding tubes. Strategies that have shown inconsistent effectiveness include instilling meat tenderizer, carbonated beverages, or cranberry juice, or flushing with small barrel syringes with or without digestive enzymes such as papain or chymotrypsin. Soda has actually been found to make the clog worse (Novartis, 2003).

TABLE 47–5 Assessing Clients Receiving Tube Feedings

ASSESSMENTS	RATIONALE
Allergies to any food in the feeding	Common allergenic foods include milk, sugar, water, eggs, and vegetable oil.
Bowel sounds before each feeding or, for continuous feedings, every 4 to 8 hours	To determine intestinal activity.
Correct placement of tube before feedings	To prevent aspiration of feedings.
Presence of regurgitation and feelings of fullness after feedings	May indicate delayed gastric emptying, need to decrease quantity or rate of the feeding, or high fat content of the formula.
Dumping syndrome: nausea, vomiting, diarrhea, cramps, pallor, sweating, heart palpitations, increased pulse rate, and fainting after a feeding	Jejunostomy clients may experience these symptoms, which result when hypertonic foods and liquids suddenly distend the jejunum. To make the intestinal contents isotonic, body fluids shift rapidly from the client's vascular system.
Abdominal distention, at least daily (Measure abdominal girth at the umbilicus.)	Abdominal distention may indicate intolerance to a previous feeding.
Diarrhea, constipation, or flatulence	The lack of bulk in liquid feedings may cause constipation. The presence of hypertonic or concentrated ingredients may cause diarrhea and flatulence.
Urine for sugar and acetone	Hyperglycemia may occur if the sugar content is too high.
Hematocrit and urine specific gravity	Both increase as a result of dehydration.
Serum BUN and sodium levels	Feeding formula may have a high protein content. If a high protein intake is combined with an inadequate fluid intake, the kidneys may not be able to excrete nitrogenous wastes adequately.

CLIENT TEACHING Tube Feedings

Clients and caregivers need the following instructions to manage these feedings:

■ Preparation of the formula. Include name of the formula and how much and how often it is to be given; the need to inspect the formula for expiration date and leaks and cracks in bags or cans; how to mix or prepare the formula, if needed; and aseptic techniques such as swabbing the container's top with alcohol before opening it, and changing the syringe administration set and reservoir every 24 hours.

■ Proper storage of the formula. Include the need to refrigerate diluted or reconstituted formula and formula that contains additives.

■ Administration of the feeding. Include proper hand washing technique, how to fill and hang the feeding bag, operation of an infusion pump if indicated, the feeding rate, and client positioning during and after the feeding.

■ Management of the enteral or parenteral access device. Include site care, aseptic precautions, dressing change, as indicated, how the site should look normally, and flushing protocols (e.g., type of irrigant and schedule).

■ Daily monitoring needs. Include temperature, weight, and intake and output.

■ Signs and symptoms of complications to report. Include fever, increased respiratory rate, decrease in urine output, increased stool frequency, and altered level of consciousness.

■ Whom to contact about questions or problems. Include emergency telephone numbers of home care agency, nursing clinician and/or primary care provider, or other 24-hour on-call emergency service.

The first strategy that should be tried is to reposition the client (this may allow a kink to straighten). Alternately flush and aspirate the tube with water. One institution has had success with a hollow catheter that allows unclogging solution to be delivered as the catheter is advanced down the clogged tube (Smith & Myers, 2005).

Parenteral Nutrition

Parenteral nutrition (PN), also referred to as total parenteral nutrition (TPN) or intravenous hyperalimentation (IVH), is provided when the gastrointestinal tract is nonfunctional because of an interruption in its continuity or because its absorptive capacity is impaired. **Parenteral** nutrition is administered intravenously such as through a central venous catheter into the superior vena cava.

Parenteral feedings are solutions of dextrose, water, fat, proteins, electrolytes, vitamins, and trace elements; they provide all needed calories. Because TPN solutions are hypertonic (highly concentrated in comparison to the solute concentration of blood), they are injected only into high-flow central veins, where they are diluted by the client's blood.

TPN is a means of achieving an anabolic state in clients who are unable to maintain a normal nitrogen balance. Such clients may include those with severe malnutrition, severe burns, bowel disease disorders (e.g., ulcerative colitis or enteric fistula), acute renal failure, hepatic failure, metastatic cancer, or major surgeries where nothing may be taken by mouth for more than 5 days.

TPN is not risk-free. Infection control is of utmost importance during TPN therapy. The nurse must always observe surgical aseptic technique when changing solutions, tubing, dressings, and filters. Clients are at increased risk of fluid, electrolyte, and glucose imbalances and require frequent evaluation and modification of the TPN mixture.

TPN solutions are 10% to 50% dextrose in water, plus a mixture of amino acids and special additives such as vitamins (e.g., B complex, C, D, K), minerals (e.g., potassium, sodium, chloride, calcium, phosphate, magnesium), and trace elements (e.g., cobalt, zinc, manganese). Additives are modified to each client's nutritional needs. Fat emulsions may be given to pro-

vide essential fatty acids to correct and/or prevent essential fatty acid deficiency or to supplement the calories for clients who, for example, have high calorie needs or cannot tolerate glucose as the only calorie source. Note that 1,000 mL of 5% glucose or dextrose contains 50 grams of sugar. Thus, a liter of this solution provides less than 200 calories!

Because TPN solutions are high in glucose, infusions are started gradually to prevent hyperglycemia. The client needs to adapt to TPN therapy by increasing insulin output from the pancreas. For example, an adult client may be given 1 liter (40 mL/hr) of TPN solution the first day; if the infusion is tolerated, the amount may be increased to 2 liters (80 mL/hr) for 24 to 48 hours, and then to 3 liters (120 mL/hr) within 3 to 5 days. Glucose levels are monitored during the infusion.

When TPN therapy is to be discontinued, the TPN infusion rates are decreased slowly to prevent hyperinsulinemia and hypoglycemia. Weaning a client from TPN may take up to 48 hours but can occur in 6 hours as long as the client receives adequate carbohydrates either orally or intravenously.

Enteral or parenteral feedings may be continued beyond hospital care in the client's home or may be initiated in the home.

Evaluating

The goals established in the planning phase are evaluated according to specific desired outcomes, also established in that phase (see Identifying Nursing Diagnoses, Outcomes, and Interventions on page 1260).

If the outcomes are not achieved, the nurse should explore the reasons. The nurse might consider the following questions:

■ Was the cause of the problem correctly identified?
■ Was the family included in the teaching plan? Are family members supportive?
■ Is the client experiencing symptoms that cause loss of appetite (e.g., pain, nausea, fatigue)?
■ Were the outcomes unrealistic for this person?
■ Were the client's food preferences considered?
■ Is anything interfering with digestion or absorption of nutrients (e.g., diarrhea)?

NURSING CARE PLAN Nutrition

ASSESSMENT DATA	NURSING DIAGNOSIS	DESIRED OUTCOMES*
Nursing Assessment Mrs. Rose Santini, a 59-year-old homemaker, attends a community hospital–sponsored health fair. She approaches the nutrition information booth, and the clinical specialist in nutritional support gathers a nutritional history. Mrs. Santini is very upset about her 9-kg (20-lb) weight gain. She relates to the nurse clinician that since the death of her husband 1 month ago she has lost interest in many of her usual physical and social activities. She no longer attends YMCA exercise and swimming sessions and has lost contact with her couple's bridge group. Mrs. Santini states she is bored, depressed, and very unhappy about her appearance. She has a small frame and has always prided herself on her petite figure. She says her eating habits have changed considerably. She snacks while watching TV and rarely prepares a complete meal.	*Imbalanced Nutrition: More than body requirements* related to excess intake and decreased activity expenditure (as evidenced by weight gain of 20 lb, triceps skin fold greater than normal, undesirable eating patterns).	**Weight Control [1612]** as evidenced by demonstrating ■ Eats three meals each day that result in a 500-calorie reduction in intake. ■ Develops a physical exercise plan that engages her in 15 to 20 minutes of exercise by day 5. ■ Identifies eating habits that contribute to weight gain by day 2.

Physical Examination

Height: 162.6 cm (5′ 4″)
Weight: 63.6 kg (140 lb)
Temperature: 37°C (98.6°F)
Pulse: 76 BPM
Respirations: 16/minute
Blood pressure: 144/84 mm Hg
Triceps skinfold: 21 mm
Small frame, weight in excess of 10% over ideal for height and frame

Diagnostic Data

CBC normal, urinalysis negative, chest x-ray negative, thyroid profile within normal limits

NURSING INTERVENTIONS*/SELECTED ACTIVITIES	RATIONALE
Weight Reduction Assistance [1280]	
Determine current eating patterns by having Mrs. Santini keep a diary of what, when, and where she eats.	*Increases awareness of activities and foods that contribute to excessive intake.*
Set a weekly goal for weight loss.	*The desirable weight loss rate is 1–2 pounds per week.*
Encourage use of internal reward systems when goals are accomplished.	*Goal setting provides motivation, which is essential for a successful weight-loss program.*
Set a realistic plan with Mrs. Santini to include reduced food intake and increased energy expenditure.	*A combined plan of calorie reduction and exercise can enhance weight loss since exercise increases caloric utilization.*
Assist client to identify motivation for eating and internal and external cues associated with eating.	*Awareness of factors that contribute to overeating will assist the individual in planning behavior modification techniques to avoid situations that prompt excess food consumption.*
Encourage attendance at support groups for weight loss and/or refer to a community weight control program.	*Overweight people are often nutritionally deprived. Intake must be reduced by 500 calories per day to obtain a one-pound-per-week weight loss.*
Develop a daily meal plan with a well-balanced diet, reduced calories, and reduced fat.	*Support groups can provide companionship, increase motivation, and offer practical solutions to problems associated with dieting.*
Nutritional Counseling [5246]	
Facilitate identification of eating behaviors to be changed.	*Increases individual's awareness of those actions that contribute to excessive intake.*
Use accepted nutritional standards to assist Mrs. Santini in evaluating adequacy of dietary intake.	*Comparing the individual's dietary history with nutritional standards will facilitate identification of nutritional deficiencies and/or excesses.*

NURSING CARE PLAN **Nutrition** *continued*

NURSING INTERVENTIONS*/SELECTED ACTIVITIES	RATIONALE
Help Mrs. Santini to consider factors of age, past eating experiences, culture, and finances in planning ways to meet nutritional requirements.	*Social, economic, physical, and psychologic factors play a role in nutrition and/or malnutrition.*
Discuss Mrs. Santini's knowledge of the basic four food groups, as well as perceptions of the needed diet modification.	*Helps to determine the client's knowledge base and identify misconceptions and/or gaps in understanding.*
Discuss food likes and dislikes.	*Incorporating Mrs. Santini's food preferences into the dietary plan will promote adherence to the weight loss program.*
Assist Mrs. Santini in stating her feelings and concerns about goal achievement.	*Fear of success, failure, or other concerns may block goal achievement.*

Behavior Modification [4360]

Assist Mrs. Santini to identify strengths and reinforce these.	*Reinforcing strengths enhances self-esteem and encourages the individual to draw on these assets during the weight-loss program.*
Encourage her to examine her own behavior.	*Involving Mrs. Santini in self-appraisal will promote identification of behaviors that may be contributing to excessive caloric intake.*
Identify the behavior to be changed in specific, concrete terms (e.g., stop snacking in front of the TV).	*Identification of specific behaviors is essential for planning behavior modification.*
Consider that it is easier to increase a behavior than to decrease a behavior (e.g., increase activities or hobbies that involve the hands such as sewing versus decreasing TV snacking).	*Habitual behaviors are difficult to change. Breaking old habits may be easier if viewed from the standpoint of increasing an enjoyable, healthy activity.*
Choose reinforcers that are meaningful to Mrs. Santini.	*Positive reinforcement is not likely to be an effective part of behavior modification if the reinforcer is meaningless to the individual.*

EVALUATION

Outcome met. Mrs. Santini kept a dietary log for 5 days and has eaten balanced meals each day, resulting in a daily deficit of 400 to 500 calories. She is aware that she eats excessively because she is bored and depressed. She has reestablished her former social contacts including her church bridge club. Mrs. Santini has purchased a stationary bicycle and exercises 20 minutes daily. She enrolled in a knitting class that meets two nights per week. She has lost 1 1/2 lb in the past week. As a reward, Mrs. Santini renewed her membership to the YMCA.

The NOC # for desired outcomes and the NIC # for nursing interventions are listed in brackets following the appropriate outcome or intervention. Outcomes, interventions, and activities selected are only a sample of those suggested by NOC and NIC and should be further individualized for each client.

APPLYING CRITICAL THINKING

1. How do Mrs. Santini's personal characteristics influence her nutritional needs?
2. What further information do you need regarding Mrs. Santini's present diet?
3. Offer suggestions for ways to modify Mrs. Santini's tendency to snack.

4. Mrs. Santini asks what her weight should be. How do you respond?

See Critical Thinking Possibilities in Appendix A. ∞

CONCEPT MAP   Nutrition

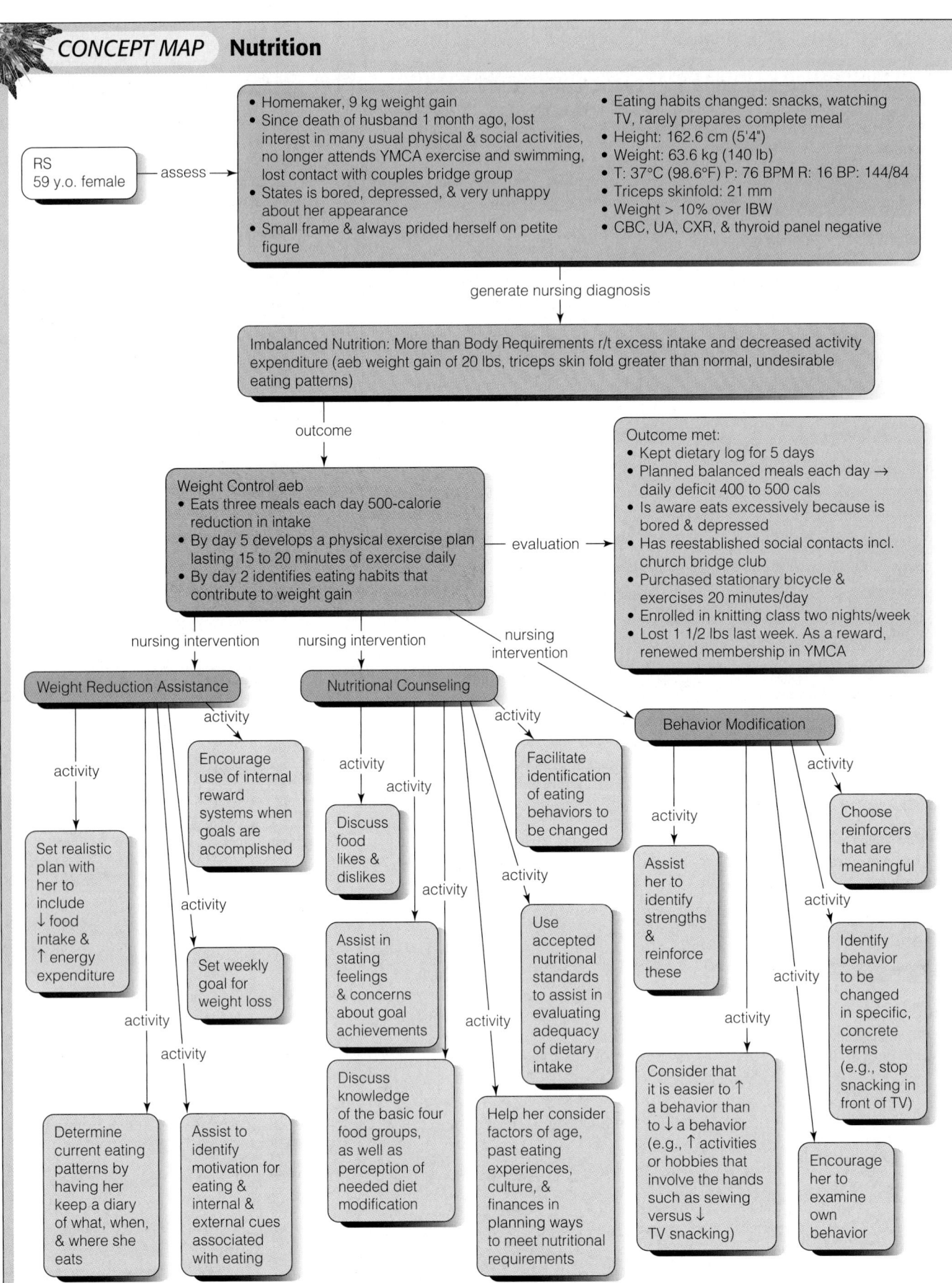

RS
59 y.o. female

— assess →

- Homemaker, 9 kg weight gain
- Since death of husband 1 month ago, lost interest in many usual physical & social activities, no longer attends YMCA exercise and swimming, lost contact with couples bridge group
- States is bored, depressed, & very unhappy about her appearance
- Small frame & always prided herself on petite figure

- Eating habits changed: snacks, watching TV, rarely prepares complete meal
- Height: 162.6 cm (5'4")
- Weight: 63.6 kg (140 lb)
- T: 37°C (98.6°F) P: 76 BPM R: 16 BP: 144/84
- Triceps skinfold: 21 mm
- Weight > 10% over IBW
- CBC, UA, CXR, & thyroid panel negative

generate nursing diagnosis

Imbalanced Nutrition: More than Body Requirements r/t excess intake and decreased activity expenditure (aeb weight gain of 20 lbs, triceps skin fold greater than normal, undesirable eating patterns)

outcome

Weight Control aeb
- Eats three meals each day 500-calorie reduction in intake
- By day 5 develops a physical exercise plan lasting 15 to 20 minutes of exercise daily
- By day 2 identifies eating habits that contribute to weight gain

— evaluation →

Outcome met:
- Kept dietary log for 5 days
- Planned balanced meals each day → daily deficit 400 to 500 cals
- Is aware eats excessively because is bored & depressed
- Has reestablished social contacts incl. church bridge club
- Purchased stationary bicycle & exercises 20 minutes/day
- Enrolled in knitting class two nights/week
- Lost 1 1/2 lbs last week. As a reward, renewed membership in YMCA

nursing intervention

nursing intervention

nursing intervention

Weight Reduction Assistance

Nutritional Counseling

Behavior Modification

activity

Encourage use of internal reward systems when goals are accomplished

activity

Set realistic plan with her to include ↓ food intake & ↑ energy expenditure

activity

Set weekly goal for weight loss

activity

Determine current eating patterns by having her keep a diary of what, when, & where she eats

activity

Assist to identify motivation for eating & internal & external cues associated with eating

activity

Discuss food likes & dislikes

activity

Assist in stating feelings & concerns about goal achievements

Discuss knowledge of the basic four food groups, as well as perception of needed diet modification

activity

Facilitate identification of eating behaviors to be changed

activity

Use accepted nutritional standards to assist in evaluating adequacy of dietary intake

activity

Help her consider factors of age, past eating experiences, culture, & finances in planning ways to meet nutritional requirements

activity

Assist her to identify strengths & reinforce these

activity

Consider that it is easier to ↑ a behavior than to ↓ a behavior (e.g., ↑ activities or hobbies that involve the hands such as sewing versus ↓ TV snacking)

activity

Choose reinforcers that are meaningful

activity

Identify behavior to be changed in specific, concrete terms (e.g., stop snacking in front of TV)

activity

Encourage her to examine own behavior

CHAPTER 47 **REVIEW**

CHAPTER HIGHLIGHTS

- Essential nutrients are grouped into categories: carbohydrates, proteins, lipids, vitamins, and minerals.
- Nutrients serve three basic purposes: forming body structures (such as bones and blood), providing energy, and helping to regulate the body's biochemical reactions.
- The amount of energy that nutrients or foods supply to the body is their caloric value. The amount of energy required to maintain basic body functions is referred to as the resting energy expenditure (REE). The basal metabolic rate (BMR) is the rate at which the body metabolizes food to maintain the energy and requirements of a person who is awake and at rest.
- A person's state of energy balance can be determined by comparing caloric intake with caloric expenditure.
- Ideal body weight (IBW) is the optimal weight recommended for optimal health.
- Body mass index (BMI) and percent body fat are indicators of changes in body fat stores. They indicate whether a person's weight is appropriate for height and may provide a useful estimate of nutrition.
- Factors influencing a person's nutrition include development, gender, ethnicity and culture, beliefs about foods, personal preferences, religious practices, lifestyle, economics, medications and therapy, health, alcohol consumption, advertising, and psychologic factors.
- Nutritional needs vary considerably according to age, growth, and energy requirements. Adolescents have high energy requirements due to their rapid growth; a diet plentiful in milk, meats, green and yellow vegetables, and fresh fruits is required. Middle-aged adults and elders often need to reduce their caloric intake because of decreases in metabolic rate and activity levels.
- Various daily food guides have been developed to help healthy people meet the daily requirements of essential nutrients and to facilitate meal planning. These include the *Dietary Guidelines for Americans* and the Food Guide Pyramid.
- Both inadequate and excessive intakes of nutrients result in malnutrition. The effects of malnutrition can be general or specific, depending on which nutrients and what level of deficiency or excess are involved.
- Assessment of nutritional status may involve all or some of the following: nursing history data, nutritional screening, physical examination, calculation of the percentage of weight loss, a dietary

history, anthropometric measurements, and laboratory data.
- Nursing diagnoses for clients with nutritional problems may be broadly stated as *Imbalanced Nutrition: Less Than Body Requirements* or *More Than Body Requirements*. Because nutritional problems may affect many other areas of human functioning, the nutritional problem may be the etiology of other diagnoses, such as *Activity Intolerance* and *Low Self-Esteem*.
- Major goals for clients with or at risk for nutritional problems include the following: maintain or restore optimal nutritional status, decrease or regain specified weight, promote healthy nutritional practices, and prevent complications associated with malnutrition.
- Assisting clients and support persons with therapeutic diets is a function shared by the nurse and the dietitian. The nurse reinforces the dietitian's instructions, assists the client to make beneficial changes, and evaluates the client's response to planned changes.
- Because many hospitalized clients have poor appetites, a major responsibility of the nurse is to provide nursing interventions that stimulate their appetites.
- Whenever possible, the nurse should help incapacitated clients to feed themselves; a number of self-feeding aids help clients who have difficulty handling regular utensils.
- The nurse can refer clients to various community programs that help special subgroups of the population meet their nutritional needs.
- Enteral feedings, administered through nasogastric, nasointestinal, gastrostomy, or jejunostomy tubes, are provided when the client is unable to ingest foods or the upper gastrointestinal tract is impaired.
- A nasogastric or nasointestinal tube is used to provide enteral nutrition for short-term use. A gastrostomy or jejunostomy tube can be used to supply nutrients via the enteral route for long-term use.
- The two most accurate methods of confirming gastrointestinal tube placement are radiographs and pH testing of aspirate.
- Aseptic technique is required during tube feedings.
- Parenteral nutrition (PN), provided when the gastrointestinal tract is nonfunctional (e.g., absorptive capacity impaired), is given intravenously into a large central vein (e.g., the superior vena cava).

TEST YOUR KNOWLEDGE

1. Which of the following nursing diagnoses is most appropriate for a client with a body mass index (BMI) of 35 would likely have?
   1. *Imbalanced Nutrition: Less Than Body Requirements*
   2. *Imbalanced Nutrition:* More *Than Body Requirements*
   3. *Risk for Imbalanced Nutrition*
   4. *Deficient Knowledge*

2. An adult reports eating, on average, the following each day: 3 cups dairy, 2 cups fruit, 2 cups vegetables, 5 ounces grains, and 5 ounces meat. The nurse would counsel the client to:
   1. Maintain the diet; the servings are adequate.
   2. Increase the number of servings of dairy.
   3. Decrease the number of servings of vegetables.
   4. Increase the number of servings of grains.

3. Which of the following are allowed on a full liquid diet? Select all that apply.
   _____ 1. Scrambled eggs
   _____ 2. Chocolate pudding
   _____ 3. Tomato juice
   _____ 4. Hard candy
   _____ 5. Mashed potatoes
   _____ 6. Cream of Wheat cereal
   _____ 7. Oatmeal cereal
   _____ 8. Fruit "smoothies"

4. Which of the following is the best indication of proper placement of a nasogastric tube in the stomach?
   1. Client is unable to speak.
   2. Client gags during insertion.
   3. pH of the aspirate is less than 5.
   4. Fluid is easily instilled into the tube.

5. What is the proper technique with gravity tube feeding?
   1. Feeding bag is hung 1 foot higher than the tube's insertion point into the client.
   2. Nurse administers the next feeding only if there is less than 25 mL of residual volume from the previous feeding.
   3. Place client in the left lateral position.
   4. Feeding is administered directly from the refrigerator.

6. A 55-year-old female is about 20 lb over her desired weight. She has been on a "low calorie" diet with no improvement. Which of the following statements reflects a healthy approach to the desired weight loss? "I need to:
   1. Increase my exercise to at least 30 minutes every day."
   2. Switch to a low-carbohydrate diet."
   3. Keep a list of my forbidden foods on hand at all times."
   4. Buy more organic and less processed foods."

7. An elderly Asian client has mild dysphagia from a recent stroke. The nurse plans the client's meals based on the need to:
   1. Have at least one serving of thick dairy (e.g., pudding, ice cream) per meal.
   2. Eliminate the beer usually ingested every evening.
   3. Include as many of the client's favorite foods as possible.
   4. Increase the calories from lipids to 40%.

8. Two (2) months ago a client weighed 195 pounds. The current weight is 182 pounds. Calculate the client's percent weight loss and determine its significance.

   _____ % weight loss

   _____ Not significant

   _____ Significant weight loss

   _____ Severe weight loss

9. Which of the sites on the diagram below indicates the correct location for the tip of a small-bore nasally placed feeding tube?

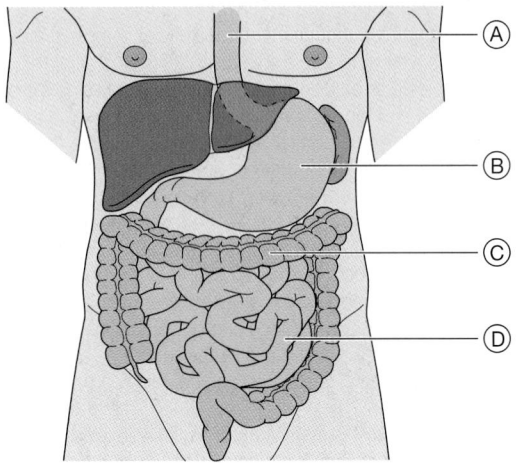

10. Which of the following meals would the nurse recommend to the client as highest in calcium, iron, and fiber?
   1. 3 ounces cottage cheese with 1/3 cup raisins and 1 banana
   2. 1/2 cup broccoli with 3 ounces chicken and 1/2 cup peanuts
   3. 1/2 cup spaghetti with 2 ounces ground beef and 1/2 cup lima beans plus 1/2 cup ice cream
   4. 3 ounces tuna plus 1 ounce cheese sandwich on whole wheat bread plus a pear

See Answers to Test Your Knowledge in Appendix A. ∞

EXPLORE MEDIALINK www.prenhall.com/berman

DVD-ROM
- Audio Glossary
- NCLEX Review
- Skills Checklists
- Videos:
     Anorexia
     Bulimia
     Eating Disorders
- Animations:
     Carbohydrates
     Proteins
     Lipids
     Inserting a Nasogastric Tube
     A & P Review

Cellular Metabolism
Organic Compounds

COMPANION WEBSITE
- Additional NCLEX Review
- Case Study: Client with PEG Tube
- Care Plan Activity: Client Experiencing Loss of Appetite
- Application Activity: Vegetarian Nutrition
- Links to Resources

READINGS AND REFERENCES

Padua, C. A., Kenny, A., Planchon, C., & Lamoureux, C. (2004). Enteral feedings: What the evidence says. *American Journal of Nursing, 104*(7), 62–70.
This continuing education article reviews the research evidence supporting the need for asepsis in the management of tube feedings. Clear do's and don'ts based on previous studies guide the nurse in preventing contamination of these systems.

RELATED RESEARCH
Evans, B., Crogan, N. L., & Shultz, J. A. (2005). The meaning of mealtimes: Connection in the social world of the nursing home. *Journal of Gerontological Nursing, 31*(2), 11–17.
Long, J. D., & Stevens, K. (2004). Using technology to promote self-efficacy for healthy eating in adolescents. *Journal of Nursing Scholarship, 36*, 134–139.
Wright, L., Cotter, D., Hickson, M., & Frost, G. (2005). Comparison of energy and protein intakes of older people consuming a texture modified diet with a normal hospital diet. *Journal of Human Nutrition and Dietetics, 18*, 213–219.

REFERENCES
American Academy of Pediatrics Section on Breastfeeding. (2005). Policy statement: Breastfeeding and the use of human milk. *Pediatrics, 115*, 496–506.

American Dietetic Association. (2003). *National dysphagia diet: Standardization for optimal care.* Chicago: Author.

American Psychological Association. (2004). *Report of the APA task force on advertising and children.* Washington, DC: Author. Retrieved June 25, 2006, from http://www.apa.org/releases/childrenads.pdf

Anonymous. (2003). Position of the American Dietetic Association and Dietitians of Canada: Vegetarian diets. *Journal of the American Dietetic Association, 103,* 748–765.

Beers, M. H., & Berkow, R. (Eds.). (2006). *The Merck manual of diagnosis and therapy* (18th ed.). New York: John Wiley & Sons. Online edition. Retrieved June 25, 2006, from http://www.merck.com/mrkshared/mmanual/section1/chapter1/1b.jsp

Centers for Disease Control and Prevention. National Center for Infectious Diseases. Division of Bacterial and Mycotic Diseases. (2005). *Botulism.* Retrieved June 25, 2006, from http://www.cdc.gov/ncidod/dbmd/diseaseinfo/botulism_g.htm

Dahan, A., & Altman, H. (2004). Food-drug interaction: Grapefruit juice augments drug bioavailability—mechanism, extent, and relevance. European Journal of Clinical *Nutrition, 58,* 1–9.

Daniels, J. (2004). Fad diets: Slim on good nutrition. *Nursing, 34*(12), 22–23.

Dochterman, J., & Bulechek, G. B. (Eds.). (2004). *Nursing interventions classification (NIC)* (4th ed.). St. Louis, MO: Mosby.

Green, S. M., & Watson, R. (2005). Nutritional screening and assessment tools for use by nurses: Literature review. *Journal of Advanced Nursing, 50,* 69–83.

Haddad, E. H., & Tanzman, J. S. (2003). What do vegetarians eat in the United States eat? *American Journal of Clinical Nutrition, 78,* 626S–632S.

Huffman, S., Jarczyk, K. S., O'Brien, E., Pieper, P., & Bayne, A. (2004). Methods to confirm feeding tube placement: Application of research to practice. *Pediatric Nursing, 30,* 10–13.

Institute of Medicine. (2003). *Dietary reference intakes: Applications in dietary planning.* Washington, DC: National Academies Press.

Kuszajewski, M. L., & Clontz, A. S. (2005). Prealbumin is best for nutritional monitoring. *Nursing, 35*(5), 70–71.

Kyle, U. G., Bosaeusb, I., De Lorenzoc, A. D., Deurenbergd, P., Elia, M., Gomez, J. M., et al. (2004). Bioelectrical impedance analysis part I: Review of principles and methods. *Clinical Nutrition, 23,* 1226–1243.

Leibovitch, E. R., Deamer, R. L., & Sanderson, L. A. (2004). Food-drug interactions: Care, drug selection and patient counseling can reduce the risk in older patients. *Geriatrics, 59,* 19–33.

Masters, J. A. (2005). Moderate drinking and cardiovascular disease. *Annual Review of Nursing Research, 23,* 65–97.

Maurer, J., Harris, M. M., Stanford, V. A., Lohman, T. G., Cussler, E., Going, S. B., et al. (2005). Dietary iron positively influences bone mineral density in postmenopausal women on hormone replacement therapy. *Journal of Nutrition, 135,* 863–869.

Metheny, N. A., & Meert, K. L. (2004). Monitoring feeding tube placement. *Nutrition in Clinical Practice, 19,* 487–495.

Moorhead, S., Johnson, M., & Maas, M. (Eds.). (2004). *Nursing outcomes classification (NOC)* (3rd ed.). St. Louis, MO: Mosby.

NANDA International (2007). *NANDA nursing diagnoses: Definitions and classification 2007–2008.* Philadelphia: Author.

National Heart, Lung, and Blood Institute. (1998). *Clinical guidelines on the identification, evaluation, and treatment of overweight and obesity in adults: The evidence report.* Washington, DC: U.S. Department of Health & Human Services. Retrieved June 25, 2006, from http://www.nhlbi.nih.gov/guidelines/obesity/ob_gdlns.htm

National Institute of Diabetes and Digestive and Kidney Diseases. (2006). *Lactose intolerance* (NIH Publication No. 06–2751). Bethesda, MD: Author. Retrieved June 25, 2006, from http://digestive.niddk.nih.gov/ddiseases/pubs/lactoseintolerance/#risk

Novartis Nutrition Corporation. (2003). *Nasogastric tube care and maintenance procedures.* New York: Author. Retrieved June 25, 2006, from http://www.novartisnutrition.com/us/productDetail?id=42

Nutrition Screening Initiative. (2003). *Determine your nutritional health.* Washington, DC: National Council on Aging.

Ogden, C. L., Carroll, M. D., Curtin, L. R., McDowell, M. A., Tabak, C. J., & Flegal, K. M. (2006). Prevalence of overweight and obesity in the United States, 1999–2004. *Journal of the American Medical Association, 295,* 1549–1555.

Pai, M. P., & Paloucek, F. P. (2000). The origin of the "Ideal" body weight equations. *The Annals of Pharmacotherapy, 34,* 1066–1069.

Pelletier, C. A. (2005). Feeding beliefs of certified nurse assistants in the nursing home: A factor influencing practice. *Journal of Gerontological Nursing, 31*(7), 5–10.

Reising, D. L., & Neal, R. S. (2005). Enteral tube flushing: What you think are the best practices may not be. *American Journal of Nursing, 105*(3), 58–64.

Rolfes, S. R., Pinna, K., & Whitney, E. (2006). *Understanding normal and clinical nutrition* (7th ed.). Belmont, CA: Thomson Wadsworth.

Sauvaget, C., Nagano, J., Hayashi, M., & Yamada, M. (2004). Animal protein, animal fat, and cholesterol intakes and risk of cerebral infarction mortality in the adult health study. *Stroke, 35,* 1531–1537.

Schettler, A. E., & Gustafson, E. M. (2004). Osteoporosis prevention starts in adolescence. *Journal of the American Academy of Nurse Practitioners, 16,* 274–282.

Smith, R. M., & Myers, S. A. (2005). Two devices that unclog feeding tubes. *RN, 68*(1), 36–41.

U.S. Department of Agriculture. (2005). *Dietary guidelines for Americans, 2005* (6th ed.). Washington, DC: Author. Retrieved August 23, 2006, from http://www.healthierus.gosdietaryguidelines

U.S. Department of Health and Human Services. (2000). *Healthy people 2010: Understanding and improving health* (2nd ed.). Washington, DC: U.S. Government Printing Office.

U.S. Food and Drug Administration (2004). How to understand and use the nutrition facts label, 2004. *Center for Food Safety & Applied Nutrition.* Retrieved September 4, 2006 from http://www.cfsan.fda.gov/~dms/foodlab.html#twoparts.

Zagaria, M. A. E. (2005). Implications of dysphagia in the elderly. *U.S. Pharmacist, 30,* 30–39. Retrieved June 25, 2006, from http://www.uspharmacist.com/index.asp?show=article&page=8_1410.htm

SELECTED BIBLIOGRAPHY

Blackwood, H. S. (2004). Obesity: A rapidly expanding challenge. *Nursing Management, 35*(5), 27–36.

DiMaria-Ghalili, R. A., & Amella, E. (2005). Nutrition in older adults: Intervention and assessment can help curb the growing threat of malnutrition. *American Journal of Nursing, 105*(3), 40–51.

Ellett, M. L. C. (2004). What is known about methods of correctly placing gastric tubes in adults and children. *Gastroenterology Nursing, 27,* 253–261.

Ellett, M. L. C., Beckstrand, J., Flueckiger, J., Perkins, S. M., & Johnson, C. S. (2005). Predicting the insertion distance for placing gastric tubes. *Clinical Nursing Research, 14,* 11–27.

Hogan, S. L. (2004). How to help wounds heal. *RN, 67*(8), 26–31.

Khair, J. (2005). Guidelines for testing the placement of nasogastric tubes. *Nursing Times, 101*(20), 26–27.

Lovegren, S. (2005). *Fashionable food: Seven decades of food fads.* Chicago: University of Chicago Press.

Metheny, N. A. (2004). Preventing aspiration in older adults with dysphagia. *Try this: Best Practices in Care to Older Adults.* Issue 20. The Hartford Institute for Geriatric Nursing. Retrieved June 25, 2006, from http://www.hartfordign.org/ resources/education/tryThis.html

Metheny, N. A. (2004). Effect of gastrointestinal motility and feeding tube site on aspiration risk in critically ill patients: A review. *Heart and Lung, 33,* 131–145.

Moyad, M. A. (2004). Fad diets and obesity—part I: Measuring weight in a clinical setting. *Urologic Nursing, 24,* 114–119.

Moyad, M. A. (2004). Fad diets and obesity—part II: An introduction to the theory behind low-carbohydrate diets. *Urologic Nursing, 24,* 210–213.

Moyad, M. A. (2004). Fad diets and obesity—part III: A rapid review of some of the more popular low-carbohydrate diets. *Urologic Nursing, 24,* 442–445.

Moyad, M. A. (2005). Fad diets and obesity—part IV: Low-carbohydrate vs. low-fat diets. *Urologic Nursing, 25,* 67–70.

Noble, K. A. (2003). Name that tube. *Nursing, 33*(3), 56–63.

Overstreet, M. (2004). How does a PEG tube stay in? *Nursing, 34*(6), 21.

Thoyre, S. (2003). Techniques for feeding preterm infants. *American Journal of Nursing, 103*(9), 69, 71–72.

U.S. Food and Drug Administration. (2003). *Reports of blue discoloration and death in patients receiving enteral feedings tinted with the dye, FD&C blue no. 1.* Retrieved June 25, 2006, from http://www.cfsan.fda.gov/~dms/col-ltr2.html

U.S. Preventive Services Task Force. (2003). Behavioral counseling in primary care to promote a healthy diet: Recommendations and rationale. *American Journal of Nursing, 103*(8), 81–90.

Walker, B. W. (2004). Beating botulism. *Nursing, 34*(6), 74.

Westhus, N. (2004). Methods to test feeding tube placement in children. *American Journal of Maternal Child Nursing, 29,* 282–287.

Williams, S. R., & Schlenker, E. (2003). *Essentials of nutrition and diet therapy* (8th ed.). St. Louis, MO: Mosby.

Williams, T. A., & Leslie, G. D. (2004). A review of the nursing care of enteral feeding tubes in critically ill adults: Part 1. *Intensive and Critical Care Nursing, 20,* 330–343.

Williams, T. A., & Leslie, G. D. (2005). A review of the nursing care of enteral feeding tubes in critically ill adults: Part 2. *Intensive and Critical Care Nursing, 21,* 5–15.

CHAPTER 48

Urinary Elimination

LEARNING OUTCOMES

After completing this chapter, you will be able to:

1. Describe the process of urination, from urine formation through micturition.

2. Identify factors that influence urinary elimination.

3. Identify common causes of selected urinary problems.

4. Describe nursing assessment of urinary function, including subjective and objective data.

5. Identify normal and abnormal characteristics and constituents of urine.

6. Develop nursing diagnoses, desired outcomes, and interventions related to urinary elimination.

7. Delineate ways to prevent urinary infection.

8. Explain the care of clients with retention catheters or urinary diversions.

Elimination from the urinary tract is usually taken for granted. Only when a problem arises do most people become aware of their urinary habits and any associated symptoms.

A person's urinary habits depend on social culture, personal habits, and physical abilities. In North America, most people are accustomed to privacy and clean (even decorative) surroundings while they urinate.

Personal habits regarding urination are affected by the social propriety of leaving to urinate, the availability of a private clean facility, and initial bladder training. Urinary elimination is essential to health, and voiding can be postponed for only so long before the urge normally becomes too great to control.

PHYSIOLOGY OF URINARY ELIMINATION

Urinary elimination depends on effective functioning of the upper urinary tract: kidneys and ureters; and the lower urinary tract: urinary bladder, urethra, and pelvic floor (Figure 48-1 ■).

Kidneys

The paired kidneys are situated on either side of the spinal column, behind the peritoneal cavity. The right kidney is slightly lower than the left due to the position of the liver. They are the primary regulators of fluid and acid–base balance in the body. The functional units of the kidneys, the nephrons, filter the blood and remove metabolic wastes. In the average adult 1,200 mL of blood, or about 21% of the cardiac output, passes through the kidneys every minute. Each kidney contains approximately 1 million nephrons. Each nephron has a **glomerulus,** a tuft of capillaries surrounded by Bowman's capsule (Figure 48-2 ■). The endothelium of glomerular capillaries is porous, allowing fluid and solutes to readily move across this membrane into the capsule. Plasma proteins and blood cells, however, are too large to cross the membrane normally. Glomerular filtrate is similar in composition to plasma, made up of water, electrolytes, glucose, amino acids, and metabolic wastes.

From Bowman's capsule the filtrate moves into the tubule of the nephron. In the proximal convoluted tubule, most of the water

and electrolytes are reabsorbed. Solutes such as glucose are reabsorbed in the loop of Henle, but in the same area, other substances are secreted into the filtrate, concentrating the urine. In the distal convoluted tubule, additional water and sodium are reabsorbed under the control of hormones such as antidiuretic hormone (ADH) and aldosterone. This controlled reabsorption allows fine regulation of fluid and electrolyte balance in the body. When fluid intake is low or the concentration of solutes in the blood is high, ADH is released from the anterior pituitary, more water is reabsorbed in the distal tubule, and less urine is excreted. By contrast, when fluid intake is high or the blood solute concentration is low,

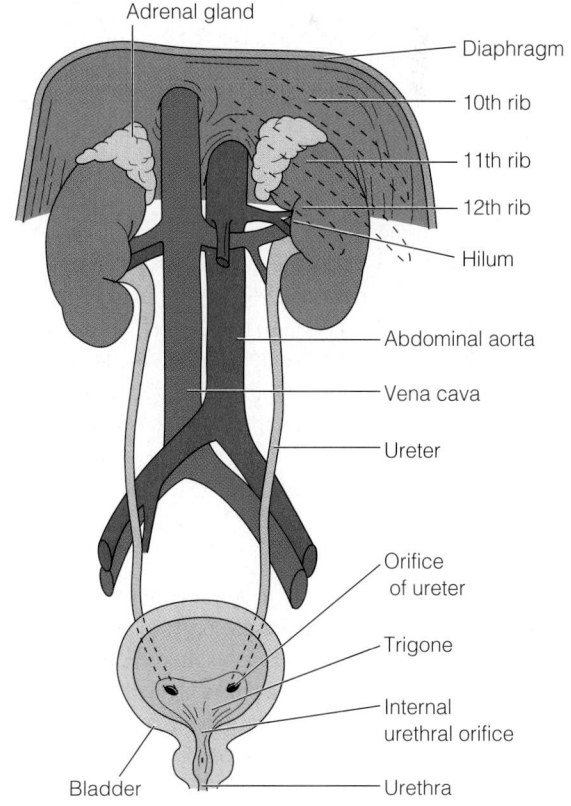

Figure 48-1 ■ Anatomic structures of the urinary tract.

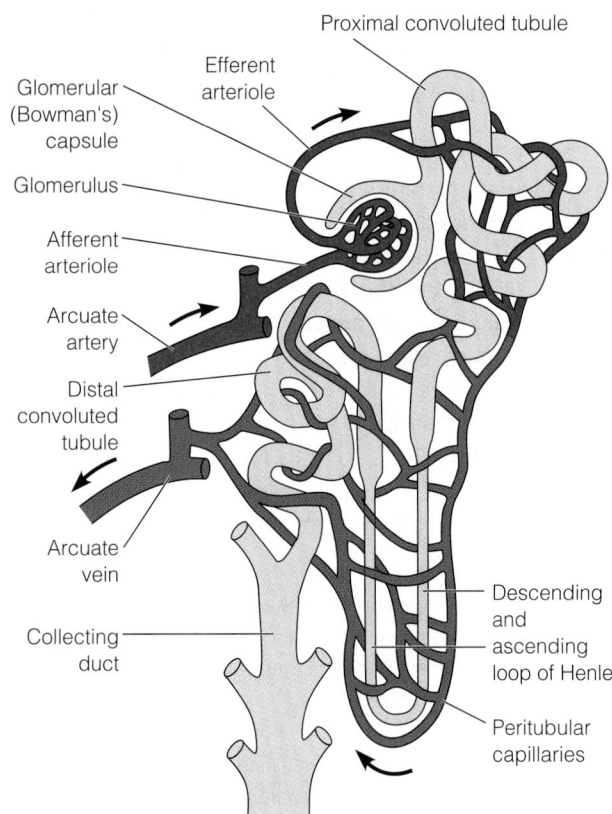

Figure 48-2 ■ The nephrons of the kidney are composed of six parts: the glomerulus, Bowman's capsule, proximal convoluted tubule, loop of Henle, distal convoluted tubule, and collecting duct.

ADH is suppressed. Without ADH, the distal tubule becomes impermeable to water, and more urine is excreted. Aldosterone also affects the tubule. When aldosterone is released from the adrenal cortex, sodium and water are reabsorbed in greater quantities, increasing the blood volume and decreasing urinary output.

Ureters

Once the urine is formed in the kidneys, it moves through the collecting ducts into the calyces of the renal pelvis and from there into the ureters. The ureters are from 25 to 30 cm (10 to 12 in.) long in the adult and about 1.25 cm (0.5 in.) in diameter. The upper end of each ureter is funnel shaped as it enters the kidney. The lower ends of the ureters enter the bladder at the posterior corners of the floor of the bladder (see Figure 48-1). At the junction between the ureter and the bladder, a flaplike fold of mucous membrane acts as a valve to prevent **reflux** (backflow) of urine up the ureters.

Bladder

The urinary bladder (vesicle) is a hollow, muscular organ that serves as a reservoir for urine and as the organ of excretion. When empty, it lies behind the symphysis pubis. In men, the bladder lies in front of the rectum and above the prostate gland (Figure 48-3 ■); in women it lies in front of the uterus and vagina (Figure 48-4 ■). The wall of the bladder is made up of four layers: (a) an inner mucous layer, (b) a connective tissue layer, (c) three layers of smooth muscle fibers, some of which extend lengthwise, some obliquely, and some more or less circularly, and (d) an outer serous layer. The

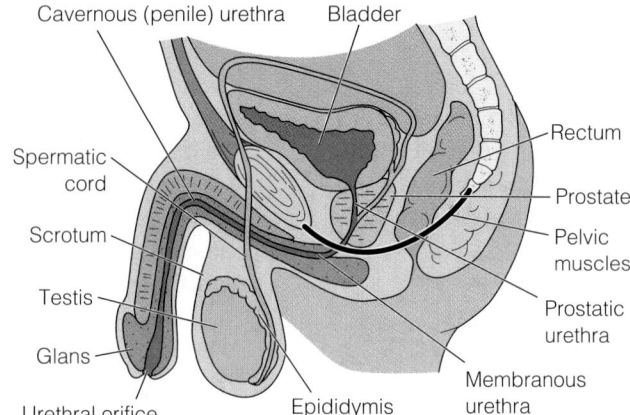

Figure 48-3 ■ The male urogenital system.

smooth muscle layers are collectively called the **detrusor muscle.** The detrusor muscle allows the bladder to expand as it fills with urine, and to contract to release urine to the outside of the body during voiding (D'Amico & Barbarito, 2007, p. 557). The **trigone** at the base of the bladder is a triangular area marked by the ureter openings at the posterior corners and the opening of the urethra at the anterior inferior corner (see Figure 48-1).

The bladder is capable of considerable distention because of rugae (folds) in the mucous membrane lining and because of the elasticity of its walls. When full, the dome of the bladder may extend above the symphysis pubis; in extreme situations, it may extend as high as the umbilicus. Normal bladder capacity is between 300 and 600 mL of urine.

Urethra

The urethra extends from the bladder to the urinary **meatus** (opening). In the adult woman, the urethra lies directly behind the symphysis pubis, anterior to the vagina, and is between 3 and 4 cm (1.5 in.) long (see Figure 48-4). The urethra serves only as a passageway for the elimination of urine. The urinary meatus is located between the labia minora, in front of the vagina and below the clitoris. The male urethra is aproximately 20 cm (8 in.) long and serves as a passageway for semen as well as urine (see Figure 48-3). The meatus is located at the distal end of the penis.

In both men and women, the urethra has a mucous membrane lining that is continuous with the bladder and the ureters. Thus, an infection of the urethra can extend through the urinary tract

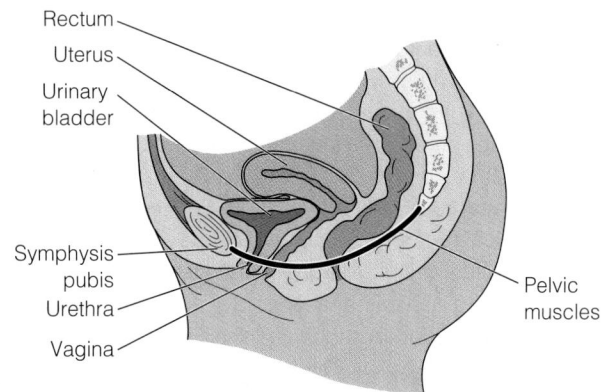

Figure 48-4 ■ The female urogenital system.

to the kidneys. Women are particularly prone to urinary tract infections because of their short urethra and the proximity of the urinary meatus to the vagina and anus.

Pelvic Floor

The vagina and the urethra and rectum pass through the pelvic floor which consists of sheets of muscles and ligaments that provide support to the viscera of the pelvis (Figures 48-3 and 48-4). They extend from the symphysis pubis to the coccyx forming a sling. Specific sphincter muscles contribute to the continence mechanism (see the Anatomy & Physiology Review). The internal sphincter muscle situated in the proximal urethra and the bladder neck is composed of smooth muscle under *involuntary* control. It provides active tension designed to close the urethral lumen. The external sphincter muscle is composed of skeletal muscle under *voluntary* control, allowing the individual to choose when urine is eliminated.

Urination

Micturition, voiding, and **urination** all refer to the process of emptying the urinary bladder. Urine collects in the bladder until pressure stimulates special sensory nerve endings in the bladder wall called stretch receptors. This occurs when the adult bladder contains between 250 and 450 mL of urine. In children, a considerably smaller volume, 50 to 200 mL, stimulates these nerves.

The stretch receptors transmit impulses to the spinal cord, specifically to the voiding reflex center located at the level of the second to fourth sacral vertebrae, causing the internal sphincter to relax and stimulating the urge to void. If the time and place are appropriate for urination, the conscious portion of the brain relaxes the external urethral sphincter muscle and urination takes place. If the time and place are inappropriate, the micturition reflex usually subsides until the bladder becomes more filled and the reflex is stimulated again.

MediaLink

A & P Review Animation

ANATOMY & PHYSIOLOGY REVIEW   Female and Male Urinary Bladders and Urethras

The pelvic floor muscles are under voluntary control and are important in controlling urination (continence). These muscles can become weakened by pregnancy and childbirth, chronic constipation, a decrease in estrogen (menopause), being overweight, aging, and lack of general fitness.

Review the figures and find the pelvic floor muscles.

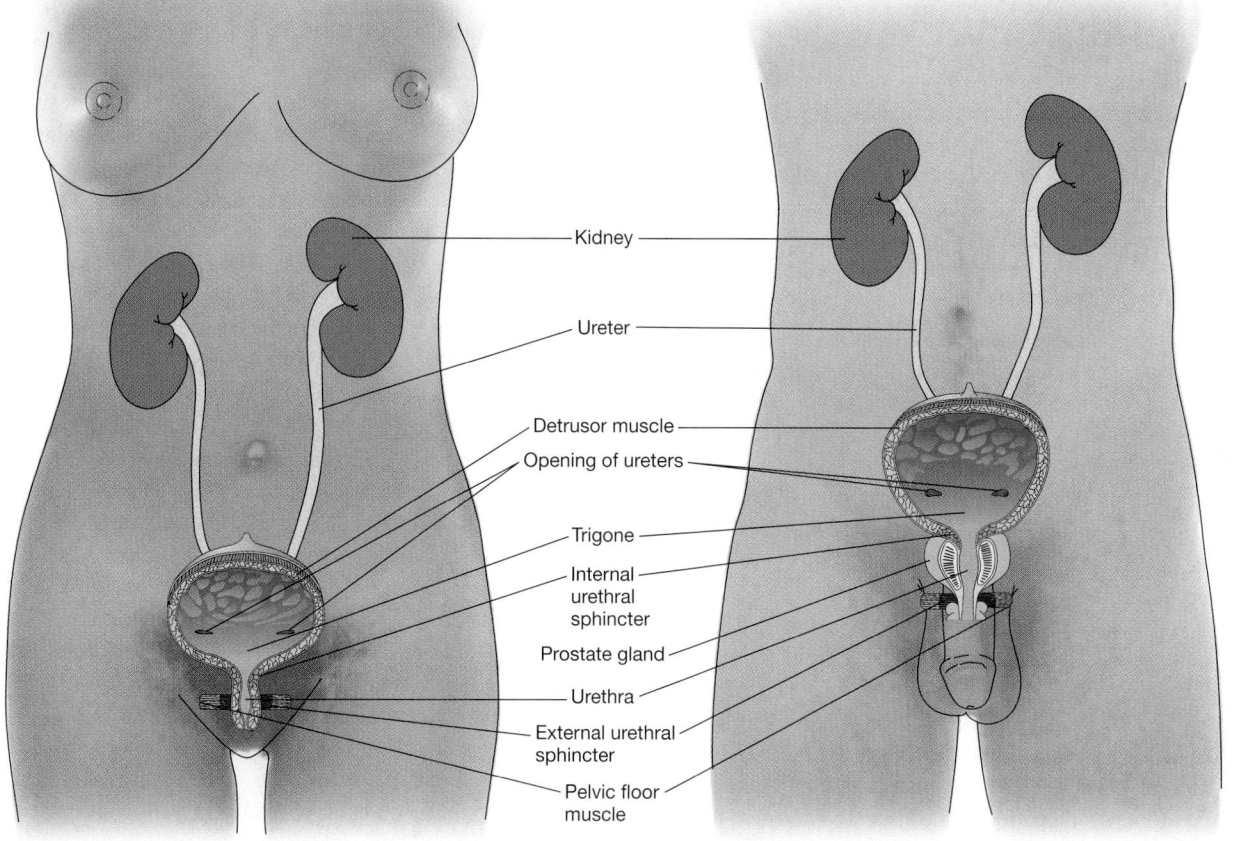

Kidney
Ureter
Detrusor muscle
Opening of ureters
Trigone
Internal urethral sphincter
Prostate gland
Urethra
External urethral sphincter
Pelvic floor muscle

(Custom Medical Stock Photo, Inc.)

QUESTIONS
1. Do you think pelvic floor muscles can be strengthened? Provide your rationale.
2. Explain how exercising the pelvic floor muscles helps to control urination.

Voluntary control of urination is possible only if the nerves supplying the bladder and urethra, the neural tracts of the cord and brain, and the motor area of the cerebrum are all intact. The individual must be able to sense that the bladder is full. Injury to any of these parts of the nervous system—for example, by a cerebral hemorrhage or spinal cord injury above the level of the sacral region—results in intermittent involuntary emptying of the bladder. Elders whose cognition is impaired may not be aware of the need to urinate or able to respond to this urge by seeking toilet facilities.

FACTORS AFFECTING VOIDING

Numerous factors affect the volume and characteristics of the urine produced and the manner in which it is excreted.

Developmental Factors

Infants

Urine output varies according to fluid intake but gradually increases to 250 to 500 mL a day during the first year. An infant may urinate as often as 20 times a day. The urine of the neonate is colorless and odorless and has a specific gravity of 1.008. Because newborns and infants have immature kidneys, they are unable to concentrate urine very effectively.

Infants are born without urinary control. Most will develop this between the ages of 2 and 5 years. Control during the daytime normally precedes nighttime control.

Preschoolers

The preschooler is able to take responsibility for independent toileting. Parents need to realize that accidents do occur and the child should never be punished or chastised for this. Children often forget to wash their hands or flush the toilet and need instruction in wiping themselves. Girls should be taught to wipe from front to back to prevent contamination of the urinary tract by feces.

School-Age Children

The school-age child's elimination system reaches maturity during this period. The kidneys double in size between ages 5 and 10 years. During this period, the child urinates six to eight times a day. **Enuresis,** which is defined as the involuntary passing of urine when control should be established (about 5 years of age), can be a problem for some school-age children. About 10% of all 6-year-olds experience difficulty controlling the bladder. **Nocturnal enuresis,** or bed-wetting, is the involuntary passing of urine during sleep. It has many causes but basically it occurs because the client fails to awaken when the bladder empties (Nield & Kamat, 2004, p. 409). Bed-wetting should not be considered a problem until after the age of 6. Nocturnal enuresis may be referred to as primary when the child has never achieved nighttime urinary control. The incidence of nocturnal enuresis declines as the child matures. Secondary enuresis is that which appears after the child has achieved dryness for a period of 6 consecutive months. It is often related to another problem such as constipation, stress, or illness and may resolve when the cause is eliminated. Recent research indicates that primary and secondary nocturnal enuresis may both be related to poor daytime voiding habits, and children should be taught to be aware of the sensation to void (Robson, Leung, & Van Howe, 2005).

Elders

The excretory function of the kidney diminishes with age, but usually not significantly below normal levels unless a disease process intervenes. Blood flow can be reduced by arteriosclerosis, impairing renal function. With age, the number of functioning nephrons decreases to some degree, impairing the kidney's filtering abilities. Conditions that alter normal fluid intake and output, such as having influenza or having surgery, can compromise the kidney's ability to filter, maintain acid–base balance, and maintain electrolyte balance in elders. It also takes a much longer time for these processes to return to normal functioning. The decrease in kidney function also places the elder at higher risk for toxicity from medications if excretion rates are longer.

The more noticeable changes with age are those related to the bladder. Complaints of urinary urgency and urinary frequency are common. In men these changes are often due to an enlarged prostate gland, and in women they may be due to weakened muscles supporting the bladder or weakness of the urethral sphincter. The capacity of the bladder and its ability to completely empty diminish with age. This explains the need for elders to arise during the night to void (**nocturnal frequency**) and the retention of residual urine, predisposing the elder to bladder infections.

See Table 48–1 for a summary of the developmental changes affecting urinary output and the Lifespan Considerations feature.

Psychosocial Factors

For many people, a set of conditions helps stimulate the micturition reflex. These conditions include privacy, normal position, sufficient time, and, occasionally, running water. Circumstances that do not allow for the client's accustomed conditions may produce anxiety and muscle tension. As a result, the person is unable to relax abdominal and perineal muscles and the external urethral sphincter, and voiding is inhibited. People also may voluntarily suppress urination because of perceived time pressures; for example, nurses often ignore the urge to void until they are able to take a break. This behavior can increase the risk of urinary tract infections.

Fluid and Food Intake

The healthy body maintains a balance between the amount of fluid ingested and the amount of fluid eliminated. When the amount of fluid intake increases, therefore, the output normally increases. Certain fluids, such as alcohol, increase fluid output by inhibiting the production of antidiuretic hormone. Fluids that contain caffeine (e.g., coffee, tea, and cola drinks) also increase urine production. By contrast, food and fluids high in sodium can cause fluid retention because water is retained to maintain the normal concentration of electrolytes.

Some foods and fluids can change the color of urine. For example, beets can cause urine to appear red; foods containing carotene can cause the urine to appear yellower than usual.

Medications

Many medications, particularly those affecting the autonomic nervous system, interfere with the normal urination process and

TABLE 48-1	**Changes in Urinary Elimination through the Life Span**
STAGE	**VARIATIONS**
Fetuses	The fetal kidney begins to excrete urine between the 11th and 12th week of development.
Infants	Ability to concentrate urine is minimal; therefore, urine appears light yellow.
	Because of neuromuscular immaturity, voluntary urinary control is absent.
Children	Kidney function reaches maturity between the first and second year of life; urine is concentrated effectively and appears a normal amber color.
	Between 18 and 24 months of age, the child starts to recognize bladder fullness and is able to hold urine beyond the urge to void.
	At approximately 2 1/2 to 3 years of age, the child can perceive bladder fullness, hold urine after the urge to void, and communicate the need to urinate.
	Full urinary control usually occurs at age 4 or 5 years; daytime control is usually achieved by age 3 years.
	The kidneys grow in proportion to overall body growth.
Adults	The kidneys reach maximum size between 35 and 40 years of age.
	After 50 years, the kidneys begin to diminish in size and function. Most shrinkage occurs in the cortex of the kidney as individual nephrons are lost.
Elders	An estimated 30% of nephrons are lost by age 80.
	Renal blood flow decreases because of vascular changes and a decrease in cardiac output.
	The ability to concentrate urine declines.
	Bladder muscle tone diminishes, causing increased frequency of urination and nocturia (awakening to urinate at night).
	Diminished bladder muscle tone and contractility may lead to residual urine in the bladder after voiding, increasing the risk of bacterial growth and infection.
	Urinary incontinence may occur due to mobility problems or neurologic impairments.

may cause retention (see Box 48–1). **Diuretics** (e.g., chlorothiazide and furosemide) increase urine formation by preventing the reabsorption of water and electrolytes from the tubules of the kidney into the bloodstream. Some medications may alter the color of the urine.

Muscle Tone

Good muscle tone is important to maintain the stretch and contractility of the detrusor muscle so the bladder can fill adequately and empty completely. Clients who require a retention catheter for a long period may have poor bladder muscle tone

LIFESPAN CONSIDERATIONS   Factors Affecting Voiding

INFANTS AND CHILDREN

- Urinary tract infections (UTIs) are the second most common infection in children, after respiratory infections. They are seen more frequently in newborn and young infant boys than girls and are most often due to obstructions or malformations of the urinary system in these children (Ball & Bindler, 2006). In older infants and children, girls have more UTIs than boys, usually due to contamination of the urethra with stool (Cavagnaro, 2005).
- Teaching proper perineal hygiene can reduce infection. Girls should learn to wipe from front to back and wear cotton underwear.
- Teach children and parents that they should go to the bathroom as soon as the sensation to void is felt and not try to hold the urine in.

ELDERS

Many changes of aging cause specific problems in urinary elimination in the older adult. Many conditions can be treated and interventions can be used to either resolve or decrease the problem. Some of the following conditions are etiological factors in problems with urinary elimination:

- Many older men have enlarged prostate glands, which can inhibit complete emptying of the bladder resulting in urinary retention and urgency which sometimes causes incontinence.

- Women past menopause have decreased estrogen, which results in a decrease in perineal tone and support of bladder, vagina, and supporting tissues. This often results in urgency and stress incontinence and can even increase the incidence of urinary tract infections.
- Increased stiffness and pain in joints, previous joint surgery, and neuromuscular problems can impair mobility and often make it difficult to get to the bathroom.
- Cognitive impairment, such as in dementia, often prevents the person from understanding the need to urinate and the actions needed to perform the activity.

Interventions that may improve these conditions include:

- Medications or surgery to relieve obstructions in men and strengthen support in the urogenital area in women.
- Behavioral training for better bladder control.
- Providing safe, easy access to the bathroom or bedside commode, whether at home or in an institution. Make sure the room is well lit, the environment is safe, and the proper assistive devices are within reach (such as walkers, canes).
- Habit training, such as taking the person to the bathroom at a regular, scheduled time. This can often work very well with cognitively impaired persons.

1290 UNIT X / Promoting Physiologic Health

BOX 48–1 Medications that May Cause Urinary Retention

- Anticholinergic and antispasmodic medications, such as atropine and papaverine
- Antidepressant and antipsychotic agents, such as phenothiazines and MAO inhibitors
- Antihistamine preparations, such as pseudoephedrine (Actifed and Sudafed)
- Antihypertensives, such as hydralazine (Apresoline) and methyldopate (Aldomet)
- Antiparkinsonism drugs, such as levodopa, trihexyphenidyl (Artane), and benztropine mesylate (Cogentin)
- Beta-adrenergic blockers, such as propranolol (Inderal)
- Opioids, such as hydrocodone (Vicodin)

TABLE 48–2 Average Daily Urine Output by Age

AGE	AMOUNT (ML)
1 to 2 days	15–60
3 to 10 days	100–300
10 days to 2 months	250–450
2 months to 1 year	400–500
1 to 3 years	500–600
3 to 5 years	600–700
5 to 8 years	700–1,000
8 to 14 years	800–1,400
14 years through adulthood	1,500
Older adulthood	1,500 or less

because continuous drainage of urine prevents the bladder from filling and emptying normally. Pelvic muscle tone also contributes to the ability to store and empty urine.

Pathologic Conditions

Some diseases and pathologies can affect the formation and excretion of urine. Diseases of the kidneys may affect the ability of the nephrons to produce urine. Abnormal amounts of protein or blood cells may be present in the urine, or the kidneys may virtually stop producing urine altogether, a condition known as renal failure. Heart and circulatory disorders such as heart failure, shock, or hypertension can affect blood flow to the kidneys, interfering with urine production. If abnormal amounts of fluid are lost through another route (e.g., vomiting or high fever), water is retained by the kidneys and urinary output falls.

Processes that interfere with the flow of urine from the kidneys to the urethra affect urinary excretion. A urinary stone (calculus) may obstruct a ureter, blocking urine flow from the kidney to the bladder. Hypertrophy of the prostate gland, a common condition affecting older men, may obstruct the urethra, impairing urination and bladder emptying.

Surgical and Diagnostic Procedures

Some surgical and diagnostic procedures affect the passage of urine and the urine itself. The urethra may swell following a cystoscopy, and surgical procedures on any part of the urinary tract may result in some postoperative bleeding; as a result, the urine may be red or pink tinged for a time.

Spinal anesthetics can affect the passage of urine because they decrease the client's awareness of the need to void. Surgery on structures adjacent to the urinary tract (e.g., the uterus) can also affect voiding because of swelling in the lower abdomen.

ALTERED URINE PRODUCTION

Although people's patterns of urination are highly individual, most people void about 5 to 6 times a day. People usually void when they first awaken in the morning, before they go to bed, and around mealtimes. Table 48–2 shows the average urinary output per day at different ages.

Polyuria

Polyuria (or **diuresis**) refers to the production of abnormally large amounts of urine by the kidneys, often several liters more than the client's usual daily output. Polyuria can follow excessive fluid intake, a condition known as **polydipsia,** or may be associated with diseases such as diabetes mellitus, diabetes insipidus, and chronic nephritis. Polyuria can cause excessive fluid loss, leading to intense thirst, dehydration, and weight loss.

Oliguria and Anuria

The terms *oliguria* and *anuria* are used to describe decreased urinary output. **Oliguria** is low urine output, usually less than 500 mL a day or 30 mL an hour for an adult. Although oliguria may occur because of abnormal fluid losses or a lack of fluid intake, it often indicates impaired blood flow to the kidneys or impending renal failure and should be promptly reported to the primary care provider. Restoring renal blood flow and urinary output promptly can prevent renal failure and its complications. **Anuria** refers to a lack of urine production.

Should the kidneys become unable to adequately function, some mechanism of filtering the blood is necessary to prevent illness and death. This filtering is done though the use of renal **dialysis,** a technique by which fluids and molecules pass through a semipermeable membrane according to the rules of osmosis. The two most common methods of dialysis are hemodialysis and peritoneal dialysis. In hemodialysis, the client's blood flows through vascular catheters, passes by the dialysis solution in an external machine, and then returns to the client. In peritoneal dialysis, the dialysis solution is instilled into the abdominal cavity through a catheter, allowed to rest there while the fluid and molecules exchange, and then removed through the catheter. Both hemodialysis and peritoneal dialysis must be performed at frequent intervals until the client's kidneys can resume the filtering function.

ALTERED URINARY ELIMINATION

Despite normal urine production, a number of factors or conditions can affect urinary elimination. Frequency, nocturia, urgency, and dysuria often are manifestations of underlying

TABLE 48–3 Selected Factors Associated with Altered Urinary Elimination

PATTERN	SELECTED ASSOCIATED FACTORS
Polyuria	Ingestion of fluids containing caffeine or alcohol
	Prescribed diuretic
	Presence of thirst, dehydration, and weight loss
	History of diabetes mellitus, diabetes insipidus, or kidney disease
Oliguria, anuria	Decrease in fluid intake
	Signs of dehydration
	Presence of hypotension, shock, or heart failure
	History of kidney disease
	Signs of renal failure such as elevated blood urea nitrogen (BUN) and serum creatinine, edema, hypertension
Frequency or nocturia	Pregnancy
	Increase in fluid intake
	Urinary tract infection
Urgency	Presence of psychologic stress
	Urinary tract infection
Dysuria	Urinary tract inflammation, infection, or injury
	Hesitancy, hematuria, pyuria (pus in the urine), and frequency
Enuresis	Family history of enuresis
	Difficult access to toilet facilities
	Home stresses
Incontinence	Bladder inflammation or other disease
	Difficulties in independent toileting (mobility impairment)
	Leakage when coughing, laughing, sneezing
	Cognitive impairment
Retention	Distended bladder on palpation and percussion
	Associated signs, such as pubic discomfort, restlessness, frequency, and small urine volume
	Recent anesthesia
	Recent perineal surgery
	Presence of perineal swelling
	Medications prescribed
	Lack of privacy or other factors inhibiting micturition

conditions such as a urinary tract infection. Enuresis, incontinence, retention, and neurogenic bladder may be either a manifestation or the primary problem affecting urinary elimination. Selected factors associated with altered patterns of urine elimination are identified in Table 48–3.

Frequency and Nocturia

Urinary frequency is voiding at frequent intervals, that is, more than 4 to 6 times per day. An increased intake of fluid causes some increase in the frequency of voiding. Conditions such as urinary tract infection, stress, and pregnancy can cause frequent voiding of small quantities (50 to 100 mL) of urine. Total fluid intake and output may be normal.

   Nocturia is voiding two or more times at night. Like frequency, it is usually expressed in terms of the number of times the person gets out of bed to void, for example, "nocturia × 4."

Urgency

Urgency is the sudden strong desire to void. There may or may not be a great deal of urine in the bladder, but the person feels a need to void immediately. Urgency accompanies psychologic

stress and irritation of the trigone and urethra. It is also common in people who have poor external sphincter control and unstable bladder contractions. It is not a normal finding.

Dysuria

Dysuria means voiding that is either painful or difficult. It can accompany a stricture (decrease in caliber) of the urethra, urinary infections, and injury to the bladder and urethra. Often clients will say they have to push to void or that burning accompanies or follows voiding. The burning may be described as severe, like a hot poker, or more subdued, like a sunburn. Often, **urinary hesitancy** (a delay and difficulty in initiating voiding) is associated with dysuria.

Enuresis

Enuresis is involuntary urination in children beyond the age when voluntary bladder control is normally acquired, usually 4 or 5 years of age. Nocturnal enuresis often is irregular in occurrence and affects boys more often than girls. Diurnal (daytime) enuresis may be persistent and pathologic in origin. It affects women and girls more frequently.

Urinary Incontinence

Urinary incontinence, or involuntary urination, is a symptom, not a disease. It can have a significant impact on the client's life, creating physical problems such as skin breakdown and possibly leading to psychosocial problems such as embarrassment, isolation, and social withdrawal. Common causes of incontinence include urinary tract infections, urethritis, pregnancy, hypercalcemia, volume overload, delirium, restricted mobility, stool impaction, and psychologic causes (Morantz, 2005, p. 175). Urinary incontinence can be broken into two categories: acute and chronic.

Acute

Many factors can contribute to acute or reversible incontinence, including polyuria, exposure to irritants, infection, urinary retention, use of pharmaceuticals, stool impaction or constipation, atrophic urethritis or vaginitis, restricted mobility or dexterity, psychologic conditions, and delirium or acute confused state. Some of these factors are readily reversible with a lessening of syptoms if not complete resolution of urinary incontinence.

Chronic

There are different types of chronic incontinence, each having a different etiology, including stress, urge, reflex, retention with overflow, and functional incontinence. NANDA categorizes five types of incontinence (see "Diagnosing" on page 1294). Although incontinence is experienced in some elders, it is *not* a normal consequence of aging and can often be treated.

The preliminary assessment and identification of the symptom of urinary incontinence is truly within the scope of nursing practice. All clients should be asked about their voiding patterns. Elders who are incontinent while in their home or who manage to contain or conceal their incontinence from others do not consider themselves incontinent. Therefore, if asked if they are incontinent, they may deny it. However, asking if they lose urine when they don't want to may provide more accurate information (Palmer & Newman, 2006). If incontinence is described, a thorough history and assessment is indicated. Treatment may include surgery, medication, or behavioral therapies. Nursing management of incontinence includes implementing individualized bladder programs, containment of urine, and meticulous skin care.

Urinary Retention

When emptying of the bladder is impaired, urine accumulates and the bladder becomes overdistended, a condition known as **urinary retention.** Overdistention of the bladder causes poor contractility of the detrusor muscle, further impairing urination. Common causes of urinary retention include prostatic hypertrophy (enlargement), surgery, and some medications (see Box 48–1).

Clients with urinary retention may experience overflow voiding or incontinence, eliminating 25 to 50 mL of urine at frequent intervals. The bladder is firm and distended on palpation and may be displaced to one side of midline.

Neurogenic Bladder

Impaired neurologic function can interfere with the normal mechanisms of urine elimination, resulting in a **neurogenic**

bladder. The client with a neurogenic bladder does not perceive bladder fullness and is unable to control the urinary sphincters. The bladder may become flaccid and distended or spastic, with frequent involuntary urination.

NURSING MANAGEMENT

Assessing

A complete assessment of a client's urinary function includes the following:

- Nursing history
- Physical assessment of the genitourinary system, hydration status, and examination of the urine
- Relating the data obtained to the results of any diagnostic tests and procedures

Nursing History

The nurse determines the client's normal voiding pattern and frequency, appearance of the urine and any recent changes, any past or current problems with urination, the presence of an ostomy, and factors influencing the elimination pattern.

Examples of interview questions to elicit this information are shown in the Assessment Interview. The number of questions asked depends on the individual and the responses to the first three categories.

Physical Assessment

Complete physical assessment of the urinary tract usually includes percussion of the kidneys to detect areas of tenderness. Palpation and percussion of the bladder are also performed. If the client's history or current problems indicate a need for it, the urethral meatus of both male and female clients is inspected for swelling, discharge, and inflammation.

Because problems with urination can affect the elimination of wastes from the body, it is important that the nurse assess the skin for color, texture, and tissue turgor as well as the presence of edema. If incontinence, dribbling, or dysuria is noted in the history, the skin of the perineum should be inspected for irritation because contact with urine can excoriate the skin.

Assessing Urine

Normal urine consists of 96% water and 4% solutes. Organic solutes include urea, ammonia, creatinine, and uric acid. Urea is the chief organic solute. Inorganic solutes include sodium, chloride, potassium, sulfate, magnesium, and phosphorus. Sodium chloride is the most abundant inorganic salt. Variations in color can occur. Characteristics of normal and abnormal urine are shown in Table 48–4.

MEASURING URINARY OUTPUT. Normally, the kidneys produce urine at a rate of approximately 60 mL per hour or about 1,500 mL per day. Urine output is affected by many factors, including fluid intake, body fluid losses through other routes such as perspiration and breathing or diarrhea, and the cardiovascular and renal status of the individual.

ASSESSMENT INTERVIEW Urinary Elimination

VOIDING PATTERN

- How many times do you urinate during a 24-hour period?
- Has this pattern changed recently?
- Do you need to get out of bed to void at night? How often?

DESCRIPTION OF URINE AND ANY CHANGES

- How would you describe your urine in terms of color, clarity (clear, transparent, or cloudy), and odor (faint or strong)?

URINARY ELIMINATION PROBLEMS

- What problems have you had or do you now have with passing your urine?
- Passage of small amounts of urine?
- Voiding at intervals that are more frequent?
- Trouble getting to the bathroom in time or feeling an urgent need to void?
- Painful voiding?
- Difficulty starting urine stream?
- Frequent dribbling of urine or feeling of bladder fullness associated with voiding small amounts of urine?
- Reduced force of stream?

- Accidental leakage of urine? If so, when does this occur (e.g., when coughing, laughing, or sneezing; at night; during the day)?
- Past urinary tract illness such as infection of the kidney, bladder, or urethra; urinary calculi; surgery of kidney, ureters, or bladder?

FACTORS INFLUENCING URINARY ELIMINATION

- Medications. Do you take any medications that could increase urinary output or cause retention of urine? Note specific medication and dosage.
- Fluid intake. What amount and kind of fluid do you take each day (e.g., six glasses of water, two cups of coffee, three cola drinks with or without caffeine)?
- Environmental factors. Do you have any problems with toileting (mobility, removing clothing, toilet seat too low, facility without grab bar)?
- Stress. Are you experiencing any major stress? If so, what are the stressors? Do you think these affect your urinary pattern?
- Disease. Have you had or do you have any illnesses that may affect urinary function, such as hypertension, heart disease, neurologic disease, cancer, prostatic enlargement, or diabetes?
- Diagnostic procedures and surgery. Have you recently had a cystoscopy or anesthetic?

TABLE 48–4 Characteristics of Normal and Abnormal Urine

CHARACTERISTIC	NORMAL	ABNORMAL	NURSING CONSIDERATIONS
Amount in 24 hours (adult)	1,200–1,500 mL	Under 1,200 mL A large amount over intake	Urinary output normally is approximately equal to fluid intake. Output of less than 30 mL/hr may indicate decreased blood flow to the kidneys and should be immediately reported.
Color, clarity	Straw, amber Transparent	Dark amber Cloudy Dark orange Red or dark brown Mucous plugs, viscid, thick	Concentrated urine is darker in color. Dilute urine may appear almost clear, or very pale yellow. Some foods and drugs may color urine. Red blood cells in the urine (hematuria) may be evident as pink, bright red, or rusty brown urine. Menstrual bleeding can also color urine but should not be confused with hematuria. White blood cells, bacteria, pus, or contaminants such as prostatic fluid, sperm, or vaginal drainage may cause cloudy urine.
Odor	Faint aromatic	Offensive	Some foods (e.g., asparagus) cause a musty odor; infected urine can have a fetid odor; urine high in glucose has a sweet odor.
Sterility	No microorganisms present	Microorganisms present	Urine in the bladder is sterile. Urine specimens, however, may be contaminated by bacteria from the perineum during collection.
pH	4.5–8	Over 8 Under 4.5	Freshly voided urine is normally somewhat acidic. Alkaline urine may indicate a state of alkalosis, urinary tract infection, or a diet high in fruits and vegetables. More acidic urine (low pH) is found in starvation, with diarrhea, or with a diet high in protein foods or cranberries.
Specific gravity	1.010–1.025	Over 1.025 Under 1.010	Concentrated urine has a higher specific gravity; diluted urine has a lower specific gravity.
Glucose	Not present	Present	Glucose in the urine indicates high blood glucose levels (>180 mg/dL) and may be indicative of undiagnosed or uncontrolled diabetes mellitus.
Ketone bodies (acetone)	Not present	Present	Ketones, the end product of the breakdown of fatty acids, are not normally present in the urine. They may be present in the urine of clients who have uncontrolled diabetes mellitus, who are in a state of starvation, or who have ingested excessive amounts of aspirin.
Blood	Not present	Occult (microscopic) Bright red	Blood may be present in the urine of clients who have urinary tract infection, kidney disease, or bleeding from the urinary tract.

Urine outputs below 30 mL per hour may indicate low blood volume or kidney malfunction and must be reported. To measure fluid output the nurse follows these steps:

- Wear clean gloves to prevent contact with microorganisms or blood in urine.
- Ask the client to void in a clean urinal, bedpan, commode, or toilet collection device ("hat") (Figure 48-5 ■).
- Instruct the client to keep urine separate from feces and to avoid putting toilet paper in the urine collection container.
- Pour the voided urine into a calibrated container.
- Holding the container at eye level, read the amount in the container. Containers usually have a measuring scale on the inside.
- Record the amount on the fluid intake and output sheet, which may be at the bedside or in the bathroom.
- Rinse the urine collection and measuring containers with cool water and store appropriately.
- Remove gloves and perform hand hygiene.
- Calculate and document the total output at the end of each shift and at the end of 24 hours on the client's chart.

Many clients can measure and record their own urine output when the procedure is explained to them.

When measuring urine from a client who has a urinary catheter, the nurse follows these steps:

- Put on clean gloves.
- Take the calibrated container to the bedside.
- Place the container under the urine collection bag so that the spout of the bag is above the container but not touching it. The calibrated container is not sterile, but the inside of the collection bag is sterile (Figure 48-6 ■).
- Open the spout and permit the urine to flow into the container.
- Close the spout, then proceed as described in the previous list.

MEASURING RESIDUAL URINE. **Residual urine** (urine remaining in the bladder following the voiding) is normally 50 to 100 mL. However, a bladder outlet obstruction (e.g., enlargement of the prostate gland) or loss of bladder muscle tone may interfere with complete emptying of the bladder during urination. Manifestations of urine retention may include frequent voiding of small amounts (e.g., less than 100 mL in an adult).

Figure 48-5 ■ A urine "hat"—a urine collection device for the toilet.

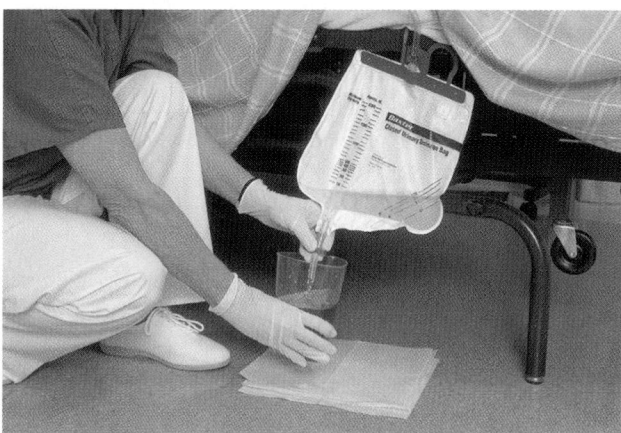

Figure 48-6 ■ Urine being measured from a urine collection bag.

Urinary stasis and urinary tract infection are possible consequences of incomplete bladder emptying. Residual urine is measured to assess the amount of retained urine after voiding and determine the need for interventions (e.g., medications to promote detrusor muscle contraction).

To measure residual urine, the nurse catheterizes or bladder scans the client after voiding. The amount of urine voided and the amount obtained by catheterization or bladder scan are measured and recorded. An indwelling catheter may be inserted if the residual urine exceeds a specified amount.

Diagnostic Tests

Blood levels of two metabolically produced substances, urea and creatinine, are routinely used to evaluate renal function. Both are normally eliminated by the kidneys through filtration and tubular secretion. Urea, the end product of protein metabolism, is measured as **blood urea nitrogen (BUN).** Creatinine is produced in relatively constant quantities by the muscles. The **creatinine clearance** test uses 24-hour urine and serum creatinine levels to determine the glomerular filtration rate, a sensitive indicator of renal function. Other tests related to urinary functions such as collecting urine specimens, measuring specific gravity, and visualization procedures are described in Chapter 34. ∞

Diagnosing

NANDA (2007) includes one general diagnostic label for urinary elimination problems and several labels that are more specific:

- *Impaired Urinary Elimination:* dysfunctional in urine elimination

Other NANDA nursing diagnoses related to urinary elimination are subcategories of this diagnosis, and include the following:

- *Functional Urinary Incontinence*
- *Reflex Urinary Incontinence*
- *Stress Urinary Incontinence*
- *Total Urinary Incontinence*
- *Urge Urinary Incontinence*
- *Overflow Urinary Incontinence*
- *Urinary Retention*

See Box 48–2 for definitions of NANDA diagnoses related to incontinence.

BOX 48–2 Definitions of NANDA Incontinence Diagnoses

- *Functional Urinary Incontinence*—Inability of usually continent person to reach toilet in time to avoid unintentional loss of urine.
- *Reflex Urinary Incontinence*—Involuntary loss of urine at somewhat predictable intervals when a specific bladder volume is reached.
- *Stress Urinary Incontinence*—Sudden leakage of urine occurring with activities that increase abdominal pressure.
- *Total Urinary Incontinence*—Continuous and unpredictable passage of urine.
- *Urge Urinary Incontinence*—Involuntary passage of urine occurring soon after a strong sense of urgency to void.

Note: Reprinted from *Nursing Outcomes Classification* (NOC), 3rd ed., by S. Moorhad, M. Johnson, & M. Meridean, Copyright © 2004 with permission from Elsevier.

Clinical examples of assessment data clusters and related nursing diagnoses, outcomes, and interventions are shown in Identifying Nursing Diagnoses, Outcomes, and Interventions on page 1296 and in the Nursing Care Plan and Concept Map at end of this chapter.

Problems of urinary elimination also may become the etiology for other problems experienced by the client. Examples include the following:

- *Risk for Infection* if the client has urinary retention or undergoes an invasive procedure such as catheterization or cystoscopic examination.
- *Low Self-Esteem* or *Social Isolation* if the client is incontinent. Incontinence can be physically and emotionally distressing to clients because it is considered socially unacceptable. Often the client is embarrassed about dribbling or having an accident and may restrict normal activities for this reason.
- *Risk for Impaired Skin Integrity* if the client is incontinent. Bed linens and clothes saturated with urine irritate and macerate the skin. Prolonged skin dampness leads to dermatitis

(inflammation of the skin) and subsequent formation of dermal ulcers.

- *Self-Care Deficit: Toileting* if the client has functional incontinence.
- *Risk for Deficient Fluid Volume* or *Excess Fluid Volume* if the client has impaired urinary function associated with a disease process.
- *Disturbed Body Image* if the client has a urinary diversion ostomy.
- *Deficient Knowledge* if the client requires self-care skills to manage (e.g., a new urinary diversion ostomy).
- *Risk for Caregiver Role Strain* if the client is incontinent and being cared for by a family member for extended periods.
- *Risk for Social Isolation* if the client is incontinent.

Planning

The goals established will vary according to the diagnosis and defining characteristics. Examples of overall goals for clients with urinary elimination problems may include the following:

- Maintain or restore a normal voiding pattern.
- Regain normal urine output.
- Prevent associated risks such as infection, skin breakdown, fluid and electrolyte imbalance, and lowered self-esteem.
- Perform toilet activities independently with or without assistive devices.
- Contain urine with the appropriate device, catheter, ostomy appliance, or absorbent product.

Appropriate preventive and corrective nursing interventions that relate to these must be identified. Specific nursing activities associated with each of these interventions can be selected to meet the client's individual needs. Examples of clinical applications of these using NANDA, NIC, and NOC designations are shown in Identifying Nursing Diagnoses, Outcomes, and Interventions and in the Nursing Care Plan and Concept Map at the end of the chapter.

DRUG CAPSULE Anticholinergic Agents   *oxybutynin ER* (Ditropan XL)

THE CLIENT WITH MEDICATIONS FOR URGE URINARY INCONTINENCE

Anticholinergic agents reduce urgency and frequency by blocking muscarinic receptors in the detrusor muscle of the bladder, thereby inhibiting contractions and increasing storage capacity. They are useful in relieving symptoms associated with voiding in clients with neurogenic bladder and reflex neurogenic bladder, and urge urinary incontinence.

NURSING RESPONSIBILITIES

- Monitor for constipation, dry mouth, urinary retention, blurred vision, and mental confusion in the elderly; symptoms may be dose related.
- Keep primary care provider informed of expected responses to therapy (e.g., effect on urinary frequency, urge incontinence, nocturia, and bladder emptying).
- Start with small doses to clients over the age of 75.
- Try using intermittently.
- Oxybutynin is contraindicated in clients with urinary retention, gastrointestinal motility problems (partial or complete GI obstruction, paralytic ileus), or uncontrolled narrow-angle glaucoma.

CLIENT AND FAMILY TEACHING

- Explain the reason for taking oxybutynin.
- Explain the side effects and the importance of reporting them to the health care provider.
- Exercise caution in hot environments. By suppressing sweating, oxybutynin can cause fever and heat stroke.
- Provide strategies for managing dry mouth.
- Instruct and advise regarding behavioral therapies for urge suppression.

Note: Prior to administering any medication, review all aspects with a current drug handbook or other reliable source.

IDENTIFYING NURSING DIAGNOSES, OUTCOMES, AND INTERVENTIONS
Clients with Urinary Elimination Disorders

DATA CLUSTER Mrs. Amy Brown, 75, reports accidental loss of urine before she is able to reach the toilet. She is aware of the urge to void but states, "Because of my stroke I sometimes can't get there soon enough."

NURSING DIAGNOSIS/ DEFINITION	SAMPLE DESIRED OUTCOMES*/ DEFINITION	INDICATORS	SELECTED INTERVENTIONS*/ DEFINITION	SAMPLE NIC ACTIVITIES
Functional Urinary Incontinence/Inability of usually continent person to reach toilet in time to avoid unintentional loss of urine	Urinary Continence [0502]/*Control of the elimination of urine from the bladder*	Consistently demonstrated: ▪ Responds to urge in timely manner ▪ Gets to toilet between urge and passage of urine ▪ Voids > 150 mL each time	Prompted Voiding [0640]/*Promotion of urinary continence through the use of timed verbal toileting reminders and positive social feedback for successful toileting*	▪ Determine client awareness of continence status by asking if wet or dry ▪ Prompt up to three times to use toilet or substitute, regardless of continence status ▪ Give positive feedback by praising desired toileting behavior ▪ Document outcomes of toileting session

DATA CLUSTER Anthony Cherry, a teenager with a spinal cord injury, has no awareness of bladder filling, the urge to void, or feelings of bladder fullness. He reports loss of urine at fairly regular intervals.

Reflex Urinary Incontinence/Involuntary loss of urine at somewhat predictable intervals when a specific bladder volume is reached	Urinary Elimination [0503]/*Collection and discharge of urine*	Not compromised: ▪ Elimination pattern ▪ Empties bladder completely ▪ Urine amount ▪ Urine clarity	Urinary Catheterization: Intermittent [0582]/*Regular periodic use of a catheter to empty the bladder*	▪ Teach client/family purpose, supplies, method, and rationale of intermittent catheterization ▪ Demonstrate procedure and have a return demonstration ▪ Determine catheterization schedule based on a comprehensive assessment

DATA CLUSTER Tammy Tyndale reports dribbling whenever she laughs, coughs, or sneezes. She is 8 months pregnant.

Stress Urinary Incontinence/Sudden loss of urine occurring with activities that increase abdominal pressure	Symptom Control [1608]/*Personal actions to minimize perceived adverse changes in physical and emotional functioning*	Consistently demonstrated: ▪ Uses preventive measures ▪ Uses available resources	Pelvic Muscle Exercise [0560]/*Strengthening and training the levator ani and urogenital muscles through voluntary repetitive contraction to decrease stress, urge, or mixed types of urinary incontinence*	▪ Instruct client to tighten, then relax, the ring of muscle around urethra and anus, as if trying to prevent urination or bowel movement ▪ Provide positive feedback for doing exercises as prescribed

DATA CLUSTER Mrs. Gail Brady reports urinary urgency, difficulty in getting to the bathroom in time, frequency (more often than every 2 hours), and leakage of urine when unable to reach the toilet in time.

Urge Urinary Incontinence/Involuntary passage of urine occurring soon after a strong sense of urgency to void	Tissue Integrity: Skin and Mucous Membranes [1101]/*Structural intactness and normal physiological function of skin and mucous membranes*	Not compromised: ▪ Skin intactness	Urinary Bladder Training [0570]/*Improving bladder function for those with urge incontinence by increasing the bladder's ability to hold urine and the patient's ability to suppress urination*	▪ Keep a continence record for 3 days to establish voiding pattern ▪ Establish interval for toileting, preferably more than 2 hours ▪ Reduce toileting interval by 1/2 hour if more than 3 incontinence episodes in 24 hours ▪ Increase interval by 1/2 hour if no incontinence episodes for 3 days until optimal 4-hour interval is reached

*The NOC # for desired outcomes and the NIC # for nursing interventions are listed in brackets following the appropriate outcome or intervention. Outcomes, indicators, interventions, and activities selected are only a sample of those suggested by NOC and NIC and should be further individualized for each client

---

HOME CARE ASSESSMENT **Urinary Elimination**

CLIENT AND ENVIRONMENT

- Self-care abilities: Ability to consume adequate fluids, to perceive bladder fullness, to ambulate and get to the toilet, to manipulate clothing for toileting, and to perform hygiene measures after toileting
- Current level of knowledge: Fluid and dietary intake modifications to promote normal patterns of urinary elimination, bladder training methods, and specific techniques to promote voiding care for indwelling catheter or ostomy (if appropriate)
- Assistive devices required: Ambulatory aids such as walker, cane, or wheelchair; safety devices such as grab bars; toileting aids such as raised toilet seat, urinal, commode, or bedpan; presence of a urinary catheter
- Physical layout of the toileting facilities: Presence of mobility aids; toilet at correct height to enable elders to get up after voiding
- Home environment factors that interfere with toileting: Distance to the bathroom from living areas or bedrooms; barriers such as stairways, scatter rugs, clutter, or narrow doorways that interfere with bathroom access; lighting (including night lighting)
- Urinary elimination problems: Type of incontinence and precipitating factors; manifestations of urinary tract infection such as dysuria,

frequency, urgency; evidence of prostatic hypertrophy and effect on urination; ability to perform self-catheterization and care for other urinary elimination devices such as indwelling catheter, urinary diversion ostomy, or condom drainage

FAMILY

- Caregiver availability, skills, and responses: Ability and willingness to assume responsibilities for care, including assisting with toileting, intermittent catheterization, indwelling catheter care, urinary drainage devices or ostomy care; ready access to laundry facilities; access to and willingness to use respite or relief caregivers
- Family role changes and coping: Effect on spousal and family roles, sleep/rest patterns, sexuality, and social interactions
- Financial resources: Ability to purchase protective pads and garments, supplies for catheterization or ostomy care

COMMUNITY

- Environment: Access to public restrooms and sanitary facilities
- Current knowledge of and experience with community resources: Medical and assistive equipment and supply companies, home health agencies, local pharmacies, available financial assistance, support and educational organizations

---

Planning for Home Care

To provide for continuity of care, the nurse needs to consider the client's needs for teaching and assistance with care in the home. Discharge planning includes assessment of the client's and family's resources and abilities for self-care, available financial resources, and the need for referrals and home health services. The above Home Care Assessment outlines an assessment of home care capabilities related to urinary elimination problems and needs. The Client Teaching box on page 1298 addresses the learning needs of the client and family.

Implementing

Maintaining Normal Urinary Elimination

Most interventions to maintain normal urinary elimination are independent nursing functions. These include promoting adequate fluid intake, maintaining normal voiding habits, and assisting with toileting.

PROMOTING FLUID INTAKE. Increasing fluid intake increases urine production, which in turn stimulates the micturition reflex. A normal daily intake averaging 1,500 mL of measurable fluids is adequate for most adult clients.

Many clients have increased fluid requirements, necessitating a higher daily fluid intake. For example, clients who are perspiring excessively (have diaphoresis) or who are experiencing abnormal fluid losses through vomiting, gastric suction, diarrhea, or wound drainage require fluid to replace these losses in addition to their normal daily intake requirements.

Clients who are at risk for urinary tract infection or urinary calculi (stones) should consume 2,000 to 3,000 mL of fluid daily. Dilute urine and frequent urination reduce the risk of urinary tract infection as well as stone formation.

Increased fluid intake may be contraindicated for some clients such as people with kidney failure or heart failure. For these clients, a fluid restriction may be necessary to prevent fluid overload and edema.

MAINTAINING NORMAL VOIDING HABITS. Prescribed medical therapies often interfere with a client's normal voiding habits. When a client's urinary elimination pattern is adequate, the nurse helps the client adhere to normal voiding habits as much as possible (see Practice Guidelines on page 1299).

ASSISTING WITH TOILETING. Clients who are weakened by a disease process or impaired physically may require assistance with toileting. The nurse should assist these clients to the bathroom and remain with them if they are at risk for falling. The bathroom should contain an easily accessible call signal to summon help if needed. Clients also need to be encouraged to use handrails placed near the toilet.

For clients unable to use bathroom facilities, the nurse provides urinary equipment close to the bedside (e.g., urinal, bedpan, commode) and provides the necessary assistance to use them.

Preventing Urinary Tract Infections

The rate of urinary tract infection (UTI) is greater in women than men because of the short urethra and its proximity to the anal and vaginal areas (Anonymous, 2004). UTIs are the most common type of nosocomial infection found in long-term care facilities (Midthun, 2004). Most UTIs are caused by bacteria common to the intestinal environment (e.g., *Escherichia coli*). These gastrointestinal bacteria can colonize the perineal area and move into the urethra, especially when there is urethral trauma, irritation, or manipulation. Women are particularly at risk.

plan of care in order to follow a program. A bladder training program may include the following:

- Education of the client and support people.
- **Bladder training,** which requires that the client postpone voiding, resist or inhibit the sensation of urgency, and void according to a timetable rather than according to the urge to void. The goals are to gradually lengthen the intervals between urination to correct the client's frequent urination, to stabilize the bladder, and to diminish urgency. This form of training may be used for clients who have bladder instability and urge incontinence. Delayed voiding provides larger voided volumes and longer intervals between voiding. Initially, voiding may be encouraged every 2 to 3 hours except during sleep and then every 4 to 6 hours. A vital component of bladder training is inhibiting the urge-to-void sensation. To do this, the nurse instructs the client to practice deep, slow breathing until the urge diminishes or disappears. This is performed every time the client has a premature urge to void.
- **Habit training,** also referred to as timed voiding or scheduled toileting, attempts to keep clients dry by having them void at regular intervals. With habit training, there is no attempt to motivate the client to delay voiding if the urge occurs. This approach can be effective in children who are experiencing urinary dysfunction. Biofeedback therapy in which the child is taught to relax the pelvic floor can also decrease incidents of wetting (Shei Dei Yang & Cheng Wang, 2005).
- **Prompted voiding** supplements habit training by encouraging the client to try to use the toilet (prompting) and reminding the client when to void.

PELVIC MUSCLE EXERCISES. Pelvic muscle exercises (PME), or Kegel exercises, help to strengthen pelvic floor muscles and can reduce or eliminate episodes of incontinence. The client can identify the perineal muscles by stopping urination midstream or by tightening the anal sphincter as if to hold a bowel movement.

CLIENT TEACHING   Pelvic Muscle Exercises (Kegels)

- First, sit or lie in a comfortable, relaxed position.
- Contract your pelvic muscles whereby you pull your rectum, urethra, and vagina up inside, and hold for a count of 3 to 5 seconds. Then relax the same muscles for a count of 3 to 5 seconds.
- Initially perform each contraction 10 times, three times daily. Gradually increase the count to a full 10 seconds for both contraction and relaxation.
- Develop a schedule that will help remind you to do these exercises, for example, before getting out of bed in the morning, when working at the kitchen sink, or at scheduled times (e.g., 0700, 1200, 1800 hours).
- To control episodes of stress incontinence, perform a pelvic muscle contraction when initiating any activity that increases intra-abdominal pressure, such as coughing, laughing, sneezing, or lifting.

The following technique is sometimes used to teach PME. Ask the client to think of the perineal muscles as an elevator. When the client relaxes, the elevator is on the first floor. To perform the exercise, contract the perineal muscles, bringing the elevator to the second, third, and fourth floors. Keep the elevator on the fourth floor for a few seconds, and then gradually relax the area. When the exercise is properly performed, contraction of the muscles of the buttocks and thighs is avoided. PME can be performed anytime, anywhere, sitting or standing—even when voiding. Specific client instructions for performing PME are summarized in Client Teaching.

MAINTAINING SKIN INTEGRITY. Skin that is continually moist becomes macerated (softened). Urine that accumulates on the skin is converted to ammonia, which is very irritating to the skin. Because both skin irritation and maceration predis-

---

PRACTICE GUIDELINES   Bladder Training

- Determine the client's voiding pattern and encourage voiding at those times, or establish a regular voiding schedule and help the client to maintain it, whether the client feels the urge or not (e.g., on awakening, every 1 or 2 hours during the day and evening, before retiring at night, every 4 hours at night). The stretching-relaxing sequence of such a schedule tends to increase bladder muscle tone and promote more voluntary control. Encourage the client to inhibit the urge-to-void sensation when a premature urge to void is experienced. Instruct the client to practice slow, deep breathing until the urge diminishes or disappears.
- When the client finds that voiding can be controlled, the intervals between voiding can be lengthened slightly without loss of continence.
- Regulate fluid intake, particularly during evening hours, to help reduce the need to void during the night.
- Encourage fluids between the hours of 0600 and 1800.

- Avoid excessive consumption of citrus juices, carbonated beverages (especially those containing artificial sweeteners), alcohol, and drinks containing caffeine because these irritate the bladder, increasing the risk of incontinence.
- Schedule diuretics early in the morning.
- Explain to clients that adequate fluid intake is required to ensure adequate urine production that stimulates the micturition reflex.
- Apply protector pads to keep the bed linen dry and provide specially made waterproof underwear to contain the urine and decrease the client's embarrassment. Avoid using diapers, which are demeaning and also suggest that incontinence is permissible.
- Assist the client with an exercise program to increase the general muscle tone and a pelvic muscle exercise program aimed at strengthening the pelvic floor muscles.
- Provide positive reinforcements to encourage continence. Praise clients for attempting to toilet and for maintaining continence.

pose the client to skin breakdown and ulceration, the incontinent person requires meticulous skin care. To maintain skin integrity, the nurse washes the client's perineal area with mild soap and water or a commercially prepared no-rinse cleanser after episodes of incontinence, rinses it thoroughly if used soap and water, dries it gently and thoroughly, and provides clean, dry clothing or bed linen. The nurse applies barrier ointments or creams to protect the skin from contact with urine. If it is necessary to pad the client's clothes for protection, the nurse should use products that absorb wetness and leave a dry surface in contact with the skin.

Specially designed incontinence drawsheets may be used that provide significant advantages over standard drawsheets for incontinent clients confined to bed. These sheets are like a drawsheet but are double layered, with a quilted upper nylon or polyester surface and an absorbent viscose rayon layer below. The rayon soaker layer generally has a waterproof backing on its underside. Fluid (i.e., urine) passes through the upper quilted layer and is absorbed and dispersed by the viscose rayon, leaving the quilted surface dry to the touch. This absorbent sheet helps maintain skin integrity; it does not stick to the skin when wet, decreases the risk of bedsores, and reduces odor.

APPLYING EXTERNAL URINARY DRAINAGE DEVICES. The application of a condom or external catheter connected to a urinary drainage system can be used for incontinent males. Use of a condom appliance is preferable to insertion of a retention catheter because the risk of urinary tract infection is minimal.

Methods of applying condoms vary. The nurse needs to follow the manufacturer's instructions when applying a condom. First the nurse determines when the client experiences incontinence. Some clients may require a condom appliance at night only, others continuously. Skill 48-1 describes how to apply and remove an external catheter.

SKILL 48-1

APPLYING AN EXTERNAL CATHETER

PURPOSES
- To collect urine and control urinary incontinence
- To permit the client physical activity while controlling urinary incontinence
- To prevent skin irritation as a result of urine incontinence

ASSESSMENT
- Review the client record to determine a pattern to voiding and other pertinent data.
- Put on clean gloves and examine the client's penis for swelling or excoriation that would contraindicate use of the condom catheter.

PLANNING
Determine if the client has had an external catheter previously and any difficulties with it. Perform any procedures that are best completed without the catheter in place, for example, weighing the client would be easier without the tubing and bag.

Delegation
Applying a condom catheter may be delegated to unlicensed assistive personnel (UAP). However, the nurse must determine if the specific client has unique needs that would require special training of the UAP in the use of the condom catheter.

Equipment
- Leg drainage bag with tubing or urinary drainage bag with tubing
- Condom sheath
- Drape (e.g., sheet or bath blanket)
- Clean gloves
- Basin of warm water and soap
- Washcloth and towel
- Elastic tape or Velcro strap

IMPLEMENTATION
Preparation
- Assemble the leg drainage bag or urinary drainage bag for attachment to the condom sheath.
- Roll the condom outward onto itself to facilitate easier application. ❶ On some models, an inner flap will be exposed. This flap is applied around the urinary meatus to prevent the reflux of urine.
- Position the client in either a supine or a sitting position.

Performance
1. Prior to performing the procedure, introduce self and verify the client's identity using agency protocol. Explain to the client what you are going to do, why it is necessary, and how he can cooperate.
2. Perform hand hygiene, apply clean gloves, and observe appropriate infection control procedures.

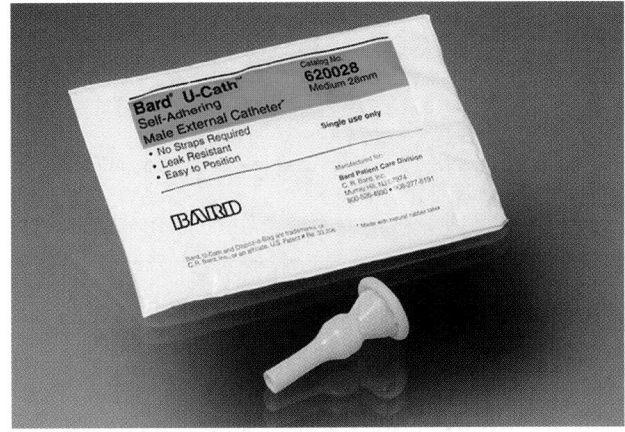

❶ Before application, roll the condom outward onto itself.
(Courtesy of Bard Medical Division.)

continued on page 1302

APPLYING AN EXTERNAL CATHETER *continued*

3. Provide for client privacy.
   * Drape the client appropriately with the bath blanket, exposing only the penis.
4. Inspect and clean the penis.
   * Clean the genital area and dry it thoroughly. **Rationale:** *This minimizes skin irritation and excoriation after the condom is applied.*
5. Apply and secure the condom.
   * Roll the condom smoothly over the penis, leaving 2.5 cm. (1 in.) between the end of the penis and the rubber or plastic connecting tube. ❷ **Rationale:** *This space prevents irritation of the tip of the penis and provides for full drainage of urine.*
   * Secure the condom firmly, but not too tightly, to the penis. Some condoms have an adhesive inside the proximal end that adheres to the skin of the base of the penis. Many condoms are packaged with special tape. If neither is present, use a strip of elastic tape or Velcro around the base of the penis over the condom. Ordinary tape is contraindicated because it is not flexible and can stop blood flow.
6. Securely attach the urinary drainage system.
   * Make sure that the tip of the penis is not touching the condom and that the condom is not twisted. **Rationale:** *A twisted condom could obstruct the flow of urine.*
   * Attach the urinary drainage system to the condom.
   * Remove the gloves and perform hand hygiene.
   * If the client is to remain in bed, attach the urinary drainage bag to the bed frame.
   * If the client is ambulatory, attach the bag to the client's leg. ❸ **Rationale:** *Attaching the drainage bag to the leg helps control the movement of the tubing and prevents twisting of the thin material of the condom appliance at the tip of the penis.*
7. Teach the client about the drainage system.
   * Instruct the client to keep the drainage bag below the level of the condom and to avoid loops or kinks in the tubing.
8. Inspect the penis 30 minutes following the condom application, and check urine flow. Document these findings.
   * Assess the penis for swelling and discoloration, *which indicates that the condom is too tight.*
   * Assess urine flow if the client has voided. Normally, some urine is present in the tube if the flow is not obstructed.
9. Change the condom daily and provide skin care.
   * Remove the elastic or Velcro strip, apply clean gloves, and roll off the condom.

❷ The condom rolled over the penis.

❸ Urinary drainage leg bags.
(Courtesy of Bard Medical Division.)

   * Wash the penis with soapy water, rinse, and dry it thoroughly.
   * Assess the foreskin for signs of irritation, swelling, and discoloration.
   * Reapply a new condom.
10. Document in the client record using forms or checklists supplemented by narrative notes when appropriate. Record the application of the condom, the time, and pertinent observations, such as irritated areas on the penis.

EVALUATION

* Perform a detailed follow-up based on findings that deviated from expected or normal for the client. Relate findings to previous assessment data if available.
* Report significant deviations from normal to the primary care provider.

Managing Urinary Retention

Interventions that assist the client to maintain a normal voiding pattern, discussed earlier, also apply when dealing with urinary retention. If these actions are unsuccessful, the primary care provider may order a cholinergic drug such as bethanechol chloride (Urecholine) to stimulate bladder contraction and facilitate voiding. Clients who have a **flaccid** bladder (weak, soft, and lax bladder muscles) may use manual pressure on the bladder to promote bladder emptying. This is known as **Credé's maneuver** or Credé's method. It is not advised without a physician or nurse practitioner's order and is used only for clients who have lost and are not expected to regain voluntary bladder control. When all measures fail to initiate voiding, urinary catheterization may be necessary to empty the bladder completely. An indwelling Foley catheter may be inserted until the underlying cause is treated. Alternatively, intermittent straight catheterization (every 3 to 4 hours) may be performed because the risk of urinary tract infection may be less than with an indwelling catheter.

Urinary Catheterization

Urinary catheterization is the introduction of a catheter into the urinary bladder. This is usually performed only when absolutely necessary, because the danger exists of introducing microorganisms into the bladder. Clients who have lowered immune resistance are at the greatest risk. Once an infection is introduced into the bladder, it can ascend the ureters and eventually involve the kidneys. The hazard of infection remains after the catheter is in place because normal defense mechanisms such as intermittent flushing of microorganisms from the urethra through voiding are bypassed. Thus, strict sterile technique is used for catheterization.

CLINICAL ALERT

The insertion of urinary catheters is one of the most common causes of hospital-acquired infections. ■

Another hazard is trauma with urethral catheterization, particularly in the male client, whose urethra is longer and more tortuous. It is important to insert a catheter along the normal contour of the urethra. Damage to the urethra can occur if the catheter is forced through strictures or at an incorrect angle. In males, the urethra is normally curved, but it can be straightened by elevating the penis to a position perpendicular to the body.

A

B

Figure 48-7 ■ Red-rubber or plastic Robinson straight catheters.

(Courtesy of Bard Medical Division.)

Figure 48-8 ■ A coudé catheter.

(Courtesy of Bard Medical Division.)

Catheters are commonly made of rubber or plastics although they may be made from latex, silicone, or polyvinyl chloride (PVC). They are sized by the diameter of the lumen using the French (Fr) scale: the larger the number, the larger the lumen. Either straight catheters, inserted to drain the bladder and then immediately removed, or retention catheters, which remain in the bladder to drain urine, may be used.

The straight catheter is a single-lumen tube with a small eye or opening about 1 1/4 cm (1/2 in.) from the insertion tip (Figure 48-7 ■). The coudé catheter is a variation of the straight catheter. It is more rigid than other straight catheters and has a tapered, curved tip (Figure 48-8 ■). This catheter may be used for men with prostatic hypertrophy because it is more easily controlled and less traumatic on insertion.

The retention, or Foley, catheter is a double-lumen catheter. The larger lumen drains urine from the bladder. A second, smaller lumen is used to inflate a balloon near the tip of the catheter to hold the catheter in place within the bladder (Figure 48-9 ■). Clients who require continuous or intermittent bladder irrigation may have a three-way Foley catheter (Figure 48-10 ■). The three-way

Figure 48-9 ■ An indwelling/retention (Foley) catheter with the balloon inflated.

(Courtesy of Bard Medical Division.)

MediaLink

Catheterization Animation

Figure 48-10 ■ A three-way Foley catheter often used for continuous bladder irrigation.
(Courtesy of Bard Medical Division.)

BOX 48–3   Selecting a Urinary Catheter

- Select the type of material in accordance with the estimated length of the catheterization period. Antimicrobial-impregnated or hydrogel/silver-coated catheters may also be used to reduce the risk of infection.
  - a. Use plastic catheters for short periods only (e.g., 1 week or less), because they are inflexible.
  - b. Use a rubber or Silastic catheter for periods of 2 or 3 weeks. Latex may be used for clients with no known latex allergy. However, because of these allergies, latex is being phased out of health care products.
  - c. Use silicone catheters for long-term use (e.g., 2 to 3 months) because they create less encrustation at the urethral meatus. However, they are expensive.
  - d. Use PVC catheters for 4- to 6-week periods. They soften at body temperature and conform to the urethra.
- Determine appropriate catheter length by the client's gender. For adult female clients, use a 22-cm catheter; for adult male clients, a 40-cm catheter.
- Determine appropriate catheter size by the size of the urethral canal. Use sizes such as #8 or #10 for children, #14 or #16 for adults. Men frequently require a larger size than women, for example, #18.
- Select the appropriate balloon size. For adults, use a 10-mL balloon to facilitate optimal urine drainage. The smaller balloons allow more complete bladder emptying because the catheter tip is closer to the urethral opening in the bladder. However, a 30-mL balloon is commonly used to achieve hemostasis of the prostatic area following a prostatectomy. Use 3-mL balloons for children.

catheter has a third lumen through which sterile irrigating fluid can flow into the bladder. The fluid then exits the bladder through the drainage lumen, along with the urine.

The balloons of retention catheters are sized by the volume of fluid used to inflate them. The two commonly used sizes are 10-mL and 30-mL balloons. The size of the balloon is indicated on the catheter along with the diameter, for example, "#18 Fr— 10 mL." Box 48–3 provides guidelines for catheter selection.

Retention catheters usually are connected to a closed gravity drainage system. This system consists of the catheter, drainage tubing, and a collecting bag for the urine. A closed system cannot be opened anywhere along the system, from catheter to collecting bag. Closed systems reduce the risk of microorganisms entering the system and infecting the urinary tract. Urinary drainage systems typically depend on the force of gravity to drain urine from the bladder to the collecting bag.

Skill 48-2 describes catheterization of females and males, using straight and retention catheters.

PERFORMING URETHRAL URINARY CATHETERIZATION

SKILL 48-2

PURPOSES
- To relieve discomfort due to bladder distention or to provide gradual decompression of a distended bladder
- To assess the amount of residual urine if the bladder empties incompletely
- To obtain a sterile urine specimen
- To empty the bladder completely prior to surgery
- To facilitate accurate measurement of urinary output for critically ill clients whose output needs to be monitored hourly
- To provide for intermittent or continuous bladder drainage and/or irrigation
- To prevent urine from contacting an incision after perineal surgery
- To manage incontinence when other measures have failed

ASSESSMENT
- Determine the most appropriate method of catheterization based on the purpose and any criteria specified in the order such as total amount of urine to be removed or size of catheter to be used.
- Use a straight catheter if only a spot urine specimen is needed, if amount of residual urine is being measured, or if temporary decompression/emptying of the bladder is required.
- Use an indwelling/retention catheter if the bladder must remain empty or continuous urine measurement/collection is needed.
- Assess the client's overall condition. Determine if the client is able to cooperate and hold still during the procedure and if the client can be positioned supine with head relatively flat.
- Determine when the client last voided or was last catheterized.
- Percuss the bladder to check for fullness or distention.
- When possible, complete a bladder scan to assess the amount of urine present in the bladder before performing a urethral catheterization.

PERFORMING URETHRAL URINARY CATHETERIZATION *continued*

PLANNING

Allow adequate time to perform the catheterization. Although the entire procedure can require as little as 15 minutes, several sources of difficulty could result in a much longer time. If possible, it should not be performed just prior to or after the client eats.

Delegation
Due to the need for sterile technique and detailed knowledge of anatomy, insertion of a urinary catheter is not delegated to UAP.

Equipment
- Sterile catheter of appropriate size (An extra catheter should also be at hand.)
- Catheterization kit ❶ or individual sterile items:
  - 1–2 pair sterile gloves
  - Waterproof drape(s)
  - Antiseptic solution
  - Cleansing balls
  - Forceps
  - Water-soluble lubricant
  - Urine receptacle
  - Specimen container
- For an indwelling catheter:
  - Syringe prefilled with sterile water in amount specified by catheter manufacturer
  - Collection bag and tubing
- 2% Xylocaine gel (if agency permits)
- Disposable clean gloves
- Supplies for performing perineal cleansing
- Bath blanket or sheet for draping the client
- Adequate lighting (Obtain a flashlight or lamp if necessary.)

❶ Catheter insertion kits: *A*, indwelling; *B*, straight.
(Courtesy of Bard Medical Division.)

IMPLEMENTATION
Preparation
If using a catheterization kit, read the label carefully to be sure all necessary items are included. Perform routine perineal care to cleanse the meatus from gross contamination. For women, use this time to locate the urinary meatus relative to surrounding structures. ❷

Performance
1. Prior to performing the procedure, introduce self and verify the client's identity using agency protocol. Explain to the client what you are going to do, why it is necessary, and how he or she can cooperate.
2. Perform hand hygiene and observe appropriate infection control procedures.
3. Provide for client privacy.
4. Place the client in the appropriate position and drape all areas except the perineum.
   a. Female: supine with knees flexed, feet about 2 feet apart, and hips slightly externally rotated, if possible
   b. Male: supine, thighs slightly abducted or apart
5. Establish adequate lighting. Stand on the client's right if you are right-handed, on the client's left if you are left-handed.

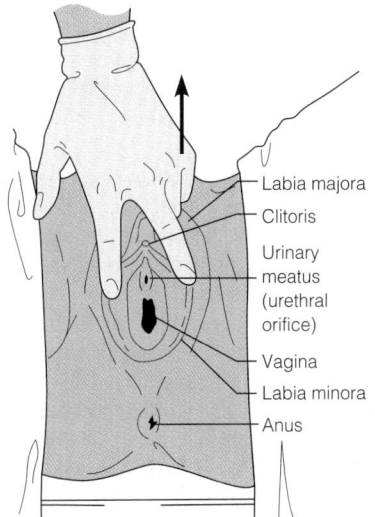

❷ To expose the urinary meatus, separate the labia minora and retract the tissue upward.

continued on page 1306

SKILL 48-2

PERFORMING URETHRAL URINARY CATHETERIZATION *continued*

6. If using a collecting bag and it is not contained within the catheterization kit, open the drainage package and place the end of the tubing within reach. **Rationale:** *Since one hand is needed to hold the catheter once it is in place, open the package while two hands are still available.*

7. If agency policy permits, apply clean gloves and inject 10 to 15 mL Xylocaine gel into the urethra of the male client. Wipe the underside of the shaft to distribute the gel up the urethra. Wait at least 5 minutes for the gel to take effect before inserting the catheter. Remove gloves.

8. Open the catheterization kit. Place a waterproof drape under the buttocks (female) or penis (male) without contaminating the center of the drape with your hands.

9. Put on sterile gloves.

10. Organize the remaining supplies:
    - Saturate the cleansing balls with the antiseptic solution.
    - Open the lubricant package.
    - Remove the specimen container and place it nearby with the lid loosely on top.

11. Attach the prefilled syringe to the indwelling catheter inflation hub and test the balloon. **Rationale:** *If the balloon malfunctions, it is important to replace it prior to use.*

12. Lubricate the catheter (1 to 2 in. for females, 6 to 7 in. for males) and place it with the drainage end inside the collection container.

13. If desired, place the fenestrated drape over the perineum, exposing the urinary meatus.

14. Cleanse the meatus. *Note:* The nondominant hand is considered contaminated once it touches the client's skin.
    a. Women:
       Use your nondominant hand to spread the labia. Establish a firm but gentle position. The antiseptic may make the tissues slippery but the labia must not be allowed to return over the cleaned meatus. Pick up a cleansing ball with the forceps in your dominant hand and wipe one side of the labia majora in an anteroposterior direction. ❸ Use great care that wiping the client does not contaminate this sterile hand. Use a new ball for the opposite side. Repeat for the labia minora. Use the last ball to cleanse directly over the meatus. *Note:* Location of the urethral meatus is best identified during the cleansing process.
    b. Men:
       Use your nondominant hand to grasp the penis just below the glans. If necessary, retract the foreskin. Hold the penis firmly upright, with slight tension. **Rationale:** *Lifting the penis in this manner helps straighten the urethra.* Pick up a cleansing ball with the forceps in your dominant hand and wipe from the center of the meatus in a circular motion around the glans. Use great care that wiping the client does not contaminate this sterile hand. Use a new ball and repeat three more times. The antiseptic may make the tissues slippery but the foreskin must not be allowed to return over the cleaned meatus nor the penis be dropped.

15. Insert the catheter.
    - Grasp the catheter firmly 2 to 3 in. from the tip. Ask the client to take a slow deep breath and insert the catheter as the client

❸ When cleaning the urinary meatus, move the swab downward.

exhales. Slight resistance is expected as the catheter passes through the sphincters. If necessary, twist the catheter or hold pressure on the catheter until the sphincter relaxes.
    - Advance the catheter 2 inches farther after the urine begins to flow through it, *to be sure it is fully in the bladder.* For male clients, some agencys' policies and procedures indicate to advance the catheter to the "Y" bifurcation of the catheter. Check your agency's policy.
    - If the catheter accidentally contacts the labia or slips into the vagina, it is considered contaminated and a new, sterile catheter must be used. The contaminated catheter may be left in the vagina until the new catheter is inserted to help avoid mistaking the vaginal opening for the urethral meatus.

16. Hold the catheter with the nondominant hand. In males, lay the penis down onto the drape, being careful that the catheter does not pull out.

17. For an indwelling catheter, inflate the retention balloon with the designated volume.
    - Without releasing the catheter, hold the inflation valve between two fingers of your nondominant hand while you attach the syringe (if not left attached earlier when testing the balloon) and inflate with your dominant hand. If the client complains of discomfort, immediately withdraw the instilled fluid, advance the catheter further, and attempt to inflate the balloon again.
    - Pull *gently* on the catheter until resistance is felt to ensure that the balloon has inflated and to place it in the trigone of the bladder. ❹

18. Collect a urine specimen if needed. Allow 20 to 30 mL to flow into the bottle without touching the catheter to the bottle.

19. Allow the straight catheter to continue draining. If necessary, attach the drainage end of an indwelling catheter to the collecting tubing and bag.

PERFORMING URETHRAL URINARY CATHETERIZATION *continued*

4 Placement of indwelling catheter and inflated balloon in *A,* female client; and *B,* male client.

20. Examine and measure the urine. In some cases, only 750 to 1,000 mL of urine are to be drained from the bladder at one time. Check agency policy for further instructions if this should occur.

21. Remove the straight catheter when urine flow stops. For an indwelling catheter, secure the catheter tubing to the inner thigh for female clients **5** or the upper thigh/abdomen for male clients **6** with enough slack to allow usual movement. Tape or a manufactured catheter-securing device should be used to secure the catheter tubing to the client. This prevents unnecessary trauma to the urethra. Also secure the collecting tubing to the bed linens and hang the bag below the level of the bladder. No tubing should fall below the top of the bag. **7**

22. Wipe the perineal area of any remaining antiseptic or lubricant. Replace the foreskin if retracted earlier. Return the client to a comfortable position.

23. Discard all used supplies in appropriate receptacles and wash your hands.

24. Document the catheterization procedure including catheter size and results in the client record using forms or checklists supplemented by narrative notes when appropriate.

5 Tape the catheter tube to the inside of a female client's thigh.

6 Tape the catheter tube to the thigh or abdomen of a male client.

7 Correct position for urine drainage bag and tubing.

continued on page 1308

PERFORMING URETHRAL URINARY CATHETERIZATION *continued*

SAMPLE DOCUMENTATION

7/24/2007 2000 Has not voided since surgery (6 hours) despite repeated attempts. C/O discomfort. Moderate distention noted above the symphysis pubis. Straight cath performed per Dr. Carpenter's order. Obtained 650 cc of clear yellow urine. Specimen sent to lab. States she "feels much better".———C. Chavez, RN

SAMPLE DOCUMENTATION

9/12/2007 1030 Explained that Dr. Rattigan ordered insertion of a Foley catheter. Stated that the doctor had discussed it with her previously. Explained the insertion process. Stated she understood and that she had one inserted on a previous admission. #16 Fr silicone catheter inserted without difficulty with 10 cc of solution added to balloon. Obtained 800 cc of yellow, clear urine. Specimen sent to lab. Tolerated procedure well. States she feels "comfortable and has no discomfort".———

——————— K. Bishop, RN.

EVALUATION

Conduct appropriate follow-up such as notifying the primary care provider of the catheterization results. Perform a detailed follow-up based on findings that deviated from expected or normal for the client. Relate findings to previous assessment data if available. Teach the client how to care for the indwelling catheter, to drink more fluids, and other appropriate instructions.

LIFESPAN CONSIDERATIONS   Catheterization

INFANTS AND CHILDREN

- Adapt the size of the catheter for pediatric clients.
- Ask a family member to assist in holding the child during catheterization, if appropriate.

ELDERS

When catheterizing elders, be very attentive to problems of limited movement, especially in the hips. Arthritis, or previous hip or knee surgery, may limit their movement and cause discomfort. Modify the position (e.g., side-lying) as needed to perform the procedure safely and comfortably. For women, obtain the assistance of another nurse to flex and hold the client's knees and hips as necessary or place her in a modified Sims' position.

HOME CARE CONSIDERATIONS   Catheterization

For intermittent catheterization, instruct the client to

- Follow instructions for clean technique.
- Wash hands well with warm water and soap prior to handling equipment or performing catheterization.
- Monitor for signs and symptoms of urinary tract infection including burning, urgency, abdominal pain, and cloudy urine; in elders, confusion may be an early sign.
- Ensure adequate oral intake of fluids.
- After each catheterization, assess the urine for color, odor, clarity, and the presence of blood.
- Wash rubber catheters thoroughly with soap and water after use, dry, and store in a clean place.

For indwelling catheters, instruct the client to

- Never pull on the catheter.
- Secure the catheter tubing to your leg using a catheter securing device.
- Ensure that there are no kinks or twists in the tubing.
- Keep the urine drainage bag below the level of the bladder (Figure 48-11 ■). A leg bag may substitute for a hanging bag for those who are upright.
- Empty the drainage bag regularly.
- Take a shower rather than a tub bath. *Sitting in a tub allows bacteria easier access into the urinary tract.*
- Monitor for signs and symptoms of urinary tract infection including burning, urgency, abdominal pain, cloudy urine; in older adults, confusion may be an early sign.

- Ensure adequate oral intake of fluids.

   Clients who have indwelling catheters for lengthy periods of time need to have the catheter and bag changed at regular intervals. Changing equipment once a month is often the standard, although agency policy may differ.

Figure 48-11 ■
Positioning the collecting bag and tubing when sitting in a chair.

Nursing Interventions for Clients with Indwelling Catheters

Nursing care of the client with an indwelling catheter and continuous drainage is largely directed toward preventing infection of the urinary tract and encouraging urinary flow through the drainage system. It includes encouraging large amounts of fluid intake, accurately recording the fluid intake and output, changing the retention catheter and tubing, maintaining the patency of the drainage system, preventing contamination of the drainage system, and teaching these measures to the client.

FLUIDS. The client with a retention catheter should drink up to 3,000 mL per day if permitted. Large amounts of fluid ensure a large urine output, which keeps the bladder flushed out and decreases the likelihood of urinary stasis and subsequent infection. Large volumes of urine also minimize the risk of sediment or other particles obstructing the drainage tubing.

DIETARY MEASURES. Acidifying the urine of clients with a retention catheter may reduce the risk of urinary tract infection and calculus formation. Foods such as eggs, cheese, meat and poultry, whole grains, cranberries, plums and prunes, and tomatoes tend to increase the acidity of urine. Conversely, most fruits and vegetables, legumes, and milk and milk products result in alkaline urine.

PERINEAL CARE. No special cleaning other than routine hygienic care is necessary for clients with retention catheters, nor is special meatal care recommended. Agency practices regarding catheter care vary considerably. The nurse should check agency practice in this regard.

CHANGING THE CATHETER AND TUBING. Routine changing of catheter and tubing is not recommended. Collection of sediment in the catheter or tubing or impaired urine drainage are indicators for changing the catheter and drainage system. When this occurs the catheter and drainage system are removed and discarded, and a new sterile catheter with a closed drainage system is inserted.

Guidelines to prevent catheter-associated urinary tract infections are given in Practice Guidelines. Ongoing assessment of clients with retention catheters is a high priority (see Box 48–4).

PRACTICE GUIDELINES Preventing Catheter-Associated Urinary Infections

- Have an established infection control program.
- Catheterize clients only when necessary, by using aseptic technique, sterile equipment, and trained personnel.
- Maintain a sterile closed-drainage system.
- Do not disconnect the catheter and drainage tubing unless absolutely necessary.
- Remove the catheter as soon as possible.
- Follow and reinforce good hand washing technique.
- Provide routine perineal hygiene, including cleansing with soap and water after defecation.
- Prevent contamination of the catheter with feces in the incontinent client.

BOX 48–4 Ongoing Assessment of Clients with Indwelling Catheters

- Ensure that there are no obstructions in the drainage. Check that there are no kinks in the tubing, the client is not lying on the tubing, and the tubing is not clogged with mucus or blood.
- Check that there is no tension on the catheter or tubing, that the catheter is securely attached to the thigh or abdomen, and that the tubing is fastened appropriately to the bedclothes.
- Ensure that gravity drainage is maintained. Make sure there are no loops in the tubing below its entry to the drainage receptacle and that the drainage receptacle is below the level of the client's bladder.
- Ensure that the drainage system is well sealed or closed. Check that there are no leaks at the connection sites in open systems.
- Observe the flow of the urine every 2 or 3 hours, and note color, odor, and any abnormal constituents. If sediment is present, check the catheter more frequently to ascertain whether it is plugged.

REMOVING INDWELLING CATHETERS. Indwelling catheters are removed after their purpose has been achieved, usually on the order of the primary care provider. If the catheter has been in place for a short time (e.g., a few days), the client usually has little difficulty regaining normal urinary elimination patterns. Swelling of the urethra, however, may initially interfere with voiding, so the nurse should regularly assess the client for urinary retention until voiding is reestablished.

Clients who have had a retention catheter for a prolonged period may require bladder retraining to regain bladder muscle tone. With an indwelling catheter in place, the bladder muscle does not stretch and contract regularly as it does when the bladder fills and empties by voiding. A few days before removal, the catheter may be clamped for specified periods of time (e.g., 2 to 4 hours), then released to allow the bladder to empty. This allows the bladder to distend and stimulates its musculature. Check agency policy regarding bladder training procedures.

To remove a retention catheter, the nurse follows these steps:

- Obtain a receptacle for the catheter (e.g., a disposable basin); a clean, disposable towel; clean gloves; and a sterile syringe to deflate the balloon. The syringe should be large enough to withdraw all the solution in the catheter balloon. The size of the balloon is indicated on the label at the end of the catheter.
- Ask the client to assume a supine position as for a catheterization.
- *Optional:* Obtain a sterile specimen before removing the catheter. Check agency protocol.
- Remove the tape or catheter securing device attaching the catheter to the client, put on gloves, and then place the towel between the legs of the female client or over the thighs of the male.
- Insert the syringe into the injection port of the catheter, and withdraw the fluid from the balloon. If not all of the fluid can be removed, report this fact to the nurse in charge before proceeding.
- Do not pull the catheter while the balloon is inflated; doing so may injure the urethra.

RESEARCH NOTE   What Guides Practice in the Nursing Care of Clients with Problems of Urinary Elimination?

When do you insert a urinary catheter? What type of urinary catheter is best for this client? Do you clamp the catheter prior to discontinuing an indwelling catheter? Is cranberry juice effective in preventing urinary tract infections? Which management strategy is most effective for urge urinary incontinence? How often should the urostomy appliance be changed? These are some of the questions faced daily by the nurse clinician when caring for clients experiencing problems with urinary elimination. A review of the literature and of systematic reviews of the literature (i.e., Cochrane Library) consistently reveal a lack of evidence from randomized or quasi-randomized controlled studies, whereby no conclusions can be made regarding the use of specific products, techniques, or interventions that support current practice. Studies that do exist are small and identify consistently the need for larger, randomized controlled studies. Documentation is needed of not only what is being done, but also how it is affecting client outcomes such as decreasing nosocomial urinary tract infections, decreasing perineal dermal ulcers, shortening hospital stays, and increasing client and caregiver independence.

IMPLICATIONS

Nurse clinicians at the bedside are aptly positioned to complete needed research trials to document evidence and client outcomes.

- After all of the fluid is withdrawn from the balloon, gently withdraw the catheter and place it in the waste receptacle.
- Dry the perineal area with a towel.
- Remove gloves.
- Measure the urine in the drainage bag, and record the removal of the catheter. Include in the recording (a) the time the catheter was removed; (b) the amount, color, and clarity of the urine; (c) the intactness of the catheter; and (d) instructions given to the client.
- Provide the client with either a urinal (men), bedpan, commode, or toilet collection device ("hat") to be used with each, subsequent unassisted void.
- Following removal of the catheter, determine the time of the first voiding and the amount voided during the first 8 hours. Compare this output to the client's intake.
- Observe for dysfunctional voiding behaviors (i.e., <100 mL per void), which might indicate urinary retention. If this occurs, perform an assessment of postvoid residuals using a bladder scanner if available. Generally postvoid residuals greater than 200 cc will require straight catheterization as needed.

Clean Intermittent Self-Catheterization

Clean intermittent self-catheterization (CISC) is performed by many clients who have some form of neurogenic bladder dysfunction, such as that caused by spinal cord injury. Clean or medical aseptic technique is used. Intermittent self-catheterization

- Enables the client to retain independence and gain control of the bladder.
- Reduces incidence of urinary tract infection.
- Protects the upper urinary tract from reflux.
- Allows normal sexual relations without incontinence.
- Reduces the use of aids and appliances.
- Frees the client from embarrassing dribbling.

The procedure for self-catheterization is similar to that used by the nurse to catheterize a client. Essential steps are outlined in the accompanying Client Teaching feature. Because the procedure requires physical and mental preparation, client assessment is important. The client should have

- Sufficient manual dexterity to manipulate a catheter.
- Sufficient mental ability.
- Motivation and acceptance of the procedure.
- For women, reasonable agility to access the urethra.
- Bladder capacity greater than 100 mL.

Before teaching CISC, the nurse should establish the client's voiding patterns, the volume voided, fluid intake, and residual amounts. CISC is easier for males to learn because of the visibility of the urinary meatus. Females need to learn initially with the aid of a mirror but eventually should perform the procedure by using only the sense of touch (as described in Client Teaching).

Urinary Irrigations

An **irrigation** is a flushing or washing-out with a specified solution. Bladder irrigation is carried out on a primary care provider's order, usually to wash out the bladder and sometimes to apply a medication to the bladder lining. Catheter irrigations may be performed to maintain or restore the patency of a catheter; for example, to remove pus or blood clots blocking the catheter.

The closed method is the preferred technique for catheter or bladder irrigation because it is associated with a lower risk of urinary tract infection. Closed catheter irrigations may be either continuous or intermittent. This method is most often used for clients who have had genitourinary surgery. The continuous irrigation helps prevent blood clots occluding the catheter. A three-way, or triple lumen, catheter (see Figure 48-10) is generally used for closed irrigations. The irrigating solution flows into the bladder through the irrigation port of the catheter and out through the urinary drainage lumen of the catheter.

Occasionally an open irrigation may be necessary to restore catheter patency. The risk of injecting microorganisms into the urinary tract is greater with open irrigations, because the connection between the indwelling catheter and the drainage tubing is broken. Strict precautions to maintain the sterility of the drainage tubing connector and interior of the indwelling catheter must be taken to minimize this risk.

The open method of catheter or bladder irrigation is performed with double-lumen indwelling catheters. It may be necessary for clients who develop blood clots and mucous fragments that occlude the catheter and when it is undesirable to change the catheter. Techniques for catheter irrigation are outlined in Skill 48-3.

CLIENT TEACHING   Clean Intermittent Self-Catheterization

- Catheterize as often as needed to maintain. At first, catheterization may be necessary every 2 to 3 hours, increasing to 4 to 6 hours.
- Attempt to void before catheterization; insert the catheter to remove residual urine if unable to void or if amount voided is insufficient (e.g., less than 100 mL).
- Assemble all needed supplies ahead of time. Good lighting is essential, especially for women.
- If a woman, remove a tampon before catheterizing. *A tampon can inhibit catheterization.*
- Wash your hands.
- Clean the urinary meatus with either a towelette or soapy washcloth, then rinse with a wet washcloth. Women should clean the area from front to back.
- Assume a position that is comfortable and that facilitates passage of the catheter, such as a semireclining position in bed or sitting on a chair or the toilet. Men may prefer to stand over the toilet; women may prefer to stand with one foot on the side of the bathtub.
- Apply lubricant to the catheter tip (1 in. [2.5 cm] for women; 2 to 6 in. [5 to 15 cm] for men).
- Insert the catheter until urine flows through.
  a. If a woman, locate the meatus using a mirror or other aid, or use the "touch" technique as follows:

  - Place the index finger of your nondominant hand on your clitoris.
  - Place the third and fourth fingers at the vagina.
  - Locate the meatus between the index and third fingers.
  - Direct the catheter through the meatus and then upward and forward.
  b. If a man, hold the penis with a slight upward tension at a 60- to 90-degree angle to insert the catheter. Return the penis to its natural position when urine starts to flow.
- Hold the catheter in place until all urine is drained.
- Withdraw the catheter slowly *to ensure complete drainage of urine.*
- Wash the catheter with soap and water; store in a clean container. Replace the catheter when it becomes difficult to clean, or too soft or hard to insert easily.
- Contact your care provider if your urine becomes cloudy or contains sediment; if you have bleeding, difficulty, or pain when passing the catheter; or if you have a fever.
- Drink at least 2,000 to 2,500 mL of fluid a day *to ensure adequate bladder filling and flushing.* To keep your urine acidic and reduce the risk of bladder infections, drink cranberry and prune juices.

PERFORMING BLADDER IRRIGATION

SKILL 48-3

PURPOSES
- To maintain the patency of a urinary catheter and tubing (closed continuous irrigation)
- To free a blockage in a urinary catheter or tubing (open intermittent irrigation)

ASSESSMENT
- Determine the client's current urinary drainage system. Review the client record for recent intake and output and any difficulties the client has been experiencing with the system. Review the results of previous irrigations.
- Assess the client for any discomfort, bladder spasms, or distended bladder.

PLANNING
Before irrigating a catheter or bladder, check (a) the reason for the irrigation; (b) the order authorizing the continuous or intermittent irrigation (in most agencies, primary care provider's order is required); (c) the type of sterile solution, the amount, and strength to be used, and the rate (if continuous); and (d) the type of catheter in place. If these are not specified on the client's chart, check agency protocol.

Delegation
Due to the need for sterile technique, urinary irrigation is generally not delegated to UAP. If the client has continuous irrigation, the UAP may care for the client and note abnormal findings. These must be validated and interpreted by the nurse.

Equipment
- Clean gloves (2 pairs)
- Retention catheter in place
- Drainage tubing and bag (if not in place)
- Drainage tubing clamp
- Antiseptic swabs
- Sterile receptacle
- Sterile irrigating solution warmed or at room temperature (Label the irrigant clearly with the words *Bladder Irrigation,* including the information about any medications that have been added to the original solution, and the date, time, and nurse's initials.)
- Infusion tubing
- IV pole

IMPLEMENTATION
Performance
1. Prior to performing the procedure, introduce self and verify the client's identity using agency protocol. Explain to the client what you are going to do, why it is necessary, and how he or she can cooperate. The irrigation should not be painful or uncomfortable. Discuss how the results will be used in planning further care or treatments.
2. Perform hand hygiene and observe appropriate infection control procedures.
3. Provide for client privacy.
4. Put on clean gloves.

continued on page 1312

PERFORMING BLADDER IRRIGATION *continued*

5. Empty, measure, and record the amount and appearance of urine present in the drainage bag. Discard urine and gloves. **Rationale:** *Emptying the drainage bag allows more accurate measurement of urinary output after the irrigation is in place or completed. Assessing the character of the urine provides baseline data for later comparison.*

6. Prepare the equipment.
   - Perform hand hygiene.
   - Connect the irrigation infusion tubing to the irrigating solution and flush the tubing with solution, keeping the tip sterile. **Rationale:** *Flushing the tubing removes air and prevents it from being instilled into the bladder.*
   - Apply clean gloves and cleanse the port with antiseptic swabs.
   - Connect the irrigation tubing to the input port of the three-way catheter.
   - Connect the drainage bag and tubing to the urinary drainage port if not already in place.
   - Remove the gloves and perform hand hygiene.

7. Irrigate the bladder.
   a. For closed continuous irrigation, open the flow clamp on the urinary drainage tubing (if present). See ❶ **Rationale:** *This allows the irrigating solution to flow out of the bladder continuously.*
      - Open the regulating clamp on the irrigating tubing and adjust the flow rate as prescribed by the primary care provider or to 40 to 60 drops per minute if not specified.
      - Assess the drainage for amount, color, and clarity. The amount of drainage should equal the amount of irrigant entering the bladder plus expected urine output.
   b. For closed intermittent irrigation, determine whether the solution is to remain in the bladder for a specified time.
      - If the solution is to remain in the bladder (a bladder irrigation or instillation), apply the flow clamp to the urinary drainage tubing. **Rationale:** *Closing the flow clamp allows the solution to be retained in the bladder and in contact with bladder walls.*
      - If the solution is being instilled to irrigate the catheter, open the flow clamp on the urinary drainage tubing. **Rationale:** *Irrigating solution will flow through the urinary drainage port and tubing, removing mucous shreds or clots.*
      - Open the flow clamp on the irrigating tubing, allowing the specified amount of solution to infuse. Clamp the tubing.
      - After the specified period the solution is to be retained, open the drainage tubing flow clamp and allow the bladder to empty.
      - Assess the drainage for amount, color, and clarity. The amount of drainage should equal the amount of irrigant entering the bladder plus expected urine output.

8. Assess the client and the urinary output.
   - Assess the client's comfort.
   - Empty the drainage bag and measure the contents. Subtract the amount of irrigant instilled from the total volume of drainage to obtain the volume of urine output.

9. Document the procedure and results in the client record using forms or checklists supplemented by narrative notes when appropriate.
   - Note any abnormal constituents such as blood clots, pus, or mucous shreds.

VARIATION: OPEN IRRIGATION USING A TWO-WAY INDWELLING CATHETER

1. Assemble the equipment. Use an irrigation tray ❷ or assemble individual items, including
   - Clean gloves
   - Sterile gloves
   - Disposable water-resistant towel
   - Sterile irrigating solution
   - Sterile irrigation set
   - Sterile basin
   - Sterile 50-mL Asepto syringe
   - Antiseptic swabs
   - Sterile protective cap (for catheter drainage tubing)

Irrigation bag

Drip chamber

Clamp

Bladder

Tubing to irrigation port

Port for inflation of catheter balloon

Tubing from bladder

Drainage bag

❶ A continuous bladder irrigation (CBI) setup.

❷ An irrigation set.

(Courtesy of Bard Medical Division.)

PERFORMING BLADDER IRRIGATION *continued*

2. Prepare the client (see steps 1–5 of main procedure for catheter irrigation).
3. Prepare the equipment.
   - Perform hand hygiene.
   - Using aseptic technique, open supplies and pour the irrigating solution into the sterile basin or receptacle. **Rationale:** *Aseptic technique is vital to reduce the risk of instilling microorganisms into the urinary tract during the irrigation.*
   - Place the disposable water-resistant towel under the catheter.
   - Put on clean gloves. Disconnect catheter from drainage tubing. Place sterile protective cap over end of drainage tubing. **Rationale:** *The end of the drainage tubing will be considered contaminated if it touches bed linens or skin surfaces.*
   - Remove clean gloves and put on sterile gloves.
   - Withdraw the prescribed amount of irrigating solution into the syringe, maintaining the sterility of the syringe and solution.

4. Irrigate the bladder.
   - Insert the tip of the syringe into the catheter opening.
   - Gently and slowly inject the solution. In adults, about 30 to 40 mL generally is instilled for catheter irrigations; 100 to 200 mL may be instilled for bladder irrigation. **Rationale:** *Gentle instillation reduces the risks of injury to bladder mucosa and of bladder spasms.*
   - Remove syringe and allow solution to drain into basin.
   - Continue to irrigate client's bladder until fluid returns are clear and/or clots are removed.
   - Remove protective cap from drainage tube and wipe with antiseptic swab or alcohol sponge.
   - Reconnect catheter to drainage tubing.
   - Assess the drainage for amount, color, and clarity. The amount of drainage should equal the amount of irrigant entering the bladder. Determine the amount of fluid used for the irrigation and subtract from total ouput on the client's I&O record.
5. Assess the client and the urinary output and document the procedure as in steps 8 and 9 above.

EVALUATION
- Perform detailed follow-up based on findings that deviated from expected or normal for the client. Relate findings to previous assessment data if available.
- Report significant deviations from normal to the primary care provider.

Suprapubic Catheter Care

A **suprapubic catheter** is inserted surgically through the abdominal wall above the symphysis pubis into the urinary bladder (Figure 48-12 ■). The physician inserts the catheter using local anesthesia or during bladder or vaginal surgery. The catheter may be secured in place with sutures if a retention balloon is not used and is then attached to a closed drainage system. The suprapubic catheter may be placed for temporary bladder drainage until the client is able to resume normal voiding (e.g., after urethral, bladder, or vaginal surgery) or it may become a permanent device (e.g., urethral or pelvic trauma).

Care of clients with a suprapubic catheter includes regular assessments of the client's urine, fluid intake, and comfort; maintenance of a patent drainage system; skin care around the insertion site; and periodic clamping of the catheter preparatory to removing it if it is not a permanent appliance. If the catheter is temporary, orders generally include leaving the catheter open to drainage for 48 to 72 hours, then clamping the catheter for 3- to 4-hour periods during the day until the client can void satisfactory amounts. Satisfactory voiding is determined by measuring the client's residual urine after voiding.

Care of the catheter insertion site involves sterile technique. Dressings around the newly placed suprapubic catheter are changed whenever they are soiled with drainage to prevent bacterial growth around the insertion site and reduce the potential for infection. A small amount of povidone-iodine ointment is frequently applied around the insertion site and the site covered with gauze dressings. For catheters that have been in place for an extended period, no dressing may be needed and the healed insertion tract enables removal and replacement of the catheter

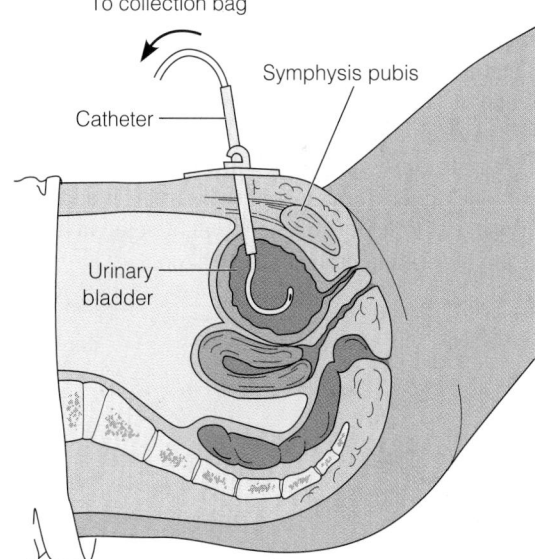

Figure 48-12 ■ A suprapubic catheter in place.

as needed. Securing the catheter tube to the abdomen helps to reduce tension at the insertion site. The nurse assesses the insertion area at regular intervals. If abdominal hair invades the insertion site, it may be carefully shaved. Any redness or discharge at the skin around the insertion site must be reported.

Urinary Diversions

A urinary diversion is the surgical rerouting of urine from the kidneys to a site other than the bladder. There are two categories of diversions: incontinent and continent.

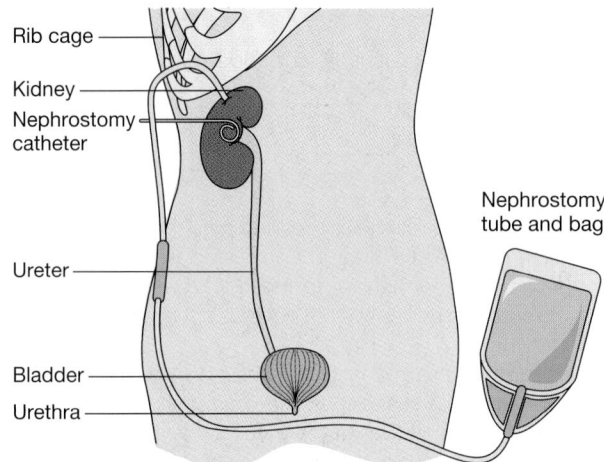

Figure 48-13 ■ A nephrostomy.

INCONTINENT. With incontinent diversions clients have no control over the passage of urine and require the use of an external ostomy appliance to contain the urine. Urinary diversions may or may not involve the removal of the bladder (cystectomy). Examples of incontinent diversions include ureterostomy, nephrostomy, vesicostomy, and ileal conduits. A **ureterostomy** is when one or both of the ureters may be brought directly to the side of the abdomen to form small stomas. This procedure, however, has some disadvantages in that the stomas provide direct access for microorganisms from the skin to the kidneys, the small stomas are difficult to fit with an appliance to collect the urine, and they may narrow, impairing urine drainage. A **nephrostomy** diverts urine from the kidney to a stoma (Figure 48-13 ■). A **vesicostomy** may be formed when the bladder is left intact but voiding through the urethra is not possible (e.g., due to an obstruction or a neurogenic bladder). The ureters remain connected to the bladder, and the bladder wall is surgically attached to an opening in the skin below the navel forming an incontinent stoma.

The most common urinary diversion is the **ileal conduit** or ileal loop (Figure 48-14 ■). In this procedure, a segment of the ileum is removed and the intestinal ends are reattached. One end of the portion removed is closed with sutures to create a pouch, and the other end is brought out through the abdominal wall to create a stoma. The ureters are implanted into the ileal pouch. The ileal stoma is more readily fitted with an appliance than ureterostomies because of its larger size. The mucous membrane lining of the ileum also provides some protection from ascending infection. Urine drains continuously from the ileal pouch.

CONTINENT. With continent diversions, a continence mechanism is created giving clients control over the passage of urine, either by intermittent catheterization of the internal reservoir (e.g., Kock pouch) or by strained voiding (neobladder).

The Kock (pronounced "coke") pouch, or continent ileal bladder conduit, also uses a portion of the ileum to form a reservoir for urine (Figure 48-15 ■). In this procedure, nipple valves are formed by doubling the tissue backward into the reservoir where the pouch connects to the skin and the ureters connect to

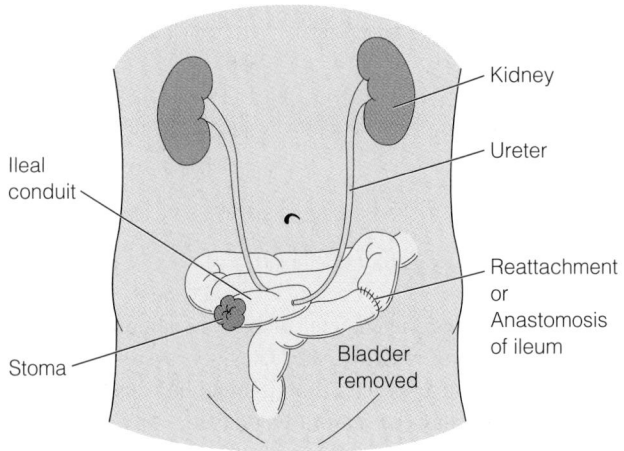

Figure 48-14 ■ An incontinent urinary diversion (ileal conduit).

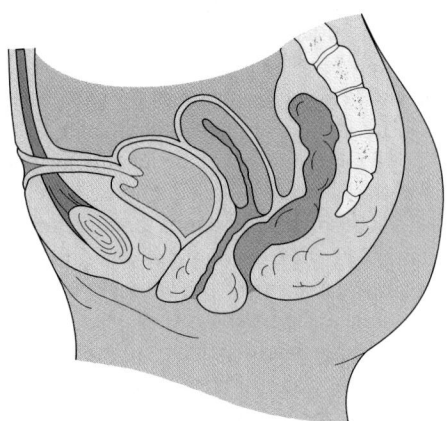

Figure 48-15 ■ The Kock pouch—a continent urinary diversion.

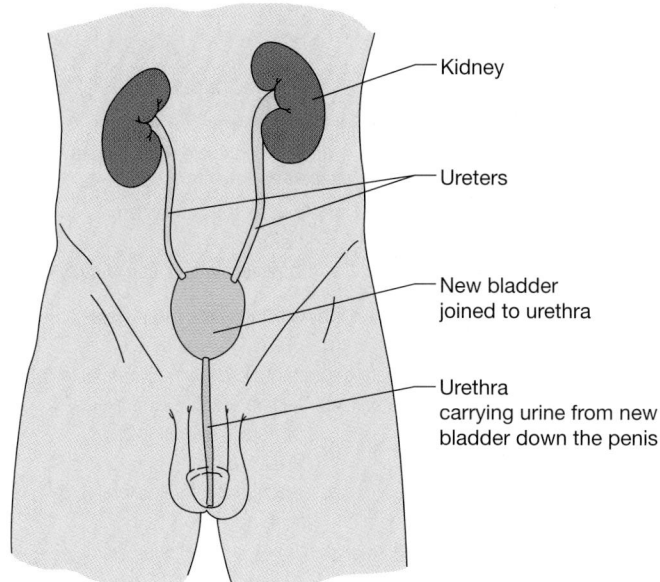

Figure 48-16 ■ A neobladder.

the pouch. These valves close as the pouch fills with urine, preventing leakage and reflux of urine back toward the kidneys. The client empties the pouch by inserting a clean catheter approximately every 4 hours. Between catheterizations, a small dressing is worn to protect the stoma and clothing.

As opposed to the vesicostomy, a neobladder replaces a diseased or damaged bladder with a piece of ileum, thus making a new bladder. This new bladder is then sutured to the functional urethra. Clients with these can control voiding (Figure 48-16 ■).

When caring for clients with a urinary diversion, the nurse must accurately assess intake and output; note any changes in urine color, odor, or clarity (mucous shreds are commonly seen in the urine of clients with an ileal diversion); and frequently assess the condition of the stoma and surrounding skin. Clients who must wear a urine collection appliance are at risk for impaired skin integrity because of irritation by urine. Well-fitting appliances are vital. The nurse should consult with the wound ostomy continence nurse (WOCN) to identify strategies for management of stoma and peristomal problems and the most appropriate appliance for the client's needs. The steps of changing a urostomy appliance are similar to those described in the procedure for changing a bowel diversion appliance (see Chapter 49 ∞). However, there are some differences, including the following: Incontinent urinary diversions drain continually. As a result the stoma must be wicked throughout the measurement and change

of the ostomy appliance. This prevents the peristomal skin from becoming wet with urine during the appliance change. Immediately following surgery, ureteral stents may be present and protruding from the stoma. They remain in place for 10 to 14 days postop and are removed by either, the surgeon or the WOCN, depending on institutional protocol. Ureteral stents are used to maintain the patency of ureters at the anastomotic sites.

Clients with urinary diversions may experience problems with their body image and sexuality and may require assistance in coping with these changes and managing the stoma. Most clients are able to resume their normal activities and lifestyle.

Evaluating

Using the overall goals and desired outcomes identified in the planning stage, the nurse collects data to evaluate the effectiveness of nursing activities. Examples of desired outcomes for the identified goals are listed in the Identifying Nursing Diagnoses, Interventions, and Outcomes box earlier in this chapter.

If the desired outcomes are not achieved, explore the reasons before modifying the care plan. For example, if the outcome "Remains dry between voidings and at night" is not met, examples of questions that need to be considered include:

■ What is the client's perception of the problem?
■ Does the client understand and comply with the health care instructions provided?
■ Is access to toilet facilities a problem?
■ Can the client manipulate clothing for toileting? Are there adjustments that can be made to allow easier disrobing?
■ Are scheduled toileting times appropriate?
■ Is there adequate transition lighting for nighttime toileting?
■ Are mobility aids such as a walker, elevated toilet seat, or grab bar needed? If currently used, are they appropriate or adequate?
■ Is the client performing pelvic floor muscle exercises appropriately as scheduled?
■ Is the client's fluid intake adequate? Does the timing of fluid intake need to be adjusted (e.g., restricted after dinner)?
■ Is the client restricting caffeine, citrus juice, carbonated beverages, and artificial sweetener intake?
■ Is the client taking a diuretic? If so, when is the medication taken? Do the times need to be adjusted (e.g., taking second dose no later than 4 PM)?
■ Should continence aids such as a condom catheter or absorbent pads be considered or used?

NURSING CARE PLAN   Urinary Elimination

ASSESSMENT DATA	NURSING DIAGNOSIS	DESIRED OUTCOMES*
Nursing Assessment Mr. John Baker is a 68-year-old shopkeeper who was admitted to the hospital with urinary retention, hematuria, and fever. The admitting nurse gathers the following information when taking a nursing history. Mr. Baker states he has noticed urinary frequency during the day for the past 2 weeks, and that he doesn't feel he has emptied his bladder after urinating. He also has to get up two or three times during the night to urinate. During the past few days, he has had difficulty starting urination and dribbles afterward. He verbalizes the embarrassment his urinary problems cause in his dealings with the public. Mr. Baker is concerned about the cause of this urinary problem. He is diagnosed with benign prostatic hypertrophy (BPH) and referred to a urologist who suggests a transurethral resection of the prostate (TURP) in several months. He is placed on antibiotic therapy.	*Impaired Urinary Elimination* (retention and overflow incontinence) related to bladder neck obstruction by enlarged prostate gland (as evidenced by dysuria, frequency, nocturia, dribbling, hesitancy, and bladder distention)	Urinary Continence [0502] as evidenced by: ■ Able to start and stop stream ■ Empties bladder completely Knowledge: Treatment Regimen [1813] as evidenced by substantial: ■ Description of self-care responsibilities for ongoing care ■ Description of self-monitoring techniques

Physical Examination	**Diagnostic Data**
Height: 185.4 cm (6'2") Weight: 85.7 kg (189 lb) Temperature: 38.1°C (100.6°F) Pulse: 88 BPM Respirations: 20/minute Blood pressure: 146/86 mm Hg Catheterization for urinary retention yielded 300 mL amber urine, Foley left in place for 2 days	CBC normal; urinalysis: amber, clear, pH 6.5, specific gravity 1.025, negative for glucose, protein, ketone, RBCs, and bacteria; IVP: evidence of enlarged prostate gland

NURSING INTERVENTIONS*/SELECTED ACTIVITIES	RATIONALE
Urinary Incontinence Care [0610]	
Monitor urinary elimination, including consistency, odor, volume, and color.	*These parameters help determine adequacy of urinary tract function.*
Help the client select appropriate incontinence garment or pad for short-term management while more definitive treatment is designed.	*Appropriate undergarments can help diminish the embarrassing aspects of urinary incontinence.*
Instruct Mr. Baker to limit fluids for 2 to 3 hours before bedtime.	*Decreased fluid intake several hours before bedtime will decrease the incidence of urinary retention and overflow incontinence, and promote rest.*
Instruct him to drink a minimum of 1,500 mL (six 8-ounce glasses) fluids per day.	*Increased fluids during the day will increase urinary output and discourage bacterial growth.*
Limit ingestion of bladder irritants (e.g., colas, coffee, tea, and chocolate).	*Alcohol, coffee, and tea have a natural diuretic effect and are bladder irritants.*
Urinary Retention Care [0620]	
Instruct Mr. Baker or a family member to record urinary output.	*Serves as an indicator of urinary tract and renal function and of fluid balance.*
Catheterize for residual urine, as appropriate.	*An enlarged prostate compresses the urethra so that urine is retained. Checking for residual urine provides information about bladder emptying.*
Implement intermittent catheterization, as appropriate.	*Helps maintain tonicity of the bladder muscle by preventing overdistention and providing for complete emptying.*

NURSING CARE PLAN Urinary Elimination *continued*

NURSING INTERVENTIONS*/SELECTED ACTIVITIES	RATIONALE
Provide enough time for bladder emptying (10 minutes).	*In addition to the effect of an enlarged prostate on the bladder, stress or anxiety can inhibit relaxation of the urinary sphincter. Sufficient time should be allowed for micturition.*
Instruct the client in ways to avoid constipation or stool impaction.	*Impacted stool may place pressure on the bladder outlet, causing urinary retention.*
Teaching: Disease Process [5602]	
Appraise Mr. Baker's current level of knowledge about benign prostatic hypertrophy.	*Assessing the client's knowledge will provide a foundation for building a teaching plan based on his present understanding of his condition.*
Explain the pathophysiology of the disease and how it relates to urinary anatomy and function.	*In this case, urinary retention and overflow incontinence are caused by obstruction of the bladder neck by an enlarged prostate gland.*
Describe the rationale behind management, therapy, and treatment recommendations.	*Adequate information about treatment options is important to diminish anxiety, promote compliance, and enhance decision making.*
Instruct Mr. Baker on which signs and symptoms to report to the health care provider (e.g., burning on urination, hematuria, oliguria).	*In the individual with prostatic hypertrophy, urinary retention and an overdistended bladder reduce blood flow to the bladder wall, making it more susceptible to infection from bacterial growth. Monitoring for these manifestations of urinary tract infection is essential to prevent urosepsis.*

EVALUATION

Outcomes partially met. Following removal of the Foley catheter, Mr. Baker reported continued difficulty initiating a urinary stream but experienced less dribbling and nocturia. He and his wife selected an undergarment that was acceptable to Mr. Baker and he reports that he feels more confident. Intermittent catheterization not indicated. Intake is approximately 200 mL in excess of output. He is able to discuss the correlation between his enlarged prostate and urinary difficulties. A transurethral resection of the prostate is scheduled in 2 weeks.

The NOC # for desired outcomes and the NIC # for nursing interventions are listed in brackets following the appropriate outcome or intervention. Outcomes, interventions, and activities selected are only a sample of those suggested by NOC and NIC and should be further individualized for each client.

APPLYING CRITICAL THINKING

1. Considering Mr. Baker's history and assessment data, what other physical conditions could explain his symptoms?
2. The primary care provider has recommended surgery. What assumptions will the nurse need to validate in helping prepare Mr. and Mrs. Baker for this surgery?
3. It does not appear that other alternatives have been considered. Why might this be so?
4. Incontinence can lead to client decisions to limit social interactions. What would be an appropriate response if Mr. Baker states that he will just stay home until he has his surgery?

See Critical Thinking Possibilities in Appendix A.

CONCEPT MAP Urinary Elimination

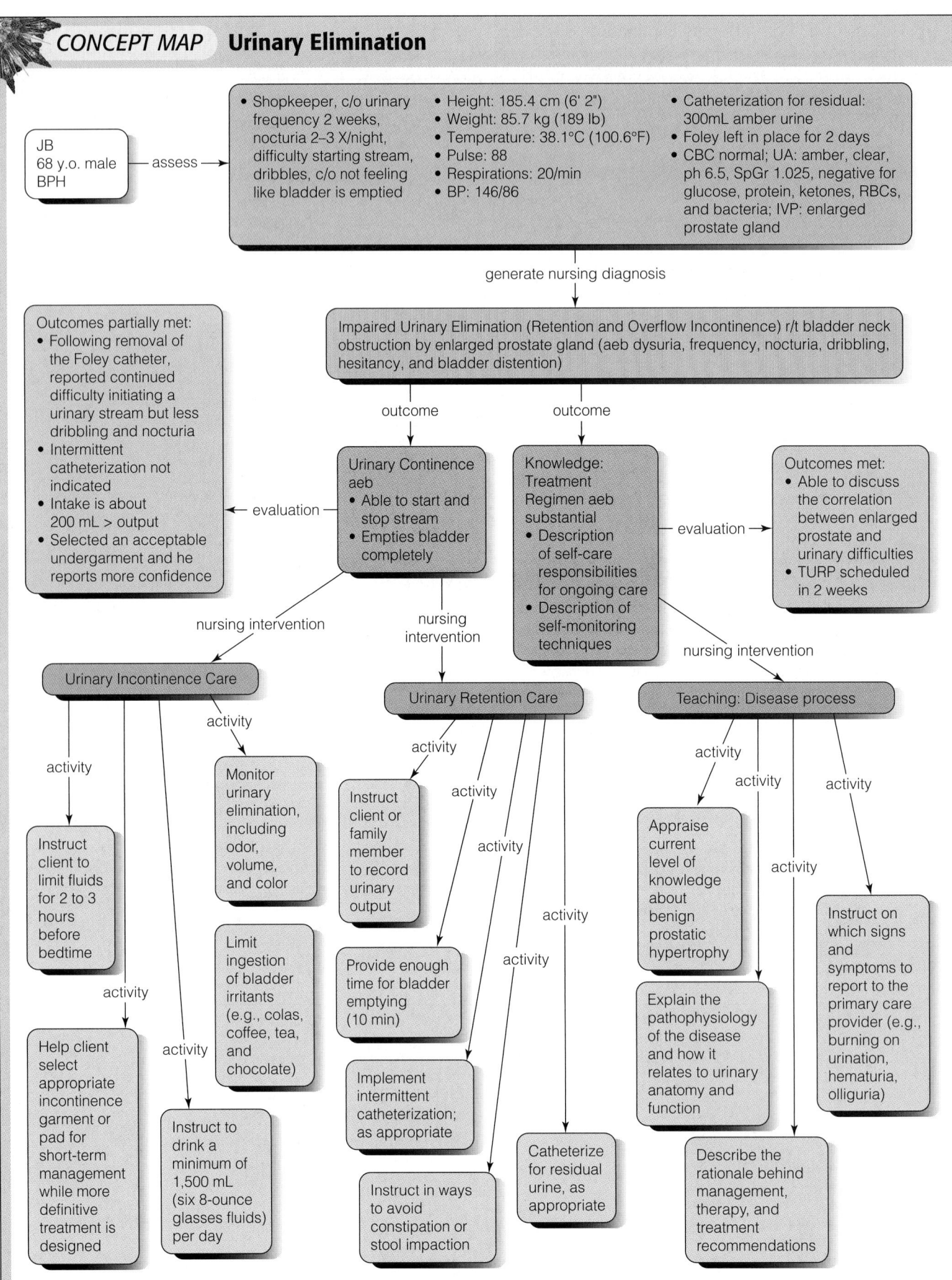

JB
68 y.o. male
BPH

— assess →

- Shopkeeper, c/o urinary frequency 2 weeks, nocturia 2–3 X/night, difficulty starting stream, dribbles, c/o not feeling like bladder is emptied

- Height: 185.4 cm (6' 2")
- Weight: 85.7 kg (189 lb)
- Temperature: 38.1°C (100.6°F)
- Pulse: 88
- Respirations: 20/min
- BP: 146/86

- Catheterization for residual: 300mL amber urine
- Foley left in place for 2 days
- CBC normal; UA: amber, clear, ph 6.5, SpGr 1.025, negative for glucose, protein, ketones, RBCs, and bacteria; IVP: enlarged prostate gland

generate nursing diagnosis

Impaired Urinary Elimination (Retention and Overflow Incontinence) r/t bladder neck obstruction by enlarged prostate gland (aeb dysuria, frequency, nocturia, dribbling, hesitancy, and bladder distention)

outcome ↓   outcome ↓

Outcomes partially met:
- Following removal of the Foley catheter, reported continued difficulty initiating a urinary stream but less dribbling and nocturia
- Intermittent catheterization not indicated
- Intake is about 200 mL > output
- Selected an acceptable undergarment and he reports more confidence

← evaluation —

Urinary Continence aeb
- Able to start and stop stream
- Empties bladder completely

Knowledge: Treatment Regimen aeb substantial
- Description of self-care responsibilities for ongoing care
- Description of self-monitoring techniques

— evaluation →

Outcomes met:
- Able to discuss the correlation between enlarged prostate and urinary difficulties
- TURP scheduled in 2 weeks

nursing intervention   nursing intervention   nursing intervention

Urinary Incontinence Care

activity   activity

activity

Instruct client to limit fluids for 2 to 3 hours before bedtime

Monitor urinary elimination, including odor, volume, and color

activity

Help client select appropriate incontinence garment or pad for short-term management while more definitive treatment is designed

activity

Limit ingestion of bladder irritants (e.g., colas, coffee, tea, and chocolate)

Instruct to drink a minimum of 1,500 mL (six 8-ounce glasses fluids) per day

Urinary Retention Care

activity   activity   activity

activity

activity

Instruct client or family member to record urinary output

Provide enough time for bladder emptying (10 min)

Implement intermittent catheterization; as appropriate

Instruct in ways to avoid constipation or stool impaction

Catheterize for residual urine, as appropriate

Teaching: Disease process

activity   activity   activity

activity

Appraise current level of knowledge about benign prostatic hypertrophy

Explain the pathophysiology of the disease and how it relates to urinary anatomy and function

Instruct on which signs and symptoms to report to the primary care provider (e.g., burning on urination, hematuria, olliguria)

Describe the rationale behind management, therapy, and treatment recommendations

CHAPTER 48 **REVIEW**

CHAPTER HIGHLIGHTS

▨ Urinary elimination depends on normal functioning of the urinary, cardiovascular, and nervous systems.

▨ Urine is formed in the nephron, the functional unit of the kidney, through a process of filtration, reabsorption, and secretion. Hormones such as antidiuretic hormone (ADH) and aldosterone affect the reabsorption of sodium and water, thus affecting the amount of urine formed.

▨ The normal process of urination is stimulated when sufficient urine collects in the bladder to stimulate stretch receptors. Impulses from stretch receptors are transmitted to the spinal cord and the brain, causing relaxation of the internal sphincter (unconscious control) and, if appropriate, relaxation of the external sphincter (conscious control).

▨ In the adult, urination generally occurs after 250 to 450 mL of urine has collected in the bladder.

▨ Many factors influence a person's urinary elimination, including growth and development, fluid intake, stress, activity, medications, and various diseases.

▨ Alterations in urine production and elimination include polyuria, oliguria, anuria, frequency, nocturia, urgency, dysuria, enuresis, hematuria, incontinence, and retention. Each may have various influencing and associated factors that need to be identified.

▨ Assessment of a client's urinary function includes (a) a nursing history that identifies voiding patterns, recent changes, past and current problems with urination, and factors influencing the elimination pattern; (b) a physical assessment of the genitourinary system; (c) inspection of the urine for amount, color, clarity, and odor; and, if indicated, (d) testing of urine for specific gravity, pH, and the presence of glucose, ketone bodies, protein, and occult blood.

▨ Many NANDA-approved nursing diagnoses may apply to clients with altered urinary elimination patterns, for example, *Functional Incontinence, Urinary Retention,* and related diagnoses such as *Risk for Infection.*

▨ Incontinence can be physically and emotionally distressing to clients because it is considered socially unacceptable.

▨ Bladder training can often reduce episodes of incontinence.

▨ Clients with urinary retention not only experience discomfort but also are at risk of urinary tract infection.

▨ The most common cause of urinary tract infection is invasive procedures such as catheterization and cystoscopic examination. Women in particular are prone to ascending urinary tract infections because of their short urethras.

▨ Goals for the client with problems with urinary elimination include maintaining or restoring normal elimination patterns and preventing associated risks such as skin breakdown.

▨ In planning for home care, the nurse considers the client's needs for teaching and assistance or assistive devices in the home.

▨ Nursing interventions related to urinary elimination are generally directed toward facilitating the normal functioning of the urinary system or toward assisting the client with particular problems.

▨ Interventions include (a) assisting the client to maintain an appropriate fluid intake, (b) assisting the client to maintain normal voiding patterns, (c) monitoring the client's daily fluid intake and output, and (d) maintaining cleanliness of the genital area.

▨ Urinary catheterization is frequently required for clients with urinary retention but is only performed when all other measures to facilitate voiding fail. Sterile technique is essential to prevent ascending urinary infections.

▨ Care of clients with indwelling catheters is directed toward preventing infection of the urinary tract and encouraging urinary flow through the drainage system.

▨ Clients with urinary retention may be taught to perform clean intermittent self-catheterization to enhance their independence, reduce the risk of infection, and eliminate incontinence.

▨ Bladder or catheter irrigations may be used to apply medication to bladder walls or maintain catheter patency.

▨ When the urinary bladder is removed, a urinary diversion is formed to allow urine to be eliminated from the body. The ileal conduit or ileal loop is the most common diversion and requires that the client wear a urine collection device continually over the stoma.

TEST YOUR KNOWLEDGE

1. The nurse recognizes that urinary elimination changes may occur even in healthy elders because:
 1. The bladder distends and its capacity increases.
 2. Elders ignore the need to void.
 3. Urine becomes more concentrated.
 4. The amount of urine retained after voiding increases.

2. During assessment of the client with urinary incontinence, the nurse is most likely to assess which of the following? Select all that apply.
 1. Perineal skin irritation
 2. Fluid intake of less than 1,500 mL/day
 3. History of antihistamine intake
 4. History of frequent urinary tract infections

3. Which of the following represents the appropriate nursing management of a client wearing a condom catheter?
 1. Ensure that the tip of the penis fits snugly against the end of the condom.
 2. Check the penis for adequate circulation 30 minutes after applying.
 3. Change the condom every 8 hours.
 4. Tape the collecting tubing to the lower abdomen.

4. During the straight catheterization of a female client, if the catheter slips into the vagina, the nurse should:
 1. Leave the catheter in place and get a new sterile catheter.
 2. Leave the catheter in place and ask another nurse to attempt the procedure.
 3. Remove the catheter and redirect it to the urinary meatus.
 4. Remove the catheter, wipe it with a sterile gauze, and redirect it to the urinary meatus.

5. Which of the following statements indicates a need for further teaching of the home care client with a long-term indwelling catheter?
   1. "I will keep the collecting bag below the level of the bladder at all times."
   2. "Intake of cranberry juice may help decrease the risk of infection."
   3. "Soaking in a warm tub bath may ease the irritation associated with the catheter."
   4. "I should use clean technique when emptying the collecting bag."

6. During shift report, the nurse learns that an older female client is unable to maintain continence after she senses the urge to void and becomes incontinent on the way to the bathroom. Which of the following nursing diagnoses is most appropriate?
   1. *Stress Urinary Incontinence*
   2. *Total Urinary Incontinence*
   3. *Functional Urinary Incontinence*
   4. *Urge Urinary Incontinence*

7. A female client has a urinary tract infection (UTI). Which of the following teaching is most appropriate? Select all that apply.
   1. Limit fluids to avoid the burning sensation on urination.
   2. Review symptoms of UTI with the client.
   3. Wipe the perineal area from back to front.
   4. Wear cotton underclothes.
   5. Take baths rather than showers.

8. The nurse will need to assess the client's performance of clean intermittent self-catheterization (CISC) for a client with which of the following?
   1. Ileal conduit
   2. Kock pouch
   3. Neobladder
   4. Vesicostomy

9. Because a client has a flaccid bladder the nurse is most likely to teach which of the following?
   1. Habit training: attempt voiding at specific time periods
   2. Bladder training: delay voiding according to a preschedule time table.
   3. Credé's maneuver: apply gentle manual pressure to the lower abdomen.
   4. Kegel exercises: contract the pelvic muscles

10. Which of the following behaviors indicates that the client on a bladder training program has met the expected outcomes? Select all that apply.
    1. Voids each time there is an urge
    2. Practices slow, deep breathing until the urge decreases
    3. Uses adult diapers, for "just in case"
    4. Drinks citrus juices and carbonated beverages
    5. Performs pelvic muscle exercises

See Answers to Test Your Knowledge in Appendix A.

EXPLORE MEDIALINK www.prenhall.com/berman

DVD-ROM
- Audio Glossary
- NCLEX Review
- Skills Checklists
- Animations:
  Kidney
  Catheterization
  A & P Review

COMPANION WEBSITE
- Additional NCLEX Review
- Case Study: Intermittent Self-Catheterization
- Care Plan Activity: Client with Urinary Retention Catheter
- Application Activity: Urinary Incontinence
- Links to Resources

READINGS AND REFERENCES

SUGGESTED READINGS

Newman, D. K., & Palmer, M. H. (Eds.). (2003). State of the science on urinary incontinence. *American Journal of Nursing, 103*(3), Suppl. 1–58.
This is a report of a consensus symposium on urinary incontinence involving nurse researchers, clinicians, educators, administrators, and industry stakeholders. Critique, review, identification of barriers to management, recommendations for future research, clinical practice, education, and policy are presented in this monumental document.

Patraca, K. (2005). Measure bladder volume without catheterization. *Nursing, 35*(4), 46–47.
This article provides step-by-step photos for performing portable ultrasound scanning of a client's bladder.

Polt, C. A. (2006). Taking the pressure off for women with stress incontinence. *Nursing, 36*(2), 49–51.
The transvaginal tape (TVT) sling has become one of the most commonly performed surgeries for stress incontinence. The author reviews the pathophysiology of stress incontinence, describes the TVT sling procedure, and presents information that the client needs to know about the procedure.

Pringle Specht, J. K. (2005). Nine myths of incontinence in older adults. Both clinicians and the over-65 set need to know more. *American Journal of Nursing, 105*(6), 58–68.
Common misconceptions of bladder health in older adults are discussed to help nurses in all settings to provide nursing care that prevents and treats incontinence.

RELATED RESEARCH

Chen, L., Hsiao, A., Moore, C. L., Dziura, J. D., & Santucci, K. A. (2005). Utility of bedside bladder ultrasound before urethral catheterization in young children. *Pediatrics, 115*(1), 108–111.

Heidrich, S. M., & Wells, T. J. (2004). Effects of urinary incontinence: Psychological well-being and distress in older community-dwelling women. *Journal of Gerontological Nursing, 30*(5), 47–54.

Lundblad, B., & Hellstrom, A. (2005). Perceptions of school toilets as a cause for irregular toilet habits among school children aged 6 to 16 years. *Journal of School Health, 75*(4), 125–128.

McGlynn, B., Al-Saffar, N., Begg, H., Gurun, M., Hollins, G., McPhee, S., et al. (2004).

Management of urinary incontinence following radical prostatectomy. *Urologic Nursing, 24*(6), 475–515.

McIntosh, L. (2005). The role of the nurse in the use of vaginal pessaries to treat pelvic organ prolapse and/or urinary incontinence: A literature review. *Urologic Nursing, 25*(1), 41–48.

Midthun, S. J., Paur, R., & Lindseth, G. (2004). Urinary tract infections: Does the smell really tell? *Journal of Gerontological Nursing, 30*(6), 4–9.

Ruff, C. C. (2005). Risk factors for urinary incontinence in African-American women. *Urologic Nursing, 25*(1), 33–39.

Simmons, S. F., & Ouslander, J. G. (2005). Resident and family satisfaction with incontinence and mobility care: Sensitivity to intervention effects? *Gerontologist, 45*(3), 318–326.

Taunton, R. L., Swagerty, D. L., & Lasseter, J. A. (2005). Continent or incontinent? That is the question. *Journal of Gerontological Nursing, 31*(9), 36–44.

REFERENCES

Anonymous. (2004). Information from your family doctor: Urinary tract infections in adults. *American Family Physician, 69*(1), 159–160.

Ball, J. W., & Bindler, R. C. (2006). *Child health nursing.* Upper Saddle River, NJ: Prentice Hall.

Cavagnaro, S. M. F. (2005). Infeccion urinaria en la infancia [Urinary infection in infancy]. *Revista Chilena de Infectologia, 22*(2), 161–168.

D'Amico, D., & Barbarito, C. (2007). *Health & physical assessment in nursing.* Upper Saddle River, NJ: Pearson Education.

Dochterman, J. M., & Bulechek, G. M. (2004). *Nursing interventions classification (NIC)* (4th ed.). St. Louis, MO: Mosby.

Midthun, S. J. (2004). Criteria for urinary tract infection in the elderly: Variables that challenge nursing assessment. *Urologic Nursing, 24*(3), 157–186.

Moorhead, S., Johnson, M., & Maas, M. (2004). *Nursing outcomes classification (NOC)* (3rd ed.). St. Louis, MO: Mosby.

Morantz, C. A. (2005). ACOG guidelines on urinary incontinence in women. *American Family Physician, 72*(1), 175–178.

NANDA International. (2007). NANDA nursing diagnoses: Definitions and classification 2007–2008. Philadelphia: Author.

Nield, L. S., & Kamat, D. (2004). Enuresis: How to evaluate and treat. *Clinical Pediatrics, 43*(5), 409–415.

Palmer, M. H., & Newman, D. K. (2006). Bladder control: Educational needs of older adults. *Journal of Gerontological Nursing, 32*(1), 28–32.

Robson, W. L. M., Leung, A.K.C., & Van Howe, R. (2005). Primary and secondary nocturnal enuresis: Similarities in presentation. *Pediatrics, 115,* 956–959.

Shei Dei Yang, S., & Cheng Wang, C. (2005). Outpatient biofeedback relaxation of the pelvic floor in treating pediatric dysfunctional voiding: A short-course program is effective. *Urologia Internationalis, 74*(2), 118–122.

Sparks, A., Boyer, D., Gambrel, A., Lovet, M., Johnson, J., Richards, T., et al. (2004). The clinical benefits of the bladder scanner: A research synthesis. *Journal of Nursing Care Quality, 19*(3), 188–192.

SELECTED BIBLIOGRAPHY

Colwell, C. C., Goldberg, M. T., & Carmel, J. E. (2004). *Fecal & urinary diversions: Management principles.* St. Louis, MO: Mosby.

Davis, K. (2004). Need urine from a catheter system? Forget the needle! *Nursing, 34*(12), 64.

Dulczak, S., & Kirk, J. (2005). Overview of the evaluation, diagnosis, and management of urinary tract infections in infants and children. *Urologic Nursing, 25*(3), 185–192.

Gray, M. (2004). Clinical practice: Stress urinary incontinence in women. *Journal of the American Academy of Nurse Practitioners, 16*(5), 188–197.

Hathaway, L. (2004). How to insert an indwelling catheter. *Nursing Made Incredibly Easy, 2*(2), 43–45.

Nix, D., & Ermer-Seltun, J. (2004). A review of perineal skin care protocols and skin barrier product use. *OstomyWound Management, 50*(12), 59–67.

Palmer, M. H., & Newman, D. K. (2004). Urinary incontinence in nursing homes: Two studies show the inadequacy of care. *American Journal of Nursing, 104*(11), 57–59.

Pomfret, I., & Tew, L. E. (2004). Urinary catheters and associated UTI's. *Journal of Community Nursing, 18*(9), 15–20.

Pullen, R. L. (2004). Inserting an indwelling urinary catheter in a male patient. *Nursing, 34*(7), 24.

Robinson, J. (2005). Clinical skills: How to remove and change a suprapubic catheter. *British Journal of Nursing, 14*(1), 30–35.

Rushing, J. (2004). Inserting an indwelling urinary catheter in a female patient. *Nursing, 34*(8), 22.

Toughill, E. (2005). Indwelling urinary catheters. Common mechanical and pathogenic problems. *American Journal of Nursing, 105*(5), 35–37.

Woods, A. (2005). Managing UTIs in older adults. *Nursing, 35*(3), 12.

CHAPTER 49

Fecal Elimination

LEARNING OUTCOMES

After completing this chapter, you will be able to:

1. Understand the physiology of defecation:

2. Identify factors that influence fecal elimination and patterns of defecation.

3. Distinguish normal from abnormal characteristics and constituents of feces.

4. Identify common causes and effects of selected fecal elimination problems.

5. Describe methods used to assess the intestinal tract.

6. Identify examples of nursing diagnoses, outcomes, and interventions for clients with elimination problems.

7. Identify measures that maintain normal fecal elimination patterns.

8. Describe the purpose and action of commonly used enema solutions.

9. Describe essentials of fecal stoma care for clients with an ostomy.

KEY TERMS

bedpan, *1337*
bowel incontinence, *1329*
carminatives, *1339*
cathartics, *1338*
chyme, *1324*
colostomy, *1330*
commode, *1337*
constipation, *1328*
defecation, *1325*
diarrhea, *1329*
enema, *1339*

fecal impaction, *1328*
fecal incontinence, *1329*
feces, *1323*
flatulence, *1330*
flatus, *1324*
gastrocolic reflex, *1326*
gastrostomy, *1330*
haustra, *1323*
haustral churning, *1324*
hemorrhoids, *1324*
ileostomy, *1330*

ingestion, *1324*
jejunostomy, *1330*
laxatives, *1327*
mass peristalsis, *1324*
meconium, *1326*
ostomy, *1330*
peristalsis, *1324*
stoma, *1331*
stool, *1323*
suppositories, *1339*

Nurses frequently are consulted or involved in assisting clients with elimination problems. These problems can be embarrassing to clients and can cause considerable discomfort. The elimination of feces is a prominent public topic in North America. For example, laxative advertisements, describing such feelings as tiredness due to irregularity, keep the subject in the public consciousness. Some elders are preoccupied with their bowels. People who have had a bowel movement once a day for 75 years can view missing one day as a serious problem.

PHYSIOLOGY OF DEFECATION

Elimination of the waste products of digestion from the body is essential to health. The excreted waste products are referred to as **feces** or **stool.**

Large Intestine

The large intestine extends from the ileocecal (ileocolic) valve, which lies between the small and large intestines, to the anus. The colon (large intestine) in the adult is generally about 125 to 150 cm (50 to 60 in.) long. It has seven parts: the cecum; ascending, transverse, and descending colons; sigmoid colon; rectum; and anus (Figure 49-1 ■).

The large intestine is a muscular tube lined with mucous membrane. The muscle fibers are both circular and longitudinal, permitting the intestine to enlarge and contract in both width and length. The longitudinal muscles are shorter than the colon and therefore cause the large intestine to form pouches, or **haustra.**

The colon's main functions are the absorption of water and nutrients, the mucoid protection of the intestinal wall, and fecal

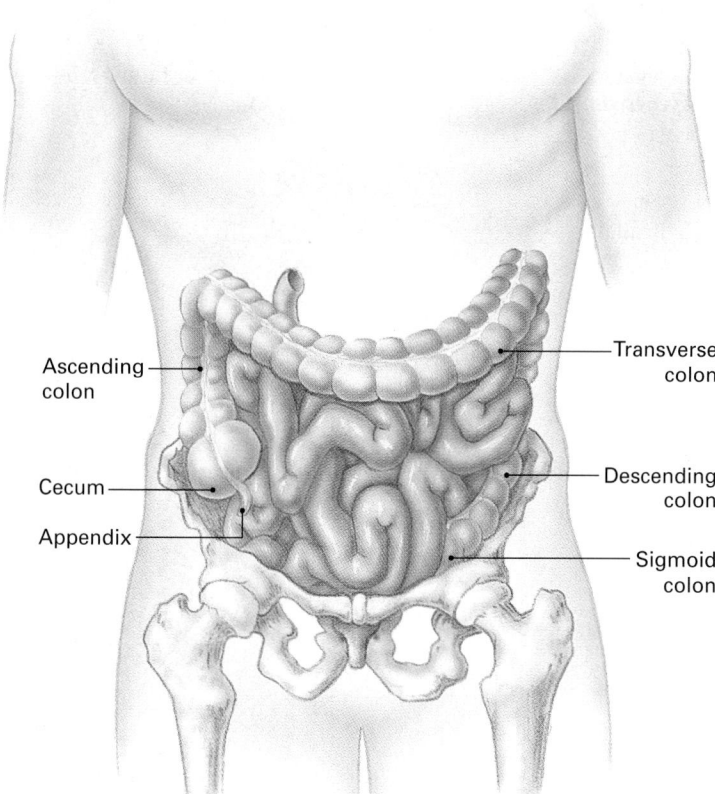

Ascending colon

Transverse colon

Cecum

Descending colon

Appendix

Sigmoid colon

Figure 49-1 ■ The large intestine.

(Fremgen, Bonnie F., Frucht, Suzanne S., *Medical Terminology: A Living Language*, 3rd ed. © 2005. Electronically reproduced with permission of Pearson Education, Inc., Upper Saddle River, New Jersey.)

elimination. The contents of the colon normally represent foods ingested over the previous 4 days, although most of the waste products are excreted within 48 hours of **ingestion** (the act of taking food). The waste products leaving the stomach through the small intestine and then passing through the ileocecal valve are called **chyme.** The ileocecal valve, located at the junction of the ileum of the small intestine and the first part of the large intestine, regulates the flow of chyme into the large intestine and prevents backflow into the ileum. As much as 1,500 mL of chyme passes into the large intestine daily, and all but about 100 mL is reabsorbed in the proximal half of the colon. The 100 mL of fluid is excreted in the feces.

The colon also serves a protective function in that it secretes mucus. This mucus contains large amounts of bicarbonate ions. The mucus secretion is stimulated by excitation of parasympathetic nerves. During extreme stimulation—for example, as a result of emotions—large amounts of mucus are secreted, resulting in the passage of stringy mucus with little or no feces. Mucus serves to protect the wall of the large intestine from trauma by the acids formed in the feces, and it serves as an adherent for holding the fecal material together. Mucus also protects the intestinal wall from bacterial activity.

The colon acts to transport along its lumen the products of digestion, which are eventually eliminated through the anal canal. These products are flatus and feces. **Flatus** is largely air and the by-products of the digestion of carbohydrates. Three types of movements occur in the large intestine: haustral churning, colon peristalsis, and mass peristalsis. **Haustral churning** involves movement of the chyme back and forth within the haustra. In addition to mixing the contents, this action aids in the absorption of water and moves the contents forward to the next haustra. **Peristalsis** is wavelike movement produced by the circular and longitudinal muscle fibers of the intestinal walls; it propels the intestinal contents forward. Colon peristalsis is very sluggish and is thought to move the chyme very little along the large intestine. **Mass peristalsis,** the third type of colonic movement, involves a wave of powerful muscular contraction that moves over large areas of the colon. Usually mass peristalsis occurs after eating, stimulated by the presence of food in the stomach and small intestine. In adults, mass peristaltic waves occur only a few times a day.

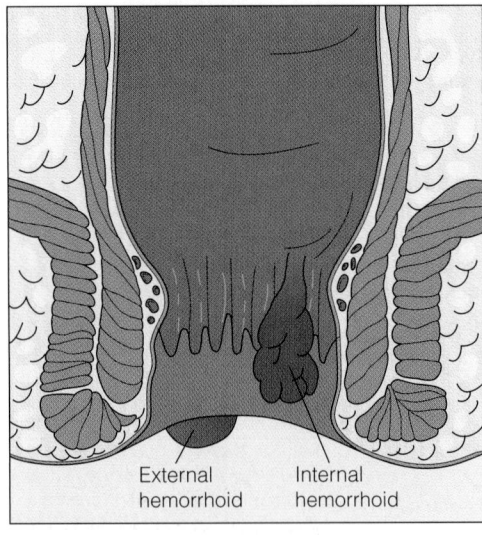

Figure 49-2 ■ Internal and external hemorrhoids.

Rectum and Anal Canal

The rectum in the adult is usually 10 to 15 cm (4 to 6 in.) long; the most distal portion, 2.5 to 5 cm (1 to 2 in.) long, is the anal canal. In the rectum are folds that extend vertically. Each of the vertical folds contains a vein and an artery. It is believed that these folds help retain feces within the rectum. When the veins become distended, as can occur with repeated pressure, a condition known as **hemorrhoids** occurs (Figure 49-2 ■).

The anal canal is bounded by an internal and an external sphincter muscle (Figure 49-3 ■). The internal sphincter is under involuntary control, and the external sphincter normally is voluntarily controlled. The internal sphincter muscle is innervated by the autonomic nervous system; the external sphincter is innervated by the somatic nervous system.

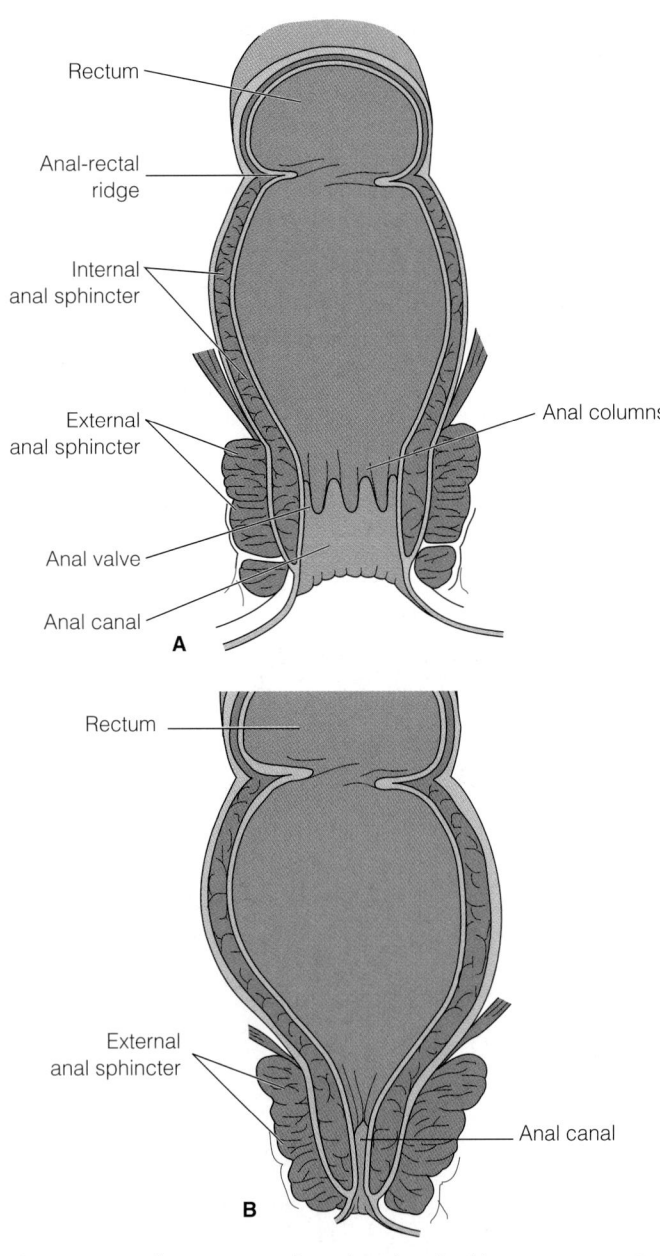

Figure 49-3 ■ The rectum, anal canal, and anal sphincters: *A,* open; *B,* closed.

Defecation

Defecation is the expulsion of feces from the anus and rectum. It is also called a *bowel movement.* The frequency of defecation is highly individual, varying from several times per day to two or three times per week. The amount defecated also varies from person to person. When peristaltic waves move the feces into the sigmoid colon and the rectum, the sensory nerves in the rectum are stimulated and the individual becomes aware of the need to defecate.

When the internal anal sphincter relaxes, feces move into the anal canal. After the individual is seated on a toilet or bedpan, the external anal sphincter is relaxed voluntarily. Expulsion of the feces is assisted by contraction of the abdominal muscles and the diaphragm, which increases abdominal pressure, and by contraction of the muscles of the pelvic floor, which moves the feces through the anal canal. Normal defecation is facilitated by (a) thigh flexion, which increases the pressure within the abdomen, and (b) a sitting position, which increases the downward pressure on the rectum.

If the defecation reflex is ignored, or if defecation is consciously inhibited by contracting the external sphincter muscle, the urge to defecate normally disappears for a few hours before occurring again. Repeated inhibition of the urge to defecate can result in expansion of the rectum to accommodate accumulated feces and eventual loss of sensitivity to the need to defecate. Constipation can be the ultimate result.

Feces

Normal feces are made of about 75% water and 25% solid materials. They are soft but formed. If the feces are propelled very quickly along the large intestine, there is not time for most of the water in the chyme to be reabsorbed and the feces will be more fluid, containing perhaps 95% water. Normal feces require a normal fluid intake; feces that contain less water may be hard and difficult to expel.

Feces are normally brown, chiefly due to the presence of stercobilin and urobilin, which are derived from bilirubin (a red pigment in bile). Another factor that affects fecal color is the action of bacteria such as *Escherichia coli* or staphylococci, which are normally present in the large intestine. The action of microorganisms on the chyme is also responsible for the odor of feces. Table 49–1 lists the characteristics of normal and abnormal feces.

TABLE 49–1 Characteristics of Normal and Abnormal Feces

CHARACTERISTIC	NORMAL	ABNORMAL	POSSIBLE CAUSE
Color	Adult: brown	Clay or white	Absence of bile pigment (bile obstruction); diagnostic study using barium
	Infant: yellow	Black or tarry	Drug (e.g., iron); bleeding from upper gastrointestinal tract (e.g., stomach, small intestine); diet high in red meat and dark green vegetables (e.g., spinach)
		Red	Bleeding from lower gastrointestinal tract (e.g., rectum); some foods (e.g., beets)
		Pale	Malabsorption of fats; diet high in milk and milk products and low in meat
		Orange or green	Intestinal infection
Consistency	Formed, soft, semisolid, moist	Hard, dry	Dehydration; decreased intestinal motility resulting from lack of fiber in diet, lack of exercise, emotional upset, laxative abuse
		Diarrhea	Increased intestinal motility (e.g., due to irritation of the colon by bacteria)
Shape	Cylindrical (contour of rectum) about 2.5 cm (1 in.) in diameter in adults	Narrow, pencil-shaped, or stringlike stool	Obstructive condition of the rectum
Amount	Varies with diet (about 100–400 g per day)		
Odor	Aromatic: affected by ingested food and person's own bacterial flora	Pungent	Infection, blood
Constituents	Small amounts of undigested roughage, sloughed dead bacteria and epithelial cells, fat, protein, dried constituents of digestive juices (e.g., bile pigments, inorganic matter)	Pus	Bacterial infection
		Mucus	Inflammatory condition
		Parasites	
		Blood	Gastrointestinal bleeding
		Large quantities of fat	Malabsorption
		Foreign objects	Accidental ingestion

An adult usually forms 7 to 10 L of flatus (gas) in the large intestine every 24 hours. The gases include carbon dioxide, methane, hydrogen, oxygen, and nitrogen. Some are swallowed with food and fluids taken by mouth, others are formed through the action of bacteria on the chyme in the large intestine, and other gas diffuses from the blood into the gastrointestinal tract.

FACTORS THAT AFFECT DEFECATION

Defecation patterns vary at different stages of life. Circumstances of diet, fluid intake and output, activity, psychologic factors, lifestyle, medications and medical procedures, and disease also affect defecation.

Development

Newborns and infants, toddlers, children, and elders are groups within which members have similarities in elimination patterns.

Newborns and Infants

Meconium is the first fecal material passed by the newborn, normally up to 24 hours after birth. It is black, tarry, odorless, and sticky. Transitional stools, which follow for about a week, are generally greenish yellow; they contain mucus and are loose.

Infants pass stool frequently, often after each feeding. Because the intestine is immature, water is not well absorbed and the stool is soft, liquid, and frequent. When the intestine matures, bacterial flora increase. After solid foods are introduced, the stool becomes less frequent and firmer.

Infants who are breast-fed have light yellow to golden feces, and infants who are taking formula will have dark yellow or tan stool that is more formed.

Toddlers

Some control of defecation starts at 1 1/2 to 2 years of age. By this time, children have learned to walk, and the nervous and muscular systems are sufficiently well developed to permit bowel control. A desire to control daytime bowel movements and to use the toilet generally starts when the child becomes aware of (a) the discomfort caused by a soiled diaper and (b) the sensation that indicates the need for a bowel movement. Daytime control is typically attained by age 2 1/2, after a process of toilet training.

School-Age Children and Adolescents

School-age children and adolescents have bowel habits similar to those of adults. Patterns of defecation vary in frequency, quantity, and consistency. Some school-age children may delay defecation because of an activity such as play.

Elders

Constipation is the most common bowel-management problem in the elder population (Mauk, 2005). This is due, in part, to reduced activity levels, inadequate amounts of fluid and fiber intake, and muscle weakness. Many older people believe that "regularity" means a bowel movement every day. Those who do not meet this criterion often seek over-the-counter preparations to relieve what they believe to be constipation. Elders should be advised that normal patterns of bowel elimination vary considerably. For some, a normal pattern may be every other day; for others, twice a day. Adequate roughage in the diet, adequate exercise, and 6 to 8 glasses of fluid daily are essential preventive measures for constipation. A cup of hot water or tea at a regular time in the morning is helpful for some. Responding to the **gastrocolic reflex** (increased peristalsis of the colon after food has entered the stomach) is also an important consideration. For example, toileting is recommended 5 to 15 minutes after meals, especially after breakfast when the gastrocolic reflex is strongest (Hinrichs & Huseboe, 2001, p. 23).

The older adult should be warned that consistent use of laxatives inhibits natural defecation reflexes and is thought to cause rather than cure constipation. The habitual user of laxatives eventually requires larger or stronger doses because the effect is progressively reduced with continual use. Laxatives may also interfere with the body's electrolyte balance and decrease the absorption of certain vitamins. The reasons for constipation can range from lifestyle habits (e.g., lack of exercise) to serious malignant disorders (e.g., colorectal cancer). The nurse should evaluate any complaints of constipation carefully for each individual. A change in bowel habits over several weeks with or without weight loss, pain, or fever should be referred to a primary care provider for a complete medical evaluation. See Clinical Manifestations.

Diet

Sufficient bulk (cellulose, fiber) in the diet is necessary to provide fecal volume. Bland diets and low-fiber diets are lacking in bulk and therefore create insufficient residue of waste products to stimulate the reflex for defecation. Low-residue foods, such as rice, eggs, and lean meats, move more slowly through the intestinal tract. Increasing fluid intake with such foods increases their rate of movement.

Certain foods are difficult or impossible for some people to digest. This inability results in digestive upsets and, in some instances, the passage of watery stools. Irregular eating can also impair regular defecation. Individuals who eat at the same times

---

CLINICAL MANIFESTATIONS
COLORECTAL CANCER

Inform clients to see their primary care provider if they have any of the following:

- A change in bowel habits such as diarrhea, constipation, or narrowing of the stool that lasts for more than a few days
- A feeling of needing to have a bowel movement that is not relieved by doing so
- Rectal bleeding or blood in the stool (often, though, the stool will look normal)
- Cramping or steady abdominal pain
- Weakness and fatigue

Note: Reprinted by permission of the American Cancer Society, Inc. from www.cancer.org. All rights reserved.

every day usually have a regularly timed, physiologic response to the food intake and a regular pattern of peristaltic activity in the colon.

Spicy foods can produce diarrhea and flatus in some individuals. Excessive sugar can also cause diarrhea. Other foods that may influence bowel elimination include the following:

- Gas-producing foods, such as cabbage, onions, cauliflower, bananas, and apples
- Laxative-producing foods, such as bran, prunes, figs, chocolate, and alcohol
- Constipation-producing foods, such as cheese, pasta, eggs, and lean meat

Fluid

Even when fluid intake is inadequate or output (urine or vomitus, for example) is excessive for some reason, the body continues to reabsorb fluid from the chyme as it passes along the colon. The chyme becomes drier than normal, resulting in hard feces. In addition, reduced fluid intake slows the chyme's passage along the intestines, further increasing the reabsorption of fluid from the chyme. Healthy fecal elimination usually requires a daily fluid intake of 2,000 to 3,000 mL. If chyme moves abnormally quickly through the large intestine, however, there is less time for fluid to be absorbed into the blood; as a result, the feces are soft or even watery.

Activity

Activity stimulates peristalsis, thus facilitating the movement of chyme along the colon. Weak abdominal and pelvic muscles are often ineffective in increasing the intra-abdominal pressure during defecation or in controlling defecation. Weak muscles can result from lack of exercise, immobility, or impaired neurologic functioning. Clients confined to bed are often constipated.

Psychologic Factors

Some people who are anxious or angry experience increased peristaltic activity and subsequent nausea or diarrhea. In contrast, people who are depressed may experience slowed intestinal motility, resulting in constipation. How a person responds to these emotional states is the result of individual differences in the response of the enteric nervous system to vagal stimulation from the brain.

Defecation Habits

Early bowel training may establish the habit of defecating at a regular time. Many people defecate after breakfast, when the gastrocolic reflex causes mass peristaltic waves in the large intestine. If a person ignores this urge to defecate, water continues to be reabsorbed, making the feces hard and difficult to expel. When the normal defecation reflexes are inhibited or ignored, these conditioned reflexes tend to be progressively weakened. When habitually ignored, the urge to defecate is ultimately lost. Adults may ignore these reflexes because of the pressures of time or work. Hospitalized clients may suppress the urge because of embarrassment about using a bedpan, because of lack of privacy, or because defecation is too uncomfortable.

Medications

Some drugs have side effects that can interfere with normal elimination. Some cause diarrhea; others, such as large doses of certain tranquilizers and repeated administration of morphine and codeine, cause constipation because they decrease gastrointestinal activity through their action on the central nervous system. Iron tablets, which have an astringent effect, act more locally on the bowel mucosa to cause constipation.

Some medications directly affect elimination. **Laxatives** are medications that stimulate bowel activity and so assist fecal elimination. Other medications soften stool, facilitating defecation. Certain medications suppress peristaltic activity and may be used to treat diarrhea.

Medications also affect the appearance of the feces. Any drug that causes gastrointestinal bleeding (e.g., aspirin products) can cause the stool to be red or black. Iron salts lead to black stool because of the oxidation of the iron; antibiotics may cause a gray-green discoloration; and antacids can cause a whitish discoloration or white specks in the stool. Pepto-Bismol, a common over-the-counter drug, causes stools to be black.

Diagnostic Procedures

Before certain diagnostic procedures, such as visualization of the colon (colonoscopy or sigmoidoscopy), the client is restricted from ingesting food or fluid. The client may also be given a cleansing enema prior to the examination. In these instances normal defecation usually will not occur until eating resumes.

Anesthesia and Surgery

General anesthetics cause the normal colonic movements to cease or slow by blocking parasympathetic stimulation to the muscles of the colon. Clients who have regional or spinal anesthesia are less likely to experience this problem.

Surgery that involves direct handling of the intestines can cause temporary cessation of intestinal movement. This condition, called ileus, usually lasts 24 to 48 hours. Listening for bowel sounds that reflect intestinal motility is an important nursing assessment following surgery.

Pathologic Conditions

Spinal cord injuries and head injuries can decrease the sensory stimulation for defecation. Impaired mobility may limit the client's ability to respond to the urge to defecate and the client may experience constipation. Or, a client may experience fecal incontinence because of poorly functioning anal sphincters.

Pain

Clients who experience discomfort when defecating (e.g., following hemorrhoid surgery) often suppress the urge to defecate to avoid the pain. Such clients can experience constipation as a result. Clients taking narcotic analgesics for pain may also experience constipation as a side effect of the medication.

FECAL ELIMINATION PROBLEMS

Four common problems are related to fecal elimination: constipation, diarrhea, bowel incontinence, and flatulence.

Constipation

Constipation may be defined as fewer than three bowel movements per week. This infers the passage of dry, hard stool or the passage of no stool. It occurs when the movement of feces through the large intestine is slow, thus allowing time for additional reabsorption of fluid from the large intestine. Associated with constipation are difficult evacuation of stool and increased effort or straining of the voluntary muscles of defecation. The person may also have a feeling of incomplete stool evacuation after defecation. However, it is important to define constipation in relation to the person's regular elimination pattern. Some people normally defecate only a few times a week; other people defecate more than once a day. Careful assessment of the person's habits is necessary before a diagnosis of constipation is made. Box 49–1 lists the frequent defining characteristics of constipation.

Many causes and factors contribute to constipation. Among them are the following:

- Insufficient fiber intake
- Insufficient fluid intake
- Insufficient activity or immobility
- Irregular defecation habits
- Change in daily routine
- Lack of privacy
- Chronic use of laxatives or enemas
- Irritable bowel syndrome (IBS)
- Pelvic floor dysfunction or muscle damage
- Poor motility or slow transit
- Neurological conditions (e.g., Parkinson's disease), stroke, or paralysis
- Emotional disturbances such as depression or mental confusion
- Medications such as opioids, iron supplements, antihistamines, antacids, and antidepressants

---

BOX 49–1   Sample Defining Characteristics for Constipation

- Decreased frequency of defecation
- Hard, dry, formed stools
- Straining at stool; painful defecation
- Reports of rectal fullness or pressure or incomplete bowel evacuation
- Abdominal pain, cramps, or distention
- Anorexia, nausea
- Headache

Constipation can cause health problems for some clients. In children it is often associated with urinary tract infections. Straining associated with constipation often is accompanied by holding the breath. This Valsalva maneuver can present serious problems to people with heart disease, brain injuries, or respiratory disease. Holding the breath, while bearing down, increases intrathoracic pressure and vagal tone, slowing the pulse rate (Lemone & Burke, 2004).

Fecal Impaction

Fecal impaction is a mass or collection of hardened feces in the folds of the rectum. Impaction results from prolonged retention and accumulation of fecal material. In severe impactions the feces accumulate and extend well up into the sigmoid colon and beyond. Fecal impaction can be recognized by the passage of liquid fecal seepage (diarrhea) and no normal stool. The liquid portion of the feces seeps out around the impacted mass. Impaction can also be assessed by digital examination of the rectum, during which the hardened mass can often be palpated.

Along with fecal seepage and constipation, symptoms include frequent but nonproductive desire to defecate and rectal pain. A generalized feeling of illness results; the client becomes anorexic, the abdomen becomes distended, and nausea and vomiting may occur.

The causes of fecal impaction are usually poor defecation habits and constipation. The barium used in radiologic exami-

---

DRUG CAPSULE   Emollient or Surfactant

docusate calcium (Surfak)
docusate sodium (Colace)

THE CLIENT WITH DRUGS FOR TREATING THE LOWER GASTROINTESTINAL TRUST

Docusates lower the surface tension of fecal material, which allows water and lipids to penetrate the stool resulting in softer fecal mass. They do not stimulate peristalsis.

Docusates are commonly used for prevention of constipation and to decrease the strain of defecation in individuals who should avoid straining during bowel movements (e.g., cardiac disease [prevent Valsalva maneuver], eye surgery, rectal surgery).

NURSING RESPONSIBILITIES

- Assess client for abdominal distention, bowel sounds, and usual bowel movement frequency.
- Evaluate effectiveness of medication.

CLIENT AND FAMILY TEACHING

- Advise client to drink a glass of fluid (e.g., water, juice, milk) with each dose.

- Explain that it may take 1 to 3 days to soften fecal material.
- Advise client not to take docusate within 2 hours of other laxatives, especially mineral oil, as it may cause increased absorption of the mineral oil.
- Discuss other forms of bowel regulation (e.g., increasing fiber intake, fluid intake, and activity).

Note: Prior to administering any medication, review all aspects with a current drug handbook or other reliable source.

REAL WORLD PRACTICE

As a Registered Nurse, your role in monitoring your client's intake and output is extremely important. Normal bowel sounds should occur in the amount of 5–30 per minute. A colon that is full of stool will feel like a firm round mass when palpated. This can sometimes be confused with a distended bladder which will feel like a smooth round mass above the symphysis pubis.

Monitoring the client's last bowel movement and monitoring the color, consistency, amount, frequency, and regularity are all part of the RN function. One method of communicating specific amounts could be by charting "1/2 cup or 1 cup." Terms such as small, medium, and large are ambiguous and should be avoided. Asking the nurse aide or the client to approximate the amount on each shift and then charting this amount may help in assessing the client's overall health.

Chronic constipation is a condition that occurs because of some of the things we do to clients while in the hospital, or while they are getting treatment for something else. If the doctor limits a client's fluids, the client can become constipated. Medications such as the following may also cause constipation:

- Methadone maintenance treatment for narcotic addiction
- Antidiarrheal medications
- Anticholinergic medications
- Pain medications

If the client has an impaction, she or he might have some stool that goes around the impaction. The stool can be watery or have some slight substance to it. Once I cared for a client who frequently become impacted. After discussing the situation with the client and the doctor, we decided on a regime that consisted of fluids, activity, and a light stool softener. It worked! Some clients will need a more aggressive program, and that can be determined after you have done an assessment.

The most important role that you will have as an RN is to monitor the client's bowel sounds, chart the last bowel movement, and get your client up and moving! I don't ask "Do you want to get up" I say "When would you like to get up, now or in 5 minutes?" This approach helps you manage your time and you can chart the client getting up and going back to bed or the chair. Doing it early in the shift allows for interventions and contacting the primary care provider if needed.

—Jane Reintges MS, RN, CRRN, APRN-bc,
Washington Hospital Healthcare Systems, Fremont, CA

---

nations of the upper and lower gastrointestinal tracts can also be a causative factor. Therefore, after these examinations, laxatives or enemas are usually taken to ensure removal of the barium.

Digital examination of the impaction through the rectum should be done gently and carefully. Although digital rectal examination is within the scope of nursing practice, some agency policies require a primary care provider's order for digital manipulation and removal of a fecal impaction.

Although fecal impaction can generally be prevented, treatment of impacted feces is sometimes necessary. When fecal impaction is suspected, the client is often given an oil retention enema, a cleansing enema 2 to 4 hours later, and daily additional cleansing enemas, suppositories, or stool softeners. If these measures fail, manual removal is often necessary.

Diarrhea

Diarrhea refers to the passage of liquid feces and an increased frequency of defecation. It is the opposite of constipation and results from rapid movement of fecal contents through the large intestine. Rapid passage of chyme reduces the time available for the large intestine to reabsorb water and electrolytes. Some people pass stool with increased frequency, but diarrhea is not present unless the stool is relatively unformed and excessively liquid. The person with diarrhea finds it difficult or impossible to control the urge to defecate for very long. Diarrhea and the threat of incontinence are sources of concern and embarrassment. Often, spasmodic cramps are associated with diarrhea. Bowel sounds are increased. With persistent diarrhea, irritation of the anal region extending to the perineum and buttocks generally results. Fatigue, weakness, malaise, and emaciation are the results of prolonged diarrhea.

When the cause of diarrhea is irritants in the intestinal tract, diarrhea is thought to be a protective flushing mechanism. It can create serious fluid and electrolyte losses in the body, however, that can develop within frighteningly short periods of time, particularly in infants, small children, and elders. Table 49–2 lists some of the major causes of diarrhea and the physiologic responses of the body.

The irritating effects of diarrhea stool increase the risk for skin breakdown. Therefore, the area around the anal region should be kept clean and dry and be protected with zinc oxide or other ointment. In addition, a fecal collector can be used (see page 1344).

Bowel Incontinence

Bowel incontinence, also called **fecal incontinence,** refers to the loss of voluntary ability to control fecal and gaseous discharges through the anal sphincter. The incontinence may occur at specific times, such as after meals, or it may occur irregularly. Two types of bowel incontinence are described: partial and major. Partial incontinence is the inability to control flatus or to prevent minor soiling. Major incontinence is the inability to control feces of normal consistency.

Fecal incontinence is generally associated with impaired functioning of the anal sphincter or its nerve supply, such as in some neuromuscular diseases, spinal cord trauma, and tumors of the external anal sphincter muscle.

The rate of fecal incontinence among elders living in the community has been reported to be 4% to 17% compared to 2% in the general community population and 20% to 54% in elderly nursing home residents (Bliss, Fischer, & Savik, 2005, p. 36). Fecal incontinence is an emotionally distressing problem that

TABLE 49–2 Major Causes of Diarrhea

CAUSE	PHYSIOLOGIC EFFECT
Psychologic stress (e.g., anxiety)	Increased intestinal motility and mucus secretion
Medications	Inflammation and infection of mucosa due to overgrowth of pathogenic intestinal microorganisms
Antibiotics	Irritation of intestinal mucosa
Iron	Irritation of intestinal mucosa
Cathartics	Incomplete digestion of food or fluid
Allergy to food, fluid, drugs	Increased intestinal motility and mucus secretion
Intolerance of food or fluid	Reduced absorption of fluids
Diseases of the colon (e.g., malabsorption syndrome, Crohn's disease)	Inflammation of the mucosa often leading to ulcer formation

can ultimately lead to social isolation. Afflicted persons withdraw into their homes or, if in the hospital, the confines of their room to minimize the embarrassment associated with soiling. Several surgical procedures are used for the treatment of fecal incontinence. These include repair of the sphincter and fecal diversion or colostomy.

Flatulence

There are three primary sources of flatus: (a) action of bacteria on the chyme in the large intestine, (b) swallowed air, and (c) gas that diffuses between the bloodstream and the intestine.

Most gases that are swallowed are expelled through the mouth by eructation (belching). However, large amounts of gas can accumulate in the stomach, resulting in gastric distention. The gases formed in the large intestine are chiefly absorbed through the intestinal capillaries into the circulation. **Flatulence** is the presence of excessive flatus in the intestines and leads to stretching and inflation of the intestines (intestinal distention). Flatulence can occur in the colon from a variety of causes, such as foods (e.g., cabbage, onions), abdominal surgery, or narcotics. If the gas is propelled by increased colon activity before it can be absorbed, it may be expelled through the anus. If excessive gas cannot be expelled through the anus, it may be necessary to insert a rectal tube to remove it.

BOWEL DIVERSION OSTOMIES

An **ostomy** is an opening for the gastrointestinal, urinary, or respiratory tract onto the skin. There are many types of intestinal ostomies. A **gastrostomy** is an opening through the abdominal wall into the stomach. A **jejunostomy** opens through the abdominal wall into the jejunum, an **ileostomy** opens into the ileum (small bowel), and a **colostomy** opens into the colon (large bowel). Gastrostomies and jejunostomies are generally performed to provide an alternate feeding route. The purpose of

---

RESEARCH NOTE   What Self-Care Practices Do Older Adults Use for Fecal Incontinence?

These researchers conducted the first systematic investigation of self-care for fecal incontinence (FI) among elderly individuals living in the community. The purpose of the study was to describe the self-care practices used and to examine factors associated with the number of self-care practices and willingness to report FI to a health care practitioner. FI was described as accidental leakage of stool during the past 12 months. A 51-item survey was distributed at four HMO primary care clinics in the Midwest. The clinic staff offered surveys to individuals 65 or older who lived in the community. Over 1,300 surveys were received, primarily from women.

The results indicated that the most common self-care practices for managing FI were changing diet (e.g., avoiding certain foods); wearing a sanitary panty liner, pad, or brief; and reducing activity or exercise. There was a significant difference in the number and types of self-care practices between men and women. Fifty-two percent of men compared to 19% of women did not use any self-care practices to manage FI. Only 43% of the respondents discussed their FI with a health care practitioner, with no significant difference between men and women. More of those who had a health problem or disability that caused FI or were not sure about the cause of FI consulted with a health professional.

The study has some limitations in that it was based on self-report rather than a more rigorous method such as observation. Also, the population included elderly individuals who visited HMO clinics and, as a result, generalizability is limited.

IMPLICATIONS

The findings indicate that nurses who care for the elderly living in the community need to routinely inquire about FI. Discussing FI with a client, especially if it is a new onset for the client, allows the health care practitioner to provide appropriate follow-up to ascertain if the FI is a symptom of a health problem. Some elderly believe that FI is a normal part of aging and may minimize its significance. If the FI is not health related, the nurse will need to assess the self-care practices of the elder and if they are effective. The authors also suggest future research be conducted to investigate the reasons for the differences between men and women in self-care practices for FI.

Note: From "Managing Fecal Incontinence: Self-Care Practices of Older Adults" by D. Bliss, L. Fischer, & K. Savik, 2005, *Journal of Gerontological Nursing,* Copyright © 2005 SLACK, Inc. Reprinted with permission.

bowel ostomies is to divert and drain fecal material. Bowel diversion ostomies are often classified according to (a) their status as permanent or temporary, (b) their anatomic location, and (c) the construction of the **stoma,** the opening created in the abdominal wall by the ostomy. A stoma is generally red in color and moist. Initially, slight bleeding may occur when the stoma is touched and this is considered normal. A person doesn't feel the stoma because there are no nerve endings in the stoma.

Permanence

Colostomies can be either temporary or permanent. Temporary colostomies are generally performed for traumatic injuries or inflammatory conditions of the bowel. They allow the distal diseased portion of the bowel to rest and heal. Permanent colostomies are performed to provide a means of elimination when the rectum or anus is nonfunctional as a result of a birth defect or a disease such as cancer of the bowel.

> ### CLINICAL ALERT
>
> Surgery to reconnect the ends of the bowel of a temporary ostomy may be called a take down. ■

Anatomic Location

An ileostomy generally empties from the distal end of the small intestine. A cecostomy empties from the cecum (the first part of the ascending colon). An ascending colostomy empties from the ascending colon, a transverse colostomy from the transverse colon, a descending colostomy from the descending colon, and a sigmoidostomy from the sigmoid colon (Figure 49-4 ■).

The location of the ostomy influences the character and management of the fecal drainage. The farther along the bowel, the

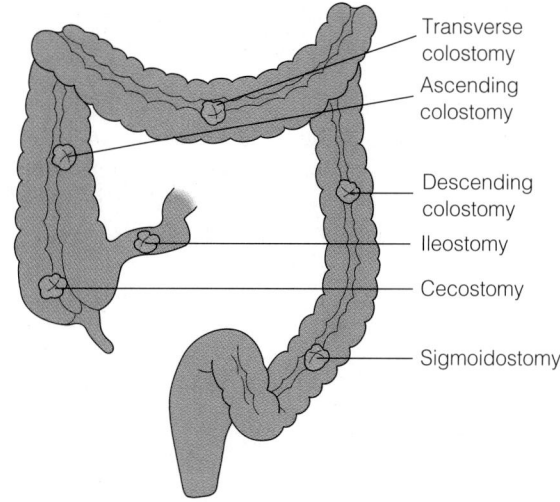

Figure 49-4 ■ The locations of bowel diversion ostomies.

Transverse colostomy
Ascending colostomy
Descending colostomy
Ileostomy
Cecostomy
Sigmoidostomy

MediaLink ■ The United Ostomy Association Application

more formed the stool (because the large bowel reabsorbs water from the fecal mass) and the more control over the frequency of stomal discharge can be established. For example:

- An ileostomy produces liquid fecal drainage. Drainage is constant and cannot be regulated. Ileostomy drainage contains some digestive enzymes, which are damaging to the skin. For this reason, ileostomy clients must wear an appliance continuously and take special precautions to prevent skin breakdown. Compared to colostomies, however, odor is minimal because fewer bacteria are present.
- An ascending colostomy is similar to an ileostomy in that the drainage is liquid and cannot be regulated, and digestive enzymes are present. Odor, however, is a problem requiring control.

LIFESPAN CONSIDERATIONS Factors in Potential Bowel Elimination Problems

CHILDREN

- Successful toilet training can prevent many problems with elimination. The family should be assessed for "readiness to train." Assess the child's physical, cognitive, and interpersonal skills, and parental readiness. Does the child have sphincter control (usually by 18 to 24 months)? Does the child understand the meaning of toileting? Is the child able to express him- or herself and does he or she demonstrate interest in learning? Are parents ready to work with the child?
- Encourage a regular toileting routine for children. When toilet training, ensure that toddlers can rest their feet comfortably on the floor or foot stool, and are not frightened or pressured while toileting.
- An acute episode of dehydration and constipation (often related to an illness) can lead to chronic stool problems. Constipation can cause painful defecation, which causes the child to withhold stool, leading to more severe constipation, more pain on defecation, more withholding, and so on. Breaking the cycle by helping ease defecation is important to prevent long-term problems.

ELDERS

- Poor fluid intake and inability to eat a high-fiber diet, due to swallowing or chewing difficulties, are often causes of constipation.
- Medications that are commonly taken by elders such as antacids, many antihypertensives, antidepressants, diuretics, and narcotics for pain also contribute to constipation.
- Clients receiving tube feedings can experience diarrhea. To alleviate it, they require a change of formula, a change in its strength, or a change in the speed or temperature of tube feeding administration.
- Clients receiving laxative preparation for x-rays or other procedures may experience fluid and electrolyte imbalances due to diarrhea.
- Persons with cognitive impairment, such as Alzheimer's disease, may be unaware of what and when they eat or drink or of their bowel habits. These should be monitored by the caregiver, whether the person is being cared for at home or in an institution, to note any special needs or concerns.
- Persons with impaired mobility may have difficulty getting to the bathroom or using a regular toilet. A raised toilet seat and other devices, such as bars to assist in ambulation, may be very helpful. The decrease in activity may also contribute to constipation.

- A transverse colostomy produces a malodorous, mushy drainage because some of the liquid has been reabsorbed. There is usually no control.
- A descending colostomy produces increasingly solid fecal drainage. Stools from a sigmoidostomy are of normal or formed consistency, and the frequency of discharge can be regulated. People with a sigmoidostomy may not have to wear an appliance at all times, and odors can usually be controlled.

The length of time that an ostomy is in place also helps to determine the consistency of the stool, particularly with transverse and descending colostomies. Over time, the stool becomes more formed because the remaining functioning portions of the colon tend to compensate by increasing water reabsorption.

Surgical Construction of the Stoma

Stoma constructions are described as single, loop, divided, or double-barreled colostomies. The *single* stoma is created when one end of bowel is brought out through an opening onto the anterior abdominal wall. This is referred to as an *end* or *terminal colostomy;* the stoma is permanent (Figure 49-5 ■).

In the *loop colostomy,* a loop of bowel is brought out onto the abdominal wall and supported by a plastic bridge, or a piece of rubber tubing (Figure 49-6 ■). A loop stoma has two openings: the proximal or afferent end, which is active, and the distal or efferent end, which is inactive. The loop colostomy is usually performed in an emergency procedure and is often situated on the right transverse colon. It is a bulky stoma that is more difficult to manage than a single stoma.

ANATOMY & PHYSIOLOGY REVIEW   Small and Large Intestines

Review the figure and reflect back on your Anatomy and Physiology courses.

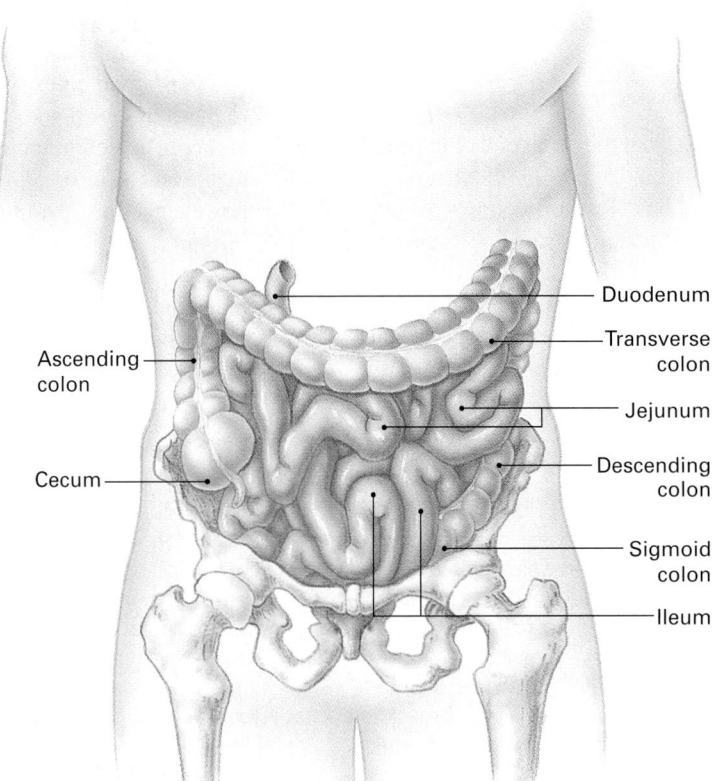

Ascending colon

Cecum

Duodenum

Transverse colon

Jejunum

Descending colon

Sigmoid colon

Ileum

From Fremgen, Bonnie F., Frucht, Suzanne S., *Medical Terminology: A Living Language,* 3rd ed. © 2005. Electronically reproduced by permission of Pearson Education, Inc., Upper Saddle River, New Jersey.

QUESTIONS
1. What are the primary functions of the small intestine?
2. What are the primary functions of the large intestine?
3. What part of the small intestine connects to the colon?
4. What consistency would the stool be in a client with an ileostomy and why?
5. Compare and contrast the consistency of stool in a transverse colostomy and a descending colostomy.
6. How would you describe the stool discharged from a sigmoidostomy?

Figure 49-5 ■ End colostomy: the diseased portion of bowel is removed and a rectal pouch remains.

The *divided colostomy* consists of two edges of bowel brought out onto the abdomen but separated from each other (Figure 49-7 ■). The opening from the digestive or proximal end is the colostomy. The distal end in this situation is often referred to as a mucous fistula, since this section of bowel continues to secrete mucus. The divided colostomy is often used in situations where spillage of feces into the distal end of the bowel needs to be avoided.

The *double-barreled colostomy* resembles a double-barreled shotgun (Figure 49-8 ■). In this type of colostomy, the proximal and distal loops of bowel are sutured together for about 10 cm (4 in.) and both ends are brought up onto the abdominal wall.

Figure 49-6 ■ Loop colostomy.
(Courtesy of Cory Patrick Hartley, San Ramon Regional Medical Center, San Ramon, CA.)

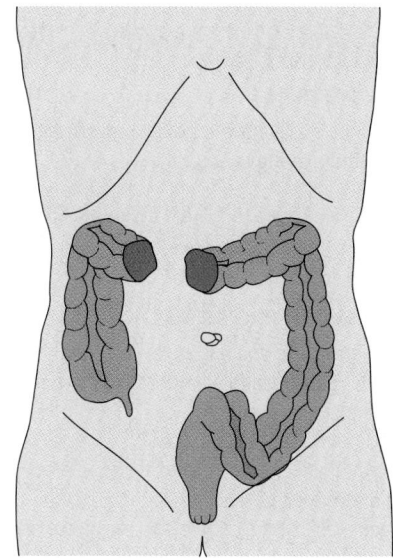

Figure 49-7 ■ Divided colostomy with two separated stomas.

Figure 49-8 ■ Double-barreled colostomy.

NURSING MANAGEMENT

Assessing

Assessment of fecal elimination includes taking a nursing history; performing a physical examination of the abdomen, rectum, and anus; and inspecting the feces. The nurse also should review any data obtained from relevant diagnostic tests.

Nursing History

A nursing history for fecal elimination helps the nurse ascertain the client's normal pattern. The nurse elicits a description of usual feces and any recent changes and collects information about any past or current problems with elimination, the presence of an ostomy, and factors influencing the elimination pattern.

Examples of questions to elicit this information are shown in the Assessment Interview. The number of questions to ask is adapted to the individual client, according to the client's responses in the first three categories. For example, questions about factors influencing elimination might be addressed only to clients who are experiencing problems.

When eliciting data about the client's defecation pattern, the nurse needs to understand that the time of defecation and the

ASSESSMENT INTERVIEW Fecal Elimination

DEFECATION PATTERN

- When do you usually have a bowel movement?
- Has this pattern changed recently?

DESCRIPTION OF FECES AND ANY CHANGES

- Have you noticed any changes in the color, texture (hard, soft, watery), shape, or odor of your stool recently?

FECAL ELIMINATION PROBLEMS

- What problems have you had or do you now have with your bowel movements (constipation, diarrhea, excessive flatulence, seepage, or incontinence)?
- When and how often does it occur?
- What do you think causes it (food, fluids, exercise, emotions, medications, disease, surgery)?
- What have you tried to solve the problem, and how effective was it?

FACTORS INFLUENCING ELIMINATION

- Use of elimination aids. What routines do you follow to maintain your usual defecation pattern? Do you use natural aids such as specific foods or fluids (e.g., a glass of hot lemon juice before breakfast), laxatives, or enemas to maintain elimination?
- Diet. What foods do you believe affect defecation? What foods do you typically eat? What foods do you avoid? Do you take meals at regular times?
- Fluid. What amount and kind of fluid do you take each day (e.g., 6 glasses of water, 2 cups of coffee)?
- Exercise. What is your usual daily exercise pattern? (Obtain specifics about exercise rather than asking whether it is sufficient; ideas of what is sufficient vary among individuals.)
- Medications. Have you taken any medications that could affect the intestinal tract (e.g., iron, antibiotics)?
- Stress. Are you experiencing any stress? Do you think this affects your defecation pattern? How?

PRESENCE AND MANAGEMENT OF OSTOMY

- What is your usual routine with your colostomy/ileostomy?
- What type of appliance do you wear and did you bring a spare with you?
- What problems, if any, do you have with it?
- How can the nurses help you manage your colostomy/ileostomy?

---

amount of feces expelled are as individual as the frequency of defecation. Often, the patterns individuals follow depend largely on early training and on convenience.

Physical Examination

Physical examination of the abdomen in relation to fecal elimination problems includes inspection, auscultation, percussion, and palpation with specific reference to the intestinal tract. Auscultation precedes palpation because palpation can alter peristalsis. Examination of the rectum and anus includes inspection and palpation. Physical examination of the abdomen, rectum, and anus is discussed in Chapter 30. ∞

Inspecting the Feces

Observe the client's stool for color, consistency, shape, amount, odor, and the presence of abnormal constituents. Table 49–1, earlier in this chapter, summarizes normal and abnormal characteristics of stool and possible causes.

Diagnostic Studies

Diagnostic studies of the gastrointestinal tract include direct visualization techniques, indirect visualization techniques, and laboratory tests for abnormal constituents (see Chapter 34 ∞).

Diagnosing

NANDA includes the following diagnostic labels for fecal elimination problems:

- *Bowel Incontinence*
- *Constipation*
- *Risk for Constipation*
- *Perceived Constipation*
- *Diarrhea*

Clinical application of selected diagnoses is shown in Identifying Nursing Diagnoses, Outcomes, and Interventions, and at the end of the chapter in the Nursing Care Plan and the Concept Map.

Fecal elimination problems may affect many other areas of human functioning and as a consequence may be the etiology of other NANDA diagnoses. Examples follow:

- *Risk for Deficient Fluid Volume* related to
  a. Prolonged diarrhea
  b. Abnormal fluid loss through ostomy
- *Risk for Impaired Skin Integrity* related to
  a. Prolonged diarrhea
  b. Bowel incontinence
  c. Bowel diversion ostomy
- *Low Self-Esteem* related to
  a. Ostomy
  b. Fecal incontinence
  c. Need for assistance with toileting
- *Disturbed Body Image* related to
  a. Ostomy
  b. Bowel incontinence
- *Deficient Knowledge (Bowel Training, Ostomy Management)* related to lack of previous experience
- *Anxiety* related to
  a. Lack of control of fecal elimination secondary to ostomy
  b. Response of others to ostomy

Planning

The major goals for clients with fecal elimination problems are to

- Maintain or restore normal bowel elimination pattern.
- Maintain or regain normal stool consistency.
- Prevent associated risks such as fluid and electrolyte imbalance, skin breakdown, abdominal distention, and pain.

IDENTIFYING NURSING DIAGNOSES, OUTCOMES, AND INTERVENTIONS
Clients With Fecal Elimination Problems

DATA CLUSTER Marvin Lombardi reports having loose, liquid, light brown stools for 2 days. Passage of stools is associated with cramping abdominal pain. Bowel sounds are hyperactive. Temperature is 38°C (100.4°F). Has not taken any medications but reports a feeling of general malaise. States he "ate at a fast-food restaurant 2 nights ago."

NURSING DIAGNOSIS/ DEFINITION	SAMPLE DESIRED OUTCOMES*/ DEFINITION	INDICATORS	SELECTED INTERVENTIONS*/ DEFINITION	SAMPLE NIC ACTIVITIES
Diarrhea/Passage of loose, unformed stools	Bowel Elimination [0501]/Formation and evacuation of stool	No ▪ Diarrhea ▪ Painful cramps	Diarrhea Management [0460]/Management and alleviation of diarrhea	▪ Obtain stool for culture and sensitivity if diarrhea continues ▪ Observe skin turgor ▪ Monitor skin in perianal region for irritation or ulceration ▪ Consult primary care provider if signs and symptoms of diarrhea persist

DATA CLUSTER Mary Kuoko has had involuntary leakage of stool. States her clothing is soiled several times a day. Says she is too embarrassed to go out with her friends because of the fecal odor. Last bowel movement was more than 3 days ago. Digital examination reveals impaction.

Bowel Incontinence/ Change in normal bowel habits, characterized by involuntary passage of stool	Bowel Continence [0500]/Control of passage of stool from the bowel	Consistently demonstrated ▪ Evacuates stool at least q 3 days ▪ Responds to urge in a timely manner ▪ Describes relationship of food intake to stool consistency	Bowel Management [0430]/Establishment and maintenance of a regular pattern of bowel elimination Bowel Incontinence Care [0410]/ Promotion of bowel continence and maintenance of perianal skin integrity	▪ Instruct on foods high in fiber, as appropriate ▪ Give warm liquids after meals, as appropriate ▪ Initiate a bowel training program as appropriate ▪ Wash perianal area with soap and water and dry it thoroughly after each stool ▪ Monitor for adequate bowel evacuation ▪ Monitor diet and fluid requirements

*The NOC # for desired outcomes and the NIC # for nursing interventions are listed in brackets following the appropriate outcome or intervention. Outcomes, indicators, interventions, and activities selected are only a sample of those suggested by NOC and NIC and should be further individualized for each client.

Appropriate preventive and corrective nursing interventions that relate to these must be identified. Specific nursing activities associated with each of these interventions can be selected to meet the client's individual needs. Examples of clinical applications of these using NANDA, NIC, and NOC designations are shown in Identifying Nursing Diagnoses, Outcomes, and Interventions and in the Nursing Care Plan.

Planning for Home Care

Clients who have bowel diversion ostomies, who wear pouches, or who have other ongoing elimination problems will need continuing care in the home setting. In preparation for discharge, the nurse needs to assess the client's and family's ability to meet specific care needs. The Home Care Assessment outlines the specific assessment data required before developing a home care plan. Using the assessment data, the nurse designs a teaching plan for the client and family (see Client Teaching on page 1336).

Implementing
Promoting Regular Defecation

The nurse can help clients achieve regular defecation by attending to (a) the provision of privacy, (b) timing, (c) nutrition and fluids, (d) exercise, and (e) positioning. See Client Teaching on page 1337 for healthy habits related to bowel elimination.

PRIVACY. Privacy during defecation is extremely important to many people. The nurse should therefore provide as much privacy as possible for such clients but may need to stay with those who are too weak to be left alone. Some clients also prefer to wipe, wash, and dry themselves after defecating. A nurse may need to provide water and a washcloth and towel for this purpose.

TIMING. A client should be encouraged to defecate when the urge is recognized. To establish regular bowel elimination, the client and nurse can discuss when mass peristalsis normally occurs and provide time for defecation. Many people have

---

HOME CARE ASSESSMENT   Fecal Elimination

CLIENT AND ENVIRONMENT

- Self-care abilities for toileting: Ability to get to the toilet, to manipulate clothing for toileting, to perform toilet hygiene, and to flush the toilet
- Mechanical aids required: Walker, cane, wheelchair, raised toilet seat, grab bars, bedpan, commode
- Mechanical barriers that limit access to the toilet or are unsafe: Poor lighting, cluttered pathway to bathroom, narrow doorway for wheelchair, and so on
- Bowel elimination problem: Alterations in characteristics of feces, diarrhea, constipation, incontinence, presence of ostomy, and methods of handling these
- Level of knowledge: Planned bowel management or training program, prescribed medications, ostomy care, dietary alterations, and fluid and exercise requirements or restrictions
- Facilities: Adequacy of bathroom facilities to facilitate toilet hygiene and ostomy care and to contain potentially infectious fecal effluent or stool

FAMILY

- Caregiver availability and skills: People able to assist with toileting, medications, ostomy care, or other prescribed therapeutic measures
- Family role changes and coping: Effect on financial status, parenting and spousal roles, sexuality, social roles
- Alternate potential primary or respite caregivers: For example, other family members, volunteers, church members, paid caregivers or housekeeping services; available community respite care (adult day care, senior centers)

COMMUNITY

- Availability of and familiarity with possible sources of assistance: Equipment and supply companies, financial assistance, home health agencies

---

well-established routines. Other activities, such as bathing and ambulating, should not interfere with the defecation time.

NUTRITION AND FLUIDS. The diet a client needs for regular normal elimination varies, depending on the kind of feces the client currently has, the frequency of defecation, and the types of foods that the client finds assist with normal defecation.

For Constipation. Increase daily fluid intake, and instruct the client to drink hot liquids and fruit juices, especially prune juice. Include fiber in the diet, that is, foods such as raw fruit, bran products, and whole-grain cereals and bread.

For Diarrhea. Encourage oral intake of fluids and bland food. Eating small amounts can be helpful because it is more easily absorbed. Excessively hot or cold fluids should be avoided because they stimulate peristalsis. In addition, highly spiced foods and high-fiber foods can aggravate diarrhea. See Client Teaching for details about managing diarrhea.

For Flatulence. Limit carbonated beverages, the use of drinking straws, and chewing gum—all of which increase the ingestion of air. Gas-forming foods, such as cabbage, beans, onions, and cauliflower, should also be avoided.

EXERCISE. Regular exercise helps clients develop a regular defecation pattern. A client with weak abdominal and pelvic muscles (which impede normal defecation) may be able to strengthen them with the following isometric exercises:

CLIENT TEACHING   Fecal Elimination

FACILITATING TOILETING

- Ensure safe and easy access to the toilet. Make sure lighting is appropriate, scatter rugs are removed or securely fastened, and so on.
- Facilitate instruction as needed about transfer techniques.
- Suggest ways that garments can be adjusted to make disrobing easier for toileting (e.g., Velcro closing on clothing).

MONITORING BOWEL ELIMINATION PATTERN

- Instruct the client, if appropriate, to keep a record of time and frequency of stool passage, any associated pain, and color and consistency of the stool.

DIETARY ALTERATIONS

- Provide information about required food and fluid alterations to promote defecation or to manage diarrhea.

MEDICATIONS

- Discuss problems associated with overuse of laxatives, if appropriate, and the use of alternatives to laxatives, suppositories, and enemas.
- Discuss the addition of a fiber supplement if the client is taking a constipating medication.

MEASURES SPECIFIC TO ELIMINATION PROBLEM

- Provide instructions associated with specific elimination problems and treatment, such as
  - a. Constipation
  - b. Diarrhea
  - c. Ostomy care

COMMUNITY AGENCIES AND OTHER SOURCES OF HELP

- Make appropriate referrals to home care or community care for assistance with resources such as installation of grab bars and raised toilet seats, structural alterations for wheelchair access, homemaker or home health aide services to assist with ADLs, and enterostomal therapy nurse for assistance with stoma care and selection of ostomy appliances.
- Provide information about companies where durable medical equipment (e.g., raised toilet seats, commodes, bedpans, urinals) can be purchased, rented, or obtained free of charge, and where medical supplies such as incontinence pads or ostomy irrigating supplies and appliances can be obtained.
- Suggest additional sources of information and help such as ostomy self-help and support groups or clubs.

- In a supine position, the client tightens the abdominal muscles as though pulling them inward, holding them for about 10 seconds and then relaxing them. This should be repeated 5 to 10 times, four times a day, depending on the client's health.
- Again in a supine position, the client can contract the thigh muscles and hold them contracted for about 10 seconds, repeating the exercise 5 to 10 times, four times a day. This helps the client confined to bed gain strength in the thigh muscles, thereby making it easier to use a bedpan.

POSITIONING. Although the squatting position best facilitates defecation, on a toilet seat the best position for most people seems to be leaning forward.

For clients who have difficulty sitting down and getting up from the toilet, an elevated toilet seat can be attached to a regular toilet. Clients then do not have to lower themselves as far onto the seat and do not have to lift as far off the seat. Elevated toilet seats can be purchased for use in the home.

Figure 49-9 ■ A commode with overlying seat.

A bedside **commode,** a portable chair with a toilet seat and a receptacle beneath that can be emptied, is often used for the adult client who can get out of bed but is unable to walk to the bathroom. Some commodes have wheels and can slide over the base of a regular toilet when the waste receptacle is removed, thus providing clients the privacy of a bathroom. Some commodes have a seat and can be used as a chair (Figure 49-9 ■). Potty chairs are available for children.

Clients restricted to bed may need to use a **bedpan,** a receptacle for urine and feces. Female clients use a bedpan for both urine and feces; male clients use a bedpan for feces and a urinal for urine.

There are two main types of bedpans: the regular high-back pan and the slipper, or fracture, pan (Figure 49-10 ■). The slipper pan has a low back and is used for clients unable to raise

Figure 49-10 ■ *Top,* The high-back or regular bedpan; *Bottom,* the slipper or fracture pan.

PRACTICE GUIDELINES   Giving and Removing a Bedpan

- Provide privacy.
- Wear disposable gloves.
- If the bedpan is metal, warm it by rinsing it with warm water.
- Adjust the bed to a height appropriate to prevent back strain.
- Elevate the side rail on the opposite side to prevent the client from falling out of bed.
- Ask the client to assist by flexing the knees, resting the weight on the back and heels, and raising the buttocks, or by using a trapeze bar, if present.
- Help lift the client as needed by placing one hand under the lower back, resting your elbow on the mattress, and using your forearm as a lever.
- Lubricate the back of the bedpan with a small amount of hand lotion or liquid soap to reduce tissue friction and shearing.
- Place a regular bedpan so that the client's buttocks rest on the smooth, rounded rim. Place a slipper pan with the flat, low end under the client's buttocks (Figure 49-11 ■).
- For the client who cannot assist, obtain the assistance of another nurse to help lift the client onto the bedpan or place the client on his or her side, place the bedpan against the buttocks (Figure 49-12 ■), and roll the client back onto the bedpan.
- To provide a more normal position for the client's lower back, elevate the client's bed to a semi-Fowler's position, if permitted. If elevation is contraindicated, support the client's back with pillows as needed to prevent hyperextension of the back.
- Cover the client with bed linen to maintain comfort and dignity.

- Provide toilet tissue, place the call light within reach, lower the bed to the low position, elevate the side rail if indicated, and leave the client alone.
- Answer the call bell promptly.
- Do not leave anyone on a bedpan longer than 15 minutes unless they are able to remove the pan themselves. Lengthy stays on a bedpan can cause pressure ulcers.
- When removing the bedpan, return the bed to the position used when giving the bedpan, hold the bedpan steady to prevent spillage of its contents, cover the bedpan, and place it on the adjacent chair.
- If the client needs assistance, don gloves and wipe the client's perineal area with several layers of toilet tissue. If a specimen is to be collected, discard the soiled tissue into a moisture-proof receptacle other than the bedpan. For female clients, clean from the urethra toward the anus to prevent transferring rectal microorganisms into the urinary meatus.
- Wash the perineal area of dependent clients with soap and water as indicated and thoroughly dry the area.
- For all clients, offer warm water, soap, a washcloth, and a towel to wash the hands.
- Assist the client to a comfortable position, empty and clean the bedpan, and return it to the bedside.
- Remove and discard your gloves and wash your hands.
- Spray the room with air freshener as needed to control odor unless contraindicated because of respiratory problems or allergies.
- Document color, odor, amount, and consistency of urine and feces, and the condition of the perineal area.

Figure 49-11 ■ Placing a slipper pan under the buttocks.

Figure 49-12 ■ Placing a regular bedpan against the client's buttocks.

their buttocks because of physical problems or therapy that contraindicates such movement. Many older adults benefit from the use of a slipper pan. See Practice Guidelines for the techniques of giving and removing a bedpan.

Teaching about Medications

The most common categories of medications affecting fecal elimination are cathartics and laxatives, antidiarrheals, and antiflatulents.

CATHARTICS AND LAXATIVES. **Cathartics** are drugs that induce defecation. They can have a strong, purgative effect. A

laxative is mild in comparison to a cathartic, and it produces soft or liquid stools that are sometimes accompanied by abdominal cramps. Examples of cathartics are castor oil, cascara, phenolphthalein, and bisacodyl. Table 49–3 describes the different types of laxatives.

Laxatives are contraindicated in the client who has nausea, cramps, colic, vomiting, or undiagnosed abdominal pain. Clients need to be informed about the dangers of laxative use. Continual use of laxatives to encourage bowel evacuation weakens the bowel's natural responses to fecal distention, resulting in chronic constipation. To eliminate chronic laxative

TABLE 49–3 Types of Laxatives

TYPE	ACTION	EXAMPLES	PERTINENT TEACHING INFORMATION
Bulk-forming	Increases the fluid, gaseous, or solid bulk in the intestines	Psyllium hydrophilic mucilloid (Metamucil), methylcellulose (Citrucel)	May take 12 or more hours to act. Sufficient fluid must be taken. Safe for long-term use.
Emollient/stool softener	Softens and delays the drying of the feces; permits fat and water to penetrate feces	Docusate sodium (Colace) Docusate calcium (Surfak)	Slow-acting, may take several days.
Stimulant/irritant	Irritates the intestinal mucosa or stimulates nerve endings in the wall of the intestine, causing rapid propulsion of the contents	Bisacodyl (Dulcolax, Correctol), senna (Senokot, Ex-Lax), cascara, castor oil	Acts more quickly than bulk-forming agents. Fluid is passed with the feces. May cause cramps. Prolonged use may cause fluid and electrolyte imbalance.
Lubricant	Lubricates the feces in the colon	Mineral oil (Haley's M-O)	Prolonged use inhibits the absorption of some fat-soluble vitamins.
Saline/osmotic	Draws water into the intestine by osmosis, distends bowel, and stimulates peristalsis	Epsom salts, magnesium citrate, sodium phosphate (Fleet phospho-soda)	May be rapid acting. Can cause fluid and electrolyte imbalance, particularly in elderly people and children with cardiac and renal disease. Should not be used by elderly clients. Prolonged use inhibits the absorption of some fat-soluble vitamins.
		Electrolyte-free polyethylene glycol 3350 (PEG 3350) (MiraLax)	A new laxative that is helpful in the treatment of constipation in children. It is a powder that is tasteless when mixed in a flavored liquid such as juice. It is a prescription drug and costs more than OTC laxatives.

use, it is usually necessary to teach the client about dietary fiber, regular exercise, taking sufficient fluids, and establishing regular defecation habits. In addition, any medication regimen should be examined to see whether it could cause constipation.

Some laxatives are given in the form of **suppositories.** These act in various ways: by softening the feces, by releasing gases such as carbon dioxide to distend the rectum, or by stimulating the nerve endings in the rectal mucosa. The best results can be obtained by inserting the suppository 30 minutes before the client's usual defecation time or when the peristaltic action is greatest, such as after breakfast.

ANTIDIARRHEAL MEDICATIONS. These medications slow the motility of the intestine or absorb excess fluid in the intestine. Guidelines for using antidiarrheals are shown in Box 49–2.

ANTIFLATULENT MEDICATIONS. Antiflatulent agents such as simethicone do not decrease the formation of flatus but they do coalesce the gas bubbles and facilitate their passage by belching through the mouth or expulsion through the anus. These agents are frequently combined with an antacid. **Carminatives** are herbal oils known to act as agents that help expel gas from the stomach and intestines. Suppositories can also be given to relieve flatus by increasing intestinal motility.

Decreasing Flatulence

There are a number of ways to reduce or expel flatus, including avoiding gas-producing foods, exercise, moving in bed, and ambulation. Movement stimulates peristalsis and the

BOX 49–2 Guidelines for Using Antidiarrheal Medications

- If the diarrhea persists for more than 3 or 4 days, determine the underlying cause. Using a medication such as an opiate when the cause is an infection, toxin, or poison may prolong diarrhea.
- Long-term use of over-the-counter medications (e.g., loperamide hydrochloride [Imodium]) can produce dependence.
- Some antidiarrheal agents can cause drowsiness (e.g., diphenoxylate hydrochloride [Lomotil]) and should not be used when driving an automobile or running machinery.
- Kaolin-pectin preparations (e.g., Kaopectate) may absorb nutrients.
- Bulk laxatives and other absorbents may be used to help bind toxins and absorb excess bowel liquid.
- Bismuth preparations (e.g., Pepto-Bismol), often used to treat "traveler's diarrhea," may contain aspirin and should not be given to children and teenagers with chickenpox, influenza, and other viral infections.

escape of flatus and reabsorption of gases in the intestinal capillaries.

Administering Enemas

An **enema** is a solution introduced into the rectum and large intestine. The action of an enema is to distend the intestine and sometimes to irritate the intestinal mucosa, thereby increasing peristalsis and the excretion of feces and flatus. Enemas are classified into four groups: cleansing, carminative, retention, and return-flow enemas.

TABLE 49–4　Commonly Used Enema Solutions

SOLUTION	CONSTITUENTS	ACTION	TIME TO TAKE EFFECT	ADVERSE EFFECTS
Hypertonic	90–120 mL of solution (e.g., sodium phosphate)	Draws water into the colon	5–10 min	Retention of sodium
Hypotonic	500–1,000 mL of tap water	Distends colon, stimulates peristalsis, and softens feces	15–20 min	Fluid and electrolyte imbalance; water intoxication
Isotonic	500–1,000 mL of normal saline	Distends colon, stimulates peristalsis, and softens feces	15–20 min	Possible sodium retention
Soapsuds	500–1,000 mL (3–5 mL soap to 1,000 mL water)	Irritates mucosa, distends colon	10–15 min	Irritates and may damage mucosa
Oil (mineral, olive, cottonseed)	90–120 mL	Lubricates the feces and the colonic mucosa	1/2–3 hr	

CLEANSING ENEMAS. Cleansing enemas are intended to remove feces. They are given chiefly to

- Prevent the escape of feces during surgery.
- Prepare the intestine for certain diagnostic tests such as x-ray or visualization tests (e.g., colonoscopy).
- Remove feces in instances of constipation or impaction.

Cleansing enemas use a variety of solutions. Table 49–4 lists commonly used solutions.

Hypertonic solutions (e.g., saline) exert osmotic pressure, which draws fluid from the interstitial space into the colon. The increased volume in the colon stimulates peristalsis and hence defecation. A commonly used hypertonic enema is the commercially prepared Fleet phosphate enema. Hypotonic solutions (e.g., tap water) exert a lower osmotic pressure than the surrounding interstitial fluid, causing water to move from the colon into the interstitial space. Before the water moves from the colon, it stimulates peristalsis and defecation. Because the water moves out of the colon, the tap water enema should not be repeated because of danger of circulatory overload when the water moves from the interstitial space into the circulatory system.

Isotonic solutions, such as physiologic (normal) saline, are considered the safest enema solutions to use. They exert the same osmotic pressure as the interstitial fluid surrounding the colon. Therefore, there is no fluid movement into or out of the colon. The instilled volume of saline in the colon stimulates peristalsis. Soapsuds enemas stimulate peristalsis by increasing the volume in the colon and irritating the mucosa. Only pure soap (i.e., castile soap) should be used in order to minimize mucosa irritation.

Some enemas are large volume (i.e., 500 to 1,000 mL) for an adult and others are small volume, including hypertonic solutions. The amount of solution administered for a high-volume enema will depend on the age and medical condition of the individual. For example, clients with certain cardiac or renal diseases would be adversely affected by significant fluid retention that might result from large-volume hypotonic enemas.

Cleansing enemas may also be described as high or low. A high enema is given to cleanse as much of the colon as possible. The client changes from the left lateral position to the dorsal recumbent position and then to the right lateral position during administration so that the solution can follow the large intestine. The low enema is used to clean the rectum and sigmoid colon only. The client maintains a left lateral position during administration.

The force of flow of the solution is governed by (a) the height of the solution container, (b) size of the tubing, (c) viscosity of the fluid, and (d) resistance of the rectum. The higher the solution container is held above the rectum, the faster the flow and the greater the force (pressure) in the rectum. During most adult enemas, the solution container should be no higher than 30 cm (12 in.) above the rectum. During a high cleansing enema, the solution container is usually held 30 to 49 cm (12 to 18 in.) above the rectum because the fluid is instilled farther to clean the entire bowel.

CARMINATIVE ENEMA. A carminative enema is given primarily to expel flatus. The solution instilled into the rectum releases gas, which in turn distends the rectum and the colon, thus stimulating peristalsis. For an adult, 60 to 80 mL of fluid is instilled.

RETENTION ENEMA. A retention enema introduces oil or medication into the rectum and sigmoid colon. The liquid is retained for a relatively long period (e.g., 1 to 3 hours). An oil retention enema acts to soften the feces and to lubricate the rectum and anal canal, thus facilitating passage of the feces. Antibiotic enemas are used to treat infections locally, anthelmintic enemas to kill helminths such as worms and intestinal parasites, and nutritive enemas to administer fluids and nutrients to the rectum.

RETURN-FLOW ENEMA. A return-flow enema is used occasionally to expel flatus. Alternating flow of 100 to 200 mL of fluid into and out of the rectum and sigmoid colon stimulates peristalsis. This process is repeated five or six times until the flatus is expelled and abdominal distention is relieved.

Skill 49-1 describes how to administer an enema.

CLINICAL ALERT

Some clients may wish to administer their own enemas. If this is appropriate, the nurse validates the client's knowledge of correct technique and assists as needed. ■

ADMINISTERING AN ENEMA

PURPOSES
- To achieve one or more of the following actions: cleansing, carminative, retention, or return-flow

ASSESSMENT
Assess the following:
- When the client last had a bowel movement and the amount, color, and consistency of the feces
- Presence of abdominal distention (the distended abdomen appears swollen and feels firm rather than soft when palpated)
- Whether the client has sphincter control
- Whether the client can use a toilet or commode or must remain in bed and use a bedpan

PLANNING
Before administering an enema, determine that there is a primary care provider's order. At some agencies, a primary care provider must order the kind of enema and the time to give it, for example, the morning of an examination. At other agencies, enemas are given at the nurses' discretion (i.e., as necessary on a prn order). In addition, determine the presence of kidney or cardiac disease that contraindicates the use of a hypotonic solution.

Delegation
Administration of some enemas may be delegated to unlicensed assistive personnel (UAP). However, the nurse must ensure the personnel are competent in the use of standard precautions. Abnormal findings such as inability to insert the rectal tip, client inability to retain the solution, or unusual return from the enema must be validated and interpreted by the nurse.

Equipment
- Disposable linen-saver pad
- Bath blanket
- Bedpan or commode
- Clean gloves
- Water-soluble lubricant if tubing not prelubricated
- Paper towel

Large-Volume Enema
- Solution container with tubing of correct size and tubing clamp
- Correct solution, amount, and temperature

Small-Volume Enema
- Prepackaged container of enema solution with lubricated tip

IMPLEMENTATION

Preparation
- Lubricate about 5 cm (2 in.) of the rectal tube (some commercially prepared enema sets already have lubricated nozzles). Lubrication facilitates insertion through the sphincters and minimizes trauma.
- Run some solution through the connecting tubing of a large-volume enema set and the rectal tube to expel any air in the tubing; then close the clamp. **Rationale:** *Air instilled into the rectum, although not harmful, causes unnecessary distention.*

Performance
1. Prior to performing the procedure, introduce self and verify the client's identity using agency protocol. Explain to the client what you are going to do, why it is necessary, and how he or she can cooperate. Discuss how the results will be used in planning further care or treatments. Indicate that the client may experience a feeling of fullness while the solution is being administered.
2. Perform hand hygiene, apply clean gloves, and observe appropriate infection control procedures.
3. Provide for client privacy.
4. Assist the adult client to a left lateral position, with the right leg as acutely flexed as possible ❶, and the linen-saver pad under the buttocks. **Rationale:** *This position facilitates the flow of solution by gravity into the sigmoid and descending colon, which are on the left side. Having the right leg acutely flexed provides for adequate exposure of the anus.*
5. Insert the enema tube.
   - For clients in the left lateral position, lift the upper buttock *to ensure good visualization of the anus.*
   - Insert the tube smoothly and slowly into the rectum, directing it toward the umbilicus. ❷ **Rationale:** *The angle follows*

❶ Assuming a left lateral position for an enema. Note the commercially prepared enema.

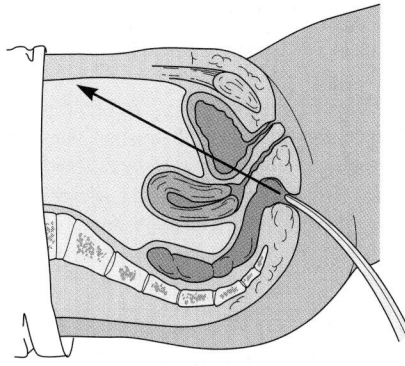

❷ Inserting the enema tube following the direction of the rectum.

continued on page 1342

ADMINISTERING AN ENEMA *continued*

the normal contour of the rectum. Slow insertion prevents spasm of the sphincter.

- Insert the tube 7 to 10 cm (3 to 4 in.). **Rationale:** *Because the anal canal is about 2.5 to 5 cm (1 to 2 in.) long in the adult, insertion to this point places the tip of the tube beyond the anal sphincter into the rectum.*
- If resistance is encountered at the internal sphincter, ask the client to take a deep breath, then run a small amount of solution through the tube *to relax the internal anal sphincter.*
- Never force tube or solution entry. If instilling a small amount of solution does not permit the tube to be advanced or the solution to freely flow, withdraw the tube. Check for any stool that may have blocked the tube during insertion. If present, flush it and retry the procedure. You may also perform a digital rectal examination to determine if there is an impaction or other mechanical blockage. If resistance persists, end the procedure and report the resistance to the primary care provider and nurse in charge.

6. Slowly administer the enema solution.
   - Raise the solution container, and open the clamp to allow fluid flow.

   or

   - Compress a pliable container by hand.
   - During most low enemas, hold or hang the solution container no higher than 30 cm (12 in.) above the rectum. **Rationale:** *The higher the solution container is held above the rectum, the faster the flow and the greater the force (pressure) in the rectum.* During a high enema, hang the solution container about 45 cm (18 in.). **Rationale:** *The fluid must be instilled farther to clean the entire bowel.* See agency protocol.
   - Administer the fluid slowly. If the client complains of fullness or pain, lower the container or use the clamp to stop the flow for 30 seconds, and then restart the flow at a slower rate. **Rationale:** *Administering the enema slowly and stopping the flow momentarily decreases the likelihood of intestinal spasm and premature ejection of the solution.*
   - If you are using a plastic commercial container, roll it up as the fluid is instilled. This prevents subsequent suctioning of the solution. ❸
   - After all the solution has been instilled or when the client cannot hold any more and feels the desire to defecate (the urge to defecate usually indicates that sufficient fluid has been administered), close the clamp, and remove the enema tube from the anus.
   - Place the enema tube in a disposable towel as you withdraw it.

7. Encourage the client to retain the enema.
   - Ask the client to remain lying down. It is easier for the client to retain the enema when lying down than when sitting or standing, because gravity promotes drainage and peristalsis.
   - Request that the client retain the solution for the appropriate amount of time, for example, 5 to 10 minutes for a cleansing enema or at least 30 minutes for a retention enema.

8. Assist the client to defecate.

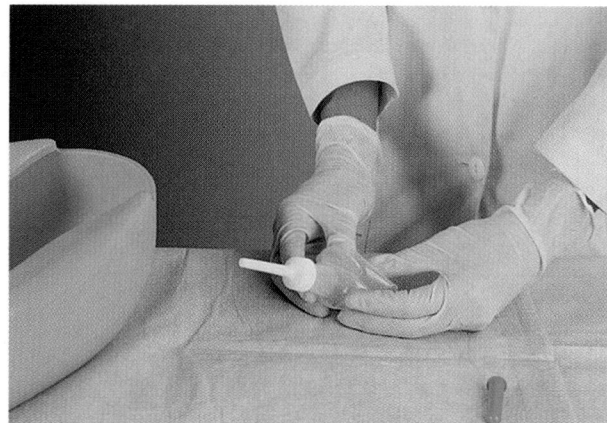

❸ Rolling up a commercial enema container.

- Assist the client to a sitting position on the bedpan, commode, or toilet. A sitting position facilitates the act of defecation.
- Ask the client who is using the toilet not to flush it. The nurse needs to observe the feces.
- If a specimen of feces is required, ask the client to use a bedpan or commode.

9. Document the type and volume, if appropriate, of enema given. Describe the results.

SAMPLE DOCUMENTATION

8/2/2007 1000. States last BM five days ago. Abdomen distended and firm. Bowel sounds hypoactive. Fleet's enema given per order resulting in large amount of firm brown stool. States he "feels better". ————————————*M. Lopez, RN*

VARIATION: ADMINISTERING AN ENEMA TO AN INCONTINENT CLIENT

Occasionally a nurse needs to administer an enema to a client who is unable to control the external sphincter muscle and thus cannot retain the enema solution for even a few minutes. In that case, after the rectal tube is inserted, the client assumes a supine position on a bedpan. The head of the bed can be elevated slightly, to 30 degrees if necessary for easier breathing, and pillows support the client's head and back.

VARIATION: ADMINISTERING A RETURN-FLOW ENEMA

For a return-flow enema, the solution (100 to 200 mL for an adult) is instilled into the client's rectum and sigmoid colon. Then the solution container is lowered so that the fluid flows back out through the rectal tube into the container, pulling the flatus with it. The inflow–outflow process is repeated five or six times (to stimulate peristalsis and the expulsion of flatus), and the solution is replaced several times during the procedure if it becomes thick with feces.

Document type of solution; length of time solution was retained; the amount, color, and consistency of the returns; and the relief of flatus and abdominal distention in the client record using forms or checklists supplemented by narrative notes when appropriate.

EVALUATION

- Perform a detailed follow-up based on findings that deviated from expected or normal for the client. Relate findings to previ-ous assessment data if available. Report significant deviations from expected to the primary care provider.

LIFESPAN CONSIDERATIONS   Administering an Enema

INFANTS/CHILDREN

- Provide a careful explanation to the parents and child before the procedure.
- The enema solution should be isotonic (usually normal saline). Some hypertonic commercial solutions (e.g., Fleet phosphate enema) can lead to hypovolemia and electrolyte imbalances. In addition, the osmotic effect of the enema may produce diarrhea and subsequent metabolic acidosis.
- Infants and small children do not exhibit sphincter control and need to be assisted in retaining the enema. The nurse administers the enema while the infant or child is lying with the buttocks over the bedpan, and the nurse firmly presses the buttocks together to prevent the immediate expulsion of the solution. Older children can usually hold the solution if they understand what to do and are not required to hold it for too long a period. It may be necessary to ensure that the bathroom is available for an ambulatory child before starting the procedure or to have a bedpan ready.
- Enema temperature should be 37.7°C (100°F) unless otherwise ordered.
- Large-volume enemas consist of 50 to 200 mL in children less than 18 months old; 200 to 300 mL in children 18 months to 5 years; and 300 to 500 mL in children 5 to 12 years old.

- Careful explanation is especially important for the preschool child. An enema is an intrusive procedure and therefore threatening.
- For infants and small children, the dorsal recumbent position is frequently used. Position them on a small padded bedpan with support for the back and head. Secure the legs by placing a diaper under the bedpan and then over and around the thighs. Place the underpad under the client's buttocks to protect the bed linen, and drape the client with the bath blanket.
- Insert the tube 5 to 7.5 cm (2 to 3 in.) in the child and only 2.5 to 3.75 cm (1 to 1.5 in.) in the infant.
- For children, lower the height of the solution container appropriately for the age of the child. See agency protocol.
- To assist a small child in retaining the solution, apply firm pressure over the anus with tissue wipes, or firmly press the buttocks together.

ELDERS

- Elders may fatigue easily.
- Elders may be more susceptible to fluid and electrolyte imbalances. Use tap water enemas with great caution.
- Monitor the client's tolerance during the procedure, watching for vagal episodes (e.g., slow pulse) and dysrhythmias.
- Protect older adults' skin from prolonged exposure to moisture.
- Assist older clients with perineal care as indicated.

HOME CARE CONSIDERATIONS   Administering an Enema

Teach the caregiver or client the following:

- To make saline solution, mix 1 teaspoon of table salt with 500 mL of tap water.

- Use enemas only as directed. Do not rely on them for regular bowel evacuation.
- Prior to administration, make sure a bedpan, commode, or toilet is nearby.

Digital Removal of a Fecal Impaction

Digital removal involves breaking up the fecal mass digitally and removing it in portions. Because the bowel mucosa can be injured during this procedure, some agencies restrict and specify the personnel permitted to conduct digital disimpactions. Rectal stimulation is also contraindicated for some people because it may cause an excessive vagal response resulting in cardiac arrhythmia. Before disimpaction it is suggested an oil retention enema be given and held for 30 minutes. After a disimpaction, the nurse can use various interventions to remove remaining feces, such as a cleansing enema or the insertion of a suppository.

Because manual removal of an impaction can be painful, the nurse may use, if the agency permits, 1 to 2 mL of lidocaine (Xylocaine) gel on a gloved finger inserted into the anal canal as far as the nurse can reach. The lidocaine will anesthetize the anal canal and rectum and should be inserted 5 minutes before the disimpaction.

For digital removal of a fecal impaction:

1. If indicated, obtain assistance from a second person who can comfort the client during the procedure.
2. Ask the client to assume a left side-lying position, with the knees flexed and the back toward the nurse.

3. Place a bedpad under the client's buttocks and a bedpan nearby to receive stool.
4. Drape the client for comfort and to avoid unnecessary exposure of the body.
5. Put on a pair of clean gloves and liberally lubricate the index finger to be inserted.
6. Gently insert the index finger into the rectum and move the finger along the length of the rectum.
7. Loosen and dislodge stool by gently massaging around it. Break up stool by working the finger into the hardened mass, taking care to avoid injury to the mucosa of the rectum.
8. Carefully work stool downward to the end of the rectum and remove it in small pieces. Continue to remove as much fecal material as possible. Periodically assess the client for signs of fatigue, such as facial pallor, diaphoresis, or change in pulse rate. Manual stimulation should be minimal.
9. Following disimpaction, assist the client to clean the anal area and buttocks. Then assist the client onto a bedpan or commode for a short time because digital stimulation of the rectum often induces the urge to defecate.

Bowel Training Programs

For clients who have chronic constipation, frequent impactions, or fecal incontinence, bowel training programs may be helpful.

The program is based on factors within the client's control and is designed to help the client establish normal defecation. Such matters as food and fluid intake, exercise, and defecation habits are all considered. Before beginning such a program, clients must understand it and want to be involved. The major phases of the program are as follows:

- Determine the client's usual bowel habits and factors that help and hinder normal defecation.
- Design a plan with the client that includes the following:
  a. Fluid intake of about 2,500 to 3,000 mL per day
  b. Increase in fiber in the diet
  c. Intake of hot drinks, especially just before the usual defecation time
  d. Increase in exercise
- Maintain the following daily routine for 2 to 3 weeks:
  a. Administer a cathartic suppository (e.g., Dulcolax) 30 minutes before the client's defecation time to stimulate peristalsis.
  b. When the client experiences the urge to defecate, assist the client to the toilet or commode or onto a bedpan. Note the length of time between the insertion of the suppository and the urge to defecate.
  c. Provide the client with privacy for defecation and a time limit; 30 to 40 minutes is usually sufficient.
  d. Teach the client to lean forward at the hips, to apply pressure on the abdomen with the hands, and to bear down for defecation. These measures increase pressure on the colon. Straining should be avoided because it can cause hemorrhoids.
- Provide positive feedback when the client successfully defecates. Refrain from negative feedback if the client fails to defecate.
- Offer encouragement to the client and convey that patience is often required. Many clients require weeks or months of training to achieve success.

Fecal Incontinence Pouch

To collect and contain large volumes of liquid feces, the nurse may place a fecal incontinence collector pouch around the anal area (Figure 49-13 ■). The purpose of the pouch is to prevent progressive perianal skin irritation and breakdown and frequent linen changes necessitated by incontinence. In many agencies, the pouch is replacing the traditional approach to this problem, that is, inserting a large Foley catheter into the client's rectum and inflating the balloon to keep it in place—a practice that may damage the rectal sphincter and rectal mucosa. A rectal catheter also increases peristalsis and incontinence by stimulating sensory nerve fibers in the rectum.

A fecal collector is secured around the anal opening and may or may not be attached to drainage. Pouches are best applied before the perianal skin becomes excoriated. If perianal skin excoriation is present, the nurse either (a) applies a dimethicone-based moisture-barrier cream or alcohol-free barrier film to the skin to protect it from feces until it heals and then applies the pouch, or (b) applies a skin barrier or hydrocolloid barrier underneath the pouch to achieve the best possible seal.

Figure 49-13 ■ A drainable fecal collector pouch.
(Permission to use this copyrighted image has been granted by the owner, Hollister Incorporated.)

Nursing responsibilities for clients with a rectal pouch include (a) regular assessment and documentation of the perianal skin status, (b) changing the bag every 72 hours or sooner if there is leakage, (c) maintaining the drainage system, and (d) providing explanations and support to the client and support people.

Some clients (e.g., post-trauma, quadriplegic, paraplegic, or post-stroke) may be treated for fecal incontinence with surgical repair of a damaged sphincter or an artificial bowel sphincter. The artificial sphincter consists of three parts: a cuff around the anal canal, a pressure-regulating balloon, and a pump that inflates the cuff (Figure 49-14 ■). The cuff is inflated to close the sphincter, maintaining continence. To have a bowel movement, the client deflates the cuff. The cuff automatically reinflates in 10 minutes. Management of this device is usually specific to the device; contact the manufacturing company for details.

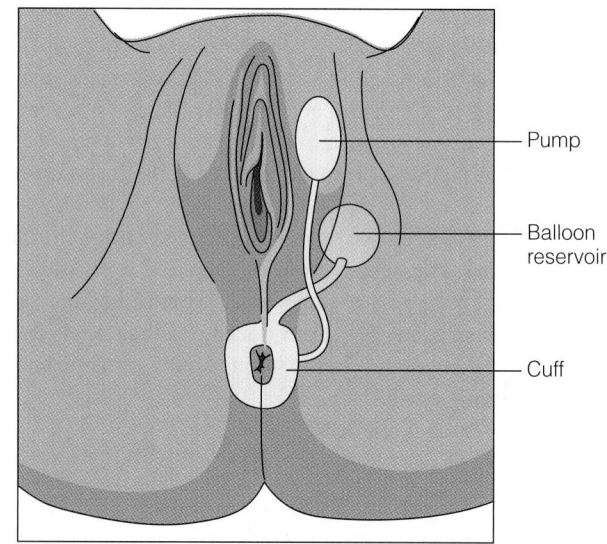

Figure 49-14 ■ Inflatable artificial sphincter.

Administering enemas and rectal medications may be harmful with this device in place. Ensure safety of these practices with the device instruction guide provided by the device manufacturer.

Ostomy Management

Clients with fecal diversions need considerable psychologic support, instruction, and physical care. This section is limited to the nurse's physical interventions of stoma assessment, application of an appliance to collect feces and protect skin, and promotion of self-care. Many agencies have access to a wound ostomy continence nurse (WOCN) to assist these clients. National organizations (e.g., United Ostomy Associations of America) have support groups whose mission is to improve the quality of life of people who have, or will have, an ostomy. Members of local chapters of such an organization have been known to meet and visit with a person who has a new ostomy. It is common for a client with a new ostomy to feel frightened and alone. Talking with another person who has gone through a similar experience may help the client realize that he or she is not alone and others are willing to listen and help.

STOMA AND SKIN CARE.   Care of the stoma and skin is important for all clients who have ostomies. The fecal material from a colostomy or ileostomy is irritating to the peristomal skin. This is particularly true of stool from an ileostomy, which contains digestive enzymes. It is important to assess the peristomal skin for irritation each time the appliance is changed. Any irritation or skin breakdown needs to be treated immediately. The skin is kept clean by washing off any excretion and drying thoroughly.

An ostomy appliance should protect the skin, collect stool, and control odor. The appliance consists of a skin barrier and a pouch. Some clients may prefer to also wear an adjustable ostomy belt which attaches to an ostomy pouch to hold the pouch firmly in place (Figure 49-15 ■). Appliances can be one piece where the skin barrier is already attached to the pouch (Figure 49-16, A ■), or an appliance can consist of two pieces: a separate pouch with a flange and a separate skin barrier with a flange where the pouch

A   **B**

Figure 49-16 ■ *A,* A one-piece ostomy appliance or pouching system, and *B,* a two-piece ostomy appliance or pouching system.
(Permission to use this copyrighted image has been granted by the owner, Hollister, Incorporated)

fastens to the barrier at the flange (Figure 49-16, *B* ■). The pouch can be removed without removing the skin barrier when using a two-piece appliance. Pouches can be closed or drainable (Figure 49-17 ■). A drainable pouch usually has a clip where the

A

B
Figure 49-17 ■ *A,* A closed pouch, and *B,* a drainable pouch.

Figure 49-15 ■ Adjustable ostomy belt.
(Permission to use this copyrighted image has been granted by the owner, Hollister, Incorporated)

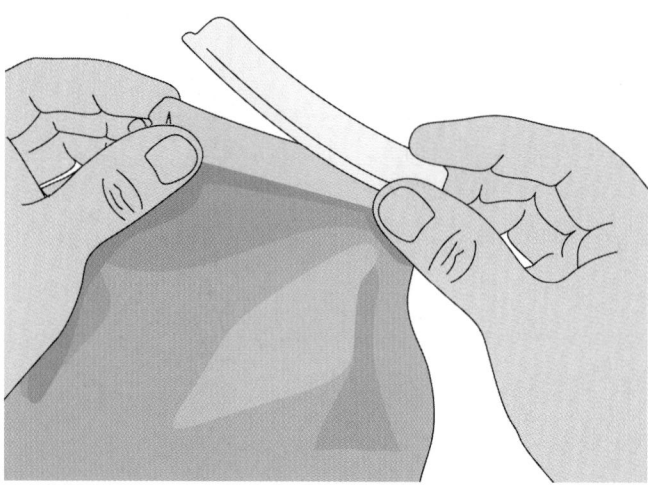

Figure 49-18 ■ Applying a pouch clamp.

end of the pouch is folded over the clamp and clipped (Figure 49-18 ■). Newer drainable pouches have an integrated closure system instead of a clamp. The client folds up the end of the pouch three times and presses firmly to seal the pouch. Drainable pouches are usually used by people who need to empty the pouch more than twice a day.

Closed pouches are often used by people who have a regular stoma discharge (e.g., sigmoid colostomy) and only have to empty the pouch 1 or 2 times a day. Some people find it easier to change a closed pouch than emptying a drainable pouch which requires some dexterity.

Odor control is essential to clients' self-esteem. As soon as clients are ambulatory, they can learn to work with the ostomy in the bathroom to avoid odors at the bedside. Selecting the appropriate kind of appliance promotes odor control. An intact appliance contains odors. Most pouches contain odor-barrier material. Some pouches also have a pouch filter which allows gas out of the pouch but not the odor.

Ostomy appliances can be applied for up to 7 days. Most clinicians agree that an ostomy appliance should be changed at least once a week (Hollister, n.d.). Some manufacturers recommend removing the pouch and skin barrier twice a week to clean and inspect the peristomal skin. They require changing whenever the stool leaks onto the peristomal skin. If the skin is erythematous, eroded, denuded, or ulcerated, the pouch should be changed every 24 to 48 hours to allow appropriate treatment of the skin. More frequent changes are recommended if the client complains of pain or discomfort.

The type of ostomy and amount of ouput influences how often the pouch is emptied. The pouch is emptied when it is one-third to one-half full. If the pouch overfills, it can cause separation of the skin barrier from the skin and stool comes in contact with the skin. This results in the entire appliance needing to be removed and a new one applied.

Skill 49-2 explains how to change a bowel diversion ostomy appliance.

SKILL 49-2

CHANGING A BOWEL DIVERSION OSTOMY APPLIANCE

PURPOSES
- To assess and care for the peristomal skin
- To collect stool for assessment of the amount and type of output
- To minimize odors for the client's comfort and self-esteem

ASSESSMENT
Determine the following:

- The type of ostomy and its placement on the abdomen. Surgeons often draw diagrams when there are two stomas. If there is more than one stoma, it is important to confirm which is the functioning stoma.
- The type and size of appliance currently used and the special barrier substance applied to the skin, according to the nursing care plan.

Assess the following:

- Stoma color: The stoma should appear red, similar in color to the mucosal lining of the inner cheek and slightly moist. Very pale or darker-colored stomas with a dusky bluish or purplish hue indicate impaired blood circulation to the area. Notify the surgeon immediately.
- Stoma size and shape: Most stomas protrude slightly from the abdomen. New stomas normally appear swollen, but swelling generally decreases over 2 or 3 weeks or for as long as 6 weeks. Failure of swelling to recede may indicate a problem, for example, blockage.
- Stomal bleeding: Slight bleeding initially when the stoma is touched is normal, but other bleeding should be reported.
- Status of peristomal skin: Any redness and irritation of the peristomal skin—the 5 to 13 cm (2 to 5 in.) of skin surrounding the stoma—should be noted. Transient redness after removal of adhesive is normal.
- Amount and type of feces: Assess the amount, color, odor, and consistency. Inspect for abnormalities, such as pus or blood.
- Complaints: Complaints of burning sensation under the skin barrier may indicate skin breakdown. The presence of abdominal discomfort and/or distention also needs to be determined.
- The client's and family members' learning needs regarding the ostomy and self-care.
- The client's emotional status, especially strategies used to cope with the body image changes and the ostomy.

CHANGING A BOWEL DIVERSION OSTOMY APPLIANCE *continued*

PLANNING

Review features of the appliance to ensure that all parts are present and function correctly.

> **Delegation**
> Care of a *new* ostomy is not delegated to UAP. However, aspects of ostomy function are observed during usual care and may be recorded by persons other than the nurse. Abnormal findings must be validated and interpreted by the nurse. In some agencies, UAP may remove and replace well-established ostomy appliances.

Equipment

- Clean gloves
- Bedpan
- Moisture-proof bag (for disposable pouches)
- Cleaning materials, including warm water, mild soap (optional), washcloth, towel
- Tissue or gauze pad
- Skin barrier (optional)
- Stoma measuring guide
- Pen or pencil and scissors
- New ostomy pouch with optional belt
- Tail closure clamp
- Deodorant for pouch (optional)

IMPLEMENTATION

Preparation

1. Determine the need for an appliance change.
   - Assess the used appliance for leakage of stool. **Rationale:** *Stool can irritate the peristomal skin.*
   - Ask the client about any discomfort at or around the stoma. **Rationale:** *A burning sensation may indicate breakdown beneath the faceplate of the pouch.*
   - Assess the fullness of the pouch. **Rationale:** *The weight of an overly full bag may loosen the skin barrier and separate it from the skin, causing the stool to leak and irritate the peristomal skin.*
2. If there is pouch leakage or discomfort at or around the stoma, change the appliance.
3. Select an appropriate time to change the appliance.
   - Avoid times close to meal or visiting hours. **Rationale:** *Ostomy odor and stool may reduce appetite or embarrass the client.*
   - Avoid times immediately after meals or the administration of any medications that may stimulate bowel evacuation. **Rationale:** *It is best to change the pouch when drainage is least likely to occur.*

Performance

1. Prior to performing the procedure, introduce self and verify the client's identity using agency protocol. Explain to the client what you are going to do, why it is necessary, and how he or she can cooperate. Discuss how the results will be used in planning further care or treatments. Changing an ostomy appliance should not cause discomfort, but it may be distasteful to the client. Communicate acceptance and support to the client. It is important to change the appliance competently and quickly. Include support persons as appropriate.
2. Perform hand hygiene, apply clean gloves, and observe appropriate infection control procedures.
3. Provide for client privacy preferably in the bathroom, where clients can learn to deal with the ostomy as they would at home.
4. Assist the client to a comfortable sitting or lying position in bed or preferably a sitting or standing position in the bathroom. **Rationale:** *Lying or standing positions may facilitate smoother pouch application, that is, avoid wrinkles.*

5. Unfasten the belt if the client is wearing one.
6. Empty the pouch and remove the ostomy skin barrier.
   - Empty the contents of a drainable pouch through the bottom opening into a bedpan or toilet. **Rationale:** *Emptying before removing the pouch prevents spillage of stool onto the client's skin.*
   - If the pouch uses a clamp, do not throw it away as it can be reused.
   - Assess the consistency, color, and amount of stool.
   - Peel the skin barrier off slowly, beginning at the top and working downward, while holding the client's skin taut. **Rationale:** *Holding the skin taut minimizes client discomfort and prevents abrasion of the skin.*
   - Discard the disposable pouch in a moisture-proof bag.
7. Clean and dry the peristomal skin and stoma.
   - Use toilet tissue to remove excess stool.
   - Use warm water, mild soap (optional), and a washcloth to clean the skin and stoma. ❶ Check agency practice on the use of soap. **Rationale:** *Soap is sometimes not advised because it can be irritating to the skin.*

      If soap is allowed, do not use deodorant or moisturizing soaps **Rationale:** *They may interfere with the adhesives in the skin barrier.*

❶ Cleaning the skin.

(Cory Patrick Hartley, San Ramon Regional Medical Center, San Ramon, CA. Reprinted with permission.)

continued on page 1348

CHANGING A BOWEL DIVERSION OSTOMY APPLIANCE *continued*

- Dry the area thoroughly by patting with a towel. **Rationale:** *Excess rubbing can abrade the skin.*
8. Assess the stoma and peristomal skin.
    - Inspect the stoma for color, size, shape, and bleeding.
    - Inspect the peristomal skin for any redness, ulceration, or irritation. Transient redness after the removal of adhesive is normal.
9. Place a piece of tissue or gauze over the stoma, and change it as needed. **Rationale:** *This absorbs any seepage from the stoma while the ostomy appliance is being changed.*
10. Prepare and apply the skin barrier (peristomal seal).
    - Use the guide ❷ to measure the size of the stoma.
    - On the backing of the skin barrier, trace a circle the same size as the stomal opening.
    - Cut out the traced stoma pattern to make an opening in the skin barrier. ❸ Make the opening no more than 1/8 to 1/4 inch larger than the stoma (Erwin-Toth, 2003). **Rationale:** *This allows space for the stoma to expand slightly when functioning and minimizes the risk of stool contacting peristomal skin.*
    - Remove the backing to expose the sticky adhesive side. The backing can be saved and used as a pattern when making an opening for future skin barriers.

    For a one-piece pouching system:
    - Center the one-piece skin barrier and pouch over the stoma, and gently press it onto the client's skin for 30 seconds. **Rationale:** *The heat and pressure help activate the adhesives in the skin barrier.* ❹, ❺

    For a two-piece pouching system:
    - Center the skin barrier over the stoma and gently press it onto the client's skin for 30 seconds.
    - Remove the tissue over the stoma before applying the pouch.
    - Snap the pouch onto the flange or skin barrier wafer.
    - For drainable pouches, close the pouch according to the manufacturer's directions.

❸ The nurse is making a stoma opening on a disposable one-piece pouch.

(Courtesy of Convatec, a Bristol-Meyers Squibb Company.)

❹ Centering the skin barrier over the stoma.

(Cory Patrick Hartley, San Ramon Regional Medical Center, San Ramon, CA. Reprinted with permission.)

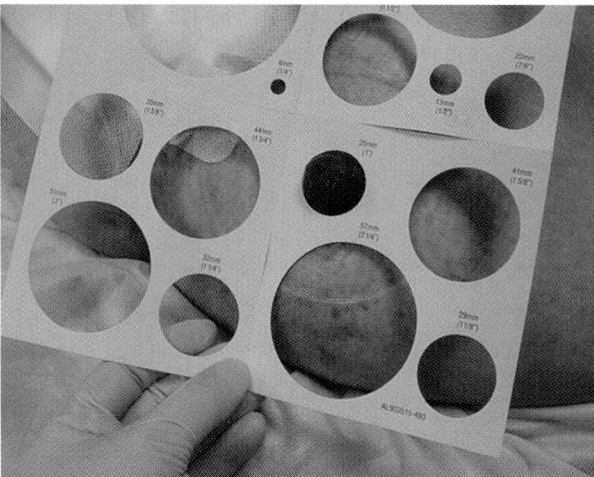

❷ A guide for measuring the stoma.

(Cory Patrick Hartley, San Ramon Regional Medical Center, San Ramon, CA. Reprinted with permission.)

❺ Pressing the skin barrier of a disposable one-piece pouch for 30 seconds to activate the adhesives in the skin barrier.

(Courtesy of Convatec, a Bristol-Meyers Squibb Company.)

CHANGING A BOWEL DIVERSION OSTOMY APPLIANCE *continued*

11. Document the procedure in the client record using forms or checklists supplemented by narrative notes when appropriate. Report and record pertinent assessments and interventions. Report any increase in stoma size, change in color indicative of circulatory impairment, and presence of skin irritation or erosion. Record on the client's chart discoloration of the stoma, the appearance of the peristomal skin, the amount and type of drainage, the client's reaction to the procedure, the client's experience with the ostomy, and skills learned by the client.

SAMPLE DOCUMENTATION

8/3/2007 0900 Colostomy bag changed. Moderate to large amount of semi-formed brown stool. Stoma reddish color. No redness or irritation around stoma. Client looked at stoma today and started asking questions as to how she will be able to change the pouch when she is home. Asked if she would like to do the next changing of the pouch. Stated "yes".

—— G. Hsu, RN

VARIATION: Emptying a Drainable Pouch

- Empty the pouch when it is 1/3 to 1/2 full of stool or gas. **Rationale:** *Emptying before it is overfull helps avoid breaking the seal with the skin and stool them coming in contact with the skin.*
- Hold the pouch outlet over a bedpan or toilet. Lift the lower edge up.
- Unclamp or unseal the pouch.
- Drain the pouch.
- Clean the inside of the tail of the pouch with a tissue or a pre-moistened towelette.
- Apply the clamp or seal the pouch.
- Dispose of used supplies.
- Remove clean gloves. Perform hand hygiene.
- Document the amount, consistency, and color of stool.

EVALUATION

- Relate findings to previous data if available. Adjust the teaching plan and nursing care plan as needed. Reinforce the teaching each time the care is performed. Encourage and support self-care as soon as possible as clients should be able to perform self-care by discharge. **Rationale:** *Client learning is facilitated by consistent nursing interventions.*
- Perform detailed follow-up based on findings that deviated from expected or normal for the client. Report significant deviations from normal to the primary care provider.

HOME CARE CONSIDERATIONS | **Changing an Ostomy Appliance**

- Provide the client with the names and phone numbers of a WOCN, supply vendor, and other resource people to contact when needed. Provide pertinent Internet resources for information and support.
- Inform the client of signs to report to a health care provider (e.g., peristomal redness, skin breakdown, and changes in stomal color).
- Provide client and family education regarding care of the ostomy and appliance when traveling.

- Educate the client and family regarding infection control precautions, including proper disposal of used pouches since these cannot be flushed down a toilet.
- Younger clients may have special concerns about odor and appearance. Provide information about ostomy care and community support groups. A visit from someone who has had an ostomy under similar circumstances may be helpful.

COLOSTOMY IRRIGATION. A colostomy irrigation, similar to an enema, is a form of stoma management used only for clients who have a sigmoid or descending colostomy. The purpose of irrigation is to distend the bowel sufficiently to stimulate peristalsis, which stimulates evacuation. When a regular evacuation pattern is achieved, the wearing of a colostomy pouch is unnecessary. Currently, colostomy irrigations are not routinely taught to most clients. Routine daily irrigations for control of the time of elimination ultimately become the client's decision. Some clients prefer to control the time of elimination through rigid dietary regulation and not be bothered with irrigations, which can take up to an hour to complete. When regulation by irrigation is chosen, it should be done at the same time each day. Control by irrigations also necessitates some control of the diet. For example, laxative foods that might cause an unexpected evacuation need to be avoided.

For most clients, a relatively small amount of fluid (300 to 500 mL) stimulates evacuation. For others, up to 1,000 mL may be needed because a colostomy has no sphincter and the fluid tends to return as it is instilled. This problem is reduced by the use of a cone on the irrigating catheter. The cone helps to hold the fluid within the bowel during the irrigation. Clients who have used irrigation for several years are more prone to peristomal hernias, bowel perforation, and electrolyte imbalance with large-volume irrigations (500 to 1,000 mL). Careful observation and assessment of this practice may be required in older, more fragile clients.

Evaluating

The goals established during the planning phase are evaluated according to specific desired outcomes, also established in that phase. Examples of these are shown in Identifying Nursing Diagnoses, Outcomes, and Interventions earlier in this chapter.

If outcomes are not achieved, the nurse should explore the reasons. The nurse might consider some or all of the following questions:

■ Were the client's fluid intake and diet appropriate?
■ Was the client's activity level appropriate?

■ Are prescribed medications or other factors affecting the gastrointestinal function?
■ Do the client and family understand the provided instructions well enough to comply with the required therapy?
■ Were sufficient physical and emotional support provided?

NURSING CARE PLAN Altered Bowel Elimination

ASSESSMENT DATA	NURSING DIAGNOSIS	DESIRED OUTCOMES
Nursing Assessment Mrs. Emma Brown is a 78-year-old widow of 9 months. She lives alone in a low-income housing complex for elders. Her two children live with their families in a city approximately 150 miles away. She has always enjoyed cooking for her family; however, now that she is alone, she does not cook for herself. As a result, she has developed irregular eating patterns and tends to prepare soup-and-toast meals. She gets little exercise and has had bouts of insomnia since her husband's death. For the past month, Mrs. Brown has been having a problem with constipation. She states she has a bowel movement about every 3 to 4 days and her stools are hard and painful to excrete. Mrs. Brown decides to attend the health fair sponsored by the housing complex and seeks assistance from the county public health nurse.	*Constipation* related to low-fiber diet and inactivity (as evidenced by infrequent, hard stools; painful defecation; abdominal distention)	Bowel Elimination [0501], as evidenced by ■ Comfort of stool passage ■ Stool soft and formed ■ Passage of stool without aids

Physical Examination

Diagnostic Data

Height: 162 cm (5'4")
Weight: 65 kg (143 lb)
Temperature: 36.2°C (97.2°F)
Pulse: 82 BPM
Respirations: 20/minute
Blood pressure: 128/74 mm Hg
Active bowel sounds, abdomen slightly distended

CBC: Hgb 10.8

Urinalysis negative

NURSING INTERVENTIONS*/SELECTED ACTIVITIES	RATIONALE
Constipation/Impaction Management [0450]	
Identify factors (e.g., medications, bed rest, diet) that may cause or contribute to constipation.	*Assessing causative factors is an essential first step in teaching and planning for improved bowel elimination.*
Encourage increased fluid intake, unless contraindicated.	*Sufficient fluid intake is necessary for the bowel to absorb sufficient amounts of liquid to promote proper stool consistency.*
Evaluate medication profile for gastrointestinal side effects.	*Constipation is a common side effect of many drugs including narcotics and antacids.*
Teach Mrs. Brown how to keep a food diary.	*An appraisal of food intake will help identify if Mrs. Brown is eating a well-balanced diet and consuming adequate amounts of fluid and fiber. Excessive meat or refined food intake will produce small, hard stools.*
Instruct Mrs. Brown on a high-fiber diet, as appropriate.	*Fiber absorbs water, which adds bulk and softness to the stool and speeds up passage through the intestines.*
Instruct her on the relationship of diet, exercise, and fluid intake to constipation and impaction.	*Fiber without adequate fluid can aggravate, not facilitate, bowel function.*

NURSING CARE PLAN **Altered Bowel Elimination** *continued*

NURSING INTERVENTIONS*/SELECTED ACTIVITIES	RATIONALE
Exercise Promotion [0200]	
Encourage verbalization of feelings about exercise or need for exercise.	*Perceptions of the need for exercise may be influenced by misconceptions, cultural and social beliefs, fears, or age.*
Determine her motivation to begin/continue an exercise program.	*Individuals who have been successful in an exercise program can assist Mrs. Brown by providing incentive and enhancing motivation. For example, a walking partner may be beneficial.*
Inform Mrs. Brown about the health benefits and physiologic effects of exercise.	*Activity influences bowel elimination by improving muscle tone and stimulating peristalsis.*
Instruct her about appropriate types of exercise for her level of health, in collaboration with a primary care provider.	*Any individual beginning an exercise program should consult a primary care provider primarily for a cardiac evaluation. Mrs. Brown's age and lack of activity should be considered in planning the level of activity.*
Assist Mrs. Brown to set short-term and long-term goals for the exercise program.	*Realistic goal setting provides direction and motivation.*

EVALUATION

Outcome not met. Mrs. Brown has kept a food diary and is able to identify the need for more fluid and fiber but has not consistently included fiber in her diet. She has started a walking program with a neighbor but is only able to walk for 10 minutes at a time twice a week. She states her last bowel movement was 3 days ago.

The NOC # for desired outcomes and the NIC # for nursing interventions are listed in brackets following the appropriate outcome or intervention. Outcomes, interventions, and activities selected are only a sample of those suggested by NOC and NIC and should be further individualized for each client.

APPLYING CRITICAL THINKING

1. You learn that Mrs. Brown's stools have been liquid, in very small amounts, and at infrequent intervals, generally occurring when she feels the urge to defecate. What additional data are important to obtain from her?
2. What nursing intervention is most appropriate before making suggestions to correct or prevent the problem she is experiencing?
3. What suggestions can you give her about maintaining a regular bowel pattern?
4. Explain why cathartics and laxatives are generally contraindicated for people in Mrs. Brown's situation.

See Critical Thinking Possibilities in Appendix A. ∞

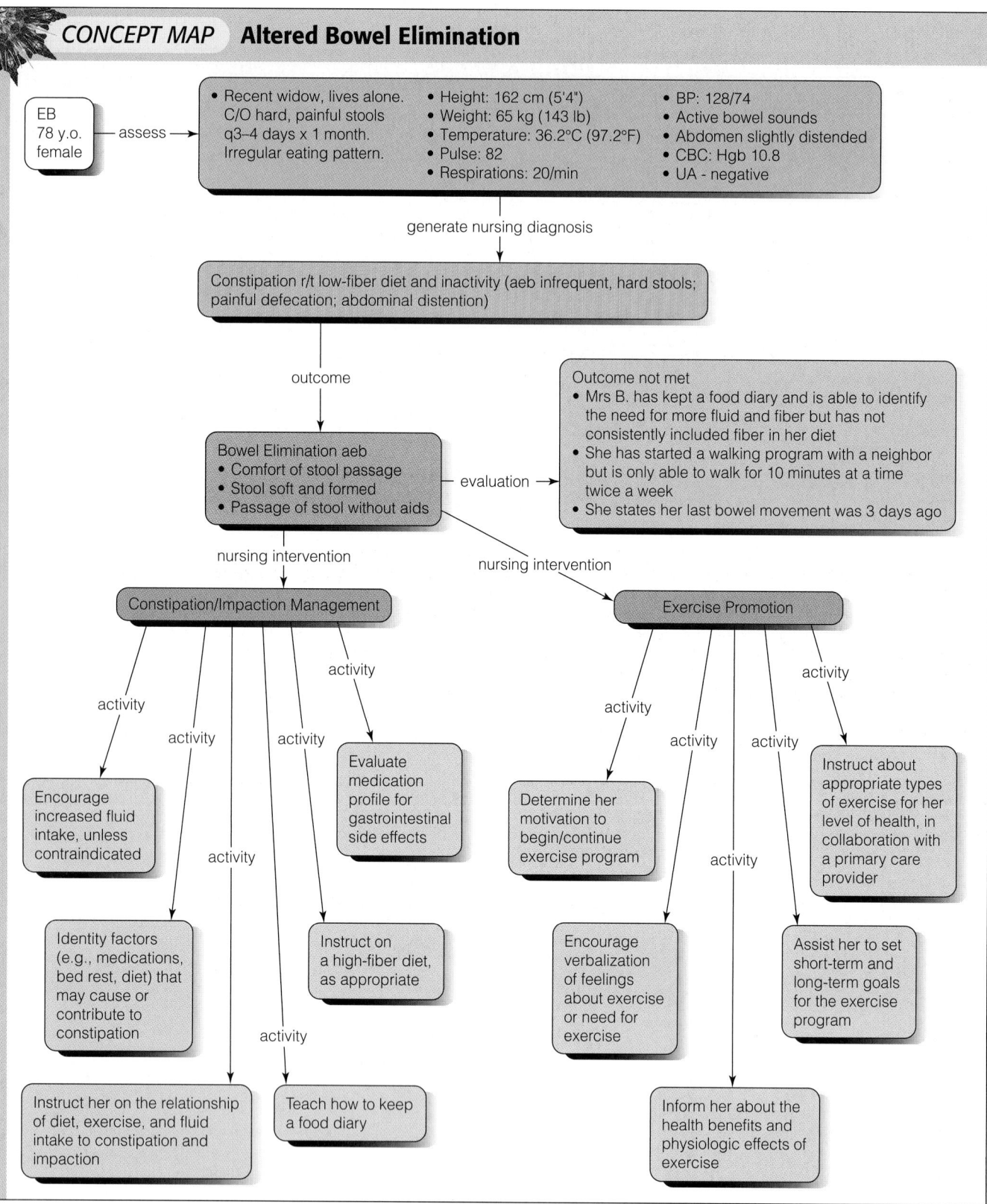

CONCEPT MAP **Altered Bowel Elimination**

EB
78 y.o.
female
—assess→

- Recent widow, lives alone. C/O hard, painful stools q3–4 days x 1 month. Irregular eating pattern.
- Height: 162 cm (5'4")
- Weight: 65 kg (143 lb)
- Temperature: 36.2°C (97.2°F)
- Pulse: 82
- Respirations: 20/min
- BP: 128/74
- Active bowel sounds
- Abdomen slightly distended
- CBC: Hgb 10.8
- UA - negative

↓ generate nursing diagnosis

Constipation r/t low-fiber diet and inactivity (aeb infrequent, hard stools; painful defecation; abdominal distention)

↓ outcome

Bowel Elimination aeb
- Comfort of stool passage
- Stool soft and formed
- Passage of stool without aids

—evaluation→

Outcome not met
- Mrs B. has kept a food diary and is able to identify the need for more fluid and fiber but has not consistently included fiber in her diet
- She has started a walking program with a neighbor but is only able to walk for 10 minutes at a time twice a week
- She states her last bowel movement was 3 days ago

↓ nursing intervention

Constipation/Impaction Management

↓ nursing intervention

Exercise Promotion

activity → Encourage increased fluid intake, unless contraindicated

activity → Identity factors (e.g., medications, bed rest, diet) that may cause or contribute to constipation

activity → Instruct her on the relationship of diet, exercise, and fluid intake to constipation and impaction

activity → Teach how to keep a food diary

activity → Instruct on a high-fiber diet, as appropriate

activity → Evaluate medication profile for gastrointestinal side effects

activity → Determine her motivation to begin/continue exercise program

activity → Encourage verbalization of feelings about exercise or need for exercise

activity → Inform her about the health benefits and physiologic effects of exercise

activity → Assist her to set short-term and long-term goals for the exercise program

activity → Instruct about appropriate types of exercise for her level of health, in collaboration with a primary care provider

CHAPTER 49 **REVIEW**

CHAPTER HIGHLIGHTS

- Primary functions of the large intestine are the excretion of digestive waste products and the maintenance of fluid balance.
- Patterns of fecal elimination vary greatly among people, but a regular pattern of fecal elimination with formed, soft stools is essential to health and a sense of well-being.
- A variety of factors affects defecation: developmental level, diet, fluid intake, activity and exercise, psychologic factors, regular defecation, medications, diagnostic procedures, anesthesia, and pathologic conditions.
- Normal defecation is often facilitated in both well and ill clients by providing privacy, teaching clients to attend to defecation urges promptly, assisting clients to normal sitting positions whenever possible, encouraging appropriate food and fluid intake, and scheduling regular exercise.
- Common fecal elimination problems include constipation, diarrhea, bowel incontinence, and flatulence. Each has specific defining characteristics and contributing causes that often relate to or are identical to the factors that affect defecation.
- Lack of exercise, irregular defecation habits, bland diets, and overuse of laxatives are all thought to contribute to constipation. Sufficient fluid and fiber intake are required to keep feces soft.
- An adverse effect of constipation is straining during defecation, during which the Valsalva maneuver may be used. Cardiac problems may ensue.
- An adverse effect of prolonged diarrhea is fluid and electrolyte imbalance.
- Assessment relative to fecal elimination includes a nursing history; physical examination of the abdomen, rectum, and anus; and in some situations, visualization studies and inspection and analysis of stool for abnormal constituents such as blood.
- A nursing history includes data about the client's defecating pattern, description of feces and any changes, problems associated with

elimination, and data about possible factors altering bowel elimination.

- When inspecting the client's stool, the nurse must observe its color, consistency, shape, amount, odor, and the presence of abnormal constituents.
- A function of the nurse is to assist clients with diet and bowel preparation before endoscopic and radiographic studies of the large intestine.
- NANDA-approved nursing diagnoses that relate specifically to altered bowel elimination include *Risk for Constipation, Constipation, Perceived Constipation, Diarrhea,* and *Bowel Incontinence.* However, because altered elimination patterns affect several areas of human functioning, diagnoses such as *Risk for Deficient Fluid Volume, Low Self-Esteem,* and *Risk for Impaired Skin Integrity* may also apply.
- Nursing strategies include administering cathartics and antidiarrheals; administering cleansing, carminative, or retention enemas; applying protective skin agents; monitoring fluid and electrolyte balance; and instructing clients in ways to promote normal defecation.
- Digital removal of an impaction should be carried out gently because of vagal nerve stimulation and subsequent depressed cardiac rate. A primary care provider's order is often necessary.
- The purpose of an enema is to increase peristalsis and the excretion of feces and flatus. Enemas are classified into four groups: cleansing, carminative, retention, and return-flow enemas.
- Clients who have bowel diversion ostomies require special care, with attention to psychologic adjustment, diet, and stoma and skin care. A variety of stoma management methods is available to these clients, depending on the type and position of the ostomy.

TEST YOUR KNOWLEDGE

1. Clients should be taught that repeatedly ignoring the sensation of needing to defecate could result in
   1. Constipation.
   2. Diarrhea.
   3. Incontinence.
   4. Hemorrhoids.

2. Which of the following statements provide evidence that an older adult who is prone to constipation is in need of further teaching?
   1. "I need to drink one and a half to two quarts of liquids each day."
   2. "I need to take a laxative such as milk of magnesia if I don't have a BM every day."
   3. "If my bowel pattern changes on its own, I should call you."
   4. "Eating my meals at regular times is likely to result in regular bowel movements."

3. Because a client is scheduled for a colonoscopy, the nurse will instruct the client to perform which of the following?
   1. Oil retention enema
   2. Return flow enema
   3. High, large volume enema
   4. Low, small volume enema

4. The nurse is most likely to report which of the following findings to the primary care provider for a client who has an established colostomy?
   1. The stoma extends 1/2 in. above the abdomen.
   2. The skin under the appliance looks red briefly after removing the appliance.
   3. The stoma color is a deep red-purple.
   4. An ascending colostomy delivers liquid feces.

5. The most appropriate goal for clients with diarrhea related to ingestion of an antibiotic for an upper respiratory infection is which of the following?
   1. The client will wear a medic-alert bracelet for antibiotic allergy.
   2. The client will return to his or her previous fecal elimination pattern.
   3. The client verbalizes the need to take an antidiarrheal medication prn.
   4. The client will increase intake of insoluble fiber such as grains, rice, and cereals.

6. A client with a new stoma who has not had a bowel movement since surgery last week reports feeling nauseous. What is the appropriate nursing action?
  1. Prepare to irrigate the colostomy.
  2. After assessing the stoma and surrounding skin, notify the surgeon.
  3. Assess bowel sounds and administer antiemetic.
  4. Administer a bulk-forming laxative, and encourage increased fluids and exercise.

7. The nurse assesses a client's abdomen several days after abdominal surgery. It is firm, distended, and painful to palpate. The client reports feeling "bloated." The nurse consults with the surgeon, who orders an enema. The nurse prepares to give what kind of enema?
  1. Soapsuds enema
  2. Retention enema
  3. Return flow enema
  4. Oil retention enema

8. Which of the following is most likely to validate that a client is experiencing intestinal bleeding?
  1. Large quantities of fat mixed with pale yellow liquid stool
  2. Brown, formed stools
  3. Semisoft tar-colored stools
  4. Narrow, pencil-shaped stool

9. Which of the following nursing diagnoses is most applicable to a client with fecal incontinence? Choose all that apply.
  1. *Bowel Incontinence*
  2. *Risk for Deficient Fluid Volume*
  3. *Disturbed Body Image*
  4. *Social Isolation*
  5. *Risk for Impaired Skin Integrity*

10. A student nurse (SN) is assigned to care for a client with a sigmoidostomy. The student will assess which of the following ostomy sites?

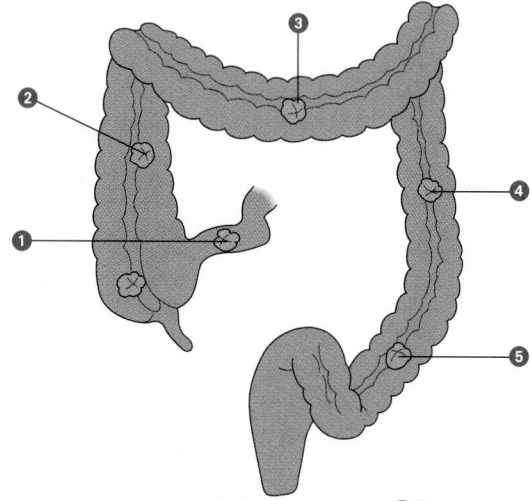

See Answers to Test Your Knowledge in Appendix A. ∞

EXPLORE MEDIALINK www.prenhall.com/berman

DVD-ROM
- Audio Glossary
- NCLEX Review
- Skills Checklists
- Animations:
    Performing an Enema
    A & P Review
        Digestive System
        Intestinal Wall

COMPANION WEBSITE
- Additional NCLEX Review
- Case Study: Client After Abdominal Surgery
- Care Plan Activity: Client Who Had a Stroke
- Application Activity:
    The United Ostomy Association
    Wound Ostomy Nurse
- Links to Resources

READINGS AND REFERENCES

Erwin-Toth, P. (2003). Ostomy pearls: A concise guide to stoma siting, pouching systems, patient education and more. *Advances in Skin & Wound Care, 16*(3), 146–152.
The author, a certified wound ostomy and continence nurse, provides clear, relevant information about stoma siting, appliance fitting, choosing a pouching system, and changing the pouch. In addition, the photos showing the ideal stoma and possible stoma complications are very helpful.

Youssef, N. N., Sanders, L., & Di Lorenzo, C. (2004). Adolescent constipation: Evaluation and management. *Adolescent Medicine Clinics, 15*(1), 37–52.
This physician-written article provides a comprehensive review of constipation (e.g., causes, tests, management) with a focus on adolescents. As the authors state, a long history of constipation is challenging to uncover in adolescents who often protect their privacy and are uncomfortable discussing their bowel habits.

RELATED RESEARCH
Dahl, W. J., Whiting, S. J., Healey, A., Zello, G. A., & Hildebrandt, S. L. (2003). Increased stool frequency occurs when finely processed pea hull fiber is added to usual foods consumed by elderly residents in long-term care. *Journal of the American Dietetic Association, 103*(9), 1199–1202.

Kinservik, M. A., & Friedhoff, M. M. (2004). The efficacy and safety of polyethylene glycol 3350 in the treatment of constipation in children. *Pediatric Nursing, 30*(3), 232–237.

Schonwald, A., Sherritt, L., Stadtler, A., & Bridgemohan, C. (2004). Factors associated with difficult toilet training. *Pediatrics, 113*(6), 1753–1757.

REFERENCES
American Cancer Society (ACS). (2006). *How is colorectal cancer diagnosed?* Retrieved June 27, 2006, from http://www.cancer.org/docroot/CRI/content/CRI_2_4_3X_How_is_colon_and_rectum_cancer_diagnosed.asp?site area=

Bliss, D. Z., Fischer, L., & Savik, K. (2005). Managing fecal incontinence: Self-care practices of older adults. *Journal of Gerontological Nursing, 31*(7), 35–44.

Dochterman, J. M., & Bulechek, G. M. (Eds.). (2004). *Nursing interventions classification (NIC)* (4th ed.). St. Louis, MO: Mosby.

Hinrichs, M., & Huseboe, J. (2001). Research-based protocol: Management of constipation. *Journal of Gerontological Nursing, 27*(2), 17–28.

Hollister, Inc. (n.d.). *Ostomy care FAQs.* Retrieved June 26, 2006, from http://www.hollister.com/us/resource/faqs.asp?id=1

Lemone, P., & Burke, K. (2004). *Medical-surgical nursing* (3rd ed.). Upper Saddle River, NJ: Pearson Prentice Hall.

Madsen, D., Sebolt, T., Cullen, L., Folkedahl, B., Mueller, T., Richardson, C., & Titler, M. (2005). Listening to bowel sounds: An evidence-based practice project. *American Journal of Nursing, 105*(12), 40–49.

Mauk, K. L. (2005). Preventing constipation in older adults. *Nursing, 35*(6), 22–23.

Moorhead, S., Johnson, M., & Maas, M. (Eds.). (2004). *Nursing outcomes classification (NOC)* (3rd ed.). St. Louis, MO: Mosby.

NANDA International. (2007). *NANDA nursing diagnoses: Definitions and Classification 2007–2008.* Philadelphia: Author.

SELECTED BIBLIOGRAPHY

Banks, N., & Razor, B. (2003). Preoperative stoma site assessment and marking: Trained RNs can improve ostomy outcomes. *American Journal of Nursing, 103*(3), 64A–64D.

Hsieh, C. (2005). Treatment of constipation in older adults. *American Family Physician, 72*(11), 2277–2284.

Peate, I. (2003). Nursing role in the management of constipation: Use of laxatives. *British Journal of Nursing, 12*(19), 1130–1136.

Ringhofer, J. (2005). Meeting the needs of your ostomy patient. *RN, 68*(8), 37–41.

Rushing, J. (2003). Administering an enema to an adult. *Nursing, 33*(11), 28.

Pullen, R. L. (2006). Teaching your patient to irrigate a colostomy. *Nursing, 36*(4), 22.

CHAPTER 50

Oxygenation

LEARNING OUTCOMES

After completing this chapter, you will be able to:

1. Outline the structure and function of the respiratory system.

2. Describe the processes of breathing (ventilation) and gas exchange (respiration).

3. Explain the role and function of the respiratory system in transporting oxygen and carbon dioxide to and from body tissues.

4. Identify factors influencing respiratory function.

5. Identify common manifestations of impaired respiratory function.

6. Describe nursing measures to promote respiratory function and oxygenation.

7. Explain the use of therapeutic measures such as medications, inhalation therapy, oxygen therapy, artificial airways, airway suctioning, and chest tubes to promote respiratory function.

8. State outcome criteria for evaluating client responses to measures that promote adequate oxygenation.

KEY TERMS

adventitious breath sounds, *1364*	hemothorax, *1393*	oxyhemoglobin, *1361*
apnea, *1363*	humidifiers, *1369*	partial pressure, *1360*
atelectasis, *1360*	hypercapnia, *1363*	pneumothorax, *1393*
Biot's (cluster) respirations, *1364*	hypercarbia, *1363*	postural drainage, *1372*
bradypnea, *1363*	hyperinflation, *1385*	respiratory membrane, *1358*
Cheyne-Stokes respirations, *1364*	hyperoxygenation, *1385*	sputum, *1364*
cyanosis, *1363*	hypoxemia, *1363*	stridor, *1364*
diffusion, *1360*	hypoxia, *1363*	suctioning, *1382*
dyspnea, *1364*	incentive spirometers, *1370*	surfactant, *1360*
emphysema, *1361*	intrapleural pressure, *1360*	tachypnea, *1363*
erythrocytes, *1361*	intrapulmonary pressure, *1360*	tidal volume, *1360*
eupnea, *1363*	Kussmaul's breathing, *1363*	torr, *1361*
expectorate, *1368*	lung compliance, *1360*	vibration, *1372*
hematocrit, *1361*	lung recoil, *1360*	
hemoglobin, *1361*	orthopnea, *1364*	

Oxygen, a clear, odorless gas that constitutes approximately 21% of the air we breathe, is necessary for proper functioning of all living cells. The absence of oxygen can lead to cellular, tissue, and organism death. Although the delivery of oxygen to body tissues is affected at least indirectly by other body systems, the respiratory system is most directly involved in this process. Impaired function of the system can significantly affect our ability to breathe, transport gases, and participate in everyday activities.

Respiration is the process of gas exchange between the individual and the environment. The process of respiration involves three components:

1. Pulmonary ventilation or breathing; the movement of air between the atmosphere and the alveoli of the lungs as we inhale and exhale
2. Gas exchange, which involves diffusion of oxygen and carbon dioxide between the alveoli and pulmonary capillaries
3. Transport of oxygen from the lungs to the tissues, and carbon dioxide from the tissues to the lungs

STRUCTURE AND FUNCTION OF THE RESPIRATORY SYSTEM

The function of the respiratory system is gas exchange. Oxygen from inspired air diffuses from alveoli in the lungs into the blood in pulmonary capillaries. Carbon dioxide produced during cell metabolism diffuses from the blood into the alveoli and is exhaled. The organs of the respiratory system facilitate this gas exchange and protect the body from foreign matter such as particulates and pathogens.

Structure of the Respiratory System

The respiratory system (Figure 50-1 ■) is divided structurally into the upper respiratory system and the lower respiratory system. The mouth, nose, pharynx, and larynx compose the upper respiratory system. The lower respiratory system includes the trachea and lungs, with the bronchi, bronchioles, alveoli, pulmonary capillary network, and pleural membranes.

Air enters through the nose, where it is warmed, humidified, and filtered. Large particles in the air are trapped by the hairs at the entrance of the nares, and smaller particles are filtered and trapped as air changes direction on contact with the nasal turbinates and septum. The sneeze reflex is initiated by irritants in nasal passages. A large volume of air rapidly exits through the nose and mouth during a sneeze, helping to clear nasal passages.

Inspired air passes from the nose through the pharynx. The pharynx is a shared pathway for air and food. It includes both the nasopharynx and the oropharynx, which are richly supplied with lymphoid tissue that traps and destroys pathogens entering with the air.

The larynx is a cartilaginous structure that can be identified externally as the Adam's apple. In addition to its role in providing for speech, the larynx is important for maintaining airway patency and protecting the lower airways from swallowed food and fluids. During swallowing, the inlet to the larynx (the epiglottis) closes, routing food to the esophagus. The epiglottis is open during breathing, allowing air to move freely into the lower airways. Below the larynx, the trachea leads to the right and left main bronchi (primary bronchi) and the other conducting airways of the lungs. Within the lungs, the primary bronchi divide repeatedly into smaller and smaller bronchi, ending with the terminal bronchioles. Together these airways are known as the bronchial tree. The trachea and bronchi are lined with mucosal epithelium. These cells produce a thin layer of mucus, the "mucous blanket," that traps pathogens and microscopic particulate matter. These foreign particles are then swept upward toward the larynx and throat by cilia, tiny hairlike projections on the epithelial cells. The cough reflex is triggered by irritants in the larynx, trachea, or bronchi and is described in Box 50–1.

Until air passes through the terminal bronchioles and enters the respiratory bronchioles and alveoli, no gas exchange occurs.

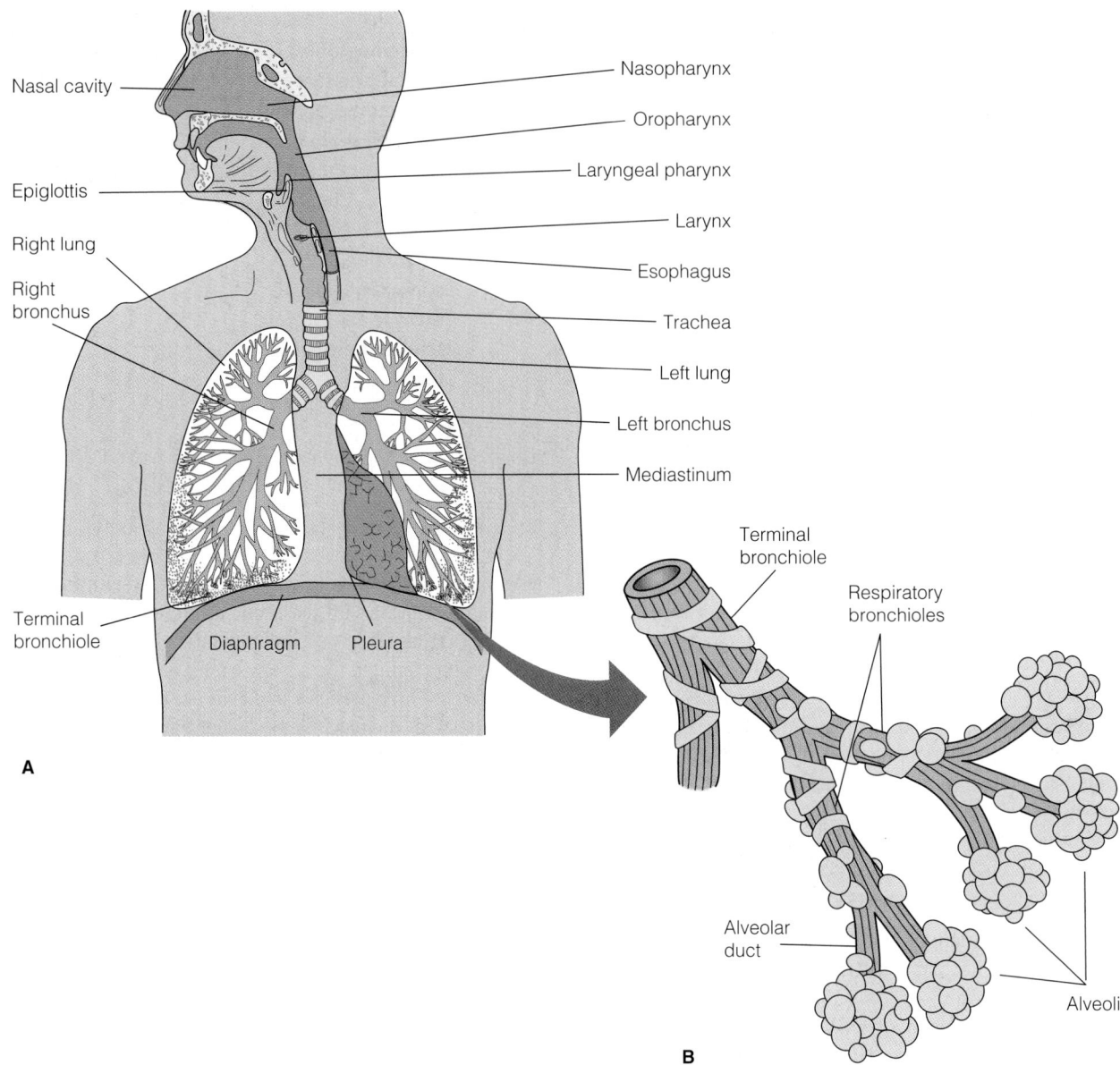

Figure 50-1 ■ *A,* Organs of the respiratory tract. *B,* Respiratory bronchioles, alveolar ducts, and alveoli.

The respiratory zone of the lungs includes the respiratory bronchioles (which have scattered air sacs in their walls), the alveolar ducts, and the alveoli (Figure 50-1). Alveoli have very thin walls, composed of a single layer of epithelial cells covered by a thick

BOX 50–1   **The Cough Reflex**

- Nerve impulses are sent through the vagus nerve to the medulla.
- A large inspiration of approximately 2.5 L occurs.
- The epiglottis and glottis (vocal cords) close.
- A strong contraction of abdominal and internal intercostal muscles dramatically raises the pressure in the lungs.
- The epiglottis and glottis open suddenly.
- Air rushes outward with great velocity.
- Mucus and any foreign particles are dislodged from the lower respiratory tract and are propelled up and out.

mesh of pulmonary capillaries. The alveolar and capillary walls form the **respiratory membrane** (also known as the alveolar/capillary membrane), where gas exchange occurs between the air on the alveolar side and the blood on the capillary side. The airways move air to and from the alveoli; the right ventricle and pulmonary vascular system transport blood to the capillary side of the membrane (Figure 50-2 ■).

The outer surface of the lungs is covered by a thin, double layer of tissue known as the pleura. The parietal pleura lines the thorax and surface of the diaphragm. It doubles back to form the visceral pleura, covering the external surface of the lungs. Between these pleural layers is a potential space that contains a small amount of pleural fluid, a serous lubricating solution. This fluid prevents friction during the movements of breathing and serves to keep the layers adherent through its surface tension.

ANATOMY & PHYSIOLOGY REVIEW   **The Respiratory System**

The larynx, trachea, bronchi, and lungs with an expanded view showing the structures of an alveolus and the pulmonary blood vessels.

From Rice, Jane, *Medical Terminology with Human Anatomy,* 5th ed., © 2005. Reproduced by permission of Pearson Education, Inc., Upper Saddle River, New Jersey.

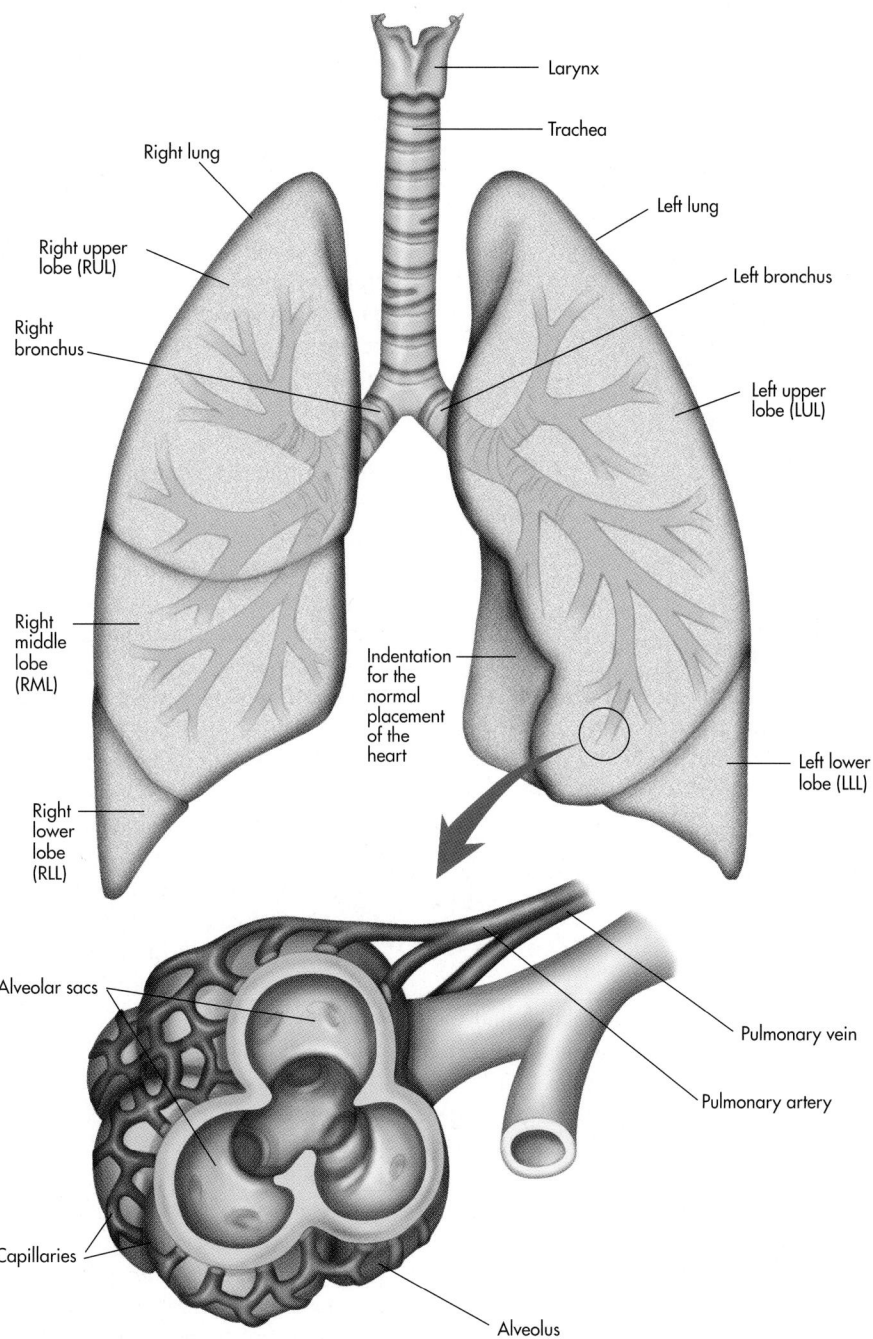

Larynx

Trachea

Right lung

Left lung

Right upper lobe (RUL)

Left bronchus

Right bronchus

Left upper lobe (LUL)

Right middle lobe (RML)

Indentation for the normal placement of the heart

Left lower lobe (LLL)

Right lower lobe (RLL)

Alveolar sacs

Pulmonary vein

Pulmonary artery

Capillaries

Alveolus

QUESTIONS

1. Pneumonia occurs when microorganisms get into the lower respiratory tract and overwhelm the body's defenses. Name at least two normal defense mechanisms present in the *upper* airway that help prevent microorganisms getting into the lower respiratory tract.
2. Microorganisms can travel past the upper respiratory tract defense mechanisms. What defense mechanisms are present in the *lower* respiratory tract that may help the client?
3. The microorganisms have quickly multiplied and overpowered the client's defense mechanisms. The client has pneumonia and the alveoli are filled with infectious fluid. How will this affect gas exchange at the respiratory or alveolar/capillary membrane?

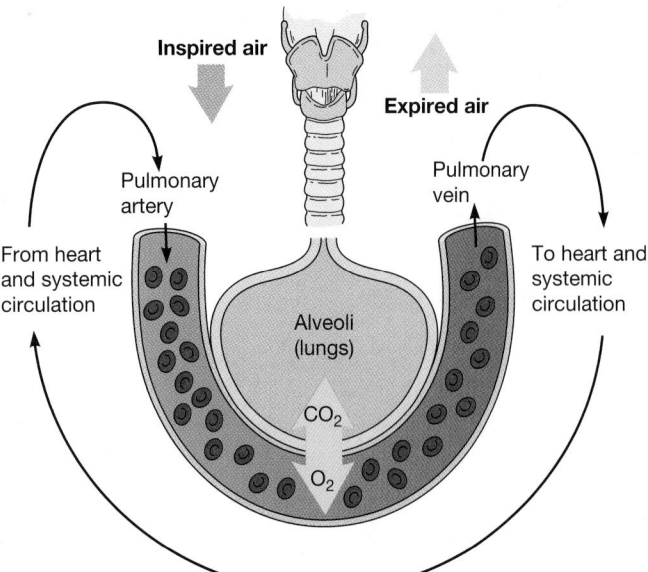

Figure 50-2 ■ Gas exchange occurs between the air on the alveolar side and the blood on the capillary side.

Pulmonary Ventilation

Ventilation of the lungs is accomplished through the act of breathing: inspiration (inhalation) when air flows into the lungs and expiration (exhalation) as air moves out of the lungs. Adequate ventilation depends on several factors:

- Clear airways
- An intact central nervous system and respiratory center
- An intact thoracic cavity capable of expanding and contracting
- Adequate pulmonary compliance and recoil

A number of mechanisms including ciliary action and the cough reflex work to keep airways open and clear. In some cases, however, these defenses may be overwhelmed. The inflammation, edema, and excess mucous production that occur with some types of pneumonia may clog small airways, impairing ventilation of distal alveoli.

The respiratory centers of the medulla and pons in the brain stem control breathing. Severe head injury or drugs that depress the central nervous system (e.g., opiates or barbiturates) can affect the respiratory centers, impairing the drive to breathe.

Expansion and recoil of the lungs occurs passively in response to changes in pressures within the thoracic cavity and the lungs themselves. The **intrapleural pressure** (pressure in the pleural cavity surrounding the lungs) is always slightly negative in relation to atmospheric pressure. This negative pressure is essential because it creates the suction that holds the visceral pleura and the parietal pleura together as the chest cage expands and contracts. The recoil tendency of the lungs is a major factor in creating this negative pressure. The intrapleural fluid also contributes by causing the pleura to adhere together, much as a film of water can cause two glass slides to adhere together.

The **intrapulmonary pressure** (pressure within the lungs) always equalizes with atmospheric pressure. Inspiration occurs when the diaphragm and intercostal muscles contract, increasing the size of the thoracic cavity. The volume of the lungs increases, decreasing intrapulmonary pressure. Air then rushes into the lungs to equalize this pressure with atmospheric pressure. Conversely, when the diaphragm and intercostal muscles relax, the volume of the lungs decreases, intrapulmonary pressure rises, and air is expelled.

The degree of chest expansion during normal breathing is minimal, requiring little energy expenditure. In adults, approximately 500 mL of air is inspired and expired with each breath. This is known as **tidal volume.** Breathing during strenuous exercise or some types of heart disease require greater chest expansion and effort. At this time, more than 1,500 mL of air may be moved with each breath. Accessory muscles of respiration, including the anterior neck muscles, intercostal muscles, and muscles of the abdomen, are employed. Active use of these muscles and noticeable effort in breathing are seen in clients with obstructive pulmonary disease.

Diseases such as muscular dystrophy, or trauma such as spinal cord injury can affect the muscles of respiration, impairing the ability of the thoracic cavity to expand and contract. A gunshot wound or other trauma to the chest wall may allow intrapleural pressure to equalize with the atmosphere, causing the lung to collapse.

Lung compliance, the expansibility or stretchability of lung tissue, plays a significant role in the ease of ventilation. At birth, the fluid-filled lungs are stiff and resistant to expansion, much as a new balloon is difficult to inflate. With each subsequent breath, the alveoli become more compliant and easier to inflate, just as a balloon becomes easier to inflate after several tries. Lung compliance tends to decrease with aging, making it more difficult to expand alveoli and increasing risk of **atelectasis,** or collapse of a portion of the lung.

In contrast to lung compliance is **lung recoil,** the continual tendency of the lungs to collapse away from the chest wall. Just as lung compliance is necessary for normal inspiration, lung recoil is necessary for normal expiration. Although elastic fibers in lung tissue contribute to lung recoil, the surface tension of fluid lining the alveoli has the greatest effect on recoil. Fluid molecules tend to draw together, reducing the size of alveoli. **Surfactant,** a lipoprotein produced by specialized alveolar cells, acts like a detergent, reducing the surface tension of alveolar fluid. Without surfactant, lung expansion is exceedingly difficult and the lungs collapse. Premature infants whose lungs are not yet capable of producing adequate surfactant develop respiratory distress syndrome.

Alveolar Gas Exchange

After the alveoli are ventilated, the second phase of the respiratory process—the diffusion of oxygen from the alveoli and into the pulmonary blood vessels—begins. **Diffusion** is the movement of gases or other particles from an area of greater pressure or concentration to an area of lower pressure or concentration.

Pressure differences in the gases on each side of the respiratory membrane obviously affect diffusion. When the pressure of oxygen is greater in the alveoli than in the blood, oxygen diffuses into the blood. The **partial pressure** (the pressure exerted by each individual gas in a mixture according to its concentration in the mixture) of oxygen (PO_2) in the alveoli is about 100 mm Hg (sometimes referred to as **torr,** which is the same as millimeters of mercury), whereas the PO_2 in the venous blood of the pulmonary arteries is about 60 mm Hg. These pressures rapidly equalize, however, so that the arterial oxygen pressure also reaches about 100 mm Hg. By contrast, carbon dioxide in the venous blood entering the pulmonary capillaries has a partial pressure of about 45 mm Hg (PCO_2), whereas that in the alveoli has a partial pressure of about 40 mm Hg. Therefore, carbon dioxide diffuses from the blood into the alveoli, where it can be eliminated with expired air. When referring to the pressure of oxygen in the arterial blood the abbreviation is PaO_2. When referring to partial pressure in venous blood there is no "a," that is, PO_2.

Transport of Oxygen and Carbon Dioxide

The third part of the respiratory process involves the transport of respiratory gases. Oxygen needs to be transported from the lungs to the tissues, and carbon dioxide must be transported from the tissues back to the lungs. Normally most of the oxygen (97%) combines loosely with **hemoglobin** (oxygen-carrying red pigment) in the red blood cells and is carried to the tissues as **oxyhemoglobin** (the compound of oxygen and hemoglobin). The remaining oxygen is dissolved and transported in the fluid of the plasma and cells.

Several factors affect the rate of oxygen transport from the lungs to the tissues:

1. Cardiac output
2. Number of erythrocytes and blood hematocrit
3. Exercise

Any pathologic condition that decreases cardiac output (e.g., damage to the heart muscle, blood loss, or pooling of blood in the peripheral blood vessels) diminishes the amount of oxygen delivered to the tissues. The heart compensates for inadequate output by increasing its pumping rate or heart rate; however, with severe damage or blood loss, this compensatory mechanism may not restore adequate blood flow and oxygen to the tissues.

The second factor influencing oxygen transport is the number of **erythrocytes** (red blood cells, or RBCs) and the hematocrit. The **hematocrit** is the percentage of the blood that is erythrocytes. In men, the number of circulating erythrocytes normally averages about 5 million per cubic milliliter of blood, and in women, about 4.5 million per cubic milliliter. Normally the hematocrit is about 40% to 54% in men and 37% to 50% in women. Excessive increases in the blood hematocrit raise the blood viscosity, reducing the cardiac output and therefore reducing oxygen transport. Excessive reductions in the blood hematocrit, such as occur in anemia, reduce oxygen transport.

Exercise also has a direct influence on oxygen transport. In well-trained athletes, oxygen transport can be increased up to 20 times the normal rate, due in part to an increased cardiac output and to increased use of oxygen by the cells.

Carbon dioxide, continually produced in the processes of cell metabolism, is transported from the cells to the lungs in three ways. The majority (about 65%) is carried inside the red blood cells as bicarbonate (HCO_3^-) and is an important component of the bicarbonate buffer system (see Chapter 52 ∞). A moderate amount of carbon dioxide (30%) combines with hemoglobin as carbhemoglobin (also known as carbaminohemoglobin) for transport. Smaller amounts (5%) are transported in solution in the plasma and as carbonic acid (the compound formed when carbon dioxide combines with water).

RESPIRATORY REGULATION

Respiratory regulation includes both neural and chemical controls to maintain the correct concentrations of oxygen, carbon dioxide, and hydrogen ions in body fluids. The nervous system of the body adjusts the rate of alveolar ventilations to meet the needs of the body so that PO_2 and PCO_2 remain relatively constant. The body's "respiratory center" is actually a number of groups of neurons located in the medulla oblongata and pons of the brain.

A chemosensitive center in the medulla oblongata is highly responsive to increases in blood CO_2 or hydrogen ion concentration. By influencing other respiratory centers, this center can increase the activity of the inspiratory center and the rate and depth of respirations. In addition to this direct chemical stimulation of the respiratory center in the brain, special neural receptors sensitive to decreases in O_2 concentration are located outside the central nervous system in the carotid bodies (just above the bifurcation of the common carotid arteries) and aortic bodies located above and below the aortic arch. Decreases in arterial oxygen concentrations stimulate these chemoreceptors, and they in turn stimulate the respiratory center to increase ventilation. Of the three blood gases (hydrogen, oxygen, and carbon dioxide) that can trigger chemoreceptors, increased carbon dioxide concentration normally has the strongest effect on stimulating respiration.

However, in clients with certain chronic lung ailments such as **emphysema,** oxygen concentrations, not carbon dioxide concentrations, play a major role in regulating respiration. For such clients, decreased oxygen concentrations are the main stimuli for respiration because the chronically elevated carbon dioxide levels that occur with emphysema "desensitize" the central chemoreceptors. This is sometimes called the hypoxic drive. Increasing the concentration of oxygen depresses the respiratory rate. Thus, only low concentrations of supplemental oxygen are administered to these clients.

CLINICAL ALERT

In clients with chronic obstructive lung disease, administering too much supplemental oxygen can actually cause the client to stop breathing. ■

FACTORS AFFECTING RESPIRATORY FUNCTION

Factors that influence oxygenation affect the cardiovascular system as well as the respiratory system. These factors include age, environment, lifestyle, health status, medications, and stress.

Age

Developmental factors are important influences on respiratory function. At birth, profound changes occur in the respiratory systems. The fluid-filled lungs drain, the PCO_2 rises, and the neonate takes a first breath. The lungs gradually expand with each subsequent breath, reaching full inflation by 2 weeks of age. Changes of aging that affect the respiratory system of elders become especially important if the system is compromised by changes such as infection, physical or emotional stress, surgery, anesthesia, or other procedures. Changes are:

- Chest wall and airways become more rigid and less elastic.
- The amount of exchanged air is decreased.
- The cough reflex and cilia action are decreased.
- Mucous membranes become drier and more fragile.
- Decreases in muscle strength and endurance occur.
- If osteoporosis is present, adequate lung expansion may be compromised.
- A decrease in efficiency of the immune system occurs.
- Gastroesophageal reflux disease is more common in older adults and increases the risk of aspiration. The aspiration of stomach contents into the lungs often causes bronchospasm by setting up an inflammatory response.

Environment

Altitude, heat, cold, and air pollution affect oxygenation. The higher the altitude, the lower the PO_2 an individual breathes. As a result, the person at high altitudes has increased respiratory and cardiac rates and increased respiratory depth, which usually become most apparent when the individual exercises.

Healthy people exposed to air pollution, such as smog or secondhand smoke, may experience stinging of the eyes, headache, dizziness, coughing, and choking. People who have a history of existing lung disease and altered respiratory function experience varying degrees of respiratory difficulty in a polluted environment. Some are unable to perform self-care in such an environment.

Lifestyle

Physical exercise or activity increases the rate and depth of respirations and hence the supply of oxygen in the body. Sedentary people, by contrast, lack the alveolar expansion and deep breathing patterns of people with regular activity and are less able to respond effectively to respiratory stressors.

Certain occupations predispose an individual to lung disease. For example, silicosis is seen more often in sandstone blasters and potters than in the rest of the population; asbestosis in asbestos workers; anthracosis in coal miners; and organic dust disease in farmers and agricultural employees who work with moldy hay.

Health Status

In the healthy person, the respiratory system can provide sufficient oxygen to meet the body's needs. Diseases of the respiratory system, however, can adversely affect the oxygenation of the blood.

LIFESPAN CONSIDERATIONS   Respiratory Development

INFANTS

- Respiratory rates are highest and most variable in newborns. The respiratory rate of a neonate is 40 to 80 breaths per minute.
- Infant respiratory rates average about 30 per minute.
- Because of rib cage structure, infants rely almost exclusively on diaphragmatic movement for breathing. This is seen as abdominal breathing, as the abdomen rises and falls with each breath.

CHILDREN

- The respiratory rate gradually decreases, averaging around 25 per minute in the preschooler and reaching the adult rate of 12 to 18 per minute by late adolescence.
- During infancy and childhood, upper respiratory infections are common and, fortunately, usually not serious. Infants and preschoolers also are at risk for airway obstruction by foreign objects such as coins and small toys. Cystic fibrosis is a congenital disorder that affects the lungs, causing them to become congested with thick, tenacious (sticky) mucus. Asthma is another chronic disease often identified in childhood. The airways of the asthmatic child react to stimuli such as allergens, exercise, or cold air by constricting, becoming edematous, and producing excessive mucus. Airflow is impaired, and the child may wheeze as air moves through narrowed air passages.

ELDERS

- Elders are at increased risk for acute respiratory diseases such as pneumonia and chronic diseases such as emphysema and chronic

bronchitis. Chronic obstructive pulmonary disease (COPD) may affect elders, particularly after years of exposure to cigarette smoke or industrial pollutants.
- Pneumonia may not present with the usual symptoms of a fever, but will present with atypical symptoms, such as confusion, weakness, loss of appetite, and increase in heart rate and respirations.

Nursing interventions should be directed toward achieving optimal respiratory effort and gas exchange:

- Always encourage wellness and prevention of disease by reinforcing the need for good nutrition, exercise, and immunizations, such as for influenza and pneumonia.
- Increase fluid intake, if not contraindicated by other problems, such as cardiac or renal impairment.
- Proper positioning and frequent changing of positions allow for better lung expansion and air and fluid movement.
- Teach the client to use breathing techniques for better air exchange (see Client Teaching boxes throughout this chapter).
- Pace activities to conserve energy.
- Encourage the client to eat more frequent, smaller meals to decrease gastric distention, which can cause pressure on the diaphragm.
- Teach the client to avoid extreme hot or cold temperatures that will further tax the respiratory system.
- Teach actions and side effects of drugs, inhalers, and treatments.

Medications

A variety of medications can decrease the rate and depth of respirations. The most common medications with this effect are the benzodiazepine sedative-hypnotics and antianxiety drugs. (e.g., diazepam [Valium], flurazepam [Dalmane], midazolam [Versed]), barbiturates (e.g., phenobarbital), and narcotics such as morphine and meperidine hydrochloride (Demerol). When administering these, the nurse must carefully monitor respiratory status, especially when the medication is begun or when the dose is increased. Although this is a safety concern, usually the importance of the medication outweighs the risk of respiratory depression.

Stress

When stress and stressors are encountered, both psychologic and physiologic responses can affect oxygenation. Some people may hyperventilate in response to stress. When this occurs, arterial PO_2 rises and PCO_2 falls. The person may experience light-headedness and numbness and tingling of the fingers, toes, and around the mouth as a result.

Physiologically, the sympathetic nervous system is stimulated and epinephrine is released during stress. Epinephrine causes the bronchioles to dilate, increasing blood flow and oxygen delivery to active muscles. Although these responses are adaptive in the short term, when stress continues they can be destructive, increasing the risk of cardiovascular disease.

ALTERATIONS IN RESPIRATORY FUNCTION

Respiratory function can be altered by conditions that affect

- The movement of air into or out of the lungs.
- The diffusion of oxygen and carbon dioxide between the alveoli and the pulmonary capillaries.
- The transport of oxygen and carbon dioxide via the blood to and from the tissue cells.

Three major alterations in respiration are hypoxia, altered breathing patterns, and obstructed or partially obstructed airway.

Hypoxia

Hypoxia is a condition of insufficient oxygen anywhere in the body, from the inspired gas to the tissues. It can be related to any of the parts of respiration—ventilation, diffusion of gases, or transport of gases by the blood—and can be caused by any condition that alters one or more parts of the process. The Clinical Manifestations box lists signs of hypoxia.

CLINICAL MANIFESTATIONS HYPOXIA

- Rapid pulse
- Rapid, shallow respirations and dyspnea
- Increased restlessness or light-headedness
- Flaring of the nares
- Substernal or intercostal retractions
- Cyanosis

Hypoventilation, that is, inadequate alveolar ventilation, can lead to hypoxia. Hypoventilation may occur because of diseases of the respiratory muscles, drugs, or anesthesia. With hypoventilation, carbon dioxide often accumulates in the blood, a condition called **hypercarbia (hypercapnia).**

Hypoxia can also develop when the diffusion of oxygen from alveoli into the arterial blood decreases, as with pulmonary edema or pneumonia, or it can result from problems in the delivery of oxygen to the tissues (e.g., anemia, heart failure, and embolism). The term **hypoxemia** refers to reduced oxygen in the blood and is characterized by a low partial pressure of oxygen in arterial blood or a low hemoglobin saturation.

Cyanosis (bluish discoloration of the skin, nailbeds, and mucous membranes, due to reduced hemoglobin-oxygen saturation) may be present when there is hypoxemia. Cyanosis requires these two conditions: The blood must contain about 5 g or more of unoxygenated hemoglobin per 100 mL of blood, and the surface blood capillaries must be dilated. Factors that interfere with either of these conditions (e.g., severe anemia or the administration of epinephrine) will eliminate cyanosis as a sign even if the client is experiencing hypoxia.

Adequate oxygenation is essential for cerebral functioning. The cerebral cortex can tolerate hypoxia for only 3 to 5 minutes before permanent damage occurs. The face of the acutely hypoxic person usually appears anxious, tired, and drawn. The person usually assumes a sitting position, often leaning forward slightly to permit greater expansion of the thoracic cavity.

With chronic hypoxia, the client often appears fatigued and is lethargic. The client's fingers and toes may be clubbed as a result of long-term lack of oxygen in the arterial blood supply. With clubbing, the base of the nail becomes swollen and the ends of the fingers and toes increase in size. The angle between the nail and the base of the nail increases to more than 180 degrees. See Figure 30-10, page 583. ∞

Altered Breathing Patterns

Breathing patterns refer to the rate, volume, rhythm, and relative ease or effort of respiration. Normal respiration (**eupnea**) is quiet, rhythmic, and effortless. **Tachypnea** (rapid rate) is seen with fevers, metabolic acidosis, pain, and hypercapnia or hypoxemia. **Bradypnea** is an abnormally slow respiratory rate, which may be seen in clients who have taken drugs such as morphine, who have metabolic alkalosis, or who have increased intracranial pressure (e.g., from brain injuries). **Apnea** is the cessation of breathing.

Hyperventilation, often called *alveolar hyperventilation,* is an increased movement of air into and out of the lungs. During hyperventilation, the rate and depth of respirations increase, and more CO_2 is eliminated than is produced. One particular type of hyperventilation that accompanies metabolic acidosis is **Kussmaul's breathing,** by which the body attempts to compensate (give off excess body acids) by blowing off the carbon dioxide through deep and rapid breathing. Hyperventilation can also occur in response to stress or anxiety.

Abnormal respiratory rhythms create an irregular breathing pattern. Two abnormal respiratory rhythms are

- **Cheyne-Stokes respirations.** Marked rhythmic waxing and waning of respirations from very deep to very shallow breathing and temporary apnea; common causes include congestive heart failure, increased intracranial pressure, and overdose of certain drugs.
- **Biot's (cluster) respirations.** Shallow breaths interrupted by apnea; may be seen in clients with central nervous system disorders.

Orthopnea is the inability to breathe except in an upright or standing position. Difficult or uncomfortable breathing is called **dyspnea.** The dyspneic person often appears anxious and may experience *shortness of breath* (SOB), a feeling of being unable to get enough air (breathlessness). Often the nostrils are flared because of the increased effort of inspiration. The skin may appear dusky; heart rate is increased. Dyspnea may have many causes, most of which stem from cardiac or respiratory disorders. It is a subjective feeling; that is, dyspnea may not be directly observed or measured but is reported by the client. Since treatment is aimed at removing the underlying cause, it is important for the nurse to conduct a thorough history of the onset, duration, and precipitating and relieving factors of the client's dyspnea plus a comprehensive physical examination.

Obstructed Airway

A completely or partially obstructed airway can occur anywhere along the upper or lower respiratory passageways. An upper airway obstruction—that is, in the nose, pharynx, or larynx—can arise because of a foreign object such as food, because the tongue falls back into the oropharynx when a person is unconscious, or when secretions collect in the passageways. In the latter instance, the respirations will sound gurgly or bubbly as the air attempts to pass through the secretions. Lower airway obstruction involves partial or complete occlusion of the passageways in the bronchi and lungs most often due to increased accumulation of mucus or inflammatory exudate.

Assessing for and maintaining an open (patent) airway is a nursing responsibility, one that often requires immediate action. Partial obstruction of the upper airway passages is indicated by a low-pitched snoring sound during inhalation. Complete obstruction is indicated by extreme inspiratory effort that produces no chest movement and an inability to cough or speak. Such a client, in an effort to obtain air, may also exhibit marked sternal and intercostal retractions. Lower airway obstruction is not always as easy to observe. **Stridor,** a harsh, high-pitched sound, may be heard during inspiration. The client may have altered arterial blood gas levels, restlessness, dyspnea, and **adventitious breath sounds** (abnormal breath sounds). See Table 30–8, page 613.

 NURSING MANAGEMENT

Assessing

Nursing assessment of oxygenation status includes a history, physical examination, and review of relevant diagnostic data.

Nursing History

A comprehensive nursing history relevant to oxygenation status should include data about current and past respiratory problems; lifestyle; presence of cough, **sputum** (coughed-up material), or pain; medications for breathing; and presence of risk factors for impaired oxygenation status. Examples of interview questions to elicit this information are shown in the Assessment Interview.

Physical Examination

In assessing a client's oxygenation status, the nurse uses all four physical examination techniques: inspection, palpation, percussion, and auscultation. The nurse first observes the rate, depth, rhythm, and quality of respirations, noting the position the client assumes for breathing. The nurse also inspects for variations in the shape of the thorax that may indicate adaptation to chronic respiratory conditions. For example, clients with emphysema frequently develop a *barrel chest.*

The nurse palpates the thorax for bulges, tenderness, or abnormal movements. Palpation is also used to detect vocal (tactile) fremitus. The thorax can be percussed for diaphragmatic excursion (the movement of the diaphragm during maximal inspiration and expiration). However, this is not commonly done in acute care and long-term care settings. And the nurse frequently auscultates the chest to assess if the client's breath sounds are normal or abnormal. See Chapter 30 ∞ , Skill 30-11 (Assessing the Thorax and Lungs) for more information.

Diagnostic Studies

The primary care provider may order various diagnostic tests to assess respiratory status, function, and oxygenation. Included are sputum specimens, throat cultures, visualization procedures (see Chapter 34 ∞), venous and arterial blood specimens, and pulmonary function tests.

Measurement of arterial blood gases is an important diagnostic procedure (see Chapter 52 ∞). Specimens of arterial blood are normally taken by specialty nurses, respiratory therapists, or medical technicians. Blood for these tests is taken directly from the radial, brachial, or femoral arteries or from catheters placed in these arteries. Because of the relatively great pressure of the blood in these arteries, it is important to prevent hemorrhaging by applying pressure to the puncture side for about 5 minutes after removing the needle. Frequently the noninvasive measurement of oxygen saturation (using a device placed on the fingertip) is sufficient for attaining a measurement of oxygenation of the arterial blood.

PULMONARY FUNCTION TESTS. Pulmonary function tests measure lung volume and capacity. Clients undergoing pulmonary function tests, which are usually carried out by a respiratory therapist, do not require an anesthetic. The client breathes into a machine. The tests are painless, but the client's cooperation is essential. It requires the ability to follow directions and some hand–eye coordination. Nurses need to explain the tests to clients beforehand and help them to rest afterward because the tests are often tiring. Table 50–1 describes the

ASSESSMENT INTERVIEW   Oxygenation

CURRENT RESPIRATORY PROBLEMS

- Have you noticed any changes in your breathing pattern (e.g., shortness of breath, difficulty in breathing, need to be in upright position to breathe, or rapid and shallow breathing)?
- If so, which of your activities might cause these symptom(s) to occur?
- How many pillows do you use to sleep at night?

HISTORY OF RESPIRATORY DISEASE

- Have you had colds, allergies, asthma, tuberculosis, bronchitis, pneumonia, or emphysema?
- How frequently have these occurred? How long did they last? And how were they treated?
- Have you been exposed to any pollutants?

LIFESTYLE

- Do you smoke? If so, how much? If not, did you smoke previously, and when did you stop?
- Does any member of your family smoke?
- Is there cigarette smoke or other pollutants (e.g., fumes, dust, coal, asbestos) in your workplace?
- Do you use alcohol? If so, how many drinks (mixed drinks, glasses of wine, or beers) do you usually have per day or per week?
- Describe your exercise patterns. How often do you exercise and for how long?

PRESENCE OF COUGH

- How often and how much do you cough?
- Is it productive, that is, accompanied by sputum, or nonproductive, that is, dry?
- Does the cough occur during certain activity or at certain times of the day?

DESCRIPTION OF SPUTUM

- When is the sputum produced?
- What is the amount, color, thickness, odor?
- Is it ever tinged with blood?

PRESENCE OF CHEST PAIN

- How does going outside in the heat or the cold affect you?
- Do you experience any pain with breathing or activity?
- Where is the pain located?
- Describe the pain. How does it feel?
- Does it occur when you breathe in or out?
- How long does it last, and how does it affect your breathing?
- Do you experience any other symptoms when the pain occurs (e.g., nausea, shortness of breath or difficulty breathing, light-headedness, palpitations)?
- What activities precede your pain?
- What do you do to relieve the pain?

PRESENCE OF RISK FACTORS

- Do you have a family history of lung cancer, cardiovascular disease (including strokes), or tuberculosis?
- The nurse should also note the client's weight, activity pattern, and dietary assessment. Risk factors include obesity, sedentary lifestyle, and diet high in saturated fats.

MEDICATION HISTORY

- Have you taken or do you take any over-the-counter or prescription medications for breathing (e.g., bronchodilator, inhalant, narcotic)?
- If so, which ones? And what are the dosages, times taken, and results, including side effects?

---

measurements taken, and Figure 50-3 ■ shows their relationships and normal adult values.

Diagnosing

NANDA includes the following diagnostic labels for clients with oxygenation problems:

- *Ineffective Airway Clearance:* Inability to clear secretions or obstructions from the respiratory tract to maintain a clear airway. A clinical example using this nursing diagnosis is

shown in the Nursing Care Plan and the Concept Map later in the chapter.

- *Ineffective Breathing Pattern:* Inspiration and/or expiration that does not provide adequate ventilation.
- *Impaired Gas Exchange:* Excess or deficit in oxygenation and/or carbon dioxide elimination at the alveolar-capillary membrane.
- *Activity Intolerance:* Insufficient physiological or psychological energy to endure or complete required or desired daily activities.

TABLE 50–1   Pulmonary Volumes and Capacities

MEASUREMENT	DESCRIPTION
Tidal volume (V_T)	Volume inhaled and exhaled during normal quiet breathing
Inspiratory reserve volume (IRV)	Maximum amount of air that can be inhaled over and above a normal breath
Expiratory reserve volume (ERV)	Maximum amount of air that can be exhaled following a normal exhalation
Residual volume (RV)	The amount of air remaining in the lungs after maximal exhalation
Total lung capacity (TLC)	The total volume of the lungs at maximum inflation; calculated by adding the V_T, IRV, ERV, and RV
Vital capacity (VC)	Total amount of air that can be exhaled after a maximal inspiration; calculated by adding the V_T, IRV, and ERV
Inspiratory capacity	Total amount of air that can be inhaled following normal quiet exhalation; calculated by adding the V_T and IRV
Functional residual capacity (FRC)	The volume left in the lungs after normal exhalation; calculated by adding the ERV and RV
Minute volume (MV)	The total volume or amount of air breathed in 1 minute

Figure 50-3 ■ The relationship of lung volumes and capacities. Volumes (mL) shown are for an average adult male; female volumes are 20% to 25% smaller.

The preceding nursing diagnoses may also be the etiology of several other nursing diagnoses. Examples follow:

- *Anxiety* related to ineffective airway clearance and feeling of suffocation
- *Fatigue* related to ineffective breathing pattern
- *Fear* related to chronic disabling respiratory illness
- *Powerlessness* related to inability to maintain independence in self-care activities because of ineffective breathing pattern
- *Insomnia* related to orthopnea and required O₂ therapy
- *Social Isolation* related to activity intolerance and inability to travel to usual social activities

Planning

The overall outcomes/goals for a client with oxygenation problems are to

- Maintain a patent airway.
- Improve comfort and ease of breathing.
- Maintain or improve pulmonary ventilation and oxygenation.
- Improve ability to participate in physical activities.
- Prevent risks associated with oxygenation problems such as skin and tissue breakdown, syncope, acid–base imbalances, and feelings of hopelessness and social isolation.

HOME CARE ASSESSMENT Oxygenation

CLIENT

- Self-care abilities: Ability to ambulate and perform ADLs independently
- Exercise and activity pattern: Type and regularity of usual exercise, perceived and actual energy for desired and required leisure activities
- Assistive devices required: Supplemental oxygen, humidifier, nebulizer treatments, or inhalers; walker, cane, or wheelchair; grab bars, shower chair, and other devices to promote safety and minimize energy expenditure; scale to monitor weight on a regular basis
- Home environment for factors that impair airway clearance, gas exchange, or activity tolerance: Indoor pollutants such as cigarette smoke, dust, and allergens such as pets; lack of humidity in the air; and barriers such as stairs
- Current level of knowledge: Importance of avoiding smoking and other pollutants; dietary salt and other restrictions (if appropriate); recommended activities; medications; need to limit exposure to respiratory infections; use of prescribed nebulizer, multidose inhaler, powdered dose inhaler, or home oxygen; activity level

FAMILY

- Caregiver availability, skills, and responses: Ability and willingness to provide care as needed (help with ADLs, providing meals, assisting with transportation and shopping, caring for dependents; performing treatments such as percussion and postural drainage)
- Family role changes and coping: Effect on financial status, parenting and spousal roles, sexuality, social roles
- Alternate potential primary or respite caregivers: For example, other family members, volunteers, church members, paid caregivers or housekeeping services; available community respite care (e.g., adult day care, senior centers)

COMMUNITY

- Environment: Usual temperature and humidity, presence of air pollutants such as automobile exhaust, industrial smoke and pollutants, smoke from field burning
- Current knowledge of and experience with community resources: Medical and assistive equipment and supply companies, respiratory and physical therapy services, home health agencies, local pharmacies, available financial assistance, support and educational organizations such as the local lung association, COPD support groups

---

CLIENT TEACHING   Home Care Oxygenation

MAINTAINING AIRWAY CLEARANCE AND EFFECTIVE GAS EXCHANGE

- Emphasize to the client and family the importance of not smoking or lighting any flammable materials (e.g., candles) in the same room. Refer them to smoking cessation programs as needed. For family members resistant to not smoking, emphasize the need to avoid smoking inside the home.
- Instruct the client in effective coughing techniques such as controlled coughing or "huff" coughing (see "Deep Breathing and Coughing" in the "Implementing" section).
- Discuss the significance of changes in sputum, including the amount and characteristics such as color, viscosity, and odor. Instruct the client when to contact a health care provider.
- Teach the client to maintain a fluid intake of 2,500 mL (2.5 qt) to 3,000 mL (3 qt) per day.
- Instruct the client of the rationale for using and how to use nebulizers or inhalers if prescribed; see Chapter 35 ∞, pages 895–898.
- Teach the client and family how to use home oxygen delivery systems.

PROMOTING EFFECTIVE BREATHING

- Teach relaxation techniques such as progressive muscle relaxation, meditation, and visualization. Use prerecorded tapes as needed.
- Help the client identify specific factors that affect breathing such as stress, and exposure to allergens or air pollution, and exposure to cold. Assist with identifying possible interventions and measures to avoid these factors.

MEDICATIONS

- Teach the client about prescribed medications, including the rationale for the medications, the dose, the desired and possible adverse effects, and any precautions about using a medication with food, beverages, or other medications.

SPECIFIC MEASURES FOR OXYGENATION PROBLEMS

- Provide instructions and rationale for specific procedures and problems such as
  a. Suctioning oropharyngeal and nasopharyngeal cavities.
  b. Caring for a temporary or permanent tracheostomy.
  c. Preventing the spread of tuberculosis and other respiratory infections to family members and others.

REFERRALS

- Make appropriate referrals to home health agencies or community social services for assistance in obtaining medical and assistive equipment such as grab bars, respiratory and physical therapy services, and home health or housekeeping services to assist with ADLs.

COMMUNITY AGENCIES AND OTHER SOURCES OF HELP

- Provide information about where durable medical equipment can be purchased, rented, or obtained free of charge; how to access home oxygen equipment and support services; physical and occupational therapy services and where to obtain supplies such as tracheostomy supplies or nutritional supplements.
- Suggest additional sources of information such as the American Lung Association and the Asthma and Allergy Foundation of America.

These outcomes provide direction for planning interventions and as criteria for evaluating client progress.

A clinical example of desired outcomes, interventions, and activities are provided in the Nursing Care Plan and the Concept Map later in the chapter.

Planning for Home Care

To provide for continuity of care, the nurse needs to consider the client's learning needs and needs for assistance with care in the home. Planning incorporates an assessment of the client's and family's knowledge and abilities for self-care, financial resources, and evaluation of the need for referrals and for home health services. The Home Care Assessment outlines a home care assessment related to the client's oxygenation problems and needs. Client Teaching: Home Care Oxygenation addresses the learning needs of the client and family.

Implementing

Examples of nursing interventions to facilitate pulmonary ventilation may include ensuring a patent airway, positioning, encouraging deep breathing and coughing, and ensuring adequate hydration. Other nursing interventions helpful to ventilation are suctioning, lung inflation techniques, administration of analgesics before deep breathing and coughing, postural drainage, and percussion and vibration. Nursing strategies to facilitate the diffusion of gases through the alveolar membrane include encouraging coughing, deep breathing, and suitable activity. A

client's nursing care plan should also include appropriate dependent nursing interventions such as oxygen therapy, tracheostomy care, and maintenance of a chest tube.

Promoting Oxygenation

Most people in good health give little thought to their respiratory function. Changing position frequently, ambulating, and exercising usually maintain adequate ventilation and gas exchange. Client Teaching lists other ways to promote healthy breathing.

CLIENT TEACHING   Promoting Healthy Breathing

- Sit straight and stand erect to permit full lung expansion.
- Exercise regularly.
- Breathe through the nose.
- Breathe in to expand the chest fully.
- Do not smoke cigarettes, cigars, or pipes.
- Eliminate or reduce the use of household pesticides and irritating chemical substances.
- Do not incinerate garbage in the house.
- Avoid exposure to secondhand smoke.
- Use building materials that do not emit vapors.
- Make sure furnaces, ovens, and wood stoves are correctly ventilated.
- Support a pollution-free environment.

When people become ill, however, their respiratory functions may be inhibited for such reasons as pain and immobility. Shallow respirations inhibit both diaphragmatic excursion and lung distensibility. The result of inadequate chest expansion is pooling of respiratory secretions, which ultimately harbor microorganisms and promote infection. Additionally, shallow respirations may potentiate alveolar collapse which may cause decreased diffusion of gases and subsequent hypoxemia. This situation is often compounded by giving narcotics for pain, because narcotics further depress the rate and depth of respiration.

Interventions by the nurse to maintain the normal respirations of clients include

- Positioning the client to allow for maximum chest expansion.
- Encouraging or providing frequent changes in position.
- Encouraging ambulation.
- Implementing measures that promote comfort, such as giving pain medications.

The semi-Fowler's or high Fowler's position allows maximum chest expansion in clients who are confined to bed, particularly those with dyspnea. The nurse also encourages clients to turn from side to side frequently, so that alternate sides of the chest are permitted maximum expansion. Dyspneic clients often sit in bed and lean over their overbed tables (which are raised to a suitable height), usually with a pillow for support. This orthopneic position is an adaptation of the high Fowler's position. It has a further advantage in that, unlike in high Fowler's, the abdominal organs are not pressing on the diaphragm. Also, a client in the orthopneic position can press the lower part of the chest against the table to help in exhaling (Figure 50-4 ■).

Figure 50-4 ■ A client using the overbed table to assist with breathing.

Deep Breathing and Coughing

The nurse can facilitate respiratory functioning by encouraging deep breathing exercises and coughing to remove secretions from the airways. When coughing raises secretions high enough, the client may either **expectorate** (spit out) or swallow them. Swallowing the secretions is not harmful but does not allow the nurse to view the secretions for documentation purposes or to obtain a specimen for testing.

Breathing exercises are frequently indicated for clients with restricted chest expansion, such as people with chronic obstructive pulmonary disease (COPD) or clients recovering from thoracic surgery.

A commonly employed breathing exercise is *abdominal (diaphragmatic)* and pursed-lip breathing. Abdominal breathing permits deep full breaths with little effort. Pursed-lip breathing helps the client develop control over breathing. The pursed lips create a resistance to the air flowing out of the lungs, thereby prolonging exhalation and preventing airway collapse by maintaining positive airway pressure. The client purses the lips as if about to whistle and breathes out slowly and gently, tightening the abdominal muscles to exhale more effectively. The client usually inhales to a count of 3 and exhales to a count of 7.

Forceful coughing is often less effective than using controlled or huff coughing techniques. Instructions for abdominal (diaphragmatic) and pursed-lip breathing and coughing techniques are provided in Client Teaching.

CLIENT TEACHING Abdominal (Diaphragmatic) and Pursed-Lip Breathing

- Assume a comfortable semi-sitting position in bed or a chair or a lying position in bed with one pillow.
- Flex your knees to relax the muscles of the abdomen.
- Place one or both hands on your abdomen, just below the ribs.
- Breathe in deeply through the nose, keeping the mouth closed.
- Concentrate on feeling your abdomen rise (expand) as far as possible; stay relaxed, and avoid arching your back. If you have difficulty raising your abdomen, take a quick, forceful breath through the nose.
- Then purse your lips as if about to whistle, and breathe out slowly and gently, making a slow "whooshing" sound without puffing out the cheeks. This pursed-lip breathing creates a resistance to air flowing out of the lungs, increases pressure within the bronchi (main air passages), and minimizes collapse of smaller airways, a common problem for people with COPD.
- Concentrate on feeling the abdomen fall or sink, and tighten (contract) the abdominal muscles while breathing out to enhance effective exhalation. Count to seven during exhalation.
- Use this exercise whenever feeling short of breath, and increase gradually to 5 to 10 minutes four times a day. Regular practice will help you do this type of breathing without conscious effort. The exercise, once learned, can be performed when sitting upright, standing, and walking.

MediaLink

Humidifier Animation

CLIENT TEACHING Controlled and Huff Coughing

- After using a bronchodilator treatment (if prescribed), inhale deeply and hold your breath for a few seconds.
- Cough twice. The first cough loosens the mucus; the second expels secretions.
- For huff coughing, lean forward and exhale sharply with a "huff" sound. This technique helps keep your airways open while moving secretions up and out of the lungs.
- Inhale by taking rapid short breaths in succession ("sniffing") to prevent mucus from moving back into smaller airways.
- Rest.
- Try to avoid prolonged episodes of coughing because these may cause fatigue and hypoxia.

Hydration

Adequate hydration maintains the moisture of the respiratory mucous membranes. Normally, respiratory tract secretions are thin and are therefore moved readily by ciliary action. However, when the client is dehydrated or when the environment has a low humidity, the respiratory secretions can become thick and tenacious. Fluid intake should be as great as the client can tolerate. See Chapter 52 ∞ for normal daily fluid intake.

Humidifiers are devices that add water vapor to inspired air. Room humidifiers provide cool mist to room air. Nebulizers are used to deliver humidity and medications. They may be used with oxygen delivery systems to provide moistened air directly to the client. Their purposes are to prevent mucous membranes from drying and becoming irritated and to loosen secretions for easier expectoration.

Medications

A number of types of medications can be used for clients with oxygenation problems.

Bronchodilators, anti-inflammatory drugs, expectorants, and cough suppressants are some medications that may be used to treat respiratory problems. Bronchodilators, including sympathomimetic drugs and xanthines, reduce bronchospasm, opening tight or congested airways and facilitating ventilation. These drugs may be administered orally or intravenously, but the preferred route is by inhalation to prevent many systemic side effects.

Since drugs used to dilate the bronchioles and improve breathing are usually drugs that enhance the sympathetic nervous system, clients must be monitored for side effects of increased heart rate, blood pressure, anxiety, and restlessness. This is especially important in elders, who may also have cardiac problems. Some over-the-counter drugs for respiratory problems have these same effects, so clients should be cautioned about taking them without checking with their primary care provider. Another class of drugs used is the *anti-inflammatory drugs,* such as glucocorticoids. They can be given orally, intravenously, or by inhaler. They work by decreasing the edema and inflammation in the airways and allowing a better air exchange. If both bronchodilators and anti-inflammatory drugs are ordered by inhaler, the client should be instructed to use the bronchodilator inhaler first and then the anti-inflammatory inhaler. If the bronchioles

---

DRUG CAPSULE Sympathomimetics   *albuterol* (Proventil, Ventolin)

THE CLIENT WITH RESPIRATORY MEDICATIONS THAT CAUSE BRONCHODILATION BY STIMULATING BETA-2 ADRENERGIC RECEPTORS IN THE LUNG

The beta-2 adrenergic agonists are called sympathomimetic drugs because they "mimic" the action of sympathetic stimulation to the beta-2 receptors in the smooth muscle of the lung. At therapeutic levels these drugs promote bronchodilation and so relieve bronchospasm.

Sympathomimetic agents are useful in the treatment of bronchospasm in reversible obstructive airway diseases such as asthma and bronchitis. They are also useful in preventing exercise-induced bronchospasm.

NURSING RESPONSIBILITIES

- Most inhaled sympathomimetics have a very rapid onset and short duration of action, so they are useful for relief of acute attacks but not for prophylaxis.
- Monitor the client's respiratory status while administering sympathomimetics. This includes respiratory rate, lung sounds, oxygen saturation, and subjective symptoms.
- These medications should be used with caution in clients with conditions such as cardiac disease, vascular disease, hypertension, hyperthyroidism, and pregnancy.
- Monitor the client for common side effects including increased heart rate (due to sympathetic stimulation of the heart) and tremors.
- Monitor for other side effects that occur with excessive dosing, which may include central nervous system stimulation, gastrointestinal upset, hypertension, and sweating.

CLIENT AND FAMILY TEACHING

- Caution the client to use the least amount of medication needed to get relief for the shortest time period necessary. This will help prevent adverse effects.
- Counsel the client to report immediately any chest pain and/or changes in heart rate or rhythm.
- Teach the client and/or family how to use the delivery system. This will most often be a metered-dose inhaler (MDI) or dry powder inhaler (DPI) or nebulizer.
- Teach the client to record the frequency and intensity of symptoms.

Note: Prior to administering any medication, review all aspects with a current drug handbook or other reliable source.

DRUG CAPSULE Glucocorticoids

Inhaled: *beclomethasone* (Beclovent)
Oral: *Prednisone*

Glucocorticoids are administered to clients with oxygenation problems to suppress inflammation. They can be administered either by inhalation, orally, or intravenously. The route of administration depends on the severity of the client's disorder and the individual's response. Glucocorticoids (steroids) are well absorbed from the respiratory tract so giving them by inhalation is often effective. Steroids suppress the inflammatory response in the airways by decreasing synthesis and release of inflammatory mediators, decreasing activity of inflammatory cells, and decreasing edema.

NURSING RESPONSIBILITIES

- Glucocorticoids are intended for preventive therapy. They will not be useful in an acute attack.
- If the client is also taking a sympathomimetic medication, delivery of the glucocorticoid to the respiratory tract may be enhanced by administering the sympathomimetic first (and waiting 3 to 5 minutes).
- It is important to monitor the client's respiratory status while administering glucocorticoids. This includes respiratory rate, lung sounds, oxygen saturation, and subjective symptoms.
- These medications should be used with caution or not at all in clients with conditions such as allergy, pregnancy, lactation, and systemic infections.
- Monitor the client for side effects of the medications. Most commonly this could be an increase in heart rate (due to sympathetic stimulation of the heart) and tremors.
- The client should be monitored for other side effects which will usually only occur with excessive dosing and may include central nervous system stimulation, gastrointestinal upset, hypertension, and sweating.

CLIENT AND FAMILY TEACHING

- Caution the client to use the least amount needed to get relief for the shortest time period necessary. This will help prevent adverse effects. Alternate day therapy may be recommended to decrease adrenal suppression.
- Make sure the client understands that these drugs are NOT for acute attacks. They are intended for preventive therapy.
- Teach the client and/or family how to use the delivery system. This will most often be a metered-dose inhaler (MDI) or dry powder inhaler (DPI) or nebulizer.
- Counsel the client to report adverse effects such as sore throat, hoarseness, and pharyngeal and laryngeal fungal infections.
- Teach the client to record the frequency and intensity of symptoms.

Note: Prior to administering any medication, review all aspects with a current drug handbook or other reliable source.

---

are dilated first, more tissue is exposed for the anti-inflammatory drugs to act upon.

A fairly new class of drugs is the *leukotriene modifiers*. These medications suppress the effects of leukotrienes on the smooth muscle of the respiratory tract. Leukotrienes cause bronchoconstriction, mucous production, and edema of the respiratory tract.

Expectorants help "break up" mucus, making it more liquid and easier to expectorate. Guaifenesin is a common expectorant found in many prescription and nonprescription cough syrups. When frequent or prolonged coughing interrupts sleep, a cough suppressant such as codeine may be prescribed.

Other medications can be used to improve oxygenation by improving cardiovascular function. The *digitalis glycosides* act directly on the heart to improve the strength of contraction and slow the heart rate. *Beta-adrenergic blocking agents* such as propranolol affect the sympathetic nervous system to reduce the workload of the heart. These drugs, however, can negatively affect people with asthma or COPD as they may constrict airways.

Incentive Spirometry

Incentive spirometers (Figure 50-5 ■), also referred to as *sustained maximal inspiration devices* (SMIs), measure the flow of air inhaled through the mouthpiece and are used to

- Improve pulmonary ventilation.
- Counteract the effects of anesthesia or hypoventilation.
- Loosen respiratory secretions.
- Facilitate respiratory gaseous exchange.
- Expand collapsed alveoli.

They offer an incentive to improve inhalation. When using an SMI, the client should be assisted into a position, preferably an upright sitting position in bed or a chair, that facilitates maximum ventilation. Client Teaching lists instructions for clients in the use of incentive spirometers.

Percussion, Vibration, and Postural Drainage

Percussion, vibration, and postural drainage (PVD) are dependent nursing functions performed according to a primary care provider's order. Percussion, sometimes called *clapping*, is forceful striking of the skin with cupped hands. Mechanical percussion cups and vibrators are also available. When the hands

---

CLIENT TEACHING Using Cough Medications

- Do not take cough medications in excessive amounts because of adverse side effects.
- If you have diabetes mellitus, avoid cough syrups that contain sugar or alcohol; these can disturb metabolism.
- When a cough medicine does not act as expected, consult a health care professional.
- Be aware of side effects (e.g., drowsiness) that can make the operation of machinery dangerous.

MediaLink

Incentive Spirometer Animation

Figure 50-5 ■ *A,* Flow-oriented SMI; *B,* volume-oriented SMI.

are used, the fingers and thumb are held together and flexed slightly to form a cup, as one would to scoop up water. Percussion over congested lung areas can mechanically dislodge tenacious secretions from the bronchial walls. Cupped hands trap the air against the chest. The trapped air sets up vibrations through the chest wall to the secretions.

CLIENT TEACHING
Using an Incentive Spirometer

- Hold or place the spirometer in an upright position. A tilted *flow-oriented* device requires less effort to raise the balls or discs; a *volume-oriented* device will not function correctly unless upright.
- Exhale normally.
- Seal the lips tightly around the mouthpiece.
- Take in a slow, deep breath to elevate the balls or cylinder, and then hold the breath for 2 seconds initially, increasing to 6 seconds (optimum), to keep the balls or cylinder elevated if possible.
- For a flow-oriented device, avoid brisk, low-volume breaths that snap the balls to the top of the chamber. Greater lung expansion is achieved with a very slow inspiration than with a brisk, shallow breath, even though it may not elevate the balls or keep them elevated while you hold your breath. Sustained elevation of the balls or cylinder ensures adequate ventilation of the alveoli (lung air sacs).
- If you have difficulty breathing only through the mouth, a nose clip can be used.
- Remove the mouthpiece and exhale normally.
- Cough after the incentive effort. Deep ventilation may loosen secretions, and coughing can facilitate their removal.
- Relax and take several normal breaths before using the spirometer again.
- Repeat the procedure several times and then four or five times hourly. Practice increases inspiratory volume, maintains alveolar ventilation, and prevents atelectasis (collapse of the air sacs).
- Clean the mouthpiece with water and shake it dry.

To percuss a client's chest, the nurse follows these steps:

- Cover the area with a towel or gown to reduce discomfort.
- Ask the client to breathe slowly and deeply to promote relaxation.
- Alternately flex and extend the wrists rapidly to slap the chest (Figure 50-6 ■).
- Percuss each affected lung segment for 1 to 2 minutes.

When done correctly, the percussion action should produce a hollow, popping sound. Percussion is avoided over the breasts, sternum, spinal column, and kidneys.

Figure 50-6 ■ Percussing the upper posterior chest.

Vibration is a series of vigorous quiverings produced by hands that are placed flat against the client's chest wall. Vibration is used after percussion to increase the turbulence of the exhaled air and thus loosen thick secretions. It is often done alternately with percussion.

To vibrate the client's chest, the nurse follows these steps:

- Place hands, palms down, on the chest area to be drained, one hand over the other with the fingers together and extended (Figure 50-7 ■). Alternatively, the hands may be placed side by side.
- Ask the client to inhale deeply and exhale slowly through the nose or pursed lips.
- During the exhalation, tense all the hand and arm muscles, and using mostly the heel of the hand, vibrate (shake) the hands, moving them downward. Stop the vibrating when the client inhales.
- Vibrate during five exhalations over one affected lung segment.
- After each vibration, encourage the client to cough and expectorate secretions into the sputum container.

Postural drainage is the drainage by gravity of secretions from various lung segments. Secretions that remain in the lungs or respiratory airways promote bacterial growth and subsequent infection. They also can obstruct the smaller airways and cause atelectasis. Secretions in the major airways, such as the trachea and the right and left main bronchi, are usually coughed into the pharynx, where they can be expectorated, swallowed, or effectively removed by suctioning.

A wide variety of positions is necessary to drain all segments of the lungs, but not all positions are required for every client. Only those positions that drain specific affected areas are used. The lower lobes require drainage most frequently because the upper lobes drain by gravity. Before postural drainage, the client may be given a bronchodilator medication or nebulization therapy to loosen secretions. Postural drainage treatments are

Figure 50-7 ■ Vibrating the upper posterior chest.

scheduled two or three times daily, depending on the degree of lung congestion. The best times include before breakfast, before lunch, in the late afternoon, and before bedtime. It is best to avoid hours shortly after meals because postural drainage at these times can be tiring and can induce vomiting.

The nurse needs to evaluate the client's tolerance of postural drainage by assessing the stability of the client's vital signs, particularly the pulse and respiratory rates, and by noting signs of intolerance, such as pallor, diaphoresis, dyspnea, nausea, and fatigue. Some clients do not react well to certain drainage positions, and the nurse must make appropriate adjustments. For example, some become dyspneic in Trendelenburg's position and require only a moderate tilt or a shorter time in that position.

The sequence for PVD is usually as follows: positioning, percussion, vibration, and removal of secretions by coughing or suction. Each position is usually assumed for 10 to 15 minutes, although beginning treatments may start with shorter times and gradually increase.

Following PVD, the nurse should auscultate the client's lungs, compare the findings to the baseline data, and document the amount, color, and character of expectorated secretions.

Oxygen Therapy

Clients who have difficulty ventilating all areas of their lungs, those whose gas exchange is impaired, or people with heart failure may benefit from oxygen therapy to prevent hypoxia.

Oxygen therapy is prescribed by the primary care provider, who specifies the concentration, method of delivery, and depending on the method, liter flow per minute. The concentration is of more importance than the liter flow per minute. When administering oxygen is an *emergency measure*, the nurse may initiate the therapy without a primary care provider's order. For clients who have COPD, a low-flow oxygen system is essential.

Safety precautions are essential during oxygen therapy (see Box 50–2). Although oxygen by itself will not burn or explode, it does facilitate combustion. For example, a bed sheet ordinarily burns slowly when ignited in the atmosphere; however, if saturated with free-flowing oxygen and ignited by a spark, it will burn rapidly and explosively. The greater the concentration of oxygen, the more rapidly fires start and burn, and such fires are difficult to extinguish. Because oxygen is colorless, odorless, and tasteless, people are often unaware of its presence.

Oxygen is supplied in several different ways. In hospitals and long-term care facilities, it is usually piped into wall outlets at the client's bedside, making it readily available for use at all times. Tanks or cylinders of oxygen under pressure are also frequently available for use when wall oxygen is either unavailable or impractical (e.g., for transporting oxygen-dependent clients between treatment areas).

Clients who require oxygen therapy in the home may use small cylinders of oxygen, oxygen in liquid form, or an oxygen concentrator. Portable oxygen delivery systems are available to increase the client's independence. Home oxygen therapy services are readily available in most communities. These services generally supply the oxygen and delivery devices, training for the client and family, equipment maintenance, and emergency services should a problem occur.

BOX 50–2 Oxygen Therapy Safety Precautions

- For home oxygen use or when the facility permits smoking, teach family members and roommates to smoke only outside or in provided smoking rooms away from the client and oxygen equipment.
- Place cautionary signs reading "No Smoking: Oxygen in Use" on the client's door, at the foot or head of the bed, and on the oxygen equipment.
- Instruct the client and visitors about the hazard of smoking with oxygen in use.
- Make sure that electric devices (such as razors, hearing aids, radios, televisions, and heating pads) are in good working order to prevent the occurrence of short-circuit sparks.
- Avoid materials that generate static electricity, such as woolen blankets and synthetic fabrics. Cotton blankets should be used, and clients and caregivers should be advised to wear cotton fabrics.
- Avoid the use of volatile, flammable materials, such as oils, greases, alcohol, ether, and acetone (e.g., nail polish remover), near clients receiving oxygen.
- Be sure that electric monitoring equipment, suction machines, and portable diagnostic machines are all electrically grounded.
- Make known the location of fire extinguishers, and make sure personnel are trained in their use.

Oxygen administered from a cylinder or wall-outlet system is dry. Dry gases dehydrate the respiratory mucous membranes. Humidifying devices that add water vapor to inspired air are thus an essential adjunct of oxygen therapy, particularly for liter flows over 2 L per minute (Figure 50-8 ■). These devices provide 20% to 40% humidity. The oxygen passes through sterile distilled water or tap water and then along a line to the device through which the moistened oxygen is inhaled (e.g., a cannula, nasal catheter, or oxygen mask).

Humidifiers prevent mucous membranes from drying and becoming irritated and loosen secretions for easier expectoration. Oxygen passing through water picks up water vapor before it reaches the client. The more bubbles created during this process, the more water vapor is produced. Very low liter flows (e.g., 1 to 2 L per minute by nasal cannula) do not require humidification. When a client is breathing very low flow oxygen, there is enough atmospheric air inhaled (which naturally has water vapor in it) to prevent mucosal drying.

Oxygen cylinders need to be handled and stored with caution and strapped securely in wheeled transport devices or stands to prevent possible falls and outlet breakages. They should be placed away from traffic areas and heaters.

To use an oxygen wall outlet, the nurse carries out these steps:

- Attach the flow meter to the wall outlet, exerting firm pressure. The flow meter should be in the off position (Figure 50-9 ■).
- Fill the humidifier bottle with distilled or tap water in accordance with agency protocol. This can be done before coming to the bedside. Some humidifier bottles come prefilled by the manufacturer.
- Attach the humidifier bottle to the base of the flow meter.
- Attach the prescribed oxygen tubing and delivery device to the humidifier.

Figure 50-8 ■ An oxygen humidifier attached to a wall outlet oxygen flow meter.

- Regulate the flow meter to the prescribed level. The line for the prescribed flow rate (e.g., 2 L/min) should be in the middle of the ball of the flow meter (Figure 50-10 ■).

Oxygen Delivery Systems

A number of systems are available to deliver oxygen to the client. The choice of system depends on the client's oxygen

Figure 50-9 ■ Insert flow meter into the wall unit.

(Shirlee Snyder)

Figure 50-10 ■ This flow meter is set to deliver 2 L/minute.

(Shirlee Snyder)

needs, comfort, and developmental considerations. With many systems, the oxygen delivered mixes with room air before being inspired. With this type of system, the amount of oxygen delivered is determined by regulating its flow rate (e.g., 2 to 6 L per minute), and precise regulation of the percentage of inspired oxygen, or fraction of inspired oxygen (FiO_2), is not possible. When it is important to regulate the percentage of oxygen received by the client more precisely, a device such as a Venturi mask may be used.

CANNULA. The nasal cannula (nasal prongs) is the most common and inexpensive device used to administer oxygen (Figure 50-11 ■).

The nasal cannula is easy to apply and does not interfere with the client's ability to eat or talk. It also is relatively comfortable, permits some freedom of movement, and is well tolerated by the client. It delivers a relatively low concentration of oxygen (24% to 45%) at flow rates of 2 to 6 L per minute. Above 6 L per minute, the client tends to swallow air and the FiO_2 is not increased. Limitations of the cannula include inability to deliver

Figure 50-12 ■ A simple face mask.

Photographer: Jenny Thomas

higher concentrations of oxygen, and that it can be drying and irritating to mucous membranes.

Administering oxygen by cannula is detailed in Skill 50-1.

FACE MASK. Face masks that cover the client's nose and mouth may be used for oxygen inhalation. Exhalation ports on the sides of the mask allow exhaled carbon dioxide to escape. A variety of oxygen masks are marketed:

■ The simple face mask delivers oxygen concentrations from 40% to 60% at liter flows of 5 to 8 L per minute, respectively (Figure 50-12 ■).
■ The partial rebreather mask delivers oxygen concentrations of 60% to 90% at liter flows of 6 to 10 L per minute, respectively. The oxygen reservoir bag that is attached allows the client to rebreathe about the first third of the exhaled air in conjunction with oxygen (Figure 50-13 ■). Thus, it increases

Figure 50-11 ■ A nasal cannula.

Figure 50-13 ■ A partial rebreather mask.

Photographer: Elena Dorfman

Figure 50-14 ■ A nonrebreather mask.
Photographer: Elena Dorfman

Figure 50-15 ■ A Venturi mask.
Photographer: Jenny Thomas

the FiO_2 by recycling expired oxygen. The partial rebreather bag must not totally deflate during inspiration to avoid carbon dioxide buildup. If this problem occurs, the nurse increases the liter flow of oxygen.

■ The nonrebreather mask delivers the highest oxygen concentration possible—95% to 100%—by means other than intubation or mechanical ventilation, at liter flows of 10 to 15 L per minute. One-way valves on the mask and between the reservoir bag and the mask prevent the room air and the client's exhaled air from entering the bag so only the oxygen in the bag is inspired (Figure 50-14 ■). To prevent carbon dioxide buildup, the nonrebreather bag must not totally deflate during inspiration. If it does, the nurse can correct this problem by increasing the liter flow of oxygen.

■ The Venturi mask delivers oxygen concentrations varying from 24% to 40% or 50% at liter flows of 4 to 10 L per minute (Figure 50-15 ■). The Venturi mask has wide-bore tubing and color-coded jet adapters that correspond to a precise oxygen concentration and liter flow. For example, a blue adapter delivers a 24% concentration of oxygen at 4 L per minute, and a green adapter delivers a 35% concentration of oxygen at 8 L per minute.

Initiating oxygen by mask is much the same as initiating oxygen by cannula, except that the nurse must find a mask of appropriate size. Smaller sizes are available for children. Administering oxygen by mask or face tent is detailed in Skill 50-1. Limitations of masks include difficulty in achieving a proper fit and poor tolerance by some clients who may complain of feeling hot or "smothering."

FACE TENT. Face tents (Figure 50-16 ■) can replace oxygen masks when masks are poorly tolerated by clients. Face tents provide varying concentrations of oxygen, for example, 30% to 50% concentration of oxygen at 4 to 8 L per minute. Frequently inspect the client's facial skin for dampness or chafing, and dry and treat as needed. As with face masks, the client's facial skin must be kept dry.

Figure 50-16 ■ An oxygen face tent.
Photographer: Jenny Thomas

MediaLink Face Mask Animation

MediaLink Nonrebreather Mask Animation

ADMINISTERING OXYGEN BY CANNULA, FACE MASK, OR FACE TENT

Before administering oxygen, check (a) the order for oxygen, including the administering device and the liter flow rate (L/min) or the percentage of oxygen; (b) the levels of oxygen (PaO_2) and carbon dioxide ($PaCO_2$) in the client's arterial blood (PaO_2 is normally 80 to 100 mm Hg; $PaCO_2$ is normally 35 to 45 mm Hg); and (c) whether the client has COPD. NOTE: If the client has not had arterial blood gases ordered, oxygen saturation should be checked using a noninvasive oximeter.

PURPOSES

Cannula
- To deliver a relatively low concentration of oxygen when only minimal O_2 support is required
- To allow uninterrupted delivery of oxygen while the client ingests food or fluids

Face Mask
- To provide moderate O_2 support and a higher concentration of oxygen and/or humidity than is provided by cannula

Face Tent
- To provide high humidity
- To provide oxygen when a mask is poorly tolerated
- To provide a high flow of O_2 when attached to a Venturi system

ASSESSMENT
See also Skill 30-11, Assessing the Thorax and Lungs on page 614. ∞

Assess
- Skin and mucous membrane color: Note whether cyanosis is present.
- Breathing patterns: Note depth of respirations and presence of tachypnea, bradypnea, or orthopnea.
- Chest movements: Note whether there are any intercostal, substernal, suprasternal, supraclavicular, or tracheal retractions during inspiration or expiration.
- Chest wall configuration (e.g., kyphosis).

- Lung sounds audible by auscultating the chest and by ear.
- Presence of clinical signs of hypoxemia: tachycardia, tachypnea, restlessness, dyspnea, cyanosis, and confusion. Tachycardia and tachypnea are often early signs. Confusion is a later sign of severe oxygen deprivation.
- Presence of clinical signs of hypercarbia (hypercapnia): restlessness, hypertension, headache, lethargy, tremor.
- Presence of clinical signs of oxygen toxicity: tracheal irritation and cough, dyspnea, and decreased pulmonary ventilation.

Determine
- Vital signs, especially pulse rate and quality, and respiratory rate, rhythm, and depth.
- Whether the client has COPD. A high carbon dioxide level in the blood is the normal stimulus to breathe. However, people with COPD may have a chronically high carbon dioxide level, and their stimulus to breathe is hypoxemia. Low flows of oxygen (2 L/min) stimulate breathing for such persons by maintaining slight hypoxemia. During continuous oxygen administration, arterial blood gas levels of oxygen (PaO_2) and carbon dioxide ($PaCO_2$) are measured periodically to monitor hypoxemia.
- Results of diagnostic studies such as chest x-ray.
- Hemoglobin, hematocrit, and complete blood count.
- Oxygen saturation levels.
- Arterial blood gases levels, if available.
- Pulmonary function tests, if available.

PLANNING
Consult with a respiratory therapist as needed in the beginning and during ongoing care of clients receiving ordered oxygen therapy. In many agencies, the therapist establishes the initial equipment and client teaching.

Delegation
Initiating the administration of oxygen is considered similar to administering a medication and is not delegated to unlicensed assistive personnel (UAP). However, reapplying the oxygen delivery device may be performed by the UAP, and many aspects of the client's response to oxygen therapy are observed during usual care and may be recorded by persons other than the nurse. Abnormal findings must be validated and interpreted by the nurse. The nurse is also responsible for ensuring that the correct delivery method is being used.

Equipment
Cannula
- Oxygen supply with a flow meter and adapter
- Humidifier with distilled water or tap water according to agency protocol
- Nasal cannula and tubing
- Tape
- Padding for the elastic band

Face Mask
- Oxygen supply with a flow meter and adapter
- Humidifier with distilled water or tap water according to agency protocol
- Prescribed face mask of the appropriate size
- Padding for the elastic band

Face Tent
- Oxygen supply with a flow meter and adapter
- Humidifier with distilled water or tap water according to agency protocol
- Face tent of the appropriate size

IMPLEMENTATION
Preparation
1. Determine the need for oxygen therapy, and verify the order for the therapy.
   - Perform a respiratory assessment to develop baseline data if not already available.

2. Prepare the client and support people.
   - Assist the client to a semi-Fowler's position if possible. **Rationale:** *This position permits easier chest expansion and hence easier breathing.*

ADMINISTERING OXYGEN BY CANNULA, FACE MASK, OR FACE TENT *continued*

- Explain that oxygen is not dangerous when safety precautions are observed. Inform the client and support people about the safety precautions connected with oxygen use.

Performance

1. Prior to performing the procedure, introduce self and verify the client's identity using agency protocol. Explain to the client what you are going to do, why it is necessary, and how he or she can cooperate. Discuss how the effects of the oxygen therapy will be used in planning further care or treatments.
2. Perform hand hygiene and observe appropriate infection control procedures.
3. Provide for client privacy, if appropriate.
4. Set up the oxygen equipment and the humidifier.
   - Attach the flow meter to the wall outlet or tank. The flow meter should be in the off position.
   - If needed, fill the humidifier bottle. (This can be done before coming to the bedside.)
   - Attach the humidifier bottle to the base of the flow meter.
   - Attach the prescribed oxygen tubing and delivery device to the humidifier.
5. Turn on the oxygen at the prescribed rate and ensure proper functioning.
   - Check that the oxygen is flowing freely through the tubing. There should be no kinks in the tubing, and the connections should be airtight. There should be bubbles in the humidifier as the oxygen flows through. You should feel the oxygen at the outlets of the cannula, mask, or tent.
   - Set the oxygen at the flow rate ordered.
6. Apply the appropriate oxygen delivery device.

Cannula
- Put the cannula over the client's face, with the outlet prongs fitting into the nares and the elastic band around the head (see Figure 50-11). Some models have a strap to adjust under the chin.
- If the cannula will not stay in place, tape it at the sides of the face.
- Pad the tubing and band over the ears and cheekbones as needed.

Face Mask
- Guide the mask toward the client's face, and apply it from the nose downward.

- Fit the mask to the contours of the client's face (see Figure 50-12). **Rationale:** *The mask should mold to the face, so that very little oxygen escapes into the eyes or around the cheeks and chin.*
- Secure the elastic band around the client's head so that the mask is comfortable but snug.
- Pad the band behind the ears and over bony prominences. **Rationale:** *Padding will prevent irritation from the mask.*

Face Tent
- Place the tent over the client's face, and secure the ties around the head (see Figure 50-16).
7. Assess the client regularly.
   - Assess the client's vital signs, level of anxiety, color, and ease of respirations, and provide support while the client adjusts to the device.
   - Assess the client in 15 to 30 minutes, depending on the client's condition, and regularly thereafter.
   - Assess the client regularly for clinical signs of hypoxia, tachycardia, confusion, dyspnea, restlessness, and cyanosis. Review oxygen saturation or arterial blood gas results if they are available.

Nasal Cannula
- Assess the client's nares for encrustations and irritation. Apply a water-soluble lubricant as required to soothe the mucous membranes.
- Assess the top of the client's ears for any signs of irritation from the cannula strap. If present, padding with a gauze pad may help relieve the discomfort.

Face Mask Or Tent
- Inspect the facial skin frequently for dampness or chafing, and dry and treat it as needed.
8. Inspect the equipment on a regular basis.
   - Check the liter flow and the level of water in the humidifier in 30 minutes and whenever providing care to the client.
   - Be sure that water is not collecting in dependent loops of the tubing.
   - Make sure that safety precautions are being followed.
9. Document findings in the client record using forms or checklists supplemented by narrative notes when appropriate.

EVALUATION
- Perform follow-up based on findings that deviated from expected or normal for the client. Relate findings to previous data if available (e.g., check oxygen saturation to evaluate adequate oxygenation).
- Report significant deviations from normal to the primary care provider.

LIFESPAN CONSIDERATIONS   Oxygen Delivery Equipment

INFANTS

Oxygen Hood

- An oxygen hood is a rigid plastic dome that encloses an infant's head. It provides precise oxygen levels and high humidity.
- The gas should not be allowed to blow directly into the infant's face, and the hood should not rub against the infant's neck, chin, or shoulder.

CHILDREN

Oxygen Tent (Figure 50-17 ■)

- The tent consists of a rectangular, clear, plastic canopy with outlets that connect to an oxygen or compressed air source and to a humidifier that moisturizes the air or oxygen.
- Because the enclosed tent becomes very warm, some type of cooling mechanism such as an ice chamber or a refrigeration unit is provided to maintain the temperature at 20°C to 21°C (68°F to 70°F).
- Cover the child with a gown or a cotton blanket. Some agencies provide gowns with hoods, or a small towel may be wrapped around the head. *The child needs protection from chilling and from the dampness and condensation in the tent.*
- Flood the tent with oxygen by setting the flow meter at 15 L/min for about 5 minutes. Then, adjust the flow meter according to or-

Figure 50-17 ■ Pediatric oxygen tent.

ders (e.g., 10 to 15 L/min). *Flooding the tent quickly increases the oxygen to the desired level.*
- The tent can deliver approximately 30% oxygen.

HOME CARE CONSIDERATIONS   Home Care Oxygen Equipment

Three major oxygen systems for home care use are available in most communities: cylinders or tanks of compressed gas, liquid (cryogenic) oxygen, and oxygen concentrators.

1. Cylinders ("green tanks"): These are the system of choice for clients who need oxygen episodically (e.g., on a prn basis). Advantages are that cylinders deliver all liter flows (1 to 15 L/min), and oxygen evaporation does not occur during storage. Disadvantages are that the cylinders are heavy and awkward to move, the supply company must be notified when a refill is needed, and they are costly for the high-use client. A size "D" tank weighs about 8 pounds and stores 425 L of oxygen; an "E" tank holds 680 L and is transported on wheels (Figure 50-18 ■). The large "H" tank weighs 150 pounds. The gauge on a full tank reads a pressure of at least 2,000 pounds per square inch (psi), and a tank is considered empty when it reads less than 500 psi.

2. Liquid oxygen: Liquid systems have two parts—a large stationary container and a portable unit with a small lightweight tank that is refilled from the stationary unit. Liquid reservoirs store oxygen at −212°C (−350°F) in a smaller amount of space than compressed gas. Advantages are that these reservoirs are lighter in weight and cleaner in appearance than cylinders and they are not as difficult to operate. Disadvantages of liquid oxygen are that many home care medical supply and service companies are not able to handle it, oxygen evaporation occurs when the unit is not used, only low flows (1 to 4 L/min) can be used or freezing occurs, and the portable unit designed to be carried over the shoulder weighs 8 to 10 pounds, a possible burden to the typical COPD client (Figure 50-19 ■). A wheeled cart can be used to carry the unit but may be awkward.

3. Oxygen concentrators: Concentrators are electrically powered systems that manufacture oxygen from room air. At 1 L/min, such

Figure 50-18 ■ An "E" cylinder oxygen tank on a wheeled stand.

a system can deliver a concentration of about 95% oxygen, but the concentration drops when the flow rate increases (e.g., 75% concentration at 4 L/min). Advantages are that they are more attractive in appearance, resembling furniture rather than medical equipment; they eliminate the need for regular delivery of oxy-

HOME CARE CONSIDERATIONS   **Home Care Oxygen Equipment—*continued***

Figure 50-19 ■ A portable liquid oxygen supply.

gen or refilling of cylinders; because the supply of oxygen is constant, they alleviate the client's anxiety about running out of oxygen; and they are the most economical system when continuous use is required. Major disadvantages of a concentrator are that it is expensive; it lacks real portability (small units weigh 28 pounds); it tends to be noisy; it is powered by electricity (an emergency backup unit, for example, an oxygen tank, must be provided for clients for whom a power failure could be life threatening); and heat produced by the concentrator motor is a problem for those who live in trailers, small houses, or warm climates, where air conditioners are required. The oxygen concentrator must also be checked periodically with an O_2 analyzer to ensure that it is providing an adequate delivery of oxygen.

Another type of oxygen concentrator is the *oxygen enricher.* It uses a plastic membrane that allows water vapor to pass through with the oxygen, thus eliminating the need for a humidifying device. It is also thought to filter out bacteria present in the air. The enricher provides an O_2 concentration of 40% at all flow rates, it tends to be quieter than the concentrator, there is less chance of combustion (since the gas is only 40% oxygen), it has only two moving parts (thus decreasing the risk of something going wrong), and a nebulizer can be operated off the enricher because of the high flow rate.

Social services or the case manager needs to ensure that the client has appropriate help in choosing a reputable home oxygen vendor. Services furnished should include

■ A 24-hour emergency service.
■ Trained personnel to make the initial delivery and instruct the client in safe, appropriate use of the oxygen and maintenance of the equipment.
■ At least monthly follow-up visits to check the equipment and reinstruct the client as necessary.
■ A regular cost review to ensure that the system is the most cost-effective one for that client, with routine notification of the physician or home care professional if it seems that another system is more appropriate.

The nurse needs to also ensure that the client knows about the financial reimbursements available from Medicare and Medicaid or other insurance agencies.

Artificial Airways

Artificial airways are inserted to maintain a patent air passage for clients whose airway has become or may become obstructed. A patent airway is necessary so that air can flow to and from the lungs. Four of the more common types of airways are oropharyngeal, nasopharyngeal, endotracheal, and tracheostomy.

OROPHARYNGEAL AND NASOPHARYNGEAL AIRWAYS. Oropharyngeal and nasopharyngeal airways are used to keep the upper air passages open when they may become obstructed by secretions or the tongue. These airways are easy to insert and have a low risk of complications. Sizes vary and should be appropriate to the size and age of the client. The airway should be well lubricated with water-soluble gel prior to inserting.

Oropharyngeal airways (Figure 50-20 ■) stimulate the gag reflex and are only used for clients with altered levels of consciousness (e.g., because of general anesthesia, overdose, or head injury). To insert the airway:

■ Place the client in a supine or semi-Fowler's position.
■ Put on clean gloves.

Figure 50-20 ■ An oropharyngeal airway in place.

■ Hold the lubricated airway by the outer flange, with the distal end pointing up.
■ Open the client's mouth and insert the airway along the top of the tongue.
■ When the distal end of the airway reaches the soft palate at the back of the mouth, rotate the airway 180 degrees downward, and slip it past the uvula into the oral pharynx.

Figure 50-21 ■ A nasopharyngeal airway in place.

■ If not contraindicated, place the client in a side-lying position or with the head turned to the side to allow secretions to drain out of the mouth.
■ The oropharynx may be suctioned as needed by inserting the suction catheter alongside the airway.
■ Do not tape the airway in place; remove it when the client begins to cough or gag.
■ Provide mouth care at least every 2 to 4 hours, keeping suction available at the bedside.
  ● As appropriate for the client's condition, remove the airway every 8 hours to assess the mouth and provide oral care. Reinsert the airway immediately.

Nasopharyngeal airways are tolerated better by alert clients. They are inserted through the nares, terminating in the oropharynx (Figure 50-21 ■). When caring for a client with a nasopharyngeal airway, provide frequent oral and nares care, repositioning the airway in the other naris every 8 hours or as ordered to prevent necrosis of the mucosa.

ENDOTRACHEAL TUBES. Endotracheal tubes are most commonly inserted for clients who have had general anesthetics or for those in emergency situations where mechanical ventilation is required. An endotracheal tube is inserted by the primary care provider, nurse, or respiratory therapist with specialized education. It is inserted through the mouth or the nose and into the trachea with the guide of a laryngoscope (Figure 50-22 ■). The tube terminates just superior to the bifurcation of the trachea into the bronchi. The tube may have an air-filled cuff to prevent air leakage around it. Because an endotracheal tube passes through the epiglottis and glottis, the client is unable to speak while it is in

nasal ET
oral ET

Figure 50-22 ■ An endotracheal tube (ET).

---

place. Nursing interventions for clients with endotracheal tubes are shown in Box 50–3.

TRACHEOSTOMY. Clients who need long-term airway support may have a tracheostomy. A tracheostomy is an opening into the trachea through the neck. A tube is usually inserted through this opening and an artificial airway is created. Tracheostomy is done using one of two techniques: the traditional open surgical method or a percutaneous insertion. The percutaneous method can be done at the bedside in a critical care unit. The open technique is done in the operating room, and a surgical incision is made in the trachea just below the larynx. A curved tracheostomy tube is inserted to extend through the stoma into the trachea (Figure 50-23 ■). Tracheostomy tubes may be either plastic or metal and are available in different sizes.

Tracheostomy tubes have an outer cannula that is inserted into the trachea and a flange that rests against the neck and allows the tube to be secured in place with tape or ties (Figure 50-24 ■). All tubes also have an obturator, which is used to insert the outer cannula and is then removed. The obturator is kept at the client's bedside in case the tube becomes dislodged and needs to be reinserted. Some tracheostomy tubes have an inner cannula that may be removed for periodic cleaning.

Figure 50-23 ■ A tracheostomy tube in place.

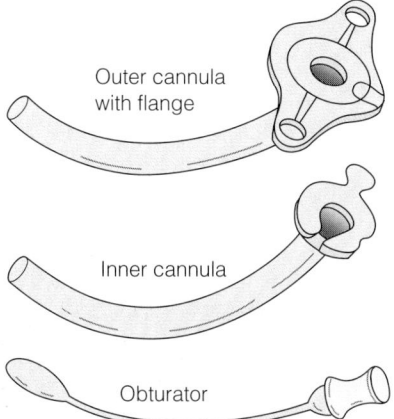

Figure 50-24 ■ Components of a tracheostomy tube.

Outer cannula with flange

Inner cannula

Obturator

Cuffed tracheostomy tubes are surrounded by an inflatable cuff that produces an airtight seal between the tube and the trachea. This seal prevents aspiration of oropharyngeal secretions and air leakage between the tube and the trachea. Cuffed tubes are often used immediately after a tracheostomy and are essential when ventilating a tracheostomy client with a mechanical ventilator. Children do not require cuffed tubes, because their tracheas are resilient enough to seal the air space around the tube.

Low-pressure cuffs (Figure 50-25 ■) are commonly used to distribute a low, even pressure against the trachea, thus decreas-

Figure 50-26 ■ A tracheostomy tube with a foam cuff.
(Courtesy of Portex Inc., Keene, NH.)

ing the risk of tracheal tissue necrosis. They do not need to be deflated periodically to reduce pressure on the tracheal wall. Foam cuffed tracheostomy tubes (Figure 50-26 ■) do not require injected air; instead, when the port is opened, ambient air enters the balloon, which then conforms to the client's trachea. Air is removed from the cuff prior to insertion or removal of the tube.

The nurse provides tracheostomy care for the client with a new or recent tracheostomy to maintain patency of the tube and reduce the risk of infection. Initially a tracheostomy may need to be suctioned (see the section on suctioning that follows) and cleaned as often as every 1 to 2 hours. After the initial inflammatory response subsides, tracheostomy care may only need to be done once or twice a day, depending on the client. Skill 50-4 describes tracheostomy care.

When the client breathes through a tracheostomy, air is no longer filtered and humidified as it is when passing through the upper airways; therefore, special precautions are necessary. Humidity may be provided with a mist collar (Figure 50-27 ■). Clients with long-term tracheostomies may wear a light scarf or

Figure 50-25 ■ A tracheostomy tube with a low-pressure cuff.

Figure 50-27 ■ A tracheostomy mist collar.

Figure 50-28 ■ Types of suction catheters: *A*, open tipped; *B*, whistle tipped.

a 4-in. × 4-in. gauze held in place with a cotton tie over the stoma to filter air as it enters the tracheostomy.

Suctioning

When clients have difficulty handling their secretions or an airway is in place, suctioning may be necessary to clear air passages. **Suctioning** is aspirating secretions through a catheter connected to a suction machine or wall suction outlet. Even though the upper airways (the oropharynx and nasopharynx) are not sterile, sterile technique is recommended for all suctioning to avoid introducing pathogens into the airways.

Suction catheters may be either open tipped or whistle tipped (Figure 50-28 ■). The whistle-tipped catheter is less irritating to respiratory tissues, although the open-tipped catheter may be more effective for removing thick mucous plugs. An oral suction tube, or Yankauer device, is used to suction the oral cavity (Figure 50-29 ■). Most suction catheters have a thumb port on the side to control the suction. The catheter is connected to suction tubing, which in turn is connected to a collection chamber and suction control gauge (Figure 50-30 ■).

The nurse decides when suctioning is needed by assessing the client for signs of respiratory distress or evidence that the client is unable to cough up and expectorate secretions. Dyspnea, bubbling or rattling breath sounds, poor skin color (cyanosis), or decreased oxygen saturation (SpO_2) levels (also called O_2 sat) may indicate the need for suctioning. Good nursing judgment is necessary, because suctioning irritates mucous membranes and can increase secretions if performed too frequently. In other words, suctioning is based on clinical need versus a fixed schedule.

Figure 50-29 ■ Oral (Yankauer) suction tube.

Figure 50-30 ■ A wall suction unit.

Photographer: Jenny Thomas

Oral and oropharyngeal suctioning removes secretions from the upper respiratory tract. Nasopharyngeal and nasotracheal suctioning provides closer access to the trachea and requires sterile technique. Skill 50-2 outlines oropharyngeal and nasopharyngeal suctioning.

SKILL 50-2

OROPHARYNGEAL, NASOPHARYNGEAL, AND NASOTRACHEAL SUCTIONING

Purposes
- To remove secretions that obstruct the airway
- To facilitate ventilation

- To obtain secretions for diagnostic purposes
- To prevent infection that may result from accumulated secretions

ASSESSMENT

Assess for clinical signs indicating the need for suctioning:

- Restlessness
- Gurgling sounds during respiration
- Adventitious breath sounds when the chest is auscultated

- Change in mental status
- Skin color
- Rate and pattern of respirations
- Pulse rate and rhythm
- Decreased oxygen saturation

OROPHARYNGEAL, NASOPHARYNGEAL, AND NASOTRACHEAL SUCTIONING *continued*

PLANNING

> **Delegation**
>
> Oral suctioning using a Yankauer suction tube and oropharyngeal suctioning using a suction catheter can be delegated to UAP and to the client or family, if appropriate, since this is not a sterile procedure. The nurse needs to review the procedure and important points such as not applying suction during insertion of the tube to avoid trauma to the mucous membrane. In contrast, nasopharyngeal and nasotracheal suctioning uses sterile technique and requires application of knowledge and problem solving and should be performed by the nurse or respiratory therapist.

Equipment

Oral and Nasopharyngeal/Nasotracheal Suctioning
- Towel or moisture-resistant pad
- Portable or wall suction machine with tubing, collection receptacle, and suction pressure gauge
- Sterile disposable container for fluids
- Sterile normal saline or water
- Goggles or face shield, if appropriate
- Moisture-resistant disposal bag
- Sputum trap, if specimen is to be collected

Oral and Oropharyngeal Suctioning
- Yankauer suction catheter or suction catheter kit
- Clean gloves

Nasopharyngeal or Nasotracheal Suctioning
- Sterile gloves
- Sterile suction catheter kit (#12 to #18 Fr for adults, #8 to #10 Fr for children, and #5 to #8 Fr for infants)
- Water-soluble lubricant
- Y-connector

IMPLEMENTATION

Performance

1. Prior to performing the procedure, introduce self and verify the client's identity using agency protocol. Explain to the client what you are going to do, why it is necessary, and how he or she can cooperate. Inform the client that suctioning will relieve breathing difficulty and that the procedure is painless but may be uncomfortable and stimulate the cough, gag, or sneeze reflex. **Rationale:** *Knowing that the procedure will relieve breathing problems is often reassuring and enlists the client's cooperation.*

2. Perform hand hygiene and observe other appropriate infection control procedures.

3. Provide for client privacy.

4. Prepare the client.
   - Position a conscious person who has a functional gag reflex in the semi-Fowler's position with the head turned to one side for oral suctioning or with the neck hyperextended for nasal suctioning. **Rationale:** *These positions facilitate the insertion of the catheter and help prevent aspiration of secretions.*
   - Position an unconscious client in the lateral position, facing you. **Rationale:** *This position allows the tongue to fall forward, so that it will not obstruct the catheter on insertion. The lateral position also facilitates drainage of secretions from the pharynx and prevents the possibility of aspiration.*
   - Place the towel or moisture-resistant pad over the pillow or under the chin.

5. Prepare the equipment.
   - Set the pressure on the suction gauge, and turn on the suction. Many suction devices are calibrated to three pressure ranges.
   - *Wall unit:*
     Adult: 100 to 120 mm Hg
     Child: 95 to 110 mm Hg
     Infant: 50 to 95 mm Hg
   - *Portable unit:*
     Adult: 10 to 15 mm Hg
     Child: 5 to 10 mm Hg
     Infant: 2 to 5 mm Hg

For Oral and Oropharyngeal Suction
- Moisten the tip of the Yankauer or suction catheter with sterile water or saline. **Rationale:** *This reduces friction and eases insertion.*
- Pull the tongue forward, if necessary, using gauze.
- Do not apply suction (that is, leave your finger off the port) during insertion. **Rationale:** *Applying suction during insertion causes trauma to the mucous membrane.*
- Advance the catheter about 10 to 15 cm (4 to 6 in.) along one side of the mouth into the oropharynx. **Rationale:** *Directing the catheter along the side prevents gagging.*
- It may be necessary during oropharyngeal suctioning to apply suction to secretions that collect in the vestibule of the mouth and beneath the tongue.

For Nasopharyngeal and Nasotracheal Suction
- Open the lubricant if performing nasopharyngeal/nasotracheal suctioning.
- Open the sterile suction package.
  a. Set up the cup or container, touching only the outside.
  b. Pour sterile water or saline into the container.
  c. Put on the sterile gloves, or put on a nonsterile glove on the nondominant hand and then a sterile glove on the dominant hand. **Rationale:** *The sterile gloved hand maintains the sterility of the suction catheter, and the unsterile glove prevents the transmission of the microorganisms to the nurse.*
- With your sterile gloved hand, pick up the catheter and attach it to the suction unit. ❶

❶ Attaching the catheter to the suction unit.

continued on page 1384

OROPHARYNGEAL, NASOPHARYNGEAL, AND NASOTRACHEAL SUCTIONING *continued*

6. Make an approximate measure of the depth for the insertion of the catheter and test the equipment.
   - Measure the distance between the tip of the client's nose and the earlobe, or about 13 cm (5 in.) for an adult.
   - Mark the position on the tube with the fingers of the sterile gloved hand.
   - Test the pressure of the suction and the patency of the catheter by applying your sterile gloved finger or thumb to the port or open branch of the Y-connector (the suction control) to create suction.
   - If needed, apply or increase supplemental oxygen.
7. Lubricate and introduce the catheter.
   - Lubricate the catheter tip with sterile water, saline, or water-soluble lubricant. **Rationale:** *This reduces friction and eases insertion.*
   - Remove oxygen with the nondominant hand, if appropriate.
   - *Without applying suction,* insert the catheter the premeasured or recommended distance into either naris and advance it along the floor of the nasal cavity. **Rationale:** *This avoids the nasal turbinates.*
   - Never force the catheter against an obstruction. If one nostril is obstructed, try the other.
8. Perform suctioning.
   - Apply your finger to the suction control port to start suction, and gently rotate the catheter. **Rationale:** *Gentle rotation of the catheter ensures that all surfaces are reached and prevents trauma to any one area of the respiratory mucosa due to prolonged suction.*
   - Apply suction for 5 to 10 seconds while slowly withdrawing the catheter, then remove your finger from the control and remove the catheter.
   - A suction attempt should last only 10 to 15 seconds. During this time, the catheter is inserted, the suction applied and discontinued, and the catheter removed.
9. Rinse the catheter and repeat suctioning as above.
   - Rinse and flush the catheter and tubing with sterile water or saline.
   - Relubricate the catheter, and repeat suctioning until the air passage is clear.
   - Allow sufficient time between each suction for ventilation and oxygenation. Limit suctioning to 5 minutes in total. **Rationale:** *Applying suction for too long may cause secretions to increase or decrease the client's oxygen supply.*
   - Encourage the client to breathe deeply and to cough between suctions. Use supplemental oxygen, if appropriate. **Rationale:** *Coughing and deep breathing help carry secretions from the trachea and bronchi into the pharynx, where they can be reached with the suction catheter. Deep breathing and supplemental oxygen provide oxygen to the alveoli.*
10. Obtain a specimen if required.
    - Use a sputum trap ❷ as follows:
    - Attach the suction catheter to the tubing of the sputum trap.
    - Attach the suction tubing to the sputum trap air vent.
    - Suction the client. The sputum trap will collect the mucus during suctioning.

❷ A sputum collection trap.

   - Remove the catheter from the client. Disconnect the sputum trap tubing from the suction catheter. Remove the suction tubing from the trap air vent.
   - Connect the tubing of the sputum trap to the air vent. **Rationale:** *This retains any microorganisms in the sputum trap.*
   - Connect the suction catheter to the tubing.
   - Flush the catheter to remove secretions from the tubing.
11. Promote client comfort.
    - Offer to assist the client with oral or nasal hygiene.
    - Assist the client to a position that facilitates breathing.
12. Dispose of equipment and ensure availability for the next suction.
    - Dispose of the catheter, gloves, water, and waste container. Wrap the catheter around your sterile gloved hand and hold the catheter as the glove is removed over it for disposal.
    - Rinse the suction tubing as needed by inserting the end of the tubing into the used water container. Empty and rinse the suction collection container as needed or indicated by protocol. Change the suction tubing and container daily.
    - Ensure that supplies are available for the next suctioning (suction kit, gloves, water or normal saline).
13. Assess the effectiveness of suctioning.
    - Auscultate the client's breath sounds to ensure they are clear of secretions. Observe skin color, dyspnea, level of anxiety, and oxygen saturation levels.
14. Document relevant data.
    - Record the procedure: the amount, consistency, color, and odor of sputum (e.g., foamy, white mucus; thick, green-tinged mucus; or blood-flecked mucus) and the client's respiratory status before and after the procedure. This may include lung sounds, rate and character of breathing, and oxygen saturation.
    - If the procedure is carried out frequently (e.g., every hour), it may be appropriate to record only once, at the end of the shift; however, the frequency of the suctioning must be recorded.

OROPHARYNGEAL, NASOPHARYNGEAL, AND NASOTRACHEAL SUCTIONING *continued*

SAMPLE DOCUMENTATION

12/12/2007 0830 Producing large amounts of thick, tenacious white mucus to back of oral pharynx but unable to expectorate into tissue. Uses Yankauer suction tube as needed.

O₂ sat increased from 89% before suctioning to 93% after suctioning. RR also decreased from 26 to 18–20 after suctioning. Continuous O₂ at 2 L/min via n/c. Will continue to reassess q hour. —————————————————*L. Webb, RN*

EVALUATION

■ Conduct appropriate follow-up, such as appearance of secretions suctioned; breath sounds; respiratory rate, rhythm, and depth; pulse rate and rhythm; and skin color.

■ Compare findings to previous assessment data if available.
■ Report significant deviations from normal to the primary care provider.

LIFESPAN CONSIDERATIONS Suctioning

INFANTS

■ A bulb syringe is used to remove secretions from an infant's nose or mouth. Care needs to be taken to avoid stimulating the gag reflex.

CHILDREN

■ A catheter is used to remove secretions from an older child's mouth or nose.

ELDERS

■ Elders often have cardiac and/or pulmonary disease, thus increasing their susceptibility to hypoxemia related to suctioning. Watch closely for signs of hypoxemia. If noted, stop suctioning and hyperoxygenate.

HOME CARE CONSIDERATIONS Suctioning

■ Teach clients and families that the most important aspect of infection control is frequent hand washing.
■ Airway suctioning in the home is considered a clean procedure.
■ The catheter or Yankauer should be flushed by suctioning recently boiled or distilled water to rinse away mucus, followed by the suctioning of air through the device to dry the internal surface and, thus, discourage bacterial growth. The outer surface of the device

may be wiped with alcohol or hydrogen peroxide. The suction catheter or Yankauer should be allowed to dry and then be stored in a clean, dry area.
■ Suction catheters treated in the manner described above may be reused. It is recommended that catheters be discarded after 24 hours. Yankauer suction tubes may be cleaned, boiled, and reused.

Following endotracheal intubation or a tracheostomy, the trachea and surrounding respiratory tissues are irritated and react by producing excessive secretions. Sterile suctioning is necessary to remove these secretions from the trachea and bronchi to maintain a patent airway. The frequency of suctioning depends on the client's health and how recently the intubation was done. Additionally, suctioning may be necessary in clients who have increased secretions because of pneumonia or inability to clear secretions because of altered level of consciousness.

Suctioning is associated with several complications: hypoxemia, trauma to the airway, nosocomial infection, and cardiac dysrhythmia, which is related to the hypoxemia. The following techniques are used to minimize or decrease these complications:

■ **Hyperinflation.** This involves giving the client breaths that are 1 to 1.5 times the tidal volume set on the ventilator through the ventilator circuit or via a manual resuscitation bag. Three to five breaths are delivered before and after each pass of the suction catheter.

■ **Hyperoxygenation.** This can be done with a manual resuscitation bag or through the ventilator and is performed by increasing the oxygen flow (usually to 100%) before suctioning and between suction attempts.

For tracheostomy and endotracheal suctioning, the outer diameter of the suction catheter should not exceed one-half the internal diameter of the tracheostomy or endotracheal tube so that hypoxia can be prevented (St. John, 2004). The nurse uses sterile techniques to prevent infection of the respiratory tract (see Skill 50-3). The traditional method of suctioning an endotracheal tube or tracheostomy is sometimes referred to as the *open method*. If a client is connected to a ventilator, the nurse disconnects the client from the ventilator, suctions the airway, reconnects the client to the ventilator, and discards the suction catheter. Drawbacks to the open airway suction system include the nurse needing to wear personal protective equipment (e.g., goggles or face shield, gown) to avoid exposure to the client's sputum and the potential cost

Client connection

T piece

Irrigation port

Ventilator connection

Labels

0.9% sodium chloride vials

Suction catheter and sleeve

Suction connection

Control valve

Figure 50-31 ▪ A closed airway suction (in-line) system.

of one-time catheter use, especially if the client requires frequent suctioning.

With the *closed airway/tracheal suction system* (*in-line suctioning*) (Figure 50-31 ▪), the suction catheter attaches to the ventilator tubing and the client does not need to be disconnected from the ventilator. The nurse is not exposed to any secretions because the suction catheter is enclosed in a plastic sheath. The catheter can be reused as many times as necessary until the system is changed. The nurse needs to inquire about the agency's policy for changing the closed suction system.

SKILL 50-3

SUCTIONING A TRACHEOSTOMY OR ENDOTRACHEAL TUBE

Purposes
▪ To maintain a patent airway and prevent airway obstructions
▪ To promote respiratory function (optimal exchange of oxygen and carbon dioxide into and out of the lungs)

▪ To prevent pneumonia that may result from accumulated secretions

ASSESSMENT
Assess the client for the presence of congestion on auscultation of the thorax. Note the client's ability or inability to remove the secretions through coughing.

PLANNING

Delegation
Suctioning a tracheostomy or endotracheal tube is a sterile, invasive technique requiring application of scientific knowledge and problem solving. This skill is performed by a nurse or respiratory therapist and is not delegated to UAP.

Equipment
▪ Resuscitation bag (Ambu bag) connected to 100% oxygen
▪ Sterile towel (optional)
▪ Equipment for suctioning (see Skill 50-2)
▪ Goggles and mask if necessary
▪ Gown (if necessary)
▪ Sterile gloves
▪ Moisture-resistant bag

IMPLEMENTATION
Preparation
Determine if the client has been suctioned previously and, if so, review the documentation of the procedure. This information can be very helpful in preparing the nurse for both the physiologic and psychologic impact of suctioning on the client.

Performance
1. Prior to performing the procedure, introduce self and verify the client's identity using agency protocol. Explain to the client what you are going to do, why it is necessary, and how he or she can cooperate. Inform the client that suctioning usually causes

some intermittent coughing and that this assists in removing the secretions.
2. Perform hand hygiene and observe other appropriate infection control procedures (e.g., gloves, goggles).
3. Provide for client privacy.
4. Prepare the client.
   • If not contraindicated because of health, place the client in the semi-Fowler's position to promote deep breathing, maximum lung expansion, and productive coughing. **Rationale:** *Deep breathing oxygenates the lungs, counteracts the hypoxic effects of suctioning, and may induce coughing. Coughing helps to loosen and move secretions.*

SUCTIONING A TRACHEOSTOMY OR ENDOTRACHEAL TUBE *continued*

- If necessary, provide analgesia before suctioning. Endotracheal suctioning stimulates the cough reflex, which can cause pain for clients who have had thoracic or abdominal surgery or who have experienced traumatic injury. **Rationale:** *Premedication can increase the client's comfort during the suctioning procedure.*

5. Prepare the equipment.
   - Attach the resuscitation apparatus to the oxygen source. ❶ Adjust the oxygen flow to 100%.
   - Open the sterile supplies in readiness for use.
   - Place the sterile towel, if used, across the client's chest below the tracheostomy.
   - Turn on the suction, and set the pressure in accordance with agency policy. For a wall unit, a pressure setting of about 100 to 120 mm Hg is normally used for adults, 50 to 95 mm Hg for infants and children.
   - Put on goggles, mask, and gown if necessary.
   - Put on sterile gloves. Some agencies recommend putting a sterile glove on the dominant hand and an unsterile glove on the nondominant hand to protect the nurse.
   - Holding the catheter in the dominant hand and the connector in the nondominant hand, attach the suction catheter to the suction tubing (see Figure ❶ in Skill 50-2).

6. Flush and lubricate the catheter.
   - Using the dominant hand, place the catheter tip in the sterile saline solution.
   - Using the thumb of the nondominant hand, occlude the thumb control and suction a small amount of the sterile solution through the catheter. **Rationale:** *This determines that the suction equipment is working properly and lubricates the outside and the lumen of the catheter. Lubrication eases insertion and reduces tissue trauma during insertion. Lubricating the lumen also helps prevent secretions from sticking to the inside of the catheter.*

7. If the client does not have copious secretions, hyperventilate the lungs with a resuscitation bag before suctioning.
   - Summon an assistant, if one is available, for this step.
   - Using your nondominant hand, turn on the oxygen to 12 to 15 L/min.
   - If the client is receiving oxygen, disconnect the oxygen source from the tracheostomy tube using your nondominant hand.
   - Attach the resuscitator to the tracheostomy or endotracheal tube. ❷
   - Compress the Ambu bag three to five times, as the client inhales. This is best done by a second person who can use both hands to compress the bag, thus, providing a greater inflation volume.
   - Observe the rise and fall of the client's chest to assess the adequacy of each ventilation.
   - Remove the resuscitation device and place it on the bed or the client's chest with the connector facing up.

Variation: Using a Ventilator to Provide Hyperventilation

If the client is on a ventilator, use the ventilator for hyperventilation and hyperoxygenation. Newer models have a mode that

❶ Attaching the resuscitation apparatus to the oxygen source.
Photographer: Jenny Thomas

❷ Attaching the resuscitator to the tracheostomy.
Photographer: Jenny Thomas

provides 100% oxygen for 2 minutes and then switches back to the previous oxygen setting as well as a manual breath or sigh button. **Rationale:** *The use of ventilator settings provides more consistent delivery of oxygenation and hyperinflation than a resuscitation device.*

8. If the client has copious secretions, do not hyperventilate with a resuscitator. *Instead:*
   - Keep the regular oxygen delivery device on and increase the liter flow or adjust the FiO_2 to 100% for several breaths before suctioning. **Rationale:** *Hyperventilating a client who has copious secretions can force the secretions deeper into the respiratory tract.*

9. Quickly but gently insert the catheter *without* applying any suction.
   - With your nondominant thumb off the suction port, quickly but gently insert the catheter into the trachea through the

continued on page 1388

SUCTIONING A TRACHEOSTOMY OR ENDOTRACHEAL TUBE *continued*

3 Inserting the catheter into the trachea through the tracheostomy tube. *Note:* Suction is not applied while inserting the catheter.

tracheostomy tube. **3** **Rationale:** *To prevent tissue trauma and oxygen loss, suction is not applied during insertion of the catheter.*

- Insert the catheter about 12.5 cm (5 in.) for adults, less for children, or until the client coughs or you feel resistance. **Rationale:** *Resistance usually means that the catheter tip has reached the bifurcation of the trachea.* To prevent damaging the mucous membranes at the bifurcation, withdraw the catheter about 1 to 2 cm (0.4 to 0.8 in.) before applying suction.

10. Perform suctioning.
- Apply suction for 5 to 10 seconds by placing the nondominant thumb over the thumb port. **Rationale:** *Suction time is restricted to 10 seconds or less to minimize oxygen loss.*
- Rotate the catheter by rolling it between your thumb and forefinger while slowly withdrawing it. **Rationale:** *This prevents tissue trauma by minimizing the suction time against any part of the trachea.*
- Withdraw the catheter completely, and release the suction.
- Hyperventilate the client.
- Suction again, if needed.

11. Reassess the client's oxygenation status and repeat suctioning.
- Observe the client's respirations and skin color. Check the client's pulse if necessary, using your nondominant hand.
- Encourage the client to breathe deeply and to cough between suctions.
- Allow 2 to 3 minutes with oxygen, as appropriate between suctions when possible. **Rationale:** *This provides an opportunity for reoxygenation of the lungs.*
- Flush the catheter and repeat suctioning until the air passage is clear and the breathing is relatively effortless and quiet.
- After each suction, pick up the resuscitation bag with your nondominant hand and ventilate the client with no more than three breaths.

12. Dispose of equipment and ensure availability for the next suction.
- Flush the catheter and suction tubing.
- Turn off the suction and disconnect the catheter from the suction tubing.

- Wrap the catheter around your sterile hand and peel the glove off so that it turns inside out over the catheter.
- Discard the glove and the catheter in the moisture-resistant bag.
- Replenish the sterile fluid and supplies so that the suction is ready for use again. **Rationale:** *Clients who require suctioning often require it quickly, so it is essential to leave the equipment at the bedside ready for use.*
- Be sure that the ventilator and oxygen settings are returned to presuctioning settings. **Rationale:** *On some ventilators this is automatic, but always check. It is very dangerous for clients to be left on 100% oxygen.*

13. Provide for client comfort and safety.
- Assist the client to a comfortable, safe position that aids breathing. If the person is conscious, a semi-Fowler's position is frequently indicated. If the person is unconscious, Sims' position aids in the drainage of secretions from the mouth.

14. Document relevant data.
- Record the suctioning, including the amount and description of suction returns and any other relevant assessments.

SAMPLE DOCUMENTATION

12/13/2007   1000   Coarse rales in RLL and LLL. Requires suctioning about every 1–2 hrs. Obtain large amount of pinkish tinged white thin mucous via ETT. Breath sounds clearer after suctioning. Pt. signals when he wants to be suctioned.
                                                    —*C. Holmes, RN*

Variation: Closed Airway/Tracheal Suction System (In-Line Catheter)

- If a catheter is not attached, put on clean gloves, aseptically open a new closed catheter set, and attach the ventilator connection on the T piece to the ventilator tubing. Attach the client connection to the endotracheal tube or tracheostomy.
- Attach one end of the suction connecting tubing to the suction connection port of the closed system and the other end of the connecting tubing to the suction device.
- Turn suction on, occlude or kink tubing, and depress the suction control valve (on the closed catheter system) to set suction to the appropriate level. Release the suction control valve.
- Use the ventilator to hyperoxygenate and hyperinflate the client's lungs.
- Unlock the suction control mechanism if required by the manufacturer.
- Advance the suction catheter enclosed in its plastic sheath with the dominant hand. Steady the T piece with the nondominant hand.
- Depress the suction control valve and apply suction for no more than 10 seconds and gently withdraw the catheter.
- Repeat as needed remembering to provide hyperoxygenation and hyperinflation as needed.
- When completed suctioning, withdraw the catheter into its sleeve and close the access valve, if appropriate. **Rationale:** *If the system does not have an access valve on the client*

SUCTIONING A TRACHEOSTOMY OR ENDOTRACHEAL TUBE *continued*

connector, the nurse needs to observe for the potential of the catheter migrating into the airway and partially obstructing the artificial airway.

- Flush the catheter by instilling normal saline into the irrigation port and applying suction. Repeat until the catheter is clear.
- Close the irrigation port and close the suction valve.

EVALUATION

- Perform a follow-up examination of the client to determine the effectiveness of the suctioning (e.g., respiratory rate, depth, and character; breath sounds; color of skin and nail beds; character and amount of secretions suctioned; changes in vital signs).
- Relate findings to previous assessment data if available.
- Report significant deviations from normal to the primary care provider.

LIFESPAN CONSIDERATIONS Suctioning a Tracheostomy or Endotracheal Tube

INFANTS AND CHILDREN

- Have an assistant gently restrain the child to keep the child's hands out of the way. The assistant should maintain the child's head in the midline position.

ELDERS

- Do a thorough lung assessment before and after suctioning to determine effectiveness of suctioning and to be aware of any special problems.

HOME CARE CONSIDERATIONS Suctioning a Tracheostomy or Endotracheal Tube

- Whenever possible, the client should be encouraged to clear the airway by coughing.
- Clients may need to learn to suction their secretions if they cannot cough effectively.
- Clean gloves should be used when endotracheal suctioning is performed in the home environment.
- The nurse needs to instruct the caregiver on how to determine the need for suctioning and the correct process and rationale underlying the practice of suctioning to avoid potential complications of suctioning.
- Stress the importance of adequate hydration as it thins secretions, which can aid in the removal of secretions by coughing or suctioning.

RESEARCH NOTE What Are Current Practices of Nurses and Respiratory Therapists Regarding Closed Suctioning Systems and Airway Management?

The purpose of this multisite survey study by Sole, Byers, Ludy, Zhang, Banta, and Brummel (2003) was to describe different institutional practices related to closed-system suctioning and airway management of intubated clients. A total of 1,665 nurses and respiratory therapists at 27 different sites in the United States responded by filling out the survey. The surveys showed that most sites had policies for management of endotracheal tube cuffs, hyperoxygenation prior to suctioning, use of gloves with closed-system suctioning, and instillation of saline solution to thin thick secretions. Only 50% of institutions had policies regarding oral care, and less had policies for oral suctioning.

IMPLICATIONS

There is a lot of variety with policies and procedures related to airway management. The survey data also suggested that practice does not always reflect the most recent research evidence related to closed-system suctioning, use of saline solution, management of endotracheal cuff pressures, and oral care. Research-based policies and procedures need to be developed and implemented. This will improve the quality of care for clients.

Note: From *American Journal of Critical Care* by M. L. Sole et al. Copyright 2003 by American Association of Critical-Care Nurses. Reproduced with permission of American Association of Critical-Care Nurses in the format Textbook via Copyright Clearance Center.

PROVIDING TRACHEOSTOMY CARE

PURPOSES
- To maintain airway patency
- To maintain cleanliness and prevent infection at the tracheostomy site
- To facilitate healing and prevent skin excoriation around the tracheostomy incision
- To promote comfort

ASSESSMENT
Assess the following:
- Respiratory status including ease of breathing, rate, rhythm, depth, lung sounds, and oxygen saturation level
- Pulse rate
- Character and amount of secretions from tracheostomy site
- Presence of drainage on tracheostomy dressing or ties
- Appearance of incision (note any redness, swelling, purulent discharge, or odor)

PLANNING

> **Delegation**
> Tracheostomy care involves application of scientific knowledge, sterile technique, and problem solving, and therefore needs to be performed by a nurse or respiratory therapist.

Equipment
- Sterile disposable tracheostomy cleaning kit or supplies including sterile containers, sterile nylon brush and/or pipe cleaners, sterile applicators, gauze squares
- Towel or drape to protect bed linens
- Sterile suction catheter kit (suction catheter and sterile container for solution)
- Sterile normal saline (Check agency protocol for soaking solution.)
- Sterile gloves (2 pairs)
- Clean gloves
- Moisture-proof bag
- Commercially prepared sterile tracheostomy dressing or sterile 4-in. × 4-in. gauze dressing
- Cotton twill ties
- Clean scissors

IMPLEMENTATION
Performance
1. Prior to performing the procedure, introduce self and verify the client's identity using agency protocol. Explain to the client what you are going to do, why it is necessary, and how he or she can cooperate. Provide for a means of communication, such as eye blinking or raising a finger, to indicate pain or distress.
2. Perform hand hygiene and observe other appropriate infection control procedures.
3. Provide for client privacy.
4. Prepare the client and the equipment.
   - Assist the client to a semi-Fowler's or Fowler's position *to promote lung expansion.*
   - Open the tracheostomy kit or sterile basins. Pour the soaking solution and sterile normal saline into separate containers.
   - Establish a sterile field.
   - Open other sterile supplies as needed including sterile applicators, suction kit, and tracheostomy dressing.
5. Suction the tracheostomy tube, if needed.
   - Put a clean glove on your nondominant hand and a sterile glove on your dominant hand (or put on a pair of sterile gloves).
   - Suction the full length of the tracheostomy tube to remove secretions and ensure a patent airway (see Skill 50-3).
   - Rinse the suction catheter and wrap the catheter around your hand, and peel the glove off so that it turns inside out over the catheter.
   - Using the gloved hand, unlock the inner cannula (if present) and remove it by gently pulling it out toward you in line with its curvature. Place the inner cannula in the soaking solution. **Rationale:** *This moistens and loosens dried secretions.*
   - Remove the soiled tracheostomy dressing. Place the soiled dressing in your gloved hand and peel the glove off so that it turns inside out over the dressing. Discard the glove and the dressing.

- Put on sterile gloves. Keep your dominant hand sterile during the procedure.
6. Clean the inner cannula. (See Variation for using a disposable inner cannula.)
   - Remove the inner cannula from the soaking solution.
   - Clean the lumen and entire inner cannula thoroughly using the brush or pipe cleaners moistened with sterile normal saline. ❶ Inspect the cannula for cleanliness by holding it at eye level and looking through it into the light.
   - Rinse the inner cannula thoroughly in the sterile normal saline.
   - After rinsing, gently tap the cannula against the inside edge of the sterile saline container. Use a pipe cleaner folded in half to dry only the inside of the cannula; do not dry the outside. **Rationale:** *This removes excess liquid from the cannula and prevents possible aspiration by the client, while leaving a film of moisture on the outer surface to lubricate the cannula for reinsertion.*

❶ Cleaning the inner cannula with a brush.
Photographer: Elena Dorfman

PROVIDING TRACHEOSTOMY CARE *continued*

7. Replace the inner cannula, securing it in place.
   - Insert the inner cannula by grasping the outer flange and inserting the cannula in the direction of its curvature.
   - Lock the cannula in place by turning the lock (if present) into position to secure the flange of the inner cannula to the outer cannula.
8. Clean the incision site and tube flange.
   - Using sterile applicators or gauze dressings moistened with normal saline, clean the incision site. ❷ Handle the sterile supplies with your dominant hand. Use each applicator or gauze dressing only once and then discard. **Rationale:** *This avoids contaminating a clean area with a soiled gauze dressing or applicator.*
   - Hydrogen peroxide may be used (usually in a half-strength solution mixed with sterile normal saline; use a separate sterile container if this is necessary) to remove crusty secretions. Check agency policy. Thoroughly rinse the cleaned area using gauze squares moistened with sterile normal saline. **Rationale:** *Hydrogen peroxide can be irritating to the skin and inhibit healing if not thoroughly removed.*
   - Clean the flange of the tube in the same manner.
   - Thoroughly dry the client's skin and tube flanges with dry gauze squares.
9. Apply a sterile dressing.
   - Use a commercially prepared tracheostomy dressing of non-raveling material or open and refold a 4-in. × 4-in. gauze dressing into a V shape as shown ❸ in, *A* through *D.* Avoid using cotton-filled gauze squares or cutting the 4-in. × 4-in. gauze. **Rationale:** *Cotton lint or gauze fibers can be aspirated by the client, potentially creating a tracheal abscess.*
   - Place the dressing under the flange of the tracheostomy tube as shown in Figure ❸, *E.*
   - While applying the dressing, ensure that the tracheostomy tube is securely supported. **Rationale:** *Excessive movement of the tracheostomy tube irritates the trachea.*
10. Change the tracheostomy ties.
    - Change as needed to keep the skin clean and dry.
    - Twill tape and specially manufactured Velcro ties are available. Twill tape is inexpensive and readily available; however, it is easily soiled and can trap moisture that leads to irritation of the skin of the neck. Velcro ties are becoming more commonly used. ❹ They are wider, more comfortable, and cause less skin abrasion (American Thoracic Society, 2006).

Two-Strip Method (Twill Tape)
   - Cut two unequal strips of twill tape, one approximately 25 cm (10 in.) long and the other about 50 cm (20 in.) long. **Rationale:** *Cutting one tape longer than the other allows them to be fastened at the side of the neck for easy access and to avoid the pressure of a knot on the skin at the back of the neck.*
   - Cut a 1-cm (0.5-in.) lengthwise slit approximately 2.5 cm (1 in.) from one end of each strip. To do this, fold the end of the tape back onto itself about 2.5 cm (1 in.), then cut a slit in the middle of the tape from its folded edge.
   - Leaving the old ties in place, thread the slit end of one clean tape through the eye of the tracheostomy flange from the bottom side; then thread the long end of the tape through

❷ Using an applicator stick to clean the tracheostomy site.
Photographer: Jenny Thomas

❸ Folding a 4-in. × 4-in. gauze to make a tracheostomy dressing.

❹ A Velcro tracheostomy tie.

continued on page 1392

PROVIDING TRACHEOSTOMY CARE *continued*

the slit, pulling it tight until it is securely fastened to the flange. **Rationale:** *Leaving the old ties in place while securing the clean ties prevents inadvertent dislodging of the tracheostomy tube. Securing tapes in this manner avoids the use of knots, which can come untied or cause pressure and irritation.*

- If old ties are very soiled or it is difficult to thread new ties onto the tracheostomy flange with old ties in place, have an assistant put on a sterile glove and hold the tracheostomy in place while you replace the ties. This is very important because movement of the tube during this procedure may cause irritation and stimulate coughing. Coughing can dislodge the tube if the ties are undone.
- Repeat the process for the second tie.
- Ask the client to flex the neck. Slip the longer tape under the client's neck, place a finger between the tape and the client's neck ⑤, and tie the tapes together at the side of the neck. **Rationale:** *Flexing the neck increases its circumference the way coughing does. Placing a finger under the tie prevents making the tie too tight, which could interfere with coughing or place pressure on the jugular veins.*
- Tie the ends of the tapes using square knots. Cut off any long ends, leaving approximately 1 to 2 cm (0.5 in.). **Rationale:** *Square knots prevent slippage and loosening. Adequate ends beyond the knot prevent the knot from inadvertently untying.*
- Once the clean ties are secured, remove the soiled ties and discard.

One-Strip Method (Twill Tape)

- Cut a length of twill tape 2.5 times the length needed to go around the client's neck from one tube flange to the other.
- Thread one end of the tape into the slot on one side of the flange.
- Bring both ends of the tape together. Take them around the client's neck, keeping them flat and untwisted.
- Thread the end of the tape next to the client's neck through the slot from the back to the front.
- Have the client flex the neck. Tie the loose ends with a square knot at the side of the client's neck, allowing for slack by placing two fingers under the ties as with the two-strip method. Cut off long ends.

11. Tape and pad the tie knot.
- Place a folded 4-in. × 4-in. gauze square under the tie knot, and apply tape over the knot. **Rationale:** *This reduces skin irritation from the knot and prevents confusing the knot with the client's gown ties.*

12. Check the tightness of the ties.
- Frequently check the tightness of the tracheostomy ties and position of the tracheostomy tube. **Rationale:** *Swelling of*

⑤ Placing a finger underneath the tie tape before tying it.

the neck may cause the ties to become too tight, interfering with coughing and circulation. Ties can loosen in restless clients, allowing the tracheostomy tube to extrude from the stoma.

13. Document all relevant information.
- Record suctioning, tracheostomy care, and the dressing change, noting your assessments.

SAMPLE DOCUMENTATION

12/11/2007 0900 Respirations 18–20/min. Lung sounds clear. Able to cough up secretions requiring little suctioning. Inner cannula changed. Trach dressing changed. Minimal amount of sero-sanguinous drainage present. Trach incision area pink to reddish in color 0.2 cm around entire opening. No broken skin noted in the reddened area ———————— J. Garcia, RN

Variation: Using a Disposable Inner Cannula

- Check policy for frequency of changing inner cannula *because standards vary among institutions.*
- Open a new cannula package.
- Using a gloved hand, unlock the current inner cannula (if present) and remove it by gently pulling it out toward you in line with its curvature.
- Check the cannula for amount and type of secretions and discard properly.
- Pick up the new inner cannula touching only the outer locking portion.
- Insert the new inner cannula into the tracheostomy.
- Lock the cannula in place by turning the lock (if present).

EVALUATION

- Perform appropriate follow-up such as determining character and amount of secretions, drainage from the tracheostomy, appearance of the tracheostomy incision, pulse rate and respiratory status compared to baseline data, and complaints of pain or discomfort at the tracheostomy site.

- Relate findings to previous assessment data if available.
- Report significant deviations from normal to the primary care provider.

LIFESPAN CONSIDERATIONS **Tracheostomy Care**

INFANTS AND CHILDREN
- An assistant should *always* be present while tracheostomy care is performed.
- Always keep a sterile, packaged tracheostomy tube taped to the child's bed so that if the tube dislodges, a new one is available for immediate reintubation (Bindler & Ball, 2003, p. 95).

ELDERS
- Older adult skin is more fragile and prone to breakdown. Care of the skin at the tracheostomy stoma is very important.

HOME CARE CONSIDERATIONS **Tracheostomy Care**

- For tracheostomies older than 1 month, clean technique (rather than sterile technique) is used for tracheostomy care.
- Stress the importance of good hand hygiene to the caregiver.
- Tap water may be used for rinsing the inner cannula.
- Teach the caregiver the tracheostomy care procedure and observe a return demonstration. Periodically reassess caregiver knowledge and/or tracheostomy care technique.
- Inform the caregiver of the signs and symptoms that may indicate an infection of the stoma site or lower airway.
- Names and telephone numbers of health care personnel who can be reached for emergencies or advice must be available to the client and/or caregiver.
- If the tracheostomy is permanent, provide contact information for available support groups.

Chest Tubes and Drainage Systems

If the thin, double-layered pleural membrane is disrupted by lung disease, surgery, or trauma, the negative pressure between the pleural layers may be lost. The lung then collapses because it is no longer drawn outward as the diaphragm and intercostal muscles contract during inhalation. When air collects in the pleural space, it is known as a **pneumothorax.** Blood or fluid in the pleural space, a **hemothorax,** places pressure on lung tissue and interferes with lung expansion. Chest tubes may be inserted into the pleural cavity to restore negative pressure and drain collected fluid or blood. Because air rises, chest tubes for pneumothorax often are placed in the upper anterior thorax, whereas chest tubes used to drain fluid generally are placed in the lower lateral chest wall.

When chest tubes are inserted, they must be connected to a sealed drainage system or a one-way valve that allows air and fluid to be removed from the chest cavity but prevents air from entering from the outside. Sterile disposable drainage systems are used to prevent outside air from entering the chest tube. These systems typically have a suction control chamber, a water seal chamber, and a closed collection chamber, for drainage (Figure 50-32 ■). With the water-seal system, when the client inhales, the water prevents air from entering the system from the atmosphere. During exhalation, however, air can exit the chest cavity, bubbling up through the water. Suction can be added to the system to facilitate removing air and secretions from the chest cavity. The drainage system should always be kept below the level of the client's chest to prevent fluid and drainage from being drawn back into the chest cavity.

A Heimlich valve may be used for ambulatory clients (Figure 50-33 ■). The Heimlich valve is a one-way flutter valve that allows air to escape from the chest cavity, but prevents air from reentering. The arrow on the housing of the valve should always point away from the client. At each assessment, observe the inner

Figure 50-32 ■ A disposable chest drainage system.
(Pleur-evac® Chest Drainage System. Reprinted with permission from Genzyme Biosurgery, Cardiothoracic Division, Fall River, MA.)

Figure 50-33 ■ Heimlich chest drain valve.

valve carefully for movement during exhalation, indicating air-flow through the device (Carroll, 2005, p. 29). The Heimlich valve is not designed to collect fluid. Another device that can at-tach to the chest tube, called the Pneumostat, also has a one-way valve and, unlike the Heimlich valve, a small built-in collection chamber. It is used exclusively for clients with a pneumothorax who usually have small amounts of fluid (Figure 50-34 ■).

Nursing responsibilities regarding drainage systems include the following:

■ Monitor and maintain the patency and integrity of the drainage system.

■ Assess the client's vital signs, oxygen saturation, cardiovascular status, and respiratory status. Check the breath sounds bilaterally and check for symmetry of breath sounds.

■ Observe the dressing site at least every 4 hours. Inspect the dressing for excessive and abnormal drainage, such as bleeding or foul-smelling discharge. Palpate around the dressing site, and listen for a crackling sound indicative of subcutaneous emphysema. *Subcutaneous emphysema, which is air in the subcutaneous tissues, can result from a poor seal at the chest tube insertion site.*

■ Determine level of discomfort with and without activity and medicate the client for pain if indicated.

■ Encourage deep breathing and coughing exercises every 2 hours (this may be contraindicated in clients who have had a

Figure 50-34 ■ The Pneumostat is an example of a device often used for clients with a pneumothorax. It uses a one-way valve and has a small collection chamber.

lung removed). Have the client sit upright to perform the exercises, and splint the chest around the tube insertion site with a pillow or with a hand to minimize discomfort.

■ Reposition the client every 2 hours. When the client is lying on the affected side, place rolled towels beside the tubing. *Frequent position changes promote drainage, prevent complications, and provide comfort. Rolled towels prevent occlusion of the chest tube by the client's weight.*

■ Assist the client with range-of-motion exercises of the affected shoulder three times per day to maintain joint mobility.

■ Ensure that the connections are securely taped and that the chest tube is secured to the client's chest wall.

■ Keep the collection device below the client's chest level.

■ Frequently check the water seal and suction control chambers. The water can evaporate and water may need to be added to the chamber. The water seal level should fluctuate with respiratory effort (Coughlin & Parchinsky, 2006).

■ Assess the drainage in the tubing and collection chamber. The drainage is measured at regularly scheduled times (check the agency policy). Mark the date and time at the fluid level on the drainage chamber. The unit is not replaced until almost full.

■ Avoid aggressive chest tube manipulation (e.g., milking or stripping the tube). Studies have shown that these techniques do not improve chest tube patency. If necessary, however, a gentle technique such as squeezing hand over hand along the tubing and releasing the tubing between squeezes may help improve patency (Coughlin & Parchinsky, 2006, p. 40).

■ Avoid clamping the chest tube as this increases the risk of a tension pneumothorax. You can clamp the tube for a moment to replace the drainage unit or to locate the source of an air leak, but never when transporting a client or for any extended period of time (Coughlin & Parchinsky, 2006, p. 40).

■ If the tube becomes disconnected from the collecting system, submerge the end in 1 in. of sterile saline or water *to maintain the seal.* If the chest tube is inadvertently pulled out, the wound should be immediately covered with a dry sterile dressing. If you can hear air leaking out the site, ensure that the dressing is not occlusive. *If the air cannot escape, this would lead to a tension pneumothorax. A tension pneumothorax occurs when there is buildup of air in the pleural space and it cannot escape, causing increased pressure. This pressure can eventually compromise cardiovascular function.*

■ When transporting and ambulating the client:
   a. Keep the water-seal unit below chest level and upright.
   b. Disconnect the drainage system from the suction apparatus before moving the client and make sure the air vent is open.

■ Use standard precautions and personal protective equipment while manipulating the system and assisting with insertion or removal.

Chest tube insertion and removal require sterile technique and must be done without introducing air or microorganisms into the pleural cavity. Removal of a chest tube is a brief but quite painful procedure. Medicate the client before the removal. Remove the dressing around the tube and prepare the dressing that will cover the insertion site. This will be an occlusive dressing if there is no purse-string suture around the insertion site to prevent air from entering the chest. Generally, the primary care provider performs the removal but, in some areas, specially trained nurses may be permitted to do so.

Evaluating

Using the goals and desired outcomes identified in the planning stage of the nursing process, the nurse collects data to evaluate the effectiveness of interventions. If outcomes are not achieved, the nurse, client, and support person if appropriate need to explore the reasons before modifying the care plan. For example, if the outcome "Respirations unlabored and rate is within expected range" is not met, examples of questions that need to be considered include the following:

- What is the client's perception of the problem?
- Is the client complaining of shortness of breath or difficulty breathing?

- Is the client taking medications or performing treatments such as percussion, vibration, and postural drainage as prescribed?
- Has the client been exposed to an upper respiratory infection that is affecting breathing?
- Do other factors need to be considered, such as the client's psychologic stress level?

Examples of questions to consider if the outcome "Able to complete ADLs without fatigue" is not met include the following:

- What other factors may be affecting the client's ability to complete ADLs?
- Is the client getting adequate sleep? If not, what is interfering with the client's rest?
- Are there assistive devices (e.g., a shower chair, clothing that is easy to put on) that could help the client achieve this goal?
- Does the client need help with housework and other ADLs?
- Is the client's diet adequate to meet nutritional needs?

NURSING CARE PLAN   For Ineffective Airway Clearance

ASSESSMENT DATA	NURSING DIAGNOSIS	DESIRED OUTCOMES*
Nursing Assessment Johti Singh is a 39-year-old secretary who was admitted to the hospital with an elevated temperature, fatigue, rapid, labored respirations; and mild dehydration. The nursing history reveals that Ms. Singh has had a "bad cold" for several weeks that just wouldn't go away. She has been dieting for several months and skipping meals. Ms. Singh mentions that in addition to her full-time job as a secretary she is attending college classes two evenings a week. She has smoked one package of cigarettes per day since she was 18 years old. Chest x-ray confirms pneumonia.	*Ineffective Airway Clearance* related to thick sputum, secondary to pneumonia (as evidenced by rapid respirations, diminished and adventitious breath sounds, thick yellow sputum)	Respiratory Status: Airway Patency [0410] as evidenced by not compromised ■ Respiratory rate ■ Moves sputum out of airway ■ No adventitious breath sounds

Physical Examination

Height: 167.6 cm (5'6")
Weight: 54.4 kg (120 lb)
Temperature: 39.4°C (103°F)
Pulse: 68 BPM
Respirations: 24/minute
Blood pressure:
118/70 mm Hg
Skin pale; cheeks flushed; chills; use of accessory muscles; inspiratory crackles with diminished breath sounds right base; expectorating thick, yellow sputum

Diagnostic Data

Chest x-ray: right lobar infiltration
WBC: 14,000
pH: 7.49
$PaCO_2$: 33 mm Hg
HCO_3^-: 20 mEq/L
PaO_2: 80 mm Hg
O_2 sat: 88%

NURSING INTERVENTIONS*/SELECTED ACTIVITIES	RATIONALE
Cough Enhancement [3250]	
Assist Ms. Singh to a sitting position with head slightly flexed, shoulders relaxed, and knees flexed.	*Lying flat causes the abdominal organs to shift toward the chest, crowding the lungs and making it more difficult to breathe.*

NURSING CARE PLAN For Ineffective Airway Clearance *continued*

NURSING INTERVENTIONS*/SELECTED ACTIVITIES	RATIONALE
Encourage her to take several deep breaths.	Deep breathing promotes oxygenation before controlled coughing.
Encourage her to take a deep breath, hold for 2 seconds, and cough two or three times in succession.	Controlled coughing is accomplished by closure of the glottis and the explosive expulsion of air from the lungs by the work of abdominal and chest muscles.
Encourage use of incentive spirometry, as appropriate.	Breathing exercises help maximize ventilation.
Promote systemic fluid hydration, as appropriate.	Adequate fluid intake enhances liquefaction of pulmonary secretions and facilitates expectoration of mucus.
Respiratory Monitoring [3350]	
Monitor rate, rhythm, depth, and effort of respirations.	Provides a basis for evaluating adequacy of ventilation.
Note chest movement, watching for symmetry, use of accessory muscles, and supraclavicular and intercostal muscle retractions.	Presence of nasal flaring and use of accessory muscles of respirations may occur in response to ineffective ventilation.
Auscultate breath sounds, noting areas of decreased or absent ventilation and presence of adventitious sounds.	As fluid and mucus accumulate, abnormal breath sounds can be heard including crackles and diminished breath sounds owing to fluid-filled air spaces and diminished lung volume.
Auscultate lung sounds after treatments to note results.	Assists in evaluating prescribed treatments and client outcomes.
Monitor client's ability to cough effectively.	Respiratory tract infections alter the amount and character of secretions. An ineffective cough compromises airway clearance and prevents mucus from being expelled.
Monitor client's respiratory secretions.	People with pneumonia commonly produce rust-colored, purulent sputum.
Institute respiratory therapy treatments (e.g., nebulizer) as needed.	A variety of respiratory therapy treatments may be used to open constricted airways and liquefy secretions.
Monitor for increased restlessness, anxiety, and air hunger.	These clinical manifestations would be early indicators of hypoxia.
Note changes in SpO_2, tidal volume, and changes in arterial blood gas values, as appropriate.	Evaluates the status of oxygenation, ventilation, and acid–base balance.

EVALUATION

Outcome partially met. Ms. Singh coughs and deep breathes purposefully q1–2h during the day. Her fluid intake is approximately 1,500 mL each day. Cough continues to be productive of moderately thick, rusty-colored sputum. Inspiratory crackles remain present in right lower lobe.

The NOC # for desired outcomes and the NIC # for nursing interventions are listed in brackets following the appropriate outcome or intervention. Outcomes, interventions and activities selected are only a sample of those by NOC and NIC and should be further individualized for each client.

APPLYING CRITICAL THINKING

1. What factors may have led the medical staff to suspect that Ms. Singh had more than a very bad cold? Would you have come to the same conclusion?
2. The care plan appropriately focuses on the acute care of this client. Once she is significantly improved, the nurse will perform discharge teaching. What areas should be included?
3. The client already has some signs of respiratory distress. What signs might indicate that her condition was deteriorating into a more emergency situation? How would you handle this?
4. It appears that the client's sputum has not been cultured. In caring for this client, what infection control guidelines would be needed?
5. Ms. Singh's oxygen order is for a face mask at 6 L/minute. She repeatedly pulls it off and you find it lying in the sheets. How might you intervene?

See Critical Thinking Possibilities in Appendix A.

CONCEPT MAP Ineffective Airway Clearance

JS
39 y.o. female
Pneumonia

→ assess →

- Increased temperature; fatigue; rapid, labored respirations; mild dehydration. "Bad cold" X several weeks. Dieting for several months and skipping meals. Works full-time job as secretary, college classes 2x/week. Smokes, 21 pack/years.

- Height: 167.6 cm (5' 6")
- Weight: 54.4 kg (120 lbs)
- TPR: 39.4°C (103°F), 68, 24
- BP: 118/70
- Skin pale; cheeks flushed; chills; use of accessory muscles, inspiratory crackles with diminished breath sounds at right base; expectorating thick, yellow sputum

- Chest x-ray: right lobar infiltrate
- WBC: 14,000
- pH: 7.49
- $PaCO_2$: 33 mm Hg
- HCO_3: 20 mEG/L
- PaO_2: 80 mm Hg

↓ generate nursing diagnosis

Ineffective Airway Clearance r/t thick sputum, secondary to pneumonia
(aeb rapid respirations, diminished and adventitious breath sounds, thick, yellow sputum)

↓ outcome

Respiratory Status: Airway Patency aeb not compromised
- Respiratory rate
- Moves sputum out of airway
- No adventitious breath sounds

→ evaluation →

Outcomes partially met:
- Coughs and deep breaths purposefully q 1–2 hr during the day
- Fluid intake approximately 1500 mL/day
- Cough productive of moderately thick, rusty-colored sputum
- Inspiratory crackles remain present in RLL

nursing intervention

Cough Enhancement

nursing intervention

Respiratory Monitoring

activity

Assist to a sitting position with head slightly flexed, shoulders relaxed, and knees flexed

activity

Promote systemic fluid hydration, as appropriate

activity

Encourage her to take several deep breaths

activity

Encourage her to take a deep breath, hold for 2 seconds, and cough two or three times in succession

activity

Encourage use of incentive spirometry, as appropriate

activity

Monitor rate, rhythm, depth, and effort of respirations

activity

Note chest movement, watching for symmetry, use of accessory muscles, and supraclavicular and intercostal muscle retractions

activity

Auscultate breath sounds, noting areas of decreased or absent ventilation and presence of adventitious sounds

activity

Monitor respiratory secretions

activity

Monitor ability to cough effectively

activity

Note changes in SpO_2, and changes in ABG values, as appropriate

CHAPTER 50 **REVIEW**

CHAPTER HIGHLIGHTS

- Respiration is the process of gas exchange between the individual and the environment.
- The respiratory system contributes to effective respiration through pulmonary ventilation (the movement of air between the atmosphere and the lungs), the diffusion of oxygen and carbon dioxide across the pulmonary membrane, and transport of oxygen from the lungs to the tissues and carbon dioxide from the tissues to the lungs.
- Alveoli and the capillaries that surround them form the respiratory membrane, where gas exchange between the lungs and the blood occurs.
- Effective pulmonary ventilation, or breathing, requires clear airways, an intact central nervous system and respiratory center, an intact thoracic cavity and musculature, and adequate pulmonary compliance (stretch) and recoil.
- Gas exchange occurs by diffusion, as gas molecules move from an area of higher concentration to an area of lower concentration. At the respiratory membrane, oxygen moves from the alveolus into the blood, while carbon dioxide moves from the blood into the alveolus.
- Most oxygen (97%) is carried to the tissues loosely combined with hemoglobin in red blood cells (RBCs). Anemia, which is too few RBCs or low hemoglobin levels, impairs oxygen transportation.
- Respiratory rates normally are highest in neonates and infants, gradually slowing to adult ranges.
- Aging affects the respiratory system: The chest wall becomes more rigid and lungs less elastic.
- Other factors affecting oxygenation include the environment, lifestyle, health status, narcotic analgesics, and stress and coping.
- Hypoxia, insufficient oxygen in the tissues, can result from impaired ventilation (hypoventilation) or diffusion, or from impaired oxygen transportation to the tissues because of anemia or decreased cardiac output.
- Normal respirations are quiet and unlabored; altered respiratory patterns include tachypnea, bradypnea, hyperventilation, hypoventilation, and dyspnea. Shortness of breath is a subjective sensation of not getting enough air.
- Airway obstruction interferes with ventilation. A low-pitched snoring sound, stridor, and abnormal breath sounds may accompany partial airway obstruction. Extreme inspiratory effort with no chest movement indicates complete upper airway obstruction.
- The nursing history includes questions about current or past respiratory problems and about lifestyle, presence of symptoms such as cough or shortness of breath, smoking and other risk factors, and medications.
- Physical assessment should include a general assessment, as well as specific examination of the respiratory system.
- Diagnostic tests that may be performed to assess oxygenation include sputum and throat culture specimens; blood tests such as arterial blood gases; pulmonary function tests; and visualization procedures such as x-rays, lung scans, laryngoscopy, and bronchoscopy.
- Nursing diagnoses for the client with problems of oxygenation include *Ineffective Airway Clearance, Ineffective Breathing Pattern, Impaired Gas Exchange,* and *Activity Intolerance.* These problems also may be the etiology for several other nursing diagnoses, including *Anxiety, Fatigue, Fear, Powerlessness, Sleep Pattern Disturbance,* and *Social Isolation.*
- In discharge and home care planning, the nurse assesses the client's self-care abilities and need for assistive devices, home environment, compliance with medical regimen, and knowledge level. The ability of the family or support people to provide assistance and financial support and to cope with the changes is also assessed, as are community factors like the environment and resources.
- The nurse teaches the client about home care activities to maintain a patent airway and gas exchange and to promote healthy breathing. Dietary modifications, prescribed medications, and specific procedures also are taught, and the nurse makes referrals to community agencies as needed.
- Nursing interventions to promote oxygenation include promoting healthy breathing and a healthy heart, deep breathing and coughing, and hydration; administering medications; implementing measures to clear secretions (e.g., incentive spirometry, percussion, vibration, and postural drainage); initiating and monitoring oxygen therapy; initiating or assisting with procedures to maintain the airway (e.g., artificial airways and suctioning); providing tracheostomy care; and monitoring chest drainage systems.
- The effectiveness of nursing interventions is evaluated by using the goals and desired outcomes identified in the planning stage of the nursing process. If a goal is not met, the nurse asks pertinent questions to assess the reason for not meeting the goal.

TEST YOUR KNOWLEDGE

1. A client with chronic pulmonary disease has a bluish tinge around the lips. Which of the following most accurately describes the client's condition?
   1. Hypoxia
   2. Hypoxemia
   3. Dyspnea
   4. Cyanosis

2. To prevent postoperative complications the nurse assists the client with coughing and deep breathing exercises. This is best accomplished by implementing which of the following?
   1. Coughing exercises 1 hour before meals and deep breathing 1 hour after meals
   2. Forceful coughing as many times as tolerated
   3. Huff coughing every 2 hours or as needed
   4. Diaphragmatic and pursed-lip breathing 5 to 10 times four times a day

3. A client with a chronic lung disorder requires some supplemental oxygen. The nurse ensures consistent and safe delivery with which of the following?
   1. 2 L/min per nasal cannula
   2. 6 L/min per face mask
   3. 8 L/min per partial rebreather mask
   4. 10 L/min per nonrebreather mask

4. Which of the following represents proper nasopharyngeal/nasotracheal suction technique?
   1. Lubricate the suction catheter with petroleum jelly before and between insertions.
   2. Apply suction intermittently while inserting the suction catheter.
   3. Rotate the catheter while applying suction.
   4. Hyperoxygenate with 100% oxygen for 30 minutes before and after suctioning.

5. The client demonstrates knowledge of the proper use of an incentive spirometer when which of the following statements is made?
   1. "I should breathe out as fast and hard as possible into the device."
   2. "I should inhale slowly and steadily to keep the balls up."
   3. "I should use the device three times a day, after meals."
   4. "The entire device should be washed thoroughly in sudsy water once a week."

6. While a client with chest tubes is ambulating, the connection between the tube and the water seal dislodges. Which of the following actions by the nurse is most appropriate?
   1. Assist the client to ambulate back to bed.
   2. Reconnect the tube to the water seal.
   3. Assess the client's lung sounds with a stethoscope.
   4. Have the client cough forcibly several times.

7. Which of the following clients is most at risk for a problem with the transport of oxygen from the lungs to the tissues?
   1. A client who has anemia
   2. A client who has an infection
   3. A client who has a fractured rib
   4. A client who has a tumor of the medulla

8. Which of the following terms is most descriptive of a client experiencing dyspnea when lying down and must assume an upright or sitting position to breathe more comfortably and effectively?
   1. Dyspnea
   2. Hyperpnea
   3. Orthopnea
   4. Acapnea

9. A client with emphysema is prescribed corticosteroid therapy on a short-term basis for acute bronchitis. What would be the rationale for the use of steroids in clients with bronchitis?
   1. Corticosteroids promote bronchodilation.
   2. Corticosteroids help the client to cough.
   3. Corticosteroids prevent respiratory infection.
   4. Corticosteroids decrease inflammation in the airways.

10. The nurse is planning to perform percussion and postural drainage. Which of following is an important aspect of planning the client's care?
   1. Percussion and postural drainage should be done before lunch.
   2. The order should be coughing, percussion, positioning, and then suctioning.
   3. A good time to perform percussion and postural drainage is in the morning after breakfast when the client is well rested.
   4. Percussion and postural drainage should always be preceded by 3 minutes of 100% oxygen.

See Answers to Test Your Knowledge in Appendix A.

EXPLORE MEDIALINK www.prenhall.com/berman

DVD-ROM
- Audio Glossary
- NCLEX Review
- Skills Checklists
- Animations:
   Gas Exchange in the Lung
   Carbon Dioxide Transport
   Oxygen Transport
   Pulmonary Diseases
   A & P Review
- Videos:
   Incentive Spirometer
   Humidifier
   Nasal Cannula
   Face Mask
   Nonrebreather Mask

COMPANION WEBSITE
- Additional NCLEX Review
- Case Study: Coping with Emphysema
- Care Plan Activity: Deep Breathing and Coughing
- Application Activities:
   Learning About Lung Disease
   Tracheostomy Nursing Care
- Links to Resources

READINGS AND REFERENCES

SUGGESTED READINGS

Celik, S. A., & Kanan, N. (2006). A current conflict: Use of isotonic sodium chloride solution on endotracheal suctioning in critically ill patients. *Dimensions of Critical Care Nursing, 25*(1), 11–14. *Instilling sterile isotonic sodium chloride solution into the endotracheal tube before suctioning has been a widespread practice* over the past few years. Researchers have demonstrated that this is a risk for the client; however, it continues to be a common practice. The authors review the literature and research and conclude with recommendations for clinical practice.

Coughlin, A. M., & Parchinsky, C. (2006). Go with the flow of chest tube therapy. *Nursing, 36*(3), 36–41.

This in-depth article describes the reasons for chest tube placement and the various types of chest drainage units. Risks, complications, and important client assessments are very helpful. It also includes steps for the nurse to assist with chest tube insertion and removal.

Pruitt, B., & Jacobs, M. (2005). Clearing away pulmonary secretions. *Nursing, 35*(7), 37–41.

The authors, an RN and a respiratory therapist, review which clients are at greatest risk for excess or retained pulmonary secretions. They also provide helpful assessments and interventions to keep airways clear.

St. John, R. E., & Malen, J. F. (2004). Contemporary issues in adult tracheostomy management. *Critical Care Nursing Clinics of North America, 16*(3), 413–430.
This excellent article provides an overview of the indications, techniques of insertion, and types of tracheostomy tubes. It then addresses specific aspects of nursing care of clients with tracheostomy tubes.

RELATED RESEARCH

Corff, K. E., & McCann, D. L. (2005). Room air resuscitation versus oxygen resuscitation in the delivery room. *Journal of Perinatal & Neonatal Nursing, 19*(4), 379–390.

Demir, F., & Dramali, A. (2005). Requirement for 100% oxygen before and after closed suction. *Journal of Advanced Nursing, 51*(3), 245–251.

Oh, H., & Seo, W. (2003). A meta-analysis of the effects of various interventions in preventing endotracheal suction-induced hypoxemia. *Journal of Clinical Nursing, 12,* 912–924.

Pitta, F., Troosters, T., Spruit, M. A., Probst, V. S., Decramer, M., & Gosselink, R. (2005). Characteristics of physical activities in daily life in chronic obstructive pulmonary disease. *American Journal of Respiratory and Critical Care Medicine, 171*(9), 972–978.

Wu, H., Wu, S., Lin, J., & Lin, L. (2004). Effectiveness of acupressure in improving dyspnea in chronic obstructive pulmonary disease. *Journal of Advanced Nursing, 45*(3), 252–259.

REFERENCES

American Thoracic Society. (2006). Tracheostomy tube care. Retrieved July 9, 2006, from http://www.thoracic.org/sections/education/care-of-the-child-with-a-chronic-tracheostomy/components-of-tracheostomy-care/tracheostomy-tube-care.html

Bindler, R. C., & Ball, J. W. (2003). *Clinical skills manual for pediatric nursing: Caring for children* (3rd ed.). Upper Saddle River, NJ: Prentice Hall Health.

Carroll, P. (2005). Keeping up with mobile chest drains. *RN, 68*(10), 26–31.

Dochterman, J. M., & McCloskey, J. C. (Eds.). (2004). *Nursing interventions classification (NIC)* (4th ed.). St. Louis, MO: Mosby.

Moorhead, S., Johnson, M., & Maas, M. (Eds.). (2004). *Nursing outcomes classification (NOC)* (3rd ed.). St. Louis, MO: Mosby.

NANDA International. (2007). *NANDA nursing diagnoses: Definitions and classification 2007–2008.* Philadelphia: Author.

Sole, M. L., Byers, J. F., Ludy, J. E., Zhang, Y., Banta, C. M., & Brummel, K. (2003). A multisite survey of suctioning techniques and airway management practices. *American Journal of Critical Care, 12*(3), 220–230.

St. John, R. E. (2004). Airway management. *Critical Care Nurse, 24*(2), 93–96.

SELECTED BIBLIOGRAPHY

Andrs, K. (2004). Chest drainage to go. *Nursing, 34*(5), 54–55.

Astle, S. M., & Caulfield, E. V. (2003). Bedside tracheostomy: A step by step guide. *RN, 66*(10), 41–45.

Coleman, P. R. (2004). Pneumonia in the long-term care setting: Etiology, management, and prevention. *Journal of Gerontological Nursing, 30*(4), 14–24.

Covey, M. K., & Larson, J. L. (2004). Exercise and COPD. *American Journal of Nursing, 104*(5), 40–43.

Dulak, S. B. (2005). Hands-on help: Removing chest tubes. *RN, 68*(8), 28ac1–28ac4.

Dulak, S. B. (2005). Hands-on help: Sputum sample collection. *RN, 68*(10), 24ac2–24ac4.

Hockman, R. H. (2004). Pharmacologic therapy for acute exacerbations of chronic obstructive pulmonary disease: A review. *Critical Care Nursing Clinics of North America, 16*(3), 293–310.

Keith, D. D., Garrett, K. M., Hickox, G., Echols, B., & Comeau, E. (2004). Ventilator-associated pneumonia: Improved clinical outcomes. *Journal of Nursing Care Quality, 19*(4), 328–344.

Lehne, R. A. (2004). *Pharmacology for nursing care* (5th ed.). St. Louis, MO: W. B. Saunders.

Puritt, B. (2005). Clear the air with closed suctioning. *Nursing, 35*(7), 4–45.

Pruitt, W. C. (2005). Teaching your patient to use a peak flowmeter. *Nursing, 35*(3), 54–55.

Pruitt, W. C., & Jacobs, M. (2003). Basics of oxygen therapy. *Nursing, 33*(10), 43–45.

Roman, M. (2005). Tracheostomy tubes. *Medsurg Nursing, 14*(2), 143–145.

Roman, M., & Mercado, D. (2006). Review of chest tube use. *Medsurg Nursing, 15*(1), 41–43.

Russell, C. (2005). Providing the nurse with a guide to tracheostomy care and management. *British Journal of Nursing, 14*(8), 428–433.

Warren, M. L., Jarrett, C., Senegal, R., Parker, A., Kraus, J., & Hartgraves, D. (2004). An interdisciplinary approach to transitioning ventilator-dependent patients to home. *Journal of Nursing Care Quality, 19*(1), 67–72.

Circulation

LEARNING OUTCOMES

After completing this chapter, you will be able to:

1. Outline the structure and function of the cardiovascular system.

2. Identify factors influencing cardiovascular function.

3. Identify major risk factors for the development of coronary heart disease.

4. Discuss the manifestations of cardiovascular disorders.

5. Identify common responses to alterations in cardiovascular status.

6. List signs of alterations in cardiovascular function.

7. Identify and describe nursing measures to promote circulation.

8. Describe the critical nature of cardiopulmonary resuscitation.

The circulatory system or cardiovascular system is responsible for transport of oxygen, fluids, electrolytes, and products of metabolism via the blood to and from tissues.

PHYSIOLOGY OF THE CARDIOVASCULAR SYSTEM

The respiratory and cardiovascular systems are closely linked and dependent on one another to deliver oxygen to the tissues of the body. Alterations in function of either system can affect the other and lead to tissue hypoxia, or lack of oxygen.

The heart and the blood vessels make up the cardiovascular system. Together with blood, it is the major transport system of the body, bringing oxygen and nutrients to the cells and removing wastes for disposal. The heart serves as the system pump, moving blood through the vessels to the tissues.

The Heart

The heart is a hollow, cone-shaped organ about the size of a fist. It is located in the mediastinum, between the lungs and underlying the sternum. It is enclosed by a double layer of fibroserous membrane known as the **pericardium.** The parietal, or outermost, pericardium serves to protect the heart and anchor it to surrounding structures. The visceral pericardium adheres to the surface of the heart, forming the heart's outermost layer, the **epicardium.** The heart wall contains two additional layers: the **myocardium,** cardiac muscle cells that form the bulk of the heart and contract with each beat, and the **endocardium,** which lines the inside of the heart's chambers and great vessels (Figure 51-1 ■).

Four hollow chambers within the heart, two upper **atria** and two lower **ventricles,** are separated longitudinally by the interventricular **septum,** forming two parallel pumps. The atria and

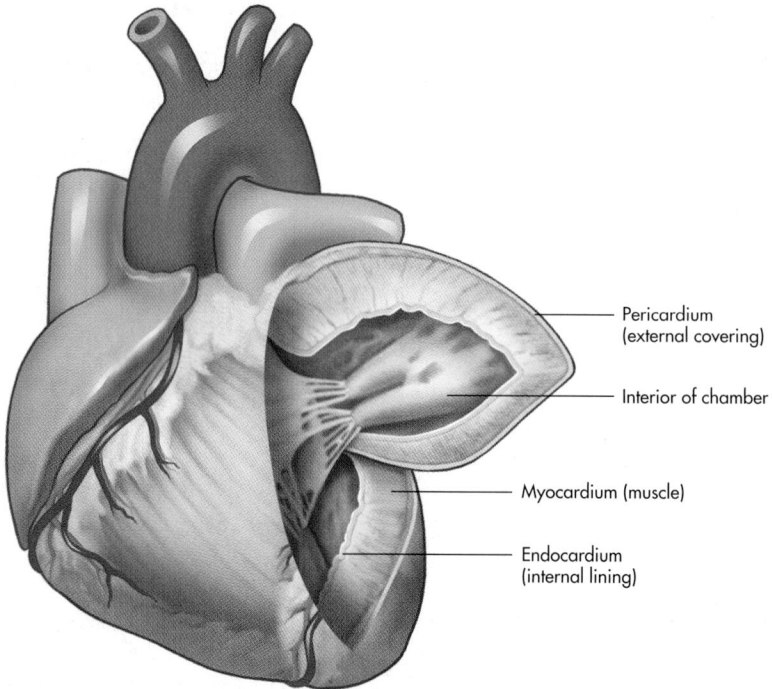

Pericardium (external covering)

Interior of chamber

Myocardium (muscle)

Endocardium (internal lining)

Figure 51-1 ■ The layers of the heart: the epicardium, the myocardium, and the endocardium.

Figure 51-2 ■ Heart valves in closed position viewed from the top.

From Rice, Jane, *Medical Terminology with Human Anatomy*, 5th ed., © 2005. Reproduced by permission of Pearson Education, Inc., Upper Saddle River, New Jersey.

ventricles are separated from one another by the **atrioventricular (AV) valves,** the tricuspid valve on the right and the bicuspid or mitral valve on the left. The valves are named for the number of cusps (or leaflets) present on the valve. The ventricles, in turn, are separated from the great vessels (the pulmonary arteries and aorta) by the **semilunar valves** (named for their crescent moon shape): the pulmonic valve on the right and the aortic valve on the left. The valves serve to direct the flow of blood, allowing it to move from the atria to the ventricles, and the ventricles to the great vessels, but preventing backflow (Figure 51-2 ■).

Deoxygenated blood from the veins enters the right side of the heart through the superior and inferior venae cavae (singular is vena cava). From there, it flows into the right ventricle, which pumps it through the pulmonary artery into the lungs for gas exchange at the alveolar/capillary membrane. Freshly oxygenated blood returns to the left atrium via the pulmonary veins. From here, the blood enters the left ventricle to be pumped out to the systemic circulation through the aorta (Figure 51-3 ■).

Coronary Circulation

The heart muscle moves blood to the lungs and peripheral tissues but receives no oxygen or nourishment from the blood within its chambers. Instead, it is supplied by a network of vessels known as the coronary circulation or more commonly the **coronary arteries.** The coronary arteries originate at the base of the aorta, branching out to encircle and penetrate the myocardium. The coronary arteries fill during ventricular relaxation, bringing oxygen-rich blood to the myocardium (Figure 51-4 ■). If these arteries become clogged with atherosclerotic plaque or are obstructed by a blood clot, the myocardium is deprived of oxygen, and the client may develop chest pain (angina) or experience a myocardial infarction (heart attack). The cardiac veins drain the deoxygenated blood from the myocardium into the coronary sinus, which empties into the right atrium.

Cardiac Cycle

With each heartbeat, the myocardium goes through a cycle of contraction (*systole*) and relaxation (*diastole*). **Systole** is when the heart ejects (propels) the blood into the pulmonary and systemic circulations. **Diastole** is when the ventricles fill with blood. The diastolic phase of the cardiac cycle is twice as long as the systolic phase. This is important because diastole (or ventricular filling) is largely a passive process. The longer diastolic phase allows this filling to occur. At the end of the diastolic phase the atria contract, adding an additional volume to the ventricles. This volume is sometimes called *atrial kick.* The relationship between the phases of the cardiac cycle and the normal heart sounds is described in Table 51–1.

Cardiac Conduction System

Cardiac muscle contraction is a mechanical event that occurs in response to electrical stimulation. Cardiac muscle is unique in that, unlike skeletal muscle, it can generate an electrical impulse and contraction independently of the nervous system. This unique property of the heart is called **automaticity.** A network of specialized cells and pathways known as the cardiac conduction system normally controls the electrical activity and contraction of the heart.

The primary pacemaker of the heart is the **sinoatrial (SA or sinus) node,** located where the superior vena cava enters the right atrium. The SA node normally initiates electrical impulses that are conducted throughout the heart and result in ventricular contraction. In adults, it usually discharges impulses at a regular rate of 60 to 100 times per minute, the "normal" heart rate. The impulse then spreads throughout the atria via the interatrial pathways. These conduction pathways converge and narrow through the **atrioventricular (AV) node,** slightly delaying transmission of the impulse to the ventricles. This delay allows the atria to contract slightly before ventricular contraction occurs. From the AV node, the impulse then progresses down through the intraventricular septum to the ventricular conduction pathways: the

Figure 51-3 ■ Blood flow through the heart. The diagram shows the vena cava, right atrium (1), tricuspid valve (2), right ventricle (3), pulmonic valve, pulmonary arteries, pulmonary veins, left atrium (4), mitral valve (5), left ventricle (6), aortic valve, and the aorta.

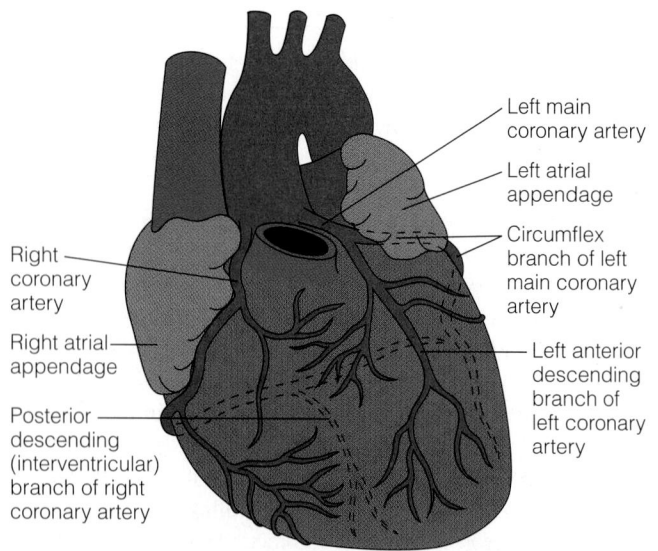

Figure 51-4 ■ The coronary arteries supply the heart muscle with oxygenated blood.

TABLE 51–1	**Cardiac Cycle and Heart Sounds**
SOUND	**PHASE OF CARDIAC CYCLE**
S$_1$—first sound	Beginning of ventricular systole; the sound is caused by closure of the atrioventricular valves—the tricuspid and the mitral
S$_2$—second sound	Beginning of ventricular diastole; the sound is caused by closure of the semilunar valves—the aortic and pulmonic

bundle of His, the right and left bundle branches, and the **Purkinje fibers.** These fibers terminate in ventricular muscle, stimulating contraction (Figure 51-5 ■).

Cardiac Output

As the ventricles contract during systole, blood flows out of the ventricles through the aorta and pulmonary artery into the systemic and pulmonic circulation. The heart muscle then relaxes (the diastolic phase), allowing the ventricles to refill and cardiac

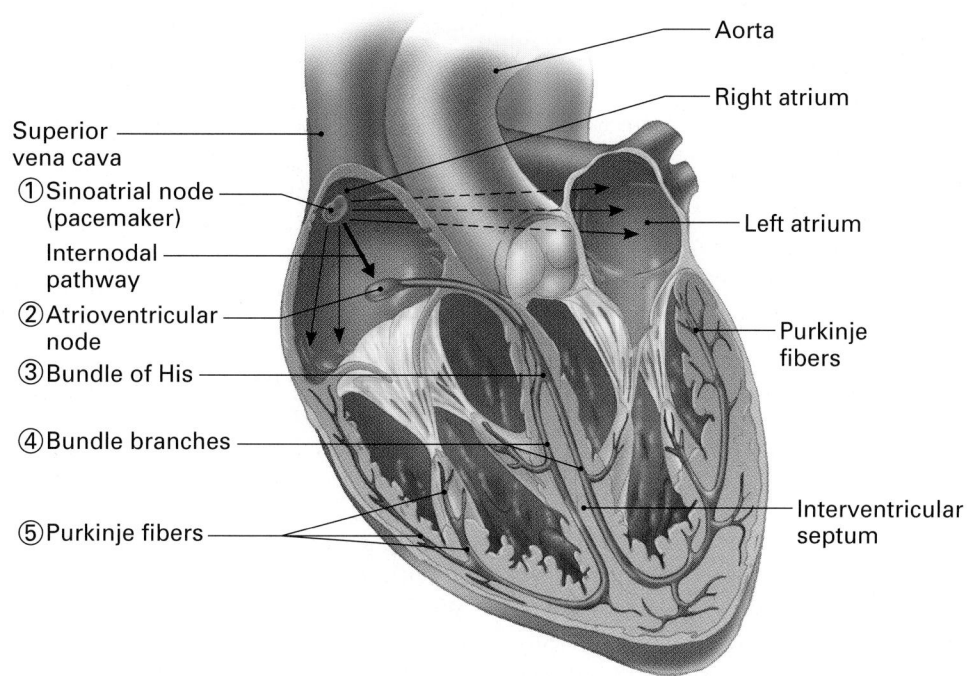

Superior vena cava

①Sinoatrial node (pacemaker)

Internodal pathway

②Atrioventricular node

③Bundle of His

④Bundle branches

⑤Purkinje fibers

Aorta

Right atrium

Left atrium

Purkinje fibers

Interventricular septum

Figure 51-5 ■ The electrical system of the heart. The impulse is initiated by the SA node, then travels to the AV node, the bundle of His, bundle branches, and finally to the Purkinje fibers.

From Fremgen, Bonnie F., Frucht, Suzanne S. *Medical Terminology: A Living Language,* 3rd ed., © 2005. Electronically reproduced by permission of Pearson Education, Inc., Upper Saddle River, New Jersey.

muscle to be perfused. This contraction and relaxation of the heart is known as the *cardiac cycle* or the *heartbeat*. The cycle is repeated 60 to 100 times a minute in the adult, stimulated by impulses generated by the SA node.

With each contraction, a certain amount of blood, known as the stroke volume, is ejected from the ventricles into the circulation. In adults, the average stroke volume is about 70 mL per beat. **Cardiac output (CO)** is the amount of blood pumped by the ventricles in 1 minute. Cardiac output is calculated by multiplying the **stroke volume (SV),** the amount of blood ejected with each contraction, times the heart rate (HR). Thus, $SV \times HR = CO$. The cardiac output is an important indicator of how well the heart is functioning as a pump. If the cardiac output is poor, tissue perfusion suffers and oxygen and nutrients do not reach the cells as needed.

Cardiac output is affected by several factors:

HEART RATE. An increased heart rate increases cardiac output, even if the stroke volume doesn't change. Conversely, cardiac output decreases when the heart rate falls if the stroke volume remains constant. There are physiologic limits to this. For example, very rapid heart rates, more than 150 beats per minute, may not allow adequate time for the ventricles to fill, causing cardiac output to fall. The heart rate is influenced by many factors including the autonomic nervous system, blood pressure, hormones such as thyroid hormone, and some medications.

PRELOAD. **Preload** is the degree to which muscle fibers in the ventricle are stretched at the end of the relaxation period (diastole). Preload largely depends on the amount of blood returning to the heart from the venous circulation: Increased volume causes increased stretch, leading to more forceful contraction of

cardiac muscle fibers. This physiologic action is referred to as the Frank-Starling law of the heart. The length of the ventricular muscle fibers (stretch) at the end of diastole directly affects the strength (force) of contraction. For example, exercise increases venous return and the amount of blood in the ventricle before contraction; therefore, the heart contracts more forcefully and stroke volume and cardiac output increase during exercise.

CONTRACTILITY. **Contractility** is the inherent ability of cardiac muscle fibers to shorten or contract. Stroke volume decreases if contractility is poor, reducing cardiac output. Contractility also is affected by the autonomic nervous system and certain drugs. Drugs that affect contractility are called inotropic drugs. Positive inotropic drugs increase contractility, and negative inotropic drugs decrease the contractile strength.

AFTERLOAD. **Afterload** is the resistance against which the heart must pump to eject the blood into the circulation. Blood flows from an area of higher pressure to an area of lower pressure. To move blood into the circulatory system, the ventricles must generate sufficient pressure to overcome vascular resistance or the pressure within the arteries, known as afterload. The right ventricle pumps blood into the low-pressure, low-resistance pulmonary vascular system; therefore, the pressures generated by the right ventricle are fairly low. The left ventricle, by contrast, pumps blood into the higher pressure systemic arterial system, generating much higher pressures and requiring more work. Systemic vasoconstriction increases the arterial blood pressure and afterload, increasing the cardiac workload; vasodilation, on the other hand, reduces arterial pressure and the workload of the heart. Table 51–2 summarizes the factors related to cardiac function.

TABLE 51–2 Factors Related to Cardiac Function

INDICATOR	DEFINITION
Cardiac output (CO)	Amount of blood ejected from the heart each minute; CO = SV × HR
Stroke volume (SV)	Amount of blood ejected from the heart with each beat
Heart rate (HR)	Number of beats each minute
Contractility	Inotropic state of the myocardium, strength of contraction
Preload	Left ventricular end diastolic volume, stretch of the myocardium
Afterload	Resistance against which the heart must pump

The Blood Vessels

With each cardiac contraction, blood is ejected into a closed system of blood vessels that transport blood to the tissues and return it to the heart. The heart supports two circulatory systems: the low-pressure pulmonary system and the higher pressure systemic circulatory system.

Deoxygenated blood from the right ventricle enters the pulmonary vascular system through the pulmonary arteries. The pulmonary arteries subdivide into lobar arteries. These lobar arteries follow the main bronchi into the lungs, then branch out to form arterioles and the dense capillary networks that encompass the alveoli. Oxygen diffuses into the blood from the alveoli, and carbon dioxide diffuses into the alveoli from the blood. This diffusion occurs across the alveolar/capillary membrane. The blood then returns to the left side of the heart via venules and the pulmonary veins. Note that the pulmonary vascular system is the only part of the circulatory system in which arteries (which transport blood away from the heart) carry deoxygenated blood, and veins (which transport blood toward the heart) contain oxygenated blood.

The muscular left ventricle of the heart pumps oxygenated blood into the aorta. The blood then moves into major arteries that branch from the aorta and into successively smaller arteries, arterioles, and finally into the thin-walled capillary beds of organs and tissues. It is in the capillary beds that oxygen and nutrients are exchanged for metabolic waste products. The deoxygenated blood then returns to the heart through a series of venules and veins that become progressively larger until they empty into the superior and inferior venae cavae.

With the exception of capillaries, blood vessel walls have three distinct layers, or tunics. The innermost layer, the tunica intima, is smooth endothelium that facilitates blood flow. The tunica media is made up of elastic fibers and smooth muscle

---

ANATOMY & PHYSIOLOGY REVIEW   Preload and Afterload

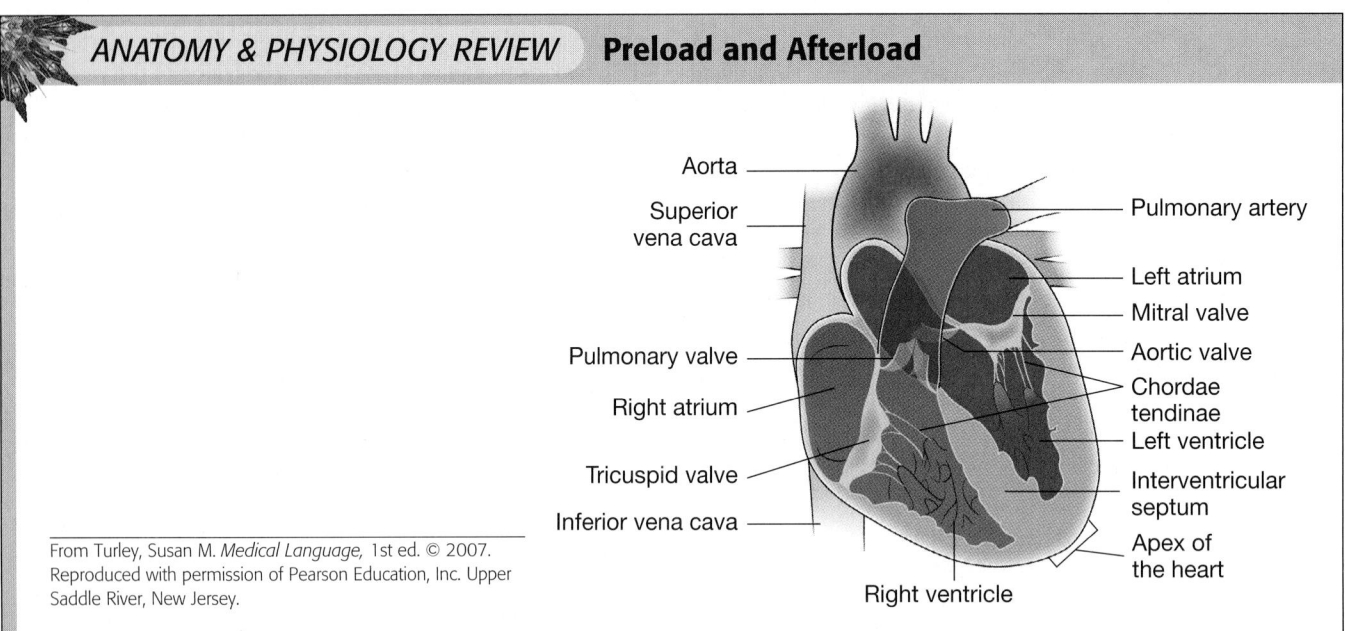

From Turley, Susan M. *Medical Language*, 1st ed. © 2007. Reproduced with permission of Pearson Education, Inc. Upper Saddle River, New Jersey.

QUESTIONS
Preload is affected by the amount of blood returning to the heart from the venous circulation. Review the figure.
1. What side of the heart is primarily affected by preload?
2. What could cause an *increase* of venous blood return to the heart?
3. When would an increase in preload have a positive effect/outcome for the client?
4. When does an increase in preload have a negative effect/outcome for the client?
5. What medication classification decreases preload? (Hint: Think about what could cause a decrease in venous return of volume to the heart.)

Afterload is the resistance against which the heart must pump. Review the figure.
6. What side of the heart is primarily affected by afterload?
7. What can cause an increase in afterload (e.g., what can cause the left side of the heart to work harder)?
8. Based on the physiology, afterload can be decreased by medications that would have what physiological result/outcome?

cells innervated by the autonomic nervous system. This allows vessels to constrict or dilate, depending on the needs of the body. The tunica media of arteries is thicker and more muscular than in veins, a feature that helps maintain blood pressure and continuous circulation to the tissues. The outermost layer of blood vessels is the tunica adventitia, a layer of connective tissue that supports, protects, and anchors the vessel to surrounding tissues. Capillaries contain only one thin layer of tunica intima, allowing gases and molecules to diffuse between the blood and the tissues.

Arterial Circulation

The arterial circulation moves blood pumped by the heart to the tissues, maintaining a constant flow to the capillary beds despite the intermittent pumping action of the heart.

Blood flow, the volume of blood flowing through a given vessel, organ, or the entire circulation over a specific period, is determined by pressure differences and resistance. Blood always moves from an area of higher pressure to an area of lower pressure. The greater the difference between pressures, the greater the blood flow. The **blood pressure (BP)** is the force exerted on arterial walls by the blood flowing within the vessel (see Chapter 29 ∞ for a further explanation of blood pressure). The *mean arterial pressure (MAP)* maintains blood flow to the tissues throughout the cardiac cycle. It is a product of the cardiac output times the **peripheral vascular resistance (PVR),** or $CO \times PVR = MAP$.

Resistance is opposition to flow; peripheral vascular resistance impedes or opposes blood flow to the tissues. PVR is determined by

- The viscosity, or thickness, of the blood.
- Blood vessel length.
- Blood vessel diameter.

Venous Return

In contrast to the high-pressure arterial system, venous pressure is too low to adequately return blood from peripheral tissues to the heart without assistance. The fall in intrathoracic pressure that occurs with breathing draws blood upward toward the heart, an adaptation known as the respiratory pump. Skeletal muscle activity contributes to the muscular pump, as muscle contractions "milk" blood toward the heart. Venous valves are vital in making these pumps work; once blood passes a valve, it cannot flow backward away from the heart. Figure 51-6 ■ depicts the relationship between arteries and veins and the entire circulatory system.

Blood

Blood serves as the transport medium within the cardiovascular system, bringing oxygen and nutrients from the environment (via the lungs and gastrointestinal system) to the cells. Blood is a complex mixture of living formed elements (the blood cells) suspended in fluid (the plasma). Its primary functions are

- Transporting oxygen, nutrients, and hormones to the cells, and metabolic wastes from the tissues for elimination.
- Regulating body temperature, pH, and fluid volume.
- Preventing infection and blood loss.

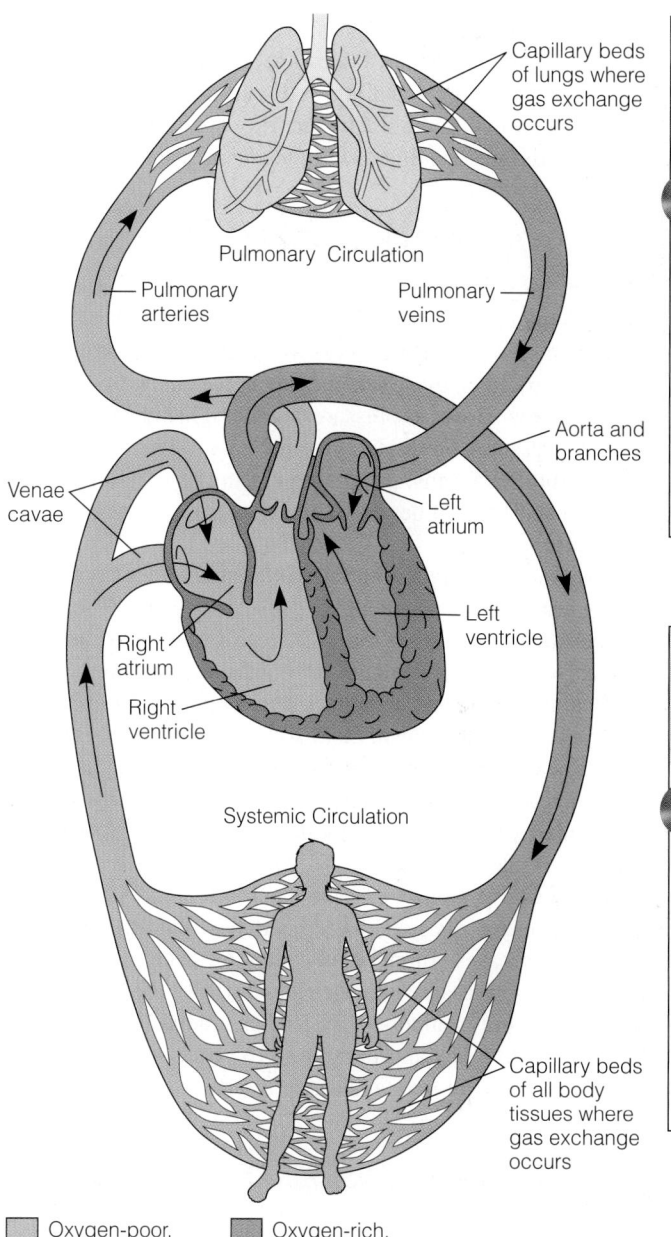

Oxygen-poor, CO_2-rich blood

Oxygen-rich, CO_2-poor blood

Figure 51-6 ■ The heart and blood vessels. The left side of the heart pumps oxygenated blood into the arteries. Deoxygenated blood returns via the venous system into the right side of the heart.

As previously noted in Chapter 50 ∞ , most oxygen is transported bound to hemoglobin. **Hemoglobin** is a major component of red blood cells (erythrocytes), the predominant cell present in blood. Hemoglobin binds easily with oxygen, releasing it in the body tissues. When all four heme groups of the hemoglobin molecule are bound to oxygen, it is said to be *fully saturated.* Oxygen binding is affected by several factors, including the PO_2, temperature, pH, and PCO_2. Up to a certain point (about 70 mm Hg), the higher the PO_2, the greater the affinity of hemoglobin for oxygen and the more saturated the hemoglobin molecules. The relationship to temperature, pH, and PCO_2 is the opposite: At higher temperatures, greater hydrogen ion concentrations (lower pH), and higher PCO_2 levels, the affinity for oxygen decreases, and hemoglobin releases its oxygen molecules. Because of hemoglobin's importance in oxygen transportation, anemia (too few red blood cells or RBCs that contain too little or abnormal hemoglobin) interferes with oxygen delivery to the tissues, leading to fatigue and activity intolerance.

LIFE SPAN CONSIDERATIONS

At birth, profound changes occur in the cardiovascular systems. As the lungs expand, pressures in the pulmonary vascular system fall, changing pressure relationships within the heart. The foramen ovale (an opening between the two atria of the fetal heart) closes as pressures on the right side of the heart fall and pressures on the left side increase. Arterial PO_2 rises and arterial PCO_2 falls, prompting closure of the ductus arteriosus (a short vessel between the pulmonary artery and aorta of the fetus).

Pulse rates are highest and most variable in newborns. The resting heart rate for a neonate ranges from 100 to 180 beats per minute immediately after birth and then stabilizes to between 120 and 160 beats per minute (Ball & Bindler, 2006, p. 303). The heart rate decreases to 80 to 130 in infants to 2 years of age and reaches the adult rate of 60 to 100 by about age 10 years. Irregular heart rates are common in infants and young children, often increasing and decreasing with each breath. This pattern of irregularity is known as sinus arrhythmia, a normal variation of the heart rate.

As the conversion from fetal circulation takes place and pressures in the left side of the heart rise, the arterial blood pressure increases. Immediately after birth (1 to 3 days of age) the blood pressure averages about 65/40. By 1 month the arterial pressure is about 90/55. It rises gradually to the adult "norm" of 120/80 by approximately 16 years of age. With aging, blood pressure may again rise as arteriosclerosis affects the blood vessels, narrowing their lumen and decreasing their compliance (ability to distend).

Congenital heart disease affects less than 1% of all live births, but is the leading cause of early death from all congenital anomalies (Hoffman, 2001). Acquired heart diseases are rare in childhood. Rheumatic fever is an inflammatory disorder that may occur following streptococcal infection (e.g., strep throat) and lead to heart valve damage. For most people, the heart continues to function effectively well into older adulthood unless the blood supply to the heart muscle is impaired by blood vessel disease. **Atherosclerosis**, the buildup of fatty plaque within the arteries, is the major contributor to cardiovascular disease, the leading cause of death in North America.

Children rarely are affected by diseases of the blood vessels. Hypertension may be associated with obesity, sedentary lifestyle, and stress in children and adolescents. During middle adulthood, the incidence of hypertension, or an elevated blood pressure, increases significantly. Hypertension, known as the silent killer because of its lack of symptoms, is a major risk factor for sudden cardiac death in middle adulthood.

FACTORS AFFECTING CARDIOVASCULAR FUNCTION

Many factors affect cardiovascular function. Some of these factors are called risk factors, because, if present, they increase the risk of cardiovascular disease. Risk factors have been identified for coronary artery disease, hypertension, and peripheral vascular disease, and the majority are the same.

Risk Factors

Major risk factors for cardiovascular disease in general are classified as *nonmodifiable* (cannot be altered) and *modifiable* (can be reduced) (Box 51–1).

LIFESPAN CONSIDERATIONS Circulation

CHILDREN
- Blood pressure should be taken routinely on children after age 3 years.
- Heart murmurs, extra sounds detected when listening to the heart, are common in children, especially in the preschool years. The vast majority are not associated with a pathology, but are due to normal blood flow or transitional physiological processes that increase cardiac output (e.g., anemia, fever, exercise) (Blosser & Freitas-Nichols, 2004).

ELDERS
Normal changes of aging may contribute to problems of circulation in elders, even when there is no actual pathology:
- Blood vessels become less elastic and have an increase in calcification. This results in a restricted blood flow and a decrease of oxygen and nutrients to tissues (heart, peripheral, and cerebral).
- Impaired valve function in the heart is often the result of increased stiffness and calcification and results in a decrease in cardiac output.
- A decrease of muscle tone in the heart results in a decrease in cardiac output.

- There is a decrease in baroreceptor response to blood pressure changes, making the heart and blood vessels less responsive to exercise and stress. This often results in dizziness, falls, orthostatic hypotension, and mental changes.
- A decrease in conduction ability in the heart also makes the heart less responsive to changes and stresses. This can also result in dizziness, falls, orthostatic hypotension, and mental changes.

All of these factors become important if the person is challenged by stressors, such as exercise, stress, fever, surgery, or other changes. If challenged, the circulatory system of elders is not as effective or as quick to return to normal. Persons living with normal changes of aging and/or pathologic conditions of the circulatory system need to learn to balance diet, medications, and exercise. Nurses have a large part in working with these clients to develop appropriate interventions and provide teaching to help them maintain optimal functioning. Teaching clients to recognize any changes or worsening of their condition is very important. They need to contact the primary care provider and make any needed changes. Changing lifestyles and fine-tuning medications can be critical, and nurses can be a part of this in every phase of the nursing process.

BOX 51–1   Risk Factors for Coronary Heart Disease

NONMODIFIABLE RISK FACTORS
  Heredity
  Age
  Gender (women's risk increases at postmenopause)

MODIFIABLE RISK FACTORS
  Elevated serum lipid level
  Hypertension
  Cigarette smoking
  Diabetes
  Obesity
  Sedentary lifestyle

OTHER RISK FACTORS
  Heat and cold
  Previous health status
  Stress and coping
  Dietary factors
  Alcohol intake
  Elevated homocysteine level

Nonmodifiable Risk Factors

The first nonmodifiable risk factor is *heredity*. There is a genetic link for the development of coronary artery disease. That is, if a client has a parent with heart disease, he or she is at higher risk. The second is *age*. Coronary heart disease is mainly a disease of people over 60. It does occur in younger people as well, but generally risk increases with age. The third nonmodifiable risk factor is *gender*. Through middle adulthood (until menopause), estrogen has a protective effect in women, slowing the progress of atherosclerosis and reducing the risk of cardiovascular disease. This effect is lost at menopause, but hormone replacement therapy (HRT) *may* be beneficial in reducing this risk later in life. Possible benefits from HRT must be weighed against possible risks. This is a complex analysis and requires thorough discussion between the woman and her primary care provider. Among people in their 40s and 50s, men have a higher incidence of hypertension than women.

The modifiable risk factors include elevated serum lipid levels, hypertension, cigarette smoking, diabetes, obesity, and sedentary lifestyle.

Elevated Serum Lipid Levels

A strong link exists between elevated serum lipid levels and the development of coronary heart disease. Lipoproteins circulate in the blood and are made up of cholesterol, triglycerides, and phospholipids. A high dietary intake of saturated fats is the most critical factor for the development of elevated serum lipids. The average American diet often contains more than 40% of its calories in fats. The American Heart Association recommends that less than 30% of total calories come from fats.

Hypertension

Hypertension (or increased blood pressure) increases the risk of coronary heart disease in several ways. First, it increases the

workload of the heart, increasing oxygen demand and coronary blood flow. The increased workload also causes hypertrophy of the ventricles. Over time this can contribute to heart failure. Secondly, hypertension causes endothelial damage to the blood vessels, which stimulates the development of atherosclerosis.

Cigarette Smoking

The cardiovascular system also is affected by cigarette smoking. Nicotine increases the heart rate, blood pressure, and peripheral vascular resistance, increasing the heart's workload. Smoking causes vasoconstriction, and in areas where vessels already are narrowed by atherosclerosis, tissue oxygenation can be impaired.

Diabetes

Diabetes mellitus increases the risk of coronary heart disease, myocardial infarction, and peripheral vascular disease. High blood sugars are linked with accelerated development of atherosclerosis as well as high levels of serum lipids and triglycerides. Closely monitoring blood sugar levels in clients with diabetes and checking blood sugar levels in all clients for the development of increased levels is an important nursing function. Control of blood sugar levels can greatly reduce risk and slow development of atherosclerosis.

Obesity

Nearly 60% of the adult population of the United States is overweight or obese (Evangelista & Miller, 2006, p. 27). Obese people have an increased risk for the development of cardiovascular disease. Obesity is often accompanied by elevated serum lipid levels, which increase risk. Additionally, obesity places an increased workload on the heart, which increases oxygen demand. Recent research data show that obese individuals have an increased risk for heart failure and death that increases in proportion to the degree of obesity (Evangelista & Miller, 2006, p. 28).

Sedentary Lifestyle

Physical activity is associated with a reduction in the risk of death due to cardiovascular disease (Richardson, Kriska, Lantz, & Hayward, 2004, p. 192). Physical exercise or activity increases the heart rate and hence the supply of oxygen in the body. With regular vigorous exercise, the heart muscle becomes more powerful and efficient. Aerobic exercise slows the atherosclerotic process, reducing the risk of cardiovascular disease. Sedentary people, by contrast, have a higher risk of cardiovascular disease.

Other Factors Influencing Cardiovascular Function

Other factors that may influence cardiovascular function include environmental factors such as heat and cold, previous health status, stress and coping, dietary factors, alcohol intake, and an elevated homocysteine level.

Heat and Cold

In response to heat, the peripheral blood vessels dilate; consequently, blood flows to the skin, increasing the amount of heat

Coronary Artery Disease Video | **MediaLink**

RESEARCH NOTE Can the Lifetime Risk for Cardiovascular Disease Be Predicted?

Prior to this research, the lifetime risk for cardiovascular disease (CVD) had not been estimated and the effect of possessing risk factors on lifetime risk for developing CVD was unknown.

The study included all of the Framingham Heart Study participants who were free of CVD (e.g., myocardial infarction, angina, stroke) at 50 years of age. They may have had risk factors but did not have CVD. The researchers then estimated the lifetime risk for CVD for men and women up to 95 years of age. They examined overall survival in the presence and absence of established risk factors.

During routine examinations of the Framingham Heart Study, the participants underwent standardized measurements for body mass index (BMI), diabetes, BP, cholesterol, and a self-report of smoking.

The results reflected that men free of CVD at age 50 had a 51.7% risk of developing CVD by 95 years of age and the overall survival was 30 years. Women had a 39.2% risk of developing CVD and a median overall survival of 36 years.

The study showed the following effect of individual risk factors:

- High blood pressure and total cholesterol were associated with increased lifetime risk for CVD and shorter survival.
- The highest single lifetime risk for CVD of all the risk factors was diabetes.
- Overweight and obesity resulted in modest increases in lifetime risk and reduction in survival.

On the other hand, those participants who had no established risk factors at age 50 were associated with very low lifetime risk for CVD and much longer survival.

The authors noted that CVD is the leading cause of morbidity and mortality in the United States. They also made the relevant point that in spite of this fact, most Americans perceive that cancer is their greatest health risk.

IMPLICATIONS

The results of this study along with the decreased awareness of CVD risk mandates health promotion activities to educate the public about CVD risk factors. Prevention efforts need to begin before age 50. Lifestyle activities focusing on diet and exercise in young adulthood and middle age can prevent many of the CVD risk factors such as obesity, hypertension, hyperlipidemia, and diabetes.

The authors caution that the lifetime risk estimates are based on a large population group and applying the results to an individual client should be done with caution. The results, however, can help health care providers focus on prevention and modification of CVD risk factors.

Note: From "Prediction of Lifetime Risk for Cardiovascular Disease by Risk Factor Burden at 50 Years of Age," by D. M. Lloyd-Jones, E. P. Leip, M. G. Larson, R. B. D'Agostino, A. Beiser, P. Wilson, et al., 2006, *Circulation, 113*(6), pp. 791–798. Copyright © 2006 Lippincott, Williams & Wilkins.

---

lost from the body surface. With vasodilation the lumens of blood vessels enlarge, thus decreasing the resistance to the blood flow. In response the heart increases output to maintain blood pressure. The increased cardiac output requires additional oxygen, which is acquired through increased rate and depth of breathing.

In response to cold environmental temperatures, the peripheral blood vessels constrict. This mechanism helps to conserve heat that is normally lost through the skin. However, the vasoconstriction also increases blood pressure which may increase the risk of a heart attack or stroke for clients with cardiac conditions.

Health Status

In the healthy person, the cardiovascular system (working together with the respiratory system) is able to provide sufficient oxygen to meet the body's needs. Diseases of the cardiovascular system will often affect the delivery of oxygen to the cells of

---

Dysrhythmia Video | **MediaLink**

CULTURALLY COMPETENT CARE Gender and Race Disparities in Clients with Cardiovascular Disease

ACUTE MYOCARDIAL INFARCTION (AMI)

Coronary heart disease is the leading cause of death in American females. Yet, they are underrepresented in the majority of cardiovascular research studies.

Women tend to have an AMI at an older age than men and are more likely to have complications. The presence of chest pain varies between men and women. More women have pain-free AMIs than men. They also tend to have more mid-back, shoulder blade, and upper-back pain than men. Research reflects that women who have an AMI have increased delays in treatment and less aggressive treatment than men. This results in increased mortality rates.

HEART FAILURE (HF)

Symptoms of heart failure occur earlier in African Americans, possibly because of the higher rate of uncontrolled hypertension. The rate of hypertension for both African Americans and Caucasians is greatest in the southeastern United States.

Studies reveal the following information about other risk factors for heart failure and other cardiovascular disease:

- African Americans have a higher average BMI than Caucasians. African Americans do not view obesity as a negative body image.
- African Americans have a higher incidence of diabetes than other populations.
- The incidence of HF is increasing in African American women. However, few studies have been completed in which they are the subjects of the research.

STROKE

African Americans have a greater incidence, greater mortality, and greater severity of strokes.

IMPLICATIONS

Research on gender differences is gradually increasing. However, research focusing on differences by race remains limited and needs to be more thoroughly investigated. In the meantime, two important areas for client education include informing women that AMI does not occur only in men, and teaching the public about how to prevent risk factors that contribute to heart failure and stroke.

the body, and when any system or tissue does not get the required oxygen for metabolic processes, cellular function will be altered. The body has "compensatory mechanisms" that are activated when oxygen decreases. These mechanisms include increased heart rate, increased strength of cardiac contraction, vasoconstriction, and the release of certain hormones such as aldosterone. The health status of a client may affect how the body tolerates the compensation and the decreased oxygen availability. A client with no significant health history and with good nutritional status will be more likely to tolerate short periods of decreased oxygen and the body's compensation than a client with multiple disorders and poor nutritional status.

Most cardiovascular conditions affect how the blood gets to the tissues. One cardiovascular condition that affects the oxygen-carrying capacity of the blood is anemia, described in the "Blood Alterations" section later in this chapter.

Stress and Coping

Stress causes a neurohormonal response. The stress response involves a number of interrelated responses and effects. One of the major effects of stress is the release of adrenal medullary hormones: epinephrine and norepinephrine. Epinephrine has several effects including causing the heart to contract more forcefully, increasing heart rate, and stimulating peripheral vasoconstriction. Norepinephrine causes widespread vasoconstriction, which increases the blood pressure.

Diet

Diet can also affect cardiovascular function. A healthy diet with adequate calories, protein, and other nutrients is important to maintain good immune function and increase resistance to disease. Along with certain vitamins and minerals, dietary protein is important to prevent anemia. High salt intake can affect blood pressure and contribute to the development of hypertension. High intake of sodium may contribute to hypertension in two ways. First, it may increase the release of a hormone called natriuretic hormone which indirectly contributes to hypertension. Additionally, sodium stimulates vasopressor mechanisms, which cause vasoconstriction. There is also evidence that other factors such as low potassium, calcium, and magnesium intake may contribute to vasoconstriction and the development of hypertension. One study showed that a high consumption of dairy products and dietary calcium reduced blood pressure levels (Ruidavets et al., 2006).

Alcohol

Recent studies suggest that moderate alcohol use (1 to 2 oz of alcohol per day) may actually reduce the risk of heart disease; however, excessive alcohol intake affects oxygenation several ways. Alcohol is a respiratory depressant, slowing respirations. Alcohol abusers often are malnourished, increasing their risk of anemia and infections. Excess alcohol intake also increases the risk of hypertension.

Elevated Homocysteine Level

Homocysteine is an amino acid that has been shown to be increased in many people with atherosclerosis. Clients with elevated homocysteine levels may have an increased risk of

myocardial infarction, coronary artery disease, cerebrovascular accidents (stroke), and peripheral vascular disease. Individuals can reduce their homocysteine level by taking a multivitamin that provides folate, vitamin B_6, vitamin B_{12}, and riboflavin (Bergen & Compher, 2006).

ALTERATIONS IN CARDIOVASCULAR FUNCTION

Cardiovascular function can be altered by conditions that affect

1. The function of the heart as a pump.
2. Blood flow to organs and peripheral tissues.
3. The composition of the blood and its ability to transport oxygen and carbon dioxide.

Three major alterations in cardiovascular function are decreased cardiac output, impaired tissue perfusion, and disorders that affect the composition or amount of blood available for transport of gases.

Decreased Cardiac Output

Although the heart normally is able to increase its rate and force of contraction to increase cardiac output during exercise, fever, or other times of need, some conditions interfere with these mechanisms.

The vessels that supply blood to the heart muscle may become occluded by atherosclerosis or a blood clot, shutting off the blood supply to a portion of the myocardium. When this happens, the tissue becomes necrotic and dies, a condition known as a **myocardial infarction (MI)** or *heart attack*. If a large portion of the heart muscle is affected, particularly in the left ventricle, cardiac output falls because the affected muscle no longer contracts. Signs and symptoms of myocardial infarction are variable and may include the following:

- Chest pain; substernal and/or radiating to the left arm, jaw
- Nausea
- Shortness of breath
- Diaphoresis

Heart failure may develop if the heart isn't able to keep up with the body's need for oxygen and nutrients to the tissues. Heart failure usually occurs because of myocardial infarction, but it may also result from chronic overwork of the heart, such as in clients with uncontrolled hypertension or extensive arteriosclerosis. In left-sided heart failure, the vessels of the pulmonary system become congested or engorged with blood. This may cause fluid to escape into the alveoli and interfere with gas exchange, a condition known as *pulmonary edema*. Signs of heart failure may include the following:

- Pulmonary congestion; adventitious lung sounds
- Shortness of breath
- Increased heart rate
- Increased respiratory rate
- Peripheral vasoconstriction; cold, pale extremities
- Distended neck veins

Other diseases such as myocarditis and cardiomyopathy also can affect the heart muscle, impairing its ability to contract and

BOX 51-3 Calculating an Ankle/Brachial Index (ABI) and Toe Brachial Pressure Index (TBPI)

Both assessments use a blood pressure (BP) cuff and a Doppler ultrasound device to measure the blood pressure using the client's brachial pulse and either the posterior tibial pulse and dorsalis pedis pulse (ABI) or the great toe's distal pulse (TBPI). The pressure index is calculated by dividing either the posterior tibial or dorsalis pedis (whichever is highest) in ABI or the toe's systolic pressure (TBPI) by the highest brachial systolic pressure. For example, for TBPI the results consist of a right brachial pressure of 130 and a left brachial pressure of 128 along with a left great toe pressure of 130 and a right great toe pressure of 60. The left TBPI is 1 (130 divided by 130) and the right TBPI is 0.46 (60 divided by 130). A TBPI less than 0.64 warrants further evaluation and testing.

Note: From "Determining the Toe Brachial Pressure Index" by P. A. Bonham, 2003, *Nursing, 33(9)*, 54–55. Copyright © 2003 by Lippincott, Williams, & Wilkins. . Reprinted with permission.

in many instances: for clients who have known or suspected cardiovascular disease, during and after surgery, to monitor responses to drug therapy, and to monitor clients at risk for serious complications such as shock. Electrodes placed on the client's chest are attached to a monitor cable and bedside monitor (Figure 51-8 ■). The monitor is equipped with alarms used to warn of potential problems such as very fast, very slow, or irregular heart rates. The alarm limits are set for 20 beats higher and lower than the client's baseline rate, often at 100 to 110 and 50 to 55, respectively, for adults. For ambulatory clients (in the hospital or at home), the electrodes connect to a transmitter unit (also called telemetry). This unit electronically sends the signal to a central monitor for display or may store the information to be retrieved later in the primary care provider's office. Another name for this type of ambulatory monitoring is the Holter monitor. Electrodes are attached and the client wears the monitor for 24 hours. A continuous ECG is recorded and later analyzed for irregularities.

Electrocardiography most commonly uses 12 "leads" or 12 different views of the heart. In contrast, cardiac monitoring uses 2 or 3 leads at any given time. See Chapter 34 ∞ for more information about ECGs.

Figure 51-8 ■ A client with cardiac monitoring.

CLINICAL ALERT

It is important to remember that ECG monitoring is a recording of the electrical activity of the heart; it does not reflect mechanical contraction and cardiac output. ALWAYS remember to check the client to assess for cardiac function. Just looking at the ECG does not give an assessment of the client's status. ■

BLOOD TESTS. Specimens of venous blood are taken for several tests that may reflect some aspect of cardiovascular functioning.

Because *hemoglobin* is the molecule that oxygen attaches to, it gives an indication of the oxygen-carrying capacity of the blood. A decreased hemoglobin increases the risk of oxygen deficit in the tissues when cardiovascular disease is present.

Measurement of serum electrolytes is important for clients with cardiovascular problems because electrolyte abnormalities such as hyperkalemia (higher than normal potassium) and hypokalemia (lower than normal potassium) can have a critical effect on the heart. Serum levels of magnesium, calcium, sodium, and phosphorus are also important to assess.

Measurement of enzyme levels in the blood is an important part of the diagnostic evaluation of clients with chest pain. Certain enzymes such as **creatine kinase (CK)** and **troponin** are released into the blood during an MI. These enzymes are released into the blood as the cell membrane is damaged. Elevated levels of these enzymes can help differentiate between an MI (when the cells actually die) and chest pain from a different cause such as angina or pleuritic pain.

HEMODYNAMIC STUDIES. *Hemodynamics* is the study of the forces or pressures involved in blood circulation. Hemodynamic studies or monitoring procedures may be performed to evaluate fluid status and cardiovascular function. Parameters evaluated in hemodynamic studies include heart rate, arterial blood pressure, central venous pressure, pressures in the pulmonary vascular system, and cardiac output. Some of these parameters—for example, heart rate, arterial blood pressure, and venous pressure—are measured directly using an arterial, central venous, or pulmonary artery catheter; others such as the stroke volume and cardiac output are calculated. Hemodynamic studies are performed in a diagnostic cardiac laboratory and require informed consent. Clients in intensive and cardiac care units may undergo continuous hemodynamic monitoring to evaluate cardiovascular status and the effect of interventions. Nurses in these units are responsible for maintaining accurate readings and the integrity of the system.

Diagnosing

NANDA includes the following diagnostic labels for clients with circulation problems:

- *Ineffective Tissue Perfusion* (Cardiopulmonary): Decrease in oxygen resulting in the failure to nourish the tissues at the capillary level
- *Decreased Cardiac Output*: Inadequate blood pumped by the heart to meet metabolic (demands) of the body
- *Activity Intolerance*: Insufficient physiological or psychological energy to endure or complete required or desired daily activities

IDENTIFYING NURSING DIAGNOSES, OUTCOMES, AND INTERVENTIONS
Client with Decreased Cardiac Output

DATA CLUSTER   Ed Wallace, a 67-year-old retired contractor, has a history of an acute myocardial infarction 1 year ago. During the last 2 weeks he has experienced a weight gain of 4 kg (9 lb). He states that he can't walk a flight of stairs without shortness of breath, and he sleeps on three pillows. His ankles are swollen, and his heart pounds at times. Physical exam reveals jugular vein distention above 3 cm; pulse (86); pitting edema in feet, ankles, and lower legs; and crackles in both lung fields.

NURSING DIAGNOSIS/ DEFINITION	SAMPLE DESIRED OUTCOMES*/ DEFINITION	INDICATORS	SELECTED INTERVENTIONS*/ DEFINITION	SAMPLE NIC ACTIVITIES
Decreased Cardiac Output/Inadequate blood pumped by the heart to meet metabolic demands of the body	Cardiac Pump Effectiveness [0400]/*Adequacy of blood volume ejected from the left ventricle per minute to support systemic perfusion pressure*	No ■ Neck vein distention ■ Peripheral edema ■ Weight gain ■ Dyspnea	Cardiac Care [4040]/ *Limitation of complications resulting from an imbalance between myocardial oxygen supply and demand for a patient with symptoms of impaired cardiac function*	■ Perform a comprehensive appraisal of peripheral circulation ■ Monitor respiratory status for symptoms of heart failure ■ Monitor fluid balance (e.g., intake/output, daily weights) ■ Arrange exercise and rest periods to avoid fatigue ■ Monitor the patient's activity tolerance

*The NOC # for desired outcomes and the NIC # for nursing interventions are listed in brackets following the appropriate outcome or intervention. Outcomes, indicators, interventions, and activities selected are only a sample of those suggested by NOC and NIC and should be further individualized for each client.

Examples of application of these using NANDA, NIC, and NOC designations are shown in Identifying Nursing Diagnoses, Outcomes, and Interventions.

Planning

When planning care the nurse identifies nursing interventions that will assist the client to achieve these broad goals:

■ Maintain or improve tissue perfusion.
■ Maintain or restore an adequate cardiac output.

Obviously, goals will vary according to the diagnosis and defining characteristics for each individual. Appropriate preventive and corrective nursing interventions that relate to these must be identified. Specific nursing activities can be selected to meet the client's individual needs. Examples of NIC interventions related to decreased cardiac output and tissue perfusion include the following:

■ Circulatory Care: Arterial Insufficiency
■ Cardiac Care
■ Hemodynamic Regulation

To promote the transport of oxygen and carbon dioxide, the nurse can optimize cardiac output by reducing stress, planning appropriate activities, and positioning the client for improved vascular blood flow (see Identifying Nursing Diagnoses, Outcomes, and Interventions).

Implementing
Promoting Circulation

Most people in good health give little thought to their cardiovascular function. Changing position frequently, ambulating, and exercising usually maintain adequate cardiovascular functioning. See Client Teaching for other ways to promote a healthy heart.

CLIENT TEACHING   Home Care and Circulation

MAINTAINING CARDIAC OUTPUT AND TISSUE PERFUSION

■ Teach the symptoms of heart failure to the client and family and emphasize when to contact the primary care provider.
■ Teach the client about the importance of maintaining regular physical activity to promote circulation and vascular health. Emphasize the need to increase activity levels gradually with the goal of exercising (walking, swimming, weight training, or aerobic exercise as recommended by the care provider) for at least 20 minutes four to five times per week.
■ Instruct the client to avoid exposure to cold, wearing warm clothing as needed.
■ Teach cardiopulmonary resuscitation or refer for instruction.

DIETARY ALTERATIONS

■ Instruct the client and family about prescribed dietary restrictions such as a low-sodium diet. Refer to a dietitian as needed for further instruction.
■ Discuss dietary measures to reduce the risk of atherosclerosis, including reducing total and saturated fats in the diet, reducing weight if obese, and increasing the intake of dietary fiber.

MEDICATIONS

■ Instruct the client and family about prescribed medications, including effects, side effects, and administration instructions.

CLIENT TEACHING   Promoting a Healthy Heart

- Exercise regularly, participating in at least 20 minutes (40 minutes is preferred) of vigorous exercise four to five times a week.
- Do not smoke.
- Maintain your ideal weight.
- Eat a diet low in total fat, saturated fats, and cholesterol.
- Drink alcohol in moderation, if at all, consuming no more than 1 cocktail or 1 to 1 1/2 glasses of wine or beer daily.
- Reduce stress and manage anger.

- Effectively manage diabetes and hypertension, maintaining blood glucose and blood pressure levels within normal limits.
- If female, discuss with your health care provider the advantages and risks of hormone replacement therapy after menopause (or after a total hysterectomy).
- Consult your primary care provider about the advisability of low-dose aspirin therapy to further reduce the risk of cardiovascular disease.

Immobility is also detrimental to cardiovascular function. Without exercise of the calf and leg muscles, blood pools in the veins of the lower extremities. This stagnant blood flow may allow clots to develop (venous thrombosis). With time, these clots can break loose and become emboli, eventually lodging in the small vessels of the pulmonary vascular system. Blood flow and gas exchange in the lungs are then impaired.

There are many nursing interventions that can help clients maintain cardiac and vascular function. They may be classified as vascular and cardiac.

VASCULAR

- Position with the legs elevated to promote venous return to the heart. This is particularly important for clients with venous dysfunction. Care should be taken to avoid this position in clients with cardiac dysfunction because it will increase preload and may stress the dysfunctional heart.
- Avoid pillows under the knees or more than 15 degrees of knee flexion to improve blood flow to the lower extremities and reduce venous stagnation.
- Encourage leg exercises (such as flexion and extension of the feet, active contraction and relaxation of calf muscles) for a client on bed rest and promote ambulation as soon as possible.
- Encourage or provide frequent position changes.

CARDIAC

- Position the client in a high Fowler's position to decrease preload and reduce pulmonary congestion.
- Monitor intake and output. Fluid restriction is usually not required for clients with mild to moderate cardiac dysfunction. With severe heart failure, a fluid restriction may be ordered.

Medications

Many classes of medications are administered to clients with cardiovascular disorders. Drugs such as nitrates, calcium channel blockers, and angiotensin-converting enzyme (ACE) inhibitors reduce the workload of the heart and prevent vasoconstriction. Various drugs are used to treat cardiac dysrhythmias. Positive inotropic drugs such as digitalis are used to increase the contractile strength of the heart. Beta adrenergic blocking agents such as propranolol or metoprolol may be given to block the sympathetic nervous system action on the heart and decrease oxygen consumption. Direct vasodilators may be used for clients with peripheral vascular disease and sometimes hypertension. Often clients are on numerous medications, and it is

an important role of the nurse to help the client understand the purposes, effects, and side effects of the different medications.

Administering medications is an important nursing function. The nurse is responsible for assessing for the effects of medications and also for potential complications. Examples include:

- When diuretics are administered, the nurse assesses intake and output and potassium level (because many diuretics can lower potassium level).
- When positive inotropic medications are administered, the nurse should assess blood pressure, heart rate, peripheral pulses, and lung sounds as indicators of cardiac output.
- When antihypertensive medications are administered, it is critical for the nurse to monitor blood pressure. Additionally, many antihypertensive medications can cause postural hypotension.

Preventing Venous Stasis

When clients have limited mobility or are confined to bed, venous return to the heart is impaired and the risk of venous stasis increases. Immobility is a problem not only for ill or debilitated

Figure 51-9 ■ The sequential venous compression device enhances venous return. They are available in knee-high or above-the-knee length.

Photographer: Elena Dorfman

clients but also for some travelers who sit with legs dependent for long periods in a motor vehicle or an airplane. Venous stasis can lead to thrombus formation and edema of the extremities.

Preventing venous stasis is an important nursing intervention to reduce the risk of complications following surgery, trauma, or major medical problems. Positioning and leg exercises are discussed in Chapter 50 ∞ and antiemboli stockings in Chapter 37 ∞ . Sequential compression devices are additional measures to help prevent venous stasis.

SEQUENTIAL COMPRESSION DEVICES. Clients who are undergoing surgery or who are immobilized because of illness or injury may benefit from a sequential compression device (SCD) to promote venous return from the legs. SCDs inflate and deflate plastic sleeves wrapped around the legs to promote venous flow. The plastic sleeves are attached by tubing to an air pump that alternately inflates and deflates portions of the sleeve to a specified pressure. The ankle area inflates first, followed by the calf region, and then the thigh area. This sequential inflation and deflation assists the leg muscles in moving blood toward the heart (Figure 51-9 ■).

The SCD is removed for ambulation and is usually discontinued when the client resumes activities. SCDs are useful in preventing thrombi and edema from venous stasis, but they are not used for clients who have arterial insufficiency, cellulitis, infection of the extremity, or preexisting venous thrombosis.

Skill 51-1 outlines how to apply a sequential compression device.

SEQUENTIAL COMPRESSION DEVICES

SKILL 51-1

PURPOSES
- To promote venous return from the legs
- To decrease risk of deep vein thrombosis and/or pulmonary embolism

ASSESSMENT
Assess for baseline data:

- Cardiovascular status, including heart rate and rhythm, peripheral pulses, and capillary refill

- Color and temperature of extremities
- Movement and sensation of feet and lower extremities and Homans' sign

PLANNING
Check the primary care provider's order for type of SCD sleeve. **Rationale:** *Both knee- and thigh-length sleeves are available.*

Delegation

UAP often remove and reapply the SCD when performing hygiene care. The nurse should check that the UAP knows the correct application process for the SCD. Remind the UAP that the client should not have the SCD removed for long periods of time because the purpose of the SCD is to promote circulation.

Equipment
- Measuring tape
- SCD, including disposable sleeves, air pump, and tubing

IMPLEMENTATION
Performance
1. Prior to performing the procedure, introduce self and verify the client's identity using agency protocol. Explain to the client what you are going to do, why it is necessary, and the procedure for applying the sequential compression device. **Rationale:** *The client's cooperation and comfort will be increased by understanding the rationale for applying the SCD.*
2. Perform hand hygiene and observe appropriate infection control procedures.
3. Provide for client privacy and drape the client appropriately.
4. Prepare the client.
   - Place the client in a dorsal recumbent or semi-Fowler's position.
   - Measure the client's legs as recommended by the manufacturer if a thigh-length sleeve is required. **Rationale:** *Knee-length sleeves come in just one size; the thigh circumference determines the size needed for a thigh-length sleeve.*
5. Apply the sequential compression sleeves.
   - Place a sleeve under each leg with the opening at the knee.
   - Wrap the sleeve securely around the leg, securing the Velcro tabs. Allow two fingers to fit between the leg and the sleeve.

Rationale: *This amount of space ensures that the sleeve does not impair circulation when inflated.* ❶
6. Connect the sleeves to the control unit and adjust the pressure as needed.
   - Connect the tubing to the sleeves and control unit, ensuring that arrows on the plug and the connector are in alignment and that the tubing is not kinked or twisted. **Rationale:** *Improper alignment or obstruction of the tubing by kinks or twists will interfere with operation of the SCD.*

❶ Applying a sequential compression device to the leg.

continued on page 1418

SEQUENTIAL COMPRESSION DEVICES *continued*

• Turn on the control unit and adjust the alarms and pressures as needed. The sleeve cooling control and alarm should be on; ankle pressure is usually set at 35 to 55 mm Hg. **Rationale:** *It is important to have the sleeve cooling control on for comfort and to reduce the risk of skin irritation from moisture under the sleeve. Alarms warn of possible control unit malfunctions.*

7. Document the procedure.
   • Record baseline assessment data and application of the SCD. Note control unit settings.
   • Assess and document skin integrity and neurovascular status at least every 8 hours while the SCD is in place. Remove the unit and notify the primary care provider if the client complains of numbness and tingling or leg pain. These may be symptoms of nerve compression.

EVALUATION

▪ Perform appropriate follow-up assessments, such as cardiovascular status including pedal pulses, skin color and temperature, skin integrity, and neurovascular status, including movement and sensation.

▪ Compare to the baseline data, if available.
▪ Report significant deviations from normal to the primary care provider.

LIFESPAN CONSIDERATIONS **Sequential Compression Devices**

CHILDREN

▪ As young children tend to be more active, the SCD is rarely necessary unless the child is immobile (e.g., comatose).

ELDERS

▪ The SCD sleeves may become loose as clients move around in bed. Check that the sleeves are secure and properly positioned.

HOME CARE CONSIDERATIONS **Sequential Compression Devices**

▪ A sequential compression device may be used in the home. Inform the client or caregiver how to apply the device correctly and how to operate the system, including how to respond to the alarm.

Sequential compression therapy often complements other preventive measures. The client's risk level for DVT or pulmonary embolism often determines the preventive measures used. For example, clients at low risk may require only antiemboli stockings. Clients at moderate risk may have both antiemboli stockings and sequential therapy as part of their treatment. The primary care provider may order antiemboli stockings, sequential therapy, and anticoagulation therapy for the high-risk client.

DRUG CAPSULE **Low-Molecular-Weight Heparin** *enoxaparin* (Lovenox)

PREVENTION OF DEEP-VEIN THROMBOSIS

The low-molecular-weight heparins are anticoagulants used to prevent deep vein thrombosis after hip, knee, or abdominal surgery. They are also used for clients at risk for thromboembolus secondary to prolonged bed rest due to acute illness. These heparins are given subcutaneously either once a day or every 12 hours. They have a predictable dose response and do not require lab test monitoring.

NURSING RESPONSIBILITIES

▪ Administration:
   • Administer deep subcutaneous. Do not give IM.
   • Client should be lying down during administration.
   • Do not expel the air bubble from the prefilled syringe. This avoids loss of the drug.
   • The manufacturer recommends injection into the right or left anterior lateral or posterior lateral aspect of the abdominal wall for best absorption.
   • Alternate between right and left abdomen sites.
   • Insert the entire length of the needle into a skinfold created by the thumb and forefinger; hold the skinfold until the needle is withdrawn.
   • Do not massage the injection site to minimize bruising.

▪ Do not mix with other injections.
▪ Lovenox and regular heparin cannot be used interchangeably.
▪ Assess baseline lab data (e.g., CBC, liver function, coagulation) and monitor.
▪ Observe for early signs/symptoms of bleeding.

CLIENT AND FAMILY TEACHING

▪ Review how to administer (see above).
▪ Administer at the same time each day.
▪ Report any unusual bleeding or bruising.
▪ Avoid aspirin or NSAIDs.

Note: Prior to administering any medications, review all aspects with a current drug handbook or other reliable source.

Cardiopulmonary Resuscitation

Cardiopulmonary resuscitation (CPR) is a combination of oral resuscitation (mouth-to-mouth breathing), which supplies oxygen to the lungs, and external cardiac massage (chest compression), which is intended to reestablish cardiac function and blood circulation. CPR is also referred to as *basic life support (BLS)*.

The American Heart Association reviews resuscitation literature to evaluate their guidelines for CPR. Table 51–3 provides highlights of the 2005 American Heart Association guidelines for CPR for the health care provider.

A cardiac arrest is the cessation of cardiac function; the heart stops beating. Often a cardiac arrest is unexpected and sudden. When it occurs, the heart no longer pumps blood to any of the organs of the body. Breathing then stops, and the person becomes unconscious and limp. Within 20 to 40 seconds of a cardiac arrest the victim is clinically dead. After 4 to 6 minutes the lack of oxygen supply to the brain causes permanent and extensive damage.

The three cardinal signs of a cardiac arrest are apnea, absence of a carotid or femoral pulse, and dilated pupils. The person's skin appears pale or grayish and feels cool. Cyanosis is evident when respiratory function fails before heart failure.

A respiratory arrest (pulmonary arrest) is the cessation of breathing. It often occurs because of a blocked airway, but it can occur following a cardiac arrest and for other reasons. A respiratory arrest may occur abruptly or be preceded by short, shallow breathing that becomes increasingly labored.

It is vital that all nurses be trained to perform CPR so resuscitation measures can be initiated immediately when a cardiac or respiratory arrest occurs. Nurses also can be instrumental in increasing community awareness of the need for CPR training and ensuring its availability.

Each health care facility has policies and procedures for announcing cardiac/respiratory arrest and initiating interventions. In many institutions this emergency is called a **Code Blue,** and the announcement is referred to as "calling a code." Each health care institution has a procedure for calling a code. There may be a special Code Blue button at the head of each bed, sometimes it is a special extension on the phone, or it may be a special phone used to announce the emergency. It is critical that each

TABLE 51–3　Changes in CPR Guidelines for the Health Care Provider

CHANGE	NEW (2005)	OLD (2000)	RATIONALE FOR CHANGE
Chest compressions	■ "Push hard and push fast." ■ Compress chest at rate of 100/minute. ■ Allow complete chest recoil after each compression. ■ Minimize interruptions in chest compression.	■ Quality and rate of compressions, importance of chest recoil and need to minimize interruptions were not emphasized.	■ Studies showed that chest compressions were too shallow, and compressions were interrupted too often during CPR.
Compression-to-ventilation ratio	■ Compression–ventilation ratio of 30:2 for single rescuer for all clients except newborns.	■ Adult CPR—15:2 ratio. ■ Infant and child—5:1 ratio.	■ Simplify training. ■ To ensure a longer series of uninterrupted chest compressions. ■ To increase blood flow to heart, brain, and vital organs.
1-second breaths	■ Each rescue breath should be given over 1 second. ■ Chest should rise with each breath. ■ Avoid delivering too many breaths or breaths too large and/or too forceful.	■ Different tidal volumes were recommended. ■ Breaths to be delivered over 1–2 seconds.	■ Blood flow to the lungs is less than normal during CPR. Thus, the victim needs less ventilation than normal. ■ Want to reduce interruptions in compression. ■ Large and forceful breaths may cause gastric inflation.
Attempted defibrillation	■ Deliver one shock followed by immediate CPR beginning with chest compressions. ■ Check rhythm after 5 cycles of CPR.	■ Deliver 3 shocks without CPR between shocks. ■ Check rhythm before and after shocks.	■ Rhythm checks resulted in delays of 37 seconds or longer before delivering compressions. ■ The first shock eliminates ventricular fibrillation (VF) more than 85% of the time. ■ Even when VF is eliminated, it takes several minutes for the heart to return to a normal rhythm. Immediate chest compressions can help deliver oxygen to the heart. ■ There is no evidence that compressions after a shock results in the reoccurrence of VF.

Note: From "Highlights of the 2005 American Heart Association Guidelines for Cardiopulmonary Resuscitation and Emergency Cardiovascular Care," by American Heart Association, 2005–2006, *Currents in Emergency Cardiovascular Care, 16*(4), pp. 1–27.

member of the client care team know the procedure for announcing a code. Calling the code summons the code team to the location of the emergency. The code team is made up of specially trained staff who can handle the emergency. Persons are needed to perform rescue breathing, deliver chest compressions, administer medications, and make a record of the code activities. One person must be designated as the code leader—the person who directs the activities of the other team members.

Some clients have designated via an advance directive that, should they arrest, they not be resuscitated. It is every person's right to make an advance directive of their wishes. If it is the client's wish, the primary care provider should designate "No Code Blue," "No CPR," or "Do Not Resuscitate (DNR)" on the medical record.

Evaluating

Using the overall goals identified in the planning stage, the nurse collects data to evaluate the effectiveness of interventions.

Examples of desired outcomes for the identified goals are found in the Identifying Nursing Diagnoses, Outcomes, and Interventions box earlier in this chapter.

If desired outcomes are not achieved, the nurse, client, and support person if appropriate need to explore the reasons before modifying the care plan. For example, if the outcome "cardiac pump effectiveness" is not achieved, questions to be considered might include the following:

- Have other outcome measures for the goal of maintaining adequate cardiac output been met?
- Are prescribed medications being taken/administered as ordered?
- Are there additional factors that are placing stress on the heart?
- Is there a balance between factors that affect cardiac output, such as preload and afterload?
- Are there signs of fluid overload such as weight gain?

CRITICAL THINKING CHECKPOINT

Mrs. Gloria Papadopolis reports that she is having increasing difficulty because she experiences severe pain in her calf muscles after walking for more than a city block. The pain subsides if she rests for a few minutes, but returns with activity. Her feet are cool and pale; pedal and posterior tibial pulses are not palpable, and femoral pulses are difficult to palpate. She lives in a downtown apartment and uses public transportation to travel across town to visit her husband's grave weekly.

1. What are the circulatory causes of her leg pain? Which risk factors would you expect to find in her history to support this conclusion?

2. Name two nursing diagnoses appropriate for Mrs. Papadopolis. Which would have the highest priority and why?

3. The primary care provider suggests that Mrs. Papadopolis cease her visits to the cemetery since she has to walk a long way there to reach the grave site. Would you agree with this plan? Why or why not? What considerations or viewpoints influence your choice?

4. Mrs. Papadopolis says that she wears support stockings because her friend told her they help the circulation in her legs. How would you respond to this information?

See Critical Thinking Possibilities in *Appendix A*.

CHAPTER 51 **REVIEW**

CHAPTER HIGHLIGHTS

- The cardiovascular system transports gases in the blood to and from the tissues and facilitates the diffusion of gases between the capillaries and body tissues.
- The heart and the blood vessels make up the cardiovascular system that, together with blood, is the major system for transporting oxygen and nutrients to the tissues, and waste products away from the tissues for elimination.
- The right side of the heart receives deoxygenated blood from the body and pumps it to the lungs via the pulmonary arteries; the left side receives oxygenated blood from the lungs and pumps it out to the body via the aorta.
- Coronary arteries supply oxygen and nutrients to the heart muscle.
- The cardiac cycle is made up of systole and diastole periods.
- The cardiac conduction system controls the electrical activity of the heart and the cardiac cycle: systole, contraction of the heart muscle and ejection of blood, and diastole, the relaxation period during which the heart fills with blood.

- Cardiac output depends on the stroke volume, or amount of blood ejected during systole, and the heart rate.
- The systemic blood vessels carry blood to the tissues through a system of arteries, arterioles, and capillaries and return it to the heart through the venules, veins, and the venae cavae.
- The blood pressure rises gradually from birth to reach the adult range in adolescence.
- Atherosclerosis causes fatty plaque to develop within arteries.
- Decreased cardiac output, impaired tissue perfusion, and disorders affecting the blood are the major cardiovascular problems that may affect oxygenation.
- Cardiac output may fall with a myocardial infarction (MI), heart failure, dysrhythmias, and structural alterations of the heart (e.g., valve deformities).

- The most common cause of impaired blood flow to tissues is atherosclerosis; this can lead to tissue ischemia and pain.
- Cardiac monitoring is used for continuous observation of the heart rate and rhythm.
- Nursing interventions to promote circulation include using antiembolic stockings and sequential compression devices to

prevent venous stasis and edema, and also administering cardiopulmonary resuscitation.
- Cardiopulmonary resuscitation (CPR) is used during cardiopulmonary arrest. Each nurse needs to be aware of the hospital's policies and procedures regarding emergencies.

TEST YOUR KNOWLEDGE

1. The home health nurse has developed a teaching guide for a client that focuses on the importance of regular physical activity with gradually increasing activity levels. This teaching guide specifically promotes:
   1. Cardiac output and tissue perfusion.
   2. Renal perfusion and formation of urine.
   3. Oxygen-carrying capacity of white blood cells.
   4. Effective breathing and airway clearance.

2. The client's ECG monitor reflects normal electrical activity through the heart's conduction system. The nurse knows that the electrical impulse travels in which sequence?
   1. Atrioventricular node
   2. Bundle branches
   3. Sinoatrial node
   4. Bundle of His
   5. Purkinje fibers

   Place the numbers in the correct sequence:_____

3. Which of the following would most likely be included in the evaluation of the client goal: "Demonstrate adequate tissue perfusion"
   1. Symmetrical chest expansion
   2. Uses pursed-lip breathing
   3. Brisk capillary refill
   4. Activity intolerance

4. A client is admitted with acute crushing chest pain that radiates down his left arm. The nurse expects which of the following blood tests to be ordered for this client? Select all that apply.
   1. Blood urea nitrogen (BUN)
   2. Hemoglobin and hematocrit
   3. Creatine kinase (CK)
   4. Serum glucose
   5. Troponin

5. Which of the following clients is most likely to experience poor cardiac output?
   1. A client who has recently completed exercising
   2. A client who has a stroke volume of 70 mL per beat and a heart rate of 70 beats/minute
   3. A client with a sustained heart rate of 150 beats/minute
   4. A client who receives a positive inotropic medication

6. The nurse is assigned to three clients with the following diagnoses: myocardial infarction (MI), heart failure (HF), and anemia. In planning for their nursing care, the nurse knows that all three clients will have which one of the following signs/symptoms?
   1. Pain
   2. Distended neck veins
   3. Shortness of breath
   4. Nausea

7. Which of the following validates that the nurse should initiate cardiopulmonary resuscitation on a comatose client?
   1. Cool, pale skin; unconsciousness; absence of radial pulse
   2. Cyanosis, slow pulse, dilated pupils
   3. Absent pulses, flushed skin, pinpoint pupils
   4. Apnea, absence of carotid or femoral pulses, dilated pupils

8. Which of the following diagnoses would be most appropriate for clients with cardiovascular disease? Select all that apply.
   1. *Ineffective Tissue Perfusion*
   2. *Acute Confusion*
   3. *Decreased Cardiac Output*
   4. *Sleep Pattern Disturbance*
   5. *Activity Intolerance*

9. The surgeon ordered SCDs to be applied postoperatively. The nurse teaches the client that the purpose of sequential compression devices is to:
   1. Promote arterial circulation.
   2. Promote venous return from the legs.
   3. Decrease afterload.
   4. Decrease postoperative pain.

10. A client with severe mitral stenosis is having surgery tomorrow. While teaching the client, the nurse shows the client a diagram of the heart. Identify with an "X" which valve the client will have replaced.

From Fremgen, Bonnie F., Frucht, Suzanne S. *Medical Terminology: A Living Language*, 3rd ed., © 2005. Electronically reproduced by permission of Pearson Education, Inc., Upper Saddle River, New Jersey.

See Answers to Test Your Knowledge in Appendix A.

EXPLORE MEDIALINK www.prenhall.com/berman

DVD-ROM
- Audio Glossary
- NCLEX Review
- Skill Checklist
- Animations:
  - Heart
  - Blood Flow Atria
  - Blood Pressure
  - Hemodynamics
  - Congenital Heart Defects
  - Dysrhythmias
  - Ventricular Contraction
  - A & P Review

- Videos:
  - Coronary Artery Disease
  - Dysrhythmia
  - Heart Attack

COMPANION WEBSITE
- Additional NCLEX Review
- Case Study: Client with Diabetes
- Care Plan Activity: Client Experiencing Pain from Walking
- Application Activity: Health Promotion for a Healthy Heart
- Links to Resources

READINGS AND REFERENCES

SUGGESTED READINGS

Crowther, M., & McCourt, K. (2004). Get the edge on deep vein thrombosis. *Nursing Management, 35*(1), 21–29.
The authors provide a comprehensive overview of the prevention, identification, and treatment of deep vein thrombosis.

Piano, M. R. (2005). The cardiovascular effects of alcohol: The good and the bad. *American Journal of Nursing, 105*(7), 87–91.
This article reviews the physiology of alcohol metabolism, provides information related to the benefits and adverse effects of alcohol consumption, and ends with helpful information about what to tell clients.

RELATED RESEARCH

Heitman, L. K. (2006). The influence of social support on cardiovascular health in families. *Family Community Health, 29*(2), 131–142.

Henderson, D. P., & Knapp, J. F. (2005). Report of the National Consensus Conference on family presence during pediatric cardiopulmonary resuscitation and procedures. *Pediatric Emergency Care, 21*(11), 787–791.

REFERENCES

American Heart Association. (2005–2006). Highlights of the 2005 American Heart Association guidelines for cardiopulmonary resuscitation and emergency cardiovascular care. *Currents in Emergency Cardiovascular Care, 16*(4), 1–27.

Ball, J. W., & Bindler, R. C. (2006). *Child health nursing.* Upper Saddle River, NJ: Prentice Hall Health.

Bergen, C., & Compher, C. (2006). Total homocysteine concentration and associated cardiovascular and renal implications in adults. *Journal of Cardiovascular Nursing, 21*(1), 40–46.

Blosser, C. G., & Freitas-Nichols, J. (2004). Cardiovascular disorders. In C. E. Burns, A. M. Dunn, M. A. Brady, M. B. Starr, & C. G. Blosser, *Pediatric primary care: A handbook for nurse practitioners.* Philadelphia: W. B. Saunders/Elsevier.

Bonham, P. A. (2003). Determing the toe brachial pressure index. *Nursing, 33*(9), 54–55.

Dochterman, J. M., & Bulechek, G. M. (Eds.). (2004). *Nursing interventions classification (NIC)* (4th ed.). St. Louis, MO: Mosby.

Evangelista, L. S., & Miller, P. S. (2006). Overweight and obesity in the context of heart failure. Implications for practice and future research. *Journal of Cardiovascular Nursing, 21*(1), 27–33.

Hoffman, J. (2001). Incidence, mortality and natural history. In R. H. Anderson, R. Anderson, E. J. Baker, F. J. McCartney, M. L. Rigby, & M. Tynan, *Paediatric cardiology* (2nd ed.). New York: Churchill Livingstone.

Lloyd-Jones, D. M., Leip, E. P., Larson, M. G., D'Agostino, R. B., Beiser, A., Wilson, P., et al. (2006). Prediction of lifetime risk for cardiovascular disease by risk factor burden at 50 years of age. *Circulation, 113*(6), 791–798.

Moorhead, S., Johnson, M., & Maas, M. (Eds.). (2004) *Nursing outcomes classification (NOC)* (3rd ed.). St. Louis, MO: Mosby.

NANDA International. (2007). *NANDA nursing diagnoses: Definitions and classification 2007–2008.* Philadelphia: Author.

Rice, K. L. (2005). How to measure ankle/brachial index. *Nursing, 35*(1), 56–57.

Richardson, C. R., Kriska, A. M., Lantz, P. M., & Hayward, R. A. (2004). Physical activity and mortality across cardiovascular disease risk groups. *Medicine & Science in Sports & Exercise, 36*(11), 1923–1929.

Ruidavets, J., Bongard, V., Simon, C., Dallongeville, J., Ducimetiere, P., Arveiler, D., et al. (2006). Independent contribution of dairy products and calcium intake to blood pressure variations at a population level. *Journal of Hypertension, 24,* 671–681.

SELECTED BIBLIOGRAPHY

Anonymous. (2003). Why a drink a day may keep heart disease at bay. *Tufts University Health & Nutrition Letter, 28*(8), 2.

Bollinger, K., & Sadar, A. M. (2003). Care and management of the patient with right heart failure secondary to diastolic dysfunction. *Critical Care Nursing Quarterly, 26*(1), 22–27.

Bolton, M. M., & Wilson, B. A. (2005). The influence of race on heart failure in African-American women. *Medsurg Nursing, 14*(1), 8–15.

Caboral, M., & Mitchell, J. (2003). B-type natriuretic peptide: A new tool in the armamentarium used to accurately diagnose heart failure. *Progress in Cardiovascular Nursing, 18*(4), 190–193.

Calver, P., Braungardt, T., Kupchik, N., Jensen, A., & Cutler, C. (2005). The big chill: Improving the odds after cardiac arrest. *RN, 68*(5), 58–62.

Craig, K. J., & Hopkins-Pepe, L. (2006). Understanding the new AHA guidelines, part I. *Nursing, 36*(3), 53–54.

Craig, K. J., & Hopkins-Pepe, L. (2006). Understanding the new AHA guidelines, part II. *Nursing, 36*(5), 52–53.

Duffy, J. R., Hoskins, L. M., & Chen, M. (2004). Nonpharmacological strategies for improving heart failure outcomes in the community: A systematic review. *Journal of Nursing Care Quality, 19*(4), 349–360.

Efre, A. J. (2004). Gender bias in acute myocardial infarction. *Nurse Practitioner, 29*(11), 42, 49–55.

Fort, C. W. (2002). Get pumped to prevent DVT. *Nursing, 32*(9), 50–53.

Hussey, L. C., & Hardin, S. (2005). Comparison of characteristics of heart failure by race and gender. *Dimensions of Critical Care Nursing, 24*(1), 41–46.

Konick-McMahan, J., Bixby, B., & McKenna, C. (2003). Heart failure in older adults. Providing nursing care to improve outcomes. *Journal of Gerontological Nursing, 29*(12), 35–41.

Lippincott Williams & Wilkins. (2004). Applying antiembolism stockings isn't just pulling on socks. *Nursing, 34*(8), 48–49.

Nicholas, M. (2004). Heart failure: Pathophysiology, treatment and nursing care. *Nursing Standard, 19*(11), 46–51.

Raymond, S. U., Leeder, S., & Greenberg, H. M. (2006). Obesity and cardiovascular disease in developing countries: A growing problem and an economic threat. *Current Opinion in Clinical Nutrition and Metabolic Care, 9,* 111–116.

Robinson, S. L. (2004). Is it an MI? What the leads tell you. *RN, 67*(5), 48–53.

Scordo, K. A. (2005). Noninvasive diagnosis of coronary artery disease in women. *Journal of Cardiovascular Nursing, 20*(6), 420–426.

Stansbury, J. P., Jia, H., Williams, L. S., Vogel, W. B., & Duncan, P. W. (2005). Ethnic disparities in stroke: Epidemiology, acute care, and postacute outcomes. *Stroke, 36,* 374–386.

Fluid, Electrolyte, and Acid–Base Balance

LEARNING OUTCOMES

After completing this chapter, you will be able to:

1. Discuss the function, distribution, movement, and regulation of fluids and electrolytes in the body.

2. Describe the regulation of acid–base balance in the body, including the roles of the lungs, the kidneys and buffers.

3. Identify factors affecting normal body fluid, electrolyte, and acid–base balance.

4. Discuss the risk factors for and the causes and effects of fluid, electrolyte, and acid–base imbalances.

5. Collect assessment data related to the client's fluid, electrolyte, and acid–base balances.

6. Identify examples of nursing diagnoses, outcomes, and interventions for clients with altered fluid, electrolyte, or acid–base balance.

7. Teach clients measures to maintain fluid and electrolyte balance.

8. Implement measures to correct imbalances of fluids and electrolytes or acids and bases such as enteral or parenteral replacements and blood transfusions.

9. Evaluate the effect of nursing and collaborative interventions on the client's fluid, electrolyte, or acid–base balance.

KEY TERMS

acid, *1432*	**hematocrit,** *1449*	**isotonic,** *1427*
acidosis, *1433*	**hemolytic transfusion reaction,** *1473*	**metabolic acidosis,** *1442*
active transport, *1428*	**homeostasis,** *1424*	**metabolic alkalosis,** *1442*
agglutinins, *1472*	**hydrostatic pressure,** *1427*	**milliequivalent,** *1425*
agglutinogens, *1472*	**hypercalcemia,** *1441*	**obligatory losses,** *1429*
alkalosis, *1433*	**hyperchloremia,** *1442*	**oncotic pressure,** *1427*
anions, *1425*	**hyperkalemia,** *1438*	**osmolality,** *1427*
antibodies, *1472*	**hypermagnesemia,** *1442*	**osmosis,** *1426*
antigens, *1472*	**hypernatremia,** *1438*	**osmotic pressure,** *1427*
arterial blood gases (ABGs), *1449*	**hyperphosphatemia,** *1442*	**overhydration,** *1437*
bases, *1432*	**hypertonic,** *1427*	**peripherally inserted central venous catheter (PICC),** *1456*
buffers, *1433*	**hypervolemia,** *1435*	**pH,** *1432*
cations, *1425*	**hypocalcemia,** *1441*	**pitting edema,** *1436*
central venous catheters, *1456*	**hypochloremia,** *1442*	**plasma,** *1424*
colloid osmotic pressure, *1427*	**hypokalemia,** *1438*	**renin-angiotensin-aldosterone system,** *1429*
colloids, *1426*	**hypomagnesemia,** *1442*	**respiratory acidosis,** *1442*
compensation, *1442*	**hyponatremia,** *1438*	**respiratory alkalosis,** *1442*
crystalloids, *1426*	**hypophosphatemia,** *1442*	**selectively permeable,** *1426*
dehydration, *1437*	**hypotonic,** *1427*	**solutes,** *1426*
diffusion, *1427*	**hypovolemia,** *1435*	**solvent,** *1426*
drip factor, *1465*	**insensible fluid loss,** *1428*	**specific gravity,** *1449*
electrolytes, *1425*	**interstitial fluid,** *1425*	**third space syndrome,** *1435*
extracellular fluid (ECF), *1424*	**intracellular fluid (ICF),** *1424*	**transcellular fluid,** *1425*
filtration, *1427*	**intravascular fluid,** *1424*	**volume expanders,** *1456*
filtration pressure, *1427*	**ions,** *1425*	
fluid volume deficit (FVD), *1435*		
fluid volume excess (FVE), *1435*		

In good health, a delicate balance of fluids, electrolytes, and acids and bases is maintained in the body. This balance, or physiologic **homeostasis,** depends on multiple physiologic processes that regulate fluid intake and output and the movement of water and the substances dissolved in it between the body compartments.

Almost every illness has the potential to threaten this balance. Even in daily living, excessive temperatures or vigorous activity can disturb the balance if adequate water and salt intake is not maintained. Therapeutic measures, such as the use of diuretics or nasogastric suction, can also disturb the body's homeostasis unless water and electrolytes are replaced.

BODY FLUIDS AND ELECTROLYTES

The proportion of the human body composed of fluid is surprisingly large. Approximately 60% of the average healthy adult's weight is water, the primary body fluid. In good health this volume remains relatively constant and the person's weight varies by less than 0.2 kg (0.5 lb) in 24 hours, regardless of the amount of fluid ingested.

Water is vital to health and normal cellular function, serving as

- A medium for metabolic reactions within cells.
- A transporter for nutrients, waste products, and other substances.

- A lubricant.
- An insulator and shock absorber.
- One means of regulating and maintaining body temperature.

Age, sex, and body fat affect total body water. Infants have the highest proportion of water, accounting for 70% to 80% of their body weight. The proportion of body water decreases with aging. In people older than 60 years of age, it represents only about 50% of the total body weight. Women also have a lower percentage of body water than men. Women and the elderly have reduced body water due to decreased muscle mass and a greater percentage of fat tissue. Fat tissue is essentially free of water, whereas lean tissue contains a significant amount of water. Water makes up a greater percentage of a lean person's body weight than an obese person's.

Distribution of Body Fluids

The body's fluid is divided into two major compartments, intracellular and extracellular. **Intracellular fluid (ICF)** is found within the cells of the body. It constitutes approximately two-thirds of the total body fluid in adults. **Extracellular fluid (ECF)** is found outside the cells and accounts for about one-third of total body fluid. It is subdivided into compartments. The two main compartments of ECF are intravascular and interstitial. **Intravascular fluid,** or **plasma,** accounts for approximately 20% of the ECF

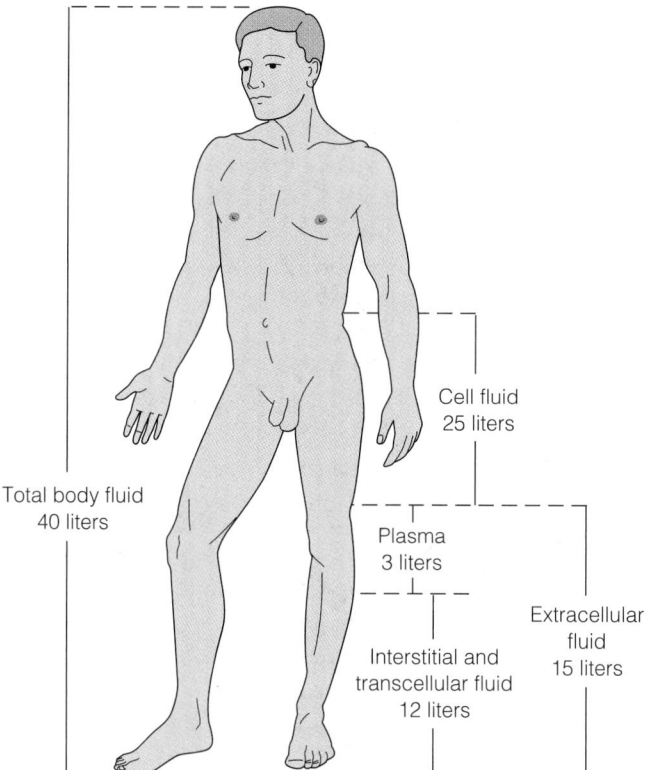

Figure 52-1 ■ Total body fluid represents 40 L in an adult male weighing 70 kg (154 lb).

and is found within the vascular system. **Interstitial fluid,** accounting for approximately 75% of the ECF, surrounds the cells. The other compartments of ECF are the lymph and transcellular fluids. Examples of **transcellular fluid** include cerebrospinal, pericardial, pancreatic, pleural, intraocular, biliary, peritoneal, and synovial fluids (Figure 52-1 ■).

Intracellular fluid is vital to normal cell functioning. It contains solutes such as oxygen, electrolytes, and glucose, and it provides a medium in which metabolic processes of the cell take place.

Although extracellular fluid is in the smaller of the two compartments, it is the transport system that carries nutrients to and waste products from the cells. For example, plasma carries oxygen from the lungs and glucose from the gastrointestinal tract to the capillaries of the vascular system. From there, the oxygen and glucose move across the capillary membranes into the interstitial spaces and then across the cellular membranes into the cells. The opposite route is taken for waste products, such as carbon dioxide going from the cells to the lungs and metabolic acid wastes going eventually to the kidneys. Interstitial fluid transports wastes from the cells by way of the lymph system as well as directly into the blood plasma through capillaries.

Composition of Body Fluids

Extracellular and intracellular fluids contain oxygen from the lungs, dissolved nutrients from the gastrointestinal tract, excretory products of metabolism such as carbon dioxide, and charged particles called **ions.**

Many salts dissociate in water, that is, break up into electrically charged ions. The salt sodium chloride breaks up into one ion of sodium (Na^+) and one ion of chloride (Cl^-). These charged particles are called **electrolytes** because they are capable of conducting electricity. The number of ions that carry a positive charge, called **cations,** and ions that carry a negative charge, called **anions,** should be equal. Examples of cations are sodium (Na^+), potassium (K^+), calcium (Ca^{2+}), and magnesium (Mg^{2+}). Examples of anions include chloride (Cl^-), bicarbonate HCO_3^-, phosphate HPO_4^{2-}, and sulfate SO_4^{2-}.

Electrolytes generally are measured in milliequivalents per liter of water (mEq/L) or milligrams per 100 milliliters (mg/100 mL). The term **milliequivalent** refers to the chemical combining power of the ion, or the capacity of cations to combine with anions to form molecules. This combining activity is measured in relation to the combining activity of the hydrogen ion (H^+). Thus, 1 mEq of any anion equals 1 mEq of any cation. For example, sodium and chloride ions are equivalent, since they combine equally: 1 mEq of Na^+ equals 1 mEq of Cl^-. However, these cations and anions are not equal in weight: 1 mg of Na^+ does not equal 1 mg of Cl^-; rather, 3 mg of Na^+ equals 2 mg of Cl^-.

Clinically, the milliequivalent system is most often used. However, nurses need to be aware that different systems of measurement may be found when interpreting laboratory results. For example, calcium levels frequently are reported in milligrams per deciliter (1 dL = 100 mL) instead of milliequivalents per liter. It also is important to remember that laboratory tests are usually performed using blood plasma, an extracellular fluid. These results may reflect what is happening in the ECF, but it generally is not possible to directly measure electrolyte concentrations within the cell.

The composition of fluids varies from one body compartment to another. In extracellular fluid, the principal electrolytes are sodium, chloride, and bicarbonate. Other electrolytes such as potassium, calcium, and magnesium are also present but in much smaller quantities. Plasma and interstitial fluid, the two primary components of ECF, contain essentially the same electrolytes and solutes, with the exception of protein. Plasma is a protein-rich fluid, containing large amounts of albumin, but interstitial fluid contains little or no protein.

The composition of intracellular fluid differs significantly from that of ECF. Potassium and magnesium are the primary cations present in ICF, with phosphate and sulfate the major anions. As in ECF, other electrolytes are present within the cell, but in much smaller concentrations (Figure 52-2 ■).

Maintaining a balance of fluid volumes and electrolyte compositions in the fluid compartments of the body is essential to health. Normal and unusual fluid and electrolyte losses must be replaced if homeostasis is to be maintained.

Other body fluids such as gastric and intestinal secretions also contain electrolytes. This is of particular concern when these fluids are lost from the body (for example, in severe vomiting or diarrhea or when gastric suction removes the gastric secretions). Fluid and electrolyte imbalances can result from excessive losses through these routes.

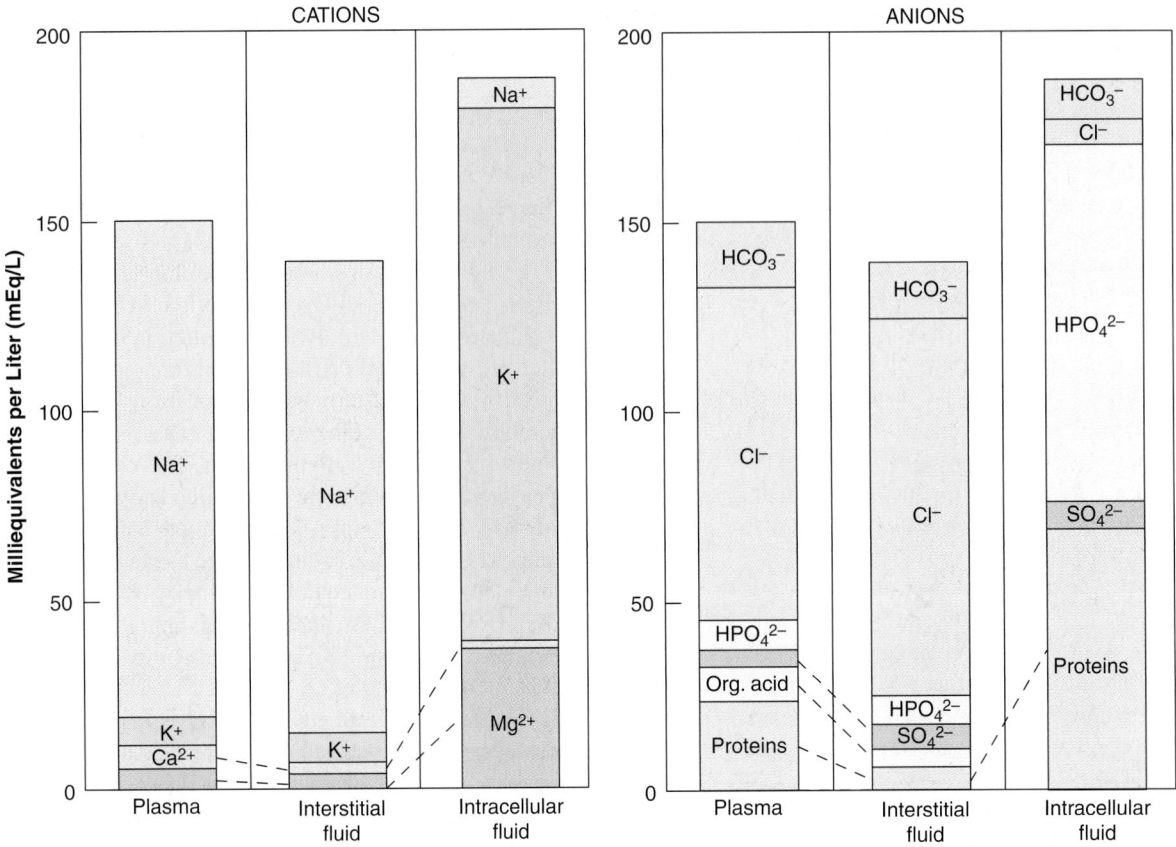

Figure 52-2 ■ Electrolyte composition (cations and anions) of body fluid compartments.

Martini, Fredric H.; Halyard, Rebecca A., *Fundamentals of Anatomy and Physiology Interactive*, (Media Edition), 4th ed., © 1998. Reproduced with permission of Pearson Education, Inc., Upper Saddle River, New Jersey.

Movement of Body Fluids and Electrolytes

The body fluid compartments are separated from one another by cell membranes and the capillary membrane. While these membranes are completely permeable to water, they are considered to be **selectively permeable** to solutes as substances move across them with varying degrees of ease. Small particles such as ions, oxygen, and carbon dioxide easily move across these membranes, but larger molecules like glucose and proteins have more difficulty moving between fluid compartments.

The methods by which electrolytes and other solutes move are osmosis, diffusion, filtration, and active transport.

Osmosis

Osmosis is the movement of water across cell membranes, from the less concentrated solution to the more concentrated solution (Figure 52-3 ■). In other words, water moves toward the higher concentration of solute in an attempt to equalize the concentrations.

Solutes are substances dissolved in a liquid. For example, when sugar is added to coffee, the sugar is the solute. Solutes may be **crystalloids** (salts that dissolve readily into true solutions) or **colloids** (substances such as large protein molecules that do not readily dissolve into true solutions). A **solvent** is the component of a solution that can dissolve a solute. In the previous example, coffee is the solvent for the sugar.

In the body, water is the solvent; the solutes include electrolytes, oxygen and carbon dioxide, glucose, urea, amino acids, and proteins. Osmosis occurs when the concentration of solutes on one side of a selectively permeable membrane, such as the capillary membrane, is higher than on the other side. For example, a marathon runner loses a significant amount of water through perspiration, increasing the concentration of solutes in the plasma because of water loss. This higher solute concentration draws water from the interstitial space and cells into the vascular compartment to equalize the concentration of solutes

Figure 52-3 ■ Osmosis: Water molecules move from the less concentrated area to the more concentrated area in an attempt to equalize the concentration of solutions on two sides of a membrane.

in all fluid compartments. Osmosis is an important mechanism for maintaining homeostasis and fluid balance.

The concentration of solutes in body fluids is usually expressed as the **osmolality.** Osmolality is determined by the total solute concentration within a fluid compartment and is measured as parts of solute per kilogram of water.

Osmolality is reported as milliosmols per kilogram (mOsm/kg). Sodium is by far the greatest determinant of *serum osmolality,* with glucose and urea also contributing. Potassium, glucose, and urea are the primary contributors to the osmolality of intracellular fluid. The term *tonicity* may be used to refer to the osmolality of a solution. Solutions may be termed isotonic, hypertonic, or hypotonic. An **isotonic** solution has the same osmolality as body fluids. Normal saline, 0.9% sodium chloride, is an isotonic solution. **Hypertonic** solutions have a higher osmolality than body fluids; 3% sodium chloride is a hypertonic solution. **Hypotonic** solutions such as one-half normal saline (0.45% sodium chloride), by contrast, have a lower osmolality than body fluids.

Osmotic pressure is the power of a solution to draw water across a semipermeable membrane. When two solutions of different solute concentrations are separated by a semipermeable membrane, the solution of higher solute concentration exerts a higher osmotic pressure, drawing water across the membrane to equalize the concentrations of the solutions. For example, infusing a hypertonic intravenous solution such as 3% sodium chloride will draw fluid out of red blood cells (RBCs), causing them to shrink. On the other hand, a hypotonic solution administered intravenously will cause the RBCs to swell as water is drawn into the cells by their higher osmotic pressure. In the body, plasma proteins exert an osmotic draw called **colloid osmotic pressure** or **oncotic pressure,** pulling water from the interstitial space into the vascular compartment. This is an important mechanism in maintaining vascular volume.

Diffusion

Diffusion is the continual intermingling of molecules in liquids, gases, or solids brought about by the random movement of the molecules. For example, two gases become mixed by the constant motion of their molecules. The process of diffusion occurs even when two substances are separated by a thin membrane. In the body, diffusion of water, electrolytes, and other substances occurs through the "split pores" of capillary membranes.

The rate of diffusion of substances varies according to (a) the size of the molecules, (b) the concentration of the solution, and (c) the temperature of the solution. Larger molecules move less

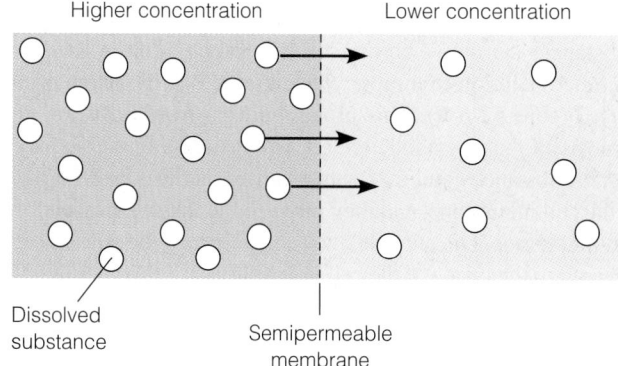

Figure 52-4 ■ Diffusion: The movement of molecules through a semipermeable membrane from an area of higher concentration to an area of lower concentration.

quickly than smaller ones because they require more energy to move about. With diffusion, the molecules move from a solution of higher concentration to a solution of lower concentration (Figure 52-4 ■). Increases in temperature increase the rate of motion of molecules and therefore the rate of diffusion.

Filtration

Filtration is a process whereby fluid and solutes move together across a membrane from one compartment to another. The movement is from an area of higher pressure to one of lower pressure. An example of filtration is the movement of fluid and nutrients from the capillaries of the arterioles to the interstitial fluid around the cells. The pressure in the compartment that results in the movement of the fluid and substances dissolved in fluid out of the compartment is called **filtration pressure.** **Hydrostatic pressure** is the pressure exerted by a fluid within a closed system on the walls of a container in which it is contained. The hydrostatic pressure of blood is the force exerted by blood against the vascular walls (e.g., the artery walls). The principle involved in hydrostatic pressure is that fluids move from the area of greater pressure to the area of lesser pressure. Using the example of the blood vessels, the plasma proteins in the blood exert a colloid osmotic or oncotic pressure (see the earlier section "Osmosis") that opposes the hydrostatic pressure and holds the fluid in the vascular compartment to maintain the vascular volume. When the hydrostatic pressure is greater than the osmotic pressure, the fluid filters out of the blood vessels. The filtration pressure in this example is the difference between the hydrostatic pressure and the osmotic pressure (Figure 52-5 ■).

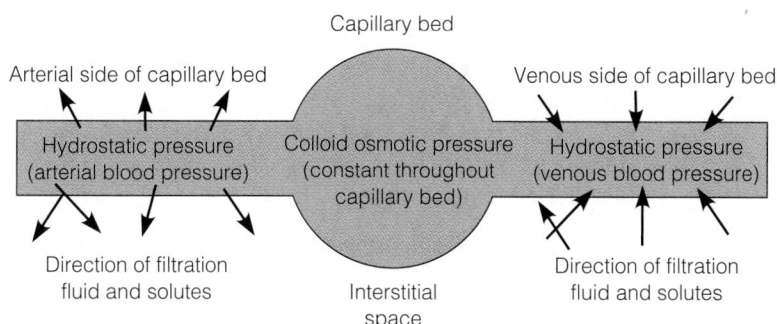

Capillary bed

Arterial side of capillary bed | Venous side of capillary bed

Hydrostatic pressure (arterial blood pressure) | Colloid osmotic pressure (constant throughout capillary bed) | Hydrostatic pressure (venous blood pressure)

Direction of filtration fluid and solutes | Interstitial space | Direction of filtration fluid and solutes

Figure 52-5 ■ Schematic of filtration pressure changes within a capillary bed. On the arterial side, arterial blood pressure exceeds colloid osmotic pressure, so that water and dissolved substances move out of the capillary into the interstitial space. On the venous side, venous blood pressure is less than colloid osmotic pressure, so that water and dissolved substances move into the capillary.

Active Transport

Substances can move across cell membranes from a less concentrated solution to a more concentrated one by **active transport** (Figure 52-6 ■). This process differs from diffusion and osmosis in that metabolic energy is expended. In active transport, a substance combines with a carrier on the outside surface of the cell membrane, and they move to the inside surface of the cell membrane. Once inside, they separate, and the substance is released to the inside of the cell. A specific carrier is required for each substance, enzymes are required for active transport, and energy is expended.

This process is of particular importance in maintaining the differences in sodium and potassium ion concentrations of ECF and ICF. Under normal conditions, sodium concentrations are higher in the extracellular fluid, and potassium concentrations are higher inside the cells. To maintain these proportions, the active transport mechanism (the sodium-potassium pump) is activated, moving sodium from the cells and potassium into the cells.

Regulating Body Fluids

In a healthy person, the volumes and chemical composition of the fluid compartments stay within narrow safe limits. Normally fluid intake and fluid loss are balanced. Illness can upset this balance so that the body has too little or too much fluid.

Fluid Intake

During periods of moderate activity at moderate temperature, the average adult drinks about 1,500 mL per day but needs 2,500 mL per day, an additional 1,000 mL. This added volume is acquired from foods and from the oxidation of these foods during metabolic processes. Interestingly, the water content of food is relatively large, contributing about 750 mL per day. The water content of fresh vegetables is approximately 90%, of fresh fruits about 85%, and of lean meats around 60%.

Figure 52-6 ■ An example of active transport. Energy (ATP) is used to move sodium molecules and potassium molecules across a semipermeable membrane against sodium's and potassium's concentration gradients (i.e., from areas of lesser concentration to areas of greater concentration).

TABLE 52–1 **Average Daily Fluid Intake for an Adult**	
SOURCE	**AMOUNT (ML)**
Oral fluids	1,200 to 1,500
Water in foods	1,000
Water as by-product of food metabolism	200
Total	2,400 to 2,700

Water as a by-product of food metabolism accounts for most of the remaining fluid volume required. This quantity is approximately 200 mL per day for the average adult. See Table 52–1.

The thirst mechanism is the primary regulator of fluid intake. The thirst center is located in the hypothalamus of the brain. A number of stimuli trigger this center, including the osmotic pressure of body fluids, vascular volume, and angiotensin (a hormone released in response to decreased blood flow to the kidneys). For example, a long-distance runner loses significant amounts of water through perspiration and rapid breathing during a race, increasing the concentration of solutes and the osmotic pressure of body fluids. This increased osmotic pressure stimulates the thirst center, causing the runner to experience the sensation of thirst and the desire to drink to replace lost fluids.

Thirst is normally relieved immediately after drinking a small amount of fluid, even before it is absorbed from the gastrointestinal tract. However, this relief is only temporary, and the thirst returns in about 15 minutes. The thirst is again temporarily relieved after the ingested fluid distends the upper gastrointestinal tract. These mechanisms protect the individual from drinking too much, because it takes from 30 minutes to 1 hour for the fluid to be absorbed and distributed throughout the body. See Figure 52-7 ■.

Fluid Output

Fluid losses from the body counterbalance the adult's 2,500-mL average daily intake of fluid, as shown in Table 52–2. There are four routes of fluid output:

1. Urine
2. Insensible loss through the skin as perspiration and through the lungs as water vapor in the expired air
3. Noticeable loss through the skin
4. Loss through the intestines in feces

URINE. Urine formed by the kidneys and excreted from the urinary bladder is the major avenue of fluid output. Normal urine output for an adult is 1,400 to 1,500 mL per 24 hours, or at least 0.5 mL per kilogram per hour. In healthy people, urine output may vary noticeably from day to day. Urine volume automatically increases as fluid intake increases. If fluid loss through perspiration is large, however, urine volume decreases to maintain fluid balance in the body.

INSENSIBLE LOSSES. **Insensible fluid loss** occurs through the skin and lungs. It is called insensible because it is usually not noticeable and cannot be measured. Insensible fluid loss through

Figure 52-7 ■ Factors stimulating water intake through the thirst mechanism.

From Lemone, Priscilla; Burke, Karen M., *Medical Surgical Nursing: Critical Thinking in Client Care,* 3rd ed © 2004. Reproduced with permission of Pearson Education, Inc., Upper Saddle River, New Jersey.

the skin occurs in two ways. Water is lost through diffusion and through perspiration (which is noticeable but not measurable). Water losses through diffusion are not noticeable but normally account for 300 to 400 mL per day. This loss can be significantly increased if the protective layer of the skin is lost as with burns or large abrasions. Perspiration varies depending on factors such as environmental temperature and metabolic activity. Fever and exercise increase metabolic activity and heat production, thereby increasing fluid losses through the skin.

Another type of insensible loss is the water in exhaled air. In an adult, this is normally 300 to 400 mL per day. When respiratory rate accelerates, for example, due to exercise or an elevated body temperature, this loss can increase.

TABLE 52–2 Average Daily Fluid Output for an Adult

ROUTE	AMOUNT (ML)
Urine	1,400 to 1,500
Insensible losses	
Lungs	350 to 400
Skin	350 to 400
Sweat	100
Feces	100 to 200
Total	2,300 to 2,600

FECES. The chyme that passes from the small intestine into the large intestine contains water and electrolytes. The volume of chyme entering the large intestine in an adult is normally about 1,500 mL per day. Of this amount, all but about 100 mL is reabsorbed in the proximal half of the large intestine.

Certain fluid losses are required to maintain normal body function. These are known as **obligatory losses.** Approximately 500 mL of fluid must be excreted through the kidneys of an adult each day to eliminate metabolic waste products from the body. Water lost through respirations, through the skin, and in feces also are obligatory losses, necessary for temperature regulation and elimination of waste products. The total of all these losses is approximately 1,300 mL per day.

Maintaining Homeostasis

The volume and composition of body fluids is regulated through several homeostatic mechanisms. A number of body systems contribute to this regulation, including the kidneys, the endocrine system, the cardiovascular system, the lungs, and the gastrointestinal system. Hormones such as antidiuretic hormone (ADH; also known as arginine vasopressin or AVP), the renin-angiotensin-aldosterone system, and atrial natriuretic factor are involved, as are mechanisms to monitor and maintain vascular volume.

KIDNEYS. The kidneys are the primary regulator of body fluids and electrolyte balance. They regulate the volume and osmolality of extracellular fluids by regulating water and electrolyte excretion. The kidneys adjust the reabsorption of water from plasma filtrate and ultimately the amount excreted as urine. Although 135 to 180 L of plasma per day is normally filtered in an adult, only about 1.5 L of urine is excreted. Electrolyte balance is maintained by selective retention and excretion by the kidneys. The kidneys also play a significant role in acid–base regulation, excreting hydrogen ion (H^+) and retaining bicarbonate.

ANTIDIURETIC HORMONE. Antidiuretic hormone, which regulates water excretion from the kidney, is synthesized in the anterior portion of the hypothalamus and acts on the collecting ducts of the nephrons. When serum osmolality rises, ADH is produced, causing the collecting ducts to become more permeable to water. This increased permeability allows more water to be reabsorbed into the blood. As more water is reabsorbed, urine output falls and serum osmolality decreases because the water dilutes body fluids. Conversely, if serum osmolality decreases, ADH is suppressed, the collecting ducts become less permeable to water, and urine output increases. Excess water is excreted, and serum osmolality returns to normal. Other factors also affect the production and release of ADH, including blood volume, temperature, pain, stress, and some drugs such as opiates, barbiturates, and nicotine. See Figure 52-8 ■.

RENIN-ANGIOTENSIN-ALDOSTERONE SYSTEM. Specialized receptors in the juxtaglomerular cells of the kidney nephrons respond to changes in renal perfusion. This initiates the **renin-angiotensin-aldosterone system.** If blood flow or pressure to the kidney decreases, renin is released. Renin causes the conversion of angiotensinogen to angiotensin I, which is then converted to angiotensin II by angiotensin-converting enzyme. Angiotensin II

Figure 52-8 ■ Antidiuretic hormone (ADH) regulates water excretion from the kidneys.

acts directly on the nephrons to promote sodium and water retention. In addition, it stimulates the release of aldosterone from the adrenal cortex. Aldosterone also promotes sodium retention in the distal nephron. The net effect of the renin-angiotensin-aldosterone system is to restore blood volume (and renal perfusion) through sodium and water retention.

ATRIAL NATRIURETIC FACTOR. Atrial natriuretic factor (ANF) is released from cells in the atrium of the heart in response to excess blood volume and stretching of the atrial walls. Acting on the nephrons, ANF promotes sodium wasting and acts as a potent diuretic, thus reducing vascular volume. ANF also inhibits thirst, reducing fluid intake.

Regulating Electrolytes

Electrolytes, charged ions capable of conducting electricity, are present in all body fluids and fluid compartments. Just as maintaining the fluid balance is vital to normal body function, so is

maintaining electrolyte balance. Although the concentration of specific electrolytes differs between fluid compartments, a balance of cations (positively charged ions) and anions (negatively charged ions) always exists. Electrolytes are important for

- Maintaining fluid balance.
- Contributing to acid–base regulation.
- Facilitating enzyme reactions.
- Transmitting neuromuscular reactions.

Most electrolytes enter the body through dietary intake and are excreted in the urine. Some electrolytes, such as sodium and chloride, are not stored by the body and must be consumed daily to maintain normal levels. Potassium and calcium, on the other hand, are stored in the cells and bone, respectively. When serum levels drop, ions can shift out of the storage "pool" into the blood to maintain adequate serum levels for normal functioning. The regulatory mechanisms and functions of the major electrolytes are summarized in Table 52–3.

TABLE 52–3   Regulation and Functions of Electrolytes

ELECTROLYTE	REGULATION	FUNCTION
Sodium (Na$^+$)	▪ Renal reabsorption or excretion ▪ Aldosterone increases Na$^+$ reabsorption in collecting duct of nephrons	▪ Regulating ECF volume and distribution ▪ Maintaining blood volume ▪ Transmitting nerve impulses and contracting muscles
Potassium (K$^+$)	▪ Renal excretion and conservation ▪ Aldosterone increases K$^+$ excretion ▪ Movement into and out of cells ▪ Insulin helps move K$^+$ into cells; tissue damage and acidosis shift K$^+$ out of cells into ECF	▪ Maintaining ICF osmolality ▪ Transmitting nerve and other electrical impulses ▪ Regulating cardiac impulse transmission and muscle contraction ▪ Skeletal and smooth muscle function ▪ Regulating acid–base balance
Calcium (Ca^{2+})	▪ Redistribution between bones and ECF ▪ Parathyroid hormone and calcitriol increase serum Ca^{2+} levels; calcitonin decreases serum levels	▪ Forming bones and teeth ▪ Transmitting nerve impulses ▪ Regulating muscle contractions ▪ Maintaining cardiac pacemaker (automaticity) ▪ Blood clotting ▪ Activating enzymes such as pancreatic lipase and phospholipase
Magnesium (Mg^{2+})	▪ Conservation and excretion by kidneys ▪ Intestinal absorption increased by vitamin D and parathyroid hormone	▪ Intracellular metabolism ▪ Operating sodium-potassium pump ▪ Relaxing muscle contractions ▪ Transmitting nerve impulses ▪ Regulating cardiac function
Chloride (Cl$^-$)	▪ Excreted and reabsorbed along with sodium in the kidneys ▪ Aldosterone increases chloride reabsorption with sodium	▪ HCl production ▪ Regulating ECF balance and vascular volume ▪ Regulating acid–base balance ▪ Buffer in oxygen–carbon dioxide exchange in RBCs
Phosphate (PO$_4^-$)	▪ Excretion and reabsorption by the kidneys ▪ Parathyroid hormone decreases serum levels by increasing renal excretion ▪ Reciprocal relationship with calcium: increasing serum calcium levels decrease phosphate levels; decreasing serum calcium increases phosphate	▪ Forming bones and teeth ▪ Metabolizing carbohydrate, protein, and fat ▪ Cellular metabolism; producing ATP and DNA ▪ Muscle, nerve, and RBC function ▪ Regulating acid–base balance ▪ Regulating calcium levels
Bicarbonate (HCO$_3^-$)	▪ Excretion and reabsorption by the kidneys ▪ Regeneration by kidneys	▪ Major body buffer involved in acid–base regulation

Sodium (Na$^+$)

Sodium is the most abundant cation in extracellular fluid and a major contributor to serum osmolality. Normal serum sodium levels are 135 to 145 mEq/L. Sodium functions largely in controlling and regulating water balance. When sodium is reabsorbed from the kidney tubules, chloride and water are reabsorbed with it, thus maintaining ECF volume. Sodium is found in many foods, such as bacon, ham, processed cheese, and table salt.

Potassium (K$^+$)

Potassium is the major cation in intracellular fluids, with only a small amount found in plasma and interstitial fluid. ICF levels of potassium are usually 125 to 140 mEq/L while normal serum potassium levels are 3.5 to 5.0 mEq/L. The ratio of intracellular to extracellular potassium must be maintained for neuromuscular response to stimuli. Potassium is a vital electrolyte for skeletal, cardiac, and smooth muscle activity. It is involved in maintaining acid–base balance as well, and it contributes to intracellular enzyme reactions. Potassium must be ingested daily because the body can't conserve it. Many fruits and vegetables, meat, fish, and other foods contain potassium (see Box 52–1).

Calcium (Ca^{2+})

The vast majority, 99%, of calcium in the body is in the skeletal system, with a relatively small amount in extracellular fluid. Although this calcium outside the bones and teeth amounts to only about 1% of the total calcium in the body, it is vital in regulating muscle contraction and relaxation, neuromuscular function, and cardiac function. ECF calcium is regulated by a complex interaction of parathyroid hormone, calcitonin, and calcitriol, a metabolite of vitamin D. When calcium levels in the

---

BOX 52–1   Potassium-Rich Foods

VEGETABLES	FRUITS
Avocado	Dried fruits (e.g., raisins and dates)
Raw carrot	Banana
Baked potato	Apricot
Raw tomato	Cantaloupe
Spinach	Orange

MEATS AND FISH	BEVERAGES
Beef	Milk
Cod	Orange juice
Pork	Apricot nectar
Veal	

ECF fall, parathyroid hormone and calcitriol cause calcium to be released from bones into ECF and increase the absorption of calcium in the intestines, thus raising serum calcium levels. Conversely, calcitonin stimulates the deposition of calcium in bone, reducing the concentration of calcium ions in the blood.

With aging, the intestines absorb calcium less effectively and more calcium is excreted via the kidneys. Calcium shifts out of the bone to replace these ECF losses, increasing the risk of osteoporosis and fractures of the wrists, vertebrae, and hips. Lack of weight-bearing exercise (which helps keep calcium in the bones) and a vitamin D deficiency because of inadequate exposure to sunlight contribute to this risk.

Milk and milk products are the richest sources of calcium, with other foods such as dark green leafy vegetables and canned salmon containing smaller amounts. Many clients benefit from calcium supplements.

Serum calcium levels are often reported in two ways, based upon the way it is circulating in the plasma. Approximately 50% of serum calcium circulates in a free, ionized, or unbound form. The other 50% circulates in the plasma bound to either plasma proteins or other nonprotein ions. The normal total serum calcium levels, which range from 8.5 to 10.5 mg/dL, represent both bound and unbound calcium. The normal ionized serum calcium, which ranges from 4.0 to 5.0 mg/dL, represents calcium circulating in the plasma in free, or unbound, form (Hayes, 2004).

Magnesium (Mg^{2+})

Magnesium is primarily found in the skeleton and in intracellular fluid. It is the second most abundant intracellular cation with normal serum levels of 1.5 to 2.5 mEq/L. It is important for intracellular metabolism, being particularly involved in the production and use of ATP. Magnesium also is necessary for protein and DNA synthesis within the cells. Only about 1% of the body's magnesium is in ECF; here it is involved in regulating neuromuscular and cardiac function. Maintaining and ensuring adequate magnesium levels is an important part of care of clients with cardiac disorders. Cereal grains, nuts, dried fruit, legumes, and green leafy vegetables are good sources of magnesium in the diet, as are dairy products, meat, and fish.

Chloride (Cl^-)

Chloride is the major anion of ECF, and normal serum levels are 95 to 108 mEq/L. Chloride functions with sodium to regulate serum osmolality and blood volume. The concentration of chloride in ECF is regulated secondarily to sodium; when sodium is reabsorbed in the kidney, chloride usually follows. Chloride is a major component of gastric juice as hydrochloric acid (HCl) and is involved in regulating acid–base balance. It also acts as a buffer in the exchange of oxygen and carbon dioxide in RBCs. Chloride is found in the same foods as sodium.

Phosphate PO_4^-

Phosphate is the major anion of intracellular fluids. It also is found in ECF, bone, skeletal muscle, and nerve tissue. Normal serum levels of phospate in adults range from 2.5 to 4.5 mg/dL. Children have much higher phosphate levels than adults, with that of a newborn nearly twice that of an adult. Higher levels of growth hormone and a faster rate of skeletal growth probably account for this difference. Phosphate is involved in many chemical actions of the cell; it is essential for functioning of muscles, nerves, and red blood cells. It is also involved in the metabolism of protein, fat, and carbohydrate. Phosphate is absorbed from the intestine and is found in many foods such as meat, fish, poultry, milk products, and legumes.

Bicarbonate HCO_3^-

Bicarbonate is present in both intracellular and extracellular fluids. Its primary function is regulating acid–base balance as an essential component of the carbonic acid–bicarbonate buffering system. Extracellular bicarbonate levels are regulated by the kidneys: Bicarbonate is excreted when too much is present; if more is needed, the kidneys both regenerate and reabsorb bicarbonate ions. Unlike other electrolytes that must be consumed in the diet, adequate amounts of bicarbonate are produced through metabolic processes to meet the body's needs.

ACID–BASE BALANCE

An important part of regulating the chemical balance or homeostasis of body fluids is regulating their acidity or alkalinity. An **acid** is a substance that releases hydrogen ions (H^+) in solution. Strong acids such as hydrochloric acid release all or nearly all their hydrogen ions; weak acids like carbonic acid release some hydrogen ions. **Bases** or *alkalis* have a low hydrogen ion concentration and can accept hydrogen ions in solution. The relative acidity or alkalinity of a solution is measured as **pH**. The pH reflects the hydrogen ion concentration of the solution: The higher the hydrogen ion concentration (and the more acidic the solution), the lower the pH. Water has a pH of 7 and is neutral; that is, it is neither acidic in nature nor is it alkaline. Solutions with a pH lower than 7 are acidic; those with a pH higher than 7 are alkaline. The pH scale is logarithmic: A solution with a pH of 5 is 10 times more acidic than one with a pH of 6.

Regulation of Acid–Base Balance

Body fluids are maintained within a narrow range that is slightly alkaline. The normal pH of arterial blood is between 7.35 and 7.45 (Figure 52-9 ■). Acids are continually produced during me-

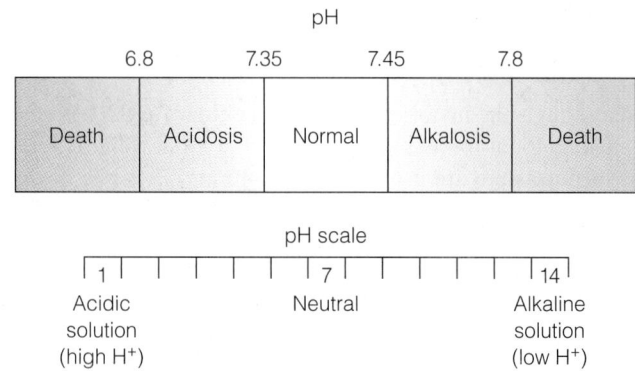

Figure 52-9 ■ Body fluids are normally slightly alkaline, between a pH of 7.35 and 7.45.

tabolism. Several body systems, including buffers, the respiratory system, and the renal system, are actively involved in maintaining the narrow pH range necessary for optimal function. Buffers help maintain acid–base balance by neutralizing excess acids or bases. The lungs and the kidneys help maintain a normal pH by either excreting or retaining acids and bases.

Buffers

Buffers prevent excessive changes in pH by removing or releasing hydrogen ions. If excess hydrogen ion is present in body fluids, buffers bind with the hydrogen ion, minimizing the change in pH. When body fluids become too alkaline, buffers can release hydrogen ion, again minimizing the change in pH. The action of a buffer is immediate, but limited in its capacity to maintain or restore normal acid–base balance.

The major buffer system in extracellular fluids is the bicarbonate (HCO_3^-) and carbonic acid (H_2CO_3) system. When a strong acid such as hydrochloric acid (HCl) is added, it combines with bicarbonate and the pH drops only slightly. A strong base such as sodium hydroxide combines with carbonic acid, the weak acid of the buffer pair, and the pH remains within the narrow range of normal. The amounts of bicarbonate and carbonic acid in the body vary; however, as long as a ratio of 20 parts of bicarbonate to 1 part of carbonic acid is maintained, the pH remains within its normal range of 7.35 to 7.45 (Figure 52-10 ■). Adding a strong acid to ECF can change this ratio as bicarbonate is depleted in neutralizing the acid. When this happens, the pH drops, and the client has a condition called **acidosis.** The ratio can also be upset by adding a strong base to ECF, depleting carbonic acid as it combines with the base. In this case the pH rises and the client has **alkalosis.**

In addition to the bicarbonate–carbonic acid buffer system, plasma proteins, hemoglobin, and phosphates also function as buffers in body fluids.

Respiratory Regulation

The lungs help regulate acid–base balance by eliminating or retaining carbon dioxide (CO_2), a potential acid. Combined with water, carbon dioxide forms carbonic acid ($CO_2 + H_2O \rightarrow H_2CO_3$). This chemical reaction is reversible; carbonic acid breaks down into carbon dioxide and water. Working together with the bicarbonate–carbonic acid buffer system, the lungs regulate acid–base balance and pH by altering the rate and depth of respirations. The response of the respiratory system to changes in pH is rapid, occurring within minutes.

Carbon dioxide is a powerful stimulator of the respiratory center. When blood levels of carbonic acid and carbon dioxide rise, the respiratory center is stimulated and the rate and depth of respirations increase. Carbon dioxide is exhaled, and carbonic acid levels fall. By contrast, when bicarbonate levels are excessive, the rate and depth of respirations are reduced. This causes carbon dioxide to be retained, carbonic acid levels to rise, and the excess bicarbonate to be neutralized.

Carbon dioxide levels in the blood are measured as the PCO_2, or partial pressure of the dissolved gas in the blood. PCO_2 refers to the pressure of carbon dioxide in venous blood. $PaCO_2$ refers to the pressure of carbon dioxide in arterial blood. The normal $PaCO_2$ is 35 to 45 mm Hg.

Renal Regulation

Although buffers and the respiratory system can compensate for changes in pH, the kidneys are the ultimate long-term regulator of acid–base balance. They are slower to respond to changes, requiring hours to days to correct imbalances, but their response is more permanent and selective than that of the other systems (Yucha, 2004).

The kidneys maintain acid–base balance by selectively excreting or conserving bicarbonate and hydrogen ions. When excess hydrogen ion is present and the pH falls (acidosis), the kidneys reabsorb and regenerate bicarbonate and excrete hydrogen ion. In the case of alkalosis and a high pH, excess bicarbonate is excreted and hydrogen ion is retained. The normal serum bicarbonate level is 22 to 26 mEq/L.

The relationship of the respiratory and renal regulation of acid–base balance is further explained in Box 52–2.

Figure 52-10 ■ Carbonic acid–bicarbonate ratio and pH.

BOX 52–2 **Physiological Regulation of Acid–Base Balance**

Lungs				*Kidneys*
$CO_2 + H_2O$	$\leftrightarrow$	H_2CO_3	$\leftrightarrow$	$H + HCO_3$
Carbon dioxide				Hydrogen
+		Carbonic acid		+
water				bicarbonate

The lungs and kidneys are the two major systems that are working on a continuous basis to help regulate the acid–base balance in the body. In the biochemical reactions above, the processes are all reversible and go back and forth as the body's needs change. The lungs can work very quickly and do their part by either retaining or getting rid of carbon dioxide by changing the rate and depth of respirations. The kidneys work much more slowly; they may take hours to days to regulate the balance by either excreting or conserving hydrogen and bicarbonate ions. Under normal conditions, the two systems work together to maintain homeostasis.

FACTORS AFFECTING BODY FLUID, ELECTROLYTES, AND ACID–BASE BALANCE

The ability of the body to adjust fluids, electrolytes, and acid–base balance is influenced by age, gender and body size, environmental temperature, and lifestyle.

Age

Infants and growing children have much greater fluid turnover than adults because their higher metabolic rate increases fluid loss. Infants lose more fluid through the kidneys because immature kidneys are less able to conserve water than adult kidneys. In addition, infants' respirations are more rapid and the body surface area is proportionately greater than that of adults, increasing insensible fluid losses. The more rapid turnover of fluid plus the losses produced by disease can create critical fluid imbalances in children much more rapidly than in adults.

In elderly people, the normal aging process may affect fluid balance. The thirst response often is blunted. Antidiuretic hormone levels remain normal or may even be elevated, but the nephrons become less able to conserve water in response to ADH. Increased levels of atrial natriuretic factor seen in older adults may also contribute to this impaired ability to conserve water. These normal changes of aging increase the risk of dehydration. When combined with the increased likelihood of heart diseases, impaired renal function, and multiple drug regimens, the older adult's risk for fluid and electrolyte imbalance is significant. Additionally, it is important to consider that the older adult has thinner, more fragile skin and veins, which can make an intravenous insertion more difficult.

Gender and Body Size

Total body water also is affected by gender and body size. Because fat cells contain little or no water, and lean tissue has a high water content, people with a higher percentage of body fat have less body fluid. Women have proportionately more body fat and less body water than men. Water accounts for approximately 60% of an adult man's weight, but only 52% for an adult woman. In an obese individual this may be even less, with water responsible for only 30% to 40% of the person's weight.

Environmental Temperature

People with an illness and those participating in strenuous activity are at risk for fluid and electrolyte imbalances when the environmental temperature is high. Fluid losses through sweating are increased in hot environments as the body attempts to dissipate heat. These losses are even greater in people who have not been acclimatized to the environment.

Both salt and water are lost through sweating. When only water is replaced, salt depletion is a risk. The person who is salt depleted may experience fatigue, weakness, headache, and gastrointestinal symptoms such as anorexia and nausea. The risk of adverse effects is even greater if lost water is not replaced. Body temperature rises, and the person is at risk for heat exhaustion or heatstroke. Heatstroke may occur in older adults or ill people during prolonged periods of heat; it can also affect athletes and

---

LIFESPAN CONSIDERATIONS Fluid and Electrolyte Imbalance

INFANTS AND CHILDREN

Infants are at high risk for fluid and electrolyte imbalance because

- Their immature kidneys cannot concentrate urine.
- They have a rapid respiratory rate and proportionately larger body surface area than adults, leading to greater insensate loss through the skin and respirations.
- They cannot express thirst, nor actively seek fluids.

Vomiting and/or diarrhea in infants and young children can lead quickly to electrolyte imbalance. Oral rehydration therapy (ORT) (e.g., electrolyte solutions such as Pedialyte) should be used to restore fluid and electrolyte balance in mild to moderate dehydration (American Medical Association et al., 2004). Prompt treatment with ORT can prevent the need for intravenous therapy and hospitalization (Spandorfer, Alessandrini, Joffe, Localio, & Shaw, 2005). Even if the child is nauseated and vomiting, small sips of ORT can be helpful.

ELDERS

Certain changes related to aging place the elder at risk for serious problems with fluid and electrolyte imbalance, if homeostatic mechanisms are compromised. Some of the changes are

- A decrease in thirst sensation.
- A decrease in ability of the kidneys to concentrate urine.
- A decrease in intracellular fluid and in total body water.
- A decrease in response to body hormones that help regulate fluid and electrolytes.

Other factors that may influence fluid and electrolyte balance in elders are

- Increased use of diuretics for hypertension and heart disease.
- Decreased intake of food and water, especially in elders with dementia or who are dependent on others to feed them and offer them fluids.
- Preparations for certain diagnostic tests that have the client NPO for long periods of time or cause diarrhea from laxative preps.
- Clients with impaired renal function, such as elders with diabetes.
- Those having certain diagnostic procedures. (Dyes used for some procedures, such as arteriograms and cardiac catheterizations, may cause further renal problems. Always see that the client is well hydrated before, during, and after the procedure to help in diluting and excreting the dye. If the client is NPO for the procedure, the nurse should check with the primary care provider to see if IV fluids are needed.)
- Any condition that may tax the normal compensatory mechanisms, such as a fever, influenza, surgery, or heat exposure.

All of these conditions increase elders' risk for fluid and electrolyte imbalance. The change can happen quickly and become serious in a short time. Astute observations and quick actions by the nurse can help prevent serious consequences. A change in mental status may be the first symptom of impairment and must be further evaluated to determine the cause.

laborers when their heat production exceeds the body's ability to dissipate heat.

Consuming adequate amounts of cool liquids, particularly during strenuous activity, reduces the risk of adverse effects from heat. Balanced electrolyte solutions and carbohydrate-electrolyte solutions such as sports drinks are recommended because they replace both water and electrolytes lost through sweat.

Lifestyle

Other factors such as diet, exercise, and stress affect fluid, electrolyte, and acid–base balance.

The intake of fluids and electrolytes is affected by the diet. People with anorexia nervosa or bulimia are at risk for severe fluid and electrolyte imbalances because of inadequate intake or purging regimens (e.g., induced vomiting, use of diuretics and laxatives). Seriously malnourished people have decreased serum albumin levels, and may develop edema because the osmotic draw of fluid into the vascular compartment is reduced. When calorie intake is not adequate to meet the body's needs, fat stores are broken down and fatty acids are released, increasing the risk of acidosis.

Regular weight-bearing physical exercise such as walking, running, or bicycling has a beneficial effect on calcium balance. The rate of bone loss that occurs in postmenopausal women and older men is slowed with regular exercise, reducing the risk of osteoporosis.

Stress can increase cellular metabolism, blood glucose concentration, and catecholamine levels. In addition, stress can increase production of ADH, which in turn decreases urine production. The overall response of the body to stress is to increase the blood volume.

Other lifestyle factors can also affect fluid, electrolyte, and acid–base balance. Heavy alcohol consumption affects electrolyte balance, increasing the risk of low calcium, magnesium, and phosphate levels. The risk of acidosis associated with breakdown of fat tissue also is greater in the person who drinks large amounts of alcohol.

DISTURBANCES IN FLUID VOLUME, ELECTROLYTE, AND ACID–BASE BALANCES

A number of factors such as illness, trauma, surgery, and medications can affect the body's ability to maintain fluid, electrolyte, and acid–base balance. The kidneys play a major role in maintaining fluid, electrolyte, and acid–base balance, and renal disease is a significant cause of imbalance. Clients who are confused or unable to communicate their needs are at risk for inadequate fluid intake. Vomiting, diarrhea, or nasogastric suction can cause significant fluid losses. Tissue trauma, such as burns, causes fluid and electrolytes to be lost from damaged cells. Decreased blood flow to the kidneys due to impaired cardiac function stimulates the renin-angiotensin-aldosterone system, causing sodium and water retention. Medications such as diuretics or corticosteroids can result in abnormal losses of electrolytes and fluid loss or retention. Diseases such as diabetes mellitus or chronic obstructive lung disease may affect acid–base balance. Diabetic ketoacidosis, cancer, and head injury may also lead to electrolyte imbalances.

Fluid Imbalances

Fluid imbalances are of two basic types: isotonic and osmolar. *Isotonic imbalances* occur when water and electrolytes are lost or gained in equal proportions, so that the osmolality of body fluids remains constant. *Osmolar imbalances* involve the loss or gain of only water, so that the osmolality of the serum is altered. Thus four categories of fluid imbalances may occur: (a) an isotonic loss of water and electrolytes, (b) an isotonic gain of water and electrolytes, (c) a hyperosmolar loss of only water, and (d) a hypo-osmolar gain of only water. These are referred to, respectively, as fluid volume deficit, fluid volume excess, dehydration (hyperosmolar imbalance), and overhydration (hypo-osmolar imbalance).

Fluid Volume Deficit

Isotonic **fluid volume deficit (FVD)** occurs when the body loses both water and electrolytes from the ECF in similar proportions. Thus, the decreased volume of fluid remains isotonic. In FVD, fluid is initially lost from the intravascular compartment, so it often is called **hypovolemia.**

FVD generally occurs as a result of (a) abnormal losses through the skin, gastrointestinal tract, or kidney; (b) decreased intake of fluid; (c) bleeding; or (d) movement of fluid into a third space. See the section on third space syndrome that follows.

For the risk factors and clinical signs related to fluid volume deficit, see Table 52–4.

THIRD SPACE SYNDROME. In **third space syndrome,** fluid shifts from the vascular space into an area where it is not readily accessible as extracellular fluid. This fluid remains in the body but is essentially unavailable for use, causing an isotonic fluid volume deficit. Fluid may be sequestered in the bowel, in the interstitial space as edema, in inflamed tissue, or in potential spaces such as the peritoneal or pleural cavities.

The client with third space syndrome has an isotonic fluid deficit but may not manifest apparent fluid loss or weight loss. Careful nursing assessment is vital to effectively identify and intervene for clients experiencing third-spacing. Because the fluid shifts back into the vascular compartment after time, assessment for manifestations of fluid volume excess or hypervolemia is also vital.

Fluid Volume Excess

Fluid volume excess (FVE) occurs when the body retains both water and sodium in similar proportions to normal ECF. This is commonly referred to as **hypervolemia** (increased blood volume). FVE is always secondary to an increase in the total body sodium content, which leads to an increase in total body water. Because both water and sodium are retained, the serum sodium concentration remains essentially normal and the excess volume of fluid is isotonic. Specific causes of FVE include (a) excessive intake of sodium chloride; (b) administering sodium-containing infusions too rapidly, particularly to clients

TABLE 52–4   Isotonic Fluid Volume Deficit

RISK FACTORS	CLINICAL MANIFESTATIONS	NURSING INTERVENTIONS
Loss of water and electrolytes from ■ Vomiting ■ Diarrhea ■ Excessive sweating ■ Polyuria ■ Fever ■ Nasogastric suction ■ Abnormal drainage or wound losses Insufficient intake due to ■ Anorexia ■ Nausea ■ Inability to access fluids ■ Impaired swallowing ■ Confusion, depression	Complaints of weakness and thirst Weight loss ■ 2% loss = mild FVD ■ 5% loss = moderate ■ 8% loss = severe Fluid intake less than output Decreased tissue turgor Dry mucous membranes, sunken eyeballs, decreased tearing Subnormal temperature Weak, rapid pulse Decreased blood pressure Postural (orthostatic) hypotension (significant drop in BP when moving from lying to sitting or standing position) Flat neck veins; decreased capillary refill Decreased central venous pressure Decreased urine volume (<30 mL/h) Increased specific gravity of urine (>1.030) Increased hematocrit Increased blood urea nitrogen (BUN)	Assess for clinical manifestations of FVD. Monitor weight and vital signs, including temperature. Assess tissue turgor. Monitor fluid intake and output. Monitor laboratory findings. Administer oral and intravenous fluids as indicated. Provide frequent mouth care. Implement measures to prevent skin breakdown. Provide for safety, e.g., provide assistance for a client rising from bed.

with impaired regulatory mechanisms; and (c) disease processes that alter regulatory mechanisms, such as heart failure, renal failure, cirrhosis of the liver, and Cushing's syndrome.

The risk factors and clinical manifestations for FVE are summarized in Table 52–5.

EDEMA. In fluid volume excess, both intravascular and interstitial spaces have an increased water and sodium content. Excess interstitial fluid is known as edema. Edema typically is most apparent in areas where the tissue pressure is low, such as around the eyes, and in dependent tissues (known as dependent edema), where hydrostatic capillary pressure is high.

Edema can be caused by several different mechanisms. The three main mechanisms are increased capillary hydrostatic pressure, decreased plasma oncotic pressure, and increased capillary permeability. It may be due to FVE that increases capillary hydrostatic pressures, pushing fluid into the interstitial tissues. This type of edema is often seen in dependent tissues such as the feet, ankles, and sacrum because of the effects of gravity. Low levels of plasma proteins from malnutrition or liver or kidney diseases can reduce the plasma oncotic pressure so that fluid is not drawn into the capillaries from interstitial tissues, causing edema. With tissue trauma and some disorders such as allergic reactions, capillaries become more permeable, allowing fluid to escape into interstitial tissues. Obstructed lymph flow impairs the movement of fluid from interstitial tissues back into the vascular compartment, resulting in edema.

Pitting edema is edema that leaves a small depression or pit after finger pressure is applied to the swollen area. The pit is caused by movement of fluid to adjacent tissue, away from the point of pressure (Figure 52-11 ■). Within 10 to 30 seconds the pit normally disappears.

TABLE 52–5   Isotonic Fluid Volume Excess

RISK FACTORS	CLINICAL MANIFESTATIONS	NURSING INTERVENTIONS
Excess intake of sodium-containing intravenous fluids Excess ingestion of sodium in diet or medications (e.g., sodium bicarbonate antacids such as Alka-Seltzer or hypertonic enema solutions such as Fleet's) Impaired fluid balance regulation related to ■ Heart failure ■ Renal failure ■ Cirrhosis of the liver	Weight gain ■ 2% gain = mild FVE ■ 5% gain = moderate ■ 8% gain = severe Fluid intake greater than output Full, bounding pulse; tachycardia Increased blood pressure and central venous pressure Distended neck and peripheral veins; slow vein emptying Moist crackles (rales) in lungs; dyspnea, shortness of breath Mental confusion	Assess for clinical manifestations of FVE. Monitor weight and vital signs. Assess for edema. Assess breath sounds. Monitor fluid intake and output. Monitor laboratory findings. Place in Fowler's position. Administer diuretics as ordered. Restrict fluid intake as indicated. Restrict dietary sodium as ordered. Implement measures to prevent skin breakdown.

2mm
1+ Barely detectable

4mm
2+ 2 to 4 mm

6mm
3+ 5 to 7 mm

12mm
4+ More than 7 mm

A **B**

Figure 52-11 ■ Evaluation of edema. *A,* Palpate for edema over the tibia as shown here and behind the medial malleolus, and over the dorsum of each foot. *B,* Four-point scale for grading edema.

Dehydration

Dehydration, or hyperosmolar imbalance, occurs when water is lost from the body leaving the client with excess sodium. Because water is lost while electrolytes, particularly sodium, are retained, the serum osmolality and serum sodium levels increase. Water is drawn into the vascular compartment from the interstitial space and cells, resulting in cellular dehydration. Older adults are at particular risk for dehydration because of decreased thirst sensation. This type of water deficit also can affect clients who are hyperventilating or have prolonged fever or are in diabetic ketoacidosis and those receiving enteral feedings with insufficient water intake.

Overhydration

Overhydration, also known as hypo-osmolar imbalance or water excess, occurs when water is gained in excess of electrolytes, resulting in low serum osmolality and low serum sodium levels. Water is drawn into the cells, causing them to swell. In the brain this can lead to cerebral edema and impaired neurologic function. Water intoxication often occurs when both fluid and electrolytes are lost, for example, through excessive sweating, but only water is replaced. It can also result from the syndrome of inappropriate antidiuretic hormone (SIADH), a disorder that can occur with some malignant tumors, AIDS, head injury, or administration of certain drugs such as barbiturates or anesthetics.

DRUG CAPSULE **Diuretic Agent** *furosemide* (Lasix)

THE CLIENT WITH FLUID VOLUME EXCESS

Furosemide inhibits sodium and chloride reabsorption in the loop of Henle and the distal renal tubule. This results in significant diuresis, with renal excretion of water, sodium chloride, magnesium, hydrogen, and calcium.

Furosemide is commonly used for the clinical management of edema secondary to heart failure, treatment of hypertension, and treatment of hepatic or renal disease. Therapeutic effects include diuresis and lowering of blood pressure.

NURSING RESPONSIBILITIES

■ Assess the client's fluid status regularly. Assessment should include daily weights, close monitoring of intake and output, skin turgor, edema, lung sounds, and mucous membranes.
■ Monitor the client's potassium levels. Furosemide is a loop diuretic which excretes potassium and may result in hypokalemia.
■ Administer in the morning to avoid increased urination during hours of sleep.
■ If the client is also taking digitalis glycosides, he or she should be assessed for anorexia, nausea, vomiting, muscle cramps, paresthesia, and confusion. The potassium-depleting effect of furosemide places the client at increased risk for digitalis toxicity.

CLIENT AND FAMILY TEACHING

■ Medication should be taken exactly as directed. If you miss a dose, take it as soon as possible; however, if a day has been missed, do not double the dose the next day.
■ Weigh on a daily basis and report weight gain or loss of more than 3 lb in 1 day to your primary care provider.
■ Contact your primary care provider immediately if you begin to experience muscle weakness, cramps, nausea, dizziness, numbness, or tingling of the extremities.
■ Some form of potassium supplementation will be needed. The primary care provider may order oral potassium supplements for you; if not, you will need to consume a diet high in potassium.
■ Make position changes slowly in order to minimize dizziness from orthostatic hypotension.

Note: Prior to administering any medication, review all aspects with a current drug handbook or other reliable source.

MediaLink

Furosemide Drug Animation

Electrolyte Imbalances

The most common and most significant electrolyte imbalances involve sodium, potassium, calcium, magnesium, chloride, and phosphate.

Sodium

Sodium (Na^+), the most abundant cation in the extracellular fluid, not only moves into and out of the body but also moves in careful balance among the three fluid compartments. It is found in most body secretions, for example, saliva, gastric and intestinal secretions, bile, and pancreatic fluid. Therefore, continuous excretion of any of these fluids, such as via intestinal suction, can result in a sodium deficit. Because of its role in regulating water balance, sodium imbalances usually are accompanied by water imbalance.

Hyponatremia is a sodium deficit, or serum sodium level of less than 135 mEq/L, and is, in acute care settings, a common electrolyte imbalance. Because of sodium's role in determining the osmolality of ECF, hyponatremia typically results in a low serum osmolality. Water is drawn out of the vascular compartment into interstitial tissues and the cells (Figure 52-12 ■, *A*), causing the clinical manifestations associated with this disorder. As sodium levels decrease, the brain and nervous system are affected by cellular edema. Severe hyponatremia, serum levels below 110 mEq/L, is a medical emergency and can lead to permanent neurological damage (Astle, 2005).

Cell swells as water is pulled in from ECF

Cell shrinks as water is pulled out into ECF

H_2O H_2O H_2O H_2O

A Hyponatremia: Na^+ less than 135 mEq/L

B Hypernatremia: Na^+ greater than 145 mEq/L

Figure 52-12 ■ The extracellular sodium level affects cell size. *A*, In hyponatremia, cells swell; *B*, in hypernatremia, cells shrink in size.

Hypernatremia is excess sodium in ECF, or a serum sodium of greater than 145 mEq/L. Because the osmotic pressure of extracellular fluid is increased, fluid moves out of the cells into the ECF (Figure 52-12 ■, *B*). As a result, the cells become dehydrated. Like hyponatremia, the primary manifestations of hypernatremia are neurological in nature.

It is important to note that a person's thirst mechanism protects against hypernatremia. For example, when an individual becomes thirsty, the body is stimulated to drink water which helps correct the hypernatremia. Clients at risk for hypernatremia are those who are unable to access water (e.g., unconscious, unable to request fluids such as infants or elders with dementia, or ill clients with an impaired thirst mechanism).

Table 52–6 lists risk factors and clinical signs for hyponatremia and hypernatremia.

Potassium

Although the amount of potassium (K^+) in extracellular fluid is small, it is vital to normal neuromuscular and cardiac function. Normal renal function is important for maintenance of potassium balance as 80% of potassium is excreted by the kidneys. Potassium must be replaced daily to maintain its balance. Normally, potassium is replaced in food. See previous Box 52–1 on page 1431 for a review of foods high in potassium.

Hypokalemia is a potassium deficit or a serum potassium level of less than 3.5 mEq/L. Gastrointestinal losses of potassium through vomiting and gastric suction are common causes of hypokalemia, as are the use of potassium-wasting diuretics, such as thiazide diuretics or loop diuretics (e.g., furosemide). Symptoms of hypokalemia are usually mild until the level drops below 3 mEq/L unless the decrease in potassium was rapid. When the decrease is gradual, the body compensates by shifting potassium from the intracellular environment into the serum.

Hyperkalemia is a potassium excess or a serum potassium level greater than 5.0 mEq/L. Hyperkalemia is less common than hypokalemia and rarely occurs in clients with normal renal function. It is, however, more dangerous than hypokalemia and can lead to cardiac arrest. As with hypokalemia, symptoms are more severe and occur at lower levels when the increase in potassium is abrupt. Table 52–6 lists risk factors and clinical signs for hypokalemia and hyperkalemia.

TABLE 52–6 Electrolyte Imbalances

RISK FACTORS	CLINICAL MANIFESTATIONS	NURSING INTERVENTIONS
Hyponatremia		
Loss of sodium	Lethargy, confusion, apprehension	Assess clinical manifestations.
■ Gastrointestinal fluid loss	Muscle twitching	Monitor fluid intake and output.
■ Sweating	Abdominal cramps	Monitor laboratory data (e.g., serum sodium).
■ Use of diuretics	Anorexia, nausea, vomiting	Assess client closely if administering
Gain of water	Headache	hypertonic saline solutions.
■ Hypotonic tube feedings	Seizures, coma	Encourage food and fluid high in sodium if
■ Excessive drinking of water	*Laboratory findings:*	permitted (e.g., table salt, bacon, ham,
■ Excess IV D5W (dextrose in water) administration	Serum sodium below 135 mEq/L	processed cheese).
	Serum osmolality below 280 mOsm/kg	Limit water intake as indicated.
Syndrome of inappropriate ADH (SIADH)		
■ Head injury		
■ AIDS		
■ Malignant tumors		
Hypernatremia		
Loss of water	Thirst	Monitor fluid intake and output.
■ Insensible water loss (hyperventilation or fever)	Dry, sticky mucous membranes	Monitor behavior changes (e.g., restlessness, disorientation).
■ Diarrhea	Tongue red, dry, swollen	Monitor laboratory findings (e.g., serum
■ Water deprivation	Weakness	sodium).
Gain of sodium	Severe hypernatremia:	Encourage fluids as ordered.
■ Parenteral administration of saline solutions	■ Fatigue, restlessness	Monitor diet as ordered (e.g., restrict intake of salt and foods high in sodium).
■ Hypertonic tube feedings without adequate water	■ Decreasing level of consciousness	
■ Excessive use of table salt (1 tsp contains 2,300 mg of sodium)	■ Disorientation	
	■ Convulsions	
Conditions such as	*Laboratory findings:*	
■ Diabetes insipidus	Serum sodium above 145 mEq/L	
■ Heat stroke	Serum osmolality above 300 mOsm/kg	
Hypokalemia		
Loss of potassium	Muscle weakness, leg cramps	Monitor heart rate and rhythm.
■ Vomiting and gastric suction	Fatigue, lethargy	Monitor clients receiving digitalis (e.g., digoxin) closely, because hypokalemia increases risk of
■ Diarrhea	Anorexia, nausea, vomiting	digitalis toxicity.
■ Heavy perspiration	Decreased bowel sounds, decreased bowel motility	Administer oral potassium as ordered with food or fluid to prevent gastric irritation.
■ Use of potassium-wasting drugs (e.g., diuretics)	Cardiac dysrhythmias	Administer IV potassium solutions at a rate no faster than 10–20 mEq/h; never administer
■ Poor intake of potassium (as with debilitated clients, alcoholics, anorexia nervosa)	Depressed deep-tendon reflexes	undiluted potassium intravenously. For clients receiving IV potassium, monitor for pain and
■ Hyperaldosteronism	Weak, irregular pulses	inflammation at the injection site.
	Laboratory findings:	Teach client about potassium-rich foods.
	Serum potassium below 3.5 mEq/L	Teach clients how to prevent excessive loss of
	Arterial blood gases (ABGs) may show alkalosis	potassium (e.g., through abuse of diuretics
	T wave flattening and ST segment depression on ECG	and laxatives).
Hyperkalemia		
Decreased potassium excretion	Gastrointestinal hyperactivity, diarrhea	Closely monitor cardiac status and ECG.
■ Renal failure	Irritability, apathy, confusion	Administer diuretics and other medications such as glucose and insulin as ordered.
■ Hypoaldosteronism	Cardiac dysrhythmias or arrest	Hold potassium supplements and K^+
■ Potassium-conserving diuretics	Muscle weakness, areflexia (absence of reflexes)	conserving diuretics.
High potassium intake	Decreased heart rate;	
	Irregular pulse	

continued on page 1440

TABLE 52–6   Electrolyte Imbalances—*continued*

RISK FACTORS	CLINICAL MANIFESTATIONS	NURSING INTERVENTIONS
Hyperkalemia–*continued* ■ Excessive use of K⁺ containing salt substitutes ■ Excessive or rapid IV infusion of potassium ■ Potassium shift out of the tissue cells into the plasma (e.g., infections, burns, acidosis)	Paresthesias and numbness in extremities *Laboratory findings:* Serum potassium above 5.0 mEq/L Peaked T wave, widened QRS on ECG	Monitor serum K⁺ levels carefully; a rapid drop may occur as potassium shifts into the cells. Teach clients to avoid foods high in potassium and salt substitutes.
Hypocalcemia *Surgical removal of the parathyroid glands* Conditions such as ■ Hypoparathyroidism ■ Acute pancreatitis ■ Hyperphosphatemia ■ Thyroid carcinoma *Inadequate vitamin D intake* ■ Malabsorption ■ Hypomagnesemia ■ Alkalosis ■ Sepsis ■ Alcohol abuse	Numbness, tingling of the extremities and around the mouth Muscle tremors, cramps; if severe can progress to tetany and convulsions Cardiac dysrhythmias; decreased cardiac output Positive Trousseau's and Chvostek's signs (see Table 52–8) Confusion, anxiety, possible psychoses Hyperactive deep tendon reflexes *Laboratory findings:* Serum calcium less than 8.5 mg/dL or 4.5 mEq/L (total) Lengthened QT intervals Prolonged ST segments	Closely monitor respiratory and cardiovascular status. Take precautions to protect a confused client. Administer oral or parenteral calcium supplements as ordered. When administering intravenously, closely monitor cardiac status and ECG during infusion. Teach clients at high risk for osteoporosis about ■ Dietary sources rich in calcium. ■ Recommendation for 1,000–1,500 mg of calcium per day. ■ Calcium supplements. ■ Regular exercise. ■ Estrogen replacement therapy for postmenopausal women.
Hypercalcemia ■ Prolonged immobilization Conditions such as ■ Hyperparathyroidism ■ Malignancy of the bone ■ Paget's disease	Lethargy, weakness Depressed deep-tendon reflexes Bone pain Anorexia, nausea, vomiting Constipation Polyuria, hypercalciuria Flank pain secondary to urinary calculi Dysrhythmias, possible heart block *Laboratory findings:* Serum calcium greater than 10.5 mg/dL or 5.5 mEq/L (total) Shortened QT intervals Shortened ST segments	Increase client movement and exercise. Encourage oral fluids as permitted to maintain a dilute urine. Teach clients to limit intake of food and fluid high in calcium. Encourage ingestion of fiber to prevent constipation. Protect a confused client; monitor for pathologic fractures in clients with long-term hypercalcemia. Encourage intake of acid-ash fluids (e.g., prune or cranberry juice) to counteract deposits of calcium salts in the urine.
Hypomagnesemia ■ Excessive loss from the gastrointestinal tract (e.g., from nasogastric suction, diarrhea, fistula drainage) ■ Long-term use of certain drugs (e.g., diuretics, aminoglycoside antibiotics) Conditions such as ■ Chronic alcoholism ■ Pancreatitis ■ Burns	Neuromuscular irritability with tremors Increased reflexes, tremors, convulsions Positive Chvostek's and Trousseau's signs (see Table 52–8) Tachycardia, elevated blood pressure, dysrhythmias Disorientation and confusion Vertigo Anorexia, dysphagia Respiratory difficulties *Laboratory findings:* Serum magnesium below 1.5 mEq/L Prolonged PR intervals, widened QRS complexes, prolonged QT intervals, depressed ST segments, broad flattened T waves, prominent U waves	Assess clients receiving digitalis for digitalis toxicity. Hypomagnesemia increases the risk of toxicity. Take protective measures when there is a possibility of seizures. ■ Assess the client's ability to swallow water prior to initiating oral feeding. ■ Initiate safety measures to prevent injury during seizure activity. ■ Carefully administer magnesium salts as ordered. Encourage clients to eat magnesium-rich foods if permitted (e.g., whole grains, meat, seafood, and green leafy vegetables). Refer clients to alcohol treatment programs as indicated.

TABLE 52–6   Electrolyte Imbalances—*continued*

RISK FACTORS	CLINICAL MANIFESTATIONS	NURSING INTERVENTIONS
Hypermagnesemia Abnormal retention of magnesium, as in ■ Renal failure ■ Adrenal insufficiency ■ Treatment with magnesium salts	Peripheral vasodilation, flushing Nausea, vomiting Muscle weakness, paralysis Hypotension, bradycardia Depressed deep-tendon reflexes Lethargy, drowsiness Respiratory depression, coma Respiratory and cardiac arrest if hypermagnesemia is severe *Laboratory findings:* Serum magnesium above 2.5 mEq/L Electrocardiogram showing prolonged QT interval, prolonged PR interval, widened QRS complexes, tall T waves	Monitor vital signs and level of consciousness when clients are at risk. If patellar reflexes are absent, notify the primary care provider. Advise clients who have renal disease to contact their primary care provider before taking over-the-counter drugs.

CLINICAL ALERT

Potassium may be given intravenously for severe hypokalemia. It must ALWAYS be diluted appropriately and NEVER be given IV push. Potassium that is to be given IV should be mixed in the pharmacy and double-checked prior to administration by two nurses. The usual concentration of IV potassium is 20 to 40 mEq/L. ■

Calcium

Regulating levels of calcium (Ca^{2+}) in the body is more complex than the other major electrolytes so calcium balance can be affected by many factors. Imbalances of this electrolyte are relatively common.

Hypocalcemia is a calcium deficit, or a total serum calcium level of less than 8.5 mg/dL or an ionized calcium level of less than 4.0 mg/dL. Severe depletion of calcium can cause tetany with muscle spasms and paresthesias (numbness and tingling around the mouth and hands and feet) and can lead to convulsions. Two signs indicate hypocalcemia: The Chvostek's sign is contraction of the facial muscles that is produced by tapping the facial nerve in front of the ear (Figure 52-13 ■, A). Trousseau's sign is a carpal spasm that occurs by inflating a blood pressure cuff on the upper arm to 20 mm Hg greater than the systolic pressure for 2 to 5 minutes (Figure 52-13 ■, B). Clients at greatest risk for hypocalcemia are those whose parathyroid glands have been removed. This is frequently associated with total thyroidectomy or bilateral neck surgery for cancer. Low serum magnesium levels (hypomagnesemia) and chronic alcoholism also increase the risk of hypocalcemia.

Hypercalcemia, or total serum calcium levels greater than 10.5 mg/dL, or an ionized calcium level of greater than 5.0 mg/dL, most often occurs when calcium is mobilized from the bony skeleton. This may be due to malignancy or prolonged immobilization.

A. Positive Chvostek's Sign

B. Positive Trousseau's Sign

Figure 52-13 ■ *A*, Positive Chvostek's sign. *B*, Positive Trousseau's sign.

The risk factors and clinical manifestations related to calcium imbalances are found in Table 52–6.

Magnesium

Magnesium (Mg^{2+}) imbalances are relatively common in hospitalized clients, although they may be unrecognized. **Hypomagnesemia** is a magnesium deficiency, or a total serum magnesium level of less than 1.5 mEq/L. It occurs more frequently than hypermagnesemia. Chronic alcoholism is the most common cause of hypomagnesemia. Magnesium deficiency also may aggravate the manifestations of alcohol withdrawal, such as delirium tremens (DTs). **Hypermagnesemia** is present when the serum magnesium level rises above 2.5 mEq/L. It is due to increased intake or decreased excretion. It is often iatrogenic, that is, a result of overzealous magnesium therapy.

Table 52–6 lists risk factors and manifestations for clients with altered magesium balance.

Chloride

Because of the relationship between sodium ions and chloride ions (Cl^-), imbalances of chloride commonly occur in conjunction with sodium imbalances. **Hypochloremia** is a decreased serum chloride level, in adults a level below 95 mEq/L, and is usually related to excess losses of chloride ion through the GI tract, kidneys, or sweating. Hypochloremic clients are at risk for alkalosis and may experience muscle twitching, tremors, or tetany.

Conditions that cause sodium retention also can lead to a high serum chloride level or **hyperchloremia,** in adults a level above 108 mEq/L. Excess replacement of sodium chloride or potassium chloride are additional risk factors for high serum chloride levels. The manifestations of hyperchloremia include acidosis, weakness, and lethargy, with a risk of dysrhythmias and coma.

Phosphate

The phosphate anion PO_4^- is found in both intracellular and extracellular fluid. Most of the phosphorus (P^+) in the body exists as PO_4^-. Phosphate is critical for cellular metabolism because it is a major component of adenosine triphosphate (ATP).

Phosphate imbalances frequently are related to therapeutic interventions for other disorders. Glucose and insulin administration and total parenteral nutrition can cause phosphate to shift into the cells from extracellular fluid compartments, leading to **hypophosphatemia,** defined in adults as a total serum phosphate level less than 2.5 mg/dL. Alcohol withdrawal, acid–base imbalances, and the use of antacids that bind with phosphate in the GI tract are other possible causes of low serum phosphate levels. Manifestations of hypophosphatemia include paresthesias, muscle weakness and pain, mental changes, and possible seizures.

Hyperphosphatemia, defined in adults as a total serum phosphate level greater than 4.5 mg/dL, occurs when phosphate shifts out of the cells into extracellular fluids (e.g., due to tissue trauma or chemotherapy for malignant tumors), in renal failure, or when excess phosphate is administered or ingested. Infants who are fed cow's milk are at risk for hyperphosphatemia, as are people using phosphate-containing enemas or laxatives. Clients who have high serum phosphate levels may experience numbness and tingling around the mouth and in the fingertips, muscle spasms, and tetany.

Acid–Base Imbalances

Acid–base imbalances generally are classified as *respiratory* or *metabolic* by the general or underlying cause of the disorder. Carbonic acid levels are normally regulated by the lungs through the retention or excretion of carbon dioxide, and problems of regulation lead to respiratory acidosis or alkalosis. Bicarbonate and hydrogen ion levels are regulated by the kidneys, and problems of regulation lead to metabolic acidosis or alkalosis. Healthy regulatory systems will attempt to correct acid–base imbalances, a process called **compensation.**

Respiratory Acidosis

Hypoventilation and carbon dioxide retention cause carbonic acid levels to increase and the pH to fall below 7.35, a condition known as **respiratory acidosis.** Serious lung diseases such as asthma and COPD are common causes of respiratory acidosis. Central nervous system depression due to anesthesia or a narcotic overdose can sufficiently slow the respiratory rate so that carbon dioxide is retained. When respiratory acidosis occurs, the kidneys retain bicarbonate to restore the normal carbonic acid to bicarbonate ratio. Recall, however, that the kidneys are relatively slow to respond to changes in acid–base balance, so this compensatory response may require hours to days to restore the normal pH.

Respiratory Alkalosis

When a person hyperventilates, more carbon dioxide than normal is exhaled, carbonic acid levels fall, and the pH rises to greater than 7.45. This condition is termed **respiratory alkalosis.** Psychogenic or anxiety-related hyperventilation is a common cause of respiratory alkalosis. Other causes include fever and respiratory infections. In respiratory alkalosis, the kidneys will excrete bicarbonate to return the pH to within the normal range. Often, however, the cause of the hyperventilation is eliminated and the pH returns to normal before renal compensation occurs.

Metabolic Acidosis

When bicarbonate levels are low in relation to the amount of carbonic acid in the body, the pH falls and **metabolic acidosis** develops. This may develop because of renal failure and the inability of the kidneys to excrete hydrogen ion and produce bicarbonate. It also may occur when too much acid is produced in the body, for example, in diabetic ketoacidosis or starvation when fat tissue is broken down for energy. Metabolic acidosis stimulates the respiratory center, and the rate and depth of respirations increase. Carbon dioxide is eliminated and carbonic acid levels fall, minimizing the change in pH. This respiratory compensation occurs within minutes of the pH imbalance.

Metabolic Alkalosis

In **metabolic alkalosis,** the amount of bicarbonate in the body exceeds the normal 20-to-1 ratio. Ingestion of bicarbonate of soda as an antacid is one cause of metabolic alkalosis. Another

ANATOMY & PHYSIOLOGY REVIEW   Gas Exchange

Pulmonary artery branch

Bronchiole

Pulmonary vein

CO_2

O_2

Alveolar wall

Capillary wall

Red blood cell

O_2 molecule

CO_2 molecule

Blood

O_2

CO_2

From Turley, Susan M., *Medical Language,* 1st ed., © 2002. Reproduced with permission of Pearson Education, Inc., Upper Saddle River, New Jersey.

QUESTIONS

1. Hypoventilation can affect gas exchange. What are some causes of hypoventilation?
2. How does the shallow breathing from hypoventilation cause the $PaCO_2$ to increase and the pH to decrease?
3. ABGs that indicate an increased $PaCO_2$ and a decreased pH reflect which acid–base imbalance?
4. Hyperventilation can also affect gas exchange. What are some causes of hyperventilation?
5. How does hyperventilation cause a decreased $PaCO_2$ and increased pH?
6. ABGs that indicate a decreased $PaCO_2$ and an increased pH reflect which acid–base imbalance?

cause is prolonged vomiting with loss of hydrochloric acid from the stomach. The respiratory center is depressed in metabolic alkalosis, and respirations slow and become more shallow. Carbon dioxide is retained and carbonic acid levels increase, helping balance the excess bicarbonate.

The risk factors and manifestations for acid–base imbalances are listed in Table 52–7.

NURSING MANAGEMENT

Assessing

Assessing clients for fluid, electrolyte, and acid–base balance and imbalances is an important nursing care function. Components of the assessment include (a) the nursing history, (b) physical assessment of the client, (c) clinical measurements, and (d) review of laboratory test results.

Nursing History

The nursing history is particularly important for identifying clients who are at risk for fluid, electrolyte, and acid–base imbalances. The current and past medical history reveal conditions such as chronic lung disease or diabetes mellitus that can disrupt normal balances. Medications prescribed to treat acute or chronic conditions (e.g., diuretic therapy for hypertension) also may place the client at risk for altered homeostasis. Functional, developmental, and socioeconomic factors must also be considered in assessing the client's risk. Older people and very young children, clients who must depend on others to meet their needs for food and fluid intake, and people who cannot afford or do not have the means to cook food for a balanced diet (e.g., homeless people) are at greater risk for fluid and electrolyte imbalances. Common risk factors are listed in Box 52–3.

When obtaining the nursing history, the nurse needs to not only recognize risk factors but also elicit data about the client's

TABLE 52–7 Acid–Base Imbalances

RISK FACTORS	CLINICAL MANIFESTATIONS	NURSING INTERVENTIONS
Respiratory Acidosis Acute lung conditions that impair alveolar gas exchange (e.g., pneumonia, acute pulmonary edema, aspiration of foreign body, near-drowning) Chronic lung disease (e.g., asthma, cystic fibrosis, or emphysema) Overdose of narcotics or sedatives that depress respiratory rate and depth Brain injury that affects the respiratory center Airway obstruction Mechanical chest injury	Increased pulse and respiratory rates Headache, dizziness Confusion, decreased level of consciousness (LOC) Convulsions Warm, flushed skin **Chronic:** Weakness Headache *Laboratory findings:* Arterial blood pH less than 7.35 $PaCO_2$ above 45 mm Hg HCO_3^- normal or slightly elevated in acute; above 26 mEq/L in chronic	Frequently assess respiratory status and lung sounds. Monitor airway and ventilation; insert artificial airway and prepare for mechanical ventilation as necessary. Administer pulmonary therapy measures such as inhalation therapy, percussion and postural drainage, bronchodilators, and antibiotics as ordered. Monitor fluid intake and output, vital signs, and arterial blood gases. Administer narcotic antagonists as indicated. Maintain adequate hydration (2–3 L of fluid per day).
Respiratory Alkalosis Hyperventilation due to ■ Extreme anxiety ■ Elevated body temperature ■ Overventilation with a mechanical ventilator ■ Hypoxia ■ Salicylate overdose Brain stem injury Fever Increased basal metabolic rate	Complaints of shortness of breath, chest tightness Light-headedness with circumoral paresthesias and numbness and tingling of the extremities Difficulty concentrating Tremulousness, blurred vision *Laboratory findings (in uncompensated respiratory alkalosis):* Arterial blood pH above 7.45 $PaCO_2$ less than 35 mm Hg	Monitor vital signs and ABGs. Assist client to breathe more slowly. Help client breathe in a paper bag or apply a rebreather mask (to inhale CO_2).
Metabolic Acidosis Conditions that increase nonvolatile acids in the blood (e.g., renal impairment, diabetes mellitus, starvation) Conditions that decrease bicarbonate (e.g., prolonged diarrhea) Excessive infusion of chloride-containing IV fluids (e.g., NaCl) Excessive ingestion of acids such as salicylates Cardiac arrest	Kussmaul's respirations (deep, rapid respirations) Lethargy, confusion Headache Weakness Nausea and vomiting *Laboratory findings:* Arterial blood pH below 7.35 Serum bicarbonate less than 22 mEq/L $PaCO_2$ less than 38 mm Hg with respiratory compensation	Monitor ABG values, intake and output, and LOC. Administer IV sodium bicarbonate carefully if ordered. Treat underlying problem as ordered.
Metabolic Alkalosis Excessive acid losses due to ■ Vomiting ■ Gastric suction Excessive use of potassium-losing diuretics Excessive adrenal corticoid hormones due to ■ Cushing's syndrome ■ Hyperaldosteronism Excessive bicarbonate intake from ■ Antacids ■ Parenteral $NaHCO_3$	Decreased respiratory rate and depth Dizziness Circumoral paresthesias, numbness and tingling of the extremities Hypertonic muscles, tetany *Laboratory findings:* Arterial blood pH above 7.45 Serum bicarbonate greater than 26 mEq/L $PaCO_2$ higher than 45 mm Hg with respiratory compensation	Monitor intake and output closely. Monitor vital signs, especially respirations, and LOC. Administer ordered IV fluids carefully. Treat underlying problem.

BOX 52–3 **Common Risk Factors for Fluid, Electrolyte, and Acid–Base Imbalances**

CHRONIC DISEASES AND CONDITIONS
- Chronic lung disease (COPD, asthma, cystic fibrosis)
- Heart failure
- Kidney disease
- Diabetes mellitus
- Cushing's syndrome or Addison's disease
- Cancer
- Malnutrition, anorexia nervosa, bulimia
- Ileostomy

ACUTE CONDITIONS
- Acute gastroenteritis
- Bowel obstruction
- Head injury or decreased level of consciousness
- Trauma such as burns or crushing injuries
- Surgery
- Fever, draining wounds, fistulas

MEDICATIONS
- Diuretics
- Corticosteroids
- Nonsteroidal anti-inflammatory drugs

TREATMENTS
- Chemotherapy
- IV therapy and total parenteral nutrition
- Nasogastric suction
- Enteral feedings
- Mechanical ventilation

OTHER FACTORS
- Age: Very old or very young
- Inability to access food and fluids independently

food and fluid intake, fluid output, and the presence of signs or symptoms suggestive of altered fluid and electrolyte balance. The Assessment Interview provides examples of questions to elicit information regarding fluid, electrolyte, and acid–base balance.

Physical Assessment

Physical assessment to evaluate a client's fluid, electrolyte, and acid–base status focuses on the skin, the oral cavity and mucous membranes, the eyes, the cardiovascular and respiratory systems, and neurologic and muscular status. Data from this physical assessment are used to expand and verify infor-

mation obtained in the nursing history. The focused physical assessment is summarized in Table 52–8 on page 1446. Refer to Tables 52–5 through 52–8 for possible abnormal findings related to specific imbalances.

Clinical Measurements

Three simple clinical measurements that the nurse can initiate without a primary care provider's order are daily weights, vital signs, and fluid intake and output.

DAILY WEIGHTS. Daily weight measurements provide a relatively accurate assessment of a client's fluid status. Significant changes in weight over a short time (e.g., more than 5 pounds

---

ASSESSMENT INTERVIEW **Fluid, Electrolyte, and Acid–Base Balance**

CURRENT AND PAST MEDICAL HISTORY
- Are you currently seeing a health care provider for treatment of any chronic diseases such as kidney disease, heart disease, high blood pressure, diabetes insipidus, or thyroid or parathyroid disorders?
- Have you recently experienced any acute conditions such as gastroenteritis, severe trauma, head injury, or surgery? If so, describe them.

MEDICATIONS AND TREATMENTS
- Are you currently taking any medications on a regular basis such as diuretics, steroids, potassium supplements, calcium supplements, hormones, salt substitutes, or antacids?
- Have you recently undergone any treatments such as dialysis, parenteral nutrition, or tube feedings or been on a ventilator? If so, when and why?

FOOD AND FLUID INTAKE
- How much and what type of fluids do you drink each day?
- Describe your diet for a typical day. (Pay particular attention to the client's intake of foods high in sodium content, of protein, and of whole grains, fruits, and vegetables.)
- Have there been any recent changes in your food or fluid intake, for example, as a result of following a weight-loss program?
- Are you on any type of restricted diet?

- Has your food or fluid intake recently been affected by changes in appetite, nausea, or other factors such as pain or difficulty breathing?

FLUID OUTPUT
- Have you noticed any recent changes in the frequency or amount of urine output?
- Have you recently experienced any problems with vomiting, diarrhea, or constipation? If so, when and for how long?
- Have you noticed any other unusual fluid losses such as excessive sweating?

FLUID, ELECTROLYTE, AND ACID–BASE IMBALANCES
- Have you gained or lost weight in recent weeks?
- Have you recently experienced any symptoms such as excessive thirst, dry skin or mucous membranes, dark or concentrated urine, or low urine output?
- Do you have problems with swelling of your hands, feet, or ankles? Do you ever have difficulty breathing, especially when lying down or at night? How many pillows do you use to sleep?
- Have you recently experienced any of the following symptoms: difficulty concentrating or confusion; dizziness or feeling faint; muscle weakness, twitching, cramping, or spasm; excessive fatigue; abnormal sensations such as numbness, tingling, burning, or prickling; abdominal cramping or distention; heart palpitations?

TABLE 52–8 Focused Physical Assessment for Fluid, Electrolyte, or Acid–Base Imbalances

SYSTEM	ASSESSMENT FOCUS	TECHNIQUE	POSSIBLE ABNORMAL FINDINGS
Skin	Color, temperature, moisture	Inspection, palpation	Flushed, warm, very dry Moist or diaphoretic Cool and pale
	Turgor	Gently pinch up a fold of skin over sternum or inner aspect of thigh for adults, on the abdomen or medial thigh for children	Poor turgor: Skin remains tented for several seconds instead of immediately returning to normal position
	Edema	Inspect for visible swelling around eyes, in fingers, and in lower extremities	Skin around eyes is puffy, lids appear swollen; rings are tight; shoes leave impressions on feet
		Compress the skin over the dorsum of the foot, around the ankles, over the tibia, in the sacral area	Depression remains (pitting): see scale for describing edema in Figure 52-11
Mucous membranes	Color, moisture	Inspection	Mucous membranes dry, dull in appearance; tongue dry and cracked
Eyes	Firmness	Gently palpate eyeball with lid closed	Eyeball feels soft to palpation
Fontanels (infant)	Firmness, level	Inspect and gently palpate anterior fontanel	Fontanel bulging, firm Fontanel sunken, soft
Cardiovascular system	Heart rate	Auscultation, cardiac monitor	Tachycardia, bradycardia; irregular; dysrhythmias
	Peripheral pulses	Palpation	Weak and thready; bounding
	Blood pressure	Auscultation of Korotkoff's sounds BP assessment lying and standing	Hypotension Postural hypotension
	Capillary refill	Palpation	Slowed capillary refill
	Venous filling	Inspection of jugular veins and hand veins	Jugular venous distention; flat jugular veins, poor venous refill
Respiratory system	Respiratory rate and pattern	Inspection	Increased or decreased rate and depth of respirations
	Lung sounds	Auscultation	Crackles or moist rales
Neurologic	Level of consciousness (LOC)	Observation, stimulation	Decreased LOC, lethargy, stupor, or coma
	Orientation, cognition	Questioning	Disoriented, confused; difficulty concentrating
	Motor function	Strength testing	Weakness, decreased motor strength
	Reflexes	Deep-tendon reflex (DTR) testing	Hyperactive or depressed DTRs
	Abnormal reflexes	*Chvostek's sign:* Tap over facial nerve about 2 cm anterior to tragus of ear	Facial muscle twitching including eyelids and lips on side of stimulus
		Trousseau's sign: Inflate a blood pressure cuff on the upper arm to 20 mm Hg greater than the systolic pressure, leave in place for 2 to 5 minutes	Carpal spasm: contraction of hand and fingers on affected side

in a week or less) are indicative of acute fluid changes. Each kilogram (2.2 lb) of weight gained or lost is equivalent to 1 L of fluid gained or lost. Such fluid gains or losses indicate changes in total body fluid volume rather than in any specific compartment, such as the intravascular compartment. Rapid losses or gains of 5% to 8% of total body weight indicate moderate to severe fluid volume deficits or excesses.

To obtain accurate weight measurements, the nurse should balance the scale before each use and weigh the client (a) at the same time each day (e.g., before breakfast and after the first void), (b) wearing the same or similar clothing, and (c) on the same scale. The type of scale (i.e., standing, bed, chair) should be documented.

Regular assessment of weight is particularly important for clients in the community and extended care facilities who are at

risk for fluid imbalance. For these clients, measuring intake and output may be impractical because of lifestyle or problems with incontinence. Regular weight measurement, either daily, every other day, or weekly, provides valuable information about the client's fluid volume status.

VITAL SIGNS. Changes in the vital signs may indicate, or in some cases precede, fluid, electrolyte, and acid–base imbalances. For example, elevated body temperature may be a result of dehydration or a cause of increased body fluid losses.

Tachycardia is an early sign of hypovolemia. Pulse *volume* will decrease in FVD and increase in FVE. Irregular pulse rates may occur with electrolyte imbalances. Changes in respiratory rate and depth may cause respiratory acid–base imbalances or act as a compensatory mechanism in metabolic acidosis or alkalosis.

Blood pressure, a sensitive measure to detect blood volume changes, may fall significantly with FVD and hypovolemia or increase with FVE. Postural, or orthostatic, hypotension may also occur with FVD and hypovolemia.

To assess for orthostatic hypotension, measure the client's blood pressure and pulse in a supine position. Allow the client to remain in that position for 3 to 5 minutes, leaving the blood pressure cuff on the arm. Stand the client up and immediately reassess the blood pressure and pulse. A drop of 10 to 15 mm Hg in the systolic blood pressure with a corresponding drop in diastolic pressure and an increased pulse rate (by 10 or more beats per minute) is indicative of orthostatic or postural hypotension.

FLUID INTAKE AND OUTPUT. The measurement and recording of all fluid intake and output (I & O) during a 24-hour period provides important data about the client's fluid and electrolyte balance. Generally, intake and output are measured for hospitalized at-risk clients.

The unit used to measure intake and output is the milliliter (mL) or cubic centimeter (cc); these are equivalent metric units of measurement. In household measures, 30 mL is roughly equivalent to 1 fluid ounce, 500 mL is about 1 pint, and 1,000 mL is about 1 quart. To measure fluid intake, nurses convert household measures such as a glass, cup, or soup bowl to metric units. Most agencies provide conversion tables, since the sizes of dishes vary from agency to agency. Such a table is often provided on or with the bedside I & O record. Examples of equivalents are given in Box 52–4.

Most agencies have a form for recording I & O, usually a bedside record on which the nurse lists all items measured and the quantities per shift (Figure 52-14 ■). Some agencies have another form for recording the specifics of intravenous fluids, such as the type of solution, additives, time started, amounts absorbed, and amounts remaining per shift.

It is important to inform clients, family members, and all caregivers that accurate measurements of the client's fluid in-

	PATIENT LABEL		
Intake and Output Record			
INTAKE	0600-1800	1800-0600	TOTAL
Oral			
Tube feeding			
IV (primary)			
IV Meds			
TPN			
Blood			
TOTAL			24-Hour Total
OUTPUT	0600-1800	1800-0600	TOTAL
Urine			
Emesis			
G.I. Suction			
Stool			
TOTAL			24-Hour Total

Figure 52-14 ■ *A sample 24-hour fluid intake and output record.*

take and output are required, explaining why and emphasizing the need to use a bedpan, urinal, commode, or in-toilet collection device (unless a urinary drainage system is in place). Instruct the client not to put toilet tissue into the container with urine. Clients who wish to be involved in recording fluid intake measurements need to be taught how to compute the values and what foods are considered fluids.

To measure fluid intake, the nurse records on the I & O form each fluid item taken (if the client has not already done so), specifying the time and type of fluid. All of the following fluids need to be recorded:

- Oral fluids. Water, milk, juice, soft drinks, coffee, tea, cream, soup, and any other beverages. Include water taken with medications. To assess the amount of water taken from a water pitcher, measure what remains and subtract this amount from the volume of the full pitcher. Then refill the pitcher.
- Ice chips. Record the fluid as approximately one-half the volume of the ice chips. For example, if the ice chips fill a cup holding 200 mL and the client consumed all of the ice chips, the volume consumed would be recorded as 100 mL.
- Foods that are or tend to become liquid at room temperature. These include ice cream, sherbert, custard, and gelatin. Do not measure foods that are pureed, because purees are simply solid foods prepared in a different form.
- Tube feedings. Remember to include the 30- to 60-mL water flush at the end of intermittent feedings or during continuous feedings.
- Parenteral fluids. The exact amount of intravenous fluid administered is to be recorded, since some fluid containers may be overfilled. Blood transfusions are included.
- Intravenous medications. Intravenous medications that are prepared with solutions such as normal saline (NS) and are

BOX 52–4 Commonly Used Fluid Containers and Their Volumes

Water glass	200 mL
Juice glass	120 mL
Cup	180 mL
Soup bowl	
Adult	180 mL
Child	100 mL
Teapot	240 mL
Creamer	
Large	90 mL
Small	30 mL
Water pitcher	1,000 mL
Jello, custard dish	100 mL
Ice cream dish	120 mL
Paper cup	
Large	200 mL
Small	120 mL

administered as an intermittent or continuous infusion must also be included (e.g., ceftazidime 1 g in 50 mL of sterile water). Most intravenous medications are mixed in 50 to 100 mL of solution.

■ Catheter or tube irrigants. Fluid used to irrigate urinary catheters, nasogastric tubes, and intestinal tubes must be measured and recorded if not immediately withdrawn.

To measure fluid output, measure the following fluids (remember to observe appropriate infection control precautions):

■ Urinary output. Following each voiding, pour the urine into a measuring container, observe the amount, and record it and the time of voiding on the I & O form. For clients with retention catheters, empty the drainage bag into a measuring container at the end of the shift (or at prescribed times if output is to be measured more often). Note and record the amount of urine output. In intensive care areas, urine output often is measured hourly. If the client is incontinent of urine, estimate and record these outputs. For example, for an incontinent client the nurse might record "Incontinent × 3" or "Drawsheet soaked in 12-in. diameter." A more accurate estimate of the urine output of infants and incontinent clients may be obtained by first weighing diapers or incontinent pads that are dry, and then subtracting this weight from the weight of the soiled items. Each gram of weight left after subtracting is equal to 1 mL of urine. If urine is frequently soiled with feces, the number of voidings may be recorded rather than the volume of urine.

■ Vomitus and liquid feces. The amount and type of fluid and the time need to be specified.

■ Tube drainage, such as gastric or intestinal drainage.

■ Wound drainage and draining fistulas. Wound drainage may be recorded by documenting the type and number of dressings or linen saturated with drainage or by measuring the exact amount of drainage collected in a vacuum drainage (e.g., Hemovac) or gravity drainage system.

Fluid intake and output measurements are totaled at the end of the shift (every 8 to 12 hours), and the totals are recorded in the client's permanent record. In intensive care areas, the nurse may record intake and output hourly. Usually the staff on night shift totals the amounts of I & O recorded for each shift and records the 24-hour total.

To determine whether the fluid output is proportional to fluid intake or whether there are any changes in the client's fluid status, the nurse (a) compares the total 24-hour fluid output measurement with the total fluid intake measurement and (b) compares both to previous measurements. Urinary output is normally equivalent to the amount of fluids ingested; the usual range is 1,500 to 2,000 mL in 24 hours, or 40 to 80 mL in 1 hour (0.5 mL/kg/hour). Clients whose output substantially exceeds intake are at risk for fluid volume deficit. By contrast, clients whose intake substantially exceeds output are at risk for fluid volume excess. In assessing the client's fluid balance it is important to consider additional factors that may affect intake and output. The client who is extremely diaphoretic or who has rapid, deep respirations has fluid losses that

BOX 52–5 Normal Electrolyte Values for Adults*	
VENOUS BLOOD	
Sodium	135–145 mEq/L
Potassium	3.5–5.0 mEq/L
Chloride	95–108 mEq/L
Calcium (total)	4.5–5.5 mEq/L or 8.5–10.5 mg/dL
(ionized)	56% of total calcium (2.5 mEq/L or 4.0–5.0 mg/dL)
Magnesium	1.5–2.5 mEq/L or 1.6–2.5 mg/dL
Phosphate (phosphorus)	1.8–2.6 mEq/L or 2.5 – 4.5 mg/dL
Serum osmolality	280–300 mOsm/kg water

*Normal laboratory values vary from agency to agency.

cannot be measured but must be considered in evaluating fluid status.

When there is a significant discrepancy between intake and output or when fluid intake or output is inadequate (for example, a urine output of less than 500 mL in 24 hours or less than 0.5 mL per kilogram per hour in an adult), this information should be reported to the charge nurse or primary care provider.

Laboratory Tests

Many laboratory studies are conducted to determine the client's fluid, electrolyte, and acid–base status. Some of the more common tests are discussed here.

SERUM ELECTROLYTES. Serum electrolyte levels are often routinely ordered for any client admitted to the hospital as a screening test for electrolyte and acid–base imbalances. Serum electrolytes also are routinely assessed for clients at risk in the community, for example, clients who are being treated with a diuretic for hypertension or heart failure. The most commonly ordered serum tests are for sodium, potassium, chloride, magnesium, and bicarbonate ions. Normal values of commonly measured electrolytes are shown in Box 52-5. Some primary care providers use a diagram format for keeping track of the client's electrolytes when documenting in their progress notes. See Figure 52-15 ■.

Figure 52-15 ■ *A*, Format for a diagram of serum electrolyte results. *B*, Example that may be seen in a primary care provider's documentation notes.

COMPLETE BLOOD COUNT (CBC). The complete blood count, another basic screening test, includes information about the hematocrit (Hct). The **hematocrit** measures the volume (percentage) of whole blood that is composed of RBCs. Because the hematocrit is a measure of the volume of cells in relation to plasma, it is affected by changes in plasma volume. Thus the hematocrit increases with severe dehydration and decreases with severe overhydration. Normal hematocrit values are 40% to 54% (men) and 37% to 47% (women).

OSMOLALITY. Serum osmolality is a measure of the solute concentration of the blood. The particles included are sodium ions, glucose, and urea (blood urea nitrogen, or BUN). Serum osmolality can be estimated by doubling the serum sodium, because sodium and its associated chloride ions are the major determinants of serum osmolality. Serum osmolality values are used primarily to evaluate fluid balance. Normal values are 280 to 300 mOsm/kg. An increase in serum osmolality indicates a fluid volume deficit; a decrease reflects a fluid volume excess.

Urine osmolality is a measure of the solute concentration of urine. The particles included are nitrogenous wastes, such as creatinine, urea, and uric acid. Normal values are 500 to 800 mOsm/kg. An increased urine osmolality indicates a fluid volume deficit; a decreased urine osmolality reflects a fluid volume excess.

URINE pH. Measurement of urine pH may be obtained by laboratory analysis or by using a dipstick on a freshly voided specimen. Because the kidneys play a critical role in regulating acid–base balance, assessment of urine pH can be useful in determining whether the kidneys are responding appropriately to acid–base imbalances. Normally the pH of the urine is relatively acidic, averaging about 6.0, but a range of 4.6 to 8.0 is considered normal. In metabolic acidosis, urine pH should decrease as the kidneys excrete hydrogen ions; in metabolic alkalosis, the pH should increase.

URINE SPECIFIC GRAVITY. **Specific gravity** is an indicator of urine concentration that can be performed quickly and easily by nursing personnel. Normal specific gravity ranges from 1.005 to 1.030 (usually 1.010 to 1.025). When the concentration of solutes in the urine is high, the specific gravity rises; in very dilute urine with few solutes, it is abnormally low.

URINE SODIUM AND CHLORIDE EXCRETION. These are indicators of renal perfusion and can provide useful information about a client's fluid status. With hypovolemia, aldosterone will be secreted. This will cause reabsorption of sodium and chloride which will result in decreased levels of sodium and chloride, less than 20 mEq/L each (Elgart, 2004).

ARTERIAL BLOOD GASES. **Arterial blood gases (ABGs)** are performed to evaluate the client's acid–base balance and oxygenation. Arterial blood is used because it provides a truer reflection of gas exchange in the pulmonary system than venous blood. Blood gases may be drawn by laboratory technicians, respiratory therapy personnel, or nurses with specialized skills. Because a high-pressure artery is used to obtain blood, it is important to apply pressure to the puncture site for 5 minutes after the procedure to reduce the risk of bleeding or bruising.

Six measurements are commonly used to interpret arterial blood gas tests (Simpson, 2004):

- pH: a measure of the relative acidity or alkalinity of the blood. The greater the number of hydrogen ions, the more acidic the solution is. The normal range for pH is narrow, and death may ensue with pH values below 6.8 or above 7.8.
- PaO_2: the pressure exerted by oxygen dissolved in the plasma of arterial blood; an indirect measure of blood oxygen content. This measure, representing one of the two forms in which oxygen is transported in the blood, accounts for only about 3% of oxygen content in the blood.
- $PaCO_2$: the partial pressure of carbon dioxide in arterial plasma; the respiratory component of acid–base determination. Carbon dioxide is regulated by the lungs, and the $PaCO_2$ is used to determine if an acid–base imbalance is respiratory in origin.
- Bicarbonate HCO_3^-: a measure of the metabolic component of acid–base balance.
- Base excess (BE): a calculated value of bicarbonate levels, also reflective of the metabolic component of acid–base balance. If the number is preceded by a plus sign, it is a base excess and indicates alkalosis; if preceded by a minus sign, it is a base deficit and indicates acidosis.
- Oxygen saturation (SpO_2): the percentage of hemoglobin saturated (combined) with oxygen. This represents the other form in which oxygen is transported in the blood and accounts for about 97% of the oxygen in the blood.

Normal ABG values are listed in Box 52–6. Changes seen in common acid–base imbalances are summarized in Table 52–9. Note that although the PaO_2 and SpO_2 are important for assessing respiratory status, they generally do not provide useful information for assessing acid–base balance and so are not included in this table.

When evaluating ABG results to determine acid–base balance, it is important to use a systematic approach such as the one outlined in Box 52–7. Nurses need to assess each measurement individually, then look at the interrelationships to determine what type of acid–base imbalance may be present.

BOX 52–6	Normal Values of Arterial Blood Gases*
pH	7.35–7.45
PaO_2	80–100 mm Hg
$PaCO_2$	35–45 mm Hg
HCO_3^-	22–26 mEq/L
Base excess	−2 to +2 mEq/L
O_2 saturation	95–98%

Some normal values will vary according to the kind of test carried out in the laboratory. Nurses are advised to use the normal values issued by the agency when interpreting laboratory results.

TABLE 52–9   Arterial Blood Gas Values in Common Acid–Base Disorders

DISORDER		ABG VALUES
Respiratory acidosis	pH	< 7.35
	$PaCO_2$	> 45 mm Hg (excess CO_2 and carbonic acid)
	HCO_3^-	Normal; or >26 mEq/L with renal compensation
Respiratory alkalosis	pH	> 7.45
	$PaCO_2$	< 35 mm Hg (inadequate CO_2 and carbonic acid)
	HCO_3^-	Normal; or < 22 mEq/L with renal compensation
Metabolic acidosis	pH	< 7.35
	$PaCO_2$	Normal; or < 35 mm Hg with respiratory compensation
		< 22 mEq/L (inadequate bicarbonate)
	HCO_3^-	
Metabolic alkalosis	pH	> 7.45
	$PaCO_2$	Normal; or > 45 mm Hg with respiratory compensation
		> 26 mEq/L (excess bicarbonate)
	HCO_3^-	

Diagnosing

NANDA includes the following diagnostic labels that relate to fluid and acid–base imbalances:

- *Deficient Fluid Volume:* Decreased intravascular, interstitial, and/or intracellular fluid. This refers to dehydration, water loss alone without change in sodium.
- *Excess Fluid Volume:* Increased isotonic fluid retention.

- *Risk for Imbalanced Fluid Volume:* At risk for a decrease, increase, or rapid shift from one to the other of intravascular, interstitial, and/or intracellular fluid. This refers to body fluid loss, gain, or both.
- *Risk for Deficient Fluid Volume:* At risk for experiencing vascular, cellular, or intracellular dehydration.
- *Impaired Gas Exchange:* Excess or deficit in oxygenation and/or carbon dioxide elimination at the alveolar-capillary membrane.

BOX 52–7   Interpreting ABGs — Do You Have a Match?

1. Look at each number separately.
   - Label the pH:
     - If the pH is less than 7.35, the problem is acidosis.
     - If the pH is greater than 7.45, the problem is alkalosis.
   - Label the $PaCO_2$:
     - If the $PaCO_2$ is less than 35 mm Hg, more carbon dioxide is being exhaled than normal and indicates alkalosis.
     - If the $PaCO_2$ is greater than 45 mm Hg, less carbon dioxide is being exhaled than normal and indicates acidosis.
   - Label the bicarbonate:
     - If the HCO_3^- is less than 22 mEq/L, bicarbonate levels are lower than normal, indicating acidosis.
     - If the HCO_3^- is greater than 26 mEq/L, bicarbonate levels are higher than normal, indicating alkalosis.
2. Determine the cause of the acid–base imbalance.
   - Look at the pH—is it acidosis or alkalosis?
3. Determine if the origin of the imbalance is respiratory or metabolic.
   - Check the $PaCO_2$ and HCO_3^- which one MATCHES the same acid–base status as the pH?

   EXAMPLE
   pH = 7.33 (acidosis)
   $PaCO_2$ = 55 (acidosis)
   HCO_3 = 29 (alkalosis)
   Cause of imbalance (hint: look at pH) = acidosis.
   $PaCO_2$ (acidosis) MATCHES the pH (acidosis) = respiratory problem
   Client has respiratory acidosis.

4. Look for evidence of compensation.
   - Look at the value that does NOT match the pH:
     - If it (e.g., $PaCO_2$ or HCO_3) is within normal range, there is no compensation.
     - If it (e.g., $PaCO_2$ or HCO_3) is above or below normal range, the body is compensating.

   EXAMPLES
   a. In respiratory acidosis (pH < 7.35, $PaCO_2$ > 45 mm Hg), if the HCO_3^- is greater than 26 mEq/L, the kidneys are retaining bicarbonate to minimize the acidosis: renal compensation.
   b. In respiratory alkalosis (pH > 7.45, $PaCO_2$ < 35 mm Hg), if the HCO_3^- is less than 22 mEq/L, the kidneys are excreting bicarbonate to minimize the alkalosis: again, renal compensation.
   c. In metabolic acidosis (pH < 7.35, HCO_3^- < 22 mEq/L), if the $PaCO_2$ is less than 35 mm Hg, carbon dioxide is being "blown off" to minimize the acidosis: respiratory compensation.
   d. In metabolic alkalosis (pH > 7.45, HCO_3^- > 26 mEq/L), if the $PaCO_2$ is greater than 45 mm Hg, carbon dioxide is being retained to compensate for excess base: again, respiratory compensation.

   Note: If the value that doesn't match (e.g., $PaCO_2$ or HCO_3) is above or below normal and the pH is within normal range, the body has completely compensated. Complete compensation takes time to develop and is the result of a chronic condition (e.g., chronic respiratory acidosis with COPD).

Clinical applications of selected diagnoses are shown in Identifying Nursing Diagnoses, Outcomes, and Interventions and in the Nursing Care Plan and the Concept Map at the end of this chapter.

Fluid, electrolyte, and acid–base imbalances affect many other body areas and as a consequence may be the etiology of other nursing diagnoses, such as

- *Impaired Oral Mucous Membrane* related to fluid volume deficit.
- *Impaired Skin Integrity* related to dehydration and/or edema.
- *Decreased Cardiac Output* related to hypovolemia and/or cardiac dysrhythmias secondary to electrolyte imbalance (K^+ or Mg^{2+}).
- *Ineffective Tissue Perfusion* related to decreased cardiac output secondary to fluid volume deficit or edema.
- *Activity Intolerance* related to hypervolemia.
- *Risk for Injury* related to calcium shift out of bones into extracellular fluids.
- *Acute Confusion* related to electrolyte imbalance.

Planning

When planning care the nurse identifies nursing interventions that will assist the client to achieve these broad goals:

- Maintain or restore normal fluid balance.
- Maintain or restore normal balance of electrolytes in the intracellular and extracellular compartments.
- Maintain or restore pulmonary ventilation and oxygenation.

- Prevent associated risks (tissue breakdown, decreased cardiac output, confusion, other neurologic signs).

Obviously, goals will vary according to the diagnosis and defining characteristics for each individual. Appropriate preventive and corrective nursing interventions that relate to these must be identified. Specific nursing activities can be selected to meet the client's individual needs. Examples of application of these using NANDA, NIC, and NOC designations are shown in Identifying Nursing Diagnoses, Outcomes, and Interventions and in the Nursing Care Plan and the Concept Map at the end of this chapter. Examples of NIC interventions related to fluid, electrolyte, and acid–base balance include the following:

- Acid–base management
- Electrolyte management
- Fluid monitoring
- Hypovolemia management
- Intravenous (IV) therapy

Specific nursing activities associated with each of these interventions can be selected to meet the individual needs of the client.

Nursing activities to meet goals and outcomes related to fluid, electrolyte, and acid–base imbalances are discussed in the next section. These include (a) monitoring fluid intake and output, cardiovascular and respiratory status, and results of laboratory tests; (b) assessing the client's weight; location and extent of edema, if present; skin turgor and skin status; specific gravity of urine; and level of consciousness and mental status;

IDENTIFYING NURSING DIAGNOSES, OUTCOMES, AND INTERVENTIONS
Clients with Fluid Volume Excess

DATA CLUSTER Tom Bricker, a 67-year-old pensioner who has a history of heart disease, has experienced a weight gain of 4 to 5 kg (9 to 11 lb) during the past month. He states his rings are too tight to remove, his ankles are swollen, his heart pounds at times, he gets breathless with exertion, and he feels bloated. Physical findings reveal jugular vein distention above 3 cm; delayed emptying of hand veins; bounding pulse (86); pitting edema in feet, ankles, and lower legs; and moist lung sounds (rales/crackles).

NURSING DIAGNOSIS/ DEFINITION	SAMPLE DESIRED OUTCOMES*/ *DEFINITION*	INDICATORS	SELECTED INTERVENTIONS*/ *DEFINITION*	SAMPLE NIC ACTIVITIES
Excess Fluid Volume/ Increased isotonic fluid retention	Fluid Balance [0601]/*Water balance in the intracellular and extracellular compartments of the body*	Not compromised: • 24-hour intake and output • Stable body weight No: • Adventitious breath sounds • Neck vein distention	Fluid Management [4120]/*Promotion of fluid balance and prevention of complications resulting from abnormal or undesired fluid levels*	• Assess location and extent of edema on scale from 1+ to 4+ • Monitor for indications of fluid overload/retention (e.g., crackles, elevated BP, edema, neck vein distention) as appropriate • Maintain accurate intake and output record • Weigh daily and monitor trends • Consult primary care provider if signs and symptoms of fluid volume excess persist or worsen

* The NOC # for desired outcomes and the NIC # for nursing interventions are listed in brackets following the appropriate outcome or intervention. Outcomes, indicators, interventions, and activites selected are only a sample of those suggested by NOC and NIC and should be further individualized for each client.

IDENTIFYING NURSING DIAGNOSES, OUTCOMES, AND INTERVENTIONS
Clients with Impaired Gas Exchange

DATA CLUSTER Fred Boysniak was admitted to emergency after being found with an empty bottle of morphine tablets by his bed. He appears very lethargic and stuporous; pulse is 120, respiration 12 and very shallow. Blood gases reveal pH of 7.28, $PaCO_2$ 49 mm Hg, and HCO_3^- 25 mEq/L.

NURSING DIAGNOSIS/ DEFINITION	SAMPLE DESIRED OUTCOMES*/ DEFINITION	INDICATORS	SELECTED INTERVENTIONS*/ DEFINITION	SAMPLE NIC ACTIVITIES
Impaired Gas Exchange/Excess or deficit in oxygenation and/or carbon dioxide elimination at the alveolar-capillary membrane	Respiratory Status: Ventilation [0403]/ *Movement of air in and out of the lungs*	Not compromised ▪ Depth of inspiration ▪ Auscultated breath sounds	Acid–Base Management: Respiratory Acidosis [1913]/ *Promotion of acid–base balance and prevention of complications resulting from serum PCO_2 levels higher than desired*	▪ Monitor respiratory pattern ▪ Monitor ABG levels for decreasing pH level, as appropriate ▪ Monitor neurological status (e.g., level of consciousness and confusion) ▪ Monitor determinants of tissue oxygen delivery (e.g., PaO_2, SaO_2, hemoglobin levels) ▪ Provide mechanical ventilatory support if necessary

*The NOC # for desired outcomes and the NIC # for nursing interventions are listed in brackets following the appropriate outcome or intervention. Outcomes, indicators, interventions, and activites selected are only a sample of those suggested by NOC and NIC and should be further individualized for each client.

(c) fluid intake modifications; (d) dietary changes; (e) parenteral fluid, electrolyte, and blood replacement; and (f) other appropriate measures such as administering prescribed medications and oxygen, providing skin care and oral hygiene, positioning the client appropriately, and scheduling rest periods.

Planning for Home Care

To provide for continuity of care, the client's needs for assistance with care in the home need to be considered. Home care planning includes assessment of the client's and family's resources and abilities for care, and the need for refer-

rals and home health services. The accompanying Home Care Assessment describes the specific assessment data required to establish a home care plan. Based on the data gathered in assessment of the home situation, the nurse tailors the teaching plan for the client and family (see Client Teaching on page 1453).

Implementing
Promoting Wellness

Most people rarely think about their fluid, electrolyte, or acid–base balance. They know it is important to drink adequate

HOME CARE ASSESSMENT   Fluid, Electrolyte, and Acid–Base Balance

CLIENT

- Risk factors for imbalances: The client's age, medications required such as diuretic therapy or corticosteroids, and presence of chronic diseases such as diabetes mellitus, heart disease, lung disease, or dementia (see Box 52–3 on p. 1445)
- Self-care abilities for maintaining food and fluid intake: Mobility; ability to chew and swallow, to access fluids and respond to thirst, to purchase food and prepare a balanced diet
- Current level of knowledge (as appropriate) about: Prescribed diet, any fluid restrictions, activity restrictions, actions and side effects of prescribed medications, regular weight monitoring, gastric tube care and enteral feedings, central line or PICC catheter care, and parenteral fluids and nutrition

FAMILY

- Caregiver availability, skills, and responses: Availability and willingness to assume responsibility for care, knowledge and ability to

provide assistance with preparing food and maintaining adequate intake of food and fluids, knowledge of risk factors and early warning signs of problems
- Family role changes and coping: Effect on financial status, parenting and spousal roles, social roles
- Alternate potential primary or respite caregivers: For example, other family members, volunteers, church members, paid caregivers or housekeeping services; available community respite care (e.g., adult day care, senior centers)

COMMUNITY

- Current knowledge of and experience with community resources: Home health agencies, organizations that offer financial assistance or assistance with food preparation, Meals on Wheels or meal services (e.g., at senior centers, homeless shelters), pharmacies, home intravenous services, respiratory care services

---

CLIENT TEACHING   Promoting Fluid and Electrolyte Balance

- Consume six to eight glasses of water daily.
- Avoid excess amounts of foods or fluids high in salt, sugar, and caffeine.
- Eat a well-balanced diet. Include adequate amounts of milk or milk products to maintain bone calcium levels.
- Limit alcohol intake because it has a diuretic effect.
- Increase fluid intake before, during, and after strenuous exercise, particularly when the environmental temperature is high, and replace lost electrolytes from excessive perspiration as needed with commercial electrolyte solutions.

- Maintain normal body weight.
- Learn about and monitor side effects of medications that affect fluid and electrolyte balance (e.g., diuretics) and ways to handle side effects.
- Recognize possible risk factors for fluid and electrolyte imbalance such as prolonged or repeated vomiting, frequent watery stools, or inability to consume fluids because of illness.
- Seek prompt professional health care for notable signs of fluid imbalance such as sudden weight gain or loss, decreased urine volume, swollen ankles, shortness of breath, dizziness, or confusion.

---

fluids and consume a balanced diet, but they may not understand the potential effects when this is not done. Nurses can promote clients' health by providing wellness teaching that will help them maintain fluid and electrolyte balance.

Enteral Fluid and Electrolyte Replacement

Fluids and electrolytes can be provided orally in the home and hospital if the client's health permits, that is, if the client is not vomiting, has not experienced an excessive fluid loss, and has

---

CLIENT TEACHING   Home Care and Fluid, Electrolyte, and Acid–Base Balance

MONITORING FLUID INTAKE AND OUTPUT

- Teach and provide the rationale for monitoring fluid intake and output to the client and family as appropriate. Include how to use a commode or collection device ("hat") in the toilet, how to empty and measure urinary catheter drainage, and how to count or weigh diapers.
- Instruct and provide the rationale for regular weight monitoring to the client and family. Weigh at the same time of day, using the same scale and with the client wearing the same amount of clothing.
- Educate and provide the rationale to the client and family on when to contact a health care professional, such as in the cases of a significant change in urine output; any change of 5 pounds or more in a 1- to 2-week period; prolonged episodes of vomiting, diarrhea, or inability to eat or drink; dry, sticky mucous membranes; extreme thirst; swollen fingers, feet, ankles, or legs; difficulty breathing, shortness of breath, or rapid heartbeat; and changes in behavior or mental status.

MAINTAINING FOOD AND FLUID INTAKE

- Instruct the client and family about any diet or fluid restrictions, such as a low-sodium diet.
- Teach family members the rationale for the importance of offering fluids regularly to clients who are unable to meet their own needs because of age, impaired mobility or cognition, or other conditions such as impaired swallowing due to a stroke.
- If the client is on enteral or intravenous fluids and feeding at home, teach and provide the underlying rationale to caregivers about proper administration and care. Contact a home health or home intravenous service to provide services and teaching.

SAFETY

- Instruct and provide the rationale to the client to change positions slowly if appropriate, especially when moving from a supine to a sitting or standing position.
- Inform and provide the rationale to the client and family about the importance of good mouth and skin care. Teach the client to change positions frequently and to elevate the feet on a stool when sitting for a long period.

- Teach the client and family how to care for intravenous access sites or gastric tubes. Include what to do if tubes become dislodged.

MEDICATIONS

- Emphasize the importance of and rationale for taking medications as prescribed.
- Instruct clients taking diuretics to take the medication in the morning. If a second daily dose is prescribed, they should take it in the late afternoon to avoid disrupting sleep to urinate.
- Inform clients about any expected side effects of prescribed medications and how to handle them (e.g., if a potassium-depleting diuretic is prescribed, increase intake of potassium-rich foods; if taking a potassium-sparing diuretic, avoid excess potassium intake such as using a salt substitute).
- Teach clients when to contact their primary care provider, for example, if they are unable to take a prescribed medication or have signs of an allergic or toxic reaction to a medication.

MEASURES SPECIFIC TO CLIENT'S PROBLEM

- Provide instructions and rationale specific to the client's fluid, electrolyte, or acid–base imbalance, such as
  a. Fluid volume deficit.
  b. Risk for fluid volume deficit.
  c. Fluid volume excess.

REFERRALS

- Make appropriate referrals to home health or community social services for assistance with resources such as meals, meal preparation and food, intravenous infusions and access, enteral feedings, and homemaker or home health aide services to help with ADLs.

COMMUNITY AGENCIES AND OTHER SOURCES OF HELP

- Provide information about companies or agencies that can provide durable medical equipment such as commodes, lift chairs, or hospital beds for purchase, for rental, or free of charge.
- Provide a list of sources for supplies such as catheters and drainage bags, measuring devices, tube feeding formulas, and electrolyte replacement drinks.
- Suggest additional sources of information and help such as the American Dietetic Association, the American Heart Association, and the American Lung Association.

PRACTICE GUIDELINES Facilitating Fluid Intake

- Explain to the client the reason for the required intake and the specific amount needed. This provides a rationale for the requirement and promotes compliance.
- Establish a 24-hour plan for ingesting the fluids. For the hospitalized or long-term care client, half of the total volume is given during the day shift, and the other half is divided between the evening and night shifts, with most of that ingested during the evening shift. For example, if 2,500 mL is to be ingested in 24 hours, the plan may specify 7–3 (1,500 mL); 3–11 (700 mL); and 11–7 (300 mL). Try to avoid the ingestion of large amounts of fluid immediately before bedtime to prevent the need to urinate during sleeping hours.
- Set short-term outcomes that the client can realistically meet. Examples include ingesting a glass of fluid every hour while awake or a pitcher of water by 12 noon.
- Identify fluids the client likes and make available a variety of those items, including fruit juices, soft drinks, and milk (if al-

lowed). Remember that beverages such as coffee and tea have a diuretic effect, so their consumption should be limited.
- Help clients to select foods that tend to become liquid at room temperature (e.g., gelatin, ice cream, sherbet, custard), if these are allowed.
- For clients who are confined to bed, supply appropriate cups, glasses, and straws to facilitate appropriate fluid intake and keep the fluids within easy reach.
- Make sure fluids are served at the appropriate temperature: hot fluids hot and cold fluids very cold.
- Encourage clients when possible to participate in maintaining the fluid intake record. This assists them to evaluate the achievement of desired outcomes.
- Be alert to any cultural implications of food and fluids. Some cultures may restrict certain foods and fluids and view others as having healing properties.

---

an intact gastrointestinal tract and gag and swallow reflexes. Clients who are unable to ingest solid foods may be able to ingest fluids.

FLUID INTAKE MODIFICATIONS. Increased fluids (ordered as "push fluids") are often prescribed for clients with actual or potential fluid volume deficits arising, for example, from mild diarrhea or mild to moderate fevers. Guidelines for helping clients increase fluid intake are shown in the above Practice Guidelines.

Restricted fluids may be necessary for clients who have fluid retention (fluid volume excess) as a result of renal failure, congestive heart failure, SIADH, or other disease processes. Fluid restrictions vary from "nothing by mouth" to a precise amount ordered by a primary care provider. The restriction of fluids can be difficult for some clients, particularly if they are experiencing thirst. Guidelines for helping clients restrict fluid intake are shown in Practice Guidelines.

DIETARY CHANGES. Specific fluid and electrolyte imbalances may require simple dietary changes. For example, clients receiving potassium-depleting diuretics need to be informed about foods with a high potassium content (e.g., bananas, oranges, and leafy greens). Some clients with fluid retention need to avoid foods high in sodium. Most healthy clients can benefit from foods rich in calcium.

ORAL ELECTROLYTE SUPPLEMENTS. Some clients can benefit from oral supplements of electrolytes, particularly when a medication is prescribed that affects electrolyte balance, when dietary intake is inadequate for a specific electrolyte, or when fluid and electrolyte losses are excessive as a result of, for example, excessive perspiration.

Corticosteroids and many diuretics can cause too much potassium to be eliminated through the kidneys. For clients taking these medications, potassium supplements may be prescribed. Instruct clients taking oral potassium supplements to

---

PRACTICE GUIDELINES Helping Clients Restrict Fluid Intake

- Explain the reason for the restricted intake and how much and what types of fluids are permitted orally. Many clients need to be informed that ice chips, gelatin, and ice cream, for example, are considered fluid.
- Help the client decide the amount of fluid to be taken with each meal, between meals, before bedtime, and with medications. For the hospitalized or long-term care client, half the total volume is scheduled during the day shift, when the client is most active, receives two meals, and most oral medications. A large part of the remainder is scheduled for the evening shift to permit fluids with meals and evening visitors.
- Identify fluids or fluidlike substances the client likes and make sure that these are provided, unless contraindicated. A client who is allowed only 200 mL of fluid for breakfast, for example, should receive the type of fluid the client favors.
- Set short-term goals that make the fluid restriction more tolerable. For example, schedule a specified amount of fluid at one

or two hourly intervals between meals. Some clients may prefer fluids only between meals if the food provided at mealtime helps relieve thirst.
- Place allowed fluids in small containers such as a 4-ounce juice glass to allow the perception of a full container.
- Periodically offer the client ice chips as an alternative to water, because ice chips when melted are approximately half of the frozen volume.
- Provide frequent mouth care and rinses to reduce the thirst sensation.
- Instruct the client to avoid ingesting or chewing salty or sweet foods (hard candy or gum), because these foods tend to produce thirst. Sugarless gum may be an alternative for some clients.
- Encourage the client when possible to participate in maintaining the fluid intake record.

take the medication with juice to mask the unpleasant taste and reduce the possibility of gastric distress. Emphasize the importance of taking the medication as prescribed and seeing their primary care provider on a regular basis. Because hyperkalemia can have serious cardiac effects, clients should never increase the amount of potassium being taken without an order to do so. In addition, inform clients that most salt substitutes contain potassium, so it is important to consult with the primary care provider before using salt substitutes.

People who ingest insufficient milk and milk products benefit from calcium supplements. The recommended daily allowance for calcium is 1,000 to 1,500 mg. It is generally recommended that postmenopausal women take 1,500 mg of calcium per day to reduce the risk of osteoporosis. Long-term use of corticosteroid drugs can also cause calcium loss from the bone, and calcium supplements may help reduce this loss. Clients who take supplemental calcium need to maintain a fluid intake of at least 2,500 mL per day (unless contraindicated) to reduce the risk of kidney stones, which are commonly composed of calcium salts.

Although routine supplements for other electrolytes generally are not recommended, clients who have poor dietary habits, who are malnourished, or who have difficulty accessing or eating fresh fruits and vegetables may benefit from electrolyte supplements. A daily multiple vitamin with minerals may achieve the desired goal. People who engage in strenuous activity in a warm environment need to be encouraged to replace water and electrolytes lost through excessive perspiration by consuming a sports drink such as Gatorade or another commercial fluid and electrolyte solution.

Liquid nutritional supplements are often given to clients who are malnourished or have poor eating habits. They are used with frequency in older adults to bolster nutritional status and caloric intake. It is very important to be a "label reader" of the product and to be aware of the contents of the supplement. Some of them are very high in protein and high in potassium, which may be contraindicated in an individual with impaired renal function.

Parenteral Fluid and Electrolyte Replacement

Intravenous (IV) fluid therapy is essential when clients are unable to take food and fluids orally. It is an efficient and effective method of supplying fluids directly into the intravascular fluid compartment and replacing electrolyte losses. Intravenous fluid therapy is usually ordered by the primary care provider. The nurse is responsible for administering and maintaining the therapy and for teaching the client and significant others how to continue the therapy at home if necessary.

INTRAVENOUS SOLUTIONS. Intravenous solutions can be classified as isotonic, hypotonic, or hypertonic. Most IV solutions are *isotonic*, having the same concentration of solutes as blood plasma. Isotonic solutions are often used to restore vascular volume. *Hypertonic* solutions have a greater concentration of solutes than plasma; *hypotonic* solutions have a lesser concentration of solutes. Table 52–10 provides examples of IV solutions and nursing implications.

IV solutions can also be categorized according to their purpose. Nutrient solutions contain some form of carbohydrate (e.g., dextrose, glucose, or levulose) and water. Water is supplied for fluid requirements and carbohydrate for calories and energy. For example, 1 L of 5% dextrose provides 170 calories. *Nutrient solutions* are useful in preventing dehydration and ketosis but do not provide sufficient calories to promote wound healing, weight gain, or normal growth in children. Common nutrient solutions are 5% dextrose in water (D5W) and 5% dextrose in 0.45% sodium chloride (dextrose in half-strength saline).

Electrolyte solutions contain varying amounts of cations and anions. Commonly used solutions are normal saline (0.9% sodium chloride solution), Ringer's solution (which contains sodium, chloride, potassium, and calcium), and lactated Ringer's solution (which contains sodium, chloride, potassium, calcium, and lactate). Lactate is metabolized in the liver to form bicarbonate HCO_3^-. Saline and balanced electrolyte solutions commonly are used to restore vascular volume, particularly

TABLE 52–10 **Selected Intravenous Solutions**	
TYPE/EXAMPLES	**COMMENTS/NURSING IMPLICATIONS**
Isotonic Solutions 0.9% NaCl (normal saline) Lactated Ringer's (a balanced electrolyte solution) 5% dextrose in water (D5W)	Isotonic solutions such as NS and lactated Ringer's initially remain in the vascular compartment, expanding vascular volume. Assess clients carefully for signs of hypervolemia such as bounding pulse and shortness of breath. D5W is isotonic on initial administration but provides free water when dextrose is metabolized, expanding intracellular and extracellular fluid volumes. D5W is avoided in clients at risk for increased intracranial pressure (IICP) because it can increase cerebral edema.
Hypotonic Solutions 0.45% NaCl (half normal saline) 0.33% NaCl (one-third normal saline)	Hypotonic solutions are used to provide free water and treat cellular dehydration. These solutions promote waste elimination by the kidneys. Do not administer to clients at risk for IICP or third-space fluid shift.
Hypertonic Solutions 5% dextrose in normal saline (D5NS) 5% dextrose in 0.45% NaCl (D5 1/2NS) 5% dextrose in lactated Ringer's (D5LR)	Hypertonic solutions draw fluid out of the intracellular and interstitial compartments into the vascular compartment, expanding vascular volume. Do not administer to clients with kidney or heart disease or clients who are dehydrated. Watch for signs of hypervolemia.

after trauma or surgery. They also may be used to replace fluid and electrolytes for clients with continuing losses, for example, because of gastric suction or wound drainage.

Lactated Ringer's solution is an *alkalinizing solution* that may be given to treat metabolic acidosis. *Acidifying solutions,* in contrast, are administered to counteract metabolic alkalosis. Examples of acidifying solutions are 5% dextrose in 0.45% sodium chloride and 0.9% sodium chloride solution.

Volume expanders are used to increase the blood volume following severe loss of blood (e.g., from hemorrhage) or loss of plasma (e.g., from severe burns, which draw large amounts of plasma from the bloodstream to the burn site). Examples of expanders are dextran, plasma, and albumin.

VENIPUNCTURE SITES. The site chosen for venipuncture varies with the client's age, the length of time the infusion is to run, the type of solution used, and the condition of veins. For adults, veins in the hand and arm are commonly used; for infants, veins in the scalp and dorsal foot veins are often used. Larger veins are preferred for infusions that need to be given rapidly and for solutions that could be irritating (e.g., certain medications).

The metacarpal, basilic, and cephalic veins are commonly used for intermittent or continuous infusions (Figure 52-16 ■, *B*). The ulna and radius act as natural splints at these sites, and the client has greater freedom of arm movements for activities such as eating. Although the basilic and median cubital veins in the antecubital space are convenient sites for venipuncture, they are usually used for blood draws, bolus injections of medication, and insertion sites for a peripherally inserted central catheter line (see Figure 52-16 ■, *A*). See Practice Guidelines for vein selection and general tips for easier IV starts.

When long-term IV therapy or parenteral nutrition is anticipated or the client is receiving IV medications that are damaging to vessels (e.g., chemotherapy), a central venous catheter may be inserted. **Central venous catheters** usually are inserted into the subclavian or jugular vein, with the distal tip of the catheter resting in the superior vena cava just above the right

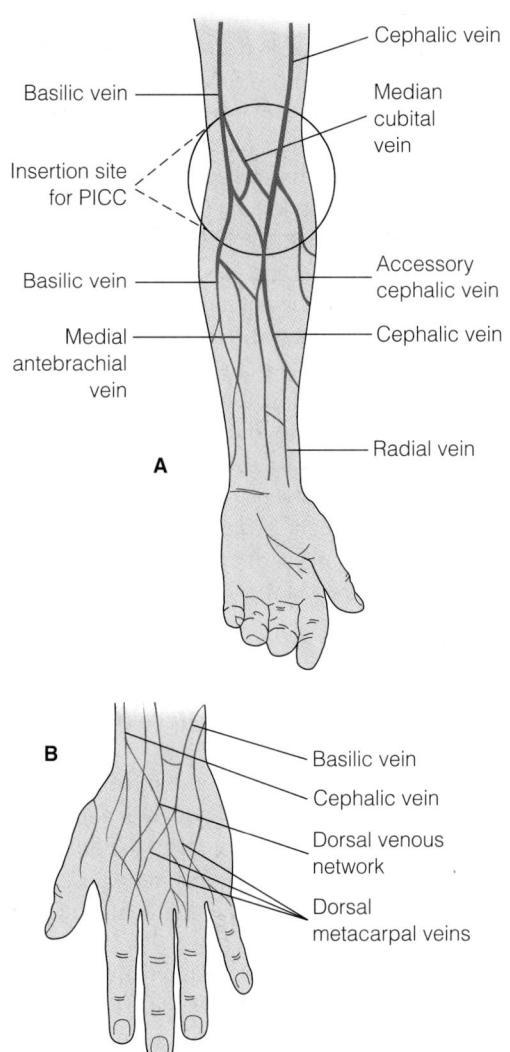

Figure 52-16 ■ Commonly used venipuncture sites of the *A*, arm; *B*, hand. *A* also shows the site used for a peripherally inserted central catheter (PICC).

atrium (Figure 52-17 ■). They may be inserted at the client's bedside or, for longer term access, surgically inserted. Subclavian central venous catheters permit freedom of movement for ambulation; however, there is greater risk of complications, including hemothorax or pneumothorax, cardiac perforation, thrombosis, and infection. Assess the client closely for manifestations such as shortness of breath, chest pain, cough, hypotension, tachycardia, and anxiety after the insertion procedure.

With a **peripherally inserted central venous catheter (PICC),** the catheter is inserted in the basilic or cephalic vein just above or below the antecubital space of the right arm. The tip of the catheter rests in the superior vena cava. The risk of pneumothorax is eliminated with PICC. These catheters frequently are used for long-term intravenous access when the client will be managing IV therapy at home.

Implantable venous access devices or ports (Figures 52-18 ■ and 52-19 ■ on page 1458) are used for clients with chronic illness who require long-term IV therapy (e.g., intermittent medications such as chemotherapy, total parenteral nutrition, and

---

PRACTICE GUIDELINES Vein Selection

- Use distal veins of the arm first.
- Use the client's nondominant arm whenever possible.
- Select a vein that is
  a. Easily palpated and feels soft and full.
  b. Naturally splinted by bone.
  c. Large enough to allow adequate circulation around the catheter.
- Avoid using veins that are
  a. In areas of flexion (e.g., the antecubital fossa).
  b. Highly visible, because they tend to roll away from the needle.
  c. Damaged by previous use, phlebitis, infiltration, or sclerosis.
  d. Continually distended with blood, or knotted or tortuous.
  e. In a surgically compromised or injured extremity (e.g., following a mastectomy), because of possible impaired circulation and discomfort for the client.

- Review the client's medical history. In general, you'll want to avoid using an arm affected by hemiplegia or with a dialysis access. Also avoid an arm on the same side as a mastectomy, sites near infections or below previous infiltrations of extravasations, and veins affected by phlebitis.

- Put gravity to work. Dangle the client's arm over the side of the bed to encourage dependent vein filling.

- Make sure the client is comfortable. Pain and anxiety stimulate the sympathetic nervous system and trigger vasoconstriction and vasovagal reactions. Have the client void before you start the IV line, make sure he or she is warm enough, and administer pain medication as ordered before the procedure. Help the patient into a comfortable prone or semi-Fowler position for the IV insertion.

- Warmth encourages vasodilation. Apply warm compresses to the site for 10 to 15 minutes before you attempt venipuncture. Unless contraindicated, the client could take a hot shower or drink warm fluids before IV insertion.

- Avoid hand veins. Because of the risk of nerve injuries, hand veins should be a last choice, especially in older clients whose skin is very thin.

- Choose the right device for the ordered therapy. If the ordered IV medication is irritating to veins and therapy is expected to last more than a few days, consult with the IV nurse or medical team to determine whether the client is a candidate for a mid-line catheter, a peripherally inserted central catheter, or another type of central venous access device.

- Use the smallest gauge cannula that will accommodate the therapy and allow good venous flow around the catheter tip. For example, for routine hydration or intermittent therapies, use 22- to 27-gauge catheters; for transfusion therapies, 20- to 24-gauge; and for therapy for neonates or clients with very small, fragile veins, 24- to 27-gauge.

- Use good body mechanics. Raise the bed or stretcher to a comfortable working height. Sit, when possible, and keep all equipment within reach. Stabilize the client's hand or arm with your nondominant arm, tucking it under your forearm if necessary to prevent a moving target.

- Display confidence in your own abilities. When you approach the client, don't say, "I'm here to try to start your IV line." Instead, confidently state, "I'm here to insert your IV line."

- If you miss, offer an honest explanation in a matter-of-fact and friendly manner. Think about what you can do to improve your next attempt, and explain what you'll do differently (if anything). Most important, limit your attempts to two. If you're not successful after two tries, ask another nurse or an anesthesia provider to try again a little later.

Note: From "Tailor Your I.V. Insertion Techniques for Special Populations," by K. Rosenthal, 2005a, *Nursing, 35*(5), 39. Copyright © 2005 Lippincott, Williams & Wilkins. Reprinted with permission.

frequent blood samples). The device is designed to provide repeated access to the central venous system, avoiding the trauma and complications of multiple venipunctures. Using local anesthesia, implantable ports are surgically placed into a small subcutaneous pocket under the skin, usually on the anterior chest near the clavicle, and no part of the port is exposed. The distal end of the catheter is placed in the subclavian or jugular vein. There are different kinds of implantable venous access devices and they may be tunneled or nontunneled (Rosenthal, 2005b).

Special precautions need to be taken with all central lines and venous access ports to ensure asepsis and catheter patency. Nursing care of clients with these devices is outlined in Practice Guidelines on page 1459.

INTRAVENOUS EQUIPMENT. Because equipment varies according to the manufacturer, the nurse must become familiar with the equipment used in each particular agency.

Solution containers are available in various sizes (50, 100, 250, 500, or 1,000 mL); the smaller containers are often used to administer medications. Most solutions are currently dispensed in plastic bags (Figure 52-20 ■). However, glass bottles may need to be used if the administered medications are incompatible with plastic. Glass bottles require an air vent so that air can enter the bottle and replace the fluid that enters the client's vein. Some have a tube inside the bottle that serves as a vent; other containers without air vents require a vent on the administration set. Air vents usually have filters to prevent contamination from the air that enters the container. Air vents are not required for plastic solution bags, because the bags collapse under atmospheric pressure when the solution enters the vein.

It is essential that the solution be sterile and in good condition, that is, clear. Cloudiness, evidence that the container has been opened previously, or leaks indicate possible contamination. Always check the expiration date on the label. Return any

Figure 52-17 ■ Central venous lines with *A*, subclavian vein insertion, and *B*, left jugular insertion.

Figure 52-18 ■ An implantable venous access device: *A*, components; *B*, the device in place.

questionable or contaminated solutions to the pharmacy or IV therapy department.

Infusion sets usually include an insertion spike, a drip chamber, a roller valve or screw clamp, tubing with secondary ports, and a protective cap over the needle adapter (Figure 52-21 ■). The insertion spike is kept sterile and inserted into the solution

Figure 52-19 ■ An implantable venous access device (right) and a Huber needle with extension tubing.

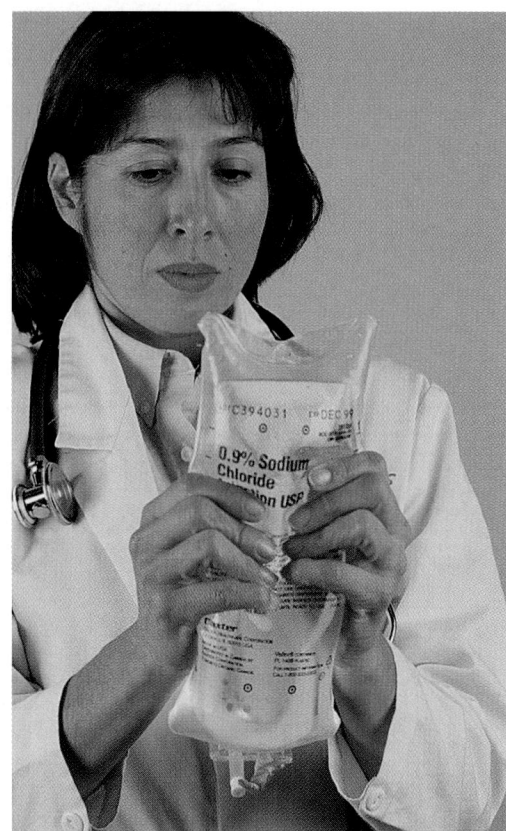

Figure 52-20 ■ A plastic intravenous fluid container.

container when the equipment is set up and ready to start. The drip chamber permits a predictable amount of fluid to be delivered. A commonly used drip chamber is the 10 to 20 drops, which delivers macrodrip per milliliter of solution. This infor-

Figure 52-21 ■ A standard IV administration set.

PRACTICE GUIDELINES   Caring for Clients with a Venous Access Device

On insertion, document the date; the site; the brand, gauge, and catheter length; the location of the catheter tip (verified by x-ray); the length of the external segment; and client teaching. Do not use the access device until correct placement has been verified by x-ray.

SITE CARE

- Use strict aseptic technique when caring for central lines and long-term venous access devices.
- The frequency of dressing changes may vary from every 3 to 7 days, depending on the site. Dressings also should be changed when loose or soiled.
- Assess the site for any redness, swelling, tenderness, or drainage. Compare the length of the external portion of the catheter with its documented length to assess for possible displacement. Obtain a chest x-ray to determine the catheter tip's position if in doubt. Report and document any position changes or signs of infection.
- Follow agency protocol for cleaning solutions and types of dressings. Isopropyl alcohol or a combination of alcohol and acetone followed by povidone-iodine are commonly used to clean the port site.
- Before accessing the port, clean an area 2 inches in diameter around the site with an alcohol-acetone solution on a sterile cotton swab. Start at the center of the port site, moving outward with a firm, circular motion. Follow with povidone-iodine solution. Allow the site to air dry.
- Secure the catheter, and cover the entry site and external portion of the catheter with an occlusive dressing.
- Provide routine care of the incision site for the implant device until it is healed. Once it heals, no care is necessary when the port is idle.

CATHETER CARE AND FLUSHING

- Change the catheter cap as indicated by protocol, usually every 3 to 7 days.
- Flush the port with normal saline, a heparin flush solution (10 units/mL or 100 units/mL), or as agency protocol recommends for the specific type of port being used. After infusing medications or solutions, again flush the port with saline before using heparinized saline.

- Using a 10-mL syringe, flush the catheter with a solution of 10 units of heparin after each use. The frequency of flushes between uses may vary from every 12 hours to once a week or less, depending on the type of catheter.
- Remember to flush all lumens for multiple-lumen catheters.
- Use a specially designed needle to access an implanted port. A needle with a 90-degree angle is generally used for infusions because it is easier to stabilize and more comfortable for the client. Stabilizing the port between the thumb and index finger of the nondominant hand, insert the needle through the center of the port until the resistance of the platform is felt.
- To remove the needle after a treatment, again stabilize the port and use even pressure to withdraw the needle. Maintain positive pressure by withdrawing the needle as the last milliliter of flush solution is being instilled.
- Flush idle implanted ports with heparinized saline in accordance with agency protocol or at least every 8 weeks.

TEACHING

Provide clients with the following instructions:

- Do not allow anyone to take a blood pressure on the arm in which a PICC line is inserted.
- Wear a medic-alert tag or bracelet if the device is to be in place for a long period.
- For a PICC, you do not need to restrict activities, except do not immerse the arm in water. Showering is allowed if the site and catheter are covered by an occlusive dressing.
- For an implanted venous port there are no activity restrictions, but remember that the port or catheter tip can become dislodged. Signs of a dislodged catheter tip include pain in the neck or ear on the affected side, swishing or gurgling sounds, or palpitations. Free movement of the port, swelling, or difficulty accessing the port may indicate port dislodgment. Notify the primary care provider should any of these occur or if symptoms of infection develop.

Note: From "Getting a Line on Central Vascular Access Devices," by S. Masoorli & T. Angeles, 2002, *Nursing, 32*(4), pp. 36–43. Copyright © 2005 Lippincott, Williams & Wilkins. Reprinted with permission.

---

mation is found on the package. There are also 60 drops sets, which deliver microdrip per milliliter of solution. The roller valve or screw clamp, which compresses the lumen of the tubing, controls the rate of the flow. The protective cap over the needle adapter maintains the sterility of the end of the tubing so that it can be attached to a sterile needle inserted in the client's vein.

Most infusion sets include one or more injection ports for administering IV medications or secondary infusions. Needleless systems are increasingly used because they reduce the risk of needlestick injury and contamination of the intravenous line. There are various types of needleless systems available, including two-piece prepierced septum and blunt cannula devices, Luer-activated devices, and three-way pressure-activated safety valves (Rosenthal, 2003). With each of these needleless systems, a blunt cannula is inserted into a special injection port or adapter on the IV tubing to administer medications or secondary infusions (Figure 52-22 ■). Many infusion sets include an

in-line filter to trap air, particulate matter, and microbes. A special infusion set may be required if the IV flow rate will be regulated by an infusion pump.

Catheters and needles are commonly used for intravenous infusions. Over-the-needle catheters, also known as angiocaths, are commonly used for adult clients. The plastic catheter fits over a needle used to pierce the skin and vein wall (Figure 52-23 ■). Once inserted into the vein, the needle is withdrawn and discarded, leaving the catheter in place. IV catheters allow the client more mobility and rarely infiltrate, that is, become dislodged from the vein and allow fluid to flow into interstitial spaces.

Safety devices on IV catheters are now common. With the original over-the-needle catheters, the sharp stylet remained exposed until placed in a sharps container. This resulted in needlestick injuries to nurses. The 2000 Needlestick Safety and Prevention Act requires the use of needle saftey devices to prevent exposure to

A   **B**

Figure 52-22 ■ Cannulae used to connect the tubing of additive sets to primary infusions: *A,* threaded-lock cannula; *B,* lever-lock cannula.
(Photographs reprinted courtesy of (BD) Becton, Dickinson and Company and courtesy of Baxter Healthcare Corporation. All rights reserved.)

Figure 52-23 ■ Schematic of an over-the-needle catheter.

bloodborne pathogens (Wilburn, 2004). The safety devices for IV catheters vary. They can be either an active safety device which requires activation by the nurse or a passive safety device where the safety feature is automatically activated after the sytlet is removed from the catheter.

Butterfly, or wing-tipped, needles with plastic flaps attached to the shaft are sometimes used (Figure 52-24 ■). The flaps are held tightly together to hold the needle securely during insertion; after insertion, they are flattened against the skin and secured with tape.

IV poles are used to hang the solution container. Some poles are attached to hospital beds; others stand on the floor or hang from the ceiling. In the home, plant hangers or robe hooks (even kitchen cabinet knobs or an S-hook over the top of a door) may be used to hang solution containers. The height of most poles is adjustable. The higher the solution container, the greater the force of the solution as it enters the client and the faster the rate of flow.

STARTING AN INTRAVENOUS INFUSION. Although the primary care provider is responsible for ordering IV therapy for clients, nurses initiate, monitor, and maintain the prescribed IV infusion. This is true not only in hospitals and long-term care facilities but increasingly in community-based settings such as clinics and clients' homes.

Before starting an infusion, the nurse determines the following:

■ The type and amount of solution to be infused
■ The exact amount (dose) of any medications to be added to a compatible solution
■ The rate of flow or the time over which the infusion is to be completed

If solutions are prepared by the pharmacy or another department, the nurse must verify that the solution supplied exactly matches that which the primary care provider ordered.

Understanding the purpose for the infusion is as important as assessing the client. For example, the nurse may question an order for 5% dextrose in water at 150 mL/h if the client has peripheral edema and other signs of fluid overload.

To perform venipuncture and start an intravenous infusion, see Skill 52-1.

Figure 52-24 ■ Schematic of a butterfly needle with adapter.

STARTING AN INTRAVENOUS INFUSION

SKILL 52-1

Before preparing the infusion, the nurse first verifies the primary care provider's order indicating the type of solution, the amount to be administered, the rate of flow of the infusion, and any client allergies (e.g., to tape or povidone-iodine).

PURPOSES
- To supply fluid when clients are unable to take in an adequate volume of fluids by mouth
- To provide salts and other electrolytes needed to maintain electrolyte balance
- To provide glucose (dextrose), the main fuel for metabolism
- To provide water-soluble vitamins and medications
- To establish a lifeline for rapidly needed medications

ASSESSMENT
Assess the following:
- Vital signs (pulse, respiratory rate, and blood pressure) for baseline data
- Skin turgor
- Allergy to latex (e.g., tourniquet), tape, or iodine
- Bleeding tendencies
- Disease or injury to extremities
- Status of veins to determine appropriate venipuncture site

PLANNING
Prior to initiating the IV infusion, consider how long the client is likely to have the IV, what kinds of fluids will be infused, and what medications the client will be receiving or is likely to receive. These factors may affect the choice of vein and catheter size.

Delegation
This procedure is done by a registered nurse and, in many states, by a licensed pratical nurse or licensed vocational nurse. Check the state's nurse practice act. Due to the use of sterile technique, intravenous infusion therapy is not delegated to unlicensed assistive personnel (UAP). UAP may care for clients receiving IV therapy, and the nurse must ensure that the UAP knows how to perform routine tasks such as bathing and positioning without disturbing the IV. The UAP should also know what complications or adverse signs, such as leakage, should be reported to the nurse. In some states a licensed vocational nurse with special IV therapy training may start intravenous infusions.

Equipment
- Infusion set
- Sterile parenteral solution
- IV pole
- Adhesive or nonallergenic tape
- Clean gloves
- Tourniquet
- Antiseptic swabs
- Antiseptic ointment (check agency policy)
- Intravenous catheter; see Variation at the end of this procedure for a butterfly (winged-tip) needle
- Sterile gauze dressing or transparent occlusive dressing
- Arm splint, if required
- Towel or pad
- Electronic infusion device or pump (The nurse decides what device is needed as appropriate to the client's condition.)

IMPLEMENTATION
Preparation
1. Prepare the client.
   - Prior to performing the procedure, introduce self and verify the client's identity using agency protocol. Explain the procedure to the client. A venipuncture can cause discomfort for a few seconds, but there should be no discomfort while the solution is flowing. Use a doll to demonstrate for children, and explain the procedure to the parents. Clients often want to know how long the process will last. The primary care provider's order may specify the length of time of the infusion, for example, 3,000 mL over 24 hours.
   - Unless initiating IV therapy is urgent, provide any scheduled care before establishing the infusion to minimize movement of the affected limb during the procedure. Moving the limb after the infusion has been established could dislodge the catheter.
   - Make sure that the client's clothing or gown can be removed over the IV apparatus if necessary. Some agencies provide special gowns that open over the shoulder and down the sleeve for easy removal.

Performance
Perform hand hygiene.
1. Open and prepare the infusion set.
   - Remove tubing from the container and straighten it out.
   - Slide the tubing clamp along the tubing until it is just below the drip chamber to facilitate its access.
   - Close the clamp.
   - Leave the ends of the tubing covered with the plastic caps until the infusion is started. **Rationale:** *This will maintain the sterility of the ends of the tubing.*
2. Spike the solution container.
   - Remove the protective cover from the entry site of the bag.
   - Remove the cap from the spike and insert the spike into the insertion site of the bag or bottle. ❶ Follow the manufacturer's instructions.
3. Apply a medication label to the solution container if a medication is added.
   - In many agencies, medications and labels are applied in the pharmacy; if they are not, apply the label upside down on the container. **Rationale:** *The label is applied upside down so it can be read easily when the container is hanging up.*

continued on page 1462

STARTING AN INTRAVENOUS INFUSION *continued*

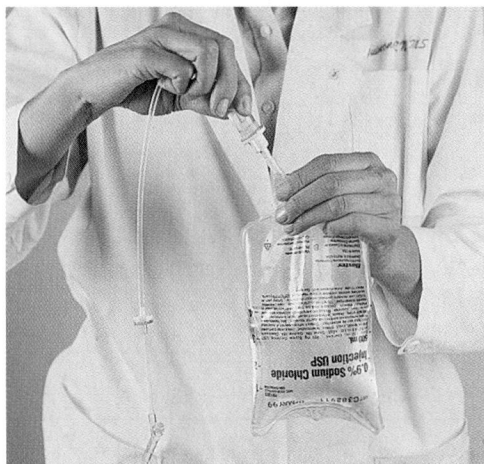

1 Inserting the spike.
Photographer: Elena Dorfman

4. Apply a timing label on the solution container.
   • The timing label may be applied at the time the infusion is started. Follow agency practice. See later discussion of regulating infusion flow rates and Figure 52-26.
5. Hang the solution container on the pole.
   • Adjust the pole so that the container is suspended about 1 m (3 ft) above the client's head. **Rationale:** *This height is needed to enable gravity to overcome venous pressure and facilitate flow of the solution into the vein.*
6. Partially fill the drip chamber with solution.
   • Squeeze the chamber gently until it is half full of solution. **2**
7. Prime the tubing.
   • Remove the protective cap and hold the tubing over a container. Maintain the sterility of the end of the tubing and the cap.
   • Release the clamp and let the fluid run through the tubing until all bubbles are removed. Tap the tubing if necessary with your fingers to help the bubbles move. **Rationale:** *The tubing is primed to prevent the introduction of air into the client.*

2 Squeezing the drip chamber.
Photographer: Elena Dorfman

Air bubbles smaller than 0.5 mL usually do not cause problems in peripheral lines.
   • Reclamp the tubing and replace the tubing cap, maintaining sterile technique.
   • For caps with air vents, do not remove the cap when priming this tubing. The flow of solution through the tubing will cease when the cap is moist with one drop of solution.
   • If an infusion control pump, electronic device, or controller is being used, follow the manufacturer's directions for inserting the tubing and setting the infusion rate.
8. Perform hand hygiene again just prior to client contact.
9. Select the venipuncture site.
   • Use the client's nondominant arm, unless contraindicated (e.g., mastectomy, fistula for dialysis). Identify possible venipuncture sites by looking for veins that are relatively straight, not sclerotic or tortuous, and avoid venous valves. The vein should be palpable, but may not be visible, especially in clients with dark skin. Consider the catheter length; look for a site sufficiently distal to the wrist or elbow that the tip of the catheter will not be at a point of flexion. **Rationale:** *Sclerotic veins may make initiating and maintaining the IV difficult. Joint flexion increases the risk of irritation of vein walls by the catheter.*
   • Check agency protocol about shaving if the site is very hairy. Shaving is not usually recommended *because of the potential for microabrasions which can increase the risk of infection.*
   • Place a towel or bed protector under the extremity *to protect linens (or furniture if in the home).*
10. Dilate the vein.
   • Place the extremity in a dependent position (lower than the client's heart). **Rationale:** *Gravity slows venous return and distends the veins. Distending the veins makes it easier to insert the needle properly.*
   • Apply a tourniquet firmly 15 to 20 cm (6 to 8 in.) above the venipuncture site. **3** Explain that the tourniquet will feel tight. **Rationale:** *The tourniquet must be tight enough to obstruct venous flow but not so tight that it occludes arterial flow. Obstructing arterial flow inhibits venous filling. If a radial pulse can be palpated, the arterial flow is not obstructed.*
     Use the tourniquet on only one client. This avoids cross-contamination to other clients.

Pull this end to untie

A

B

3 Applying a tourniquet.

STARTING AN INTRAVENOUS INFUSION *continued*

- If the vein is not sufficiently dilated:
  a. Massage or stroke the vein distal to the site and in the direction of venous flow toward the heart. **Rationale:** *This action helps fill the vein.*
  b. Encourage the client to clench and unclench the fist. **Rationale:** *Contracting the muscles compresses the distal veins, forcing blood along the veins and distending them.*
  c. Lightly tap the vein with your fingertips. **Rationale:** *Tapping may distend the vein.*
- If the preceding steps fail to distend the vein so that it is palpable, remove the tourniquet and wrap the extremity in a warm, moist towel for 10 to 15 minutes. **Rationale:** *Heat dilates superficial blood vessels, causing them to fill.* Then repeat step 10.

11. Put on clean gloves and clean the venipuncture site. **Rationale:** *Gloves protect the nurse from contamination by the client's blood.*
    - Clean the skin at the site of entry with a topical antiseptic swab (e.g., 2% chlorhexidine, or alcohol). Some institutions may use an anti-infective solution such as povidone-iodine (check agency protocol). Check for allergies to iodine or shellfish before cleansing skin with Betadine or iodine products.
    - Use a circular motion, moving from the center outward for several inches. **Rationale:** *This motion carries microorganisms away from the site of entry.*
    - Permit the solution to dry on the skin. Povidone-iodine should be in contact with the skin for 1 minute to be effective.

12. Insert the catheter and initiate the infusion.
    - If desired and permitted by policy, inject 0.05 mL of 1% lidocaine intradermally over the site where you plan to insert the IV needle. Allow 5 to 10 seconds for the anesthetic to take effect. Transdermal analgesic creams (e.g., ELA-Max, EMLA) may also be used, depending on policy. Allow 30 minutes for the transdermal analgesic to take effect.
    - Use the nondominant hand to pull the skin taut below the entry site. **Rationale:** *This stabilizes the vein and makes the skin taut for needle entry. It can also make initial tissue penetration less painful.*

- Holding the over-the-needle catheter at a 15- to 30-degree angle with bevel up, insert the catheter through the skin and into the vein. Sudden lack of resistance is felt as the needle enters the vein. Jabbing, stabbing, or quick thrusting should be avoided because it may cause rupture of delicate veins (Phillips, 2005).
- Once blood appears in the lumen of the needle or you feel the lack of resistance, lower the angle of the catheter until it is almost parallel with the skin, and advance the needle and catheter approximately 0.5 to 1 cm (about 1/4 in.) farther. Holding the needle portion steady, advance the catheter until the hub is at the venipuncture site. The exact technique depends on the type of device used. **Rationale:** *The catheter is advanced to ensure that it, and not just the metal needle, is in the vein. The exact technique depends on the type of catheter used.*
- Release the tourniquet.
- Put pressure on the vein proximal to the catheter to eliminate or reduce blood oozing out of the catheter. Stabilize the hub with thumb and index finger of the nondominant hand.
- Remove the protective cap from the distal end of the tubing and hold it ready to attach to the catheter, maintaining the sterility of the end.
- Carefully remove the needle, engage the needle safety device, and attach the end of the infusion tubing to the catheter hub.
- Initiate the infusion.

13. Tape the catheter.
    - Tape the catheter by the "U" method or according to the manufacturer's instructions. Using three strips of adhesive tape, each about 7.5 cm (3 in.) long:
      a. Place one strip, sticky side up, under the catheter's hub.
      b. Fold each end over so that the sticky sides are against the skin. ❹
      c. Place the second strip, sticky side down, over the catheter hub.
      d. Place the third strip, sticky side down, over the tubing hub.

14. Dress and label the venipuncture site and tubing according to agency policy.
    - Unless there is an allergy, a sterile transparent occlusive dressing is applied. ❺ This permits assessment of the site

❹ Taping an intravenous catheter by the "U" method.

❺ Cover insertion site with transparent dressing.
(Patrick Watson)

continued on page 1464

SKILL 52-1

STARTING AN INTRAVENOUS INFUSION *continued*

6 Label IV site with date, time, size of catheter, and initials.
(Patrick Watson)

without disturbing the dressing. This type of dressing can be left on for 72 hours, then changed.

- Discard the tourniquet. Remove soiled gloves and discard appropriately.
- Loop the tubing and secure it with tape. **Rationale:** *Looping and securing the tubing prevent the weight of the tubing or any movement from pulling on the needle or catheter.*
- Label the dressing with the date and time of insertion, type, gauge of catheter used, and your initials. **6**

15. Ensure appropriate infusion flow.
    - Apply a padded arm board to splint the joint, as needed.
    - Adjust the infusion rate of flow according to the order.
16. Label the IV tubing.
    - Label the tubing with the date and time of attachment and your initials. **7** This labeling may also be done when the infusion is started. **Rationale:** *The tubing is labeled to ensure*

that it is changed at regular intervals (i.e., every 24 to 96 hours according to agency policy).

17. Document relevant data, including assessments.
    - Record the start of the infusion on the client's chart. Some agencies provide a special form for this purpose. Include the date and time of the venipuncture; amount and type of solution used, including any additives (e.g., kind and amount of medications); container number; flow rate; type, length, and gauge of the needle or catheter; venipuncture site, how many attempts were made, and location of each attempt; the type of dressing applied; and the client's general response.

SAMPLE DOCUMENTATION

1/15/2008 0600 Inserted 20 gauge angiocath in (L) forearm on first attempt. IV infusing at 125 mL/hour. Explained reason for IV. Stated understanding.————————A. Luis, RN

VARIATION: INSERTING A BUTTERFLY (WINGED-TIP) NEEDLE

- Hold the needle, pointed in the direction of the blood flow, at a 30-degree angle, with the bevel up, and pierce the skin beside the vein about 1 cm (1/2 in.) below the site planned for piercing the vein.
- Once the needle is through the skin, lower the needle so that it is almost parallel with the skin. **Rationale:** *Lowering the needle reduces the chances of puncturing both sides of the vein.*

Follow the course of the vein, and pierce one side of the vein. Sudden lack of resistance can be felt as blood enters the needle.

- When blood flows back into the needle tubing, insert the needle to its hub.
- Release the tourniquet, attach the infusion, and initiate flow as quickly as possible. **Rationale:** *Attaching the tubing quickly prevents blood from clotting and obstructing the needle.*
- Secure the butterfly needle by taping it securely by the crisscross (chevron) method. **8** Place a small gauze square under the needle, if required. **Rationale:** *The gauze keeps the needle in position in the vein.*

8 Taping the butterfly needle by the chevron method.

| I.V. SET– 72 HRS.–ONLY |
| START DATE 9/11 HR. 0800 |
| DISCARD DATE 9/14 HR. 0800 |
| R.N. INITIAL LA |

7 Tubing labeled with date, time of attachment, and nurse's initials. Also shown is a preprinted label.

Photographer: Elena Dorfman

STARTING AN INTRAVENOUS INFUSION *continued*

EVALUATION
Evaluate the following:

- Skin status at IV site (warm temperature and absence of pain, redness, and swelling)
- Status of dressing

- IV flow rate consistent with that ordered
- Ability to perform self-care activities; understanding of any mobility limitations
- Vital signs compared to baseline level

REGULATING AND MONITORING INTRAVENOUS INFUSIONS.
Orders for IV infusions may take several forms: "3,000 mL over 24 hours"; "1,000 mL every 8 hours × 3 bags"; "125 mL/h until oral intake is adequate." The nurse initiating the IV calculates the correct flow rate, regulates the infusion, and monitors the client's responses. Unless an infusion control device is used, the nurse manually regulates the drops per minute of flow using the roller clamp to ensure that the prescribed amount of solution will be infused in the correct time span. If the flow is incorrect, problems such as hypervolemia, hypovolemia, or inadequate medication administration can result.

The number of drops delivered per milliliter of solution varies with different brands and types of infusion sets. This rate, called the **drip factor** (sometimes called the *drop factor*), generally is printed on the package of the infusion set. Macrodrops commonly have drop factors of 10, 12, 15, or 20 drops/mL; the drop factor for microdrip is always 60 drops/mL (Figure 52-25 ■).

To calculate flow rates, the nurse must know the volume of fluid to be infused and the specific time for the infusion. Two commonly used methods of indicating flow rates are designating the number of milliliters to be administered in 1 hour (mL/h) and the number of drops to be given in 1 minute (gtt/min). Because 1 milliliter of fluid displaces 1 cubic centimeter of space, the volume to be infused in the first method may also be designated as cubic centimeters per hour (cc/h).

Milliliters per Hour. Hourly rates of infusion can be calculated by dividing the total infusion volume by the total infusion time

in hours. For example, if 3,000 mL is infused in 24 hours, the number of milliliters per hour is

$$\frac{3{,}000 \text{ mL (total infusion volume)}}{24 \text{ h (total infusion time)}} = 125 \text{ mL/h}$$

Nurses need to check infusions at least every hour to ensure that the indicated milliliters per hour have infused and that IV patency is maintained. A strip of adhesive marking the exact time and/or amount to be infused may be taped to the solution container. Some agencies make premarked labels available (Figure 52-26 ■).

Drops per Minute. The nurse initiating and monitoring an infusion must regulate the drops per minute to ensure that the prescribed amount of solution will infuse. Drops per minute are calculated by the following formula:

$$\text{Drops per minute} = \frac{\text{Total infusion volume} \times \text{drop factor}}{\text{Total time of infusion in } minutes}$$

If the requirements are 1,000 mL in 8 hours and the drip factor is 20 drops/mL, the drops per minute should be

$$\frac{1{,}000 \text{ mL} \times 20}{8 \times 60 \text{ min (480 min)}} = 41 \text{ drops/min}$$

Approximating this rate as 40 drops/min, the nurse regulates the drops per minute by tightening or releasing the IV tubing clamp and counting the drops for 15 seconds, then multiplying that number by 4 (e.g., 10 drops/15 sec).

A number of factors influence flow rate (see Box 52–8).

Figure 52-25 ■ Infusion set spikes and drip chambers: nonvented macrodrip, vented macrodrip, nonvented microdrip.

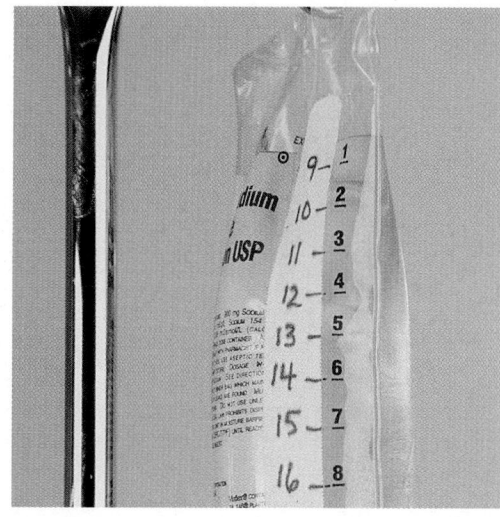

Figure 52-26 ■ Timing label on an intravenous container. The first time marked (0900 hours) would be correct for a bag hung at 0800 hours with a rate of 100 mL per hour.

Photographer: Elena Dorfman

BOX 52–8 Factors Influencing Flow Rates

- The position of the forearm. Sometimes a change in the position of the client's arm decreases flow. Slight pronation, supination, extension, or elevation of the forearm on a pillow can increase flow.
- The position and patency of the tubing. Tubing can be obstructed by the client's weight, a kink, or a clamp closed too tightly. The flow rate also diminishes when part of the tubing dangles below the puncture site.
- The height of the infusion bottle. Elevating the height of the infusion bottle a few inches can speed the flow by creating more pressure.
- Possible infiltration or fluid leakage. Swelling, a feeling of coldness, and tenderness at the venipuncture site may indicate infiltration.
- Relationship of the size of the angiocath to the vein. A catheter that is too large may impede the infusion flow.

DEVICES TO CONTROL INFUSIONS. A number of devices are used to control the rate of an infusion. *Electronic infusion devices* (EIDs) regulate the infusion rate at preset limits. They also have an alarm that is triggered when the solution in the IV bag is low, when there is air in the tubing, or when the tubing is not high enough. The *Dial-A-Flo* in-line device (Figure 52-27 ■) is a regulator that controls the amount of fluid to be administered. Hospitals may stock the Dial-A-Flo for use in situations where a pump is not required, but prevention of fluid overload is important. It is preset at the volume to be infused and can be attached at the time the infusion is set up or when the tubing is changed. Another variation is a *volume-control set,* or *Volutrol,* which is used if the volume of fluid administered is to be carefully controlled. The set, which holds a maximum of 100 mL of solution, is attached below the solution container, and the drip chamber is placed below the set. Volume-control sets are frequently used in pediatric settings, where the volume administered is critical.

CLINICAL ALERT

A flow rate control device should be used when administering IV fluid to elderly or pediatric clients. Both of these age groups are especially at risk for complications of fluid overload, which can occur with rapid infusion of IV fluids. ■

Figure 52-27 ■ The Dial-A-Flo in-line device.
Photographer: Elena Dorfman

Figure 52-28 ■ An intravenous infusion pump.
Photographer: Jenny Thomas

An infusion pump (Figures 52-28 ■ and 52-29 ■) delivers fluids intravenously by exerting positive pressure on the tubing or on the fluid. In situations where the fluid flow is unrestricted, the pump pressure is comparable to that of gravity flow. However, if restrictions develop (increased venous resistance), the pump can maintain the fluid flow by increasing the pressure applied to the fluid.

A controller, by contrast, operates solely by gravitational force. The delivery pressure depends on the height of the container in relation to the venipuncture site. The container must be at least 76 cm (30 in.) above the venipuncture site for a controller to work. A controller does not have the ability to add pressure to the line and to overcome resistances to fluid flow.

Skill 52-2 outlines the steps involved in monitoring an intravenous infusion.

Figure 52-29 ■ Programmable infusion pumps.
(Courtesy of ALARIS Medical Systems, Inc., San Diego, California.)

MONITORING AN INTRAVENOUS INFUSION

PURPOSES
- To maintain the prescribed flow rate
- To prevent complications associated with IV therapy

ASSESSMENT
Assess the following:

- Appearance of infusion site; patency of system
- Type of fluid being infused and rate of flow
- Response of the client

PLANNING
Review the type of equipment used outside the client's room. Read all appropriate materials and confirm the type of tubing, controller, or pump being used.

Delegation
This procedure should be done by the nurse because it is an important part of assessment and complications may occur.

IMPLEMENTATION
Preparation
1. Gather the pertinent data.
   - From the primary care provider's order, determine the type and sequence of solutions to be infused.
   - Determine the rate of flow and infusion schedule.

Performance
1. Ensure that the correct solution is being infused.
   - If the solution in incorrect, slow the rate of flow to a minimum to maintain the patency of the catheter. **Rationale:** *Stopping the infusion may allow a thrombus to form in the IV catheter. If this occurs, the catheter must be removed and another venipuncture performed before the infusion can be resumed.*
   - Change the solution to the correct one. Document and report the error according to agency protocol.
2. Observe the rate of flow every hour.
   - Compare the rate of flow regularly, for example, every hour, against the infusion schedule. **Rationale:** *Infusions that are off schedule can be harmful to a client.*
   - If the rate is too fast, slow it so that the infusion will be completed at the planned time. **Rationale:** *Solution administered too quickly may cause a significant increase in circulating blood volume (which is about 6 L in an adult). Hypervolemia may result in pulmonary edema and cardiac failure. Assess the client for manifestations of hypervolemia and its complications, including dyspnea; rapid, labored breathing; cough; crackles (rales) in the lung bases; tachycardia; and bounding pulses.*
   - If the rate is too slow, check agency practice. Some agencies permit nursing personnel to adjust a rate of flow by a specified amount. Adjustments above this rate require a primary care provider's order. **Rationale:** *Solution that is administered too slowly can supply insufficient fluid, electrolytes, or medication for a client's needs.*
   - If the rate of flow is 150 mL/h or more, check the rate of flow more frequently, for example, every 15 to 30 minutes.
3. Inspect the patency of the IV tubing and catheter.
   - Observe the position of the IV solution. If it is less than 1 m (3 ft) above the IV site, readjust it to the correct height of the pole. **Rationale:** *If the IV bag/bottle is too low, the solution may not flow into the vein because there is insufficient grav-*

itational pressure to overcome the pressure of the blood within the vein.
   - Observe the drip chamber. If it is less than half full, squeeze the chamber to allow the correct amount of fluid to flow in.
   - Open the drip regulator and observe for a rapid flow of fluid from the solution container into the drip chamber. Then partially close the drip regulator to reestablish the prescribed rate of flow. **Rationale:** *Rapid flow of fluid into the drip chamber indicates patency of the IV line. Closing the drip regulator to the prescribed rate of flow prevents fluid overload.*
   - Inspect the tubing for pinches or kinks or obstructions to flow. Arrange the tubing so that it is lightly coiled and under no pressure. Sometimes the tubing becomes caught under the client's body and the weight blocks the flow.
   - Observe the position of the tubing. If it is dangling below the venipuncture, coil it carefully on the surface of the bed. **Rationale:** *The solution may not flow upward into the vein against the force of gravity.*
   - Lower the solution container below the level of the infusion site and observe for a return flow of blood from the vein. **Rationale:** *A return flow of blood indicates that the needle is patent and in the vein. Blood returns in this instance because venous pressure is greater than the fluid pressure in the IV tubing. Absence of blood return may indicate that the needle is no longer in the vein or that the tip of the catheter is partially obstructed by a thrombus, the vein wall, or a valve in the vein.*
   - Determine whether the bevel of the catheter is blocked against the wall of the vein. If it is blocked, pull back gently, turn it slightly, or carefully raise or lower the angle of insertion slightly, using a sterile gauze pad underneath to protect the skin and change the position of the catheter bevel.
   - If there is leakage, locate the source. If the leak is at the catheter connection, tighten the tubing into the catheter. If the leak cannot be stopped, slow the infusion as much as possible without stopping it, and replace the tubing with a new sterile set. Estimate the amount of solution lost, if it was substantial.
4. Inspect the insertion site for fluid infiltration.
   - When an IV needle becomes dislodged from the vein, fluid flows into interstitial tissues, causing swelling. This is known

continued on page 1468

MONITORING AN INTRAVENOUS TRANSFUSION *continued*

as *infiltration* and is manifested by localized swelling, cool-ness, pallor, and discomfort at the IV site.

- If an infiltration is present, stop the infusion and remove the catheter. Restart the infusion at another site.
- Apply a warm compress to the site of the infiltration. **Rationale:** *Warmth promotes comfort and vasodilation, facilitating absorption of the fluid from interstitial tissues.*

5. If the infiltration involves a vesicant drug, it is called extravasa-tion and other measures may be indicated. Extravasated vesi-cant drugs can cause severe tissue injury or destruction. The extravasation of a vesicant drug should be considered an emer-gency (Hadaway, 2004).
   - Stop the infusion immediately. Disconnect the tubing as close to the catheter hub as possible and attempt to aspirate any drug remaining in the hub. If an injectable antidote is available, the catheter should remain in place.
   - The primary care provider should be notified and if ordered, the antidote administered.
   - The affected arm should be elevated and depending on the drug, heat or cold therapy should be implemented.
6. If infiltration is not evident but the infusion is not flowing, de-termine whether the needle is dislodged from the vein.
   - Gently pinch the IV tubing adjacent to the needle site. This will cause blood to flow (flash back) into the tubing if the needle is in the vein.
   - Use a sterile syringe of saline to withdraw fluid from the port near the venipuncture site. If blood does not return, discon-tinue the intravenous solution.
7. Inspect the insertion site for phlebitis (inflammation of a vein).
   - Inspect and palpate the site at least every 8 hours. Phlebitis can occur as a result of injury to a vein, for example, because

of mechanical trauma or chemical irritation. Chemical injury to a vein can occur from intravenous electrolytes (especially potassium and magnesium) and medications. The clinical signs are redness, warmth, and swelling at the intravenous site and burning pain along the course of a vein.
   - If phlebitis is detected, discontinue the infusion, and apply warm compresses to the venipuncture site. Do not use this injured vein for further infusions.
8. Inspect the intravenous site for bleeding.
   - Oozing or bleeding into the surrounding tissues can occur while the infusion is freely flowing but is more likely to occur after the needle has been removed from the vein.
   - Observation of the venipuncture site is extremely important for clients who bleed readily, such as those receiving antico-agulants.
9. Teach the client ways to maintain the infusion system, for example:
   - Avoid sudden twisting or turning movements of the arm with the needle or catheter.
   - Avoid stretching or placing tension on the tubing.
   - Try to keep the tubing from dangling below the level of the needle.
   - Notify a nurse if
     a. The flow rate suddenly changes or the solution stops dripping.
     b. The solution container is nearly empty.
     c. There is blood in the IV tubing.
     d. Discomfort or swelling is experienced at the IV site.
10. Document all relevant information.

EVALUATION

Evaluate the following:

- Amount of fluid infused according to the schedule
- Intactness of IV system

- Appearance of IV site (e.g., dry, tissue infiltration, discomfort)
- Urinary output compared to urinary intake
- Tissue turgor; specific gravity of urine
- Vital signs and lung sounds compared to baseline data

CHANGING INTRAVENOUS CONTAINERS, TUBING, AND DRESSINGS. Intravenous solution containers are changed when only a small amount of fluid remains in the neck of the container and fluid still remains in the drip chamber. However,

all IV bags should be changed every 24 hours, regardless of how much solution remains, to minimize the risk of contami-nation. IV tubing is changed every 48 to 96 hours, depending on agency protocol, as is the site dressing. Skill 52-3 provides

CHANGING AN INTRAVENOUS CONTAINER, TUBING, AND DRESSING

PURPOSES

- To maintain the flow of required fluids
- To maintain sterility of the IV system and decrease the incidence of phlebitis and infection

- To maintain patency of the IV tubing
- To prevent infection at the IV site and the introduction of mi-croorganisms into the bloodstream

ASSESSMENT

Assess the following:

- Presence of fluid infiltration, bleeding, or phlebitis at IV site
- Allergy to tape or iodine
- Infusion rate and amount absorbed

- Blockages in IV system
- Appearance of the dressing for integrity, moisture, and need for change
- The date and the time of the previous dressing change

CHANGING AN INTRAVENOUS CONTAINER, TUBING, AND DRESSING *continued*

PLANNING

Review primary care provider's orders for changes in fluid administration.

> **Delegation**
>
> This procedure includes assessment of the IV site and should be completed by a registered nurse. In many states, licensed vocational nurses with IV certification may complete the procedure.

Equipment

- Container with the correct kind and amount of sterile solution
- Administration set, including sterile tubing and drip chamber
- Timing label
- Sterile gauze square for positioning the needle

For the Dressing

- Clean gloves
- Sterile 2-in. × 2-in. or 4-in. × 4-in. gauze or transparent dressing
- Adhesive remover
- Chlorhexidine swabs
- Alcohol swabs
- Tape
- Towel

IMPLEMENTATION

Preparation

1. Obtain the correct solution container.
   - Read the label of the new container.
   - Verify that you have the correct solution, correct client, correct additives (if any), and correct dose (number of bags or total volume ordered).

Performance

1. Perform hand hygiene.
2. Set up the intravenous equipment with the new container and label all. See Skill 52-1, steps 1 to 8.
   - Apply a timing label to the container.
   - Prime the tubing.
   - Label the tubing as shown in Figure ❷ in Skill 52-1.
3. Prepare the IV needle or catheter, tape, and the dressing equipment near the client.
   - Prepare strips of tape as needed for the type of needle or catheter. For the butterfly needle, two or three strips of 1.25-cm (1/2-in.) tape are needed. For a catheter, three strips of 1.25-cm (1/2-in.) tape are needed. These will be used later to secure the needle or catheter without covering the insertion site.
   - Hang the pieces of tape from the edge of a table. **Rationale:** *This places the tape in readiness for use without disrupting the adhesive.* Ensure that the table is clean *to avoid contaminating the tape.*
   - Open all equipment: swabs, dressing and adhesive bandage, and ointment. **Rationale:** *This facilitates access to supplies after gloves are donned.*
   - Place a towel under the extremity. **Rationale:** *This prevents soiling of bed linens.*
   - Apply clean gloves.
4. Remove the soiled dressing and all tape, except the tape holding the catheter or IV needle in place.
   - Remove tape and gauze from the old dressing one layer at a time. **Rationale:** *This prevents dislodgment of the catheter or needle in case tubing becomes entangled between layers of dressing.*
   - Remove adhesive dressings in the direction of the client's hair growth when possible. **Rationale:** *This minimizes discomfort when adhesive is removed from the skin.*
   - Discard the used dressing materials in the appropriate container.

5. Assess the IV site.
   - Inspect the IV site for the presence of infiltration or inflammation. **Rationale:** *Inflammation or infiltration necessitates removal of the IV needle or catheter to avoid further trauma to the tissues.*
   - Go to step 6, or discontinue and relocate the IV site if indicated. See Skills 52-1 and 52-4.
6. Disconnect the used tubing.
   - Place a sterile swab under the hub of the catheter. **Rationale:** *This absorbs any leakage that might occur when the tubing is disconnected.*
   - Clamp the tubing. With the fourth or fifth finger of the nondominant hand, apply pressure to the vein above the end of the catheter. **Rationale:** *This helps prevent blood from coming out of the needle during the change of tubing.*
   - Holding the hub of the catheter with the thumb and index finger of the nondominant hand, loosen the tubing with the dominant hand, using a twisting, pulling motion. **Rationale:** *Holding the catheter firmly but gently maintains its position in the vein.*
   - Remove the used IV tubing.
   - Place the end of the tubing in the basin or other receptacle.
7. Connect the new tubing, and reestablish the infusion.
   - Continue to hold the catheter and grasp the new tubing with the dominant hand.
   - Remove the protective tubing cap and, maintaining sterility, insert the tubing end securely into the needle hub. Twist it to secure it.
   - Open the clamp to start the solution flowing.
8. Remove the tape securing the needle or catheter.
   - When removing this tape and while cleaning the site, stabilize the needle or catheter hub with one hand. **Rationale:** *This prevents inadvertent dislodgment of the needle or catheter.*
9. Clean the IV site.
   - Start with adhesive remover to remove adhesive residue. **Rationale:** *Removal of adhesive residue facilitates adherence of the new dressing.*
   - Then, using chlorhexidine swabs or alcohol swabs, clean the site, beginning at the catheter or needle and cleaning outward in a 2-in. diameter. **Rationale:** *Cleaning in this manner prevents contamination of the IV site from bacteria on the peripheral skin areas. Antiseptics reduce the number of*

continued on page 1470

SKILL 52-3

CHANGING AN INTRAVENOUS CONTAINER, TUBING, AND DRESSING *continued*

microorganisms present at the site, thus reducing the risk of infection.

- Follow agency protocol about cleaning procedures.

10. Retape the needle or catheter.
    - For a butterfly needle, apply strips of tape to the wings of the butterfly using the crisscross (chevron) method (Figure ❽ in Skill 52-1).
    - For a catheter; apply the tape using the U method (Figure ❹ in Skill 52-1).
    - Apply a sterile transparent dressing over the site.
    - Remove gloves.

11. Label the dressing and secure IV tubing.

- Place the date and time of the dressing change and your initials either on the label provided or directly over the top of the dressing.
- Secure IV tubing with additional tape as required.

12. Regulate the rate of flow of the solution according to the order on the chart.

13. Document all relevant information.
    - Record the change of the solution container, tubing, and/or dressing in the appropriate place on the client's chart. Also record the fluid intake according to agency practice. Record the number of the container if the containers are numbered at the agency. Also record your assessments.

EVALUATION
Evaluate the following:

- Status of IV site
- Patency of IV system
- Accuracy of flow

---

guidelines for changing an IV solution container, tubing, and the IV site dressing.

When an IV infusion is no longer necessary to maintain the client's fluid intake or to provide a route for medication administration, the infusion is either discontinued and the catheter re-

moved or the catheter is left in place and converted to a saline or heparin lock. Guidelines for discontinuing an IV infusion or converting the catheter to a lock are outlined in Skills 52-4 and 52-5, respectively.

SKILL 52-4

DISCONTINUING AN INTRAVENOUS INFUSION

PURPOSE
- To discontinue an intravenous infusion when the therapy is complete or when the IV site needs to be changed

ASSESSMENT
Assess the following:

- Appearance of the venipuncture site
- Any bleeding from the infusion site
- Amount of fluid infused
- Appearance of IV catheter

PLANNING
Review the primary care provider's orders.

Delegation
This procedure should be done by a registered nurse. In many states, licensed vocational nurses may initiate and discontinue IV therapy.

Equipment
- Clean gloves
- Dry or antiseptic-soaked swabs, according to agency practice
- Small sterile dressing and tape

IMPLEMENTATION
Performance

1. Prepare the equipment.
   - Clamp the infusion tubing. **Rationale:** *Clamping the tubing prevents the fluid from flowing out of the needle onto the client or bed.*
   - Loosen the tape at the venipuncture site while holding the needle firmly and applying countertraction to the skin. **Rationale:** *Movement of the needle can injure the vein and*

cause discomfort to the client. Countertraction prevents pulling the skin and causing discomfort.

   - Put on clean gloves and hold a sterile gauze above the venipuncture site.

2. Withdraw the needle or catheter from the vein.
   - Withdraw the needle or catheter by pulling it out along the line of the vein. **Rationale:** *Pulling it out in line with the vein avoids injury to the vein.*

DISCONTINUING AN INTRAVENOUS INFUSION *continued*

- Immediately apply firm pressure to the site, using sterile gauze, for 2 to 3 minutes. **Rationale:** *Pressure helps stop the bleeding and prevents hematoma formation.*
- Hold the client's arm above the body if any bleeding persists. **Rationale:** *Raising the limb decreases blood flow to the area.*

3. Examine the catheter removed from the client.
- Check the catheter to make sure it is intact. **Rationale:** *If a piece of tubing remains in the client's vein it could move centrally (toward the heart or lungs) and cause serious problems.*
- Report a broken catheter to the nurse in charge or primary care provider immediately.
- If a broken piece can be palpated, apply a tourniquet above the insertion site. **Rationale:** *Application of a tourniquet de-creases the possibility of the piece moving until a primary care provider is notified.*

4. Cover the venipuncture site.
- Apply the sterile dressing. **Rationale:** *The dressing continues the pressure and covers the open area in the skin, prevent-ing infection.*
- Discard the IV solution properly, if infusions are being discon-tinued, and discard the used supplies appropriately.

5. Document all relevant information.
- Record the amount of fluid infused on the intake and output record and on the chart, according to agency practice. In-clude the container number, type of solution used, time of discontinuing the infusion, and the client's response.

EVALUATION

Evaluate the following:

- Appearance of the venipuncture site
- The pulse
- Respirations, skin color, edema, sputum, cough, and urine output
- How the person feels physically and psychologically

CHANGING AN INTRAVENOUS CATHETER TO AN INTERMITTENT INFUSION LOCK

PURPOSE

- To permit IV administration of medications or fluids on an intermittent basis

ASSESSMENT

Assess the following:

- Patency of the IV catheter
- Appearance of the site (evidence of inflammation or infiltration)

PLANNING

Review the primary care provider's order.

- A specific order may be written to convert an intravenous access to a heparin or saline lock. The order also may be implied, for example, IV fluids are to be discontinued but the client has or-ders for an IV antibiotic every 6 hours or is receiving analgesics intravenously.

Delegation

Due to the need for sterile technique and technical complexity, this procedure is not delegated to UAP. UAP may care for clients with such devices, and the nurse must ensure that the UAP knows what complications or adverse signs should be reported to the nurse.

Equipment

- Intermittent infusion cap or device
- Clean gloves
- Sterile 2-in. × 2-in. or 4-in. × 4-in. gauze
- Sterile saline for injection (without preservative) or heparin flush solution (10 units/mL or 100 units/mL) in a prefilled syringe, a 3-mL syringe with a needleless infusion device
- Isopropyl alcohol wipe
- Tape
- Clean emesis basin

IMPLEMENTATION

Preparation

1. Prepare the client.
- Prior to performing the procedure, introduce self and verify the client's identity using agency protocol. Explain the proce-dure to the client and the reason for leaving the IV catheter in place. Changing an IV to a heparin or saline lock should cause no discomfort other than that associated with remov-ing tape from the IV tubing.

Performance

1. Prepare the equipment.
- Perform hand hygiene.
- Assess the IV site (if visible) and determine the patency of the catheter (see Skill 52-2). If the catheter is not fully patent or there is evidence of phlebitis or infiltration, discontinue the catheter and establish a new IV site.

CHANGING AN INTRAVENOUS CATHETER TO AN INTERMITTENT INFUSION LOCK *continued*

- Expose the IV catheter hub and loosen any tape that is holding the IV tubing in place or that will interfere with insertion of the intermittent infusion plug into the catheter.
- Clamp the IV tubing to stop the flow of IV fluid.
- Open the gauze pad and place it under the IV catheter hub.
- Open the alcohol wipe and intermittent infusion plug, leaving the plug in its sterile package.

2. Remove the IV tubing and insert the intermittent infusion plug into the IV catheter.
 - Put on gloves.
 - Stabilize the IV catheter with your nondominant hand and use the little finger to place slight pressure on the vein above the end of the catheter. Twist the IV tubing adapter to loosen it from the IV catheter and remove it, placing the end of the tubing in a clean emesis basin.
 - Pick up the intermittent infusion plug from its package and remove the protective sleeve from the male adapter, maintaining its sterility. Insert the plug into the IV catheter, twisting it to seat it firmly or engage the Luer lock.

3. Instill saline or heparin solution per agency policy. **Rationale:** *Saline or heparin are used to maintain patency of the IV catheter when fluids are not infusing through the catheter.*

4. Tape the intermittent infusion plug in place using a chevron or U method. **Rationale:** *Tape provides added security to prevent the infusion plug from coming out of the intravenous catheter. It also promotes comfort, preventing the plug from catching on clothing or bedding.*

5. Teach the client how to maintain the lock.
 - Avoid manipulating the catheter or infusion plug and protect it from catching on clothing or bedding. A gauze bandage such as Kerlix or Kling may be wrapped over the plug when it is not in use to protect it.
 - Cover the site with an occlusive dressing when showering; avoid immersing the site.
 - Flush the catheter with saline or heparin solution as directed.
 - Notify the nurse or primary care provider if the plug or catheter comes out; if the site becomes red, inflamed, or painful; or if any drainage or bleeding occurs at the site.

6. Document all relevant information.

EVALUATION
Evaluate the following:

- Patency of the catheter
- Appearance of the site
- Ease of flushing

Blood Transfusions

Intravenous fluids can be effective in restoring intravascular (blood) volume; however, they do not affect the oxygen-carrying capacity of the blood. When red and white blood cells, platelets, or blood proteins are lost because of hemorrhage or disease, it may be necessary to replace these components to restore the blood's ability to transport oxygen and carbon dioxide, to clot, to fight infection, and to keep extracellular fluid within the intravascular compartment. A blood transfusion is the introduction of whole blood or blood components into the venous circulation.

BLOOD GROUPS. Human blood is commonly classified into four main groups (A, B, AB, and O). The surface of an individual's red blood cells contains a number of proteins known as **antigens** that are unique for each person. Many blood antigens have been identified, but the antigens A, B, and Rh are the most important in determining blood group or type. Because antigens promote *agglutination* or clumping of blood cells, they are also known as **agglutinogens.** The A antigen or agglutinogen is present on the RBCs of people with blood group A, the B antigen is present in people with blood group B, and both A and B antigens are found on the RBC surface in people with group AB blood. Neither antigen is present in people with group O blood.

Preformed **antibodies** to RBC antigens are present in the plasma; these antibodies are often called **agglutinins.** People with blood group A have B antibodies (agglutinins); A antibodies are present in people with blood group B; and people with blood group O have antibodies to both A and B antigens. People with group AB blood do not have antibodies to either A or B antigens (Table 52–11). When blood is transfused, the blood

TABLE 52–11 The Blood Groups with Their Constituent Agglutinogens and Agglutinins

BLOOD TYPES	RBC ANTIGENS (AGGLUTINOGENS)	PLASMA ANTIBODIES (AGGLUTININS)
A	A	B
B	B	A
AB	A and B	—
O	—	A and B

group of the donor and recipient must match to avoid an antigen-antibody reaction and destruction (hemolysis) of RBCs.

RHESUS (RH) FACTOR. The Rh factor antigen is present on the RBCs of approximately 85% of the people in the United States. Blood that contains the Rh factor is known as Rh-positive (Rh$^+$); when it is not present the blood is said to be Rh-negative (Rh$^-$). In contrast to the ABO blood groups, Rh$^-$ blood does not naturally contain Rh antibodies. However, on exposure to blood containing Rh factor (e.g., an Rh$^-$ mother carrying a fetus with Rh$^+$ blood, or transfusion of Rh$^+$ blood into a client who is Rh$^-$), Rh antibodies develop. Subsequent exposures to Rh$^+$ blood place the client at risk for an antigen–antibody reaction and hemolysis of RBCs.

BLOOD TYPING AND CROSSMATCHING. To avoid transfusing incompatible red blood cells, both blood donor and recipient are typed and their blood crossmatched. *Blood typing* is done to determine the ABO blood group and Rh factor status. This test is also performed on pregnant women and neonates to assess for possible intrauterine exposure of either to an incompatible blood type (particularly Rh factor incompatibilities).

Because blood typing only determines the presence of the major ABO and Rh antigens, *crossmatching* also is necessary prior to transfusion to identify possible interactions of minor antigens with their corresponding antibodies. RBCs from the donor blood are mixed with serum from the recipient; a reagent (Coombs' serum) is added, and the mixture is examined for visible agglutination. If no antibodies to the donated RBCs are present in the recipient's serum, agglutination does not occur and the risk of transfusion reaction is small.

SELECTION OF BLOOD DONORS. Screening of blood donors is rigorous. Criteria have been established to protect the donor from possible ill effects of donation and to protect the recipient from exposure to diseases transmitted through the blood. Blood donors are unpaid volunteers. Potential donors are eliminated by a history of hepatitis, HIV infection (or risk factors for HIV infection), heart disease, most cancers, severe asthma, bleeding disorders, or convulsions. Donation may be deferred for people with malaria or who have been exposed to malaria or hepatitis or in situations of pregnancy, surgery, anemia, high or low blood pressure, and certain drugs.

BLOOD AND BLOOD PRODUCTS FOR TRANSFUSION. Most clients do not require transfusion of whole blood. It is more common for clients to receive a transfusion of a particular blood component specific to their individual needs. Table 52–12 lists some of the common blood products that may be transfused.

TRANSFUSION REACTIONS. Transfusion of ABO- or Rh-incompatible blood can result in a **hemolytic transfusion reaction** with destruction of the transfused RBCs and subsequent risk of kidney damage or failure. Other forms of transfusion reaction also may occur, including febrile, allergic, circulatory overload, and sepsis. Because the risk of an adverse reaction is high when blood is transfused, clients must be frequently and carefully assessed before and during transfusion. Many reactions become evident within 5 to 15 minutes of initiating the transfusion but they can develop any time during a transfusion; clients are closely monitored during the initial period of the transfusion. Stop the transfusion immediately if signs of a reaction develop. Possible transfusion reactions, their clinical signs, and nursing implications are listed in Table 52–13.

ADMINISTERING BLOOD. Special precautions are necessary when administering blood.

When a transfusion is ordered, obtain the blood from the blood bank just before starting the transfusion. Do not store the blood in the refrigerator on the nursing unit; lack of temperature control may damage the blood. Once blood or a blood product is removed from the refrigerator, there is a limited amount of time to administer it (e.g., packed RBCs should not hang for more than 4 hours after being removed from the refrigerator). Follow agency policies

TABLE 52–12 Blood Products for Transfusion

PRODUCT	USE
Whole blood	Not commonly used except for extreme cases of acute hemorrhage. Replaces blood volume and all blood products: RBCs, plasma, plasma proteins, fresh platelets, and other clotting factors.
Packed red blood cells (PRBCs)	Used to increase the oxygen-carrying capacity of blood in anemias, surgery, and disorders with slow bleeding. One unit of PRBCs has the same amount of oxygen-carrying RBCs as a unit of whole blood (Rosenthal, 2004, p. 23). One unit raises hematocrit by approximately 2% to 3%.
Autologous red blood cells	Used for blood replacement following planned elective surgery. Client donates blood for autologous transfusion 4–5 weeks prior to surgery.
Platelets	Replaces platelets in clients with bleeding disorders or platelet deficiency. Fresh platelets most effective. Each unit should increase the average adult client's platelet count by about 5,000 platelets/microliter (Rosenthal, 2004, p. 24).
Fresh frozen plasma	Expands blood volume and provides clotting factors. Does not need to be typed and crossmatched (contains no RBCs). Each unit will increase the level of any clotting factor by 2% to 3% in the average adult (Rosenthal, 2004, p. 26).
Albumin and plasma protein fraction	Blood volume expander; provides plasma proteins.
Clotting factors and cryoprecipitate	Used for clients with clotting factor deficiencies. Each provides different factors involved in the clotting pathway; cryoprecipitate also contains fibrinogen.

TABLE 52–13 Transfusion Reactions

REACTION: CAUSE	CLINICAL SIGNS	NURSING INTERVENTION*
Hemolytic reaction: incompatibility between client's blood and donor's blood	Chills, fever, headache, backache, dyspnea, cyanosis, chest pain, tachycardia, hypotension	1. Discontinue the transfusion immediately. **NOTE:** When the transfusion is discontinued, the blood tubing must be removed as well. Use *new* tubing for the normal saline infusion. 2. Maintain vascular acess with normal saline, or according to agency protocol. 3. Notify the primary care provider immediately. 4. Monitor vital signs. 5. Monitor fluid intake and output. 6. Send the remaining blood, bag, filter, tubing, a sample of the client's blood, and a urine sample to the laboratory.
Febrile reaction: sensitivity of the client's blood to white blood cells, platelets, or plasma proteins	Fever; chills; warm, flushed skin; headache; anxiety; muscle pain	1. Discontinue the transfusion immediately. 2. Give antipyretics as ordered. 3. Notify the primary care provider. 4. Keep the vein open with a normal saline infusion.
Allergic reaction (mild): sensitivity to infused plasma proteins	Flushing, itching, urticaria, bronchial wheezing	1. Stop or slow the transfusion, depending on agency protocol. 2. Notify the primary care provider. 3. Administer medication (antihistamines) as ordered.
Allergic reaction (severe): antibody–antigen reaction	Dyspnea, chest pain, circulatory collapse, cardiac arrest	1. Stop the transfusion. 2. Keep the vein open with normal saline. 3. Notify the primary care provider immediately. 4. Monitor vital signs. Administer cardiopulmonary resuscitation if needed. 5. Administer medications and/or oxygen as ordered.
Circulatory overload: blood administered faster than the circulation can accommodate	Cough, dyspnea, crackles (rales), distended neck veins, tachycardia, hypertension	1. Place the client upright, with feet dependent. 2. Stop or slow the transfusion. 3. Notify the primary care provider. 4. Administer diuretics and oxygen as ordered.
Sepsis: contaminated blood administered	High fever, chills, vomiting, diarrhea, hypotension	1. Stop the transfusion. 2. Keep the vein open with a normal saline infusion. 3. Notify the primary care provider. 4. Administer IV fluids, antibiotics. 5. Obtain a blood specimen from the client for culture. 6. Send the remaining blood and tubing to the laboratory.

*Nurses should follow the agency's protocol regarding interventions. These may vary among agencies.

for verifying that the unit is correct for the client. The U.S. Food and Drug Administration (FDA) requires blood products to have bar codes to allow for scanning and machine-readable information on blood and blood component container labels to help reduce medication errors (FDA, 2004). Blood is usually administered through a #18- to #20-gauge intravenous needle or catheter; using a smaller needle may slow the infusion and damage blood cells (although a smaller gauge needle may be necessary for small children or clients with small, fragile veins). A Y-type blood transfusion set with an in-line or add-on filter is used when administering blood (Figure 52-30 ■). One arm of the administration set connects to the blood; normal saline (0.9% NaCl) is attached to the other arm of the Y-type set. Saline is used to prime the set and flush the needle before administering blood. It also provides a means to keep the vein open should a transfusion reaction occur. No other IV solu-

tions should be administered with blood; they may cause the blood cells to clump or cause clotting. A transfusion should be completed within 4 hours of initiation. The risk of sepsis increases if blood hangs for a longer period. Blood tubing is changed after every 4 to 6 units per agency policy; new intravenous tubing is used following a transfusion.

CLINICAL ALERT

Normal saline should always be used when giving a blood transfusion. If the client has an infusion of dextrose, stop that infusion and flush the line with saline prior to initiating the transfusion. Solutions other than saline can cause damage to the blood components. ■

To initiate, maintain, and terminate a blood transfusion, see Skill 52-6.

To saline solution

To blood

Spikes

Upper clamps

Drip chamber

Blood filter chamber

Main flow rate clamp

Slide clamp

Y-Injection site

Adapter

Figure 52-30 ■ Schematic of a Y-set for blood administration.

INITIATING, MAINTAINING, AND TERMINATING A BLOOD TRANSFUSION USING A Y-SET

SKILL 52-6

PURPOSES
- To restore blood volume after severe hemorrhage
- To restore the oxygen-carrying capacity of the blood
- To provide plasma factors, such as antihemophilic factor (AHF) or factor VIII, or platelet concentrates, *which prevent or treat bleeding*

ASSESSMENT
Assess the following:

- Clinical signs of reaction (e.g., sudden chills, fever, nausea, itching, rash, low back pain, dyspnea)
- Manifestations of hypervolemia
- Status of infusion site
- Any unusual symptoms

PLANNING
- Verify the primary care provider order for transfusion.
- Verify client consent and obtain baseline data before the transfusion.
- Verify that a signed consent form was obtained.
- Assess vital signs for baseline data, including blood pressure, pulse, respiratory rate and depth, and temperature.
- Determine any known allergies or previous adverse reactions to blood.
- Note specific signs related to the client's pathology and the reason for the transfusion. For example, for an anemic client, note the hemoglobin and hematocrit levels.

continued on page 1476

INITIATING, MAINTAINING, AND TERMINATING A BLOOD TRANSFUSION USING A Y-SET *continued*

Delegation

Due to the need for sterile technique and technical complexity, blood transfusion is not delegated to UAP. The nurse must ensure that the UAP knows what complications or adverse signs can occur and should be reported to the nurse.

Equipment

- Blood product
- Blood administration set
- 250 mL normal saline for infusion
- IV pole
- Venipuncture set containing a #18- to #20-gauge needle or catheter (if one is not already in place) or, if blood is to be administered quickly, a larger catheter
- Chlorhexidine solution
- Alcohol swabs
- Tape
- Clean gloves

IMPLEMENTATION

Preparation

1. Prepare the client.
   - Prior to performing the procedure, introduce self and verify the client's identity using agency protocol.
   - Explain the procedure and its purpose to the client. Instruct the client to report promptly any sudden chills, nausea, itching, rash, dyspnea, back pain, or other unusual symptoms.
   - If the client has an intravenous solution infusing, check whether the needle and solution are appropriate to administer blood. The preferred needle size is from #18 to #20 gauge, and the solution *must* be normal saline. Dextrose (which causes lysis of RBCs), Ringer's solution, medications and other additives, and hyperalimentation solutions are incompatible. Refer to step 5 below if the infusing solution is not compatible.
   - If the client does not have an IV solution infusing, check agency policies. In some agencies an infusion must be running before the blood is obtained from the blood bank. In this case, you will need to perform a venipuncture on a suitable vein (see Skill 52-1) and start an IV infusion of normal saline.

Performance

1. Obtain the correct blood component for the client.
   - Check the primary care provider's order with the requisition.
   - Check the requisition form and the blood bag label with a laboratory technician or according to agency policy. Specifically, check the client's name, identification number, blood type (A, B, AB, or O) and Rh group, the blood donor number, and the expiration date of the blood. Observe the blood for abnormal color, RBC clumping, gas bubbles, and extraneous material. Return outdated or abnormal blood to the blood bank.
   - With another nurse (most agencies require an RN), compare the laboratory blood record with
     a. The client's name and identification number.
     b. The number on the blood bag label.
     c. The ABO group and Rh type on the blood bag label.
   - If any of the information does not match exactly, notify the charge nurse and the blood bank. Do not administer blood until discrepancies are corrected or clarified.
   - Sign the appropriate form with the other nurse according to agency policy.
   - Make sure that the blood is left at room temperature for no more than 30 minutes before starting the transfusion. **Rationale:** *RBCs deteriorate and lose their effectiveness after 2 hours at room temperature. Lysis of RBCs releases potassium into the bloodstream, causing hyperkalemia.*

Agencies may designate different times at which the blood must be returned to the blood bank if it has not been started. **Rationale:** *As blood components warm, the risk of bacterial growth also increases.* If the start of the transfusion is unexpectedly delayed, return the blood to the blood bank. Do not store blood in the unit refrigerator. **Rationale:** *The temperature of unit refrigerators is not precisely regulated and the blood may be damaged.*

2. Verify the client's identity according to agency protocol.
   - Check the client's arm band for name and ID number. Do not administer blood to a client without an arm band.

3. Set up the infusion equipment.
   - Ensure that the blood filter inside the drip chamber is suitable for whole blood or the blood components to be transfused. Attach the blood tubing to the blood filter, if necessary. **Rationale:** *Blood filters have a surface area large enough to allow the blood components through easily but are designed to trap clots.*
   - Put on gloves.
   - Close all clamps on the Y-set: the main flow rate clamp and both Y-line clamps.
   - Using a twisting motion, insert the piercing pin (spike) into a container of 0.9% saline solution.
   - Hang the container on the IV pole about 1 m (36 in.) above the venipuncture site.

4. Prime the tubing.
   - Open the upper clamp on the normal saline tubing and squeeze the drip chamber until it covers the filter and one-third of the drip chamber above the filter.
   - Tap the filter chamber to expel any residual air in the filter.
   - Remove the adapter cover at the tip of the blood administration set.
   - Open the main flow rate clamp, and prime the tubing with saline.
   - Close both clamps.

5. Start the saline solution.
   - If an IV solution incompatible with blood is infusing, stop the infusion and discard the solution and tubing according to agency policy.
   - Attach the blood tubing primed with normal saline to the intravenous catheter.
   - Open the saline and main flow rate clamps and adjust the flow rate. Use only the main flow rate clamp to adjust the rate.
   - Allow a small amount of solution to infuse to make sure there are no problems with the flow or with the venipuncture site. **Rationale:** *Infusing normal saline before initiating the transfusion also clears the IV catheter of incompatible solutions or medications.*

INITIATING, MAINTAINING, AND TERMINATING A BLOOD TRANSFUSION USING A Y-SET *continued*

6. Prepare the blood bag.
   - Invert the blood bag gently several times to mix the cells with the plasma. **Rationale:** *Rough handling can damage the cells.*
   - Expose the port on the blood bag by pulling back the tabs. ❶
   - Insert the remaining Y-set spike into the blood bag.
   - Suspend the blood bag.
   - Close the upper clamp below the IV saline solution on the Y-set.
   - Open the clamp on the blood arm of the Y-set and prime the tubing.
7. Establish the blood transfusion.
   - The blood will run into the saline-filled drip chamber. If necessary, squeeze the drip chamber to reestablish the liquid level with drip chamber one-third full. (Tap the filter to expel any residual air within the filter.)
   - Readjust the flow rate with the main clamp.
8. Observe the client closely for the first 5 to 10 minutes.
   - Run the blood slowly for the first 15 minutes at 20 drops per minute.
   - Note adverse reactions, such as chilling, nausea, vomiting, skin rash, or tachycardia. **Rationale:** *The earlier a transfusion reaction occurs, the more severe it tends to be. Identifying such reactions promptly helps to minimize the consequences.*
   - Remind the client to call a nurse immediately if any unusual symptoms are felt during the transfusion.
   - If any of these reactions occur, report these to the nurse in charge and take appropriate nursing action (see Table 52–13).
9. Document relevant data.
   - Record starting the blood, including vital signs, type of blood, blood unit number, sequence number (e.g., no. 1 of three ordered units), site of the venipuncture, size of the needle, and drip rate.

   SAMPLE DOCUMENTATION

   1/21/2008 1400 1 unit of PRBCs (#65234) hung to be infused over 3 hours. IV site in (L) forearm with 19 G angiocath. VS taken (see transfusion record). Informed to contact nurse if begins to experience any discomfort during transfusion. Stated he would use the call light.

   ——————————————————————— C. Jones, RN.

10. Monitor the client.
    - Fifteen minutes after initiating the transfusion, check the vital signs of the client. If there are no signs of a reaction, establish the required flow rate. Most adults can tolerate receiving one unit of blood in 1 1/2 to 2 hours. Do not transfuse a unit of blood for longer than 4 hours.
    - Assess the client including vital signs every 30 minutes or more often, depending on the health status, until 1 hour post-transfusion. If the client has a reaction and the blood is discontinued, send the blood bag and tubing to the laboratory for investigation of the blood.
11. Terminate the transfusion.
    - Put on clean gloves.

❶ Exposing the port on the blood bag by pulling back the tabs.

   - If no infusion is to follow, clamp the blood tubing and remove the needle. If another transfusion is to follow, clamp the blood tubing and open the saline infusion arm. Blood administration sets are changed within 24 hours or after 4 to 6 units of blood per agency protocol.
   - If the primary IV is to be continued, flush the maintenance line with saline solution. Disconnect the blood tubing system and reestablish the intravenous infusion using new tubing. Adjust the drip to the desired rate. Often a normal saline or other solution is kept running in case of delayed reaction to the blood.
   - Discard the administration set according to agency practice. Needles should be placed in a labeled, puncture-resistant container designed for such disposal. Blood bags and administration sets should be bagged and labeled before being sent for decontamination and processing. See agency policy.
   - Remove gloves.
   - Again monitor vital signs.
12. Follow agency protocol for appropriate disposition of the blood bag.
    - On the requisition attached to the blood unit, fill in the time the transfusion was completed and the amount transfused.
    - Attach one copy of the requisition to the client's record and another to the empty blood bag.
    - Return the blood bag and requisition to the blood bank.
13. Document relevant data.
    - Record completion of the transfusion, the amount of blood absorbed, the blood unit number, and the vital signs. If the primary intravenous infusion was continued, record connecting it. Also record the transfusion on the IV flow sheet and I & O record.

    SAMPLE DOCUMENTATION

    1/21/2008 1410 C/O feeling warm, headache and backace. Skin flushed. Temp. 102.6, BP. 140/90, P. 112, R. 28. Approximately 50–100 cc infused. Infusion stopped. Tubing changed and NS infusing at 15 cc/hr. Dr. Riley notified. ————————————— C. Jones, RN

continued on page 1478

INITIATING, MAINTAINING, AND TERMINATING A BLOOD TRANSFUSION USING A Y-SET *continued*

EVALUATION

Evaluate the following:

- Changes in vital signs or health status
- Presence of chills, nausea, vomiting, or skin rash

Evaluating

Using the overall goals identified in the planning stage of maintaining or restoring fluid balance, maintaining or restoring pulmonary ventilation and oxygenation, maintaining or restoring normal balance of electrolytes, and preventing associated risks of fluid, electrolyte, and acid–base imbalances, the nurse collects data to evaluate the effectiveness of interventions. Examples of desired outcomes for the identified goals are found in Identifying Nursing Diagnoses, Outcomes, and Interventions on pages 1451 and 1452.

If desired outcomes are not achieved, the nurse, client, and support person if appropriate need to explore the reasons before modifying the care plan. For example, if the outcome "Urine output is greater than 1,300 mL per day and within 500 mL of intake" is not achieved, questions to be considered might include

- Have other outcome measures for the goal of achieving fluid balance been met?
- Does the client understand and comply with planned fluid intake?
- Is all urinary output being measured?
- Are unusual or excessive amounts of fluid being lost by another route (e.g., gastric suction, excessive perspiration, fever, rapid respiratory rate, wound drainage)?
- Are prescribed medications being taken or administered as ordered?

NURSING CARE PLAN   Deficient Fluid Volume

ASSESSMENT DATA	NURSING DIAGNOSIS	DESIRED OUTCOMES*
Nursing Assessment Merlyn Chapman, a 27-year-old sales clerk, reports weakness, malaise, and flu-like symptoms for 3–4 days. Although thirsty, she is unable to tolerate fluids because of nausea and vomiting, and she has liquid stools 2–4 times per day.	*Deficient Fluid Volume* related to nausea, vomiting, and diarrhea as evidenced by decreased urine output, increased urine concentration, weakness, fever, decreased skin/tongue turgor, dry mucous membranes, increased pulse rate, and decreased blood pressure	Electrolyte & Acid/Base Balance [0600] as evidenced by not compromised: • Serum electrolytes • Muscle strength Fluid Balance [0601] as evidenced by not compromised: • 24-hour intake and output balance • Urine specific gravity • Blood pressure, pulse, and body temperature • Skin turgor • Moist mucous membranes

Physical Examination	**Diagnostic Data**
Height: 160 cm (5′3″) Weight: 66.2 kg (146 lb) Mild fever: 38.6°C (101.5°F) Pulse: 86 BPM Respirations: 24/minute Scant urine output BP: 102/84 mm Hg Dry oral mucosa, furrowed tongue, cracked lips	Urine specific gravity: 1.035 Serum sodium 155 mEq/L Serum potassium 3.2 mEq/L Chest x-ray negative

NURSING INTERVENTIONS*/SELECTED ACTIVITIES	RATIONALE
Electrolyte Management: Hypokalemia [2007]	
Obtain specimens for analysis of altered potassium levels (e.g., serum and urine potassium) as indicated.	*Urine and serum analysis provides information about extracellular levels of potassium. There is no practical way to measure intracellular K^+.*
Administer prescribed supplemental potassium (PO, NG, or IV) per policy.	*Low potassium levels are dangerous and Mrs. Chapman may require supplements.*
Monitor for neurologic and neuromuscular manifestations of hypokalemia (e.g., muscle weakness, lethargy, altered level of consciousness).	*Potassium is a vital electrolyte for skeletal and smooth muscle activity.*

NURSING CARE PLAN Deficient Fluid Volume *continued*

NURSING INTERVENTIONS*/SELECTED ACTIVITIES	RATIONALE
Monitor for cardiac manifestations of hypokalemia (e.g., hypotension, tachycardia, weak pulse, rhythm irregularities).	*Many cardiac rhythm disorders can result from hypokalemia. It is critical to monitor cardiac function with hypokalemia.*

Electrolyte Management: Hypernatremia [2004]

Obtain specimens for analysis of altered sodium levels (e.g., serum and urine sodium, urine osmolality, and urine specific gravity) as indicated.	*Urine analysis provides information about retention or loss of sodium and the ability of the kidneys to concentrate or dilute urine in response to fluid changes.*
Provide frequent oral hygiene.	*Oral mucous membranes become dry and sticky due to loss of fluid in the interstitial spaces.*
Monitor for neurologic and neuromuscular manifestations of hypernatremia (e.g., lethargy, irritability, seizures, and hyperreflexia).	*Hypernatremia, as a result of low fluid volume, creates a hypertonic vascular space, which causes water to move out of the cells, including brain cells. This accounts for neurologic symptoms.*
Monitor for cardiac manifestations of hypernatremia (e.g., tachycardia, orthostatic hypotension).	*The heart responds to a loss of fluid by increasing the heart rate to compensate with an increase in cardiac output. Low fluid volume leads to a fall in blood pressure.*

Fluid Management [4120]

Weigh daily and monitor trends.	*Weight helps to assess fluid balance.*
Maintain accurate I & O record.	*Accurate records are critical in assessing the patient's fluid balance.*
Monitor vital signs as appropriate.	*Vital sign changes such as increased heart rate, decreased blood pressure, and increased temperature indicate hypovolemia.*
Give fluids as appropriate.	*As her nausea decreases encourage her oral intake of fluids as tolerated, again to replace lost volume.*
Administer IV therapy as prescribed.	*Mrs. Chapman has signs of severe fluid volume deficit. She will probably require intravenous replacement of fluid. This is especially true because her oral intake is limited because of nausea and vomiting.*

EVALUATION

Outcomes met. Mrs. Chapman remained hospitalized for 48 hours. She required fluid replacement of a total of 5 liters. Her blood pressure increased to 122/74, pulse rate decreased to a resting level of 74, and respirations decreased to 12/minute. Her urine output increased as the fluid was replaced and was adequate at > 0.5 mL/kg/hour by the time of discharge. The urine specific gravity was 1.015. Lab work on the day of discharge was: K+: 3.8 and Na+: 140. She had elastic skin turgor and moist mucous membranes. She was taking oral fluids and was able to discuss symptoms of deficient fluid volume that would necessitate her calling her health care provider.

* The NOC # for desired outcomes and the NIC # for nursing interventions and seleted activities are listed in brackets following the appropriate outcome or intervention. Outcomes, interventions, and activities selected are only a sample of those suggested by NOC and NIC and should be further individualized for each client.

APPLYING CRITICAL THINKING

1. What action would you take if Mrs. Chapman's heart became irregular?
2. Mrs. Chapman is responding inappropriately to your questions; she seems to be confused. What do you think is happening?
3. Offer suggestions for ways to help Mrs. Chapman increase her oral intake.
4. Mrs. Chapman asks why you weigh her every morning. How do you respond?

See Critical Thinking Possibilities in Appendix A.

CONCEPT MAP **Deficient Fluid Volume**

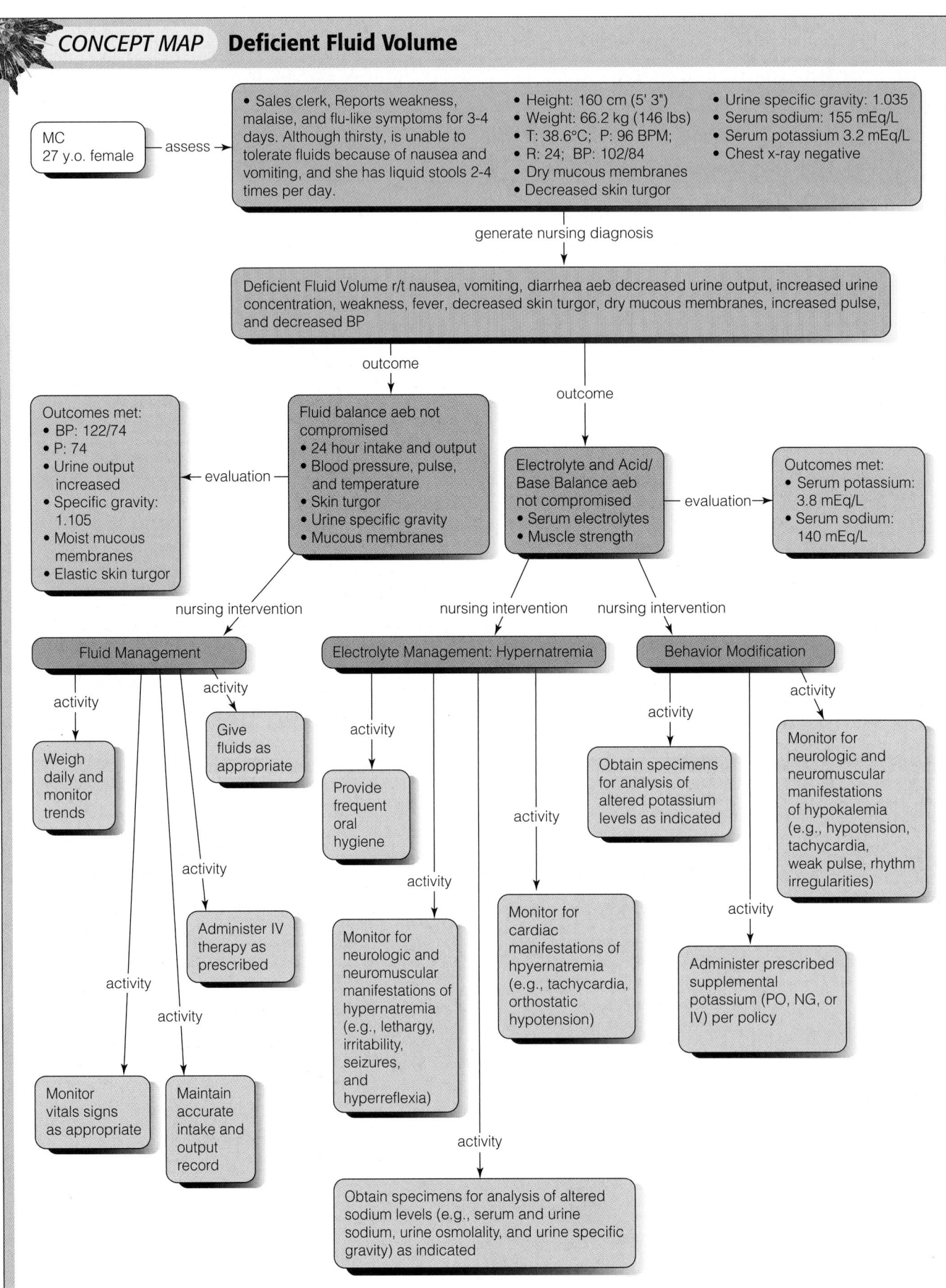

MC
27 y.o. female

→ assess →

- Sales clerk, Reports weakness, malaise, and flu-like symptoms for 3-4 days. Although thirsty, is unable to tolerate fluids because of nausea and vomiting, and she has liquid stools 2-4 times per day.

- Height: 160 cm (5' 3")
- Weight: 66.2 kg (146 lbs)
- T: 38.6°C; P: 96 BPM;
- R: 24; BP: 102/84
- Dry mucous membranes
- Decreased skin turgor

- Urine specific gravity: 1.035
- Serum sodium: 155 mEq/L
- Serum potassium 3.2 mEq/L
- Chest x-ray negative

generate nursing diagnosis

Deficient Fluid Volume r/t nausea, vomiting, diarrhea aeb decreased urine output, increased urine concentration, weakness, fever, decreased skin turgor, dry mucous membranes, increased pulse, and decreased BP

outcome

outcome

Outcomes met:
- BP: 122/74
- P: 74
- Urine output increased
- Specific gravity: 1.105
- Moist mucous membranes
- Elastic skin turgor

← evaluation ←

Fluid balance aeb not compromised
- 24 hour intake and output
- Blood pressure, pulse, and temperature
- Skin turgor
- Urine specific gravity
- Mucous membranes

Electrolyte and Acid/ Base Balance aeb not compromised
- Serum electrolytes
- Muscle strength

→ evaluation →

Outcomes met:
- Serum potassium: 3.8 mEq/L
- Serum sodium: 140 mEq/L

nursing intervention

nursing intervention

nursing intervention

Fluid Management

Electrolyte Management: Hypernatremia

Behavior Modification

activity

activity

activity

activity

activity

Weigh daily and monitor trends

Give fluids as appropriate

Provide frequent oral hygiene

Obtain specimens for analysis of altered potassium levels as indicated

Monitor for neurologic and neuromuscular manifestations of hypokalemia (e.g., hypotension, tachycardia, weak pulse, rhythm irregularities)

activity

activity

activity

Administer IV therapy as prescribed

Monitor for neurologic and neuromuscular manifestations of hypernatremia (e.g., lethargy, irritability, seizures, and hyperreflexia)

Monitor for cardiac manifestations of hpyernatremia (e.g., tachycardia, orthostatic hypotension)

Administer prescribed supplemental potassium (PO, NG, or IV) per policy

activity

activity

Monitor vitals signs as appropriate

Maintain accurate intake and output record

activity

Obtain specimens for analysis of altered sodium levels (e.g., serum and urine sodium, urine osmolality, and urine specific gravity) as indicated

CHAPTER 52 **REVIEW**

CHAPTER HIGHLIGHTS

- A balance of fluids, electrolytes, acids, and bases in the body is necessary for health and life.
- The body fluid is divided into two major compartments: the intracellular fluid (ICF) inside the cells and extracellular fluid (ECF) outside the cells.
- Extracellular fluid is subdivided into two compartments: intravascular (plasma) and interstitial. It constitutes about one-fourth to one-third of total body fluid.
- ECF is in constant motion throughout the body. It is the transport system that carries nutrients to and waste products from the cells.
- The percentage of total body fluids varies according to the individual's age, body fat, and sex. The younger the person, the higher the proportion of water in the body. The less body fat present, the greater the proportion of body fluid. Postadolescent females have a smaller percentage of fluid in relation to total body weight than do men.
- There are two types of body electrolytes (ions): positively charged ions (cations) and negatively charged ions (anions).
- The principal ions of ECF are sodium and chloride; the principal ions of ICF are potassium and phosphate.
- Fluids and electrolytes move among the body compartments by osmosis, diffusion, filtration, and active transport.
- The major fluid pressures exerted as part of the movement of fluid and electrolytes from one compartment to another are osmotic pressure and hydrostatic pressure.
- The three sources of body fluid are fluids taken orally, food ingested, and the oxidation of food. Fluid intake is regulated by the thirst mechanism.
- Fluid output occurs chiefly through excretion of urine, although body fluid is also lost through sweat, feces, and insensible vapor loss.
- In healthy adults, measurable fluid intake and output should balance (about 1,500 mL per day). The output of urine normally approximates the oral intake of fluids. Water from food and oxidation is balanced by fluid loss through the skin, respiratory process, and feces.
- A number of body systems and organs are involved in regulating the volume and composition of body fluids: the kidneys, the endocrine system, the cardiovascular system, the lungs, and the gastrointestinal system. The kidneys are the primary regulator of fluid and electrolyte balance.
- Substances such as the antidiuretic hormone, the renin-angiotensin-aldosterone system, and the atrial natriuretic factor are also involved in maintaining fluid balance.
- Fluid imbalances include
  a. Fluid volume deficit (FVD), also referred to as hypovolemia.
  b. Fluid volume excess (FVE), also referred to as hypervolemia.
  c. Dehydration, a deficit in water and increase in serum sodium level.
  d. Overhydration, an excess of water and decrease in serum sodium level.
- The most common electrolyte imbalances are deficits or excesses in sodium, potassium, and calcium.
- The acid–base balance (pH range) of body fluids is maintained within a precise range of 7.35 to 7.45.

- Acid–base balance is regulated by buffers that neutralize excess acids or bases; the lungs, which eliminate or retain carbon dioxide, a potential acid; and the kidneys, which excrete or conserve bicarbonate and hydrogen ions.
- Acid–base imbalance occurs when the normal 20-to-1 ratio of bicarbonate to carbonic acid is upset. Imbalances may be either respiratory or metabolic in origin; either can result in acidosis or alkalosis.
- Factors that influence an individual's fluid, electrolyte, and acid–base balance include age, gender and body size, environmental temperature, and lifestyle. Illness, trauma, surgery, and certain medications can place individuals at risk for fluid, electrolyte, and acid–base imbalances.
- Fluid, electrolyte, and acid–base imbalance is most accurately determined through laboratory examination of blood plasma.
- Assessment relative to fluid, electrolyte, and acid–base balances includes (a) a nursing history; (b) physical examination of the skin, oral cavity, eyes, jugular vein, veins of the hand, and the neurologic system; (c) measurement of body weight, vital signs, and fluid intake and output; and (d) various diagnostic studies of blood and urine.
- A nursing history includes data about the client's fluid and food intake; fluid output; signs of fluid, electrolyte, and acid–base imbalances; and medications, therapies, or disease processes that may disrupt these balances.
- NANDA-approved nursing diagnoses that relate specifically to fluid, electrolyte, and acid–base imbalances include *Deficient Fluid Volume, Excess Fluid Volume, Risk for Imbalanced Fluid Volume, Risk for Deficient Fluid Volume,* and *Impaired Gas Exchange.* Other diagnoses that may be relevant are *Impaired Oral Mucous Membrane, Impaired Skin Integrity, Decreased Cardiac Output, Impaired Tissue Perfusion, Activity Intolerance, Risk for Injury,* and *Acute Confusion.*
- In many instances, fluids and electrolytes can be provided orally to clients who are experiencing or at risk of developing fluid deficits. The nurse needs to establish with the client a 24-hour plan for ingesting the necessary fluids and to respect the client's fluid preferences.
- For clients with fluid retention, fluids may need to be restricted; a schedule and short-term goals that make the fluid restriction more tolerable need to be developed.
- For clients experiencing excessive fluid losses, the administration of fluids and electrolytes intravenously is necessary. Meticulous aseptic technique is required when caring for clients with intravenous infusions.
- Preventing complications such as infiltration, phlebitis, hypervolemia (circulatory overload), and infection is an important aspect of intravenous therapy.
- The administration of blood transfusions involves accurately matching and identifying the blood for the individual, correctly identifying the recipient, and monitoring the client throughout the procedure for transfusion reactions.

TEST YOUR KNOWLEDGE

1. An elderly nursing home resident has refused to eat or drink for several days and is admitted to the hospital. The nurse should assess for which of the following?
   1. Increased blood pressure
   2. Weak, rapid pulse
   3. Moist mucous membranes
   4. Jugular vein distention

2. A man brings his elderly wife to the emergency department. He states that she has been vomiting and has had diarrhea for the past 2 days. She appears lethargic and is complaining of leg cramps. What should the nurse do first?
   1. Start an IV.
   2. Review the results of serum electrolytes.
   3. Offer the woman foods that are high in sodium and potassium content.
   4. Administer an antiemetic.

3. The nurse administers an IV solution of D5 ½ NS to a postoperative client. This is classified as what type of intravenous solution? _____

4. An older client comes to the emergency department experiencing chest pain and shortness of breath. An arterial blood gas is ordered. Which of the following ABG results indicates respiratory acidosis?
   1. pH 7.54; $PaCO_2$ 28 mm Hg; HCO_3 22 mEq/L
   2. pH 7.32; $PaCO_2$ 46 mm Hg; HCO_3 24 mEq/L
   3. pH 7.31; $PaCO_2$ 35 mm Hg; HCO_3 20 mEq/L
   4. pH 7.50; $PaCO_2$ 37 mm Hg; HCO_3 28 mEq/L

5. The intake and output (I & O) record of a client with a nasogastric tube that has been attached to suction for two (2) days shows greater output than input. Which nursing diagnoses are most applicable? Select all that apply.
   1. *Deficient Fluid Volume*
   2. *Risk for Deficient Fluid Volume*
   3. *Impaired Oral Mucous Membranes*
   4. *Impaired Gas Exchange*
   5. *Decreased Cardiac Output*

6. Which of the following client statements indicates a need for further teaching regarding treatment for hypokalemia?
   1. "I will use avocado in my salads."
   2. "I will be sure to check my heart rate before I take my digoxin."
   3. "I will take my potassium in the morning after eating breakfast."
   4. "I will stop using my salt substitute."

7. An elderly man is admitted to the medical unit with a diagnosis of dehydration. Which of the following signs or symptoms are most representative of a sodium imbalance?
   1. Hyperreflexia
   2. Mental confusion
   3. Irregular pulse
   4. Muscle weakness

8. The client's arterial blood gas results are: pH 7.32; $PaCO_2$ 58; HCO_3 32. The nurse knows that the client is experiencing which acid–base imbalance?
   1. Metabolic acidosis
   2. Respiratory acidosis
   3. Metabolic alkalosis
   4. Respiratory alkalosis

9. A client is admitted to the hospital for hypocalcemia. Nursing interventions relating to which system would have the highest priority?
   1. Renal
   2. Cardiac
   3. Gastrointestinal
   4. Neuromuscular

10. The nurse would assess for signs of hypomagnesemia in which of the following clients? Select all that apply.
    1. A client with renal failure
    2. A client with pancreatitis
    3. A client taking magnesium-containing antacids
    4. A client with excessive nasogastric drainage
    5. A client with chronic alcoholism

See Answers to Test Your Knowledge in Appendix A.

EXPLORE MEDIALINK www.prenhall.com/berman

DVD-ROM
- Audio Glossary
- NCLEX Review
- Skills Checklists
- Animations:
  Membrane Transport
  Filtration Pressure
  Fluid Balance
  Acid–Base Balance
  Furosemide Drug
  Applying a Central Venous Line

COMPANION WEBSITE
- Additional NCLEX Review
- Case Study: Client with Suspected Electrolyte Imbalance
- Care Plan Activity: Client with Heart Failure
- Application Activities:
  Determining Body Fluid Problems
  Arterial Blood Gases and Acid–Base Balance
- Links to Resources

READINGS AND REFERENCES

SUGGESTED READINGS

Billings, D., & Kowalski, K. (2005). Do your CATS PRRR? A mnemonic device to teach safety checks for administering intravenous medications. *Journal of Continuing Education in Nursing, 36*(3), 104–106.
The authors suggest using this mnemonic (CATS PRRR) to help nurses remember the important safety checks of IV medication administration. Having this mnemonic written on the nurse's clipboard will help the nurse to stay focused on the task in a hectic and stressful working environment. The article explains how each letter pertains to important safety checks when administering IV medications.

Davidhizar, R., Dunn, C. L., & Hart, A. N. (2004). A review of the literature on how important water is to the world's elderly population. *International Nursing Review, 51*(3), 159–167.
These authors discuss the importance of water to the elderly population and provide strategies to promote health related to water intake.

Mentes, J. (2006). Oral hydration in older adults. *American Journal of Nursing, 106*(6), 40–49.
This article reviews age-related changes, risk factors, assessment measures, and nursing interventions for dehydration.

Rosenthal, K. (2003). Keeping I.V. therapy safe with needleless systems. *Nursing, 33*(10), 16–20.
This article details how needleless systems reduce the health care professional's risk of injury and exposure to bloodborne pathogens.

Rosenthal, K. (2004). The new look of I.V. therapy: Improvements to existing products and technology enhance patient care, satisfaction, and outcomes. *Nursing Management, 35*(12), 66–70.
This article provides information about the new infusion devices that are now available. This author provides information on an array of anesthetics and needleless IV devices.

RELATED RESEARCH

Berk, D. R., Conti, P. M., & Sommer, B. R. (2004/2005). Orange juice-induced hyperkalemia in schizophrenia. *International Journal of Psychiatry in Medicine, 34*(1), 79–82.

Crawford, A. (2004). An audit of the patient's experience of arterial blood gas testing. *British Journal of Nursing, 13*(9), 529–532.

Da Silva, L. (2004). The use & abuse of parenteral nutrition: Can we change practice? *Canadian Journal of Dietetic Practice and Research, 26,* 3.

Mentes, J. C. (2006). A typology of oral hydration: Problems exhibited by frail nursing home residents. *Journal of Gerontological Nursing, 32*(1), 13–19.

Oh, H., Suh, Y., Hwang, S., & Seo, W. (2005). Effects of nasogastric tube feeding on serum sodium, potassium, and glucose levels. *Journal of Nursing Scholarship, 37*(2), 141–147.

Wathen, J. E., MacKenzie, T., & Bothner, J. P. (2004). Usefulness of the serum electrolyte panel in the management of pediatric dehydration treated with intravenously administered fluids. *Pediatrics, 114*(5), 1227–1234.

REFERENCES

American Medical Association, American Nurses Association–American Nurses Foundations, Centers for Disease Control and Prevention, Center for Food Safety and Applied Nutrition, Food and Drug Administration, Food Safety and Inspection Service, U.S. Department of Agriculture. (2004). Diagnosis and management of foodborne illnesses: A primer for physicians and other health care professionals. *Morbidity and Mortality Weekly Report, 53* (RR-4), 1–33.

Andrews, M. M., & Boyle, J. S. (2003). *Transcultural concepts in nursing care* (4th ed.). Philadelphia: Lippincott Williams & Wilkins.

Astle, S. M. (2005). Restoring electrolyte balance. *RN, 68*(5), 34–39.

Bennett, J. A., Thomas, V., & Riegel, B. (2004). Unrecognized chronic dehydration in older adults. Examining prevalence rate and risk factors. *Journal of Gerontological Nursing, 30*(1), 22–28.

Dochterman, J. M., & Bulechek, G. M. (Eds.). (2004). *Nursing interventions classification (NIC)* (4th ed.). St. Louis, MO: Mosby.

Elgart, H. N. (2004). Assessment of fluids and electrolytes. *AACN Clinical Issues, 15*(4), 607–621.

Food and Drug Administration (FDA). (2004). Bar code label requirements for human drug products and biological products. *Federal Register, 69*(38), 9119–9171.

Hadaway, L. C. (2004). Preventing and managing peripheral extravasation. *Nursing, 34*(5), 66–67.

Hayes, D. D. (2004). Calcium in the balance. *Nursing Made Incredibly Easy, 2*(2), 46–53.

Masoorli, S., & Angeles, T. (2002). Getting a line on central vascular access devices. *Nursing, 32*(4), 36–43.

Moorhead, S., Johnson, M., & Maas, M. (Eds.). (2004). *Nursing outcomes classification (NOC)* (3rd ed.). St. Louis, MO: Mosby.

NANDA International. (2007). *NANDA nursing diagnoses: Definitions and classification 2007–2008.* Philadelphia: Author.

Phillips, L. D. (2005). *Manual of I.V. therapeutics* (4th ed.). Philadelphia: F. A. Davis.

Rosenthal, K. (2004). Avoiding bad blood: Key steps to safe transfusions. *Nursing Made Incredibly Easy, 2*(5), 20–29.

Rosenthal, K. (2005a). Tailor your I.V. insertion techniques for special populations. *Nursing, 35*(5), 37–41.

Rosenthal, K. (2005b). Ports: The gateway to central lines. *Nursing Made Incredibly Easy, 3*(1), 53–56.

Simpson, H. (2004). Interpretation of arterial blood gases: A clinical guide for nurses. *British Journal of Nursing, 13*(9), 522–528.

Spandorfer, P. R., Alessandrini, E. A., Joffe, M. D., Localio, R., & Shaw, K. N. (2005). Oral versus intravenous rehydration of moderately dehydrated children: A randomized, controlled trial. *Pediatrics, 115*(2), 295–301.

Wilburn, S. Q. (2004). Needlestick and sharps injury prevention. *Online Journal of Issues in Nursing, 9*(3), manuscript 4. Retrieved July 15, 2006, from http://www.nursingworld.org/ojin/topic25/tpc25_4.htm

Yucha, C. (2004). Renal regulation of acid–base balance. *Nephrology Nursing Journal, 31*(2), 201–208.

SELECTED BIBLIOGRAPHY

Allen, K. (2005). Four-step method of interpreting arterial blood gas analysis. *Nursing Times, 101*(1), 42–45.

Anderson, N. R. (2005). When to use a midline catheter. *Nursing, 35*(4), 28.

Bunce, M. (2003). Troubleshooting central lines. *RN, 66*(12), 28–33.

Burger, C. M. (2004). Hyperkalemia: When serum K+ is not okay. *American Journal of Nursing, 104*(10), 66–70.

Burger, C. M. (2004). Hypokalemia: Averting crisis with early recognition and intervention. *American Journal of Nursing, 104*(11), 61–65.

Centers for Disease Control and Prevention. (2002). Guidelines for the prevention of intravascular catheter-related infections. *Morbidity and Mortality Weekly Report, 51*(10), 1–29.

Corbett, J. V. (2004). *Laboratory tests and diagnostic procedures with nursing diagnoses* (6th ed.). Upper Saddle River, NJ: Pearson Prentice Hall.

Deglin, J. H., & Vallerand, A. H. (2004). *Davis's drug guide for nurses* (9th ed.). Philadelphia: F. A. Davis.

Dulak, S. B. (2005). Technology today: Smart IV pumps. *RN, 68*(12), 38–43.

Hadaway, L. C. (2003). Infusing without infecting. *Nursing, 33*(10), 58–64.

Hadaway, L. C. (2005). Reopen the pipeline for I.V. therapy. *Nursing, 35*(8), 54–61.

Hadaway, L. C. (2006). Keeping central line infection at bay. *Nursing, 36*(4), 58–63.

Hayes, D. D. (2004). Balancing act: What happens when sodium and water are off-kilter? *Nursing Made Incredibly Easy, 2*(1), 52–57.

Hayes, D. D. (2004). Magnesium's balancing act. *Nursing Made Incredibly Easy, 2*(4), 44–50.

Hayes, D. D. (2004). Phosphorus: Here, there, everywhere. *Nursing Made Incredibly Easy, 2*(6), 36–41.

Hogan, M. A., & Wane, D. (2003). *Fluids, electrolytes, & acid-base balance: Reviews & rationales.* Upper Saddle River, NJ: Prentice Hall.

Just the facts: Fluids & electrolytes. (2005). Philadelphia: Lippincott Williams & Wilkins.

Lynes, D. (2003). Respiratory care skills: An introduction to blood gas analysis. *Nursing Times, 99*(11), 54–55.

Pruitt, W. C., & Jacobs, M. (2004). Interpreting arterial blood gases: Easy as ABC. *Nursing, 34*(8), 50–53.

Marders, J. (2005). Sounding the alarm for I.V. infiltration. *Nursing, 35*(4), 19–20.

Moureau, N. L. (2003). Is your skin-prep technique up-to-date? *Nursing, 33*(11), 17.

Moureau, N. L. (2004). Tips for inserting an I.V. in an older patient. *Nursing, 34*(7), 18.

Newberry, N. (Ed.). (2003). *Sheehy's emergency nursing* (5th ed.). St. Louis, MO: Mosby.

Quillen, T. F. (2005). Myths & facts: About hypercalcemia. *Nursing, 35*(7), 74.

Rosenthal, K. (2004). It's not magic! The tricks to cannulating difficult veins. *Nursing Made Incredibly Easy, 2*(2), 4–7.

Rosenthal, K. (2004). The line—for central venous access—forms here. *Nursing Made Incredibly Easy, 2*(5), 4–7.

Rosenthal, K. (2004). What you should know about needleless I.V. systems. *Nursing, 34*(9), 76.

Rosenthal, K. (2005). Documenting peripheral I.V. therapy. *Nursing, 35*(7), 28.

Sweeney, J. (2005). What causes sudden hypokalemia? *Nursing, 35*(4), 12.

Sweeney, J. (2005). What causes hyponatremia? *Nursing, 35*(6), 18.

Trimble, T. (2003). Peripheral I.V. starts: Securing and removing the catheter. *Nursing, 33*(9), 26.

Woodrow, P. (2004). Arterial blood gas analysis. *Nursing Standard, 18*(21), 45–52.

Answers to *Anatomy & Physiology Review, Critical Thinking Possibilities,* and *Answers to Test Your Knowledge*

CHAPTER 1

TEST YOUR KNOWLEDGE

1. *Answer*: 1, 4, and 5 *Rationale*: Option 2, Florence Nightingale, contributed to the nursing care of soldiers in the Crimean War. Option 3, Fabiola, used her wealth to provide houses of caring and healing during the Roman Empire. *Cognitive Level*: Knowledge *Client Need*: Not Applicable *Nursing Process*: Not Applicable

2. *Answer*: 3 *Rationale*: Health promotion focuses on maintaining normal status without consideration of diseases. Option 1 is an example of illness prevention. Option 2 is aesthetic (i. e., not needed for health promotion or disease prevention). Option 4 focuses on disease detection. *Cognitive Level*: Knowledge *Client Need*: Not Applicable *Nursing Process*: Not Applicable

3. *Answer*: 3 *Rationale*: All are noted nurses. Linda Richards was America's first trained nurse, and Mary Mahoney was America's first black trained nurse. *Cognitive Level*: Knowledge *Client Need*: Not Applicable *Nursing Process*: Not Applicable

4. *Answer*: 2 *Rationale*: Option 1, the advanced beginner, demonstrates marginally acceptable performance. Option 3, the proficient practitioner, has 3 to 5 years of experience and has developed a holistic understanding of the client. Option 4, the expert practitioner, demonstrates highly skilled intuitive and analytic ability in new situations. *Cognitive Level*: Knowledge *Client Need*: Not Applicable *Nursing Process*: Not Applicable

5. *Answer*: 4 *Rationale*: The National Student Nurses' Association developed the Code of Academic and Clinical Conduct for nursing students in 2001. Option 1, ANA, developed Standards of Nursing Practices. Option 2, NLN, focuses on nursing education. Option 3, the American Association of Colleges of Nursing (AACN), is the national organization that focuses on the advancement and maintenance of America's baccalaureate- and higher-degree nursing education programs. *Cognitive Level*: Knowledge *Client Need*: Not Applicable *Nursing Process*: Not Applicable

6. *Answer*: 1 *Rationale*: All will impact nursing but not necessarily the supply and demand issue. The aging population contributes to more elders needing specialized care (increasing the demand). Fewer nursing faculty to educate students and fewer nurses practicing because of retirement contribute to the decreasing supply. *Cognitive Level*: Analysis *Client Need*: Not Applicable *Nursing Process*: Not Applicable

CHAPTER 2

CRITICAL THINKING POSSIBILITIES

1. It will be important to gather the following information to allow you to give the person the best response:
    *   What is their knowledge of nursing? Is it accurate or based on a stereotype or the media's image of nursing? Do they know the differences between the types of nursing education?
    *   Do they have any experience with the health care system? If yes, how has that experience influenced them?
    *   Do they have prior educational experience or degrees? For example, if they have a baccalaureate degree they may be interested in a generic master's program.
    *   What are their professional goals and what kind of time frame are they considering?
    *   What is their personal situation? For example, some students have a professional goal of becoming a nurse practitioner; however, they wish to enter the nursing field as soon as possible. They elect to first complete a practical nursing program to allow them to work in nursing while completing course work for an RN program and finally advancing to a graduate program.
    *   What is the availability and accessibility to nursing programs in their area? People in rural areas may not have as many choices as individuals who live in an urban area.

    Obtaining answers to these questions will provide you needed information that will enable you to provide direction for the individual.

2. Consider influences on your decision making such as other nurses you have known and similar role models, experiences with the health care system prior to applying to nursing school, feedback you have received from teachers and friends regarding your skills, your views of health and illness, and similar inspiring situations.

3. Research studies examining the outcomes of different types and locations of nursing programs might be useful in choosing a school. For example, how do the NCLEX pass rates, graduation rates, and class sizes compare? Where do graduates tend to work? Consider the importance of how recently the study was done and how frequently curricula and accreditation standards change.

TEST YOUR KNOWLEDGE

1. *Answer*: 3 *Rationale*: Continuing education refers to formalized experiences designed to enlarge the knowledge or skills of practitioners. The other answers are examples of in-service education, which is designed to upgrade the knowledge or skills of current employees with regard to the specific setting and is usually less formal in presentation. *Cognitive Level*: Analysis *Client Need*: Safe, Effective Care Environment *Nursing Process*: Not Applicable

2. *Answer*: 2 *Rationale*: Since the primary purpose of research is to improve the quality of client care, the nurse should determine if published research results are applicable to the specific client population. Published studies may have flawed designs, data collection, or analysis. Although more than one well-conducted study with similar findings supports usefulness of the results, applicability must still be determined for the specific client population. It is not realistic for the nurse to rerun the data to check the results of the study. *Cognitive Level*: Application *Client Need*: Not Applicable *Nursing Process*: Not Applicable

3. *Answer*: 1 *Rationale*: Quantitative research collects numerical data. Sleep deprivation can be defined by X number of hours without sleep, and wound healing can be measured by size of wound in relation to the period of time. While some of the other options may be calculated using sophisticated numerical processes, they

are not as easily measured and may be more appropriate for qualitative research methods. *Cognitive Level*: Analysis *Client Need*: Not Applicable *Nursing Process*: Not Applicable

4. *Answer*: 3 *Rationale*: This study investigates the subjective experience of stress and would be collected through narrative data. The other answers are examples of quantitative research using numbers and values. *Cognitive Level* Analysis *Client Need*: Not Applicable *Nursing Process*: Not Applicable

5. *Answer*: 4 *Rationale*: The right of self-determination means that subjects feel free of constraints, coercion, or any undue influence to participate in a study. There is not enough information given to indicate if any of the other rights have been violated. *Cognitive Level*: Comprehension *Client Need*: Safe, Effective Care Environment *Nursing Process*: Diagnosis

CHAPTER 3

CRITICAL THINKING POSSIBILITIES

1. Some of the many concepts that can be identified are illness, disease, wellness, and nutrition.

2. The physician seems to view Tony as someone who has some choices in his own care. He also appears to be making a statement related to quality of life (wellness) that reflects a belief that the client would not be getting better and intravenous nutrition was, therefore, not indicated. The nurse appears to have expanded the definition of client to include family and friends and has a different prognosis in mind.

3. Florence Nightingale would focus Tony's care on the need for a clean environment, good water, and light as necessary for his health.

4. All nursing models recognize an interdependence of systems and relationships that would make controlling diarrhea a top priority. None of the nursing models is any more powerful than the others as a foundation for the nurse's plan of care.

TEST YOUR KNOWLEDGE

1. *Answer*: 3 *Rationale*: A supposition or system of ideas proposed to explain a given phenomenon is a theory. Concepts are mental images which are included within a theory; a conceptual framework is a group of related ideas, statements, or concepts; and a paradigm is a pattern of shared understandings and assumptions about reality and the world. *Cognitive Level*: Knowledge *Client Need*: Not Applicable *Nursing Process*: Not Applicable

2. *Answer*: 2 *Rationale*: A group of related ideas or statements is a conceptual framework. A philosophy is a belief system; a supposition or system of ideas proposed to explain a given phenomenon is a theory; and a paradigm is a pattern of shared understandings and assumptions about reality and the world. *Cognitive Level*: Knowledge *Client Need*: Not Applicable *Nursing Process*: Not Applicable

3. *Answer*: 4 *Rationale*: A set of shared understandings and assumptions about reality and the world is a paradigm. Concepts are mental images; a conceptual framework is a group of related ideas, statements, or concepts; and a practice discipline is a field of study in which the central focus is performance of a professional role. *Cognitive Level*: Knowledge *Client Need*: Not Applicable *Nursing Process*: Not Applicable

4. *Answer*: 1 *Rationale*: Practice disciplines are fields of study in which the central focus is performance of a professional role. Time and experience are necessary for developing proficiency in any profession or career. Research and theory development do not

have performance as their primary focus. The primary focus of nursing is providing quality service to humans. Team or group practice can be a part of a career in humanities, computer science, or rocket science. *Cognitive Level*: Analysis *Client Need*: Not Applicable *Nursing Process*: Not Applicable

5. *Answer*: 2 *Rationale*: Person/client, environment, health, and nursing are relevant when providing care for any client whether in the hospital, at home, in the community, or in elementary school systems. These elements can be used to understand diseases, conduct and apply research, develop nursing theories, as well as implement the nursing process. *Cognitive Level*: Application *Client Need*: Not Applicable *Nursing Process*: Not Applicable

CHAPTER 4

CRITICAL THINKING POSSIBILITIES

1. The nurse needs to verify that the client received information from the primary care provider and that she understands the information. Can the client explain in her own words what the doctor told her? Does she have any questions?

2. The three exceptions of people who cannot provide consent are minors, persons who are unconscious or injured in such a way that they are unable to give consent, and mentally ill persons judged to be incompetent. If this client is an alert, competent adult, she can provide consent.

3. The nurse will need to read the form to the client.

4. Unless the husband is the appointed guardian or has power of attorney for health care decisions, the client should sign the form. The client will need assistance as to where to sign the form. The client could even mark an "X." Remember, the nurse witnesses that the client gave her consent voluntarily and that the signature is authentic.

5. The nurse needs to include the following:

   • The consent form was read to the client before she signed it.

   • A reference to the client's understanding of the procedure (e.g., "able to state reasons for surgery, pros and cons of surgery. Stated she had no questions. Aware that she can change her mind").

   • If the husband helped the client sign (e.g., guided her hand), this information should be documented.

   • Record any teaching as a result of nursing-related questions by the client (e.g., "discussed and demonstrated techniques for coughing and deep breathing after surgery").

TEST YOUR KNOWLEDGE

1. *Answer*: 3 *Rationale*: This is the best answer because the nurse is assessing the client's level of knowledge as a result of the discussion with the primary care provider. Based on this assessment, the nurse may initiate other actions (e.g., call the primary care provider if the client has many questions). In option 1, the nurse is not assessing if the client received enough information to give consent. Option 2 is one way to assess the client's level of knowledge regarding the procedure. However, it is not the best approach because it is a closed-ended question, asking for only a "yes" or "no" response. Option 3 provides more information from the client in his or her own words. The statement in option 4 is true; however, the nurse should first verify if the client received enough information to give consent. After the assessment, this statement may be appropriate but the assessment needs to be done first. *Cognitive Level*: Application *Client Need*: Safe, Effective Care Environment *Nursing Process*: Assessment

2. *Answer*: 4 *Rationale*: Battery is the willful touching of a person without permission. Another name for an unintentional tort is malpractice. This situation is an intentional tort because the nurse executed the act on purpose. Assault is the attempt or threat to touch another person unjustifiably or without permission. Invasion of privacy injures the feelings of the person and does not take into consideration how revealing information or exposing the client will affect the client's feelings. *Cognitive Level*: Analysis *Client Need*: Safe, Effective Care Environment *Nursing Process*: Not Applicable

3. *Answer*: 2 *Rationale*: The nurse should call the person who wrote the order for clarification. Administering the medication is incorrect because knowing the dose is outside the normal range and not questioning the order could lead to client harm and liability for the nurse. Calling the pharmacist is not the best answer because it will not solve the problem, and the nurse needs to seek clarification from the person who wrote the order. The nurse should suspend administration but not refuse to administer the medication until the issue is resolved. *Cognitive Level*: Application *Client Need*: Safe, Effective Care Environment *Nursing Process*: Implementation

4. *Answer*: 1 *Rationale*: All elements such as duty, foreseeability, causation, harm/injury, and damages much be present for malpractice to be proven. The nurse is a licensed professional responsible for individual actions. Notifying the primary care provider does not exempt the nurse from liability. Since it is apparent the standard of practice was not performed, a breach of duty does exist. Violation/omission of the standard of practice resulted in an excessive dosage. Therefore foreseeability is present; however, no harm occurred to the client. *Cognitive Level*: Analysis *Client Need*: Safe, Effective Care Environment *Nursing Process*: Evaluation

5. *Answer*: 4 *Rationale*: A sterile, invasive procedure which places the client at significant risk for infection is generally outside the scope of practice of a UAP. Even though the UAP is a nursing student, the agency job description should be followed. The job description is the standard of care in this situation. *Cognitive Level*: Application *Client Need*: Safe, Effective Care Environment *Nursing Process*: Implementation

6. *Answer*: 3 *Rationale*: A DNR order only controls CPR and similar lifesaving treatments. All other care continues as previously ordered. Competent clients can still decide about their own care (including the DNR order). Nothing about the DNR order is related to when the client may die. Because clients' medical conditions and their views of their lives can change, a new DNR order is required for each admission to a health care agency. Once admitted, that order stands until changed or until it expires according to agency policy. *Cognitive Level*: Application *Client Need*: Psychosocial Integrity *Nursing Process*: Planning

7. *Answer*: 3 *Rationale*: The only person entitled to information without written consent is the client and those providing direct care. The nurse has open access to information regarding assigned clients only. *Cognitive Level*: Application *Client Need*: Safe, Effective Care Environment *Nursing Process*: Implementation

8. *Answer*: 1, 2, and 5 *Rationale*: The nurse is subject to the limitation of the state law and should be familiar with the Good Samaritan laws in the specific state. Gross negligence would be described by the individual state law. Unless there is another equally or more qualified person present, the nurse needs to stay until the injured person leaves. The nurse should ask someone else to call or go for additional help. Since there was no prior agreement, the nurse cannot accept compensation. Also, the nurse is not

employed by the accident victim. The same client rights apply at the scene of an accident as well as those in the workplace. *Cognitive Level*: Application *Client Need*: Safe, Effective Care Environment *Nursing Process*: Planning

9. *Answer*: 1, 3, and 4 *Rationale*: Interacting with others (versus isolating self from others) and setting limits on the number of hours working are positive behaviors and not indicative of possible impairment. The other options are warning signs for impairment. *Cognitive Level*: Analysis *Client Need*: Safe, Effective Care Environment *Nursing Process*: Evaluation

10. *Answer*: 2 and 3 *Rationale*: Standards of practice require a complete assessment. A nurse needs to be sure the client's needs have been met. They both can impact client safety and do not follow standards of care. The other options meet the standards of practice. *Cognitive Level*: Analysis *Client Need*: Safe, Effective Care Environment *Nursing Process*: Implementation

CHAPTER 5
CRITICAL THINKING POSSIBILITIES

1. Personal values are often based on family, cultural, religious, or other beliefs and attitudes. The nurse must not assume any particular values based on these characteristics, however. They must be validated with the individual. What appear to be the client's values must be confirmed with him through open and supportive discussion.

2. The nurse needs to review the variety of factors influencing the client's values and decisions such as family support, previous experience with health care situations, the meaning of illness (and of the foot) to the person, and his personal goals. The surgeon has information about the client's overall health status, possibly previous experiences with this client, and personal values and beliefs about the impact of an amputation.

   Conduct a thorough health history on the client if not already completed, and review the content related to the factors influencing the client's values and decision. Review the medical history and physical examination for additional data. Gather missing information from the client or surgeon as indicated.

3. The nurse's responsibility is to ensure that the client has all the accurate information required for him to make an informed decision. This may include information beyond his physiologic condition such as facts about his health insurance coverage for acute and rehabilitative care. The nurse's personal beliefs about what the client should do or what the surgeon should recommend must not influence the nurse in carrying out this responsibility.

4. It is sometimes difficult to find the middle ground between advocating for the client and interfering in the client physician relationship. Also, the client's informed decision may be counter to standard or recommended medical practice.

5. The Code of Ethics for Nurses or a patient bill of rights can help the nurse recall the standards that apply in guiding nurse decision making during possible ethical dilemmas. The nurse's actions should be based on ethical theory and standards, not on personal opinion.

TEST YOUR KNOWLEDGE

1. *Answer*: 1 *Rationale*: A nurse's actions in an ethical dilemma must be defensible according to moral and ethical standards. The nurse may have strong personal beliefs but distancing oneself from the situation does not serve the client. A team is not always required to reach decisions and the nurse is not obligated to fol-

low the client's wishes automatically when they may have negative consequences for self or others. *Cognitive Level*: Application *Client Need*: Safe, Effective Care Environment *Nursing Process*: Planning

2. *Answer*: 2 *Rationale*: The nurse has an ethical responsibility to act only when actions are safe or risks minimized. This nurse is putting the client at unnecessary risk for a medication error. Many medical practices are controversial but not necessarily unethical (Option 1). The nurse should follow the agency policy. Although some may view nurses' strikes as unethical, supporting others who are striking is a personal decision (Option 3). Although a client statement in confidence to a nurse may have ethical overtones, it does not automatically constitute an ethical dilemma. Since the assigned health care provider is a member of the team, principles of confidentiality do not include him or her (Option 4). *Cognitive Level*: Analysis *Client Need*: Safe, Effective Care Environment *Nursing Process*: Not Applicable

3. *Answer*: 1 *Rationale*: Autonomy is the client's (or surrogate's) right to make his or her own decision. The nurse is obliged to respect a client's or significant others' informed decision. These parents may modify their decision as time goes on and the child's condition, or their feelings, change. This situation is not clearly one of nonmaleficence (do no harm) or beneficence (do good) since there are many aspects of both. If the child appeared to be suffering or an effective treatment was being denied, these principles might apply. Justice (fairness) generally applies when the rights of one client are being balanced against those of another client. *Cognitive Level*: Application *Client Need*: Safe, Effective Care Environment *Nursing Process*: Not Applicable

4. *Answer*: 3 *Rationale*: In values clarification, clients are assisted to think about the factors that influence their beliefs and decisions. Any judgmental statement that reflects the rightness or wrongness of the client's thoughts or actions will impede this process. *Cognitive Level*: Application *Client Need*: Safe, Effective Care Environment *Nursing Process*: Implementation

5. *Answer*: 4 *Rationale*: A major role of the client advocate is to mediate between conflicting parties. The nurse needs to assess the situation before offering an intervention. Informing the family is an intervention without assessment. If the primary care provider sends the client home, the nurse has not acted to assist in resolving or reducing the conflict. If the nurse assists in resolving or reducing the conflict, the added expense of an attorney may not be needed. However, legal action should be a last resort. *Cognitive Level*: Analysis *Client Need*: Safe, Effective Care Environment *Nursing Process*: Implementation

CHAPTER 6

CRITICAL THINKING POSSIBILITIES

1. It does not seem as though the client has used many health promotion or prevention services. He would have used secondary prevention services extensively in seeing the primary care provider for his blood pressure and joint problems and having surgery. His time at the skilled nursing facility, with the home health nurse, and the physical therapist visits were tertiary preventive care.

2. He has visited the primary care provider's office, which is useful for monitoring existing problems and screening for new ones; the hospital has the expert staff for performing his surgery and the nursing personnel for caring for him during the perioperative period. They have laboratories, therapeutic services (e.g., physical therapy), and nutrition services to meet his needs. Examples of

other agencies would include the skilled nursing facility and home health care.

3. This client has health care needs in a variety of areas. His age and health problems suggest that he will continue to need health care for the foreseeable future. The case manager can become very familiar with the client and family situation so that the appropriate levels of care can be provided when he needs them and within his insurance coverage. He would have Medicare but may also have supplemental coverage. Should he become unable to continue living in the current house, the case manager may assist with determining the type of living facility most appropriate. If the client needs to be readmitted to the hospital, the case manager serves as an excellent facilitator in the communication needed among the physician, hospital, rehabilitative setting, and home health care personnel.

4. Examples include these: Pharmacist—elders often take many different medications. During an acute illness there is a particular need to ensure that newly ordered medications that may be required for the current condition do not interfere with medications used for chronic conditions. Spiritual support—although we do not know Mr. Mendel's religious preference, he may be experiencing some spiritual concerns, for example, about dying. If he and his wife have a relationship with a church or other similar institution, it would be important to include this aspect in his care. Many other professionals may be included on the team.

TEST YOUR KNOWLEDGE

1. *Answer*: 3 *Rationale*: Actions such as diet modification that help to prevent an illness or detect it in its early stages are primary prevention. Treatment of a disease such as antibiotic therapy or surgery is secondary prevention, while rehabilitation efforts following an illness are considered tertiary prevention. *Cognitive Level*: Analysis *Client Need*: Health Promotion and Maintenance *Nursing Process:* Not Applicable

2. *Answer*: 2 *Rationale*: City, county, state, or federal government funds pay for health department and agency activities aimed at the global health of the community. Hospitals may provide a variety of wellness and clinic programs in addition to inpatient services. Surgery may be performed in outpatient surgery centers and physicians' offices in addition to within hospitals. Skilled nursing, extended care, and long-term care facilities provide care to persons of all ages who require rehabilitation or subacute care. This is not necessarily related to insurance coverage for hospital stays. *Cognitive Level*: Analysis *Client Need*: Not Applicable *Nursing Process*: Not Applicable

3. *Answer*: 1 *Rationale*: Primary care providers are limited to generalist physicians and advanced practice nurses. In some cases a gynecologist may qualify as a primary care provider and in other cases not. Physical therapists do not have a scope of practice broad enough to serve as primary care providers. Pharmacists and case managers/discharge planners are not responsible for providing direct client care. *Cognitive Level*: Analysis *Client Need*: Safe, Effective Care Environment *Nursing Process*: Planning

4. *Answer*: 2 *Rationale*: When people have inadequate insurance for health costs, they tend to avoid early and preventive care. This results in eventual use of much more costly resources such as emergency rooms. Methods to provide minimum levels of insurance coverage have been successful in other countries. The number of children is increasing, but in the United States and Canada this is a nonmodifiable factor. Also, the majority of health care costs are incurred by adults and elders who tend to have multiple

and chronic health conditions. There is currently a significant shortage of nurses and maldistribution of physicians so reducing their numbers would only worsen the problem. Competition among manufacturers is more likely to cause costs to fall than to rise. *Cognitive Level*: Application *Client Need*: Not Applicable *Nursing Process:* Diagnosis

5. *Answer*: 4 *Rationale*: A health maintenance organization involves a set monthly membership fee and predictable visit or deductible costs. Medicare covers a minimal number of preventive and outpatient services so the cost cannot be anticipated. Individual fee-for-service insurance is perhaps the most costly to the client, with potentially large differences between the amount of coverage the insurance company pays and the provider's charges. PPOs are less costly than fee-for-service but more expensive than HMOs. *Cognitive Level*: Analysis *Client Need*: Safe, Effective Care Management *Nursing Process*: Planning

CHAPTER 7

CRITICAL THINKING POSSIBILITIES

There can be no traditional answers to these questions. What follow below are aspects to consider.

1. Overall, decreasing the time clients spend in dependent situations such as being in acute care hospitals is consistent with the agenda's aims at health care reform. However, the nurse must also consider the culture of the client and the environment. Active decision making by the client is a Western view that may not be shared by clients from Eastern, African American, or Latino backgrounds. In European health care systems, clients often spend as much as five times longer in a hospital than do American clients. The client may not be accustomed to community-based care and have very different views of the health care professionals who provide community-based care. Also, the scenario does not address outcomes. A primary concern would be to measure the incidence of complications, need for rehospitalization, and client satisfaction with the short stays.

2. Individuals will have unique responses to this question. Answers should reflect consideration of the views and skills of nurses, clients, and systems.

3. In an integrated health care system, the client would move easily from the diagnostic phase through treatment and rehabilitation— possibly using a case manager to assess the client and family and follow her though the entire episode. A community coalition would focus more on the risk factors leading to the health problem and initiatives to educate the population on wellness, prevention, and early detection.

4. Communication with the client, family, and other health care providers would be key to determining that a particular client is appropriate for this "fast-track" approach to the surgery. If the parties disagree, shared decision making should be used in establishing the details of how the care will actually be provided. Mutual respect and trust are key—that the health care providers are skilled and knowledgeable about the procedure and that the client and family can carry out their respective roles once the decisions have been made and communicated. Collaboration with third-party payers can be more complex. Investigate their chain of command and try to find nurses with whom to discuss the case.

TEST YOUR KNOWLEDGE

1. *Answer*: 3 *Rationale*: *Nursing's Agenda for Healthcare Reform* (ANA, 1991) called for case management of those with ongoing health care needs. It also proposed that primary care be commu-

nity based but that essential services be paid for by a combination of public and private funding sources (not just public funds) and be phased in gradually. *Cognitive Level*: Application *Client Need*: Not Applicable *Nursing Process*: Not Applicable

2. *Answer*: 1 *Rationale*: The Pew Commission identified the need for modern health care providers to be proficient in the use of technology. No mention is made of financial competencies beyond the attention to cost-effective care. The commission also identified the need for contemporary (not traditional) clinical strategies and for collaborative decision making with clients. *Cognitive Level*: Analysis *Client Need*: Not Applicable *Nursing Process*: Not Applicable

3. *Answer*: 2 *Rationale*: In community-based health care, clients are cared for according to their geographical locations such as where they live or work, rather than at a major medical center or similar provider setting, which facilitates access. Emphasis is more on client wellness and prevention than on illness and may be paid for through any of the usual forms of insurance or payment (including managed care, private pay, or welfare). *Cognitive Level*: Analysis *Client Need*: Safe, Effective Care Environment *Nursing Process*: Not Applicable

4. *Answer*: 2 *Rationale*: In collaboration, each member of the team, including the client, participates in sharing ideas and reaching consensus on the best plan of care. The team is generally led by the health care professional most skilled in the client's specific areas of need. Once the plan is established, it may be implemented by any member of the team or a designate at an appropriate time and place. It not necessarily delegated by the nurse. *Cognitive Level*: Analysis *Client Need*: Safe, Effective Care Environment *Nursing Process*: Not Applicable

5. *Answer*: 4 *Rationale*: Effective discharge planning would have included an assessment of home care needs prior to the client leaving the hospital. The kind of care is determined before the client leaves the current setting. That is why it is called discharge "planning." Following a thorough assessment, the client would be taught self-care strategies and a basic plan of care for the coming days. Obtaining medications and a ride home does not indicate the client possesses the knowledge and skills needed to manage care after discharge. If the client will need care at home, those referrals would be made by the discharge planner and communicated to the client. Option 4 indicates the client knows and accepts these referrals. *Cognitive Level*: Analysis *Client Need*: Safe, Effective Care Environment *Nursing Process*: Evaluation

6. *Answer*: 4 *Rationale*: The home health nurse more commonly works with single persons or families at one time—addressing their particular needs that may be similar to or different from those of others. The community health nurse will focus on activities that influence the larger group of individuals affected. These include prevention and monitoring of infectious disease plus actions that will promote health for multiple affected persons (e.g., food, water, and shelter). *Cognitive Level*: Comprehension *Client Need*: Safe, Effective Care Environment *Nursing Process*: Implementation

CHAPTER 8

CRITICAL THINKING POSSIBILITIES

1. Many aspects of the nurse's role will be the same. The techniques such as intravenous medication administration will have the same steps but they may need to be modified to apply in situations where not all usual supplies or equipment are available (e.g., us-

ing a door hook for an IV pole). More so than in the acute care setting, the nurse needs to consider the client's family as a client in addition to the client.

2. The client has all the same rights of any client but, in addition, has the right to direct that care be administered in a way that is acceptable within his or her environment, to decline to accept the nurse's recommendations, and to decline the nurse's assistance and care.

3. Safety issues: any aspects of his home or daily activities that could worsen his diabetes (e.g., inadequate heating/cooling) or potentially cause injury (unsafe railings). Infection control issues: lack of access to needed hygiene facilities, inability to participate in dressing changes and wound care due to poor vision, reduced dexterity, or other factors. Lack of adequate caregiver support.

4. In addition to the intangible savings of emotional comfort provided by being in one's own home, the client is able to maintain many of his personal contacts and activities—including such important tasks as paying bills and caring for pets. While home, the client avoids large hospital room charges and does not incur extra costs of having someone care for things at home.

TEST YOUR KNOWLEDGE

1. *Answer*: 3 *Rationale*: Although hospitals have recently become more welcoming to families, a major strength of home care is the involvement and proximity of loved ones. Curative and lifesaving approaches may be used both at home and in the hospital. An asset of home care nurses is their ability to manage complex symptoms. This includes expertise in pain management, but the same legal strategies are available in either in-home care or hospitals. *Cognitive Level*: Application *Client Need*: Not Applicable *Nursing Process*: Not Applicable

2. *Answer*: 1 *Rationale*: Assuming the client is medically stable, feeding and bathing are tasks within the aide's abilities. Teaching the client about or adjusting medications (and oxygen is considered a medication) and performing assessments are duties restricted to the registered nurse. *Cognitive Level*: Application *Client Need*: Safe, Effective Care Environment *Nursing Process*: Planning

3. *Answer*: 2 *Rationale*: The nurse needs to encourage the client to express feelings or thoughts that led to the refusal so that misunderstandings can be clarified and other possible solutions explored. The nurse should apply the principle that all behavior has meaning. Otherwise, the nurse is intervening before assessing the situation. In option 3, that approach did not work the first time. A reason for the refusal needs to be explored. Option 4 is almost a threat and has a paternalistic implication. Clients are entitled to make informed decisions to perform or not perform recommended activities. Notifying the primary care provider is implementing an intervention before the nurse has done an assessment. *Cognitive Level*: Application *Client Need*: Health Promotion and Maintenance *Nursing Process*: Implementation

4. *Answer*: 1 *Rationale*: If the caregiver's own health is becoming threatened, it may be a sign of overload. It would be appropriate for the caregiver to ask for assistance from others or to ask for clarification of ways he or she can assist the client. Sadness related to a poor prognosis would be a normal and expected response as long as it does not evolve into depression. *Cognitive Level*: Application *Client Need*: Psychosocial Integrity *Nursing Process*: Diagnosis

5. *Answer*: 4 *Rationale*: A physician's authorization of the plan of care is needed before home health care by a nurse can be initiated. Insurance coverage is not required although the agency may need proof of the client's ability to pay if insurance is not available or adequate. Many clients benefit from home health care even if there is no in-home caregiver present or needed. The health problem for which home care is needed may be chronic or acute and may necessitate preventive, curative, or palliative therapy. *Cognitive Level*: Application *Client Need*: Safe, Effective Care Environment *Nursing Process*: Planning

CHAPTER 9

CRITICAL THINKING POSSIBILITIES

1. Consider the uses of the computer in the following areas: searching the Internet and literature for research or case studies that might relate; sending queries to experts identified through university medical centers of excellence; e-mailing colleagues from relevant professional nursing organizations.

2. Ask the client to share exactly the nature of the concern. Discuss with the client whether any unique identifiers will be associated with the photos or query, for example, name, address. Suggest that your colleagues will be asked to delete the photo files as soon as the consultation is complete. Would the client find fax or hard copies more acceptable?

3. Use one of the documents available to critique the website yourself. Share with the client the criteria for determining the usefulness of the information found on health websites and discuss how they apply to the specific site. Also provide the client with other reliable sources of health information such as printed pamphlets or referenced articles.

4. Consider issues such as the ability to do your studying and assignments at a time (and place) of your choosing rather than in a classroom on specific days and times; whether you prefer to work alone or in "real place" groups (online programs also use groups that may do synchronous or asynchronous work); how self-directed you are; the availability of local quality education programs; concern about privacy regarding your academic records and financial aid information; and so on.

TEST YOUR KNOWLEDGE

1. *Answer*: 1 *Rationale*: Most CD-ROMs cannot be changed by the user although some CDs are "rewriteable." RAM is random-access memory that is emptied when the computer is turned off. A floppy diskette is more fragile than a CD, and even files on a locked disk are easily erased since it can be unlocked by any person. A network is a communication method and not data storage. *Cognitive Level*: Knowledge *Client Need*: Not Applicable *Nursing Process*: Not Applicable

2. *Answer*: 3 *Rationale*: Control over who has access to confidential computerized data is the greatest concern. Computer hackers can bypass codes and gain access to personal information which could result in identity theft. The benefits often outweigh cost. Computerized data can be much more accurate than paper and pencil. Due to ease of making copies and backups, electronic data can last forever. *Cognitive Level*: Analysis *Client Need*: Safe, Effective Care Environment *Nursing Process*: Not Applicable

3. *Answer*: 4 *Rationale*: Since learners may do their online work at different times and do much of their work offline, it is harder for them to feel and act like a class group. The courses are often self-paced. Communication is possible because through audio and video file sharing, learners can see and hear the faculty as well as each other. For many courses, learners may log on at their convenience. *Cognitive Level*: Comprehension *Client Need*: Not Applicable *Nursing Process*: Not Applicable

4. *Answer*: 3 *Rationale*: Although all steps of the research process can be accomplished without computers, electronic data analysis helps ensure accuracy and speeds the analysis immensely. *Cognitive Level*: Analysis *Client Need*: Not Applicable *Nursing Process*: Not Applicable

5. *Answer*: 1 *Rationale*: Each website is different and the practitioner is compelled to evaluate the site and the treatment to determine if it is safe and appropriate for the client. Some websites are advertising but many are sponsored by legitimate organizations such as the National Cancer Institute (option 4). They often report results of extensive research (option 2). One of the most important purposes of posting treatment information and results on the Internet is so that many different people can determine if the treatment is useful for other clients (option 3). *Cognitive Level*: Application *Client Need*: Health Promotion and Maintenance *Nursing Process*: Implementation

CHAPTER 10
CRITICAL THINKING POSSIBILITIES

1. Examples include these: What evidence supports the assumption? What are other possible explanations for his condition? What might another nurse who sees this situation differently think? What evidence would suggest a different assumption?

2. This attitude says that critical thinking will lead to appropriate conclusions. It requires that you trust yourself, examine the influence of emotions on your thinking, and use logic to reach conclusions. Suggest how you can show that you have considered these things.

3. If your conclusion is correct and acted on, you have helped keep the client's problems at a minimum through early intervention. He can receive proper treatment and the nurse can develop a plan of care to assist the client and family with the impact of the condition. If you are incorrect in your assumption and do not consider what the correct conclusion was, time may be wasted and the real condition could worsen. Increased cost, emotional frustration, and other negative outcomes may result.

4. How does the client feel about his recent retirement? What is the impact of his retirement while his wife continues to work? Do the coming holidays play a role in his illness?

TEST YOUR KNOWLEDGE

1. *Answer*: 2 *Rationale*: The nurse has inferred and concluded something that is beyond the available information (and in this case may not be accurate). The prescription and the diarrhea are facts. It would be judgment and opinion if the nurse stated that the laxative would make the diarrhea worse and should not be given. (Note: Critical thinking will cause this nurse to examine the assumptions made and gather more data before acting.) *Cognitive Level*: Analysis *Client Need*: Not Applicable *Nursing Process*: Evaluation

2. *Answer*: 1 *Rationale*: The nurse recognizes that many assumptions (beliefs) could interfere with the client eating—such as that the food presented is not culturally appropriate. These assumptions must be clarified. Options 2 and 3 reach conclusions not supported by the facts. In option 4, the nurse has made a judgment or has an opinion that may not be accurate. Also, the nurse is acting without assessment. Implementation should be preceded by assessment. *Cognitive Level*: Application *Client Need*: Physiologic Integrity *Nursing Process*: Planning

3. *Answer*: 4 *Rationale*: The critical-thinking approach should include perseverance until a reasonable solution or answer is deter-

mined. Giving in (option 1), overquestioning self or poor trust in one's own beliefs (option 2), or bypassing normal routes of authority (option 3) violate the desirable attitudes of integrity, intellectual courage, and confidence in reason. *Cognitive Level*: Application *Client Need*: Not Applicable *Nursing Process*: Not Applicable

4. *Answer*: 1 *Rationale*: The scientific method uses a research study-based approach to problem solving. Trial and error and intuition would involve unstructured approaches resulting in less predictable results. The nursing process generally uses application of known interventions, previously determined by the scientific (research) process. *Cognitive Level*: Application *Client Need*: Not Applicable *Nursing Process*: Not Applicable

5. *Answer*: 4 *Rationale*: It is important to project what problems might interfere with the plan and have appropriate responses prepared to prevent the interferences. The purpose for the decision should have been clear enough at the outset as to not require reexamination at this point. Clients and families should be consulted early—in the purpose-setting and criteria-setting steps. Criteria should not be set until all significant participants have an opportunity to present their point of view. Considering various means for reaching the outcomes is the same as examining alternatives. *Cognitive Level*: Application *Client Need*: Not Applicable *Nursing Process*: Planning

CHAPTER 11
CRITICAL THINKING POSSIBILITIES

1. Extremely important areas to include are allergies, comorbidities (other health problems or diseases), and previous experience with surgery.

2. Because the musculoskeletal system is the reason she is in the hospital, it would be given priority. Due to her age and the immobility that will follow surgery, other priority systems would be cardiopulmonary and integumentary.

3. Many answers may be correct. The question should be open-ended and prompt for the desired information (for example, it would not be helpful to ask her where she lives). One example would be "It may not be possible for you to be alone when you go home from the hospital. Tell me about who might be available to assist you?"

4. Consider family, friends, clergy, and her old charts.

TEST YOUR KNOWLEDGE

1. *Answer*: 1 *Rationale*: Identifying problems/needs is part of nursing diagnosis. For example, a client with difficulty breathing would have *Impaired Gas Exchange* related to constricted airways as manifested by shortness of breath (dyspnea) as a nursing diagnosis. Organizing the family history is part of the assessment phase. Establishing goals is a part of the planning phase. Administering an antibiotic is part of the implementation phase. *Cognitive Level*: Application *Client Need*: Not Applicable *Nursing Process*: Diagnosis

2. *Answer*: 3 *Rationale*: During assessment, data are collected, organized, validated, and documented. Hypotheses are generated during diagnosing; outcomes are set during planning; and documentation occurs throughout the nursing process. *Cognitive Level*: Application *Client Need*: Not Applicable *Nursing Process*: Assessment

3. *Answer*: 2 *Rationale*: Primary data come from the client (option 4), whereas secondary data come from any other source (chart, family). Subjective data are covert (reported or an opinion),

whereas objective data can be measured or validated (weight—option 1, edema—option 3). If the spouse had stated that the client had eaten only toast and tea, this would be secondary objective (measured) data. *Cognitive Level*: Application *Client Need*: Not Applicable *Nursing Process*: Assessment

4. *Answer*: 3 *Rationale*: Eliciting feelings requires an open-ended question that does more than seek factual information (option 1) and cannot be answered with a single word (option 2). The family can provide indirect information about the client but is not most likely to provide the most accurate information (option 4). *Cognitive Level*: Analysis *Client Need*: Not Applicable *Nursing Process*: Assessment

5. *Answer*: 4 *Rationale*: Frameworks help the nurse be systematic in data collection. Other members of the health care team may use very different conceptual organizing frameworks so data may not correlate (option 1). Cost-effective care (option 2) is more likely to occur with systematic application of the nursing process, but use of a framework for assessment alone may not accomplish this goal. Because the framework is structured and because of the nature of client needs/problems, creativity and intuition in care planning are not assured (option 3). *Cognitive Level*: Application *Client Need*: Not Applicable *Nursing Process*: Assessment

CHAPTER 12
CRITICAL THINKING POSSIBILITIES

1. Examples would include insomnia; fidgeting; dry mouth; increased pulse, blood pressure, and respirations; and poor attention span.

2. Examples include the uncertainty of his prognosis, lack of knowledge about his condition and its treatment, and fear of pain.

3. *Ineffective Airway Clearance* or *Breathing Pattern*, *Ineffective Coping*, *Spiritual Distress*, *Hopelessness*, (*Readiness in Enhanced Comport*,) *Grieving*.

4. Although this may be a true statement, lung cancer is a medical diagnosis—not a nursing diagnosis, which is a response to health status or a health problem. In addition, the stressor (related to) should be something the nurse can treat independently.

TEST YOUR KNOWLEDGE

1. *Answer*: 2 *Rationale*: In diagnosing, data from assessment (option 1) are analyzed and problems, risks, and strengths are identified before diagnostic statements can be established. Interventions (option 3) are more commonly part of the planning and implementing phases of the nursing process. Cost (option 4) is an important consideration but would be estimated in the planning phase. *Cognitive Level*: Application *Client Need*: Not Applicable *Nursing Process*: Diagnosis

2. *Answer*: 2 *Rationale*: Because the venous return is impaired, fluid is static, resulting in swelling. Therefore, decreased venous return is the cause (etiology) of the problem. *Excess Fluid Volume* is the nursing diagnosis, and edema of the lower extremity is the sign/symptom or critical attribute. The cause is known. *Cognitive Level*: Application *Client Need*: Not Applicable *Nursing Process*: Diagnosis

3. *Answer*: 1 *Rationale*: States the relationship between the stem (caregiver role strain) and the cause of the problem. Option 2: the diagnostic statement says the same thing as the related factor (falls and collapse). Option 3: It is inappropriate to use medical diagnoses such as stroke within a nursing diagnosis statement. Option 4 is vague. The statement must be specific and guide the plan of care (fatigue may be a result of sleep deprivation and does not di-

rect intervention). *Cognitive Level*: Application *Client Need*: Not Applicable *Nursing Process*: Diagnosis

4. *Answer*: 4 *Rationale*: The PES format assists with comprehensive and accurate organization of client data. More efficient planning may or may not reduce health care cost. Nursing diagnostic statements should be confirmed with the client but using PES does not ensure this. PES statements can be wellness or illness focused. *Cognitive Level*: Application *Client Need*: Not Applicable *Nursing Process*: Diagnosis

5. *Answer*: 1 *Rationale*: A collaborative (multidisciplinary) problem is indicated when both medical and nursing interventions are needed to prevent or treat the problem. If nursing care alone (whether that care involves independent or dependent nursing actions) can treat the problem, a nursing diagnosis is indicated. If medical care alone can treat the problem, a medical diagnosis is indicated. *Cognitive Level*: Application *Client Need*: Not Applicable *Nursing Process*: Diagnosis

CHAPTER 13
CRITICAL THINKING POSSIBILITIES

1. The nurse assumes that the standardized care plan is comprehensive enough for this client with the individualization that is applied to it.

2. The last outcome for *Anxiety*, "Freely expressing concerns and possible solutions about work and parenting roles," and the associated interventions are examples because the roles described occur between the client and her family in the home rather than in the hospital setting.

3. Several possibilities exist. The nurse needs to set aside time to discuss the plan with the client, alone or with other family and health care team members. The plan can be presented verbally or in writing. It can be initiated by the nurse who seeks validation from the client. Or the problem list, nursing diagnoses, goals, outcomes, and interventions can be decided on by the client and nurse together after the nurse presents assessment data.

4. If agency guidelines delineate the frequency of nursing interventions and the care plan does not require these more often than specified, no time frame is required. Also, if the intervention is performed during every interaction (e.g., the nurse remains calm and appears confident) no frequency need be written.

5. Nursing diagnoses related to airway are often highest priority since they represent life-threatening conditions. In reassessing priorities, the nurse considers new problems as well as progress toward meeting existing goals. If the airway problem is in the process of improving, other diagnoses may become higher priority.

TEST YOUR KNOWLEDGE

1. *Answer*: 4 *Rationale*: Strategic planning is an ongoing process focused on organizational change rather than individual clients so it is least useful and not relevant in this case. The client requires initial planning since he has just arrived on the orthopedic unit for the first time. Of the three types of planning that need to be done at this time, initial is the highest priority since he has just had surgery. The client also requires the ongoing type of planning necessary to determine the care appropriate for this shift. Discharge planning needs to start on admission to ensure adequate client preparation for management of health needs outside the health agency. *Cognitive Level*: Application *Client Need*: Safe, Effective Care Environment *Nursing Process*: Planning

2. *Answer*: 1 *Rationale*: Policy and procedure documents provide data about how certain situations are handled. Standardized care

plans and standards of care are written for groups of clients with similar medical or nursing diagnoses. They generally do not address questions such as hospital routines and nonmedical client needs. Note: Even hospital policies are not absolute. Each situation must be analyzed and responded to individually. Orthopedic protocols would address elements specifically associated with the surgery, not whether or the family slept in the room. *Cognitive Level*: Application *Client Need*: Psychosocial Integrity *Nursing Process*: Planning

3. *Answer*: 2 *Rationale*: A more detailed assessment data and consultation with the client would be needed to absolutely confirm the priority. Postoperative nausea to the level of inhibiting oral intake has the greatest likelihood of leading to complications and requires nursing intervention now. The client's pain level is not extreme considering the recency of the surgery, and pain intervention can be assumed to be effective. Although the constipation is probably bordering abnormal, nursing intervention would most likely begin with oral treatment, which is not possible due to the nausea. More invasive interventions such as an enema or suppository would not be commonly administered the first day postoperative. Wound infection can occur but there are no data to indicate that this requires a change in the current plan.

4. *Answer*: 3 *Rationale*: The goal or outcome should state the opposite of the nursing diagnosis stem, and thus healthy intact skin is the reverse condition of impaired skin integrity. Turning in bed, applying lotion, and using a special mattress are all interventions that may result in achieving the goal. *Cognitive Level*: Application *Client Need*: Physiological Integrity *Nursing Process*: Planning

5. *Answer*: 3 *Rationale*: Although there may be standard policies or routines for measuring intake and output, the nursing intervention should specify if this is to be done "routinely" or at specific intervals (e.g., q4h). The nurse is also aware, however, that critical thinking indicates that the intake and output should be monitored more frequently than ordered if assessment reveals abnormal findings. *Cognitive Level*: Comprehension *Client Need*: Physiological Integrity *Nursing Process*: Planning

CHAPTER 14

CRITICAL THINKING POSSIBILITIES

1. For *Ineffective Airway Clearance*, the overall outcome is not met. Although the client is able to cough productively, the care plan requires modification and continuation in order to achieve all of the goals. For *Anxiety*, the overall outcome is mostly met. Ongoing assessment and data collection are indicated.

2. Some possibilities are that the interventions have not been adequately implemented (and still are needed) or more time is needed for their effects to be apparent.

3. It might be good to keep the diagnosis so it can be followed in case it reoccurs. On the other hand, the outcomes remaining may be accomplished through plans for other nursing diagnoses (such as respiratory rate) or are ongoing (teaching).

4. Data collected are recorded in the chart on graphic records and nurses' notes (see Chapter 15 ∞).

TEST YOUR KNOWLEDGE

1. *Answer*: 3 *Rationale*: The first step of implementing is reassessing the client to determine that the activity is still indicated and safe. The next action would be to determine if assistance is required, and then implement the intervention (delegating if appro-

priate), and last document the intervention. *Cognitive Level*: Comprehension *Client Need*: Not Applicable *Nursing Process*: Implementation

2. *Answer*: 4 *Rationale*: It is never acceptable practice for the nurse to document a nursing activity before it is carried out. This would be very unsafe because many things can cause an activity to be postponed or canceled and prior charting would be inaccurate, misleading, and potentially dangerous. In a few situations, it may be permissible to chart frequent or routine activities some time following the activities such as at the end of a shift or after a particular interval (e.g., every 4 hours) rather than immediately following the activity. *Cognitive Level*: Application *Client Need*: Not Applicable *Nursing Process*: Implementation

3. *Answer*: 1 *Rationale*: The desired outcomes and indicator statements reflect the parameters by which success will be measured. The goal can be met even if the nursing activities were not carried out or were ineffective. Although the desired outcome, by definition, indicates a change in the client's condition (behavior, knowledge, or attitude), only specific changes (desired outcomes) reflect the success of the care plan. *Cognitive Level*: Comprehension *Client Need*: Not Applicable *Nursing Process*: Evaluation

4. *Answer*: 2 *Rationale*: There is no reason to delete or modify the nursing diagnosis or demote its priority since the risk factors that prompted it are still present. *Cognitive Level*: Analysis *Client Need*: Safe, Effective Care Environment *Nursing Process*: Evaluation

5. *Answer*: 2 *Rationale*: Because this assessment focuses on how care is provided, it is a process evaluation. A structure evaluation would focus on the setting (e.g., how well equipment functions), and outcome evaluations focus on changes in client status (e.g., whether reported satisfaction levels vary with type of person who answers the call light). An audit would be a chart or document review. *Cognitive Level*: Analysis *Client Need*: Not Applicable *Nursing Process*: Evaluation

CHAPTER 15

CRITICAL THINKING POSSIBILITIES

1. No date. Do not know if the hospital policy requires military time. Showed assumption and bias with use of the term "complainer." Not complete (e.g., what did the nurse listen to . . . would that information be helpful in the care of the client? Were the BPs taken in two different positions or two different times?). No information as to why the client refused lunch. Another assumption that client fell out of bed . . . did the nurse see it or walk in and find the client lying on the floor? No evidence of using the nursing process as a framework for documentation.

2. Use the nursing process as a framework. Document assessment findings that relate to the defining characteristics of pain. Chart those interventions that were done to help relieve the pain. Document the client's response to those interventions. If any teaching was done, be sure to document what the teaching was and the client's response.

3. 6/6/03 #1 Pain

   S: "sharp, stabbing pain in lower back that radiates to left leg"

   States pain is 8 out of 10

   "I didn't sleep last night"

   "I feel better" (after interventions)

   O: BP 210/90, P. 72, R. 18

Last medicated 5 hours previously

Medicated with ordered analgesic

Heating pad applied to lower back

Positioned on side with pillows behind back

A: Continues to need narcotic medication to progress toward goal of pain relief

P: Add to plan of care to offer analgesic around the clock q4hr versus Prn

4. 6/6/03 Pain

D: "sharp, stabbing pain in lower back that radiates to left leg"

States pain is 8 out of 10

"I didn't sleep last night"

BP 210/90, P. 72, R. 18

Last medicated 5 hours previously

Continues to need narcotic medication to progress toward goal of pain relief

A: Medicated with ordered analgesic

Heating pad applied to lower back

Positioned on side with pillows behind back

Add to plan of care to offer analgesic around the clock q4hr versus Prn

R: "I feel better" (after interventions)

TEST YOUR KNOWLEDGE

1. *Answer*: 3 *Rationale*: All of the other answers endanger the client's confidentiality. *Cognitive Level*: Application *Client Need*: Safe, Effective Care Environment *Nursing Process*: Implementation

2. *Answer*: 1 *Rationale*: Critical pathways work best for clients with one diagnosis. Option 2 is a possibility; however, there may be many individualized needs. Because that information is not available, the best answer is 1. Options 3 and 4 have too many diagnoses to work well with a critical pathway. *Cognitive Level*: Application *Client Need*: Safe, Effective Care Environment *Nursing Process*: Assessment

3. *Answer*: 4 *Rationale*: It is the most complete answer. The client's record is a legal record and should not be altered with correcting liquid. You may see "error" written above a mistake even though many authors suggest not writing it. It is important to also put your name or initials next to the words of the mistaken entry. *Cognitive Level*: Application *Client Need*: Safe, Effective Care Environment *Nursing Process*: Implementation

4. *Answer*: 4 *Rationale*: 4 is the "best" answer although it could be more complete by adding the response of the primary care provider. Option 1 is too vague because it is not clear if the nurse found the client or was present when the client fell. Also, there is no need to write the word *client* because it is the client's chart. Option 2 is judgmental revealing a negative attitude toward the person. It would be better to describe specific signs and symptoms such as staggering, slurred speech, and smell of alcohol on breath. Option 3 is too general and can be more specific by charting "2 cm × 3 cm purplish bruise on mid-inner thigh along with color." *Cognitive Level*: Analysis *Client Need*: Safe, Effective Care Environment *Nursing Process*: Evaluation

5. *Answer*: 1. No known allergies; 2. Bathroom privileges; 3. When necessary; 4. Diet as tolerated. *Cognitive Level*: Knowledge *Client Need*: Safe, Effective Care Environment *Nursing Process*: Implementation

6. *Answer*: 2 *Rationale*: The graphic record provides the trend of the vital signs. Option 1, verbal information, is not appropriate for validation assessment that is measurable. This is more appropriate for pain or dizziness. The medication record would not include documentation of blood pressure ranges (option 3). The progress notes (option 4) provide information about how the client is progressing. It may have information about the client's BP if it was a problem. The best answer is option 2. *Cognitive Level*: Application *Client Need*: Safe, Effective Care Environment *Nursing Process*: Assessment

7. *Answer*: 1, 2, and 4 *Rationale*: Option 3 is incorrect as it could be a HIPAA violation if others hear health protected information. Option 5 is not needed unless it is a concern and it would not be done for every client. *Cognitive Level*: Analysis *Client Need*: Safe, Effective Care Environment *Nursing Process*: Implementation

8. *Answer*: 2, 3 and 5 *Rationale*: Option 1: MS is on the "Do Not Use" list—the nurse needs to write out morphine sulfate. Option 4 has three errors—should not have a trailing zero after the decimal point; u and SQ are on the "Do Not Use" list. *Cognitive Level*: Analysis *Client Need*: Safe, Effective Care Environment *Nursing Process*: Implementation

9. *Answer*: 1 *Rationale*: 1 is the most specific, nonassuming, and nonjudgmental charting. Option 2 could be more specific by describing the lesions and not calling them "burns." Option 3 is making a judgment of elder abuse, and option 4 is also making an assumption that the lesions are from cigarette burns. *Cognitive Level*: Analysis *Client Need*: Safe, Effective Care Environment *Nursing Process*: Evaluation

10. *Answer*: 1, 2, and 4 *Rationale*: Military time is commonly used; documenting worries or concerns provides clues to other nurses; gossip, unprofessional comments or thoughts, or personnel issues should not be recorded in the client's chart. Option 3 is incorrect as charting should be done as events occur. Waiting till the end of the shift increases the chance of forgetting something. *Cognitive Level*: Application *Client Need*: Safe, Effective Care Environment *Nursing Process*: Implementation

CHAPTER 16
CRITICAL THINKING POSSIBILITIES

1. Key points to remember include, but are not limited to, the following:
   - Active listening is very important because it strengthens the rapport between the client and nurse. Careful listening can help check your understanding of what the client is saying or meaning with the responses.
   - It is important to emphasize that the client has personal choice and control. The client should decide what behavior, if any, to focus on.
   - Readiness to change, including importance and confidence, needs to be continually assessed.
   - It is not unusual for individuals to recycle through the stages of change.

2. Questions to consider include these:
   - "Take me through a typical day in your life and tell me where your [behavior] fits in."
   - "You have mentioned smoking, exercise, food, and losing weight. Would you like to talk about one of these topics or is there something else you would prefer to talk about?" (This gives clients the opportunity to choose the topic most important to them at the time.)

- "Which of these behaviors do you feel most ready to think about changing?"
- "Sometimes it can be helpful to examine the pros and cons of [behavior]—would this be helpful?"
- "What concerns you the most about [behavior]?"
- "Would you like to know more about [behavior]?"
- "How do you see the connection between [behavior] and [behavior]?"

3. Mr. W. is in the contemplation stage, because he wonders about changing and is willing to discuss it. Contemplators want to change; however, at the same time, they have a resistance to change. Consciousness raising is important during this stage. Find out if the client wants more information. Assist the client to increase his awareness of the behavior—why does he want to change, the pros and cons of changing, and so on.

TEST YOUR KNOWLEDGE

1. *Answer*: 3 *Rationale*: Holism implies consideration of all aspects of the client's life. Although arranging for home care, facilitating spirituality, and offering coping resources may be appropriate, the nurse begins a holistic approach to care by examining, with the client, in what ways the illness influences the various segments of her life. The client is the best source of information regarding personal needs. Assessment should always precede intervention. *Cognitive Level*: Application *Client Need*: Psychosocial Integrity *Nursing Process*: Implementation

2. *Answer*: 4 *Rationale*: Child's behavior results in a change in the father's behavior. It is considered feedback. It is also a type of negative feedback in that, the more the child cries, the less the father leaves. In some ways, the child's behavior is also input because it is used by the father in making a decision (throughput). *Cognitive Level*: Application *Client Need*: Health Promotion/Maintenance and Psychosocial Integrity *Nursing Process*: Assessment

3. *Answer*: 2 *Rationale*: Choices are often related to learned experiences, lifestyle, and values. The client obviously values the business more than physical health. When a person feels strongly enough, a lower level need (rest) can be postponed until a higher level need (success, safety) is met. It is very likely that no one else can meet that need for him and the lower need must still be met eventually. *Cognitive Level*: Application *Client Need*: Health Promotion and Maintenance *Nursing Process*: Assessment

4. *Answer*: 3 *Rationale*: A person in this stage recognizes there is a problem, is seriously considering changing, actively gathers information, and verbalizes plans to change in the near future. Option 1 reflects the precontemplation stage in which the person denies there is a problem. Option 2 reflects the planning stage in which the person makes final plans to accomplish the change, and option 4 is the maintenance stage in which the person made the change and demonstrates the appropriate behavioral change. *Cognitive Level*: Analysis *Client Need*: Health Promotion and Maintenance *Nursing Process*: Assessment

5. *Answer*: 2 *Rationale*: Perceived self-efficacy is the confidence the person has for achieving the desired outcome. Option 1 is a person's perceptions about available time, inconvenience, expense, and difficulty performing the activity. Option 3 is the person's perceptions concerning the behaviors, beliefs, or attitudes of others. Option 4 refers to the person's perception of the environment and how it assists or detracts from the healthy behavior. *Cognitive Level*: Application *Client Need*: Health Promotion and Maintenance *Nursing Process*: Planning

6. *Answer*: 4 *Rationale*: See Box 16–8. ∞ The death of a spouse is a score of 100 on the Life-Change Index by Holmes and Rahe (1967). Option 1 is a score of 50, option 2 is a score of 47, and option 3 is a score of 26. *Cognitive Level*: Analysis *Client Need*: Health Promotion and Maintenance *Nursing Process*: Assessment

7. *Answer*: 1 *Rationale*: Option 2 is a strategy for the contemplation stage, option 3 is a strategy for the preparation stage, and option 4 is a strategy for the maintenance stage. *Cognitive Level*: Application *Client Need*: Health Promotion and Maintenance *Nursing Process*: Implementation

8. *Answer*: 4 *Rationale*: Change is a complex process and a nurse should not give up or assume that the client doesn't want to change. People often resist a tough approach because it can make them feel cornered. This approach may work for some people but not for everyone. The goal of teaching is to try to help the client become the expert as well. *Cognitive Level*: Application *Client Need*: Health Promotion and Maintenance *Nursing Process*: Implementation

9. *Answer*: 1 *Rationale*: The compensatory mechanism of increasing the heart rate is the body's way of trying to balance an ineffective cardiac output since the BP has decreased. Decompensation (option 2) occurs when the compensatory mechanism is ineffective. Self-regulation (option 3) refers to the homeostatic mechanisms that come into play automatically in the healthy person. Equilibrium (option 4) is balance through adaptation to the environment. *Cognitive Level*: Application *Client Need*: Health Promotion and Maintenance *Nursing Process*: Assessment

10. *Answer*: 3 *Rationale*: Option 1 is a physiological need. Option 2 is a love and belonging need, and option 4 is a safety and security need. *Cognitive Level*: Analysis *Client Need*: Health Promotion and Maintenance *Nursing Process*: Assessment

CHAPTER 17

CRITICAL THINKING POSSIBILITIES

1. Jerry has a positive outlook and views himself as "well" while Joe has a negative outlook and views himself as "ill." Identify and compare data indicating the psychologic dimension (self-concept, mind–body interactions, and emotional response to health) for both clients. Speculate about how their differences in perception may affect their continuing recovery process.

2. Jerry is most likely an "internal" because he has taken charge of his own health by changing his diet, initiating an exercise program, and attempting to lower his stress. Joe is more likely an "external" because he has been unable to take control of his health. Joe may believe that his health is largely controlled by outside forces and is beyond his control.

3. At least one external factor is Jerry's physician's advice. Another may come from his work environment colleagues.

4. Joe's perception of his illness, and thus his ability to respond in a positive manner, may be affected by a family history of heart disease and his perception that he is at high risk and there is nothing he can do to change his pattern of health.

- Joe's perceived barriers to action (cost, time, lack of social support).
- Perhaps the benefit of assuming the sick role outweighs the benefit of recovery.

5. Verifying that Joe values the planned outcome achieved from smoking cessation; verifying Joe's knowledge about the effects of smoking and providing needed information or correcting miscon-

ceptions; demonstrating genuine concern for Joe and positively reinforcing positive changes that he does make; allowing Joe to make his own decisions, thereby demonstrating trust and respect. Many other interventions are possible.

TEST YOUR KNOWLEDGE

1. *Answer*: 3 *Rationale*: Frustration is an example of an emotion. The client who chooses healthy foods (option 1) represents the physical component, taking parenting classes enhances the intellectual component (option 2), and the bowling league (option 4) enhances both the physical and social components. *Cognitive Level*: Comprehension *Client Need*: Health Promotion and Maintenance *Nursing Process*: Assessment

2. *Answer*: 2 *Rationale*: The mother has taken on the sick role by expecting to be excused from her usual role responsibilities. The sick role states that persons are not answerable for their illness, contrary to the obese client's perspective. In the sick role, the client tries to get better as opposed to the man who misses his physical therapy appointments. The elder is not following the sick role expectation to rely on competent help. *Cognitive Level*: Application *Client Need*: Health Promotion and Maintenance, and Physiological Adaptation *Nursing Process*: Assessment

3. *Answer*: 1 *Rationale*: The behavior is most representative of health promotion, which is the central focus of the health belief model. The clinical model focuses on relieving signs and symptoms of illness. The role performance model emphasizes social activities such as fulfilling a particular role. The agent–host–environment model focuses on predicting illness. *Cognitive Level*: Analysis *Client Need*: Health Promotion and Maintenance *Nursing Process*: Analysis

4. *Answer*: 2, 3, and 4 *Rationale*: Significant evidence exists that a trusting relationship with the provider, effectiveness of the medication, and a less complex dosing regime are important predictors of adherence with the medical regimen. Neither education nor gender has been shown to be a predictive factor. *Cognitive Level*: Application *Client Need*: Health Promotion and Maintenance *Nursing Process*: Planning

5. *Answer*: 1 *Rationale*: Although not always practical, direct observation is the best method to measure adherence (for example, watching heroin addicts actually take their methadone dose). Since lack of adherence may be life threatening or damaging to the client as well as others, waiting until the client displays illness or until laboratory values reflect lack of adherence are not the best methods. Client report or recall is not always accurate, even if the client believes he or she is telling the truth. *Cognitive Level*: Analysis *Client Need*: Health Promotion and Maintenance *Nursing Process*: Evaluation

CHAPTER 18

CRITICAL THINKING POSSIBILITIES

1. Rachel's culture (values, beliefs, norms, and life practices that guide thinking, decisions, and actions) is mixed and can be referred to as bicultural because she has integrated practices and values from both her mother and father who were of different backgrounds.
   - Rachel's ethnicity (consciousness of belonging to a group that is differentiated from others by symbolic markers) is most strongly associated with her Jewish background as evidenced by her return to the Jewish religion as an adult and by her obvious connection with this group.
   - Rachel's race (shared biologic characteristics, genetic markers, or features) is unknown since we do not know the race of her parents. Jewish persons who come from similar national origins (e.g., Eastern Europe or the Middle East) may share racial traits.

2. Cultural values often determine the roles of family members, their interactions, who has authority to make decisions on the client's behalf, and family involvement in the client's care. Without clear guidelines on the cultural practices Rachel adheres to, it may be difficult to provide culturally sensitive care.

3. Rachel's beliefs and values will strongly affect her approach to death and the way her family reacts toward her before and during the death process.
   - Rachel's culture may dictate her choice of dying with family members present, rites, or rituals to be performed, and the degree of knowledge she wishes about the dying process.
   - Rachel's religion is likely to strongly influence the care of her body after death and burial procedures.

4. A cultural assessment is particularly important at this time in Rachel's life so that her death can be congruent with her beliefs and traditions. It is also important to determine her primary support systems, to preserve her preferences, and to offer support to Rachel and her family in culturally acceptable ways.

5. All aspects of client care are influenced by the nurses' and the clients' cultures. When the beliefs are different, misunderstandings can occur, the relationship can suffer, and client outcomes may be adversely affected. Self-awareness can enable nurses to successfully cope with client practices they themselves might not believe in or value.

TEST YOUR KNOWLEDGE

1. *Answer*: 3 *Rationale*: There is an ongoing shift in the North American population which includes a decreasing number of Caucasian Americans (formerly the majority population) and increasing numbers of other cultural groups. The birth rate is actually decreasing, immigration has increased, and limited access to health care is a complex issue that is not the major factor here. *Cognitive Level*: Comprehension *Client Need*: Psychosocial Integrity *Nursing Process*: Not Applicable

2. *Answer*: 2 *Rationale*: Cultural differences may result in various interpretations of a medical regime. Cultural sensitivity results in recognition of the right "not to fit." This is a standard of practice and should be initiated with all clients. Teaching or explaining the effects of lack of adherence would be more appropriate than warning. Asking a person of the same culture to assist may be helpful after the nurse discusses the matter with the client. *Cognitive Level*: Application *Client Need*: Psychosocial Integrity *Nursing Process*: Not Applicable

3. *Answer*: 3 *Rationale*: The nurse should indicate that he or she is open to diverse views and practices. Option 1 assumes the client follows this particular cultural practice, which may not be the case. The nurse should assess before intervening. It may be good to learn more about the culture (option 2), but that is not the best starting place to care for the client. Subcultures exist among all cultures. Reading books is helpful, but assessment of individual situations is the best approach. Option 4 reflects an incorrect approach to culturally appropriate care. The nurse needs to assess which customs and practices the individual client performs before drawing conclusions. *Cognitive Level*: Application *Client Need*: Psychosocial Integrity *Nursing Process*: Not Applicable

4. *Answer*: 3 *Rationale*: Culturally competent implies that, within the delivered care, the nurse understands and attends to the total

context of the client's situation, including awareness of immigration, stress factors, and cultural differences. Options 1 and 2 do not show that the nurse needs to respect the choices made by the clients. Option 4 shows bias or stereotyping. *Cognitive Level*: Application *Client Need*: Psychosocial Integrity *Nursing Process*: Not Applicable

5. *Answer*: 3 *Rationale*: Culture involves socially inherited characteristics of a group. Race usually addresses shared physical characteristics among a group of individuals. *Cognitive Level*: Comprehension *Client Need*: Psychosocial Integrity *Nursing Process*: Not Applicable

CHAPTER 19

CRITICAL THINKING POSSIBILITIES

1. Tim's name suggests that he may be of Asian descent (and cancer of the stomach is more common in Asian populations than in some other ethnic groups). Tim's parents do not speak English and this suggests that they are not from a North American culture. Many Asian people use CAM as a regular part of their health activities. Tim's gastric cancer appears to be quite serious. Often, cancer clients whose disease is not responding to conventional therapy seek CAM to treat the disease or to cope with symptoms.

2. Certainly, touch, biofeedback, prayer, music, meditation, and similar CAM therapies might help Tim's ability to cope with his pain and even increase his nutritional intake. There may also be herbs, homeopathic, and TCM products that are safe to use with his Western therapy although the nurse must investigate these carefully. Where would you look for this information?

3. The nurse may ignore finding the bags of "tea," but there is a risk that the substance could be contraindicated with other medications Tim currently takes. The nurse can ask Tim or his wife what is in the bags and determine the safety of their use.

4. If the nurse is strongly in favor of or opposed to CAM, this may color interactions with the client and family. The nurse should review these biases and ensure that he or she can still provide professional care considering personal perspectives. The nurse should be open-minded to hearing the client's beliefs and supporting the client's right to act in accordance with his beliefs.

TEST YOUR KNOWLEDGE

1. *Answer*: 3 *Rationale*: Although the effectiveness of alternative therapies is sometimes not scientifically established, many people report significant benefit from them for a wide variety of conditions. Alternative therapies often cost less, but this is not a primary consideration. Clients often seek alternative therapies because traditional therapies are ineffective, but this is not the primary difference. Both traditional therapies utilize products from nature. *Cognitive Level*: Application *Client Need*: Physiological Integrity *Nursing Process*: Not Applicable

2. *Answer*: 1 *Rationale*: Spirituality gives us purpose and meaning in life; involves a relationship with oneself, others, and a higher power; and involves finding significant meaning in the entirety of life. Spirituality is a much broader concept than religion and religious services. Responsibility to life patterns is a concept of humanism. *Cognitive Level*: Application *Client Need*: Psychological Integrity *Nursing Process*: Not Applicable

3. *Answer*: 2 *Rationale*: Healing environments help empower clients to make healthy decisions. They are not dependent on technology or physicians' orders. Aquariums are environmental interventions, not a general approach to clients. *Cognitive Level*:

Application *Client Need*: Health Promotion and Maintenance, and Psychosocial Integrity *Nursing Process*: Implementation

4. *Answer*: 4 *Rationale*: Naturopathy focuses on the total person. The primary focus is disease prevention. Naturopathy may be the best choice in decreasing disease rates by empowering and educating people about ways to stay healthy. Belief in a higher being is not a core principle. *Cognitive Level*: Analysis *Client Need*: Health Promotion and Maintenance *Nursing Process*: Not Applicable

5. *Answer*: 2 *Rationale*: Qi is the flow of energy in the body that must be uninterrupted for a person to be in a healthy state. All the other imbalances may result from an imbalance in the flow of qi or flow of vital energy through specific anatomical points along the surface of the body. *Cognitive Level*: Comprehension *Client Need*: Health Promotion and Maintenance *Nursing Process*: Not Applicable

CHAPTER 20

CRITICAL THINKING POSSIBILITIES

1. Chloe is in early adolescence. She is entering Erikson's stage of identity versus role confusion, in which she will develop a stronger, more well-defined sense of self, especially as she relates to others around her. In this process she will explore future goals, experiment with looks and manners, practice different social roles (e.g., dating, volunteering for social service agencies, baby-sitting and child care), and increase her cognitive and intellectual capacity.

2. She appears to be a shy, quiet individual and is likely to acquiesce to her mother's demand and allow her to be present for the exam. However, doing so may cause feelings of confusion, embarrassment, or even resentment.

3. Chloe appears to have a slow-to-warm up, sensitive temperament. Evaluation of temperament cannot be made on the basis of one observation alone, and further discussion and interaction with Chloe and her mother, plus observation of Chloe's behavior in different settings, would allow for a more definitive judgment.

TEST YOUR KNOWLEDGE

1. *Answer*: 3 *Rationale*: The sequence of each stage of development is predictable, although the time of onset, the length of the stage, and the effects of each stage vary with the person. *Cognitive Level*: Application *Client Need*: Health Promotion and Maintenance *Nursing Process*: Implementation

2. *Answer*: 4 *Rationale*: The study of growth (physical) and development (function and skills) is correct because the answer needs to have both components to be complete. Option 1 addresses only the growth aspects. Option 2 addresses only developmental aspects, and option 3 addresses only the environmental factors that might influence growth and development. *Cognitive Level*: Knowledge *Client Need*: Health Promotion and Maintenance *Nursing Process*: Assessment

3. *Answer*: 3 *Rationale*: Toddlers typically demonstrate negative behavior and are hesitant around strangers, resisting close contact with people they do not know well. They do not have sophisticated language skills and often use crying or fussing to communicate. Older school-age children and adolescents are likely to cooperate without complaint in many health procedures (option 1). School-age children, engaged in the task of industry versus inferiority, display curiosity about how things work, asking many questions of nurses (option 2). Preschool-age children, who are in a stage of fantasy, curiosity, and exploration, like to manipulate

objects and play "pretend" (option 4). *Cognitive Level*: Analysis *Client Need*: Health Promotion and Maintenance *Nursing Process*: Planning

4. *Answer*: 4 *Rationale*: Adolescents need to establish identity, which involves developing a more mature sense of independence and responsibility. Providing her with school work keeps her connected to her peer group and gives a sense of accomplishment. Also, it prevents the client from "worrying" about getting behind in school assignments. Interaction with peers is very important during this stage, but they are likely to be attending school during the day (option 1); an infant's sense of trust is reinforced if parents room-in, and older infants and toddlers experience less separation anxiety if parents are nearby (option 2); and preschool and school-age children would benefit from the distraction and social interaction of others in the recreation room (option 3). *Cognitive Level*: Application *Client Need*: Health Promotion and Maintenance *Nursing Process*: Implementation

5. *Answer*: 2 *Rationale*: The client is in Erikson's stage of integrity versus despair. Finding meaning and purpose in his life after retirement is a sign of achievement. His comments regarding visits to his family and being asked by friends to help with their projects indicate that he is actively involved and purposeful (options 1 and 4). His comment regarding needing medication for knee pain can be expected in many older people, especially those who have been laborers or suffered injury when younger (option 3). *Cognitive Level*: Analysis *Client Need*: Health Promotion and Maintenance *Nursing Process*: Evaluation

6. *Answer*: 2 *Rationale*: This stage includes the preadolescent period. The peer group increasingly influences behavior. Physical, cognitive, and social development increases and communication skills improve. One needs to allow time and energy for the school-age child to pursue hobbies and school activities and to recognize and support the child's achievement. Option 1 is a judgmental statement as this is not unusual and not indicative of problems in the home. It is good to be supportive of the school-age child; however, making her stay home with her family might cause anger and resentment (option 3). Option 4 is also a judgmental statement. Even though this is normal development, calling the father "silly" is not therapeutic communication. *Cognitive Level*: Application *Client Need*: Health Promotion and Maintenance *Nursing Process*: Implementation

7. *Answer*: 2 *Rationale*: Erikson's late childhood stage focuses on initiative versus guilt. During this stage, the children are beginning to have the ability to evaluate one's own behavior and are learning the degree to which assertiveness and purpose influence the environment. Option 1 is incorrect because Fowler's focus is spiritual development. Both options 3 and 4 are adult theorists. *Cognitive Level*: Application *Client Need*: Health Promotion and Maintenance *Nursing Process*: Planning

8. *Answer*: 1 *Rationale*: Piaget identifies this phase as the intuitive thought phase with the significant behaviors as: egocentric thinking diminishes, thinks of one idea at a time, includes others in the environment, words express thoughts. Erikson identifies this developmental stage as industry versus inferiority, and the children are learning the degree to which assertiveness and purpose influence the environment. They have the beginning ability to evaluate their own behavior. Fowler identifies this stage as intuitive-projective, a combination of images and beliefs given by trusted others, mixed with the child's own experience and imagination. Therefore, the nurse knows that this child has a normal imagination and needs to explore and learn about this new

piece of equipment in language appropriate to his age. For option 2, imagination is normal for this age group, and stating that he needs to be "a big boy" is counterproductive. Option 3 is incorrect because his language skills are developing and he needs to understand the world around him. Option 4 is incorrect because adding to his fears will only increase his anxiety level and decrease his trust in you as a nurse. *Cognitive Level*: Application *Client Need*: Health Promotion and Maintenance *Nursing Process*: Implementation

CHAPTER 21

CRITICAL THINKING POSSIBILITIES

1. Sean is at Erikson's stage of initiative versus guilt. He is learning what he is capable of doing and should be given opportunities to explore, play with, and successfully master his environment.

2. Sean's cringing behavior is of concern. That, combined with the fact that he is very quiet and does not resist or protest, may be an indication that he feels fearful but has learned that resistance is not effective. A "typical" 3-year-old would be likely to cry aggressively with pain; be frightened of nurses or doctors, resist treatment, and seek comfort from a parent.

3. The presence of multiple bruises in various stages of healing on the torso and buttocks is suspicious. Most bruising in children at this age is on the extremities and/or head from falls and bumping into things. The story that Sean injured his arm and shoulder by falling out of bed is also suspicious. A fall from the upper bunk of a bed would not typically fracture a bone or cause a dislocation. If the history of how the injury occurred is not consistent with the severity of the injury, one should be suspicious of child abuse.

4. As a mandatory reporter, the nurse must report suspected child abuse to the proper authorities. Based on the report, an investigation may be made to determine if the child is in danger, and what, if any, intervention should be taken. In the emergency department, additional assessment information should be collected both directly (e.g., asking Sean's mother questions about family dynamics, how the child is disciplined, what stressors the family is under) and by observation (e.g., what attitude does the mother demonstrate toward the child, how does the child respond to the mother). Reporting can be done anonymously, or the mother could be informed that a report will be made. Some families resent and are threatened by the possibility of an investigation. If aware that a report will be made, they may "run" (i.e., flee the area so they cannot be located). This is a difficult problem, and the nurse must keep in mind that the outcome goals are first and foremost the safety of the child. In addition, the "cause" of abuse must be addressed, with goals of reducing stressors on the family, developing successful coping skills, educating families about child development and appropriate discipline, and, ideally, creating positive family systems.

TEST YOUR KNOWLEDGE

1. *Answer*: 4 *Rationale*: Providing opportunities for the parent to express worries and discuss facts about SIDS gives more control over the situation. The nurse can also provide her with information about the Back to Sleep campaign. Option 1: The highest incidence of SIDS occurs between 2 and 4 months of age, but it does occur in older infants. It is not the best response because it provides facts but does not address the parent's immediate concerns. Option 2: SIDS affects boys more than girls. However, information is likely to increase anxiety and does not address the concerns of the parent. Option 3: There is no known cause of

SIDS, although respiratory problems may be present in some infants. This response is insensitive to the needs of the mother. *Cognitive Level*: Application *Client Need*: Psychosocial Integrity *Nursing Process*: Implementation

2. *Answer*: 3 *Rationale*: Preschool-age children use fantasy and make-believe to learn about, understand, and master their environment, including their concepts of death. The child's conceptualization of death is consistent with her cognitive development. The response in option 1 negates the child's understanding and limits her ability to develop fuller understanding and adapt to the loss. Option 2 negates the child's attempts to understand and deal with the loss. Option 4 is incorrect because at 4 years of age, children can hear explanations such as "when people get old they will die" but these children do not have a firm grasp of the meaning of time and age, and probably will not understand. *Cognitive Level*: Application *Client Need*: Health Promotion and Maintenance, and Psychosocial Integrity *Nursing Process*: Implementation

3. *Answer*: 1 *Rationale*: It is the responsibility of adults to supervise children constantly and closely when around water. Option 2, learning water safety and how to swim, is important and should be encouraged at an early age, but that still does not ensure a child's safety. Option 3 is incorrect because young children are at risk near any amount of water that can cover the nose and mouth. With option 4, infants and toddlers can drown in a very small amount of water, even several inches in a bathtub or "kiddie pool." *Cognitive Level*: Application *Client Need*: Safe, Effective Care Environment, and Health Promotion and Maintenance *Nursing Process*: Planning

4. *Answer*: 2 *Rationale*: Children begin shedding teeth at about age 6 to 7 years and continue through the school-age years. Option 1: Birth weight triples by about 12 months. Children enter school age weighing about 45 pounds and gain about 5 to 7 pounds per year. Option 3: There is significant physical change during the school-age years. Option 4: Fat deposits do not normally appear until puberty. *Cognitive Level*: Comprehension *Client Need*: Health Promotion and Maintenance *Nursing Process*: Assessment

5. *Answer*: 1 *Rationale*: Increased fat deposits are normal as girls begin hormonal changes of puberty. During this stage of development, females become very sensitive about their appearance and need reassurance. Option 2: Puberty is a period when children become more self-conscious of their appearance. They need to be reassured that normal weight gain and body changes with fat deposits are to be expected. The nurse would need to perform further individual assessments before determining a weight problem existed. Option 3: Regular strenuous exercise should be a part of the healthy adolescent's lifestyle, but its goal should be to provide energy and strength, not to control weight. Option 4: Dieting and efforts to lose weight can threaten the health of adolescents. This intervention lacks scientific evidence. Unless an actual or potential disease process exists, a balanced diet is most appropriate. *Cognitive Level*: Application *Client Need*: Health Promotion and Maintenance *Nursing Process*: Planning

6. *Answer*: 2 *Rationale*: Many newborn babies have a misshapen head because of the molding made possible by fontanels in the bone structure of the skull and overriding of the sutures. This asymmetry is usually corrected within the first 7 to 10 days. Option 1: The client is crying and upset; the nurse's response needs to be more sensitive and caring. Option 3: Educational materials are not appropriate for a client who is crying and emotionally upset. Option 4: The client is concerned about the misshapen head right now. The most appropriate intervention should focus on relieving the current emotional state. *Cognitive Level*: Application *Client Need*: Psychosocial Integrity *Nursing Process*: Implementation

7. *Answer*: 1 *Rationale*: Although toddlers like to explore the environment, they always need to have a significant person nearby. Parents need to know that young children experience acute separation anxiety and that abandonment is their greatest fear. Option 2: This is normal toddler development. Option 3: Child is probably not old enough to perform manipulative type strategies. Option 4: This is normal behavior for this age group. *Cognitive Level*: Application *Client Need*: Health Promotion and Maintenance *Nursing Process*: Assessment

8. *Answer*: 3 *Rationale*: The child can perform regular activities as long as the injury arm and the cast are not placed in jeopardy. Option 1: A competent nurse could answer this question. Option 2: A 5-year-old needs to be physically active. This would be more appropriate for health problems in which moving about could prevent healing or cause injury. Limiting a preschooler to only sitting activities is unrealistic. Option 4: Riding a bike and jumping rope could place the client at risk for injury. *Cognitive Level*: Application *Client Need*: Health Promotion and Maintenance *Nursing Process*: Implementation

9. *Answer*: 1 *Rationale*: During the phase of concrete operations, children change from egocentric interactions to cooperative interactions. They also develop an increased understanding of concepts that are associated with specific objects. They learn to add and subtract and understand cause-and-effect relationships. Option 2 action is indicative of the preconceptual phase—an egocentric approach that uses magical thinking. Option 3 action is indicative of the formal operations phase—reasoning is deductive and futuristic. Option 4 is indicative of physical growth. *Cognitive Level*: Application *Client Need*: Health Promotion and Maintenance *Nursing Process*: Assessment

10. *Answer*: 1 *Rationale*: Often the first noticeable sign of puberty in females is the appearance of the breast bud, although the appearance of hair along the labia may precede this. Option 2: The growth spurt in girls is between ages 10 and 14, but is too vague to be noticeable. Option 3: The eccrine glands are found over most of the body and produce sweat. The apocrine glands develop in the axillae, anal and genital areas, external auditory canals, and around the umbilicus and the areola of the breasts. Option 4: Mood swings are not as definitive as physical changes. *Cognitive Level*: Analysis *Client Need*: Health Promotion and Maintenance *Nursing Process*: Assessment

CHAPTER 22

CRITICAL THINKING POSSIBILITIES

1. Health promotion for the young, or emerging, adult should include a comprehensive health assessment (including physical exam) at least every 5 years. Mr. Jones stated he had not seen a health care provider since high school. The nurse should attempt to get the name of the previous provider, and ask if Mr. Jones has participated in any workplace health fairs or screenings, such as blood pressure, hearing, or blood glucose. Young adults need regular dental care, so the nurse should ask Mr. Jones when he last saw a dentist, what took place at the visit, and if he has another visit scheduled. If he does not, the nurse can suggest he sets up dental appointments for every 6 months, and may supply him with the names and phone numbers of local dentists if Mr. Jones does not have a regular source of dental care.

Several aspects of Mr. Jones's occupation put him at risk for injury and/or illness, so it is important to ask how he manages these threats. Particularly, his work exposes him to noise, sun, and falls. He should be asked about use of sunscreen, ear protection, and hard hat. Exercise is not a major concern if he is engaged in strenuous physical labor on his job, but he should be asked about nutrient and water intake. It is important that he take in adequate amounts of protein, iron, fruits, and vegetables. His fluid intake should be at LEAST 64 ounces per day, more if he is perspiring heavily.

Mr. Jones has made several comments that bear further discussion in relation to his health promotion. His intake of alcohol should be investigated for the amount and frequency of intake, as well as signs of alcohol abuse. He should also be asked about the use of a designated driver, or other strategy for travel when he has been using alcohol. His statement about "chasing women" should also be followed up on. He may be at risk for STIs (see below) and should be referred for STI testing and treatment. His ability to form mature and intimate relationships should also be investigated.

2. Sexual activity is a risk factor for STIs. If Mr. Jones is sexually active, the nurse should explain the rationale for asking questions that he may find embarrassing or intrusive. In a nonjudgmental manner, the nurse should ask the age at which Mr. Jones became sexually active, how many sexual partners he has had, and whether the partners have been men, women, or both. He should also be asked how many partners he currently has, and if he has engaged in oral or anal sex. Mr. Jones should be asked if he uses condoms with every sexual activity. The nurse should be careful not to lead Mr. Jones into a politically correct answer, so might ask "How often do you use condoms?" The nurse should then ask him to explain how he applies the condom, and instruct him on correct technique, if needed.

The nurse is promoting safe sexual practices. If the nurse identifies high-risk sexual behaviors that place Mr. Jones at risk for having an STI, the nurse needs to refer him for testing and possible treatment.

3. Young adults are typically very healthy, and the health risks they are exposed to are primarily from behavior. In addition, health problems in middle and old age may be prevented by health habits started now, and Mr. Jones should be advised of this fact.

Violence and substance abuse are major threats to the health of young adults. Mr. Jones should be asked if he feels safe at work and home, and if he has firearms in his possession. The presence of a gun in the home is strongly correlated with accidental injury and suicide. The risk of injury increases if alcohol or other substances are abused, so these practices are important to query. Tobacco, although not usually a cause of imminent injury, may precipitate health problems, particularly respiratory ones, later in life. Risks for STI and alcohol-related motor vehicle accidents have been discussed in #1 and #2, above. Finally, Mr. Jones should be apprised of the heightened risk for suicide in young adults. He should be asked about suicidal ideation (particularly given his accident at work) and be given the telephone number of a suicide prevention hotline, if appropriate.

4. Young adults should have a comprehensive physical exam at least every 5 years, with testicular exam, hearing and vision assessment, blood pressure and cholesterol measurement, tuberculin test, and administration of needed immunizations. Monthly testicular self-exam is no longer recommended (ACS, 2005), and nurses do not need to teach this skill to men, unless the client specifically asks for this information. Even then, the nurse may explain that this self-exam does not improve health outcomes (USPSTF, 2004). Since Mr. Jones has not seen a health care provider in several years, by his report, it is important to conduct all these assessments today, including the testicular examination. The American Cancer Society recommends that a testicular exam be a part of the annual physical exam. His work-related risks of noise and sun exposure indicate a need for a careful hearing screening and examination of the skin for sun damage. The purpose for conducting these exams is to identify signs of developing disease or dysfunction, as well as to reveal any areas where health promotion or protection is needed.

5. The developmental milestones of psychosocial function in young adults are feeling independent, having a realistic self-image, having positive regard for self and life direction, coping with stress, interacting well with one's family, being responsible for one's self, and developing lasting relationships with others. Mr. Jones has displayed some bravado about drinking with friends and interacting with women, but it is difficult to ascertain the quality of the relationships. The nurse should ask more about these friendships, as well as if Mr. Jones has close friends, either male or female. Furthermore, although Mr. Jones has a job, there is no information about its adequacy to meet his financial needs, or how responsibly Mr. Jones manages his employment. No information is given about how Mr. Jones interacts with his family. He should be asked about the use of alcohol or other substances as coping mechanisms. He should also be asked if he is satisfied with his life and occupation. If he is not, the nurse should ask if Mr. Jones has the plans and resources needed to make a change.

TEST YOUR KNOWLEDGE

1. *Answer*: 3 *Rationale*: The average age for the onset of menopause in American women is 47 years. Therefore, there is nothing abnormal about ongoing menses in a 45-year-old woman, and gynecological care is not warranted (option 1). As a woman nears menopause, ovulation may become irregular and difficult to predict. Conception remains a possibility, and the lack of predictable ovulation may actually increase the likelihood of unintended pregnancy (option 2). Many women have no negative symptoms of menopause, and the experience of menopause is highly culturally determined (option 4). *Cognitive Level*: Analysis *Client Need*: Health Promotion and Maintenance *Nursing Process*: Implementation

2. *Answer*: 2 *Rationale*: Generation X is characterized by both skepticism and resentment of persons in authority (such as a nurse). Baby Boomers tend to be interested in improving themselves, and health teaching may be viewed as self-improvement. Generation Y and Millennials are the same cohort, and are most likely to receive their health information from technological sources, such as the Internet. *Cognitive Level*: Analysis *Client Need*: Health Promotion and Maintenance *Nursing Process*: Implementation

3. *Answer*: 3 *Rationale*: Lung cancer, once primarily a man's disease, is now increasingly common in women. Cervical cancer is most prevalent in younger women, and is detected with the Pap smear (option 1). Lymphoma and colon cancer are significant diseases for both men and women (options 2 and 4). *Cognitive Level*: Analysis *Client Need*: Health Promotion and Maintenance *Nursing Process*: Assessment

4. *Answer*: 4 *Rationale*: Although HIV and syphilis may have more disastrous health effects, chlamydia is the most prevalent infectious disease in the United States. Gonorrhea is still common, and its prevalence may vary geographically, but chlamydia is more common and therefore the most likely contracted STI. *Cognitive Level*: Analysis *Client Need*: Health Promotion and Maintenance *Nursing Process*: Implementation

5. *Answer*: 2 *Rationale*: Kohlberg's initial work indicated that moral development was completed by adulthood, but more recent research has demonstrated that moral development continues throughout adulthood. Moral development refers to a decision-making process of right and wrong, and proceeds in a series of predictable stages. Moral development and spirituality are unrelated, and represent very different spheres of human thought and behavior. *Cognitive Level*: Analysis *Client Need*: Psychosocial Integrity *Nursing Process*: Assessment

6. *Answer*: 2 *Rationale*: The middle-aged person is generally attempting to relate to adult children and grandchildren as well as assisting aging parents. Hence, continuous efforts to meet the needs of others occur. Selecting a life partner is the developmental task for young adults. Reviewing the life course is the task for older adulthood. Establishing a sense of self is usually achieved during adolescence. *Cognitive Level*: Analysis *Client Need*: Health Promotion and Maintenance *Nursing Process*: Assessment

7. *Answer*: 3 *Rationale*: Because individuals over 50 years tend to have multiple chronic illnesses as well as an aging immune system, the influenza vaccine is highly recommended. Influenza can lead to serious complications in these persons. The pneumococcal vaccine protects against the most common pathogens that cause pneumonia, a very serious disease in elders. The vaccine must be given every 10 years. Tetanus is appropriate for all ages and must be renewed every 10 years. Immunization for pertussis is only appropriate in children, and meningococcal vaccine is appropriate in adolescents and young adults living in congregate housing. *Cognitive Level*: Application *Client Need*: Health Promotion and Maintenance *Nursing Process*: Implementation

8. *Answer*: 1, 2, 3, and 5 *Rationale*: Hypertension (elevated blood pressure) forces the heart to work harder resulting in decreased function of the heart; the electrocardiogram assesses cardiac rhythm and rate; high cholesterol levels are directly related to a decrease in arterial size, which decreases circulation blood to the cardiac tissue; activity level (e.g., dyspnea on exertion) can indicate cardiovascular disease. While cardiac impairment may decrease sexual performance, which is important to assess, the others would have priority given the limitations for the screening program. *Cognitive Level*: Analysis *Client Need*: Health Promotion and Maintenance *Nursing Process*: Assessment

9. *Answer*: 1 *Rationale*: Asking the woman if she is afraid of someone at home, or if someone hurt her, is a critical step in a comprehensive assessment. Domestic violence is a serious problem for women of all ages, cultures, and socioeconomic levels. The nurse should suspect it in women whose injuries are not consistent with the history they give, women who "hospital shop"—going to multiple emergency rooms, and women who are socially isolated. Referring the woman to a shelter without completing a thorough assessment may lead to inappropriate care; the nursing process requires assessment before intervention. Collaboration with other health care professionals may be very helpful. Documentation of the assessment does not directly address, reduce, nor solve the problem. *Cognitive Level*: Analysis *Client Need*: Safe, Effective Environment *Nursing Process*: Assessment

10. *Answer*: 3 *Rationale*: Each of these activities indicates achievement of a developmental task, but the nurse must know which task is appropriate for the client's chronological age. Creating a scrapbook is an important strategy to enhance ego integrity, the developmental task for older adults. Working with philanthropic groups is a hallmark of generativity, the developmental task for those in midlife. Obtaining and decorating a place to live is an ac-tivity that establishes independence from parents, a task for young adults, while considering career paths is more appropriate to the identity task of adolescence. *Cognitive Level*: Application *Client Need*: Health Promotion and Maintenance *Nursing Process*: Assessment

CHAPTER 23

CRITICAL THINKING POSSIBILITIES

1. Osteoporosis means "porous bone," or bone that has gotten thinner and greatly increases the risk of fractures, particularly in older women. Pictures or actual x-rays can be shown to the client to facilitate learning the basics of osteoporosis. The seriousness of the condition should be stressed. At the same time, it should be stressed that following preventive measures and participating in treatment regimes, if this is indicated, will help to maintain bone health.

2. Risk factors should include physical factors such as early menopause, small thin frame, use of steroids, history of rheumatoid arthritis, family history of disease, or history of fractures.

3. Some risk factors are considered to be modifiable, including smoking, diet low in calcium, lack of exposure to sun (sunlight helps to increase vitamin D), increased intake of caffeine and alcohol, and lack of exercise.

4. Most of the medications used to treat osteoporosis help to reduce bone resorption, which means that bone mass is at least maintained. Some of these medications have serious gastrointestinal side effects and some increase the risk of formation of blood clots. It is essential for the client to know the possible side effects and call the physician if any unusual symptoms are experienced. If the medication is an experimental medication, bone density scans may be done at regular intervals to determine effectiveness of the treatment.

5. Measures to discuss for a decreased risk of fractures include these: assessment of home environment to see what safety measures need to be instituted, making sure that hallways and stairwells are well lit, wearing well-fitting shoes with nonskid soles, removing loose rugs in the house, and keeping the floor free of cords (electrical and telephone) to prevent tripping over them. Measures to maintain bone mass include increasing calcium in the diet and taking a calcium supplement, increasing the amount of weight-bearing exercise, and taking medications to prevent further bone loss.

TEST YOUR KNOWLEDGE

1. *Answer*: 2 *Rationale*: Grieving is a normal behavior after the death of a loved one, and the behaviors listed in the other answers would indicate signs of normal grieving. When the behavior becomes extreme, and signs of self-neglect are obvious, ineffective coping may be a problem. Then it would be the responsibility of the nurse to be attentive to the problem and engage appropriate resources for her, if needed. *Cognitive Level*: Application *Client Need*: Psychosocial Integrity *Nursing Process*: Assessment

2. *Answer*: 3 *Rationale*: Since the hearing loss occurs in the ability to distinguish high-pitched tones, speaking in a low and distinctive voice tone is the most appropriate method of communicating with the clients. Hearing loss in the elder includes a loss of the ability to discern higher frequencies, and speaking slowly at a particular volume is not the best way to communicate with the clients. The stem indicates the clients have noticeable hearing loss, but does not indicate the clients are deaf; large lettering is appropriate if the client has a visual problem; hearing aids are not

usually effective when the problem is related to neural damage. *Cognitive Level*: Analysis *Client Need*: Health Promotion and Maintenance *Nursing Process*: Assessment

3. *Answer*: 2 *Rationale*: Reminiscence about past life events, doing a "life review" of past experiences, especially if they were positive, is considered to be a normal psychosocial activity of elders. It helps them focus on past accomplishments and contributions to society, thus increasing their self-concept. If behavioral or significant memory problems had been noted, then a geriatric psychiatric consult would be appropriate, but not in this situation. Other activities and conversations should certainly be encouraged, but not to the point of demeaning the importance of his life stories. *Cognitive Level*: Application *Client Need*: Health Promotion and Maintenance *Nursing Process*: Assessment

4. *Answer*: 3 and 4 *Rationale*: When clients with dementia become agitated, the main interventions are to decrease the stimuli, but not to leave them alone. Distracting them, staying with them, and the use of a calm, gentle manner will usually decrease the agitation. Touching must be done in a gentle way, not to surprise or alarm them. *Cognitive Level*: Application *Client Need*: Psychosocial Integrity *Nursing Process*: Implementation

5. *Answer*: 3 *Rationale*: This option will provide the nurse with the most information for potential intervention. Urinary incontinence is not normal and it is something the nurse should investigate. *Cognitive Level*: Analysis *Client Need*: Physiological Integrity *Nursing Process*: Assessment

6. *Answer*: 1 *Rationale*: The client has loss of muscle strength. Strengthening exercises will improve his mobility and lessen the possibility of a fall. Option 2: Information indicates the client has difficulty rising from a seating position, not standing after he reaches the position; further assessment is needed before implementing this intervention. Option 3: Praise should come after the proper intervention is implemented and a plan is in place so that the praise is focused toward a goal to resolve the problem. Option 4 resolves the problem immediately but does nothing to resolve the underlying problem. *Cognitive Level*: Application *Client Need*: Safe, Effective Care Environment *Nursing Process*: Implementation

7. *Answer*: 4 *Rationale*: Sexual activity is possible for older adults although the responses are slower. Option 1: The clients would need a health history and physical assessment of the cardiovascular system before drawing this conclusion. Option 2: With the introduction of Viagra older men are more able to perform than in the past. Option 3: Older men's interest tends to decline, but it is not known whether it is related to impotence; apparently this elder is interested in sexual activity. *Cognitive Level*: Analysis *Client Need*: Health Promotion and Maintenance *Nursing Process*: Implementation

8. *Answer*: 3 *Rationale*: Presbyopia is loss of near vision related to aging. Option 1 is loss of hearing ability related to aging. Option 2 is dry mouth related to a decrease in saliva, and option 4 is a decrease in the motility of the esophagus related to aging. *Cognitive Level*: Application *Client Need*: Health Promotion and Maintenance *Nursing Process*: Assessment

9. *Answer*: 2 *Rationale*: Genetics, interests, careers, marital status, and economic status vary as much among elders as among other age groups. The elderly are a heterogeneous group. *Cognitive Level*: Application *Client Need*: Health Promotion and Maintenance *Nursing Process*: Assessment

10. *Answer*: 4 *Rationale*: This response reflects an understanding of the different stages of independence and control an older adult ex-periences when admitted to the hospital and the need for the nurse to assess the elder's need for control and autonomy. After admission, the client willingly gives up autonomy to the hospital routine because the client wants to get better (option 4). As the elder's health improves and progresses, he or she wants to increase autonomy (option 1). Before discharge they are thinking about if they can go home (option 2). Option 3 is not realistic given the usual hospital routine. *Cognitive Level*: Analysis *Client Need*: Psychosocial Integrity *Nursing Process*: Planning

CHAPTER 24

CRITICAL THINKING POSSIBILITIES

1. Many illnesses can be affected by the client's emotional state. If her arthritis is the type called rheumatoid, it can flare when the client is under stress. Also, some medications used to treat arthritis can cause mood changes and other distressing adverse effects. Any aspect of the illness that interferes with daily functioning of a family member will affect the coping of all members.

2. The family is affected because Linda's role functioning is impaired. Others might need to take on additional tasks Linda would normally perform. In addition, Linda's emotional response to her illness can interfere with her ability to provide psychological support to her children and spouse and thus cause them severe distress.

3. Facing illness as a family often draws the members, including those normally at some physical or emotional distance, closer together. A disadvantage of facing an illness with the family is the additional stress, cost, and responsibilities members may have to take on. The ill member may feel great guilt about the extra work that falls to others. Members may become fatigued and be unable or unwilling to support the ill person.

4. Each family member exists as a part of the whole. They interact with each other and with their human and nonhuman environment. The family has become a more closed system (and with thicker boundaries) than usual due to the parents' desire to avoid assistance or interference from previous spouses. Linda's biological systems may be malfunctioning, leading to altered function of her other systems and those of the family. For example, feedback in the form of pain will serve as input to her in deciding how much and what types of physical activity she can perform.

TEST YOUR KNOWLEDGE

1. *Answer*: 1 *Rationale*: Grandparents, aunts, and uncles are considered extended family members. Parents and spouse are considered immediate family members. Children who no longer live at home are considered immediate family members. Roommates and close family friends may be considered extended family members if grandparents, aunts, and uncles do not exist. *Cognitive Level*: Analysis *Client Need*: Psychosocial Integrity *Nursing Process*: Assessment

2. *Answer*: 4 *Rationale*: Because the child's behavior results in a change in the father's behavior, it is considered feedback. It is also a type of negative feedback in that the more the child cries, the less the father leaves. In some ways, the child's behavior is also input because it is used by the father in making a decision (throughput) about his behavior (output). *Cognitive Level*: Application *Client Need*: Psychosocial Integrity *Nursing Process*: Not Applicable

3. *Answer*: 1 *Rationale*: The health history of the client's current living partners is critical information since many illnesses are communicable or environmental. Giving this advice, the nurse also validates that family is whoever the client says they are. History of illness data of blood relatives is also extremely valuable

and should always be included, whether or not the client lives with them. Neither the history nor the physical exam is more important than the other—both are necessary for a complete plan of care. *Cognitive Level*: Application *Client Need*: Psychosocial Integrity *Nursing Process*: Assessment

4. *Answer*: A visual representation of family members by gender, age, health status, and lines of relationships through the generations is referred to as a genogram. *Cognitive Level*: Knowledge *Client Need*: Psychosocial Integrity *Nursing Process*: Assessment

5. *Answer*: 1, 2, and 4 *Rationale*: It is essential that the nurse determine the duration of the illness, the meaning of the illness to the family and its significance to family systems, and the financial impact of the illness in order to completely assess the impact of the illness on the family as a whole. Duration of the illness will determine the degree of disruption and adaptation required. These factors affect the members of the family in addition to the ill client. Option 3: Coping mechanisms used by other families with similar illnesses may not be relevant since families vary greatly in their makeup and function patterns. Option 5: Knowing the incidence of the illness in the community at large is an important factor for the community health nurse in exploring epidemiological issues such as prevention strategies and public health policies but is not as relevant for assisting the particular family. *Cognitive Level*: Comprehension *Client Need*: Psychosocial Integrity *Nursing Process*: Assessment

6. *Answer*: 1 *Rationale*: Presenting to the clinic indicates the family is probably ready to face the health challenges caused by the previous activities. There is no evidence that the adult child or parent is experiencing disabling coping (option 2). *Impaired Parenting* applies when the parent is unable to care for a child rather than the reverse. Although some strain must be experienced by the child evidence does not indicate that *Caregiver Role Strain* is the most important aspect of the situation. *Cognitive Level*: Analysis *Client Need*: Psychosocial Integrity *Nursing Process*: Diagnosis

7. *Answer*: 3 *Rationale*: Establishing trust allows for effective communication and confirms that there is mutual commitment to the goals. Meetings with the family as a group should be goal-oriented. A trusting relationship is important for communication as well as accepting and implementing a plan. While considering the cost of health care is important, it does not take priority over a trusting relationship with the nurse. A detailed history and examination of each family member is relevant but family members or the family as a whole will need to trust the nurse before providing the information. *Cognitive Level*: Application *Client Need*: Psychosocial Integrity *Nursing Process*: Planning

8. *Answer*: 4 *Rationale*: The focus of activity on personal purposes does not promote effective family functioning. A family system that functions efficiently focuses primarily on purposes involving the *total* system, allows input from the outside, personal boundaries are well-defined, and family members are interdependent. *Cognitive Level*: Analysis *Client Need*: Psychosocial Integrity *Nursing Process*: Evaluation

CHAPTER 25

CRITICAL THINKING POSSIBILITIES

1. Possible examples describing which aspect of the nurse's approach relates to each of the following "SIX Cs of Caring in Nursing" as outlined by Roach:
   - Compassion: The nurse prioritizes care to alleviate pain before continuing to other tasks.

- Competence: The nurse draws up the correct dose of morphine and administers it safely.
- Confidence: The nurse does not hesitate to provide essential care, and expresses her belief in this treatment to the client.
- Conscience: The nurse follows safety procedures and protocols at all times, putting the welfare of the client first.
- Commitment: The nurse has made arrangements in her personal life (for her own child), so that she can focus on her professional role.
- Comportment: The nurse dresses and acts in a professional manner, communicating who she is to the child and mother.

2. Possibilities for descriptions of how each type of knowing prepared the nurse, Megan, for her caring approach:
   - Personal knowing: The nurse is aware of her own strengths and limitations. She has made arrangements for her own child's care so that she can focus on her clients.
   - Empirical knowing: The nurse combines knowledge of growth and development, pathophysiology, medical treatments, and nursing process to provide competent nursing care.
   - Aesthetic knowing: By knowing this client and what motivates him, the nurse can plan activities that he understands and appreciates, and that lead to healing and comfort.
   - Ethical knowing: The nurse appreciates the need to "do no harm" to the client and to promote health and healing.

3. Possible descriptions of how each of the following aspects from Ray's theory influences the nurse's care:
   - Spiritual-ethical-caring: The importance of providing holistic, respectful, safe care that maintains the client's integrity and promotes healing
   - Physical: The client's acute illness (ruptured appendix) and his physical deviations from health
   - Technological: The skills involved in nursing care, such as intravenous (IV) therapy, NG tube to suction, IV medications
   - Social-cultural: The child's developmental level, family and peer relationships, and cultural background
   - Educational: The child's level of understanding as well as individual factors that motivate him to ambulate and participate in other aspects of care
   - Legal: Practice guidelines that serve as standards of care for this medical diagnosis, as well as nursing policies and procedures that guide the nurse's actions

TEST YOUR KNOWLEDGE

1. *Answer*: 2 *Rationale*: This assessment activity gathers more information to help the nurse know the client's usual self-care practices. Option 1 aims to provide comfort. Option 3 is a therapeutic, not an assessment, activity. Option 4 does not meet the aim of knowing the client. *Cognitive Level*: Application *Client Need*: Psychosocial Integrity *Nursing Process*: Implementation

2. *Answer*: 1 *Rationale*: Teaching the client to make self-care decisions at home empowers him to care for his illness. Empowerment is not the primary goal for the other options. *Cognitive Level*: Application *Client Need*: Health Promotion and Maintenance *Nursing Process*: Implementation

3. *Answer*: 3 *Rationale*: Mayeroff defines patience as "allowing the other to grow in his own way and time." The other options are not clearly the goal. *Cognitive Level*: Knowledge *Client Need*: Psychosocial Integrity *Nursing Process*: Planning

4. *Answer*: 1 *Rationale*: In this situation, culture care diversity addresses the differences between Indonesian medical practices and

traditional American practices. Universality addresses the similar-ities among the cultures. Since Leininger's theory addresses cul-tural elements relevant to nursing, options 2, 3, and 4 are incorrect. *Cognitive Level*: Analysis *Client Need*: Psychosocial Integrity *Nursing Process*: Evaluation

5. *Answer*: 3 *Rationale*: This represents an ethical dilemma. The other options are ways of knowing less clearly related to the situ-ation. *Cognitive Level*: Application *Client Need*: Psychosocial Integrity *Nursing Process*: Assessment

6. *Answer*: 1 *Rationale*: The nurse's presence is most significant in this situation. Assessment (option 2), knowing the client (option 3), and empowering the client (option 4) are not the focus of the nurse's action. *Cognitive Level*: Application *Client Need*: Psy-chosocial Integrity *Nursing Process*: Implementation

7. *Answer*: 2 *Rationale*: As depicted in Figure 25-1, this is the model for the theory of bureaucratic caring. *Cognitive Level*: Knowledge *Client Need*: Psychosocial Integrity *Nursing Process*: Assessment

8. *Answer*: 1 *Rationale*: Empirical knowing is gained from study-ing scientific models and theories. Aesthetic knowing arises from application in practice (option 2). Personal knowing arises from self-examination (option 3). Ethical knowing arises from con-fronting conflicting values (option 4). *Cognitive Level*: Applica-tion *Client Need*: Not Applicable *Nursing Process*: Not Applicable

9. *Answer*: 4 *Rationale*: Meditation involves the described behav-iors. Storytelling involves communication with others (option 1). Yoga combines various postures with breathing practices (option 2). Music therapy involves listening to music (option 3). *Cognitive Level*: Analysis *Client Need*: Not Applicable *Nursing Process*: Not Applicable

10. *Answer*: 3 *Rationale*: This is the recommendation for a healthy lifestyle. Option 1: More sustained activity has more positive physiological benefits. Options 2 and 4: This amount of activity exceeds baseline requirements and may be more difficult to main-tain. *Cognitive Level*: Application *Client Need*: Health Promo-tion and Maintenance *Nursing Process*: Implementation

CHAPTER 26

CRITICAL THINKING POSSIBILITIES

1. Mrs. Manasovitz's nonverbal behavior may include changes in posture, facial expression, lack of verbal expression, and so on. Mrs. Manasovitz's nonverbal communication most likely repre-sents fear, disappointment, loss, anxiety, devastation, and so on.

2. The nurse conveyed the following caring actions: sitting with Mrs. Manasovitz, listening to her, and giving her undivided atten-tion. The nurse also conveyed comforting actions: using a sooth-ing voice, reassuring, touching, offering presence, and offering a cup of coffee. The nurse's actions did communicate caring and comforting as evidenced by Mrs. Manasovitz's willingness to share her feelings.

3. It is important to provide essential information and establish a trusting relationship during emotionally stressful times. Other ad-vantages of effective communication are helping families with stress reduction, helping them understand treatment options, and helping them with decision making.

4. The nurse conveyed attentive listening by sitting with Mrs. Man-asovitz, paying attention to both her verbal and nonverbal lan-guage, remaining silent, and focusing solely on Mrs. Manasovitz.

Other examples may include not interrupting the client, noting the congruency between verbal and nonverbal language, encouraging the client to talk, and thinking before responding.

TEST YOUR KNOWLEDGE

1. *Answer*: 3 *Rationale*: Nonverbal, gentle touch is an important tool; overstimulation may affect the client in a negative way. Op-tion 1: Written communication requires a higher level of con-sciousness than verbal. Option 2: The client does not have a hearing problem but the ability to interpret and understand com-munication. Option 4: Lack of facial expression may increase fear. *Cognitive Level*: Application *Client Need*: Psychosocial In-tegrity *Nursing Process*: Implementation

2. *Answer*: 3, 1, 2, 4 *Rationale*: During the preinteraction phase (op-tion 3), the nurse gathers information about the client before meet-ing the client. During the introductory phase (option 1), the nurse usually engages in some social interaction to put the client at ease. During the working phase (option 2), the nurse helps the client to explore feelings and helps the client plan a program. During the termination phase (option 4), the nurse summarizes or reviews the process that took place. *Cognitive Level*: Analysis *Client Need*: Psychosocial Integrity *Nursing Process*: Planning

3. *Answer*: Options 1 and 3 are listening behaviors; the others are barriers to listening. *Cognitive Level*: Application *Client Need*: Psychosocial Integrity *Nursing Process*: Implementation

4. *Answer*: 1 *Rationale*: Respect is correct because the nurse is val-idating the client's feeling. It is not genuineness (option 2) be-cause the nurse is giving information versus being genuine. Concreteness (option 3) is giving a specific example. The nurse is not confronting (option 4) but supporting through respect for the client's feelings. *Cognitive Level*: Application *Client Need*: Psy-chosocial Integrity *Nursing Process*: Implementation

5. *Answer*: 2 *Rationale*: Because anxiety and low self-esteem pre-cede powerlessness which results in indecisiveness, it is the most correct answer; nursing management always deals with the client's current display of needs. Option 1 and option 3: Anxiety and low self-esteem may cause a sense of powerlessness that re-sults in indecisiveness. Option 4: There is no evidence that the client's social interactions are less than adequate. *Cognitive Level*: Application *Client Need*: Psychosocial Integrity *Nursing Process*: Diagnosis

6. *Answer*: 2 and 3 *Rationale*: Assessing possible visual or hearing problems allows the nurse to provide appropriate interventions (e.g., inserting hearing aid). Communicating what will be occur-ring at a stressful time helps the client feel more secure and can reduce anxiety. Option 1 is not the best answer as the client could say yes/no or nod the head and the nurse will not know if the client fully understands. It would be better to ask the client to tell you where he or she is. Option 4 is important to do; however, im-mediately after surgery is not the best time as the client may be in pain and/or groggy from the anesthesia. *Cognitive Level*: Ap-plication *Client Need*: Psychosocial Integrity *Nursing Process*: Implementation

7. *Answer*: 3 *Rationale*: All of the other options are forms of elder-speak. *Cognitive Level*: Analysis *Client Need*: Psychosocial In-tegrity *Nursing Process*: Implementation

8. *Answer*: 4 *Rationale*: Option 4 is a therapeutic technique using an open-ended question that allows the client to elaborate. The other options are barriers to communication. In option 1 the client did not ask about the abilities of the surgeon and is not focusing on the client. Option 2 is changing the subject, and option 3 is giving advice.

Cognitive Level: Analysis *Client Need*: Psychosocial Integrity *Nursing Process*: Implementation

9. *Answer*: 2 *Rationale*: Option 2 uses an "I" statement which is assertive communication and is clear and direct. The message includes only the necessary information. Option 1 contains inflammatory language ("ineffective" and "you prescribed"). Options 3 and 4 do not provide the health care provider with specific information and could stimulate defensive behaviors. *Cognitive Level*: Analysis *Client Need*: Safe, Effective Care Environment *Nursing Process*: Assessment

10. *Answer*: 1 *Rationale*: It encourages the client to verbalize and choose the topic of the conversation. Option 2 is used when the nurse is unsure of the message and asks the client to repeat or restate the message. Option 3 is used to help a client differentiate the real from the unreal, and there is no information available to indicate this is a concern in this situation. Option 4 is used at the end of an interview or teaching session. *Cognitive Level*: Application *Client Need*: Psychosocial Integrity *Nursing Process*: Assessment

CHAPTER 27
CRITICAL THINKING POSSIBILITIES

1. Mrs. Yorty seems preoccupied, so this may not be the ideal time to proceed with teaching. She needs time to adjust to the news that she has received and to come to terms with how her heart condition is going to affect her life. When she is ready to learn, she will give you her full attention, ask questions, talk to others, and show interest.

2. A needs assessment provides information about numerous factors that affect learning, not just cognitive ability. Don't assume that well-educated persons have all the information they need to make decisions about their health, or that persons who are not as well educated do not have the capacity to understand.

   • A needs assessment would provide such information as Mrs. Yorty's baseline knowledge of cardiac disease, any health beliefs or cultural factors that may impact her acceptance or rejection of needed changes, the method of learning she prefers to use, and the support systems available to her.

3. Using your learning needs assessment, consider how Mrs. Yorty prefers to learn.

   • Consider leaving material for Mrs. Yorty to read or videos for her to view.

   • Schedule short learning sessions rather than overwhelmingly long sessions, use teaching aids, repeat information often, and allow active learning. Allow Mrs. Yorty to set the pace.

4. If Mrs. Yorty is able to accurately select foods in accordance with her prescribed diet, is able to accurately plan an exercise program, and can offer suggestions for stress reduction, your teaching has most likely been effective.

   • Don't confuse the client's lack of compliance with ineffective teaching. Clients may choose not to follow a prescribed regimen even though they have thorough knowledge of the regimen.

5. Teaching strategies may differ depending on the availability of equipment; however, the principles of teaching would be similar.

   • A learning needs assessment would still be useful. The person's learning readiness and motivation remain important, and learning objectives would continue to serve as evaluation criteria.

   • The client and family would be more in control of the teaching setting, including scheduling, time limits, and place.

TEST YOUR KNOWLEDGE

1. *Answer*: 2 *Rationale*: Options 1 and 3 are psychomotor, and 4 is under the cognitive domain. *Cognitive Level*: Comprehension *Client Need*: Health Promotion and Maintenance *Nursing Process*: Implementation

2. *Answer*: 3 *Rationale*: Options 1 and 2 are passive learning strategies. Learning is faster and retention better when the learner is actively involved. Option 4 promotes affective learning about adapting to a chronic health condition and is important. However, the question asks about learning diet information. *Cognitive Level*: Application *Client Need*: Physiological Integrity *Nursing Process*: Implementation

3. *Answer*: 2 *Rationale*: The client most ready to learn is experiencing or has recently experienced the least amount of stress or is the least preoccupied with other concerns. There will be no separation anxiety because the parents are present. The story book may allow the child to learn information about the hospital and ask questions. The client in option 1 will be preoccupied by his illness. The client in option 3 is most likely still in pain. It would be better to wait until the pain is resolved. It would also be important to check if the client is too sleepy because pain medication can have that effect also. The client in option 4 may be too tired after his physical therapy treatment. This would need to be assessed. *Cognitive Level*: Application *Client Need*: Psychosocial Integrity *Nursing Process*: Assessment

4. *Answer*: 1 *Rationale*: Individuals learn in various ways, such as visually, group learning, auditory, participatory, etc. The individual knows how learning has occurred in the past. Option 2 is a component of the implementation phase of teaching, and the question is asking how to assess a client's style of learning. Options 3 and 4 involve others and it is best to ask the client. *Cognitive Level*: Knowledge *Client Need*: Health Promotion and Maintenance *Nursing Process*: Assessment

5. *Answer*: 3 *Rationale*: Option 1 is an old diagnosis, which has been changed. Option 2 is a wellness nursing diagnosis; the data would need to address that the client is seeking health information and why in order to be the correct answer. The diagnosis of *Noncompliance* is associated with the intent to comply, but situational factors make it difficult. The data in the question do not support option 4. *Cognitive Level*: Knowledge *Client Need*: Physiological Integrity *Nursing Process*: Diagnosis

6. *Answer*: 2 and 3 *Rationale*: Both options 2 and 3 are open-ended questions that will give the client the opportunity to ask questions. Options 1 and 4 are closed-ended (yes/no) questions. A "no" answer may cause a discussion but it will be difficult for the nurse to assess if it is the information the client really wants to know. *Cognitive Level*: Application *Client Need*: Psychosocial Integrity *Nursing Process*: Assessment

7. *Answer*: 1, 2, 3, and 4 *Rationale*: All of the statements could indicate a low literacy skill. The nurse will need to assess which teaching strategies will be most appropriate and will also need to carefully evaluate if the client has learned the skill and necessary information. *Cognitive Level*: Analysis *Client Need*: Physiological Integrity *Nursing Process*: Assessment

8. *Answer*: 3 *Rationale*: All are important factors to assess. The priority, however, would be the potential economic factor as the medications can be very expensive and the client may not take them if he or she cannot afford them. *Cognitive Level*: Application *Client Need*: Physiological Integrity *Nursing Process*: Assessment

9. *Answer*: 3 *Rationale*: This option is the easiest for the nurse to evaluate. Option 1 is difficult to evaluate because "understand" is

too vague. Option 2 refers more to an affective outcome and the question is asking about a cognitive outcome. Option 4 is telling more about the husband than the client. *Cognitive Level*: Analysis *Client Need*: Health Promotion and Maintenance *Nursing Process*: Evaluation

10. *Answer*: 2 *Rationale*: This is the only option that clearly reflects the teaching process, evaluation method, and the response of the client indicating evidence of learning. *Cognitive Level*: Analysis *Client Need*: Physiological Integrity *Nursing Process*: Evaluation

CHAPTER 28

CRITICAL THINKING POSSIBILITIES

1. Mr. Caruso has characteristics of democratic or participative leadership. He is complimentary of his staff's ability to set goals and make decisions. He encourages your input and ideas. Mrs. Turner has characteristics of the autocratic leader. She explains her expectations and speaks of implementing her programs.

2. Not sure which characteristics of your admired manager/leader you might want for yourself? If you didn't already, consider how they influence people; their interest in exploring new ideas; their ability to relate to others; how much freedom they allow or control they exert over others; their use of authoritarian, democratic, or laissez-faire style; their energy level; and their creativity.

3. Strategies for dealing with change may include acknowledging that some resistance to change is normal, examining the reasons for the change, focusing on the positive impact of the change, forming a support group, and examining the steps of the change process. Review Boxes 28–4 ∞ and 28–5 ∞ for more ideas.

4. In both primary care and team nursing, registered nurses may delegate tasks to other nurses or to UAPs. However, in primary nursing, the nurse generally provides as much direct care as possible while present, accepts supervisory responsibility for the client's 24-hour care, and, by definition, delegates care to the other shifts. In team nursing, a designated set or pair of providers is assigned to care for a group of clients. These members will share care for the clients according to agreed-on assignments that include delegation of appropriate tasks by the nurse.

TEST YOUR KNOWLEDGE

1. *Answer*: 1 *Rationale*: This is a situation in which urgent decisions are needed, and one person provides instructions without input from others (authoritarian). This is especially appropriate if the rest of the group is not functioning at an appropriate level. Option 2 would be found in shared governance structures when the risks are low and there is time for collaboration. Option 3 is most effective in groups with high levels of professional and personal maturity and where cooperation and coordination are not significant. Option 4 involves the rigid use of rules; since managing casualties is a highly unpredictable activity, enforcement of rules is not appropriate. *Cognitive Level*: Analysis *Client Need*: Safe, Effective Care Environment *Nursing Process*: Not Applicable

2. *Answer*: 1 *Rationale*: Transformational leaders are creative and use collaboration and group empowerment. Subgroups or task forces (option 2) would be found in shared governance structures (democratic leadership). Transactional leaders use rewards such as paying the cost of continuing education as incentives. Situational leaders vary their approach depending on the context. *Cognitive Level*: Comprehension *Client Need*: Safe, Effective Care Environment *Nursing Process*: Not Applicable

3. *Answer*: 2 *Rationale*: The manager is responsible for evaluating the staff (accountable) but has no authority to terminate staff who do not meet the standards nor promote staff with outstanding performance. In option 1 the manager has authority to carry out the reduction, but is not accountable because the actions were delegated and not initiated independently. In option 3, the manager has only responsibility; in option 4, both authority and accountability. *Cognitive Level*: Analysis *Client Need*: Safe, Effective Care Environment *Nursing Process*: Planning

4. *Answer*: 3 *Rationale*: A fresh postoperative client is, by definition, in a somewhat unstable condition and the nurse must assess and supervise this initial transfer. A UAP should be able to perform the transfer safely with a new wheelchair or elderly client; the scenario does not indicate that the wheelchair had special features. Age does not determine need for assistance. The task is simple and can be easily recalled safely after an absence. *Cognitive Level*: Analysis *Client Need*: Safe, Effective Care Environment *Nursing Process*: Planning

5. *Answer*: 4 *Rationale*: Interaction between the two groups may lead to a compromise. Option 1: Although explaining the reasons for the desired change is useful, overemphasis on the rationale may not be useful since resistance is often more emotional than rational. Option 2: This situation does not meet the criteria for an autocratic leadership style. There is no urgency and the task primarily involves the staff. Option 3: If the manager were not solidly committed to the proposal, it should not have been introduced, resulting in unnecessary disturbance; the manager should be open to modification of the proposal if justified. *Cognitive Level*: Application *Client Need*: Safe, Effective Care Planning *Nursing Process*: Implementing

CHAPTER 29

CRITICAL THINKING POSSIBILITIES

1. You need to determine the source of the client's concern. Is this just a bad time for her? Inquire if she has ever had her blood pressure taken previously. If so, what was the experience like for her? What does she imagine will happen if you take her blood pressure?

   • Discuss factors that influence clients' views of having vital signs measured—especially factors such as setting: long-term care, hospitals, clinics, primary care providers' offices.

2. Each nurse develops his or her own style for addressing problems such as this with clients. You need to develop yours or it will sound insincere. As a general rule, however, explain the situation without assigning fault. For example, you might say, "I wasn't able to hear your blood pressure that time," rather than "I'm really new at this and not very good yet."

   • If you are confident that your equipment is functioning properly, you may wish to retake the pressure using palpation rather than auscultation since you will be able to establish the presence of the peripheral pulse before you begin.

   • If you are very new at taking blood pressures, you may wish to ask another nurse to take the blood pressure for you this time. If a teaching stethoscope is available, use it so both of you can listen at the same time.

   • Role-play this situation with fellow students or friends. Try several different responses until you feel comfortable and the "client" expresses trust in your approach.

3. When you take a client's blood pressure for the first time, you need to relate it to previous or expected values. Determine the client's most recent BP—although this reading is elevated, it

might actually be lower than previous readings. Also assess for any stressors or medications that might currently be influencing the reading.

4. The oxygen saturation value is inconsistent with her other vital signs. Begin by determining if the pulse oximeter equipment is functioning properly and you have applied it to an appropriate location correctly.

TEST YOUR KNOWLEDGE

1. *Answer*: 2 *Rationale*: Although the temperature is slightly lower than expected for the morning, it would be best to determine the client's previous temperature range next. This may be a normal range for this client. Depending on that finding, you might want to retake it in a few minutes (no need to wait 15 minutes) or with another thermometer to see if the initial thermometer was functioning properly. Chart after determining that the temperature has been measured properly. *Cognitive Level*: Application *Client Need*: Health Maintenance and Promotion *Nursing Process*: Assessment

2. *Answer*: 3 *Rationale*: The apical rate would confirm the rate and determine the actual cardiac rhythm for a client with an abnormal rhythm; a radial pulse would only reveal the heart rate and suggest an arrhythmia. For clients in shock, use the carotid or femoral pulse (option 1). The radial pulse is adequate for determining change in orthostatic heart rate (option 2). The radial pulse is appropriate for routine postoperative vital sign checks for clients with regular pulses (option 4). *Cognitive Level*: Comprehension *Client Need*: Health Maintenance and Promotion *Nursing Process*: Planning

3. *Answer*: 4 *Rationale*: Since the client's needs are always considered first, the measurement should be delayed unless the client is in distress or there are other urgent reasons. Option 1: Respirations should be measured for 30 seconds to 1 minute and are affected by talking. Option 2: There needs to be an important reason for interrupting the client. Option 3: It is inappropriate to wait and listen to the client's conversation. *Cognitive Level*: Comprehension *Client Need*: Health Maintenance and Promotion *Nursing Process*: Planning

4. *Answer*: 2 *Rationale*: If the cuff is inflated to about 30 mm Hg over previous systolic pressure, that would be 168. To ensure that the diastolic has been determined, the cuff should be released slowly until the mid-60s mm Hg (and then completely) for someone with a previous reading of 74. The cuff should be deflated at a rate of 2 to 3 mm per second. Thus, a range of 90 mm Hg will require 30 to 45 seconds. *Cognitive Level*: Analysis *Client Need*: Health Maintenance and Promotion *Nursing Process*: Implementation

5. *Answer*: 1 *Rationale*: Vital signs measurement may be delegated to UAP if the client is in stable condition, the findings are expected to be predictable, and the technique requires no modification. Only the preoperative client meets these requirements. In addition, UAP are not delegated to take apical pulse measurements for the client with an irregular pulse as would be the case with the client newly started on antiarrhythmic medication. *Cognitive Level*: Application *Client Need*: Health Maintenance and Promotion *Nursing Process*: Planning

6. *Answer*: 3, 4, and 5 *Rationale*: For this client, the nurse could take an axillary, tympanic, or temporal artery temperature. Due to the facial drooping and difficulty swallowing, the oral route is not recommended. Although the rectal route could be used, it would require unnecessary moving and positioning of a client who cannot assist, and it would not provide a significant advantage over the other

routes. *Cognitive Level*: Application *Client Need*: Health Maintenance and Promotion *Nursing Process*: Assessment

7. *Answer*: 4 *Rationale*: The posterior tibial and pedal pulses in the foot are considered peripheral and at least one of them should be palpable in normal individuals. Option 1: A bounding radial pulse is more indicative that perfusion exists. Options 2 and 3: Apical and carotid pulses are central and not peripheral. *Cognitive Level*: Analysis *Client Need*: Health Promotion and Maintenance *Nursing Process*: Diagnosing

8. *Answer*: 3 *Rationale*: Dyspnea, difficult or labored breathing, is commonly related to inadequate oxygenation. Therefore, the client is likely to experience shortness of breath, that is, a sense that none of the breaths provide enough oxygen and an immediate second breath is needed. Shallow respirations are seen in tachypnea (rapid breathing). Wheezing is a high-pitched breathing sound that may or may not occur with dyspnea. The medical term for coughing up blood is *hemoptysis* and is unrelated to dyspnea. *Cognitive Level*: Application *Client Need*: Health Promotion and Maintenance *Nursing Process*: Evaluating

9. *Answer*: This blood pressure should be recorded as 180/105/95 using the systolic/1st diastolic/2nd diastolic convention. Rationale: Phase 1 first sound is a clear tapping when deflation of the cuff begins. Phase 2 has a muffled, swishing sound. In phase 3, blood is flowing freely via an increasingly open artery; sounds are more crisp and more intense but softer than phase 1. Phase 4 sounds become muffled and have a soft blowing quality. In phase 5 the last sound is heard followed by silence. *Cognitive Level*: Analysis *Client Need*: Health Promotion and Maintenance *Nursing Process*: Assessment

10. *Answer*: 4 The SpO_2 in this case is 97%. Option 1 indicates the systolic blood pressure of 121 mm Hg, option 2 the mean arterial pressure of 95 mm Hg, option 3 the pulse of 87, and option 5 the diastolic blood pressure of 84 mm Hg. In addition, the client's temperature is shown. *Cognitive Level*: Comprehension *Client Need*: Health Maintenance and Promotion *Nursing Process*: Assessment

CHAPTER 30

CRITICAL THINKING POSSIBILITIES

1. A focused neurologic system assessment must be conducted, including determining her mental status, motor and sensory function, and pupillary reactions. The client may have had a stroke or have injured her head when/if she fell. The musculoskeletal system is also a priority since she may have injured herself or broken a hip either before or after falling. In an older adult who has apparently been injured, the integumentary system is a priority because of the high risk for skin damage, bruising, and skin breakdown. Assessment of other systems may also be justifiable.

2. Be sure that you are asking open-ended questions that cannot be answered with yes or no. Open-ended questions often begin with the words "how" or "what" or "tell me about." Use good nonverbal communication skills such as being at her level when you speak and making eye contact.

3. Although you should still use the head-to-toe approach, it may be best to do all of the anterior assessment first and then turn her to perform posterior assessments. You can assess her upper extremities and much of her lower extremities without turning her at all. Do not omit the posterior assessment, however, just to reduce her discomfort. It is extremely important to determine if abnormal findings are there such as lung consolidation or skin breakdown.

4. Begin with family members. Although she lives alone, there may be children, grandchildren, or other relatives who are in contact with her regularly. Also, ask about the source of her regular health care. Other community sources may be neighbors or organizations with which she is affiliated (e.g., church, social groups). If she has a primary care provider, ensure that he or she has been notified of the client's admission and determine if she was seen recently or if the office can provide pertinent medical history data.

TEST YOUR KNOWLEDGE

1. *Answer*: 2 *Rationale*: Resonance is a normal sound over the lung. Tympany would be heard over the stomach (air filled), hyperresonance is never a normal finding, and dullness would be heard below (not above) the 10th intercostal space. *Cognitive Level*: Knowledge *Client Need*: Health Promotion and Maintenance *Nursing Process*: Evaluating

2. *Answer*: 4 *Rationale*: The client should sit for examination of the head and neck. For palpation of the abdomen, genitals, and breast, the client should be supine. *Cognitive Level*: Application *Client Need*: Health Promotion and Maintenance *Nursing Process*: Planning

3. *Answer*: 1 *Rationale*: A bruit suggests abnormal turbulence in the aorta, and the primary care provider must be notified. In order for absence of bowel sounds to be considered abnormal, they must be silent for 3 to 5 minutes. Continuous bowel sounds are normally heard over the ileocecal valve following meals. Bowel sounds are more commonly irregular than they are regular. *Cognitive Level*: Comprehension *Client Need*: Health Promotion and Maintenance *Nursing Process*: Evaluating

4. *Answer*: 1 *Rationale*: If a pedal pulse, which is more distal than the popliteal, is present, then adequate arterial circulation to the leg is present even though the popliteal artery has not been located. Presence of a femoral pulse would not provide confirmation that arterial flow exists below that point. Taking a thigh BP requires locating the popliteal pulse. Since the purpose of finding the popliteal pulse is to provide information about arterial circulation to the leg, checking the distal pulse before requesting assistance from another nurse is appropriate. *Cognitive Level*: Analysis *Client Need*: Health Promotion and Maintenance *Nursing Process*: Planning

5. *Answer*: 2 *Rationale*: Visual acuity often lessens with age. Facial hair is likely to become coarser, not finer. The sense of smell becomes less, rather than more acute. The respiratory rate and rhythm is regular at rest. However, both may change quickly with activity and be slow to return to the resting level. *Cognitive Level*: Analysis *Client Need*: Health Promotion and Maintenance *Nursing Process*: Evaluating

6. Answers include color, turgor, temperature, moisture, lesions, odor, and edema. *Cognitive Level*: Knowledge *Client Need*: Health Promotion and Maintenance *Nursing Process*: Assessing

7. *Answer*: 3 *Rationale*: Recent memory includes events of the current day. Recalling a series of numbers tests immediate recall. Recalling childhood events tests remote (long-term) memory and subtracting backwards from 100 tests attention span and calculation skills. *Cognitive Level*: Application *Client Need*: Health Promotion and Maintenance *Nursing Process*: Planning

8. *Answer*: 4 *Rationale*: Row 6 indicates normal vision of 20/20. If the client can only read line 4, vision is impaired and could lead to falls or other injuries. This impaired vision is not related to deficient knowledge or memory and may or may not be related to circulation. *Cognitive Level*: Analysis *Client Need*: Health Promotion and Maintenance *Nursing Process*: Diagnosing

9. *Answer*: 3 *Rationale*: Use the pads of two fingers and a gentle rotating motion over the nodes. None of the other options is proper palpation of lymph nodes. *Cognitive Level*: Application *Client Need*: Health Promotion and Maintenance *Nursing Process*: Implementing

10. *Answer*: Of the terms listed, only equal, symmetrical, and firm are normal findings. Atrophied, flaccid, contractured, hypertrophied, crepitation, spastic, and tremor are abnormal findings. Review the terms in the glossary to go over their meanings. *Cognitive Level*: Comprehension *Client Need*: Health Promotion and Maintenance *Nursing Process*: Evaluating

CHAPTER 31

CRITICAL THINKING POSSIBILITIES

1. Examples include age (reduced immune defenses), dehydration, nutritional deficit (decreased ability to synthesize antibodies), and the chronic respiratory problem.

2. A full history and physical assessment are indicated.
   - In particular, explore her immunization status, chronic illnesses, exposure to others who may have had an infection, medications that could increase susceptibility to infection, stress level, and history of previous infections of any kind.
   - Assess her skin and mucous membranes and check vital signs that could indicate infection.
   - Determine spiritual, cultural, and educational characteristics that may influence her beliefs and understandings, care preferences, and practices.

3. Use of standard precautions (SP) alone will not prevent transmission of her respiratory infection (if contagious) to others since SP are designed to prevent the transmission of bloodborne pathogens. As such, SP do not apply to sputum, nasal secretions, or urine unless contaminated with blood.

4. Depending on the type of organism infecting Mrs. Cortez's respiratory tract, she may need to be placed on specific isolation precautions. Identification of the organism will determine the type of mask and other precautions needed.
   - Interventions that protect all clients from the spread of disease include consistent and thorough hand cleansing, encouraging clients to cover their mouths with tissues when coughing or sneezing, disposal of soiled tissues in an appropriate bedside receptacle, making sure that reusable equipment is cleaned or sterilized appropriately, and handling soiled linens to prevent cross-contamination.

5. The assistant should be complimented on knowing the need to wash/cleanse her hands after contact with the client. However, her technique could be improved through the use of paper towels on the faucet handles and increasing the time spent washing to at least 10 seconds.

TEST YOUR KNOWLEDGE

1. *Answer*: 2 *Rationale*: Blocking the movement of the organism from the reservoir will succeed in preventing the infection of any other persons. Since the carrier person is the reservoir and the condition is chronic, it is not possible to eliminate the reservoir. Blocking the entry into a host or decreasing the susceptibility of the host will be effective for only that one single individual and, thus, is not as effective as blocking exit from the reservoir. *Cognitive Level*: Comprehension *Client Need*: Safe, Effective Care Environment *Nursing Process*: Planning

2. *Answer*: 1 *Rationale*: Since the hands are frequently in contact with clients and equipment, they are the most obvious source of transmission. Regular and routine hand cleansing is the most effective way to prevent movement of potentially infective materials. PPE (gloves and masks) is indicated for situations requiring Standard Precautions. Isolation precautions are used for clients with known communicable diseases. Routine use of antibiotics is not effective and can be harmful due to the incidence of superinfection and development of resistant organisms. *Cognitive Level*: Application *Client Need*: Safe, Effective Care Environment *Nursing Process*: Implementing

3. *Answer*: 3 *Rationale*: Standard Precautions include all aspects of contact precautions with the exception of placing the client in a private room. A mask is indicated when working over a sterile wound rather than an infected one. Disposable food trays are not necessary for clients with infected wounds unlikely to contaminate the client's hands. Sterile technique (surgical asepsis) is not indicated for all contact with the client. The nurse would utilize clean technique when dressing the wound to prevent introduction of additional microbes. *Cognitive Level*: Application *Client Need*: Safe, Effective Care Environment *Nursing Process*: Implementing

4. *Answer*: 1 *Rationale*: Unless overly contaminated by material that has splashed in the nurse's face and cannot be effectively rinsed off, goggles may be worn repeatedly. Since gowns are at high risk for contamination, they should be used only once and then discarded or washed. Surgical masks and gloves are never washed or reused. *Cognitive Level*: Comprehension *Client Need*: Safe, Effective Care Environment *Nursing Process*: Implementing

5. *Answer*: 4 *Rationale*: It should not be necessary to unroll this small edge of the cuff. The most important consideration is the sterility of the fingers and hand that will be used to perform the sterile procedure. The rolled-under portion is now contaminated and should not be unrolled by the nurse or colleague since it would then touch the remaining sterile portion of the glove. *Cognitive Level*: Application *Client Need*: Safe, Effective Care Environment *Nursing Process*: Implementing

6. *Answer*: 2, 3, and 4 *Rationale*: All adults should receive a tetanus booster every 10 years (or sooner if injured). Flu shots are recommended for all adults over age 50. Only persons at risk need to receive hepatitis B and A vaccine. *Cognitive Level*: Knowledge *Client Need*: Safe, Effective Care Environment *Nursing Process*: Assessing

7. *Answer*: Because a malnourished client with a wound is less able to resist an infection, *Risk for Infection* is the most likely nursing diagnosis. Others may include *Pain* or *Imbalanced Nutrition* but they are less focused on the immediate health risk. *Cognitive Level*: Application *Client Need*: Safe, Effective Care Environment *Nursing Process*: Diagnosing

8. *Answer*: 2 *Rationale*: Raw foods touched by human hands can carry significant infectious organisms and must be washed or peeled. Antimicrobial soap is not indicated for regular use and may lead to resistant organisms. Hand cleansing should occur as needed. Hot water can dry and harm skin, increasing the risk of infection. Clients should learn all the signs of inflammation and infection (e.g., redness, swelling, pain, heat) and not rely on the presence of pus to indicate this. Persons should not share washcloths or towels. *Cognitive Level*: Analysis *Client Need*: Safe, Effective Care Environment *Nursing Process*: Evaluating

9. *Answer*: 1 *Rationale*: Sterile objects are considered unsterile if placed lower than the waist. Only area 1 in this situation would be considered sterile. Above the neck, higher than 2 inches above the

elbow, below the waist/table, and the back are all considered unsterile. *Cognitive Level*: Application *Client Need*: Physiologic Integrity *Nursing Process*: Planning

10. *Answer*: 3 *Rationale*: All items within 1 inch of the edge of the sterile field are considered contaminated because the edge of the field is in contact with unsterile areas. When hands are ungloved, forceps tips are to be held downward to prevent fluid from becoming contaminated by the hands and then returned to the sterile field. Fields should be established immediately before use to prevent accidental contamination when not observed closely. Reaching over a sterile field increases the chances of dropping an unsterile item onto or touching the sterile field. *Cognitive Level*: Application *Client Need*: Safe, Effective Care Environment *Nursing Process*: Evaluating

CHAPTER 32
CRITICAL THINKING POSSIBILITIES

1. Restraints should only be used as a last resort. Some of the reasons include, but are not limited to, the following: Research has not proven that restraining clients prevents falls or injury; they lessen the client's movement and independence, which infringes on their rights; restraints can increase agitation of the client; the restraints can cause injury (pressure ulcers, skin tears, or death); restraints can interfere with the client's treatment; restraints can potentially cause health problems such as poor circulation; and restraints can be embarrassing to both client and family members.

2. Several factors that could affect Mr. Moore's safety include, but are not limited to, the following.
   - He is older than age 65; he has a history of falls; recent surgery for a hip fracture may impair his mobility; he may be weaker now than before his surgery; and his medications may affect his safety (e.g., antihypertensives, diuretics, analgesics).
   - Mr. Moore may resume normal activities before he is strong enough.
   - Mr. Moore may not be able to meet his nutritional needs because he will need to prepare all but one meal per day. He is at greater risk for injury while preparing his own food.
   - Mr. Moore may not understand the precautions necessary to protect his own safety.

3. You need to perform a home hazard appraisal. Suggestions for safety enhancement include the following:
   - Because the majority of adult injuries stem from falls, caution Mr. Moore about using area rugs and to be aware of where his pets are when he is up moving about.
   - Use grip handles in the bathtub and toilet.
   - All rooms should be well lighted. Use night-lights.
   - Carpets should be in good condition and hardwood floors should not be waxed.
   - The house should have smoke alarms; telephones should be easily accessible in case of emergency.

4. He has been physically and socially active and independent; he has a strong family support system (his son will visit daily); he has access to community resources; his rooms are on one level and his house is small; he has pets to decrease his loneliness; he has no other chronic illnesses that would interfere with his healing process.

TEST YOUR KNOWLEDGE

1. *Answer*: 3, 1, 4, 2 *Cognitive Level*: Knowledge *Client Need*: Safe, Effective Care Environment *Nursing Process*: Implementation

2. *Answer*: 1 *Rationale*: Option 2 is the leading cause for school-age children, option 3 is the leading cause for older adults, and option 4 relates to adolescents. *Cognitive Level*: Analysis *Client Need*: Safe, Effective Care Environment *Nursing Process*: Assessment

3. *Answer*: 3 *Rationale*: A bedside commode decreases the number of steps required to reach the goal. Leaving the light on would assist the client in locating the bathroom, but would not reduce the risk of falling when rushing to the bathroom. The nurse cannot withhold a client's medication without consultation with the physician. Rails up would increase the risks of falls as well as falling from a greater distance. *Cognitive Level*: Application *Client Need*: Safe, Effective Care Environment *Nursing Process*: Implementation

4. *Answer*: 3 *Rationale*: Remember that toddlers are active, like to explore, and are unable to use discretion about what they place in their mouths and as a result are at risk for poisoning (e.g., lead poisoning, toxic substances under the sink or in a drawer). The risk for suffocation (option 1) could happen but is more likely with a newborn or infant, which is the reason parents are taught not to prop the bottle, to cut food in small pieces, and to use toys with no small detachable pieces. Option 2 is too vague to address risks associated with a specific group of clients. Option 4 is more applicable to the elder who is on total bed rest. *Cognitive Level*: Analysis *Client Need*: Safe, Effective Care Environment *Nursing Process*: Diagnosis

5. *Answer*: 4 *Rationale*: Answer 4 is an intervention that can allow the client to feel independent and also alert the nurse and nursing staff when the client needs assistance. It is the most realistic answer that promotes client safety. Option 1 can increase agitation and confusion and removes the client's independence. Option 2 would help but transfers the responsibility to the family member. Option 3: Client could fall during the unobserved interval and is also not a realistic answer for a nurse. *Cognitive Level*: Analysis *Client Need*: Safe, Effective Care Environment *Nursing Process*: Implementation

6. *Answer*: 2 and 5 *Rationale*: These are measures needed to keep the client safe in the event of another seizure. Option 1 is incorrect because the current nursing literature states to not put anything in the client's mouth during a seizure. Options 3 and 4 are more relevant after the cause of the seizure is known. Not all seizures are caused by epilepsy. *Cognitive Level*: Application *Client Need*: Safe, Effective Care Environment *Nursing Process*: Planning

7. *Answer*: 4 *Rationale*: Placing the bed in the lowest position results in a client falling the shortest distance. The client is least likely to fall when getting up if the bed is at an appropriate height. Option 1 can cause a fall with injury because the client may fall from a higher distance when trying to get over the rail. Option 2 is important to do as certain meds can increase a risk of a fall (e.g., tranquilizers, analgesics). The nurse would discuss this with the primary care provider. While it may be a priority, placing the bed in the lowest position would be a higher priority in the hospital setting. Option 3 would help the nurse assess if a client is at risk for a fall. *Cognitive Level*: Analysis *Client Need*: Safe, Effective Care Environment *Nursing Process*: Implementation

8. *Answer*: 3, 4, and 5 *Rationale*: Reviewing near misses could identify flaws in the system or practices that placed the client at risk. Communication among staff and with clients will increase efficiency and create an atmosphere where nurses are willing to discuss errors openly so that the flaws in the system can be corrected.

Options 1 and 2: A competent nurse may make medication errors. Evidence is needed to support these conclusions. *Cognitive Level*: Comprehension *Client Need*: Safe, Effective Care Environment *Nursing Process*: Planning

9. *Answer*: 3 *Rationale*: Suicide and homicide are two leading causes of death among teenagers, and adolescent males commit suicide at a higher rate than adolescent females. Options 1 and 2 are true; however, they would not be as high a priority as preventing suicide. Option 4 is not true. A driver's education course is certainly encouraged; however, completing a course does not ensure safe practice. *Cognitive Level*: Analysis *Client Need*: Health Promotion and Maintenance *Nursing Process*: Planning

10. *Answer*: 1, 3, 4, and 5 *Rationale*: Standards require documentation of the necessity of the restraints. Range of motion prevents joint stiffness and pain from disuse. Orienting the client helps the nurse determine the necessity of the restraint. Option 2 is inappropriate because it can cause injury if the side rail is lowered without untying the restraint. *Cognitive Level*: Analysis *Client Need*: Safe, Effective Care Environment *Nursing Process*: Implementation

CHAPTER 33
CRITICAL THINKING POSSIBILITIES

1. After reviewing the defining characteristics and related factors, there is little data to support that the client actually has an impaired ability to perform her own bathing and hygiene. She has been providing for her own needs, has been ambulating, and has no physical impairments.
   - The following factors influence an individual's hygienic practices: culture, religion, environment, developmental level, health and energy, and personal preference.

2. Assess the client for discomfort/pain, fatigue, embarrassment, cultural beliefs, or personal preferences that may affect her decision to omit her personal care.
   - Suggested questions for the client: "Are you uncomfortable?" "Are you more tired today than yesterday?" "Do you want to wait until you go home?"

3. In general, bathing and personal care are essential for maintenance of skin integrity and mucous membranes, decreasing potential for infections, enhancing comfort, fostering a feeling of well-being, enhancing relaxation, minimizing odor, increasing circulation, and so on.
   - Benefits of personal care to the client include, but are not limited to, decreasing her risk of surgical wound infection and enhancing her comfort and ability to relax. Cleaning her teeth decreases the risk for infection and enables her to enjoy her food.

4. Offer the client several explanations regarding the benefits of proceeding with her bath and personal care, emphasizing the need to prevent infections.
   - Offer to assist her and seek her input on where she wants to bathe (e.g., at the bedside or in the bathroom); gather her toiletries and provide for privacy.
   - Make sure she has warm water and clean linens.
   - Provide intervention, if appropriate, depending on her reason for not wanting to perform personal care (e.g., pain medication).

5. You can gather information and perform assessments during the bathing process.
   - You can convey to clients that you have the time and the interest to make them feel better.

TEST YOUR KNOWLEDGE

1. *Answer*: 3 *Rationale*: The client fits the descriptors for semi-dependent functional level (see Table 33–2). *Cognitive Level*: Application *Client Need*: Physiological Integrity *Nursing Process*: Assessment

2. *Answer*: 3 *Rationale*: The client will be positioned in a side-lying position with the head of the bed lowered because the client is at risk for aspiration. The absence of gag reflex lets the nurse know that the client has no natural defense (cough) and is at a higher risk for aspiration. All other answers are assessments more appropriate prior to bathing the client. *Cognitive Level*: Application *Client Need*: Physiological Integrity *Nursing Process*: Assessment

3. *Answer*: 2 *Rationale*: A lotion will help moisten the skin. Perfumed lotions contain alcohol, which is drying to the skin. Soaking the feet for a long time or frequently also causes dry skin. Applying foot powder is appropriate to prevent or control unpleasant foot odor. Elastic stockings may decrease circulation. *Cognitive Level*: Application *Client Need*: Physiological Integrity *Nursing Process*: Implementation

4. *Answer*: 1 *Rationale*: Check that the battery is in the hearing aid. Turn off the hearing aid and make sure the volume is turned all the way down because a too loud volume is distressing. An in-the-ear hearing aid is cleaned with a damp cloth. Make sure the device is functioning. Removing cerumen without a prescription is beyond the UAP scope of practice as well as the nurse. Hearing aids are cleansed with a moist cloth. *Cognitive Level*: Application *Client Need*: Physiological Integrity *Nursing Process*: Implementation

5. *Answer*: 4 *Rationale*: Both the placement of the linens for a surgical bed and placing the bed in a high position facilitate the client's transfer from a stretcher into the bed. The linens for a closed bed are drawn up to the top of the bed and under the pillows. *Cognitive Level*: Knowledge *Client Need*: Physiological Integrity *Nursing Process*: Implementation

6. *Answer*: 1, 2, and 4 *Rationale*: Moving quickly may agitate the client. Protesting, screaming, and crying are not normal. Stop the bath and approach again later. *Cognitive Level*: Application *Client Need*: Physiological Integrity *Nursing Process*: Implementation

7. *Answer*: 4 *Rationale*: It is important to retract the foreskin to remove the smegma that collects under the foreskin and can cause bacterial growth. *Cognitive Level*: Analysis *Client Need*: Physiological Integrity *Nursing Process*: Evaluation

8. *Answer*: 1, 3, and 5 *Rationale*: The developmental level warrants supervision. If the bottle is given during naps or bed time, the solution has continuous contact with the toddler's teeth. The first visit to the dentist should be about 2 or 3 years old. Over 50% of older adults have their own teeth. *Cognitive Level*: Application *Client Need*: Health Promotion and Maintenance *Nursing Process*: Planning

9. *Answer*: 2 *Rationale*: The client needs to avoid walking barefoot as that could cause injury which may result in an infection. Also, neurological impairment is likely which may result in decreased sensation. The client would be unaware of an injury. *Cognitive Level*: Analysis *Client Need*: Health Promotion and Maintenance *Nursing Process*: Evaluation

10. *Answer*: 1 *Rationale*: Fowler's is a semi-sitting position which should ease the client's breathing. The head of the bed (HOB) in semi-Fowler's is lower. The HOB is lowered in the Trendelenburg position. While the HOB is raised in the reverse Trendelenburg position, it is a straight tilt and may not be as comfortable as Fowler's. *Cognitive Level*: Application *Client Need*: Safe, Effective Care Environment *Nursing Process*: Implementation

CHAPTER 34

CRITICAL THINKING POSSIBILITIES

1. Consider the possible causes. Is the finger vasoconstricted because of decreased blood volume? Would warming it with a warm cloth and having the client hold her hand in a dependent position help? Check the equipment (e.g., lancet injector) to see that it is operating correctly. Was it poor technique? Frequently, a novice nurse does not use enough force to press the injector firmly against the skin and/or have the injector in a perpendicular position relative to the skin. Both are needed to obtain a deep, clean puncture. After you have ascertained the cause, you will need to do another finger stick to obtain a large enough drop of blood to obtain an accurate reading.

2. The lab results suggest an infection is present and dehydration. Having a previous Hct for comparison would be helpful. Nursing interventions would relate to both infection and dehydration: VS TPR, check for orthostatic hypotension, obtain urine for C&S, interventions to promote hydration.

3. Consider that Ms. Angyal has had no fluids for 3 days. There is no information about the antibiotic (e.g., route and classification), which can also be a factor. Some antibiotics can be nephrotoxic. It is important to obtain a specimen for C&S before starting antibiotics, otherwise the results may not be accurate. Therefore, priorities would be to first start the IV fluids, because this will begin rehydrating her and may also help with obtaining the urine specimen. Second, obtain the urine specimen. You will need to assess how much assistance she may need with providing the clean-catch urine specimen because of expected weakness as a result of not eating or drinking for 3 days. Assistance may include placing her on a bedpan with the nurse doing the cleansing of the area and collecting the sample. Finally, the third priority would be administration of the antibiotic. All of these priorities would take place quickly because they are all important as is the order of the priorities.

4. The reduction in Hct reflects that she was dehydrated and the first Hct was elevated due to hemoconcentration. After being rehydrated, this Hct is more accurate. The WBC indicates that the infectious process is subsiding.

5. Assess her knowledge about an MRI and explain, if necessary, the purpose, procedure, benefits, and risks. Sedation is provided if the client is claustrophobic or unable to lie still during the procedure. Assure her that two-way communication is provided so that the client can provide feedback and be monitored. Inform her that there is a loud knocking noise during the procedure and earplugs are available if she desires. Document her concerns and the teaching you provided. If she continues to be anxious, inform the primary care provider.

TEST YOUR KNOWLEDGE

1. *Answer*: 2 *Rationale*: Option 2 is very low and can lead to death. Red blood cells participate in oxygenation. All of the other options are within normal range. *Cognitive Level*: Application *Client Need*: Physiological Integrity *Nursing Process*: Implementation

2. *Answer*: 3 *Rationale*: Communication of the test to all staff is likely to result in completing the collection. Option 1 is incorrect because you want to discard the first voiding. A clean re-

ceptacle, not a sterile one, is used to collect the urine; the purpose of the test will determine if refrigeration is needed. *Cognitive Level*: Application *Client Need*: Physiological Integrity *Nursing Process*: Implementation

3. *Answer*: 2 *Rationale*: This is an x-ray of the kidneys, ureters, and bladder. An IVP and retrograde pyelography use injections of contrast media. A cystoscopy uses a lighted instrument (cystoscope) inserted through the urethra resulting in direct visualization. *Cognitive Level*: Comprehension *Client Need*: Physiological Integrity *Nursing Process*: Assessment

4. *Answer*: 4 *Rationale*: A nuclear scan demonstrates ability of tissue to absorb the chemical. All of the other answers provide anatomic information. *Cognitive Level*: Knowledge *Client Need*: Physiological Integrity *Nursing Process*: Assessment

5. *Answer*: 3 *Rationale*: Bone marrow aspiration includes deep penetration into soft tissue and large bones such as the sternum and iliac crest, resulting in an increased risk for bleeding. Option 1 pertains to a liver biopsy, 2 to a thoracentesis, and 4 a lumbar puncture. *Cognitive Level*: Application *Client Need*: Physiological Integrity *Nursing Process*: Implementation

6. *Answer*: 1 and 4. *Rationale*: ALT is an enzyme that contributes to protein and carbohydrate metabolism. An increase in the enzyme indicates damage to liver. The liver contributes to the metabolism of protein which results in the production of ammonia. If the liver is damaged, the ammonia level will increase. Myoglobin, cholesterol, and BNP are relevant for heart disease. *Cognitive Level*: Application *Client Need*: Physiological Integrity *Nursing Process*: Assessment

7. *Answer*: 3 *Rationale*: Options 1 and 2 will provide information about the current blood glucose level. Option 4 is used to determine if a client has diabetes. *Cognitive Level*: Knowledge *Client Need*: Physiological Integrity *Nursing Process*: Planning

8. *Answer*: 2, 3, and 5 *Rationale*: The reagent is placed on the stool smear after it is applied to the card. A pink color would be considered negative and does not require verification. *Cognitive Level*: Application *Client Need*: Physiological Integrity *Nursing Process*: Planning

9. *Answer*: 2 *Rationale*: Puncture site is usually on the posterior chest. Leaning forward separates the ribs, allowing for exposure of the site. The site would not be exposed when supine in the Trendelenburg position. Vital sign changes and pain are not commonly associated with this procedure. *Cognitive Level*: Analysis *Client Need*: Physiological Integrity *Nursing Process*: Planning

10. *Answer*: 2, 4, and 5 *Rationale*: A sputum specimen is often collected in the morning. "Spit" is usually saliva—the client needs to cough up or expectorate mucus or sputum. *Cognitive Level*: Application *Client Need*: Physiological Integrity *Nursing Process*: Planning

CHAPTER 35
ANATOMY & PHYSIOLOGY REVIEW
GI System

1. A liquid medication is absorbed faster because it does not need to dissolve.

2. Diarrhea may decrease absorption because the drug is moving too rapidly through the small intestine to be absorbed.

3. The presence of food in the stomach will slow the rate of absorption and may decrease the amount of drug absorbed.

Cardiovascular System

1. The distribution of the drug depends on cardiac output and adequate blood flow to the organs and tissues of the body. The distribution of the oral medication may be hindered with a low cardiac output.

Liver

1. Age, especially the very young (immature organ) and the very old (diminished function), history of liver disease, chronic alcohol consumption.

2. If it is a hepatotoxic drug, the nurse would need to be vigilant about assessing the client and the client's lab values (e.g., liver enzymes) to avoid further organ dysfunction.

Kidneys

1. The very young have immature kidney function, and the elder has diminished organ function.

2. Monitor urine output, check lab values (e.g., BUN and creatinine levels), and assess for signs of edema or fluid overload.

CRITICAL THINKING POSSIBILITIES

1. Differences between an allergic reaction and a drug side effect can include:
   • Side effects are not related to an allergic reaction and do not produce the same symptoms as are produced by allergies. Allergic reactions have a distinct pattern of reaction (e.g., skin rash, pruritus, angioedema, rhinitis, tearing, nausea, vomiting, wheezing, dyspnea, or diarrhea).
   • A severe reaction is called *anaphylaxis* and can produce respiratory collapse if emergency treatment is not immediately instituted.
   • Drug hypersensitivity or drug allergy is often listed as a systemic side effect in drug handbooks.

2. Mr. Ketron may have allergies to either of the drugs; he may be on another prescribed drug, tobacco, alcohol, or nonprescription drug that interferes with or potentiates one of the prescribed drugs; he may have a medical condition that limits the kinds of drugs he can take safely, he could be allergic to penicillin, and so on.

3. Make the following assessments:
   • Inspect and palpate the IV insertion site for signs of infection, infiltration, or a dislocated catheter.
   • Inspect the surrounding skin for redness, pallor, or swelling.
   • Palpate the surrounding tissues for coldness and the presence of edema, which could indicate leakage of the IV fluid into the tissues.
   • Take vital signs for baseline data, especially respiratory rate.
   • Determine if the client has allergies to the medication.
   • Check the compatibility of the medication and IV fluid.
   • Determine specific drug action, side effects, normal dosage, recommended administration time, and peak action time of the morphine.
   • Check patency of the IV line by assessing flow rate.

4. All the same precautions should be taken with intravenous medications as with other medications: correct client, correct dose, correct route, and so on. Additional precautions include, but are not limited to, confirming that the antibiotic is compatible with the intravenous fluid infusing, verifying sterility of the system and integrity of the medication bag, verifying that there is no air in the system, cleaning the port prior to placing a needle, and reviewing Mr. Ketron's medication history for possible allergies.

5. Some drugs are better absorbed when given on an empty stomach, whereas others cause gastrointestinal irritation and should be given with meals or after meals.

TEST YOUR KNOWLEDGE

1. *Answer*: 2 *Rationale*: If there is any doubt, the medication administration process should be interrupted until the question is clarified. Medications should never be left unattended. Listen to the client. Find out any other information the client may have about that certain medication. For example, does he know the dosage of the medication taken at home? Do not administer the medication. Inform the client that you will check the chart first. Do not leave medications at the bedside. Review the chart to make sure there is no discrepancy between the physician's order and the MAR. Review the physician's progress notes because the medication may have been increased or reduced as part of the treatment plan. Check with the pharmacist because sometimes a pill may be a different color or shape based on the pharmaceutical company. Inform the client of your findings. The client will appreciate that you took the time to make sure that he received the correct medication. While it takes time to check out the client's statement, you will be glad that you avoided a potential medication error. *Cognitive Level*: Application *Client Need*: Physiological Integrity *Nursing Process*: Implementation

2. *Answer*: 4 *Rationale*: The dosage is missing from this order. *Cognitive Level*: Application *Client Need*: Physiological Integrity *Nursing Process*: Evaluation

3. *Answer*: 2 *Rationale*: Five milliliters is too great an amount to inject into one site. The nurse needs to divide the amount into two 2.5-mL injections. A 3-mL syringe could be used. The length of the needle will depend on the muscle development of the client. The nurse needs to assess the client. The presumption, based on the information provided, is that this client's muscle mass is within normal limits. The needle length would need to be 1 1/2 inches because the medication is ordered to be given "deep IM." This also suggests that the medication should be given in the preferred site for IM injections—the ventrogluteal site—because it provides the greatest thickness of gluteal muscle. The gauge of the needle for an IM injection into the ventrogluteal muscle can range between #20 and #23. The nurse needs to assess the viscosity of the medication. Smaller gauges (e.g., #23) produce less tissue trauma; however, viscous solutions may require a larger gauge (e.g., #20–#21). *Cognitive Level*: Analysis *Client Need*: Physiological Integrity *Nursing Process*: Implementation

4. *Answer*: 3 *Rationale*: The type of syringe for subcutaneous injections depends on the medication to be given. This situation does not indicate that the medication is insulin and, thus, another syringe is needed. Generally a 2-mL syringe is used for most subcutaneous injections. Generally, a #20 to #23 gauge needle is used for IM injections. Needle size and length are based on the client's body mass, the intended angle of insertion, and the site of the injection. Generally, a #25-gauge, 5/8-inch needle is used for adults of normal weight and the needle is inserted at a 45-degree angle. Because 2 inches of tissue can be grasped or pinched at the site of the injection, the nurse should administer the medication at a 90-degree angle to ensure the medication reaches subcutaneous tissue. *Cognitive Level*: Analysis *Client Need*: Physiological Integrity *Nursing Process*: Implementation

5. *Answer*: 1 *Rationale*: A tuberculin test is given by intradermal injection. A tuberculin syringe is used because the dosage will most likely be 0.1 mL. A short, fine needle is needed to avoid entering the subcutaneous tissue. The needle should have a short bevel and usually be between #25 and #27 gauge. The needle should be between 1/4- to 5/8-inch long. *Cognitive Level*: Analysis *Client Need*: Physiological Integrity *Nursing Process*: Implementation

6. *Answer*: 4 *Rationale*: If the nurse goes by the amount of the medication (0.5 mL) only, the deltoid muscle would be the site. However, knowing and assessing the client is critical. The muscles of an elderly, emaciated client will most likely be diminished or atrophied. The nurse should consider the ventrogluteal site because that site will have the most muscle mass. *Cognitive Level*: Analysis *Client Need*: Physiological Integrity *Nursing Process*: Implementation

7. *Answer*: 1 *Rationale*: Due to renal insufficiency, the dose of the medication would need to be decreased in order to avoid accumulation of the medication and the risk of toxicity. *Cognitive Level*: Application *Client Need*: Physiological Integrity *Nursing Process*: Assessment

8. *Answer*: 2 *Rationale*: In order to straighten the ear canal in children less than 3 years of age, the ear must be pulled down and back. In individuals over 3 years of age, the ear is pulled up and back. *Cognitive Level*: Application *Client Need*: Physiological Integrity *Nursing Process*: Implementation

9. *Answer*: 0.375 or rounded to 0.38 mL *Rationale*: After converting to like numbers, the formula would be set up as follows:

    400 micrograms = 1 mL

    150 micrograms = X mL

    Cross multiply (400 X = 150)

    Divide by 400

    $X = 0.375$

    Cognitive Level: Application *Client Need*: Physiological Integrity *Nursing Process*: Implementation

10. *Answer*: 3, 4, 1, 5, 2, 6, 7, 8 *Rationale*: This is the correct order for this skill—first the nurse mixes the insulin, assesses the skin, and cleanses the skin. The nurse would then pinch the skin, insert the needle, inject the medication, count to five, and remove the syringe. *Cognitive Level*: Application *Client Need*: Physiological Integrity *Nursing Process*: Implementation

CHAPTER 36

CRITICAL THINKING POSSIBILITIES

1. Mr. Johns's age, his decreased activity and mobility, his decreased sensation on the right, his incontinence, and his nutritional status (thin for his height) suggest he is vulnerable. In fact, he has evidence of a stage I pressure ulcer over his hips and coccyx.

2. You should assess the degree of his loss of sensation, his ability to recognize if he is incontinent, the frequency of his incontinence, how often he ambulates and his capacity for ambulation, his serum protein as an indicator of his nutritional status, and his ability to attend to his own needs.

3. You should undertake measures that include, but are not limited to, providing nutritious meals and snacks, assisting him if necessary, changing his position every 2 hours, avoiding shearing or friction when moving and positioning him, keeping his skin clean and dry, using pressure-relieving support devices, and encouraging activity. Ongoing skin assessment and evaluation of the effectiveness of his overall treatment plan are also essential. Discuss the benefit of each of these measures. Consider their cost and the amount of caregiver time required. Prioritize the measures and include rationales.

4. Although the skin is not yet broken, he meets the description of having a stage I ulcer and will progress to further stages (and probably more areas of breakdown) if interventions are not initiated.

TEST YOUR KNOWLEDGE

1. *Answer*: 2 *Rationale*: A score ranging from 15 to 18 is considered at risk and a turning schedule is appropriate. Option 1 requires a

score above 18 (normal and ongoing assessment is indicated). Option 3, moderate risk, for which a transparent barrier would be appropriate, is applied to persons with scores of 13 to 14. Option 4, very high risk, is assigned for those with a score of 9 or less. *Cognitive Level*: Application *Client Need*: Safe, Effective Care Management *Nursing Process*: Implementing

2. *Answer*: 1 *Rationale*: Wound culture specimens should be obtained from a cleaned area of the wound. Microbes responsible for the infection are more likely to be found in viable tissue. Collected drainage contains old and mixed organisms. An appropriate specimen can be obtained without causing the client the discomfort of debriding. The nurse does not generally debride the wound to obtain a specimen. Once systemic antibiotics have been begun, the interval following a dose will not significantly affect the concentration of wound organisms. *Cognitive Level*: Application *Client Need*: Physiological Integrity *Nursing Process*: Implementing

3. *Answer*: 3 *Rationale*: Hydrocolloid dressings protect shallow ulcers and maintain an appropriate healing environment. Alginates (option 1) are used for wounds with significant drainage; dry gauze (option 2) will stick to new granulation tissue, causing more damage. A dressing is needed to protect the wound and enhance healing. *Cognitive Level*: Application *Client Need*: Physiological Integrity *Nursing Process*: Implementing

4. *Answer*: 1 *Rationale*: The heating pad needs to be removed. After 30 minutes of heat application, the blood vessels in the area will begin to exhibit the rebound effect resulting in vasoconstriction. Lowering the temperature, but still delivering heat—dry or moist—will not prevent the rebound effect. The visual appearance of the site on inspection (option 3) does not indicate if rebound is occurring. *Cognitive Level*: Analysis *Client Need*: Physiological Integrity *Nursing Process*: Planning

5. *Answer*: 3 *Rationale*: Immobile and dependent persons should be repositioned at least every 2 hours, not every 4, so this client or family member requires further teaching. Warm water and moisturizing damp skin are correct techniques for skin care. Red areas that do not return to normal skin color should be reported. It would also be correct to use a foam pad to help relieve pressure. *Cognitive Level*: Analysis *Client Need*: Physiological Integrity *Nursing Process*: Evaluating

6. *Answer*: Potential pressure ulcer sites for side-lying clients include ankles, knees, trochanters, ilia, shoulders, and ears. *Cognitive Level*: Knowledge *Client Need*: Health Promotion and Maintenance *Nursing Process*: Assessing

7. *Answer*: 2 *Rationale*: This client has an actual impairment of the integrity of the skin due to the rash and the scratching so is no longer "at risk." Because the damage is at the skin level, it is not impaired tissue integrity (option 3) since that would involve deeper tissues. Surface excoriation is also not prone to becoming infected. *Cognitive Level*: Analysis *Client Need*: Physiological Integrity *Nursing Process*: Diagnosing

8. *Answer*: 1, 3, and 4 *Rationale*: Risk factors for pressure ulcers include low-protein diet, lengthy surgical procedures, and fever. Protein is needed for adequate skin health and healing. During surgery, the client is on a hard surface and may not be well protected from pressure on bony prominences. Fever increases skin moisture which can lead to skin breakdown, plus the stress on the body from the cause of the fever could impair circulation and skin integrity. Insomnia (option 5) would generally involve restless sleeping which transfers pressure to different parts of the body and would reduce the chances of skin breakdown. A waterbed (option 5) distributes pressure more evenly than a regular mattress

and, thus, actually reduces the chances of skin breakdown. *Cognitive Level*: Knowledge *Client Need*: Health Promotion and Maintenance *Nursing Process*: Assessing

9. *Answer*: 1, 2, and 4 *Rationale*: To irrigate a wound, the nurse uses clean gloves to remove the old dressing and to hold the basin collecting the irrigating fluid plus sterile gloves to apply the new dressing. A 60-mL syringe is the correct size to hold the volume of irrigating solution plus deliver safe irrigating pressure. The irrigation fluid should be room or body temperature—certainly not refrigerated. *Cognitive Level*: Knowledge *Client Need*: Physiological *Nursing Process*: Planning

10. *Answer*: 2 *Rationale*: The knot of the triangle sling must be kept off the spinal processes as this would be uncomfortable and put unnecessary pressure on the vertebrae. The elbow should be flexed slightly less than 80 degrees (not >90 as in option 1) so the hand is above the elbow to prevent dependent swelling. The sling must extend past the wrist in order to support the hand. Although the sling must be removed to check for circulation and skin integrity, every 2 hours (option 4) is unnecessarily frequent and impractical. *Cognitive Level*: Knowledge *Client Need*: Physiological *Nursing Process*: Evaluating

CHAPTER 37

ANATOMY & PHYSIOLOGY REVIEW

1. Assess skin integrity and the presence or absence of any breakdown and/or bruises. Assess the musculoskeletal, neurological, and circulatory systems for previous injury or limitations. Assessment for positioning needs is done before the client is transferred to the operating table.

2. The potential pressure areas are the occiput, scapula, olecranon, sacrum, coccyx, and calcaneus. Special attention is paid to previously damaged tissues and diseased joints to prevent breakdown or deterioration due to positioning during the surgical procedure.

3. Nursing diagnoses: *Risk for Injury* related to sustained pressure and *Misalignment of Specific Body Areas During Surgery*.

   Outcome: Client will be free from injury related to positioning.

CRITICAL THINKING POSSIBILITIES

1. Factors that may increase Mr. Teng's risk include, but are not limited to, the following: he is 77 years old, placing him at greater risk than younger adults; his respiratory status is compromised and he runs a greater risk for developing postoperative atelectasis or lung infection; and he may be taking medications that will slow healing, such as corticosteroids.

2. A major disadvantage of general anesthesia is that it depresses the respiratory and circulatory systems, so the surgeon and anesthesiologist probably chose not to further complicate Mr. Teng's respiratory status. A client's preference for a particular anesthesia is also considered when selecting the type of anesthesia to use.

3. Mr. Teng's preoperative preparation most likely included, but was not limited to, preoperative teaching regarding preparation for surgery; what to expect following surgery; deep-breathing, coughing, and leg exercises; how to splint his abdomen when moving or coughing; fluid and nutritional support; a bath or shower; antiemboli stockings; and medications to enhance rest the night prior to the scheduled surgery.

4. Even though Mr. Teng had spinal anesthesia and is awake, the same general assessments will be made to detect actual or potential problems. He will not go through the stages of anesthesia arousal or experience altered gag reflexes. He will be assessed for

return of feeling to his lower extremities to evaluate remaining spinal anesthesia effect. His postoperative monitoring will not differ from that of other clients.

5. Specific precautions may include, but are not limited to, promoting adequate hydration to replace fluids lost during surgery or fluid limitations prior to surgery, early movement and ambulation to foster maximum lung expansion and prevent lung infection, deep-breathing exercises to remove mucus and prevent stasis of lung secretions, pain control so that he can ambulate and cough more effectively, and leg exercises to prevent thrombophlebitis.

TEST YOUR KNOWLEDGE

1. *Answer*: 3 *Rationale*: These tests are specific to liver function. Option 1 evaluates fluid and electrolyte status. Option 2 evaluates renal status; option 4 evaluates nutritional status. *Cognitive Level*: Analysis *Client Need*: Physiological Integrity *Nursing Process*: Assessment

2. *Answer*: 2 *Rationale*: Anticipatory grieving is the state in which an individual experiences reactions in response to an expected significant loss. The definition for option 1 is "confusion in mental picture of one's self" and is often characterized by negative responses such as shame, embarrassment, guilt, or revulsion. Option 3, fear, is usually characterized by feelings of dread, fright, apprehension, or alarm. Ineffective coping, option 4, is usually characterized by verbalization of inability to cope or ask for help, inappropriate use of defense mechanisms, or inability to meet role expectations. *Cognitive Level*: Application *Client Need*: Psychological Integrity *Nursing Process*: Diagnosis

3. *Answer*: 4 *Rationale*: Option 1 is incorrect because of the ASA guidelines for preoperative fasting. Option 2 is incorrect because clients are taught how to cough and also how to splint their incision to prevent complications. Option 3 is incorrect because anticoagulants are discontinued a few days before surgery to avoid excessive bleeding postoperatively. *Cognitive Level*: Application *Client Need*: Physiological Integrity *Nursing Process*: Evaluation

4. *Answer*: 2 *Rationale*: The symptoms describe decreased cardiac output and not any of the other listed complications. *Cognitive Level*: Application *Client Need*: Physiological Integrity *Nursing Process*: Assessment

5. *Answer*: 3 *Rationale*: Options 1 and 2 are incorrect because the client is still recovering from the anesthesia used during surgery. Option 4 is incorrect because pain usually decreases after the second or third postoperative day. *Cognitive Level*: Application *Client Need*: Physiological Integrity *Nursing Process*: Implementation

6. *Answer*: Splinting *Rationale*: If the incision is painful when the client coughs, splinting the abdomen may reduce the pain while coughing. *Cognitive Level*: Knowledge *Client Need*: Physiological Integrity *Nursing Process*: Implementation

7. *Answer*: 4 *Rationale*: The tongue can obstruct the airway in a semiconscious client. Repositioning in the side-lying position with the face slightly down will help prevent occlusion of the pharynx and also allow drainage of mucus out of the mouth. A pillow under the head increases the risk of aspiration or airway obstruction. Since the problem is airway obstruction, actions to promote an open airway are most appropriate. The nurse would want to keep the airway in place. The problem is obstruction, not percentage of available oxygen. *Cognitive Level*: Application *Client Need*: Physiological Integrity *Nursing Process*: Implementation

8. *Answer*: 1 and 3 *Rationale*: The nurse would also assess bowel sounds—for presence and degree of activity. Anesthetics, narcotics, fasting, and inactivity all inhibit peristalsis. Oral fluids and food are started after the return of peristalsis. The client may feel hungry but peristalsis may not be present. The other options are important but not related specifically to advancing the client's diet. *Cognitive Level*: Application *Client Need*: Physiological Integrity *Nursing Process*: Assessment

9. *Answer*: Safety *Rationale*: The client's protective reflexes are compromised, especially with general anesthesia. Thus the perioperative nurse needs to maintain the client's safety during surgery. *Cognitive Level*: Analysis *Client Need*: Safe, Effective Care Environment *Nursing Process*: Planning

10. *Answer*: 2, 3, and 5: *Rationale*: Sterile technique is used. The suture material that is visible is in contact with bacteria and must not be pulled beneath the skin during removal. Removal of alternate sutures prevents dehiscence. *Cognitive Level*: Application *Client Need*: Physiological Integrity *Nursing Process*: Implementation

CHAPTER 38

ANATOMY & PHYSIOLOGY REVIEW

1. Open
2. Closed
3. Figure 38-3, *B*
4. Figure 38-3, *C*
5. Optic Nerve (review Figure 38-3 ∞)

CRITICAL THINKING POSSIBILITIES

1. Mrs. Dodd is at greatly increased risk for sensory overload due to her environment (critical care unit). She is being bombarded by the noise of her monitors and ventilator, which may be distorted and meaningless due to the sedation she is receiving. Her pain and inability to communicate also contribute to her sensory overload because they contribute to her feelings of being overwhelmed and out of control.

2. Signs of sensory overload may include, but are not limited to, restlessness, agitation, confusion, disorientation, hallucinations, or inability to sleep or rest. Signs of sensory deprivation may include apathy, emotional detachment, and depression. Many times the signs of sensory deprivation and overload are the same; consequently, the nurse must assess the client for factors that may be contributing to one problem over the other.

3. Interventions include, but are not limited to, reducing and dimming lights; decreasing noise to the degree possible (close doors or curtains); providing comfort measures; explaining all procedures; orienting the client to person, place, and time; speaking in a soft, unhurried manner; and limiting visitors.

4. Clients cared for at home may experience either sensory deprivation or overload depending on the environment. If it is a busy, active environment with several family members, they may experience overload. If clients live alone, have few supportive family members, or are seldom contacted, they are more likely to experience social isolation and become withdrawn or uncommunicative, or lose interest in their usual activities. Interventions for home care or ICU clients are similar and adapted to the specific needs of the client, regardless of setting.

TEST YOUR KNOWLEDGE

1. *Answer*: 4 *Rationale*: A sudden, unexpected admission for surgery may involve many experiences (e.g., lab work, x-rays, signing of forms) while the client is in pain or some form of discomfort. The time for orientation will thus be lessened. After surgery, the client may be in pain and possibly in a critical care

setting. Options 1 and 2 reflect a greater risk for sensory depriva- tion, and 3 is a normal activity for a teenager. *Cognitive Level*: Application *Client Need*: Psychosocial Integrity *Nursing Process*: Evaluation

2. *Answer*: 3 *Rationale*: The transfer to a different setting can change the amount or patterning of incoming stimuli accompa- nied by a diminished, exaggerated, distorted, or impaired re- sponse to such stimuli. Options 1 and 2: There is no evidence of long-standing or progressive deterioration of intellect and person- ality. Option 4: *Disturbed Thought Processes* is applied when cog- nitive abilities (e.g., dementia) interfere with the ability to accurately interpret stimuli. *Cognitive Level*: Application *Client Need*: Psychosocial Integrity *Nursing Process*: Diagnosis

3. *Answer*: 2 *Rationale*: Because of the paraplegia (paralysis of lower body), the client is unable to feel discomfort. The client will be taught to lift self using chair arms every 10 minutes if possible. Option 1 is an actual problem versus a potential problem. In op- tion 3, the client wears glasses that help correct the poor vision. Option 4 is more of a *Risk for Injury* diagnosis. *Cognitive Level*: Application *Client Need*: Psychosocial Integrity *Nursing Process*: Diagnosis

4. *Answer*: 2 *Rationale*: This client could use an assistive device that flashes a light when the doorbell rings. Option 1 relates to safety of the environment rather than sensory alteration. Options 3 and 4 reflect how the client adapts to the sensory alteration. *Cognitive Level*: Analysis *Client Need*: Safe, Effective Care En- vironment *Nursing Process*: Evaluation

5. *Answer*: 4 *Rationale*: Option 4 is the only response that helps ori- ent the client and treats the client with respect. *Cognitive Level*: Application *Client Need*: Psychosocial Integrity *Nursing Process*: Implementation

6. *Answer*: 1, 3, and 4 *Rationale*: Options 2 and 5 relate to interven- tions for a client with a hearing impairment. *Cognitive Level*: Ap- plication *Client Need*: Psychosocial Integrity *Nursing Process*: Implementation

7. *Answer*: 3 *Rationale*: A disorganized, cluttered environment in- creases confusion. Option 1: Keeping the room well lit during waking hours promotes adequate sleep at night. It is important to eliminate unnecessary noise (option 2). Client does not meet the standard criteria for restraint application (option 4). *Cognitive Level*: Application *Client Need*: Safe, Effective Care Environ- ment *Nursing Process*: Implementation

8. *Answer*: 2, 4, and 5 *Rationale*: Options 1 and 3 are clinical signs of sensory overload. *Cognitive Level*: Knowledge *Client Need*: Psychosocial Integrity *Nursing Process*: Assessment

9. *Answer*: a) 5, b) 3, c) 1, d) 4, e) 2 *Cognitive Level*: Knowledge *Client Need*: Health Promotion and Maintenance *Nursing Process*: Assessment

10. *Answer*: 1 *Rationale*: The amplified telephone helps with hear- ing and provides a means for communicating with others. Option 2 refers to a tactile impairment. Option 3 relates to a visual impair- ment, and option 4 an olfactory impairment. *Cognitive Level*: Ap- plication *Client Need*: Psychosocial Integrity *Nursing Process*: Planning

CHAPTER 39
CRITICAL THINKING POSSIBILITIES

1. Because of his age, Craig's basic self-concept should be fairly well set and is not likely to be negatively affected. Body image

and self-esteem, however, may be altered by his amputation. Body image is at risk because the amputation will change the way he views his body. Personal identity is at risk because he sees him- self as an athlete.

2. If Craig's mood, inability to look at the stump, and unwillingness to discuss rehabilitation continue or new negative responses de- velop, a negative change in his self-esteem may be occurring. Since his father is also having difficulty with the loss, a strong source of support is unavailable to Craig.

3. There are many possibilities, including his nurses' attitudes; reha- bilitation team and primary caregiver abilities; family and friends' support; and his internal ability to be adaptable, revise his goals, and use his resources. Craig's mother's presence is likely to be support- ive unless she offers assistance while encouraging dependency.

4. Adapting to change may be more difficult for elders. Elders fear dependence more than younger clients; therefore, a large loss such as this puts them at greater risk for altered self-esteem. In addi- tion, elders do not heal and progress as quickly as younger clients—the additional time required may seem to them a negative factor. Much care, however, will be similar: encouragement and support, participation in their own care, identifying personal strengths, and so on.

5. Clients with chronic mental illnesses, cancer, socially stigmatized diseases (AIDS, TB, obesity, sexually transmitted diseases), and other sources of disfigurement.

TEST YOUR KNOWLEDGE

1. *Answer*: 1 *Rationale*: Sally has an inappropriate view of her physical self which is body image. Personal identity is a sense of uniqueness; self-expectation consists of those things one believes the self should be able to do; and core self-concept includes the most vital central beliefs about one's identity. *Cognitive Level*: Application *Client Need*: Psychosocial Integrity *Nursing Process*: Diagnosing

2. *Answer*: 3 *Rationale*: This is role conflict—several different roles are competing for the person's time, energy, and abilities. Role ambiguity results when there are unclear expectations of the role. Role strain exists when there are feelings of inadequacy in performing a role. Role enhancement is a nursing intervention. *Cognitive Level*: Comprehension *Client Need*: Psychosocial In- tegrity *Nursing Process*: Diagnosing

3. *Answer*: 2 *Rationale*: This is a realistic and measurable outcome. Restored self-esteem is vague and not measurable. Teaching is an intervention, not an outcome. Decreased preoccupation with al- tered self relates to body image rather than self-esteem. *Cognitive Level*: Application *Client Need*: Psychosocial Integrity *Nursing Process*: Planning

4. *Answer*: 1 *Rationale*: This response encourages the client to say more and focuses on the positive. Option 2 is condescending and closes the discussion. Both options 3 and 4 ignore the emotional component of the client's statement and do not address the person's feelings of worthlessness. *Cognitive Level*: Application *Client Need*: Psychosocial Integrity *Nursing Process*: Implementing

5. *Answer*: 4 *Rationale*: A person who follows the crowd is demon- strating unsuccessful resolution of this task. Successful resolution would result in assertion of independence. Inability to express de- sires is symptomatic of unresolved toddlerhood autonomy versus shame and doubt, while difficulty being a team player suggests unresolved early school-age industry versus inferiority. *Cognitive Level*: Comprehension *Client Need*: Psychosocial Integrity *Nursing Process*: Assessing

that either option 2 or 3 is the best diagnosis. The mother is experiencing distress versus being at risk for it (option 4). *Cognitive Level*: Application *Client Need*: Psychosocial Integrity *Nursing Process*: Diagnosis

CHAPTER 42

CRITICAL THINKING POSSIBILITIES

1. It is difficult to know whether Ruby's coping would differ if only a portion of the breast were going to be removed or whether this is merely the focus of her difficulty in coping with the diagnosis and need for surgery. It might depend on how large her breasts are and if the lump represented a significant portion of the breast. Persons may have very different emotional reactions to situations in which they can or cannot hide their condition or if the impact is directly linked to their role (such as the fact that she is a dress designer).

2. Ruby's situation fits with a stimulus-based model since the stressors of diagnosis, surgery, and implications of having cancer serve as stress stimuli causing physical and emotional outcomes (such as her ineffective mothering). However, her situation would also fit the response model since the surgery and any further cancer treatment required plus her alcohol use would create stress reactions in the mind and body.

3. The nurse will validate that she cannot know exactly what Ruby is experiencing (assuming the nurse has not actually had a mastectomy), but has worked with many clients undergoing extremely distressful and possibly life-threatening conditions. One of the interventions will include making a connection with other women who have had breast cancer, but that is a response to the content of her message. The nurse first needs to respond to the emotional part of the message—Ruby's anger, frustration, and lack of control.

4. The suddenness of this diagnosis and Ruby's extreme reaction of alcohol abuse and neglecting her children certainly may qualify the situation as a crisis. Her inability to discuss her feelings or plans supports the presence of a crisis situation. Under these circumstances, caregivers may need to be more assertive in providing her care and making decisions. She may benefit from referral for psychological therapy/counseling.

5. Many answers may be correct. She does not appear to be using denial. She might use projection in attempting to find a cause of her cancer, which could be maladaptive since, most commonly, the cause of breast cancer is unknown.

TEST YOUR KNOWLEDGE

1. *Answer*: 3 *Rationale*: Taking on additional work would only serve as an additional stressor. In addition, a nurse who has not begun resolution of feelings is unlikely to be able to meet clients' emotional needs. Effective coping may include verbalizing feelings (one-on-one or in groups) or initiating distractions. Of course, the nurse may not disclose confidential information to her partner or others who would not already have this information. *Cognitive Level*: Analysis *Client Need*: Psychosocial Integrity *Nursing Process*: Evaluating

2. *Answer*: 4 *Rationale*: Wearing glasses is another example of beginning a new strategy to assist with what will be a lifelong health need even though it is not necessarily a desired change. Interviewing for a job (option 1) is a very short-lived situational stressor. Coping strategies effective while a teenager may not be relevant at age 50 (option 2). Experiencing the stress of a divorce is a so-

cial/role stressor quite unlike that of a health problem (option 3). *Cognitive Level*: Analysis *Client Need*: Psychosocial Integrity *Nursing Process*: Assessing

3. *Answer*: 1 *Rationale*: In the transaction model, stress is a very personal experience and varies widely among individuals. Option 2 represents the stimulus model, and 3 represents the response model of stress. In option 4, external resources and support are a factor in determining stress levels but omit the key aspects of internal/personal influences. *Cognitive Level*: Application *Client Need*: Psychosocial Integrity *Nursing Process*: Assessing

4. *Answer*: 3 *Rationale*: With stress, respirations increase, pupils dilate, peripheral blood vessels constrict, and the heart rate increases. *Cognitive Level*: Application *Client Need*: Psychosocial Integrity Integrative Process *Nursing Process*: Assessing

5. *Answer*: 2 *Rationale*: It is too soon for *Caregiver Role Strain* to be an appropriate nursing diagnosis—especially since the child is not at home. *Ineffective Denial* and *Fear* are common reactions to this type of threat. The father demonstrates *Compromised Family Coping* by his difficulty in being supportive. *Cognitive Level*: Application *Client Need*: Psychosocial Integrity *Nursing Process*: Diagnosing

6. *Answer*: 1, 3, and 4 *Rationale*: Common stressors among young adults include marriage, starting a new job, and leaving the parental home. Stressors from aging parents are more common among middle-aged adults; decreased physical abilities is a stressor in elders; and changing body structure serves as a stressor in both children and older adults. *Cognitive Level*: Comprehension *Client Need*: Psychosocial Integrity *Nursing Process*: Planning

7. *Answer*: 2 *Rationale*: All of the four areas of health promotion strategies may be important but for this client sleep is likely to be the most adversely affected by travel in which changing time zones and unfamiliar sleeping quarters are common. It is easier for clients to adapt to modifying exercise, nutrition, and time management during travel than it is to control sleep. Thus, it becomes the most important area requiring intervention to avoid worsening the existing stress. *Cognitive Level*: Application *Client Need*: Psychosocial Integrity *Nursing Process*: Implementing

8. *Answer*: 4 *Rationale*: Unless the nurse feels in physical danger, it is important to remain with the client, allow the anger to dissipate, and then begin assessing the cause. Leaving the room provides no therapeutic action. Option 2 may be considered setting limits, which can be helpful, but cannot occur until the client is calmer. All behavior is meaningful; it is inappropriate to ignore the client's behavior (option 3). *Cognitive Level*: Application *Client Need*: Psychosocial Integrity *Nursing Process*: Implementing

CHAPTER 43

CRITICAL THINKING POSSIBILITIES

1. The eldest son most nearly approximates the "awareness of loss" phase. He is experiencing the loss but is able to resume normal activities. The middle son has characteristics of the "conservation/withdrawal" phase. He has a need to be alone, and is experiencing both physical and psychologic symptoms of bereavement. The younger son is experiencing "shock." He is having difficulty believing that his mother is dead and is experiencing several physical symptoms.

2. Factors include amount of conflict or closeness each brother felt to the mother, amount of time/caring each was able to provide,

significance/meaning of the mother to each, spiritual beliefs and practices, and the amount of guilt each felt related to meeting the mother's needs during her later years or illness.

3. Cues might include wanting to talk about death, reminiscing or reviewing one's life, emotional withdrawal or becoming quiet and pensive, allowing others to take over physical care, voicing a sense of urgency about seeing loved ones, and so on.

4. One significant need she may have is for relief of shortness of breath. Both from the pneumonia and the dying process, normal respirations are impaired and she may feel as though she cannot get enough air. In addition, shortness of breath may instill fear — an important need the nurse must attend to. Although this client was not diagnosed as terminally ill, as she approached death, many of the physiological needs identified in Table 43–5 would occur.

5. If you have had mostly positive experiences, or ones similar to those the client is experiencing, these can be shared with others. Consider characteristics of the losses (e.g., if they were expected or unexpected, your age and that of the deceased) and effectiveness of sources of support during grieving.

TEST YOUR KNOWLEDGE

1. *Answer*: 1, 2, and 3 *Rationale*: Correct answers include abbreviated (normal grief that is briefly experienced), anticipatory grief (experienced before the loss/death but appropriate), and disenfranchised grief (the emotions are felt privately, just not expressed in public). Unhealthy/abnormal types of grief include complicated grief in several different forms: Unresolved grief is extended in length and severity. With inhibited grief, symptoms are suppressed, and other effects, including somatic, are experienced instead. *Cognitive Level*: Knowledge *Client Need*: Psychosocial Integrity *Nursing Process*: Diagnosing

2. *Answer*: 2 *Rationale*: When possible, modifications of policy that demonstrate respect for individual differences should be explored. The primary care provider is in no position to modify the implementation of hospital policy. Utilizing an empty room and a staff member for a deceased client is an inappropriate use of resources. *Cognitive Level*: Analysis *Client Need*: Psychosocial Integrity *Nursing Process*: Planning

3. *Answer*: 1 *Rationale*: This statement acknowledges the family's grief simply. Avoid statements that may be interpreted as overly impersonal (option 2), false support (option 3), or harsh (option 4). Other responses may also be correct. *Cognitive Level*: Application *Client Need*: Psychosocial Integrity *Nursing Process*: Implementing

4. *Answer*: 3 *Rationale*: Until children are about 5 years old, they believe that death is reversible. Between ages 5 and 9, the child knows death is irreversible but believes it can be avoided. Between 9 and 12 years of age, the child recognizes that he, too, will someday die. At 12 to 15 years old, the child builds on previous beliefs and may fear death, but often pretends not to care about it. *Cognitive Level*: Knowledge *Client Need*: Psychosocial Integrity *Nursing Process*: Assessing

5. *Answer*: 4 *Rationale*: Adaptive responses indicate the client can put the loss into perspective and begin to develop strategies for coping with the loss. Although the other options are responses the client might likely give and feel, and are not pathologic, they do not demonstrate movement toward a goal of adaptation nor problem solving. *Cognitive Level*: Application *Client Need*: Psychosocial Integrity *Nursing Process*: Evaluating

6. *Answer*: 1 *Rationale*: The nurse needs to assess and explore the meaning of the client's crying. Options 2 and 4 leap to assumptions about the meaning of the tears and ignore the possibility of the client's distress. Option 3 suggests that the client has the same feelings as the nurse, which may not be correct. *Cognitive Level*: Application *Client Need*: Psychosocial Integrity *Nursing Process*: Implementing

7. *Answer*: 4 *Rationale*: Quality of life is determined by the client and expressed in terms of his or her satisfaction with a variety of aspects of life. Although being able to pay for care, apparent spiritual peace, and absence of physiological complications may appear to contribute to good quality of life, only the client's expression of satisfaction can provide the data the nurse requires to evaluate the goal. *Cognitive Level*: Analysis *Client Need*: Psychosocial Integrity *Nursing Process*: Evaluating

8. *Answer*: 4 *Rationale*: In order for the nurse to plan with and assist the family, the nurse needs more data regarding the family's reactions to their loss. Information on issues such as insurance coverage can wait until later and may be more appropriately the responsibility of social services rather than the nurse. It is important for the nurse to determine their understanding of their injuries but they are stated as minor. Once the nurse has assessed the family's responses it will be important to determine availability of outside resources to assist them. *Cognitive Level*: Analysis *Client Need*: Psychosocial Integrity *Integrative Process*: Assessing

CHAPTER 44

ANATOMY & PHYSIOLOGY REVIEW

1. Because the upper and lower body are connected, any change in gait such as a limp will affect general alignment, and therefore affect musculoskeletal functioning in the back. Improper alignment throughout the body can lead to discomfort and injury.

2. When the right arm swings forward at the same time as the left leg swings through, a natural rotation of the hips and shoulders is demonstrated. This is a more energy efficient gait, and makes use of the natural movement in the low back for locomotion. When people hold themselves "stiffly" as they walk, either not moving their shoulders or hips in a rhythmic, swinging fashion, they are interrupting the normal flow of energy through the spine and into the legs, and will likely become tired more quickly, or develop various discomforts throughout their body.

CRITICAL THINKING POSSIBILITIES

1. His dyspnea on mild exertion is a worrisome sign, and his activity intolerance will worsen if he remains immobile. His edema indicates inadequate venous return, especially with his amount of time spent sitting, and will lead to other problems.

2. Check environment for possible safety hazards, get a walker light enough to handle easily and be sure it has been adjusted for proper height, keep the tips in good shape, do exercises to keep strength in the hands and arms.

3. Being overweight certainly contributes to his difficulties and should be addressed. More assessment is needed regarding how long he has been overweight and his eating patterns.

4. There is a relationship between physical and emotional health; that the client "wants" to be healthier.

5. With chronic illness, because the condition has existed for a longer time, the outcomes may require more time to achieve than with acute illnesses. Outcomes should be in smaller increments.

Lower levels of expectations are often appropriate since full return to earlier levels of health is unlikely.

TEST YOUR KNOWLEDGE

1. *Answer*: 2 *Rationale*: A key word in the question is "base," and the feet provide this foundation. Leaning backward actually decreases balance, and tensing abdominal muscles alone or bending the knees does not affect the base of support. *Cognitive Level*: Application *Client Need*: Health Promotion and Maintenance *Nursing Process*: Implementation

2. *Answer*: 1, 3, and, 5 *Rationale*: Isotonic exercise increases muscle tone, mass, and strength and maintains joint flexibility and circulation. During isotonic exercise, both heart rate and cardiac output quicken to increase blood flow to all parts of the body. Little or no change in blood pressure occurs. *Cognitive Level*: Knowledge *Client Need*: Physiological Integrity *Nursing Process*: Planning

3. *Answer*: 1 *Rationale*: Vital signs that do not return to baseline 5 minutes after exercising indicate intolerance of exercise at that time. This is a real problem, not "at risk for." There is no evidence that the client requires assistance (impaired mobility) or is immobile (disuse syndrome). *Cognitive Level*: Analysis *Client Need*: Physiological Integrity *Nursing Process*: Diagnosis

4. *Answer*: 3 *Rationale*: Although the crutches (or cane) are always used along with the weaker leg, the weaker leg should go down the stairs first. The stronger leg can support the body as the weaker leg moves forward. All of the other statements are correct. *Cognitive Level*: Analysis *Client Need*: Physiological Integrity *Nursing Process*: Evaluation

5. *Answer*: 2 *Rationale*: The benzodiazepines (e.g., Valium) impair the function of the central nervous system resulting in unstable ambulation or movement. *Cognitive Level*: Comprehension *Client Need*: Safe, Effective Care Environment *Nursing Process*: Assessment

6. *Answer*: 1 *Rationale*: Normal gait involves a level gaze, an initial rotation beginning in the spine, heel strike with follow through to the toes, and opposite arm and leg swinging forward. *Cognitive Level*: Application *Client Need*: Physiological Integrity *Nursing Process*: Assessment

7. *Answer*: 1, 4, and 5 *Rationale*: Eating and bathing will flex the elbow joint, and grasping and manipulating utensils to eat and write will take the thumb through its normal ROM, Walking flexes the hip. Writing brings the fingers toward the inner aspect of the forearm, thus flexing the wrist joint. *Cognitive Level*: Application *Client Need*: Health Promotion and Maintenance *Nursing Process*: Implementation

8. *Answer*: 3 *Rationale*: It is prudent for nurses to understand and use proper body mechanics at all times to decrease risk, while keeping in mind the importance of assistive devices and help from other staff. While it is generally accepted that proper body mechanics alone will not prevent injury, many work settings do not yet have "no manual lift" and "no solo lift" policies and resources in place. *Cognitive Level*: Analysis *Client Need*: Safe, Effective Care Environment *Nursing Process*: Implementation

9. *Answer*: 4 *Rationale*: Placing the client in a safe position is the best maneuver. Leaving the client creates unsafe conditions as the client may faint before being able to return to her room. Rapid, shallow breathing (hyperventilation) may increase the dizziness. *Cognitive Level*: Application *Client Need*: Safe, Effective Care Environment *Nursing Process*: Implementation

10. *Answer*: 2 *Rationale*: The reddened area of the skin can lead to skin breakdown. The other options are within normal limits. *Cognitive Level*: Application *Client Need*: Physiological Integrity *Nursing Process*: Assessment

CHAPTER 45
ANATOMY & PHYSIOLOGY REVIEW

1. When preparing for sleep, people close their eyes, place themselves into a relaxing position, turn out the lights, etc. This decreases the amount of sensory stimuli to the RAS which, in turn, relays few stimuli to the cerebral cortex which promotes sleep.

2. The sensory stimuli (auditory from the noise of the alarm clock and light in the room) activates the RAS which sends stimuli to the cerebral cortex and causes wakefulness.

3. Brain stem (location of reticular formation and RAS), cerebral cortex (an intact cerebral cortex is necessary for the regulation of sleep and waking states), and the hypothalamus. Injury to the hypothalamus may cause a person to sleep for abnormally long periods.

CRITICAL THINKING POSSIBILITIES

1. Other data that may be helpful include, but are not limited to, activities and bedtime habits, degree of noise in the environment, what foods or drinks he consumes just prior to bedtime, if he uses over-the-counter medications to help him sleep, if he has a regular pattern of arising, and whether he is a smoker.

2. Suggest that he read a book or other quiet activity (not watching TV or exercising) before going to sleep, maintain regular sleep and waking hours, explore nonpharmacologic sleep remedies, and so on.

3. Common causes of difficulty in sleeping are physical distress, noisy environment, severe fatigue, changing work shifts, emotional distress, alcohol and other stimulants, weight loss, and smoking.

TEST YOUR KNOWLEDGE

1. *Answer*: 2 *Rationale*: This is the brain stem where the reticular formation (and RAS) is located and which integrates sensory information from the peripheral nervous system and relays the information to the cerebral cortex. An intact cerebral cortex and reticular formation are necessary for the regulation of sleep and waking states. *Cognitive Level*: Knowledge *Client Need*: Physiological Integrity *Nursing Process*: Assessment

2. *Answer*: 4 *Rationale*: Most clients with sleep apnea report excessive daytime sleepiness. If they don't volunteer this, clients should be asked if they fall asleep or struggle to stay awake at work. Although cardiac arrhythmias may occur, they are usually only detectable during a sleep study, and thus the client would not be aware of them. Nasal obstruction is rarely the cause of sleep apnea or a complaint of clients with sleep apnea. There are many causes of chest pain, and this is unlikely to be something reported by clients with sleep apnea unless they have underlying cardiac disease. *Cognitive Level*: Analysis *Client Need*: Physiological Integrity *Nursing Process*: Assessment

3. *Answer*: 2 *Rationale*: Falling asleep within 20 to 30 minutes is normal for adults and would represent substantial improvement in the client's difficulties. Most adults do not need to sleep 8 to 10 hours per day. Although it would be ideal to remove the source of the client's stress, he is unlikely to have a plan to pay all his bills within 5 days. Distraction or keeping busy until bedtime will not prevent the client from worrying about his bills at bedtime.

Cognitive Level: Analysis *Client Need*: Physiological Integrity *Nursing Process*: Planning

4. *Answer*: 4 *Rationale*: Suddenly stopping barbiturate sleeping pills can precipitate a dangerous withdrawal. Doses should be tapered gradually and the tapering process supervised by the client's primary care provider. *Cognitive Level*: Analysis *Client Need*: Physiological Integrity *Nursing Process*: Implementation

5. *Answer*: 1 *Rationale*: Preschool children require 10 to 12 hours of sleep/night. Young children often rise early, so it is more appropriate to put the child to bed earlier in the evening. *Cognitive Level*: Analysis *Client Need*: Health Promotion and Maintenance *Nursing Process*: Implementation

6. *Answer*: 1 and 3 *Rationale*: It is important to find out if he is obtaining sufficient sleep. If his sleep is greater on weekends than weekdays, insufficient sleep may be the cause of his difficulties staying awake in class. It is important to determine if his symptoms are chronic (e.g., longer than 3 months) or if they are of recent onset. Although alcohol abuse or binge drinking can cause health problems, neither is likely to cause excessive daytime sleepiness. Unless the person is sleep deprived, boring classes will not induce sleep. *Cognitive Level*: Analysis *Client Need*: Health Promotion and Maintenance *Nursing Process*: Assessment

7. *Answer*: 4 *Rationale*: The client's symptoms, combined with his weight, suggest that he has obstructive sleep apnea and should be referred to a sleep disorders specialist for further evaluation. It would not be wrong to refer him to a dietitian for weight loss counseling, but being evaluated by a sleep disorders specialist is more critical. Drinking alcohol or taking sleeping pills is not advised in clients with sleep apnea because they reduce the client's ability to get around. *Cognitive Level*: Analysis *Client Needs*: Physiological Integrity *Nursing Process*: Intervention

8. *Answer*: 1 *Rationale*: Reducing exposure to bright light in the morning, driving home, and when going to sleep will make it easier to fall asleep after work. Exercising before going to bed will increase arousal. Caffeine consumed at the beginning of a 12-hour shift will not assist the nurse in remaining awake during the later part of the shift. Although working in a brightly lit area will reduce drowsiness, this strategy is rarely available to nurses working the night shift; lights are often dimmed in hospital corridors and client rooms. *Cognitive Level*: Analysis *Client Need*: Health Promotion and Maintenance *Nursing Process*: Implementation

9. *Answer*: 3 *Rationale*: Napping frequently reappears in elders. Unless the person has difficulty falling asleep at night, there is no reason an individual should not be allowed to take a 15 to 20-minute nap in the early afternoon. *Cognitive Level*: Analysis *Client Need*: Health Promotion and Maintenance *Nursing Process*: Implementation

10. *Answer*: 1, 3, and 4 *Rationale*: Reducing environmental noise, as well as the number of times she is disturbed for medications and vital signs, will reduce the likelihood that she will awaken during the night. Since it is unlikely that all the noise in the environment can be eliminated, using a fan to generate a steady background noise may help mask sounds of people talking, carts being moved through the halls, etc. Music is not recommended because it can be interesting to listen to, thus encouraging wakefulness (option 2). *Cognitive Level*: Analysis *Client Need*: Physiological Integrity *Nursing Process*: Implementation

CHAPTER 46

CRITICAL THINKING POSSIBILITIES FOR CRITICAL THINKING CHECKPOINT

1. There are subjective data (rating her pain as 5) and objective data (vital signs, position, holding abdomen, lying in rigid position) to support that Mrs. Lundahl is experiencing pain; however, no conclusions can be drawn about the intensity, location, quality, or pattern of Mrs. Lundahl's pain.

2. It would be incorrect to assume that Mrs. Lundahl needs no interventions for her pain. People rate their pain differently based on their past pain experiences, their pain tolerance, their ethnic/cultural values, and so on. Mrs. Lundahl should be asked if she needs pain intervention.

3. Mrs. Lundahl is most likely experiencing acute pain from her surgery. Depending on the amount of manipulation of bowel, blood vessels, and so on, within her abdomen, she may also be experiencing visceral pain.

4. Numerous interventions may be helpful, such as changing her body position, a back massage, use of a cutaneous stimulator, distraction (e.g., soft music), and so on.

5. The most reliable method of determining that Mrs. Lundahl's pain has been relieved is for her to tell you that her pain has been relieved. Objective data may include decreased pulse, blood pressure, and respirations when compared to preintervention values; Mrs. Lundahl resting quietly or sleeping; pink color; absence of nausea or perspiration; and relaxed facial expression.

CRITICAL THINKING POSSIBILITIES

1. Obtaining information regarding factors that affect a person's pain experience. For example, has he been hospitalized before, previous pain experiences, cultural values regarding pain, support people, effect of the environment, and his anxiety and stress levels.

2. Consider ATC analgesia the first few days postoperatively. Make his pain assessment the fifth vital sign—assess each time you take vital signs. Assess his sense of control over his pain management.

3. Breakthrough pain even with ATC. Mr. C. needing to have more of a sense of control over his pain management.

TEST YOUR KNOWLEDGE

1. *Answer*: 3 *Rationale*: During the transduction phase, tissue injury triggers the release of biochemical mediators such as prostaglandin. Ibuprofen works by blocking the production of prostaglandin. The co-analgesic medication in option 1 would affect the modulation phase because they inhibit the reuptake of norepinephrine and serotonin, which increases the modulation phase that helps inhibit painful ascending stimuli. In option 2, opioids block the release of neurotransmitters, particularly substance P, which stops the pain at the spinal level that occurs during the transmission phase. In option 4, distraction is best used during the perception phase when the client becomes conscious of the pain. Distraction (e.g., music, guided imagery, TV) can help direct the client's attention away from the pain. *Cognitive Level*: Application *Client Need*: Physiological Integrity *Nursing Process*: Implementation

2. *Answer*: 2 *Rationale*: Options 1 and 3 are also appropriate but you need to assess the client's pain intensity for effective pain management. Option 1 is important and many now consider pain intensity as the fifth vital sign. Option 2, however, is the best answer because it specifically addresses pain intensity. In a postoperative client it is important to assess pain intensity frequently to

manage the acute pain experience. Option 3: Location of pain is important, but you need to know the client's pain intensity first for effective pain management. Option 4: This information is important but not for a client in acute pain. The priority would be to assess the pain intensity. Clients in acute pain may not want to answer pain history questions. You can ask when they are more comfortable. *Cognitive Level*: Analysis *Client Need*: Safe, Effective Care Environment *Nursing Process*: Assessment

3. *Answer*: 3 *Rationale*: A rating of 6 is considered moderate-severe and demands immediate attention. *Cognitive Level*: Application *Client Need*: Physiological Integrity *Nursing Process*: Assessment

4. *Answer*: 1 *Rationale*: This indicates an increasing level of sedation, which can be an early sign of impending respiratory depression. Option 2 is normal. Option 3 can indicate increasing sedation; however, option 1 describes a higher level of sedation and an intervention such as notifying the primary care provider. Option 4 indicates pain management that may be tolerable for the client. *Cognitive Level*: Application *Client Need*: Safe, Effective Care Environment *Nursing Process*: Implementation

5. *Answer*: 4 *Rationale*: The client's perception/intensity rating of his pain is the most important even though other signs may suggest he is not having pain. His pain rating warrants a higher dose of the as-needed (prn) morphine. With option 1, you would be undermedicating the client based on the most important data when assessing a client's pain, his perception or rating of the pain. Option 2: Research shows that few clients become addicted, plus there is no information to indicate signs of addiction. This answer, based on the data, would be undermedicating the client. Option 3 does not address the intensity as well as 4. *Cognitive Level*: Analysis *Client Need*: Physiological Integrity *Nursing Process*: Evaluation

6. *Answer*: 4 *Rationale*: Options 2 and 3 are subcategories of physiological pain. A clue to the answer is that the client has diabetes which often leads to diabetic peripheral neuropathy. *Cognitive Level*: Analysis *Client Need*: Physiological Integrity *Nursing Process*: Assessment

7. *Answer*: 2, 4, and 5 *Rationale*: Massage, heat, and cold are topical therapies that can "close" the gates and inhibit the transmission of further pain. Client education and anticipatory guidance address the client's mood and goals which can also inhibit further pain by reducing fear and anxiety. Options 1 and 3 are pharmacological interventions which are important; however, they inhibit the pain during the transmission phase of nociception. *Cognitive Level*: Application *Client Need*: Physiological Integrity *Nursing Process*: Implementation

8. *Answer*: 2 *Rationale*: The words "pain" or "complain" may have emotional or sociocultural meanings. It is better to ask clients if they are having any discomfort—they can then elaborate in their own words. Option 3 is too general and expects clients to report their pain without being asked. *Cognitive Level*: Application *Client Need*: Safe Effective Care Environment *Nursing Process*: Assessment

9. *Answer*: 3 and 5 *Rationale*: Older clients may withhold complaints of pain because it may indicate a worsening of their condition that may threaten their independence. Elders may describe pain differently—using words other than "pain." Although many perceive pain as a natural outcome of aging, pain is not a natural part of aging. Pain perception may decrease and narcotics can be used with careful monitoring by the nurse. *Cognitive Level*: Com-

prehension *Client Need*: Physiological Integrity *Nursing Process*: Planning

10. *Answer*: 1 *Rationale*: Based on the information provided, the nurse needs to gather more information about the client's understanding about the effects of pain on recovery and if the client has misconceptions about pain. Option 2 usually pertains more to chronic pain and fatigue. Options 3 and 4 could be true but the priority is option 1. Movement enhances respiratory, cardiovascular, and gastrointestinal recovery from general anesthesia and the outcomes associated with a surgical procedure. *Cognitive Level*: Analysis *Client Need*: Physiological Integrity *Nursing Process*: Diagnosis

CHAPTER 47
ANATOMY & PHYSIOLOGY REVIEW

1. Salivary glands secrete enzymes that begin the digestion of carbohydrates.

2. If the pyloric sphincter is obstructed, food cannot move from the stomach into the small intestine.

3. If the gall bladder has been removed bile is not stored, although it is still made by the liver. The client may have difficulty digesting fats.

4. If the colon is removed, most of the water and many minerals will not be reabsorbed from the chyme into the body. What is eliminated from the small intestine will be very liquid and still contain many enzymes.

CRITICAL THINKING POSSIBILITIES

1. Being a woman means that her distribution of fat is generally higher than a man's. At age 59, she is beginning to enter the age range when the body configuration changes somewhat, fewer calories are needed to maintain weight, but nutrients are still very important. Being alone contributes to poor eating habits since meals are often a social event. We do not know her ethnicity but this can influence her view of nutrition and weight.

2. What were her eating patterns before her husband died? What foods does she like and dislike most? What kinds of snacks is she eating? Does she have the financial means to buy food? Does her living situation allow her to make and store food?

3. Suggestions may be many, such as keeping busy with her hands while watching TV (e.g., folding laundry), choosing healthy snacks like carrot and celery sticks, and not buying snacks at the store.

4. Although there are many ways to determine her ideal weight from tables, charts, and calculators, her best weight is influenced by many other factors that are difficult to include in these (specific activity level, BMR, body configuration). Since she states she formerly was "petite," she may wish to return to this state—as much as is possible as she ages. It is important that the nurse not tell her a specific weight that she should achieve. Goal setting must be collaborative.

TEST YOUR KNOWLEDGE

1. *Answer*: 2 *Rationale*: A BMI of 31 to 40 indicates moderate to severe obesity. A BMI of less than 20 indicates underweight. BMI is calculated using the client's weight in kilograms/(height meters). The client is not at risk for imbalance since it already exists. There is no evidence to support a diagnosis of *Deficient Knowledge*. *Cognitive Level*: Application *Client Need*: Health Promotion and Maintenance *Nursing Process*: Diagnosing

2. *Answer*: 4 *Rationale*: This client needs more grains in the diet. The food pyramid indicates that the client should have 6 to 7 oz

grains per day, 3 cups/week dark green vegetables, 2 cups/week orange vegetables, 3 cups/week legumes, 3 cups/week starchy vegetables, 1.5 to 2 cups fruit per day, 5 to 6 oz meat and beans per day, and 3 cups milk, yogurt, and cheese per day. *Cognitive Level*: Application *Client Need*: Health Promotion and Maintenance *Nursing Process*: Planning

3. *Answer*: 2, 3, 4, 6, and 8 *Rationale*: A full liquid diet contains only liquids or foods that turn to liquid at body temperature. Pudding, juices, hard candy, Cream of Wheat cereal, and fruit smoothies are permitted on a full liquid diet. Scrambled eggs, mashed potatoes, and oatmeal cereal are not permitted until the client advances to a soft diet. *Cognitive Level*: Application *Client Need*: Physiological Integrity *Nursing Process*: Implementing

4. *Answer*: 3 *Rationale*: Gastric secretions are acidic as evidenced by a pH of less than 6. If the tube were in the client's airway, speaking would usually be impaired. Gagging during insertion is common and does not indicate that the tube is in the stomach. Ability to easily instill fluid into the tube does not relate to its placement. The lungs would offer no resistance to the flow of liquid. *Cognitive Level*: Analysis *Client Need*: Physiological Integrity *Nursing Process*: Evaluating

5. *Answer*: 1 *Rationale*: For proper flow, the feeding container hangs 1 foot above the tube insertion. Feedings may be administered if there is less than 90 to 100 mL of residual volume (unless agency policy specifies otherwise). To prevent or reduce the risk of aspiration, the client should be placed in Fowler's position during feeding. The feeding should be warmed to room temperature before administration to decrease cramping and diarrhea. *Cognitive Level*: Application *Client Need*: Physiological Integrity *Nursing Process*: Implementing

6. *Answer*: 1 *Rationale*: The Dietary Guidelines recommend 30 minutes of physical activity on most days of the week to achieve optimal weight. Some persons benefit from a low-carbohydrate diet, but no particular diet is the solution for all persons. A reasonable diet emphasizes balance and portion control rather than forbidding or requiring any specific foods. Fresh and chemical-free foods may be healthier than preserved foods but do not automatically assist with weight loss. *Cognitive Level*: Analysis *Client Need*: Health Promotion and Maintenance *Nursing Process*: Evaluating

7. *Answer*: 3 *Rationale*: Always inquire into the client's favorite foods when planning a diet. Dairy may not be indicated for this client due to the high incidence of lactose intolerance in individuals of Asian heritage. Beer can be a source of calories and, in moderation, is not harmful and may maintain the client's satisfaction with the dietary changes. The nurse will need to assess the ability to swallow beer safely, however. Calories from lipid sources should be kept below 35% and, when enhanced wound healing is indicated (not so with a stroke), increased protein and carbohydrates are needed rather than fats. *Cognitive Level*: Application *Client Need*: Health Promotion and Maintenance *Nursing Process*: Planning

8. *Answer*: This client has lost 13 pounds which is 6.7%: $(195-182)/195$. If the weight loss has been steady over the past 2 months, that would indicate a 3.3% loss per month. Less than 5% loss in 1 month is not significant but if this loss continues, the client will reach a 10% loss in 3 months which is a severe loss. A more detailed assessment is indicated to determine the client's nutritional status. *Cognitive Level*: Application *Client Need*: Health Promotion and Maintenance *Nursing Process*: Assessing

9. *Answer*: 2 *Rationale*: A small-bore nasal feeding tube tip is most commonly placed in the stomach. Option 1 indicates the esophagus. A tube tip placed there can lead to aspiration. Option 3 indicates the post-pyloric duodenum. Small-bore nasal tubes can be advanced to this location if desired but is less common than gastric placement. Option 4 indicates the jejunum where feeding tubes can be placed but usually not from a nasally placed tube. *Cognitive Level*: Comprehension *Client Need*: Physiological Integrity *Nursing Process*: Evaluating

10. *Answer*: 4 *Rationale*: 3 ounces tuna + 2 slices whole wheat bread = 3.1 mg Fe; 1 ounce cheese = ~200 mg Ca++; pear = 4.2 gm fiber. Option 1: 1/3 cup raisins = 1.75 mg Fe; 3 ounces cottage cheese = 90 mg Ca++; 1 banana = 2.1 gm fiber. Option 3: 1/2 cup spaghetti + 2 ounces ground beef = 2.3 mg Fe; 1/2 cup ice cream = 97 mg Ca++; 1/2 cup lima beans = 3.2 gm fiber. Option 2: 3 ounces chicken + 1/2 cup peanuts = 2.9 mg Fe; 1/2 cup broccoli = ~158 mg Ca++; 1/2 cup broccoli = 2.4 gm fiber. *Cognitive Level*: Application *Client Need*: Health Promotion and Maintenance *Nursing Process*: Implementing

CHAPTER 48

ANATOMY & PHYSIOLOGY REVIEW

1. Yes. They are under voluntary control and they are just like any other muscles. Exercise can make them stronger.

2. When the pelvic floor muscles are weak, urine can leak from the bladder. The pelvic floor muscles help control the external urethral sphincter that closes the urethra so urine does not leak. Exercise can strengthen the pelvic muscles and decrease bladder control problems. See "Managing Urinary Incontinence" later in this chapter.

CRITICAL THINKING POSSIBILITIES

1. Urinary frequency could be a sign of infection due to causes other than prostate hypertrophy. No other data are given about his other health problems including medications that might be contributing factors. A thorough assessment is indicated.

2. The nurse needs to ensure that the client completely understands what is proposed and the intended outcomes. There is always a balance between the expected positive result and the risk of the intervention. Is this surgery considered culturally appropriate? Although you may not know a great deal about the actual surgery, you realize that not every procedure is completely successful. How would the client react if he continued to have some incontinence following the operation?

3. Often, there is a medical standard of care that is followed unless there are contraindications. If the physician determines that the hypertrophy is severe, and knows that this is not a reversible condition, surgery may be the only logical option. Investigate what other treatments may be used in this situation and propose why they may be seen as less desirable than surgery.

4. The nurse should fully explore the client's understanding of his condition and what measures can be taken to diminish its impact on his ADLs and quality of life. If the client truly understands and makes this informed choice, it is the nurse's responsibility to support the client.

TEST YOUR KNOWLEDGE

1. *Answer*: 4. *Rationale*: The capacity of the bladder may decrease with age but the muscle is weaker and can cause urine to be retained. Elders do not ignore the urge to void and may have difficulty

in getting to the toilet in time. The kidney becomes less able to concentrate urine with age. *Cognitive Level*: Knowledge *Client Need*: Physiological Integrity *Nursing Process*: Assessment

2. *Answer*: 1, 2, and 4 *Rationale*: The perineum may become irritated by the frequent contact with urine. Normal fluid intake is at least 1,500 mL/day and clients often decrease their intake to try to minimize urine leakage. Urinary tract infections can contribute to incontinence. Antihistamines can cause urinary retention rather than incontinence. *Cognitive Level*: Analysis *Client Need*: Physiological Integrity *Nursing Process*: Assessment

3. *Answer*: 2 *Rationale*: The penis and condom should be checked one-half hour after application to ensure that it is not too tight. A 1-in. space should be left between the penis and the end of the condom. The condom is changed every 24 hours, and the tubing is taped to the leg or attached to a leg bag. An indwelling catheter is taped to the lower abdomen or upper thigh. *Cognitive Level*: Application *Client Need*: Safe, Effective Care Environment *Nursing Process*: Implementation

4. *Answer*: 1 *Rationale*: The catheter in the vagina is contaminated and cannot be reused. If left in place, it may help avoid mistaking the vaginal opening for the urinary meatus. A single failure to catheterize the meatus does not indicate that another nurse is needed although sometimes a second nurse can assist in visualizing the meatus. *Cognitive Level*: Application *Client Need*: Safe, Effective Care Environment *Nursing Process*: Implementation

5. *Answer*: 3 *Rationale*: Soaking in a bathtub can increase the risk of exposure to bacteria. The bag should be below the level of the bladder to promote proper drainage. Intake of cranberry juice creates an environment nonconducive to infection. Clean technique is appropriate for touching the exterior portions of the system. *Cognitive Level*: Analysis *Client Need*: Health Promotion and Maintenance *Nursing Process*: Evaluation

6. *Answer*: 4 *Rationale*: The key phrase is "the urge to void." Option 1: occurs when the client coughs, sneezes, or jars the body resulting in accidental loss of urine. Option 2: absence of control. Option 3: involuntary loss of urine related to impaired function. *Cognitive Level*: Application *Client Need*: Physiological Integrity *Nursing Process*: Diagnosis

7. *Answer*: 2 and 4 *Rationale*: Validates diagnosis. Cotton underwear promotes appropriate exposure to air, resulting in decreased bacterial growth. In option 1, increased fluids decrease concentration and irritation. In option 3, the client should wipe the perineal area from front to back to prevent spread of bacteria from rectal area to urethra. In option 5, showers reduce exposure of area to bacteria. *Cognitive Level*: Application *Client Need*: Health Promotion and Maintenance *Nursing Process*: Implementation

8. *Answer*: 2 *Rationale*: The ileal conduit and vesicostomy (Options 1 and 4) are incontinent urinary diversions, and clients are required to use an external ostomy appliance to contain the urine. Clients with a neobladder can control their voiding. (Option 3) *Cognitive Level*: Analysis *Client Need*: Health Promotion and Maintenance *Nursing Process*: Assessment

9. *Answer*: 3 *Rationale*: Since the bladder muscles will not contract to increase the intra-bladder pressure to promote urination, the process is initiated manually. Options 1, 2, and 4: To promote continence, bladder contractions are required for habit training, bladder training, and increasing the tone of the pelvic muscles. *Cognitive Level*: Application *Client Need*: Physiological Integrity *Nursing Process*: Implementation

10. *Answer*: 2 and 5 *Rationale*: It is important for the client to inhibit the urge-to-void sensation when a premature urge is experienced. Some clients may need diapers, this is not the BEST indicator of a successful program. Citrus juices may irritate the bladder. Carbonated beverages increase diuresis, increasing the risk of incontinence. *Cognitive Level*: Application *Client Need*: Health Promotion and Maintenance *Nursing Process*: Evaluation

CHAPTER 49

ANATOMY & PHYSIOLOGY REVIEW

1. The primary functions of the small intestine are the chemical breakdown of food (digestion) and the absorption of digested foods.

2. The primary functions of the large intestine are absorbing water from indigestible food residue and eliminating the residue in the form of feces.

3. Ileum. The ileocecal valve is between the ileum and the beginning of the large intestine.

4. The stool would be liquid because it has not entered the large intestine and the water has not been reabsorbed.

5. The transverse colostomy would discharge mushy, paste-like stool. The descending colostomy would have semi-solid feces because more water has been reabsorbed.

6. Solid, formed feces.

CRITICAL THINKING POSSIBILITIES

1. Ask her about the number and amount of stool she has in order to determine if she is actually having diarrhea or has an impaction. Assess her usual diet, daily fluid intake, amount of fiber in the diet, daily activities, medications, or other factors that could be contributing to constipation and possible impaction.

2. A digital examination may be performed to verify or rule out the presence of a fecal impaction. Other interventions may include administering an oil retention enema followed by a cleansing enema, suppositories, or stool softeners. If all else fails, manual removal of the fecal impaction may be necessary.

3. Consider interventions to promote regular defecation such as increasing intake of fluids, maintaining a regular schedule for defecation, paying attention to the urge to defecate, encouraging warm liquids with breakfast to stimulate the gastrocolic reflex, and so on. To add more fiber to the diet, teach the client about foods that are high in fiber; go through her kitchen with her pointing out what foods qualify. Suggest she interface with others in her complex to plan good menus, eat together, and so on. Also consider referral to physical therapy or other resources to increase activity appropriate for elders, such as water exercises.

4. The chronic use of laxatives will actually make her more prone to constipation and impaction because she loses muscle tone. Increased fiber, fruits, and vegetables and other ways of naturally dealing with constipation are safer and more appropriate.

TEST YOUR KNOWLEDGE

1. *Answer*: 1 *Rationale*: Habitually ignoring the urge to defecate can lead to constipation through loss of the natural urge and the accumulation of feces. Diarrhea will not result—if anything, there is increased opportunity for water reabsorption because the stool remains in the colon, leading to firmer stool (Option 2). Ignoring the urge shows a strong voluntary sphincter, not a weak one that could result in incontinence (Option 3). Hemorrhoids would occur only if severe drying out of the stool occurs and, thus, repeated

need to strain to pass stool (Option 4). *Cognitive Level*: Comprehension *Client Need*: Physiological Integrity *Nursing Process*: Implementation

2. *Answer*: 2 *Rationale*: The standard of practice in assisting elders to maintain normal function of the gastrointestinal tract is regular ingestion of a well-balanced diet, adequate fluid intake, and regular exercise. If the bowel pattern is not regular with these activities, this abnormality should be reported. Stimulant laxatives can be very irritating and are not the preferred treatment for occasional constipation in older adults. In addition, a normal stool pattern for an elder may not be daily elimination. *Cognitive Level*: Analysis *Client Need*: Physiological Integrity *Nursing Process*: Evaluation

3. *Answer*: 4 *Rationale*: Small-volume enemas along with other preparations are used to prepare the client for this procedure. An oil retention enema is used to soften hard stool (option 1). Return flow enemas help expel flatus (option 2). Because of the risk of loss of fluid and electrolytes, high, large-volume enemas are seldom used (option 3). *Cognitive Level*: Analysis *Client Need*: Health Promotion and Maintenance *Nursing Process*: Planning

4. *Answer*: 3 *Rationale*: An established stoma should be dark pink like the color of the buccal mucosa and is slightly raised above the abdomen. The skin under the appliance may remain pink/red for a while after the adhesive is pulled off. Feces from an ascending ostomy are very liquid, less so from a transverse ostomy, and more solid from a descending or sigmoid stoma. *Cognitive Level*: Application *Client Need*: Physiological Integrity *Nursing Process*: Assessment

5. *Answer*: 2 *Rationale*: Once the cause of diarrhea has been identified and corrected, the client should return to his or her previous elimination pattern. This is not an example of an allergy to the antibiotic but a common consequence of overgrowth of bowel organisms not killed by the drug. Antidiarrheal medications are usually prescribed according to the number of stools, not routinely around the clock. Increasing intake of soluble fiber such as oatmeal or potatoes may help absorb excess liquid and decrease the diarrhea, but insoluble fiber will not. *Cognitive Level*: Analysis *Client Need*: Physiological Integrity *Nursing Process*: Planning

6. *Answer*: 2 *Rationale*: The client has assessment findings consistent with complications of surgery. Option 1: Irrigating the stoma is a dependent nursing action, and is also intervention without appropriate assessment. Option 3: Assessing the peristomal skin area is an independent action, but administering an antiemetic is an intervention without appropriate assessment. Antiemetics are generally ordered to treat immediate postop nausea, not several days postop. Option 4: Administering a bulk-forming laxative to a nauseated postoperative client is contraindicated. *Cognitive Level*: Analysis *Client Need*: Physiological Integrity *Nursing Process*: Implementation

7. *Answer*: 3 *Rationale*: This provides relief of postoperative flatus, stimulating bowel motility. Options 1, 2, and 4 manage constipation and do not provide flatus relief. *Cognitive Level*: Application *Client Need*: Physiological Integrity *Nursing Process*: Implementation

8. *Answer*: 3 *Rationale*: Bleeding into the upper GI tract is black and tarry. Option 1 can be a sign of malabsorption in an infant, option 2 is normal stool, and option 4 is characteristic of an obstructive condition of the rectum. *Cognitive Level*: Analysis *Client Need*: Health Promotion and Maintenance *Nursing Process*: Assessment

9. *Answer*: 1, 3, 4, and 5 *Rationale*: Option 1 is the most appropriate. The client is unable to decide when stool evacuation will occur. In option 3, client thoughts about self may be altered if unable to control stool evacuation. In option 4, client may not feel as comfortable around others. In option 5, increased tissue contact with fecal material may result in impairment. Option 2 is more appropriate for a client with diarrhea. Incontinence is the inability to control feces of normal consistency. *Cognitive Level*: Analysis *Client Need*: Physiological Integrity *Nursing Process*: Diagnosis

10. *Answer*: 5 *Rationale*: Option 5 is a sigmoidostomy site. Option 1 is an ileostomy site, option 2 is ascending colostomy, option 3 is transverse colostomy, and option 4 is descending colostomy. *Cognitive Level*: Application *Client Need*: Physiological Integrity *Nursing Process*: Assessment

CHAPTER 50
ANATOMY & PHYSIOLOGY REVIEW

1. a) Hairs in the nose filter the air as it enters and traps particles to prevent them from traveling to the lower respiratory tract; b) the sneeze reflex clears nasal passages; c) lymph tissue in the nasopharynx and oropharynx trap and destroy pathogens entering with the inhaled air; d) the epiglottis closes when swallowing to prevent food particles from entering the lungs.

2. Defense mechanisms present in the lower respiratory tract include the thin layer of mucus (the "mucous blanket") that traps pathogens. The cilia on the epithelial cells then "sweep" the foreign particles toward the throat. The cough reflex helps dislodge the mucus and foreign particles and propel them out.

3. Because the alveoli are filled with fluid, the gases (oxygen and carbon dioxide) cannot diffuse across the respiratory membrane. The client will have less oxygen in his blood and will experience symptoms of hypoxemia. One of the medical interventions will include administration of oxygen to increase the diffusion gradient from the alveoli so the oxygen molecules will diffuse faster, and hopefully improve oxygenation in the blood.

CRITICAL THINKING POSSIBILITIES

1. The physical assessment reveals fever, use of accessory muscles, adventitious lung sounds, and yellow sputum all of which suggest more than an average cold. The nurse certainly would have suspected a more significant underlying condition.

2. Ms. Singh has quite a stressful lifestyle with work and school plus her physical stressors of a poor diet and smoking for more than 20 years. The nurse should perform discharge teaching that includes examination of which of these modifiable risk factors may be addressed in both short- and long-term plans.

3. Alteration in mental status may be a very useful sign that the client is hypoxic. Also, increased respiratory and cardiac rates and substantial shortness of breath would be negative signs. If not already in place, continuous oxygen saturation monitoring should be initiated. Frequent assessments and notification of the primary care provider are required. The nurse should have nasotracheal suction equipment available. The client may require transfer to a higher acuity nursing station.

4. Standard precautions must always be in place. The nurse is careful to glove whenever coming into direct contact with the client's secretions. The nurse will also wear a mask if the client is unable to control her secretions and may cough or spit in the nurse's face.

5. A face mask may be uncomfortable or cause the client to feel confined or claustrophobic. If she is not wearing it, it cannot help her.

Discuss the face mask with her and determine why she is taking it off. Reassure her and provide measures to decrease her anxiety. If the mask cannot be modified to address these reasons, consider contacting the primary care provider for assistance (e.g., arranging for her to have oxygen by nasal cannula instead, with an appropriate change in the flow rate).

TEST YOUR KNOWLEDGE

1. *Answer*: 4 *Rationale*: A bluish tinge to mucous membranes is called cyanosis. This is most accurate because it is what the nurse observes. The nurse can only observe signs/symptoms of hypoxia. More information is needed to validate this conclusion. Hypoxemia requires blood oxygen saturation data to be confirmed, and dyspnea is difficult breathing. *Cognitive Level*: Application *Client Need*: Physiological Integrity *Nursing Process*: Assessment

2. *Answer*: 3 *Rationale*: Huff coughing helps keep the airways open and secretions mobilized. Deep breathing and coughing should be performed at the same time. Only at meal times is not sufficient. Extended forceful coughing fatigues the client. Diaphragmatic and pursed-lip breathing are techniques used for clients with obstructive airway disease. *Cognitive Level*: Application *Client Need*: Health Promotion and Maintenance *Nursing Process*: Planning

3. *Answer*: 1 *Rationale*: Clients with chronic lung disease may have only low levels of supplemental oxygen, generally not over 2 liters per minute. *Cognitive Level*: Application *Client Need*: Safe, Effective Care Environment *Nursing Process*: Implementation

4. *Answer*: 3 *Rationale*: Rotating the catheter prevents pulling of tissue into the opening on the catheter tip and side. Suction catheters may only be lubricated with water or water-soluble lubricant (petroleum jelly, e.g., Vaseline is an oil base). No suction should ever be applied while the catheter is being inserted because this can traumatize tissues. The client should be hyperoxygenated for only a few minutes before and after suctioning and this is generally limited to clients who are intubated or have a tracheostomy. *Cognitive Level*: Analysis *Client Need*: Safe, Effective Care Environment *Nursing Process*: Implementation

5. *Answer*: 2 *Rationale*: Proper use of an SMI requires the client to take slow, steady inhalations, every hour or two, 5 to 10 breaths each time. Only the mouthpiece can be successfully rinsed or wiped. The device should not be submerged in water. *Cognitive Level*: Analysis *Client Need*: Health Promotion and Maintenance *Nursing Process*: Evaluation

6. *Answer*: 2 *Rationale*: The tube should be reconnected to the water seal as quickly as possible. Assisting the client back to bed and assessing the client's lungs are possible actions after the system is reconnected. *Cognitive Level*: Application *Client Need*: Safe, Effective Care Environment *Nursing Process*: Implementation

7. *Answer*: 1 *Rationale*: Anemia is a condition of decreased red blood cells and decreased hemoglobin. Hemoglobin is how the oxygen molecules are transported to the tissues. Option 2 would depend on where the infection is located. Option 3: A fractured rib would interrupt transport of oxygen from the atmosphere to the airways. Option 4: Damage to the medulla would interfere with neural stimulation of the respiratory system. *Cognitive Level*: Application *Client Need*: Safe, Effective Care Environment *Nursing Process*: Assessment

8. *Answer*: 3 *Rationale*: Respiratory difficulty related to a reclining position without other physical alterations is defined as orthopnea. *Cognitive Level*: Knowledge *Client Need*: Safe, Effective Care Environment *Nursing Process*: Diagnosis

9. *Answer*: 4 *Rationale*: Glucocorticoids are prescribed because of the anti-inflammatory effect. *Cognitive Level*: Analysis *Client Need*: Physiological Integrity *Nursing Process*: Assessment

10. *Answer*: 1 *Rationale*: Postural drainage results in expectoration of large amounts of mucus. Clients sometimes ingest part of the secretions. The secretions may also produce an unpleasant taste in the oral cavity which could result in nausea/vomiting. This procedure should be done on an empty stomach to decrease client discomfort which could include nausea and vomiting. *Cognitive Level*: Application *Client Need*: Safe, Effective Care Environment *Nursing Process*: Planning

CHAPTER 51

ANATOMY & PHYSIOLOGY REVIEW

1. Right side of the heart.

2. Exercise, hypervolemia, mitral valve regurgitation or insufficiency.

3. It has a positive effect or outcome when it increases cardiac output. For example, during exercise there is an increased venous return which causes the heart to contract more forcefully with the result that stroke volume and cardiac output increase to supply the body with needed oxygen and nutrients.

4. The increase in the "stretch" of the heart muscle increases the contractility of the heart but only to a certain point (Frank-Starling law of the heart). Once it reaches that point, contractility decreases and cardiac output decreases.

5. Diuretics decrease circulating volume, which decreases preload (the volume returning to the heart).

6. The left ventricle.

7. High blood pressure (hypertension)—the left ventricle has to create a pressure above the client's diastolic pressure to pump blood into the circulation.

   Arterial vasoconstriction—the left heart works harder when it has to pump blood through narrowed vessels as opposed to wide or dilated vessels.

8. Decrease blood pressure (e.g., antihypertensives).

   Decrease peripheral resistance or vasoconstriction (e.g., vasodilators).

CRITICAL THINKING POSSIBILITIES

1. This client has decreased arterial circulation to her feet. When the tissues become ischemic, lactic acid builds up and causes the discomfort. The pain she describes is consistent with the medical condition *intermittent claudication*. Risk factors for peripheral vascular disease include cigarette smoking, high fat intake, obesity, sedentary lifestyle, hypertension, and diabetes.

2. *Ineffective Tissue Perfusion (Peripheral)* and *Activity Intolerance* are two likely diagnoses. Of these two, *Activity Intolerance* may be of highest priority for the nurse since there is a greater likelihood of developing a nursing care plan that can substantially affect her desired level of function and quality of life. Desired outcomes and interventions for the *Ineffective Tissue Perfusion* will focus on implementing the medical treatment plan and protection from injury. However, remember that for a care plan to be effective, the client must be an active participant in the process. Thus, the diagnoses of highest priority can only be suggested without her input.

3. The physiological impact of the plan must be weighed against the psychological impact—always a difficult thing to do. The nurse must explore the client's response to the recommendation. If it is unacceptable to her, consider if any compromises such as less frequent visits or use of a wheelchair are more agreeable.

4. Support stockings help increase venous return. This client has impaired arterial circulation. If the stockings are tight, they could actually interfere with the flow of arterial blood to her extremities. She requires client teaching explaining the differences at a level she can comprehend.

TEST YOUR KNOWLEDGE

1. *Answer*: 1 *Rationale*: Regular physical activity will help promote healthy cardiac functioning and will also promote tissue perfusion. Option 2: Improving tissue perfusion may also improve renal perfusion but it is not the primary goal. Option 3: Red blood cells carry oxygen. Option 4: Cardiac output and tissue perfusion improve the respiratory system performance. *Cognitive Level*: Application *Client Need*: Health Promotion and Maintenance *Nursing Process*: Planning

2. *Answer*: 3, 1, 4, 2, 5 *Cognitive Level*: Knowledge *Client Need*: Health Promotion and Maintenance *Nursing Process*: Assessment

3. *Answer*: 3 *Rationale*: Capillary refill is an assessment of capillary blood flow and thus tissue perfusion. Symmetrical chest expansion (Option 1) is an assessment of respiratory function, and pursed-lip breathing (Option 2) is a technique used to assist clients with obstructive lung diseases to keep alveoli open during respirations. Activity intolerance (Option 4) can occur because of low cardiac output (e.g., heart failure). Activity tolerance would indicate adequate tissue perfusion. *Cognitive Level*: Application *Client Need*: Physiological Integrity *Nursing Process*: Planning

4. *Answer*: 3 and 5 *Rationale*: These are enzymes that are released into the blood when there is hypoxia and myocardial damage. Option 1 reflects renal function. Option 2 reflects number of red blood cells. Option 4 reflects glucose levels. Altered levels 1, 2, and 4 do cause chest pain. *Cognitive Level*: Application *Client Need*: Physiological Integrity *Nursing Process*: Planning

5. *Answer*: 3 *Rationale*: Very rapid heart rates do not allow adequate time for the ventricles to fill, causing cardiac output to fall. Option 1 is normal. Option 2 is a normal cardiac output of 4900 mL/min. The formula is $SV \times HR = CO$ is about 5 L/min. Option 4: Positive inotropic drugs (e.g., digoxin) increase contractility of the cardiac muscle and thus increase stroke volume, which increases cardiac output. *Cognitive Level*: Application *Client Need*: Physiological Integrity *Nursing Process*: Assessment

6. *Answer*: 3 *Rationale*: Because the clients would experience impaired tissue perfusion resulting in respiratory compensation, they are most likely to experience the sign/symptom of shortness of breath. The client with the MI will experience cardiac impairment resulting in decreased cardiac output as well as severe chest pain resulting in increased oxygen demand with decreased availability. Clients will have decreased pumping ability of the cardiac muscle resulting in pulmonary congestion and decreased cardiac output. Clients with anemia have fewer RBCs to carry the oxygen to the tissues, resulting in hypoxia. Options 1 and 4 would be signs for the client with the MI. Option 2 is seen in heart failure. *Cognitive Level*: Analysis *Client Need*: Physiological Integrity *Nursing Process*: Planning

7. *Answer*: 4 *Rationale*: The three cardinal signs of cardiac arrest are absence of heart beat, cessation of breathing (apnea), and the absence of circulation reflected in dilated pupils. *Cognitive Level*: Application *Client Need*: Health Promotion and Maintenance *Nursing Process*: Implementation

8. *Answer*: 1, 3, and 5 *Rationale*: Option 1: An example of ineffective tissue perfusion is a decrease in arterial circulation in the legs related to atherosclerosis. Option 3: Examples of decreased car-

diac output are clients with MI, heart failure, or tachycardia. Option 5: Not enough blood is being pumped by the heart to meet the demands of the body. Activity intolerance is when the client doesn't have physiological energy for ADLs. Common reasons can be anemias and heart failure. Options 2 and 4: Acute confusion and sleep pattern disturbance are not directly related to cardiovascular disease. *Cognitive Level*: Application *Client Need*: Physiological Integrity *Nursing Process*: Diagnosing

9. *Answer*: 2 *Rationale*: The sequential compression devices promote venous return from the legs to the heart. They inflate and deflate plastic sleeves wrapped around the legs to promote venous flow. This sequential inflation and deflation counteract blood stasis in the lower extremities. Option 1: Arterial flow is from the heart to the general circulation. Option 3: Afterload is related to the ventricles' ability to eject blood forward. These devices affect peripheral circulation. Option 4: No relationship between pain and the purpose of the devices. *Cognitive Level*: Application *Client Need*: Health Promotion and Maintenance *Nursing Process*: Implementation

10. *Cognitive Level*: Knowledge *Client Need*: Physiological Integrity *Nursing Process*: Implementation

CHAPTER 52

ANATOMY & PHYSIOLOGY REVIEW

1. Respiratory problems such as pneumonia, atelectasis, narcotic overdose, central nervous system depression due to anesthesia.

2. With shallow respirations, the CO_2 is not eliminated by the lungs which causes two results: an increase in $PaCO_2$ and an increase in CO_2 in the blood which reacts with H_2O to form carbonic acid which increases the number of hydrogen ions causing a decrease in pH.

3. Respiratory acidosis.

4. Anxiety, fear, fever, respiratory infections.

5. The increase in respirations causes more carbon dioxide than normal to be exhaled. This results in a loss of CO_2 in the blood causing a low $PaCO_2$. Because of the low CO_2 in the blood, there is a reduction of carbonic acid in the blood resulting in an increased pH.

6. Respiratory alkalosis.

CRITICAL THINKING POSSIBILITIES

1. Cardiac dysrhythmias can be a result of hypokalemia. If cardiac irregularities occur, it is an emergency and requires notifying the primary care provider and the charge nurse immediately. Emergency orders may be instituted. As you are assessing her cardiac irregularity, notice whether there is a pattern to the irregularity and the rate. It is also important to assess blood pressure as an indicator of cardiac function and the effects of the dysrhythmia.

2. Fluid volume deficit creates a hypertonic vascular space, which causes water to move out of the cells, including brain cells. This is what causes neurologic symptoms—intracellular dehydration.

3. Suggestions may be many, such as finding a fluid that she likes or helps her nausea, making sure fluids are served at the appropriate temperature, using a straw, and starting with small amounts. Administering an antiemetic medication as ordered may also help improve her oral intake.

4. Although there are many indicators of fluid balance, daily weights are an important way to provide more data about fluid. You can explain that a loss of 1 kg (2.2 lb) indicates a fluid loss of approximately 1 liter. It is an easy, quick way to get more information about fluid balance.

TEST YOUR KNOWLEDGE

1. *Answer*: 2 *Rationale*: All other options are indicative of fluid volume excess. A client that has not eaten or drunk anything for several days would be experiencing fluid volume deficit. *Cognitive Level*: Application *Client Need*: Physiological Integrity *Nursing Process*: Assessment

2. *Answer*: 2 *Rationale*: Further assessment is needed to determine appropriate action. While the nurse may perform some of the other interventions, assessment is needed initially. *Cognitive Level*: Application *Client Need*: Physiological Integrity *Nursing Process*: Assessment

3. *Answer*: Hypertonic *Cognitive Level*: Knowledge *Client Need*: Physiological Integrity *Nursing Process*: Implementation

4. *Answer*: 2 *Rationale*: Because of the retention of CO_2, the clinical profile of respiratory acidosis includes decreased pH <7.35, $PaCO_2$>42 mm Hg with varying levels of HCO_3 related to hypoventilation. Option 1 is respiratory alkalosis which occurs because of blowing off of CO_2 resulting in a decreased level of acid and retention or production of bicarbonate resulting in pH>7.45, $PaCO_2$ <38 mm Hg, HCO_3 >26 mEq/mL related to hyperventilation. Option 3: Metabolic acidosis occurs because of a gain of hydrogen ions or a loss of HCO_3 with a pH <7.35, normal $PaCO_2$ 35–45 mm Hg, and HCO_3<22 mEq/mL, often caused by diarrhea, bicarbonate infusion, or retention related to kidney failure. Option 4: Metabolic alkalosis caused by gain of bicarbonate or loss of hydrogen ions related to vomiting, gastric suction, or loss of upper gastrointestinal secretions by various other methods. *Cognitive Level*: Application *Client Need*: Physiological Integrity *Nursing Process*: Assessment

5. *Answer*: 1, 3, and 5 *Rationale*: Options 1, 3, and 5 relate to fluid volume deficit. The data indicate an actual problem which excludes option 2. Option 4 relates more to fluid volume excess. *Cognitive Level*: Analysis *Client Need*: Physiological Integrity *Nursing Process*: Nursing Diagnosis

6. *Answer*: 4 *Rationale*: Salt substitutes contain potassium. The client can still use it within reason. Avocado is higher in potassium than most foods. Hypokalemia can potentiate digoxin toxicity and checking the pulse will help the client to avoid this; it is important to take potassium with food to avoid gastric upset. *Cognitive Level*: Application *Client Need*: Physiological Integrity *Nursing Process*: Evaluation

7. *Answer*: 2 *Rationale*: Sodium contributes to the function of neural tissue. Because calcium contributes the function of voluntary muscle contraction, 1 and 4 are more appropriate for calcium imbalances. Because potassium and calcium contribute to cardiac function, irregular pulse is more likely to be associated with those alterations. *Cognitive Level*: Application *Client Need*: Physiological Integrity *Nursing Process*: Assessment

8. *Answer*: 2 *Rationale*: Because of CO_2 retention the $PaCO_2$ is elevated. CO_2 is involved in production of acid which will result in a decreased pH. HCO_3 will vary. Option 1: Metabolic acidosis involves a loss of bicarbonate but no retention of CO_2. Option 3: Metabolic alkalosis involves a loss of acid or retention of HCO_3, but no retention of CO_2. Option 4: Respiratory alkalosis involves a loss of CO_2 resulting in an increased pH. *Cognitive Level*: Application *Client Need*: Physiological Integrity *Nursing Process*: Assessment

9. *Answer*: 4 *Rationale*: The major clinical signs and symptoms of hypocalcemia are due to increased neuromuscular activity. *Cognitive Level*: Analysis *Client Need*: Physiological Integrity *Nursing Process*: Implementation

10. *Answer*: 2, 4, and 5 *Rationale*: Options 1 and 3 relate to hypermagnesemia. *Cognitive Level*: Analysis *Client Need*: Physiological Integrity *Nursing Process*: Assessment

Scale Number*					
a	Severely compromised	Substantially compromised	Moderately compromised	Mildly compromised	Not compromised
b	Severe deviation from normal range	Substantial deviation from normal range	Moderate deviation from normal range	Mild deviation from normal range	No deviation from normal range
f	Not adequate	Slightly adequate	Moderately adequate	Substantially adequate	Totally adequate
g	10 and over	7–9	4–6	1–3	None
h	Extensive	Substantial	Moderate	Limited	None
i	None	Limited	Moderate	Substantial	Extensive
k	Never positive	Rarely positive	Sometimes positive	Often positive	Consistently positive
l	Very weak	Weak	Moderate	Strong	Very strong
m	Never demonstrated	Rarely demonstrated	Sometimes demonstrated	Often demonstrated	Consistently demonstrated
n	Severe	Substantial	Moderate	Mild	None
r	Poor	Fair	Good	Very good	Excellent
s	Not at all satisfied	Somewhat satisfied	Moderately satisfied	Very satisfied	Completely satisfied
t	Consistently demonstrated	Often demonstrated	Sometimes demonstrated	Rarely demonstrated	Never demonstrated

*Scale numbers (letters) are not continuous due to retirement of previous scales.

Note: From *Nursing Outcomes Classification (NOC)*, 3rd ed., by S. Moorhead, M. Johnson, and M. Maas, Eds., St. Louis, MO: Mosby, 2004, pp. 44–45. Used with permission.

Activity Intolerance
Activity Intolerance, Risk for
Airway Clearance, Ineffective
Anxiety
Anxiety, Death
Aspiration, Risk for
Attachment, Parent/Infant/Child, Risk for
    Impaired
Autonomic Dysreflexia
Autonomic Dysreflexia, Risk for
Blood Glucose, Risk for Unstable
Body Image, Disturbed
Body Temperature: Imbalanced, Risk for
Bowel Incontinence
Breastfeeding, Effective
Breastfeeding, Ineffective
Breastfeeding, Interrupted
Breathing Pattern, Ineffective
Cardiac Output, Decreased
Caregiver Role Strain
Caregiver Role Strain, Risk for
Comfort, Readiness for Enhanced
Communication: Impaired, Verbal
Communication, Readiness for Enhanced
Confusion, Acute
Confusion, Acute, Risk for
Confusion, Chronic
Constipation
Constipation, Perceived
Constipation, Risk for
Contamination
Contamination, Risk for
Coping: Community, Ineffective
Coping: Community, Readiness for Enhanced
Coping, Defensive
Coping: Family, Compromised
Coping: Family, Disabled
Coping: Family, Readiness for Enhanced
Coping (Individual), Readiness for Enhanced
Coping, Ineffective
Decisional Conflict
Decision Making, Readiness for Enhanced
Denial, Ineffective
Dentition, Impaired
Development: Delayed, Risk for
Diarrhea
Disuse Syndrome, Risk for
Diversional Activity, Deficient
Energy Field, Disturbed
Environmental Interpretation Syndrome, Impaired
Failure to Thrive, Adult
Falls, Risk for
Family Processes, Dysfunctional: Alcoholism
Family Processes, Interrupted
Family Processes, Readiness for Enhanced
Fatigue
Fear
Fluid Balance, Readiness for Enhanced
Fluid Volume, Deficient
Fluid Volume, Deficient, Risk for

Fluid Volume, Excess
Fluid Volume, Imbalanced, Risk for
Gas Exchange, Impaired
Grieving
Grieving, Complicated
Grieving, Risk for Complicated
Growth, Disproportionate, Risk for
Growth and Development, Delayed
Health Behavior, Risk-Prone
Health Maintenance, Ineffective
Health-Seeking Behaviors (Specify)
Home Maintenance, Impaired
Hope, Readiness for Enhanced
Hopelessness
Human Dignity, Risk for Compromised
Hyperthermia
Hypothermia
Immunization Status, Readiness for Enhanced
Infant Behavior, Disorganized
Infant Behavior: Disorganized, Risk for
Infant Behavior: Organized, Readiness for
    Enhanced
Infant Feeding Pattern, Ineffective
Infection, Risk for
Injury, Risk for
Insomnia
Intracranial Adaptive Capacity, Decreased
Knowledge, Deficient (Specify)
Knowledge (Specify), Readiness for Enhanced
Latex Allergy Response
Latex Allergy Response, Risk for
Liver Function, Impaired, Risk for
Loneliness, Risk for
Memory, Impaired
Mobility: Bed, Impaired
Mobility: Physical, Impaired
Mobility: Wheelchair, Impaired
Moral Distress
Nausea
Neurovascular Dysfunction: Peripheral, Risk for
Noncompliance (Specify)
Nutrition, Imbalanced: Less than Body
    Requirements
Nutrition, Imbalanced: More than Body
    Requirements
Nutrition, Imbalanced: More than Body
    Requirements, Risk for
Nutrition, Readiness for Enhanced
Oral Mucous Membrane, Impaired
Pain, Acute
Pain, Chronic
Parenting, Impaired
Parenting, Readiness for Enhanced
Parenting, Risk for Impaired
Perioperative Positioning Injury, Risk for
Personal Identity, Disturbed
Poisoning, Risk for
Post-Trauma Syndrome
Post-Trauma Syndrome, Risk for
Power, Readiness for Enhanced

Powerlessness
Powerlessness, Risk for
Protection, Ineffective
Rape-Trauma Syndrome
Rape-Trauma Syndrome: Compound Reaction
Rape-Trauma Syndrome: Silent Reaction
Religiosity, Impaired
Religiosity, Readiness for Enhanced
Religiosity, Risk for Impaired
Relocation Stress Syndrome
Relocation Stress Syndrome, Risk for
Role Conflict, Parental
Role Performance, Ineffective
Sedentary Lifestyle
Self-Care, Readiness for Enhanced
Self-Care Deficit: Bathing/Hygiene
Self-Care Deficit: Dressing/Grooming
Self-Care Deficit: Feeding
Self-Care Deficit: Toileting
Self-Concept, Readiness for Enhanced
Self-Esteem, Chronic Low
Self-Esteem, Situational Low
Self-Esteem, Risk for Situational Low
Self-Mutilation
Self-Mutilation, Risk for
Sensory Perception, Disturbed (Specify: Auditory,
    Gustatory, Kinesthetic, Olfactory Tactile,
    Visual)
Sexual Dysfunction
Sexuality Pattern, Ineffective
Skin Integrity, Impaired
Skin Integrity, Risk for Impaired
Sleep Deprivation
Sleep, Readiness for Enhanced
Social Interaction, Impaired
Social Isolation
Sorrow, Chronic
Spiritual Distress
Spiritual Distress, Risk for
Spiritual Well-Being, Readiness for Enhanced
Spontaneous Ventilation, Impaired
Stress, Overload
Sudden Infant Death Syndrome, Risk for
Suffocation, Risk for
Suicide, Risk for
Surgical Recovery, Delayed
Swallowing, Impaired
Therapeutic Regimen Management: Community,
    Ineffective
Therapeutic Regimen Management, Effective
Therapeutic Regimen Management: Family,
    Ineffective
Therapeutic Regimen Management, Ineffective
Therapeutic Regimen Management, Readiness for
    Enhanced
Thermoregulation, Ineffective
Thought Processes, Disturbed
Tissue Integrity, Impaired
Tissue Perfusion, Ineffective (Specify: Cerebral,
    Cardiopulmonary, Gastrointestinal, Renal)

Tissue Perfusion, Ineffective, Peripheral
Transfer Ability, Impaired
Trauma, Risk for
Unilateral Neglect
Urinary Elimination, Impaired
Urinary Elimination, Readiness for Enhanced
Urinary Incontinence, Functional

Urinary Incontinence, Overflow
Urinary Incontinence, Reflex
Urinary Incontinence, Stress
Urinary Incontinence, Total
Urinary Incontinence, Urge
Urinary Incontinence, Risk for Urge

Urinary Retention
Ventilatory Weaning Response, Dysfunctional
Violence: Other-Directed, Risk for
Violence: Self-Directed, Risk for
Walking, Impaired
Wandering

Source: NANDA Nursing Diagnoses: Definitions and Classification, 2007–2008. Philadelphia: North American Nursing Diagnosis Association. Used with permission.

Glossary

24-hour food recall client recall of all the food and beverages consumed during a typical 24-hour period

Abdominal paracentesis removal of fluids from the peritoneal cavity

Absorption the process by which a drug passes into the bloodstream

Accommodation a process of change whereby cognitive processes mature sufficiently to allow a person to solve problems that were previously unsolvable

Accountability the ability and willingness to assume responsibility for one's actions and to accept the consequences of one's behavior

Acculturation the involuntary process that occurs when people adapt to or borrow traits from another culture

Acid a substance that releases hydrogen ions (H+) in solution

Acidosis a condition that occurs with increases in blood carbonic acid or with decreases in blood bicarbonate; blood pH below 7.35

Acquired immunity *see* Passive immunity

Action stage occurs when a person actively implements behavioral and cognitive strategies to interrupt previous behavior patterns and adopt new ones; this stage requires a great commitment of time and energy

Active euthanasia actions that directly bring about the client's death with or without consent

Active immunity a resistance of the body to infection in which the host produces its own antibodies in response to natural or artificial antigens

Active ROM exercises isotonic exercises in which the client moves each joint in the body through its complete range, maximally stretching all muscle groups within each plane over the joint

Active transport movement of substances across cell membranes against the concentration gradient

Activity theory the best way to age is to stay active physically and mentally

Activity tolerance the type and amount of exercise or daily activities an individual is able to perform

Activity-exercise pattern refers to a person's pattern of exercise, activity, leisure, and recreation

Actual loss can be identified by others and can arise either in response to or in anticipation of a situation

Acupressure a form of healing in which the therapist exerts finger pressure on specific sites

Acupuncture a form of healing in which the therapist applies needles to stimulate specific sites of the body

Acute confusion also called *delirium;* abrupt onset of confusion and a reversible cause

Acute illness typically characterized by severe symptoms of relatively short duration

Acute infection those that generally appear suddenly or last a short time

Acute pain pain that lasts only through the expected recovery period (less than 6 months), whether it has a sudden or slow onset and regardless of the intensity

Adaptation the process of modifying to meet new, changing, or different conditions

Adaptive mechanism learned behaviors that assist an individual to adjust to the environment

Adherence the extent to which an individual's behavior (for example, taking medications, following diets, or making lifestyle changes) coincides with medical or health advice; commitment or attachment to a regimen

Adolescence the period during which a person becomes physically and psychologically mature and acquires a personal identity

Adolescent growth spurt the period during puberty when sudden and dramatic physical changes occur

Adult day care a day care center that provides health and social services to the older person

Advance health care directive a variety of legal and lay documents that allow persons to specify aspects of care they wish to receive should they become unable to make or communicate their preferences

Adventitious breath sounds abnormal or acquired breath sounds

Adverse effects more severe side effects that may justify the discontinuation of a drug

Advocate individual who pleads the cause of another or argues or pleads for a cause or proposal

Aerobic living only in the presence of oxygen

Aerobic exercise any activity during which the body takes in more or an equal amount of oxygen than it expends

Aesthetic knowing providing care and meeting the needs of clients through creativity and style

Afebrile absence of a fever

Affective domain known as the "feeling" domain and is divided into categories that specify the degree of a person's depth of emotional response to tasks; includes feelings, emotions, interests, attitudes, and appreciations

Afterload the resistance against which the heart must pump to eject blood into the circulation

Ageism deep and profound prejudice in American society against older adults

Agglutinins specific antibodies formed in the blood

Agglutinogens a substance that acts as an antigen and stimulates the production of agglutinins

Agnostic a person who doubts the existence of God or a supreme being or believes the existence of God has not been proved

Agonist a drug that interacts with a receptor to produce a response

Agonist analgesic full agonists which are pure opioid drugs that bind tightly to mu receptor sites, producing maximum pain inhibition, an agonist effect

Agonist-antagonist analgesic mixed agonist-antagonist drugs that can act like opioids and relieve pain (agonist effect) when given to a client who has not taken any pure opioids

Airborne precautions methods used to reduce exposure to infectious agents transmitted by airborne droplet nuclei smaller than 5 microns

Alarm reaction the initial reaction of the body to stress, which alerts the body's defenses

Algor mortis the gradual decrease of the body's temperature after death

Alkalosis a condition that occurs with increases in blood bicarbonate or decreases in blood carbonic acid; blood pH above 7.45

Allodynia where nonpainful stimuli (e.g., contact with linen, water, or wind) produces pain or dysthesia, which is an unpleasant abnormal sensation

Allopathic medicine term used to describe Western medical practice

Alopecia the loss of scalp hair (baldness) or body hair

Alternative medicine an unrelated group of nonorthodox practices, often with explanatory systems that do not follow conventional biomedical explanations

Alzheimer's disease disease that involves progressive dementia, memory loss, and inability to care for self

Amblyopia reduced visual acuity in one eye

Ambulation the act of walking

Ampule a small glass container for individual doses of liquid medications

Anabolism a process in which simple substances are converted by the body's cells into more complex substances (e.g., building tissue, positive nitrogen balance)

Anaerobic living only in the absence of oxygen

Anaerobic exercise involves activity in which the muscles cannot draw out enough oxygen from the bloodstream; used in endurance training

Anal stimulation stimulation applied to anus for sexual pleasure

Anaphylactic reaction a severe allergic reaction that usually occurs immediately after the administration of a drug

Andragogy the art and science of helping adults learn

Androgyny belief that most characteristics and behaviors are human qualities and not limited to a gender

Anemia a condition in which the blood is deficient in red blood cells or hemoglobin

Anger an emotional state consisting of a subjective feeling of animosity or strong displeasure

Animal-assisted therapy the use of specifically selected animals as a treatment modality in health and human service settings

Angiography a diagnostic procedure enabling x-ray visual examination of the vascular system after injection of a radiopaque dye

Angle of Louis the junction between the body of the sternum and the manubrium; the starting point for locating the ribs anteriorly

Anions ions that carry a negative charge; includes chlorine (Cl^-), bicarbonate (HCO_3^-), phosphate (HPO_4^{2-}), and sulfate (SO_4^-)

Ankylosed permanently immobile joints

Anorexia lack of appetite

Anorexia nervosa a disease characterized by a prolonged inability or refusal to eat, rapid weight loss, and emaciation in persons who continue to believe they are fat

Anoscopy visual examination of the anal canal using an anoscope (a lighted instrument)

Answer (legal) a written response made by the defendant

Antagonist drug that inhibits cell function by occupying the drug's receptor sites

Antibodies immunoglobulins, part of the body's plasma proteins, defend primarily against the extracellular phases of bacterial and viral infections

Anticipatory grief grief experienced in advance of the event

Anticipatory loss the experience of loss before the loss actually occurs

Antigen a substance capable of inducing the formation of antibodies

Antihelix the anterior curve of the auricle's upper aspect

Antiseptics agents that inhibit the growth of some microorganisms

Anuria the failure of the kidneys to produce urine, resulting in a total lack of urination or output of less than 100 mL per day in an adult

Anxiety a state of mental uneasiness, apprehension, or dread producing an increased level of arousal caused by an impending or anticipated threat to self or significant relationships

Apgar scoring system a scoring system to assess newborn babies

Aphasia any defects in or loss of the power to express oneself by speech, writing, or signs, or to comprehend spoken or written language due to disease or injury of the cerebral cortex

Apical pulse a central pulse located at the apex of the heart

Apical-radial pulse measurement of the apical beat and the radial pulse at the same time

Apnea a complete absence of respirations

Apocrine glands sweat glands located largely in the axillae and anogenital areas; they begin to function at puberty under the influence of androgens

Approximated closed tissue surfaces

Aromatherapy therapeutic use of essential oils of plants in which odor or fragrance plays an important part

Arrhythmia a pulse with an abnormal rhythm

Arterial blood gases specimen of arterial blood that assesses oxygenation, ventilation, and acid–base status

Arterial blood pressure the measure of the pressure exerted by the blood as it pulsates through the arteries

Arteriosclerosis a condition in which the elastic and muscular tissues of the arteries are replaced with fibrous tissue

Ascites the accumulation of fluid in the abdominal cavity

Asepsis freedom from infection or infectious material

Asphyxiation lack of oxygen due to interrupted breathing

Aspiration the withdrawal of fluid that has abnormally collected (e.g., pleural cavity, abdominal cavity) or to obtain a specimen (e.g., cerebral spinal fluid)

Assault an attempt or threat to touch another person unjustifiably

Assessing the process of collecting, organizing, validating, and recording data (information) about a client's health status

Assignment a downward or lateral transfer of both the responsibility and accountability of an activity from one individual to another

Assimilation the process by which an individual develops a new cultural identity and becomes like the members of the dominant culture

Assisted living facility with various degrees of personal care assistance designed to meet the needs of an older person

Assisted suicide a form of active euthanasia in which clients are given the means to kill themselves

Astigmatism an uneven curvature of the cornea that prevents horizontal and vertical rays from focusing on the retina

Atelectasis a condition that occurs when ventilation is decreased and pooled secretions accumulate in a dependent area of a bronchiole and block it

Atheist one who denies the existence of God

Atherosclerosis buildup of fatty plaque within the arteries

Atria two upper hollow chambers of the heart

Atrioventricular (AV) node conduction pathways that slightly delay transmission of the impulse from the atria to the ventricles of the heart

Atrioventricular (AV) valves between the atria and ventricles of the heart, the tricuspid valve on the right and the bicuspid or mitral valve on the left

Atrophy wasting away; decrease in size of organ or tissue (e.g., muscle)

Attentive listening listening actively, using all senses, as opposed to listening passively with just the ear

Attitudes mental stance that is composed of many different beliefs; usually involving a positive or negative judgment toward a person, object, or idea

Audit examination or review of records

Auditory related to or experienced through hearing

Auricle flap of the ear

Auscultation the process of listening to sounds produced within the body

Auscultatory gap the temporary disappearance of sounds normally heard over the brachial artery when the sphygmomanometer cuff pressure is high and the sounds reappear at a lower level

Authoritarian leader the individual who makes decisions for the group

Authority the power given by an organization to direct the work of others; the right to act

Autoantigen an antigen that originates in a person's own body

Autocratic leader *see* Authoritarian leader

Automaticity an electrical impulse and contraction independent of the nervous system and generated by the cardiac muscle

Autonomy the state of being independent and self-directed, without outside control, to make one's own decisions

Autopsy an examination of the body after death to determine the cause of death and to learn more about a disease process

Awareness the ability to perceive environmental stimuli and body reactions and to respond appropriately through thought and action

Ayurveda Indian system of medicine where illness is viewed as a state of imbalance among the body's systems

Baby Boomers generation that includes those born in years 1945–1964

Bacteremia bacteria in the blood

Bacteria the most common infection-causing microorganisms

Bactericidal bacteria-killing action

Balance concept of equilibrium between mental, physical, emotional, spiritual, and environmental components to achieve optimum wellness

Bandage a strip of cloth used to wrap some part of the body

Basal metabolic rate (BMR) the rate of energy utilization in the body required to maintain essential activities such as breathing

Base of support the area on which an object rests

Bases (alkalis) have low hydrogen ion concentration and can accept hydrogen ions in solution

Battery (legal) the willful or negligent touching of a person (or the person's clothes or even something the person is carrying), which may or may not cause harm

Bed rest strict confinement to bed (complete bed rest), or the client may be allowed to use a bedside commode or have bathroom privileges

Bedpan a receptacle for urine and feces for clients who are restricted to bed

Behaviorist theory includes the careful identification of what is to be taught and the immediate identification of and reward for correct responses

Beliefs interpretations or conclusions that one accepts as true

Beneficence the moral obligation to do good or to implement actions that benefit clients and their support persons

Bereavement a subjective response of a person who has experienced the loss of a significant other through death

Bevel the slanted part at the tip of a needle

Bicultural used to describe a person who crosses two cultures, lifestyles, and sets of values

Bier block *see* Intravenous block

Binder a type of bandage applied to large body areas (abdomen or chest) or for a specific body part (arm sling); used to provide support

Bioelectromagnetics science that studies how living organisms interact with electromagnetic fields

Bioethics ethical rules or principles that govern right conduct concerning life

Biofeedback a stress management technique that brings under conscious control bodily processes normally thought to be beyond voluntary command

Biomedical health belief *see* Scientific health belief

Biomedicine term used to describe Western medical practice

Biopsy the removal and examination of tissue from the living body

Biorhythms inner rhythms that appear to control a variety of biologic processes

Bioterrorism intentional attack using biological weapons such as viruses, bacteria, or other germs

Biotransformation process by which a drug is converted to a less active form; also called *detoxification*

Biot's respirations shallow breaths interrupted by apnea

Bladder training client postpones voiding, resists or inhibits the sensation of urgency, and voids according to a timetable rather than according to the urge to void

Blanch test a test during which the client's fingertip is temporarily pinched to assess capillary refill and peripheral circulation

Blood chemistry a number of tests performed on blood serum (the liquid portion of the blood)

Blood pressure (BP) the force exerted on arterial walls by blood flowing within the vessel

Blood urea nitrogen (BUN) a measure of blood level of urea, the end product of protein metabolism

Bloodborne pathogens those microorganisms carried in blood and body fluids that are capable of infecting other persons with serious and difficult-to-treat viral infections, namely, hepatitis B virus, hepatitis C virus, and HIV

Body image how a person perceives the size, appearance, and functioning of his or her body and its parts

Body mass index (BMI) indicates whether weight is appropriate for height

Body substance isolation (BSI) generic infection control precautions for all clients except those with diseases transmitted through the air

Body temperature the balance between the heat produced by the body and the heat lost from the body

Bodymind a state of integration that includes body, mind, and spirit

Boomerang kids slang term used for young adults who move back into their parents' homes after an initial period of independent living

Bottle mouth syndrome describes the decay of an infant's teeth caused by constant contact with sweet liquid from a bottle

Boundary the real or imaginary lines that differentiate one system from another system or a system from its environment

Bowel (fecal) incontinence loss of voluntary ability to control fecal and gaseous discharges through the anal sphincter

Bradycardia abnormally slow pulse rate, less than 60 beats per minute

Bradypnea abnormally slow respiratory rate, usually less than 10 respirations per minute

Brand name the name given to a drug by the drug's manufacturer

Breach of duty a standard of care that is expected in the specific situation but that the nurse did not observe; this is the failure to act as a reasonable, prudent nurse under the circumstances

Bronchoscopy visual examination of the bronchi using a bronchoscope

Bruit a blowing or swishing sound created by turbulence of blood flow

Buccal pertaining to the cheek

Buffers prevent excessive changes in pH by removing or releasing hydrogen ions

Bulimia an uncontrollable compulsion to eat large amounts of food and then expel it by self-induced vomiting or by taking laxatives

Bundle of His the right and left bundle branches of the ventricular conduction pathways

Burden of proof the duty of proving an assertion

Bureaucratic leader does not trust self or others to make decisions and instead relies on the organization's rules, policies, and procedures to direct the group's work efforts

Burn results from excessive exposure to thermal, chemical, electric, or radioactive agents

Burnout a complex syndrome of behaviors that can be likened to the exhaustion stage of the general adaptation syndrome; an overwhelming feeling that can lead to physical and emotional depletion, a negative attitude and self-concept, and feelings of helplessness and hopelessness

Calculi renal stones

Callus a thickened portion of the skin

Caloric value the amount of energy that nutrients or foods supply to the body

Calorie (c, cal, kcal) a unit of heat energy equivalent to the amount of heat required to raise the temperature of 1 kg of water 1°C

Cancer pain pain associated with cancers; can be related or unrelated to the disease or its treatment

Cannula a tube with a lumen (channel) that is inserted into a cavity or duct and is often fitted with a trocar during insertion

Carbon monoxide an odorless, colorless, tasteless gas that is very toxic

Cardiac arrest the cessation of heart function

Cardiac output (CO) the amount of blood ejected by the heart with each ventricular contraction

Cardinal signs *see* Vital signs

Caregiver a role that has traditionally included those activities that assist the client physically and psychologically

Caregiver burden responses to long-term stress, such as chronic fatigue, sleeping difficulties, and high blood pressure, in family members who undertake the care of a person in the home for a long period

Caregiver role strain physical, emotional, social, and financial burdens that can seriously jeopardize the caregiver's own health and well-being

Caries tooth cavities

Caring intentional action that conveys physical and emotional security and genuine connectedness with another person or group of people

Caring practice nursing care that includes connection, mutual recognition, and involvement

Carminative an agent that promotes the passage of flatus from the colon

Carrier a person or animal that harbors a specific infectious agent and serves as a potential source of infection, yet does not manifest any clinical signs of disease

Case management a method for delivering nursing care in which the nurse is responsible for a caseload of clients across the health care continuum

Case manager a nurse who works with the multidisciplinary health care team to measure the effectiveness of the case management plan and monitor outcomes

Catabolism a process in which complex substances are broken down into simpler substances (e.g., breakdown of tissue)

Cataracts opacity of the lens or capsule of the eye

Cathartics drugs that induce defecation

Cations ions that carry a positive charge; includes sodium (Na^+), potassium (K^+), calcium (Ca^{2+}), and magnesium (Mg^{2+})

Causation a fact that must be proven that the harm occurred as a direct result of the nurse's failure to follow the standard of care and the nurse could have (or should have) known that failure to follow the standard of care could result in such harm

Cell-mediated defenses *see* Cellular immunity

Cellular immunity also known as cell-mediated defenses, occur through the T-cell system

Center of gravity the point at which the mass (weight) of the body is centered

Central neuropathic pain pain resulting from malfunctioning nerves in the central nervous system

Central processing unit (CPU) the processor/microprocessor that performs the computer program instructions, located in the box that contains the computer hardware

Central venous catheter catheter that is usually inserted into the subclavian or jugular vein, with the distal tip of the catheter resting in the superior vena cava just above the right atrium

Cephalocaudal proceeding in the direction from head to toe

Cerebral death the higher brain center or cerebral cortex is irreversibly destroyed

Cerumen the wax-like substance secreted by glands in the external ear canal

Change process of making something different from what it was

Change agents persons (or groups) who initiate change or who assist others in making modifications in themselves or in the system

Change-of-shift report a report given to nurses on the next shift

Charismatic leader characterized by an emotional relationship between the leader and the group members; personality of the leader evokes strong feelings of commitment to both the leader and the leader's cause and beliefs

Chart a formal, legal document that provides evidence of a client's care

Charting the process of making an entry on a client record

Charting by exception (CBE) a documentation system in which only significant findings or exceptions to norms are recorded

Chemical name the name by which a chemist knows a drug; describes the constituents of the drug precisely

Chemical restraints medications used to control socially disruptive behavior

Chemical thermogenesis the stimulation of heat production in the body through increased cellular metabolism caused by increases in thyroxine output

Cheyne-Stokes respirations rhythmic waxing and waning of respirations from very deep breathing to very shallow breathing with periods of temporary apnea, often associated with cardiac failure, increased intracranial pressure, or brain damage

Chiropractic from the Greek meaning "done by hand"; involves adjustments of the spine and joints and is grounded in the assumption that maintaining the alignment of the spine and joints facilitates the flow of energy throughout the body, including the nervous, circulatory, respiratory, gastrointestinal, and limbic systems

Cholesterol a lipid that does not contain fatty acid but possesses many of the chemical and physical properties of other lipids

Chronic illness illness that lasts for an extended period of time, usually greater than 6 months

Chronic infection infection that occurs slowly, over a very long period, and may last months or years

Chronic pain prolonged pain, usually recurring or persisting over 6 months or longer, and interferes with functioning

Chyme digested products that leave the stomach through the small intestine and then pass through the ileocecal valve

Circulating immunity *see* Humoral immunity

Circulating nurse assists scrub nurses and surgeons during surgery

Civil action deals with the relationship between individuals in society

Civil law the body of law that deals with relationships among private individuals; also known as *private law*

Clara Barton a schoolteacher who volunteered as a nurse during the Civil War. Most notably, she organized the American Red Cross, which linked with the International Red Cross when the U.S. Congress ratified the Geneva Convention in 1882

Clean free of potentially infectious agents

Clean voided specimen urine specimens for routine urinalysis

Clean-catch specimen urine specimens for urine culture

Cleaning bath a type of bath given chiefly for hygiene purposes

Client a person who engages the advice or services of another person who is qualified to provide this service

Client record *see* Chart

Climacteric the point in development when reproduction capacity in the female terminates (menopause) and the sexual activity of the male decreases (andropause)

Clinical aromatherapy the controlled use of essential oils for specific measurable outcomes

Closed awareness a type of awareness in which the client is unaware of impending death

Closed questions restrictive question requiring only a short answer

Closed system system that does not exchange energy, matter, or information with its environment

Closed wound drainage system consists of a drain connected to either an electric suction or a portable drainage suction, such as a Hemovac or Jackson-Pratt

Clubbing elevation of the proximal aspect of the nail and softening of the nail bed

Co-analgesic medication that is not classified as a pain medication; however, it has properties that may reduce pain alone, or in combination with other analgesics; relieve other discomforts; potentiate the effect of pain medication; or reduce the pain medication's side effects

Cochlea a seashell-shaped structure found in the inner ear; essential for sound transmission and hearing

Code blue emergency announcing cardiac/respiratory arrest and initiating interventions

Code of ethics a formal statement of a group's ideals and values; a set of ethical principles shared by members of a group, reflecting their moral judgments and serving as a standard for professional actions

Cognitive development refers to the manner in which people learn to think, reason, and use language

Cognitive domain the "thinking" domain, includes six intellectual abilities and thinking processes beginning with knowing, comprehending, and applying to analysis, synthesis, and evaluation

Cognitive skills intellectual skills that include problem solving, decision making, critical thinking, and creativity

Cognitive theory recognition of developmental levels of learners, and acknowledgments of the learner's motivation and environment

Coinsurance an insurance plan in which the client pays a percentage of the payment and some other group (e.g., employer, government) pays the remaining percentage

Collaboration a collegial working relationship with another health care provider in the provision of client care

Collaborative care plans *see* Critical pathways

Collaborative interventions actions the nurse carries out in collaboration with other health team members, such as physical therapists, social workers, dietitians, and physicians

Collagen a protein found in connective tissue; a whitish protein substance that adds tensile strength to a wound

Colloid osmotic pressure a pulling force exerted by colloids that help maintain the water content of blood

Colloids substances such as large protein molecules that do not readily dissolve into true solutions

Colonization the presence of organisms in body secretions or excretions in which strains of bacteria become resident flora but do not cause illness

Colonoscopy visual examination of the interior of the colon with a colonoscope

Colostomy an opening into the colon (large bowel)

Commode a portable, chairlike structure used as a toilet

Common law the body of principles that evolves from court decisions

Communicable disease a disease that can spread from one person to another

Communication a two-way process involving the sending and receiving of messages

Communicator nurses identify client problems and then communicate these verbally or in writing to other members of the health team

Community a collection of people who share some attribute of their lives

Community health nursing the synthesis of nursing and public health practice as applied to promoting and preserving the health of populations

Community nursing centers (CNCs) provide primary care to specific populations and are staffed by nurse practitioners and community health nurses

Community-based health care (CBHC) a system that provides health-related services within the context of people's daily lives; that is, in places where people spend their time in the community

Community-based nursing (CBN) nursing care directed toward a specific population or group within the community; primary, secondary, or tertiary care may be provided to individuals or groups

Compensation defense mechanism in which a person substitutes an activity for one that he or she would prefer doing or cannot do

Compensatory counterbalancing

Complaint (legal) a document filed by a plaintiff

Complementary and alternative medicine (CAM) those practices that do not form part of the dominant system for managing health and disease

Complementary medicine *see* Alternative medicine

Complementary therapies therapeutic practices that are not currently considered an integral part of conventional allopathic medical practice

Complete blood count (CBC) specimens of venous blood; includes hemoglobin and hematocrit measurements, erythrocyte (RBC) count, leukocyte (WBC) count, red blood cell indices, and a differential white cell count

Complete proteins a protein that contains all of the essential amino acids as well as many nonessential ones

Compliance the extent to which an individual's behavior coincides with medical or health advice

Complicated grief pathologic grief; exists when coping strategies are maladaptive

Compress a moist gauze dressing applied frequently to an open wound, sometimes medicated

Compromised host any person at increased risk for an infection

Computed tomography (CT) a painless, noninvasive x-ray procedure that has the unique capability of distinguishing minor differences in the density of tissues

Computer-based patient records (CPRs) electronic client data retrievable by caregivers, administrators, accreditors, and other persons who require the data

Concept map a visual tool in which ideas or data are enclosed in circles or boxes of some shape and relationships between these are indicated by connecting lines or arrows

Concepts abstract ideas or mental images of phenomena or reality

Conceptual framework a group of related concepts

Conceptual model a graphic illustration of the relationships among concepts

Concurrent audit evaluation of a client's health care while the client is still receiving care from the agency

Conduction the transfer of heat from one molecule to another in direct contact

Conduction hearing loss the result of interrupted transmission of sound waves through the outer and middle ear structures

Confidentiality any information a subject relates will not be made public or available to others without the subject's consent

Congruent communication the verbal and nonverbal aspects of the message match

Conjunctivitis inflammation of the bulbar and palpebral conjunctiva

Conscious sedation a minimal depression of level of consciousness during which the client retains the ability to consciously maintain a patent airway and respond appropriately to verbal and physical stimuli

Consequence-based (teleological) theories the ethics of judging whether an action is moral

Constant fever a state in which the body temperature fluctuates minimally but always remains above normal

Constipation passage of small, dry, hard stool or passage of no stool for an abnormally long time

Consultative leader *see* Democratic leader

Consumer an individual, a group of people, or a community that uses a service or commodity

Contact precautions methods used to reduce exposure to infectious agents easily transmitted by direct client contact or by contact with items in the client's environment

Contemplation stage stage in which a person acknowledges having a problem, seriously considers changing a specific behavior, actively gathers information, and verbalizes plans to change the behavior in the near future

Continuing education (CE) formalized experiences designed to enlarge the knowledge or skills of practitioners

Continuity of care the coordination of health care services by health care providers for clients moving from one health care setting to another and between and among health care professionals

Continuity theory people maintain their values, habits, and behavior in old age

Contract a written or verbal agreement between two or more people to do or not do some lawful act

Contract law the enforcement of agreements among private individuals or the payment of compensation for failure to fulfill the agreement

Contractility the inherent ability of cardiac muscle fibers to shorten or contract

Contractual obligations duty of care established by the presence of an expressed or implied contract

Contractual relationships vary among practice settings; may be as an independent or employer-employee relationship

Contracture permanent shortening of a muscle and subsequent shortening of tendons and ligaments

Convection the dispersion of heat by air currents

Conventional medicine term used to describe Western medical practice

Coordinating the process of ensuring that plans are carried out and evaluating outcomes

Coping dealing with change

Coping mechanism an innate or acquired way of responding to a changing environment or specific problem or situation

Coping strategy *see* Coping mechanism

Core self-concept the beliefs and images that are most vital to the person's identity

Core temperature the temperature of the deep tissues of the body (e.g., thorax, abdominal cavity); relatively constant at 37°C (98.6°F)

Corn a conical, circular, painful, raised area on the toe or foot

Coronary arteries a network of vessels known as the coronary circulation

Coroner a public official, not necessarily a physician, appointed or elected to inquire into the causes of death

Costal (thoracic) breathing use of the external intercostal muscles and other accessory muscles, such as the sternocleidomastoid muscles

Counseling the process of helping a client to recognize and cope with stressful psychologic or social problems, to develop improved interpersonal relationships, and to promote personal growth

Countershock phase second part of the alarm reaction in which the changes the body experienced during the shock phase are reversed

Covert data (systems, subjective data) information (data) apparent only to the person affected that can be described or verified only by that person

Creatine kinase (CK) enzyme that is released into the blood during a myocardial infarction (MI)

Creatinine a nitrogenous waste that is excreted in the urine

Creatinine clearance a test uses 24-hour urine and serum creatinine levels to determine the glomerular filtration rate, a sensitive indicator of renal function

Creativity thinking that results in the development of new ideas and products

Credentialing the process of determining and maintaining competence in practice; includes licensure, registration, certification, and accreditation

Credé's maneuver manual exertion of pressure on the bladder to force urine out

Crepitation (1) a dry, crackling sound like that of crumpled cellophane, produced by air in the subcutaneous tissue or by air moving through fluid in the alveoli of the lungs; (2) a crackling, grating sound produced by bone rubbing against bone

Crime an act committed in violation of public (criminal) law and punishable by a fine and/or imprisonment

Criminal actions deal with disputes between an individual and the society as a whole

Criminal law deals with actions against the safety and welfare of the public

Crisis counseling therapy focused on solving immediate problems involving individuals, groups, or families in crisis

Crisis intervention a short-term helping process of assisting clients to work through a crisis to its resolution and restore their precrisis level of functioning

Critical analysis a set of questions one can apply to a particular situation or idea to determine essential information and ideas and discard superfluous information and ideas

Critical pathways multidisciplinary guidelines for client care based on specific medical diagnoses designed to achieve predetermined outcomes

Critical theory describes theories that help elucidate how social structures affect a wide variety of human experiences from art to social practices

Critical thinking a cognitive process that includes creativity, problem solving, and decision making

Cross-dresser Individual of one gender (typically male) who dresses in clothing specific to the opposite gender

Crystalloids salts that dissolve readily into true solutions

Cues any piece of information or data that influences decisions

Cultural care deprivation lack of culturally assistive, supportive, or facilitative acts

Cultural deprivation *see* Cultural care deprivation

Culturally appropriate application of underlying background knowledge that must be possessed to provide a given client with the best possible health care

Culturally competent within the delivered care the nurse understands and attends to the total context of the client's situation and uses a complex combination of knowledge, attitudes, and skills

Culturally sensitive care that demonstrates basic knowledge of and constructive attitudes toward the health traditions observed among the diverse cultural groups found in the setting

Culture a world view and set of traditions used and transmitted from generation to generation by a particular group, includes related attitudes and institutions

Culture shock a disorder that occurs in response to transition from one cultural setting to another

Cultures laboratory cultivations of microorganisms in a special growth medium

Cumulative effect the increasing response to repeated doses of a drug that occurs when the rate of administration exceeds the rate of metabolism or excretion

Curanderismo cultural healing tradition found in Latin America that uses Western medicine beliefs, treatments, and practices at three levels of care: material level, spiritual level, and mental level

Cyanosis bluish discoloration of the skin and mucous membranes caused by reduced oxygen in the blood

Cystoscope a lighted instrument used to visualize the interior of the urinary bladder

Cystoscopy visual examination of the urinary bladder with a cystoscope

Dacryocystitis inflammation of the lacrimal sac

Damages if malpractice caused the injury, the nurse is held liable for damages that may be compensated

Dandruff a dry or greasy, scaly material shed from the scalp

Data information

Data warehousing the accumulation of large amounts of data that are stored over time

Database all information about a client, includes nursing health history and physical assessment, physician's history, physical examination, and laboratory and diagnostic test results

Debridement removal of infected and necrotic tissue

Decision (legal) outcome made by a judge

Decision making the process of establishing criteria by which alternative courses of action are developed and selected

Decode to relate the message perceived to the receiver's storehouse of knowledge and experience and to sort out the meaning of the message

Decubitus ulcers *see* Pressure ulcers

Deductive reasoning making specific observations from a generalization

Defamation (legal) a communication that is false, or made with careless disregard for the truth, and results in injury to the reputation of another

Defecation expulsion of feces from the rectum and anus

Defendant (legal) person against whom a plaintiff files a complaint

Defense mechanism any reaction that serves to protect against something physically or psychologically harmful

Defining characteristics client signs and symptoms that must be present to validate a nursing diagnosis

Dehiscence the partial or total rupturing of a sutured wound; usually involves an abdominal wound in which the layers below the skin also separate

Dehydration insufficient fluid in the body

Delegation the transfer of responsibility for the performance of an activity from one person to another while retaining accountability for the outcome

Delirium also called *acute confusion;* abrupt onset of confusion and a reversible cause

Demand feeding child is fed when hungry

Dementia a global impairment of cognitive function that usually is progressive and may be permanent; interferes with normal social and occupational activities

Democratic leader encourages group discussion and decision making

Demography the study of population, including statistics about distribution by age and place of residence, mortality, and morbidity

Dental caries tooth decay

Denver Developmental Screening Test (DDST) a screening test used to assess children from birth to 6 years of age

Dependent functions with regard to medical diagnoses, physician-prescribed therapies and treatments nurses are obligated to carry out

Dependent interventions those activities carried out on the order of a physician, under a physician's supervision, or according to specified routines

Dependent variable the behavior, characteristic, or outcome that the researcher wishes to explain or predict

Depression feelings of sadness and dejection, often accompanied by physiologic change such as decreased functional activity

Descriptive statistics procedures that summarize large volumes of data; used to describe and synthesize data, showing patterns and trends

Desire phase part of the response cycle, which starts in the brain, with conscious sexual desires

Desired effect *see* Therapeutic effect

Detoxification *see* Biotransformation

Detrusor muscle the smooth muscle layers of the bladder

Development an individual's increasing capacity and skill in functioning, related to growth

Developmental stage level of achievement for a particular segment of a person's life

Developmental task skill or behavior pattern learned during stages of development

Diagnosis a statement or conclusion concerning the nature of some phenomenon

Diagnosis-related groups (DRGs) a Medicare payments system to hospitals and physicians that establishes fees according to diagnosis

Diagnostic labels title used in writing a nursing diagnosis; taken from the North American Nursing Diagnosis Association (NANDA) standardized taxonomy of terms

Dialysis a technique by which fluids and molecules pass through a semipermeable membrane according to the rules of osmosis

Diaphragmatic (abdominal) breathing contraction and relaxation of the diaphragm, observed by the movement of the abdomen, which occurs as a result of the diaphragm's contraction and downward movement

Diarrhea defecation of liquid feces and increased frequency of defecation

Diastole the period during which the ventricles relax

Diastolic pressure the pressure of the blood against the arterial walls when the ventricles of the heart are at rest

Diet history a comprehensive assessment of a client's food intake that involves an extensive interview by a nutritionist or dietitian

Differentiated practice a system in which the best possible use of nursing personnel is based on their educational preparation and resultant skill sets

Diffusion the mixing of molecules or ions of two or more substances as a result of random motion

Directing a management function that involves communicating the task to be completed and providing guidance and supervision

Directive interview a highly structured interview that uses closed questions to elicit specific information

Dirty denotes the likely presence of microorganisms, some of which may be capable of causing infection

Disaccharides sugars that are composed of double molecules

Discharge planning the process of anticipating and planning for client needs after discharge

Discovery (legal) pretrial activities to gain all of the facts of a situation

Discrimination the differential treatment of individuals or groups

Discussion an informal oral consideration of a subject by two or more health care personnel to identify a problem or establish strategies to resolve a problem

Disease an alteration in body function resulting in a reduction of capacities or shortening of the normal life span

Disease prevention behavior motivated by a desire to actively avoid illness, detect it early, or maintain functioning within the constraints of illness (also called *health protection*)

Disengagement theory aging involves mutual withdrawal (disengagement) between the older person and others in the elderly person's environment

Disinfectants agents that destroy pathogens other than spores

Dissatisfaction problems dissatisfaction with sexual encounters despite desire, arousal, and orgasm

Distance learning learning in which people communicate effectively across long distances

Distribution the transportation of a drug from its site of absorption to its site of action

Diuresis the production of large amounts of urine by the kidneys without an increased fluid intake

Diuretics agents that increase urine secretion

Diversity the fact or state of being different

Documenting *see* Charting or Recording

Do-not-resuscitate (DNR) order a physician's order that specifies no effort be made to resuscitate the client with terminal or irreversible illness in the event of a respiratory or cardiac arrest

Dorothea Dix woman leader who provided nursing care during the Civil War

Dorsal (supine) position a back-lying position without a pillow

Dorsal recumbent position a back-lying position with the head and shoulders slightly elevated

Drip factor (drop factor) the number of drops per milliliter of solution delivered for a particular drip chamber

Droplet nuclei residue of evaporated droplets that remains in the air for long periods of time

Droplet precautions methods used to reduce exposure to infectious agents transmitted by particle droplets larger than 5 microns

Drug a chemical compound taken for disease prevention, diagnosis, cure, or relief or to affect the structure or function of the body

Drug abuse excessive intake of a substance either continually or periodically

Drug allergy an immunologic reaction to a drug

Drug dependence inability to keep the intake of a drug or substance under control

Drug habituation a mild form of psychologic dependence on a drug

Drug half-life (Elimination half-life) the time required for the elimination process to reduce the concentration of a drug to one-half what it was at initial administration

Drug interaction the beneficial or harmful interaction of one drug with another drug

Drug tolerance a condition in which successive increases in the dosage of a drug are required to maintain a given therapeutic effect

Drug toxicity the quality of a drug that exerts a deleterious effect on an organism or tissue

Dullness a thudlike sound produced during percussion by dense tissue of body organs such as the liver, spleen, or heart

Durable medical equipment (DME) companies companies that provide health care equipment for the client at home

Duration the length of time that a sound is heard

Duty the nurse must have (or should have had) a relationship with the client that involves providing care and following an acceptable standard of care

Dysesthesia unpleasant abnormal sensation

Dysmenorrhea painful menstruation

Dyspareunia difficult or painful intercourse

Dysphagia difficulty or inability to swallow

Dyspnea difficult or labored breathing

Dysrhythmia a pulse with an irregular rhythm

Dysuria painful or difficult voiding

Eccrine glands glands that produce sweat; found over most of the body

Echocardiogram a noninvasive test that uses ultrasound to visualize structures of the heart and evaluate left ventricular function

Ectoderm the outer layer of tissue formed in the second week of life

Edema the presence of excess interstitial fluid in the body

Effectiveness a measure of the quality or quantity of services provided

Efficiency a measure of the resources used in the provision of nursing services

Effleurage a stroking massage technique

Ego includes consciousness and memory, which serve to mediate between primitive instinctual drives (id), internal social prohibitions (superego), and reality

Ego defense mechanisms (Freud) mental mechanisms that develop as the personality attempts to defend itself, establish compromises among conflicting impulses, and allay inner tensions

Ejaculation expulsion of seminal fluid and sperm

Elasticity of the arterial wall expansibility or stretching of the vessels

Elderspeak speech style similar to babytalk; gives the message of dependence and incompetence to older adults

Elective surgery performed when surgical intervention is the preferred treatment for a condition that is not imminently life threatening or to improve the client's life

Electric shock occurs when a current travels through the body to the ground rather than through electric wiring, or from static electricity that builds up on the body

Electrocardiogram (ECG, EKG) a graph of the electric activity of the heart

Electrocardiography provides a graphic recording of the heart's electrical activity

Electroencephalogram (EEG) a graph of the electrical activity of the brain

Electromyogram (EMG) a graph of the electrical activity of muscles

Electro-oculogram (EOG) a graph of the electrical activity of eye to eye movement

Electrolytes chemical substances that develop an electric charge and are able to conduct an electric current when placed in water; ions

Electronic communication communication involving computers and technology (i.e., e-mail)

Electronic medical records (EMRs) *see* Computer-based patient records (CPRs)

Elimination half-life *see* Drug half-life

Embolus a blood clot (or a substance such as air) that has moved from its place of origin and is causing obstruction to circulation elsewhere (plural: *emboli*)

Embryonic phase the phase during which the fertilized ovum develops into an organism with most of the features of a human

Emergency surgery surgery that is performed immediately to preserve function or the life of the client

Emmetropic normal refraction so that the eyes focus images on the retina

Empathy the ability to discriminate what the other person's world is like and to communicate to the other this understanding in a way that shows that the helper understands the client's feelings and the behavior and experience underlying these feelings

Emphysema a chronic pulmonary condition in which the alveoli are dilated and distended

Empirical data information collected from the observable world

Empirical knowing knowledge that comes from science; ranges from factual, observable phenomena to theoretical analysis

Encoding involves the selection of specific signs or symbols (codes) to transmit the message, such as which language and words to use, how to arrange the words, and what tone of voice and gestures to use

Endocardium a layer of the heart wall lining the inside of the heart's chambers and great vessels

Endoderm the inner layer of tissue formed in the second week of life

End-of-life care care provided in the final weeks before death

Endogenous developing from within

Enema a solution introduced into the rectum and sigmoid colon to remove feces and/or flatus

Energy the force that integrates the body, mind, and spirit

Enteral through the gastrointestinal system

Entoderm *see* Endoderm

Enuresis bed-wetting; involuntary passing of urine in children after bladder control is achieved

Environment all of the conditions, circumstances, and influences surrounding and affecting the development of an organism or person

Enzymes biologic catalysts that speed up chemical reactions

Epicardium the visceral pericardium adhering to the surface of the heart, forming the heart's outermost layer

Epidural commonly used route for parenteral administration into the epidural space (the area inside the spinal column but outside the dura mater)

Epidural anesthesia the injection of an anesthetic agent into the epidural space

Equianalgesia equal analgesia; used when referring to the doses of various opioid analgesics that provide approximately the same pain relief

Equilibrium a state of balance

Erectile dysfunction the inability to achieve or maintain an erection sufficient for sexual satisfaction for oneself or one's partner

Erythema a redness associated with a variety of skin rashes

Erythrocytes red blood cells, or RBCs

Eschar thick necrotic tissue produced by burning, by a corrosive application, or by death of tissue associated with loss of vascular supply, bacterial invasion, and putrefaction

Essential amino acids amino acids that cannot be manufactured in the body and must be supplied as part of the protein ingested in the diet

Ethical knowing knowledge that focuses on matters of obligation or what ought to be done

Ethics the rules or principles that govern right conduct

Ethnic belonging to a specific group of individuals who share a common social and cultural heritage

Ethnocentrism the belief that one's own culture or way of life is better than that of others

Ethnography research that provides a framework to focus on the culture of a group of people

Ethnopharmacology study of the effect of ethnicity on responses to prescribed medicines

Etiology the causal relationship between a problem and its related or risk factors

Eupnea normal, quiet breathing

Eustachian tube the part of the middle ear that connects the middle ear to the nasopharynx; stabilizes air pressure between the external atmosphere and the middle ear

Euthanasia the act of painlessly putting to death persons suffering from incurable or distressing disease

Evaluating a planned ongoing, purposeful activity in which clients and health care professionals compare expected outcomes to actual outcomes

Evaluation statement a statement that consists of two parts: a conclusion and supporting data

Evidence-based practice (EBP) the use of some form of substantiation in making clinical decisions

Evisceration extrusion of the internal organs

Exacerbation the period during a chronic illness when symptoms reappear after remission

Excitement/plateau phase part of the response cycle, involves vasocongestion and myotonia

Excoriation loss of the superficial layers of the skin

Excretion elimination of a waste product produced by the body cells from the body

Exercise a type of physical activity; a planned, structured, and repetitive bodily movement done to improve or maintain one or more components of physical fitness

Exhalation (expiration) the movement of gases from the lungs to the atmosphere

Exogenous developing from outside sources

Exophthalmus a protrusion of the eyeballs with elevation of the upper eyelids, resulting in a startled or staring expression

Expectorate to cough and spit up mucus or other materials

Expert witness one who has special training, experience, or skill in a relevant area and is allowed by the court to offer an opinion on some issue within that area of expertise

Expiration *see* Exhalation

Express consent an oral or written agreement

Extended family family that includes the relatives of the nuclear family (e.g., grandparents, aunts, uncles)

External auditory meatus the entrance to the ear canal

Extinction the failure to perceive touch on one side of the body when two symmetric areas of the body are touched simultaneously

Extracellular fluid (ECF) fluid found outside the body cells

Exudate material, such as fluid and cells, that has escaped from blood vessels during the inflammatory process and is deposited in tissue or on tissue surfaces

Fabiola a wealthy Roman matron; viewed by some as the patron saint of early nursing who used her position and wealth to establish hospitals for the sick

Fad a widespread but short-lived interest, or a practice followed with considerable zeal

Failure to thrive a unique syndrome in which an infant falls below the fifth percentile for weight and height on a standard growth chart or is falling in percentiles on a growth chart

Faith an active "mode of being-in-relation" to another or others in which we invest commitment, belief, love, and hope

False imprisonment the unlawful restraint or detention of another person against his or her wishes

Family the basic unit of society that consists of those individuals, male or female, youth or adult, legally or not legally related, genetically or not genetically related, who are considered by others to represent their significant persons

Family-centered nursing nursing that considers the health of the family as a unit in addition to the health of individual family members

Fats lipids that are solid at room temperature

Fat-soluble vitamins A, D, E, and K vitamins that the body can store

Fatty acids the basic structural units of most lipids made up of carbon chains and hydrogen

Fear an emotional response to an actual, present danger

Feasibility the availability of time as well as the material and human resources needed to investigate a research problem or question

Febrile pertaining to a fever; feverish

Fecal impaction a mass or collection of hardened, putty-like feces in the folds of the rectum

Fecal incontinence *see* Bowel incontinence

Feces (stool) body wastes and undigested food eliminated from the bowel

Feedback the response or message that the receiver returns to the sender during communication

Felony a crime of a serious nature, such as murder, punishable by a term in prison

Female orgasmic disorder when the female sexual response stops before orgasm occurs

Female sexual arousal disorder when lack of vaginal lubrication causes discomfort or pain during intercourse

Fetal phase characterized by a period of rapid growth in the size of the fetus; both genetic and environmental factors affect its growth

Fever elevated body temperature

Fever spike a temperature that rises to fever level rapidly following a normal temperature and then returns to normal within a few hours

Fibrin an insoluble protein formed from fibrinogen during the clotting of blood

Fidelity a moral principle that obligates the individual to be faithful to agreements and responsibilities one has undertaken

Fifth vital sign pain assessment

Filtration process whereby fluid and solutes move together across a membrane from one compartment to another

Filtration pressure the pressure in a compartment that results in the movement of fluid and substances dissolved in fluid out of the compartment

First-level manager a manager responsible for managing the work of nonmanagerial personnel and the day-to-day activities of a specific work group or groups

Fissures deep grooves that occur as a result of dryness and cracking of the skin

Fixation immobilization or the inability of the personality to proceed to the next developmental stage because of anxiety

Flaccid weak or lax

Flatness an extremely dull sound produced, during percussion, by very dense tissue, such as muscle or bone

Flatulence the presence of excessive amounts of gas in the stomach or intestines

Flatus gas or air normally present in the stomach or intestines

Florence Nightingale considered the founder of modern nursing, she was influential in developing nursing education, practice, and administration

Flow sheet a record of the progress of specific or specialized data such as vital signs, fluid balance, or routine medications; often charted in graph form

Fluid volume deficit (hypovolemia) loss of both water and electrolytes in similar proportions from the extracellular fluid

Fluid volume excess (FVE) (hypervolemia) retention of both water and sodium in similar proportions to normal extracellular fluid (ECF)

Focus charting a method of charting that uses key words or foci to describe what is happening to the client

Folk medicine beliefs and practices relating to illness prevention and healing that derive from cultural traditions rather than from modern medicine's scientific base

Fontanels unossified membranous gaps in the bone structure of the skull of a newborn that make molding of the head possible

Food diary a detailed record of measured amounts (portion sizes) of all food and fluids a client consumes during a specified period, usually 3 to 7 days

Food frequency record a checklist that indicates how often general food groups or specific foods are eaten

Foot drop plantar flexion contracture

Foreseeability a link that must exist between the nurse's act and the injury suffered

Formal leader an appointed leader selected by an organization and given official authority to make decisions and act

Formal nursing care plan a written or computerized guide that organizes information about the client's care

Fowler's position a bed-sitting position with the head of the bed raised to 45 degrees

Friction rubbing; the force that opposes motion

Full disclosure a basic right, which means that deception, either by withholding information about a client's participation in a study or by giving the client false or misleading information about what participating in the study will involve, must not occur

Functional strength ability of the body to perform work

Fungi infection-causing microorganisms that include yeasts and molds

Gait the way a person walks

Gastrocolic reflex increased peristalsis of the colon after food has entered the stomach

Gastrostomy an opening through the abdominal wall into the stomach

Gastrostomy tube a tube that is surgically placed directly into the client's stomach and provides a route for administering nutrition and medications

Gauge diameter of a shaft

Gender indicates biologic male or female status

Gender identity a person's sense of being masculine or feminine, as distinct from being male or female

Gender-role behavior outward expression of a person's sense of maleness or femaleness

General adaptation syndrome (GAS) (Selye) a general arousal response of the body to a stressor characterized by certain physiologic events and dominated by the sympathetic nervous system

General anesthesia the induced loss of all sensation and consciousness

Generation X generation that includes those born in years 1965–1978

Generation Y generation that includes those born in years 1979–2000

Generativity concern for establishing and guiding the next generation

Generic name a drug name not protected by trademark and usually describing the chemical structure of the drug

Genital intercourse penile/vaginal intercourse (coitus)

Geragogy the term used to describe the process involved in stimulating and helping elderly persons to learn

Geriatrics medical care of the elderly

Gerontology the study of aging and older adults

Gingival of or relating to the gums

Gingivitis red, swollen gingiva (gums)

Glaucoma a disturbance in the circulation of aqueous fluid; causes an increase in intraocular pressure

Global self refers to the collective beliefs and images one holds about oneself; the most complete description that individuals can give of themselves at any one time

Global self-esteem how much one likes one's perceived self as a whole

Glomerulus a tuft of capillaries in the kidney surrounded by Bowman's capsule

Glossitis inflammation of the tongue

Glycerides the most common form of lipids consisting of a glycerol molecule with up to three fatty acids

Glycogen the chief carbohydrate stored in the body, particularly in the liver and muscles

Glycogenesis the process of glycogen formation

Goals/desired outcomes a part of a care plan that describes, in terms of observable client responses, what the nurse hopes to achieve by implementing the nursing interventions

Goniometer a device used to measure the angle of a joint in degrees

Governance the establishment and maintenance of social, political, and economic arrangements by which practitioners control their practice, self-discipline, working conditions, and professional affairs

Grand theories articulate a broad range of the significant relationships among the concepts of a discipline

Granulation tissue young connective tissue with new capillaries formed in the wound healing process

Grief emotional suffering often caused by bereavement

Gross negligence involves extreme lack of knowledge, skill, or decision making that the person clearly should have known would put others at risk for harm

Grounded theory research to understand social structures and social processes; this method focuses on the generation of categories or hypotheses that explain patterns of behavior of people in the study

Group two or more people with shared purposes and goals

Group dynamics forces that determine the behavior of the group and the relationships among the group members

Growth physical change and increase in size

Guaiac test a test performed for occult (hidden) blood to detect gastrointestinal bleeding not visible to the eye

Guided imagery state of focused attention that encourages changes in attitudes, behavior, and physiologic reactions

Gustatory referring to the sense of taste

Habit training attempts to keep clients dry by having them void at regular intervals; also referred to as *timed voiding* or *scheduled toileting*

Hardware the physical parts of a computer

Harm (Injury) the client or plaintiff must demonstrate some type of harm or injury (physical, financial, or emotional) as a result of the breach of duty owed the client; the plaintiff will be asked to document physical injury, medical costs, loss of wages, "pain and suffering," and any other damages

Harriet Tubman known as "the Moses of Her People" for her work with the Underground Railroad; during the Civil War she nursed the sick and suffering of her own race

Haustra pouches that form in the large intestine when the longitudinal muscles are shorter than the colon

Haustral churning (shuffling) movement of the chyme back and forth within the haustra in the large intestine

Health behaviors the actions a person takes to understand his or her health state, maintain an optimal state of health, prevent illness and injury, and reach his or her maximum physical and mental potential

Health beliefs concepts about health that an individual believes are true

Health care proxy a legal statement that appoints a proxy to make medical decisions for the client in the event the client is unable to do so

Health care system the totality of services offered by all health disciplines

Health literacy ability to read, understand, and act on provided health information

Health maintenance organization (HMO) a group health care agency that provides basic and supplemental health maintenance and treatment services to voluntary enrollees

Health promotion any activity undertaken for the purpose of achieving a higher level of health and well-being

Health protection behavior motivated by a desire to actively avoid illness, detect it early, or maintain functioning within the constraints of illness

Health risk assessment (HRA) an assessment and educational tool that indicates a client's risk for disease or injury during the next 10 years by comparing the client's risk with the mortality risk of the corresponding age, sex, and racial group

Health status the health of a person at a given time

Heart failure a condition that develops if the heart cannot keep up with the body's need for oxygen and nutrients to the tissues; usually occurs because of myocardial infarction, but it may also result from chronic overwork of the heart

Heart-lung death the traditional clinical signs of death: cessation of the apical pulse, respirations, and blood pressure

Heat balance the state a person is in when the amount of heat produced by the body exactly equals the amount of heat lost

Heat exhaustion condition that is the result of excessive heat and dehydration

Heat stroke life-threatening condition with body temperature greater than 106°F

Heimlich maneuver subdiaphragmatic abdominal thrusts used to clear an obstructed airway

Helix the posterior curve of the auricle's upper aspect

Helping relationships the nurse–client relationship

Hematocrit the proportion of red blood cells (erythrocytes) to the total blood volume

Hematoma a collection of blood in a tissue, organ, or space due to a break in the wall of a blood vessel

Hemoglobin (Hg) the red pigment in red blood cells that carries oxygen

Hemoglobin A_{1c} measurement of blood glucose that is bound to hemoglobin

Hemolytic transfusion reaction destruction of red blood cells as a result of transfusion of incompatible blood

Hemoptysis the presence of blood in the sputum

Hemorrhage excessive loss of blood from the vascular system

Hemorrhagic exudate *see* Sanguineous exudate

Hemorrhoids distended veins in the rectum

Hemostasis cessation of bleeding

Hemothorax a collection of blood in the pleural cavity

Herbal medicine treating illness with herbs

Heritage consistency the degree to which one's lifestyle reflects his or her respective tribal culture

Heritage inconsistency the observance of the beliefs and practices of one's acculturated belief system

Hernia a protrusion (such as of the intestine through the inguinal wall or canal)

High Fowler's position a bed-sitting position in which the head of the bed is elevated 90 degrees

Higher brain death *see* Cerebral death

Hirsutism abnormal hairiness, particularly in women

Holism all living organisms are seen as interacting, unified wholes that are more than the sums of their parts

Holistic health a model of health based on the belief that the whole is more than the sum of its parts

Holistic health belief holds that the forces of nature must be maintained in balance or harmony

Holistic health care a system that considers all components of health: health promotion, health maintenance, health education and illness prevention, and restorative–rehabilitative care

Holistic nursing nursing practice that has as its goal the healing of the whole person

Holy day a day set aside for special religious observance

Homans' sign calf pain produced by dorsiflexion of the foot

Home care providing care in the client's home

Home health care nursing services and products provided to clients in their homes that are needed to maintain, restore, or promote their physical, psychologic, and social well-being

Homeopathy an alternative therapy based on the theory that the cure for the disease lies in the disease itself; thus, treatment is with highly diluted amounts of substances that at a higher concentration would produce the same symptoms as the disease

Homeostasis the tendency of the body to maintain a state of balance or equilibrium while continually changing; a mechanism in which deviations from normal are sensed and counteracted

Hope a multidimensional concept that includes perceiving realistic expectations and goals, having motivation to achieve goals, anticipating outcomes, establishing trust and interpersonal relationships, relying on internal and external resources, having determination to endure, and being oriented to the future

Hordeolum (sty) a redness, swelling, and tenderness of the hair follicle and glands that empty at the edge of the eyelids

Horticultural therapy also called *gardening* or *healing garden;* adjunct therapy to occupational and physical therapy that may involve viewing nature, visiting a healing garden or wander garden, or actively gardening

Hospice the delivery of care for terminally ill clients either in health care facilities or in the client's home

Hospice nursing care frequently given to terminally ill clients in their home; often considered a subspecialty of public health nursing

Hospital information system (HIS) computer software program suite used to manage client, financial, and administrative data

Hub the part of a needle that fits onto a syringe

Humanism learning that focuses on the feelings and attitudes of learners, the importance of the individual in identifying learning needs and taking responsibility for them, and the self-motivation of the learners to work toward self-reliance and independence

Humanist a perspective that includes propositions such as the mind and body are indivisible, people have the power to solve their own problems, and people are responsible for their lives and well-being

Humidifiers devices that add water vapor to inspired air

Humoral immunity antibody-mediated defense; resides ultimately in the B lymphocytes and is mediated by the antibodies produced by B cells

Hydrostatic pressure the pressure a liquid exerts on the sides of the container that holds it; also called *filtration force*

Hygiene the science of health and its maintenance

Hyperalgesia extreme sensitivity to pain

Hypercalcemia an excess of calcium in the blood plasma

Hypercapnia a condition in which carbon dioxide accumulates in the blood

Hypercarbia *see* Hypercapnia

Hyperchloremia an excess of chloride in the blood plasma

Hyperemia increased blood flow to an area

Hyperinflation giving the client breaths that are 1 to 1.5 times the tidal volume through the ventilator circuit or via a manual resuscitation bag

Hyperkalemia an excess of potassium in the blood plasma

Hypermagnesemia an excess of magnesium in the blood plasma

Hypernatremia an excess of sodium in the blood plasma

Hyperopia abnormal refraction in which light rays focus behind the retina, farsightedness

Hyperoxygenation done with a manual resuscitation bag or through a ventilator; increases oxygen flow (usually to 100%) before suctioning and between suction attempts

Hyperpathia heightened response to a painful stimulus; hyperalgesia

Hyperphosphatemia an excess of phosphate in the blood plasma

Hyperpyrexia *see* Hyperthermia

Hyperresonance an abnormal booming sound produced during percussion of the lungs

Hypersomnia excessive sleep

Hypertension an abnormally high blood pressure; over 140 mm Hg systolic and/or 90 mm Hg diastolic

Hyperthermia an extremely high body temperature (e.g., 41°C [105.8°F])

Hypertonic solutions that have a higher osmolality than body fluids

Hypertrophy enlargement of a muscle or organ

Hyperventilation very deep, rapid respirations

Hypervolemia increased blood volume

Hypnotherapy application of hypnosis (trance state or altered state of consciousness) to a medical or psychologic disorder

Hypoactive sexual desire disorder involves a persistent or recurring absence of sexual thoughts or disinterest in sexual activity

Hypocalcemia deficiency of calcium in the blood plasma

Hypochloremia deficiency of chloride in the blood plasma

Hypodermic under the skin

Hypodermic syringe a type of syringe that comes in 2-, 2.5-, and 3-mL sizes; the syringe usually has two scales marked on it: the minim and the milliliter

Hypokalemia deficiency of potassium in the blood plasma

Hypomagnesemia deficiency of magnesium in the blood plasma

Hyponatremia deficiency of sodium in the blood plasma

Hypophosphatemia deficiency of phosphate in the blood plasma

Hypotension an abnormally low blood pressure; less than 100 mm Hg systolic in an adult

Hypothalamic integrator the center in the brain that controls the core temperature; located in the preoptic area of the hypothalamus

Hypothermia a core body temperature below the lower limit of normal

Hypothesis a prediction of the relationship among two or more variables

Hypotonic solutions that have a lower osmolality than body fluids

Hypoventilation very shallow respirations

Hypovolemia an abnormal reduction in blood volume

Hypoxemia reduced oxygen in the blood

Hypoxia insufficient oxygen anywhere in the body

Iatrogenic disease disease caused unintentionally by medical therapy

Iatrogenic infections infections that are the direct result of diagnostic or therapeutic procedures

Id the source of instinctive and unconscious psychologic urges

Ideal body weight (IBW) the optimal weight recommended for optimal health

Ideal self how we would prefer to be; the individual's perception of how one should behave based on certain personal standards, aspirations, goals, or values

Identification perceiving one's self as similar to and behaving like another person

Idiosyncratic effect a different, unexpected, or individual effect from the normal one usually expected from a medication; the occurrence of unpredictable and unexplainable symptoms

Ileal conduit channel created when a segment of the ileum is removed and the intestinal ends reattached

Ileostomy an opening into the ileum (small bowel)

Illicit drugs drugs that are sold illegally; street drugs

Illness a highly personal state in which the person feels unhealthy or ill, may or may not be related to disease

Illness behavior the course of action a person takes to define the state of his or her health and pursue a remedy

Imagery the internal experience of memories, dreams, fantasies, and visions that serve as a bridge connecting body, mind, and spirit

Imagination an important part of preschoolers' life (the preschooler has an active imagination and fantasizes in play)

Imitation copying the behaviors and attitudes of another person

Immobility prescribed or unavoidable restriction of movement in any area of a person's life

Immune defenses *see* Specific (immune) defenses

Immunity a specific resistance of the body to infection; it may be natural, or resistance may develop after exposure to a disease agent

Immunoglobulins *see* Antibodies

Impaired nurse a nurse whose practice has deteriorated because of chemical abuse

Implementing the phase of the nursing process in which the nursing care plan is put into action

Implied consent consent that is assumed in an emergency when consent cannot be obtained from the client or a relative

Implied contract a contract that has not been explicitly agreed to by the parties but that the law nevertheless considers to exist

Incentive spirometers devices that measure the flow of air inhaled through the mouthpiece

Incomplete proteins protein that lacks one or more essential amino acids; usually derived from vegetables

Incus the anvil bone of the middle ear

Independent variable the presumed cause or influence on the dependent variable

Independent functions areas of health care unique to nursing, separate and distinct from medical management

Independent interventions activities that the nurse is licensed to initiate as a result of the nurse's own knowledge and skills

Independent practice associations (IPAs) provide care in offices; clients pay a fixed prospective payment and IPA pays the provider; earnings or losses are assumed by the IPA

Indicator an observable patient state, behavior, or self-reported perception or evaluation; similar to desired outcomes in traditional language

Individualized care plan a plan tailored to meet the unique needs of a specific client—needs that are not addressed by the standardized plan

Individualized exercise prescription exercise mode and dose tailored to a specific individual to ensure greater adherence to the exercise program

Inductive reasoning making generalizations from specific data

Infection the disease process produced by microorganisms

Inferences interpretations or conclusions made based on cues or observed data

Inflammation local and nonspecific defensive tissue response to injury or destruction of cells

Infrared photoenergy therapy treatment to improve sensory impairment associated with peripheral neuropathy

Influence an informal strategy used to gain the cooperation of others without exercising formal authority

Informal nursing care plan a strategy for action that exists in the nurse's mind

Informal leader an individual selected by the group as its leader because of seniority, age, special abilities, or charisma

Informed consent a client's agreement to accept a course of treatment or a procedure after receiving complete information, including the risks of treatment and facts relating to it, from the physician

Ingestion the act of taking in food or medication

Ingrown toenail the growing inward of the nail into the soft tissues around it, most often results from improper nail trimming

Inhalation (inspiration) the act of breathing in; the intake of air or other substances into the lungs

Inhibiting effect the decreased effect of one or both drugs

Injury *see* Harm

Input consists of information, material, or energy that enters a system

Inquest a legal inquiry into the cause or manner of a death

Insensible fluid loss fluid loss that is not perceptible to the individual

Insensible heat loss heat loss that occurs from evaporation (vaporization) of moisture from the respiratory tract, mucosa of the mouth, and the skin

Insensible water loss continuous and unnoticed water loss

In-service education education that is designed to upgrade the knowledge or skills of employees

Insomnia inability to obtain a sufficient quality or quantity of sleep

Inspection the visual examination, that is, assessment by using the sense of sight

Inspiration *see* Inhalation

Insulin syringe similar to a hypodermic syringe, but the scale is specially designed for insulin: a 100-unit calibrated scale intended for use with U-100 insulin

Integrated delivery system (IDS) a system that incorporates acute care services, home health care, extended and skilled care facilities, and outpatient services

Integrated health care system one that makes all levels of care available in an integrated form—primary care, secondary care, and tertiary care

Intensity the loudness or softness of a sound, amplitude

Intention tremor involuntary trembling when an individual attempts a voluntary movement

Intermittent fever a body temperature that alternates at regular intervals between periods of fever and periods of normal or subnormal temperatures

Internet a worldwide computer network

Interpersonal skills all verbal and nonverbal activities people use when communicating directly with one another

Interpreter an individual who mediates spoken communication between people speaking different languages without adding, omitting, or distorting meaning or editorializing

Intersex ambiguous gender

Interstate compact an agreement between two or more states

Interstitial fluid fluid that surrounds the cells, includes lymph

Interview a planned communication; a conversation with a purpose

Intracellular fluid (ICF) fluid found within the body cells, also called *cellular fluid*

Intractable pain pain that is resistant to cure or relief

Intradermal under the epidermis (into the dermis)

Intradermal (ID) injection the administration of a drug into the dermal layer of the skin just beneath the epidermis

Intramuscular into the muscle

Intramuscular (IM) injections injections into muscle tissue that are absorbed more quickly than subcutaneous injections because of the greater blood supply to the body muscles

Intraoperative phase begins when the client is transferred to the operating table and ends when the client is admitted to the postanesthesia care unit

Intrapleural pressure pressure in the pleural cavity surrounding the lungs

Intrapulmonary pressure pressure within the lungs

Intraspinal into the spinal cord

Intrathecal *see* Intraspinal

Intravascular fluid plasma

Intravenous within a vein

Intravenous block anesthesia used most often for procedures involving the arm, wrist, and hand

Intravenous pyelography (IVP) x-ray filming of the kidney and ureters after injection of a radiopaque material into the vein

Intimacy a close friendship

Introjection the assimilation of the attributes of others

Intuition the understanding or learning of things without the conscious use of reasoning

Invasion of privacy a direct wrong of a personal nature, it injures the feelings of the person and does not take into account the effect of revealed information on the standing of the person in the community

Ions atoms or group of atoms that carry a positive or negative electric charge; electrolytes

Iron deficiency anemia a form of anemia caused by inadequate supply of iron for synthesis of hemoglobin

Irrigation (lavage) a flushing or washing-out of a body cavity, organ, or wound with a specified solution that may or may not be medicated

Ischemia deficiency of blood supply caused by obstruction of circulation to the body part

Isokinetic (resistive) exercises muscle contraction or tension against resistance

Isolation practices that prevent the spread of infection and communicable disease

Isometric (static or setting) exercise tensing of a muscle against an immovable outer resistance that does not change muscle length or produce joint motion

Isotonic solutions that have the same osmolality as body fluids

Isotonic (dynamic) exercise exercise in which muscle tension is constant and the muscle shortens to produce muscle contraction and active movement

Jaundice a yellowish color of the sclera, mucous membranes, and/or skin

Jejunostomy an opening through the abdominal wall into the jejunum

Justice fairness

Kardex the trade name for a method that makes use of a series of cards to concisely organize and record client data and instructions for daily nursing care—especially care that changes frequently and must be kept up to date

Keloid a hypertrophic scar containing an abnormal amount of collagen

Kidneys/ureters/bladder (KUB) x-ray of the kidneys, ureters, and bladder

Kilocalorie (kcal) *see* Calorie

Kilojoule (kJ) a metric measurement referring to the amount of energy required when a force of 1 newton (N) moves 1 kg of weight 1 m of distance

Kinesthetic refers to awareness of the position and movement of body parts

Knights of Saint Lazarus an order of knights that dedicated themselves to the care of people with leprosy, syphilis, and chronic skin conditions

Korotkoff's sounds a series of five sounds produced by blood within the artery with each ventricular contraction

Kosher acceptable or prepared according to Jewish law

Kussmaul's breathing hyperventilation that accompanies metabolic acidosis in which the body attempts to compensate (give off excess body acids) by blowing off carbon dioxide through deep and rapid breathing

Kyphosis excessive convex curvature of the thoracic spine

Laissez-faire (nondirective, permissive) leader recognizes the group's need for autonomy and self-regulation

Lanugo the fine, woolly hair or down on the shoulders, back, sacrum, and earlobes of the unborn child that may remain for a few weeks after birth

Large calorie (Calorie, kilocalorie [kcal]) *see* Calorie

Laryngoscopy visual examination of the larynx with a laryngoscope

Lateral position a side-lying position

Lavage an irrigation or washing of a body organ, such as the stomach

Lavinia L. Dock a nursing leader and suffragist who was active in the protest movement for women's rights that resulted in the U.S. Constitution amendment allowing women to vote in 1920

Law a rule made by humans that regulates social conduct in a formally prescribed and binding manner

Laxatives medications that stimulate bowel activity and assist fecal elimination

Leader a person who influences others to work together to accomplish a specific goal

Leadership style describes traits, behaviors, motivations, and choices used by individuals to effectively influence others

Leading question a question that influences the client to give a particular answer

Learning a change in human disposition or capability that persists over a period of time and cannot be solely accounted for by growth

Learning need a desire or a requirement to know something that is currently unknown to the learner

Leukocytes white blood cells

Leukocytosis an increase in the number of white blood cells

Liability the quality or state of being legally responsible for one's obligations and action and to make financial restitution for wrongful acts

Libel defamation by means of print, writing, or pictures

Libido urge or desire for sexual activity

License a legal permit granted to individuals to engage in the practice of a profession and to use a particular title

Licensed vocational (practical) nurse (LVN/LPN) a nurse who practices under the supervision of a registered nurse, providing basic direct technical care to clients

Lifestyle the values and behaviors adopted by a person in daily life

Lift an abnormal anterior movement of the chest related to enlargement of the right ventricle

Lillian Wald founder of the Henry Street Settlement and Visiting Nurse Service, which provided nursing and social services and organized educational and cultural activities; considered the founder of public health nursing

Linda Richards America's first trained nurse

Line of gravity an imaginary vertical line running through the center of gravity

Lipids organic substances that are greasy and insoluble in water but soluble in alcohol or ether

Lipoproteins soluble compounds made up of various lipids

Litigation the action of a lawsuit

Living will a document that states medical treatments(s) the client chooses to omit or refuse in the event that the client is unable to make these decisions

Livor mortis discoloration of the skin caused by breakdown of the red blood cells; occurs after blood circulation has ceased; appears in the dependent areas of the body

Lobule earlobe

Local adaptation syndrome (LAS) the reaction of one organ or body part to stress

Local anesthesia an anesthetic agent used for minor surgical procedures that is injected into a specific area

Local area network (LAN) personal computers (PCs) linked directly to nearby PCs and servers by wires or wireless communication devices

Local infection an infection that is limited to the specific part of the body where the microorganisms remain

Locus of control (LOC) a concept about whether clients believe their health status is under their own or others' control

Logrolling a technique used to turn a client whose body must at all times be kept in straight alignment (like a log)

Long-term memory the repository for information stored for periods longer than 72 hours and usually weeks and years

Lordosis an exaggerated concavity in the lumbar region of the vertebral column

Loss an actual or potential situation in which a valued ability, object, or person is inaccessible or changed so that it is perceived as no longer valuable

Low Fowler's position a bed-sitting position in which the head of the bed is elevated between 15 and 45 degrees, with or without knee flexion

Lumbar puncture a procedure where cerebrospinal fluid (CSF) is withdrawn through a needle that is inserted into the subarachnoid space of the spinal canal between the third and fourth lumbar vertebrae or between the fourth and fifth lumbar vertebrae

Lung compliance expansibility of the lung

Lung recoil the tendency of lungs to collapse away from the chest wall

Lung scan records the emissions from radioisotopes that indicate how well gas and blood are traveling through the lungs; also known as a *V/Q (ventilation/perfusion) scan*

Maceration the wasting away or softening of a solid as if by the action of soaking; often used to describe degenerative changes and eventual disintegration

Macrominerals any of the minerals that people require daily in amounts over 100 mg

Macronutrients refers to carbohydrates, fats, and protein because they are needed in large amounts (e.g., hundreds of grams) to provide energy

Magico-religious health belief a belief system in which people attribute the fate of the world and those in it to the actions of God, the gods, or other supernatural forces for good or evil

Magnetic resonance imaging (MRI) a noninvasive diagnostic scanning technique in which the client is placed in a magnetic field

Maintenance stage stage at which a person integrates newly adopted behavior patterns into his or her lifestyle

Major surgery surgery that involves a high degree of risk for a variety of reasons; it may be complicated or prolonged; large losses of blood may occur; vital organs may be involved; postoperative complications may occur

Male erectile disorder when a man has erection problems during 25% or more of his sexual interactions

Male orgasmic disorder disorder where a man can maintain an erection but has difficulty ejaculating

Malleus hammer bone of the middle ear

Malnutrition a disorder of nutrition; insufficient nourishment of the body cells

Malpractice the negligent acts of persons engaged in professions or occupations in which highly technical or professional skills are employed

Managed care a method of organizing care delivery that emphasizes communication and coordination of care among all health care team members

Management information system (MIS) software designed to facilitate the organization and application of data used to manage an organization or department

Manager one who is appointed to a position in an organization that gives the power to guide and direct the work of others

Mandated reporters a role of the nurse in which he or she identifies and assesses cases of violence against others, and in every case the situation must be reported to the proper authorities

Manometer an instrument used to measure the pressure of fluids or gases

Manslaughter second-degree murder

Manubrium the handle-like superior part of the sternum that joins with the clavicles

Margaret Higgins Sanger considered the founder of Planned Parenthood, was imprisoned for opening the first birth control information clinic in Baltimore in 1916

Mary Breckinridge a nurse who practiced midwivery in England, Australia, and New Zealand; founded the Frontier Nursing Service in Kentucky in 1925 to provide family-centered primary health care to rural populations

Mary Mahoney first African American professional nurse

Mass peristalsis involves a wave of powerful muscular contraction that moves over large areas of the colon; usually occurs after eating

Mastoid a bony prominence behind the ear

Masturbation sexual self-stimulation

Maturity the state of maximal function and integration; the state of being fully developed

Mean a measure of central tendency, computed by summing all scores and dividing by the number of subjects; commonly symbolized as X or M

Measures of central tendency measures that describe the center of a distribution of data, denoting where most of the subjects lie; include the mean, median, and mode

Measures of variability measures that indicate the degree of dispersion or spread of the data; include range, variance, and standard deviation

Meatus an opening, passage, or channel

Meconium the first fecal material passed by the newborn, normally up to 24 hours after birth

Median a measure of central tendency, representing the exact middle score or value in a distribution of scores; the median is the value above and below which 50% of the scores lie

Medicaid a U.S. federal public assistance program paid out of general taxes and administered through the individual states to provide health care for those who require financial assistance

Medical asepsis all practices intended to confine a specific microorganism to a specific area, limiting the number, growth, and spread of microorganisms

Medical examiner a physician who usually has advanced education in pathology or forensic medicine who determines causes of death

Medicare a national and state health insurance program for U.S. residents older than 65 years of age

Medication a substance administered for the diagnosis, cure, treatment, or relief of a symptom or for prevention of disease

Medication reconciliation comparison of medications client is taking to physician's admission, transfer, and/or discharge orders

Meditation mental exercise that directs the mind to think inwardly by closing the sense organs to external stimulation

Menarche onset of menstruation

Meniscus the crescent-shaped upper surface of a column of fluid

Menopause cessation of menstruation

Menstruation the monthly discharge of blood through the vagina occurring in nonpregnant women from puberty to menopause

Mentor a person who serves as an experienced guide, adviser, or advocate and assumes responsibility for promoting the growth and professional advancement of a less experienced individual

Mesoderm middle layer of the embryonic tissue that forms during the first 3 weeks of life

Metabolic acidosis a condition characterized by a deficiency of bicarbonate ions in the body in relation to the amount of carbonic acid in the body; the pH falls to less than 7.35

Metabolic alkalosis a condition characterized by an excess of bicarbonate ions in the body in relation to the amount of carbonic acid in the body; the pH rises to greater than 7.45

Metabolism the sum of all physical and chemical processes by which a living substance is formed and maintained and by which energy is made available for use by the organism

Metabolites end products or enzymes

Metaparadigm originates from the Greek *meta*, meaning "with," and *paradigm*, meaning "pattern"; based on four theoretical concepts of nursing: person, environment, health, and nursing

Metered-dose inhaler (MDI) a handheld nebulizer, which is a pressurized container of medication that can be used by the client to release the medication through a mouthpiece

Microminerals a vitamin or mineral

Micronutrients vitamins and minerals that are needed in small amounts (e.g., milligrams or micrograms) to metabolize energy-providing nutrients

Micturition *see* Urination

Mid-arm circumference (MAC) a measure of fat, muscle, and skeleton

Mid-arm muscle circumference (MAMC) calculated by using reference tables or by using a formula that incorporates the triceps skinfold and the MAC

Middle-level manager a manager who supervises a number of first-level managers and is responsible for the activities in the departments supervised

Midlevel theories focus on exploration of concepts such as pain, self-esteem, learning, and hardiness

Midstream urine specimen *see* Clean-catch specimen

Milliequivalent one-thousandth of an equivalent, which is the chemical combining power of a substance

Minerals a substance found in organic compounds, as inorganic compounds and as free ions

Minor surgery surgery that involves little risk, produces few complications, and is often performed in a "day surgery" facility

Miosis constricted pupils

Misdemeanor a legal offense usually punishable by a fine or a short-term jail sentence, or both

Mixed hearing loss a combination of conduction and sensorineural loss

Mobility ability to move about freely, easily, and purposefully in the environment

Mode the score or value that occurs most frequently in a distribution of scores

Modeling observing the behavior of people who have successfully achieved a goal that one has set for oneself and, through observing, acquiring ideas for behavior and coping strategies

Monosaccharides sugars that are composed of single molecules

Monotheism belief in the existence of one God

Monounsaturated fatty acids a fatty acid with one double bond

Moral relating to right and wrong

Moral behavior the way a person perceives the requirements necessary for people to live together and how he or she responds to them

Moral development process of learning to tell the difference between right and wrong and of learning what ought and ought not to be done

Moral rules specific prescriptions for actions

Morality a doctrine or system denoting what is right and wrong in conduct, character, or attitude

Mortician a person trained in the care of the dead; also called an *undertaker*

Motivation the desire to learn

Mourning the process through which grief is eventually resolved or altered

Multidisciplinary care plan a standardized plan that outlines the care required for clients with common, predictable—usually medical—conditions

Music therapy the behavioral science concerned with the systematic application of music to produce relaxation and desired changes in emotions, behavior, and physiology

Mutual pretense a type of awareness in which the client, family, and health personnel know that the prognosis is terminal but do not talk about it and make an effort not to raise the subject

Mutual recognition model a regulatory model developed by the National Council of State Boards of Nursing (NCSBN), which allows for multistate licensure

Mydriasis enlarged pupils

Myocardial infarction (MI) heart attack; cardiac tissue necrosis owing to obstruction of blood flow to the heart

Myocardium a layer of the heart wall; cardiac muscle cells that form the bulk of the heart and contract with each beat

Myopia abnormal refraction in which light rays focus in front of the retina (nearsightedness)

Narcolepsy an uncontrollable desire for sleep or attacks of sleep during the day

Narrative charting a descriptive record of client data and nursing interventions, written in sentences and paragraphs

Nasoenteric tube a tube inserted through one of the nostrils, down the nasopharynx, and into the alimentary tract

Nasogastric tube a tube inserted by way of the nasopharynx and placed into the client's stomach for the purpose of feeding the client or to remove gastric secretions

Naturopathic medicine practice that focuses on nutrition, herbs, homeopathy, acupuncture, hydrotherapy, physical medicine, counseling, and minor surgical interventions

Negative feedback feedback that inhibits change

Negligence failure to behave in a reasonable and prudent manner; an unintentional tort

Nephrostomy diversion of urine from a kidney to a stoma

Nerve block chemical interruption of a nerve pathway effected by injecting a local anesthetic

Network linkages

Networking a process by which people develop linkages throughout the profession to communicate, share ideas and information, and offer support and direction to each other

Neurectomy surgery in which peripheral or cranial nerves are interrupted to alleviate localized pain

Neurogenic bladder interference with the normal mechanisms of urine elimination in which the client does not perceive bladder fullness and is unable to control the urinary sphincters; the result of impaired neurologic function

Neuropathic pain the result of a disturbance of the peripheral or central nervous system that results in pain that may or may not be associated with an ongoing tissue-damaging process

Neutral question a question that does not direct or pressure a client to answer in a certain way

Nitrogen balance a measure of the degree of protein anabolism and catabolism; net result of intake and loss of nitrogen

Nociception the physiologic processes related to pain perception

Nociceptor a pain receptor

Nocturia voiding two or more times at night

Nocturnal emissions orgasm and emission of semen during sleep

Nocturnal enuresis involuntary urination at night

Nocturnal frequency the need for older adults to arise during the night to urinate

Nondirective interview an interview using open-ended questions and empathetic responses to build rapport and learn client concerns

Nondirective leader *see* Laissez-faire (nondirective, permissive) leader

Nonessential amino acids an amino acid that the body can manufacture

Nonmaleficence the duty to do no harm

Nonspecific defenses bodily defenses that protect a person against all microorganisms, regardless of prior exposure

Nonsteroidal anti-inflammatory drugs (NSAIDs) drugs that relieve pain by acting on the peripheral nerve endings to inhibit the formation of the prostaglandins that tend to sensitize nerves to painful stimuli; have analgesic, antipyretic, and anti-inflammatory effects; include aspirin and ibuprofen

Nonverbal communication communication other than words, including gestures, posture, and facial expressions

Norm an ideal or fixed standard; an expected standard of behavior of group members

Normocephalic normal head size

Normocephaly normal head circumference at birth; usually 35 cm (14 in.)

Nosocomial infections infections associated with the delivery of health care services in a health care facility

NPO from the Latin *nil per os* meaning "nothing by mouth"

NREM (non-REM) sleep a deep restful sleep rate; also called *slow wave sleep*

Nuclear family a family of parents and their offspring

Nurse informaticist an expert who combines computer, information, and nursing science to develop policies and procedures that promote effective use of computerized records by nurses and other health care professionals

Nursing the attributes, characteristics, and actions of the nurse providing care on behalf of, or in conjunction with, the client

Nursing diagnosis the nurse's clinical judgment about individual, family, or community responses to actual and potential health problems/life processes to provide the basis for selecting nursing interventions to achieve outcomes for which the nurse is accountable

Nursing ethics ethical issues that occur in nursing practice

Nursing informatics the science of using computer information systems in the practice of nursing

Nurse informaticist expert who combines computer, information, and nursing science

Nursing intervention any treatment, based on clinical judgment and knowledge, that a nurse performs to enhance patient/client outcomes

Nursing Interventions Classification (NIC) a taxonomy of nursing actions each of which includes a label, a definition, and a list of activities

Nursing Outcomes Classification (NOC) a taxonomy for describing client outcomes that respond to nursing interventions

Nursing process a systematic rational method of planning and providing nursing care

Nutrients organic or inorganic substances found in food

Nutrition the sum of all interactions between an organism and the food it consumes

Nutritive value the nutrient content of a specified amount of food

Nystagmus rapid involuntary rhythmic eye movement

Obese (obesity) when body mass index (BMI) is greater than 30 kg/m^2

Objective data information (data) that is detectable by an observer or can be tested against an accepted standard; can be seen, heard, felt, or smelled

Obligatory losses essential fluid losses required to maintain body functioning

Occult blood hidden blood

Occupational exposure skin, eye, mucous membrane, or parenteral contact with blood or other potentially infectious materials that may result from the performance of an employee's duties

Official name the name under which a drug is listed in one of the official publications (e.g., the *United States Pharmacopeia*)

Oils lipids that are liquid at room temperature

Olfactory related to smell

Oliguria production of abnormally small amounts of urine by the kidney

Oncotic pressure *see* Colloid osmotic pressure

One-point discrimination the ability to sense whether one or two areas of the skin are being stimulated by pressure

Online connected to a computer network

Onset of action the time after drug administration when the body initially responds to the drug

Open awareness a type of awareness in which a client and people around know about the impending death

Open system system in which energy, matter, and information move into and out of the system through the system boundary

Open-ended questions questions that specify only the broad topic to be discussed and invite clients to discover and explore their thoughts and feelings about the topic

Operational definitions definitions that specify the instruments or procedures by which concepts will be measured

Ophthalmic referring to the eye

Opportunistic pathogen a microorganism causing disease only in a susceptible individual

Oral referring to the mouth

Oral-genital sex oral stimulation of either female or male genitals

Organizing determining responsibilities, communicating expectations, and establishing the chain of command for authority and communication

Orgasmic phase part of the response cycle, the involuntary climax of sexual tension, accompanied by physiologic and psychologic release

Orthopnea ability to breathe only when in an upright position (sitting or standing)

Orthopneic position a sitting position that relieves respiratory difficulty; the client leans over and is supported by an overbed table across the lap

Orthostatic hypotension decrease in blood pressure related to positional or postural changes from lying to sitting or standing positions

Osmolality the concentration of solutes in body fluids

Osmosis passage of a solvent through a semipermeable membrane from an area of lesser solute concentration to one of greater solute concentration

Osmotic pressure pressure exerted by the number of nondiffusible particles in a solution; the amount of pressure needed to stop the flow of water across a membrane

Ossicles the three middle ear bones of sound transmission

Osteoporosis demineralization of the bone

Ostomy a suffix denoting the formation of an opening or outlet such as an opening on the abdominal wall for the elimination of feces or urine

Otic referring to the ear

Otoscope an instrument used to examine the ears

Outcome evaluation focuses on demonstrable changes in the client's health status as result of nursing care

Output energy, matter, or information from a system given out by the system as a result of its processes

Overhydration occurs when water is gained in excess of electrolytes, resulting in low serum osmolality and low serum sodium levels, also known as *hypo-osmolar imbalance* or *water intoxication*

Overnutrition a caloric intake in excess of daily energy requirements, resulting in storage of energy in the form of adipose tissue

Overweight a BMI of 26–30 kg/m^2

Oxyhemoglobin the compound of oxygen and hemoglobin

Pace number of steps taken per minute or the distance taken in one step when walking

Packing filling an open wound or cavity with a material such as gauze

Pain whatever the experiencing person says it is, existing whenever he or she says it does

Pain threshold the amount of pain stimulation a person requires before feeling pain

Pain tolerance the maximum amount and duration of pain that an individual is willing to endure

Palliative care symptom care of clients for whom disease no longer responds to cure-focused treatment

Pallor the absence of underlying red tones in the skin; may be most readily seen in the buccal mucosa

Palpation the examination of the body using the sense of touch

Papanicolaou (Pap) test a method of taking a sample of cervical cells for microscopic examination to detect malignancy

Paradigm a pattern of shared understandings and assumptions about reality and the world

Parasites microorganisms that live in or on another from which it obtains nourishment

Parasomnia a cluster or pattern of waking behavior that appears during sleep, such as somnambulism (sleepwalking), sleeptalking, and enuresis (bed-wetting)

Parenteral drug administration occurring outside the alimentary tract; injected into the body through some route other than the alimentary canal (e.g., intramuscularly)

Paresis slight or incomplete paralysis

Parotitis inflammation of the parotid salivary gland

Partial pressure the pressure exerted by each individual gas in a mixture according to its percentage concentration in the mixture

Partially complete proteins proteins that contain less than the required amount of one or more essential amino acids; cannot alone support continued growth

Participative leader *see* Democratic leader

Passive euthanasia allowing a person to die by withholding or withdrawing measures to maintain life

Passive (Acquired) immunity a resistance of the body to infection in which the host receives natural or artificial antibodies produced by another source

Passive ROM exercises another person moves each of a client's joints through its complete range of movement, maximally stretching all muscle groups within each plane over each joint

Pathogenicity the ability to produce disease; a pathogen is a microorganism that causes disease

Pathologic fractures spontaneous fractures to which elderly persons are prone

Patient a person who is waiting for or undergoing medical treatment and care

Patient Self-Determination Act (PSDA) legislation requiring that every competent adult be informed in writing on admission to a health care institution about his or her rights to accept or refuse medical care and to use advance directives

Patient-controlled analgesia (PCA) a pain management technique that allows the client to take an active role in managing pain

Patient-focused care delivery model that brings all services and care providers to the client

Peak level indicates the highest concentration of the drug in the blood serum

Peak plasma level the concentration of a drug in the blood plasma that occurs when the elimination rate equals the rate of absorption

Pedagogy the discipline concerned with helping children learn

Pediculosis infestation with head lice

Peer groups assume great importance and have a number of functions: provide a sense of belonging, pride, social learning, and sexual roles; most peer groups have well-defined, sex-specific modes of acceptable behavior and in adolescence, the peer groups change with age

Penrose drain a flexible rubber drain

Perceived loss the loss experienced by a person that cannot be verified by others

Perception the ability to interpret the environment through the senses

Percutaneous through the skin

Percussion a method in which the body surface is struck to elicit sounds that can be heard or vibrations that can be felt

Percutaneous endoscopic gastrostomy (PEG) feeding catheter inserted into the stomach through the skin and subcutaneous tissues of the abdomen

Percutaneous endoscopic jejunostomy (PEJ) feeding catheter inserted into the jejunum through the skin and subcutaneous tissues of the abdomen

Perfusion passage of blood constituents through the vessels of the circulatory system

Pericardium double layer of fibroserous membrane of the heart; the parietal, or outermost, pericardium serves to protect the heart and anchor it to surrounding structures

Peridural anesthesia *see* Epidural anesthesia

Periodontal disease disorder of the supporting structures of the teeth

Perioperative period refers to the three phases of surgery: preoperative, intraoperative, and postoperative

Peripheral pulse a pulse located in the periphery of the body (e.g., foot, wrist)

Peripheral vascular resistance (PVR) impedance or opposition to blood flow to the tissues; determined by viscosity, or thickness, of the blood; blood vessel length; blood vessel diameter

Peripherally inserted central venous catheter (PICC) catheter inserted in the basilic or cephalic vein just above or below the antecubital space

Peripheral neuropathic pain pain (e.g., phantom limb pain, postherpetic neuralgia, carpal tunnel syndrome) that follows damage and/or sensitization of peripheral nerves

Peripherals at the edge or outward boundary

Peristalsis wavelike movements produced by circular and longitudinal muscle fibers of the intestinal walls; the movement propels the intestinal contents onward

Permissive leader *see* Laissez-faire leader

Personal computers (PCs) individual microcomputer systems referred to as a desktop, portable, laptop, notebook, or handheld computer

Personal knowing promotes wholeness and integrity in the personal encounter to achieve engagement

Personal space the distance people prefer in interactions with others

Personal values values internalized from the society or culture in which one lives

Personality the outward expression of the inner self

PES format the three essential components of nursing diagnostic statements including the terms describing the *problem*, the *etiology* of the problem, and the defining characteristics or cluster of *signs* and *symptoms*

pH a measure of the relative alkalinity or acidity of a solution; a measure of the concentration of hydrogen ions

Phagocytes cells that ingest microorganisms, other cells, and foreign particles

Pharmacist a person licensed to prepare and dispense drugs and prescriptions

Pharmacodynamics the process by which a drug alters cell physiology

Pharmacogenetics process by which the effect of a drug is influenced by genetic variations such as gender, size, and body composition

Pharmacokinetics the study of the absorption, distribution, biotransformation, and excretion of drugs

Pharmacology the scientific study of the actions of drugs on living animals and humans

Pharmacopoeia a book containing a list of drug products used in medicine, including their descriptions and formulas

Pharmacy the art of preparing, compounding, and dispensing drugs; also refers to the place where drugs are prepared and dispensed

Phenomenology research that investigates people's life experiences and how they interpret those experiences

Philosophy an early effort to define phenomena that serves as the basis for later theoretical formulations

Phlebotomist a person from a laboratory who performs venipuncture, collecting the blood specimen for the tests ordered by the physician

Physical activity bodily movement produced by skeletal muscles that requires energy expenditure and produces progressive health benefits

Physical restraints any manual method or physical or mechanical device, material, or equipment attached to the client's body that restrict the client's movement

Physiologic dependence biochemical changes occurring in the body as a result of excessive use of a drug

Physiologic pain pain experienced when an intact properly functioning nervous system sends signals that tissues are damaged

PIE an acronym for a charting model that follows a recording sequence of *problems*, *interventions*, and *evaluation* of the effectiveness of the interventions

Piggyback secondary IV setup where the second IV set connects the second container to the tubing of the primary container at the upper port

Pilates method of physical movement and exercise designed to stretch, strengthen, and balance the body, in particular the core of the body

Pinna *see* Auricle

Pitch the frequency or number of vibrations heard during auscultation

Pitting edema edema in which firm finger pressure on the skin produces an indentation (pit) that remains for several seconds

Placebo any form of treatment (e.g., medication) that produces an effect in the client because of its intent rather than its chemical or physical properties

Placenta a flat, disc-shaped organ that is highly vascular and normally forms in the upper segment of the endometrium of the uterus; exchanges nutrients and gases between the fetus and the mother

Plaintiff a person claiming infringement of legal rights by one or more persons

Planned change an intended, purposive attempt by an individual, group, organization, or larger social system to influence its own status quo or that of another organism or situation

Planning an ongoing process that involves (a) assessing a situation, (b) establishing goals and objectives based on assessment of a situation or future trends, and (c) developing a plan of action that identifies priorities, delineates who is responsible, determines deadlines, and describes how the intended outcome is to be achieved and evaluated

Plantar wart a wart on the sole of the foot

Plaque an invisible soft film consisting of bacteria, molecules of saliva, and remnants of epithelial cells and leukocytes that adhere to the enamel surface of teeth

Plasma the fluid portion of the blood in which the blood cells are suspended

Plateau a maintained concentration of a drug in the plasma during a series of scheduled doses

Pleximeter in percussion, the middle finger of the nondominant hand placed firmly on the client's skin

Plexor in percussion, the middle finger of the dominant hand or a percussion hammer used to strike the pleximeter

Pneumothorax collection of air in the pleural space

Point of maximal impulse (PMI) the point where the apex of the heart touches the anterior chest wall

Policies rules developed to govern the handling of frequently occurring situations

Polycythemia a condition in which clients with chronic hypoxia may develop higher than normal counts of red blood cells

Polydipsia excessive thirst

Polypnea abnormally fast respirations

Polysaccharides a branched chain of dozens, sometimes hundreds, of glucose molecules; starches

Polysomnography a cluster or pattern of waking behavior that appears during sleep, such as somnambulism (sleepwalking), sleeptalking, and enuresis (bed-wetting)

Polytheism the belief in more than one God

Polyunsaturated fatty acids fatty acid with more than one double bond (or many carbons not bonded to a hydrogen atom)

Polyuria *see* Diuresis

Population includes all possible members of a group who meet the criteria for a study

Positive feedback feedback that stimulates change

Positive reinforcement giving rewards such as praise for a learner's achievements

Positron emission tomography (PET) a noninvasive radiologic study that involves the injection or inhalation of a radioisotope

Possible nursing diagnosis one in which evidence about a health problem is incomplete or unclear

Postmortem examination *see* Autopsy

Postoperative phase begins with the admission of the client to the postanesthesia area and ends when healing is complete

Postural drainage the drainage, by gravity, of secretions from various lung segments

Potentiating effect the increased effect of one or both drugs

Practice discipline field of study in which the central focus is performance of professional role (nursing, teaching, management, making music)

Prayer human communication with divine and spiritual entities

Preceptor an experienced nurse who assists the novice nurse in improving nursing skill and judgment

Precontemplation stage a person typically denies having a problem and instead views others as having a problem and therefore wants to change the other person's behavior

Precordium an area of the chest overlying the heart

Preemptive analgesia the administration of analgesics prior to an invasive or operative procedure in order to treat pain before it occurs

Preferred provider arrangements (PPAs) similar to PPOs, but PPAs can contract with individual health care providers; the plan can be limited or unlimited

Preferred provider organization (PPO) a group of physicians or a hospital that provides companies with health services at a discounted rate

Prefilled unit-dose system injectable medications that are disposable and are available as (a) prefilled syringes ready for use or (b) prefilled sterile cartridges and needles that require the attachment of a reusable holder (injection system) before use

Prejudice a negative belief or preference that is generalized about a group and that leads to "prejudgment"

Preload the degree to which muscle fibers in the ventricle are stretched at the end of diastole

Preoperative phase begins when the decision to have surgery is made and ends when the client is transferred to the operating table

Preparation stage occurs when the person undertakes cognitive and behavioral activities that prepare the person for change

Presbycusis loss of hearing related to aging

Presbyopia loss of elasticity of the lens and thus loss of ability to see close objects as a result of the aging process

Prescription the written direction for the preparation and administration of a drug

Presencing being present, being there, or just being with a client

Pressure a compressing downward force on a body area

Pressure ulcers any lesion caused by unrelieved pressure that results in damage to underlying tissue; formerly called decubitus ulcers, bed sores, pressure sores

Primary care (PC) the point of entry into the health care system at which initial health care is given

Primary health care (PHC) essential health care based on practical, scientifically sound and socially acceptable methods and technology made universally accessible to individuals and families in the community through their full participation and at a cost that the community and country can afford to maintain at every stage of their development in the spirit of self-reliance and self-determination

Primary intention healing tissue surfaces are approximated (closed) and there is minimal or no tissue loss, formation of minimal granulation tissue and scarring

Primary prevention activities directed toward the protection from or avoidance of potential health risks

Primary sexual characteristics relate to the organs necessary for reproduction, such as the testes, penis, vagina, and uterus

Principles-based (deontological) theories emphasize individual rights, duties, and obligations

Priority setting the process of establishing a preferential order for nursing strategies

Private (civil) law the body of law that deals with relationships between private individuals

Prn order "as needed order"; permits the nurse to give a medication when, in the nurse's judgment, the client requires it

Problem solving obtaining information that clarifies the nature of the problem and suggests possible solutions

Problem-oriented medical record (POMR) data about the client are recorded and arranged according to the client's problems, rather than according to the source of the information

Problem-oriented record (POR) *see* Problem-oriented medical record (POMR)

Procedures steps used in carrying out policies or activities

Process evaluation a component of quality assurance that focuses on how care was given

Process recording the verbatim (word-for-word) account of a conversation

Proctoscopy the viewing of the rectum

Proctosigmoidoscopy the viewing of the rectum and sigmoid colon

Productivity in health care, frequently measured by the amount of nursing resources used per client or in terms of required versus actual hours of care provided

Profession an occupation that requires extensive education or a calling that requires special knowledge, skill, and preparation

Professional values values acquired during socialization into nursing from codes of ethics, nursing experiences, teachers, and peers

Professionalism a set of attributes, a way of life that implies responsibility and commitment

Professionalization the process of becoming professional; acquiring characteristics considered to be professional

Progress notes chart entries made by a variety of methods and by all health professionals involved in a client's care for the purpose of describing a client's problems, treatments, and progress toward desired outcomes

Prompted voiding supplements habit training by encouraging the client to try to use the toilet (prompting) and reminding the client when to void

Prone position face-lying position, with or without a small pillow

Proprioception awareness of posture, movement, and changes in equilibrium; knowledge of position, weight, and resistance of objects in relation to body

Proprioceptors sensory receptors that are sensitive to movement and the position of the body

Protein-calorie malnutrition problem of clients with long-term deficiencies in caloric intake; characteristics include depressed visceral proteins (e.g., albumin), weight loss, and visible muscle and fat wasting

Protocols a predetermined and preprinted plan specifying the procedure to be followed in a particular situation

Proxemics the study of distance between people in their interactions

Psychologic dependence a state of emotional reliance on a drug to maintain one's well-being; a feeling of need or craving for a drug

Psychologic homeostasis emotional or psychologic balance or state of mental well-being

Psychomotor domain the "skill" domain; includes motor skills such as giving an injection

Puberty the first stage of adolescence in which sexual organs begin to grow and mature

Public law refers to the body of law that deals with relationships between individuals and the government and governmental agencies

Pulse the wave of blood within an artery that is created by contraction of the left ventricle of the heart

Pulse deficit the difference between the apical pulse and the radial pulse

Pulse oximeter a noninvasive device that measures the arterial blood oxygen saturation by means of a sensor attached to the finger

Pulse pressure the difference between the systolic and the diastolic blood pressure

Pulse rhythm the pattern of the beats and intervals between the beats

Pulse volume the strength or amplitude of the pulse, the force of blood exerted with each heart beat

Pureed diet a modification of the soft diet; liquid may be added to the food, which is then blended to a semisolid consistency

Purkinje fibers fibers of the ventricular conduction pathways that terminate in ventricular muscle, stimulating contraction

Purulent exudates an exudate consisting of leukocytes, liquefied dead tissue debris, and dead and living bacteria

Pus a thick liquid associated with inflammation and composed of cells, liquid, microorganisms, and tissue debris

Pyogenic bacteria bacteria that produce pus

Pyorrhea purulent periodontal disease

Pyrexia a body temperature above the normal range, fever

Qi body's vital energy reflexology

Qi gong breathing and mental exercises combined with body movements

Qualifiers words that have been added to some NANDA labels to give additional meaning to the diagnostic statement

Quality a subjective description of a sound (e.g., whistling, gurgling)

Quality improvement an organizational commitment and approach used to continuously improve all processes in the organization with the goal of meeting and exceeding customer expectations and outcomes; also known as *total quality management* (TQM) and *continuous quality improvement* (CQI)

Quality-assurance (QA) program an ongoing systematic process designed to evaluate and promote excellence in the health care provided to clients

Race classification of people according to shared biologic characteristics and physical features

Radiation the transfer of heat from the surface of one object to the surface of another without contact between the two objects

Radiopharmaceutical a pharmaceutical (targeted to a specific organ) labeled with a radioisotope, administered through various routes, to determine hyperfunction or hypofunction of the organ

Random access memory (RAM) data and instructions stored on chips; RAM storage is temporary and cleared when the computer is turned off

Range a measure of variability, consisting of the difference between the highest and lowest values in a distribution of scores

Range of motion (ROM) the degree of movement possible for each joint

Rapport a relationship between two or more people of mutual trust and understanding

Rationale the scientific reason for selecting a specific action

RBC indices may be performed as part of the CBC to evaluate the size, weight, and hemoglobin concentration of red blood cells

Retrograde pyelography a radiographic study used to evaluate the urinary tract

Reactive hyperemia a bright red flush on the skin occurring after pressure is relieved

Readiness behaviors or cues that reflect a learner's motivation to learn at a specific time

Reagent substance used in a chemical reaction to detect a specific substance

Recent memory deals with activities of the recent past of minutes to a few hours

Receptor a location on the surface of a cell membrane or within a cell (usually a protein) to which a drug chemically binds

Reconstitution the technique of adding a solvent to a powdered drug to prepare it for injection

Record a written communication providing formal, legal documentation of a client's progress

Recording the process of making written entries about a client on the medical record

Red blood cell (RBC) count number of red blood cells per cubic millimeter of whole blood

Red blood cell (RBC) indices evaluate size, weight, and hemoglobin concentrations of RBCs

Referred pain pain perceived to be in one area but whose source is another area

Reflection thinking from a critical point of view, analyzing why one acted in a certain way, and assessing the results of one's actions

Reflex an automatic response of the body to a stimulus

Reflexology a treatment based on massage of the feet to relieve symptoms in other parts of the body

Reflux backward flow

Regeneration renewal, regrowth, the replacement of destroyed tissue cells by cells that are identical or similar in structure and function

Regional anesthesia the temporary interruption of the transmission of nerve impulses to and from a specific area or region of the body; the client loses sensation in an area of the body but remains conscious

Registry private duty agency which contracts with individual practioners

Regression a defense mechanism in which one adapts behavior that was comforting earlier in life to overcome the discomfort and insecurity of the present situation

Regurgitation the spitting up or backward flow of undigested food

Relapsing fever the occurrence of short febrile periods of a few days interspersed with periods of 1 or 2 days of normal temperature

Relationship-based (caring) theories stress courage, generosity, commitment, and the need to nurture and maintain relationships

Relaxation response physiologic state achieved through deep relaxation breathing

Reliability the degree to which an instrument produces consistent results on repeated use

Religion an organized system of worship

REM sleep sleep during which the person experiences *rapid eye movements*

Remission a period during a chronic illness when there is a lessening of severity or cessation of symptoms

Remittent fever the occurrence of a wide range of temperature fluctuations, more than 2°C (3.6°F) over the 24-hour period, all of which are above normal

Renin-angiotensin-aldosterone system system initiated by specialized receptors in the juxtaglomerular cells of the kidney nephrons that respond to changes in renal perfusion

Report whether oral or written, it should be concise, including pertinent information but no extraneous detail

Repression a defense mechanism in which painful thoughts, experiences, and impulses are removed from awareness

Res ipsa loquitur "the thing that speaks for itself"; a legal doctrine that relates to negligence in which the harm cannot be traced to a specific health care provider or standard but does not normally occur unless there has been a negligent act

Researchability the problem can be subjected to scientific investigation

Reservoir a source of microorganisms

Resident flora microorganisms that normally reside on the skin and mucous membranes, and inside the respiratory and gastrointestinal tracts

Residual urine the amount of urine remaining in the bladder after a person voids

Resolution phase the part of the response cycle period of return to the unaroused state, which may last 10 to 15 minutes after orgasm, or longer if there is no orgasm

Resonance a low-pitched, hollow sound produced over normal lung tissue when the chest is percussed

Respiration the act of breathing; transport of oxygen from the atmosphere to the body cells and transport of carbon dioxide from the cells to the atmosphere

Respiratory acidosis (hypercapnia) a state of excess carbon dioxide in the body

Respiratory alkalosis a state of excessive loss of carbon dioxide from the body

Respiratory character *see* Respiratory quality

Respiratory membrane where gas exchange occurs between the air on the alveolar side and the blood on the capillary side; the alveolar and capillary walls form the respiratory membrane

Respiratory quality refers to those aspects of breathing that are different from normal, effortless breathing, includes the amount of effort exerted to breathe and the sounds produced by breathing

Respiratory rhythm refers to the regularity of the expirations and the inspirations

Respondeat superior a legal term meaning "let the master answer"; the employer assumes responsibility for the conduct of the employee and can also be held responsible for malpractice by the employee

Responsibility the specific accountability or liability associated with the performance of duties of a particular role

Resting energy expenditure (REE) the amount of energy required to maintain basic body functions

Resting tremor a tremor that is apparent when the client is at rest and diminishes with activity

Restraints protective devices used to limit physical activity of the client or a part of the client's body

Retrograde pyelography radiographic study of the urinary tract where contrast medium is instilled directly into the kidney pelvis via the urethra, bladder, and ureters

Retrospective audit evaluation of a client's record after discharge from an agency

Review of systems *see* Screening examination

Rhizotomy interruption of the anterior or posterior nerve root between the ganglion and the cord; generally performed on cervical nerve roots to alleviate pain of the head and neck

Right (legal) a privilege or fundamental power to which an individual is entitled unless it is revoked by law or given up voluntarily

Right of self-determination subjects feel free from constraints, coercion, or any undue influence to participate in a study

Rigor mortis the stiffening of the body that occurs after death

Risk factors factors that cause a client to be vulnerable to developing a health problem

Risk management having in place a system to reduce danger to clients and staff

Risk nursing diagnosis clinical judgment that a problem does not exist, but the presence of risk factors indicates that a problem is likely to develop unless nurses intervene

Risk of harm exposure to the possibility of injury going beyond everyday situations

Role the set of expectations about how a person occupying a specific position behaves

Role ambiguity unclear role expectations; people do not know what to do or how to do it and are unable to predict the reactions of others to their behavior

Role conflict a clash between the beliefs or behaviors imposed by two or more roles fulfilled by one person

Role development involves socialization into a particular role

Role mastery performance of role behaviors that meet social expectations

Role model providing an example of acceptable behavior(s) through demonstration

Role performance what a person does in a particular role in relation to the behaviors expected of that role

Role strain a generalized state of frustration or anxiety experienced with the stress of role conflict and ambiguity

Root cause analysis process for identifying factors that bring about deviations in practices that lead to an event

S_1 the first heart sound; occurs when the atrioventricular valves (mitral and tricuspid) close

S_2 the second heart sound; occurs when the semilunar valves (aortic and pulmonic) close

Safety monitoring device a position-sensitive switch that triggers an audio alarm when a client attempts to get out of the bed or chair

Sairy Gamp a character in the Charles Dickens book *Martin Chizzlewit* who represented the negative image of nurses in the early 1800s

Saliva the clear liquid secreted by the salivary glands in the mouth, sometimes referred to as *spit*

Sample segment of the population from whom data will actually be collected

Sanguineous exudate an exudate containing large amounts of red blood cells

Sarcopenia steady decrease in muscle fibers

Saturated fatty acids those in which all carbon atoms are filled to capacity (i.e., saturated) with hydrogen

Scabies a contagious skin infestation caused by an arachnid, the itch mite

Scald a burn from a hot liquid or vapor, such as steam

Scientific health belief based on the belief that life and life processes are controlled by physical and biochemical processes that can be manipulated by humans

Screening examination (review of systems) a brief review of essential functioning of various body parts or systems

Scrub person person who assists the surgeon

Sebaceous glands active under the influence of androgens in both males and females, which secrete sebum and become most active on the face, neck, shoulder, upper back, and chest; are often the cause of an increased incidence of acne

Sebum the oily, lubricating secretion of sebaceous glands in the skin

Secondary intention healing wound in which the tissue surfaces are not approximated and there is extensive tissue loss; formation of excessive granulation tissue and scarring

Secondary prevention activities designed for early diagnosis and treatment of disease or illness

Secondary sexual characteristics physical characteristics that differentiate the male from the female but do not relate directly to reproduction

Seizure a sudden onset of a convulsion or other paroxysmal motor or sensory activity

Seizure precautions safety measures taken by the nurse to protect clients from injury should they have a seizure

Selectively permeable cell membranes that allow substances to move across them with varying degrees of ease

Self-awareness the relationship between one's perception of oneself and others' perceptions of oneself

Self-concept the collection of ideas, feelings, and beliefs one has about oneself

Self-esteem the value one has for oneself; self-confidence

Self-regulation homeostatic mechanisms that come into play automatically in the healthy person

Semicircular canals in the inner ear; contain the organs of equilibrium

Semi-Fowler's position *see* Low Fowler's position

Semilunar valves crescent moon-shaped valves between the cardiac ventricles and the pulmonary artery (pulmonic valve) and the aorta (aortic valve)

Sensorineural hearing loss the result of damage to the inner ear, the auditory nerve, or the hearing center in the brain

Sensoristasis the need for sensory stimulation

Sensory deficit partial or complete impairment of any sensory organ

Sensory deprivation insufficient sensory stimulation for a person to function

Sensory memory momentary perception of stimuli by the senses

Sensory overload an overabundance of sensory stimulation

Sensory perception the organization and translation of stimuli into meaningful information

Sensory reception process of receiving environmental stimuli

Sentinel event an unexpected occurrence involving death or serious physical or psychological injury, or the risk thereof

Separation anxiety the fear and frustration experienced by young children that comes with parental absences

Sepsis the presence of pathogenic organisms or their toxins in the blood or body tissues

Septicemia occurs when bacteremia results in systemic infection

Septum a dividing structure such as that between the cardiac chambers or between the two sides of the nose

Serosanguineous exudate inflammatory material consisting of a combination of clear and blood-tinged drainage

Serous exudates inflammatory material composed of serum (clear portion of blood) derived from the blood and serous membranes of the body such as the peritoneum, pleura, pericardium, and meninges; watery in appearance and has few cells

Serum osmolality a measure of the solute concentration of the blood

Sexual aversion disorder severe distaste for sexual activity or thought of sexual activity

Sexual health the integration of the somatic, emotional, intellectual, and social aspects of sexuality, in ways that are positively enriching and that enhance personality, communication, and love

Sexual orientation the preference of a person for one sex or the other

Sexual pain disorders include dyspareunia, vaginismus, and genital pain

Sexual self-concept how one values oneself as a sexual being

Shaft the part of a needle that is attached to the hub

Shaken baby syndrome (SBS) violent shaking of the infant by the arms or shoulders causing a whiplash, which can lead to severe injury in infants

Shared governance a method that aims to distribute decision making among a group of people

Shared leadership a contemporary theory of leadership that recognizes the leadership capabilities of each member in a professional group and assumes that appropriate leadership will emerge in relation to the challenges that confront the group

Shearing force a combination of friction and pressure that, when applied to the skin, results in damage to the blood vessels and tissues

Shock phase first part of the alarm reaction in which the stressor may be perceived consciously or unconsciously by the person

Short-term memory information held in the brain for immediate use or what one has in mind at a given moment

Shroud a large piece of plastic or cotton material used to enclose a body after death

Side effect the secondary effect of a drug that is unintended; usually predictable and may be either harmless or potentially harmful

Significance the potential to contribute to nursing science by enhancing client care, testing or generating a theory, or resolving a day-to-day clinical problem

Signs *see* Overt data

Sims' position side-lying position with lowermost arm behind the body and uppermost leg flexed

Single order common medication order that is a "one-time order"; medication is to be given once at a specified time

Sinoatrial (SA or sinus) node the primary pacemaker of the heart located where the superior vena cava enters the right atrium

Situational leader adapts style according to consideration of the staff members' abilities, knowledge of the nature of the task to be done, and sensitivity to the context or environment in which the task takes place

Sitz bath used to soak a client's pelvic area; also referred to as a *hip bath*

Skinfold measurement an indicator of the amount of body fat, the main form of stored energy

Slander defamation by the spoken word, stating unprivileged (not legally protected) or false words by which a reputation is damaged

Sleep an altered state of consciousness in which the individual's perception of and reaction to the environment are decreased

Sleep apnea periodic cessation of breathing during sleep

Sleep architecture basic organization of normal sleep

Sleep hygiene refers to interventions used to promote sleep

Small calorie (c, cal) the amount of heat required to raise the temperature of 1 g of water 1°C

SOAP an acronym for a charting method that follows a recording sequence of *subjective* data, *objective* data, *assessment*, and *planning*

Socialization a process by which a person learns the ways of a group or society in order to become a functioning participant

Socratic questioning a technique one can use to look beneath the surface, recognize and examine assumptions, search for inconsistencies, examine multiple points of view, and differentiate what one knows from what one merely believes

Sojourner Truth an abolitionist, Underground Railroad agent, preacher, and women's rights advocate, she was a nurse for more than 4 years during the Civil War and worked as a nurse and counselor for the Freedman's Relief Association after the war

Solutes substances dissolved in a liquid

Solvent the liquid in which a solute is dissolved

Somatic pain pain that originates in the skin, muscles, bone, or connective tissue

Somnology the study of sleep

Sordes accumulation of foul matter (food, microorganisms, and epithelial elements) on the teeth and gums

Source-oriented clinical record a record in which each person or department makes notations in a separate section or sections of the client's chart

Spastic describing the sudden, prolonged involuntary muscle contractions of clients with damage to the central nervous system

Specific defenses immune functions directed against identifiable bacteria, viruses, fungi, or other infectious agents

Specific gravity the weight or degree of concentration of a substance compared with that of an equal volume of another, such as distilled water, taken as a standard

Specific self-esteem how much one approves of a certain part of oneself

Spinal anesthesia anesthesia produced by injecting an anesthetic agent into the subarachnoid space surrounding the spinal cord; also referred to as a *subarachnoid block (SAB)*

Spinal cord stimulation (SCS) involves the insertion of a cable that allows the placement of an electrode directly on the spinal cord and is used with nonmalignant pain that has not been controlled with less invasive therapies

Spiritual distress a disturbance in or a challenge to a person's belief or value system that provides strength, hope, and meaning to life

Spiritual health *see* Spiritual well-being

Spiritual well-being a feeling of inner peace and of being generally alive, purposeful, and fulfilled; the feeling is rooted in spiritual values and/or specific religious beliefs

Spirituality belief in or relationship with some higher power, creative force, driving being, or infinite source of energy

Spreadsheet programs that manipulate primarily numbers

Sputum the mucous secretion from the lungs, bronchi, and trachea

Stage of exhaustion the third stage in the adaptation syndromes that occurs when the adaptation that the body made during the second stage cannot be maintained

Stage of resistance the second stage in the adaptation syndromes when the body's adaptation takes place

Standard a generally accepted rule, model, pattern, or measure

Standard deviation the most frequently used measure of variability, indicating the average to which scores deviate from the mean; commonly symbolized as SD or S

Standardized care plan formal plan that specifies the nursing care for groups of clients with common needs (e.g., all clients with myocardial infarction)

Standards of care the skills and learning commonly possessed by members of a profession

Standards of practice descriptions of the responsibilities for which nurses are accountable

Standards of professional performance as set by the American Nurses Association (ANA), describe behaviors expected in the professional nursing role

Standing order a written document about policies, rules, regulations, or orders regarding client care; gives nurses the authority to carry out specific actions under certain circumstances

Stapes stirrups bone of the middle ear

Stat order common medication order which indicates that the medication is to be given immediately and only once

Statistically significant term applied after data have been analyzed to determine whether the results had a probability less than 0.05, which is considered the acceptable level of significance

Statutory law a law enacted by any legislative body

Steatorrhea an excessive amount of fat in the stool, which can indicate faulty absorption of fat from the small intestine

Stereognosis the ability to recognize objects by touching and manipulating them

Stereotyping assuming that all members of a culture or ethnic group are alike

Sterile field a specified area that is considered free from microorganisms

Sterile technique practices that keep an area or object free of all microorganisms

Sterilization a process that destroys all microorganisms, including spores and viruses

Sternum the breastbone

Stimulus-based stress model stress is defined as a stimulus, life event, or set of circumstances that arouses physiologic and/or psychologic reactions that may increase the individual's vulnerability to illness

Stoma an artificial opening in the abdominal wall; it may be permanent or temporary

Stool *see* Feces

Strabismus squinting or crossing of the eyes; uncoordinated eye movements

Stress an event or set of circumstances causing a disrupted response; the disruption caused by a noxious stimulus or stressor

Stress electrocardiography uses ECGs to assess a client's response to an increased cardiac workload during exercise

Stressor any factor that produces stress or alters the body's equilibrium

Stridor a harsh, crowing sound made on inhalation caused by constriction of the upper airway

Strike an organized work stoppage by a group of employees to express a grievance, enforce a demand for changes in condition of employment, or solve a dispute with management

Stroke volume (SV) the amount of blood ejected with each cardiac contraction

Structure evaluation focuses on the setting in which care is given

Subarachnoid block (SAB) *see* Spinal anesthesia

Subculture usually composed of people who have a distinct identity and yet are related to a larger cultural group

Subcutaneous beneath the layers of the skin; hypodermic

Subjective data data that are apparent only to the person affected; can be described or verified only by that person

Sublingual under the tongue

Subsystems system components

Suctioning the aspiration of secretions by a catheter connected to a suction machine or wall outlet

Sudden infant death syndrome (SIDS) the sudden and unexpected death of an infant

Sudoriferous sweat glands glands of the dermis that secrete sweat

Superego the conscience of personality; the source of feelings of guilt, shame, and inhibition

Supine position *see* Dorsal position

Supplemental Security Income (SSI) special payments for people with disabilities, those who are blind, and people who are not eligible for Social Security; these payments are not restricted to health care costs

Suppositories solid, cone-shaped, medicated substances inserted into the rectum, vagina, or urethra

Suppuration the formation of pus

Suprapubic catheter catheter inserted through the abdominal wall above the symphysis pubis into the urinary bladder

Suprasystem the system above another system

Surface anesthesia *see* Topical anesthesia

Surface temperature the temperature of tissue, the subcutaneous tissue, and fat

Surfactant a surface-active agent (e.g., soap or a synthetic detergent); in pulmonary physiology, a mixture of phospholipids secreted by alveolar cells into the alveoli and respiratory air passages that reduces the surface tension of pulmonary fluids and thus contributes to the elastic properties of pulmonary tissue

Surgical asepsis *see* Sterile technique

Suture a thread used to sew body tissues together

Sutures junction lines of the skull bones

Sweat glands *see* Sudoriferous glands

Sympathectomy severance of the pathways of the sympathetic division of the autonomic nervous system; eliminates vasospasm, improves peripheral blood supply, and is effective in treating painful vascular disorders

Sympathetically maintained pain pain that occurs with abnormal connections between pain fibers and the sympathetic nervous system

Symptoms *see* Covert data

Syndrome diagnosis a diagnosis that is associated with a cluster of other diagnoses

Synergistic when two different drugs increase the action of one or another drug

System a set of interacting identifiable parts or components

Systemic infection occurs when pathogens spread and damage different parts of the body

Systole the period during which the ventricles contract

Systolic pressure the pressure of the blood against the arterial walls when the ventricles of the heart contract

T'ai chi discipline that combines physical fitness, meditation, and self-defense

Tachycardia an abnormally rapid pulse rate; greater than 100 beats per minute

Tachypnea abnormally fast respirations; usually more than 24 respirations per minute

Tactile related to touch

Tandem secondary IV setup in which the second container is attached to the line of the first container at the lower, secondary port

Tartar a visible, hard deposit of plaque and dead bacteria that forms at the gum lines

Taxonomy a classification system or set of categories, such as nursing diagnoses, arranged on the basis of a single principle or consistent set of principles

Teacher a nurse who helps clients learn about their health and the health care procedures they need to perform to restore or maintain their health

Teaching system of activities intended to produce learning

Team nursing the delivery of individualized nursing care to clients by a team led by a professional nurse

Technical skills "hands-on" skills such as those required to manipulate equipment, administer injections, and move or reposition patients

Telecommunications the transmission of information from one site to another, using equipment to transmit information in the forms of signs, signals, words, or pictures by cable, radio, or other systems

Telemedicine technology used to transmit electronic medical data about clients to persons at distant locations

Temperament the way individuals respond to their external and internal environment

Teratogen anything that adversely affects normal cellular development in the embryo or fetus

Termination stage the ultimate goal where the individual has complete confidence that the problem is no longer a temptation or threat

Territoriality a concept of the space and things that individuals consider their own

Tertiary intention healing that occurs in wounds left open for 3 to 5 days and then closed with sutures, staples, or adhesive skin closures

Tertiary prevention activities designed to restore individuals with disabilities to their optimal level of functioning

Theory a system of ideas that is proposed to explain a given phenomenon (e.g., theory of gravity)

Therapeutic baths given for physical effects, such as to soothe irritated skin or to treat an area (e.g., the perineum)

Therapeutic communication an interactive process between nurse and client that helps the client overcome temporary stress, to get along with other people, to adjust to the unalterable, and to overcome psychologic blocks that stand in the way of self-realization

Therapeutic effect the primary effect intended of a drug; reason the drug is prescribed

Third space syndrome fluid shifts from the vascular space into an area where it is not readily accessible as extracellular fluid

Thoracentesis insertion of a needle into the pleural cavity for diagnostic or therapeutic purposes

Thrill a vibrating sensation over a blood vessel that indicates turbulent blood flow

Thrombophlebitis inflammation of a vein followed by formation of a blood clot

Thrombus a solid mass of blood constituents in the circulatory system; a clot (plural: *thrombi*)

Throughput a transformation that occurs after input is absorbed by the system and is then processed in a way that is useful to the system

Ticks small gray-brown parasites that bite into tissue and suck blood and transmit several diseases to people, in particular Rocky Mountain spotted fever, Lyme disease, and tularemia.

Tidal volume the volume of air that is normally inhaled and exhaled

Tinea pedis athlete's foot (ringworm of the foot), which is caused by a fungus

Tissue perfusion passage of fluid (e.g., blood) through a specific organ or body part

Top-level manager organizational executive primarily responsible for establishing goals and developing strategic plans

Topical applied externally (e.g., to the skin or mucous membranes)

Topical anesthesia (surface anesthesia) applied directly to the skin and mucous membranes, open skin surfaces, wounds, and burns

Torr millimeters of mercury

Tort a civil wrong committed against a person or a person's property

Tort law law that defines and enforces duties and rights among private individuals that are not based on contractual agreements

Trade name name given a drug by the manufacturer

Traditional observance of the beliefs and practices of one's heritage or cultural belief system

Traditional Chinese medicine (TCM) based on the premise that the body's vital energy circulates through pathways or meridians and can be accessed and manipulated through specific anatomical points along the surface of the body

Tragus the cartilaginous protrusion at the entrance to the ear canal

Transactional leader a contemporary theory of leadership in which resources are exchanged as an incentive for loyalty and performance

Transactional stress theory a theory that encompasses a set of cognitive, affective, and adaptive (coping) responses that arise out of person–environment transactions; the person and the environment are inseparable and affect each other

Transcellular fluid compartment of extracellular fluids; includes cerebrospinal, pericardial, pancreatic, pleural, intraocular, biliary, peritoneal, and synovial fluids

Transcendence a person's recognition that there is something other or greater than the self and a seeking and valuing of that greater other, whether it is an ultimate being, force, or value

Transcultural nursing providing care within the differences and similarities of the beliefs, values, and patterns of cultures

Transcutaneous electrical nerve stimulation (TENS) a noninvasive, nonanalgesic pain control technique that allows the client to assist in the management of acute and chronic pain

Transdermal patch a particular type of topical or dermatologic medication delivery system

Transgenderism gradation of human characteristics that run from female to male

Transformational leader leader who fosters creativity, risk taking, commitment, and collaboration by empowering the group to share in the organization's vision

Translator a person who converts written material (such as patient education pamphlets) from one language into another

Transsexual individual who feels his or her sexual anatomy is not consistent with his or her gender identity

Tremor an involuntary trembling of a limb or body part

Trial the period during which all relevant facts are presented to a jury or judge

Triangular fossa a depression of the antihelix

Triglycerides substances that have three fatty acids; they account for more than 90% of the lipids in food and in the body

Trigone a triangular area at the base of the bladder marked by the ureter openings at the posterior corners and the opening of the urethra at the anterior corner

Trimesters the 3-month periods during pregnancy marking certain landmarks for developmental changes in mother and the fetus; three trimesters occur during a pregnancy

Tripod (triangle) position the proper standing position with crutches; crutches are placed about 15 cm (6 in.) in front of the feet and out laterally about 15 cm (6 in.), creating a wide base of support

Trocar a sharp pointed instrument that fits inside a cannula and is used to pierce body tissues

Troponin enzyme that is released into the blood during a myocardial infarction (MI)

Trough level represents the lowest concentration of a drug in the blood serum

Tuberculin syringe originally designed to administer tuberculin; a narrow syringe, calibrated in tenths and hundredths of a milliliter (up to 1 mL) on one scale and in sixteenths of a minim (up to 1 minim) on the other scale

Two-point discrimination *see* One-point discrimination

Tympanic membrane the eardrum

Tympany a musical or drumlike sound produced during percussion over an air-filled stomach and abdomen

Ultrasonography the use of ultrasound to produce an image of an organ or tissue

Unconscious mind the mental life of a person of which the person is unaware

Undernutrition an intake of nutrients insufficient to meet daily energy requirements because of inadequate food intake or improper digestion and absorption of food

Undertaker *see* Mortician

Universal precautions (UP) techniques to be used with all clients to decrease the risk of transmitting unidentified pathogens; currently, Standard Precautions incorporate UP and BSI

Unplanned change haphazard change that occurs without control by any person or group

Unprofessional conduct one of the grounds for action against the nurse's license; includes incompetence or gross negligence, conviction of practicing without a license, falsification of client records, and illegally obtaining, using, or possessing controlled substances

Unsaturated fatty acid a fatty acid that could accommodate more hydrogen atoms than it currently does

Upper-level managers organizational executives who are primarily responsible for establishing goals and developing strategic plans

Urea a substance found in urine, blood, and lymph; the main nitrogenous substance in blood

Ureterostomy type of urinary diversion that involves surgery of the ureters

Urgency the feeling that one must urinate

Urinary frequency the need to urinate often

Urinary hesitancy a delay and difficulty in initiating voiding; often associated with dysuria

Urinary incontinence a temporary or permanent inability of the external sphincter muscles to control the flow of urine from the bladder

Urinary reflux backward flow of urine

Urinary retention the accumulation of urine in the bladder and inability of the bladder to empty itself

Urinary stasis stagnation of urinary flow

Urination (micturition, voiding) the process of emptying the bladder

Urine osmolality a measure of the solute concentration of urine, a more exact measurement of urine concentration than specific gravity

Utilitarianism a specific, consequence-based, ethical theory that judges as right the action that does the most good and least amount of harm for the greatest number of persons; often used in making decisions about the funding and delivery of health care

Utility *see* Utilitarianism

Vaginismus involuntary spasm of outer one-third of vaginal muscles; makes penetration of vagina painful

Validation the determination that the diagnosis accurately reflects the problem of the client, that the methods used for data gathering were appropriate, and that the conclusion or diagnosis is justified by the data

Validity the degree to which an instrument measures what it is intended to measure

Valsalva maneuver forceful exhalation against a closed glottis, which increases intrathoracic pressure and thus interferes with venous blood return to the heart

Value set all of the values (e.g., personal, professional, religious) that a person holds

Value system the organization of a person's values along a continuum of relative importance

Values something of worth; a belief held dearly by a person

Values clarification a process by which individuals define their own value

Vaporization continuous evaporation of moisture from the respiratory tract and from the mucosa of the mouth and from the skin

Variance a variation or deviation from a critical pathway; goals not met or interventions not performed according to the time frame

Vasoconstriction a decrease in the caliber (lumen) of blood vessels

Vasodilation an increase in the caliber (lumen) of blood vessels

Vector-borne transmission a vector is an animal or flying or crawling insect that serves as an intermediate means of transporting the infectious agent

Vehicle-borne transmission a vehicle is any substance that serves as an intermediate means to transport and introduce an infectious agent into a susceptible host through a suitable portal of entry

Venipuncture puncture of a vein for collection of a blood specimen or for infusion of therapeutic solutions

Ventilation the movement of air in and out of the lungs; the process of inhalation and exhalation

Ventricles two lower chambers of the heart

Veracity a moral principle that holds that one should tell the truth and not lie

Verbal communication use of verbal language to send and receive messages

Verdict the outcome made by a jury

Vernix caseosa a protective covering that develops over the unborn fetus's skin; a white, cheese-like substance that adheres to the skin and can become 1/8-inch thick by birth

Vesicostomy surgical production of an opening into the bladder

Vestibule contains the organs of equilibrium; found in the inner ear

Vestibulitis severe pain on touch or attempted vaginal entry

Vial a medication container with a sealed rubber cap, for single or multiple doses

Vibration a series of vigorous quiverings produced by hands that are placed flat against the chest wall to loosen thick secretions

Virulence ability to produce disease

Viruses nucleic acid-based infectious agents

Visceral internal organs

Visceral pain results from stimulation of pain receptors in the abdominal cavity, cranium, and thorax

Viscous thick, sticky

Vision the mental image of a possible and desirable future state

Visiting nursing delivery of services in the client's home

Visual related to sight

Visual acuity the degree of detail the eye can discern in an image

Visual fields the area an individual can see when looking straight ahead

Vital capacity the maximum amount of air that can be exhaled after a maximum inhalation

Vital signs measurements of physiologic functioning, specifically body temperature, pulse, respirations, and blood pressure; may include pain and pulse oximetry

Vitamin an organic compound that cannot be manufactured by the body and is needed in small quantities to catalyze metabolic processes

Vitiligo patches of hypopigmented skin, caused by the destruction of melanocytes in the area

Voiding *see* Urination

Volume control infusion set small fluid containers (100 to 150 mL in size) attached below the primary infusion container so that the medication is administered through the client's IV line

Volume expanders used to increase the blood volume following severe loss of blood (e.g., from hemorrhage) or loss of plasma (e.g., from severe burns, which draw large amounts of plasma from the bloodstream to the burn site)

Vulvodynia constant and unremitting burning of vulva

Water-soluble vitamins vitamins that the body cannot store, so people must get a daily supply in the diet; include C and B-complex vitamins

Well-being a subjective perception of balance, harmony, and vitality

Wellness a state of well-being; engaging in attitudes and behaviors that enhance quality of life and maximize personal potential

Wellness diagnosis (NANDA) describes human responses to levels of wellness in an individual, family, or community that have a readiness for enhancement

White blood cells (WBCs) body cells that are part of the body's defense against infection and disease

Wide area network (WAN) computers linked across large distances

World Wide Web (WWW) refers to the complex links among webpages or websites, accessed through "addresses" called *universal resource locators* (URLs)

Xenophobia the fear or dislike of people different from one's self

Xerostomia dry mouth

Yoga a type of meditation that is a system of exercises for attaining bodily or mental control and well-being

Index

Page numbers followed by *f* indicate figures and those followed by *t* indicate tables, boxes, or special features. The titles of special features (e.g., Anatomy and Physiology Review; Lifespan Considerations; Skills) are also capitalized.

Pearson Education, Inc.

YOU SHOULD CAREFULLY READ THE TERMS AND CONDITIONS BEFORE USING THE CD-ROM PACKAGE. USING THIS CD-ROM PACKAGE INDICATES YOUR ACCEPTANCE OF THESE TERMS AND CONDITIONS.

Pearson Education, Inc. provides this program and licenses its use. You assume responsibility for the selection of the program to achieve your intended results, and for the installation, use, and results obtained from the program. This license extends only to use of the program in the United States or countries in which the program is marketed by authorized distributors.

LICENSE GRANT

You hereby accept a nonexclusive, nontransferable, permanent license to install and use the program ON A SINGLE COMPUTER at any given time. You may copy the program solely for backup or archival purposes in support of your use of the program on the single computer. You may not modify, translate, disassemble, decompile, or reverse engineer the program, in whole or in part.

TERM

The License is effective until terminated. Pearson Education, Inc. reserves the right to terminate this License automatically if any provision of the License is violated. You may terminate the License at any time. To terminate this License, you must return the program, including documentation, along with a written warranty stating that all copies in your possession have been returned or destroyed.

LIMITED WARRANTY

THE PROGRAM IS PROVIDED "AS IS" WITHOUT WARRANTY OF ANY KIND, EITHER EXPRESSED OR IMPLIED, INCLUDING, BUT NOT LIMITED TO, THE IMPLIED WARRANTIES OR MERCHANTABILITY AND FITNESS FOR A PARTICULAR PURPOSE. THE ENTIRE RISK AS TO THE QUALITY AND PERFORMANCE OF THE PROGRAM IS WITH YOU. SHOULD THE PROGRAM PROVE DEFECTIVE, YOU (AND NOT PRENTICE-HALL, INC. OR ANY AUTHORIZED DEALER) ASSUME THE ENTIRE COST OF ALL NECESSARY SERVICING, REPAIR, OR CORRECTION. NO ORAL OR WRITTEN INFORMATION OR ADVICE GIVEN BY PRENTICE-HALL, INC., ITS DEALERS, DISTRIBUTORS, OR AGENTS SHALL CREATE A WARRANTY OR INCREASE THE SCOPE OF THIS WARRANTY.

SOME STATES DO NOT ALLOW THE EXCLUSION OF IMPLIED WARRANTIES, SO THE ABOVE EXCLUSION MAY NOT APPLY TO YOU. THIS WARRANTY GIVES YOU SPECIFIC LEGAL RIGHTS AND YOU MAY ALSO HAVE OTHER LEGAL RIGHTS THAT VARY FROM STATE TO STATE.

Pearson Education, Inc. does not warrant that the functions contained in the program will meet your requirements or that the operation of the program will be uninterrupted or error-free.

However, Pearson Education, Inc. warrants the diskette(s) or CD-ROM(s) on which the program is furnished to be free from defects in material and workmanship under normal use for a period of ninety (90) days from the date of delivery to you as evidenced by a copy of your receipt.

The program should not be relied on as the sole basis to solve a problem whose incorrect solution could result in injury to person or property. If the program is employed in such a manner, it is at the user's own risk and Pearson Education, Inc. explicitly disclaims all liability for such misuse.

LIMITATION OF REMEDIES

Pearson Education, Inc.'s entire liability and your exclusive remedy shall be:

1. the replacement of any diskette(s) or CD-ROM(s) not meeting Pearson Education, Inc.'s "LIMITED WARRANTY" and that is returned to Pearson Education, or

2. if Pearson Education is unable to deliver a replacement diskette(s) or CD-ROM(s) that is free of defects in materials or workmanship, you may terminate this agreement by returning the program.

IN NO EVENT WILL PRENTICE-HALL, INC. BE LIABLE TO YOU FOR ANY DAMAGES, INCLUDING ANY LOST PROFITS, LOST SAVINGS, OR OTHER INCIDENTAL OR CONSEQUENTIAL DAMAGES ARISING OUT OF THE USE OR INABILITY TO USE SUCH PROGRAM EVEN IF PRENTICE-HALL, INC. OR AN AUTHORIZED DISTRIBUTOR HAS BEEN ADVISED OF THE POSSIBILITY OF SUCH DAMAGES, OR FOR ANY CLAIM BY ANY OTHER PARTY.

SOME STATES DO NOT ALLOW FOR THE LIMITATION OR EXCLUSION OF LIABILITY FOR INCIDENTAL OR CONSEQUENTIAL DAMAGES, SO THE ABOVE LIMITATION OR EXCLUSION MAY NOT APPLY TO YOU.

GENERAL

You may not sublicense, assign, or transfer the license of the program. Any attempt to sublicense, assign or transfer any of the rights, duties, or obligations hereunder is void.

This Agreement will be governed by the laws of the State of New York.

Should you have any questions concerning this Agreement, you may contact Pearson Education, Inc. by writing to:

Director of New Media
Higher Education Division
Pearson Education, Inc.
One Lake Street
Upper Saddle River, NJ 07458

Should you have any questions concerning technical support, you may contact:

Product Support Department: Monday–Friday 8:00 A.M. –8:00 P.M. and Sunday 5:00 P.M.-12:00 A.M. (All times listed are Eastern). 1-800-677-6337

You can also get support by filling out the web form located at http://247.prenhall.com

YOU ACKNOWLEDGE THAT YOU HAVE READ THIS AGREEMENT, UNDERSTAND IT, AND AGREE TO BE BOUND BY ITS TERMS AND CONDITIONS. YOU FURTHER AGREE THAT IT IS THE COMPLETE AND EXCLUSIVE STATEMENT OF THE AGREEMENT BETWEEN US THAT SUPERSEDES ANY PROPOSAL OR PRIOR AGREEMENT, ORAL OR WRITTEN, AND ANY OTHER COMMUNICATIONS BETWEEN US RELATING TO THE SUBJECT MATTER OF THIS AGREEMENT.

NURSING EXCELLENCE

Success in Skills, Review, & Test Preparation

Excellence in Nursing Skills

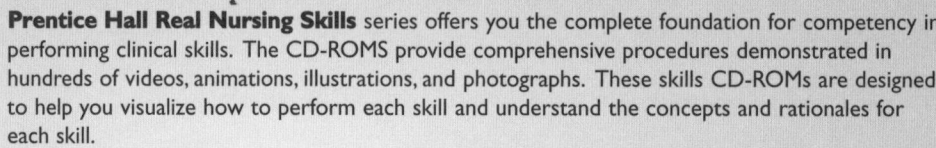

Prentice Hall's Real Nursing Skills on CD-ROMS

Prentice Hall Real Nursing Skills series offers you the complete foundation for competency in performing clinical skills. The CD-ROMS provide comprehensive procedures demonstrated in hundreds of videos, animations, illustrations, and photographs. These skills CD-ROMs are designed to help you visualize how to perform each skill and understand the concepts and rationales for each skill.

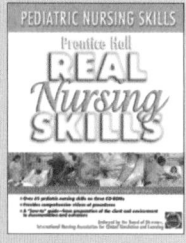

Basic Nursing Skills:
94 skills on 5 CD-ROMs. 2005, ISBN: 0-13-191526-6
Intermediate & Advanced Nursing Skills:
84 skills on 5 CD-ROMs. 2005, ISBN: 0-13-119344-9
Physical & Health Assessment Nursing Skills:
25 skills on 5 CD-ROMs. 2006, ISBN: 0-13-191525-8
Maternal-Newborn & Women's Health Nursing Skills:
24 skills on 2 CD-ROMs. 2005, ISBN: 0-13-191527-4
Pediatric Nursing Skills:
65 skills on 3 CD-ROMs. 2006, ISBN: 0-13-191524-X
Critical Care Nursing Skills:
35 skills on 2 CD-ROMs. 2005, ISBN: 0-13-119264-7

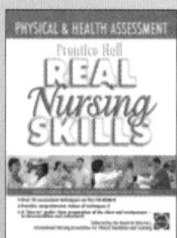

Excellence in NCLEX-RN® Review

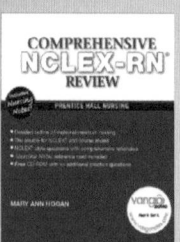

Prentice Hall's Comprehensive NCLEX-RN® Review is designed specifically to help you achieve nursing excellence by simplifying your review and making the most of your valuable study time. This review book is uniquely organized according to the April 2007 NCLEX-RN® Test Plan, providing you with both a comprehensive content review and practice questions in sections covering * Safe, Effective Care Environment * Health Promotion * Physiological Integrity, and * Psychosocial Integrity. Throughout this book, you will find:

• **Memory Aids** that help you remember key concepts.
• **NCLEX® Alerts** that identify critical concepts you are likely to see on the NCLEX-RN®.
• **Check Your NCLEX® IQ** boxes that help you to assess your readiness for the NCLEX-RN® on the topics covered in the chapter.
2008, ISBN 0-13-119599-9 • **Practice Tests** at the end of the chapter that review the concepts from that chapter and provide comprehensive rationales and test-taking strategies to help you find the right answers.

The **NCLEX-RN® Test Prep CD-ROM** that comes with your book simulates the test-taking environment by allowing you to practice questions on the computer. It contains all the questions in the book PLUS thousands of additional questions. You can choose to practice in Study, Quiz, or Exam modes, and you will receive detailed reports that will help you focus your preparation for NCLEX-RN®.

For additional information and resources